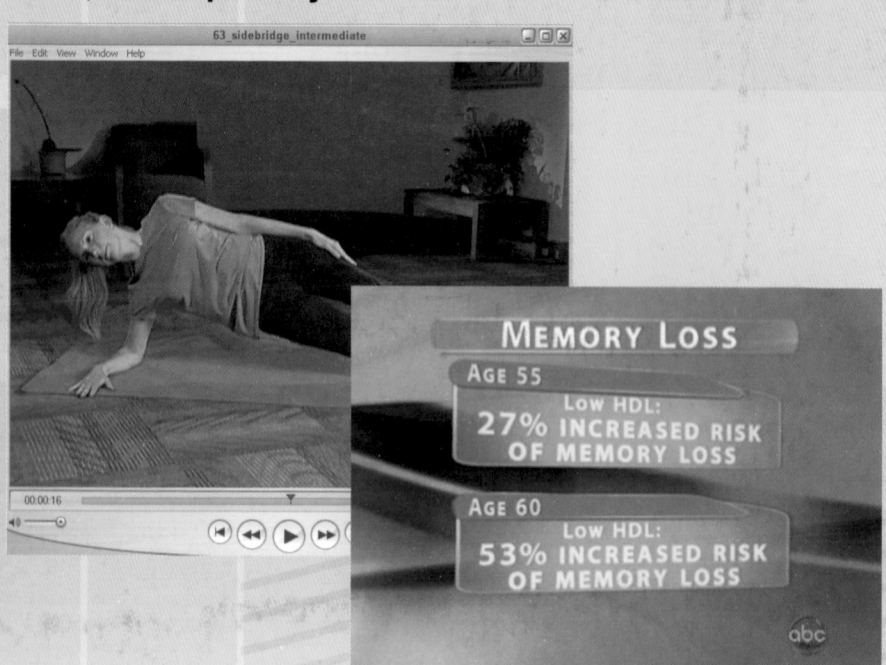

Stop!

Did you register?
Don't miss out!

Turn back one page
to register and get help
preparing for exams...
whenever and wherever
you need it.

www.pearsonhighered.com/hopson

PRE-COURSE/POST-COURSE ASSESSMENT

Name: _____ Date: _____

As you complete the key fitness/wellness lab assessments in this course, record your results in the "Pre-Course Assessment" column. At the end of the course, re-do the labs, record your results in the "Post-Course Assessment" column, and see the progress you have made!

Lab	Pre-Course Assessment	Post-Course Assessment

Lab 3.2: Assessing Your Cardiorespiratory Fitness Level	**3-minute step test**
	  1 minute recovery HR:_____ (bpm)
	  Fitness rating: _____
	1-mile walk test
	  VO$_2$ max: _____ Fitness rating: _____
	1.5-mile run test
	  VO$_2$ max: _____ Fitness rating: _____
		3-minute step test
		  1 minute recovery HR:_____ (bpm)
		  Fitness rating: _____
		1-mile walk test
		  VO$_2$ max: _____ Fitness rating: _____
		1.5-mile run test
		  VO$_2$ max: _____ Fitness rating: _____

Lab 4.1: Assessing Your Muscular Strength	**Chest press**
	  S/BW ratio: _____ Rating: _____
	Leg press
	  S/BW ratio: _____ Rating: _____
		Chest press
		  S/BW ratio: _____ Rating: _____
		Leg press
		  S/BW ratio: _____ Rating: _____

Lab 4.2: Assessing Your Muscular Endurance	**20RM assessment**
	  Chest press 20RM weight lifted: _____
	  Leg press 20RM weight lifted: _____
	Push-up assessment
	  Repetitions: _____ Rating: _____
	Curl-up assessment
	  Repetitions: _____ Rating: _____
		20RM assessment
		  Chest press 20RM weight lifted: _____
		  Leg press 20RM weight lifted: _____
		Push-up assessment
		  Repetitions: _____ Rating: _____
		Curl-up assessment
		  Repetitions: _____ Rating: _____

Lab 5.1: Assessing Your Flexibility	**Sit-and-reach test**
	  Reach distance (in or cm): _____
	  Rating: _____
		Sit-and-reach test
		  Reach distance (in or cm): _____
		  Rating: _____

Lab 6.1: How to Calculate Your BMI	BMI: _____ kg/m² Weight classification: _____	BMI: _____ kg/m² Weight classification: _____
Lab 6.2: Measure and Evaluate Your Body Circumferences	Waist: _____ Hip: _____ WHR Ratio: _____ Upper arm: _____ (right) _____ (left) Forearm: _____ (right) _____ (left) Thigh: _____ (right) _____ (left) Calf: _____ (right) _____ (left) Neck: _____ Disease risk rating for WHR: _____ Disease risk rating for WC: _____	Waist: _____ Hip: _____ WHR Ratio: _____ Upper arm: _____ (right) _____ (left) Forearm: _____ (right) _____ (left) Thigh: _____ (right) _____ (left) Calf: _____ (right) _____ (left) Neck: _____ Disease risk rating for WHR: _____ Disease risk rating for WC: _____
Lab 6.3: Estimate Your Percent Body Fat (Skinfold Test)	Sum of 3 skinfolds: _____ % body fat estimate: _____ Rating: _____	Sum of 3 skinfolds: _____ % body fat estimate: _____ Rating: _____
Lab 7.2: Keeping a Food Diary and Analyzing Your Daily Nutrition **Lab 7.3:** Improving Your Nutrition	Milk intake: _____ cups Meat and beans intake: _____ oz. Vegetables intake: _____ cups Fruits intake: _____ cups Grains intake: _____ oz.	Milk intake: _____ cups Meat and beans intake: _____ oz. Vegetables intake: _____ cups Fruits intake: _____ cups Grains intake: _____ oz.
Lab 8.1: Calculating Energy Balance and Setting Energy Balance Goals	Estimated calorie intake: _____ Estimated calorie expenditure: _____ Calorie balance (intake minus expenditure): _____	Estimated calorie intake: _____ Estimated calorie expenditure: _____ Calorie balance (intake minus expenditure): _____
Lab 8.2: Your Weight Management Plan	% body fat: _____ Weight: _____ lb. BMI: _____ kg/m²	% body fat: _____ Weight: _____ lb. BMI: _____ kg/m²
Lab 9.1: How Stressed Are You?	Sum of negative scores: _____ Interpretation: _____	Sum of negative scores: _____ Interpretation: _____
Lab 10.1: Understanding Your CVD Risk	Family risk for CVD, total points: _____ Lifestyle risk for CVD, total points: _____ Additional risks for CVD, total points: _____	Family risk for CVD, total points: _____ Lifestyle risk for CVD, total points: _____ Additional risks for CVD, total points: _____
Lab 12.1: Assessing Your Personal Risk of Cancer	Breast cancer risk, total points: _____ Skin cancer risk, total points: _____ Reproductive cancer risk, total points: _____ General cancer risk, total points: _____	Breast cancer risk, total points: _____ Skin cancer risk, total points: _____ Reproductive cancer risk, total points: _____ General cancer risk, total points: _____
Lab 13.1: Assessing Your Alcohol Use and Risk of Abuse	Drinking patterns and abuse risk score: _____ How risky is your alcohol use?_____	Drinking patterns and abuse risk score: _____ How risky is your alcohol use?_____

BEHAVIOR CHANGE CONTRACT

Choose a health behavior that you would like to change, starting this quarter or semester. Sign the contract at the bottom to affirm your commitment to making a healthy change and ask a friend to witness it.

My behavior change will be:

_____

My long-term goal for this behavior change is:

_____

Barriers I must overcome to make this behavior change are (things I am currently doing or situations that contribute to this behavior or make it harder to change):

1. _____

2. _____

3. _____

The strategies I will use to overcome these barriers are:

1. _____

2. _____

3. _____

Resources I will use to help me change this behavior include:

A friend/partner/relative _____

A school-based resource _____

A community-based resource _____

A book or reputable website _____

In order to make my goal more attainable, I have devised these short-term goals:

Short-Term Goal _____ **Target Date**_____ **Reward** _____

Short-Term Goal _____ **Target Date**_____ **Reward** _____

Short-Term Goal _____ **Target Date**_____ **Reward** _____

When I make the long-term behavior change described above, my reward will be:

Short-Term Goal _____ **Target Date**_____ **Reward** _____

I intend to make the behavior change described above, I will use the strategies and rewards to achieve the goals that will contribute to a healthy behavior change.

Signed _____ **Date**_____

Witness _____ **Date**_____

Coaching for Your Students 24/7

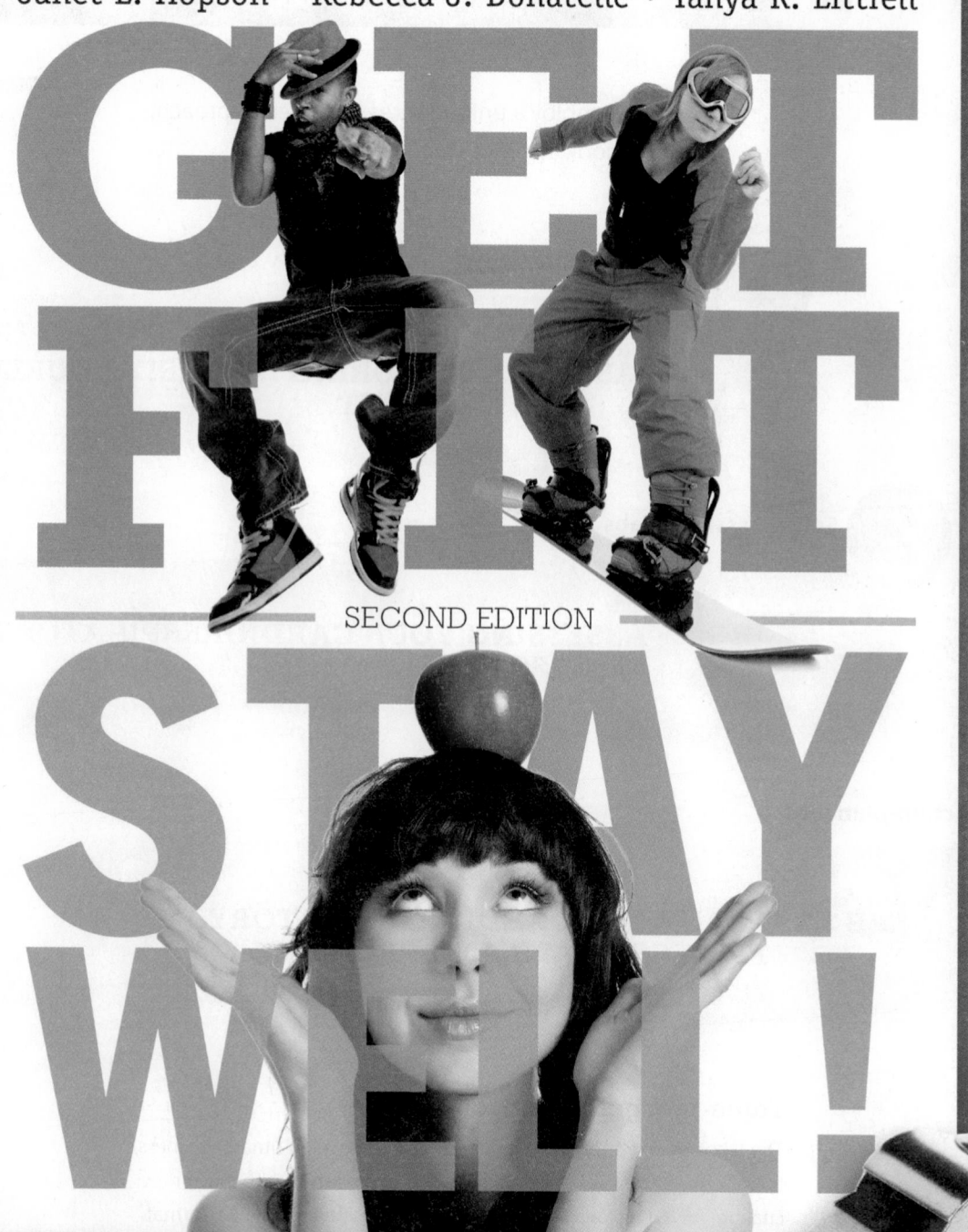

Janet L. Hopson · Rebecca J. Donatelle · Tanya R. Littrell

GET FIT

SECOND EDITION

STAY WELL!

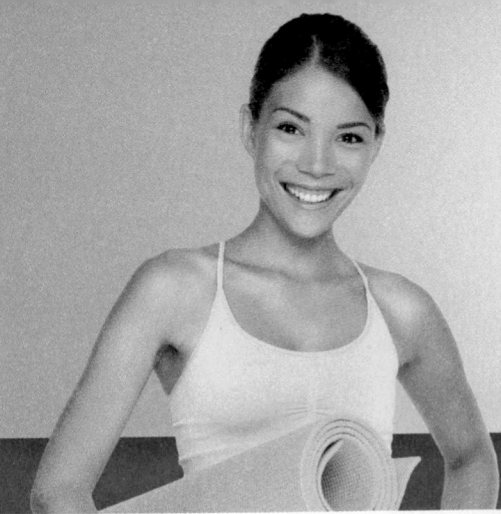

Student Coaching for the Gym

Labs employ a unique three-pronged approach.
The book includes three types of labs:

1 Skill-acquisition labs

DO IT! ONLINE
LEARN A SKILL
LAB 3.1 • MONITORING INTENSITY DURING A WORKOUT

2 Self-assessment labs

DO IT! ONLINE
ASSESS YOURSELF
LAB 3.2 • ASSESSING YOUR CARDIORESPIRATORY FITNESS LEVEL

3 Action-plan labs

DO IT! ONLINE
PLAN FOR CHANGE
LAB 3.3 • PLAN YOUR CARDIORESPIRATORY FITNESS GOALS AND PROGRAM

Three-pronged Approach to Labs

The labs not only measure a student's current level of fitness/wellness, but also teach practical lifelong skills and encourage real behavior change. All labs are also available in an online interactive PDF format.

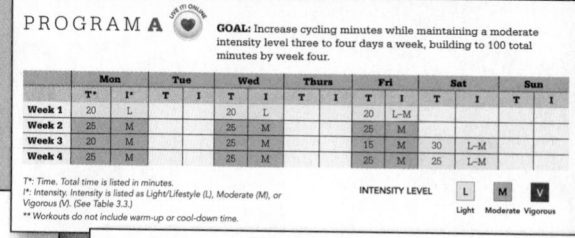

PROGRAM A

GOAL: Increase cycling minutes while maintaining a moderate intensity level three to four days a week, building to 100 total minutes by week four.

	Mon		Tue		Wed		Thurs		Fri		Sat		Sun	
	T*	I*	T	I	T	I	T	I	T	I	T	I	T	I
Week 1	20	L			20	L			20	L-M				
Week 2	25	M			25	M			25	M				
Week 3	20	M			25	M			15	M	30	L-M		
Week 4	25	M			25	M			25	M	25	L-M		

T*: Time. Total time is listed in minutes.
I*: Intensity. Intensity is listed as Light/Lifestyle (L), Moderate (M), or Vigorous (V). (See Table 3.3.)
** Workouts do not include warm-up or cool-down time.

INTENSITY LEVEL L M V — Light Moderate Vigorous

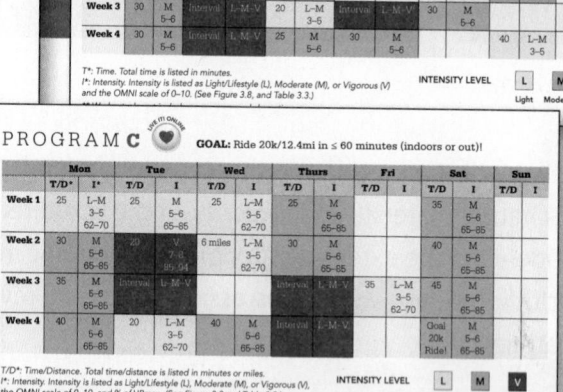

PROGRAM B

GOAL: Cycle at a moderate intensity level three to five days a week, build to a 40-minute ride, and incorporate vigorous interval training sessions each week.

	Mon		Tue		Wed		Thurs		Fri		Sat		Sun	
	T*	I*	T	I	T	I	T	I	T	I	T	I	T	I
Week 1	25	L-M 3-5			25	L-M 3-5			25	M 5-6	25	M 5-6		
Week 2	25	M 5-6			30	M 5-6			25	L-M 3-5	35	M 5-6		
Week 3	30	M 5-6	Interval	L-M-V	20	L-M 3-6	Interval	L-M-V	30	M 5-6				
Week 4	30	M 5-6	Interval	L-M-V	25	M 5-6	30	M 5-6			40	L-M 3-5		

T*: Time. Total time is listed in minutes.
I*: Intensity. Intensity is listed as Light/Lifestyle (L), Moderate (M), or Vigorous (V) and the OMNI scale of 0-10. (See Figure 3.8, and Table 3.3.)

INTENSITY LEVEL L M V — Light Moderate Vigorous

PROGRAM C

GOAL: Ride 20k/12.4mi in ≤ 60 minutes (indoors or out)!

	Mon		Tue		Wed		Thurs		Fri		Sat		Sun	
	T/D*	I*	T/D	I	T/D	I	T/D	I	T/D	I	T/D	I	T/D	I
Week 1	25	L-M 3-5 62-70	25	M 5-6 65-85	25	L-M 3-5 62-70	25	M 5-6 65-85			35	M 5-6 65-85		
Week 2	30	M 5-6 65-85	20	V 7-8 95-94	6 miles	L-M 5-6 62-70	30	M 5-6 65-85			40	M 5-6 65-85		
Week 3	35	M 5-6 65-85	Interval	L-M-V	Interval	L-M-V			35	L-M 3-5 62-70	45	M 5-6 65-85		
Week 4	40	M 5-6 65-85	20	L-M 3-5 62-70	40	M 5-6 65-85	Interval	L-M-V			Goal 20k Ride!	M 5-6 65-85		

T/D*: Time/Distance. Total time/distance is listed in minutes or miles.
I*: Intensity. Intensity is listed as Light/Lifestyle (L), Moderate (M), or Vigorous (V), the OMNI scale of 0-10, and % of HRmax. (See Figure 3.8 and Table 3.3.)
** Workouts do not include warm-up or cool-down time.

INTENSITY LEVEL L M V — Light Moderate Vigorous

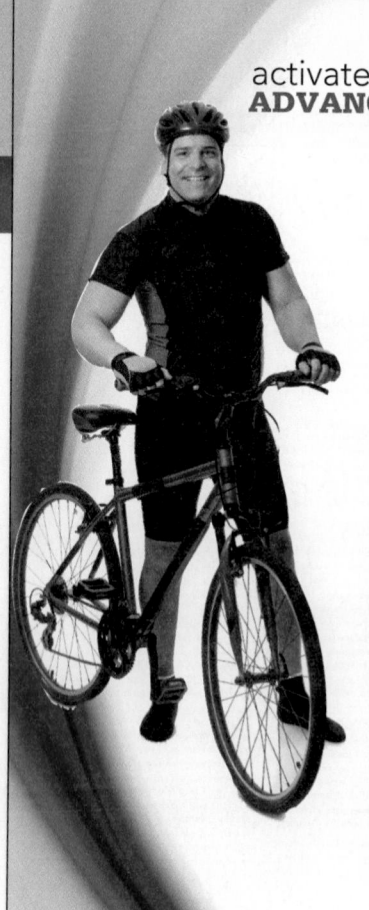

activate, motivate, & ADVANCE YOUR FITNESS

A CYCLING PROGRAM

ACTIVATE!
Whether you cycle indoors or take your bike out on the road or trail, you can get a fun and amazing workout.

Cycling Program Preparation & Safety
Sure, cycling can be an intense, calorie-burning workout, but it can also be a simple way to take care of errands, commute, meet up with friends, or just enjoy the great out doors. Follow the programs below to get started. As you get stronger, you can increase your mileage and speed.

What Do I need for Cycling?
GEAR: Safe cycling requires quite a bit of equipment (helmet padded cycling shorts, gloves, shoes, reflective gear, racks) and, of course, the bike. You can start on almost any style of bicycle, but most importantly, you need a bike that fits. Visit your local bike shop to get the right bike for you. When indoor cycling, adjust both seat and handlebar height to create a comfortable and safe fit. If you are new to indoor cycling or unfamiliar with the stationary bikes at your facility, be sure to ask a trained instructor to assist you with proper bike setup.

How Do I Start a Cycling Program?
TECHNIQUE: Work on developing a smooth and efficient pedaling technique. Lighten up, pedal in a smooth circle, and pull through the back of the stroke. Cadence is pedaling speed in revolutions per minute (RPM). A cadence of 60 RPM means that one pedal makes a complete revolution 60 times in one minute. Monitor your cadence with periodic cadence checks. Count the revolution of one leg for 15 seconds and then multiply by four. The cadence range is 80-110 RPM for cycling on a flat road and 60-80 RPM for climbing hills.

ETIQUETTE: Participating in group rides will teach you the etiquette for road cycling and mountain biking. Inquire about weekly rides or a beginners' cycling group at your local bike shop.

Cycling Tips
INDOOR CYCLING: Weather, traffic, flat tires ... with indoor cycling you won't have these excuses for missing your workout. Indoor cycling also allows you to precisely control your workout and mix periods of higher-intensity cycling with resting pedal strokes.

OUTDOOR CYCLING: Whether you choose streets, bike paths, or trails, plan safe routes that take into consideration

NEW! Activate/Motivate/Advance Sample Fitness Programs

These new programs, appearing at the ends of Chapters 2–5 and 8–9, are like having a personal trainer built into the book. Each program contains guidance on three parts of a fitness or wellness program: getting started, motivating to continue, and modifying/taking to the next level. The customizable "pre-fab" programs and the related tracking features and technique videos on the website make it easy to jump into a fitness behavior change project. These sample fitness programs are also accessible by mobile phone.

Exercise Videos

More than 100 videos of exercises are available on the Companion Website at www.pearsonhighered.com/hopson—allowing students access to additional instruction on their own time, and giving them the ability to exercise from the comfort of their own homes. Selected videos with assignable quiz questions that report to the gradebook are available in MyFitnessLab.™

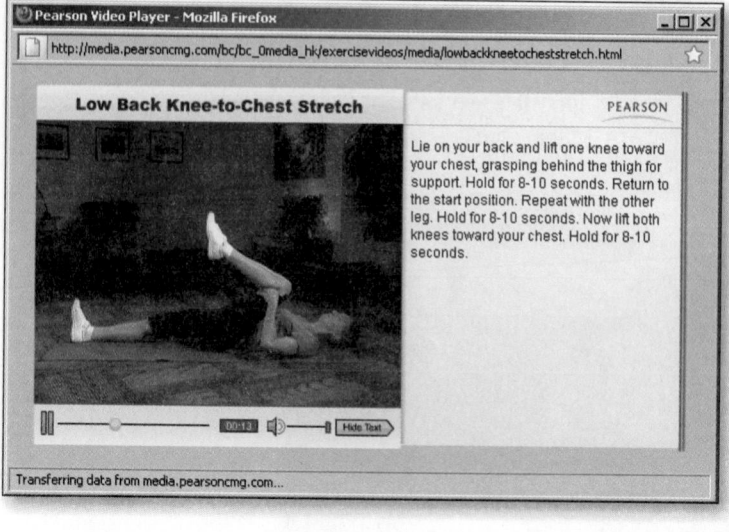

Pearson Video Player - Mozilla Firefox

http://media.pearsoncmg.com/bc/bc_0media_hk/exercisevideos/media/lowbackkneetocheststretch.html

Low Back Knee-to-Chest Stretch   PEARSON

Lie on your back and lift one knee toward your chest, grasping behind the thigh for support. Hold for 8-10 seconds. Return to the start position. Repeat with the other leg. Hold for 8-10 seconds. Now lift both knees toward your chest. Hold for 8-10 seconds.

00:13   Hide Text

Transferring data from media.pearsoncmg.com...

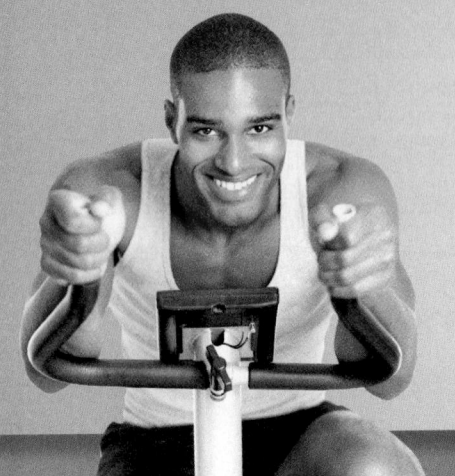

Students can pace themselves when studying

New Media Callouts in the chapter openers, end-of-chapter material, and throughout the text direct students to the extensive supporting electronic media, including videos, audio files, assignments, and review materials.

casestudy

CARLOS

"I know that my life is pretty good. I'm in college, studying what interests me, and I'm excited about the future. I just constantly feel behind. I fall asleep in class sometimes, eat a lot of junk food, and I'm not exercising—who has time? Then I got this cold, partly because I have been stressed out and not sleeping much. I've made some friends in my dorm, and it helps to know that a lot of them are going through the same thing. Talking to Liz every night on the phone helps, too."

THINK! In which dimensions of wellness could Carlos be stronger? Where would you place him on the wellness continuum? How do you compare to Carlos?

ACT! Identify your strongest wellness dimensions as well as the ones you could improve. Create a wellness balance chart and plan the balance you would like to achieve (Lab 1.2).

spectrum of existence; and promote feelings of love, joy, peace, contentment, and wonder over life's experiences.

Environmental Wellness

Our home, work, community, and school environments can be relaxing, safe havens or toxic, threatening, and stressful places to be. **Environmental wellness** entails understanding how the environment can positively or negatively affect you; the role you play in preserving, protecting, and improving the world around you; and what you can do to conserve dwindling resources for future generations.

Related Dimensions of Wellness

Occupational and financial wellness overlap with other wellness areas, and are sometimes considered their own dimensions. Your wellness in these areas can dramatically affect your overall wellness and add to your life's balance (or lack thereof). If you ask family members and friends about their current problems, many will identify their jobs or finances as the top stressors in their lives.

Occupational Wellness
Occupational wellness is the level of happiness and fulfillment you experience in your work. An important component of occupational wellness is finding a non-toxic, hazard-free work environment that provides contact with managers and co-workers who value your skills and opinions. Contrary to what people often think, job satisfaction is not closely tied to high wages.[2] You can reach optimal occupational wellness when your personal goals align closely with those of your employer, and when you feel that you are making significant contributions to both sets of goals.

environmental wellness An appreciation of how the external environment can affect oneself, and an understanding of the role one plays in preserving, protecting, and improving it

occupational wellness A level of happiness and fulfillment in work, including harmony with personal goals, appreciation from bosses and co-workers, and a safe workplace

financial wellness The ability to balance and manage financial needs and wants with your income, debts, savings, and investments

Financial Wellness **Financial wellness** is the ability to successfully balance and manage your financial needs and wants with your income, debts, savings, and investments. If you cannot pay your bills, it can be hard to think of much else and this dimension can overshadow and unbalance the others. People who are managing their finances but just breaking even will still need to make wise consumer choices, carefully control debt, and continually prioritize expenses (see the box How Can I Handle My Finances Better?).

Balancing Your Wellness Dimensions
You may have healthy relationships, but no fondness for exercise. Perhaps your spiritual life is rich, but you have trouble juggling academic demands. Virtually everyone is stronger in some dimensions of wellness than others. Striving for improvement in all six wellness dimensions is a lifelong process. One good approach is to concentrate on those dimensions that present the most pressing need, while working on the others in a steady but relaxed and motivated way. Over time, a balance of work on all the dimensions—one or two now, others later—will eventually promote overall wellness. Your brain and body, your thoughts and emotions, your actions and reactions, your relationship to yourself and others—all are interconnected and integrated. Likewise, the dimensions of wellness are interrelated. For example, increasing your exercise and general activity will also help you manage stress, mood, body composition, and so on.

NEW! Media Callouts in Book

The printed text shows you exactly where the associated media is.

Active Media Callouts—Pearson eText Version

In the eText version, media callouts provide direct links to the media resources.

Good Wellness Habits Benefit Society as a Whole
The higher a population's levels of wellness, the happier and more productive are its people and the less money it spends on health care. Accordingly, achieving better wellness and combating today's chronic diseases are important national priorities.

National public health priorities cited by the Office of the Surgeon General of the United States are summarized in a set of objectives titled *Healthy People 2020*, which has four broad goals: 1) attain high-quality, longer lives free of preventable disease, disability, injury, and premature death; 2) achieve health equity, eliminate disparities, and improve the health of all groups; 3) create social and physical environments that promote good health for all; and 4) promote quality of life, healthy development, and healthy behaviors across all life stages.[13] In order to address some of these major public health priorities, the Surgeon General advises Americans to eat healthier, be more physically active, not smoke, limit alcohol, and avoid drugs—all of which are wellness behaviors.[14]

The high cost of health care and health insurance is a major concern for Americans. In 2009, Americans spent $2.5 trillion on health care, or 17.6 percent of the gross domestic product (GDP).[15] Employer health insurance premiums increased by 131 percent between 1999 and 2009 at four times the rate of inflation.[16] Nearly 49 million Americans lack health insurance, largely due to the high cost of coverage.[17] This makes them less likely to seek preventive care and adopt wellness behaviors early enough to prevent illness down the line. Such concerns led to sweeping new health legislation in 2010 to increase the percentage of Americans with health coverage.[18]

How Can I Change My Behavior to Increase My Wellness?
If you are like most people, you have made a New Year's resolution on January 1, have worked hard to adopt some new behavior until about the 10th, have started slipping back to your old habits by the 15th, and have forgotten about the whole thing by the 31st. Your resolution may well have been a new wellness behavior—lots of resolutions are. Perhaps it was an easy one, such as "eat more fruit," and you succeeded. More likely, it was a harder one—"start lifting weights three times a week," or "lose 20 pounds," or "give up junk food"—and despite your good intentions, it just didn't stick.

People often see change as a singular event instead of a process that requires preparation, has several stages, and takes time to succeed. Classic research shows that we must go through a series of mental and emotional stages over a period of months to adequately prepare ourselves for **behavior change**. The rest of this chapter takes you through a series of practical steps inspired by a blueprint for change called the *transtheoretical model of behavior change* developed by psychologists James Prochaska and Carlo DiClemente.[19]

Step One: Understand the Stages of Behavior Change
The transtheoretical model of behavior change delineates six **stages of behavior change**: precontemplation, contemplation, preparation, action, maintenance, and termination. The model shows that changing behaviors usually involves a gradual process of awareness, preparation, and then action. Understanding this process can help you proceed more deliberately to identify and successfully change a problem behavior. Keep in mind that the steps of this model are general and people often backtrack as they work on them.

behavior change An organized, deliberate effort to alter or replace an existing habit or pattern of activity

stages of behavior change From the transtheoretical model, a set of states most people pass through in their awareness of, determination to alter, and efforts to replace existing habits or actions

New Year's Resolutions

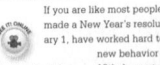

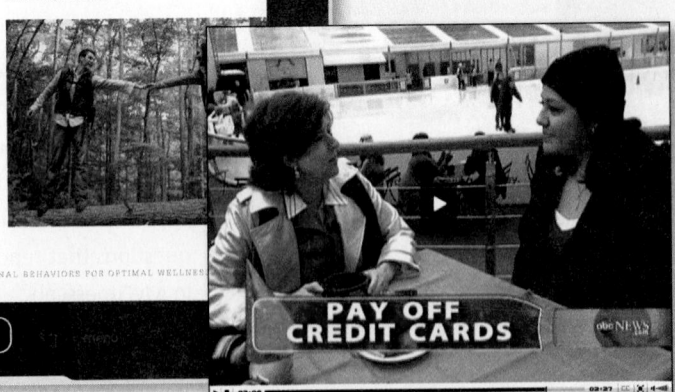

PAY OFF CREDIT CARDS

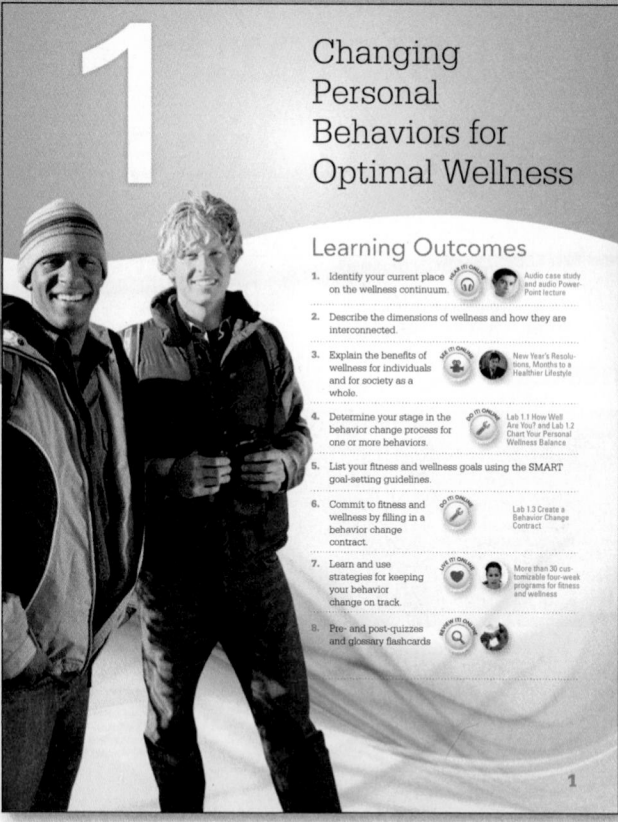

The **Second Edition** better addresses student questions and needs within the course through learning outcomes, and in their fitness/wellness behavior choices through the Question Boxes and Think!/Act! features.

NEW! Learning Outcomes

Learning Outcomes replace Chapter Objectives in the chapter openers.

Question Boxes

These boxes investigate common questions and concerns students may have about applying chapter topics to improve their own fitness & wellness.

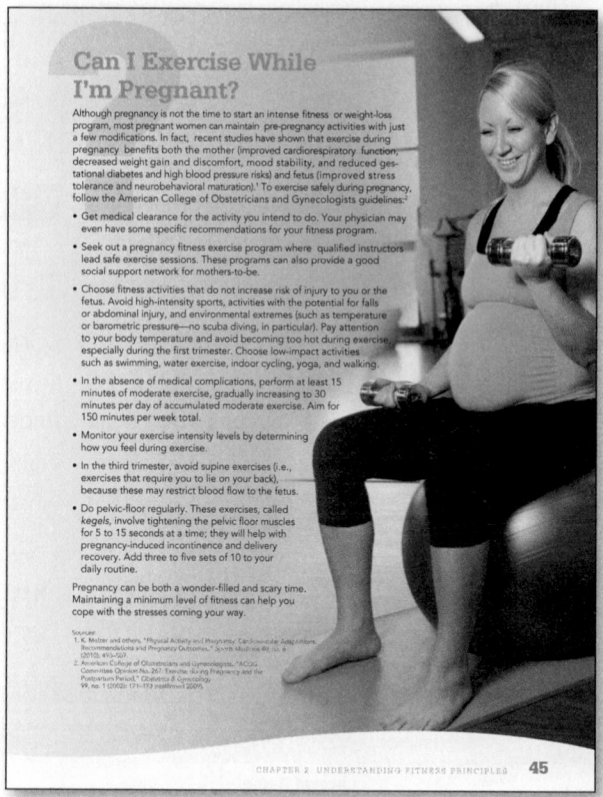

casestudy

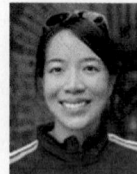

ANGELA

"I thought I would kick-start my plan to get back into shape by doing one of the workouts my tennis coach had us do in high school. I jogged for a mile, did some calisthenics on the court, and then played two sets of tennis with a friend. That was a mistake. My friend has a killer serve—it's like a bullet coming at you. She won every point she served because I couldn't move fast enough to return the ball. Also, I was surprised at how much that jog tired me out. I used to run a mile with no problem at all! By the end of the first set, I was completely exhausted. My friend won 6-1, 6-1."

THINK! Which energy system do you think Angela's friend relied on most while hitting her explosive serves?

ACT! Write out activities you would do for a 10-minute cardiorespiratory warm-up. Now, try your 10-minute warm up and think about how the three energy systems are providing fuel to keep your muscles moving.

NEW! Think!/Act!

These questions at the end of the case studies and other points within the chapters are designed to encourage critical thinking and to help students reflect on how the material applies to their own lives.

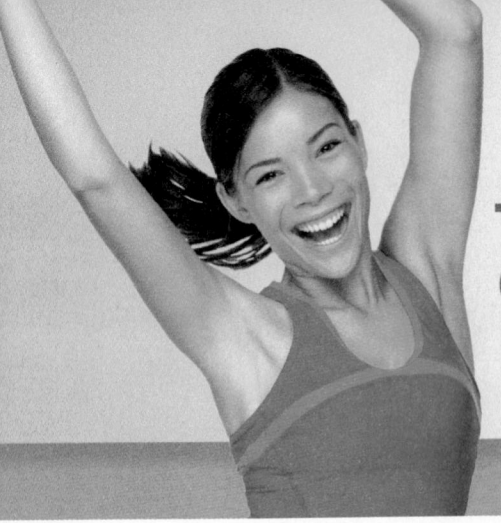

Add an assistant coach to your line up

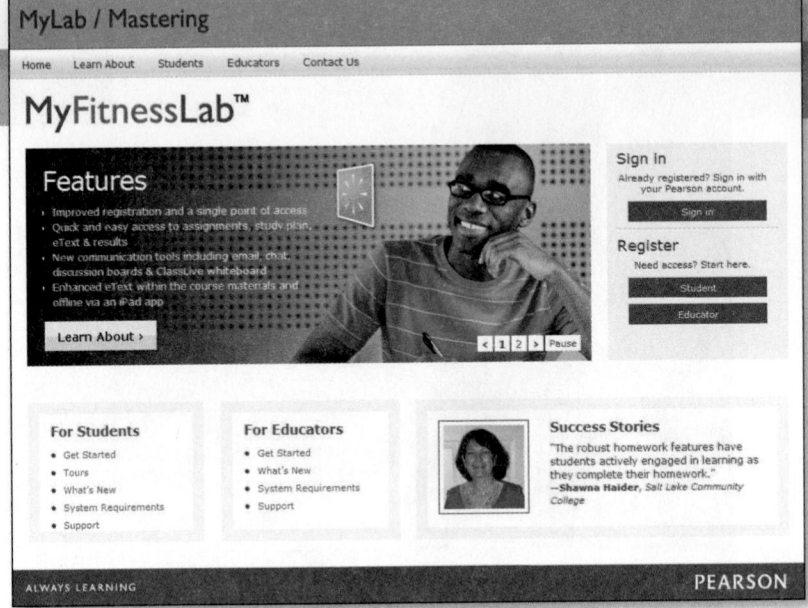

Engaging experience

MyFitnessLab™ provides a one-stop spot for accessing a wealth of preloaded content and tools, while giving you the ability to customize your course as much (or as little) as you'd like.

NEW! *ABC News* Videos

These videos bring fitness & wellness topics to life and are available on the Instructor Resource DVD, MyFitnessLab, and the Companion Website.

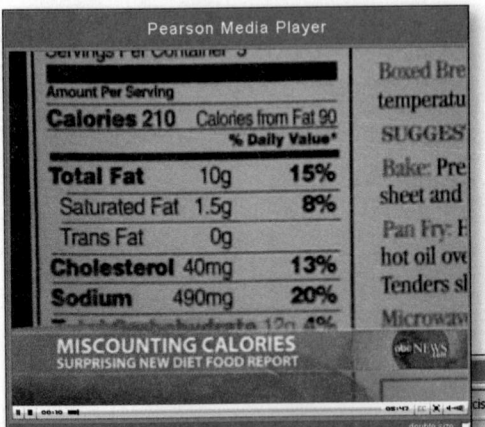

Trusted partner

MyFitnessLab delivers engaging, dynamic learning opportunities—focused on instructor learning objectives and responsive to each student's progress—with improved registration and instructor support.

• Quick Start Videos demonstrate MyFitnessLab basics for instructors giving just-in-time help.

• Dedicated instructor and student support via internet chat at **http://247pearsoned.custhelp.com** or dedicated customer service line at 800-677-6337.

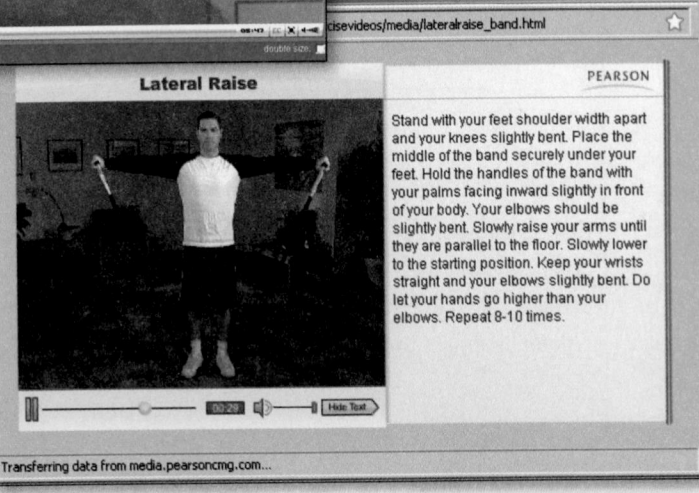

Exercise Videos

More than 100 videos of exercises are available; selected videos with assignable, gradable quiz questions make assigning homework on proper forms, technique, and safety easy to do.

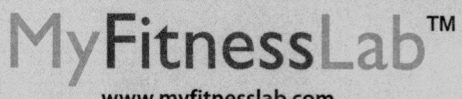
MyFitnessLab™

www.myfitnesslab.com

The new MyFinessLab from Pearson has been designed and refined with a single purpose in mind: to help educators create that moment of understanding with their students. The MyFitnessLab system helps instructors maximize class time with customizable, easy-to-assign, and automatically graded assignments that motivate students to learn outside of class and arrive prepared for lecture. By complementing your teaching with our engaging technology and content, you can be confident your students will arrive at that moment—the moment of true understanding.

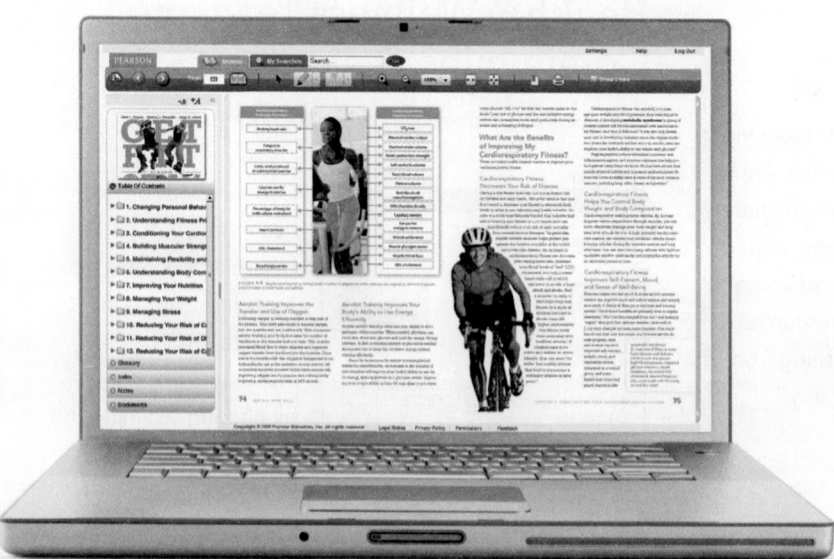

NEW! Active Media Callouts on Pearson eText

New media callouts in the chapter openers, end-of-chapter material, and throughout the text, provide direct links to the extensive supporting electronic media, including videos, audio files, assignments, and review materials.

Proven Results

MyFitnessLab has a consistently positive impact on the quality of learning in higher education fitness & wellness instruction. MyFitnessLab can be successfully implemented in any environment—lab-based, hybrid, fully online, traditional—and demonstrates the quantifiable difference that integrated usage of these products has on student retention, subsequent success, and overall achievement.

NEW! Pre- and Post-Evaluations

You can now easily measure before and after results for both Student Learning Outcomes and Fitness Evaluations. A 50-question exam can be assigned at the start of the course, and again at the end, to effectively measure Student Learning Outcomes. Additionally, an editable version of the Pre-/Post-Fitness assessment from the beginning of the book is available so students can track before and after results.

NEW! Over 180 Pre-built Assignments

Instructors can lessen their prep time and simplify their lives with preloaded quiz and test questions (specific to the textbook) that they can assign and/ or edit, a gradebook that automatically records student results from assigned tests, and the ability to customize the course as much (or as little) as desired.

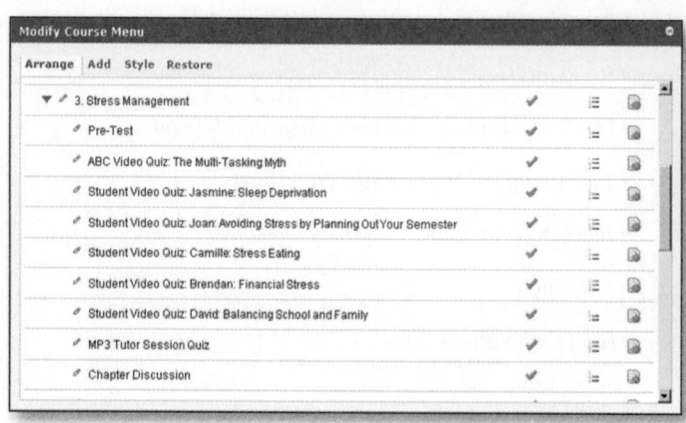

Tools to Help You Coach Better

Teaching Tool Box

978-0-321-78043-0 • 0-321-78043-4

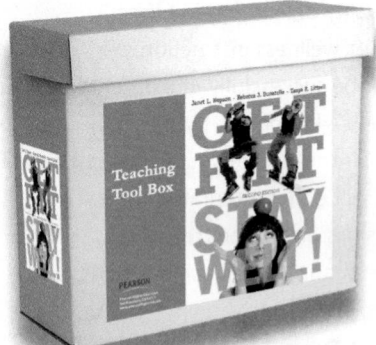

Save hours of valuable planning time with one comprehensive course planning kit. In one handy box, adjuncts, part-time, and full-time faculty will find a wealth of supplements and resources that reinforce key learning from the text and suit virtually any teaching style.

The Teaching Tool Box includes:

• Instructor Resource DVD

• Instructor Resource and Support Manual

• Test Bank

• User's Quick Guide reference guide

• Access to MyFitnessLab™ course management website

• *Great Ideas: Active Ways to Teach Health and Wellness*

• *Behavior Change Log Book and Wellness Journal*

• *Eat Right! Healthy Eating in College and Beyond*

• *Live Right! Beating Stress in College and Beyond*

• *Take Charge of Your Health!* Worksheets

• *Teaching with Student Learning Outcomes*

• *Teaching with Web 2.0*

• *Food Composition Table*

Health & Wellness Teaching Community

www.pearsonhighered.com/healthcommunity

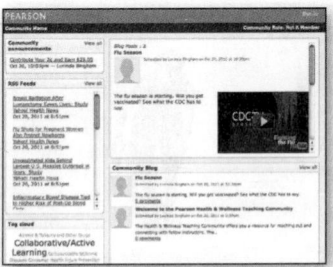

Connect with other health instructors! The Health & Wellness Teaching Community website serves instructors like you by offering teaching tips and ideas, and by providing a forum for you to discuss health-related issues with your peers.

Student Supplements

MyFitnessLab
www.myfitnesslab.com

Behavior Change Log Book and Wellness Journal
978-0-321-80317-7 • 0-321-80317-5

Live Right! Beating Stress in College and Beyond
978-0-321-49149-7 • 0-321-49149-1

Eat Right! Healthy Eating in College and Beyond
978-0-8053-8288-4 • 0-8053-8288-7

Take Charge of Your Health! Worksheets
978-0-321-49942-4 • 0-321-49942-5

Food Composition Table
978-0-321-66793-9 • 0-321-66793-X

Companion Website
www.pearsonhighered.com/hopson

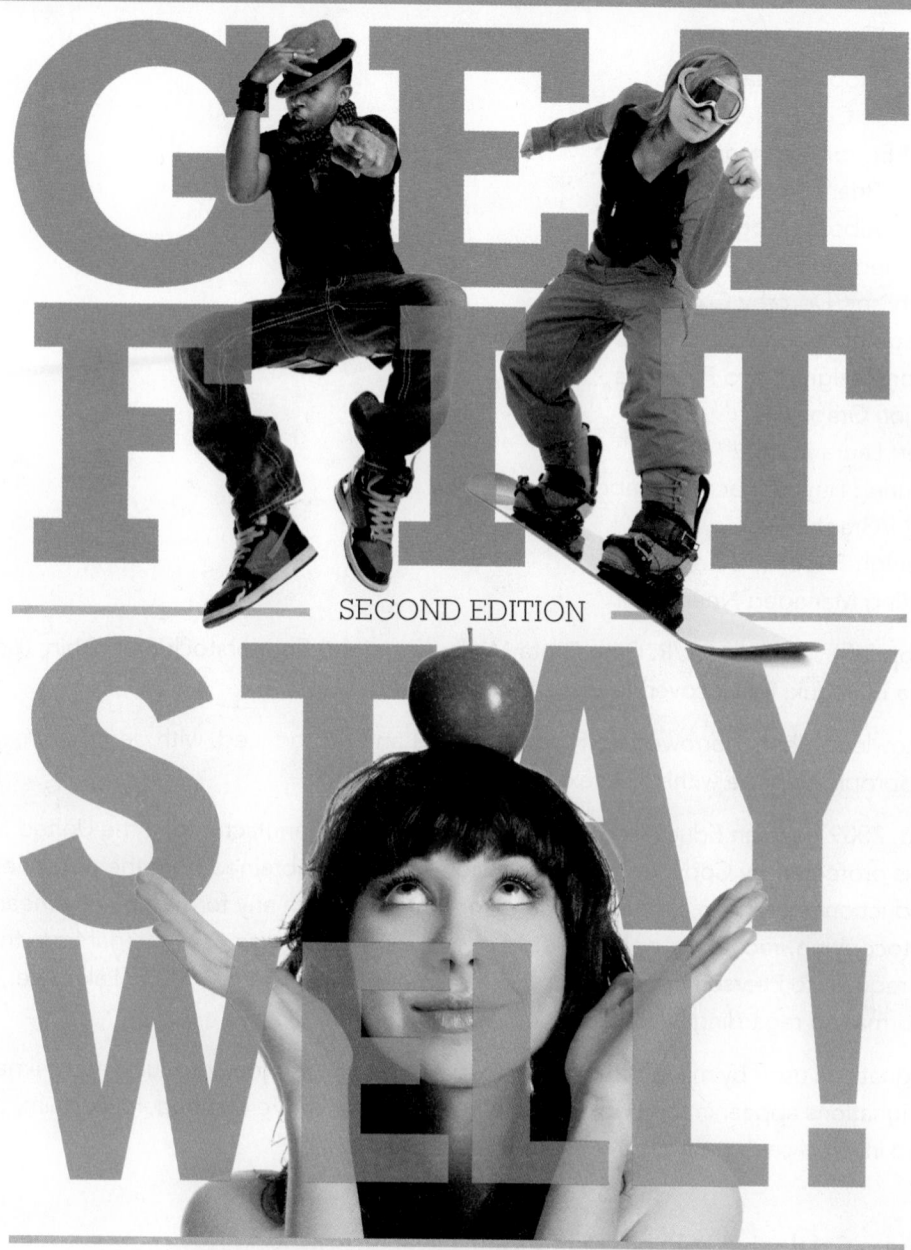

GET FIT STAY WELL!

SECOND EDITION

BRIEF EDITION

Janet L. Hopson, M.A.
San Francisco State University

Rebecca J. Donatelle, Ph.D.
Oregon State University

Tanya R. Littrell, Ph.D.
Portland Community College

PEARSON

Boston   Columbus   Indianapolis   New York   San Francisco   Upper Saddle River
Amsterdam   Cape Town   Dubai   London   Madrid   Milan   Munich   Paris   Montréal   Toronto
Delhi   Mexico City   São Paulo   Sydney   Hong Kong   Seoul   Singapore   Taipei   Tokyo

Executive Editor: Sandra Lindelof
Project Editor: Kari Hopperstead
Development Editor: Claire Alexander
Art Development Editor: Kari Hopperstead
Editorial Assistant: Briana Verdugo
Managing Editor: Deborah Cogan
Assistant Editor: Meghan Zolnay
Production Supervisor: Dorothy Cox
Production Management and Compositor: PreMediaGlobal
Cover and Interior Designer: Yvo Riezebos
Illustrator: Precision Graphics
Photo Researcher: Laura Murray
Senior Manufacturing Buyer: Stacey Weinberger
Text Printer: Quad/Graphics
Cover Printer: Lehigh-Phoenix Color
Executive Marketing Manager: Neena Bali

Cover Photos: (top left) Shutterstock/R. Gino Santa Maria; (top right) Shutterstock/Samokhin; (bottom) Shutterstock/Inga Marchuk; (back cover) Shutterstock/ULKASTUDIO

Credits and acknowledgments borrowed from other sources and reproduced, with permission, in this textbook appear on the appropriate page within the text [or on p. C-1–C-2].

Library of Congress Cataloging-in-Publication Data
Hopson, Janet L.
  Get fit, stay well! / Janet L. Hopson, Donatelle, Rebecca J., Tanya R. Littrell.
  —2nd ed.
    p. cm.
  ISBN 978-0-321-75433-2
  1. Physical fitness—Textbooks. 2. Health—Textbooks.
  I. Donatelle, Rebecca J., 1950- II. Littrell, Tanya R. III. Title.
  RA781.H65 2011
  613.7—dc23   2011042231

ISBN 10: 0-321-75433-6; ISBN 13: 978-0-321-75433-2 (Student edition)
ISBN 10: 0-321-78036-1; ISBN 13: 978-0-321-78036-2 (Brief Edition)
ISBN 10: 0-321-78041-8; ISBN 13: 978-0-321-78041-6 (Exam Copy)
ISBN 10: 0-321-80229-2; ISBN 13: 978-0-321-80229-3 (a la Carte edition)

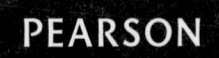

www.pearsonhighered.com   1 2 3 4 5 6 7 8 9 10—QGD—15 14 13 12 11

To the memory of Ruth and David Hopson, who taught me, by example and encouragement, to love fitness activity.—**JLH**

To the strong, intelligent, loving, and hard-working women who have motivated me and taught me to care about the important things—especially my mom, Agnes E. Donatelle.—**RJD**

To my mom, whose continued unconditional support and encouragement of her children is an inspiration.—**TRL**

About the Authors

Janet L. Hopson, M.A.

A full-time author and lecturer, Janet L. Hopson has written or co-authored nine books, including two popular nonfiction books on human pheromones and human brain development, and eight textbooks on general biology and wellness for college and high school students. Ms. Hopson currently teaches science writing at San Francisco State University and the University of California at Santa Cruz. She holds B.A. and M.A. degrees from Southern Illinois University and the University of Missouri. She has won awards for magazine writing, and her articles have appeared in *Smithsonian, Psychology Today, Science Digest, Science News, Outside,* and others. She is married and enjoys golfing, swimming, reading, traveling, competitive tennis, and teaching horseback riding.

Rebecca J. Donatelle, Ph.D.

Dr. Rebecca J. Donatelle is a Professor Emeritus in Public Health at Oregon State University, having served as the Department Chair, Coordinator of the Public Health Promotion and Education Programs, and faculty member and researcher in the College of Health and Human Sciences. She has a Ph.D. in Community Health/Health Education, a M.S. in Health Education, and a B.S. with majors in both Health/Physical Education and English. Her main research and teaching focus has been on the factors that increase risk for chronic diseases and the use of incentives and social supports in developing effective interventions for high-risk women and families. Her research has been published in numerous journals, and she has been a guest speaker and presenter at professional conferences throughout the country. Dr. Donatelle is also the author of the highly successful introductory health textbooks *Access to Health* and *Health: The Basics,* as well as the new *My Health: An Outcomes Approach.*

Tanya R. Littrell, Ph.D.

Dr. Tanya R. Littrell is a full-time faculty member in Fitness Technology and Physical Education at Portland Community College in Portland, Oregon. Dr. Littrell worked as a fitness director for many years before attending graduate school at Oregon State University, where she earned both a master's degree in Human Performance/Exercise Physiology and a doctoral degree in Exercise Science/Exercise Physiology. Dr. Littrell has been teaching lifetime fitness classes for undergraduates since 1998. When she is not teaching, preparing to teach, or writing, you can find Dr. Littrell on the trails running or mountain biking, rock climbing, traveling, or spending quality time with her family.

Brief Contents

Contents

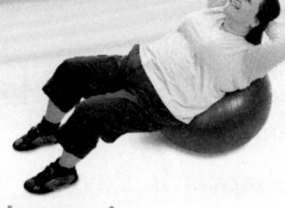
3 Conditioning Your Cardiorespiratory System 67

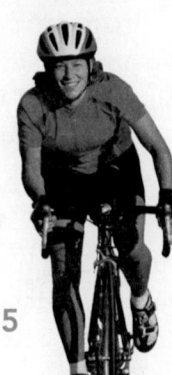

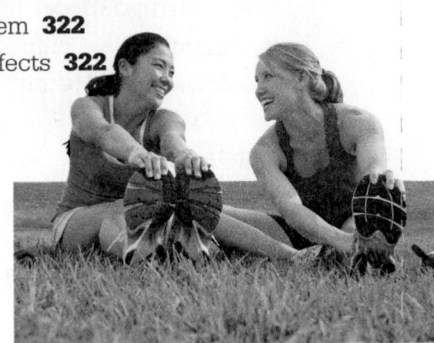

10 Reducing Your Risk of Cardiovascular Disease 347

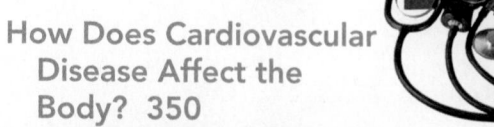

Feature Boxes

Labs and Programs

You may have noticed that health, fitness, and wellness are highly popular topics! Open a newspaper, turn on the TV, or surf the Internet and you will undoubtedly find articles about the benefits of exercise, the health risks associated with obesity, or the results of a recent nutritional study. At the same time, if you are a college student taking a fitness and wellness course, you may feel a sense of disconnect between those stories and your own life. You might wonder: What has any of this got to do with me?

Our primary goal in writing this textbook was simple: to get students to realize that the lifestyle choices you make now—regardless of your current age—have real and lasting effects on your lifelong wellness. We also wanted to write a textbook that takes into account the many challenges facing today's students and offers you maximum flexibility and options for creating a fitness and wellness program that you can personalize for your own goals and time demands. Finally, we wanted this textbook to address a common fact of life: the gap between knowing what we *ought* to do (for example, exercise more, eat healthier foods, quit smoking, etc.) and actually *doing it*. Throughout this textbook, we emphasize that effective behavior change is a gradual process, based on having realistic expectations and setting achievable short-term and long-term goals.

With these aims in mind, the following are some of the unique features you'll find in *Get Fit, Stay Well!: Brief Edition.*

New to This Edition

- *The nutrition chapter has been updated per the 2010 USDA guidelines* and the book draws upon the latest exercise recommendations from American College of Sports Medicine, American Heart Association, and U. S. Department of Health and Human Services.

- *New Activate, Motivate, & Advance sample fitness and wellness programs* placed at the ends of Chapters 2–5, 8, and 9 are like having your own personal trainer built into the book. Each program contains guidance on 3 parts of a fitness or wellness program: getting started, motivating to continue, and taking it to the next level. The customizable "pre-fab" programs and the related tracking features and technique videos on the website make it easy to jump into a behavior change project.

- *New Learning Outcomes* replace Chapter Objectives in the chapter openers.

- *New exercise photos* expand options for alternate equipment and exercises, and replace those photos identified by reviewers as showing less than optimal form or atypical equipment.

- *New media callouts* in the chapter openers, end-of-chapter material, and throughout the text direct students to the extensive supporting electronic media, including videos, audio files, assignments, and review materials. In the eText versions, these callouts provide direct links to the media assets.

- *New Think!/Act!* questions at the end of the case studies and throughout the text are designed to encourage critical thinking and to help students reflect on how the material applies to their own lives.

Updates to the Media Program Include:

- *MyFitnessLab™* has been redesigned and now contains more assignable, gradable content for every chapter. Assigning and grading homework has never been easier! More than 180 assignments, including interactive lab worksheets, pre- and post-chapter quizzes, Case Study quizzes, video quizzes, and discussion questions are available for instructors to assign with the a click of a button.

- *New ABC News videos* with accompanying quizzes and discussion questions are available on the instructor resource DVD, MyFitnessLab, and Companion Website.

- *Revised and expanded exercise videos* include new options for stability ball exercises and demonstration videos for fitness assessment labs—over 100 videos in all!

- *New sample fitness and wellness programs* link to demonstration videos and related tracking tools for customizing and logging a behavior change project.

Other Key Features

- *Unique Case Studies presented in each chapter* introduce a "character" who reflects the concerns, questions, and thought processes that students are likely to have themselves. Think!/Act! questions at the end of the case studies encourage critical thinking and help students consider how the material applies to their own lives.

- *Labs employ a unique three-pronged approach:* 1) skill-acquisition labs, 2) self-assessment labs, and 3) action-plan labs. The labs not only measure a student's current level of fitness/wellness, but also teach practical lifelong skills and encourage real behavior change. Many additional labs are offered online on the book's website. All labs are also available online in interactive PDF format and are assignable through MyFitnessLab.

- *The most modern strength-training presentation available* includes photos of more 80 strength-training and flexibility exercises featuring actual college students, modern gym equipment, and options for students with limited access to equipment. Videos of the exercises in the book, as well as many alternate exercises, are available online at the Companion Website and MyFitnessLab—allowing students access to additional instruction on their own time.

- *A separate chapter on diabetes and other chronic diseases* makes this text a valuable reference for fitness and wellness courses, as it emphasizes one of today's national health epidemics.

- *A strong emphasis is placed on behavior change throughout the text*. Think!/Act! features provide suggestions for immediate action and Tools for Change boxes provide tools for longer-term change. The "Plan for Change" labs ask students to write out an action plan for behavior change.

- *Questions boxes* investigate common questions and concerns students may have in relation to chapter topics.

- *Diversity boxes* address topics relevant to diverse student populations, acknowledging that age, race, gender, disability, and individual life circumstances can result in specific fitness and wellness needs.

- *A running glossary* helps students easily review and master key terms.

- *End-of-chapter review questions and critical thinking questions* encourage students to evaluate material they have just learned.

- *Research citations* demonstrate the accuracy, currency, and scientific grounding for information presented in the text.

- *A pre- and post-course progress worksheet* included at the beginning of the book and available online allows students to assess their progress on key fitness/wellness assessments.

Instructor Supplements

This textbook comes with unparalleled supplemental resources to assist instructors with classroom preparation and presentation.

Teaching Tool Box

Save hours of valuable planning time with one comprehensive course planning box containing a wealth of supplements and resources that reinforce key learning from the text and suit virtually any teaching style. The Teaching Tool Box includes:

- *Instructor Resource DVD* with all art, photos, and tables from the text; PowerPoint® lecture slides; a computerized test bank; *ABC News* videos; exercise demonstration videos, Active Lecture (clicker) Questions; Quiz Show Game PowerPoint slides; interactive PDF lab worksheets; PDF transparency masters, Instructor Resource and Support Manual PDFs, and Test Bank Word files

- *Instructor Resource and Support Manual* with detailed chapter outlines incorporating IR-DVD assets, in-class discussion questions, and activities, additional resources, first-time teaching tips, sample syllabi, and tips for using MyFitnessLab

- *Test Bank* with over 1000 questions in multiple-choice, true/false, and short-essay formats

- *User's Quick Start Guide* for getting up and running using the materials in the Teaching Tool Box

- *Access to MyFitnessLab™* course management website with more than 180 separate assignments, a gradebook, and an annotatable eText

- *Great Ideas: Active Ways to Teach Health and Wellness*, a manual of ideas for classroom activities related to fitness and wellness topics, including activities that can be adapted to various topics and class sizes

- *New Teaching with Student Learning Outcomes* publication containing useful suggestions and examples for successfully incorporating outcomes into a fitness and wellness course

- *New Teaching with Web 2.0* handbook introducing popular new online tools and offering ideas for incorporating them into a fitness and wellness course

- *Behavior Change Log Book with Wellness Journal*, newly revised to include updated worksheets, nutrition information, journals, and fitness logs

- *New Food Composition Table* containing detailed nutrition information about thousands of foods

- *Live Right! Beating Stress in College and Beyond* booklet on handling life's challenges including sleep, finances, time management, academic pressure, and relationships

- *Eat Right! Healthy Eating in College and Beyond* booklet of guidelines, tips, and recipes for healthy eating

- *Take Charge of Your Health!* self-assessment worksheets

MyFitnessLab

www.pearsonhighered.com/myfitnesslab

This redesigned online course management program is loaded with valuable teaching resources that make it easy to give assignments and track student progress. The preloaded content in MyFitnessLab includes unsurpassed resources for teaching online or hybrid courses and is arranged into five learning areas.

In the Read It area:

- *New Pearson eText* gives students access to the text whenever and wherever they have access to the Internet. The powerful functionality of the eText includes the ability to create notes, highlight text in different colors, create bookmarks, zoom, click on hyperlinked words and phrases to view definitions, and view in single-page or two-page view.

- *New RSS feeds* provide students easy, online access to news and spotlights about hot fitness and wellness topics, updated daily.

- *New chapter learning outcomes* reiterate the important points in each chapter.

In the See It area:

- *More than 100 exercise videos* demonstrate strength-training and flexibility exercises with resistance bands, stability balls, free weights, and gym machines, as well as lab assessment techniques. The videos are also available for download onto iPods® or other media players, and some have related quizzing.

- *New ABC News video clips* bring fitness and wellness topics to life. Related quizzing is available for assigning and automatic grading.

In the Hear It area:

- *New audio cases studies* from the text pertain to each chapter's content. All are available for download as MP3 files and have related assignable and gradable quizzing.

- *Audio PowerPoint lectures* support classroom lectures and enhance self-study options.

In the Do It area:

- *Pre-course/Post-course assessment* lets students evaluate their own fitness and wellness status both before and after taking the course.

- *New interactive labs* automatically perform calculations on students' input. Completed labs can be submitted to instructors by digital dropbox, e-mail, or print. More than 55 labs guide students through assessing fitness and wellness levels, learning core skills, and developing behavior change plans. Additional labs available only online are designed to accommodate varying skill levels, differing access to equipment, and the specific needs of students with disabilities.

In the Review It area:

- *Multiple-choice and true/false self-study quizzes* for every chapter are automatically scored, so students can get feedback and check their understanding. Quizzes can also be assigned by instructors and feed to the gradebook.

- *Online glossary* is a quick and easy resource for definitions of key terms.

- *Interactive flashcards* allow students to build a deck of flashcards from the key terms in every chapter, review them online, print them out, or even export them to a mobile phone.

- *New Activate, Motivate, & Advance programs* from the text help students commit to and track a new fitness or wellness routine. Links to exercise demonstration and technique videos provide further guidance for students just getting started on a new fitness program.

- *Behavior Change Logbook and Wellness Journal* is provided in interactive PDF format for easy assigning and submitting.

- *Take Charge of Your Health! worksheets* in interactive PDF format offer more options for self-assessment and developing behavior change plans.

Student Supplements

A wealth of materials is available to help students review and explore course content and enact behavior change in their own lives.

MyFitnessLab

www.pearsonhighered.com/myfitnesslab

This online course management program has been redesigned for greater usability and is loaded with valuable resources. The preloaded content includes unsurpassed resources for online or hybrid courses; see the full description under Instructor Supplements above.

Companion Website

www.pearsonhighered.com/hopson

The *Get Fit, Stay Well!* companion website offers hundreds of practice quiz questions, interactive labs, 50 additional health self-assessment worksheets, web links, glossary and flashcards of key terms, audio case studies and audio PowerPoint lectures, more than 30 ABC News videos, and more than 100 exercise demonstration videos.

Behavior Change Log Book and Wellness Journal
978-0-321-80317-7 / 0-321-80317-5

This booklet helps students track their daily exercise and nutritional intake and create a personalized long-term nutrition and fitness program. It has been newly revised to include updated worksheets, nutrition information, journals, and fitness logs

Eat Right! Healthy Eating in College and Beyond
978-0-8053-8288-4 / 0-8053-8288-7

This handy, full-color booklet provides practical guidelines, tips, shopper's guides and recipes for putting healthy eating principles into action. Topics include healthy eating in the cafeteria, dorm room, and fast food restaurants; eating on a budget; weight management tips; vegetarian alternatives; and guidelines on alcohol and health.

Take Charge of Your Health! Worksheets
978-0-321-49942-4 / 0-321-49942-5

Twelve new worksheets have been added to this edition's collection of self-assessment activities, providing a total of 50 self-assessment exercises in a gummed pad that can be packaged with the text.

New Lifestyles Pedometer
978-0-321-51803-3 / 0-321-51803-9

Take strides to better health with this pedometer, a first step toward overall health and wellness. This pedometer measures steps, distance (miles), activity time, and calories, and provides a time clock.

MyDietAnalysis

Powered by ESHA Research, Inc., MyDietAnalysis features a database of nearly 20,000 foods. This easy-to-use program allows students to track their diet and activity for up to three profiles and to assess the nutritional value of their food consumption.

Food Composition Table
978-0-321-66793-9 / 0-321-66793-X

This comprehensive booklet provides detailed nutritional information on thousands of foods and is correlated with MyDietAnalysis.

Acknowledgments

From Janet Hopson

Preparing a new edition of a college program such as *Get Fit, Stay Well!*—including the book and all of its accompanying study and instructional materials—is an enormous undertaking. The authors' efforts are just part of a complex, well-integrated team effort. We would like to thank the following members of the Pearson book team: Kari Hopperstead, who so ably, tirelessly, and cheerfully coordinated and managed the second edition text and ancillary revision effort; Barbara Yien, Frank Ruggirello, Sandra Lindelof, and Deirdre Espinoza, who all championed this book in its early stages; Claire Alexander, our dedicated and very able development editor; our superb marketing manager Neena Bali; Dorothy Cox and Tracy Duff, our production coordinators; art lead Mimi Bickel and all her colleagues at Precision Graphics; the talented composition and production team at PreMedia Global; photo researcher Laura Murray; Yvo Riezebos and Riezebos Holzbaur Design Group, who are responsible for this book's dynamic design; permissions editor Jennifer Bevington; Sade McDougal, who managed the online supplements; ancillary production managers Miriam Adrianowicz and Megan Power; and editorial *wunderkinds* Meghan Zolnay and Briana Verdugo. Finally, and in many ways primarily, I would like to personally thank my coauthors Becky and Tanya for their years of effort and their superb knowledge and experience.

From Rebecca Donatelle

After working on several college textbooks over the years, one thing has become very clear to me: the publishing house you choose to work with is the single most important factor in producing a quality textbook that is going to be successful in the marketplace. Pearson has assembled a truly remarkable group of top-notch acquisition, editorial, production, marketing, sales, and ancillary staff to help nurture a text through its development and growth. I am fortunate to have had the opportunity to work with individuals who worry the details and possess an incredible degree of creativity and professionalism. You are truly THE BEST . . . thank you so much to each and every one of you. A special thank you to Kari Hopperstead, who, in usual fashion, exemplified all that any publisher and author would want in an outstanding project editor. Additionally, I would like to thank my co-authors, Jan and Tanya. From conceptualization to final product, this text would not have happened without your efforts.

From Tanya Littrell

I would like to first and foremost thank my family for all of their support through the long hours of creating and revising this textbook. Thank you to my co-authors, Jan and Becky, whose expertise and experience have really guided this textbook. Working with the staff at Pearson has been a great experience. Thank you to Sandra Lindelof for bringing me into this project, Barbara Yien for her unending patience on the first edition, and Kari Hopperstead for keeping me on track with the many second edition updates. I would

Acknowledgments *(continued)*

also like to thank fellow faculty members at Portland Community College who have been supportive throughout this project; in particular, Janeen Hull, a faculty peer and friend. Ms. Hull was the knowledgeable and creative mind behind the new fitness programs for this edition. My graduate work and teaching at Oregon State University really set the stage for my work on this project, and so I would like to thank Anthony Wilcox, department chair of Nutrition and Exercise Sciences, for having faith in me as an instructor and giving me teaching and supervisory experience that lead to this opportunity.

From The Publisher

For their work on the ancillary materials, we thank Denise Wright and Rebecca Hendricks of Southern Editorial and David Payne. Many thanks go to Janeen Hull of Portland Community College and Ven. Dhammadinna of Bodhiheart Sangha for their contributions to the new Activate, Motivate, & Advance programs. Special thanks go to the participants in our second edition photo shoots: photographer Elena Dorfman; C. J. Jones, Fitness Center Coordinator at De Anza College in Cupertino, California; and models Crystaldawn Bell, Manuela Cortez, Maureen Healy, Sandra Jasso, Jodece Mason, Roy Nutt, Jaehyun Park, Philip Saneski, and Janie Zapata-Wilson. In addition, we thank the participants in our second edition exercise video shoot: Dr. Stephen Ball of the University of Missouri; Dan Desloge and Tim Donsbach from Bad Dog Pictures; and models Celsi Cowan, Dakota Evans, Marshida Harris, Marcus Johnson, Erick King, and Jordan Kroell. Dr. Tom LaFontaine deserves special recognition for facilitating our filming at Optimus: The Center for Health in Columbia, Missouri (www.optimushealth.com). The mission of Optimus is to provide research-based, lifestyle interventions designed to reduce the risks for chronic diseases. Optimus strives to provide a positive, safe, and comfortable atmosphere and environment to assist clients in achieving their personal health, fitness, and wellness goals.

Reviewers

Many thanks to the hundreds of instructors and students who reviewed and class-tested the first edition of this text, and to the following reviewers who contributed feedback for this revision:

George J. Abboud, Salem State College

Kym Y. Atwood, University of West Florida

Stephen D. Ball, University of Missouri

Diana Carey, Rockland Community College

Mandi Dupain, Millersville University

Robert Femat, El Paso Community College

Jennifer L. Gordon, Manchester Community College

Megan Granquist, University of La Verne

Carol Kennedy-Armbruster, Indiana University

Angela Baldwin Lanier, Berry College

Michelle Lesperance, Greensboro College

David Mann, Darton College

Mike Manning, Indiana Wesleyan University

Holly Molilla, Dutchess Community College

Laurie Moris, William Paterson University

Catherine R. Nolan, Moraine Valley Community College

William J. Papin, Western Carolina University

Rod Porter, San Diego Miramar College

Edgar Reed, Hardin-Simmons University

Jenifer Hudman Roberts, Northwest Vista College

Amanda Salyer Funk, Ball State University

Jay Douglas Seelbach, Anderson University

Robin Siara, Rio Hondo College

Jennifer Spry-Knutson, Des Moines Area Community College

Susan M. Tendy, United States Military Academy

Virginia L. Trummer, University of Texas at San Antonio

Michael Webster, University of Southern Mississippi

Mary Winfrey-Kovell, Ball State University

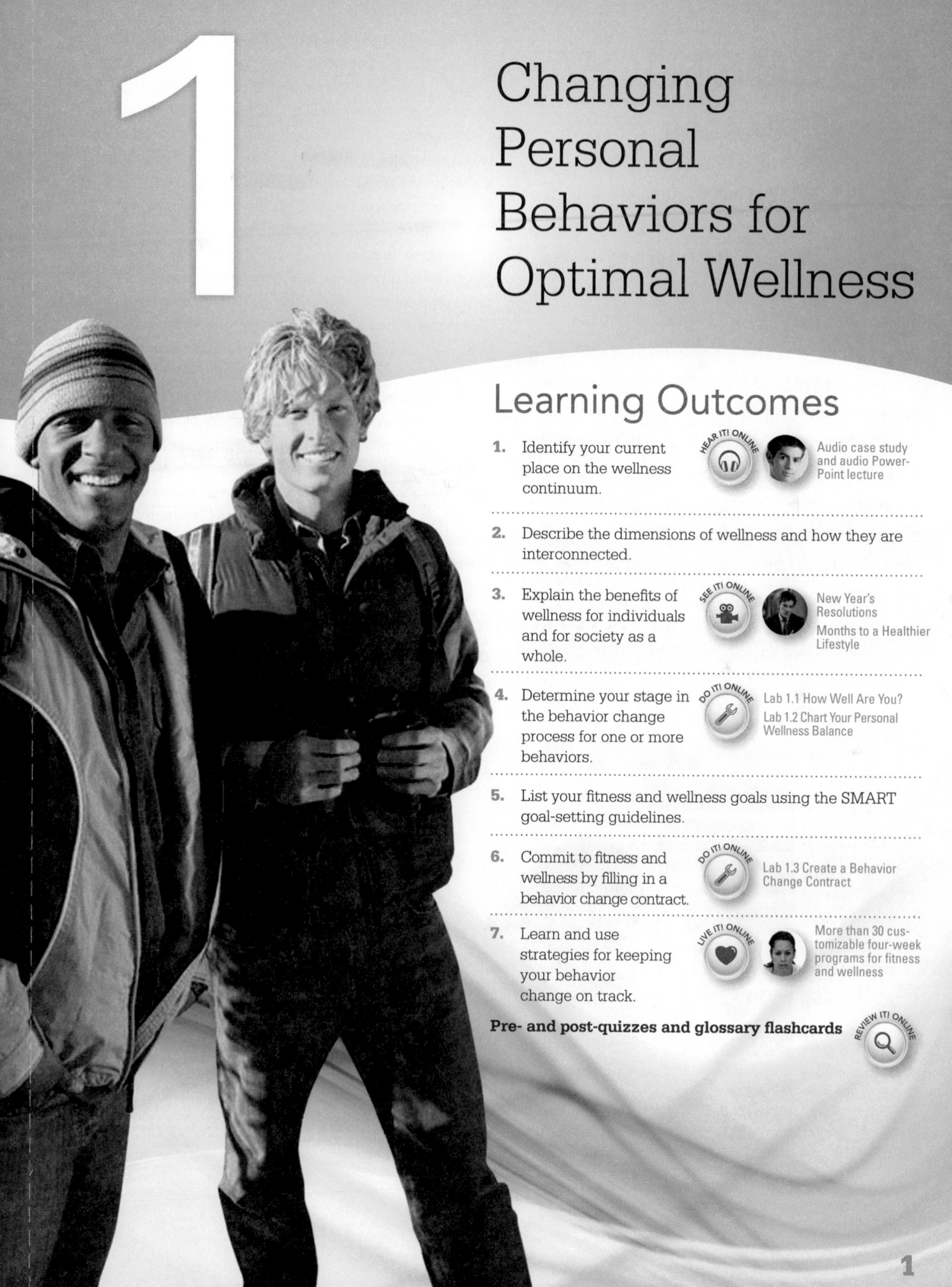

1

Changing Personal Behaviors for Optimal Wellness

Learning Outcomes

1. **Identify your current place on the wellness continuum.**

   HEAR IT! ONLINE — Audio case study and audio PowerPoint lecture

2. **Describe the dimensions of wellness and how they are interconnected.**

3. **Explain the benefits of wellness for individuals and for society as a whole.**

   SEE IT! ONLINE — New Year's Resolutions — Months to a Healthier Lifestyle

4. **Determine your stage in the behavior change process for one or more behaviors.**

   DO IT! ONLINE — Lab 1.1 How Well Are You? — Lab 1.2 Chart Your Personal Wellness Balance

5. **List your fitness and wellness goals using the SMART goal-setting guidelines.**

6. **Commit to fitness and wellness by filling in a behavior change contract.**

   DO IT! ONLINE — Lab 1.3 Create a Behavior Change Contract

7. **Learn and use strategies for keeping your behavior change on track.**

   LIVE IT! ONLINE — More than 30 customizable four-week programs for fitness and wellness

Pre- and post-quizzes and glossary flashcards

REVIEW IT! ONLINE

casestudy

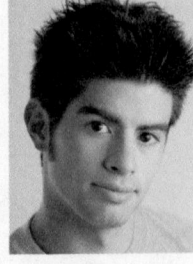

CARLOS

"Hi, I'm Carlos. I just started my freshman year in college. It's my first time living away from home, and I'm getting used to lots of new things. I know my family had to sacrifice for me to be here, so I feel pressure to do well. I also miss my girlfriend, Liz—she's a senior in high school and it's been really hard being away from her. I like my classes so far, but I am never caught up with my reading, and I haven't had a good night's sleep in about a month. To top it all off, I caught a cold that has been going around, and I feel miserable! What can I do to better manage my life?"

HEAR IT! ONLINE

Can you relate to any of Carlos's problems? If so, you are not alone. Many college students report that stress, depression, inadequate sleep, frequent colds, and relationship problems negatively affect their academic performance (Figure 1.1).[1] When asked to rate their overall **wellness,** at least one-third of college students described it as only "good" compared to "very good" or "excellent." About 10 percent rated it as just "fair" or "poor."

Wellness is an optimal soundness of body and mind. To understand wellness, it helps to first consider the concept of "health." While historically the term *health* meant merely the absence of disease, experts today view it as an inclusive term that encompasses everything from environmental health to the health of populations. The term *wellness* conveys a more personalized definition of health. It is the achievement of the highest level of health possible in physical, social, intellectual, emotional, spiritual, and environmental dimensions. It describes a vibrant state in which a person enjoys life to the fullest, adapts relatively easily to life's many challenges, feels that life is meaningful, and functions effectively in society. In this book, we will sometimes use the terms *health* and *wellness* interchangeably, but *wellness* always refers to a more individualized, dynamic concept, requiring significant personal effort, but with the potential to bring great rewards.

Central to wellness is **physical fitness**, or simply *fitness*, the ability to perform moderate to vigorous levels of physical activity without undue fatigue. Fitness is just one dimension of wellness, but we give it special attention in this book because it influences so many of the other dimensions and because the tools for improving fitness are readily available while you are a college student—a period in your life when you can establish personal habits that will benefit you for a lifetime.

Impediment	Percentage
Stress	27.4%
Sleep difficulties	20.0%
Cold/flu/sore throat	18.3%
Anxiety	18.0%
Work	13.7%
Internet use/computer games	12.3%
Depression	11.7%
Concern for friend/family member	11.1%
Relationship difficulties	11.0%
Extracurricular activities	9.1%

Percentage of students reporting impediment

FIGURE **1.1** The top 10 wellness impacts on college performance.

Data from: American College Health Association, *American College Health Association—National College Health Assessment II: Reference Group Executive Summary Spring 2010* (Linthicum, Maryland: American College Health Association, 2010).

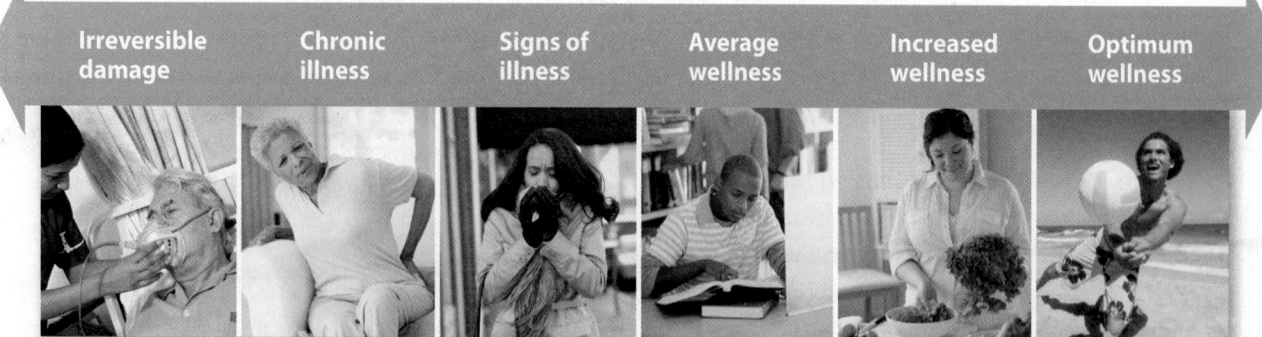

| Irreversible damage | Chronic illness | Signs of illness | Average wellness | Increased wellness | Optimum wellness |

FIGURE **1.2** The double-headed arrow depicts the continuum of wellness states.

Where Am I on the Wellness Continuum?

Improving your wellness—moving toward that vibrant multidimensional state—is an ambitious but achievable goal. The wellness patterns you establish during this course can change how you live each day and can positively affect your quality of life for years to come. However, no single college course can address every health concern or guarantee a lifetime of wellness. Your age, personal history, genetic susceptibility to medical conditions, and your physical environment all affect your wellness. So does access to high-quality medical care, nutritious food, good exercise facilities, and social support networks.

The first step in achieving optimal wellness is assessing how close you are at present to that long-term goal. We can picture wellness as a continuum of greater or lesser total soundness of body and mind (Figure 1.2). Understanding your current place on the **wellness continuum** is important for changing wellness behaviors.

What Are the Dimensions of Wellness?

We can think of wellness as consisting of six primary dimensions (physical, social, intellectual, emotional, spiritual, and environmental) (Figure 1.3). Wellness is a process, and at times you may experience faster growth in one dimension than in others. The dimensions are interconnected, however, so positive effort in one area can help you make progress in others and move you toward greater overall health and well-being.

Physical Wellness

Physical wellness encompasses all aspects of a sound body, including body size, shape, and

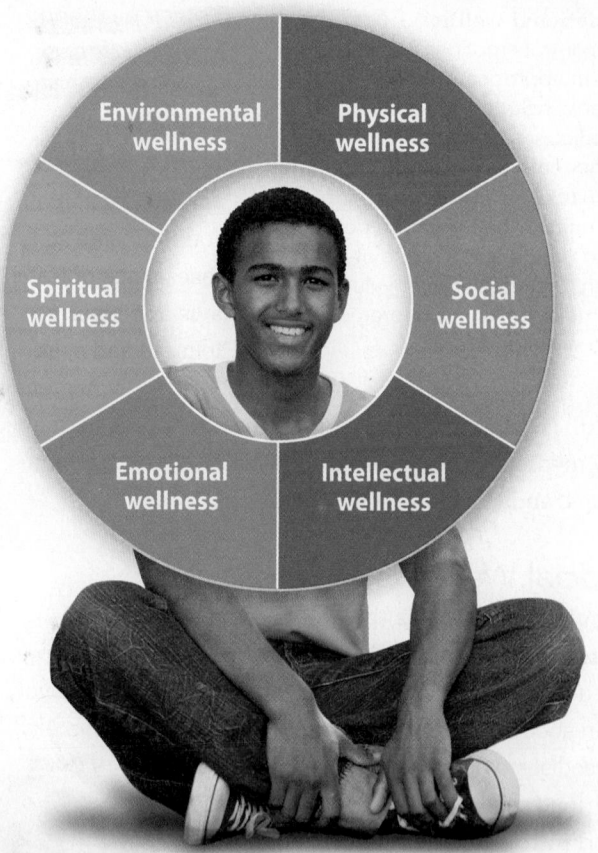

FIGURE **1.3** Wellness is an optimal level of health in six interconnected dimensions of human experience.

composition; sensory sharpness and responsiveness; body functioning; physical strength, flexibility, and endurance; resistance to diseases and disorders; and recuperative abilities. The physical

wellness Achieving the highest level of health possible in each of several dimensions

physical fitness The ability to perform moderate to vigorous levels of physical activity without undue fatigue

wellness continuum A spectrum of wellness states from pre-mature death to optimum wellness

physical wellness A state of physical health and well-being that includes body size and shape, body functioning, measures of strength and endurance, and resistance to disease

social wellness A person's degree of social connectedness and skills, leading to satisfying interpersonal relationships

intellectual wellness The ability to think clearly, reason objectively, analyze, and use brain power to solve problems and meet life's challenges

emotional wellness The ability to control emotions and express them appropriately at the right times; includes self-esteem, self-confidence, self-efficacy, and other emotional qualities

spiritual wellness A feeling of unity or oneness with people and nature and a sense of life's purpose, meaning, or value; for some, a belief in a supreme being or religion

state we call fitness includes measures of physical wellness and allows a person to exert physical effort without undue stress, strain, or injury. Many of your day-to-day choices and habits can support or undermine your physical wellness, including your diet; amount and types of exercise; sleep patterns; level of stress; use of tobacco, drugs, or alcohol; participation in unsafe sex; observance of traffic laws and wearing helmets and seat belts; daily hygiene (e.g., flossing and brushing teeth); and access to quality medical attention (e.g., regular checkups, vaccinations, and treatment).

Social Wellness

Social wellness is the ability to have satisfying interpersonal relationships and maintain connections in a diverse range of social networks. This means you can successfully interact with others, adapt to a variety of social situations, and act appropriately in various settings. Whether you are shy and introverted or outgoing and extroverted, social wellness includes the ability to communicate clearly and effectively; the capacity to establish intimacy through trust and acceptance; a willingness to ask for and give support; the ability to maintain friendships over time; and skills for interacting within groups, such as on the job or in the community.

Intellectual Wellness

Intellectual wellness is the ability to use your brain power effectively to solve problems and meet life's challenges. It allows you to think clearly, quickly, creatively, and critically; use good reasoning and make careful decisions; continually learn from your successes and mistakes; organize and streamline your tasks; and maintain a sense of humor.

Emotional Wellness

Emotional wellness means being able to control your emotions and express them appropriately at the right times. Social and emotional concerns,—such as stress, anxiety, depression, and relationship problems—are increasingly common on college campuses and can impede academic success. Improving emotional wellness requires developing good self-esteem; gaining self-confidence; being able to cope with sadness, anger, resentment, and negativity; and developing an appropriate balance of emotional dependence and independence.

Spiritual Wellness

For some people, **spiritual wellness** may involve a belief in a supreme being or a way of life prescribed by a particular religion. For others, spiritual wellness is a feeling of unity or oneness with others and with nature, and a sense of meaning or value in life. Developing greater spiritual wellness may deepen one's understanding of life's purpose; allow a person to feel a part of a greater

casestudy

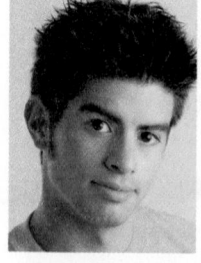

CARLOS

"I know that my life is pretty good. I'm in college, studying what interests me, and I'm excited about the future. I just constantly feel behind. I fall asleep in class sometimes, eat a lot of junk food, and I'm not exercising—who has time? Then I got this cold, partly because I have been stressed out and not sleeping much. I've made some friends in my dorm, and it helps to know that a lot of them are going through the same thing. Talking to Liz every night on the phone helps, too."

THINK! In which dimensions of wellness could Carlos be stronger? Where would you place him on the wellness continuum? How do you compare to Carlos?

ACT! Identify your strongest wellness dimensions as well as the ones you could improve. Create a wellness balance chart and plan the balance you would like to achieve (**Lab 1.2**).

DO IT! ONLINE HEAR IT! ONLINE

. . . .

spectrum of existence; and promote feelings of love, joy, peace, contentment, and wonder over life's experiences.

Environmental Wellness

Our home, work, community, and school environments can be relaxing, safe havens or toxic, threatening, and stressful places to be. **Environmental wellness** entails understanding how the environment can positively or negatively affect you; the role you play in preserving, protecting, and improving the world around you; and what you can do to conserve dwindling resources for future generations.

Related Dimensions of Wellness

Occupational and financial wellness overlap with other wellness areas, and are sometimes considered their own dimensions. Your wellness in these areas can dramatically affect your overall wellness and add to your life's balance (or lack thereof). If you ask family members and friends about their current problems, many will identify their jobs or finances as the top stressors in their lives.

Occupational Wellness **Occupational wellness** is the level of happiness and fulfilment you experience in

your work. An important component of occupational wellness is finding a non-toxic, hazard-free work environment that provides contact with managers and co-workers who value your skills and opinions. Contrary to what people often think, job satisfaction is not closely tied to high wages.[2] You can reach optimal occupational wellness when your personal goals align closely with those of your employer, and when you feel that you are making significant contributions to both sets of goals.

Financial Wellness **Financial wellness** is the ability to successfully balance and manage your financial needs and wants with your income, debts, savings, and investments. If you cannot pay your bills, it can be hard to think of much else and this dimension can overshadow and unbalance the others. People who are managing their finances but just breaking even will still need to make wise consumer choices, carefully control debt, and continually prioritize expenses (see the box How Can I Handle My Finances Better?).

Balancing Your Wellness Dimensions

You may have healthy relationships, but no fondness for exercise. Perhaps your spiritual life is rich, but you have trouble juggling academic demands. Virtually everyone is stronger in some dimensions of wellness than others. Striving for improvement in all six wellness dimensions is a lifelong process. One good approach is to concentrate on those dimensions that present the most pressing need, while working on the others in a steady but relaxed and motivated way. Over time, a balance of work on all the dimensions—one or two now, others later—will eventually promote overall wellness. Your brain and body, your thoughts and emotions, your actions and reactions, your relationship to yourself and others—all are interconnected and integrated. Likewise, the dimensions of wellness are interrelated. For example, increasing your exercise and general activity will also help you manage stress, mood, body composition, and so on.

> **environmental wellness** An appreciation of how the external environment can affect oneself, and an understanding of the role one plays in preserving, protecting, and improving it
>
> **occupational wellness** A level of happiness and fulfilment in work, including harmony with personal goals, appreciation from bosses and co-workers, and a safe workplace
>
> **financial wellness** The ability to balance and manage financial needs and wants with income, debts, savings, and investments

How Can I Handle My Finances Better?

Figuring out how to manage one's money can be tough for college students—especially for traditional-age students who are living apart from their families for the first time and perhaps also learning to use credit cards. Here are some tips that can help you handle credit and finances:

Buy only the items you truly need—and pay cash when you can.

Resist the urge to buy things on impulse. Do the research, find out a reasonable price for your major purchases, and wait a day or so before buying to make sure you really need the thing.

Watch for signs you are too deep in debt.

If you are borrowing money to pay off other loans, paying bills late on purpose, or putting off health care or other important activities because you can't cover the costs, there is a good chance you are in over your head. If you think this describes you, aim to pay off your credit cards or other high-interest loans as soon as you can, even cutting up your credit card, if needed, to save yourself from adding to the problem.

Pay bills on time.

Your actions now affect your ability to get loans later. If you want to have a good financial reputation in the future, start now. Pay your credit card, loans, rent, and other commitments on time to establish your reputation as a reliable consumer.

Keep a minimum of credit cards, and use them wisely.

Carrying more than two credit cards leaves you susceptible to impulse buying and makes you look like a bad risk to creditors. Don't fall prey to tempting credit card offers; just get the one or two cards you need and ignore the rest. Before you make your purchase, think! Will you be able to pay the bill off in full when it comes? If not, interest will start to build up and you may end up paying more in interest charges than what the item originally cost.

Watch your expenses.

Whether you use an online budgeting tool or handwritten notes, keep track of what you spend and make sure it's in line with your long-term goals.

Save for your future.

Before you pay your bills each month, put away money for your future, even if it is only 25 or 50 dollars.

Avoid fees whenever you can.

To avoid costly fees, use your own financial institution's ATMs and watch your checking account balance so you don't "bounce" checks or overdraw your account with your debit card, incurring more fees.

Take responsibility for your finances.

Review your bills and bank statements as soon as possible after they are issued each month. Be sure to check for errors, unauthorized charges, or indications of identity theft. Get errors or problems corrected immediately. Remember—it's your financial reputation on the line!

Start now!

Start small, and stretch yourself a bit to pay off your credit cards and put away money for the future. Even small changes make a big difference!

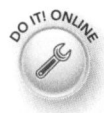
DO IT! ONLINE

Lab 1.1 and **Lab 1.2** at the end of the chapter will help you assess your wellness in each of the primary dimensions and analyze the areas that need improvement.

Why Does Wellness Matter?

Wellness has many benefits for individuals, as well as for society as a whole.

Good Wellness Habits Can Help You Live a Longer, Healthier Life

SEE IT! ONLINE

Months to a Healthier Lifestyle.

In the United States, federal health experts consider the average life expectancy at birth for males to be 76 years, and for females to be 81 years.[3] The precise numbers depend on the methods used for calculating, and some experts project a slight decline in those numbers in coming years.[4] A more important issue is average healthy life expectancy—the years a person can expect to live without disability or major illness: about 68 for males and 72 for females (Figure 1.4).[5] Maintaining good wellness habits can help extend your overall life expectancy, as well as your healthy life expectancy.

Consider the leading causes of death among Americans ages 20–24 (Figure 1.5).[6] Note that accidents kill more young adults than almost all the other causes combined. By making better wellness choices—such as wearing seat belts and bike helmets, and avoiding dangerous behaviors such as driving under the influence of drugs or alcohol—you can reduce your risk of premature death in an accident.

FIGURE 1.4 Healthy life expectancy is a subset of overall life expectancy. Lengthening the span of your healthy years is an important wellness goal.

Data from: World Health Organization, *World Health Statistics 2010.* www.who.int /whosis/whostat/2010/en/index.html.

The leading causes of death for Americans overall are heart disease and cancer (Figure 1.6).[7] Adults contribute greatly to their own risk for these diseases through poor diets, inactivity, and smoking.[8] *Modifiable* risk factors for heart disease and cancer—that is, *risk factors* that are within your control—include high blood pressure, tobacco use, alcohol use, high cholesterol, obesity, low fruit and vegetable intake, and physical inactivity.

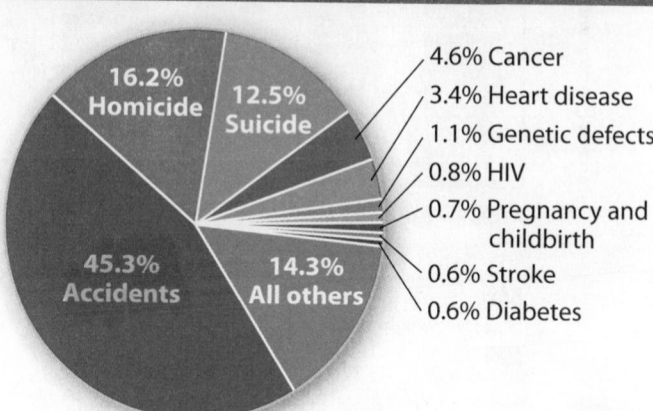

Leading causes of death among Americans ages 20–24

- 16.2% Homicide
- 12.5% Suicide
- 45.3% Accidents
- 14.3% All others
- 4.6% Cancer
- 3.4% Heart disease
- 1.1% Genetic defects
- 0.8% HIV
- 0.7% Pregnancy and childbirth
- 0.6% Stroke
- 0.6% Diabetes

FIGURE 1.5 The leading causes of death among Americans ages 20–24.

Data from: *National Vital Statistics Reports* 58, no. 14 (March 31, 2010).

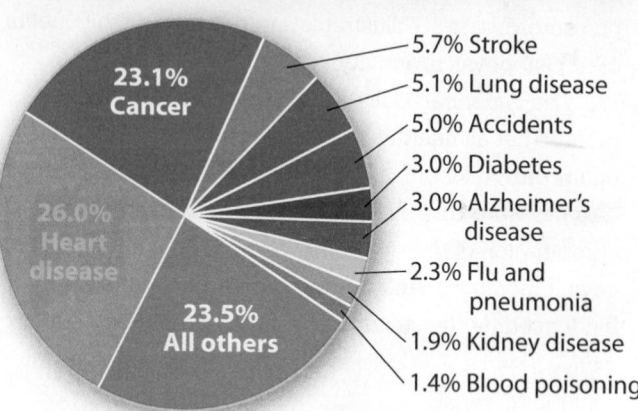

Leading causes of death among Americans overall

- 23.1% Cancer
- 26.0% Heart disease
- 23.5% All others
- 5.7% Stroke
- 5.1% Lung disease
- 5.0% Accidents
- 3.0% Diabetes
- 3.0% Alzheimer's disease
- 2.3% Flu and pneumonia
- 1.9% Kidney disease
- 1.4% Blood poisoning

FIGURE 1.6 The leading causes of death among Americans overall.

Data from: *National Vital Statistics Reports* 58, no. 14 (March 31, 2010).

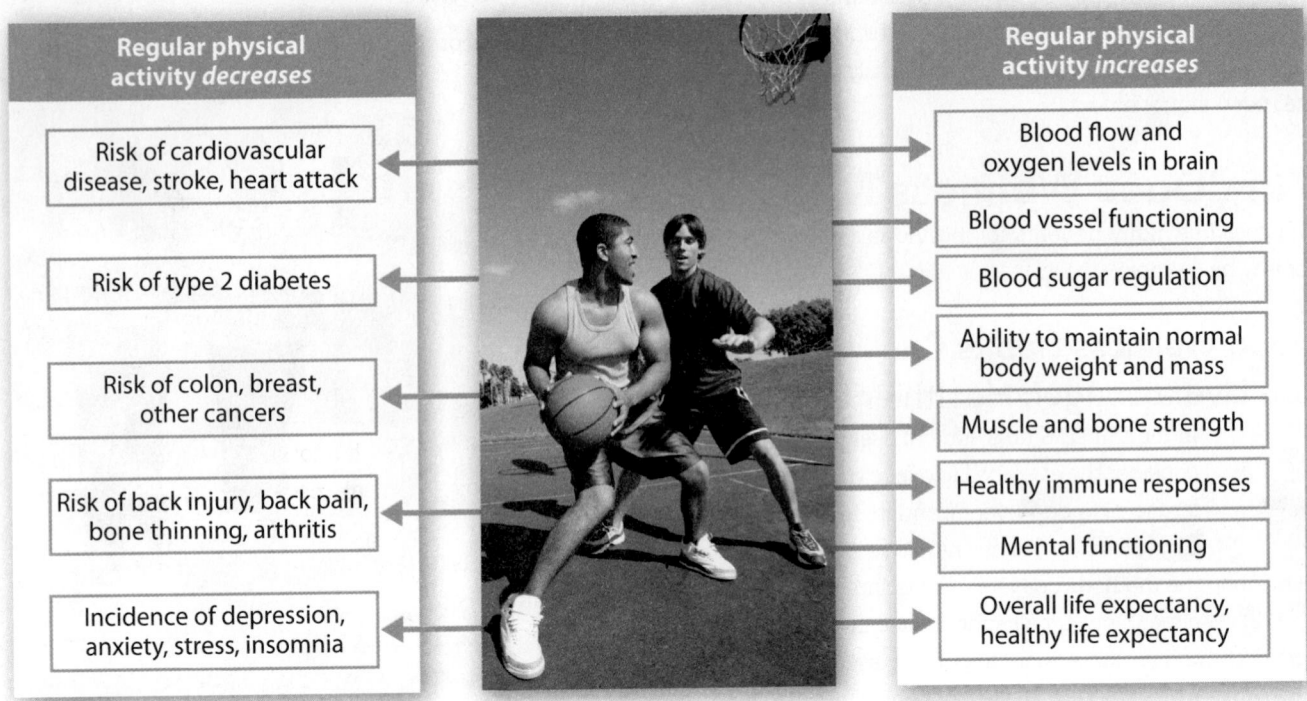

Regular physical activity *decreases*	Regular physical activity *increases*
Risk of cardiovascular disease, stroke, heart attack	Blood flow and oxygen levels in brain
Risk of type 2 diabetes	Blood vessel functioning
Risk of colon, breast, other cancers	Blood sugar regulation
Risk of back injury, back pain, bone thinning, arthritis	Ability to maintain normal body weight and mass
Incidence of depression, anxiety, stress, insomnia	Muscle and bone strength
	Healthy immune responses
	Mental functioning
	Overall life expectancy, healthy life expectancy

FIGURE **1.7** Regular physical activity results in many health benefits.

Researchers have made a compelling case for the role of physical activity in decreasing the risk of chronic disease. Medical researchers have shown in hundreds of studies that the vast majority of all illnesses of middle age and later years (including heart disease, cancer, and type 2 diabetes) are related to, and exacerbated by, a lack of physical activity.[9] Living a **sedentary** life also increases the danger of *hypokinetic diseases*—conditions that can be triggered or worsened by too little movement or activity, such as obesity, back pain, arthritis, and high blood pressure. Figure 1.7 illustrates some of the health benefits of regular physical activity.

The American College of Sports Medicine recommends that all healthy adults between the ages of 18 and 65 strive for at least 150 minutes of moderate exercise per week (or 75 minutes of vigorous exercise or a combination of the two).[10] However, recent national surveys indicate that most Americans are too inactive, as evidenced by the steady climb in percentages of overweight and obese adults (Figure 1.8).[11] Indeed, we are one of the most sedentary and overweight nations on earth.[12]

sedentary Physically inactive; exerting physical effort only for required daily tasks and not for leisure-time exercise

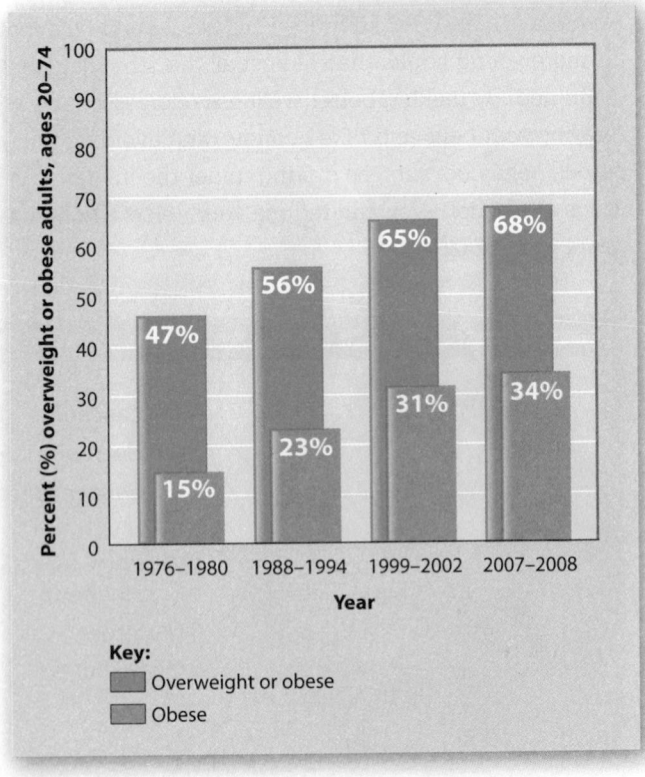

FIGURE **1.8** Overweight and obese adults are now the clear majority, with percentages rising steadily in the past 30 years.

Data from: K. Flegal and others, "Prevalence and Trends in Obesity Among US Adults, 1999–2008." *JAMA* 3003, no. 3 (2010): 235–41.

Good Wellness Habits Benefit Society as a Whole

The higher a population's levels of wellness, the happier and more productive are its people and the less money it spends on health care. Accordingly, achieving better wellness and combating today's chronic diseases are important national priorities.

National public health priorities cited by the Office of the Surgeon General of the United States are summarized in a set of objectives titled *Healthy People 2020*, which has four broad goals: 1) attain high-quality, longer lives free of preventable disease, disability, injury, and premature death; 2) achieve health equity, eliminate disparities, and improve the health of all groups; 3) create social and physical environments that promote good health for all; and 4) promote quality of life, healthy development, and healthy behaviors across all life stages.[13] In order to address some of these major public health priorities, the Surgeon General advises Americans to eat healthier, be more physically active, not smoke, limit alcohol, and avoid drugs—all of which are wellness behaviors.[14]

The high cost of health care and health insurance is a major concern for Americans. In 2009, Americans spent $2.5 trillion on health care, or 17.6 percent of the gross domestic product (GDP).[15] Employer health insurance premiums increased by 131 percent between 1999 and 2009 at four times the rate of inflation.[16] Nearly 49 million Americans lack health insurance, largely due to the high cost of coverage.[17] This makes them less likely to seek preventive care and adopt wellness behaviors early enough to prevent illness down the line. Such concerns led to sweeping new health legislation in 2010 to increase the percentage of Americans with health coverage.[18]

How Can I Change My Behavior to Increase My Wellness?

New Year's Resolutions

If you are like most people, you have made a New Year's resolution on January 1, have worked hard to adopt some new behavior until about the 10th, have started slipping back to your old habits by the 15th, and have forgotten about the whole thing by the 31st. Your resolution may well have been a new wellness behavior—lots of resolutions are. Perhaps it was an easy one, such as "eat more fruit," and you succeeded. More likely, it was a harder one—"start lifting weights three times a week," or "lose 20 pounds," or "give up junk food"— and despite your good intentions, it just didn't stick.

People often see change as a singular event instead of a process that requires preparation, has several stages, and takes time to succeed. Classic research shows that we must go through a series of mental and emotional stages over a period of months to adequately prepare ourselves for **behavior change**. The rest of this chapter takes you through a series of practical steps inspired by a blueprint for change called the *transtheoretical model of behavior change* developed by psychologists James Prochaska and Carlo DiClemente.[19]

Step One: Understand the Stages of Behavior Change

The transtheoretical model of behavior change delineates six **stages of behavior change**: precontemplation, contemplation, preparation, action, maintenance, and termination. The model shows that changing behaviors usually involves a gradual process of awareness, preparation, and then action. Understanding this process can help you proceed more deliberately to identify and successfully change a problem behavior. Keep in mind that the steps of this model are general and people often backtrack as they work on them.

> **behavior change** An organized, deliberate effort to alter or replace an existing habit or pattern of activity
>
> **stages of behavior change** From the transtheoretical model, a set of states most people pass through in their awareness of, determination to alter, and efforts to replace existing habits or actions

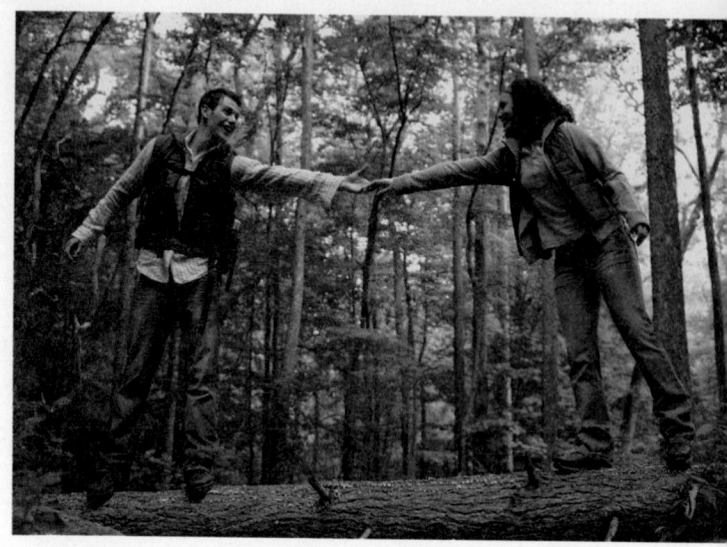

Precontemplation People in the precontemplation stage have no current intention of changing. They may have tried to change an old habit and given up, or they may be in denial and unaware of the problem.

Contemplation In this stage, people recognize that they have a problem and begin to contemplate the need to change within six months or so. People can languish in this stage for months or years, however, realizing that they have a negative wellness pattern, yet lacking the time, energy, or commitment to make the change.

Preparation Most people at this stage are within a month or so of taking action. They have thought about what they might do and may even have come up with a plan. Rather than thinking about why they can't begin, they have started to focus on what they can do.

Action In this stage, people begin to execute their action plans. Unfortunately, many people try to take shortcuts; they start behavior change here rather than going through the earlier stages. However, without making a plan, publicly stating the desire to change, enlisting other people's help, and setting realistic goals, they are likely to fail.

Maintenance In the maintenance stage, people work to prevent a relapse into old habits through a conscious application of wellness tools and techniques. Maintenance requires vigilance, attention to detail, and long-term commitment. You are in the maintenance stage after you have incorporated the new action and have continued it for six months or longer without relapse into old habits.

Relapse While not an original stage of behavior change, relapse is something that happens periodically for most people trying to change behaviors. Common causes of relapse include overconfidence, daily temptations, stress or emotional distractions, and putting yourself down.

Termination At the termination stage, the new behavior is ingrained; you are maintaining it and are no longer at risk for relapse. The new behavior has become a part of the way you live and thus the temptation to return to former behaviors is greatly reduced.

casestudy

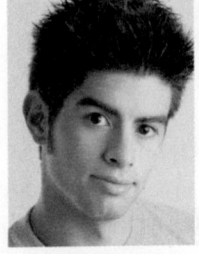

CARLOS

"In an ideal world I'd reduce my stress by sleeping eight hours a night, eating healthier food, and exercising more. Maybe then I would ace my exams and still have time for a social life. But I know I can't just snap my fingers and make all of that happen. Right now, I *really* have to get more sleep—it doesn't do me any good to stay up all night studying and then fall asleep in class. Some of my friends take 'power naps' in the afternoon. I might try that! I'm also thinking of signing up for a gym class next quarter. That way I can be sure to work some exercise into my schedule. Beyond that—well, I think I should probably take things one at a time."

THINK! What are Carlos's main wellness goals? What is his current stage of behavior change for each goal?

ACT! Name a wellness behavior that you would like to change and write down your stage of behavior change for that item. Tape this up where you can see it each morning.

HEAR IT! ONLINE

Step Two: Increase Your Awareness

LIVE IT! ONLINE

Worksheet 1
Health
Behavior Self
Assessment

Wellness behaviors that are important to college students can be simple to think about but are often challenging to achieve. An important starting point is to become aware of what is required to achieve wellness in each of the following areas.

Staying Physically Fit Nowhere does the phrase "Use it or lose it" apply more fully than to your physical fitness. Much of the decline people expect with advancing age is, in fact, a reflection of inactivity and its toll on the body. Staying active every day is probably the single most important wellness behavior you can adopt.

Eating Healthy Foods The American diet tends to be light on nutrition and heavy on calories. Most Americans consume more calories than they burn off each day. We also tend to eat too much protein, salt, sugar, animal fat, and solidified vegetable oils (trans fats). We consume too little fiber and too few helpings of fruits and vegetables.[20] Good nutrition has many wellness benefits, including increased energy, greater stamina, better weight management, stronger disease resistance, and reduced risk of chronic illness.

Managing Your Weight As we saw in Figure 1.8, 68 percent of American adults have a body weight and mass (fat-to-lean ratio) above recommended ranges. Overweight and obesity are correlated with arthritis, bone and joint problems, back pain, decreased physical performance, more chronic illness, and a shorter life expectancy. Modifying your activity level, exercise habits, eating habits, and stress levels can all contribute to maintaining a healthy weight.

Managing Your Stress Most students find college stressful. Whether you are fresh out of high school or returning to school later in life (see the box Nontraditional Students and Wellness), the lifestyle changes and the competing demands of academics, work, and social life associated with college can take an emotional and physical toll. Research shows that high levels of unrelieved stress can disrupt thinking and memory, disturb sleep, increase depression, impair our immunity to infections, and even contribute to weight gain and abdominal fat.[21] Over many years, unrelieved stress may also contribute to higher blood pressure, premature aging, and increased risk for chronic illnesses.

DIVERSITY

Nontraditional Students and Wellness

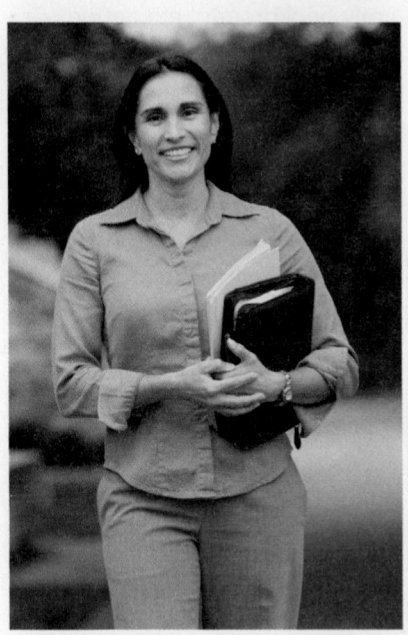

Since the 1980s, there has been a steady decline in the percentages of *traditional students* at colleges and universities—that is, 18- to 24-year-olds who go right on to college after high school with financial support from their parents.[1] During the same time period, schools have welcomed more and more *nontraditional students*—those who are 25 or older and who have spent time working, doing military service, or engaging in other activities before returning to post–high school education, full- or part-time. Nontraditional students are usually employed, self-supporting, and often married with children. They represent at least 40 percent of today's college students. And they broaden our discussion of student wellness.

The wellness needs of nontraditional students tend to differ from those of younger students for several reasons. 1) Many of them juggle work, school, and family, and thus they often derive special benefit from learning stress management skills.[2] 2) They tend to have more life experience but also to cope with more demands on their time; this can narrow their focus to educational and career goals and exclude much time for exercise. As a result, many need encouragement and creative ideas for increasing activity. 3) Nontraditional students make meals for themselves and for children more often than do traditional students and thus have broader nutritional considerations. Many also want to model good eating habits for their children, thus they tend to be receptive to nutritional improvements. 4) Many nontraditional students see themselves as unprepared for vigorous college work and are more likely to be stressed and insecure about their academic performances.[3] At the same time, most nontraditional students report having strong social support from family and friends, and thus appear to be richer in social wellness than younger students.

Sources:
1. L. G. Lunsford, "Post Secondary Education for Non-Traditional Students—The New Majority," North Carolina State University (2003).
2. J. E. Myers and A. K. Mobley, "Wellness of Undergraduates: Comparisons of Traditional and Non-traditional Students," *Journal of College Counseling* 7, no. 1 (2004): 40–49.
3. S. San Miguel Barriman and others, "Non-Traditional Student's Service Needs and Social Support Resources. A Pilot Study," *Journal of College Counseling* 7, no. 1 (2004): 13–17.

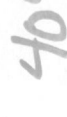

Avoiding Drugs, Smoking, and Alcohol Abuse Using drugs, smoking, and abusing alcohol are all ways of manipulating the brain chemically. Unfortunately, the use and abuse of these substances carry high risks for illness and injury and can undermine multiple dimensions of wellness.

Practicing Accident, Injury, and Disease Prevention Prevention has several practical meanings for wellness behavior. It can mean preventing injuries and the accidents that account for most deaths among young adults. It can mean self-care such as daily dental hygiene and regular prostate or breast self-exams. And it can mean preventing disease through medical checkups and vaccinations.

Step Three: Contemplate Change

Habits are usually deeply ingrained, and even minor habits can be surprisingly hard to change. As we have discussed, research has confirmed that people are more successful when they prepare for change emotionally and mentally rather than starting right in on the change itself. Contemplating change can include examining your current patterns, identifying your beliefs and attitudes, solidifying your motivation, and choosing a realistic target for your efforts to change.

Examine Current Habits and Patterns What current behavior should you work on changing? The assessment in **Lab 1.1** will help you identify habits that lower your wellness. When considering a habit, ask yourself the following:

- How long has it been going on?
- How often does it happen?
- How serious are the consequences of the habit or problem?
- What are some of your reasons for continuing this problematic behavior?
- What kinds of situations trigger the behavior?
- Are other people involved in this habit? If so, in what way?

Habits involve elements of deliberate choice but are also influenced by demographics, personal attitudes and beliefs, and many other factors. Age, sex, race, income, family background, education, and access to health care all increase or decrease the likelihood of developing certain health habits. If your parents smoke, for instance, you are 90 percent more likely to start smoking than someone whose parents don't smoke.[22] If your peers smoke, you are 80 percent more likely to smoke. Identifying factors that may encourage negative behaviors or block positive ones can help you prepare for behavior change. Analyzing the factors that reinforce your current habit pattern can also help you understand why you developed and maintained unwanted habits and where you need to make changes in order to succeed.

Assess Current Beliefs and Attitudes Your attitudes about health and wellness affect your daily choices. When reaching for another cigarette, smokers, for example, sometimes tell themselves, "I'll stop tomorrow" or "They'll have a cure for lung

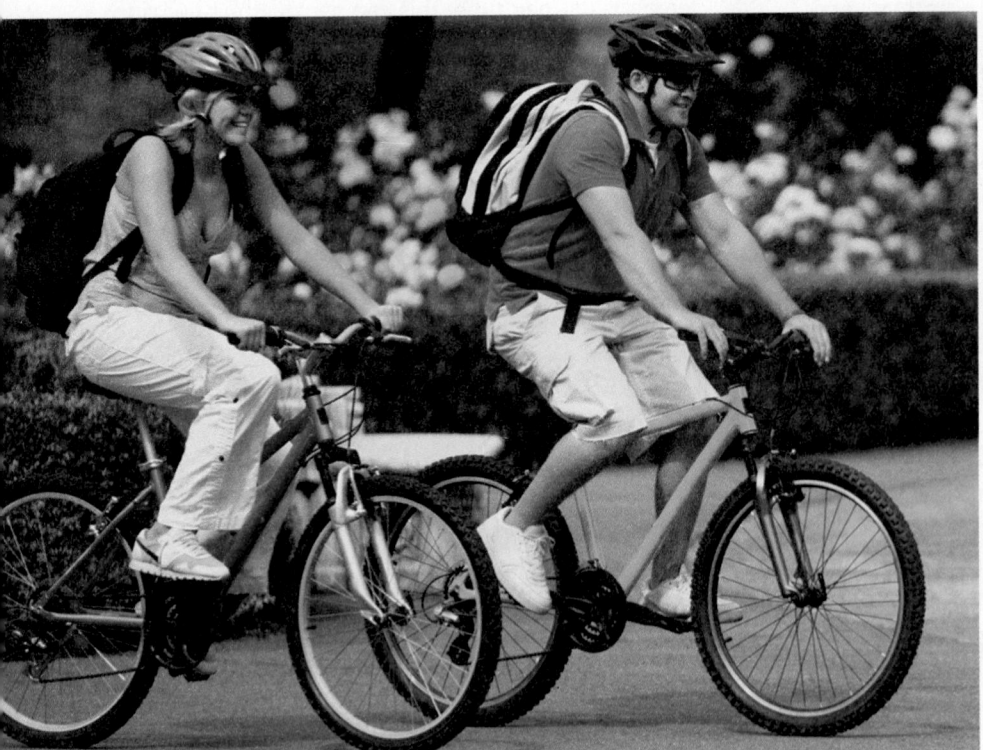

What Moves You?

Like many students, you may need powerful motivation to start a fitness program and follow it through. Researchers have discovered several interesting facets of student motivation to be active and fit that you can apply to your own wellness plan.

Studies have found that college students who participated in repetitive exercises such as weight lifting, swimming laps, or jogging around the track usually had *external* motivations for their participation. Many, but not all, tended to focus on their appearance, weight, or stress management and on the improvements that exercise could promote.[1] Conversely, college students who participated in recreational sports such as tennis, softball, and rowing usually had *internal* motivations for participating. They tended to focus on enjoyment and challenge.

If you have trouble sticking with exercise programs, you might find fitness easier if you were to choose a sport—even a mildly aerobic one such as badminton, horseback riding, ping-pong, or bowling—that provides fun and social opportunities as well as physical activity. As long as you spend enough

hours at an activity each week, you will benefit. Researchers have also confirmed that the social aspect of sports and activities—a sense of belonging to a team, a gym, or simply a group of friends who like to take bike rides or play Frisbee in the park—helps people enjoy fitness activities and stick with them.

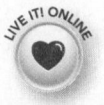

THINK! What are your main motivations for fitness and physical activity? Are they primarily external or internal? Do you participate in sports? Why or why not? Which of your activities are the most fun, and what makes them so?

ACT! If increasing your physical fitness is a goal, make a list of new activities that you could add for: a) more social contact; b) more fun and enjoyment, and c) more time willingly spent participating.

Sources:
1. M. Kilpatrick, E. Hebert, and J. Bartholomew, "College Students' Motivation for Physical Activity: Differentiating Men's and Women's Motives for Sport Participation and Exercise," *Journal of American College Health* 54, no. 2 (2005): 87–94.
2. C. J. Hale, J. W. Hannum, and D. L. Espelage, "Social Support and Physical Health: The Importance of Belonging," *Journal of American College Health* 53, no. 6 (2005): 276–84.

● ●

cancer by the time I get it." These beliefs allow them to continue smoking. One model suggests that several factors must be in place before you successfully change a habit that diminishes wellness.[23] Among these factors are the following:

- You must believe that your current pattern could lead you to a serious problem. The more severe the consequences, the more likely you are to change the behavior. For example, smoking can cause cancer and emphysema and promote heart disease. The fear of developing those diseases can help a person stop smoking.

- You must believe that you personally are quite susceptible to developing the health problem. For example, losing a parent to lung cancer could make a person work harder to stop smoking.

What beliefs underlie your current pattern of wellness habits, both positive and negative?

Assess Your Motivation What is your **motivation**, or inducement, to change a wellness behavior? For some, a rewarding result, such as looking better, can motivate change. For others, a feeling of accomplishment or just feeling better every day may do it. See the box What Moves You? to explore recent research on exercise motivation in students.

Motivations can be external (come from someone or something else) or internal (come from inside yourself), but in either case are part of your sense of self. The degree to which you believe in your own abilities is your **self-efficacy**. Your conviction that you can control events and factors in your life is your **locus of control**. An *internal* locus of control usually gives you a strong belief in your

LIVE IT! ONLINE

Worksheet 3
Health Locus
of Control

---

motivation One's inducement to do something such as change a current behavior

self-efficacy The degree to which one believes in his or her ability to achieve something

ability to effect change. An _external_ locus of control usually leads you to see other people and things as controlling what you do and whether you can change.

A person with a strong sense of self-efficacy and a largely internal locus of control has a better chance of following through with a decision to change wellness behavior. For example, suppose you wish to bring your weight down to a healthy range. If your parents are both overweight, you may think, "My weight is controlled by my genes," and thus be resigned to being overweight. By gathering information about weight management, however; by identifying behaviors that are within your power to change (such as food choices, eating habits, and exercise); and by acknowledging their importance, you can shift to a more internalized locus of control and increase your chances of successful weight management. Likewise, you can help boost your own self-efficacy through this shift to more internalized control.

• •

THINK! Where is your locus of control? Are you motivated by external factors (e.g., your genes) or internal factors (e.g., your own power)?

ACT! Write down three things you can control about the behavior you want to change. For example, if you want to lose weight, one thing you can control is rerouting your walk to class so that you don't pass tempting vending machines.

• •

Choose a Target Behavior The last preparatory step is to choose one well-defined habit, or **target behavior**, as your initial focus for change. It is a much better strategy to start small and build on success than to try for too much and end up failing. To choose potential target behaviors, ask yourself these questions:

• _What do I want?_ What is your ultimate goal? To lose weight? Exercise more? Reduce stress? Have a lasting relationship? Whatever it is, you need a clear picture of your target outcome.

• _Which change is my greatest priority at this time?_ People often decide to change several

---

locus of control Belief that control over life events and changes comes primarily from outside of oneself (external locus of control) or from within (internal locus of control)

target behavior One well-defined habit chosen as a primary focus for change

---

things at once. Suppose you are gaining unwanted weight. Rather than saying, "I need to eat less and start exercising," identify one specific behavior that contributes significantly to your greatest problem and tackle that first.

• _Why is this important to me?_ Think through why you want to change. Are you doing it because of your health? To improve your academic performance? To look better? To win someone else's approval? It's best to target a behavior because it's right for you rather than because you think it will help you win others' approval.

• _Fill in the details._ Rather than using a generality ("I need to eat better"), consider specific behaviors that relate to the general problem. What are your unhealthy eating habits? Do you eat too few fruits and vegetables? Do you have fast food for lunch every day? Identifying the specific behavior you would like to change will help you set clear goals.

Step Four: Prepare for Change

Once you have assessed your current status and chosen a target behavior, you are ready to make specific preparations, including observing role models, setting realistic goals, anticipating barriers, and making a commitment to change.

Observe Role Models Watching others successfully change their behavior can give you ideas and encouragement for your own changes. This process of modeling, or learning from role models, can be very helpful. Suppose you have trouble talking to strangers or new acquaintances and want to improve your communication skills. Try observing friends whose social skills you admire and note how they make conversation. What techniques help make them successful communicators? If you see behaviors that work well, separate their components so you can model your behavior change on a proven approach.

Set Realistic Goals and Objectives Your wellness goals and objectives should be both achievable for you and in line with what you truly want.[24] Achievable, truly desired goals increase motivation, and this, in turn, leads to a better chance of success at behavior change.

To set successful goals, try using the SMART system. SMART goals are _s_pecific, _m_easurable, _a_ction-oriented, _r_ealistic, and _t_ime-oriented. A vague goal would be "Get into better shape by exercising more." A SMART goal would be

S.M.A.R.T

- *Specific*—"Start weight training";

- *Measurable*—"Increase the amount of weight I can safely lift";

- *Action-oriented*—"Go to the gym three times per week";

- *Realistic*—"Increase the weight I can lift by 20 percent [not 200 percent]";

- *Time-oriented*—"Try my new weight program for 8 weeks, then reassess."

Anticipate and Overcome Barriers to Change Anticipating **barriers to change**, or possible stumbling blocks, will help you prepare for behavior change. A majority of students, for example, want to lose or gain weight but have failed to do so permanently.[25] Diet failure is based on several barriers to change, including internal drives to eat high-calorie foods and external temptations such as snacks and fast foods on sale in most campus buildings. The following are a few general barriers to wellness change:

1-at a time

- *Overambitious goals* can derail behavior change. Most people cannot lose weight, stop smoking, and begin running three miles a day all at the same time. It tends to be equally unsuccessful to try for dramatic change within an unrealistically short time frame—such as losing 20 pounds in one month. Habits are best changed one at a time, taking small, progressive steps; rewarding successes; and being patient with yourself.

- *Self-defeating beliefs and attitudes* can impede successful change. Believing that you are too young to worry about fitness and wellness can bar you from making a solid commitment to change.

Likewise, thinking you are helpless to change your weight, smoking, or fitness habits could undermine your efforts. Greater self-efficacy and more positive expectations may help.

barriers to change Stumbling blocks faced in the efforts to alter a current behavior

behavior change contract A formal document that clarifies the goals and steps needed to change a current habit or habit pattern

- *Failing to accurately assess your current state of wellness* could block progress. You might assume that you are strong and flexible, for example, when you are actually below average for your age. Failing to gather enough data on wellness risks and benefits can also be a barrier that leaves you with weakened motivation and commitment.

- *Lack of support and guidance* can act as a barrier. Supportive friends are a good start. You should also seek guidance from your fitness and wellness instructor; from counselors and other campus resources; from up-to-date, trusted health sources on the Internet (see the box How Can I Find Reliable Wellness Information?); and from health professionals.

Make a Commitment The more strongly you state an intention to change a wellness habit, either verbally or on paper, the more likely it is you will succeed. A formal written document called the **behavior change contract** functions as a promise to yourself

- as a public declaration of intent,

- as an organized plan that lays out start and end dates and daily actions,

- as a listing of barriers or obstacles you may encounter,

- as a place to brainstorm strategies for overcoming those impediments,

- as a collected set of sources of support, and

- as a reminder of the rewards you plan to give yourself for sticking with the program.

Writing a behavior change contract will help you clarify your goals, make a commitment to change, and, if you wish, announce your intentions to supportive friends and family. In **Lab 1.3** you will create

DO IT! ONLINE

a behavior change contract as part of your fitness and wellness plan.

Step Five: Take Action to Change

Now that you've put some thought into it, and made a plan for change, it's time to take action! The following are some strategies to keep your behavior change process on track.

Visualize New Behavior Athletes often use a form of mental practice called *imagined rehearsal* or simply *visualization* to reach their performance goals. Picturing themselves accomplishing an action in their minds ahead of time helps prepare them for real competition. Visualization can help you imagine the way a current negative behavior unfolds, and then allows you to practice in advance what you will say and do to counter it.

Control Your Environment If you are trying to quit drinking, going to a bar could lead you to resume an undesired behavior. Going to dinner and a movie with a sympathetic friend, on the other hand, could help reinforce your abstinence. Think about which people and settings tend to trigger your unwanted behavior, then stay away from them as much as possible and set up supportive situations instead.

Change Your Self-Talk Your *self-talk*—that is, the way you think and talk to yourself—matters. Think about what you say to yourself when something goes badly or when something succeeds. Purposely blocking or stopping negative thoughts and replacing them with positive ones can help you change a habit.

Learn to "Counter" **Countering** is another term for substituting a desired behavior for an undesirable one. You may want to stop eating junk food, for example, but "cold turkey" just isn't realistic—unless the turkey is on a

countering Substituting a desired behavior for an undesirable one

journaling Keeping a written record of personal experiences, interpretations, and results

sandwich! Instead, compile a list of substitute foods and places to get them and have this ready before your mouth starts watering at the smell of burgers and fries.

Practice "Shaping" *Shaping* is a stepwise process of making a series of small changes, starting slowly and mastering one step before moving on to the next. Suppose you want to start jogging three miles every other day, but right now you get tired and winded after half a mile. Shaping would dictate a process of slow, progressive steps such as walking one hour every other day at a slow, relaxed pace for the first week; walking for an hour every other day but at a faster pace the second week; and speeding up to a slow run the third week. Regardless of the change you plan, remember that current habits did not develop overnight, and they will not change overnight, either.

Reward Yourself Setting up a system of rewards can help you keep new behavior on track. Rewards can be consumable, like cookies or gourmet meals. They can be active, like going to a concert or playing Frisbee. They can be possessional, like getting a new MP3 player or buying a new CD. A reward can be an incentive, like being taken to a special event by a friend. It can be social, like receiving praise or a hug. And it can be intrinsic, meaning a new behavior feels so enjoyable it becomes its own reward. Whatever your motivating rewards may be, build a few (but not too many) into your program.

Use Writing as a Wellness Tool Throughout the labs in this textbook, you will examine your current wellness habits and analyze them through writing. **Journaling**, or writing personal experiences, interpretations, and results in a journal or notebook, is an important skill for behavior change. Journaling can help you monitor your daily efforts, measure how much you have learned, record how you feel about your progress, and note ideas for improving your program.

LIVE IT! ONLINE

Worksheet 2
Weekly Behavior Change
Evaluation

How Can I Find Reliable Wellness Information?

Fitness and wellness are important American preoccupations—and major industries as well. It can be hard to distinguish legitimate information from thinly disguised advertising for products and services. Here are some general tips and specific sources of reliable information.

Look for organizations without a direct interest in your wallet.

Examples are health-related agencies of the state and federal government (e.g., CDC or FDA); major colleges and universities; big-name hospitals and medical centers (e.g., Mayo Clinic or Cooper Institute); and well-known nonprofit organizations (e.g., American College of Sports Medicine or American Medical Association). Cross-check any information you gather from other sources against these kinds of known and reliable sources to see whether facts and figures are consistent.

If a newspaper or magazine quotes a research report, look up the research itself.

Consider details of the study, noting whether the researcher works for a large, recognizable university, government agency, or research institute; whether the study had human subjects or inferred conclusions from lab animals; and whether the conclusions were based on dozens or hundreds of research subjects or just a few.

Take fitness advice only from experts who represent reliable sources.

Well-meaning friends often have misinformation, and promoters of products and services are usually strongly biased.

Read consumer health newsletters published by distinguished universities, research institutes, and nonprofit organizations.

Examples include Harvard Health Letter; Mayo Clinic Health Letter, and Nutrition Action Health Letter.

Finally, use approved websites such as the following to learn more about fitness and wellness topics:

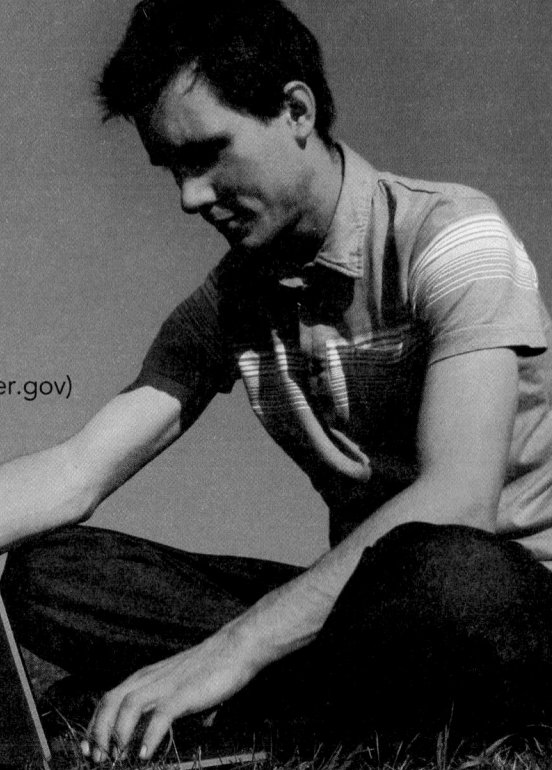

CDC Wonder (wonder.cdc.gov)

Mayo Clinic (www.mayoclinic.com)

National Center for Health Statistics (www.cdc.gov/nchs)

National Health Information Center (www.health.gov/nhic)

Harvard School of Public Health, World Health News (www.worldhealthnews.harvard.edu)

American Heart Association (www.americanheart.org)

American Medical Association (www.ama-assn.org)

Healthy People 2020 (www.healthypeople.gov)

U.S. Department of Health and Human Services (www.healthfinder.gov)

American College of Sports Medicine (www.acsm.org)

President's Council on Physical Fitness and Sports (www.fitness.gov)

FDA Information for Consumers (www.fda.gov/opacom/morecons.html)

Note: Web links are always subject to change. Visit this book's website at www.pearsonhighered.com /hopson to view updated Web links for each chapter.

chapterinreview

videos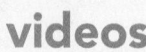

Log on to **www.pearsonhighered.com/hopson** or MyFitnessLab to view these chapter-related videos.

New Year's Resolutions   Months to a Healthier Lifestyle

onlineresources

Log on to **www.pearsonhighered.com/hopson** or MyFitnessLab for access to these book-related resources, and for links to other useful websites.

Audio case study
Audio PowerPoint lecture

Customizable 4-week fitness and wellness programs
Take Charge of Your Health! Worksheets:
   Worksheet 1 Health Behavior Self-Assessment
   Worksheet 2 Weekly Behavior Change
     Evaluation
   Worksheet 3 Multidimensional Health
     Locus of Control
Behavior Change Log Book and Wellness Journal

Lab 1.1 How Well Are You?
Lab 1.2 Chart Your Personal Wellness Balance
Lab 1.3 Create a Behavior Change Contract

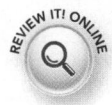
Pre- and post-quizzes
Glossary flashcards

reviewquestions

1. How does *wellness* differ from *health*?
   a. Wellness is the absence of disease.
   b. Wellness is the achievement of the highest level of health possible in physical, social, intellectual, emotional, environmental, and spiritual dimensions.
   c. Wellness and health are equivalent.
   d. Health is a more individualized, dynamic concept than wellness.

2. Which dimension of wellness includes good organizational skills?
   a. Social
   b. Intellectual
   c. Emotional
   d. Environmental

3. Which of the following is a modifiable risk factor for disease?
   a. Age
   b. Race
   c. Genetics
   d. Tobacco use

4. The American College of Sports Medicine recommends that all healthy adults between the ages of 18 and 65 strive for
   a. at least 150 minutes of moderate exercise per week.
   b. 30 minutes of exercise once a week.
   c. 50 minutes of moderate exercise per week.
   d. 20 minutes of walking once a week.

5. Which of the following is a top cause of death among Americans 20 to 24?
   a. Accidents
   b. Heart disease
   c. Stroke
   d. Lung Disease

6. Which of the following is a stage of the transtheoretical model of behavior change?
   a. Increased wellness
   b. Preparation
   c. Social wellness
   d. Motivation

7. What is meant by the term *healthy life expectancy*?
   a. How many years a person can expect to live
   b. How many years a person can expect to live without disability or major illness
   c. A realistic attitude toward how long a person can expect to live
   d. How many years a person believes he or she has to live

8. Imagined rehearsal is a form of
   a. countering.
   b. modeling.
   c. rewarding.
   d. visualization.

9. What is "shaping"?
   a. A stepwise process of change, designed to change one small piece of a target behavior at a time
   b. A model of behavior change that uses mental imaging to reshape the brain's signals
   c. A journaling strategy
   d. A way of learning behaviors by watching others perform them

10. Which of the following would be a poor reason to incorporate journaling into your wellness program?
   a. It helps you monitor your daily efforts.
   b. It helps you measure how much you have learned.
   c. It helps you record how you feel about your progress.
   d. It provides good material for blogging or tweeting.

critical**thinking**questions

1. What does it mean to be well? What are the benefits of wellness?
2. Why is it important to find your current place on the wellness continuum?
3. Describe the SMART goal-setting guidelines.
4. Name the dimensions of wellness and assign yourself a score (1 to 5) for your degree of wellness in each dimension. Identify your place on the wellness continuum in Figure 1.2.
5. Which risk-lowering choices do you incorporate into your lifestyle? Choose two or three of them and discuss the personal attitudes and beliefs that underlie your present behavior.
6. Using the stages of change (transtheoretical) model, discuss what you might do (in stages) to help a friend stop smoking. Why is it important that a person be ready to change before trying to change?
7. Which habits (wellness-related or not) have you tried to change in the past? Why do you think your efforts succeeded or failed? Using the skills for behavior change from this chapter, write a plan that will help you approach each habit more successfully.
8. Describe your current level of exercise motivation.
9. Discuss your current commitment to fitness and wellness.

references

1. American College Health Association, *American College Health Association—National College Health Assessment II (ACHA-NCHA II): Reference Group Executive Summary Spring 2010* (Linthicum, Maryland: American College Health Association, 2010).
2. G. D. A. Brown and others, "Does Wage Rank Affect Employees' Well-Being?" *Industrial Relations: A Journal of Economy and Society* 47, no. 3 (2008): 355–89.
3. World Health Organization, "World Health Statistics 2010." www.who.int/whosis /whostat/2010/en/index.html (2010).
4. Ibid.
5. Ibid.
6. M. Heron, "Deaths: Leading Causes for 2006," *National Vital Statistics Reports* 58, no. 14 (Hyattsville, MD: National Center for Health Statistics, 2010).
7. Ibid.
8. Centers for Disease Control and Prevention, "Nationwide Trend," Health-Related Quality of Life; National Center for Chronic Disease Prevention and Health Promotion,
www.cdc.gov/hrqol (accessed October 29, 2007).
9. World Health Organization, "Diet and Physical Activity: A Public Health Priority," Global Strategy on Diet, Physical Activity and Health, www.who.int/dietphysicalactivity (accessed January 31, 2011).
10. C. E. Garner and others, "American College of Sports Medicine Position Stand: Quantity and Quality of Exercise for Developing and Maintaining Cardiorespiratory, Musculoskeletal, and Neuromotor Fitness in Apparently Healthy Adults: Guidance for Prescribing Exercise," *Medicine and Science in Sports and Exercise* 43, no. 7 (2011): 1334–59.
11. K. Flegal and others, "Prevalence and Trends in Obesity Among US Adults, 1999–2008." *Journal of the American Medical Association* 3003, no. 3 (2010): 235–41.
12. C.L. Ogden and M. D. Carroll, "NCHS Health E-Stat: Prevalence of Overweight, Obesity, and Extreme Obesity Among Adults: United States, Trends 1976–1980 through 2007–2008," Centers for Disease
Control and Prevention, www.cdc.gov /nchs/data/hestat/obesity_adult_07_08 /obesity_adult_07_08.htm (updated June 2011).
13. Healthy People 2020, Framework: The Vision, Mission, and Goals of Healthy People 2020, www.healthypeople.gov /2020/consortium/HP2020Framework.pdf.
14. U. S. Department of Health and Human Services, Office of the Surgeon General, "Public Health Priorities," www.surgeongeneral .gov/publichealthpriorities.html#disease (accessed January, 31 2011).
15. National Coalition on Health Care, "Health Care Facts: Costs" September 2009. http://nchc.org/sites/default/files /resources/Fact%20Sheet%20-%20Cost .pdf (accessed January 2011).
16. Ibid.
17. B. W. Ward and others, "Early Release of Selected Estimates Based on Data from the January–June 2010 National Health Interview Survey," National Center for Health Statistics, www.cdc.gov/nchs/nhis /released201012.htm (December 2010).

18. U.S. Department of Health and Human Services, "Understanding the Affordable Health Care Act: Introduction," www .healthcare.gov/law/introduction/index .html (accessed January 31, 2011).

19. J. Prochaska, C. DiClemente, and J. Norcross, "In Search of How People Change: Application to Addictive Behaviors," *American Psychologist* 47, no. 9 (1983): 1102–14.

20. U. S. Department of Agriculture, "Report of the Dietary Guidelines Advisory Committee on the Dietary Guidelines for Americans, 2010," www.cnpp.usda.gov /DGAs2010-DGACReport.htm (January 2011).

21. V. Vicennati and others, "Stress-Related Development of Obesity and Cortisol in Women," Obesity 17, no. 9 (2009): 1678–83; E. Dias-Ferreira and others, "Chronic Stress Causes Frontostriatal Reorganization and Affects Decision-Making," *Science* 325, no. 5940 (2009): 621–25.

22. M. Yanai and others, "Smoking Incidence and the Effect of Smokefree Education Programs in Juveniles," *Chest* 128, no. 4 (2005): 205S.

23. E. P. Sarafino, *Health Psychology* (New York: Wiley, 1990) 189–91.

24. University of Iowa Advising Center, "Motivation, Goal Setting, and Success," www.uiowa.edu/web/advisingcenter /motivation.htm (accessed January 31, 2011).

25. American College Health Association, *ACHA-NCHA II: Reference Group Executive Summary Spring 2010* (2010).

LAB 1.1 • HOW WELL ARE YOU?

Name: _____ Date: _____

Instructor: _____ Section: _____

Purpose: This lab will help you assess your current level of wellness in each of the six dimensions and identify which wellness areas to target for behavior change.

Directions: Complete sections I–VII. For each item, indicate how often you think the statements describe you by checking the box under the relevant score. After each section, total your scores for that section and write your score in the space provided. After completing all sections, you will summarize and analyze your results.

SECTION I: PHYSICAL WELLNESS

	Never 1	Rarely 2	Sometimes 3	Often 4	Always 5
1. I listen to my body and make adjustments or seek professional help when something is wrong.					
2. I do moderate activity every day, such as taking the stairs instead of riding the elevator.					
3. I engage in vigorous exercise three to four times per week.					
4. I do exercise for muscular strength and endurance at least two times per week.					
5. I do stretching and limbering exercises at least five times per week.					
6. I do yoga, Pilates, tai chi, or other exercises for balance and core strength two or three times per week.					
7. I feel good about the condition of my body. I have lots of energy and can get through the day without being overly tired.					
8. I get adequate rest at night and wake on most mornings feeling ready for the day ahead.					
9. My immune system is strong, and my body heals quickly when I get sick or injured.					
10. I eat nutritious foods daily and avoid junk food.					

Total for Section I: Physical Wellness = _____

SECTION II: SOCIAL WELLNESS

	Never 1	Rarely 2	Sometimes 3	Often 4	Always 5
1. I am open, honest, and get along well with others.					
2. I participate in a wide variety of social activities and enjoy all kinds of people.					
3. I try to be a "better person" and work on behaviors that have caused friction in the past.					
4. I am open and accessible to a loving and responsible relationship.					
5. I have someone I can talk to about private feelings.					
6. When I meet people, I feel good about the impression they have of me.					
7. I get along well with members of my family.					
8. I consider the feelings of others and do not act in hurtful or selfish ways.					
9. I try to see the good in my friends and help them feel good about themselves.					
10. I am good at listening to friends and family who need to talk.					

Total for Section II: Social Wellness = _____

SECTION III: INTELLECTUAL WELLNESS

	Never 1	Rarely 2	Sometimes 3	Often 4	Always 5
1. I carefully consider options and possible consequences as I make choices.					
2. I am alert and ready to respond to life's challenges in ways that reflect thought and sound judgment.					
3. I learn from my mistakes and try to act differently the next time.					
4. I actively learn all I can about products and services before buying them.					
5. I manage my time well rather than letting time manage me.					
6. I follow directions or recommended guidelines and act in ways likely to keep myself and others safe.					
7. I consider myself to be a wise health consumer and check for reliable sources of information before making decisions.					

	Never 1	Rarely 2	Sometimes 3	Often 4	Always 5
8. I have at least one personal-growth hobby that I make time for every week.					
9. My credit card balances are low, and my finances are in good order.					
10. I examine my own perceptions and then check evidence to see whether I was correct.					

Total for Section III: Intellectual Wellness = _____

SECTION IV: EMOTIONAL WELLNESS

	Never 1	Rarely 2	Sometimes 3	Often 4	Always 5
1. I find it easy to laugh, cry, and show emotions such as love, fear, and anger and I try to express them in positive ways.					
2. I avoid using alcohol or drugs as a means to forget my problems or relieve stress.					
3. My friends regard me as a stable, well-adjusted person whom they trust and rely on for support.					
4. When I am angry, I try to resolve issues in nonhurtful ways rather than stewing about them.					
5. I try not to worry unnecessarily, and I try to talk about my feelings, fears, and concerns rather than letting them build up.					
6. I recognize when I'm stressed and take steps to relax through exercise, quiet time, or calming activities.					
7. I view challenging situations and problems as opportunities for growth.					
8. I feel good about myself and believe others like me for who I am.					
9. I try not to be too critical or judgmental of others.					
10. I am flexible and adapt to change in a positive way.					

Total for Section IV: Emotional Wellness =_____

SECTION V: SPIRITUAL WELLNESS

	Never 1	Rarely 2	Sometimes 3	Often 4	Always 5
1. I take time alone to think about life's meaning and where I fit in to the greater whole.					
2. I believe life is a gift we should cherish.					
3. I look forward to each day as an opportunity for further growth.					
4. I experience life to the fullest.					
5. I take time to enjoy nature and the beauty around me.					
6. I have faith in a greater power, nature, or the connectedness of all living things.					
7. I engage in acts of care and goodwill without expecting something in return.					
8. I look forward to each day as an opportunity to grow and be challenged in life.					
9. I work for peace in my interpersonal relationships, my community, and the world at large.					
10. I have a great love and respect for all living things and regard animals as important links in a vital living chain.					

Total for Section V: Spiritual Wellness = _____

SECTION VI: ENVIRONMENTAL WELLNESS

	Never 1	Rarely 2	Sometimes 3	Often 4	Always 5
1. I am concerned about environmental pollution and actively try to preserve and protect natural resources.					
2. I buy recycled paper and purchase biodegradable products whenever possible.					
3. I recycle my garbage, reuse containers, and try to minimize the amount of paper and plastics that I use.					
4. I try to wear my clothes for longer periods of time between washings to save on water and reduce detergent in our water sources.					
5. I try to reduce my use of gasoline and oil by limiting my driving.					
6. I write my elected leaders about environmental concerns.					

7. I turn down the heat and wear warmer clothes at home in the winter and use the air conditioner only when really necessary.

8. I am aware of potential hazards in my area and try to reduce my exposure whenever possible.

9. I use both sides of the paper when taking notes and doing assignments.

10. I try not to leave the water running too long when I shower, shave, or brush my teeth.

Total for Section VI: Environmental Wellness = _____

SECTION VII: REFLECTION—YOUR PERSONAL WELLNESS CONTINUUM

1. Enter your totals for sections I–VI below:

Physical Wellness _____

Social Wellness _____

Intellectual Wellness _____

Emotional Wellness _____

Spiritual Wellness _____

Environmental Wellness _____

2. Understanding your scores:

Scores of 35–50: Outstanding! Your answers show that you are aware of the importance of these behaviors in your overall wellness, and that you are putting your knowledge to work by practicing good habits that should reduce your overall risks.

Scores of 30–34: Your wellness practices in these areas are very good, but there is room for improvement. What changes could you make to improve your score?

Scores of 20–29: Your wellness risks are showing. Find information about the risks you face and why it is important to change these behaviors.

Scores below 20: You may be taking unnecessary risks. Identify each risk area and, whenever possible, seek additional resources, either on your campus or through your local community health resources.

LAB 1.2 • CHART YOUR PERSONAL WELLNESS BALANCE

Name: _____ Date: _____

Instructor: _____ Section: _____

Purpose: To learn how to chart your current personal wellness balance and identify the wellness areas in which you would like to improve.

Materials: Results from Lab 1.1

Directions: Follow the instructions below.

SECTION I: YOUR PERSONAL WELLNESS BALANCE

1. Create a personal wellness balance chart with your scores from sections I–VI of Lab 1.1. Allocate a larger "piece of the pie" for dimensions of wellness where your scores are higher and a smaller slice for dimensions with lower scores. Another option: allocate a larger slice for areas where you spend most of your time during a week.

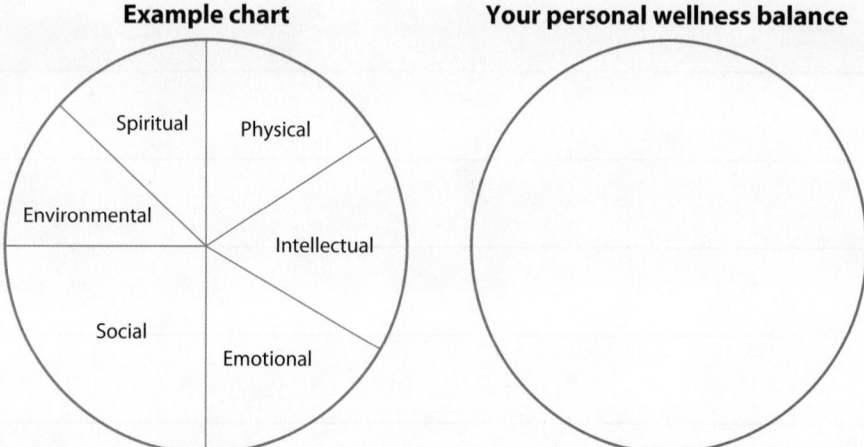

Example chart   **Your personal wellness balance**

2. Now create your **goal wellness balance chart.** Change your current balance chart to reflect your desired scores in each wellness dimension, or to reflect the optimal percentage of time you would like to allocate to each dimension.

Goal wellness balance chart

SECTION II: REFLECTION

Reflect on your answers, your wellness balance charts, and your wellness continuum (from the *Think! Act!* on page 5). What are your major areas of concern regarding your wellness? What two or three behaviors could you change easily to improve your wellness? Which one needs attention first?

_____

_____

_____

_____

_____

_____

_____

_____

_____

_____

_____

_____

_____

_____

LAB 1.3 • CREATE A BEHAVIOR CHANGE CONTRACT

Name: _____ Date: _____

Instructor: _____ Section: _____

Purpose: To introduce students to the process of writing a behavior change contract and planning for new lifestyle behaviors. This introduction will serve as a model for other behavior change plans in subsequent chapters.

Directions: Complete the following sections.

SECTION I: PERSONAL WELLNESS REVIEW

1. Review your answers from Lab 1.1 and Lab 1.2.

2. Consider the stages of change (precontemplation, contemplation, preparation, action, maintenance) and evaluate your readiness to make a behavior change.

3. Choose a target behavior to change. For this behavior, you should be in the contemplation or preparation stages. Write the behavior below.

My behavior to change is _____

SECTION II: SHORT- AND LONG-TERM GOALS

1. **Long-Term Goal:** Long-term goals are those set for six months to a year or more. These goals should be achievable and may take many steps and an extended time to reach. Be sure to use SMART (specific, measurable, action-oriented, realistic, time-oriented) goal-setting guidelines when creating your long-term goal. After writing out your long-term goal, choose an appropriate target date and a reward for completing your goal.

    a.   Long-Term Goal: _____

    b.   Target Date: _____

    c.   Reward: _____

2. **Short-Term Goals:** Short-term goals are those you want to achieve in less than six months. These goals will often help you reach your long-term goal. They may also be part of your long-term goal. Again, use SMART goal-setting guidelines when setting short-term goals. After writing out your short-term goals, choose appropriate target dates and rewards.

    a.   Short-Term Goal #1: _____

    b.   Target Date: _____

    c.   Reward: _____

    a.   Short-Term Goal #2: _____

    b.   Target Date: _____

    c.   Reward: _____

SECTION III: BEHAVIOR CHANGE OBSTACLES AND STRATEGIES

1. These are **three obstacles** to changing this behavior (things I am currently doing or situations that contribute to this behavior or make it harder to change):

a. _____

b. _____

c. _____

2. Here are **three strategies** I will use to overcome these obstacles:

a. _____

b. _____

c. _____

SECTION IV: GETTING SUPPORT

1. Resources I will use to help me change this behavior:

a. A friend/partner/relative: _____

b. A school-based resource: _____

c. A community-based resource: _____

d. A book or reputable website: _____

2. How will you use these supportive resources to help you with your goals?

_____

_____

SECTION V: CONTRACT, TRACKING, AND FOLLOW-UP

1. Contract: I intend to make the behavior change described above. I will use the strategies and rewards to achieve the goals that will contribute to a healthy behavior change.

Signed _____ Date _____

Witness _____ Date _____

2. Tracking: Tracking progress toward your goals is very important to ensure successful behavior change. As you move through this course, you will be asked to monitor your progress on several of your health, wellness, and fitness goals. Accurate and regular record-keeping is important.

3. Follow-up: When reaching your target date, it is important to follow up and reassess your program. During this course, you will be answering questions such as, Did you accomplish your goal? Do you need to set a new and more challenging goal? Do you need to alter your goals or program to make it more realistic? This section in your labs is important to modify your goals and your program and to set future goals.

2

Understanding Fitness Principles

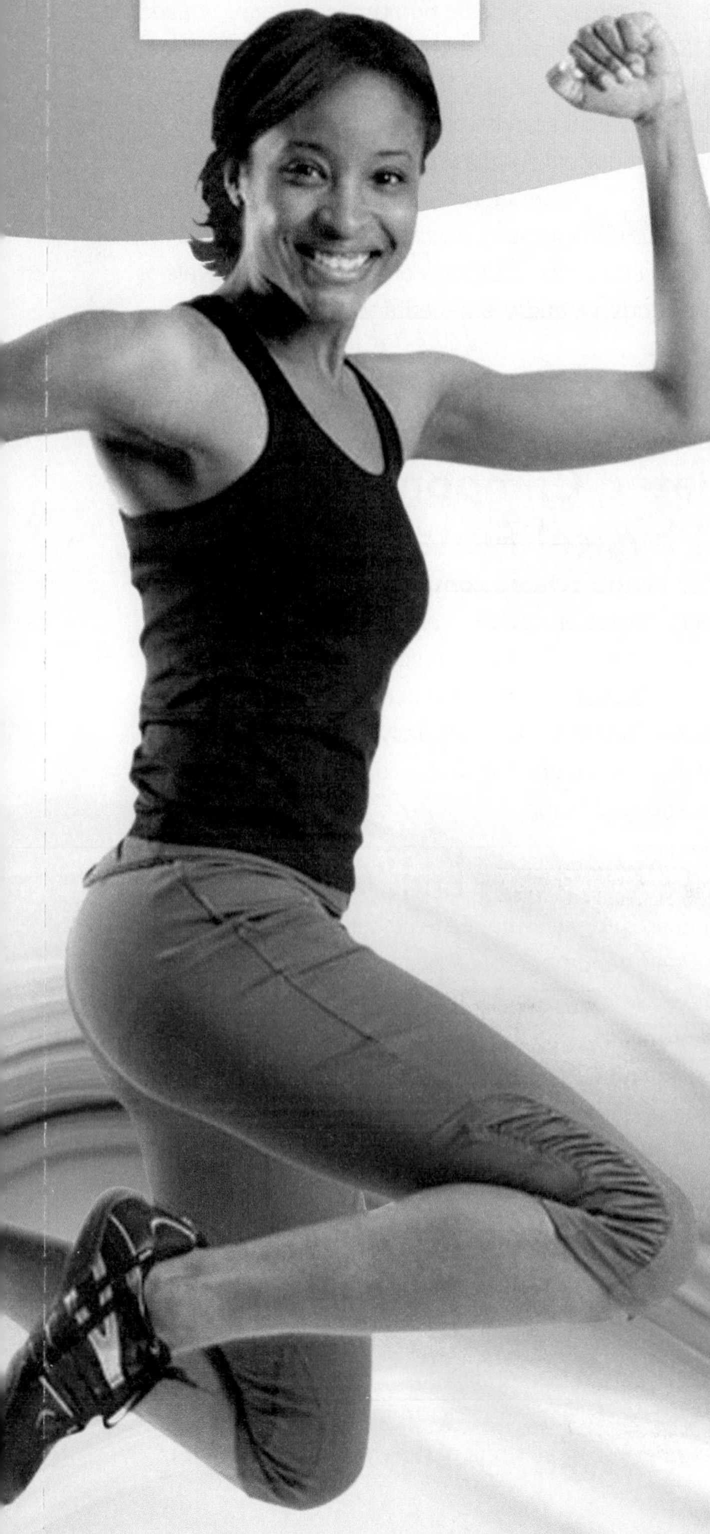

Learning Outcomes

1. Describe the three primary levels of physical activity and their benefits.

2. Articulate the importance of each health-related component of fitness.

    HEAR IT! ONLINE Audio case study and audio Power-Point lecture

3. Identify the role that the skill-related components of fitness play in overall physical fitness.

4. Explain how following the fitness principles of overload, progression, specificity, reversibility, individuality, and recovery will increase your fitness program success.

5. Describe how much and the types of physical activity you should do for optimal health and wellness.

    SEE IT! ONLINE Personal Fitness and Exercise

6. Incorporate general strategies for exercising safely.

7. Identify individual attributes that should be taken into account before beginning a fitness program.

    DO IT! ONLINE Lab 2.1 Assess Your Physical Activity Readiness
   Lab 2.2 Identify Your Physical Activity Motivations and Obstacles

8. Individualize and implement strategies that will help you get started on your fitness and exercise goals.

    DO IT! ONLINE Lab 2.3 Changing Your Sedentary Time into Active Time

    LIVE IT! ONLINE Customizable 4-week starter walking programs

Pre- and post-quizzes and glossary flashcards  REVIEW IT! ONLINE

casestudy

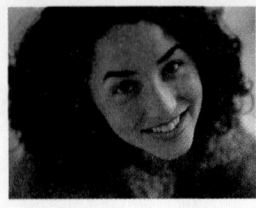

LILY

"Hi, I'm Lily. I just started my junior year, and after a summer of lazing around, I want to get back into shape. I'm ready to put some serious time and energy into it, but the last time I started exercising, I tried to do too much and ended up injured. How do I keep from doing the same thing this time? How much exercise do I really need? And what does it actually mean to be fit, anyway—does it just mean being able to run a certain distance, or is there more to it than that?"

HEAR IT! ONLINE

Fitness is a critical component of overall wellness. Being physically fit can improve your mood, give you more energy for daily activities, help you maintain a healthy weight, and reduce your risk of developing chronic diseases. All of these benefits can, in turn, help you live a longer, healthier life.

In this chapter, we cover the basic principles of fitness, address the question of how much exercise you need, introduce general guidelines for exercising safely, and discuss individual factors you should consider when designing your personal fitness program. Also, we go over strategies to help you get started exercising, including overcoming common obstacles to success.

physical fitness A set of attributes that relate to one's ability to perform moderate to vigorous levels of physical activity without undue fatigue

physical activity Any bodily movement produced by skeletal muscles that results in an expenditure of energy

exercise Physical activity that is planned or structured, done to improve or maintain one or more of the components of fitness

What Are the Three Primary Levels of Physical Activity?

Physical fitness is the ability to perform moderate to vigorous levels of physical activity without undue fatigue. Note that *physical activity* and *exercise* are not the same thing: **physical activity** technically means any bodily movement produced by skeletal muscles that results in an expenditure of energy, whereas **exercise** specifically refers to planned or structured physical activity done to achieve and maintain fitness.

Physical activity is often measured in metabolic equivalents, or **MET** levels. A MET level of 1 is equivalent to the energy you use at rest or while sitting quietly. A MET level of 2 equals two times the energy used at a MET level of 1, while a MET level of 3 equals three times the energy used at a MET level of 1, and so forth. Levels of physical activity can be grouped into three primary categories: (1) *light/lifestyle/physical activities* (<3 METS), (2) *moderate physical activities* (3 to 6 METS), and (3) *vigorous physical activities* (>6 METS). Figure 2.1 illustrates examples of each of these levels of physical activity, and the benefits that are associated with them.

What Are the Health-Related Components of Physical Fitness?

The five **health-related components of physical fitness** are *cardiorespiratory endurance, muscular strength, muscular endurance, flexibility,* and *body composition.* Minimal competence in each of these areas is necessary for you to carry out daily activities, lower your risk of developing chronic diseases, and optimize your health and well-being.

Cardiorespiratory Endurance

Cardiorespiratory endurance (also called *cardiovascular fitness/endurance, aerobic fitness,* and *cardiorespiratory fitness*) is the ability of the cardiovascular and respiratory systems to provide oxygen to working muscles during sustained exercise. Achieving adequate cardiorespiratory endurance decreases your risk of diabetes, heart disease, obesity, and other chronic diseases.[1] Increased cardiorespiratory endurance also improves your ability to enjoy recreational activities, such as bicycling and hiking, and to participate in them for extended periods of time.

Muscular Strength

Muscular strength is the ability of your muscles to exert force. You may think of it as your ability to lift a

Light/Lifestyle Physical Activities (<3 METS)	**Examples:**	**Benefits:**
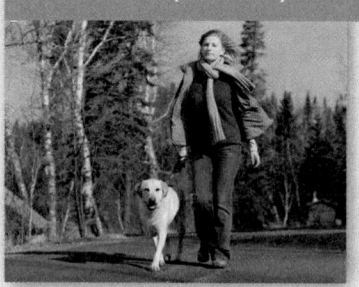	Light yard work and housework, leisurely walking, self-care and bathing, light stretching, light occupational activity	A moderate increase in health and wellness in those who are completely sedentary; reduced risk of some chronic diseases
Moderate Physical Activities (3–6 METS)	**Examples:**	**Benefits:**
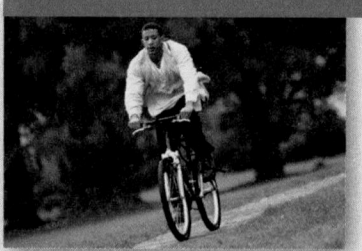	Walking 3–4.5 mph on a level surface, weight training, hiking, climbing stairs, bicycling 5–9 mph on a level surface, dancing, softball, recreational swimming, moderate yard work and housework	Increased cardiorespiratory endurance, lower body fat levels, improved blood cholesterol and pressure, better blood glucose management, decreased risk of disease, increased overall physical fitness
Vigorous Physical Activities (>6 METS)	**Examples:**	**Benefits:**
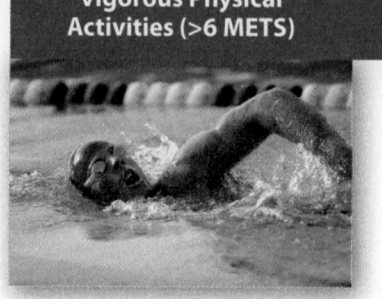	Jogging, running, circuit training, backpacking, aerobic classes, competitive sports, swimming laps, heavy yard work or housework, hard physical labor/construction, bicycling over 10 mph up steep terrain	Increased overall physical fitness, decreased risk of disease, further improvements in overall strength and endurance

FIGURE **2.1** Examples and benefits of light/lifestyle physical activity, moderate physical activity, and vigorous physical activity.

heavy weight. Improved muscular strength decreases your risk of low bone density and musculoskeletal injuries.[2] In order to improve muscular strength, you need to tax your muscles in a controlled setting. This typically involves a weight room, as well as supervision to avoid injury.

Muscular Endurance

Muscular endurance is the ability of your muscles to contract repeatedly over time. Along with cardiorespiratory endurance, muscular endurance allows you to participate in recreational sports without undue fatigue. For example, in order to play a continuous game of basketball, you need to have good cardiorespiratory endurance to move up and down the court for the entire 90 minutes—and you need to have good muscular endurance to keep guarding, blocking, and shooting the ball effectively.

Flexibility

Flexibility is the ability to move your joints in a full range of motion. This component of fitness is often overlooked but maintaining a minimal level of flexibility is important for overall wellness. Flexibility in

MET The standard metabolic equivalent used to estimate the amount of energy (oxygen) used by the body during physical activity; 1 MET = resting or sitting quietly

health-related components of physical fitness Components of physical fitness that have a relationship with good health

stretching reduces overall injury rates, it may reduce specific muscle and tendon injuries.[3] Having an adequate joint range of motion can be especially important to prevent neck and back pain when you are older[4] and help prevent the decreased physical function that often occurs with aging.[5]

Body Composition

Body composition refers to the relative amounts of fat and lean tissue in your body. Lean tissue consists of muscle, bone, organs, and fluids. A healthy body composition has adequate muscle tissue with moderate to low amounts of fat tissue. The recommendations for fat

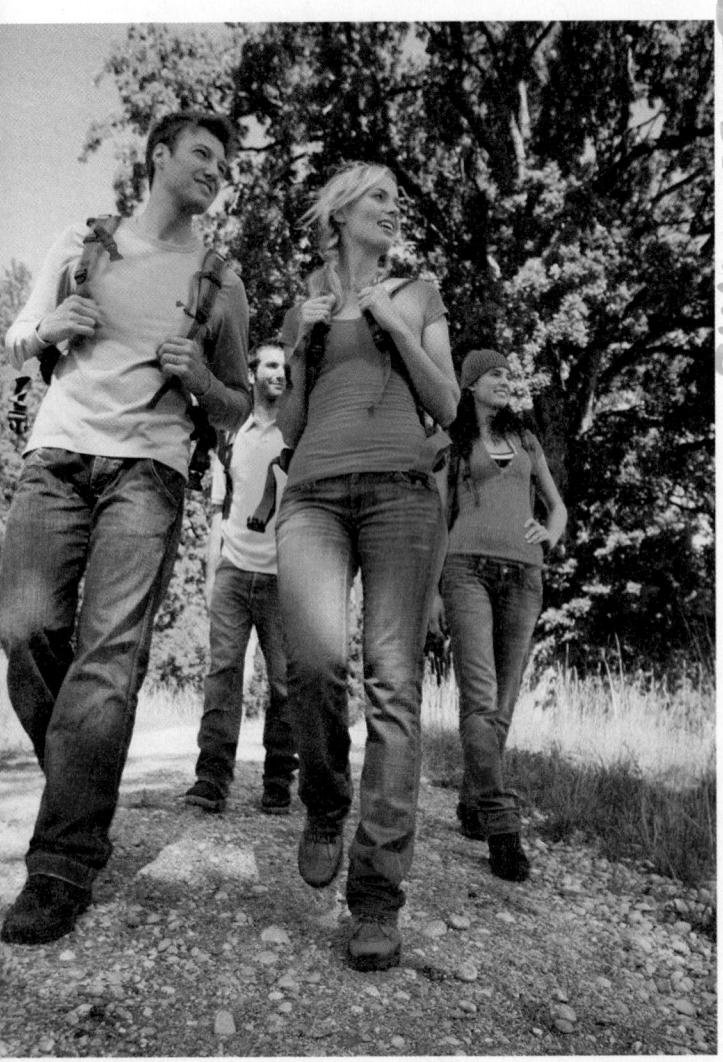

your joints increases your ability to do the activities you enjoy and work toward specific fitness goals. Although we don't know whether

percentages will vary based upon your gender and age. Increased levels of fat will put you at risk for diabetes, heart disease, and certain cancers.

What Are the Skill-Related Components of Physical Fitness?

In addition to the five health-related components of fitness, physical fitness also involves attributes that improve your ability to perform athletic and exercise tasks. These attributes are called the **skill-related components of fitness.** Often termed *sport skills,* these are qualities that athletes aim to improve in order to gain a competitive edge. Recreational athletes and general exercisers can also benefit from improving these skills. The six skill-related components of fitness are:

- *Agility*: The ability to rapidly change the position of your body with speed and accuracy
- *Balance*: The maintenance of equilibrium while you are stationary or moving
- *Coordination*: The ability to use both your senses and your body to perform motor tasks smoothly and accurately
- *Power*: The ability to perform work or contract muscles with high force quickly
- *Speed*: The ability to perform a movement in a short period of time
- *Reaction time*: The time between a stimulus and the initiation of your physical reaction to that stimulus

Although skill-related fitness is largely determined by heredity,[6] regular training can result in significant improvements. In order to improve skill-related components of fitness, athletes and exercisers first need to target the skills that will be important to their specific sport or exercise. For instance, a runner can benefit from increasing power for hill running and speed for winning races, whereas a tennis player can benefit from increased agility and reaction time.

Improving your fitness skills can be as easy as participating regularly in any sport or activity. Playing football will increase reaction time and power, while dancing will increase balance, agility, and coordination. Another way to increase these skills is to perform drills that mimic a sport-specific skill, or work specifically on any of the skill-related components of fitness. You can practice drills in group exercise classes, or you can work with a personal trainer. Specialized equipment is often used in such drills: for example, exercises utilizing obstacles such as hurdles or cones can help you improve your speed, agility, and coordination, while using balance boards or exercise balls can help you improve your balance.

What Are the Principles of Fitness?

In order to design an effective fitness program, you need to take into account the basic **principles of fitness** (also called *principles of exercise training*). These guiding principles explain how the body responds or adapts to exercise training.

Overload

The principle of **overload** states that in order to see improvements in your physical fitness, the amount or dose of training you undertake must be more than your body or specific body system is accustomed to. This applies to any of the components of physical fitness discussed earlier. For example, in order to increase your flexibility, you must stretch a little farther than you are used to.

Training Effects Consistent overloads or stresses on a body system will cause an *adaptation* to occur (Figure 2.2). An adaptation is a change in the body as a result of an overload. In exercise training this is called a *training effect*. For example, if you normally run two laps around a track each day but gradually increase this to four laps each day, the overload to your cardiorespiratory and muscular systems will cause adaptations in those systems. While you may feel tired and out of breath the first time you run four laps, after a few weeks of running those four laps the adaptations in your body will allow you to cover that distance with greater ease.

Dose-Response The amount of adaptation you can expect is directly related to the amount of overload or training dose that you complete. This is called the *dose-response relationship*. An increase in your "dose," or amount of training, will result in increased responses or adaptations to that training. How much response or adaptation you can expect is dependent upon the body system trained, the health or fitness outcome measured, and your individual physical and genetic characteristics.

Diminished Returns According to the concept of *diminished returns* (also called the *initial values principle*), the rate of fitness improvement diminishes over time

(margin note: IN ORDER TO IMPROVE:)

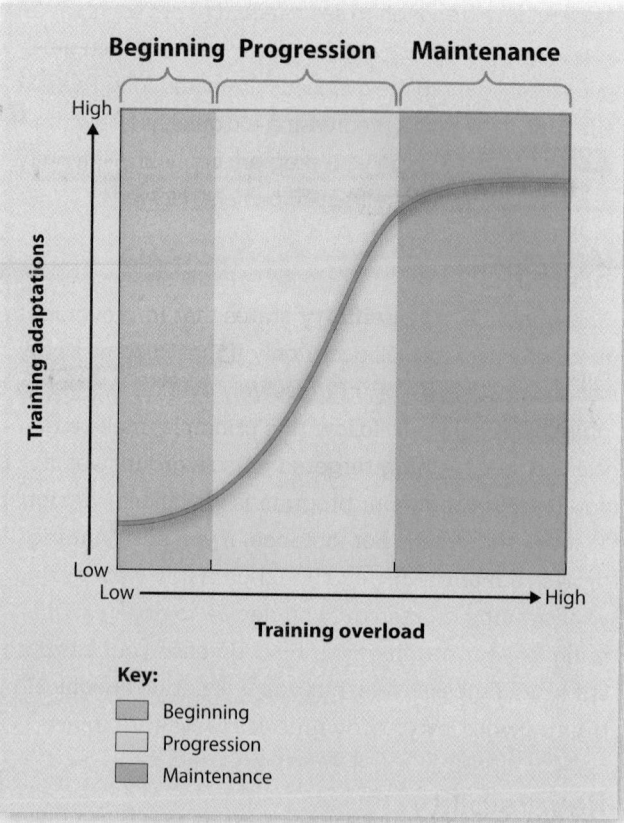

FIGURE **2.2** After adjusting to new training overloads at the beginning of your exercise program, you will see larger adaptations and improvements during the progression phase. As you approach your goal or genetic limits, your increases in overload will not result in further adaptations. This is a sign that you have reached a plateau and should maintain (if satisfied) or adjust your program for further improvement.

as fitness levels approach genetic limits. Initial fitness levels determine the amount of improvement that you can achieve from exercise training overloads. If you are sedentary and far from your genetic limits, you might experience large increases in fitness levels from moderate amounts of training. If you are active and closer to your genetic limits already, you may gain only small increases in fitness from larger amounts of training.

Progression

The principle of **progression** states that in order to effectively and safely increase fitness, you need to apply an optimal level of overload to the body within a certain time period. Simply stated, you need to increase your

principles of fitness General principles of exercise adaptation that guide fitness programming

overload Subjecting the body or body system to more physical activity than it is accustomed to

progression A gradual increase in a training program's intensity, frequency, and/or time

workout levels enough to see results, but not so much that you increase your risk of injury. Your body will then progressively adapt to the overloads presented to it. To make sure that you are not progressing too quickly, follow the "10 percent rule": increase your program frequency, intensity, or duration by no more than 10 percent per week.

Specificity

The principle of **specificity** states that improvements in a body system will occur only if that specific body system is stressed or progressively overloaded by the physical activity. To follow this principle, make sure that you are training targeted muscle groups specific to your sport or that your program is specifically designed to meet your goals. For instance, if you are planning to walk a marathon, you should primarily *walk* during your training. If, instead, you decide to do lap swimming as your training, you may increase your cardiorespiratory fitness levels, but you will not be specifically training your lower body muscles to walk 26 miles.

Reversibility

All fitness gains are reversible, according to the principle of **reversibility**. This is the "use it or lose it" principle. If you do not maintain a minimal level of physical activity and exercise, your fitness levels will slip. Unfortunately, you cannot accumulate fitness or workout sessions in a "bank" for later. Doing a great deal of exercise in one week will not compensate for a subsequent month of doing no exercise. Whenever you stop exercising, it only takes one to two weeks to start losing fitness gains you may have made while training. Most of your improvements could be gone in a few months.[7] For example, if you spent four months running four miles three times a week, you could lose any fitness gains from those four months within two months of *no* training.

specificity The principle that only the body systems worked during training will show adaptations

reversibility The principle that training adaptations will revert toward initial levels when training is stopped

individuality Refers to the variable nature of physical activity dose-response or adaptations in different persons

rest and recovery Taking a short time off from physical activities to allow the body to recuperate and improve

overtraining Excessive volume and intensity of physical training leading to diminished health, fitness, and performance

Individuality

The principle of **individuality** states that adaptations to a training overload may vary greatly from person to person. Genetics influence all individual differences in training adaptations. Two people may participate in the same training program but have very different responses. While you cannot control your genetic makeup, understanding how you respond to exercise is important in designing your personal fitness plan. A person who responds well to a training program is considered a *responder*. One who does not respond well is considered a *nonresponder*. Of those individuals who show improvements, some may respond better to increases in total amount of physical activity, while others may show more improvement with increases in exercise intensity. Figuring out your individual responses to certain exercise programs is a trial-and-error process. Complete regular fitness assessments and training logs to track your progress and then adjust your program accordingly to meet your goals.

casestudy

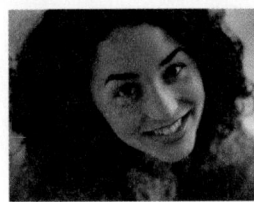

LILY

"The last time I decided to start exercising, I started off slowly, jogging about half an hour twice a week. That went well. Then I got busy with school and stopped jogging for a whole month. To make up for it, I decided to run a 10k. It was a gorgeous day, and there were tons of other people running it. There were kids, and older people, and people who looked way more out of shape than I was—so even though I hadn't trained for it, I thought it'd be no problem. Well, three miles into it, my knees started to hurt. The pain came and went, and I managed to finish the six-mile race, but my knees hurt for two weeks afterward. That was the end of my big exercise plans."

THINK! What principles of fitness would you advise Lily to keep in mind before she attempts a new exercise routine? What mistakes did Lily make?

ACT! Tell a friend about or describe in your journal a past experience with exercise that was similar to Lily's. Tell your friend or write down what you intend to do differently this time around.

HEAR IT! ONLINE

Rest and Recovery

The principle of **rest and recovery** (also called the *principle of recuperation*) is critical to ensuring continued progress toward your fitness goals. As you will recall, the overload principle states that you must subject your body to more exercise than it is accustomed to doing. However, your body also needs time to recover from the increased physiological and structural training stresses that you place on it. In *resistance training* (also called *weight training*) in particular, most of the training adaptations actually take place during the rest periods between workouts.

Constant training day after day with insufficient rest periods can result in reduced health benefits and can eventually lead to **overtraining**. If you are exercising consistently and start feeling more fatigue and muscle soreness than usual during and after exercise, you could be doing too much. Reduce the duration or intensity of your exercise and rest for a day or two. To prevent overtraining and to gain optimal benefits from your training program, schedule regular rest days (one to three per week) in any cardiorespiratory endurance program and every other day for any strength training program. Another important tip to avoid overtraining and injury is to alternate hard workout days with easier workout days during your weekly plan.

How Much Exercise Is Enough?

How much exercise or physical activity do you really need? The answers will vary, depending on which sources you turn to and on your individual fitness goals. Most agree that the first step is to avoid inactivity. *Any* amount of physical activity can confer basic health benefits. For

Worksheet 26
How Much Do
I Move?

increased health benefits, follow the minimal activity level recommendations below. For additional health benefits and fitness improvements, follow the guidelines outlined in the Physical Activity Pyramid and the FITT Principle.

Minimal Physical Activity Level Guidelines

Personal
Fitness and
Exercise

Guidelines for physical activity and exercise are issued by various organizations that rely on credible scientific research in developing their recommendations. These organizations can be *government agencies* (such as the President's Council on Physical Fitness and Sports), *professional organizations* (such

as the American College of Sports Medicine), or *private organizations* (such as the American Heart Association). In 2008, the U.S. Department of Health and Human Services issued the first ever national physical activity guidelines designed to "provide achievable steps for youth, adults, and seniors, as well as people with special conditions to live healthier and longer lives."[8] The recommendations are echoed by other leading organizations, such as the World Health Organization[9] and American College of Sports Medicine.[10]

As a nation we are doing better meeting these guidelines, but we can still improve. When the guidelines were released in 2008, 32 percent of adults reported participating in regular moderate physical activity and 24 percent of adults reported participating in regular vigorous physical activity.[11] Of these, 43 percent were meeting the recommended minimum physical activity levels (moderate or vigorous) and the goal is to increase that number to 48 percent by 2020.[12] Take a look at the guidelines in Table 2.1. How close are you to meeting these recommendations?

The Physical Activity Pyramid Guides Weekly Choices

The Physical Activity Pyramid (Figure 2.3) visually summarizes minimal physical activity and exercise guidelines for optimal health and wellness. The Physical Activity Pyramid's bottom layer represents light or lifestyle activities that you should strive to incorporate into your everyday life. Light physical activity every day, such as walking and gardening, is a great way to start and to ensure a strong "base" to your pyramid! The next layer of the pyramid represents moderate-to-vigorous aerobic and/or sports activities that you should try to do three to five times per week in order to build cardiorespiratory endurance and fitness. Aim to accumulate at least 150 minutes of moderate physical activity each week, such as quick walking or flat bicycling, or 75 minutes of vigorous activity each week, such as swimming or jogging. The third layer of the pyramid represents strength-training and flexibility-building exercises that you should try to incorporate at least two days per week. The top layer of the pyramid represents the activities that should ideally receive the least amount of your time—sedentary activities such as watching TV or surfing the Web—in favor of more active pursuits.

The box Six Easy Ways to Get More Active provides suggestions for how to incorporate more physical activity into your daily life.

TABLE 2.1 Physical Activity Guidelines for Americans			
	Key Guidelines for Health*	For Additional Fitness or Weight Loss Benefits*	PLUS
Adults	150 min/week moderate-intensity OR 75 min/week of vigorous-intensity OR Equivalent combination of moderate- and vigorous-intensity (i.e., 100 min moderate-intensity + 25 min vigorous-intensity)	300 min/week moderate-intensity OR 150 min/week of vigorous-intensity OR Equivalent combination of moderate- and vigorous-intensity (i.e., 200 min moderate-intensity + 50 min vigorous-intensity) OR More than the previously described amounts	Muscle strengthening activities for all the major muscle groups at least 2 days/week
Older Adults	If unable to follow above guidelines, then as much physical activity as your condition allows	If unable to follow above guidelines, then as much physical activity as your condition allows	In addition to muscle strengthening activities, those with limited mobility should add exercises to improve balance and reduce risk of falling
Children and Adolescents	60 min or more of moderate- or vigorous-intensity physical activity daily	Add vigorous-intensity physical activities within the 60 daily minutes at least 3 days/week	Include muscle and bone strengthening activities within the 60 daily minutes at least 3 days/week Activities should be age-appropriate, enjoyable, and varied

*Notes: Avoid inactivity, some activity is better than none; accumulate physical activity in sessions of 10 minutes or more at one time; and spread activity throughout the week.

Source: Office of Disease Prevention and Health Promotion, U.S. Department of Health and Human Services, *2008 Physical Activity Guidelines for Americans: Be Active, Healthy, and Happy!* ODPHP Publication no. U0036 (Washington, D.C.: U.S. Department of Health and Human Services, 2008), Available at www.health.gov .paguidelines.

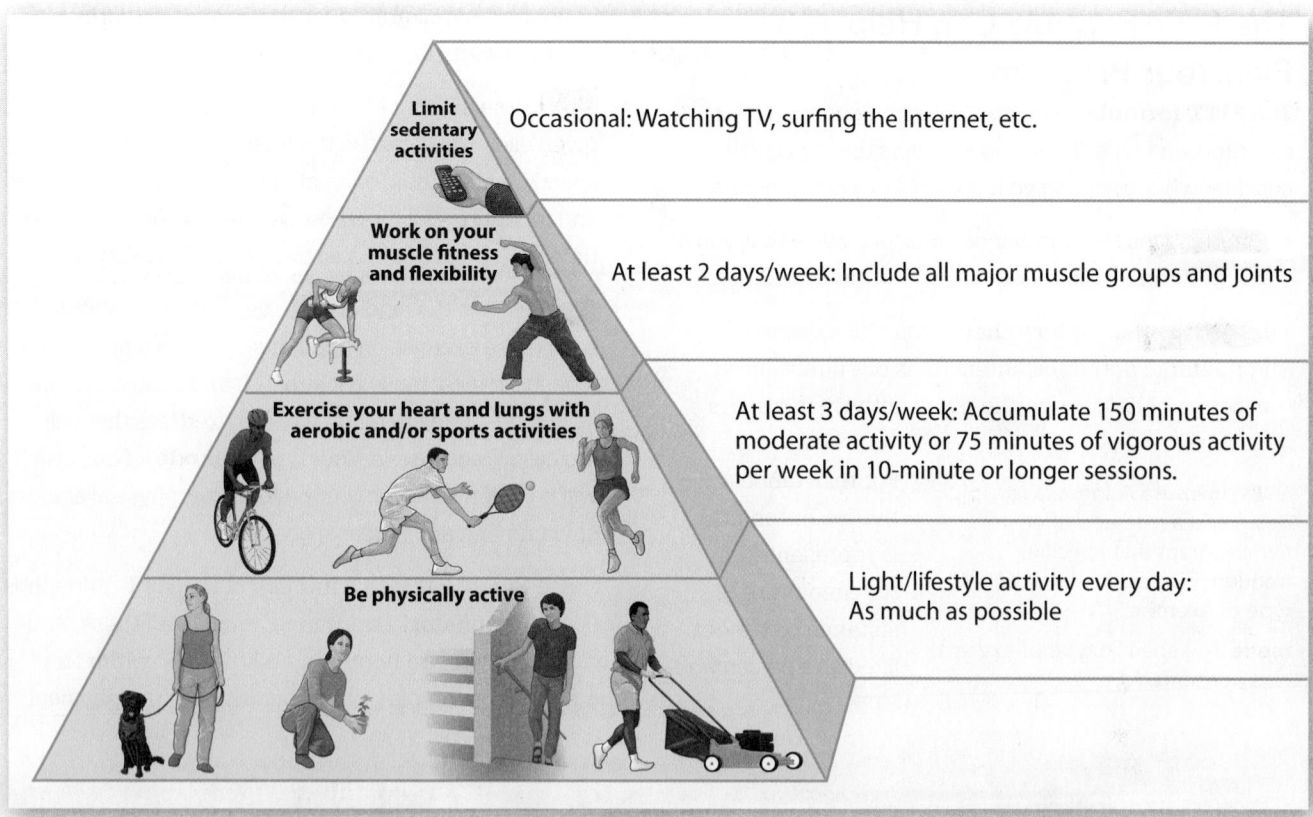

FIGURE **2.3** The Physical Activity Pyramid presents recommended levels of activity for optimal health and wellness.

TOOLS FOR **CHANGE** ●

Six Easy Ways to Become More Active

You can improve your fitness level simply by adding more physical activity to your daily life. Below are a few ways you can incorporate more physical activity:

- Instead of driving your car to campus, ride your bike or walk.

- If you must drive to campus, park your car farther from your destination than usual.

- If you have a dog, walk it daily. If you already do that, add a second daily walk—your dog will love you for it!

- Carry a handbasket while grocery shopping instead of pushing a cart (assuming your grocery list is not very long).

- If you have children, play actively with them.

- If you have a desk job, get up, stretch, and walk around often.

THINK! Examine the Physical Activity Pyramid. How does your weekly physical activity match up to its recommendations? In which areas of the pyramid could you improve?

ACT! Draw your current physical activity pyramid. Now draw your physical activity pyramid incorporating the simple suggestions above. List the activities you could add to your week to become more active.

Source: U.S. Department of Health and Human Services, "Choices," Small Step Program, www.smallstep.gov/ga/choices.html (accessed September 2011).

● ●

The FITT Formula Can Help You Plan Your Program

The **FITT formula** acronym stands for *frequency, intensity, time,* and *type.* These are all factors that you should consider when planning your personal exercise program.

- *Frequency* is the number of times per week that you will perform an exercise.

- *Intensity* refers to how "hard" you will exercise. For aerobic activities, intensity is often measured in terms of how much the given activity increases your heart rate. For resistance activities, intensity is represented in the amount of resistance or weight lifted as a percentage of your maximal ability for that exercise (percent of 1RM or repetition maximum).

- *Time* is the amount of time that you will devote to a given exercise. It can be the total amount of time you spend on an aerobic or sport activity, the number of sets and repetitions for a resistance exercise, or the amount of time you spend holding a stretch for a flexibility exercise.

- *Type* refers to the kind of exercise you will do. Within each of the exercise components of fitness (cardiorespiratory endurance, muscular strength and endurance, and flexibility), there are many types of exercises that will increase fitness levels. Your type, or **mode**, of exercise will be determined by your preferences, physical abilities, environment, and personal goals.

See Figure 2.4 for a summary of the FITT guidelines for cardiorespiratory endurance, muscular fitness, and flexibility. If you are beginning a fitness program for the first time, you may want to start with the physical

> **FITT formula** A formula for designing a safe and effective program that specifies frequency, intensity, time, and type of exercise
>
> **mode** The specific type of exercise performed

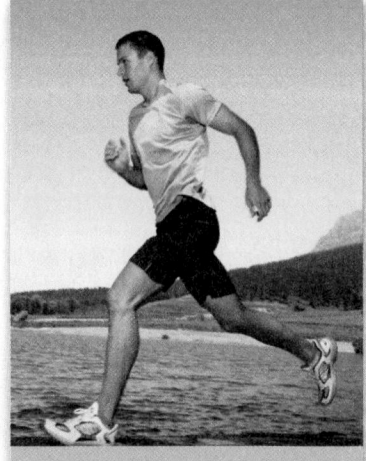 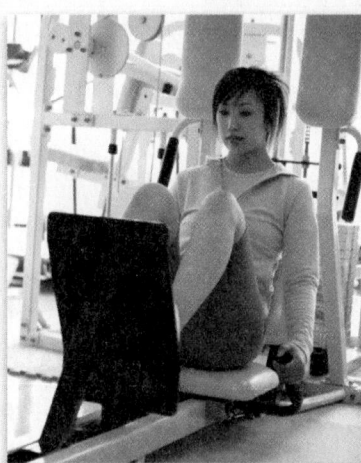 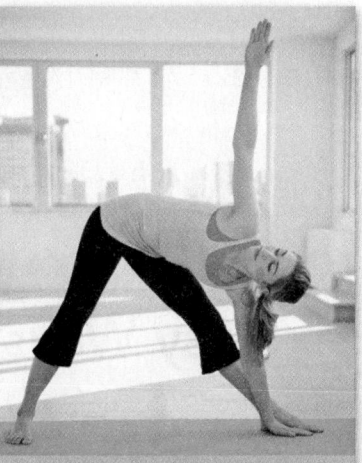

	Cardiorespiratory Endurance	Muscular Fitness	Flexibility
Frequency	3–5 days per week	2–3 days per week	Minimally 2–3 days per week
Intensity	64%–95% of maximum heart rate	60%–80% of 1RM	To the point of mild tension
Time	20–60 minutes	8–10 exercises, 2–4 sets, 8–12 reps	10–30 seconds per stretch, 2–4 reps
Type	Any rhythmic, continuous, large muscle group activity	Resistance training (with body weight and/or external resistance) for all major muscle groups	Stretching, dance, or yoga exercises for all major muscle groups

FIGURE **2.4** The FITT principle applied to summary guidelines for cardiorespiratory endurance, muscular fitness, and flexibility.

Data from: C. E. Garner and others, "American College of Sports Medicine Position Stand: Quantity and Quality of Exercise for Developing and Maintaining Cardiorespiratory, Musculoskeletal, and Neuromotor Fitness in Apparently Healthy Adults: Guidance for Prescribing Exercise," *Medicine and Science in Sports and Exercise* 43, no. 7 (2011): 1334–59.

activity guidelines in Table 2.1. When you are ready, add appropriate levels of the Physical Activity Pyramid and then customize your program using the FITT formula to suit your personal goals.

What Does It Take to Exercise Safely?

Exercise-related injuries have risen in recent decades. More than seven million Americans receive medical attention for sports-related injuries each year, with the greatest numbers of injuries affecting 5- to 24-year-olds.[13] To reduce your risk of exercise injury, follow the guidelines below.

Warm Up Properly Before Your Workout

A proper warm-up consists of two phases: a general warm-up and a specific warm-up. In a *general warm-up,* your goal is to warm up the body by doing three to ten minutes of light physical activity similar to the activities you will be performing during exercise. During this period of time (called the *rest-to-exercise transition*), you are preparing your body to withstand the more vigorous exercise to come. Your core body temperature should rise a few degrees, and you should break a slight sweat. This movement and temperature rise will increase your overall blood flow, ready the joint fluid and structures, and improve muscle elasticity.

During a *specific warm-up,* your goal is to focus on the particular muscle groups and joints that you will be using during the activity set. This part of the warm-up should consist of three to five minutes of **range-of-motion** movements. You should move the joints involved in your exercise through the range of motion that they will experience during the activity. Move joints through a full range of motion in a relaxed and controlled manner. If you want to add light stretching to your warm-up, do so at the end of your specific warm-up.

> **range-of-motion** The movement limits that limbs have around a specific joint

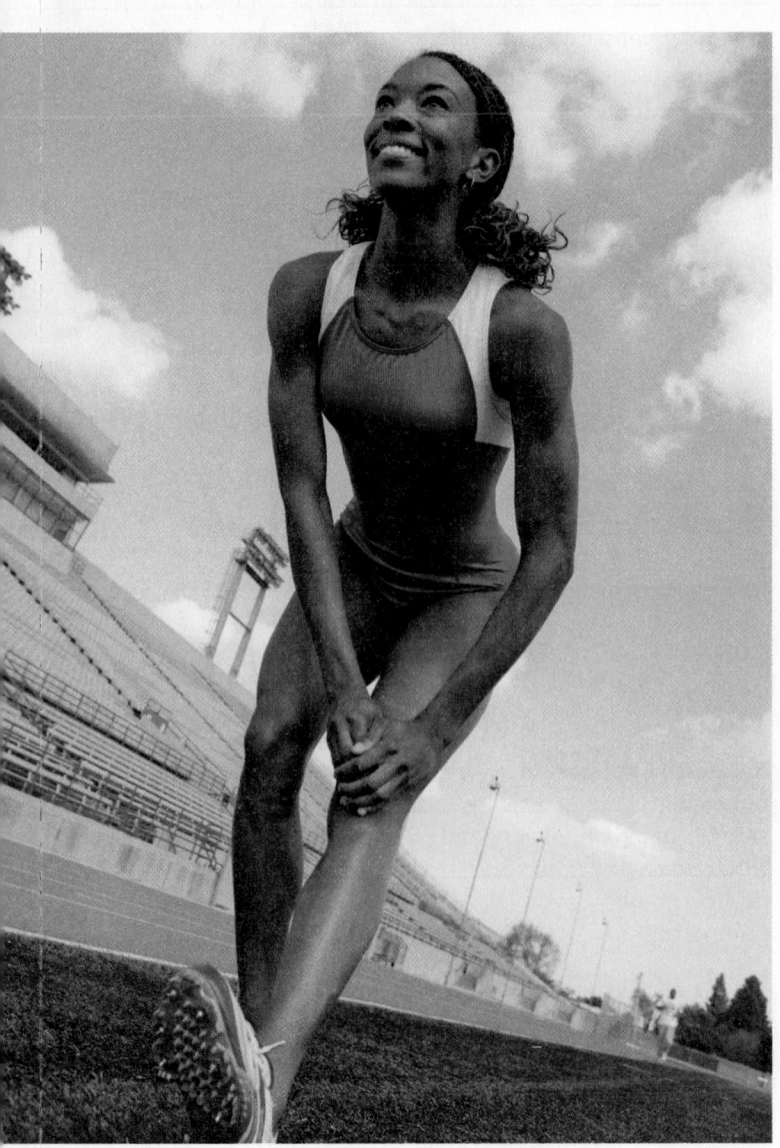

Cool Down Properly After Your Workout

After you finish your workout, cool down in a manner that is appropriate to the activity that you performed. This *exercise-to-rest transition* should last anywhere from five to fifteen minutes. If your heart rate and temperature rose during your workout, you should perform a *general cool-down* in which your goal is to bring your heart rate, breathing rate, and temperature closer to resting levels. This cool-down is usually a less vigorous version of the activity you just performed. For example, if you jogged for 25 minutes, your general cool-down may consist of 10 minutes of walking.

If you have just finished a resistance-training program and your heart rate is not elevated, you should perform a *specific cool-down* for the joints and muscles you have exercised. A specific cool-down can be performed after a general cool-down for aerobic activities and right after exercise for resistance training activities. During a specific cool-down, you should stretch the muscle groups worked during the activity.

Take the Time to Properly Learn the Skills for Your Chosen Activity

There are hundreds of different activities that you can do to increase your health and fitness, each with a specific set of physical skills required for participation. You might choose simple activities such as walking or jogging, which require little skill and have short learning curves, or you might focus on activities that require more complex skills, such as fencing or hockey. Whatever you choose, properly learn the physical skills required for the activity to enhance your enjoyment and to avoid injury. If you are just beginning a sport for the first time—for example, skiing—do not immediately approach the sport the way a more experienced athlete would. Take lessons, start on the beginner slopes, and give yourself time to safely perform your chosen activity.

Consume Enough Energy and Water for Exercise

Deciding how much to eat and drink prior to exercise can be tricky. You need enough energy to work out, but you should not exercise on a full stomach. Eating a small meal 1 1/2 to 2 hours before exercise is a good way to make sure that you have energy (but not an upset stomach) during the workout. A light snack 30 to 60 minutes before your workout is acceptable as well.

Dehydration is more likely than food intake to affect your exercise performance. During the hours before your workout, be sure to drink enough water so that you do not feel thirsty as you go into your exercise session. Guidelines for drinking before, during, and after exercising should be tailored to the individual and the exercise session.[14] General guidelines are 17 to 20 oz. of fluid two to three hours before exercise and 7 to 10 oz. of fluid ten to twenty minutes prior to exercise.[15] During your workout, hydrate when you feel thirsty, and increase the amount of water you consume as you start to sweat more profusely.

Select Appropriate Footwear and Clothing

Consider this: Your feet will typically strike the ground 1,000 times during one mile of running. Over weeks of training, that translates to a great deal of wear and tear on your feet and lower body. Needless to say, proper footwear is critical to a safe and successful training program—regardless of the activity you choose.

While some sports require specialized footwear, most beginning exercisers just need one pair of good, all-around cross-trainers or running shoes. The most important aspect of footwear is proper fit and cushioning. Always try on shoes before purchasing them, and if possible, spend a few minutes mimicking the activity you will be doing in them. The best shoes are not always the most expensive ones, but you should aim to purchase the highest quality footwear you can afford. Ask for assistance from a knowledgeable salesperson—let him or her know what activities you are planning to pursue, and ask which shoes would be most appropriate for your plans.

Clothing for exercise can be very simple (e.g., shorts and a T-shirt) or very technical (e.g., clothing with wicking fibers or special treatments for protection against harsh weather). The most important thing is to dress appropriately for your chosen activity. Make sure that your clothing is comfortable and does not restrict your range of motion. Women may wish to wear supportive athletic bras, and men may want to consider wearing supportive compression shorts or undergarments. If you are planning to exercise outdoors, take temperature into consideration and dress accordingly. The longer you plan to exercise, the more carefully you should think about what to wear for a successful workout.

casestudy

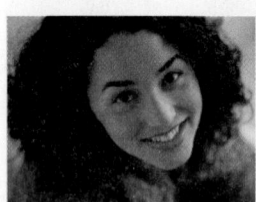

LILY

"I've started jogging again! I'm back to jogging 30 minutes twice a week and thinking of bumping things up to three times a week. I'm hoping to eventually work my way up to jogging for 45 minutes straight, each time I go out. I'm not tempted to run a 10k again any time soon, but if I can keep this new routine going, maybe I will be ready for a 5k—without hurting my knees this time."

THINK! What kinds of things would you advise Lily to do, in order to reduce her chances of injury?

ACT! Describe Lily's exercise routine, using the FITT formula, and figure out what you might do the same or different from her.

What Individual Factors Should I Consider When Designing a Fitness Program?

There is no such thing as a "one-size-fits-all" physical fitness program. Different individuals have different needs, and general recommendations often need to be adapted to fit those individual needs. Your age, weight, current fitness level, and any disabilities and special health concerns are all factors that should be considered in order to design a safe and effective exercise routine.

Age

Older adults may require additional precautions in order to prevent injury while exercising. Men over age 45 and women over age 55 should obtain medical clearance before beginning an exercise program.[16] Moderate aerobic activity, muscle-strengthening exercises, and flexibility work are all recommended activities for older adults. In addition, balance exercises should be included to help prevent the risk of falls and injury.

Weight

Overweight individuals are at higher risk of musculo-skeletal injuries due to increased stress on their muscles and joints, and they should take precautions to ensure safe workouts. If you are overweight, consider a cross-training routine with a mix of moderate weight-bearing (e.g., walking, stair-climbing) and non-weight-bearing (e.g., bicycling, water exercise) activities. If you feel pain in your lower-body joints during exercise, shift to more non-weight-bearing activities during your workout.

Underweight individuals, on the other hand, should perform more strength-training and weight-bearing activities to ensure proper muscle and bone maintenance.

Current Fitness Level

Design a program that is appropriate to your current fitness level. If you already exercise regularly, consider gradually increasing the frequency or intensity of your workouts to realize more fitness gains.

If you are currently sedentary and are just beginning to think about starting an exercise routine, do not just suddenly attempt to participate in a triathlon! Pick an activity that you find enjoyable, start at a level that is comfortable for you, and proceed from there.

Disabilities

If you have mobility restrictions, poor balance, dizziness, or other conditions that are physically limiting, you can still incorporate activity into your daily life with alternative or adaptive exercises. Many colleges, community centers, parks and recreation facilities, and fitness centers offer adaptive courses, equipment, and instructors who are specially trained to help you meet your fitness goals. After obtaining medical clearance, seek out such facilities; your physician or a physical therapist may have good recommendations. The box Getting Active Despite Disability provides additional suggestions.

Special Health Concerns

Certain medical conditions may require you to exercise under medical supervision. Individuals with asthma, heart disease, hypertension, and diabetes all need medical clearance prior to beginning exercise and may need to be monitored by medical personnel

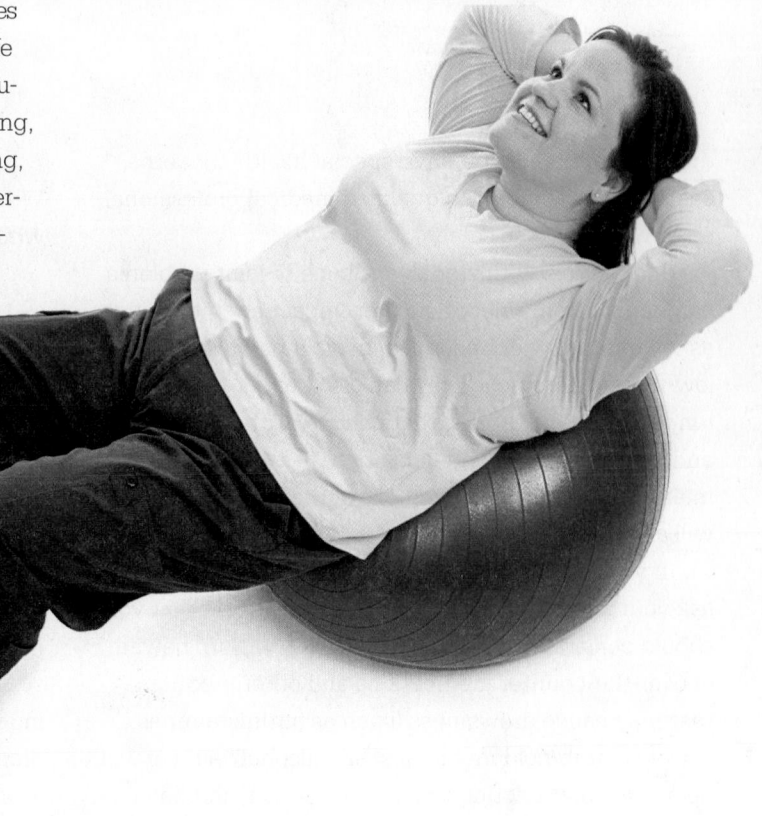

Getting Active Despite Disability

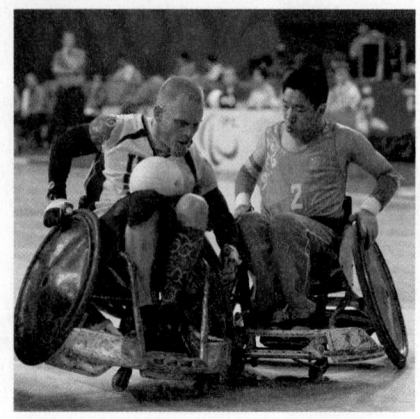

In the documentary film *Murderball*, muscular, aggressive rugby players compete in fierce, international competitions alongside other world-class athletes—all of them in wheelchairs. Their stories are an inspiration to disabled and nondisabled people alike, and demonstrate that while disability does pose undeniable obstacles, it does not have to hinder the achievement of even the highest levels of physical fitness.

With personal motivation, support from friends and family, and assistance from medical and fitness professionals, persons with disability can make exercise part of their daily routine and live physically active lives. In fact, the U.S. Department of Health and Human Services recommends that adults with disabilities follow the 2008 Physical Activity Guidelines for Americans, adjusting as necessary for varying abilities and physician recommendations.

There are various options available for modifying physical activities and helping all people achieve their health and fitness goals. For example, most strength-training machines are used from a seated position and can be operated by people in wheelchairs. Rubber exercise bands, meanwhile, can serve as alternative strength-building aids. Many companies offer modified sports equipment for people with disabilities: Handcycles allow people to ride bikes using arm power, and wakeboards and flotation devices enable waterskiing and swimming activities. Several kinds of seated skis make downhill skiing accessible to those with physical handicaps. And disabled people can play a long list of sports—with modified rules and equipment—including volleyball, tennis, golf, soccer, basketball, bowling, bocci, archery, tai chi, and karate.

during exercise. If you have special health concerns, seek out the advice of a qualified medical professional on how to exercise safely.

Individuals with significant bone or joint problems can benefit from selecting lower-impact activities such as swimming, water exercise, bicycling, walking, or low-impact aerobics. They can also benefit from resistance training exercises that can strengthen muscles and joint structures and contribute to bone-density maintenance and improvement (if their joint limitations will allow it).

If you are taking any prescription medications, ask your doctor whether there are side effects that you should consider before exercising. In addition, beware of over-the-counter medications and other products that may cause drowsiness (such as antihistamines, certain cough/cold medicines, and alcohol), as this will decrease your reaction time, coordination, and balance.

If you are pregnant, read the box Can I Exercise While I'm Pregnant? for advice on exercising safely while expecting.

How Can I Get Started Improving My Fitness Behaviors?

You know that exercise is good for you, but starting a fitness program and sticking with it over the long term can be a real challenge! According to a recent national survey, only 34 percent of adults in the United States participate in regular leisure-time physical activity.[17] College-aged adults (18 to 24 years) fared better, with 42 percent reporting regular physical activity patterns. The percentages drop as people age: Fewer than 27 percent of people 65 years and older reported regular leisure-time physical

Can I Exercise While I'm Pregnant?

Although pregnancy is not the time to start an intense fitness or weight-loss program, most pregnant women can maintain pre-pregnancy activities with just a few modifications. In fact, recent studies have shown that exercise during pregnancy benefits both the mother (improved cardiorespiratory function, decreased weight gain and discomfort, mood stability, and reduced gestational diabetes and high blood pressure risks) and fetus (improved stress tolerance and neurobehavioral maturation).[1] To exercise safely during pregnancy, follow the American College of Obstetricians and Gynecologists guidelines:[2]

- Get medical clearance for the activity you intend to do. Your physician may even have some specific recommendations for your fitness program.

- Seek out a pregnancy fitness exercise program where qualified instructors lead safe exercise sessions. These programs can also provide a good social support network for mothers-to-be.

- Choose fitness activities that do not increase risk of injury to you or the fetus. Avoid high-intensity sports, activities with the potential for falls or abdominal injury, and environmental extremes (such as temperature or barometric pressure—no scuba diving, in particular). Pay attention to your body temperature and avoid becoming too hot during exercise, especially during the first trimester. Choose low-impact activities such as swimming, water exercise, indoor cycling, yoga, and walking.

- In the absence of medical complications, perform at least 15 minutes of moderate exercise, gradually increasing to 30 minutes per day of accumulated moderate exercise. Aim for 150 minutes per week total.

- Monitor your exercise intensity levels by determining how you feel during exercise.

- In the third trimester, avoid supine exercises (i.e., exercises that require you to lie on your back), because these may restrict blood flow to the fetus.

- Do pelvic-floor exercises regularly. These exercises, called *kegels*, involve tightening the pelvic floor muscles for 5 to 15 seconds at a time; they will help with pregnancy-induced incontinence and delivery recovery. Add three to five sets of 10 to your daily routine.

Pregnancy can be both a wonder-filled and scary time. Maintaining a minimum level of fitness can help you cope with the stresses coming your way.

Sources:
1. K. Melzer and others, "Physical Activity and Pregnancy: Cardiovascular Adaptations, Recommendations and Pregnancy Outcomes," *Sports Medicine* 40, no. 6 (2010): 493–507.
2. American College of Obstetricians and Gynecologists, "ACOG Committee Opinion No. 267: Exercise during Pregnancy and the Postpartum Period," *Obstetrics & Gynecology* 99, no. 1 (2002): 171–173 (reaffirmed 2009).

activity. Despite the statistics, making fitness part of your daily life is within your reach—and can be tremendously fun and rewarding. However, preparing to exercise for the first time (or after a long sedentary period) can be daunting. If you are unsure how to start, what to do, or how much to exercise, you may have the impulse to just jump right in, do something your friends are doing, or try something you saw on TV or in a magazine. This haphazard approach often leads to disappointment and frustration—not to mention muscle soreness and even injury. A better approach is to think carefully about your exercise motivations, goals, and needs, select activities that will meet those needs (and that you enjoy!), apply the FITT formula to each of those activities, and then make a conscious long-term commitment to your exercise program.

As you plan your fitness program, ask yourself: what motivates you? What obstacles are in your way? What are reasonable fitness goals you can set for yourself? Are you prepared to commit to a fitness program? To begin, fill out **Lab 2.1** to assess your current readiness for a physical activity behavior change and to determine whether you need medical clearance to begin an exercise program.

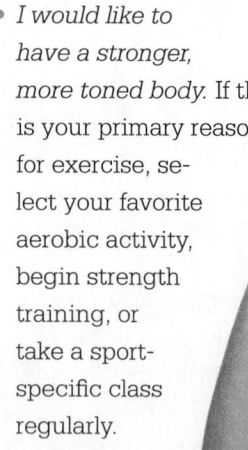

Understand Your Motivations for Beginning a Fitness Program

If you understand your motivations for participating in a fitness program, you can plan activities in a way that makes you more likely to stick with the program. Below are some of the most common reasons people decide to exercise, along with tips for how to maximize your chances of long-term fitness success.

- *I want to gain health benefits.* If this is your main motivation, try to design a program centered on physical activities that you find enjoyable and easy to incorporate in your day-to-day life. If you don't like gyms, don't sign up for one! Instead, select an activity in which you genuinely take pleasure, such as walking with a friend or family member.

- *I want to have fun.* If your main motivation is fun, consider joining an intramural sports team on campus, or going on regular outdoor trips with friends. Seek out activities that, first and foremost, you know you will enjoy, and that have the beneficial "side effect" of fitness.

- *I want to meet new people or exercise with friends.* Participating in a fitness program can be a great way to socialize. Even if you do not consider this one of your main reasons to start exercising, social motivations can often keep you coming back. Look for activity classes, clubs, or teams that you can join with friends or where you can meet new people with similar interests.

- *I like the challenge of setting goals and doing well in competition.* If this sounds like you, regardless of what activity you choose, be sure to set realistic, attainable goals. You may find a clearly defined target—such as an upcoming 5K race—to be just what you need to get started, so sign up!

- *I want to lose some weight.* If weight loss is your main motivation, you will need to consider your nutrition and diet plan along with your fitness plan. Choose fitness activities that burn plenty of calories and that you will enjoy doing often.

- *I would like to have a stronger, more toned body.* If this is your primary reason for exercise, select your favorite aerobic activity, begin strength training, or take a sport-specific class regularly.

Anticipate and Overcome Obstacles to Exercise

If you are not currently physically active, why not? Are you too busy? Do you simply dislike exercise? You can probably immediately identify several things that keep you from being

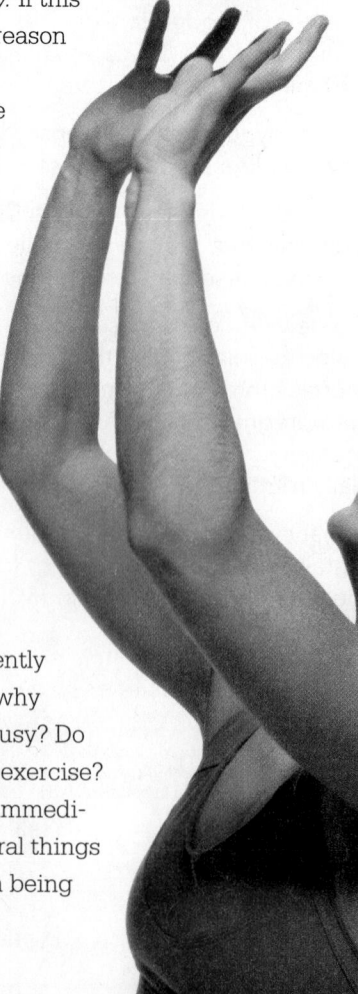

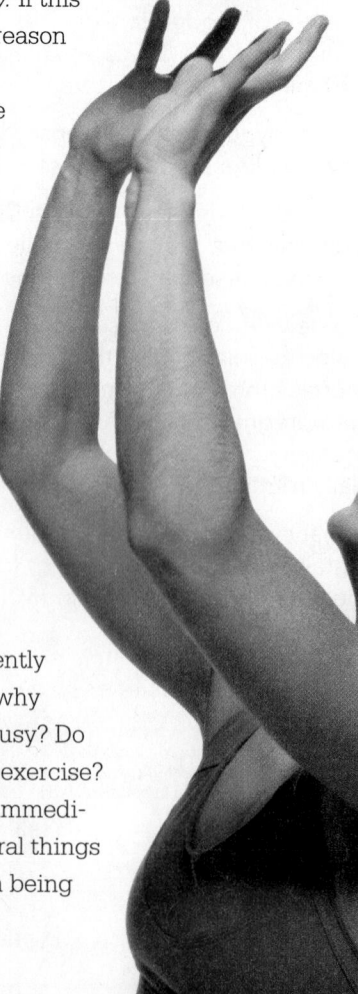

as active as you want to be. Obstacles, or **barriers to physical activity**, can be categorized as either environmental or personal. *Environmental barriers* include both external/physical factors and social/interpersonal factors that may make it harder or easier for you to exercise. Do you feel safe exercising on the streets around your campus? Is the weather conducive to exercising? Are facilities open during the hours that you need them? Do you have friends who exercise and who might be interested in exercising with you? These external factors can greatly affect your exercise habits.

Likewise, *personal barriers* can play a role in whether you are successful in sticking to an exercise plan. Typical personal barriers include lack of self-motivation, injury, starting fitness levels and weight, disability, relationship difficulties, or psychological problems such as depression or anxiety. Older-than-average students, students with children, and those who work long hours while attending school often face unique challenges as they work to improve their fitness levels. The box Overcoming Common Obstacles to Exercise provides strategies for overcoming specific obstacles. **Lab 2.2** helps you assess your motivations for exercise and identify your obstacles to beginning a fitness program.

> **barriers to physical activity** Personal or environmental issues that hinder your participation in regular physical activity

DO IT! ONLINE

Make Time for Exercise

People often state that they don't exercise because they don't have enough time. That might be the case—or they may simply be assigning exercise a lesser priority in their life than other activities, such as watching TV or text-messaging friends. While socializing and scheduling downtime in a busy life *are* important, consider how much time you spend in your life on sedentary activities. Then consider the benefits to your health and sense of

---

TOOLS FOR **CHANGE** •

Overcoming Common Obstacles to Exercise

Below are lists of strategies for overcoming common obstacles to exercise.

Obstacle: Lack of Time

- Monitor your daily activities for one week. Identify at least three 30-minute time slots you could use for physical activity.

- Add physical activity to your daily routine. For example, walk or ride your bike to work or shopping, walk the dog, exercise while you watch TV, park farther away from your destination, and so on.

- Select activities requiring minimal time, such as walking, jogging, or stair-climbing.

Obstacle: Lack of Social Support

- Explain your interest in physical activity to friends and family. Ask them to support your efforts.

- Invite friends and family members to exercise with you. Plan social activities involving exercise.

- Develop new friendships with physically active people. Join a group, such as the YMCA or a hiking club.

Obstacle: Lack of Energy

- Schedule physical activity for times in the day or week when you feel energetic.

- Convince yourself that if you give it a chance, physical activity will increase your energy level; then try it.

Obstacle: Lack of Willpower

- Plan ahead. Make physical activity a regular part of your schedule and write it on your calendar.

- Invite a friend to exercise with you on a regular basis and write it on your calendar.

- Join an exercise group or class.

Obstacle: Fear of Injury

- Learn how to warm up and cool down to prevent injury.

- Learn how to exercise appropriately considering your age, fitness level, skill level, and health status.

- Choose activities involving minimum risk.

(Continued)

Obstacle: Lack of Skill

- Select activities requiring no new skills, such as walking, climbing stairs, or jogging.

- Exercise with friends who are at your skill level.

- Find a friend who is willing to teach you some new skills.

- Take a class to develop new skills.

Obstacle: Lack of Resources

- Select activities that require minimal facilities or equipment, such as walking, jogging, jumping rope, or calisthenics.

- Identify inexpensive, convenient resources available in your community (community education programs, park and recreation programs, worksite programs, etc.).

Obstacle: Weather Conditions

- Develop a set of regular activities that are always available regardless of weather (indoor cycling, aerobic dance, indoor swimming, stair-climbing, mall-walking, dancing, gymnasium games, etc.).

Obstacle: Travel

- Put a jump rope and resistance bands in your suitcase.

- Walk the halls and climb the stairs in hotels.

- Stay in places with swimming pools or exercise facilities.

- Join the YMCA or YWCA.

- Visit the local shopping mall and walk for half an hour or more.

- Pack your favorite aerobic exercise DVD.

Obstacle: Family Obligations

- Trade babysitting time with a friend, neighbor, or family member who also has small children.

- Exercise with the kids—go for a walk together, play tag or other running games, get an aerobic dance or exercise tape for kids and exercise together.

- Hire a babysitter and look at the cost as a worthwhile investment in your health.

- Jump rope, do calisthenics, ride a stationary bicycle, or use other home gymnasium equipment while the kids are busy playing or sleeping.

- Try to exercise when the kids are not around (e.g., during school hours or their nap time).

THINK! What are your main motivations to exercise? What are obstacles that you can anticipate?

ACT! For each obstacle, write down how you will get around it. Post reminders around your home and work to help you "stick" to your plan.

Source: Adapted from CDC, National Center for Chronic Disease Prevention and Health Promotion, Division of Nutrition, Physical Activity and Obesity, "Physical Activity for Everyone: Overcoming Barriers to Physical Activity," www.cdc.gov /physicalactivity/everyone/getactive/barriers.html (accessed January 2011).

well-being that would result if you replaced some of that sedentary time with physical activity.

To successfully stick with a fitness program, you need to prioritize exercise the same way that you prioritize your classes, homework, job, and social life. Schedule your exercise sessions into your calendar/ appointment book. Prove to yourself that you are serious about getting fit by making the time for exercise.

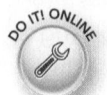 Get started by completing **Lab 2.3**, where you will make a plan to incorporate more physical activity into your daily life.

Select Fun and Convenient Activities

Even if you have committed to set aside time to exercise, you may not always *want* to. If you are accustomed to a sedentary lifestyle, it can be difficult to tear yourself away from the computer or to get off the couch. One way to counter a lack of motivation is to choose fun activities. If your workout is a form of play, you will look forward to it time and time again.

Choosing the best type of exercise is often also about convenience. Despite your good intentions and high level of motivation when starting a new activity, if it's not convenient for your existing lifestyle and commitments, you will have a hard time sticking with it. Look for activities, facilities, and workout times that make sense for your schedule.

Activities can be classified into three general categories or types: lifestyle physical activities, exercise training options, and sports and recreational activities.

Figure 2.5 illustrates sample moderate to vigorous lifestyle, exercise, and sports activities that you can choose from to meet activity guidelines and increase your fitness level.

Lifestyle Physical Activities Lifestyle physical activities are those that you perform during daily life. These include things such as walking the dog, bicycling to work, and so on. Lifestyle physical activities can be light, moderate, or vigorous, depending on what the task is and how long it takes you. For instance, watering your garden for 15 minutes may be a light activity, but raking leaves for four hours can be vigorous.

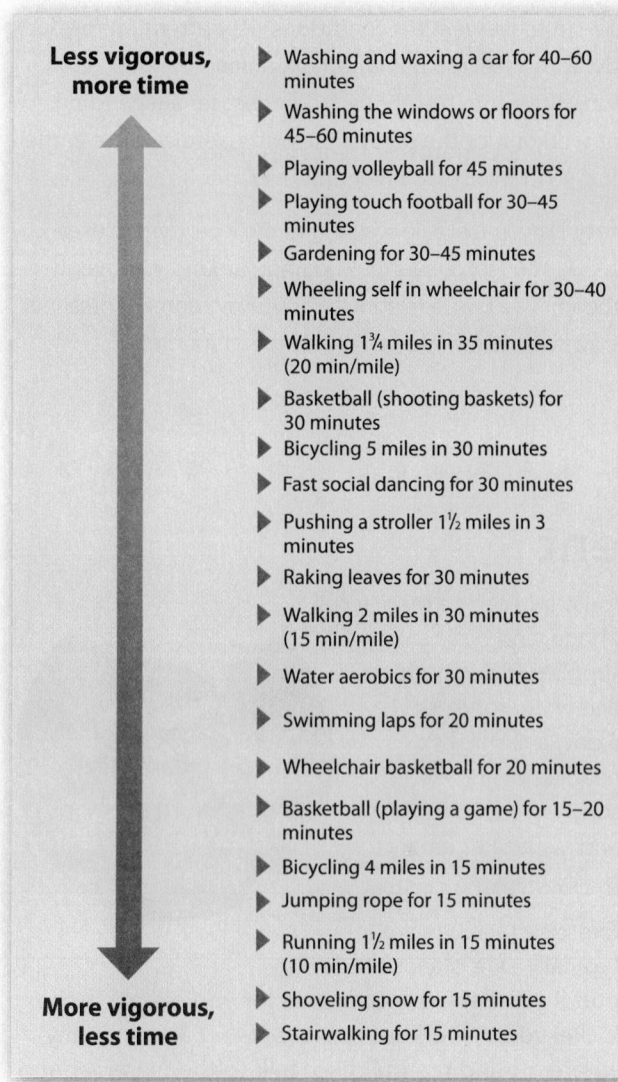

Less vigorous, more time

- Washing and waxing a car for 40–60 minutes
- Washing the windows or floors for 45–60 minutes
- Playing volleyball for 45 minutes
- Playing touch football for 30–45 minutes
- Gardening for 30–45 minutes
- Wheeling self in wheelchair for 30–40 minutes
- Walking 1¾ miles in 35 minutes (20 min/mile)
- Basketball (shooting baskets) for 30 minutes
- Bicycling 5 miles in 30 minutes
- Fast social dancing for 30 minutes
- Pushing a stroller 1½ miles in 3 minutes
- Raking leaves for 30 minutes
- Walking 2 miles in 30 minutes (15 min/mile)
- Water aerobics for 30 minutes
- Swimming laps for 20 minutes
- Wheelchair basketball for 20 minutes
- Basketball (playing a game) for 15–20 minutes
- Bicycling 4 miles in 15 minutes
- Jumping rope for 15 minutes
- Running 1½ miles in 15 minutes (10 min/mile)
- Shoveling snow for 15 minutes
- Stairwalking for 15 minutes

More vigorous, less time

FIGURE **2.5** Sample moderate to vigorous physical activities.

Source: Centers for Disease Control and Prevention, "Physical Activity and Health: A Report of the Surgeon General," www.cdc.gov/nccdphp/sgr/ataglan.htm.

Exercise Training Options Most people think of typical exercise options when asked how they are going to increase their fitness. These include aerobics classes, jogging or running, weight training, indoor cardio workouts, yoga, tai chi, lap swimming, and water aerobics. These activities are great for specifically increasing your fitness. However, consider including a variety of activities to counter the boredom that may come from doing the same exercise week after week. Add a few sports and recreational activities every now and then to keep yourself motivated and your body challenged.

Sports and Recreational Activities Traditional team sports offer a great deal of fun, motivation, and fitness. Most cities have sports leagues for adult soccer, softball, basketball, ultimate Frisbee, and other team sports. If you like the camaraderie of working with a team and enjoy the challenge of team sports, strongly consider this option. You may be able to find team sports classes on campus, at community centers, and in sports clubs.

Individual sports activities can offer great fitness benefits as well. Court sports such as tennis, squash, and racquetball will increase your cardiorespiratory fitness and muscle endurance and will improve your agility, coordination, and reaction time. Many sports are recreational for some people but a competitive pastime for others.

If you are going to rely on a sport or recreational activity for your regular fitness routine, just make sure that it really is regular. For instance, skiing is great, but does not constitute a good fitness program if you only get to the mountain a few times a year. Golf, mountain biking, hiking, ice skating, and rock climbing are additional examples of recreational and competitive sports that can maintain or increase fitness if done regularly.

Choose Environments Conducive to Regular Exercise

A major obstacle to exercise for many people is having a suitable, convenient place to work out. The following are some factors to consider when deciding where to exercise.

Exercise Facility Options Exercise facilities are often located at colleges, community centers, health and fitness clubs, athletic and tennis clubs, parks and recreation facilities, YMCAs, corporate fitness centers, and schools. Choosing a facility based upon its location is a good idea because the farther away a facility is from your home, the less likely you are to use it. Other things to consider when choosing a basic exercise facility are ease of parking (if you drive), variety of classes, quality of cardio and weight equipment, and hours that are compatible with your schedule. Additionally, you may be interested in facilities with a swimming pool, basketball and racquetball courts, locker rooms, showers, and spa.

Cost can be a big factor. Larger facilities with more offerings will likely be more expensive per month than a basic fitness center. Community centers and parks facilities often offer reasonable day use or multiday use fees. Almost all facilities offer day use passes for a fee, or even one-time free passes to check out the facility. Be sure to try the facility for several days to see whether you like the atmosphere, the equipment, and the instructors, and whether you feel safe and comfortable using the facility.

If you have not taken advantage of your college facilities yet, you may be missing out on a good deal. As a student, you can typically get access to classes, courts, leagues, equipment, and even personal trainers. College is the perfect time to try out new sports and activities.

Neighborhood When people live in safe neighborhoods where it is easy to exercise, they are more likely to be active.[18] This is becoming a bigger issue as growing cities and suburbs lead to a dramatic increase in urban sprawl. Some experts even suggest that urban sprawl is partially to blame for the rise in obesity in the United States in recent years. For example, researchers in New Jersey found that residents of sprawling counties were less likely to walk during leisure time, weighed more, and had high blood pressure more often than residents living in compact urban areas.[19] Living near streets that are conducive to physical activity (with sidewalks, bike lanes, street lights, slower traffic) and parks with bike and walking paths might make the difference between whether you stay regularly active or not.

Weather If you are an outside exerciser, the weather can create obstacles to regular physical activity. The impact of weather will, of course, depend on where you live and the time of year. If you are prepared, you can exercise in most weather conditions. Pay attention to your body. If you feel too hot when exercising outside, slow down, move into the shade, and consider suspending your workout for the day. Limit your exercise time in the rain if you become too wet and cold.

Safety Do you feel safe walking to the local gym to exercise? Do you feel comfortable jogging around your neighborhood? The box Adjusting to Your Environment presents tips for exercising safely in different environments.

TOOLS FOR **CHANGE** •

Adjusting to Your Environment

In order to maintain a regular exercise routine, you need to feel safe and comfortable in your surroundings. Below are some suggestions for exercising safely in different environments:

- If your neighborhood is not safe, consider exercising with a friend or training group, or consider driving to a different nearby neighborhood to exercise.

- If you are exercising where there are many cars, wear bright clothing and face traffic when walking or running. Seek out areas that are less busy and where speed limits are lower.

- If you are heading into a wilderness area for a hike, trail run, or mountain-bike ride, plan your outing with a friend, or at least let someone know specifically where you are going and when you will return. Know your route and carry a map, a cell phone, and basic safety supplies, including food and water for at least a day, a flashlight or headlamp, first-aid supplies, a pocketknife, and a space or emergency blanket.

- Exercise facilities are typically safe places to work out. If you have any concerns for your safety in the locker room, workout areas, parking areas, or anywhere around the building, talk to the manager and get an escort to your car at night.

casestudy

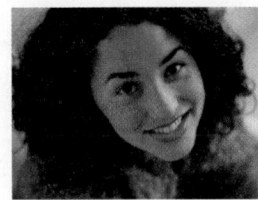

LILY

"I've been following my new jogging routine for three weeks, but now the weather is cold and I cannot get motivated to run! I don't want to give up running but I don't live close to a gym and cannot afford a home treadmill. I just heard about a running group that uses the local track once a week and I know the school has a jogging and running class. Maybe I should try one of those to keep my motivation up and my running program on track? Perhaps I will meet someone I can run with that is just my speed."

THINK! What is Lily doing to increase her chances of sticking to her new exercise plans? What are three things you can do to make exercise a regular part of your life?

ACT! At the beginning of the chapter Lily asked ". . . *what does it actually mean to be fit?*" Given what you have explored in this chapter, write an answer to that question for yourself.

Set Reasonable Goals for Increased Fitness

Setting appropriate, realistic goals can mean the difference between success and failure in fitness programming. People often start a fitness program and think they can train to run a 10k in three weeks—an unrealistic goal for a beginning exerciser. Make sure your goals are realistic; you may want to start with the sample plans in Activate, Motivate, & Advance Your Fitness: A Walking Program in this chapter (page 64). As you begin a fitness program, your progress may initially be slow, while your body adjusts to the new activity. Setting reasonable goals includes considering everything that you have assessed about yourself: your fitness level when you begin, your reasons for exercise, your motivations and attitudes about physical activity, and the constraints that other aspects of your life may impose.

Plan Your Rewards If you find yourself unmotivated to become active, try coming up with goal-related rewards to motivate yourself. Rewards can be highly individual; after all, different things motivate different people. The key is to come up with rewards that reinforce your new,

more active lifestyle. A common reward for people trying to lose weight, for example, is to shop for new clothes. But rewards do not necessarily have to be material. If competition or personal challenge motivate you, for example, you may find the exhilaration of finishing a half-marathon or completing a race in the top 10 percent of contenders to be considerable reward of its own.

Rewards can be internal or external. **Internal exercise rewards** commonly involve feeling better about yourself, feeling healthier, and having better life satisfaction from exercising. Long-term exercisers often report that internal exercise rewards are their primary motivation. Studies have shown that exercise releases endorphins in your body that can fill you with a sense of well-being.[20] For many long-term exercisers, the physical activity itself is truly its own reward. New exercisers, however, often rely on **external exercise rewards**—at least initially. External exercise rewards can be anything from a new workout wardrobe to a celebratory dinner to the admiration and praise of your peers or fitness instructor.

As you incorporate regular physical activity and exercise into your lifestyle, you may find that just having fun and feeling good while exercising is reward enough. If this switch to an internal reward motivation does not happen right away, keep setting external rewards to keep yourself motivated until it does. Don't be surprised if the switch happens faster than you think.

Make a Personal Commitment to Regular Exercise
Deciding that you are going to lead a more physically active lifestyle is the first step to changing your exercise behaviors. The harder step is to commit to that decision. Examine what a more active lifestyle would mean to you and write out your personal commitment statement: a list of reasons to commit to fitness. Review this list regularly until your new behaviors become routine.

Remember that changing behavior takes perseverance. If you feel your commitment flagging, reread your personal commitment statement and remind yourself of the reasons you began your program in the first place.

> **internal exercise rewards**
> Rewards for exercise that are based upon how one is feeling physically and mentally (sense of accomplishment, relaxation, increased self-esteem)
>
> **external exercise rewards**
> Rewards for exercise that come from outside of a person (trophy, compliment, day at the spa)

chapterin**review**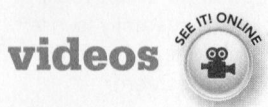

videos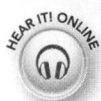

Log on to **www.pearsonhighered.com/hopson** or MyFitnessLab to view these chapter-related videos.

Personal Fitness and Exercise

onlineresources

Log on to **www.pearsonhighered.com/hopson** or MyFitnessLab for access to these book-related resources, and for links to other useful websites.

 Audio case study
Audio PowerPoint lecture

Customizable 4-week walking programs
Take Charge of Your Health! Worksheets:
  Worksheet 26 How Much Do I Move?
Behavior Change Log Book and Wellness
Journal

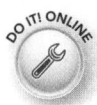 Lab 2.1 Assess Your Physical Activity Readiness
Lab 2.2 Identify Your Physical Activity Motivations and Obstacles
Lab 2.3 Changing Your Sedentary Time into Active Time

Pre- and post-quizzes
Glossary flashcards

reviewquestions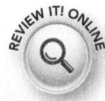

1. Moderate physical activity is best defined as activity that is
   a. less than 3 METS.
   b. 3–6 METS.
   c. 7–9 METS.
   d. over 10 METS.
2. Which health-related component of fitness involves moving your joints through a full range of motion?
   a. Cardiorespiratory fitness
   b. Muscular endurance
   c. Flexibility
   d. Body composition
3. Which skill-related component of fitness is most involved in braking quickly when a car in front of you stops suddenly?
   a. Agility
   b. Power
   c. Coordination
   d. Reaction time

4. The principle of individuality with respect to fitness states that
   a. adaptations to training overload may vary widely from person to person.
   b. all individuals respond the same way to exercise.
   c. genetic makeup has nothing to do with individual responses to exercise.
   d. nonresponders are individuals who do not benefit from exercise.
5. The 2008 Physical Activity Guidelines for Americans emphasize
   a. vigorous physical activity every day of the week.
   b. moderate physical activity for 150 minutes per week or vigorous physical activity for 75 minutes per week.
   c. resistance training for 300 minutes per week.
   d. limiting the amount of time you spend walking.
6. A proper warm-up consists of
   a. a few quick side bends.
   b. stretches that you hold for one minute or more.
   c. quick stair climbing.
   d. a gradual increase in body temperature and easy movements in the muscles and joints.

7. Experiencing knee pain can be categorized as having a(n) _____ barrier to physical activity.
   a. social
   b. scheduling
   c. environmental
   d. personal

8. Which of the following is an example of an internal exercise reward?
   a. Buying new workout clothing
   b. Having fun while exercising
   c. Placing third in your age group in the local 5K race
   d. Taking a celebratory trip after meeting an exercise goal

9. Which of the following is least likely to result in a successful long-term exercise routine?
   a. Making exercise a priority in your weekly schedule
   b. Setting up rewards for yourself
   c. Selecting fun and convenient activities
   d. Forcing yourself to go to a gym even though you don't enjoy it

10. Which fitness principle refers to subjecting the body or body system to more physical activity than it is accustomed to?
    a. Overload
    b. Adaptation
    c. Dose-response
    d. Specificity

critical**thinking**questions

1. Give an example of how a training overload can lead to adaptations and training effects.
2. Describe the similarities and differences between the principle of diminished returns and the principle of progression.
3. Imagine you are about to begin a fitness program centered on bicycling. Apply the FITT formula to describe how you might set up your program.

4. If you are reluctant to increase your activity level due to fear of injury, what are five strategies that will help you overcome those fears and avoid injury?
5. Explain the difference between internal and external exercise rewards.

references

1. M. R. Carnethon, M. Gulati, and P. Greenland, "Prevalence and Cardiovascular Disease Correlates of Low Cardiorespiratory Fitness in Adolescents and Adults," *The Journal of the American Medical Association* 294, no. 23 (2005): 2981–88.
2. H. Suominen, "Muscle Training for Bone Strength," Aging *Clinical and Experimental Research* 18, no. 2 (2006): 85–93.
3. K. Small, L. McNaughton, and M. Matthews, "A Systematic Review Into the Efficacy of Static Stretching as Part of a Warm-Up for the Prevention of Exercise-Related Injury," *Research in Sports Medicine* 16, no. 3 (2008): 213–31.
4. L. O. Mikkelsson and others, "Adolescent Flexibility, Endurance Strength, and Physical Activity as Predictors of Adult Tension Neck, Low Back Pain, and Knee Injury: A 25 Year Follow Up Study," *British Journal of Sports Medicine* 40, no. 2 (2006): 107–13.
5. M. J. Spink and others, "Foot and Ankle Strength, Range of Motion, Posture, and Deformity Are Associated with Balance and Functional Ability in Older Adults," *Archives of Physical Medicine and Rehabilitation* 92, no. 1 (2011): 68–75.
6. T. D. Brutsaert and E. J. Parra. "What Makes a Champion? Explaining Variation in Human Athletic Performance." *Respiratory Physiology and Neurobiology* 151, no. 2–3 (2006): 109–23.
7. W. D. McArdle, F. I. Katch, and V. L. Katch, *Exercise Physiology: Energy, Nutrition,*

and Human Performance, 7th Edition, (Baltimore: Lippincott Williams & Wilkins, 2010); K. Kubo and others, "Time Course of Changes in Muscle and Tendon Properties During Strength Training and Detraining," *Journal of Strength and Conditioning Research* 24, no. 2 (2010): 322–31.
8. Office of Disease Prevention and Health Promotion, U.S. Department of Health and Human Services, *2008 Physical Activity Guidelines for Americans: Be Active, Healthy, and Happy!* ODPHP Publication no. U0036 (Washington, DC: U.S. Department of Health and Human Services, 2008).
9. World Health Organization, "Global Recommendations on Physical Activity for Health," Global Strategy on Diet, Physical Activity and Health, www.who.int/dietphysicalactivity/factsheet_recommendations/en/index.html (accessed January 31, 2011).
10. C. E. Garner and others, "American College of Sports Medicine Position Stand: Quantity and Quality of Exercise for Developing and Maintaining Cardiorespiratory, Musculoskeletal, and Neuromotor Fitness in Apparently Healthy Adults: Guidance for Prescribing Exercise," *Medicine and Science in Sports and Exercise* 43, no. 7 (2011): 1334–59.
11. National Center for Health Statistics, Health Promotion Statistics Branch, CDC Wonder, *DATA2010 … the Healthy People*

2010 Database (Hyattsville, MD: Centers for Disease Control, 2009) http://wonder.cdc.gov/data2010/focus.htm (accessed January 2011).
12. Office of Disease Prevention and Health Promotion, U.S. Department of Health and Human Services, Healthy People 2020, "2020 Objectives and Goals: Physical Activity," http://healthypeople.gov/2020/topicsobjectives2020/objectiveslist.aspx?topicId=33 (2011).
13. J. M. Conn, J. L. Annest, and J. Gilchrist, "Sports and Recreation Related Injury Episodes in the U.S. Population, 1997–99," *Injury Prevention* 9, no. 2 (2003): 117–23.
14. M. N. Sawka and others, "American College of Sports Medicine Position Stand: Exercise and Fluid Replacement," *Medicine and Science in Sports and Exercise* 39, no. 2 (2007): 377–90.
15. H. H. Fink, A. E. Mikesky, and L. A. Burgoon, *Practical Applications in Sports Nutrition*. 2nd Edition (Sudbury, MA: Jones and Bartlett Publishers, 2009).
16. American College of Sports Medicine, *ACSM's Guidelines for Exercise Testing and Prescription*, 8th Edition (Baltimore: Lippincott Williams & Wilkins, 2010).
17. B. W. Ward and others, "Early Release of Selected Estimates Based on Data from the January–June 2010 National Health Interview Survey," National Center for Health Statistics, www.cdc.gov/nchs/nhis/released201012.htm (December 2010).

18. J. F. Sallis and K. Glanz, "The Role of Built Environments in Physical Activity, Eating, and Obesity in Childhood," *The Future of Children* 16, no. 1 (2006): 89–108; H. M. Grow and others, "Where Are Youth Active? Roles of Proximity, Active Transport, and Built Environment," *Medicine and Science in Sports and Exercise* 40, no. 12 (2008): 2071–9.

19. R. Ewing and others, "Relationship between Urban Sprawl and Physical Activity, Obesity, and Morbidity," *American Journal of Health Promotion* 18, no. 1 (2003): 47–57.

20. L. Carrasco, C. Villaverde, and C. M. Oltras, "Endorphin Responses to Stress Induced by Competitive Swimming Event," *The Journal of Sports Medicine and Physical Fitness* 47, no. 2 (2007): 239–45.

LAB 2.1 • ASSESS YOUR PHYSICAL ACTIVITY READINESS

Name: _____   Date: _____

Instructor: _____   Section: _____

SECTION I: THE PHYSICAL ACTIVITY READINESS QUESTIONNAIRE

Physical Activity Readiness
Questionnaire - PAR-Q
(revised 2002)

PAR-Q & YOU

(A Questionnaire for People Aged 15 to 69)

Regular physical activity is fun and healthy, and increasingly more people are starting to become more active every day. Being more active is very safe for most people. However, some people should check with their doctor before they start becoming much more physically active.

If you are planning to become much more physically active than you are now, start by answering the seven questions in the box below. If you are between the ages of 15 and 69, the PAR-Q will tell you if you should check with your doctor before you start. If you are over 69 years of age, and you are not used to being very active, check with your doctor.

Common sense is your best guide when you answer these questions. Please read the questions carefully and answer each one honestly: check YES or NO.

YES	NO	
☐	☐	1. Has your doctor ever said that you have a heart condition <u>and</u> that you should only do physical activity recommended by a doctor?
☐	☐	2. Do you feel pain in your chest when you do physical activity?
☐	☐	3. In the past month, have you had chest pain when you were not doing physical activity?
☐	☐	4. Do you lose your balance because of dizziness or do you ever lose consciousness?
☐	☐	5. Do you have a bone or joint problem (for example, back, knee or hip) that could be made worse by a change in your physical activity?
☐	☐	6. Is your doctor currently prescribing drugs (for example, water pills) for your blood pressure or heart condition?
☐	☐	7. Do you know of <u>any other reason</u> why you should not do physical activity?

If

you

answered

YES to one or more questions

Talk with your doctor by phone or in person BEFORE you start becoming much more physically active or BEFORE you have a fitness appraisal. Tell your doctor about the PAR-Q and which questions you answered YES.

• You may be able to do any activity you want — as long as you start slowly and build up gradually. Or, you may need to restrict your activities to those which are safe for you. Talk with your doctor about the kinds of activities you wish to participate in and follow his/her advice.

• Find out which community programs are safe and helpful for you.

NO to all questions

If you answered NO honestly to <u>all</u> PAR-Q questions, you can be reasonably sure that you can:
• start becoming much more physically active – begin slowly and build up gradually. This is the safest and easiest way to go.
• take part in a fitness appraisal – this is an excellent way to determine your basic fitness so that you can plan the best way for you to live actively. It is also highly recommended that you have your blood pressure evaluated. If your reading is over 144/94, talk with your doctor before you start becoming much more physically active.

→

DELAY BECOMING MUCH MORE ACTIVE:
• if you are not feeling well because of a temporary illness such as a cold or a fever – wait until you feel better; or
• if you are or may be pregnant – talk to your doctor before you start becoming more active.

PLEASE NOTE: If your health changes so that you then answer YES to any of the above questions, tell your fitness or health professional. Ask whether you should change your physical activity plan.

<u>Informed Use of the PAR-Q</u>: The Canadian Society for Exercise Physiology, Health Canada, and their agents assume no liability for persons who undertake physical activity, and if in doubt after completing this questionnaire, consult your doctor prior to physical activity.

No changes permitted. You are encouraged to photocopy the PAR-Q but only if you use the entire form.

NOTE: If the PAR-Q is being given to a person before he or she participates in a physical activity program or a fitness appraisal, this section may be used for legal or administrative purposes.

"I have read, understood and completed this questionnaire. Any questions I had were answered to my full satisfaction."

NAME _____

SIGNATURE _____   DATE _____

SIGNATURE OF PARENT _____   WITNESS _____
or GUARDIAN (for participants under the age of majority)

Note: This physical activity clearance is valid for a maximum of 12 months from the date it is completed and becomes invalid if your condition changes so that you would answer YES to any of the seven questions.

CSEP
SCPE © Canadian Society for Exercise Physiology   Supported by: 🍁 Health Canada Santé Canada

Source: *Physical Activity Readiness Questionnaire (PAR-Q)* © 2002. Used with permission from the Canadian Society for Exercise Physiology. www.csep.ca.

SECTION II: HEALTH/FITNESS PRE-PARTICIPATION SCREENING QUESTIONNAIRE

Assess your health status by indicating all TRUE statements:

History—You have had:

_____ a heart attack

_____ heart surgery

_____ cardiac catheterization

_____ coronary angioplasty

_____ pacemaker/implantable cardiac defibrillator

_____ heart rhythm disturbance

_____ heart valve disease

_____ heart failure

_____ heart transplantation

_____ congenital heart disease

Symptoms:

_____ You experience chest discomfort with exertion.

_____ You experience unreasonable breathlessness.

_____ You experience dizziness, fainting, or blackouts.

_____ You take heart medications.

Other Health Issues:

_____ You have diabetes.

_____ You have asthma or other lung disease.

_____ You have burning or cramping sensations in your lower legs when walking short distances.

_____ You have musculoskeletal problems that limit your physical activity.

_____ You have concerns about the safety of exercise.

_____ You take prescription medication(s).

_____ You are pregnant.

If any of the above statements are true for you, consult your physician or other appropriate health care provider before engaging in exercise. You may need to use a facility with a medically qualified staff.

Cardiovascular Risk Factors:

_____ You are a man older than 45 years old.

_____ You are a woman older than 55 years, have had a hysterectomy, or are postmenopausal.

_____ You smoke, or quit smoking within the previous six months.

_____ Your blood pressure is higher than 140/90 mmHg.

_____ You do not know your blood pressure.

_____ You take blood pressure medication.

_____ Your blood cholesterol level is higher than 200 mg/dL.

_____ You do not know your cholesterol level.

_____ You have a close blood relative who had a heart attack or heart surgery before age 55 (father or brother) or age 65 (mother or sister).

_____ You are physically inactive (i.e., you get less than 30 minutes of physical activity on at least 3 days/week).

_____ You are more than 20 pounds overweight.

If you marked two or more of the statements in this section, you should consult your physician or other appropriate health care provider before engaging in exercise. You might benefit from using a facility with a professionally qualified exercise staff to guide your exercise program.

If you did not mark any of the above statements, you should not need medical clearance to exercise safely in a properly designed self-guided exercise program.

Source: American College of Sports Medicine, *ACSM's Guidelines for Exercise Testing and Prescription,* 8th ed. Lippincott Williams & Wilkins, Baltimore, MD, 2010.

SECTION III: PHYSICAL ACTIVITY STAGES OF CHANGE QUESTIONNAIRE

1. After carefully reading each of the following statements, please answer **YES** or **NO**.

			NO	YES
(1)	I am currently physically active.*		NO	YES
(2)	I intend to become more physically active in the next six months.		NO	YES
(3)	I currently engage in regular** physical activity.		NO	YES
(4)	I have been regularly physically active for the past six months.		NO	YES

* Physical activity or exercise: Activities such as walking briskly, jogging, bicycling, swimming, or any other activity in which the exertion is at least as intense as these activities.

** Regular activity: Activity that adds up to a total of 30 minutes or more per day and is done at least five days per week.

2. Identify your physical activity stage of change (circle your stage):

→ If you answered NO to questions 1 and 2, you are in **PRECONTEMPLATION.**

(To move toward behavior change, it is important at this stage to start thinking about physical activity and its benefits.)

→ If you answered NO to question 1 and YES to question 2, you are in **CONTEMPLATION.**

(In order to move into preparation, you must gain information about how to get started moving toward your goal.)

→ If you answered YES to question 1 and NO to question 3, you are in **PREPARATION.**

(In this stage, it is important to remove barriers that are preventing regular physical activity.)

→ If you answered YES to questions 1 and 3, but NO to question 4, you are in **ACTION.**

(In order to maintain your new behavior, in this stage you need to track your progress, maintain your motivation, and head off potential relapses before they occur.)

→ If you answered YES to questions 1, 3, and 4, you are in **MAINTENANCE.**

(To keep your active lifestyle habits, try new activities and cross-training, make it fun, and strive to keep a consistent program despite life's obstacles.)

Source: B. H. Marcus and B. A. Lewis, "Physical Activity and the Stages of Motivational Readiness for Change Model," *President's Council on Physical Fitness and Sports Research Digest* 4, no.1 (2003): 1–8.

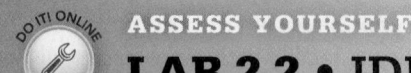

LAB 2.2 • IDENTIFY YOUR PHYSICAL ACTIVITY MOTIVATIONS AND OBSTACLES

Name: _____ Date: _____

Instructor: _____ Section: _____

Purpose: To identify your motivations for starting a physical activity, exercise, or sport (or maintaining your current fitness routine) and your obstacles to exercise, plus learn how to set up exercise-specific rewards to overcome those obstacles.

SECTION I: WHAT MOTIVATES YOU?

Assign a rating of 1–7 for each of the motivations listed below, using the following scale: 1 = not at all true, 7 = very true

I participate (or want to participate) in my physical activity or sport because:

_____ **1.** I want to be physically fit.

_____ **2.** It's fun.

_____ **3.** I like engaging in activities that physically challenge me.

_____ **4.** I want to obtain new skills.

_____ **5.** I want to maintain my weight and/or look better.

_____ **6.** I want to be with my friends.

_____ **7.** I like to do this activity.

_____ **8.** I want to improve existing skills.

_____ **9.** I like the challenge.

_____ **10.** I want to define my muscles so that I look better.

_____ **11.** It makes me happy.

_____ **12.** I want to keep up my current skill level.

_____ **13.** I want to have more energy.

_____ **14.** I like activities which are physically challenging.

_____ **15.** I like to be with others who are interested in this activity.

_____ **16.** I want to improve my cardiovascular fitness.

_____ **17.** I want to improve my appearance.

_____ **18.** I think it's interesting.

_____ **19.** I want to maintain my physical strength to live a healthy life.

_____ **20.** I want to be attractive to others.

_____ **21.** I want to meet new people.

_____ **22.** I enjoy this activity.

_____ **23.** I want to maintain my physical health and well-being.

_____ **24.** I want to improve my body shape.

_____ **25.** I want to get better at my activity.

_____ **26.** I find this activity stimulating.

_____ **27.** I will feel physically unattractive if I don't.

_____ **28.** My friends want me to.

_____ **29.** I like the excitement of participation.

_____ **30.** I enjoy spending time with others doing this activity.

SECTION II: SCORING MOTIVATIONS

Fill in your scores for the questions above in the appropriate boxes (for example, in the box for "Q 2," enter the numerical value you answered for question #2). Then add the totals for each type of motivation. Your total scores reflect which category motivates you the most.

Motivation Type	Interest/ Enjoyment	Competence	Appearance	Fitness	Social
	Q 2:	Q 3:	Q 5:	Q 1:	Q 6:
	Q 7:	Q 4:	Q 10:	Q 13:	Q 15:
	Q 11:	Q 8:	Q 17:	Q 16:	Q 21:
	Q 18:	Q 9:	Q 20:	Q 19:	Q 28:
	Q 22:	Q 12:	Q 24:	Q 23:	Q 30:
	Q 26:	Q 14:	Q 27:		
	Q 29:	Q 25:			
Totals:					

Source: R. M. Ryan, C. M. Frederick, D. Lepes, N. Rubio, and K. M. Sheldon, "Intrinsic Motivation and Exercise Adherence," *International Journal of Sport Psychology* 28 (1997): 335–354; C. M. Frederick and R. M. Ryan, "Differences in Motivation for Sport and Exercise and Their Relationships with Participation and Mental Health," *Journal of Sport Behavior* 16 (1993): 125–145.

SECTION III: WHAT KEEPS YOU FROM BEING ACTIVE?

Listed below are common reasons that people give to describe why they do not get as much physical activity as they would like. Read each statement and indicate how likely you are to state the same reason.

How likely are you to say:	Very likely	Somewhat likely	Somewhat unlikely	Very unlikely
1. My day is so busy now, I just don't think I can make the time to include physical activity in my regular schedule.	3	2	1	0
2. None of my family members or friends like to do anything active, so I don't have a chance to exercise.	3	2	1	0
3. I'm just too tired after work to get any exercise.	3	2	1	0
4. I've been thinking about getting more exercise, but I just can't seem to get started.	3	2	1	0
5. I'm getting older, so exercise can be risky.	3	2	1	0
6. I don't get enough exercise because I have never learned the skills for any sport.	3	2	1	0
7. I don't have access to jogging trails, swimming pools, bike paths, etc.	3	2	1	0
8. Physical activity takes too much time away from other commitments—work, family, etc.	3	2	1	0
9. I'm embarrassed about how I will look when I exercise with others.	3	2	1	0
10. I don't get enough sleep as it is. I just couldn't get up early or stay up late to get some exercise.	3	2	1	0
11. It's easier for me to find excuses not to exercise than to go out to do something.	3	2	1	0
12. I know of too many people who have hurt themselves by overdoing it with exercise.	3	2	1	0
13. I really can't see learning a new sport at my age.	3	2	1	0
14. It's just too expensive. You have to take a class or join a club or buy the right equipment.	3	2	1	0
15. My free periods during the day are too short to include exercise.	3	2	1	0
16. My usual social activities with family or friends do not include physical activity.	3	2	1	0
17. I'm too tired during the week, and I need the weekend to catch up on my rest.	3	2	1	0
18. I want to get more exercise, but I just can't seem to make myself stick to anything.	3	2	1	0
19. I'm afraid I might injure myself or have a heart attack.	3	2	1	0
20. I'm not good enough at any physical activity to make it fun.	3	2	1	0
21. If we had exercise facilities and showers at work, then I would be more likely to exercise.	3	2	1	0

Source: Centers for Disease Control and Prevention, "Barriers to Being Active Quiz," www.cdc.gov/nccdphp/dnpa/physical/life/barriers_quiz.pdf (accessed May 2, 2011).

SECTION IV: SCORING OBSTACLES

Follow these instructions to score your answers in Section III:

- Enter the circled number in the spaces provided, putting together the number for statement 1 on line 1, statement 2 on line 2, and so on.

- Add the three scores on each line. Your obstacles to physical activity fall into one or more of seven categories below. Circle any physical activity obstacles category with a score of 5 or above, because this is an important obstacle for you to overcome.

_____ +	_____ +	_____ =	_____
1	8	15	**Lack of time**
_____ +	_____ +	_____ =	_____
2	9	16	**Social influence**
_____ +	_____ +	_____ =	_____
3	10	17	**Lack of energy**
_____ +	_____ +	_____ =	_____
4	11	18	**Lack of willpower**
_____ +	_____ +	_____ =	_____
5	12	19	**Fear of injury**
_____ +	_____ +	_____ =	_____
6	13	20	**Lack of skill**
_____ +	_____ +	_____ =	_____
7	14	21	**Lack of resources**

SECTION V: OVERCOME OBSTACLES TO EXERCISE

1. Do the results surprise you? Explain why or why not.

_____

_____

_____

2. How can you use these results to increase your likelihood of starting or sticking with an exercise program? What strategies can you think of to overcome your personal obstacles to exercise?

_____

_____

_____

DO IT! ONLINE

LAB 2.3 • CHANGING YOUR SEDENTARY TIME INTO ACTIVE TIME

Name: _____ **Date:** _____

Instructor: _____ **Section:** _____

Purpose: To create a plan for reducing your sedentary time and replacing it with active time.

Directions:

1. On Worksheet A, list your typical activity for each hour of your day in the column labeled "Activity."

Worksheet A

Time of Day	Activity	Revised Activity
6:00 AM		
7:00 AM		
8:00 AM		
9:00 AM		
10:00 AM		
11:00 AM		
12:00 PM		
1:00 PM		
2:00 PM		
3:00 PM		
4:00 PM		
5:00 PM		
6:00 PM		
7:00 PM		
8:00 PM		
9:00 PM		
10:00 PM		
11:00 PM		

2. Now examine your list. What are your major sedentary activities? Highlight or circle them on Worksheet A.

3. List three physical activities that you would like to do but typically don't have time to do:

_____

_____

_____

4. Go back to Worksheet A and examine the sedentary activities you highlighted or circled in #2. Can you replace some of these sedentary activities with any of the physical activities you listed in #3? If so, write in the revised activity (in the "Revised Activity" column) next to the sedentary activity it is replacing.

5. If the physical activities you'd like to add to your schedule won't work in the time slots you have allotted for sedentary activity (for example, it may not be possible or safe to go out running at 11:30 PM), what are alternative physical activities you can safely pursue? Write them in.

activate, motivate, & ADVANCE YOUR FITNESS

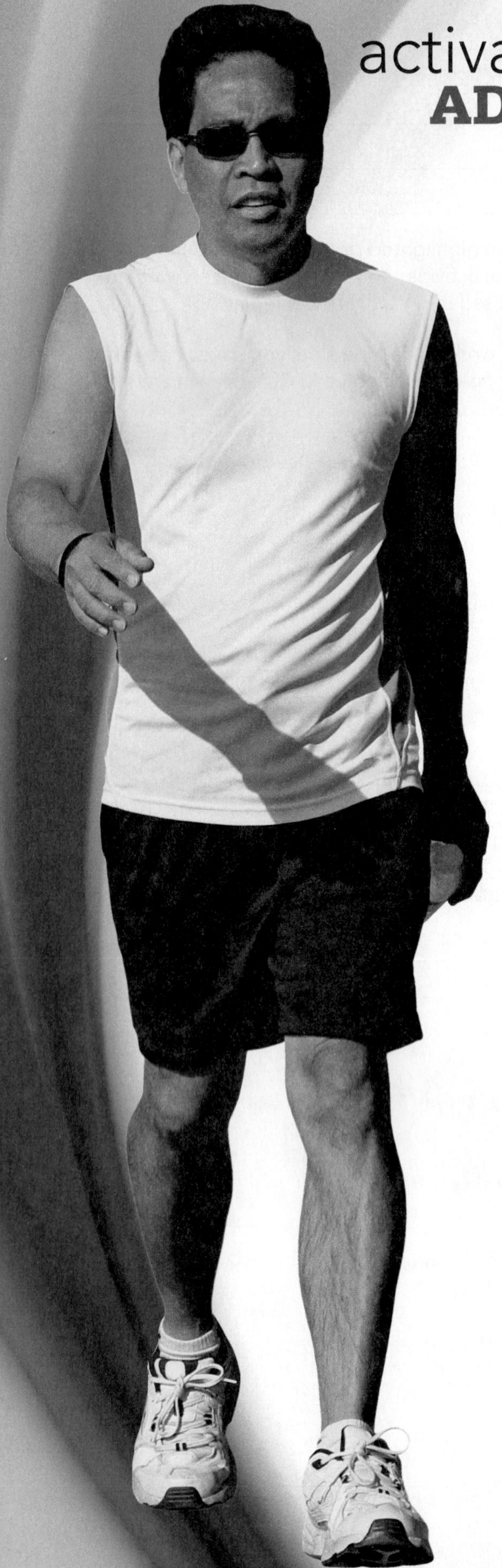

A WALKING PROGRAM

A C T I V A T E !

Walking is the most popular fitness activity in the United States and worldwide. If you are not currently active, walking is one of the best ways to start; you can participate at your own level, minimal equipment is required, and you can do the activity just about anywhere!

What Do I need for Walking?

SHOES: Obtain good-quality shoes. Visit a local running and walking store to get fitted for walking shoes or running shoes (which also work well for walking). A good fit is one of the most important determinants of the right shoe for you.

CLOTHING: Wear comfortable, non-restrictive clothing and cushioned socks that prevent blisters (avoid all-cotton socks). If you are walking outside, wear the right clothing for the weather, be it light clothing in the heat, waterproof clothing in the rain and snow, or warm clothing in the winter; dressing in layers is always a good idea. During the daytime wear sunscreen, sunglasses, and a hat; if you are walking outside at sunrise, dusk, or dark, wear reflective clothing and/or vest and lights.

How Do I Start a Walking Program?

HEALTH WALKING TECHNIQUE & SKILLS: Walking for *health* involves a basic walking stride with a focus on posture. Keep your head up and look straight ahead. Make sure that your shoulders are over your hips and you are not leaning too far forward or backward. Swing your arms easily at your sides, keeping your shoulders down and relaxed. Take natural strides and avoid overstriding (stepping out too far). Focus on being "light" on your feet; particularly avoid slapping your toes down. Instead, control your feet and roll your foot forward.

FITNESS WALKING TECHNIQUE & SKILLS: Increasing your walking pace for *fitness* involves a few adjustments to your walking stride. Follow the basic posture and foot recommendations above but add the following changes. Bend your elbows at ninety degrees and swing your arms in time with your stride. Avoid letting your elbows "chicken-wing" out to the side; instead, keep your elbows close to you. Your hands (in a loose fist) should swing from your lower chest back to your hips. Remember that the faster you swing your arms, the faster your legs will go to keep up! Shorten your stride and take faster steps instead of longer steps. Keep your light heel strike but exaggerate the roll through your foot even more.

Forcefully press off your toes with each stride to propel you forward.

Walking Tips

STREET AND TRAIL WALKING: Plan safe and interesting walking routes considering traffic and available walking paths. You can use an online mapping program to figure out your distance or to create a new route and calculate the distance. Carry a cell phone, ID, a few dollars, and a water bottle. Walk with a partner, if possible, and avoid wearing headphones or wear only one earpiece at a time. Always be aware of your surroundings and walk on the left facing traffic if possible. Follow traffic laws and do not assume that a car or bike operator has seen you.

TRACK WALKING: Walking on a track provides a nice flat, stable surface with a measured distance to walk. If you have a track near you, ensure that it is safe and that you have access to it. Most tracks are 400 meters around, with 4 laps being equal to a mile (on the innermost lane). When on the track, follow track etiquette by utilizing outside lanes for most of your training and leaving the inside lane (lane 1) for runners and sprinters or for timing yourself on a distance. If you are using the inside lane and a faster individual approaches behind you, move out to lane 2 or 3 to allow the person to pass on the inside.

TREADMILL WALKING: Walking inside on a treadmill can be a great option when the weather outside prohibits safe walking. When using the treadmill be sure to familiarize yourself with the controls before starting out. Learn to use the shut-off button (usually a large red button) and as a back-up wear the emergency shut-off clip on your clothing. Keep your body upright and avoid using the handrails or leaning forward too much. Keep your body in the center of the treadmill near the console. Most treadmills have pre-programmed workouts but you can also adjust the speed and incline manually. Start and stop by gradually increasing and decreasing the speed. When you finish, be careful exiting the treadmill; your legs may feel strange on the "non-moving" ground.

Walking Warm-Up and Cool-Down

A walking warm-up and cool-down include walking at a slower pace for three to ten minutes. After breaking a slight sweat in the warm-up, you can add range of motion exercises and 10- to 15-second light stretches. When you finish your walk, you can hold stretches longer for improved flexibility. In particular, focus on stretching the following muscle groups: quadriceps, hamstrings, gluteals, lower back, abductors, gastrocnemius, tibialis anterior, and the pectorals (see Chapter 5 for specific stretches to perform).

Four-Week Starter Walking Program

If you have been sedentary for a long time and need to start slowly, start with Program A below. If you are already able to walk 10–15 minutes continuously on three days a week, start with Program B below. Adjust time, intensity, and days of the walks to suit your personal fitness level and schedule; visit the companion website for customizable versions of these programs.

PROGRAM A **GOAL:** To walk 15–20 minutes continuously, 3–4 days a week

	Mon		Tue		Wed		Thurs		Fri		Sat		Sun	
	T*	I*	T	I	T	I	T	I	T	I	T	I	T	I
Week 1	5	L			5	L			8	M				
Week 2	5	L			8	M			10	M	8	M		
Week 3	10	M			12	M			10	M	12	M		
Week 4	15	M			15	M			20	M	15	M		

T*: Time. Total time is listed in minutes. Time does not include warm-up or cool-down time.
I*: Intensity. Intensity is listed as Light/Lifestyle (L), Moderate (M), or Vigorous (V) (see Figure 2.1).

PROGRAM B **GOAL:** To walk 25–30 minutes continuously, 4–5 days a week

	Mon		Tue		Wed		Thurs		Fri		Sat		Sun	
	T*	I*	T	I	T	I	T	I	T	I	T	I	T	I
Week 1	15	M			15	M			20	M				
Week 2	18	M			20	M			22	V	20	M		
Week 3	22	M	20	M	18	M			25	V	20	M		
Week 4	25	M	22	V	28	M			30	V	25	M		

T*: Time. Total time is listed in minutes. Time does not include warm-up or cool-down time.
I*: Intensity. Intensity is listed as Light/Lifestyle (L), Moderate (M), or Vigorous (V) (see Figure 2.1).

MOTIVATE!

Creating a plan and monitoring your progress are key motivators for any fitness program or behavior change project. Use an exercise log to track your walking program—make note of dates, times, distances, and intensity. Depending on your personal goals and the equipment available to you, you may also choose to keep track of heart rate, steps taken, or calories burned.

Sticking to a fitness plan can be tough, but there are plenty of things you can do to motivate yourself and overcome the obstacles that prevent you from achieving your goals. Here are a few; see the Tools for Change box: Overcoming Common Obstacles to Exercise on pages 47 and 48 for more ideas.

- **Is lack of time an obstacle for you?** If so, monitor your daily activities for 1 week to identify time slots of 15 minutes to half an hour that you could use for walking. Can you incorporate walking into any of your daily activities, such as walking between classes or when running errands? Figure out the timing in advance, and write your walking "appointments" into your schedule.

- **Do you need concrete numbers and immediate targets to keep you motivated?** If so, purchase a pedometer and start keeping track of the number of steps you take. Challenge yourself with mini-goals to increase your step count.

- **Is lack of willpower an obstacle for you?** If so, enlist a friend to join you on your walks, and schedule it into both of your calendars. Committing to another person can be a great motivator.

- **Is boredom an obstacle for you?** If so, look for ways to switch up your route or walk in places that offer sensory stimulation, such as a shopping mall or a wilderness trail. If you are walking on a treadmill, plan your walks to coincide with a favorite radio or television program (if your treadmill has a TV monitor) or download podcasts or audiobooks to listen to while you walk.

- **Is lack of energy or dislike of exertion an obstacle for you?** If so, create a special playlist of music to listen to while you walk, choosing up-tempo songs that will energize you, distract you from the minor discomforts of physical exertion, and help you keep pace.

- **Do you feel a need for more challenge or a long term goal?** If so, sign up for an upcoming charity walk and join a group that is training for it.

ADVANCE!

Ready for the next step? Once you have established your walking program, you may want to challenge yourself to try something new or take your activities to the next level. Below is a more advanced 4-week program you can follow; visit the companion website to personalize this or any of the programs in this book.

PROGRAM C **Goal:** To walk 40–45 minutes continuously, 5 days a week

	Mon		Tue		Wed		Thurs		Fri		Sat		Sun	
	T*	I*	T	I	T	I	T	I	T	I	T	I	T	I
Week 1	20	M			25	M			25	M				
Week 2	28	M			25	V			30	M	28	M		
Week 3	30	V	28	M	35	M			38	M	35	V		
Week 4	40	M	30	V	42	M			45	V	40	M		

T*: Time. Total time is listed in minutes. Time does not include warm-up or cool-down time.
I*: Intensity. Intensity is listed as Light/Lifestyle (L), Moderate (M), or Vigorous (V) (see Figure 2.1).

Disclaimer: These programs are designed for beginners and assume that all participants have been medically cleared for exercise via the procedures outlined in this chapter. Please also be sure that you have read and understand the basic fitness principles and procedures for starting a fitness program outlined in this chapter. This program is focused on the cardiorespiratory component of fitness, but remember that a well-rounded program will also include muscle strength, muscle endurance, flexibility, and back health components.

3

Conditioning Your Cardiorespiratory System

Learning Outcomes

1. Explain how cardiorespiratory fitness is a key component of your overall fitness and wellness.

   HEAR IT! ONLINE — Audio case study and audio PowerPoint lecture

2. Identify the key structures of the cardiorespiratory system and state how they work together to provide oxygen to the body.

3. Outline how the three metabolic systems provide energy for exercise.

4. Describe the fitness and wellness benefits you can get from cardiorespiratory training.

5. Assess your cardiorespiratory fitness level on a regular basis using a variety of methods.

   DO IT! ONLINE — Lab 3.1 Monitoring Intensity during a Workout

   Lab 3.2 Assessing Your Cardiorespiratory Fitness Level

6. Set and work toward appropriate cardiorespiratory fitness goals.

   DO IT! ONLINE — Lab 3.3 Plan Your Cardiorespiratory Fitness Goals and Program

7. Implement a cardiorespiratory exercise plan compatible with your goals and lifestyle.

   LIVE IT! ONLINE — Customizable 4-week starter running, cycling, and swimming cardiorespiratory fitness programs

8. Incorporate strategies to prevent injuries during cardiorespiratory training.

Pre- and post-quizzes and glossary flashcards

REVIEW IT! ONLINE

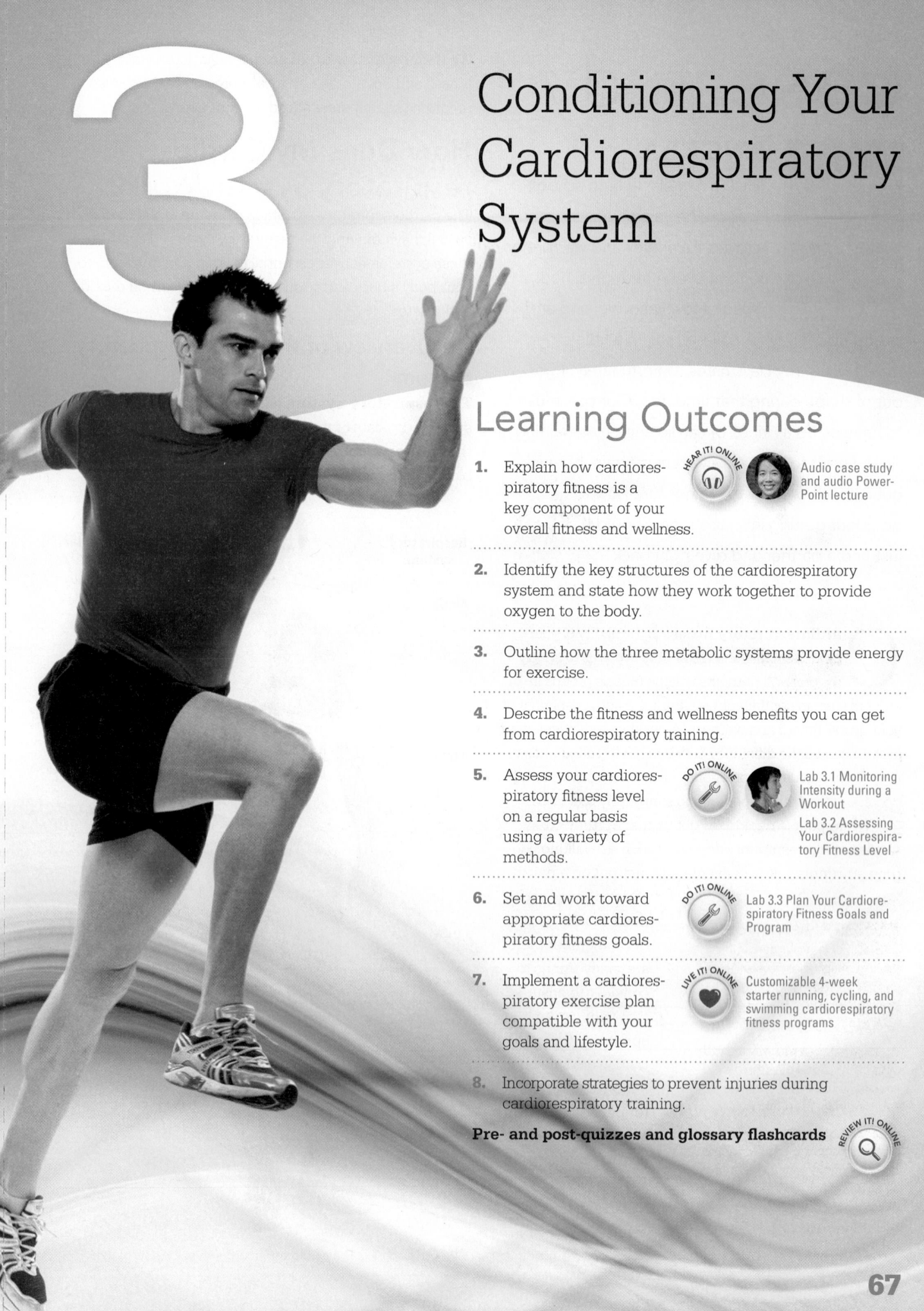

casestudy

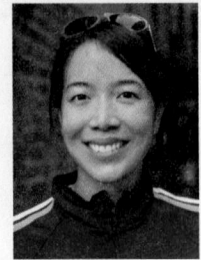

ANGELA

"Hi, I'm Angela. In high school, I was on the varsity tennis team; I played #2 singles and was pretty competitive! After high school, I spent a few years working and saving up money for college, so I'm a little older than most of my classmates. Unfortunately, I got out of shape during that time, too. Our coach used to have us do all kinds of cardio and cross-training drills. I want to start playing tennis again, but without a coach or a team, I'm not sure how to go about getting in shape for it. Should I just find a partner and dive right back in?"

HEAR IT! ONLINE

Cardiorespiratory fitness is the ability of your cardiovascular and respiratory systems to supply oxygen and nutrients to large muscle groups in order to sustain continuous activity. It is a key component of your overall fitness and wellness. A healthy cardiorespiratory system can be the difference between having adequate energy to sustain daily, recreational, and sports activities and becoming tired out by performing simple physical tasks.

When people decide to "get in shape," they often choose cardiorespiratory activities such as walking, jogging, or running. It is convenient to just put on a pair of athletic shoes and head out the door, but remember there are many things to consider to ensure that your cardiorespiratory fitness activities are safe and effective. This chapter provides a brief overview of how the cardiorespiratory system works. We discuss the benefits of regular cardiorespiratory training.

cardiorespiratory fitness The ability of your cardiovascular and respiratory systems to supply oxygen and nutrients to large muscle groups in order to sustain dynamic activity

respiratory system The body system responsible for the exchange of gases between the body and the air

cardiovascular system The body system responsible for the delivery of oxygen and nutrients to body tissues and the delivery of carbon dioxide and other wastes back to the heart and lungs

We then cover how to set goals for cardiorespiratory fitness and how to design a cardiorespiratory exercise program that is personalized for your needs.

How Does My Cardio-respiratory System Work?

The cardiorespiratory system is made up of the cardiovascular system and the respiratory system. Together, these systems deliver essential oxygen and nutrients to your body's cells and tissues and remove carbon dioxide and wastes.

An Overview of the Cardiorespiratory System

The **respiratory system** (also called the *pulmonary system*) consists of the air passageways and the lungs; the **cardiovascular system** consists of the heart and blood vessels (see Figure 3.1).

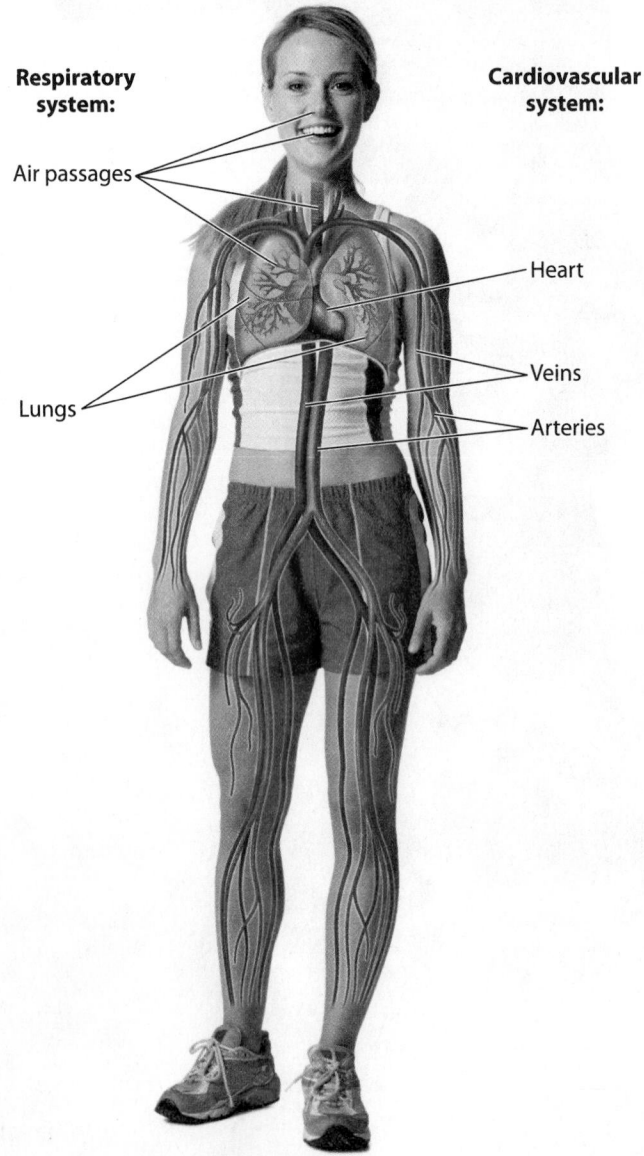

Respiratory system:
- Air passages
- Lungs

Cardiovascular system:
- Heart
- Veins
- Arteries

FIGURE **3.1** The cardiorespiratory system consists of the cardiovascular and respiratory systems.

Air Passageways Air enters your body via your nose and mouth. It then continues through your throat (*pharynx*), voice box (*larynx*), and windpipe (*trachea*) (see Figure 3.2). These upper respiratory passageways warm, humidify, and filter the air, promoting optimal gas exchange. Mucus and small, hairlike projections called *cilia* filter out unwanted particles in the air; you expel these particles through your nose or mouth, or you swallow them. The inspired air travels down through the lower respiratory tract—the lower trachea, *bronchi*, and *bronchioles*—eventually reaching air sacs (*alveoli*) in the lungs, where gas exchange (i.e., the delivery of oxygen and the removal of carbon dioxide) occurs.

Lungs The air passageways in the lungs have extensive branching, similar to the branches on a large tree. At the very ends of the smallest branches (the bronchioles) are alveoli, which are surrounded by small blood vessels called *capillaries*. Because the walls of the alveoli and capillaries are very thin, oxygen moves easily from the alveolar sacs into the capillary blood. Vessels then transport oxygen to the heart and the rest of the body. Meanwhile, carbon dioxide moves from the capillaries into the alveoli and exits the body when you exhale. This exchange of oxygen and carbon dioxide is called **respiration**.

Heart The heart is a fist-sized pump consisting of four chambers: the *right atrium*, the *right ventricle*, the *left atrium*, and the *left ventricle* (Figure 3.3 on page 70). Small *valves* regulate the steady, rhythmic flow of blood between chambers and prevent the blood from flowing backward.

respiration The exchange of gases in the lungs or in the tissues

atria Upper chambers of the heart that collect blood from the rest of the body

ventricles Lower chambers of the heart that pump blood to the rest of the body

pulmonary circulation Blood circulation from the heart to the lungs and back

systemic circulation Blood circulation from the heart to the rest of the body and back

pulmonary artery The artery that carries blood from the right ventricle to the lungs

aorta The artery that carries blood from the left ventricle to the rest of the body

The two **atria** are collecting chambers that receive blood from the rest of the body. The two **ventricles** pump blood out again. With each beat of the heart, the atria and ventricles fill and contract. The heart pumps blood through two different circulatory systems: in **pulmonary circulation**, blood circulates from the heart to the lungs and back; in **systemic circulation**, blood circulates from the heart to the rest of the body and back.

Blood returning to the heart from the body enters the heart through the right atrium. The right atrium pumps blood into the right ventricle. The right ventricle pumps blood through the **pulmonary artery** into the lungs. Blood returning from the lungs enters the heart through the left atrium. The left atrium pumps blood into the left ventricle. The left ventricle fills and contracts, pumping the blood out of the heart via the **aorta** and transporting it to the cells of the heart, brain, and body.

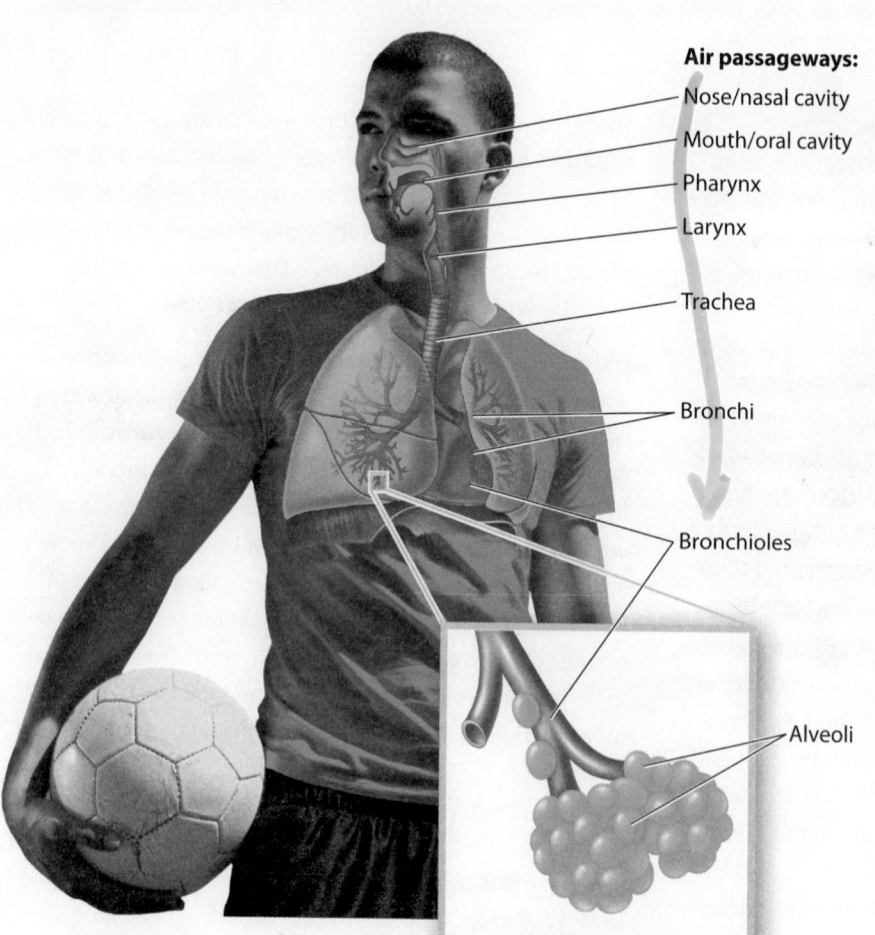

Air passageways:
- Nose/nasal cavity
- Mouth/oral cavity
- Pharynx
- Larynx
- Trachea
- Bronchi
- Bronchioles
- Alveoli

FIGURE **3.2** The respiratory system consists of the air passageways and the lungs.

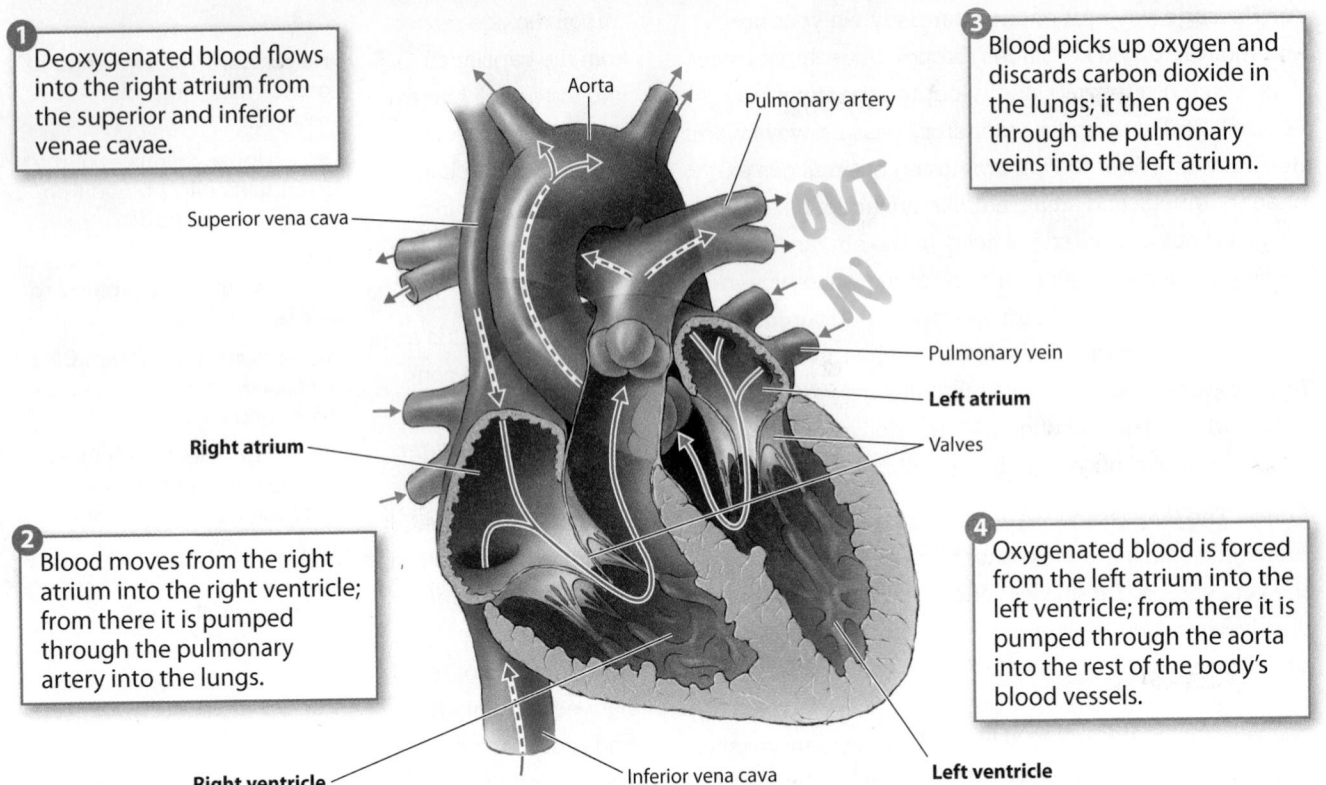

1 Deoxygenated blood flows into the right atrium from the superior and inferior venae cavae.

3 Blood picks up oxygen and discards carbon dioxide in the lungs; it then goes through the pulmonary veins into the left atrium.

Aorta

Pulmonary artery

Superior vena cava

OUT
IN

Pulmonary vein

Left atrium

Right atrium

Valves

2 Blood moves from the right atrium into the right ventricle; from there it is pumped through the pulmonary artery into the lungs.

4 Oxygenated blood is forced from the left atrium into the left ventricle; from there it is pumped through the aorta into the rest of the body's blood vessels.

Right ventricle

Inferior vena cava

Left ventricle

FIGURE **3.3** The heart is a four-chambered pump. The right atrium and left atrium collect blood from the rest of the body. The right and left ventricles pump blood back out. In pulmonary circulation, blood circulates from the heart to the lungs and back. In systemic circulation, blood circulates from the heart to the rest of the body and back.

Contraction of the ventricle chambers must be forceful enough to send blood out of the heart. In order to accomplish this task the ventricles are more muscular than the atria. The left ventricle is the most muscular chamber, because it must contract forcefully enough to send blood to the rest of the body.

The heart cycle consists of two phases: systole and diastole. During **systole**, the ventricles contract and blood is pumped out of the heart. During **diastole**, the ventricles relax and fill back up with blood from the right and left atria. Specialized heart tissue involuntarily and automatically starts the heart cycle. This tissue, located in the right atrium, is called the *pacemaker;* it determines how fast your heart beats. One "beat" of your heart consists of a full heart cycle. Through a stethoscope, you can hear your heartbeat as a "lub dub." The "lub" signals the end of the diastole phase (ventricular relaxation), and the "dub" signals the end of the systole phase (vertricular contraction). The number of times your heart beats in one minute is your **heart rate**.

Blood Vessels Blood vessels transport blood throughout your body. There are two types of blood vessels: **arteries**, which carry blood away from the heart, and **veins**, which carry blood back toward the heart. As arteries branch off from the heart, they divide into smaller blood vessels called *arterioles,* and then into even smaller blood vessels known as *capillaries.* As mentioned earlier, capillaries have thin walls that permit the exchange of substances between cells and the blood. Oxygen and nutrients move from the blood to body cells, while carbon dioxide and waste products move from body cells to the blood for transport to the lungs and kidneys through veins and *venules* (small veins).

The pressure that blood exerts on the walls of blood vessels is called **blood pressure**. The blood pressure in arteries must be high in order to drive the flow of blood to all your cells. (In veins, blood pressure is close to zero.) Due to the strength of the heart contraction, pressure in the arteries is higher during systole. The pressure

systole The contraction phase of the heart cycle

diastole The relaxation phase of the heart cycle

heart rate The number of beats of the heart in one minute

arteries High-pressure blood vessels that carry blood away from the heart to the lungs or cells

veins Low-pressure blood vessels that carry blood from the cells or lungs back to the heart

blood pressure The pressure that blood in the arteries exerts on the arterial walls

measured in the arteries during this phase is called **systolic blood pressure**. When the heart is relaxed, pressure in the arteries drops; this pressure is called **diastolic blood pressure**. In addition to oxygen, working muscles need energy to keep contracting. The three primary energy systems are discussed next.

Three Metabolic Systems Deliver Essential Energy

All of the cells in your body need energy to function. The cellular form of energy is called *adenosine triphosphate,* or **ATP**. ATP must be constantly regenerated from energy stored in your body and from food. The energy stores in your body consist of fat in adipose tissues and muscles, glucose in the muscles and liver, and protein and **creatine phosphate** in muscles. The energy in food comes from fat, carbohydrates, and protein. Your body breaks down stored and consumed nutrients to ATP via three metabolic energy systems: the *immediate, nonoxidative* (anaerobic), and *oxidative* (aerobic) systems. To varying extents, your body draws upon all three systems while you are active, depending on the duration of the activity. Let's examine each of these systems in detail.

The Immediate Energy System When it needs quick, immediate access to energy, your body first draws upon the ATP stored in your muscles. "Explosive" activities such as a basketball jump shot, a 50-meter sprint, or a dive off a diving board are all examples of actions fueled by this immediate energy system. However, your body depletes energy stored in your muscles within a matter of seconds: ATP in muscle cells is typically used up in less than 10 seconds, and creatine phosphate (which is used to make more ATP) is typically gone within 30 seconds. As a result, your body must rely on other energy systems in order to sustain longer activities.

The Nonoxidative (Anaerobic) Energy System As soon as you start moving, the nonoxidative energy system begins breaking down glucose for energy. This system breaks down glucose quickly and *anaerobically* (without oxygen) in order to produce ATP. Although this system starts working immediately, it does not supply the majority of your needed ATP until about 30 seconds into an activity. Examples of nonoxidative, **anaerobic** activities include a sprint down a soccer field, running up a steep hill, and swimming a 100-meter sprint in the pool.

You may experience muscular fatigue with activities that use the nonoxidative energy system, because your body has a limited glucose supply and because the process of breaking down glucose can produce high levels of **lactic acid**. Lactic acid accumulation in the muscles and blood can produce a burning sensation in the muscles during intense activity. The increase in lactic acid is temporary; contrary to popular belief, your body clears lactic acid from muscles within minutes or hours of exercise. Lactic acid does *not* cause the muscle soreness you may feel a day or two after an exercise session. In fact, during and after exercise, lactic acid cleared from the muscles and blood is reused for energy.

systolic blood pressure Blood pressure during the systole phase of the heart cycle

diastolic blood pressure Blood pressure during the diastole phase of the heart cycle

ATP Adenosine triphosphate; the cellular form of energy

creatine phosphate A molecule that is stored in muscle cells and used in the immediate energy system to donate a phosphate to make ATP

anaerobic Without oxygen (nonoxidative)

lactic acid An end-product of the nonoxidative breakdown of glucose that can increase acidity in muscles and the blood and cause muscular fatigue

casestudy

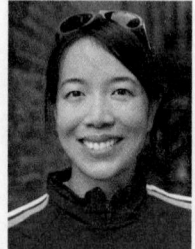

ANGELA

"I thought I would kick-start my plan to get back into shape by doing one of the workouts my tennis coach had us do in high school. I jogged for a mile, did some calisthenics on the court, and then played two sets of tennis with a friend. That was a mistake. My friend has a killer serve—it's like a bullet coming at you. She won every point she served because I couldn't move fast enough to return the ball. Also, I was surprised at how much that jog tired me out. I used to run a mile with no problem at all! By the end of the first set, I was completely exhausted. My friend won 6-1, 6-1."

THINK! Which energy system do you think Angela's friend relied on most while hitting her serves?

ACT! Write out activities you would do for a 10-minute cardiorespiratory warm-up. Now, try your 10-minute warm up and think about how the three energy systems are providing fuel to keep your muscles moving.

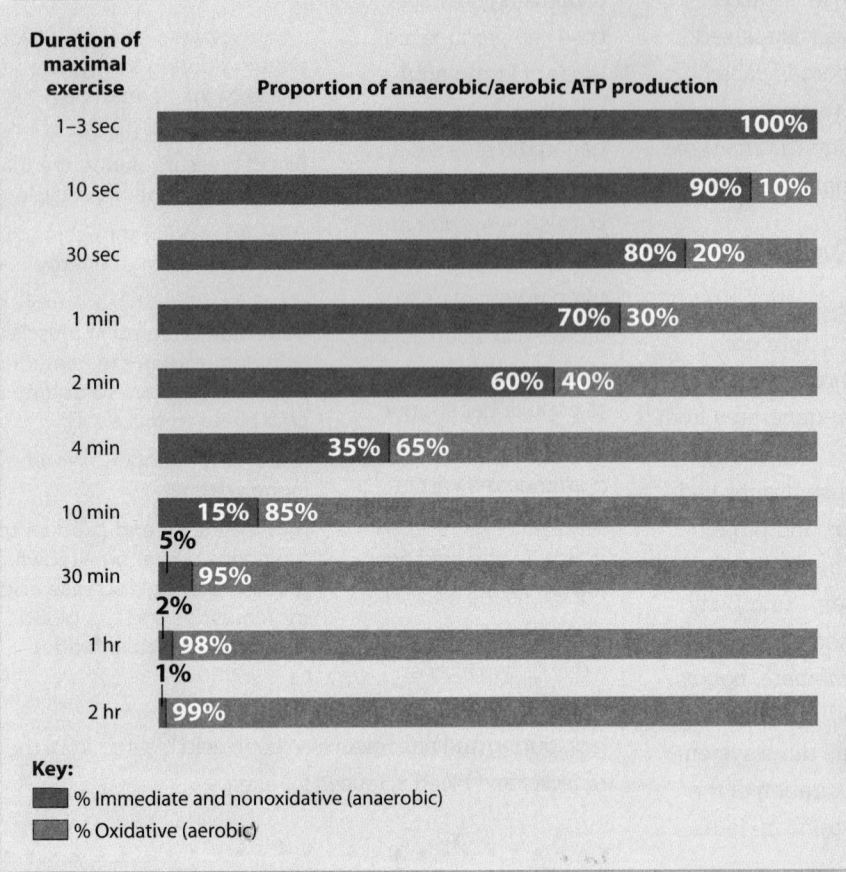

Duration of maximal exercise | **Proportion of anaerobic/aerobic ATP production**

Duration	Anaerobic	Aerobic
1–3 sec	100%	
10 sec	90%	10%
30 sec	80%	20%
1 min	70%	30%
2 min	60%	40%
4 min	35%	65%
10 min	15%	85%
30 min	5%	95%
1 hr	2%	98%
2 hr	1%	99%

Key:
■ % Immediate and nonoxidative (anaerobic)
■ % Oxidative (aerobic)

FIGURE **3.4** In the first two minutes of exercise, a body primarily uses ATP generated by the two nonoxidative (anaerobic) energy systems. After about three minutes into the exercise, a body begins to primarily use ATP generated by the oxidative (aerobic) energy system.

The nonoxidative energy system supplies your body with most of its needed ATP until about three minutes into an activity. At that point, the oxidative energy system becomes the primary provider of ATP.

The Oxidative (Aerobic) Energy System During the first three minutes of activity (when the immediate and nonoxidative systems are supplying most of the ATP you need), your body is also gradually increasing its *oxidative* production of ATP using oxygen in the **mitochondria** of your cells. The oxidative energy system is also called the **aerobic** energy system (*aerobic* means "with oxygen"). Mitochondria are often referred to as the "powerhouses of the cell," because most energy production occurs in these structures. The *complete* breakdown of fat, glucose, and protein occurs only in the mitochondria and the oxidative energy

mitochondria Cellular structures where oxidative energy production takes place

aerobic Dependent on oxygen (oxidative)

homeostasis A stable, constant internal environment

system yields more ATP from each energy source than any other system.

Aerobic activities are low- to moderate-intensity activities that are usually sustained for 20 minutes or longer. Examples of aerobic activities include cycling, treadmill walking, jogging, and water aerobics.

Figure 3.4 illustrates how the proportion of each energy system's contribution of ATP changes, depending on the duration of a given activity.

The Cardiorespiratory System at Rest and during Exercise

Your cardiorespiratory system must adapt in order to meet your body's needs during exercise.

Resting Conditions At rest, your body works to maintain **homeostasis**, a stable, constant internal environment. If you're healthy, your resting heart rate is between 50 to 90 beats per minute, your breathing rate is around 12 to 20 breaths per minute, and your resting blood pressure is below 120 systolic and below 80 diastolic. During homeostasis, your oxygen and nutrient delivery matches the needs of your cells. Your body breaks down fat via the oxidative energy system in order to supply ATP to the body. Although you "burn" fat for energy, your total energy expenditure is low.

Response to Exercise Physical activity disrupts your body's homeostasis. During exercise, your body must increase blood flow to working muscles in order to maintain adequate oxygen and nutrient delivery. Your heart rate increases, and stronger heart contractions result in an increase in **cardiac output**—the amount of blood exiting your heart in one minute. Your breathing rate also increases to ensure that adequate oxygen is transferred into the blood for working muscles.

The increased volume of blood moving from your heart into your blood vessels in exercise results in an increase in systolic blood pressure. The body directs this increased blood to contracting muscles and the vessels *dilate* (open up wider) to accommodate the increased blood flow. This arterial dilation allows diastolic blood pressure to stay the same or even decrease during aerobic exercise. In addition, capillaries that were not open at rest open up to allow for oxygen and nutrient exchange with muscles.

When you begin to exercise, it takes a few minutes for your body to increase blood flow and to fully engage the oxidative energy system. This is why your body must rely on the faster immediate and nonoxidative energy systems in the first few minutes of exercise. The slower ATP production of the oxidative system also means that during your exercise session, you may have to draw upon the nonoxidative energy system more than once. For example, if you are jogging and suddenly sprint to the end of the street, your oxidative energy system may not be able to supply ATP quickly enough. Your body will then draw upon the nonoxidative system (which breaks down glucose quickly) to supply the additional ATP you need.

How Does Aerobic Training Condition My Cardiorespiratory System?

Recall that aerobic activities are low- to moderate-intensity activities performed for an extended period of time (i.e., 20 minutes or longer). Regular aerobic training conditions your cardiorespiratory system by improving your body's ability to (1) deliver large amounts of oxygen to working muscles, (2) transfer and use oxygen efficiently in the muscles, and (3) use energy sources for sustained muscular contractions. Figure 3.5 summarizes these and other adaptations that occur over time with aerobic training.

Aerobic Training Increases Oxygen Delivery to Your Muscles

With regular aerobic training, your body gets better at delivering oxygen to working muscles. Your respiratory muscles become more efficient and you experience less fatigue in an extended workout. You can carry more oxygen in your blood, due to an increase in **hemoglobin**, the oxygen-carrying protein. Since the fluid portion of your blood, the **plasma**, also increases with aerobic training, you will see an increase in your total blood volume. Your heart will adapt to this greater volume by increasing the blood-holding capacity of your left ventricle. The ventricle will not only hold more blood, but (with training) it will also have stronger contractions. All of this will allow you to pump more blood out of your heart with every heartbeat, thus increasing your heart's **stroke volume**.

cardiac output The volume of blood ejected from the heart in one minute; expressed in liters or milliliters per minute

hemoglobin A four-part globular, iron-containing protein that carries oxygen in red blood cells

plasma The yellow-colored fluid portion of blood that contains water, proteins, hormones, ions, energy sources, and blood gases

stroke volume The volume of blood ejected from the heart in one heartbeat; expressed in liters or milliliters per beat

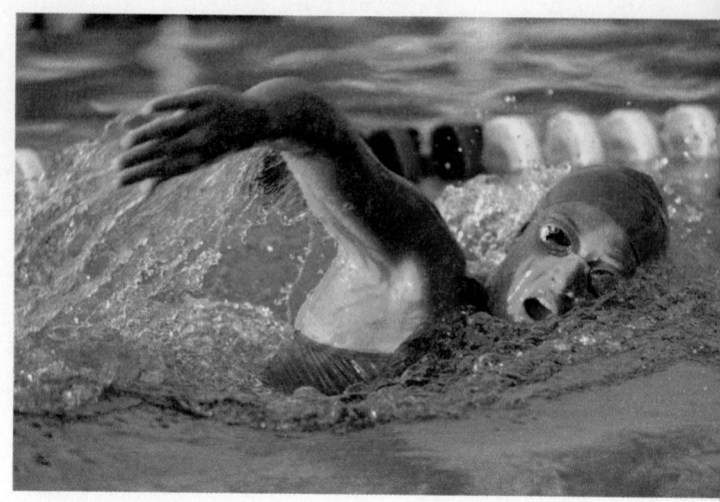

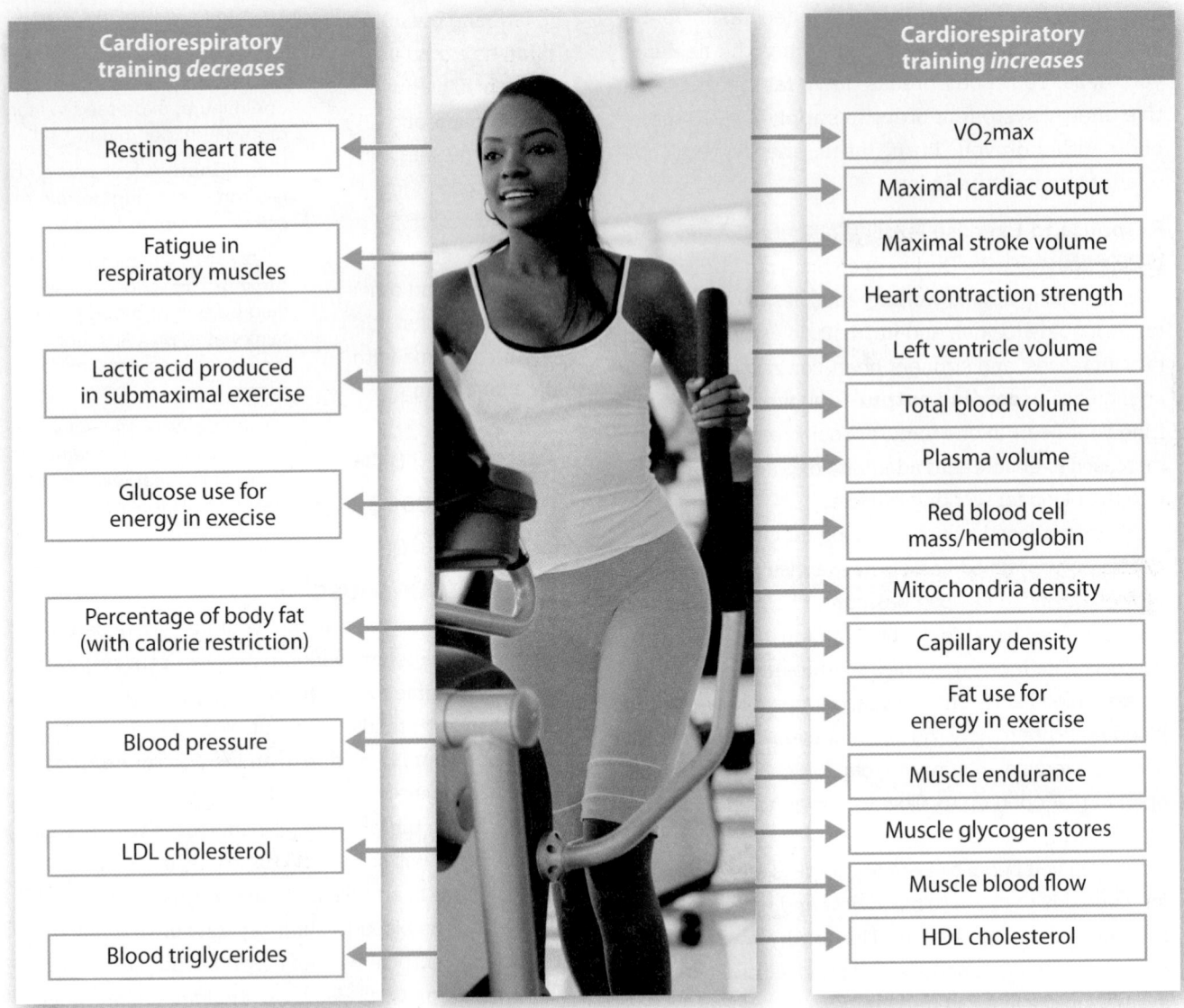

Cardiorespiratory training *decreases*		Cardiorespiratory training *increases*
Resting heart rate		VO₂max
Fatigue in respiratory muscles		Maximal cardiac output
Lactic acid produced in submaximal exercise		Maximal stroke volume
Glucose use for energy in execise		Heart contraction strength
Percentage of body fat (with calorie restriction)		Left ventricle volume
Blood pressure		Total blood volume
LDL cholesterol		Plasma volume
Blood triglycerides		Red blood cell mass/hemoglobin
		Mitochondria density
		Capillary density
		Fat use for energy in exercise
		Muscle endurance
		Muscle glycogen stores
		Muscle blood flow
		HDL cholesterol

FIGURE **3.5** Regular cardiorespiratory training results in numerous adaptations to the cardiovascular, respiratory, and muscle systems and an increase in overall health and wellness.

Aerobic Training Improves the Transfer and Use of Oxygen

Delivering oxygen to working muscles is only part of the picture. Your body also needs to transfer oxygen into the muscles and use it efficiently. With consistent aerobic training, your body increases the number of capillaries in the muscles that you train. This enables increased blood flow to these muscles and improves oxygen transfer from the blood into the muscles. Once inside the muscle cells, the oxygen is transported to mitochondria for use in the oxidative energy system. Mitochondria numbers increase within each muscle cell, improving oxygen use by muscles and subsequently improving oxidative production of ATP as well.

Aerobic Training Improves Your Body's Ability to Use Energy Efficiently

Regular aerobic training enhances your ability to store glycogen within muscles. When needed, glycogen can be broken down into glucose and used for energy during exercise. In fact, a minimal amount of glucose is needed during exercise to keep the oxidative energy system running efficiently.

Since fat breakdown for energy is accomplished within the mitochondria, an increase in the number of mitochondria will improve your body's ability to use fat for energy, sparing glucose and glycogen stores. Improving your body's ability to burn fat may allow you to have some glucose "left over" for that last-minute sprint to the finish! Less use of glucose and the nonoxidative energy system also means less lactic acid production during exercise and a delaying of fatigue.

What Are the Benefits of Improving My Cardiorespiratory Fitness?

There are many health-related reasons to improve your cardiorespiratory fitness.

Cardiorespiratory Fitness Decreases Your Risk of Disease

Having a low fitness level can put you at higher risk for disease and early death. The good news is that you don't need to increase your fitness to extremely high levels in order to see risk-reducing health benefits. Results of a multi-year federally funded trial indicate that just increasing your fitness to a moderate level can significantly reduce your risk of early mortality from several chronic diseases.[1] In particular, regular aerobic exercise helps protect you against the number-one killer in the world: cardiovascular disease. An increase in cardiorespiratory fitness can decrease your resting heart rate, decrease your blood levels of "bad" (LDL) cholesterol, and help prevent blood clots—all of which can lower your risk of heart attack and stroke. And it is never too early to start improving your fitness: in a study of children just nine to eleven years old, higher cardiorespiratory fitness levels were associated with healthier arteries.[2] If children learn to be active and sustain an active lifestyle, they can avoid the stiffer, less healthy arteries that tend to accompany a sedentary lifestyle in later years.[3]

Cardiorespiratory fitness can also help you manage your weight and blood pressure, thus reducing your chances of developing **metabolic syndrome** (a group of obesity-related risk factors associated with cardiovascular disease and type 2 diabetes).[4] It can also help lessen your risk of developing diabetes, since the regular rhythmic muscular contractions that occur in aerobic exercise improve your body's ability to use insulin and glucose.[5]

Regular physical activity stimulates hormones, anti-inflammatory agents, and immune responses that help protect against many forms of cancer. Studies have shown that regular physical activity and increased cardiorespiratory fitness can lower mortality rates in some of the most common cancers, including lung, colon, breast, and prostate.[6]

Cardiorespiratory Fitness Helps You Control Body Weight and Body Composition

Cardiorespiratory training burns calories. By increasing your calorie expenditure through exercise, you can more effectively manage your body weight and keep your level of body fat low. A high-intensity aerobic exercise session can elevate your metabolic rate for hours,[7] burning calories during the exercise session and long afterward. You can also burn many calories with light-to-moderate aerobic exercise by performing the activity for an extended period of time.

Cardiorespiratory Fitness Improves Self-Esteem, Mood, and Sense of Well-Being

Exercise makes you feel good! A single aerobic exercise session can improve mood and reduce tension and anxiety as a result of chemical changes in the brain and nervous system.[8] Since these benefits are primarily seen in regular exercisers,[9] don't be discouraged if you don't feel instantly "happy" after your first exercise session– stick with it! Long-term changes are even more dramatic. One study has shown that over the course of a 12-week aerobic fitness program, men and women reported improved self-concept, anxiety, mood, and depression scores, compared to a control group, and maintained their improved psychological health for

> **metabolic syndrome**
> A clustering of three or more heart disease and diabetes risk factors in one person (high blood pressure, impaired glucose tolerance, insulin resistance, decreased HDL cholesterol, elevated triglycerides, overweight with fat mostly around the waist)

resting heart rate The number of times your heart beats in a minute while the body is at rest; typically 50 to 90 beats per minute

pulse The pressure wave felt in the arteries due to blood ejection with each heartbeat

maximal oxygen consumption (VO₂max) The highest rate of oxygen consumption your body is capable of during maximal exercise; expressed in either liters per minute (L/min) or milliliters per minute per kilogram of body weight (ml/kg·min)

a year.[10] Numerous studies point to the importance of exercise in reducing symptoms of depression.[11,12]

Cardiorespiratory Fitness Improves Immune Function

Light to moderate exercise can boost your immune system.[13] Regular, moderate aerobic exercise can reduce stress and improve the quality of your sleep (stress and sleep are both tied to immune system health). Research has also shown that regularly participating in aerobic exercise can slow the reduction in immune system function that tends to occur as you get older.[14]

Cardiorespiratory Fitness Improves Long-Term Quality of Life

Cardiorespiratory fitness has a protective effect against age-related cognitive declines.[15] Research even suggests that aerobic exercise training can increase brain volume and thus *improve* cognitive function and memory as you age.[16,17]

Increased cardiorespiratory fitness can also improve the quality of life for individuals with chronic diseases or other medical conditions. Research has shown that after a six-month exercise program, men living with HIV improved their scores in cardiorespiratory fitness and in cognitive function and overall health.[18] Cardiorespiratory fitness has also been linked to better quality of life for survivors of breast cancer[19] and heart attacks.[20] Of course, the best time to incorporate a cardiorespiratory program into your life is *before* you show signs of disease.

How Can I Assess My Cardiorespiratory Fitness?

How fit is your cardiorespiratory system? Chances are, you already have a general idea. If you get easily winded after walking up a short flight of stairs or have trouble walking quickly for more than 10 minutes or so, you likely have a low cardiorespiratory fitness level.

Monitoring your **resting heart rate** is one way to keep track of general changes in your fitness level. Recall that your heart rate is the number of times your heart beats in one minute. Your resting heart rate decreases as your cardiorespiratory system becomes more conditioned. With an increase in stroke volume, your heart does not have to beat as many times per minute to deliver the same amount of blood to the body; at rest, your heart can slow down and still deliver adequate oxygen to all your cells.

When the heart contracts and pushes blood out, that wave of blood can be felt moving through the arteries. This is your **pulse**. To determine your heart rate, feel for your pulse at specific arteries around the body. The most common arteries to use for checking an exercise pulse are the *carotid* and the *radial* arteries (see Figure 3.6). Press your index and middle fingers gently against your skin and count the number of beats that you feel. Avoid using your thumb when taking your pulse, because the pulse in your thumb can interfere with your ability to count accurately. **Lab 3.1** walks you through how to take an accurate heart rate reading at rest and during exercise.

Understand Your Maximal Oxygen Consumption

Your body's maximal ability to utilize oxygen during exercise is called **maximal oxygen consumption** or **VO₂max**. Your VO₂max is the measure of your body's ability to deliver oxygen to the muscles and the muscles' ability to consume or use the oxygen. VO₂max numbers range from 20 to 94 ml/kg·min, with male athletes typically ranging from 50 to 70 ml/kg·min and female athletes ranging from 40 to 60 ml/kg·min. Your maximal oxygen consumption is largely determined by genetics and tends to decrease as

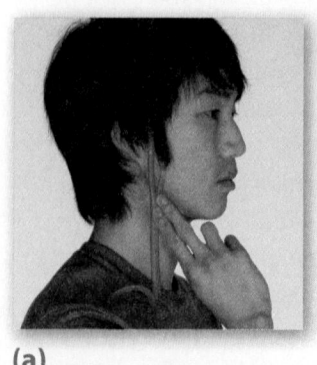 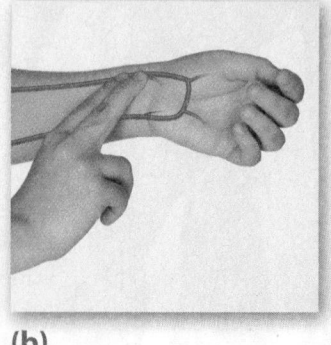

(a) **(b)**

FIGURE **3.6** To determine your heart rate, feel for your pulse at either (a) the carotid artery, or (b) the radial artery.

you get older. That said, you can typically improve your VO_2max an average of 15 to 20 percent with training. The more deconditioned you are before beginning a training program, the more dramatic an improvement you can achieve with training.

The most accurate measurements of VO_2max are performed in a laboratory setting (see Figure 3.7). The test is usually completed on a treadmill or stationary bike and requires specialized equipment and technicians to ensure safety. The technicians measure the precise amount of oxygen that enters and exits the body during a maximal exercise session.

Test Your Submaximal Heart Rate Responses

An alternative to testing your true maximal oxygen consumption is to perform a *submaximal* test. Submaximal tests do not test your body's maximal oxygen

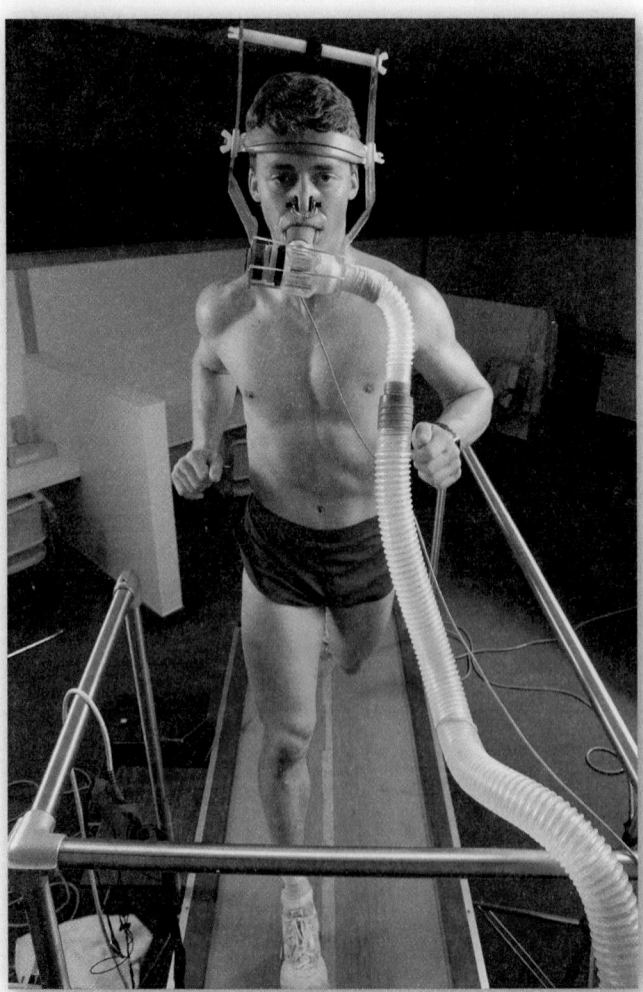

FIGURE **3.7** VO_2max can be most accurately measured in a laboratory setting, where direct gas analysis can determine the volume of oxygen a person's body is using while exercising at maximum capacity.

consumption but rather test for submaximal values that can be compared against norm charts or used to predict maximal values. Submaximal tests are safer, require less equipment and expertise, and are performed either in a laboratory or in a field/classroom setting.

Submaximal tests in the laboratory are usually performed on a stationary bike or treadmill. These tests predict your maximal effort level and oxygen consumption by assessing your heart rate response. A higher heart rate means higher oxygen consumption. By testing your heart rate response to different exercise intensities, an exercise technician can use your predicted **maximal heart rate (HRmax)** to estimate your maximal exercise intensity and oxygen consumption. Your maximal heart rate is the fastest your heart will beat in exhaustive exercise (a number that will decrease as you get older). One way to predict your HRmax is to subtract your age from the number 220. For example, if you are 18 years old, your predicted HRmax would be $220 - 18 = 202$ beats per minute. This formula is not as accurate as maximal laboratory tests, but it is used in many submaximal tests and heart rate training equations.

Test Your Cardiorespiratory Fitness in the Field/Classroom

Most classes in health and fitness enroll too many students to perform laboratory testing. More appropriate for these classes are classroom or field tests of cardiorespiratory fitness. Like laboratory tests, these tests either predict your maximal oxygen consumption from submaximal test results or allow you to compare your results with norm tables. In **Lab 3.2** you will perform three different assessments of cardiorespiratory fitness: the 3-minute step test, the 1-mile walking test, and the 1.5-mile running test.

DO IT! ONLINE

Three-Minute Step Test In this test, you will step up and down on a 12-inch-high step bench. At the end of three minutes, take your one-minute recovery heart rate and compare this to norm charts for your age and sex. The faster your heart recovers from exercise, the better conditioned you are.

One-Mile Walking Test In this test, you will walk as fast as you can for one mile. Record your finish time and your heart rate at the end of the one mile. Use your results to calculate an

> **maximal heart rate (HRmax)** The highest heart rate you can achieve during maximal exercise

estimated VO$_2$max and determine your fitness level for your age and sex. A faster time and lower heart rate indicate a higher level of fitness.

1.5-Mile Running Test In this test, you will run 1.5 miles as fast as you can. If you cannot run the entire course, you may take walking breaks. Use your finish time to calculate your estimated VO$_2$max and determine your fitness level for your age and sex. A faster time indicates a higher level of fitness.

How Can I Create My Own Cardiorespiratory Fitness Program?

Having a plan is one of the most important things you can do before beginning a personalized cardiorespiratory fitness program. Careful planning will help you reach your goals, prevent injuries, and ensure that you have fun while exercising!

Set Appropriate Cardiorespiratory Fitness Goals

Goal-setting for cardiorespiratory fitness should follow the SMART goal-setting guidelines (first introduced in Chapter 1). Recall that SMART goals are *s*pecific, *m*easurable, *a*ction-oriented, *r*ealistic, and *t*ime-oriented. Setting a vague goal such as "Build a stronger cardiorespiratory system" is not as useful as setting a specific goal that follows the SMART guidelines, such as "Improve my cardiorespiratory fitness from a 'fair' rating on my three-minute step test to a 'good' rating, by exercising on the elliptical machine three days a week for 30 minutes for the next two months."

In **Lab 3.3** you will set your own short- and long-term goals for cardiorespiratory fitness. Review the training adaptations and benefits of cardiorespiratory training discussed earlier to guide your goal-setting. Be realistic: If your goal is to run a marathon but you hate running, you will likely be setting yourself up for failure (unless your attitude toward running changes!). Choose goals that you can achieve, doing the types of activities that you enjoy most.

Learn about Cardiorespiratory Training Options

There are a wide variety of cardiorespiratory training options available to you.

Classes If you enjoy the company of other people and like the motivating aspect of an instructor leading a workout, consider enrolling in a group exercise class. Classes that incorporate a continuous, rhythmic activity lasting more than 20 minutes will help you maintain or improve your cardiorespiratory fitness. Such classes can be found in colleges, recreational centers, and fitness centers in almost every community. Class formats and instructors can vary widely, so consider sampling a few different classes and instructors before deciding on a regular class. Choose classes where the instructors are not only motivating, but also experienced, certified, and knowledgeable about your current health/fitness levels.

Indoor Workouts If you are not sure about working out in a group or with an instructor, you can design your own cardiorespiratory workout using indoor cardio equipment. You can find cardio equipment at most gyms or fitness centers or purchase it for home use. Indoor cardio workout equipment includes stationary bicycles, treadmills, elliptical trainers, stair-climbing machines,

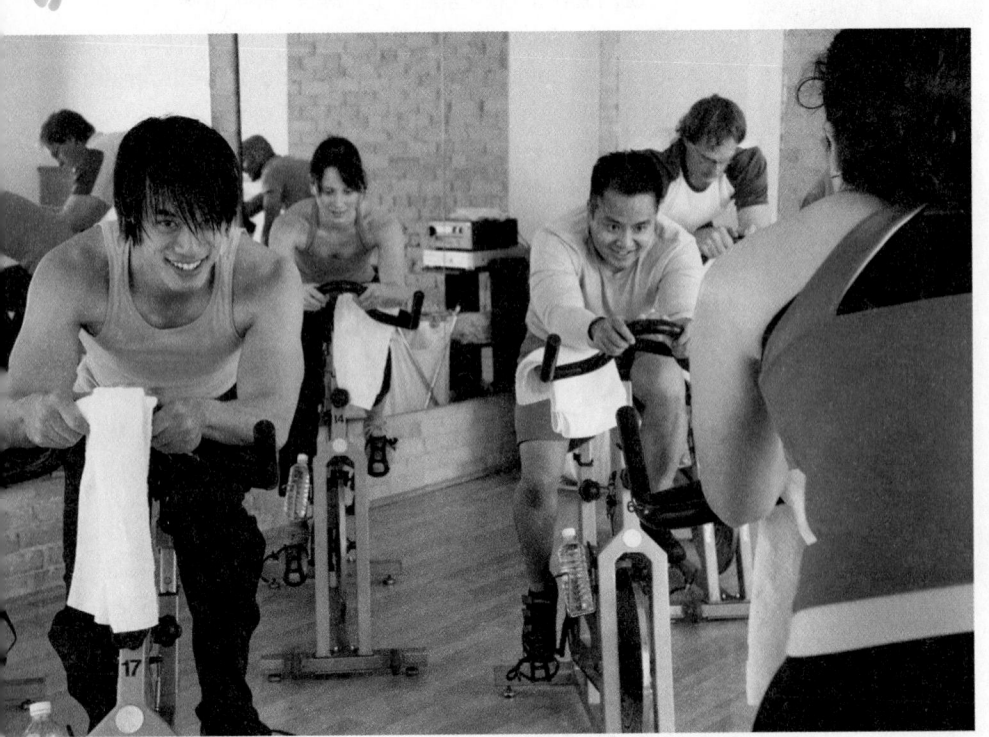

recumbent bikes, arm cycle ergometers, rowing machines, and jump ropes. If you are using a machine in a fitness facility, get an introduction to the features, use, and safety from a facility employee. In addition, consider running on an indoor track, swimming in a pool, deep-water jogging, or participating in a racquet sport.

Outdoor Workouts If you like to be outside, explore outdoor options for a cardiorespiratory workout. It is not uncommon to pursue a combination of indoor and outdoor exercise routines, depending on the weather and the facility options available to you. Exercising outdoors can be very rewarding if you live in an area with interesting sights, safe routes, and beautiful trails. The options for outdoor cardio workouts are endless. Here are just a few ideas: walking, jogging, running, cycling, track workouts, trail running, hiking, tennis, cross-country skiing, open-water swimming, and inline skating.

Differing Workout Formats (Continuous, Interval, Circuit) Aerobic training is a type of *continuous* training—i.e., you perform a rhythmic activity and sustain it for a period of time (ideally 20 minutes or more). While aerobic training should be the cornerstone of your cardiorespiratory training program, other workout formats can add variety, intensity, and other fitness benefits.

An **interval workout** alternates periods of higher-intensity exercise with periods of lower-intensity exercise or rest. An interval workout method allows you to increase the intensity of your workout to a level that you might not otherwise be able to sustain for a long period of time. If done correctly, this type of workout can further develop your body's aerobic training adaptations. High intensity anaerobic intervals improve anaerobic conditioning but also have a greater injury potential.

A **circuit-training workout** involves moving from location to location in a circuit-training room and exercising for a certain amount of time (or number of repetitions) at each "station." You can enroll in a circuit-training class or circuit-train on your own. The circuit can contain alternating aerobic and weight-training activities, just weight stations, or just aerobic stations. The best circuit for cardiorespiratory conditioning is one with all aerobic exercise stations.

Apply FITT Principles to Cardiorespiratory Fitness

After setting goals and selecting the types of cardiorespiratory exercise that you want to do, you must decide how much, how hard, and how long to exercise. Recall the FITT principles (introduced in Chapter 2): *f*requency, *i*ntensity, *t*ime, and *t*ype. Let's look at how each of these principles applies to a cardiorespiratory fitness program.

Frequency According to the American College of Sports Medicine, you should spend three to five days per week on cardiorespiratory conditioning. If you are exercising at higher intensity levels, you can improve or maintain your VO_2max by working out only three days per week. If you are exercising at lower intensity levels, you may need more than three days per week (five is recommended) to improve cardiorespiratory fitness.

If your goals include weight loss or disease prevention, you will benefit from exercising more often but at a lower intensity in order to prevent injuries and overtraining.

Intensity Your workouts should be intense enough to tax your cardiorespiratory system, but not so difficult as to discourage you or increase your chances of injury. You can measure the intensity of your exercise by various methods, including determining your heart rate, assessing your **perceived exertion**, and self-administering a **talk test**.

Determining Your Heart Rate Your heart rate provides a good indication of how hard your cardiorespiratory system is working, since it is related to the amount of oxygen that your body is consuming. You can determine your heart rate by using a heart rate monitor or (as we discussed earlier) by counting your pulse.

Heart rate monitors can be found on cardio equipment and merely require you to place your hands on the receiving pads for a few seconds. Personal heart rate monitors, which consist of a chest strap transmitter and a wrist receiver, are also widely available.

Counting your pulse while you are exercising is an easy and low-cost way to measure your heart rate. Your heart rate decreases rapidly after stopping exercise, especially after 15 seconds; therefore, count your pulse for only 10 seconds, and try to keep moving as you count. Then multiply your 10-second count by six to convert to the number of beats per minute (bpm).

interval workout A workout that alternates periods of higher-intensity exercise with periods of lower-intensity exercise or rest

circuit-training workout A workout where exercisers move from one exercise station to another after a certain number of repetitions or amount of time

perceived exertion A subjective assessment of exercise intensity

talk test A method of measuring exercise intensity based on assessing your ability to speak during exercise

TABLE 3.1 ACSM's Training Guidelines for Cardiorespiratory Fitness

Recommendations for the General Adult Population	
Frequency (days/week)	Moderate: 5 Vigorous: 3
Intensity (how hard)	Moderate: 64–76% of HRmax Vigorous: 77–95% of HRmax
Time (how long)	Moderate: 30–60 min (150 min/week) Vigorous: 20–60 min (75 min/week)
Type (exercises)	Large muscle group, dynamic activity

Data from: C. E. Garner and others, "American College of Sports Medicine Position Stand: Quantity and Quality of Exercise for Developing and Maintaining Cardiorespiratory, Musculoskeletal, and Neuromotor Fitness in Apparently Healthy Adults: Guidance for Prescribing Exercise," *Medicine & Science in Sports & Exercise* 43, no. 7 (2011): 1334–59.

What **target heart rate** should you aim for in a workout? The answer depends on your goals and fitness level. As you can see in Table 3.1, the American College of Sports Medicine's recommendations for exercise intensity level cites a wide range of target heart rates: 64 to 95 percent of HRmax. Use the following guidelines to determine where within this range you should aim:

- If your fitness level is low, you should follow the guidelines for moderate cardiorespiratory exercise or 64–76 percent of your HRmax. Start below or at the low end of this range if you are very deconditioned or brand new to exercise.

- If your fitness level is moderate, aim for the vigorous exercise guidelines or 77–95 percent of your HRmax or choose to do a mix of moderate and vigorous exercise.

Table 3.2 also provides target heart rate guidelines for exercise, using the HRmax method based on your age. Another method of determining your target heart rate is to measure your **heart rate reserve (HRR)**, the difference between your resting and maximum heart rates. **Lab 3.1** walks you through how to determine your HRR.

Perceived Exertion Another way to assess the intensity of your workout is by determining your perceived exertion; which is simply your perception of how hard you are working during exercise. One of the most well-known perceived exertion scales was developed by Gunnar Borg in 1970. His Rating of Perceived Exertion (RPE) scale is a subjective 15-point scale, from 6–20, that is related to heart rate responses to exercise.[21] The Borg RPE Scale can be a very valuable tool when it is not easy or appropriate to use heart rate monitoring to check your workout intensity. For example, if you participate in a water sport such as swimming, heart rate monitoring can be misleading; heart rates tend to slow down while exercising in water due to increased hydrostatic pressure and decreased temperature. For this reason, you may prefer to use RPE to determine your exercise intensity.

Another perceived exertion scale is the OMNI Scale of Perceived Exertion. Although originally developed for children, adult versions now exist and these provide a simple way to assess workout intensity on a 1-10 scale (see Figure 3.8). The OMNI Scale is correlated with the Borg RPE scale and heart rate responses.[22,23] As you become more experienced with a

target heart rate The heart rate you are aiming for during an exercise session; often a range with high and low heart rates called your *training zone*

heart rate reserve (HRR) The number of beats per minute available or in reserve for exercise heart rate increases; maximal heart rate minus resting heart rate

TABLE 3.2 Target Heart Rate Guidelines*

Age	Target HR Range (bpm)	10-Sec Count
18–24	139–179	23–30
25–29	135–174	22–29
30–34	132–169	22–28
35–39	129–165	21–28
40–44	125–160	21–27
45–49	122–156	20–26
50–54	118–151	20–25
55–59	114–147	19–25
60–64	110–142	18–24
65+	108–140	18–23

*Based upon the *HRmax method*, where 220 − age = HRmax and the training zone is 70 to 90% of HRmax (moderate to vigorous). Individuals with low fitness levels should start below or at the low end of these ranges.

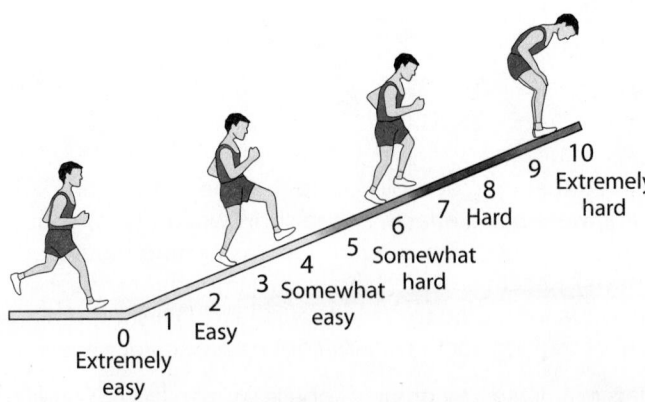

FIGURE **3.8** One method to determine your exercise intensity involves utilizing the OMNI Scale of Perceived Exertion for walking and running.

Source: A.C. Utter and others, "Validation of the Adult OMNI Scale of Perceived Exertion for Walking/Running Exercise," *Medicine & Science in Sports & Exercise* 36, no. 10 (2004): 1777. Used by permission of Wolters Kluwer/Lippincott, Williams & Wilkins.

particular cardiorespiratory activity and become more attuned to how your body feels during exercise, your ability to use the perceived exertion scales accurately will improve.

The Talk Test The talk test method of measuring exercise intensity is based on assessing how easily you can talk during exercise. While exercising at a *light* intensity, you should be able to talk easily and continuously. If you are exercising at a *moderate* intensity, you should be able to talk easily, but not continuously, during the activity. If you are too out of breath to carry on a conversation easily, you are working at a high or *vigorous* intensity. If you cannot talk at all, you are probably doing an anaerobic interval or sprinting.

To increase cardiorespiratory fitness, aim for at least a moderate intensity level for most of your workout or the highest level you can comfortably sustain for 20 to 30 minutes. You can incorporate short periods of light and vigorous activity for workout variety or interval training. Table 3.3 summarizes the most common intensity scales for cardiorespiratory endurance exercise. Use the one that works best for you and the type of exercise you have chosen.

Time For optimal cardiorespiratory conditioning, your exercise sessions should be 20 to 30 minutes long. If you are just starting out, exercise continuously for as long as you can, and then work your way up to the minimum guideline of 20 minutes. The box Can Shorter Workouts Benefit My Health? examines how workouts as short as 10 to 15 minutes can benefit health.

TABLE **3.3** Cardiorespiratory Intensity Scales*

General	Talk Test	OMNI	Borg RPE	% HRR	% HRmax
Light	Easy conversation	0	6	30	57
		1	7	35	60
		2	8		
			9		
		3	10	40	
		4	11	44	64
Moderate	Brief sentences and words	5	12	45	65
			13		
		6	14	64	84
Vigorous	A few words	7	15	65	85
			16		
		8	17	84	94
Anaerobic	Barely or not able to talk	9	18	85	95
		10	19		
			20	100	100

*The various methods to quantify exercise intensity in this table may not be equivalent to one another.

Data are from: American College of Sports Medicine, *ACSM's Guidelines for Exercise Testing and Prescription*, 8th Edition (Baltimore, MD: Lippincott Williams & Wilkins, 2010); Office of Disease Prevention and Health Promotion, U.S. Department of Health and Human Services, *2008 Physical Activity Guidelines for Americans: Be Active, Healthy, and Happy!* ODPHP Publication no. U0036 (Washington, DC: U.S. Department of Health and Human Services, 2008), Available at: www.health.gov.paguidelines; R. J. Robertson and others, "Validation of the Adult OMNI Scale of Perceived Exertion for Cycle Ergometer Exercise," *Medicine & Science in Sports & Exercise* 36, no. 1 (2004): 102–108; A. C. Utter and others, "Validation of the Adult OMNI Scale of Perceived Exertion for Walking/Running Exercise," *Medicine & Science in Sports & Exercise* 36, no. 10 (2004): 1776–1780; G. Borg, *Borg's Perceived Exertion and Pain Scales* (Champaign, IL: Human Kinetics, 1998): 27–38.

Do Short Workouts Do Me Any Good?

The short answer is *yes*, they do! Experts once believed that long aerobic workouts, where the heart rate stays continuously in the target training zone, were more effective than short workouts for your health. Naturally, getting motivated for a long exercise session is not as easy as getting motivated for a short one. The good news? Recent research shows two important concepts: 1) you don't have to work out a long time to get benefits, and 2) a short *time* but a high *intensity* level of training can have a major impact on your health.

In one study, researchers instructed one group of obese women to walk briskly for 30 minutes three times per week and another group to walk intermittently for two 15-minute sessions five days per week.[1] The intermittent walkers gained nearly as much aerobic capacity as the continuous walkers—and in both groups, blood fats and insulin measurements improved significantly. The continuous walkers lost weight, however, while the intermittent walkers did not.

In another study, young (around 25 years old) but sedentary people were instructed to eat a high-fat meal and then exercise.[2] Half of the eaters then ran for 30 minutes on a treadmill, while the other half ran for three 10-minute stretches separated by rest periods. Intermittent exercise proved to be *better* at lowering fats in the bloodstream than continuous exercise. The experimenters speculate that this may happen because each exercise session independently speeds the metabolic rate, adding up to a greater overall effect than longer, single sessions.[3]

Newer research tells us that metabolic changes from 10 minutes of exercise persist for 60 minutes, providing a better blood glucose/insulin balance and catabolic (or calorie burning, lipolysis-fat breakdown) state as opposed to the anabolic state after eating.[4] The effects were more pronounced in individuals in the study who were more fit; if you get fit, you get even more metabolic benefits from intermittent exercise!

In addition to doing shorter bouts of exercise, you can also get a lot more out of your short exercise time by employing interval training as part of your exercise strategy. High intensity interval training means you exercise at almost maximum capacity for several shorts bursts and rest between bursts. Short amounts of interval training can be as effective as longer amounts of conventional training, so you can achieve your fitness goals in less time![5] Note that you shouldn't start doing intervals until after you have reached a minimal level of fitness. Your chance of injury increases with high intensity exercise and your body needs to be ready.

So squeeze in 10 minutes of aerobic exercise whenever you can, and remember the bottom line: Get moving, whether for short periods or long!

Sources:
1. J. E. Donnelly and others, "The Effects of 18 Months of Intermittent vs. Continuous Exercise on Aerobic Capacity, Body Weight and Composition, and Metabolic Fitness in Previously Sedentary, Moderately Obese Females," *International Journal of Obesity* 24, no. 5 (2000): 566–72.
2. T. S. Altena and others, "Single Sessions of Intermittent and Continuous Exercise and Postprandial Lipemia," *Medicine & Science in Sports & Exercise* 36, no. 8 (2004): 1364–71.
3. American College of Sports Medicine, "Short Bouts of Exercise Reduce Fat in the Bloodstream After Meals," News release, August 5, 2004, www.acsm.org.
4. J. P. Little and others, "A Practical Model of Low-Volume High-Intensity Interval Training Induces Mitochondrial Biogenesis in Human Skeletal Muscle: Potential Mechanisms," *The Journal of Physiology* 588, no. 6 (2010): 1011–22.

Type For optimal motivation, training adaptation, and injury prevention, choose activities that you enjoy. Alternate your participation in these activities by the day or week for a **cross-training** effect. Cross-training can help you maintain muscle balance by working different muscle groups.

Include a Warm-up and Cool-down Phase in Your Workout Session

A cardiorespiratory workout session should consist of three components: the **warm-up** phase, the main cardiorespiratory endurance conditioning set, and the **cool-down** phase. Figure 3.9 illustrates a sample workout for a moderately fit 20-year-old showing each of these components. Remember that your warm-up should ideally consist of light physical activity that mimics the movements of your main exercise set. For example, if your main exercise set is jogging, an ideal warm-up would be to walk briskly. Likewise, your cool-down should ideally be a less-vigorous version of your main exercise set. (Review Chapter 2 for more guidelines on warming up and cooling down.) Keep in mind that when you are starting an exercise program, you should generally perform longer warm-up (15 to 20 minutes) and cool-down (10 minutes or more) segments.

> **cross-training** The practice of using different exercise modes or types in your cardiorespiratory training program
>
> **warm-up** The initial 5- to 20-minute preparation phase of a workout
>
> **cool-down** The ending phase of a workout where the body is brought gradually back to rest

Plan for Proper Progression of Your Program

When you are starting a new exercise program, it is easy to attempt to do too much too soon. A fitness program needs to be *progressive* in order for you to achieve results and avoid injury. As you begin a fitness program, your progress may initially be slow, while your body adjusts to the new activity. Eventually, consistent exercise will result in noticeable improvement.

In order to avoid injuring yourself, increase your workout by no more than 10 percent per week (the *10 percent rule*). That means that your weekly increases in frequency, intensity, and/or time should not total more than 10 percent. For example, if you are jogging for 30 minutes per exercise session, next week you could safely increase each session to 33 minutes (10 percent increase in time).

How Can I Maintain My Cardiorespiratory Program?

How many times have you started a fitness program only to quit after a few weeks? For many people, the biggest challenge to improving cardiorespiratory fitness is not beginning a program, but keeping it up. Next we discuss the stages of progression and the importance of tracking your progress and reassessing your needs.

Understand the Stages of Progression

Start-up In the *start-up* phase of a cardiorespiratory program, you will be adjusting to the new activity in your weekly routine. During this stage, it is important to pay attention to how you feel during exercise so that you can make adjustments if necessary. Do you prefer

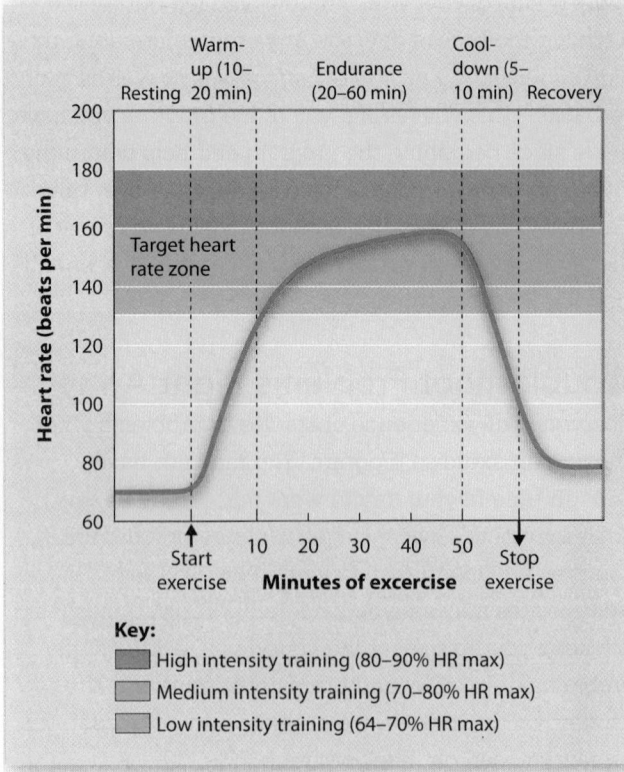

FIGURE 3.9 This graph charts the progression of a sample cardiorespiratory workout for a moderately fit 20-year-old. Note that it consists of a warm-up phase, an endurance phase, and a cool-down phase.

Adapted from *ACSM's Guidelines for Exercise Testing and Prescription*, 7th Edition (Baltimore, MD: Lippincott Williams & Wilkins, 2010).

casestudy

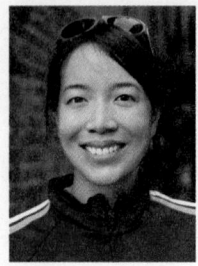

ANGELA

"After practically killing myself on the tennis court last week, I did some research into exactly what it means to 'get in shape.' I was really interested to learn about things like target heart rates and the different ways to measure cardiorespiratory fitness. I took the 1.5-mile run test and found out that my current fitness rating is only 'fair.' So my plan is to design a cardio workout that will get my rating up to 'good' or 'excellent' before challenging my friend to another match!"

THINK! Pretend you are Angela's fitness trainer and decide on an appropriate target goal for Angela. Does the goal you outlined for Angela follow the SMART guidelines?

ACT! Become your own personal fitness trainer and write yourself a target cardio-respiratory goal incorporating the SMART guidelines.

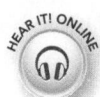

exercising in the morning or in the evening? Is that aerobics class really right for you? In this first stage, your main concern should be fine-tuning your program until you settle on an activity and routine that is comfortable for you. Depending on your fitness level and exercise experience, this stage can last anywhere from two to four weeks.

Improvement Once you have the "kinks" worked out of your program, you are ready to move into the *improvement* phase. In this stage, your body starts adapting to the cardiorespiratory exercise. Some of these changes will be evident to you; some will not (refer to Figure 3.5). You should, however, start feeling better during exercise, have more energy when not exercising, and feel that you can exercise for longer periods of time without fatigue. As in the initial stage, listen to your body so that you can make changes as needed. The improvement stage can last anywhere from three to eight months, depending on your program and goals.

Maintenance After months of hard work you are at the fitness level you desire and you feel great! You

have reached the *maintenance* stage. The key to this stage is to keep your program consistent. If you stop exercising, you can lose your newly achieved fitness level in only half the time it took you to acquire it. In fact, athletes can start losing cardiorespiratory fitness within just two weeks of inactivity. If you need to cut back but don't want to lose your hard-earned improvements, cut back on exercise time but not intensity level. It is easier to maintain cardiorespiratory fitness with shorter but more intense workouts. The maintenance stage lasts for as long as you continue your program.

Record and Track Your Fitness Progress

Do you remember how you felt during that spinning workout three weeks ago? What was the speed and incline of your treadmill workout last week? One of the best ways to make sure that you stay on track with your fitness program is to record your activity and track your progress over time. Keeping a workout journal or log will encourage you to write down things such as the FITT components of your workout, how you felt during the workout, the time of day, and any other information that may be relevant. Record your successes as well as your setbacks—this will remind you of the progress you have made since beginning the program and help determine if your goals or workouts should be adjusted over time. The box Fitness Tracking Technology explains some of the technology and websites you can use to assess and log your fitness progress.

Troubleshoot Problems Right Away

Everyone will experience obstacles or problems when starting an exercise program. You may not have enough time in your day to work out, it may be difficult for you to physically get to your workout facility, you may be feeling pain in your knee, and so on. While these issues may set you back temporarily, they should not keep you from reaching your goals. Address the problems right away and brainstorm solutions; the sooner you acknowledge a problem and address it, the sooner you can get back on track.

Periodically Reassess Your Cardiorespiratory Fitness Level

Although you will certainly feel your progress by how your body responds to exercise, it is always nice to

Fitness Tracking Technology

There are countless electronic tools out there for tracking exercise, diet and nutrition, and weight management. Wearable monitors containing tiny motion sensors can track your baseline activity levels and workouts. The Fitbit tracker, for example, clips to your clothes and lets you count the number of steps you take in an exercise session or a day. It then calculates your mileage and total calories burned. With the DirectLife monitor, you assess your normal activity for a week or so, then dial up a 12-week activity plan and download it from a website. Before you buy a pedometer, heart rate monitor, or any other such device, ask your fitness instructor or you friends for recommendations, and consult equipment reviews in newspapers and on consumer websites.

If fussing with a gadget isn't for you, you can still take advantage of some useful online programs that help you log your physical activity online, track your progress, and access information about recommended guidelines for physical activity. For example, you can choose from thousands of smart phone applications to help you log miles run or laps swum, count calories taken in and burned, keep food diaries, calculate body fat and fat grams in foods, and track and share your weight via a social site. Many websites offer similar tools; below are just a few:

Lose It!: www.loseit.com/

LiveStrong.com: www.livestrong.com/

MyPyramid Tracker: www.mypyramidtracker.gov

Nike+: http://nikerunning.nike.com/nikeos /p/nikeplus/en_US/plus/#//runs/

President's Challenge: www.presidentschallenge.org

Runner's World Training Log: http://traininglog .runnersworld.com/landingpage.aspx

These high tech tools can't substitute for your own motivation and adherence. They can, however, offer portability and ease of tracking your personal data accurately. People often find these gadgets and programs fun to use and a way to give and receive support through social media connections.

---

have quantitative measures of your progress as well. Complete the assessments in **Lab 3.2** at least twice—once after three months of your new program and again at six months. Keep in mind that you will see the most improvements in assessments that are similar to your chosen workout activity (e.g., if you are doing step aerobics, you will probably see more improvement in the step test than in the 1.5-mile run test). If you have not improved, look at your program again and figure out whether you need to redesign it.

Reassess Your Goals and Program as Needed

Once a target date arrives, review your goals for that date. Did you achieve what you set out to do? If not, list the reasons why. You may need to set more realistic goals with more realistic target dates, or select a different activity. If you need more motivation, consider finding a workout partner or working with a personal trainer. If you did reach your goal, set a new goal for maintenance or a more challenging goal to improve your fitness level even more. The sample running, cycling, and swimming programs in Activate, Motivate, & Advance Your Fitness at the end of this chapter (pages 105–114) can help you set new goals and develop new fitness plans.

How Can I Avoid Injury During Cardiorespiratory Exercise?

The fastest way to disrupt a training program is to get injured. Reduce your injury risk by understanding and following common exercise injury prevention methods.

Design a Personalized, Balanced Cardiorespiratory Program

The most common injuries from cardiorespiratory fitness programs are from overuse, such as strains and tendonitis, particularly in the lower body. If you attempt to do too much too soon, you put yourself at risk for such injuries. Make sure your exercise program considers your current level of fitness and make your FITT targets realistic and achievable. You may also want to consider incorporating cross-training into your program, since doing one activity exclusively can result in uneven muscle development, making you more vulnerable to injury.

Wear Appropriate Clothing and Footwear

Use common sense when you are dressing for your chosen cardiorespiratory activity. If you are cycling, a helmet and bright clothing are essential. If you are running, walking, taking a group fitness class, or participating in a racquet sport, pay particularly close attention to your footwear. You need shoes that will protect your feet and provide the right amount of support and cushioning. Here are some tips for finding the right shoes:[24]

- Shop for shoes after a workout or at the end of the day when your feet are their biggest.

- Wear the socks that you will use when you exercise.

- Be sure you can freely wiggle all of your toes.

- The shoes should feel comfortable as soon as you try them on.

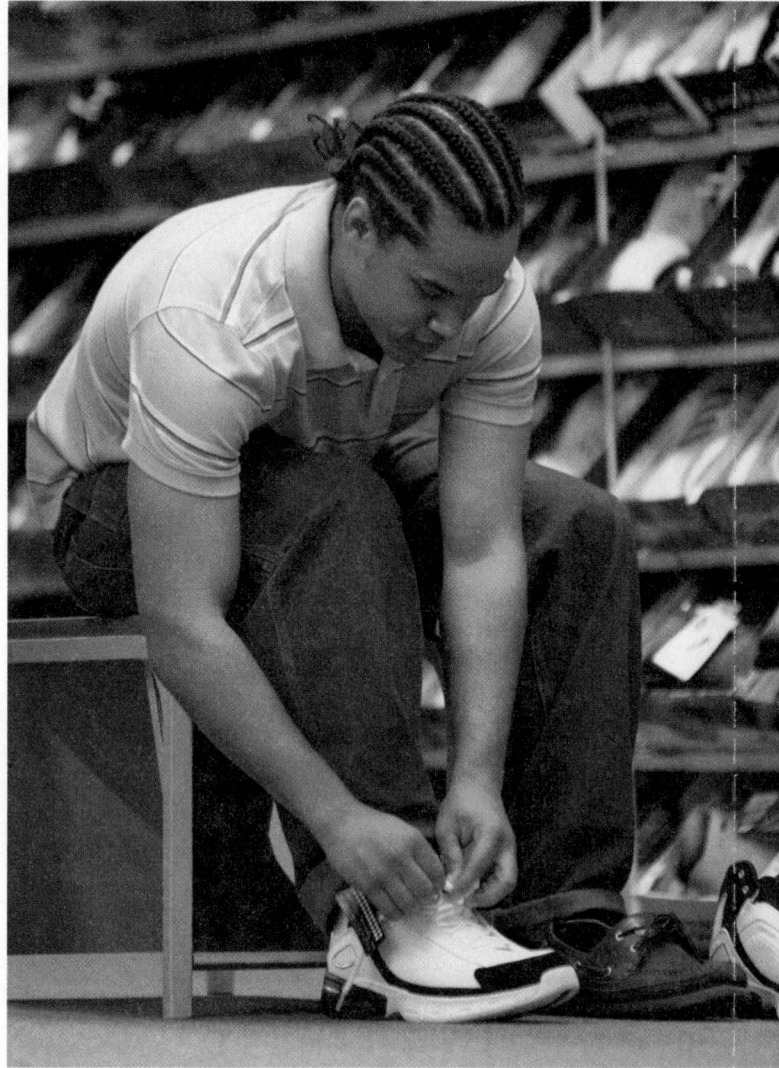

- Try them out! Lace them up correctly and then walk or run around the store.

- Your heel should not slide up and down as you walk or run.

- If you participate in a sport three or more times a week or will be doing high-intensity workouts, choose a sport-specific shoe. Ask a knowledgeable salesperson for advice on purchasing sport-specific shoes.

What about those people you see running in bare feet, or with minimalist shoes? The box Barefoot Running: Is It Safe for Me? provides an overview of this style of running.

Pay Attention to Your Exercise Environment

Prevent Heat-Related Illness When exercising indoors, be sure the exercise room is well-ventilated and cool enough to prevent your body from overheating. When exercising outdoors in hot weather, take precautions to avoid heat-related illnesses such as **heat cramps**, **heat exhaustion**, or **heat stroke**. Your risk of heat-related illness increases if you (1) exercise too hard for your fitness level, (2) exercise in high heat, humidity, and sunshine, (3) have a low fitness level overall, (4) are lacking in adequate sleep, (5) are not

heat cramps Severe cramping in the large muscle groups and abdomen caused by high fluid and electrolyte loss in sustained exertion in the heat

heat exhaustion An elevated core body temperature, headache, fatigue, profuse sweating, nausea, and clammy skin brought on by sustained exertion in the heat with dehydration and electrolyte losses

heat stroke A core body temperature above 104°F, headache, nausea, vomiting, diarrhea, rapid pulse, cessation of sweating, and disorientation resulting from extreme exertion in very hot conditions

Is Barefoot Running Safe for Me?

Have you noticed people out on the street running without shoes or wearing "FiveFingers"—those funny-looking shoes with toes? What are these people up to? They are part of a new and growing trend: barefoot running. What's behind this trend? And should you be running barefoot?

Advocates of barefoot running point out that humans have been running without shoes or with minimal shoes since they stood up on two legs and indicate several perceived advantages to doing so. One claimed benefit is that the shorter stride in barefoot running reduces the number of running injuries.[1] Advocates say the less support you give to your arch, the stronger your arch becomes—barefoot activity builds up the muscles of the foot. And, they say, running barefoot makes you more aware of the terrain you are running through, encouraging a connection with the environment.[2] Researchers have shown that runners who run barefoot tend to strike the ground with their forefoot or midfoot rather than their heel;[3] there is anecdotal evidence that forefoot or midfoot striking can help avoid and/or mitigate repetitive stress injuries, especially stress fractures, plantar fasciitis, and runner's knee.[4]

Critics of the trend, though, point out that this is still a theory. As yet, there is no evidence that barefoot or minimalist running reduces injuries. Critics concede there is no evidence that running shoes reduce injuries either.[5] More research is needed before conclusions can be drawn about any of these opinions, pro or con. However, critics do point out that, unlike running in shoes, barefoot running can result in puncture wounds from sharp objects on the ground.

So, where does that leave you? Scientists do say that some barefoot running as a part of an overall training plan can be beneficial in strengthening the bones, ligaments, muscles, and tendons in the feet. And, using a barefoot *style* of running—striking the ground with the midfoot rather than the heel even when you're wearing running shoes—may also be beneficial.[6] The benefits of barefoot running in the sand or grass, for example, have been noted as a training tool, but not for every run. There is some validity to letting your foot move in a more natural way and steering away from shoes that don't allow your foot to move at all. Increasing the actual strength of your foot muscles is another benefit.

If you want to incorporate barefoot or "barefoot-like" running into your workout, some solid advice is to make the change slowly. Don't just throw out your running shoes and do a five-mile run! Start out by doing activities around the house barefoot, and walking barefoot to build up your foot and calf muscles slowly. Check with your doctor before adding barefoot running to your exercise program; people who have circulatory or nerve issues should not attempt to run barefoot, as they are at increased risk for injury. If your doctor clears you for incorporating barefoot running, you may want to try shoes with more flexibility and less cushioning and then gradually work your way to minimalist shoes for part of your weekly workout time. Then, do a portion of your running in bare feet to allow your feet to develop calluses for running on rough surfaces. As your muscles strengthen you can build on the time you spend running barefoot.[7]

Sources:
1. M. Warburton, "Barefoot Running," *Sportscience* 5, no. 3 (2001) www.sportsci.org/jour/0103/mw.htm.
2. R. Collier, "The Rise of Barefoot Running," *Canadian Medical Association Journal* 183, no. 1 (2011): E37–38.
3. D. E. Lieberman and others, "Foot Strike Patterns and Collision Forces in Habitually Barefoot Versus Shod Runners," *Nature* 463, no. 7280 (2010): 531–35.
4. D. E. Lieberman and others, "Running Barefoot, Forefoot Striking and Training Tips," www.barefootrunning.fas.harvard.edu/5BarefootRunning&TrainingTips.html (accessed February 2011).
5. R. Collier, "The Rise of Barefoot Running."
6. D. E. Lieberman and others, "Foot Strike Patterns and Collision Forces."
7. C. Pauls and L. Kravitz, "Barefoot Running," *IDEA Fitness Journal* 7, no. 5 (2010): 14–17.

accustomed to the environment, (6) have an underlying infection, or (7) are overweight.[25] You can decrease your risk by being more fit, wearing light, sweat-wicking clothing, picking cooler times of the day to exercise, avoiding hazardous conditions, letting your body gradually become accustomed to the environment, and increasing your workout slowly.

If you suspect you are developing a heat-related illness, act immediately. For heat cramps, cease activity, seek a cool environment, and restore your body's fluid and electrolyte balances by drinking water or a sports drink. For heat exhaustion, rest in a cool environment, apply cold packs to your head and neck, drink water or a sports drink, and seek medical attention. If you suspect heatstroke, you will need medical attention immediately; untreated heatstroke is very serious and can lead to death. In heatstroke illness the body can no longer cool itself and ice-water immersion and IV fluids may be necessary right away. Because exercise increases your core body temperature, your risk of heat illness is greater when you are active, even in lower temperatures. Take extra precautions during difficult workouts to take breaks and drink fluids.

Prevent Cold-Related Illness Exercising in extreme cold also presents risks. If you like to ski, hike in the mountains, swim in cold water, or just exercise in snowy, windy, rainy environments, you should take precautions to prevent **hypothermia**, a condition in which the body's internal temperature drops so low that it can no longer warm itself back up. If untreated, hypothermia leads to death. To avoid hypothermia, (1) minimize heat loss by wearing a warm hat and clothing, (2) keep yourself dry by wearing sweat-wicking clothing and changing out of wet clothes as quickly as possible, (3) exercise with a workout partner who can help recognize early warning signs of cold-related illness, (4) avoid exercising in poor weather conditions, (5) warm up thoroughly, (6) drink fluids to stay hydrated, and (7) get out of the cold and warm up if you start shivering.

The early warning signs of hypothermia include shivering, goose bumps, and fast, shallow breathing. The next stage involves violent shivering, muscle incoordination, mild confusion, pale skin, and potentially blue lips, ears, fingers, and toes. In the most dangerous and potentially fatal stage of hypothermia, shivering will

hypothermia A condition where the core temperature of the body drops below the level required for sustaining normal bodily functions

stop and the person will have trouble thinking, speaking, walking, and using his or her hands. If you suspect you are at risk of hypothermia, get dry and warm as soon as possible. If you are in an advanced stage of hypothermia, you will need medical attention immediately.

Be Aware of the Impact of Air Quality Air pollution can irritate your air passageways and lungs, particularly if you have asthma, allergies, bronchitis, or other pulmonary disorders. If you experience a disruption in your breathing pattern, irritated eyes, or a headache, stop exercising and go indoors. Avoid exercising outdoors when the air quality is poor, particularly if you have a smog or air-quality alert in your city that day. If you exercise outside on a regular basis, take measures to reduce your intake of air pollution. Exercise in wilderness areas, in parks, or on low-traffic streets. Try to exercise at times when the air quality is better, such as early in the morning and on weekends.

Watch for Hazards Watch for hazards in your exercise environment that may cause you to trip and fall. When exercising indoors, seek out a space with a well-maintained floor and where you can work out without obstructions. When exercising outdoors, seek out lower-impact surfaces such as a school track, running or bike path, or a dirt trail. Use your common sense: avoid slippery or muddy surfaces and areas with heavy vehicle traffic. If you exercise outdoors at night, wear reflective clothing and clip a light somewhere on your body so that drivers can easily see you.

• •

THINK! What hazards do you face in your exercise routine? Can cars really see you when you are running on the road at night? Do your shoes have decent soles, so you don't slip?

ACT! List three things about your workout routine, your clothing, or your environment that might put you at risk for injury or illness. For each thing, list what steps you need to take to reduce your risk.

• •

Drink Enough Water

If you sweat profusely and do not replace the lost fluid, you will become dehydrated. Your body needs a certain amount of water in order to function. Loss of body water will decrease your blood volume and will subsequently decrease the blood flow to muscles, lowering exercise performance. **Dehydration** will also slow your sweat

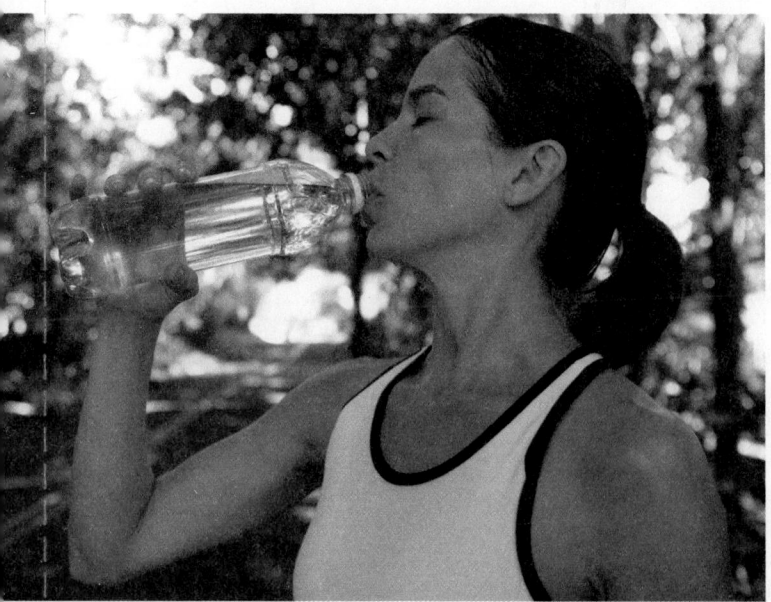

drinking additional fluid several hours before an exercise session and drink during exercise as

well. If you are exercising for more than an hour, you may benefit from drinking fluid with sugars and electrolytes (salts) in it, such as a sports drink.

Understand How to Prevent and Treat Common Injuries

Below are some of the most common exercise injuries, as well as guidelines for how to prevent and treat them. See also Table 3.4 for a summary of these and other common exercise injuries.

Delayed-Onset Muscle Soreness *Delayed-onset muscle soreness* (DOMS) is the muscle tightness and tenderness you may feel a day or two after a hard workout session. This soreness is due to microscopic tears in your muscle fibers and connective tissues; it occurs when the body sustains excessive overloads. Most people experience DOMS at one point or another and typically recover quickly. DOMS is a sign that you did too much too soon. If you experience DOMS (especially common when starting an exercise program), examine your program design. Find ways to decrease the time, intensity, resistance, or repetitions of the exercise.

rate and significantly increase your susceptibility for heat-related illness.

According to the ACSM, you should lose no more than two percent of your body weight in fluid during an exercise session. A loss of fluid equivalent to one percent of your body weight will cause you to feel thirsty; losses over three percent may start to affect your exercise performance. Weigh yourself before and after exercise to determine how much water weight you have lost and adjust your fluid intake accordingly. Water loss is an individual issue. Everyone sweats at different rates in response to exercise. To decrease water loss, start

TABLE **3.4** Common Exercise Injuries, Treatments, and Prevention		
Injury	Description	Treatment and Prevention
Delayed-Onset Muscle Soreness (DOMS)	Muscle tenderness and stiffness 24–48 hours after strenuous exercise	*Treatment:* Reduce exercise to light activity until the pain stops, gently stretch the area; for some, heat and anti-inflammatory medications help as well *Prevention:* Follow proper exercise programming guidelines
Back Pain	Sharp or dull pain and stiffness in the mid to lower back	*Treatment:* Reduce exercise until the acute pain stops; gently stretch the area; use ice, heat, anti-inflammatory medications *Prevention:* Strengthen abdominal and back muscles, stretch back and hip muscles, maintain a healthy body weight, have good posture and lifting techniques
Blisters	Red, fluid- or blood-filled pockets of skin, often on the feet after a long exercise session	*Treatment:* Change shoes that may have caused the blister, keep the area clean, and cover if needed; do not purposefully pop blisters *Prevention:* Use comfortable shoes that fit well and sweat-wicking socks (avoid all-cotton socks)
Muscle Cramps	Muscle pain, tightness, and uncontrollable spasms	*Treatment:* Stop activity; massage and stretch the affected area until the cramp releases *Prevention:* Follow warm-up, cool-down, and general exercise guidelines; stay fully hydrated for exercise

(Continued)

TABLE **3.4** (*Continued*)

Injury	Description	Treatment and Prevention
Muscle Strain	Damage to the muscle or tendon fibers due to injury or overtraining resulting in pain, swelling, and decreased function; varying levels of severity	*Treatment:* Reduce painful activity; apply ice or heat after a few days; use anti-inflammatory medications if desired; stretching *Prevention:* Follow warm-up, cool-down, and general exercise guidelines; reduce or stop activity if muscles feel overly weak and fatigued
Joint Sprain	Damage to ligaments or joint structures; the result of an acute injury resulting in pain, swelling, and loss of function; varying levels of severity	*Treatment:* Stop activity; use ice, compression, elevation; seek medical attention *Prevention:* Avoid high joint-stress activities, strengthen joint-supporting muscles, wear supportive bracing if necessary
Dislocation	Separation of bones in a joint causing structural alterations and potential ligament and nerve damage	*Treatment:* Stop activity; use ice, immobilization; seek medical treatment *Prevention:* Avoid high joint-stress activities, strengthen joint-supporting muscles, wear supportive bracing if necessary
Tendonitis	Chronic pain and swelling in tendons as a result of overuse	*Treatment:* Reduce exercise to light activity until the pain stops; apply ice, gently stretch the area; anti-inflammatory medications may help *Prevention:* Follow proper exercise programming guidelines, work for muscle balance in strength and flexibility
Plantar Fasciitis	Irritation, pain, and swelling of the fascia under the foot	*Treatment:* Reduce painful activities, gently stretch the area; for some people, ice, heat, and/or anti-inflammatory medications help *Prevention:* Wear good athletic shoes with adequate arch support and cushioning; warm up and stretch the plantar fascia prior to exercise
Runner's Knee	Patella-femoral pain syndrome where there is chronic pain behind or around the kneecap	*Treatment:* Reduce exercises that cause pain; use ice, anti-inflammatory medications if needed for pain and swelling *Prevention:* Work for balance in strength and flexibility in all of the knee-supporting muscles; wear good athletic shoes with support and foot control; exercise on softer surfaces; control weight
Shin Splints	Chronic pain in the front of the lower leg (the shins); can also occur as pain on the sides of the lower leg	*Treatment:* Reduce painful exercise; apply ice, gently stretch the area, switch to less weight-bearing activities *Prevention:* Work for balance in strength and flexibility in the lower-leg muscles, wear good athletic shoes with support and cushioning, exercise on softer surfaces
Stress Fracture	Small crack or breaks in the bone in overused areas of the body causing chronic pain; must be medically diagnosed via X-ray	*Treatment:* Perform non-weight-bearing exercise until the acute pain stops, seek medical attention, rest *Prevention:* Follow proper exercise programming guidelines to avoid overtraining, wear good athletic shoes with support and cushioning, exercise on softer surfaces

Muscle and Tendon Strains A muscle or tendon strain is a soft-tissue injury that can be acute or chronic. An acute, sudden strain occurs due to a trauma or sudden movement/force that you are not accustomed to. A chronic, perpetual strain occurs from overstressed muscles that are worked in the same way over and over. Muscle strains involve damage to the muscle fibers; tendon strains involve damage to the tissue that connects muscles to bones. The primary symptoms of a strain are muscle pain, spasms, and weakness. In addition, there may be swelling of the area, cramping, and difficulty moving the muscle involved. Commonly strained areas of the body are the lower back and the back of the thighs (hamstrings).

Ligament and Joint Sprains A sudden movement or trauma can cause a sprain (damage to joint structures.) A *mild* or *first-degree sprain* involves overstretching or slight tearing of the ligament(s), resulting in some pain and swelling but little or no decrease in joint stability. In a *moderate* or *second-degree sprain,* ligaments are partially torn, and the area is painful, swollen, and bruised. In this level of sprain, mobility is limited and medical attention should be sought to determine the true severity of the injury. A *severe* or *third-degree sprain* involves a complete tearing or rupturing of the ligament or joint structures. Excessive pain, swelling, bruising, and an inability to move or put any weight on the joint are symptoms of a third-degree sprain. Immediate medical attention is necessary to determine whether bones were broken during the injury process. The most common sprains occur in the ankle while landing from a jump, in the knee from a fall or a blow to the side, and in the wrist during a fall.

Overuse Injuries Overuse injuries are due to repetitive use. You are at an increased risk of an overuse injury if you are new to sports and exercise, if you dramatically change your exercise routine, or if you do the same type of activity day in and day out.

Tendonitis is a typical overuse injury that can result from overusing the lower- or upper-body muscles. The repetitive contractions of skeletal muscles can cause pain and swelling in the tendons near joints. Common tendonitis locations are the elbow, ankle, and shoulder; these often result from tennis ("tennis elbow"), running, and weight-lifting, respectively.

A frequent overuse injury in runners and walkers is *plantar fasciitis,* or inflammation in the fascia on the underside of the foot. Pain in the arch and the heel of the foot, particularly when you are not warmed up (stepping out of bed in the morning), is the hallmark of this overuse injury.

Another injury common in runners is "runner's knee," or *patella-femoral pain syndrome.* Pain behind the kneecap (patella), inflammation, and tenderness can result from an imbalance in knee-stabilizing muscles that will cause the patella to get "off track" with your other knee joint structures. Women tend to have more problems with this syndrome than men due to the greater dynamic flexibility of their hips and knees.

Shin splints is the general term used to describe any pain that occurs in the front or sides of the lower legs. It may be tendonitis, a muscle strain, connective tissue inflammation, or a stress fracture. In response to repetitive stresses on hard surfaces, the muscles, tendons, and connective tissues of your lower leg muscles become inflamed and painful. Shin splints are common in runners and high-mileage walkers. Over time, repeated stress to the lower leg can lead to a *stress fracture*, a small crack or break in a bone. If you think you have shin splints but the pain won't go away with rest, ice, and therapy, you should get medical attention to rule out a stress fracture.

Treating Injuries with RICE The **RICE** treatment for injuries involves *rest, ice, compression, and elevation.* After an injury, you should *rest* or stop using that body part and allow for treatment and recovery. Most injuries will require *ice* immediately to reduce blood flow, acute inflammation, and pain. Apply ice or an ice pack for 10 to 30 minutes at a time, three to five times a day until symptoms lessen. *Compression* or applying pressure to the injury can be helpful for injuries that are bleeding or swelling. Using an elastic bandage around the injury will reduce swelling but still allow for adequate blood flow to the area. Tingling or discolored skin can be a sign that your wrapping is too tight. In order to promote blood flow back to the heart and lower the amount of swelling, *elevate* the injury above heart level. Following the RICE treatment is a good start for most exercise and sports-related injuries. Seek further medical attention if you are unsure how injured you are or if symptoms do not cease within a few hours.

> **RICE** Acronym for *rest, ice, compression, and elevation;* a method of treating common exercise injuries

chapterin**review**

videos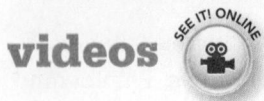

Log on to **www.pearsonhighered.com/hopson** or MyFitnessLab to view these chapter-related videos.

Personal Fitness and Exercise   3-Minute Step Test Assessment   Heart Rate: Carotid Pulse
Heart Rate: Radial Pulse

online resources

Log on to **www.pearsonhighered.com/hopson** or MyFitnessLab for access to these book-related resources and for links to other useful websites.

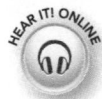 Audio case study
Audio PowerPoint lecture

 Customizable four-week running programs
Customizable four-week biking programs
Customizable four-week swimming programs
Take Charge of Your Health! Worksheets
Behavior Change Log Book and Wellness Journal

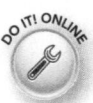 Lab 3.1 Monitoring Intensity during a Workout
Lab 3.2 Assessing Your Cardiorespiratory Fitness Level
Lab 3.3 Plan Your Cardiorespiratory Fitness Goals and Program
Alternate Aerobic Fitness Assessment: 2-Minute Marching Test
Alternate Aerobic Fitness Assessment: Adapted for Swimming
Alternate Aerobic Fitness Assessment: Adapted for Wheelchair Users

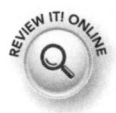 Pre- and post-quizzes
Glossary flashcards

review questions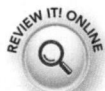

1. Cardiorespiratory fitness would be most improved by which of the following?
   a. Stretching your leg muscles every day
   b. A 90-minute yoga class, three times per week
   c. Vigorously riding your bicycle every day for 30 minutes
   d. Walking to and from classes across campus

2. Regular cardiorespiratory fitness activities reduce your chance of developing
   a. metabolic syndrome.
   b. HIV.
   c. athlete's foot.
   d. dehydration.

3. Which circulation delivers blood to the lungs?
   a. Pulmonary
   b. Systemic
   c. Hepatic
   d. Cardiac

4. Which energy system will provide most of the ATP during an hour-long bicycle ride?
   a. The immediate energy system
   b. The nonoxidative energy system
   c. The creatine phosphate energy system
   d. The oxidative energy system

5. Which of the following will decrease with regular aerobic training?
   a. Muscle cell size
   b. Blood volume
   c. Resting heart rate
   d. Maximal cardiac output

6. Which of the following is an example of vigorous exercise?
   a. Gardening
   b. Running a fast mile
   c. A one-mile leisurely walk
   d. Bowling

7. The bulk of your cardiorespiratory training program should include
   a. interval training.
   b. circuit training.
   c. hill run training.
   d. continuous target heart rate training.
8. Which OMNI Scale of Perceived Exertion value is associated with training in your target heart rate range?
   a. 1
   b. 3
   c. 7
   d. 9

9. Which of the following is the *best* way to plan for cardiorespiratory program progression?
   a. Follow the 10 percent rule
   b. Increase your exercise duration each time you work out
   c. Schedule re-assessments of your cardiorespiratory fitness every four weeks
   d. Increase your exercise intensity with every work-out session
10. What is the most common type of injury or illness in cardiorespiratory exercisers?
    a. Heat illness
    b. Hypothermia
    c. Overuse injuries
    d. Head injuries

critical**thinking**questions

REVIEW IT! ONLINE

1. Name three benefits of having a high level of cardiorespiratory fitness and explain how each impacts your overall health and wellness.

2. What are the pros and cons of each method of intensity monitoring: target heart rate, perceived exertion, and the talk test?

references

1. J. L. Johnson and others, "Exercise Training Amount and Intensity Effects on Metabolic Syndrome," *American Journal of Cardiology* 100, no. 12 (2007): 1759–66.
2. K. E. Reed and others, "Arterial Compliance in Young Children: The Role of Aerobic Fitness," *European Journal of Cardiovascular Prevention and Rehabilitation* 12, no. 5 (2005): 492–97.
3. J. M. McGavock, T. J. Anderson, and R. Z. Lewanczuk, "Sedentary Lifestyle and Antecedents of Cardiovascular Disease in Young Adults," *American Journal of Hypertension* 19, no. 7 (2006): 701–07.
4. C. E. Finley and others, "Cardiorespiratory Fitness, Macronutrient Intake, and the Metabolic Syndrome: The Aerobics Center Longitudinal Study," *Journal of the American Dietetic Association* 106, no. 5 (2006): 673–79.
5. C. R. Bruce and others, "Endurance Training in Obese Humans Improves Glucose Tolerance and Mitochondrial Fatty Acid Oxidation and Alters Muscle Lipid Content," *American Journal of Physiology: Endocrinology and Metabolism* 291, no. 1 (2006): E99–E107.
6. X. Sui and others, "Influence of Cardiorespiratory Fitness on Lung Cancer Mortality," *Medicine and Science in Sports and Exercise* 42, no. 5 (2010): 872-8; S. W. Farrell and others, "Cardiorespiratory Fitness, Different Measures of Adiposity, and Total Cancer Mortality in Women," *Obesity (Silver Spring)* (Feb 2011). [Epub ahead of print].

7. G. R. Hunter and others, "Increased Resting Energy Expenditure after 40 Minutes of Aerobic but Not Resistance Exercise," *Obesity (Silver Spring)* 14, no. 11 (2006): 2018–25.
8. S. M. Markowitz and S. M. Arent, "The Exercise and Affect Relationship: Evidence for the Dual-Mode Model and a Modified Opponent Process Theory," *Journal of Sport & Exercise Psychology* 32, no. 5 (2010): 711–30.
9. M. D. Hoffman and D. R. Hoffman, "Exercisers Achieve Greater Acute Exercise-Induced Mood Enhancement than Nonexercisers," *Archives of Physical Medicine and Rehabilitation* 89, no. 2 (2008): 358–63.
10. T. M. DiLorenzo and others, "Long-Term Effects of Aerobic Exercise on Psychological Outcomes," *Preventative Medicine* 28, no. 1 (1999): 75–85.
11. P. J. Carek, S. E. Laibstain, and S. M. Carek, "Exercise for the Treatment of Depression and Anxiety," *International Journal of Psychiatry in Medicine* 41, no. 1 (2011): 15–28.
12. V. S. Conn, "Depressive Symptom Outcomes of Physical Activity Interventions: Meta-Analysis Findings," *Annals of Behavioral Medicine* 39, no. 2 (2010): 128–38.
13. J. Romeo and others, "Physical Activity, Immunity and Infection," *The Proceedings of the Nutrition Society* 69, no. 3 (2010): 390–99.
14. M. H. Arai, A. J. Duarte, and V. M. Natale, "The Effects of Long-Term Endurance

Training on the Immune and Endocrine Systems of Elderly Men: The Role of Cytokines and Anabolic Steroid Hormones," *Immunity and Aging* 3 (2006): 9.
15. R. S. Newson and E. B. Kemps, "Cardiorespiratory Fitness as a Predictor of Successful Cognitive Ageing," *Journal of Clinical and Experimental Neuropsychology* 28, no. 6 (2006): 949–67.
16. S. J. Colcome and others, "Aerobic Exercise Training Increases Brain Volume in Aging Humans," *Journal of Gerontology Series A: Biological Sciences and Medical Sciences* 61, no. 11 (2006): 1166–70.
17. K. I. Erickson and others, "Exercise Training Increases Size of Hippocampus and Improves Memory," *Proceedings of the National Academy of Sciences U.S.A.,* 108, no. 7 (2011): 3017–22.
18. S. Fillipas and others, "A Six-Month, Supervised, Aerobic and Resistance Exercise Program Improves Self-Efficacy in People with Human Immunodeficiency Virus: A Randomized Controlled Trial," *Australian Journal of Physiotherapy* 52, no. 3 (2006): 185–90.
19. M. McNeely and others, "Effects of Exercise on Breast Cancer Patients and Survivors," *Canadian Medical Association Journal* 175, no. 1 (2006): 34–41.
20. M. Benetti, C. L. Araujo, and R. Z.Santos, "Cardiorespiratory Fitness and Quality of Life at Different Exercise Intensities after Myocardial Infarction," *Arquivos Brasileiros de Cardiologia* 95, no. 3 (2010): 399–404.

21. G. Borg, *Borg's Perceived Exertion and Pain Scales.* (Champaign: Human Kinetics, 1998) 27–38.

22. R. J. Robertson and others, "Validation of the Adult OMNI Scale of Perceived Exertion for Cycle Ergometer Exercise," *Medicine & Science in Sports & Exercise* 36, no. 1 (2004): 102–108.

23. A. C. Utter and others, "Validation of the Adult OMNI Scale of Perceived Exertion for Walking/Running Exercise," *Medicine & Science in Sports & Exercise* 36, no. 10 (2004): 1776–1780.

24. American Academy of Orthopaedic Surgeons, "Your Orthopaedic Connection: Athletic Shoes," http://orthoinfo.aaos.org /topic.cfm?topic=A00318 (accessed September 2011).

25. M. Rav-Acha and others, "Fatal Exertional Heat Stroke: A Case Series," *American Journal of the Medical Sciences* 328, no. 2 (2004): 84–87.

LAB 3.1 • MONITORING INTENSITY DURING A WORKOUT

DO IT! ONLINE

Name: _____ **Date:** _____

Instructor: _____ **Section:** _____

Materials: Calculator and a stopwatch

Purpose: (1) To measure your resting heart rate (RHR); (2) to calculate your personal target heart rate range for exercise; (3) to assess the intensity of your workout

SECTION I: DETERMINING YOUR RESTING HEART RATE

SEE IT! ONLINE

1. **Practice Taking Your Pulse** Press your middle and index fingers gently on the side of your throat to take your *carotid pulse*. You can also take a *radial pulse* by placing your middle and index fingers at the thumb side of your wrist. Measure your resting heart rate (RHR) by counting your pulse for 60 seconds, then 30 seconds, then 10 seconds. Record your counts and complete the calculations below.

Pulse Rate #1 (60 sec) _____ × 1 = _____ 1 full minute RHR

Pulse Rate #2 (30 sec) _____ × 2 = _____ 1 calculated minute RHR

Pulse Rate #3 (10 sec) _____ × 6 = _____ 1 calculated minute RHR

2. **Determine Your True Resting Heart Rate**
Take your pulse first thing in the morning on four different days. Record and average the results below. For an accurate resting heart rate, always count your pulse for a full minute. Ideally, you should take your pulse after waking up *without an alarm* and after a good night's rest.

	Resting Heart Rate (RHR)	Time of Day
Day 1		
Day 2		
Day 3		
Day 4		

Average RHR = _____

SECTION II: CALCULATE YOUR TARGET HEART RATE RANGE FOR EXERCISE

Calculate your personal target heart rate range for exercise using two methods: the maximum heart rate (HRmax) method and the heart rate reserve (HRR) method. Your target heart rate will provide a guideline for how many beats per minute (bpm) your heart should be beating during exercise, in order to achieve improvements in cardiorespiratory fitness. Note that you must count your pulse within 15 seconds of stopping exercise in order for your heart rate to reflect the exercise rate. Thus, if you take five seconds to find your pulse and start counting, that leaves you 10 seconds to take an exercise heart rate.

Method #1: Maximum Heart Rate (HRmax)

1. Find your predicted HRmax = 220 − _____ = _____
  (age)   (predicted HRmax)

2. Find your low HR target = _____ × .70 = _____ bpm ÷ 6 = _____
  (predicted HRmax)   *Low HR target*   *Low 10 sec target*

3. Find your high HR target = _____ × .90 = _____ bpm ÷ 6 = _____
  (predicted HRmax)   *High HR target*   *High 10 sec target*

Method #2: Heart Rate Reserve (HRR)

1. Find your HRR = _____ – _____ = _____
           (predicted HRmax)   RHR   HRR
                          (from Section I)

2. Find 50% of HRR = (_____ × .50) = _____ – _____ bpm ÷ 6 = _____
                    HRR   RHR   ***Low HR target***   ***Low 10 sec target***

3. Find 80% of HRR = (_____ × .80) = _____ – _____ bpm ÷ 6 = _____
                    HRR   RHR   ***High HR target***   ***High 10 sec target***

SECTION III: MONITOR YOUR WORKOUT INTENSITY LEVEL

Practice monitoring your workout intensity during a 30-minute exercise session. You can choose any form of individual exercise that allows you to easily monitor your heart rate via a pulse check.

1. Calculate your estimated heart rate goal as a 10-second count for each time interval in the chart below.

2. Conduct your exercise session. Take your pulse and record your actual exercise heart rates.

3. In the last column of the chart, write your perceived exertion scores (1–10 OMNI Scale) scores 30 seconds before the end of the time period indicated on the workout schedule.

Time	Planned Intensity	Calculated HR 10 sec Count	Actual 10 sec HR	Perceived Exertion (1–10)
5 min warm-up	Slowly up to 55% HRmax	Predicted HRmax × .55 = _____ ÷ 6 = _____		
5 min	65% HRmax	Predicted HRmax × .65 = _____ ÷ 6 = _____		
4 min	75% HRmax	Predicted HRmax × .75 = _____ ÷ 6 = _____		
3 min	85% HRmax	Predicted HRmax × .85 = _____ ÷ 6 = _____		
4 min	75% HRmax	Predicted HRmax × .75 = _____ ÷ 6 = _____		
5 min	65% HRmax	Predicted HRmax × .65 = _____ ÷ 6 = _____		
4 min cool-down	55% HRmax	Predicted HRmax × .55 = _____ ÷ 6 = _____.		

SECTION IV: REFLECTION

1. How close were your calculated and actual heart rates during your 30-minute exercise session?

2. Did the intensity levels feel higher or lower than you thought they would at each percentage of HRmax?

LAB 3.2 • ASSESSING YOUR CARDIORESPIRATORY FITNESS LEVEL

Name: _____ **Date:** _____

Instructor: _____ **Section:** _____

Materials: Calculator, 12-inch step, stopwatch, metronome

Purpose: To measure (1) recovery from physical activity, (2) walking speed, and (3) current level of cardiorespiratory fitness.

SECTION I: THE THREE-MINUTE STEP TEST

For this test, you will be stepping on a 12-inch high step bench for three minutes and then measuring your recovery pulse for one full minute.

1. Setup and preparation. Set up a 12-inch-high step bench in a place that will be safe to perform the test. Set the metronome to a pace of 96 beats per minute, which means you will be doing 24 steps up and down in a minute. Listen to the metronome and do a couple of practice steps to ensure that you can step with the right cadence ("up, up, down, down"). One foot will be stepping up or down with each beat of the metronome. Have a stopwatch available to time your three minutes on the step and your one minute HR afterward.

2. Step up and down for three minutes. Start the metronome and march in place to the beat. Start stepping up on the bench and down to the floor after starting the stopwatch. Maintain this exact pace for the entire three minutes.

3. Stop and count your pulse for one full minute. At the end of three minutes, stop stepping, turn off the metronome, sit down on your bench, and find your carotid or radial pulse immediately. Within five seconds of stopping the exercise, start counting your recovery pulse and count for one full minute.

4. Record your results and your fitness rating. Record your recovery heart rate below in beats per minute (bpm). Locate your fitness rating on the chart below and record that as well.

The 3-Minute Step Test RESULTS

1-Minute Recovery HR: _____ **(bpm)** **Fitness Rating:** _____

YMCA 3-Minute Step Test Ratings (bpm)							
Men	Excellent	Good	Above Average	Average	Below Average	Poor	Very Poor
18–25 yrs	50–76	79–84	88–93	95–100	102–107	111–119	124–157
26–35 yrs	51–76	79–85	88–94	96–102	104–110	114–121	126–161
36–45 yrs	49–76	80–88	92–98	100–105	108–113	116–124	130–163
46–55 yrs	56–82	87–93	95–101	103–111	113–119	121–126	131–159
56–65 yrs	60–77	86–94	97–100	103–109	111–117	119–128	131–154
66+ yrs	59–81	87–92	94–102	104–110	114–118	121–126	130–151

YMCA 3-Minute Step Test Ratings (bpm)							
Women	Excellent	Good	Above Average	Average	Below Average	Poor	Very Poor
18–25 yrs	52–81	85–93	96–102	104–110	113–120	122–131	135–169
26–35 yrs	58–80	85–92	95–101	104–110	113–119	122–129	134–171
36–45 yrs	51–84	89–96	100–104	107–112	115–120	124–132	137–169
46–55 yrs	63–91	95–101	104–110	113–118	120–124	126–132	137–171
56–65 yrs	60–92	97–103	106–111	113–118	119–127	129–135	141–174
66+ yrs	70–92	96–101	104–111	116–121	123–126	128–133	135–155

SECTION II: THE ONE-MILE WALK TEST

You will walk one mile and determine your heart rate response to the exercise immediately after. IMPORTANT REMINDERS: The accuracy of this test depends on three things: (1) Walk during this test. Do not run. (2) Walk the mile as fast as you can. (3) Keep a steady pace throughout the mile. Do not "sprint" at the end.

1. **Preparation and warm-up.** Make sure that you have an accurate one-mile course to complete (four laps around a standard track) and a stopwatch. Warm up with three to five minutes of light walking and range-of-motion activities.

2. **Walk one full mile as fast as you can.** After completing the one mile, record your finish time (from your watch, stopwatch, or someone calling out the time) below. Convert the time from minutes and seconds to minutes with a decimal fraction.

3. **Immediately take an exercise heart rate and cool-down.** Within five seconds of finishing the walk, find your carotid or radial pulse and count your pulse for 10 seconds. Multiply the number by 6 and record your HR below. After recording your finish time and your HR, cool down by walking slowly for another five minutes and doing some light stretching.

4. **Calculate your estimated maximal oxygen consumption (VO_2max).** Use the formula below to calculate your estimated VO_2max. This number will more accurately reflect your fitness level if you followed the test instructions carefully.

5. **Find the cardiorespiratory fitness level that corresponds to your predicted VO_2max.** Use the chart at the end of Section III to determine your cardiorespiratory fitness level, as determined by this one-mile walking test.

The One-Mile Walk Test RESULTS

One-Mile Walk Time: _____ (min:sec); divide sec by 60 = _____ (min w/decimal)

Exercise HR: _____ (beats) × 6 = _____ (bpm)
(10 sec count)

Estimated VO_2max: Use the following equation to estimate VO_2max, where gender = 0 for female and 1 for male; time = walk time to the nearest hundredth of a minute; and HR = heart rate (bpm) at the end of the walking test. Plug in your weight and numbers from above and calculate the numbers in parentheses first. Complete the calculation to find your estimated VO_2max.

- VO_2max = 132.853 − [0.0769 × body weight (lb)] − [0.3877 × age (yr)] + [6.3150 × gender] − [3.2649 × time (min)] − [0.1565 × HR (bpm)]

- $VO_2max = 132.853 - [0.0769 \times \underline{\hspace{1cm}} \text{ (lb)}] - [0.3877 \times \underline{\hspace{1cm}} \text{ (yr)}] + [6.3150 \times \underline{\hspace{1cm}}$ (gender)] $- [3.2649 \times \underline{\hspace{1cm}} \text{ (min)}] - [0.1565 \times \underline{\hspace{1cm}} \text{ (bpm)}]$

- $VO_2max = 132.853 - \underline{\hspace{1cm}} - \underline{\hspace{1cm}} = \underline{\hspace{1cm}} - \underline{\hspace{1cm}} - \underline{\hspace{1cm}}$

- $VO_2max = \underline{\hspace{1cm}} \text{ (ml/kg·min)}$

Walk Test VO₂max Fitness Rating: _____

SECTION III: 1.5-MILE RUN TEST

1. **Preparation and warm-up.** Make sure that you have an accurate 1.5-mile course to complete (six laps around a standard track) and a stopwatch. Warm up with 5 to 10 minutes of walking/jogging and range-of-motion activities.

2. **Run (with walk breaks if needed) 1.5 miles as fast as you can.** After reaching 1.5 miles, mark your finish time (from your watch, stopwatch, or someone calling out the time) below. Convert the time from minutes and seconds to minutes with a decimal fraction.

3. **Cool-down.** After recording your finish time, cool down by walking for five minutes and doing some light stretching.

4. **Calculate your estimated maximal oxygen consumption (VO₂max).** Use the formula below to calculate your estimated VO₂max.

5. **Find your cardiorespiratory fitness level that corresponds to your predicted VO₂max.** Use the chart at the end of this section to determine your cardiorespiratory fitness level, as determined by this 1.5-mile running test.

The 1.5-Mile Run Test RESULTS

1.5-Mile Run Time: _____ (min:sec); divide sec by 60 = _____ (min w/decimal)

Estimated VO₂max: You will use the following equation to estimate VO₂max, where time = run time to the nearest hundredth of a minute. Plug in your time from above, compute the number in parentheses first, and complete the calculation to find your estimated VO₂max.

- $VO_2max = [483 \div \text{time (min)}] + 3.5$
- $VO_2max = [483 \div \underline{\hspace{2cm}} \text{ (min)}] + 3.5$
- $VO_2max = \underline{\hspace{2cm}} + 3.5$
- $VO_2max = \underline{\hspace{2cm}} \text{ (ml/kg·min)}$

Run Test VO₂max Fitness Rating: _____

Estimated VO₂max Fitness Ratings (ml/kg·min)						
Men	Superior	Excellent	Good	Fair	Poor	Very Poor
18–29 yrs	>56.1	51.1–56.1	45.7–51.0	42.2–45.6	38.1–42.1	<38.1
30–39 yrs	>54.2	48.9–54.2	44.4–48.8	41.0–44.3	36.7–40.9	<36.7
40–49 yrs	>52.8	46.8–52.8	42.4–46.7	38.4–42.3	34.6–38.3	<34.6
50–59 yrs	>49.6	43.3–49.6	38.3–43.2	35.2–38.2	31.1–35.1	<31.1
60–69 yrs	>46.0	39.5–46.0	35.0–39.4	31.4–34.9	27.4–31.3	<27.4

Estimated VO$_2$max Fitness Ratings (ml/kg·min)						
Women	Superior	Excellent	Good	Fair	Poor	Very Poor
18–29 yrs	>50.1	44.0–50.1	39.5–43.9	35.5–39.4	31.6–35.4	<31.6
30–39 yrs	>46.8	41.0–46.8	36.8–40.9	33.8–36.7	29.9–33.7	<29.9
40–49 yrs	>45.1	38.9–45.1	35.1–38.8	31.6–35.0	28.0–31.5	<28.0
50–59 yrs	>39.8	35.2–39.8	31.4–35.1	28.7–31.3	25.5–28.6	<25.5
60–69 yrs	>36.8	32.3–36.8	29.1–32.2	26.6–29.0	23.7–26.5	<23.7

Reprinted with permission from The Cooper Institute, Dallas, Texas, from Physical Fitness Assessments and Norms for Adults and Law Enforcement, available online at www.CooperInstitute.org.

You may also use the chart below to estimate your fitness level using only your run time.

Estimated Run Time Ratings				
Men	Excellent	Good	Fair	Poor
Ages 20–29	<10:10	10:10–11:29	11:30–12:38	>12:38
Ages 30–39	<10:47	10:47–11:54	11:55–12:58	>12:58
Ages 40–49	<11:16	11:16–12:24	12:25–13:50	>13:50
Ages 50–59	<12:09	12:09–13:35	13:36–15:06	>15:06
Ages 60–69	<13:24	13:24–15:04	15:05–16:46	>16:46
Women	Excellent	Good	Fair	Poor
Ages 20–29	<11:59	11:59–13:24	13:25–14:50	>14:50
Ages 30–39	<12:25	12:25–14:08	14:09–15:43	>15:43
Ages 40–49	<13:24	13:24–14:53	14:54–16:31	>16:31
Ages 50–59	<14:35	14:35–16:35	16:36–18:18	>18:18
Ages 60–69	<16:34	16:34–18:27	18:28–20:16	>20:16

Reprinted with permission from The Cooper Institute, Dallas, Texas, from Physical Fitness Assessments and Norms for Adults and Law Enforcement, available online at www.CooperInstitute.org.

LAB 3.3 • PLAN YOUR CARDIORESPIRATORY FITNESS GOALS AND PROGRAM

Name: _____ Date: _____

Instructor: _____ Section: _____

Materials: Results from cardiorespiratory fitness assessments, calculator, lab pages.

Purpose: To learn how to set appropriate cardiorespiratory fitness goals and create a personal cardiorespiratory fitness program designed to meet those goals.

SECTION I: SHORT- AND LONG-TERM GOALS

Create short- and long-term goals for cardiorespiratory fitness. Be sure to use SMART goal-setting guidelines (specific, measurable, action-oriented, realistic, time-oriented). Select appropriate target dates and rewards for completing your goals.

Short-Term Goal (3–6 Months)

_____

_____

Target Date: _____

Reward: _____

Long-Term Goal (12+ Months)

_____

_____

Target Date: _____

Reward: _____

SECTION II: CARDIORESPIRATORY FITNESS OBSTACLES AND STRATEGIES

1. What **barriers or obstacles** might hinder your plan to improve your cardiorespiratory fitness? Indicate your top three obstacles below:

a. _____

b. _____

c. _____

2. Overcoming these barriers/obstacles to change will be an important step in reaching your goals. Write down three **strategies** for overcoming the obstacles listed above:

a. _____

b. _____

c. _____

SECTION III: GETTING SUPPORT

1. List resources you will use to help you change your cardiorespiratory fitness:

Friend/partner/relative: _____

School-based resource: _____

Community-based resource: _____

Other: _____

2. How will you use these supportive resources to help you meet your cardiorespiratory fitness goals?

_____

_____

_____

_____

_____

_____

_____

_____

_____

SECTION IV: CARDIORESPIRATORY FITNESS PROGRAM REFLECTIONS

1. How realistic are the short- and long-term target dates you have set for achieving your cardiorespiratory fitness goals?

_____

_____

_____

2. How many days per week are you planning to work on your cardiorespiratory fitness program? _____

3. What types of workouts are you planning to try?

_____

_____

_____

4. Do you have a workout partner? Do you plan to work with a workout partner, personal trainer, or instructor to help get you started?

_____

_____

_____

SECTION V: CARDIORESPIRATORY TRAINING PROGRAM DESIGN

Plan a four-week cardiorespiratory training program, using resources available to you (facility, instructor, text) and completing the following training calendar (A = activity, I = intensity, T = time).

Four-Week Cardiorespiratory Training Program						
Sun	Mon	Tues	Wed	Thurs	Fri	Sat
Date: _____	Date: _____	Date: _____	Date: _____	Date: _____	Date: _____	Date: _____
A:	A:	A:	A:	A:	A:	A:
I:	I:	I:	I:	I:	I:	I:
T:	T:	T:	T:	T:	T:	T:
Date: _____	Date: _____	Date: _____	Date: _____	Date: _____	Date: _____	Date: _____
A:	A:	A:	A:	A:	A:	A:
I:	I:	I:	I:	I:	I:	I:
T:	T:	T:	T:	T:	T:	T:
Date: _____	Date: _____	Date: _____	Date: _____	Date: _____	Date: _____	Date: _____
A:	A:	A:	A:	A:	A:	A:
I:	I:	I:	I:	I:	I:	I:
T:	T:	T:	T:	T:	T:	T:
Date: _____	Date: _____	Date: _____	Date: _____	Date: _____	Date: _____	Date: _____
A:	A:	A:	A:	A:	A:	A:
I:	I:	I:	I:	I:	I:	I:
T:	T:	T:	T:	T:	T:	T:

SECTION VI: TRACKING YOUR PROGRAM AND FOLLOWING THROUGH

1. **Goal and Program Tracking:** Use the following chart to monitor your progress. Change the activity, intensity, or time of your workout plan to reflect your progress as needed.

2. **Goal and Program Follow-up:** At the end of the course or at your short-term goal target date, reevaluate your cardiorespiratory fitness and ask yourself the following questions:

   a. Did you meet your short-term goal or your goal for the course? If so, what positive behavioral changes contributed to your success? If not, which obstacles blocked your success?

   b. Was your short-term goal realistic? What would you change about your goals or training plan?

	Five-Week Cardiorespiratory Training Log				
	Dates	Activity	Time	Av. HR	RPE	Comments
Week 1						
Week 2						
Week 3						
Week 4						
Week 5						

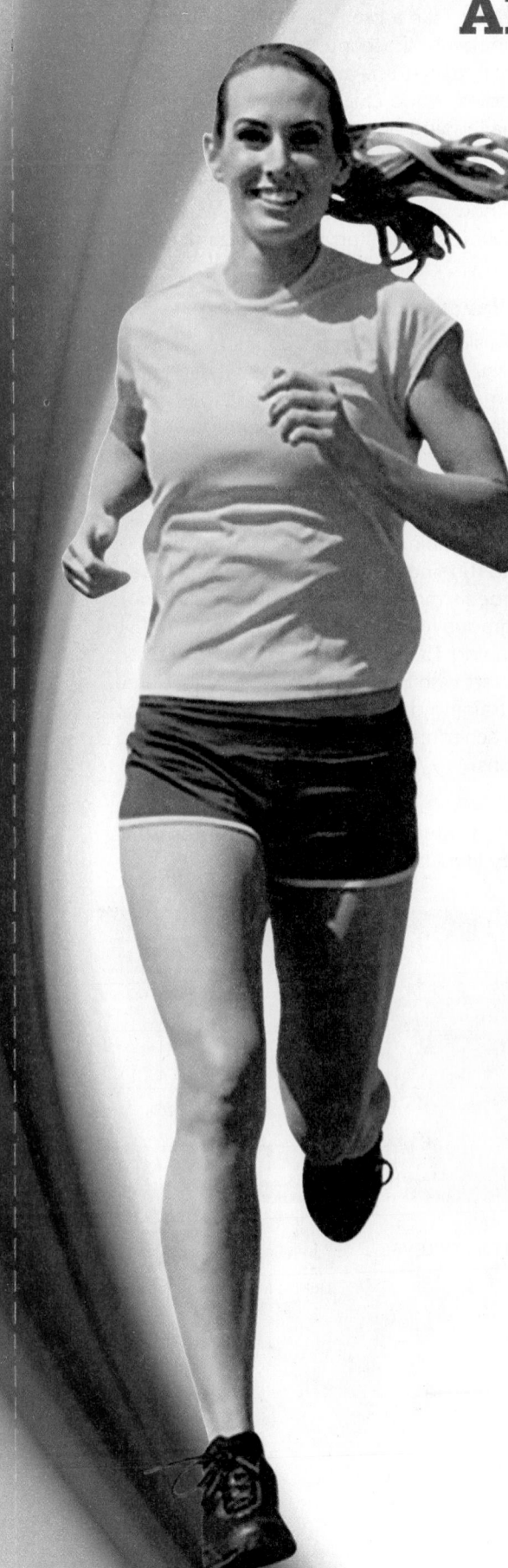

activate, motivate, & ADVANCE YOUR FITNESS

A RUNNING PROGRAM

ACTIVATE!

Whether this is your first attempt at running or you want to take your current run workouts to the next level, there is a program built just for you.

Running Program Preparation & Safety

Going too far or too fast right away is the number-one cause of injury among new runners. Focus on the minutes instead of miles, and use these programs to gradually increase your run time.

What Do I need for Running?

SHOES: Visit your local running store to find your most important running tool, your shoes! The employees are generally experienced runners who can assist you in finding a good fit for your foot, running style, gait, running surface and, of course, your goals.

CLOTHING: Wear comfortable and supportive clothing. Choose materials that wick moisture away from your skin. In cold weather, wear layers. In the sun, wear sunscreen, sunglasses, and a hat or visor. At sunrise, dusk, or night, wear reflective clothing and/or a vest and lights.

How Do I Start a Running Program?

TECHNIQUE: Relax your shoulders and gently swing your arms (90-degree elbow) up to your chest and down to your hips. Keep hands loose and relaxed. Look forward, rather than down at the ground. Stay light on your feet and use shorter, quicker steps. Land on the mid-foot or balls of your feet and push off. Aim for a stride rate (your turnover) of 180 steps per minute. Count the number of times your right foot strikes the ground in a minute and multiply that by two.

ETIQUETTE: Follow a few basic guidelines whether you are running alone or with a group, especially if you run in a high-traffic area. On a sidewalk or a multi-use path or trail, run on the right and pass on the left, after alerting others you are passing. Say, "On your left" as you approach. No matter where you run, remember to never run more than two abreast. If you need to stop, step off to the right to allow others to get by.

Running Tips

ROAD RUNNING: Plan safe and interesting routes that consider both traffic and available running paths. Check with your local running store or club for routes and running partners. Let someone know where you are going and when you will return. Carry a cell phone, ID, a few dollars, and a water bottle. Stay aware of your surroundings by wearing only one piece of your earphones. Run facing traffic and pay attention to traffic signals and signs.

TRACK RUNNING: A track will give you a stable and soft running surface. Other benefits? Tracks are usually well lit and you won't have to plan a route. Plus, you may have access to a rest room and a place to keep your water bottle and phone nearby. On a track, you can test pacing, adjust your run/walk ratios, and re-test your cardiorespiratory fitness level regularly. Most tracks are 400 meters; four laps on the inner lane equal a mile. Follow track etiquette by utilizing outside lanes for most of your training and leave the inside lane (lane 1) for faster runners and sprinters and for timing yourself on a specific distance. If you are using the inside lane and a faster individual approaches behind you, move out to lane 2 or 3 to allow the person to pass. Finally, try to change your running direction every few runs to vary the stresses on your body of going around turns.

TREADMILL RUNNING: Treadmills offer convenience, efficiency, and a safe environment when the weather is less than ideal. Be sure to familiarize yourself with the controls before starting out. Remember to maintain good form and avoid both the handrails and the back of the treadmill belt.

TRAIL RUNNING: Take a break from the asphalt jungle to run in nature. Ease into trail running by starting with flat, soft, easy-to-navigate trails (dirt, bark dust, pine needles, wood chips) and work your way up to more challenging ones. Take smaller steps, slow down, and constantly scan the trail to find the best footing. If possible, trail run with a buddy. If not, be sure that you know your route, take water, and tell someone of your location, start time, and anticipated end time.

Running Warm-Up and Cool-Down

Walk or jog at a slower pace for 5–10 minutes to warm-up or cool-down. After breaking a light sweat in your warm-up, you may want to add dynamic range-of-motion exercises. After you finish your cool-down, you can hold static stretches longer for improved flexibility.

Four-Week Running Programs

If you are new to running, if you want to transition from walking to running, or if you have taken a break from running for six months or more, then build your run program gradually and start with Program A. If you are already running 15 minutes continuously on two days a week, start with Program B below. Adjust time, intensity, and training days to suit your personal fitness level and schedule; visit the companion website for more options.

PROGRAM A 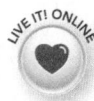
GOAL: Transition from walking to running. Increase run minutes while maintaining a moderate intensity level three to four days a week.

	Mon		Tue		Wed		Thurs		Fri		Sat		Sun	
	T*	I*	T	I	T	I	T	I	T	I	T	I	T	I
Week 1	20 1/4	L			20 1/4	L			20 1/4	L–M				
Week 2	24 1/5	M			24 1/5	M			24 1/5	M				
Week 3	32 1/7	M			32 1/7	M			32 1/7	M				
Week 4	24 2/10	M			24 2/10	M			24 2/10	M	24 2/10	M		

T*: Time. Total time is listed in minutes with the Walk/Run minute ratio below.
I*: Intensity. Intensity is listed as Light/Lifestyle (L), Moderate (M), or Vigorous (V). (See Table 3.3.)
** Workouts do not include warm-up or cool-down time.

INTENSITY LEVEL
L	M	V
Light	Moderate	Vigorous

PROGRAM B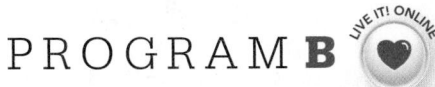

GOAL: Run at a moderate to vigorous intensity level three to five days a week, complete a 30-minute continuous run, and incorporate vigorous interval training sessions.

	Mon		Tue		Wed		Thurs		Fri		Sat		Sun	
	T*	I*	T	I	T	I	T	I	T	I	T	I	T	I
Week 1	20	L–M 3–5	20	M 5–6	20	M 5–6			20	L–M 3–5				
Week 2	20	M 5–6			25	M 5–6			20	M 5–6	25	L–M 3–5		
Week 3	25	M 5–6			20	M 5–6	Interval	L–M–V			30	M 5–6		
Week 4	25	M 5–6	Interval	L–M–V	20	L–M 3–5	Interval	L–M–V			30	L–M 3–5		

T: Time. Total time is listed in minutes.*
I: Intensity. Intensity is listed as Light/Lifestyle (L), Moderate (M), or Vigorous (V) and the OMNI scale of 0–10. (See Figure 3.8 and Table 3.3.)*
*** Workouts do not include warm-up or cool-down time.*

INTENSITY LEVEL    L M V

Light Moderate Vigorous

Program B Interval Workout—3 Miles

800m (.5 mile) at 7–8 on the OMNI scale (V)
800m (.5 mile) recovery (easy jog or walk/jog) at 2–5 on the OMNI scale (L–M)
**REPEAT this 1:1 ratio two more times for a total of 4800m or 3 miles.

MOTIVATE!

Create your own exercise log to track your running program—make note of dates, times, distances, intensity level—or use the one on the companion website. Here are a few tips to keep you running:

MORNING WORKOUTS: Try running first thing in the morning. That way, you can check it off your to-do list, and nothing can push your run off your day's schedule. Tip for success: organize your running clothes, shoes, gear, water bottle, and breakfast the night before.

DON'T PUT AWAY YOUR GEAR: Place your workout log, shoes, workout clothes, water bottle, and stretching mat in plain sight, in your work bag, or your car. Visual cues can help you remember your goals and prioritize your run.

DO IT FOR CHARITY: Need a reason or just more support? Name your cause and chances are there is a local run or race to raise awareness and funds for it. Committing to run for worthy causes reminds you that you are fortunate to be healthy and able to run. Fuel your motivation by knowing you're doing good for more than just yourself.

ADVANCE!

Now that you have established your running program, challenge yourself to try something new or take your running to the next level. How about participating in your first 5k? If you've been there, done that, how about actually racing (picking up your pace to set a new personal record)? On the next page is a more advanced four-week program you can follow; visit the companion website to find more options or simply to personalize this or any of the programs in this book.

PROGRAM C GOAL: Run 5k/3.1miles!

	Mon		Tue		Wed		Thurs		Fri		Sat		Sun	
	T/D*	I*	T/D	I	T/D	I	T/D	I	T/D	I	T/D	I	T/D	I
Week 1	25	L–M 3–5 62–70	25	L–M 3–5 62–70			25	M 5–6 65–85	25	M 5–6 65–85				
Week 2	25	M 5–6 65–85			Interval	L–M–V			2 miles	M 5–6 65–85	30	M 5–6 65–85		
Week 3	25	M 5–6 65–85	Interval	L–M–V	2.5 miles	L–M 3–5 62–70	Interval	L–M–V	3 miles	M 5–6 65–85				
Week 4	30	M 5–6 65–85			35	L–M 3–5 62–70					Goal 5k Run!			

T/D*: Time/Distance. Total time/distance is listed in minutes or miles.
I*: Intensity. Intensity is listed as Light/Lifestyle (L), Moderate (M), or Vigorous (V), the OMNI scale of 0–10, and % of HRmax. (See Figure 3.8 and Table 3.3.)
** Workouts do not include warm-up or cool-down time

INTENSITY LEVEL

Light   Moderate   Vigorous

Program C Interval Workout

Alternate two minutes hard and two minutes easy for one mile:

2 minutes at 85% HRmax or 7–8 on the OMNI scale (V)
2 minutes at <60% HRmax or 2–3 on the OMNI scale (L)
5 minutes at 65–84% HRmax or 5–6 on the OMNI scale (M)
**REPEAT twice more (total of three sets)

activate, motivate, & ADVANCE YOUR FITNESS

A CYCLING PROGRAM

ACTIVATE!

Whether you cycle indoors or take your bike out on the road or trail, you can get a fun and amazing workout.

Cycling Program Preparation & Safety

Sure, cycling can be an intense, calorie-burning workout, but it can also be a simple way to take care of errands, commute, meet up with friends, or just enjoy the great outdoors. Follow the programs below to get started. As you get stronger, you can increase your mileage and speed.

What Do I Need for Cycling?

GEAR: Safe cycling requires quite a bit of equipment (helmet, padded cycling shorts, gloves, shoes, reflective gear, racks) and, of course, the bike. You can start on almost any style of bicycle, but most importantly, you need a bike that fits. Visit your local bike shop to get the right bike for you. When indoor cycling, adjust both seat and handlebar height to create a comfortable and safe fit. If you are new to indoor cycling or unfamiliar with the stationary bikes at your facility, be sure to ask a trained instructor to assist you with proper bike setup.

How Do I Start a Cycling Program?

TECHNIQUE: Work on developing a smooth and efficient pedaling technique. Lighten up, pedal in a smooth circle, and pull through the back of the stroke. *Cadence* is pedaling speed in revolutions per minute (RPM). A cadence of 60 RPM means that one pedal makes a complete revolution 60 times in one minute. Monitor your cadence with periodic cadence checks. Count the revolution of one leg for 15 seconds and then multiply by four. The cadence range is 80–110 RPM for cycling on a flat road and 60–80 RPM for climbing hills.

ETIQUETTE: Participating in group rides will teach you the etiquette for road cycling and mountain biking. Inquire about weekly rides or a beginners' cycling group at your local bike shop.

Cycling Tips

INDOOR CYCLING: Weather, traffic, flat tires … with indoor cycling you won't have these excuses for missing your workout. Indoor cycling also allows you to precisely control your workout and mix periods of higher-intensity cycling with resting pedal strokes.

OUTDOOR CYCLING: Whether you choose streets, bike paths, or trails, plan safe routes that take into consideration both traffic and terrain. Try using a mapping program or stop by your local bike shop to learn more about the routes and popular riding areas in your neighborhood. Safety tips: brush up on your cycling skills, have proper reflective equipment, learn how to use a bike repair kit (fixing flat tires), and know local traffic laws and trail usage rules.

Cycling Warm-Up and Cool-Down

Cycle at a slow cadence for 5 to 15 minutes to warm-up or cool-down. After the cool-down portion of your ride, perform a few light stretches that focus on your low back muscles, hamstrings, quadriceps, and calves.

Four-Week Cycling Programs

If you are new to cycling or are coming back after time off, start with Program A to build your cardiorespiratory fitness base. If you are already riding for 15 or more continuous minutes at least twice a week, then start with Program B. Adjust time, intensity, and training days to suit your personal fitness level and schedule; visit the companion website for more options.

PROGRAM A

GOAL: Increase cycling minutes while maintaining a moderate intensity level three to four days a week, building to 100 total minutes by week four.

	Mon		Tue		Wed		Thurs		Fri		Sat		Sun	
	T*	I*	T	I	T	I	T	I	T	I	T	I	T	I
Week 1	20	L			20	L			20	L–M				
Week 2	25	M			25	M			25	M				
Week 3	20	M			25	M			15	M	30	L–M		
Week 4	25	M			25	M			25	M	25	L–M		

T*: Time. Total time is listed in minutes.
I*: Intensity. Intensity is listed as Light/Lifestyle (L), Moderate (M), or Vigorous (V). (See Table 3.3.)
** Workouts do not include warm-up or cool-down time.

INTENSITY LEVEL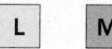
Light   Moderate   Vigorous

PROGRAM B

GOAL: Cycle at a moderate intensity level three to five days a week, build to a 40-minute ride, and incorporate vigorous interval training sessions each week.

	Mon		Tue		Wed		Thurs		Fri		Sat		Sun	
	T*	I*	T	I	T	I	T	I	T	I	T	I	T	I
Week 1	25	L–M 3–5			25	L–M 3–5			25	M 5–6	25	M 5–6		
Week 2	25	M 5–6			30	M 5–6			25	L–M 3–5	35	M 5–6		
Week 3	30	M 5–6	Interval	L–M–V	20	L–M 3–5	Interval	L–M–V	30	M 5–6				
Week 4	30	M 5–6	Interval	L–M–V	25	M 5–6	30	M 5–6			40	L–M 3–5		

T*: Time. Total time is listed in minutes.
I*: Intensity. Intensity is listed as Light/Lifestyle (L), Moderate (M), or Vigorous (V) and the OMNI scale of 0–10. (See Figure 3.8, and Table 3.3.)
** Workouts do not include warm-up or cool-down time.

INTENSITY LEVEL
Light   Moderate   Vigorous

Program B Interval Workout—25 Minutes

2 minutes of flat cycling (cadence 80–110 RPM) at 7–8 on the OMNI scale (V)
1 minute of recovery (pedal easy, below 80 RPM) at 3 on the OMNI scale (L)
**REPEAT this 2:1 ratio four more times for a total of 15 minutes
30 seconds of hill work (increase tension and drop cadence to 60–80 RPM) at 7–8 on the OMNI scale (V)
90 seconds of recovery (pedal easy, below 80 RPM with little or no resistance) at 3 on the OMNI scale (L)
**REPEAT this 1:3 ratio four more times for a total of 10 minutes

MOTIVATE!

Create your own exercise log to track your cycling program—note dates, times, distances, cadence, intensity level—or use the one on the companion website. Here are a few tips to keep you cycling:

RIDE FOR 10: If you lack energy or motivation for a spin, give yourself 10 minutes. Tell yourself that you can quit after 10 minutes if you still don't feel like riding. Chances are that once you have made the effort to start, you'll complete your workout. If not, at least you managed a solid 10 minutes and you can feel good about listening to your body and taking a rest day.

REWARD YOURSELF: Promise yourself a healthy treat or fun experience at week's end if you stick to your cycling program. Maybe a pedicure or a massage or a scoop of frozen yogurt; hard work makes a reward that much more satisfying.

INDOOR GROUP RIDE: Sometimes just knowing that others are expecting you is enough to help you show up for your workout. Try an indoor cycling class at your gym. You'll develop new friendships with other physically active people and increase your cardiorespiratory fitness. Win-Win!

ADVANCE!

Ready to be challenged in your cycling program or try a new approach? Below is a more advanced four-week program you can follow. Visit the companion website to find more options or to personalize this or any of the programs in this book.

PROGRAM C  GOAL: Ride 20k/12.4mi in ≤ 60 minutes (indoors or out)!

	Mon		Tue		Wed		Thurs		Fri		Sat		Sun	
	T/D*	I*	T/D	I	T/D	I	T/D	I	T/D	I	T/D	I	T/D	I
Week 1	25	L–M 3–5 62–70	25	M 5–6 65–85	25	L–M 3–5 62–70	25	M 5–6 65–85			35	M 5–6 65–85		
Week 2	30	M 5–6 65–85	20	V 7–8 85–94	6 miles	L–M 3–5 62–70	30	M 5–6 65–85			40	M 5–6 65–85		
Week 3	35	M 5–6 65–85	Interval	L–M–V			Interval	L–M–V	35	L–M 3–5 62–70	45	M 5–6 65–85		
Week 4	40	M 5–6 65–85	20	L–M 3–5 62–70	40	M 5–6 65–85	Interval	L–M–V			Goal 20k Ride!	M 5–6 65–85		

T/D*: Time/Distance. Total time/distance is listed in minutes or miles.
I*: Intensity. Intensity is listed as Light/Lifestyle (L), Moderate (M), or Vigorous (V), the OMNI scale of 0–10, and % of HRmax. (See Figure 3.8 and Table 3.3.)
** Workouts do not include warm-up or cool-down time

INTENSITY LEVEL | L | M | V |
Light Moderate Vigorous

Program C Interval Workout—30 Minutes

3 minutes of flat cycling (cadence 80–110 RPM) at 85% HRmax or 7–8 on the OMNI scale (V)
1 minute of recovery (pedal easy, below 80 RPM) at 3 on the OMNI scale (L)
**REPEAT this 3:1 ratio four more times for a total of 20 minutes
1 minute of hill work (increase tension and drop cadence to 60–80 RPM) at 85% HRmax or 7–8 on the OMNI scale (V)
1 minute of recovery (pedal easy, below 80 RPM with little or no resistance) at 3 on the OMNI scale (L)
**REPEAT this 1:1 ratio four more times for a total of 10 minutes

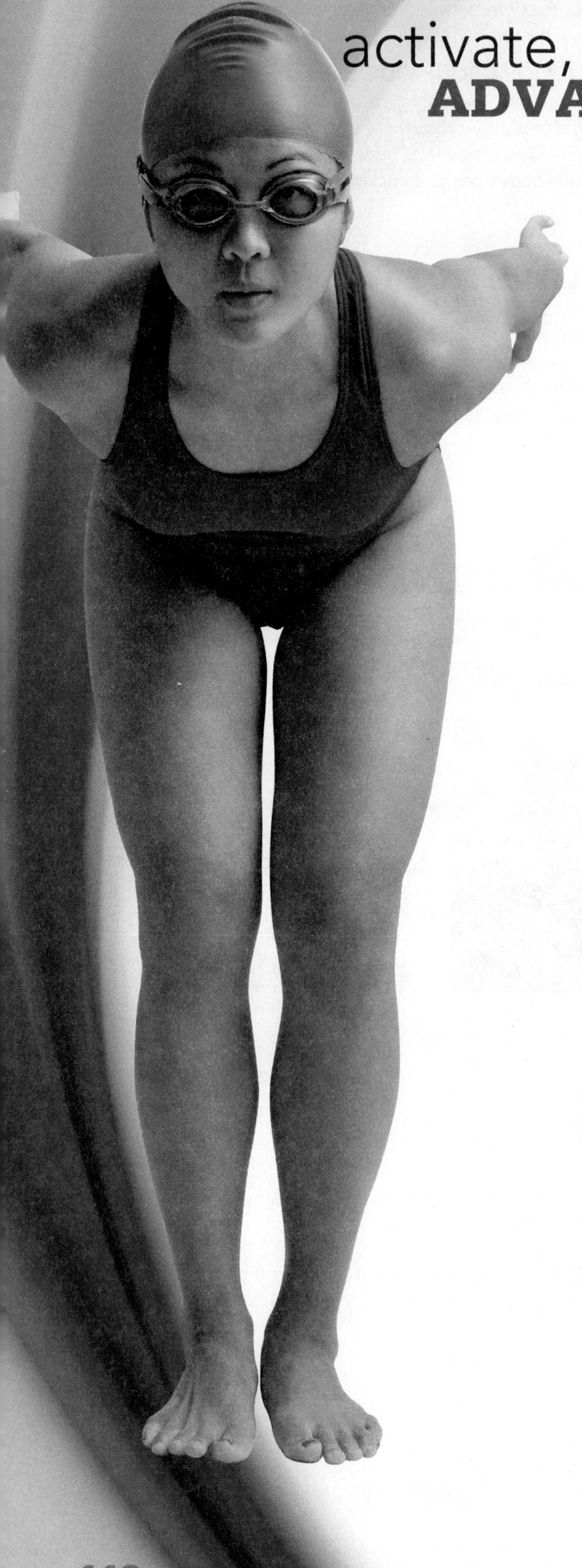

activate, motivate, & ADVANCE YOUR FITNESS

A SWIMMING PROGRAM

ACTIVATE

Low-impact and fun, swimming is an excellent way to improve your overall fitness!

Swimming Program Preparation & Safety:

If you have access to a pool, all you really need are two key items—swimsuit and goggles—and you're set to hit the water. Start and build slowly, focusing on minutes, not laps, and, as you gain strength, you will swim further and faster.

What Do I Need for Swimming?

GEAR: Look for a swimsuit that stays in place and moves with you, and be sure to try on goggles to ensure a good fit. You may want a swim cap to keep your hair out of your face. In addition, various pieces of equipment are commonly used to help swimmers improve technique and performance: kickboards, pull buoys, fins, and a stopwatch or the pool's pace clock. Lastly, don't forget your shatter-proof water bottle.

How Do I Start a Swimming Program?

TECHNIQUE: Taking a lesson is the best way to become more comfortable in the water and develop a more efficient technique. Inquire at your local college or American Red Cross chapter about adult swim classes or private swim coaches in your area.

ETIQUETTE: Pools are busy at open swim times and you will rarely get a lane to yourself. Aim to share a lane with other swimmers close to your same speed. You will most likely encounter *circle swimming* (swimming in a counter clockwise direction in the pool lane). Allow faster swimmers to take the lead, make sure there is a five second gap between you and the person in front of you, and avoid swimming in the middle of the lane. If you need to take a break at the wall, keep to the side of the lane so that others can turn or rest as well.

Swimming Tips

OPEN WATER: Although it takes strong skills, open-water swimming can be exciting and invigorating! Check with your local swim store or a swim or triathlon club to find swim partners and learn more about safe open water swim areas. Remember, the water temperature is generally much cooler than a pool; many open-water swimmers wear neoprene wetsuits to stay warm. Practice "sighting" (looking up to see where you are in relation to land, buoys, docks) and swimming in a straight line before heading out.

Swimming Warm-Up and Cool-Down

A swimming warm-up and cool-down consists of slow water walking, water jogging, or swimming at a slower pace for 5–10 minutes. You can also warm-up on deck with light, dynamic full range movements. After your cool-down, you can hold basic stretches for 10–30 seconds to improve flexibility.

Four-Week Swimming Programs

As you start a new swimming program, rest often, use resting swim strokes (elementary backstroke, sidestroke) as needed, and monitor your intensity periodically. Heart rates are typically 10–13 beats per minute lower when swimming than when performing exercise on land, so evaluate intensity using perceived exertion level. If even one length of the pool is tiring for you, start with Program A and focus on swim time, not distance or number of laps. If you are already able to swim comfortably at a moderate intensity level for close to 15 minutes (continuously or with minimum rest) and you are swimming at least twice a week, then start with Program B. Adjust time, intensity, and days of the swims to suit your personal fitness level and schedule; visit the companion website for more options.

PROGRAM A

GOAL: Increase continuous swim minutes at a light-to-moderate intensity level three to four days a week, building to 100 total minutes by week four.

	Mon		Tue		Wed		Thurs		Fri		Sat		Sun	
	T*	I*	T	I	T	I	T	I	T	I	T	I	T	I
Week 1	15	L			20	L			20	M				
Week 2	20	M			25	M			25	M				
Week 3	25	M			20	M			15	M	25	M		
Week 4	25	M			25	M			25	M	25	M		

T: Time. Total time is listed in minutes.*
I: Intensity. Intensity is listed as Light/Lifestyle (L), Moderate (M), or Vigorous (V). (See Table 3.3.)*
*** Workouts do not include warm-up or cool-down time.*

INTENSITY LEVEL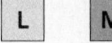

Light Moderate Vigorous

PROGRAM B

GOAL: Increase continuous swim minutes at a moderate intensity level three to five days a week, build to a 30-minute swim, and incorporate vigorous interval training sessions each week.

	Mon		Tue		Wed		Thurs		Fri		Sat		Sun	
	T*	I*	T	I	T	I	T	I	T	I	T	I	T	I
Week 1	25	L–M 3–5			25	M 5–6			25	M 5–6	25	M 5–6		
Week 2	25	M 5–6			Intervals	L–M–V			25	M 5–6				
Week 3	20	M 5–6			25	M 5–6			20	M 5–6	30	L–M 3–5		
Week 4	25	M 5–6	Intervals	L–M–V	30	M 5–6	Intervals	L–M–V	25	M 5–6				

T: Time. Total time is listed in minutes.*
I: Intensity. Intensity is listed as Light/Lifestyle (L), Moderate (M), or Vigorous (V) and the OMNI scale of 0–10. (See Figure 3.8 and Table 3.3.)*
*** Workouts do not include warm-up or cool-down time.*

INTENSITY LEVEL

Light Moderate Vigorous

Program B Interval Workout—700 m/yds

3 × 100 m/yds with 60 seconds of rest between [100s at 7–8 on the OMNI scale (V) and rest at 0–2 (L)]
2 × 75 m/yds with 45 seconds of rest between [75s at 7–8 on the OMNI scale (V) and rest at 0–2 (L)]
3 × 50 m/yds with 30 seconds of rest between [50s at 7–8 on the OMNI scale (V) and rest at 0–2 (L)]
4 × 25 m/yds with 15 seconds of rest between [25s at 7–8 on the OMNI scale (V) and rest at 0–2 (L)]

MOTIVATE!

Create your own exercise log to track your swimming program—note dates, times, laps, intensity level—or use the one on the companion website. Here are a few tips to keep you swimming:

LEARN SOMETHING NEW: Taking a lesson can help you develop confidence, which leads to more efficient swimming and increased enjoyment. The more you enjoy your workout, the better the results will be and the more likely you are to stick with it.

JOIN A TEAM: Lacking the support you need to swim regularly? Masters Swimming is a national program where adults 18 and older can swim in a team setting. You can swim at your own pace and be competitive or non-competitive—your choice! There are teams and clubs in communities across the country and all of them offer multiple practice options, workouts, and

coaching; you will gain a new group of friends who will be expecting you at the pool.

TRY A WATER EXERCISE CLASS: Getting bored? Mix things up, make new friends, and take a break from swimming laps while still getting a great workout in the water. Most pools have different types of group water exercise classes; chances are one will be right for you.

ADVANCE!

Congratulations! You have established your swim fitness program. Are you ready to challenge yourself with a new goal and take your swimming to the next level? Below is a more advanced four-week program that you can follow; visit the companion website to find more options or to personalize this or any of the programs in this book.

PROGRAM C

GOAL: Swim a mile, continuous (or with minimum rest)! (1650 yards/1508 meters)

	Mon		Tue		Wed		Thurs		Fri		Sat		Sun	
	T/D*	I*	T/D	I	T/D	I	T/D	I	T/D	I	T/D	I	T/D	I
Week 1	25	L–M 3–5 62–70	700	M 5–6 65–85	25	L–M 3–5 62–70	700	M 5–6 65–85	25	M 5–6 65–85				
Week 2	30	M 5–6 65–85	1000	M 5–6 65–85	Interval	L–M–V	1000	M 5-6 65–85	30	L–M 3–5 62–70				
Week 3	25	M 5–6 65–85	Interval	L–M–V	30	L–M 3–5 62–70	Interval	L–M–V			35	M 5–6 65–85		
Week 4	30	M 5–6 65–85	1500	M 5–6 65–85	Interval	L–M–V	20	L–M 3–5 62–70			Goal Mile Swim!			

T/D*: Time/Distance. Total time/distance is listed in minutes or yards/meters.
I*: Intensity. Intensity is listed as Light/Lifestyle (L), Moderate (M), or Vigorous (V), the OMNI scale of 0–10, and % of HRmax. (See Figure 2.1, Figure 3.8, and Table 3.3.)

** Workouts do not include warm-up or cool-down time
*** Heart rates are typically 10–13 beats per minute lower when swimming, than when performing exercise on land, adjust heart rate targets accordingly.

INTENSITY LEVEL  V

Light Moderate Vigorous

Program C Interval Workout—1200 m/yds

3 × 100 m/yds with 60 seconds of rest between [100s at 65–84% HRmax, 5–6 on the OMNI scale (M), and rest at 0–2 (L)]
2 × 200 m/yds with 2 minutes of rest between [200s at 85% HRmax, 7–8 on the OMNI scale (V), and rest at 0–2 (L)]
1 × 500 m/yds [at 65–84% HRmax, 5–6 on the OMNI scale (M)]

4

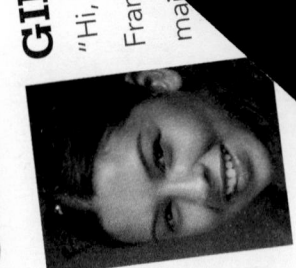

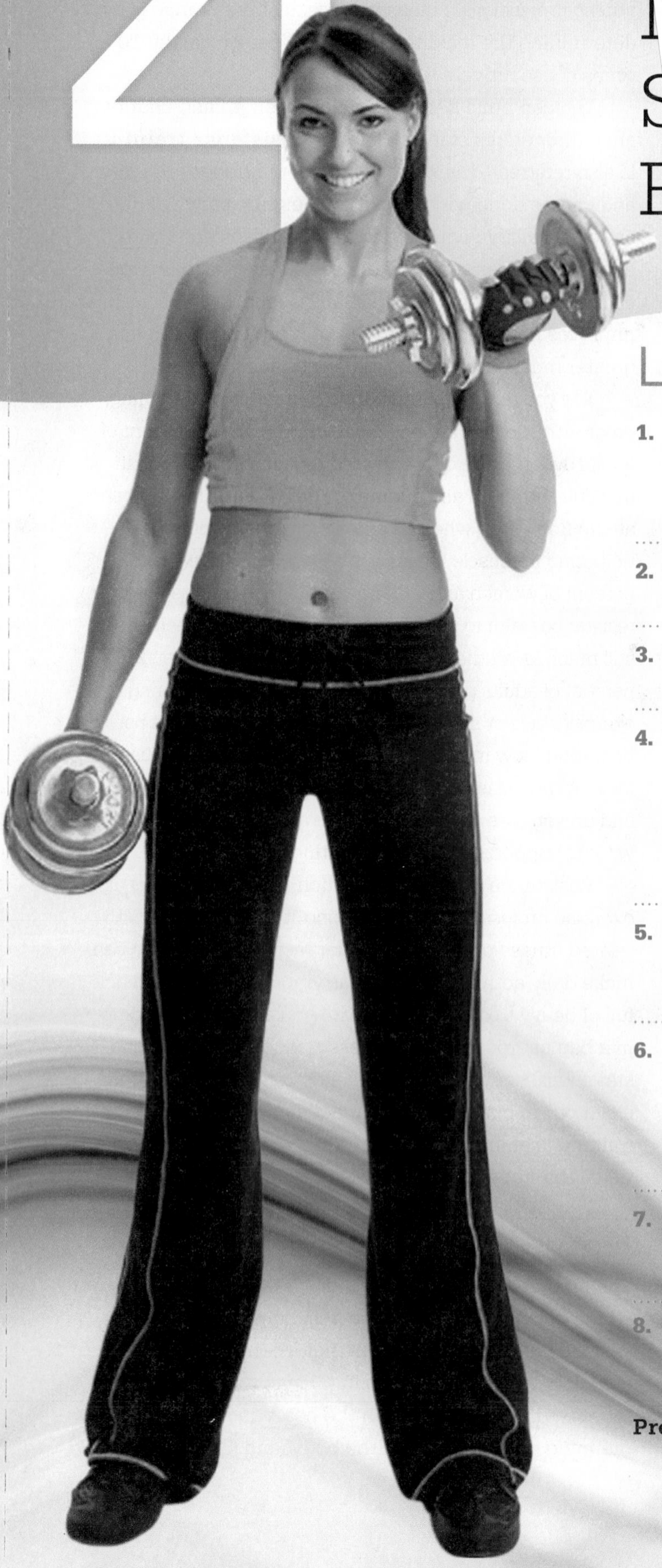

casestudy

GINA

"Hi, I'm Gina...
Francisc...
maj...

starting...
abo...

Lea...

Audio case study
and audio Power-
Point lecture

1. Exp...
   stre... ...cular
   endurance relate to lifelong fitness and wellness.

2. Identify key skeletal muscle structures and explain how
   they work together to allow for basic muscle function.

3. Articulate the fitness and wellness improvements you
   can make with regular resistance training.

4. Evaluate your changes
   in muscle fitness over
   time by assessing your
   muscular strength and
   muscular endurance at
   regular intervals.

   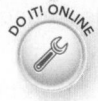
   DO IT! ONLINE

   Lab 4.1 Assessing
   Your Muscular
   Strength

   Lab 4.2 Assessing
   Your Muscular
   Endurance

5. Set and work toward
   appropriate muscular
   fitness goals.

   DO IT! ONLINE

   Lab 4.3 Setting Muscular
   Fitness Goals

   Lab 4.4 Your Resistance-
   Training Workout Plan

6. Implement a safe and
   effective resistance-
   training exercise
   program compatible
   with your goals and lifestyle.

   LIVE IT! ONLINE

   Customizable 4-week starter
   and intermediate resistance-
   training programs

7. Observe safety
   precautions when
   resistance training.

   SEE IT! ONLINE

   More than 100 videos
   demonstrating proper
   technique and resistance-
   training safety

8. Incorporate strategies
   to avoid the risks associated with supplement use.

   SEE IT! ONLINE

   The Mitchell Re-
   port on Steroids
   in Baseball

Pre- and post-quizzes and glossary flashcards

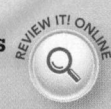
REVIEW IT! ONLINE

...a. I'm from San
...o and I'm a sophomore
...joring in economics. I'm taking
...a fitness and wellness class this
...semester, and this week we're
...the section on muscular fitness. I'm curious
...ut it because I've never lifted weights before!
I like to go hiking and I take yoga classes from time
to time, but I wouldn't call myself an athlete. Does
it really make sense for someone like me
to start a strength-training program?"

HEAR IT! ONLINE

. . . .

Whether you're a beginner like Gina or an athlete interested in conditioning, this chapter
answers common questions about muscular
fitness, explains the benefits of resistance training, and
gives you the tools for designing a program that is cus-
tom-made for you.

Muscular fitness is the ability of your musculoskeletal system to perform daily and recreational activities
without undue fatigue and injury. Muscular fitness
involves having
adequate muscular
strength and endur-
ance. **Muscular
strength** is the
ability of a muscle
or group of muscles
to contract with
maximal force.
It describes how
strong a muscle
is or how much
force it can exert.
Exercise profession-
als often measure
muscular strength
by determining the
maximum weight

muscular fitness The ability of
your musculoskeletal system to
perform daily and recreational
activities without undue fatigue
and injury

muscular strength The ability of
a muscle to contract with maximal
force

muscular endurance The
ability of a muscle to contract
repeatedly over an extended
period of time

resistance training Controlled
and progressive stressing of the
body's musculoskeletal system
using resistance (i.e., weights,
resistance bands, body weight)
exercises to build and maintain
muscular fitness

a person can lift at one time. **Muscular endurance** is
the ability of a muscle to contract repeatedly over an
extended period of time. It describes how long you can
sustain a given type of muscular exertion. One way that
fitness professionals measure muscular endurance is by
determining the maximum weight a person can lift 20
times consecutively.

You can build better muscular strength and endurance through resistance training. **Resistance training**
is also referred to as *weight training* or *strength training*
and can be done with measured weights, body weight,
or other resistive equipment (i.e., exercise bands or exercise balls). Resistance exercises stress the body's musculoskeletal system, which enlarges muscle fibers and
improves neural control of muscle function, resulting in
greater muscular strength and endurance.

Are you already participating in a resistance-training
program? If so, you are not alone. In 2008, 22–27 percent of
adults over the age of 18 reported regular participation in
muscular strength and endurance activities.[1] The numbers
are up from 1998, when 18 percent of adults reported participating in muscle fitness activities and 2004, when 17.5
percent of women and 21.5 percent of men reported regular
resistance training.[2] However, participation numbers are
still much lower than the *Healthy People 2020* target: 30
percent of adults participating in muscle strengthening
exercises two or more times per week.[3] If you are not participating, now may be the perfect time to start because
facilities and classes are readily available at most colleges
and universities and you may have a group of peers who
want to support each other in getting fit and healthy.

Resistance training offers such varied benefits that
exercise professionals recommend it in nearly all health-
related fitness programs. Regular resistance training can
make daily activities easier: carrying around a backpack
full of heavy textbooks won't tire you as much; bringing
in a bag of groceries will be less taxing; and taking the
stairs will seem natural and feel better than riding in an
elevator. No matter what your age or goals, resistance
training is an important part of staying healthy and functional throughout your life.

How Do My Muscles Work?

The human body contains hundreds of muscles, each of
which belongs to one of three basic types: (1) voluntary
skeletal muscle, which allows movement of the skeleton and generates body heat; (2) involuntary *cardiac
muscle*, which exists only in the heart and facilitates the
pumping of blood through the body; and (3) involuntary

smooth muscle, which lines some internal organs and moves food through the stomach and intestines. Resistance training and cardiorespiratory exercises benefit your skeletal and cardiac muscles. Here we focus on skeletal muscles and the signals from the nervous system that coordinate and control their contraction.

An Overview of Skeletal Muscle

Each skeletal muscle is surrounded by a sheet of connective tissue that draws together at the ends of the muscle, forming the **tendons** (see Figure 4.1). Muscular contractions allow for skeletal movement because muscles are attached to bones via tendons. These attached muscles pull the bones, which pivot at joints, creating a specific body movement.

Within each skeletal muscle are individual muscle cells called **muscle fibers**. Bundles of muscle fibers are called *fascicles.* Each muscle fiber extends the full length of the muscle. Within each muscle fiber are many **myofibrils**, each containing contractile protein filaments. These filaments are made up of two kinds of protein—*actin* and *myosin*—which partially overlap at rest and give the whole cell a striped appearance. The microscopic structure and function of actin and myosin

allow them to slide across each other and shorten the muscle. You can picture this sliding and shortening as similar to the way your forearms can slide past each other inside the front pocket of a hooded sweatshirt, pulling your elbows closer together. Simultaneous shortening of the many fibers within a whole muscle causes the pattern of muscular tension we call *contraction*. It is this whole-muscle contraction that moves bones and surrounding body parts.

Every muscle fiber can be categorized as either *slow* or *fast,* depending on how quickly it can contract. **Slow-twitch muscle fibers** (Type I) depend on oxygen and contract relatively slowly, but can contract for longer periods of time without fatigue. In slow-twitch fibers, the energy for contraction primarily comes from the breakdown of fat from the blood, muscle cells, and adipose

tendons The connective tissues attaching muscle to bone

muscle fibers The cells of the muscular system

myofibrils Thin strands within a single muscle fiber that bundle the skeletal muscle protein filaments and span the length of the fiber

slow-twitch muscle fibers Muscle fiber type that is oxygen dependent and can contract over long periods of time

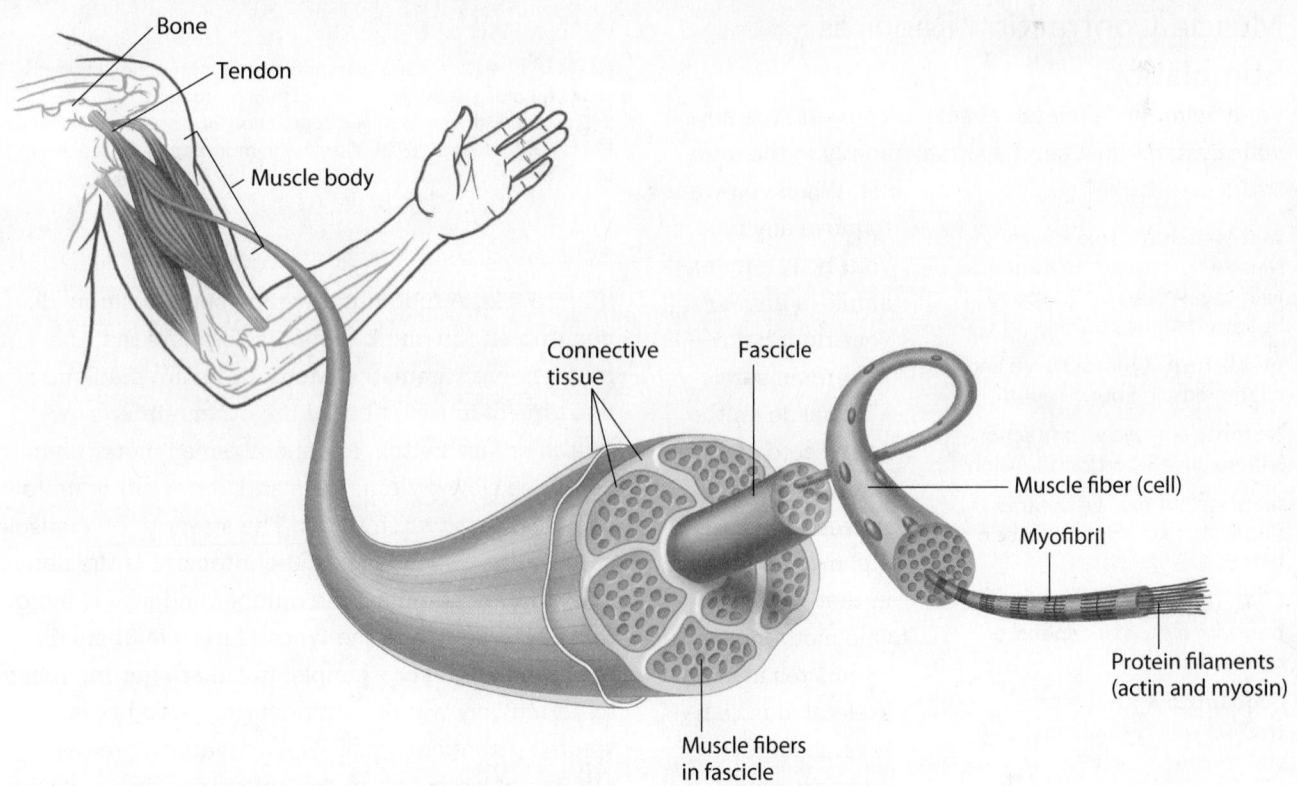

FIGURE 4.1 Muscle is attached to bones via tendons. Tendons are a continuation of the connective tissue that surrounds the entire muscle as well as each muscle bundle (fascicle). A fascicle is made up of many muscle cells (muscle fibers). Within each muscle fiber, myofibril strands contain actin and myosin proteins.

tissue. For efficient fat breakdown, oxygen and minimal levels of glucose breakdown are required. **Fast-twitch muscle fibers** (Type II) are not oxygen-dependent and contract more rapidly than slow-twitch fibers, but tire relatively quickly (they also produce greater muscle power). In fast-twitch fibers, the energy for contraction primarily comes from phosphocreatine and glycogen reserves within the muscles, glycogen stored within the liver, and glucose in the blood.

All fiber types exist in skeletal muscles, but some muscles within the body (such as postural trunk muscles) have more slow-twitch fibers, while other muscles (such as those in the calves) have more fast-twitch fibers. The proportion of muscle fiber types varies from person to person based on both genetics and training. Elite athletes have muscle fiber compositions that complement their sport. Marathoners, for instance, have higher levels of slow-twitch fibers that supply them with optimal muscular endurance. Power weight lifters, on the other hand, have more fast-twitch fibers that allow feats of enormous muscular strength over short periods of time. Sedentary individuals and people who do general resistance training typically have 50 percent slow-twitch and 50 percent fast-twitch fiber composition.

Muscle Contraction Requires Stimulation

For a voluntary skeletal muscle to contract, the nervous system must send a signal directly to the muscle. When you want to move any part of your body—for example, a finger on your right hand—your brain sends a signal down the spinal cord and through motor nerves to the skeletal muscle fibers in that finger. One motor nerve stimulates many skeletal muscle fibers, together creating a functional unit called a **motor unit**

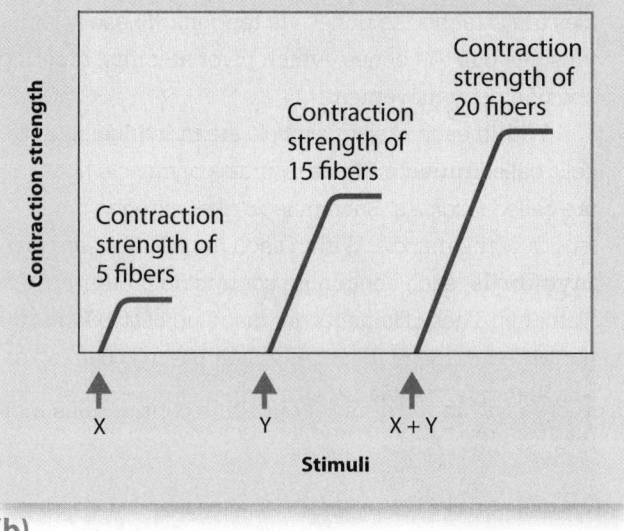

(a)

(b)

FIGURE **4.2** Motor units and muscle contraction strength. (a) Motor unit X is smaller (5 fibers) than motor unit Y (15 fibers). (b) The strength of a muscular contraction increases with increased fibers per motor unit (X vs. Y) and with more motor units activated (X + Y).

(Figure 4.2). A motor unit can be small or large, depending on the number of muscle fibers that the motor nerve stimulates. Motor units are made up of one type of muscle fiber or the other, either slow-twitch or fast-twitch. In general, small motor units comprise slow-twitch fibers and larger motor units comprise fast-twitch fibers. The strength of a muscle contraction depends upon the intensity of the nervous system stimulus, the number and size of motor units activated, and the types of muscle fibers that are stimulated. For example, if you are getting ready to lift a heavy weight, your central nervous system sends a stronger signal. This activates a greater number of large, fast motor units, resulting in a more forceful muscle contraction than if you were merely picking up an apple.

fast-twitch muscle fibers Muscle fiber type that contracts with greater force and speed but also fatigues quickly

motor unit A motor nerve and all the muscle fibers it controls

isotonic A muscle contraction with relatively constant tension

isometric A muscle contraction with no change in muscle length

isokinetic A muscle contraction with a constant speed of contraction

concentric A muscle contraction with overall muscle shortening

eccentric A muscle contraction with overall muscle lengthening

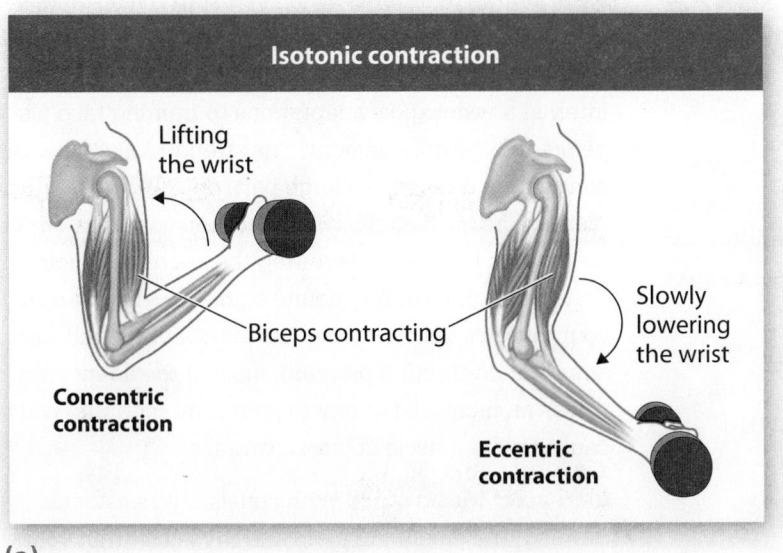

Isotonic contraction

Lifting the wrist

Biceps contracting

Concentric contraction

Slowly lowering the wrist

Eccentric contraction

(a)

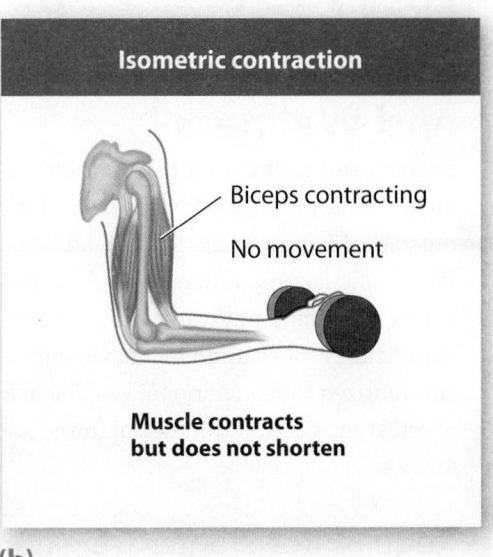

Isometric contraction

Biceps contracting

No movement

Muscle contracts but does not shorten

(b)

FIGURE **4.3** (a) Isotonic contractions include concentric (shortening) and eccentric (lengthening) contractions. (b) Isometric contractions produce force in the muscle with no movement.

Three Primary Types of Muscle Contractions

Muscle contractions all result in an increase in tension or force within the muscle, but some contractions move body parts while others do not. There are three primary types of contractions: isotonic, isometric, and isokinetic. **Isotonic** contractions are characterized by a consistent muscle tension as the contraction proceeds and a resulting movement of body parts (Figure 4.3a). An arm curl with a 10-pound hand weight involves isotonic contractions throughout your arm. **Isometric** contractions are characterized by a consistent muscle length throughout the contraction with no visible movement of body parts. An example of an isometric contraction occurs when you hold a hand weight at arm's length in front of you; your arm is not moving, but you feel tension in your arm muscles (Figure 4.3b). **Isokinetic** contractions are characterized by a consistent muscle contraction speed within a moving body part. In order to perform isokinetic contractions, you need specialized equipment that holds the speed of movement constant as your arm, leg, or other muscles contract with varying forces.

Isotonic contractions are the most common in exercise programs. Lifting free weights, working on machines, and doing push-ups are all examples of isotonic contractions. Isotonic contractions can be either concentric or eccentric. **Concentric** contractions occur when force is developed in the muscle as the muscle is shortening—for example, when you curl a free weight up toward your shoulder. In **eccentric** muscle

contractions, force remains in the muscle while the muscle is lengthening. This occurs as you lower a free weight back to its original position. Figure 4.3a illustrates these muscular contractions, using a bicep-curl exercise as an example.

casestudy

GINA

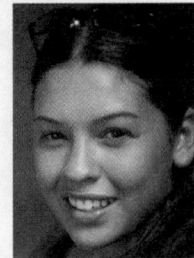

"I love to go on short hikes. There are some gorgeous trails in the San Francisco Bay Area. Some of them are hilly but I don't mind—the views from the top are always worth it. My calves definitely get a workout! I'd like to be able to do longer hikes, but the truth is that I usually get tired after about three miles. I know there are some longer hikes with spectacular views, but I don't feel ready for them yet."

THINK! Given what you've learned so far, what would you tell Gina about how resistance training can benefit her? Which type of muscle fibers would you guess that Gina has more of: slow-twitch fibers or fast-twitch fibers?

ACT! Go outside and enjoy a favorite activity. During the activity, name the muscle contractions that occur: are they isotonic or isometric contractions?

HEAR IT! ONLINE

How Can Regular Resistance Training Improve My Fitness and Wellness?

People used to think that weight lifting was solely a means of improving body shape and producing bigger muscles. We now know that, in addition to improving physical appearance, resistance training can also result in specific physiological changes that have significant fitness and wellness benefits. Figure 4.4 summarizes these changes. We discuss the benefits of resistance training in detail in the section that follows.

Regular Resistance Training Increases Your Strength

Regular resistance training with an adequate load, or amount of weight lifted, will result in an increase in muscle strength. Although men tend to realize greater gains in muscle size due to higher testosterone levels, women often have a larger capacity to improve relative strength over time.[4] Stronger lower- and upper-body muscles benefit both men and women.

hypertrophy An increase in muscle cross-sectional area

Neural Improvements When you start a resistance-training program, you will gain muscular strength before noticing any increase in muscle size. This is because internal physiological adaptations to training take place before muscle enlargement. The strength of a muscular contraction depends, in large part, on effective recruitment of the motor units needed for that contraction. The better your body is at recruiting the necessary motor units through voluntary neural signaling, the stronger your muscles will be. In the first few weeks or months of a resistance-training program, most of the adaptation involves an increased ability to recruit motor units, which causes more muscle fibers to contract.

Increased Muscle Size With consistent resistance training, the amount of actin and myosin within your muscle fibers increases. This results in **hypertrophy**, an increase in the size or cross-sectional area of the protein filaments. With more contractile proteins, a muscle can contract more forcefully; in other words, larger muscles are stronger muscles. While both slow- and fast-twitch muscles will increase in size with resistance training, greater increases in strength will result from hypertrophy of fast-twitch muscle fibers.

Muscle hypertrophy in response to resistance training takes longer than neural improvements, but

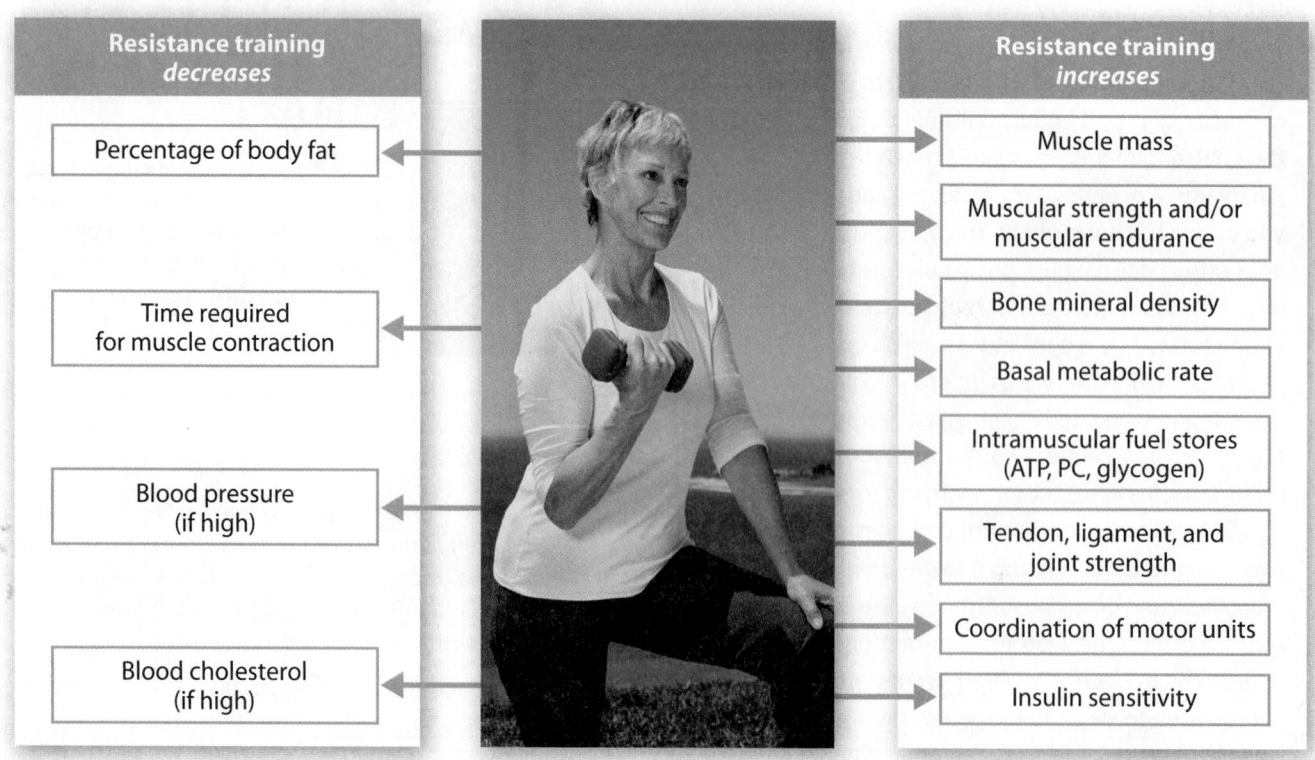

Resistance training *decreases*		Resistance training *increases*
Percentage of body fat		Muscle mass
Time required for muscle contraction		Muscular strength and/or muscular endurance
		Bone mineral density
		Basal metabolic rate
Blood pressure (if high)		Intramuscular fuel stores (ATP, PC, glycogen)
		Tendon, ligament, and joint strength
		Coordination of motor units
Blood cholesterol (if high)		Insulin sensitivity

FIGURE **4.4** Physiological changes from resistance training.

is the most important contributor to strength gains over time. The degree of hypertrophy or enlargement you can expect with weight training depends upon your gender, age, genetics, and how you design your training program. Some individuals will develop larger muscles more quickly than others; some will experience only limited hypertrophy. In particular, women and men with smaller builds will realize less muscle development than those with larger builds, even with identical training programs (see the box What Are the Benefits of Strength Training for Women?). Older individuals will also have slower progress and overall less muscle development, though they can still see significant improvements.

A program with heavier weights, longer durations, or more frequent training can produce greater gains than a more standard fitness-training program. People who stop resistance training will experience some degree of **atrophy**, a shrinking of the muscle to its pretraining size and strength. To avoid atrophy, you need to make a long-term commitment to resistance training.

Regular Resistance Training Increases Your Muscular Endurance

Muscular endurance helps you perform both cardiorespiratory activities, such as hiking and running, and muscular fitness activities, such as circuit or sports training. In fact, just doing these activities will improve your muscular endurance. Muscular endurance exercises trigger physiological adaptations that improve your ability to regenerate ATP efficiently and thus sustain muscular contractions for a longer period of time. The end result will be the ability to snowboard a long run instead of having to rest halfway down; to walk up three flights of stairs with ease; or to rake leaves vigorously for an hour without difficulty.

Regular Resistance Training Improves Your Body Composition, Weight Management, and Body Image

Improved body composition is an important outcome of resistance training: the amount of lean muscle tissue increases, the amount of fat tissue decreases, and thus the ratio of lean to fat improves. Research has demonstrated that such higher lean-to-fat ratios improve your overall health profile and reduce your risk of heart attack, diabetes, and death from cardiovascular diseases.[5] Fat does not turn into muscle or vice versa; the number of fat and muscle cells remains the same, with cells merely enlarging or shrinking depending on food intake and activity levels.

atrophy A decrease in muscle cross-sectional area

More muscle means a faster metabolic rate; pound for pound, muscle tissue expends more energy than fat tissue.[6] With more total calories being expended during the day, weight control becomes easier and more effective.[7] Resistance training should be combined with aerobic exercise for overall weight loss,[8] but resistance training during weight loss helps ensure that you will lose fat and not precious muscle tissue;[9] your body can be lighter, stronger, and leaner (i.e., more toned) instead of just lighter (and potentially still flabby), as often happens with traditional diet-only weight-loss methods.

When you begin a resistance-training program, you may experience a slight initial weight gain as muscle tissue grows. If you focus only on the scale, this can be discouraging. It is better to focus on how much stronger and more toned your muscles feel. With a consistent fitness and nutrition program, fat loss will eventually "catch up" to muscle gain and will be reflected in weight loss as well. Since muscle tissue is more compact than fat tissue, your body size will gradually decrease over time as muscles become toned and fat tissues shrink. This, in turn, can improve your body image. In one study, college students realized measurable increases in overall body image after circuit weight training (a form of resistance training) for six weeks.[10]

Regular Resistance Training Strengthens Your Bones and Protects Your Body from Injuries

Bone health is an important issue for everyone, from children to older adults. Osteoporosis-related fractures are common among older women and men and can cause dramatic decreases in a person's mobility, independence, and quality of life. By putting stress and controlled-weight loads on the muscles, joint structures, and supporting bones, resistance training

What Are the Benefits of Strength Training for Women?

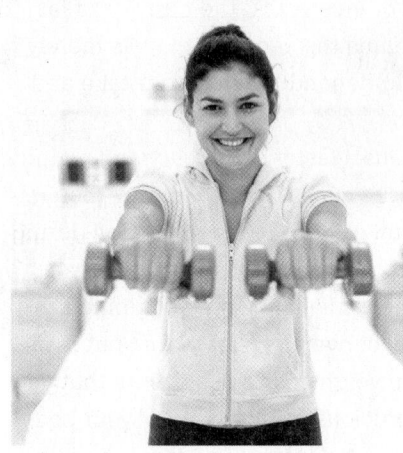

College-age men are much more likely to participate in strength training than college-age women (47% for men and 28% for women, ages 18–24).[1] Although fewer women in the United States engage in strength-training than men overall, the gap narrows as people age; 16 percent of men and 11 percent of women over 75 years of age report strength training activities. Despite this gender gap, the benefits of strength training for women are just as great as men. Many of these benefits are especially appealing to women for reasons that may differ from men. For example, strength training promotes stronger bones and this helps prevent osteoporosis in the long-term, something women are at a greater risk for than men.[2,3] In addition, the maintenance of lean tissue helps you keep your functional independence as you age; this is another long-term risk for women.[4,5] Immediate benefits of weight training include reduced body fat and greater ability to control body weight; improved stamina and decreased fatigue; better sleep and less insomnia; and increased self-confidence, body image, and sense of well-being. Plus, there is a bonus for your weekend and vacation plans! People who strength train also find that their ability to enjoy recreational activities and sports—playing ultimate Frisbee, for example—improves.

Now let's address common myths about strength training for women.

Myth 1: Women don't benefit much from resistance exercise. It's true that on average, men's muscles are larger and more powerful than women's; men produce 5 to 10 times more testosterone, which promotes muscle development. Men's nervous systems also signal muscle contraction more rapidly, producing greater power. Because they have more total muscle tissue, men's absolute strength is greater than women's. However, when muscle mass is compared pound for pound, women are equally strong. Women will increase strength and muscle endurance through strength training, just as men do.

Myth 2: Strength training will cause women to "bulk up." In truth, women who do regular resistance training rarely look heavily muscled. Very few women build large, bulky muscles without major effort (or the use of dangerous steroid drugs) because they have different natural hormone levels than men. Strength training will make your muscles leaner and, with additional strategies for fat loss, you can even "slim down" if that is your goal!

Myth 3: The weight room is a place primarily for men. Some women find it intimidating to go to a weight room. It is true that weight rooms can be dominated by men who seem to know exactly what they are doing. Although men typically lift greater amounts of weight and seem to have different training strategies than most women, many will welcome new weight training participants of both genders. Once you are comfortable, ask to join in on a set of exercises with a group. Many women also find it helpful to go to the gym with a friend (man or woman) who has similar resistance-training goals. This is a great motivation tip for everyone. You can also go to the gym when it's less busy, find an instructor for guidance, do strength training at home, or try a gym exclusively for women. Whatever it takes, begin strength training to experience the amazing benefits throughout your life, it's worth it!

THINK! What's keeping you from strength training? What obstacles are preventing you from going to the weight room?

ACT! Write down your obstacles to strength training (in a weight room or at home). Now figure out and write down a way you can tackle each one!

Sources:
1. Centers for Disease Control (CDC), "QuickStats: Percentage of Adults Aged ≥18 Years Who Engaged in Leisure-Time Strengthening Activities, by Age Group and Sex—National Health Interview Survey, United States, 2008," *Morbidity and Mortality Weekly Report* 58, no. 34 (2009): 955.
2. A. Guadalupe-Grau and others, "Exercise and Bone Mass in Adults," *Sports Medicine* 39, no. 6 (2009): 439–68.
3. J. E. Layne and M. E. Nelson, "The Effects of Progressive Resistance Training on Bone Density: A Review," *Medicine and Science in Sports and Exercise* 31, no. 1 (1999): 25–30.
4. K. Ogawa and others, "Resistance Exercise Training-Induced Muscle Hypertrophy Was Associated with Reduction of Inflammatory Markers in Elderly Women" *Mediators of Inflammation* 2010 (2010).
5. M. D. Phillips and others, "Resistance Training at Eight-Repetition Maximum Reduces the Inflammatory Milieu in Elderly Women," *Medicine and Science in Sports and Exercise* 42, no. 2 (2010): 314–25.

stimulates muscle tissue growth and the generation of harder, stronger bones, thereby reducing the risk of fracture.

Building strong bones is especially important in the period starting with childhood skeletal growth and development and ending at about age 30. The "reservoir" of bone tissue you lay down in those years and then maintain throughout life will help prevent weak, brittle bones as you age. Even the bones of older individuals can benefit from strength training; in one study, eight months of resistance training positively affected hip bone density in older women, whereas no change occurred with moderate-impact aerobic exercise over the same time period.[11]

Getting hurt will put you on the sidelines. Whether you exercise for fun, fitness, or competition, preventing injuries is a key to continued participation. Injury prevention tips are often specific to your chosen activity; however, strong muscles, bones, and connective tissues are the common denominator for preventing injury in any activity. Regular resistance training improves not only muscular strength and endurance, but also the strength of tendons, ligaments, and other supporting structures around each joint. As they grow stronger, the joints themselves are better protected from injury. A stronger body can handle the physical stresses of everyday life (carrying heavy books or groceries, lifting laundry baskets, moving furniture, etc.)

with less chance of injury. A strong, pain-free back and proper posture are crucial to daily functioning without injury. Individuals who participate in regular resistance-training exercise have stronger postural muscles and report less low back pain.

Imbalanced muscles around a joint may result in a change in joint alignment with subsequent pain or injury. Muscular balance will reduce this risk. A well-designed muscle fitness program will work toward improving strength and muscle endurance in opposing muscular groups, promoting overall muscle balance.

Regular Resistance Training Helps Maintain Your Physical Function with Aging

Starting between the ages of 25 and 30, men and women begin to lose muscle mass. As they age, they lose up to one-third of their muscle mass due to changes in hormones, activity levels, and nutrition. Injury and chronic diseases can cause people to exercise less and accelerate typical muscle loss. **Sarcopenia**, literally "poverty of flesh," is the term applied to this age-related loss in skeletal muscle (see Figure 4.5).

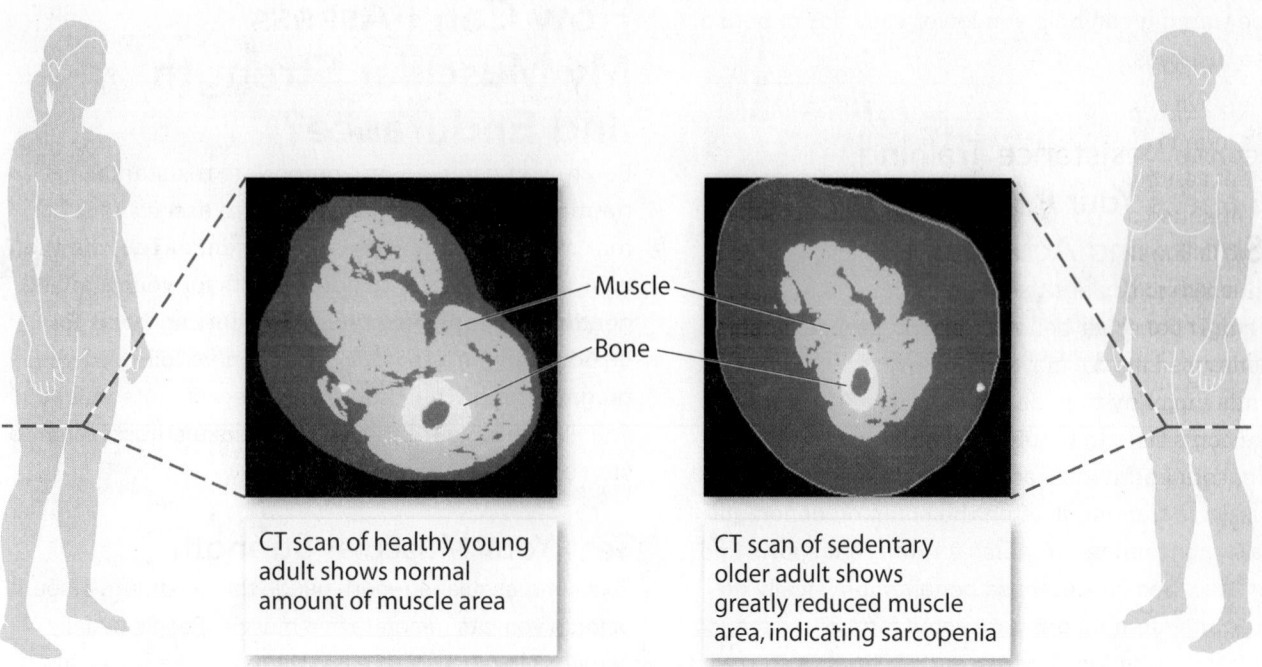

CT scan of healthy young adult shows normal amount of muscle area

CT scan of sedentary older adult shows greatly reduced muscle area, indicating sarcopenia

Muscle
Bone

FIGURE **4.5** CT scans showing the difference in muscle mass in a healthy young adult vs. an older adult with sarcopenia. Age-related muscle loss can be slowed with resistance training.

Sarcopenia reduces overall physical functioning by decreasing muscular strength and endurance and causing losses in **muscle power**, or the capacity to exert force rapidly. While no one is immune from the aging process, resistance training throughout one's life can significantly slow natural muscle loss. In fact, older individuals who do resistance training can show a rate of improvement equal to that of younger people. The increase in muscular fitness and the improvements it brings to everyday physical functioning help individuals live independently for a longer portion of their lives.

Regular Resistance Training Helps Reduce Your Cardiovascular Disease Risk

Regular resistance training can lower your risk of cardiovascular disease by increasing blood flow to working muscles and vital tissues throughout your body. In fact, people who perform regular resistance-training exercise have lower blood pressure and blood cholesterol readings than sedentary people. Since being overfat (having a higher than recommended percentage of body fat) increases your risk of cardiovascular disease and adult-onset diabetes, an improved body composition achieved through resistance training can help you lower your risk of both of these diseases.

Regular Resistance Training Enhances Your Performance in Sports and Activities

Achieving muscular fitness through resistance training has yet another benefit: A stronger body is more resistant to fatigue, moves more quickly, and recovers more quickly from illness or injury. All of these traits contribute to better performance in sports, recreational activities, and other fitness pursuits. Resistance training is often the common denominator among training programs for different sports and activities. Because of these benefits, physically active adults often incorporate some form of resistance training that builds strength and endurance in the muscle groups most crucial to their sport.

casestudy

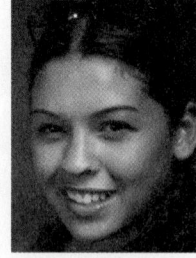

GINA

"I've always wanted to hike to the top of Nevada Falls in Yosemite National Park. I'm told that it can be done as a day hike, but it is about seven miles round trip. There is also a steep section of rocks near another waterfall along the way— apparently you get completely soaked while hiking that part of the trail! Even on dry trails, I'm always extra careful hiking downhill, because I once sprained my ankle on a hike, which was not fun.

If resistance training can help me take on Nevada Falls, I'm interested. I've also always wished I had better muscle tone, but to be honest, I don't want to 'bulk up' . . . "

THINK! Name at least two ways that resistance training can help Gina realize her goal of safely hiking to the top of Nevada Falls. How would you respond to Gina's concerns about "bulking up"?

ACT! What's your "Nevada Falls"? That is, what is something you have always wanted to do, if only you were in better physical shape? Write down your ideas and post the note somewhere you can see it each day for motivation. Start an action plan to reach your goal!

HEAR IT! ONLINE

How Can I Assess My Muscular Strength and Endurance?

Before you can plan an appropriate resistance-training program, it is important to assess your current muscular strength and endurance. You can then compare the results to norm charts for your age and gender, or simply use them as a starting point for designing your program. After you've followed your program for a while, follow-up assessments will help you evaluate your progress and make adjustments to stay on track.

Test Your Muscular Strength

Tests of muscular strength gauge the maximum amount of force you can generate in a muscle. People usually carry out these tests in a weight room where measured weights of all sizes are readily available.

1 RM Tests **One repetition maximum (1 RM)** tests are the most common tool fitness instructors and personal trainers use to assess their clients' muscular strength. To participate in the tests safely, you must be medically cleared to lift heavier weights than you have in the past, have detailed instructions for the test procedure, know general weight-training guidelines, have a few weeks of weight-training experience, and have qualified **spotters** standing nearby to watch and assist if necessary. If you are weight training on campus or at a gym, an instructor will be able to help you through these preliminary steps.

These 1 RM tests are performed by discovering the maximum amount of weight you can lift one time on a particular exercise. You must accurately determine your 1 RM within three to five trials so that muscle fatigue from repetitions does not change your result. In general health and fitness classes or beginning weight-training programs, instructors often tell students to predict their 1 RM instead of actually attempting a maximum lift. This is particularly true when students are new to resistance training and unfamiliar with weight-training guidelines. To predict your 1 RM, you will lift, press, or pull a weight that will fully fatigue your upper- or lower-body muscles in 2 to 10 repetitions. You can then use a formula that

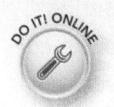

converts actual weight lifted and real number of repetitions to a prediction of your 1 RM capacity for that exercise. In **Lab 4.1** (at the back of this chapter), you will use chest-press and leg-press exercises to determine your predicted 1 RM. You can perform these tests for any weight-training exercise and then convert to the predicted 1 RM value. Many weight-training programs use a percentage of your 1 RM or predicted 1 RM to determine a safe starting level for weight lifting.

Grip Strength Test Another common test of muscle strength is the hand grip strength test using a piece of equipment called a *grip strength dynamometer*. As you squeeze the dynamometer (with one hand at a time), it measures the static or isometric strength of your grip-squeezing muscles in pounds or kilograms (kg).

Test Your Muscular Endurance

Muscular endurance tests evaluate a muscle's ability to contract for an extended period of time. Some of these tests must be performed in a weight room, whereas others require only your body weight for resistance and can be performed anywhere.

20 RM Tests You can use any weight-training exercise to find your **20 repetition maximum (20 RM).** This test determines the maximal amount of weight you can lift exactly 20 times in a row before the muscle becomes too fatigued to continue. Twenty repetition maximum tests are particularly useful for setting muscular endurance goals and then tracking your progress. Try to discover your 20 RM within one to three tries to avoid fatiguing your muscles and altering your results. **Lab 4.2** walks you through the steps of finding your 20 RM for the chest-press and leg-press exercises.

Calisthenic Tests **Calisthenics** are conditioning exercises that use your body weight for resistance. Calisthenic tests use sit-ups, curl-ups, pull-ups, push-ups, and flexed arm support/hang exercises to assess muscular endurance. The procedures for these tests vary. You will learn how to perform curl-up and push-up assessments in Lab 4.2. Calisthenic tests allow you to test yourself outside of a weight-training facility and to compare your results to well-established physical fitness norms.

How Can I Design My Own Resistance-Training Program?

Designing an effective resistance-training program takes some knowledge, and many people enlist the help of a personal trainer or fitness professional. You can become your own personal trainer, however, by using the guidelines in this section to plan a safe and effective muscular fitness program.

Set Appropriate Muscular Fitness Goals

Remember to use SMART goal-setting guidelines: Goals should be *specific*, *measurable*, *action-oriented*, and *realistic* and should have a *timeline*. Your goals may be appearance-based, function-based, or a combination of the two.

Appearance-Based Goals Many people have appearance-based goals for muscular fitness: they want larger muscles, or muscles that are more toned and less flabby. "Spot reduction" (i.e., trimming down just one area of the body) is another often-voiced goal. Researchers have proven spot-reduction to be a myth. Several carefully controlled studies show that fat doesn't disappear through repeated exercise to one area.[12]

In order to judge your progress toward appearance-based goals, be sure to include some sort of measure of progress in your resistance-training plan. For muscle size, measure the circumference of your biceps or calves, for example, and then set a goal to increase or decrease this number. For overall body size, your goal may be to increase lean tissue weight but decrease fat tissue and percentage of body fat. If your goal is to become more "toned," quantify this in some way. Look in the mirror and make notes about the way your body looks and moves. After you reach the target date for your plan, reread your notes, look in the mirror, and then reevaluate whether your muscle tone has improved.

Function-Based Goals Include some specific goals for improving muscle function in your fitness plan. Function-based goals focus on your muscular capabilities and include gaining better muscular strength, greater muscular endurance, or both. **Lab 4.3** will guide you in setting goals for realistic changes in muscle function, and then help you to assess your improvements.

Explore Your Equipment Options

Should you use weight machines in your resistance-training program? Free weights? Other equipment? No equipment at all? These are important decisions, and they will be determined by your fitness goals, the type of equipment available to you, your experience with weight-training exercises, and your preferences.

dumbbells Weights intended for use by one hand; typically one uses a dumbbell in each hand

barbells Long bars with weight plates on each end

many others allow you to isolate and strengthen specific muscle groups as well as to train without a spotting partner.

Free Weights Personal trainers and exercise physiologists consider free-weight exercises to be a more advanced approach to weight training than machine-weight exercises. Free-weight exercises use **dumbbells**; **barbells**; incline, flat, or decline benches; squat racks; and related equipment. Free-weight exercises allow your body to move through its natural range of motion instead of the path predetermined by a weight machine. This both requires and promotes development of more muscle control. Some athletes prefer free-weight exercises because the balance and movement patterns needed to successfully lift free weights are closer to their sport movement patterns, whether that be tossing a football, putting a shot, or doing the breaststroke. Since workout facilities often have both free weights and weight machines, many people start their resistance-training program exclusively with machine-weight exercises and then progress to free weights within the first few months. Table 4.1 compares machine-weight training and free-weight training.

Alternate Equipment You can increase resistance on your body with equipment other than machines or free weights. Resistance bands made of tubing or flat strips of rubber allow you to simultaneously increase resistance throughout a range of motion and to improve muscular endurance. You can perform many different exercises with these bands. They fold up and pack perfectly in a suitcase or gym bag for a portable workout. Stability balls (also called Swiss, fitness, or exercise balls) are 18-inch to 30-inch diameter vinyl balls that have various uses for muscular fitness, endurance, and balance. Ball routines involve performing exercises while sitting, lying, and/or balancing on the ball. The ball exerciser must use core trunk muscles to counteract the natural instability of the ball, which enhances overall body function. People sometimes use heavily weighted balls called medicine balls to increase resistance, either individually, with a partner, or in a group. You can hold a medicine ball while doing calisthenic or free-weight exercises or pass a ball from partner to partner for a functional increase in muscle endurance.

No-Equipment Training Calisthenics such as push-ups, pull-ups, lunges, squats, leg lifts, and curl-ups do not involve equipment. Instead, they use your body weight to provide the resistance. Like resistance bands, these exercises are perfect for maintaining muscular strength and endurance while traveling.

Machines If you are new to resistance training, weight machines can be very useful. Systems such as Cybex®, Nautilus®, Life Fitness®, and

TABLE 4.1 Machine-Weight vs. Free-Weight Training	
Machine Weights	Free Weights
PROS	PROS
Safe and less intimidating for beginners	Can be tailored for individual workouts
Quicker to set up and use	Range of motion set by lifter, not machine
Spotters not typically needed	Some exercises can be done anywhere
Support of standing posture not needed	Standing and sitting postural muscles worked
Adaptable for those with limitations	Movements can transfer to daily activities
Variable resistance is possible	Good for strength and power building
Good isolation of specific muscle groups	Additional stabilizer muscles worked
Only good option for some muscle groups	Lower cost and more available for home use
CONS	CONS
Machine sets range of motion	More difficult to learn
May not fit every body size and type	A spotter may be needed
Some people lack access to weight machines	Incorrect form may lead to injuries
Posture supporting muscles used less	More time may be needed to change weights
Limited number of exercises/machines	More training needed to create program

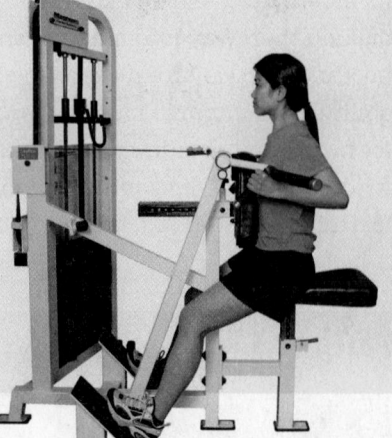
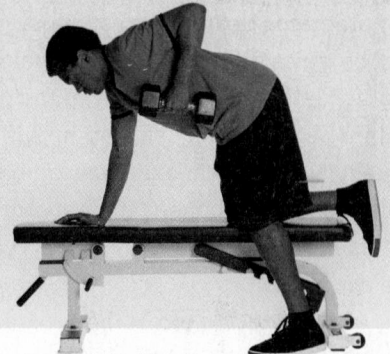

Understand the Different Types of Resistance-Training Programs

You can plan a resistance-training program with various types of equipment and numerous exercise routines. The right program for you will be determined by your goals, experience, and personal preference.

Traditional Weight Training Traditional weight training takes place in a weight room and usually includes a combination of machine-weight, free-weight, and calisthenic exercises. Individuals may work alone or with a partner and will usually perform multiple **sets** and **repetitions** of a particular exercise before moving on to the next exercise. Guidelines for setting up your traditional weight training program are outlined in the next section and sample traditional weight training programs are available at the end of the chapter.

Circuit Weight Training Circuit weight training is done in a specialized circuit-training room, a general workout room, or a weight room. Exercisers move from one station to another in a set pattern (the "circuit") after a certain amount of time at a station or after performing a certain number of repetitions of an exercise such as a biceps curl, leg press, or chest press. Some circuits include only resistance-training exercises and have the single goal of improving muscular fitness. Some circuits involve cardiorespiratory or aerobic training equipment, such as stair-steppers or stationary bicycles, mixed in with the resistance exercises to improve both cardiorespiratory and muscular fitness.

sets Single attempts at an exercise that include a fixed number of repetitions

repetitions The number of times an exercise is performed within one set

In circuit training, it is important to remember the specificity training principle: In order to get optimal muscle fitness benefits, you must focus on the resistance exercises; in order to realize added cardiorespiratory benefits, you must spend a minimal amount of time on the cardio machines (20 to 30 minutes total per exercise session).

Circuit exercises should be organized properly in order to ensure a safe and effective exercise session. For example, multi-joint exercises (bench press, leg press) are often performed before single-joint exercises (bicep curl, leg extension) and muscle groups worked are spread out to allow recovery between sets. Exercises that stress the core postural muscles are reserved for the end of the workout because these muscles provide important trunk support during seated and standing exercises.

Plyometrics and Sports Training Resistance-training programs designed to support specific sports can be quite different from general resistance training. Athletes may use many of the general weight-training exercises illustrated in this chapter, but they usually also perform exercises or exercise methods that specifically benefit their sports performance. Plyometrics, power lifts, and speed and agility drills are examples.

A **plyometric exercise** program incorporates explosive exercises that mimic the quick transition movements needed in many sports (e.g., basketball, wrestling, and gymnastics). These exercises are characterized by a landing and slowing down of the body mass followed immediately by a rapid movement in the opposite direction (for instance, jumping down off of a box and then immediately jumping back up as high as you can). Plyometrics is a highly specialized training method that should be performed under proper direction and only by individuals who have achieved a high level of muscular fitness.

Power lifting is a type of resistance training that incorporates fast and forceful actions to improve strength and speed. Lifting for **power** stresses the nervous system to act quickly and the tendons, ligaments, and joint structures to become more stable. Sports that require high levels of explosive movement and power (football, wrestling, gymnastics, and track-and-field events) may require power-lifting training to build strength with speed. Power lifting is a competitive sport in itself. Competitive power lifts include the bench press, the squat, the dead lift, and the Olympic lifts (the clean and jerk and the snatch). Like plyometrics, power lifting should be practiced only by experienced athletes or those with comparable weight-training experience.

The training regimens for certain athletes may include **speed** and **agility** drills. These drills are making their way into mainstream sports training and boot-camp-style group exercise classes. Speed and agility drills improve muscle responsiveness, speed, footwork, and coordination. Typical speed and agility drills include line sprints, high-knee runs, fast-foot-turnover running, and hopping quickly through

plyometric exercise An exercise that is characterized by a rapid deceleration of the body followed by a rapid acceleration of the body in the opposite direction

power The ability to produce force quickly

speed The ability to rapidly accelerate; exercises for speed will increase stride length and frequency

agility The ability to rapidly change body position or body direction without losing speed, balance, or body control

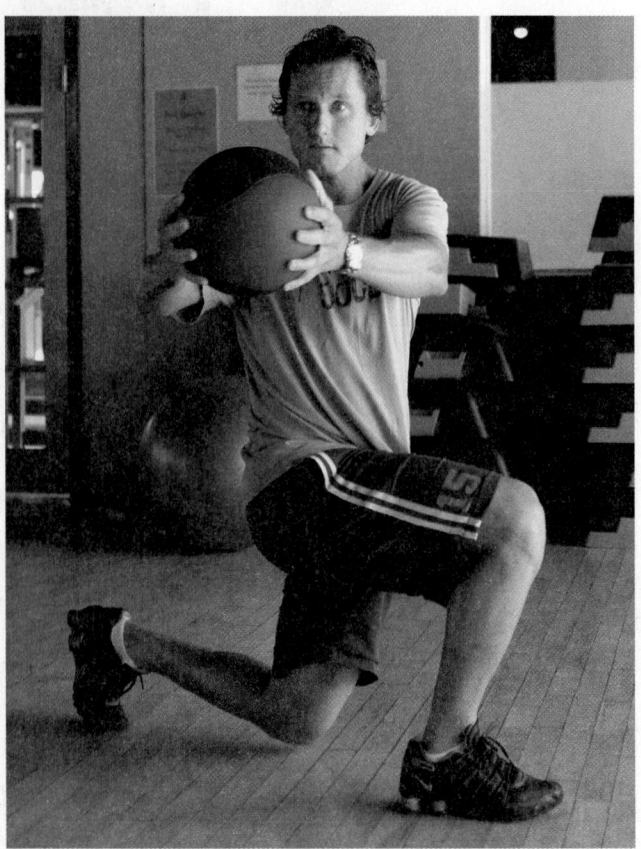

varying foot patterns (using agility dots or other markers). Speed and agility drills can be performed by anyone who is physically fit enough to learn and perform the skills. Proper instruction and modification of the drills for differing ability levels is essential to prevent injuries.

Whole-Body Exercise Programs The increasing popularity of "functional" training, training that carries over to life activities, has given rise to exercise programs that focus on whole-body exercises. These programs, such as CrossFit and kettlebell, focus on exercises that integrate various muscle groups into one exercise rather than isolate a muscle group, as do some traditional weight-room exercises. The exercises aim to address three planes of movement (forward and back, side to side, and rotational) for increased crossover into daily activities and enhanced sports and recreation performance. There has been initial evidence that this type of training can reduce neck and back pain.[13] It's not necessary to join a special gym or exercise class (although those are available) to take advantage of this type of training. Take the concepts presented in the previous section on plyometrics and sports training, think about your current resistance-training program, and integrate the concepts to add more whole-body and functional exercises. For instance, instead of limit-ing yourself to stationary lunges, add a walking forward movement with a twist to the opposite side to every lunge step.

Learn and Apply FITT Principles

FITT stands for *f*requency, *i*ntensity, *t*ime, and *t*ype. The acronym represents a checklist for determining how often, how hard, and how long to exercise, and what types of exercise to choose at your current level of muscular fitness.

Frequency of Training Your goals and your schedule determine how often you will train each week. At a minimum, you should work each muscle group twice per week. A full-body muscle workout means two sessions in the weight room each week. If you split your muscle workouts (for example, into upper body and lower body), then you would go to the weight room four times per week. Table 4.2 presents American College of Sports Medicine (ACSM) guidelines for muscular fitness programs.

It is important to let each muscle group rest for 48 hours before taxing it again with resistance training. Especially when you are just beginning, schedule your workouts so that they are at least two days apart.

When you perform an intense weight-training session, micro-damage occurs within the muscle cells

TABLE 4.2 ACSM's Guidelines for Resistance Training in Healthy Adults

Goal	Level	Intensity (% 1 RM)	Repetitions	Sets	Rest (min between sets)[b]	Frequency (days/week)[c]	Number and Types of Exercises
Improve Muscular Fitness[a]	Beginner/ novice	40–70	8–12	1–3	2–3	2–3	8–10+ emphasiz-ing multiple-joint exercises for oppos-ing muscle groups in the lower body, upper body, and trunk; add single-joint exercises as needed for muscle balance
	Intermediate/ advanced	60–80	8–12	2–4	2–3	2–3	
Increase Muscular Endurance	All levels	<50	15–25	1–2	2–3	2–3	
Further Increase Muscular Strength	Intermediate	70–80	1–12	2–4	2–3	2–5	
	Advanced	>80	1–6	2–4	2–3	2–5	

[a]Muscular strength, mass, and to some extent, muscular endurance.

[b]Rest a particular muscle group 48 hours between workout sessions

[c]2–3 days/week = total body workouts, 4–5 days/week = split routine to train each major muscle group twice per week

Data from: American College of Sports Medicine. *ACSM's Guidelines for Exercise Testing and Prescription.* 8th Edition. Baltimore, MD: Lippincott Williams & Wilkins, 2010; and Ratamess N. A., Alvar B. A., Evetovich T. K., et al. "ACSM Position Stand: Progression Models in Resistance Training for Healthy Adults," *Medicine and Science in Sports and Exercise* 341, no. 3 (2009): 687–708; C. E. Garner and others, "American College of Sports Medicine Position Stand: Quantity and Quality of Exercise for Developing and Maintaining Cardiorespiratory, Musculoskeletal, and Neuromotor Fitness in Apparently Healthy Adults: Guidance for Prescribing Exercise," *Medicine and Science in Sports and Exercise* 43, no. 7 (2011): 1334–59.

and rest time is needed for muscle repair and adaptation. Your muscles will adapt by constructing new actin and myosin contractile proteins and other supporting structures. Over time, this adaptation results in stronger, leaner, larger muscles. Intense workouts of the same muscle group on subsequent days will disrupt the repair and adaptation process. Rather than faster muscle development, this overtraining is more likely to cause injuries, muscle fatigue, and weakening. An exception can be made for lower intensity muscular fitness classes or calisthenics, which can be done daily as long as they are not overly fatiguing.

Muscle soreness that sets in within a day or two is called delayed-onset muscle soreness (DOMS); it is a sign that your body was not ready for the amount of overload you applied. Contrary to popular belief, it is not lactic acid that causes DOMS; accumulated lactic acid is cleared from the muscle cells within hours of exercise. If you choose weight amounts correctly, your muscles will sustain small amounts of micro-damage that does not result in soreness and that your body can repair within 48 hours after the workout.

Intensity of Training The intensity of a weight-training program refers to the amount of **resistance** you apply through any given exercise. For each exercise, the intensity you choose will depend on your fitness goals for that particular muscle group or your body as a whole. The ACSM guidelines in Table 4.2 for muscular fitness can help you choose weight-training

intensities (shown as a percentage of your 1 RM or percentage of predicted 1 RM).

The intensity or weight chosen for each exercise should be enough to overload the muscle group you are working; that means you should feel slight discomfort or muscle fatigue near the end of your exercise set. If you feel no fatigue during the entire set of repetitions and feel you could lift the weight another 3 to 10 times, then the intensity is too low. Aim for muscle fatigue but not complete exhaustion.

Resting between sets will affect your weight-training intensity and performance on subsequent exercises. The greater the weight you lift for strength building, the longer the rest period you may want between sets. Resting periods can be shorter for muscular endurance-building exercises. In fact, shorter rests may help build better muscular endurance.

Time: Sets and Repetitions Choosing the appropriate number of repetitions or lifts within each set is yet another important part of setting up your resistance-training program. Once again, your fitness goals help determine the number of sets you will execute for each exercise and the number of repetitions within each set. Your weight-training experience and the time you have available to work out will affect your planning as well. ACSM recommends that you perform two to four sets of each exercise during a given workout session (see Table 4.2). However, if you are new to resistance training, you will see progress with just one set per muscle group. As you progress in your resistance-training program, you can increase your sets from one to two, and eventually to three or more. You can execute two, three, or four sets for all your exercises, or perform two sets of certain exercises, three of

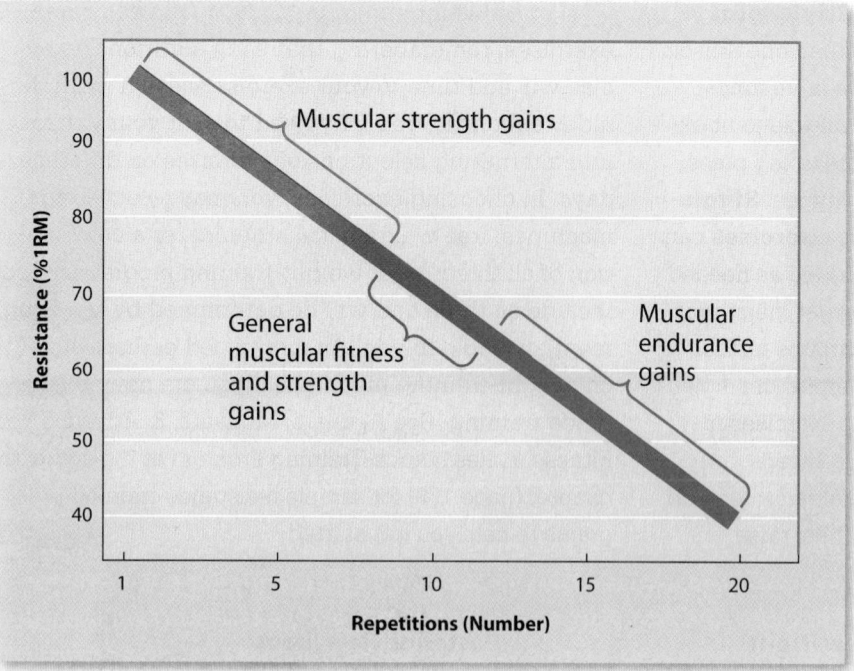

FIGURE **4.6** Fewer repetitions with higher resistance will produce gains in muscular strength. More repetitions with lower resistance will produce gains in muscular endurance.

others, and so on. Keep in mind, however, that overtraining one particular muscle group can lead to muscle imbalance and injury.

Intensity and repetitions have an inverse relationship relative to muscular strength and endurance (see Figure 4.6): For muscular strength development, you will lift heavier weights and do fewer repetitions; for muscular endurance, you will lift lighter weights with more repetitions.

Type: Choosing Appropriate Exercises Which exercises should you do during each workout session? The final part of designing a muscular fitness program is choosing exercises that will help you achieve your goals and muscle balance. Create your own muscular fitness goals in Lab 4.3 and use Figure 4.7 to start planning your resistance-training program. Next, decide which specific exercises will help you attain your muscular fitness goals: Complete **Lab 4.4** to plan a muscular fitness program using Figures 4.8 and 4.9 to assist you in exercise selection.

Muscle balance requires a selection of upper-body exercises, trunk exercises, and lower-body exercises. Choose exercises from Figure 4.9 that work *opposing muscle groups*, muscles on both the front and back of your

Determine muscular fitness goal

Increase muscular strength	Improve general muscular fitness and strength	Increase muscular endurance
Choose 5–10 key weight training exercises to do in a gym	Choose 8–10 basic resistance training exercises (full body) to do in a gym or at home	Choose 8–10 basic resistance training exercises (full body) to do in a gym or at home
Write out your plan per exercise: 60–80% 1RM 2–4 sets 8–10 reps 2–3 min rests	Write out your plan per exercise: 50–70% 1RM 1–3 sets 10–12 reps 2–3 min rests	Write out your plan per exercise: 40–50% 1RM 1–2 sets 15–20 reps 2–3 min rests

FIGURE **4.7** Use this flowchart as you design your muscular fitness program. Just starting? Begin at the lower end of all recommended ranges (for rest periods, begin at the upper end).

body. Emphasize exercises that are **multiple-joint exercises**—exercises that affect more than one muscle group—since these exercises tend to be more functional and time-efficient. Examples of multiple-joint exercises include chest press, overhead press, leg press, and lunges. **Single-joint exercises** can be added as needed to target major muscle groups further. Examples of single-joint exercises include biceps curl, lateral raise, leg curl, and heel raise.

multiple-joint exercises
Exercises that involve multiple joints and muscle groups to achieve an overall movement

single-joint exercises
Exercises that involve a single joint and typically focus on one muscle group

For a starting program, choose between 8 and 10 exercises, remembering that each additional exercise will add time to your exercise session; with too many exercises, you may need to split your workout into alternating selections of exercises on different days. In choosing exercises, you may select weight machines, free weights, calisthenics, or a combination of all three. Most weight-training programs will include all three and will be determined by the equipment available to you. As mentioned earlier, focus on weight-training machines if you are new to resistance training. See Activate, Motivate, & Advance Your Fitness: A Resistance-Training Program at the end of the chapter (page 169) for sample resistance-training programs to help you get started.

Anterior view (front)   **Posterior view (back)**

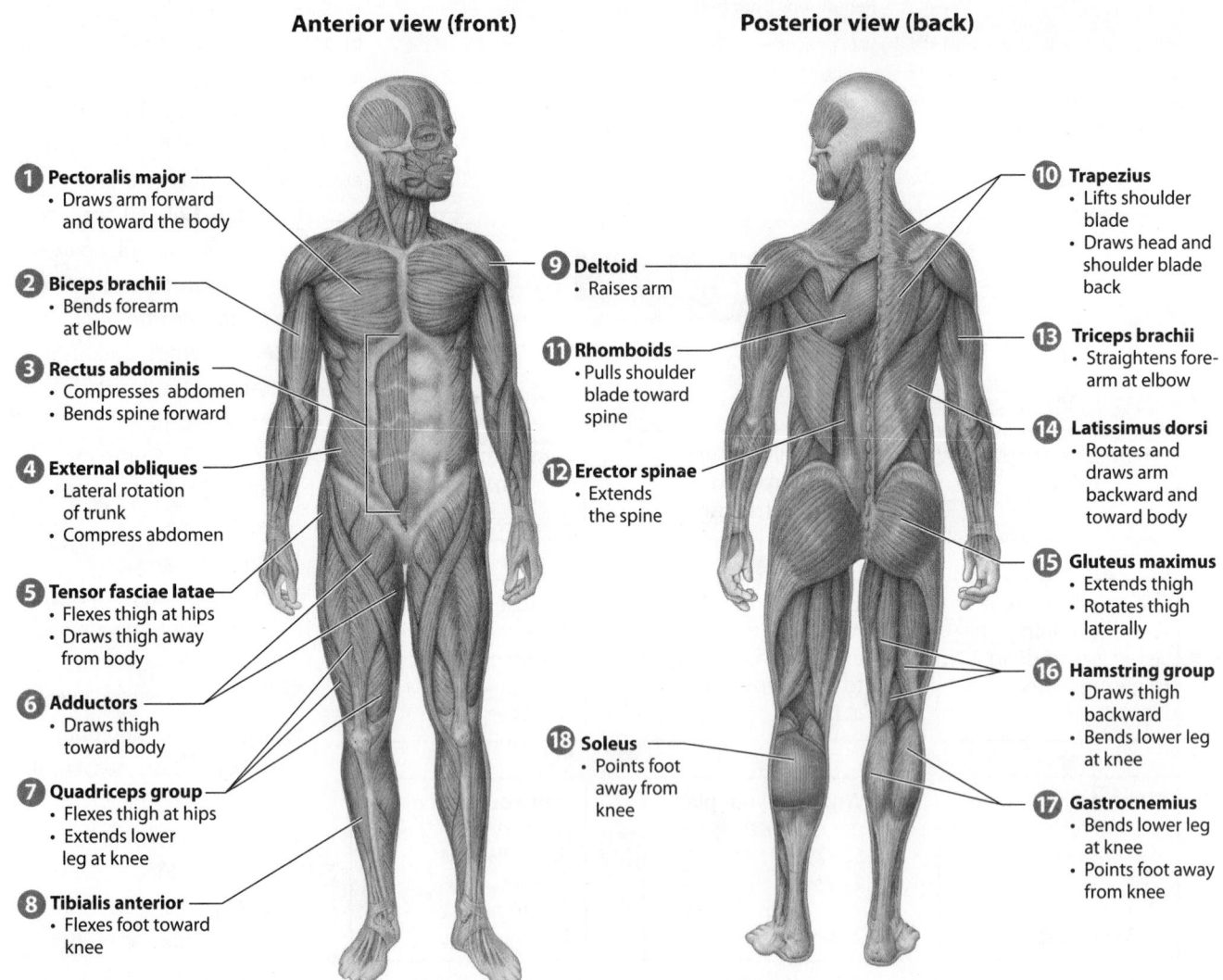

1 Pectoralis major
• Draws arm forward and toward the body

2 Biceps brachii
• Bends forearm at elbow

3 Rectus abdominis
• Compresses abdomen
• Bends spine forward

4 External obliques
• Lateral rotation of trunk
• Compress abdomen

5 Tensor fasciae latae
• Flexes thigh at hips
• Draws thigh away from body

6 Adductors
• Draws thigh toward body

7 Quadriceps group
• Flexes thigh at hips
• Extends lower leg at knee

8 Tibialis anterior
• Flexes foot toward knee

9 Deltoid
• Raises arm

11 Rhomboids
• Pulls shoulder blade toward spine

12 Erector spinae
• Extends the spine

18 Soleus
• Points foot away from knee

10 Trapezius
• Lifts shoulder blade
• Draws head and shoulder blade back

13 Triceps brachii
• Straightens forearm at elbow

14 Latissimus dorsi
• Rotates and draws arm backward and toward body

15 Gluteus maximus
• Extends thigh
• Rotates thigh laterally

16 Hamstring group
• Draws thigh backward
• Bends lower leg at knee

17 Gastrocnemius
• Bends lower leg at knee
• Points foot away from knee

FIGURE **4.8**   These muscles or muscle groups are commonly used in resistance-training exercises. Figure 4.9 illustrates exercises you can use to work the muscle groups shown.

FIGURE **4.9**

RESISTANCE-TRAINING EXERCISES

Videos for these exercises and more are available online at www.pearsonhighered.com/hopson and on MyFitnessLab.

Lower-Body Exercises

1. Squat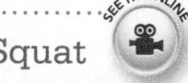

(a) **Free weight squat** and

(b) **Machine squat:** Place the barbell or pad on your upper back and shoulders. Stand with feet shoulder-width apart, toes pointing forward, hips and shoulders lined up, abdominals pulled in. Looking forward and keeping your chest open, bend your knees and press your hips back. Lower until the angle created between your thigh and calf is between 45 degrees and 90 degrees. Keep your knees behind the front of your toes. To return to the start position, contract your abdominals, press hips forward, and extend your legs until they are straight.

(c) **Ball squat:** Place the ball between your mid-back and a smooth wall. Your feet should be six to twelve inches in front of your hips, shoulder-width apart, and toes pointing forward. Contract your abdominals, look forward, and keep your shoulders and hips lined up as you lower your torso. Lower until the angle created between your thigh and calf is about 90 degrees. Your knees should be just above your toes (but not in front of them) or directly above your ankles depending upon your starting position, strength, and ankle flexibility. If not, reposition your feet before the next repetition. Return to the starting position by contracting your legs and pushing the ball into and back up the wall.

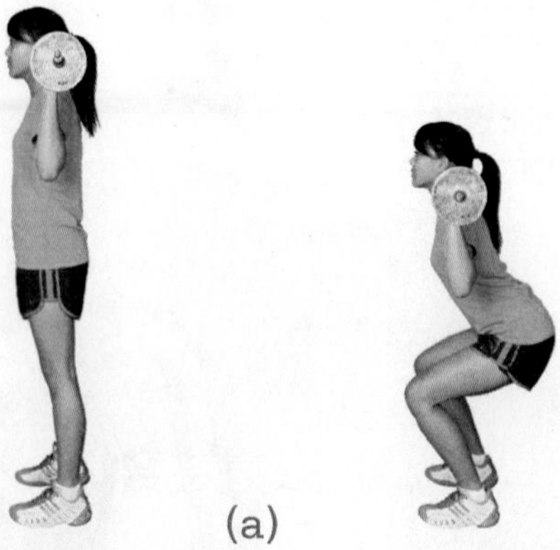

(a)

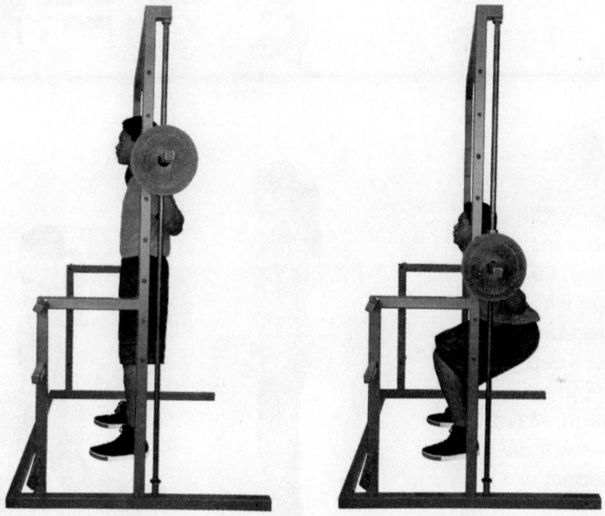

(b)

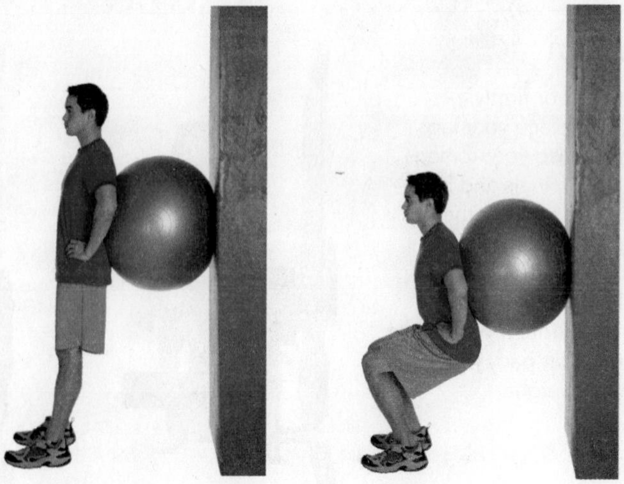

(c)

Muscles targeted:

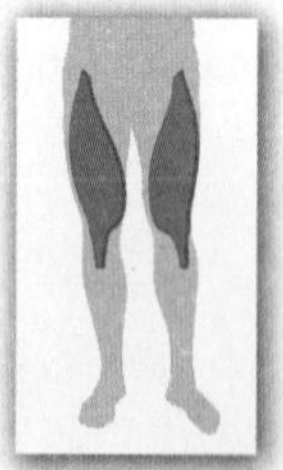

7 Quadriceps

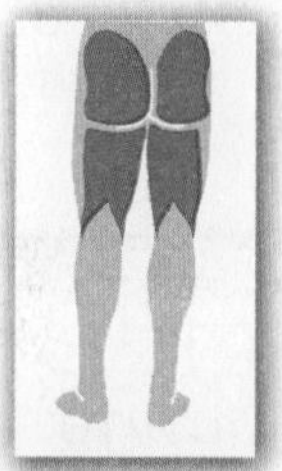

15 Gluteus maximus
16 Hamstrings

2. Leg Press

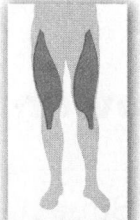

Sit with your back straight or firmly against the backrest. Place your feet on the foot pads so that your knees create a 60- to 90-degree angle. Stabilize your torso by contracting your abdominals and holding the hand grips or seat pad. Press the weight by extending your legs slowly outward to a straight position without locking your knees. Return the weight slowly back to the starting position. If your buttocks rise up off of the seat pad, you may be lifting too much weight.

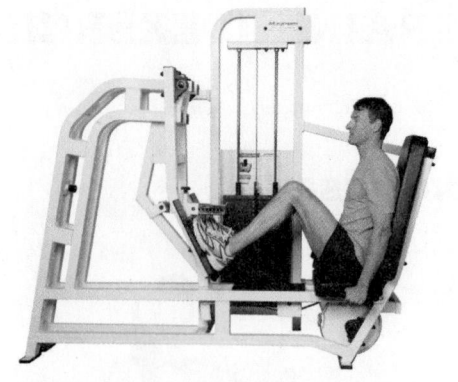

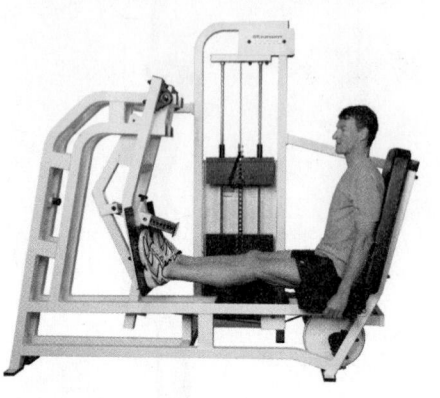

Muscles targeted:

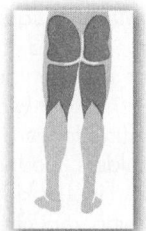

7 Quadriceps

15 Gluteus maximus
16 Hamstrings

---

3. Lunge

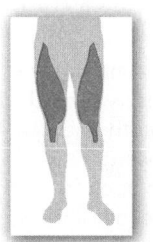

Stand with feet shoulder-width apart. Step forward and transfer weight to the forward leg. Lower your body straight down with your weight evenly distributed between the front and back legs. Keep your front knee in line with your ankle by striding out far enough. Make sure the front knee does not extend over your toes. Repeat with the other leg.

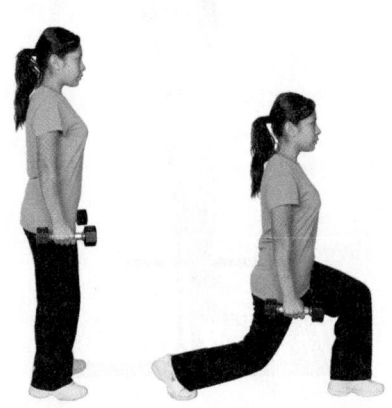

Muscles targeted:

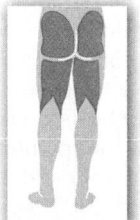

7 Quadriceps

15 Gluteus maximus
16 Hamstrings

---

4. Leg Extension

Sit with your back straight or firmly against the backrest and place your legs under the foot pad. Stabilize your torso by contracting your abdominals and holding the handgrips or seat pad. Lift the weight by extending your legs slowly upward to a straight position without locking your knees. Return the weight slowly to the starting position. If your buttocks rise up off the seat pad, you may be lifting too much weight.

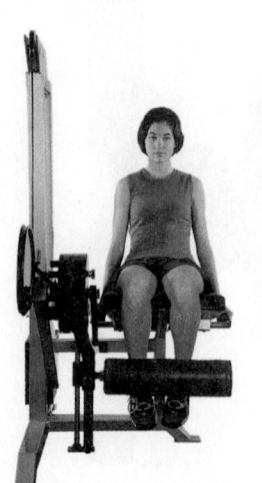

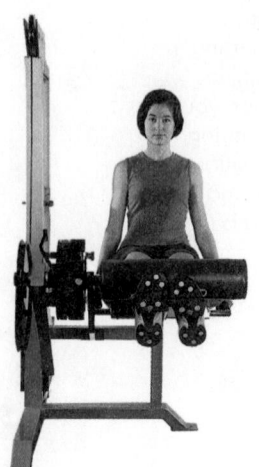

Muscles targeted:

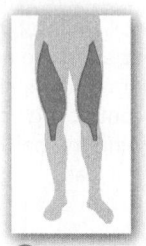

7 Quadriceps

5. Leg Curl

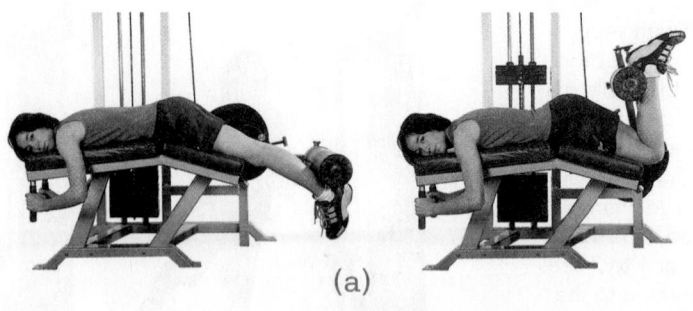

(a) Machine: Lie on your stomach so that your knees are placed at the machine's axis of rotation and the roller pad is just above your heel. Keep your head on the machine pad. Grasping the hand grips for support, lift the weight by contracting your hamstrings and pulling your heels toward your buttocks. Slowly lower the weight back to the start position.

(b) Calisthenics with ball: Lie on your stomach with knees bent and place the ball between your feet. Keep your head on the mat. Lower the ball to the ground and lift it back up by contracting your hamstrings and pulling your heels toward your buttocks.

(a)

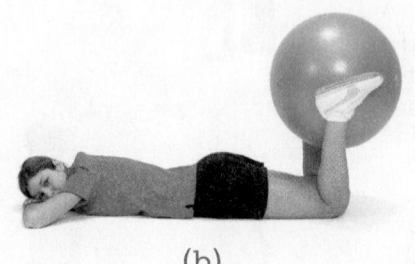

(b)

Muscles targeted:

16 Hamstrings

6. Hip Abduction

(a) Machine: Sit with your back straight or firmly against the backrest and place your legs against the pads. Grasping the hand grips or seat pad for support, press your legs outward slowly by contracting your outer thighs or hip abductors. Be careful not to extend the legs further than your normal range of motion. Slowly lower the machine weight by bringing your legs back together.

(b) Calisthenics with resistance band: Connect the resistance band to a low point on a machine and attach the free end to your outside leg. Stand with good posture and hold onto a wall or machine for support. Contract your hip abductors and extend your leg out to the side of your body. Slowly release the outside leg back to the starting position beside or crossed slightly in front of the standing leg.

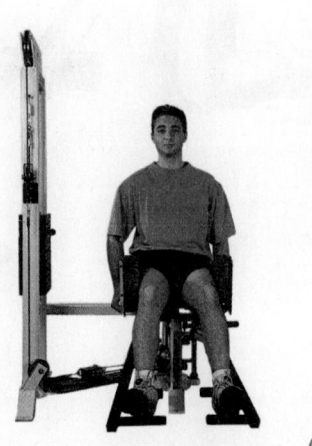
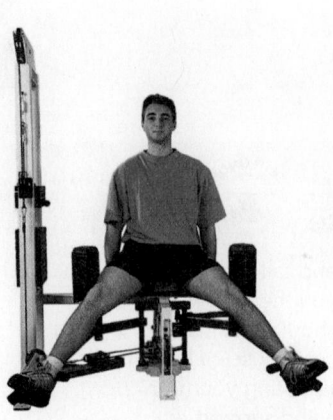
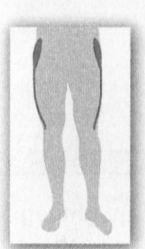

(a)

Muscles targeted:

5 Tensor fasciae latae

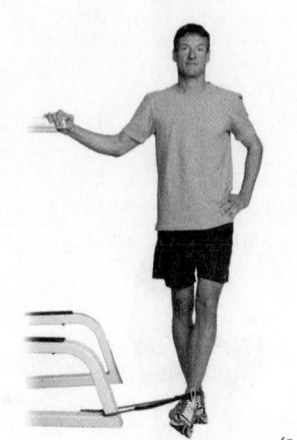
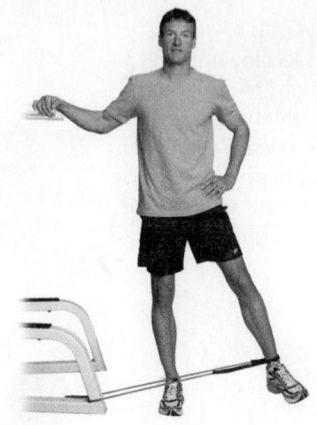

(b)

7. Hip Extension

(a) Machine: Stand tall with your working leg extended in front of you and connected to the cable machine. Support yourself by contracting your abdominals and holding on to the machine or handrails. Press the working leg behind you, contracting the gluteals and hamstrings. Hold the end position for 1 to 3 seconds before slowly returning to the starting position.

(b) Calisthenics with resistance band: Connect the resistance band to a low point on a machine and attach the free end to your lower leg. Stand with good posture and hold on to a wall or machine for support. Contract your gluteals and hamstrings and extend the working leg behind your body. Slowly release the leg back to the starting position slightly in front of the standing leg.

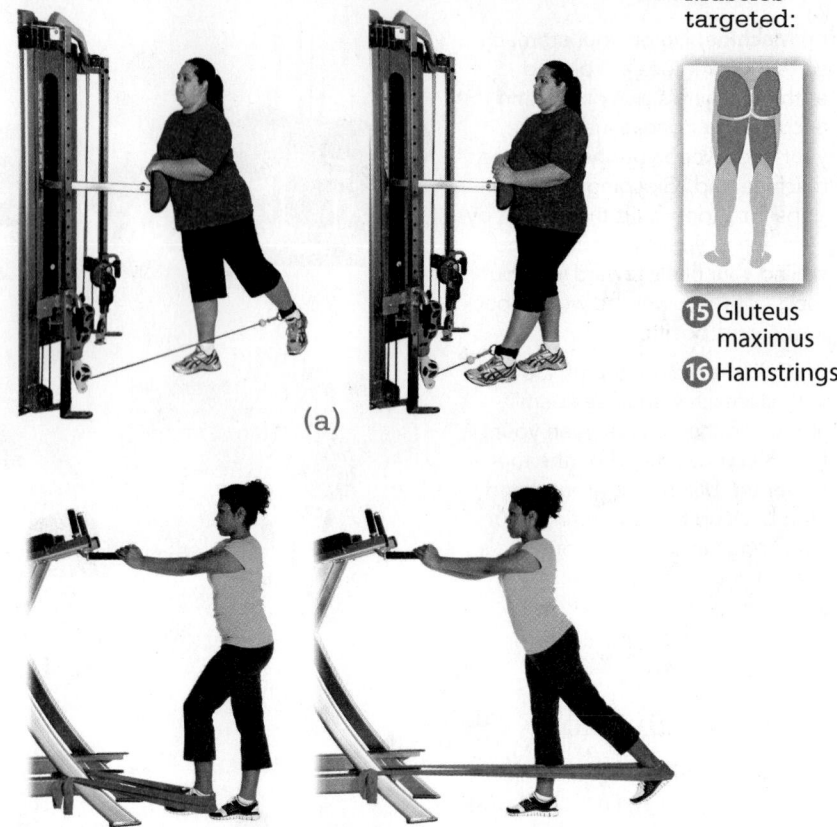

(a)

(b)

Muscles targeted:

🔟5 Gluteus maximus
🔟6 Hamstrings

8. Heel Raise

(a) Straight-leg: Stand tall with good posture and place your heels lower than the toes (you should feel just a slight stretch in the calf muscle). Looking forward and contracting your trunk muscles for balance and support, lift your heels up by contracting your gastrocnemius muscle. Be sure to do a full range of motion and slow, controlled repetitions.

(b) Bent-leg: Place your body in the machine with your heels lower than the toes and the weight pad placed comfortably on your thighs. Lift your heels up slightly and release the weight support bar with your hand. Slowly lower and lift the weight by contracting your soleus calf muscle through its full range of motion.

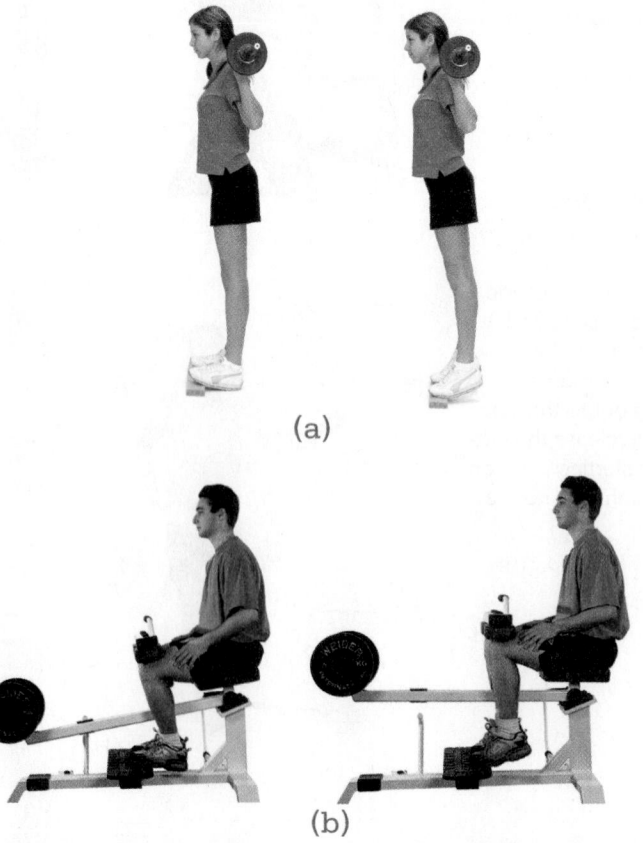

(a)

(b)

Muscles targeted:

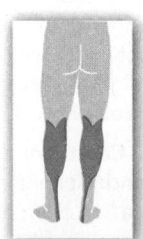

🔟7 Gastrocnemius

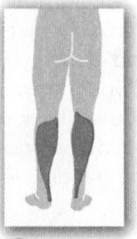

🔟8 Soleus

9. Hip Adduction

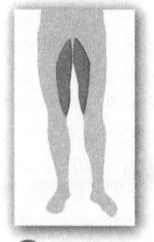

(a) Machine: Sit with your back straight or firmly against the backrest and place your legs against the pads set at a comfortable range of motion. Grasping the hand grips or seat pad for support, press your legs together slowly by contracting your inner thighs or hip adductors. Slowly return your legs to the starting position.

(b) Calisthenics with resistance band: Connect the resistance band to a low point on a machine and attach the free end to your inside leg. Stand with good posture and hold onto a wall or machine for support. Contract your hip adductors and cross your leg in front of your body to the opposite side of your body. Slowly release the leg back to the starting position beside or slightly to the side of the standing leg.

(c) Calisthenics with ball: Lie on your back with a ball pressed between your knees. Press your knees firmly together, squeezing the ball. Hold the squeeze for 3 to 10 seconds and release.

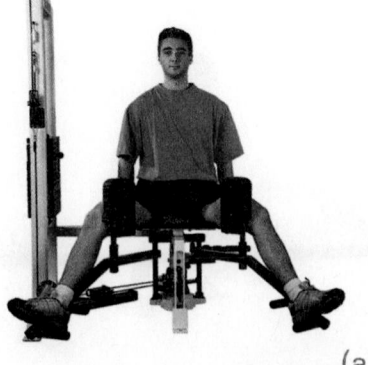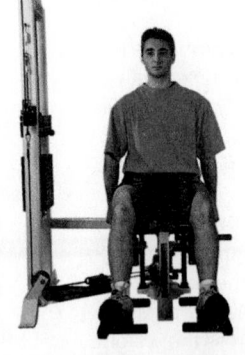

(a)

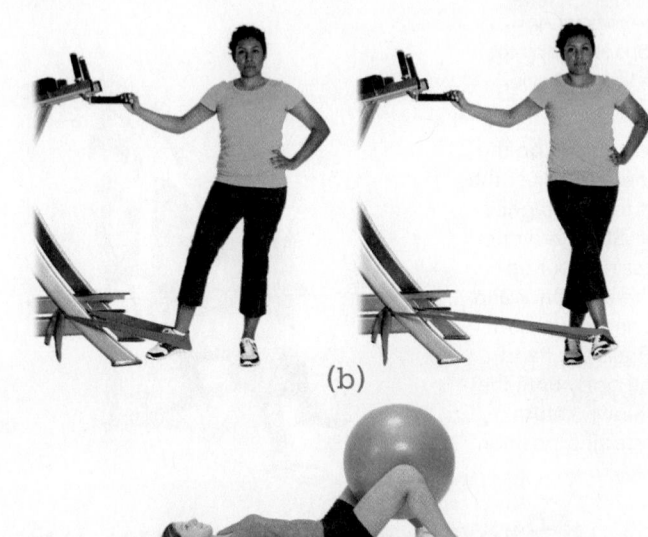

(b)

(c)

Muscles targeted:

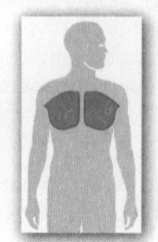

6 Adductors

Upper-Body Exercises

10. Push-Up

(a) Full push-ups and

(b) Modified push-ups: Support yourself in push-up position (from the knees or feet) by contracting your trunk muscles so that your neck, back, and hips are completely straight. Place hands slightly wider than shoulder-width apart. Slowly lower your body toward the floor, being careful to keep a straight body position. Your elbows will press out and back as you lower to a 90-degree elbow joint angle. Press yourself back up to the start position. Be careful not to let your trunk sag in the middle or your hips lift up during the exercise. Continually contract the abdominals to keep a strong, straight body position.

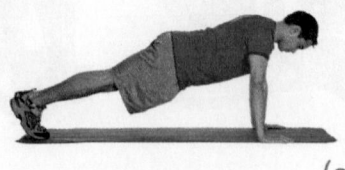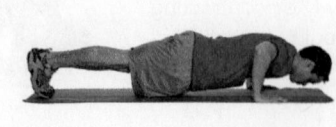

(a)

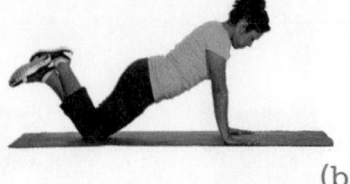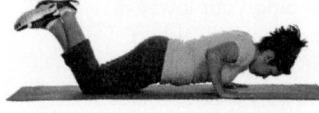

(b)

Muscles targeted:

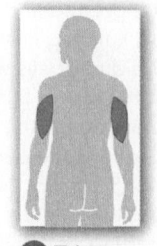

1 Pectoralis major

13 Triceps brachii

11. Chest Press

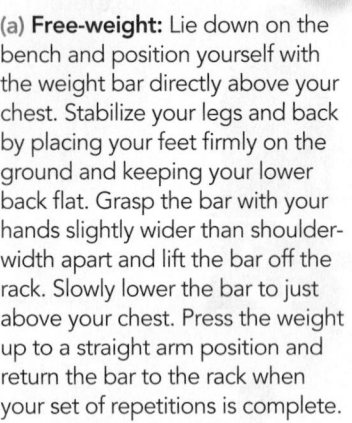

(a) **Free-weight:** Lie down on the bench and position yourself with the weight bar directly above your chest. Stabilize your legs and back by placing your feet firmly on the ground and keeping your lower back flat. Grasp the bar with your hands slightly wider than shoulder-width apart and lift the bar off the rack. Slowly lower the bar to just above your chest. Press the weight up to a straight arm position and return the bar to the rack when your set of repetitions is complete. Use a spotter when lifting heavier free weights.

(b) **Machine:** Place yourself on the chest press machine and adjust the seat height so that the hand grips are at chest height. Stabilize your torso by firmly pressing your upper back against the seat back and planting your feet on the ground or foot supports. Press the hand grips away from the body until the arms are straight. Slowly return your hands to the starting position.

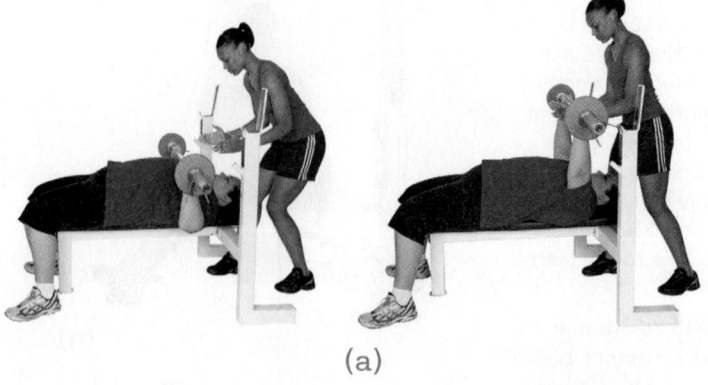
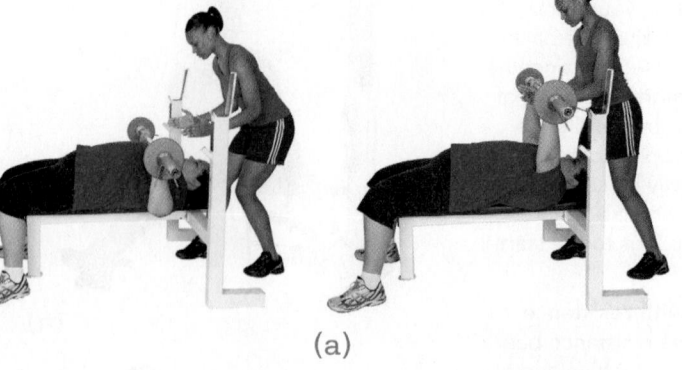
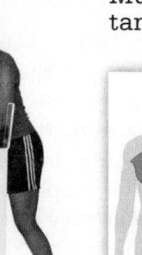

(a)

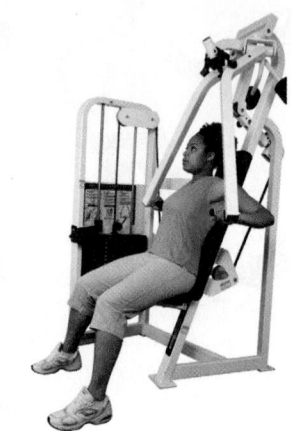
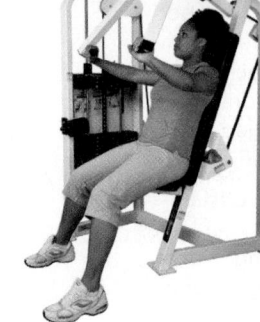

(b)

Muscles targeted:

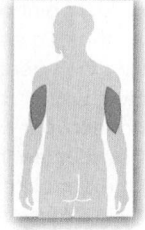

❶ Pectoralis major

⓭ Triceps brachii

12. Chest Fly

(a) **Machine:** Sit with your back straight or firmly against the back-rest, plant your feet on the ground or place on the foot pads, and grab the handles or place your arms behind the machine pads. Your arms should be directly to the side but not behind your body. Press your arms together slowly by contracting your chest and shoulder muscles. Slowly return your arms to the starting position.

(b) **Bench chest flys:** Lie down on the bench and position yourself with the dumbbells directly above your chest. Stabilize your legs and back by placing your feet firmly on the ground and keeping your lower back flat against the bench. Holding the dumbbells with a slight bend in the elbow joint, slowly lower them out to the side until your upper arms are parallel with the floor. Don't extend the arms beyond this position. Return your arms to the starting position by contracting your chest and shoulder muscles.

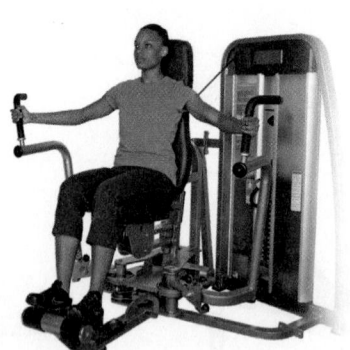
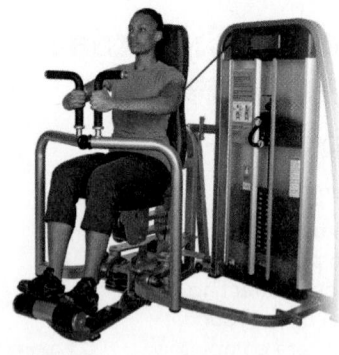

(a)

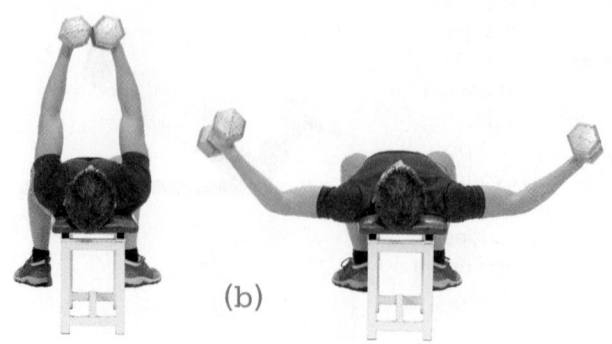

(b)

Muscles targeted:

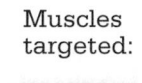
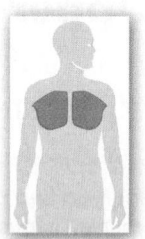

❶ Pectoralis major

13. Lat Pull-Down

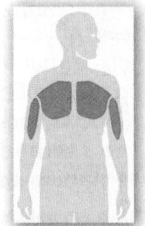

(a) Machine: Position the seat and leg pad on the lat pull-down machine so that your thighs are snug under the pad while your feet are flat on the ground. Grab the pull-down bar with a wide overhand grip on your way down to a seated position. Sitting directly under the cable, pull the bar down to your upper chest. Focus on contracting the mid-back first and then the arms by pulling the shoulder blades and elbows back and down. Slowly straighten your arms back to the starting position.

(b) Calisthenics with resistance band: Hold the resistance band above your head with your arms straight up and your hands shoulder-width apart. Pull down and outward with your hands. Focus on contracting the mid-back first and then the arms by pulling the shoulder blades and elbows back and down. End with the band at the top of your chest, hold for 1 to 3 seconds, then slowly straighten your arms back to the starting position.

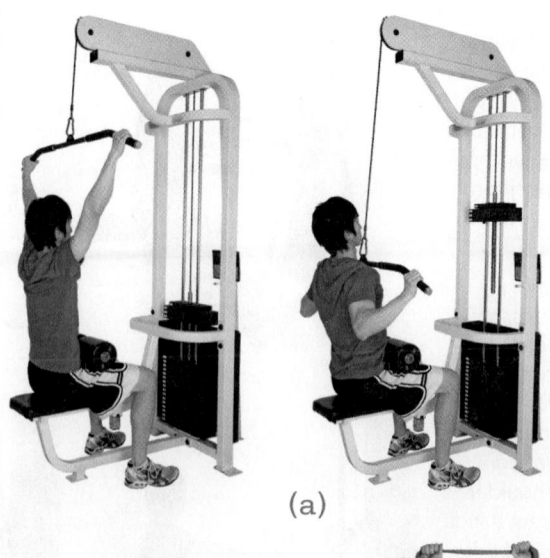

(a)

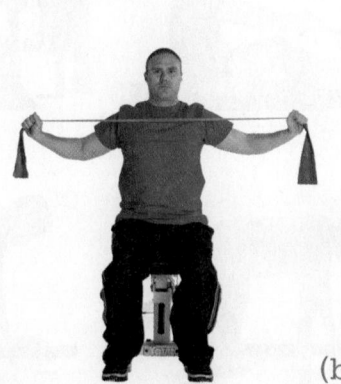 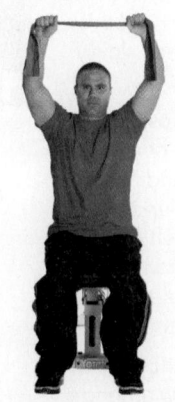

(b)

Muscles targeted:

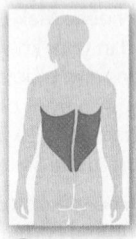

❶ Pectoralis major
❷ Biceps brachii

⓮ Latissimus dorsi

14. Assisted Pull-Up

Grab the pull-up bar with a wide overhead grip. Contract the back and arms in order to pull your body up until the bar is at chin height. Slowly straighten your arms back to the starting position.

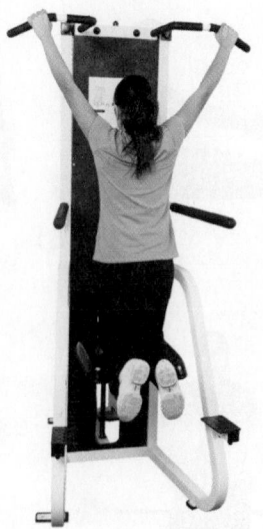 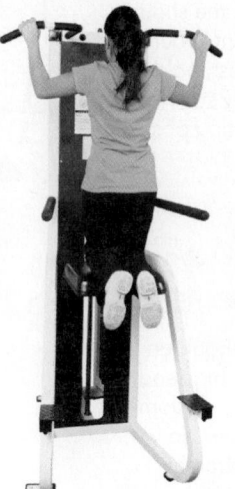

Muscles targeted:

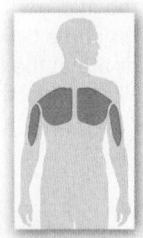

❶ Pectoralis major
❷ Biceps brachii

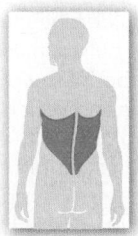

⓮ Latissimus dorsi

15. Row

(a) Machine compound row: Position the seat height until the handles are at the level of your shoulders. Sit upright and place your feet on the ground or foot pads. Grab the handgrips and pull your elbows back. Hold this position for 1 to 3 seconds, then slowly return to the starting position.

(b) Row on cable machine: Grab the cable machine handles, ropes, or bar. Make sure that you are seated so that your arms and shoulders are fully extended forward. Position your feet on foot pedals or firmly on the ground with your heels. Make sure there is a slight bend in your knees. Pull your shoulder blades and elbows back until your hands are just in front of your chest. Hold this position for 1 to 3 seconds, then slowly return to the starting position.

(c) Free-weight dumbbell: Position right hand and right knee on bench as shown. Keep your back flat and head in a straight line. Pull dumbbell up to the side of your chest with your left hand, contracting your mid-back and leading with your elbow. Return to starting position and repeat on other side.

(d) Calisthenics with resistance band: Wrap the resistance band low around a weight machine or around your feet in the seated position. Hold the resistance band with your arms straight out and initial tension on the band. Pull back with your hands, focusing on contracting the mid-back first. Pull the shoulder blades and elbows back until your hands are at the lower chest, hold for 1 to 3 seconds, then slowly straighten your arms back to the starting position.

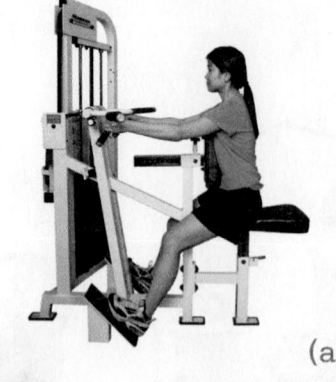
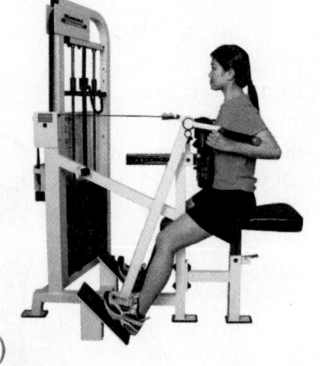
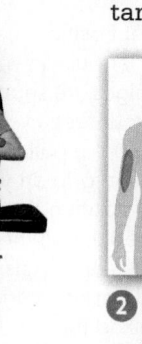
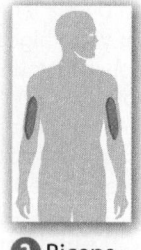

(a)

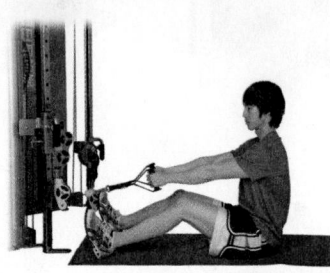

(b)

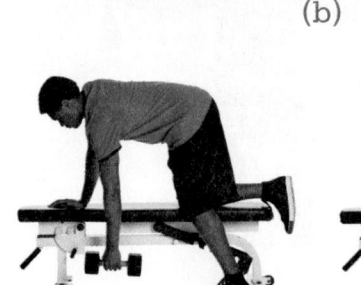
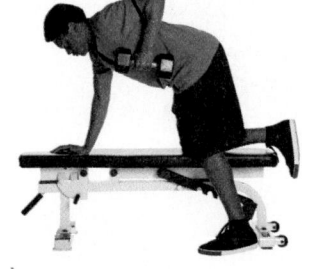

(c)

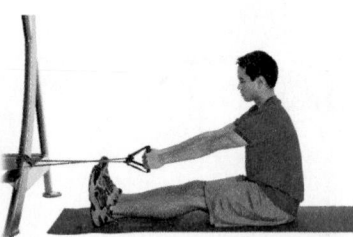
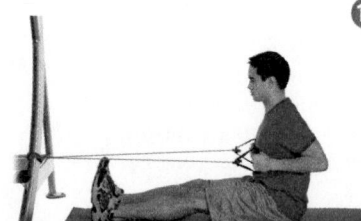

(d)

Muscles targeted:

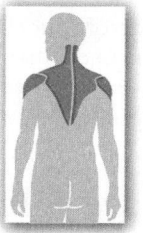

❷ Biceps brachii

❶❶ Rhomboids
❶❹ Latissimus dorsi

❾ Deltoids (posterior)
❿ Trapezius

16. Upright Row

Stand with your feet in a shoulder-width position. Keep your hips and shoulders aligned and your abdominals pulled in. Hold a barbell down in front of the body with straight arms and your hands positioned shoulder-width apart. Lift the weight to chest height keeping your elbows out, wrists straight, shoulders down. Return slowly to the starting position and repeat.

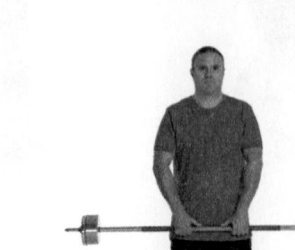
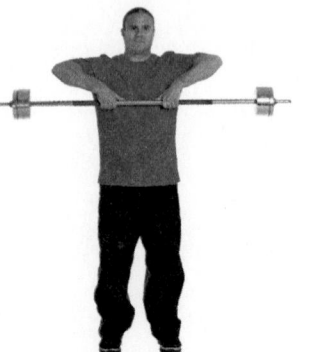

Muscles targeted:

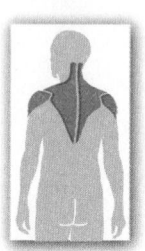

❾ Deltoids (posterior)
❿ Trapezius

17. Overhead Press

(a) **Machine** and

(b) **Free-weight dumbbell:** Sit with your back straight or firmly against the backrest, plant your feet firmly on the ground, and pull in your abdominals. Position your hands just wider than shoulder-width width and just above the shoulders. Carefully press the weight over your head until your arms are straight but your elbows are not locked out. Slowly return the weight to the starting position and repeat.

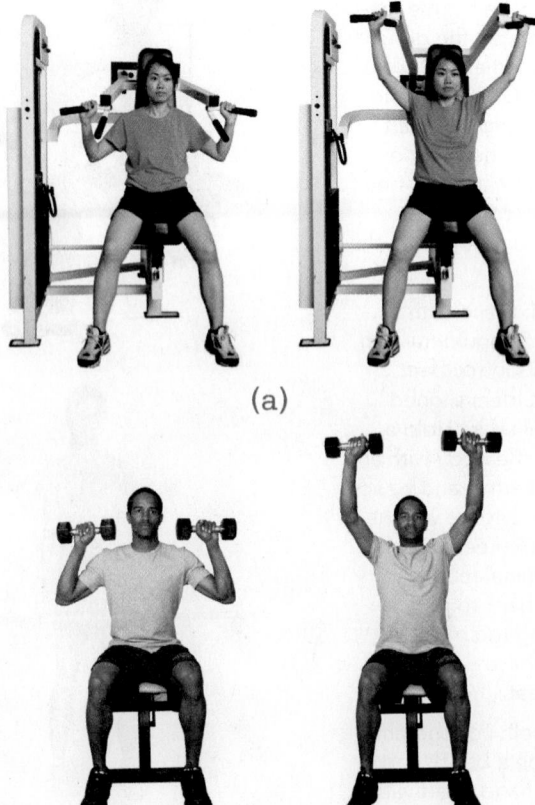

(a)

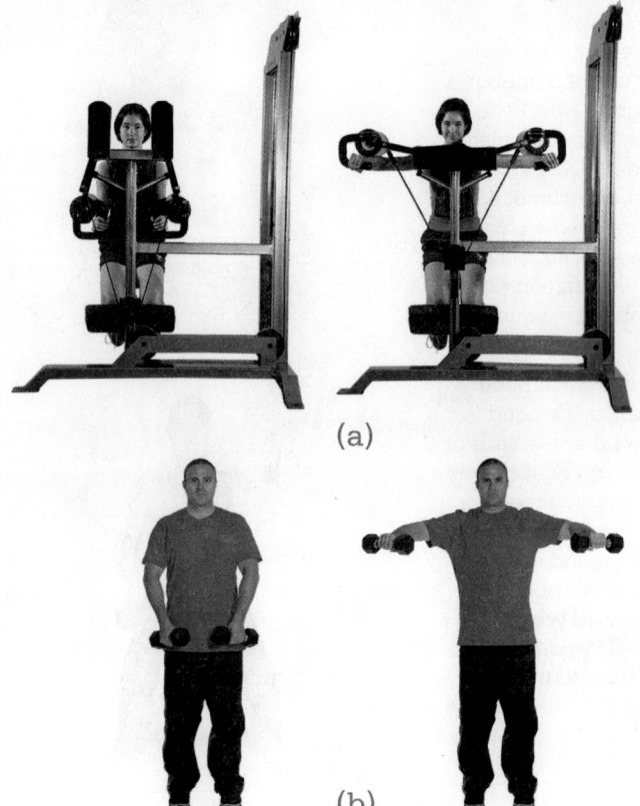

(b)

Muscles targeted:

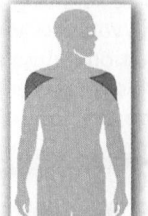

9 Deltoids (anterior and medial)

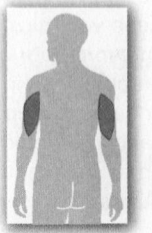

13 Triceps brachii

18. Lateral Raise

(a) **Machine:** Position yourself in the machine and sit with a tall, straight back. Contract your shoulders and lift your arms out to the side until they are parallel with the ground. Slowly lower your arms back down to your sides.

(b) **Free-weight dumbbell:** Stand with your feet shoulder-width apart. Hold the dumbbells to your sides or slightly in front of you. Lift your arms out to the side until they are parallel with the ground. While lifting, your elbows should have a slight bent to avoid over-extension of the elbow joint. Keep the weights at the same height as your elbows and keep your shoulders down. Slowly return the dumbbells back down to the starting position.

(a)

(b)

Muscles targeted:

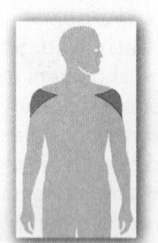

9 Deltoids (anterior and medial)

19. Biceps Curl

SEE IT! ONLINE

(a) **Machine:** Position yourself in the machine so that your feet are on the ground and your elbows are placed at the axis of rotation for the exercise. Grab the hand grips with an underhand grip and start with your arms straight but not over-extended. Lift your hands toward your head until your biceps are fully contracted. Slowly lower the weight back down to the starting position.

(b) **Free-weight barbell:** Stand with your feet either in a stride or a shoulder-width position and your knees slightly bent. Keep your hips and shoulders aligned and your abdominals pulled in. Hold a barbell down in front of the body with an underhand grip, straight arms, and your hands at shoulder-width. Lift the weight up to your shoulders while keeping your back straight and abdominal muscles tight. If you are leaning back to perform the lift, you may be lifting too much weight. Return the weight to the starting position slowly and repeat.

(c) **Free-weight dumbbell:** For one-arm concentration curls, sit on a bench and hold a dumbbell in one hand. Start with the working arm extended toward the ground and your elbow pressed into your inner thigh. Lift the dumbbell up to the shoulder and then return slowly to the starting position.

(d) **Alternating free-weight dumbbell:** Sit on a bench or chair with a dumbbell in each hand. Sit with good posture (ears and shoulders over hips and abdominals contracted) and your feet planted on the ground for balance. Lift one dumbbell up to your shoulder turning your palm toward your shoulder as you lift. Slowly lower the dumbbell to the starting position as you lift the dumbbell in your other hand.

(e) **Calisthenics with resistance band:** Place the center of a resistance band under one foot and grab the free ends of the band with a straight arm on the same side. Stand tall with your feet either in a stride or a side-to-side position and your knees soft. Keep your hips and shoulders aligned and your abdominals pulled in. Lift the resisted hand toward your shoulder until the biceps are fully contracted. Slowly lower the hand back to the starting position and repeat.

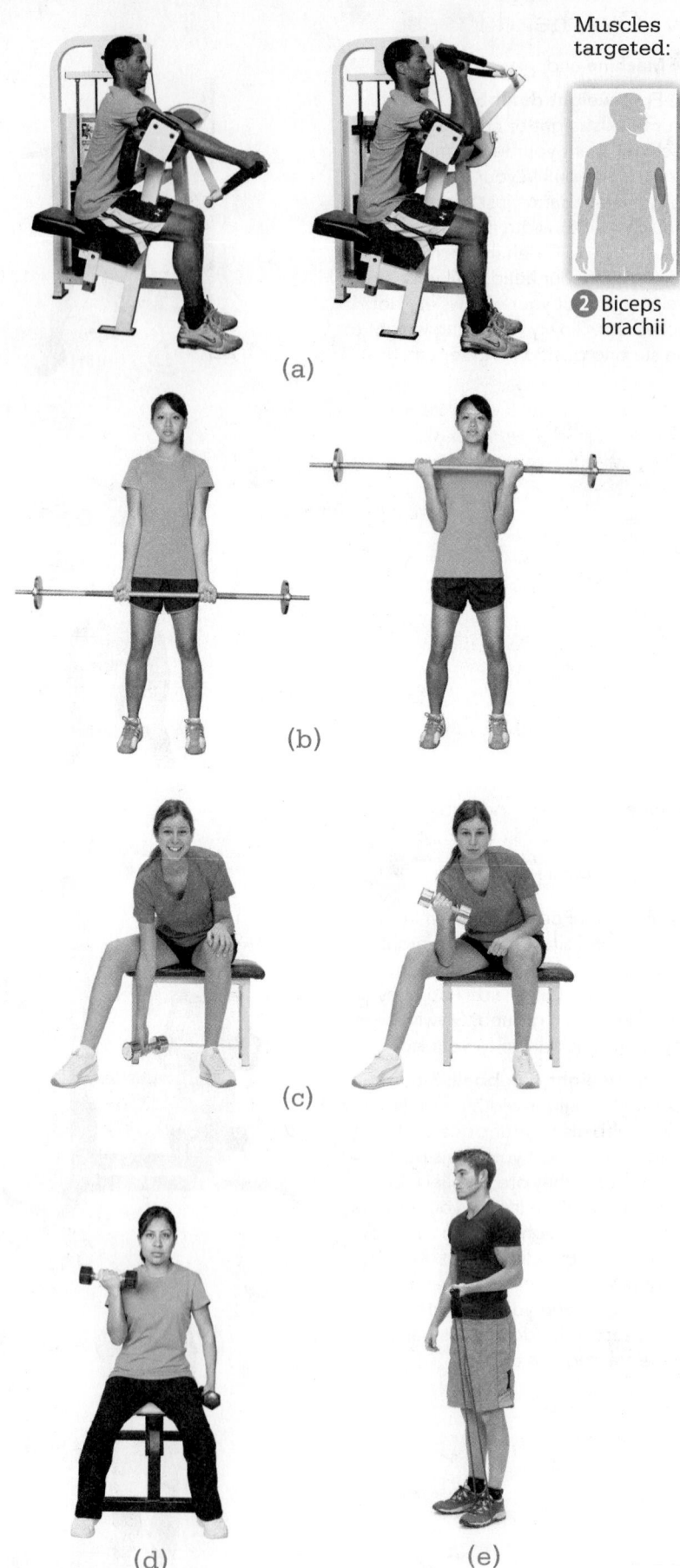

Muscles targeted:

2 Biceps brachii

(a)

(b)

(c)

(d)   (e)

20. Pullover

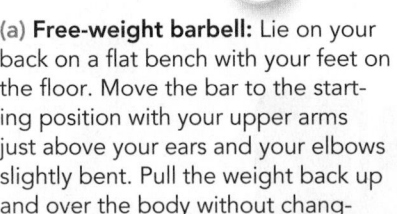

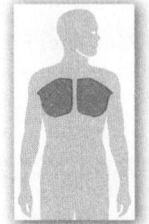

(a) Free-weight barbell: Lie on your back on a flat bench with your feet on the floor. Move the bar to the starting position with your upper arms just above your ears and your elbows slightly bent. Pull the weight back up and over the body without changing your elbow angle. Stop when the weight bar is directly over the chest.

(b) Machine: Adjust seat so that the machine pivots at your shoulder joints. Sit with your elbows against the pads and grasp the bar behind your head. Press forward and down with your arms until the bar is in front of your chest or abdomen. Slowly return to the starting position.

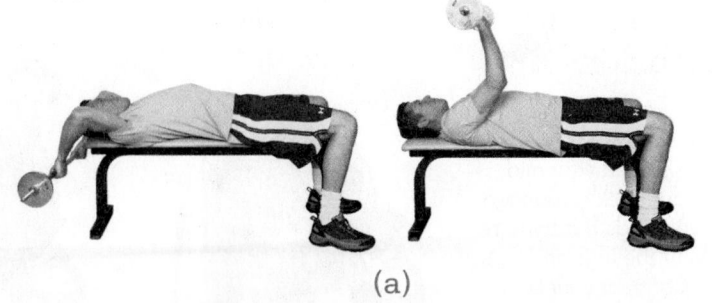

(a)

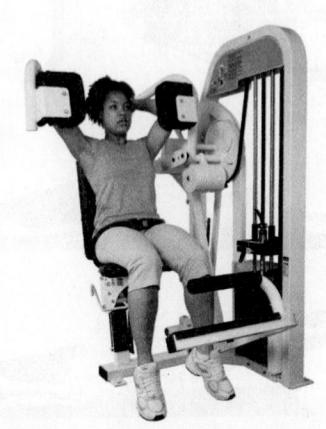 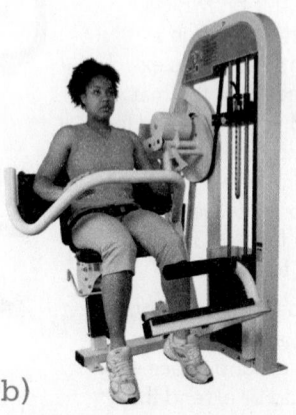

(b)

Muscles targeted:

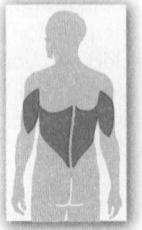

❶ Pectoralis major

⓭ Triceps brachii

⓮ Latissimus dorsi

21. Triceps Extension

(a) Machine: Grab the hand grips and start with your arms bent to at least 90 degrees. Press your hands away and down until your elbows are straight but not locked out. Slowly release the weight back to the starting position.

(b) Free-weight dumbbell: Start with the weight behind your head and your elbows lifted to the ceiling. Contract the triceps muscles to lift the weight over the head until the arms are straight. Slowly return to the starting position and repeat.

(c) Calisthenics with resistance band: Grasp the middle of a resistance band with one hand and the free ends with the other hand. Place one hand behind you and "anchor" the band at your hips or low back. Press the hand near your head upward by contracting the triceps muscle and extend the arm until straight. Slowly return the working arm to the starting position and repeat.

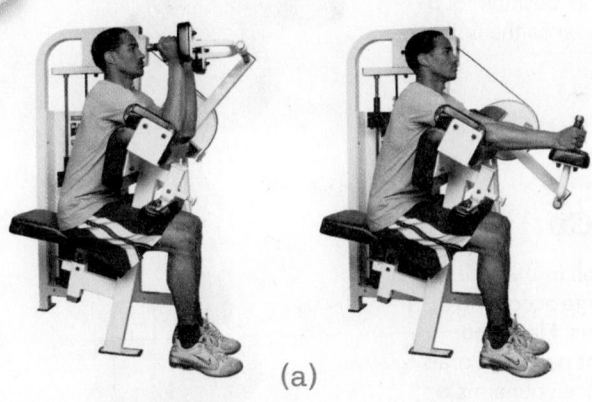

(a)

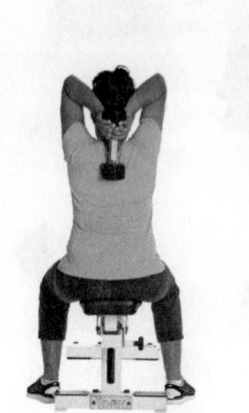 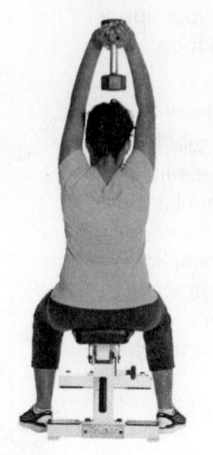 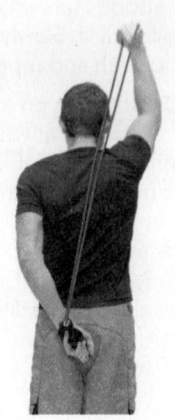

(b) (c)

Muscles targeted:

⓭ Triceps brachii

Trunk Exercises

22. Back Extension

(a) **Machine:** Position yourself in the machine so that your hips are pressed all the way back, the back pad is on your mid to upper back, and your back is rounded over. Stabilize with your legs but try to refrain from pushing with the legs and hips during the exercise. Contract your back extensors and straighten out your back until you are in an upright position.

(b) **Calisthenics on a mat:** Start in a prone position with arms and legs extended and your forehead on the mat. Lift and further extend your arms and legs using your back and hip muscles. If you are free of low-back problems, you can lift a little further up for increased intensity. Hold the position for 3 to 5 seconds and then slowly lower to the mat.

(c) **Calisthenics on a ball:** Lie with your stomach over the ball, anchoring your feet and knees on the ground. Place your hands behind your head or extend the arms out straight for increased exercise intensity. Lift the head, shoulders, arms, and upper back until you have a slight curve in the back. Hold this position for 3 to 5 seconds and then lower to the ball.

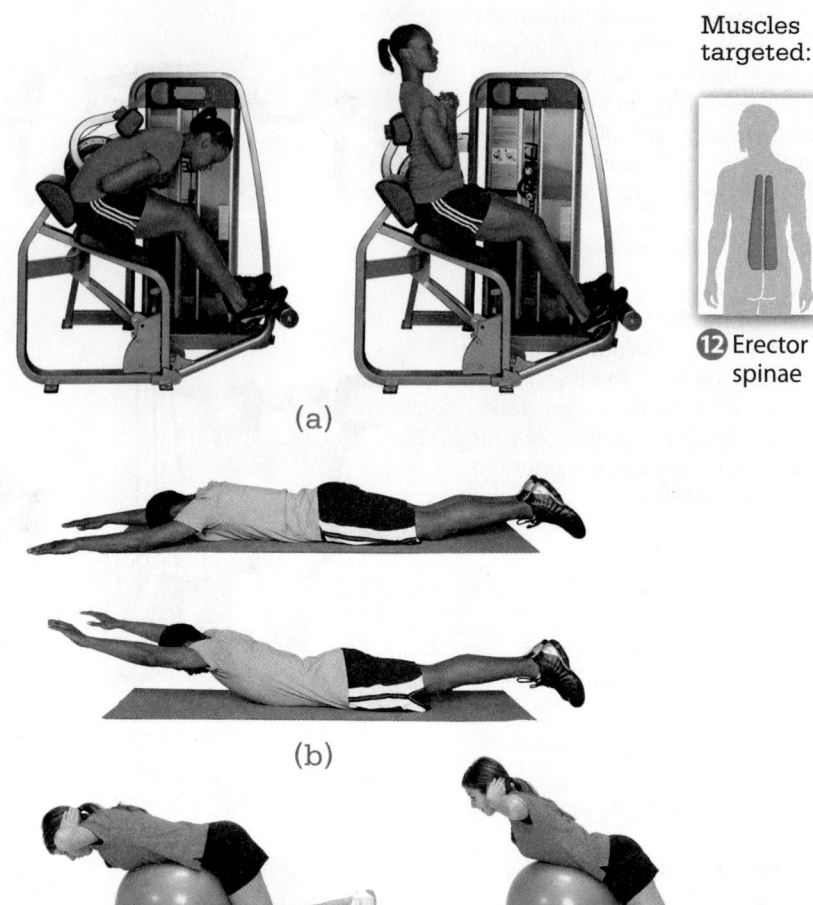

(a)

(b)

(c)

Muscles targeted:

⑫ Erector spinae

23. Abdominal Curl

(a) **Machine:** Place yourself in the sitting or lying abdominal machine according to the machine instructions. Place your feet on the ground or foot pads and grab the hand grips and/or place your arms or chest behind the machine pads. Contract your abdominals while flexing your upper torso forward. Slowly return to the starting position and repeat.

(b) **Calisthenics on a ball:** Lie back with the ball placed at your low- to mid-back region. Place your feet shoulder-width apart on the ground so that your knees are bent at about 90 degrees. Cross your hands at your chest or place them lightly behind your head. Contract your abdominals while flexing your upper torso forward. Slowly return to the starting position and repeat.

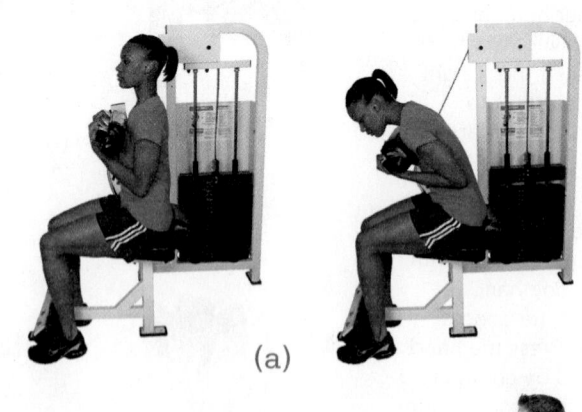

(a)

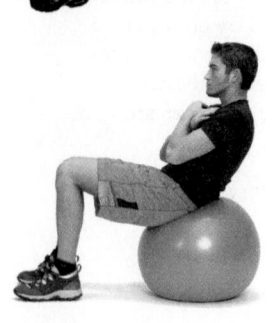

(b)

Muscles targeted:

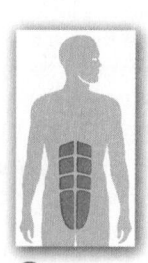

❸ Rectus abdominis

24. Reverse Curl

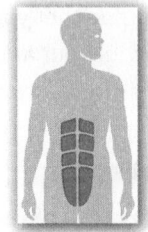

Lie on your back and place your hands near your hips. Lift your legs up so that your body creates a 90-degree angle to the floor. Your knees may be bent or straight for this exercise. Contract your abdominals while lifting your hips up off the mat. Slowly return to the starting position and repeat. Be careful not to rock the hips and legs back and forth when doing this exercise; instead, perform a controlled lifting of the hips upward.

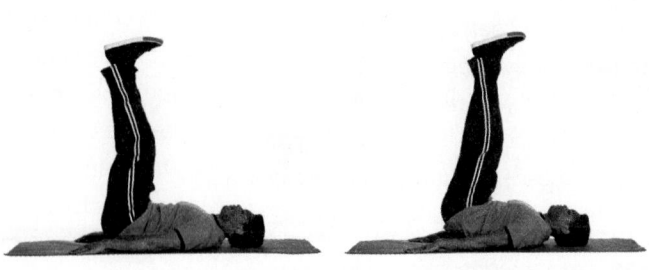

Muscles targeted:

3 Rectus abdominis

25. Oblique Curl

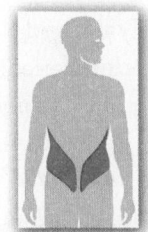

Lie on your back with one foot on the mat and knee bent to 90 degrees. Rest the opposite ankle on the bent knee. With one arm providing support on the ground and the other hand behind the head, contract your oblique abdominals and lift your opposite shoulder toward the lifted knee (elbow stays out). Keep the supporting arm and elbow on the floor and refrain from pulling on the head and neck with your hand. Return to the starting position slowly and repeat on the other side.

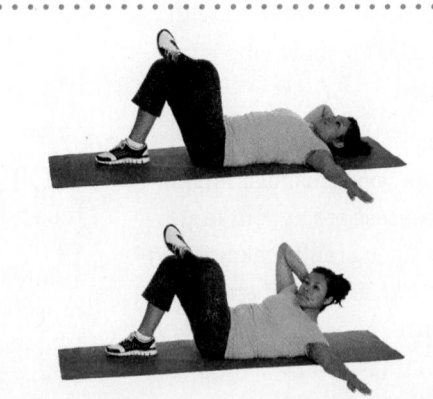

Muscles targeted:

4 External obliques

26. Side Bridge

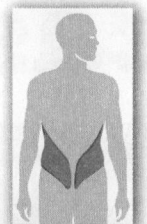

(a) Modified side bridge and

(b) Forearm side bridge and

(c) Intermediate side bridge:
Lie on your side with your legs together and straight or bent behind you at 90 degrees. Support your body weight with your forearm or a straight arm. Lift your torso to a straight body position by contracting your abdominal and back muscles. Hold this position for a number of seconds or slowly drop the hip to the mat and lift back up for repeated repetitions.

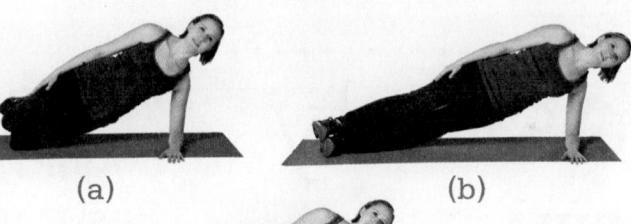

(a)   (b)

(c)

Muscles targeted:

4 External obliques

27. Plank

(a) Modified plank and

(b) Forearm plank and

(c) Push-up position plank: Lie on your stomach and support yourself in plank position (from the forearms or hands) by contracting your trunk muscles so that your neck, back, and hips are completely straight. Your forearms or hands should be under your chest and placed slightly wider than shoulder-width apart. Hold this position for 5 to 60 seconds, increasing duration as you gain muscular endurance.

(a)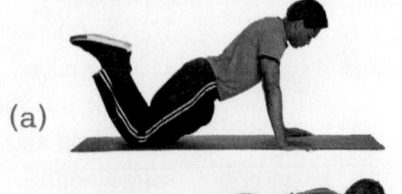

(b)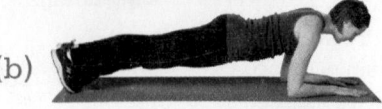

(c)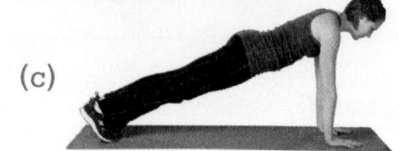

Muscles targeted:

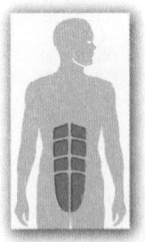 **3** Rectus abdominis

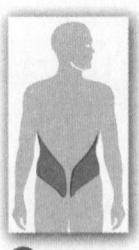 **4** External obliques

What If I Don't Reach My Goals?

Once you've applied FITT principles, chosen training levels, designed a program, and set target dates, you may find that your muscular development is not keeping up with your ambitions or that you cannot follow through consistently with training sessions. What other steps can you take to ensure success in your muscular fitness program?

Track Your Progress Use a weight-training log or a notebook to track your progress. Lab 4.4 provides you with a log that allows you to (1) see your week-to-week progress, (2) stay motivated, (3) detect problems with your program design or goals, and (4) know where to redesign your program if needed.

Evaluate and Redesign Your Program as Needed Periodically reevaluate your muscular fitness program. Common times to reassess are at your target completion date, when you feel you aren't making progress, when your improvement rate is faster than anticipated, and when you feel overtraining fatigue or injury. First, retake the initial tests for muscular strength and endurance. Second, reassess your goals: accomplished or not? Third, evaluate your overall program and write out what you like and don't like about it. If you have met your goals and enjoy your program, continue but set more challenging goals based on FITT parameters. If you have not met your goals or don't like your program, rewrite the goals and target dates, redesigning to solve your issues. Get help from an exercise professional if needed. Evaluating and redesigning should allow you, once again, to move toward your muscular fitness goals successfully. Lab 4.4 provides practice at evaluation and redesign.

- - - - - - - - - - - - - - - - - - -

THINK! Many people find group exercise classes to be motivating. Do you?

ACT! Find classes that will help you meet your muscular fitness goals (such as Pilates, fitness "boot camp," or muscle pump). Some classes are designed solely for muscular fitness, while others address both muscular fitness and cardiovascular training. Be sure to use enough resistance or weight to elicit a muscle training response.

- - - - - - - - - - - - - - - - - - -

casestudy

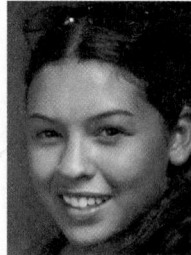

GINA

"My main goals in resistance training are to improve my muscle endurance so that I can go on longer hikes and to strengthen my muscles and joints so that I can reduce the chance I'll be injured on the trail. I live close to campus and there is a gym with weight equipment available, but how do I decide what equipment to use and what exercises to focus on?"

THINK! What would you say to Gina about the benefits of using free weights versus machines? What would you tell her about the differences between traditional weight training, circuit weight training, and plyometrics programs? Which would you advise her to begin with?

ACT! Verbalize your own resistance-training goals. Are they appearance based or function based? Write out your initial ideas for applying the FITT principles to your goals.

HEAR IT! ONLINE

What Precautions Should I Take to Avoid Resistance-Training Injuries?

Greater muscular fitness achieved through resistance training helps prevent general injury during sports or daily activity. However, weight training itself can cause injuries such as muscle or tendon strains, ligament sprains, fractures, dislocations, and other joint problems. This is especially true if the lifter pushes for an unrealistic overload. Injuries tend to occur while using free weights, but you can prevent them by getting proper instruction and guidance and by heeding a few basic suggestions.

Follow Basic Weight-Training Guidelines

When starting your resistance-training program, be conservative. Resist the temptation to begin with too many exercises or sets or with too much weight! Before increasing your resistance-training intensity or duration, observe how your body responds to the training over a few weeks. After that, you can safely increase the number of repetitions and/or the amount of weight. The safest approach is to follow the "10 percent rule." Limit increases in exercise frequency, intensity, or time to no more than 10 percent per week. Gentle increases will help prevent injury, overtraining, or soreness. Break this rule only if the initial intensity you selected was very low or a certified fitness professional instructs you to do otherwise.

Be Sure to Warm Up and Cool Down Properly

Weight-training guidelines include a warm-up and a cool-down before and after training sessions. A proper weight-training warm-up includes a general warm-up and a specific warm-up. The general warm-up consists of 3 to 10 minutes of cardiorespiratory exercises—walking, jogging (on or off a treadmill), biking, stationary biking, elliptical trainer use, or any activity that increases body temperature (breaking a light sweat) and blood flow to muscles. The specific warm-up should include range-of-motion exercises that mimic (without weight added) the resistance exercises you'll be performing. Move your limbs through a full range of motion before using a given weight machine or lifting free weights. Then, do a warm-up set with very light resistance. Now you are ready to perform your serious sets.

Some people also like to stretch before weight training. If you want to add stretching to your warm-up, do so only after a general warm-up to be sure your body has been adequately warmed up in preparation for stretching. Pre-exercise stretching should be light, and you should hold each stretch no more than 10 to 15 seconds. A proper cool-down for resistance training includes general range-of-motion exercises and stretches for the muscle groups applied during the weight-training session.

Know How to Train with Weights Safely

Get a proper introduction to weight training before you begin. Learn the proper grips and postures; the right way to isolate some muscle groups and stabilize others; the correct way to adjust machines for your height; and the safe way to sit, stand, and move during weight lifting to prevent injury. Learn the proper use of weights and weight machines. Use safety collars at the ends of weight bars to secure the weights on the bar.

When lifting free weights, use a spotter to watch, guide, and assist you. Perform all exercises in a slow and controlled manner. Some personal trainers recommend using a count of two up and four down to control the weight-lowering phase. Ask the spotter to watch your control and to make sure you are lifting safely and can return the bar safely after the lift. The object is to avoid fast, jerky, or bouncy motions that can injure your muscles or allow the weight to get away from you and cause injury.

Spotters typically assist when a weight lifter is attempting to lift a weight near his or her maximal fatigue level and the lift requires full-body balance. Exercises such as squats and the bench press require the weight to be lifted over the head or in a position that could present a danger to the lifter. When performing these exercises, always work out with a spotter.

Perform all exercises through a full range of motion. With free weights, you must determine the range yourself. Be sure to request extra training and attention if you need help.

Stay balanced: Set up in a relaxed, balanced position and maintain that position after a lift or set of lifts. Lifting while off balance is an easy way to create strain on one side and to pull or tear a muscle. Balance your exercise to build equal strength on both sides and from front to back.

Breathe in deeply in preparation for a lift and breathe out continuously as you lift. Some weight lifters use a **Valsalva maneuver** (that is, they exhale forcibly with a closed throat so no air exits) as a way to stabilize the trunk during a lift. However, holding your breath this way can cause an unhealthy blood pressure increase and slow blood flow to the heart, lungs, and brain. Breathe out during the push or pull part of a lift, particularly while lifting heavy weights, to avoid a Valsalva maneuver.

Use lighter weights when attempting new lifts or after taking time off from your routine. You can build up by three to five percent per session or 10 percent per week. Don't assume

Valsalva maneuver The process of holding one's breath while lifting heavy weight; this practice can increase chest cavity pressure and result in light-headedness during the lift; excessively increased blood pressure can result after the lift and breath are released

you can pick up where you left off before a break in your training; that's asking for muscle strain or injury.

Do not continue resistance training if you are in pain. Learn to differentiate the effort of lifting from the pain of an injury, particularly to a joint.

Muscle strains are common among people who use improper lifting techniques and machine setups. Eccentric contractions, in particular, tend to cause microtears in the muscle fibers and connective tissue within and surrounding the muscles. Eccentric contractions typically take place during the lowering of a weight, so it is important not to "drop" a weight to its starting position, whether lifting free weights or using a machine.[14] Wear gym shoes to protect your feet and wear gloves to improve your grip and protect your hands.

Get Advice from a Qualified Exercise Professional

A qualified trainer can help you learn the proper head and body position for lifting each type of weight (with or without the help of a spotter) and for using weight machines of each type. Learning to adjust the machines properly is part of this training. Seek out people qualified to provide accurate resistance-training information, especially if you are just getting started or before significantly changing aspects of your routine, such as amount of weight, number of repetitions, speed of movement, or body posture.

How can you recognize a qualified exercise professional? Ask any potential personal trainer or instructor questions such as the following:

- Are you certified as a personal trainer or fitness instructor by a reputable, nationally recognized organization such as ACSM, National Strength and Conditioning Association (NSCA), and the American Council on Exercise (ACE)?

- Do you have a certificate or degree in exercise science from an accredited two- or four-year college?

- What types of experience have you had as an instructor or personal trainer?

- How long have you been working in the field of fitness and wellness?

- What are your references from employers and past/present clients?

ergogenic aids Any nutritional, physical, mechanical, psychological, or pharmacological procedure or aid used to improve athletic performance

- How current are you with the changing guidelines and emerging trends in exercise and fitness, and how can you demonstrate this currency?

You'll want to look at practical details such as how much the personal trainer charges, whether he or she has liability insurance, and how well his or her schedule will accommodate yours. Intangibles are equally important: How well do you get along with this potential trainer, and how motivated does he or she help you feel?

Consider enrolling in a specific weight-training class at your college or university. Instructors in such courses are already screened for the qualifications listed here, and the cost will be significantly lower than hiring your own personal trainer.

Persons with Disabilities May Have Different Weight-Training Guidelines

Weight-training programs benefit virtually everyone, including people with some limitations or disabilities. Resistance training can decrease pain and increase mobility in people with joint and muscle disabilities and orthopedic conditions such as arthritis, multiple sclerosis, or osteoarthritis.

Safety guidelines and appropriate exercises will vary and will be determined by the disability or limitation of each person. Everyone will need medical clearance before beginning a resistance-training program, and those with certain chronic conditions and muscle disorders may need specific exercise recommendations and directions from a physician. If your gym lacks specialized equipment, look for a trainer who can help you perform modified exercises on the available machines. Wheelchair exercisers can perform many seated resistance-training exercises in the gym or at home. Visit this book's website to view demonstrations of easily adaptable resistance-training exercises for people of all abilities.

Is It Risky to Use Supplements for Muscular Fitness?

Dietary supplements marketed as promoters of muscle conditioning are called performance aids or dietary **ergogenic aids**. Some supplements are safe but ineffective; some are both unsafe and ineffective. Few, if any, are worth the risk and expense. Manufacturers of nutritional supplements need not prove their products are safe or effective before offering them for sale on the open market. The FDA may remove unsafe products, but this occurs after the product is "tested" on the buying public. To avoid being an inadvertent subject in an uncontrolled experiment, look into the risks of a supplement very carefully before considering its use. Some ergogenic aids, such as anabolic steroids, are controlled substances. This means they require a prescription for legal use and should not be used for nonprescription purposes. Their use can get you banned from athletic competitions.

Anabolic Steroids

The Mitchell Report on Steroids in Baseball

Anabolic steroids are synthetic drugs that are chemically related to the hormone testosterone. Physicians sometimes prescribe small doses within a medical setting for people with muscle diseases, burns, some cancers, and pituitary disorders. Some athletes and recreational weight trainers take anabolic steroids—illegally, outside of a medical setting, and without a prescription—to increase muscle mass, strength, and power. Anabolic steroids can produce some of these results in some users, but with overwhelmingly negative side effects that far outweigh the benefits. Besides being illegal, steroids increase the risk of liver and heart disease, cancer, acne, breast development in men, and masculinization in women. Because dramatically stronger muscles may exert more force than the body can handle, anabolic steroid use can also promote connective tissue and bone injuries. Steroid use can also be habit forming, lead to other drug addictions, and even cause death, as explained in the box Why Are Steroids Dangerous?

Creatine

Creatine is a legal nutritional supplement containing amino acids. It is most often sold as creatine monohydrate in powder, tablet, capsule, or liquid form. The body's natural form of creatine (phosphocreatine) is generated by the kidneys and stored in muscle cells. You can also consume creatine in the diet by eating meat products.

Creatine taken at recommended levels can improve performance by temporarily increasing the body's normal muscle stores of phosphocreatine. Since this natural energy substance powers bursts of activity lasting less than 60 seconds, creatine users sometimes find they can train more effectively in power activities and may be able to maintain higher forces during lifting. This can result in increased training adaptations such as strength and muscle size. Creatine intake also causes a temporary retention of water in muscle tissue that produces a small temporary increase in size, strength, and ability to generate power. Creatine has no effect on performance of aerobic endurance exercise.

So far, there have been few serious side effects reported in studies of people using creatine for up to four years. Since the long-term effects of creatine use are unknown, however, potential users should proceed with caution.

Adrenal Androgens (DHEA, Androstenedione)

Dehydroepiandrosterone (DHEA) is the body's most common hormone; it occurs naturally in the body and acts as a weak steroid chemical messenger (a conveyor of internal control signals and information).

casestudy

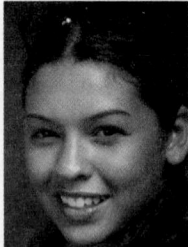

GINA

"I'm a big baseball fan. While growing up in San Francisco, I went to Giants and A's games all the time. So I was shocked to hear about the allegations of steroid and drug use among professional baseball players. I'm confused about the health risks of steroids and supplements. Are they all dangerous? What about the products you can buy in a health store, like creatine?"

THINK! How would you answer Gina's questions about steroids and creatine? Give two other examples of ergogenic supplements. How safe are they?

ACT! Talk with a friend or your instructor about ergogenic supplements. Outline the pros and cons of taking certain supplements.

Why Are Steroids Dangerous?

Why are government drug regulators—not to mention parents, educators, and coaches—so worried about steroid use in young people? Steroid use in teens and young adults is a problem for several major reasons:

1. Steroid use can lead to the abuse of other drugs. Some of the side effects of steroid use are so disruptive that people turn to opiate drugs such as cocaine and heroin to relieve their distress.
2. Anabolic steroids can permanently disrupt normal development. A person's body and brain are still developing during adolescence and into their early twenties. Steroids interfere with the normal effects of sex hormones. Most of these changes are irreversible.
3. Steroid use can lead to behavioral changes, including irritability, hostility, aggression, and depression. These changes can continue even after the user stops using steroids.[1,2]
4. Steroids promote heart disease, heart attacks, and strokes, even in athletes younger than thirty. The drugs also cause blood-filled cysts in the liver that can burst and cause serious internal bleeding.
5. Injecting steroids and sharing needles with other users can lead to the transmission of dangerous infections. The disease risks include hepatitis, HIV, and endocarditis, a bacterial infection of the heart.

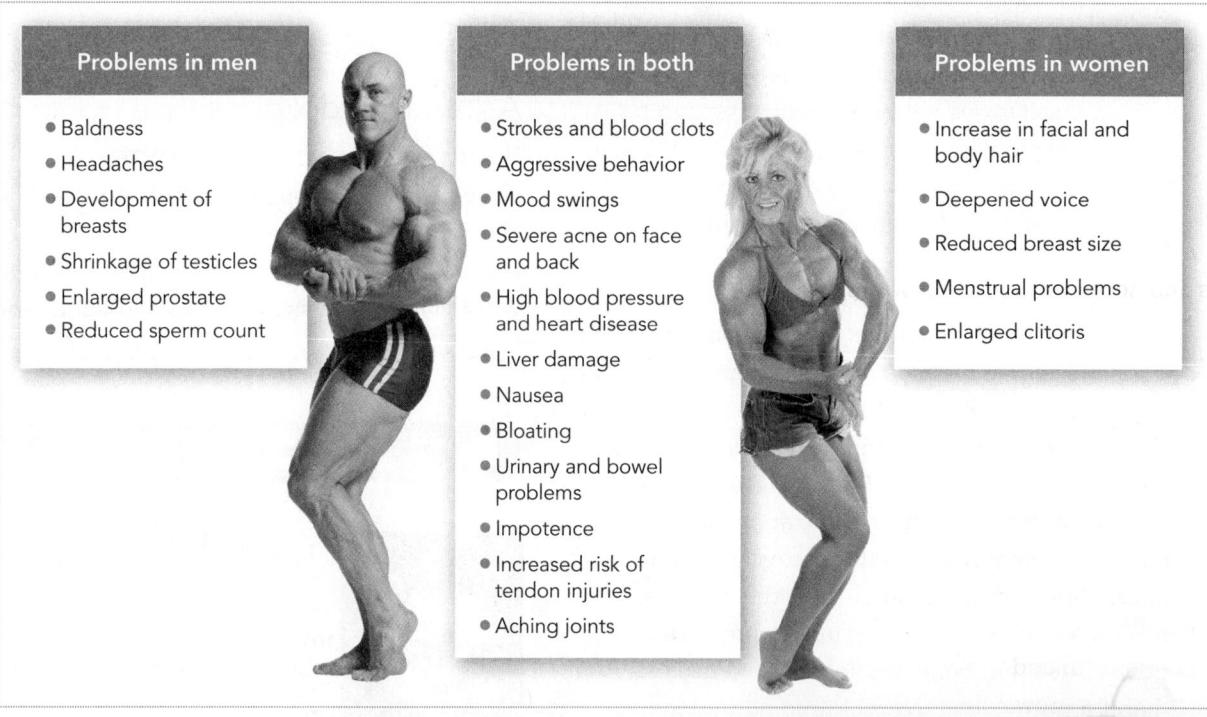

Problems in men

- Baldness
- Headaches
- Development of breasts
- Shrinkage of testicles
- Enlarged prostate
- Reduced sperm count

Problems in both

- Strokes and blood clots
- Aggressive behavior
- Mood swings
- Severe acne on face and back
- High blood pressure and heart disease
- Liver damage
- Nausea
- Bloating
- Urinary and bowel problems
- Impotence
- Increased risk of tendon injuries
- Aching joints

Problems in women

- Increase in facial and body hair
- Deepened voice
- Reduced breast size
- Menstrual problems
- Enlarged clitoris

Sources:
1. American Psychological Association (APA), Press Release, "Animal Models Show that Anabolic Steroids Flip the Adolescent Brain's Switch for Aggressive Behavior," www.apa.org/news/press/releases/2006/02/steroids.aspx (February 26, 2006).
2. J. M. Grimes and others, "Plasticity in Anterior Hypothalamic Vasopressin Correlates with Aggression during Anabolic–Androgenic Steroid Withdrawal in Hamsters," *Behavioral Neuroscience* 120, no. 1 (2006): 115–24.

Manufacturers produce and sell it as a supplement in a synthetic concentrated form despite the lack of definitive proof of its safety or effectiveness. DHEA proponents claim that it increases muscle mass and strength, lowers body fat, alters natural hormone levels, slows aging, and boosts immune functions. However, research studies have produced conflicting results on DHEA and overall do not provide strong evidence of a large positive effect on muscle mass and strength or on body fat levels.

Androstenedione (nickname "andro") is another naturally occurring steroid hormone with a structure related to both DHEA and testosterone. It is found naturally in meats and some plants. Even though manufacturers claim "andro" will increase testosterone levels, one pivotal study found that it actually lowered the body's natural production of testosterone, did not increase the body's adaptations to resistance training, and increased heart disease risk in men.[15] Androstenedione was ordered off the market by the FDA in 2004, and its use is dwindling. Both DHEA and androstenedione appear to decrease HDL or "good" cholesterol, which helps explain why these substances increase heart attack risks and other cardiovascular problems.[16] Both also increase the risk of developing certain cancers and accelerating the growth of existing cancers. These serious side effects strongly argue against the use of DHEA or "andro."

Growth Hormone (GH)

Your body's pituitary gland produces human growth hormone (GH), which promotes bone growth and muscle growth and decreases fat stores. Drug manufacturers produce GH synthetically for medical use in children and young adults with abnormally slow or reduced growth and related disorders. Although the FDA regulates growth hormone, athletes wanting to gain an edge over their competitors sometimes obtain and use it illegally. Marketers claim that growth hormone supplementation will counteract the muscle mass lost with disuse and aging, among other alleged benefits. However, GH side effects include irreversible bone growth (acromegaly/gigantism), increased risk of cardiovascular disease and diabetes, and decreased sexual desire, among others.

Marketers of oral GH supplements claim the same positive benefits to lean muscle mass and fat mass, but this is not borne out in tests or actual use. Oral GH, in fact, cannot even be absorbed from your digestive tract into your bloodstream! A far better way to increase natural levels of growth hormone is to perform regular exercise. In a study of women who ran for exercise, baseline resting GH levels increased by 50 percent in those training at higher compared to lower intensities.[17]

Amino Acid and Protein Supplements

Many bodybuilders and weight lifters take amino acid supplements because they believe that consuming protein or its building blocks (amino acids) will lead to enhanced muscle development. However, evidence is mixed that high intake of protein or taking protein-based supplements will improve training or exercise performance or build muscle mass beyond the levels achieved through normal dietary protein. When combined with resistance training, moderate increases in protein intake may lead to small increases in lean muscle mass and strength beyond resistance training alone.[18] In contrast, supplementation with the amino acid glutamine produces no beneficial effect above and beyond resistance training itself.[19] Taking moderate doses of these supplements has no dramatic side effects, but large doses of either the supplements or protein itself can create amino acid imbalances, alter protein and bone metabolism, and be dangerous to individuals with liver or kidney disease.[20] See the box Should I Increase My Protein Intake Immediately after Resistance Training? for more on protein supplementation.

Should I Increase My Protein Intake Immediately after Resistance Training?

If you are looking to increase muscle strength and size, then definitely YES! Even if your goals are health and muscle maintenance, a balanced recovery meal or drink is beneficial. After resistance training, the muscles worked are depleted of nutrients and are in a state of muscle breakdown from the exercise. Providing muscles with nutrients and correcting protein imbalances helps repair breakdown damage and promotes recovery.[1] Eating protein after exercise, particularly essential amino acids, promotes protein synthesis.[2] Protein synthesis is even more pronounced when protein consumption is accompanied by easily digestible carbohydrates.[3] Carbohydrates will increase the release of insulin into the blood, which will in turn enhance protein storage in cells.[4]

Timing is important. Immediately after resistance training the muscles are receptive to bringing protein into cells. That increased protein helps with repair and recovery and promotes increases in the strength and size of the muscle. Increasing your intake a little bit right *before* exercise can also help.[5] In one study, subjects who took protein supplements immediately before and after resistance training had 86 percent greater increase in lean tissue mass and 30 percent greater overall strength after 10 weeks of resistance training than those who had the same supplements in the morning and night (not close to the exercise session).[6]

Tips for post–resistance-training nutrition:

- Consume 100–500 calories—depending upon your body size, workout length and intensity, and goals.

- Consume something that is digested rapidly—a liquid source is great!

- Drink or eat something with essential amino acids for your protein source—whey protein is a great source and you can get this in milk and chocolate milk.

- Make sure your snack is easily digested and has high-glycemic load carbohydrates—again, chocolate milk fills the bill!

- Consume about two parts carbohydrate to one part protein. Healthy fats can also be included.

- For the greatest effect, consume your post-exercise drink or snack within an hour, preferably within 30 minutes, of stopping your exercise session.

- After an hour or later in the day, eat a full recovery meal with a balance of protein, carbohydrates, and healthy fats.

Sources:
1. S. M. Phillips, J. W. Hartman, and S. B. Wilkinson, "Dietary Protein to Support Anabolism with Resistance Exercise in Young Men," *Journal of the American College of Nutrition* 24, no. 2 (2005): 134S–9S.
2. S. L. Miller and others, "Independent and Combined Effects of Amino Acids and Glucose after Resistance Exercise," *Medicine and Science in Sports and Exercise* 35, no. 3 (2003): 449–55.
3. K. Pritchett and others, "Acute Effects of Chocolate Milk and a Commercial Recovery Beverage on Postexercise Recovery Indices and Endurance Cycling Performance," *Applied Physiology, Nutrition, and Metabolism* 34, no. 6 (2009): 1017–22.
4. S. M. Phillips, "Physiologic and Molecular Bases of Muscle Hypertrophy and Atrophy: Impact of Resistance Exercise on Human Skeletal Muscle (Protein and Exercise Dose Effects)," *Applied Physiology, Nutrition, and Metabolism* 34, no. 3 (2009): 403–10.
5. K. D. Tipton and others, "Stimulation of Net Muscle Protein Synthesis by Whey Protein Ingestion before and after Exercise," *American Journal of Physiology: Endocrinology and Metabolism* 292, no. 1 (2006): E71–6.
6. P. J. Cribb and A. Hayes, "Effects of Supplement Timing and Resistance Exercise on Skeletal Muscle Hypertrophy," *Medicine and Science in Sports and Exercise* 38, no. 11 (2006): 1918–25.

chapterinreview

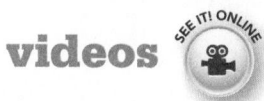

videos

Log on to **www.pearsonhighered.com/hopson** or MyFitnessLab to view these chapter-related videos.

Free-Weight Exercises
Safety Tips: Dumbbells
Bench/Chest Press
Biceps Curl
Dumbbell Flys
Dumbbell Row
Front Raise
Lateral Raise
Lunges
Pullover
Shoulder Press
Shoulder Shrugs
Squats
Straight-Leg Heel Raise
Triceps Extension
Triceps Kickback
Upright Rows
Walking Lunges

Resistance Band Exercises
Safety Tips: Resistance Bands
Bench/Chest Press
Biceps Curl
Flys
Front Raise
Lat Pull-Down
Lateral Raise
Leg Abduction
Leg Adduction
Leg Curl
Leg Press
Seated Row

Shoulder Press
Shoulder Shrug
Squats
Triceps Extension
Triceps Kickback
Upright Row

Stability Ball Exercises
Safety Tips: Stability Balls
Abdominal Curl
Abdominal Tuck
Back Extension
Bridge Leg Curl
Bridge Up
Dumbbell Fly/Press
Hip Adduction
Lat Roll-Out
Leg Curl
Oblique Side Crunch
Pike-Up
Plank
Reverse Dumbbell Fly
Wall Squat

Strength Exercises Requiring No Equipment
Arm/Leg Extensions
Back Bridge
Bench Dips
Modified Push-Ups
Oblique Curl
Pelvic Tilt
Plank (Forearm Position)

Plank (Push-Up Position)
Push-Ups
Reverse Curl
Side Bridge (Beginner)
Side Bridge (Intermediate)
Side Bridge (Advanced)

Machine Exercises
Abdominal Curl
Assisted Pull-Up
Biceps Curl
Chest Flys
Chest Press
Hip Extension
Lat Pull-Down
Lateral Raise
Leg Curl
Leg Extension
Leg Press
Machine Row
Overhead Press
Smith Machine Squat
Triceps Extension

Assessments
Curl-Up Assessment
Grip Strength Assessment
One Repetition Maximum (1RM)
    Prediction Assessment
Push-Up Assessment

The Mitchell Report on
Steroids in Baseball

onlineresources

Log on to **www.pearsonhighered.com/hopson** or MyFitnessLab for access to these book-related resources and for links to other useful websites.

Audio case study
Audio PowerPoint lecture

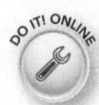
Lab 4.1 Assessing Your Muscular Strength
Lab 4.2 Assessing Your Muscular Endurance
Lab 4.3 Setting Muscular Fitness Goals
Lab 4.4 Your Resistance-Training Workout Plan
Alternate Lab: Assessing Grip Strength

Customizable 4-week resistance-training programs
Behavior Change Log Book and Wellness Journal

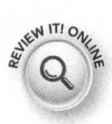
Pre- and post-quizzes
Glossary flashcards

review questions

1. Muscular strength is the ability to
   a. contract your muscles repeatedly over time.
   b. run a six-minute mile.
   c. look "toned" in a swimsuit.
   d. contract your muscle with maximal force.
2. Which of the following benefits of resistance training will reduce your risk of cardiovascular diseases?
   a. Increased bone density
   b. Increased muscle power
   c. Reduced body fat levels
   d. Better sports recovery
3. What is a single muscle cell called?
   a. Muscle fiber
   b. Muscle fascia
   c. Fascicle
   d. Contractile bundle
4. Which of the following will result in a stronger muscle contraction?
   a. Eating more protein before your workout
   b. Activating slow, smaller motor units
   c. Taking DHEA before your workout
   d. Activating more motor units overall
5. Sitting down in a chair and standing up again is an example of which type of exercise?
   a. Isotonic
   b. Isokinetic
   c. Isometric
   d. Isostatic
6. Muscle strength improvements in the first few weeks of a program are due to
   a. increased size of muscle fibers.
   b. increased activation and coordination of motor units
   c. increased ability of muscles to move through a full range of motion.
   d. increased blood flow to working muscles.
7. A test of muscular endurance includes
   a. a 1 RM test.
   b. a grip-strength test.
   c. a 20 RM test.
   d. a pull-up test.
8. One disadvantage of using machines for resistance-training exercises is
   a. it takes time to adjust the machine for your height and desired resistance level.
   b. the machine does not promote the use of postural and stabilizing muscles during the exercise.
   c. spotters are needed.
   d. it can be hard to isolate specific muscle groups.
9. Which of the following is part of the criteria you should use when selecting a personal trainer?
   a. Certified by ACSM, NSCA, or ACE
   b. Looks like someone who works out a lot
   c. Recommended by a friend who was sore after a workout with the trainer
   d. Able to provide dietary supplements at a reduced cost
10. Which of the following supplements/drugs promotes irreversible bone growth, cardiovascular disease, diabetes, and decreased sexual desire?
    a. Anabolic steroids
    b. Creatine
    c. Growth hormone
    d. Androstenedione

critical **thinking** questions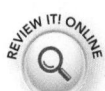

1. Why is weight training a popular activity among college students and adults of all ages?
2. Define sarcopenia and discuss how it can be reversed through exercise. How are sarcopenia and atrophy different?
3. What is the predominant fiber type in the postural trunk muscles and why does this make sense?
4. Discuss the role of resistance training in preventing injuries.
5. How does circuit weight training differ from regular weight training? What are the specific benefits of doing circuit weight training?

references

1. Centers for Disease Control and Prevention (CDC), "QuickStats: Percentage of Adults Aged ≥ 18 Years Who Engaged in Leisure-Time Strengthening Activities, by Age Group and Sex—National Health Interview Survey, United States, 2008," *Morbidity and Mortality Weekly Report* 58, no. 34 (2009): 955; National Center for Health Statistics, Health Promotion Statistics Branch, CDC Wonder, *DATA2010…the Healthy People 2010 Database* (Hyattsville, MD; Centers for Disease Control, 2010), http://wonder.cdc.gov/data2010/focus.htm (accessed May 2011).

2. National Center for Health Statistics, CDC Wonder, *DATA2010…the Healthy People 2010 Database*, 2010; CDC, "Trends in Strength Training: United States, 1998–2004," *Morbidity and Mortality Weekly Report* 55, no. 28 (2006): 769–72.

3. Office of Disease Prevention and Health Promotion, U.S. Department of Health and Human Services, "Healthy People 2020 Topics and Objectives: Physical Activity," http://healthypeople.gov/2020/topicsobjectives2020/objectiveslist.aspx?topicid=33 (accessed April 2011).

4. M. J. Hubal and others, "Variability in Muscle Size and Strength Gain after Unilateral Resistance Training," *Medicine and Science in Sports and Exercise* 37, no. 6 (2005): 964–72.

5. K. Davison and others, "Relationships between Obesity, Cardiorespiratory Fitness, and Cardiovascular Function," *Journal of Obesity* 2010 (2010); M. Fogelholm, "Physical Activity, Fitness and Fatness: Relations to Mortality, Morbidity and Disease Risk Factors. A Systematic Review," *Obesity Reviews* 11 no. 3 (2010): 202–21; J.G. Stegger and others, "Body Composition and Body Fat Distribution in Relation to Later Risk of Acute Myocardial Infarction: A Danish Follow-up Study," *International Journal of Obesity* (February 2011) [Epub ahead of print].

6. Z. Wang and others, "Specific Metabolic Rates of Major Organs and Tissues across Adulthood: Evaluation by Mechanistic Model of Resting Energy Expenditure," *American Journal of Clinical Nutrition* 92, no. 6 (2010): 1369–77.

7. S. M. Fernando and others, "Myocyte Androgen Receptors Increase Metabolic Rate and Improve Body Composition by Reducing Fat Mass," *Endocrinology* 151 no. 7 (2010): 3125–32; R. R. Wolfe, "The Underappreciated Role of Muscle in Health and Disease," *American Journal of Clinical Nutrition* 84, no. 3 (2006): 475–82.

8. J. E. Donnelly and others, "American College of Sports Medicine Position Stand: Appropriate Physical Activity Intervention Strategies for Weight Loss and Prevention of Weight Regain for Adults," *Medicine and Science in Sports and Exercise* 41 no. 2 (2009): 459–71; B. L. Marks and others, "Fat-free Mass Is Maintained in Women Following a Moderate Diet and Exercise Program," *Medicine and Science in Sports and Exercise* 27, no. 9 (1995): 1243–51.

9. W. W. Campbell and others, "Resistance Training Preserves Fat-free Mass without Impacting Changes in Protein Metabolism after Weight Loss in Older Women," *Obesity* 17, no. 7 (2009): 1332–9.

10. P. A. Williams and T. F. Cash, "Effects of a Circuit Weight Training Program on the Body Images of College Students," *International Journal of Eating Disorders* 30, no. 1 (2001): 75–80.

11. E. A. Marques and others, "Effects of Resistance and Aerobic Exercise on Physical Function, Bone Mineral Density, OPG, and RANKL in Older Women," *Experimental Gerontology* 46, no. 7 (2011): 524–32.

12. American Council on Exercise (ACE), ACE FitnessMatters, "Why Is the Concept of Spot Reduction Considered a Myth?" www.acefitness.org/fitnessqanda /fitnessqanda_display.aspx?itemid=341 (2004).

13. K. Jay and others, "Kettlebell Training for Musculoskeletal and Cardiovascular Health: A Randomized Controlled Trial," *Scandinavian Journal of Work, Environment, and Health* 37, no. 3 (2010): 196–203.

14. M. Bird, American College of Sports Medicine, "Building Strength Safely" *Fit Society Page* (Fall 2002): 3.

15. C. E. Brodeur and others, "The Andro Project: Physiological and Hormonal Influences of Androstenedione Supplementation in Men 35–65 Years Old Participating in a High-Intensity Resistance Training Program," *Archives of Internal Medicine* 160, no. 20, (2000): 3093–104.

16. M. L. Kohut and others, "Ingestion of a Dietary Supplement Containing Dehydroepiandrosterone (DHEA) and Androstenedione Has Minimal Effect on Immune Function in Middle-Aged Men," *Journal of the American College of Nutrition* 22, no. 5 (2003): 363–71.

17. A. Weltman and others, "Endurance Training Amplifies the Pulsatile Release of Growth Hormone: Effects of Training Intensity," *Journal of Applied Physiology* 72, no. 6 (1992): 2188–96.

18. D. G. Candow and others, "Effect of Whey and Soy Protein Supplementation Combined with Resistance Training in Young Adults," *International Journal of Sport Nutrition and Exercise Metabolism* 16, no. 3 (2006): 233–44.

19. D. G. Candow and others, "Effect of Glutamine Supplementation Combined with Resistance Training in Young Adults," *European Journal of Applied Physiology* 86, no. 2 (2001): 142–9.

20. E. L. Knight and others, "The Impact of Protein Intake on Renal Function Decline in Women with Normal Renal Function or Mild Renal Insufficiency," *Annals of Internal Medicine* 138, no. 6 (2003): 460–7.

LAB 4.1 • ASSESSING YOUR MUSCULAR STRENGTH

Name: _____ **Date:** _____

Instructor: _____ **Section:** _____

Materials: Calculator, leg press machine, chest press machine

Purpose: To assess your current level of muscular strength

Note: This lab should be performed in the presence of an instructor to ensure proper form and safety.

MUSCULAR STRENGTH ASSESSMENT

One Repetition Maximum (1 RM) Prediction Assessment

ACSM recommends measuring muscular strength by performing one repetition maximum (1 RM) or multiple RM assessments. This lab estimates 1 RM for the chest press and leg press by finding the amount of weight you can maximally lift 2 to 10 times.

1. **Warm up.** Complete 3 to 10 minutes of light cardiorespiratory activity to warm the muscles. Perform range-of-motion exercises and light stretches for the joints and muscles that you will be using.

2. **Use proper form while executing the chest press and leg press exercises.** For the chest press, position yourself so the bar or handles are across the middle of your chest. Spread your hands slightly wider than shoulder width. Bring the handles/bar to just above your chest and then press upward/outward until your arms are straight. For the leg press, position yourself so that your knees are at a 90-degree angle. Press the weight away from your body until your legs are straight.

3. **Perform one light warm-up set.** Set the machine at a very light weight and lift this weight about 10 times as a warm-up for your assessment.

4. **Find the appropriate strength-assessment weight and number of repetitions.** Set a weight that you think you can lift at least 2 times but no more than 10 times. Perform the lift as many times as you can (to complete fatigue) up to 10 repetitions. If you can lift more than 10 repetitions, try again using heavier weight. Repeat until you find a weight you cannot lift more than 2 to 10 times. In order to prevent muscle fatigue from affecting your results, attempt this assessment no more than three times to find the proper weight and number of repetitions. If you experience muscle fatigue, rest and perform the test again on another day. Record your results in the Muscular Strength Results section (see step 7).

5. **Find your predicted 1 RM.** Predict your 1 RM based upon the number of repetitions you performed. If the weight you lifted was between 20 and 250 pounds, use the 1 RM Prediction Table to find your predicted 1 RM. If you lifted over 250 pounds, use the Multiplication Factor Table to find your predicted 1 RM. You can find these tables at the end of this lab.

6. **Find your strength-to-body weight ratio.** Divide your predicted 1 RM by your body weight for your strength-to-body-weight ratio (S/BW). Since heavier people often have more muscle, this is a better indicator of muscular strength than just the weight lifted alone. Record your results in the Muscular Strength Results section.

7. **Find your muscle strength rating by using the Strength-to-Body Weight Ratio chart provided on the last page of this lab.** Finding your rating tells you how you compare to others who have completed this test in the past. Record your results on the next page.

Muscular Strength Results

Chest Press: Weight lifted _____ Repetitions _____

_____ × _____ = _____

Weight lifted (lb)   Multiplication factor*   Predicted 1 RM (lb)

_____ ÷ _____ = _____

Predicted 1 RM (lb)   Body weight (lb)   S/BW ratio

Rating _____

Leg Press: Weight lifted _____ Repetitions _____

_____ × _____ = _____

Weight lifted (lb)   Multiplication factor*   Predicted 1 RM (lb)

_____ ÷ _____ = _____

Predicted 1 RM (lb)   Body weight (lb)   S/BW ratio

Rating _____

*Multiplication factor from the Multiplication Factor Table on the last page of this lab.

1 RM Prediction Table

Wt (lb)	Repetitions									
	1	2	3	4	5	6	7	8	9	10
20	20	21	21	22	23	23	24	25	26	27
25	25	26	26	27	28	29	30	31	32	33
30	30	31	32	33	34	35	36	37	39	40
35	35	36	37	38	39	41	42	43	45	47
40	40	41	42	44	45	46	48	50	51	53
45	45	46	48	49	51	52	54	56	58	60
50	50	51	53	55	56	58	60	62	64	67
55	55	57	58	60	62	64	66	68	71	73
60	60	62	64	65	68	70	72	74	77	80
65	65	67	69	71	73	75	78	81	84	87
70	70	72	74	76	79	81	84	87	90	93
75	75	77	79	82	84	87	90	93	96	100
80	80	82	85	87	90	93	96	99	103	107
85	85	87	90	93	96	99	102	106	109	113
90	90	93	95	98	101	105	108	112	116	120
95	95	98	101	104	107	110	114	118	122	127
100	100	103	106	109	113	116	120	124	129	133
105	105	108	111	115	118	122	126	130	135	140
110	110	113	116	120	124	128	132	137	141	147
115	115	118	122	125	129	134	138	143	148	153

(Continued)

1 RM Prediction Table (Continued)

Wt (lb)	1	2	3	4	5	6	7	8	9	10
					Repetitions					
120	120	123	127	131	135	139	144	149	154	160
125	125	129	132	136	141	145	150	155	161	167
130	130	134	138	142	146	151	156	161	167	173
135	135	139	143	147	152	157	162	168	174	180
140	140	144	148	153	158	163	168	174	180	187
145	145	149	154	158	163	168	174	180	186	193
150	150	154	159	164	169	174	180	186	193	200
155	155	159	164	169	174	180	186	192	199	207
160	160	165	169	175	180	186	192	199	206	213
165	165	170	175	180	186	192	198	205	212	220
170	170	175	180	185	191	197	204	211	219	227
175	175	180	185	191	197	203	210	217	225	233
180	180	185	191	196	203	209	216	223	231	240
185	185	190	196	202	208	215	222	230	238	247
190	190	195	201	207	214	221	228	236	244	253
195	195	201	206	213	219	226	234	242	251	260
200	200	206	212	218	225	232	240	248	257	267
205	205	211	217	224	231	238	246	255	264	273
210	210	216	222	229	236	244	252	261	270	280
215	215	221	228	235	242	250	258	267	276	287
220	220	226	233	240	248	256	264	273	283	293
225	225	231	238	245	253	261	270	279	289	300
230	230	237	244	251	259	267	276	286	296	307
235	235	242	249	256	264	273	282	292	302	313
240	240	247	254	262	270	279	288	298	309	320
245	245	252	259	267	276	285	294	304	315	327
250	250	257	265	273	281	290	300	310	322	333

Multiplication Factor Table for Predicting 1 RM

Repetitions	1	2	3	4	5	6	7	8	9	10
Multiplication Factor	1.0	1.07	1.11	1.13	1.16	1.20	1.23	1.27	1.32	1.36

Table and multiplication factors generated using the Bryzcki equation:
1 RM = weight (kg) /[1.0278−(0.0278 × repetitions)].

Source: Adapted from M. Brzycki, "Strength Testing: Predicting a One-Rep Max from a Reps-to-Fatigue," *Journal of Physical Education, Recreation, and Dance* 64, no. 1 (1993): 88–90.

Strength-to-Body Weight Ratio Ratings

			Chest Press			
Men	**Superior**	**Excellent**	**Good**	**Fair**	**Poor**	**Very Poor**
<20 yrs	1.75	1.34–1.75	1.19–1.33	1.06–1.18	0.89–1.05	0.89
20–29 yrs	1.62	1.32–1.62	1.14–1.31	0.99–1.13	0.88–0.98	0.88
30–39 yrs	1.34	1.12–1.34	0.98–1.11	0.88–0.97	0.78–0.87	0.78
40–49 yrs	1.19	1.00–1.19	0.88–0.99	0.80–0.87	0.72–0.79	0.72
50–59 yrs	1.04	0.90–1.04	0.79–0.89	0.71–0.78	0.63–0.70	0.63
>60 yrs	0.93	0.82–0.93	0.72–0.81	0.66–0.71	0.57–0.65	0.57
Women	**Superior**	**Excellent**	**Good**	**Fair**	**Poor**	**Very Poor**
<20 yrs	0.87	0.77–0.87	0.65–0.76	0.58–0.64	0.53–0.57	0.53
20–29 yrs	1.00	0.80–1.00	0.70–0.79	0.59–0.69	0.51–0.58	0.51
30–39 yrs	0.81	0.70–0.81	0.60–0.69	0.53–0.59	0.47–0.52	0.47
40–49 yrs	0.76	0.62–0.76	0.54–0.61	0.50–0.53	0.43–0.49	0.43
50–59 yrs	0.67	0.55–0.67	0.48–0.54	0.44–0.47	0.39–0.43	0.39
>60 yrs	0.71	0.54–0.71	0.47–0.53	0.43–0.46	0.38–0.42	0.38
			Leg Press			
Men	**Superior**	**Excellent**	**Good**	**Fair**	**Poor**	**Very Poor**
<20 yrs	2.81	2.28–2.81	2.04–2.27	1.90–2.03	1.70–1.89	1.70
20–29 yrs	2.39	2.13–2.39	1.97–2.12	1.83–1.96	1.63–1.82	1.63
30–39 yrs	2.19	1.93–2.19	1.77–1.92	1.65–1.76	1.52–1.64	1.52
40–49 yrs	2.01	1.82–2.01	1.68–1.81	1.57–1.67	1.44–1.56	1.44
50–59 yrs	1.89	1.71–1.89	1.58–1.70	1.46–1.57	1.32–1.45	1.32
>60 yrs	1.79	1.62–1.79	1.49–1.61	1.38–1.48	1.25–1.37	1.25
Women	**Superior**	**Excellent**	**Good**	**Fair**	**Poor**	**Very Poor**
<20 yrs	1.87	1.71–1.87	1.59–1.70	1.38–1.58	1.22–1.37	1.22
20–29 yrs	1.97	1.68–1.97	1.50–1.67	1.37–1.49	1.22–1.36	1.22
30–39 yrs	1.67	1.47–1.67	1.33–1.46	1.21–1.32	1.09–1.20	1.09
40–49 yrs	1.56	1.37–1.56	1.23–1.36	1.13–1.22	1.02–1.12	1.02
50–59 yrs	1.42	1.25–1.42	1.10–1.24	0.99–1.09	0.88–0.98	0.88
>60 yrs	1.42	1.18–1.42	1.04–1.17	0.93–1.03	0.85–0.92	0.85

Source: Reprinted with permission from The Cooper Institute, Dallas, Texas from PHYSICAL FITNESS ASSESSMENTS AND NORMS FOR ADULTS AND LAW ENFORCEMENT, available online at www.CooperInstitute.org.

LAB 4.2 • ASSESSING YOUR MUSCULAR ENDURANCE

Name: _____ **Date:** _____

Instructor: _____ **Section:** _____

Materials: Leg press machine, bench press machine, exercise mat, yardstick or ruler, tape

Purpose: To assess your current level of muscular endurance

Note: This lab should be performed in the presence of an instructor to ensure proper form and safety.

SECTION I: MUSCULAR ENDURANCE WEIGHT-LIFTING ASSESSMENT

Twenty Repetition Maximum (20 RM) Assessment

The 20 RM assessment is a weight-lifting assessment of your muscular endurance. By performing the assessments before and after completing 8 to 12 weeks of muscular fitness exercises, you can measure your improvement.

1. Prepare for the muscle endurance assessments. If you have just completed the muscular strength assessments in Lab 4.1, you will already be warmed up. If not, follow the position, form, and warm-up instructions for bench press and leg press in Lab 4.1.

2. Find your 20 RM for chest press and leg press. Set a weight that you think you can lift a maximum of 20 times. Perform the lift to see whether you were correct. If not, increase or decrease the weight and try again until you find your 20 RM. In order to be sure that muscle fatigue does not affect your results, try to find your 20 RM within three tries. If it takes longer, rest and perform the test again on another day. Record your results below.

Muscular Endurance Weight Lifting Results

Chest Press: 20 RM weight lifted _____

Leg Press: 20 RM weight lifted _____

SECTION II: MUSCULAR ENDURANCE CALISTHENIC ASSESSMENT

Push-Up Assessment

In this muscular endurance assessment, you will perform as many push-ups as you can. This test will assess the muscular endurance of your pectoralis major, anterior deltoid, and triceps brachii muscles. If you work with a partner, your partner can check your positioning and form and count your repetitions.

1. Get into the correct push-up position on an exercise mat. Support the body in a push-up position from the knees (women) or from the toes (men). The hands should be just outside the shoulders and the back and legs straight.

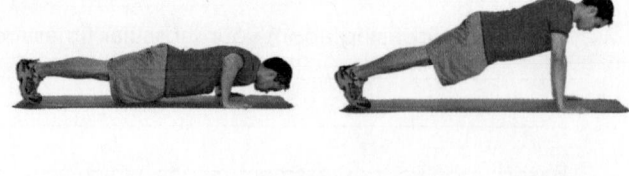

2. Start in the "down" position with your elbow joint at a 90-degree angle, your chest just above the floor, and your chin barely touching the mat. Push your body up until your arms are straight and then lower back to the starting position (count one repetition). Complete the push-ups in a slow and controlled manner.

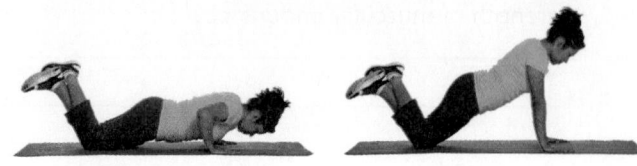

3. Complete as many correct technique push-ups as you can without stopping and record your results in the Muscular Endurance Calisthenic Results section below.

4. Find your muscle endurance rating for push-ups in the chart at the end of this lab and record your results.

Curl-Up Assessment

In this muscular endurance assessment, you will perform as many curl-ups as you can (up to 25). This test will assess the muscular endurance of your abdominal muscles.

1. Lie on a mat with your arms by your sides, palms flat on the mat, elbows straight, and fingers extended. Bend your knees at a 90-degree angle. Mark the start and end positions with tape. Your instructor or partner will mark your starting finger position with a piece of tape under each hand. He or she will then mark the ending position 10 cm (or close to 4 inches) away from the first piece of tape, one ending position tape for each hand. Your goal is to rise far enough on the curl-up to achieve a 30-degree trunk elevation.

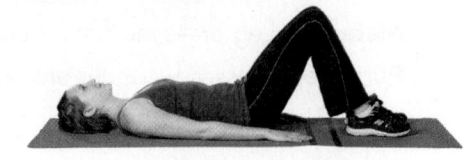

2. Your instructor or partner will set a metronome to 50 beats/min and you will complete the curl-ups at this slow, controlled pace: one curl-up every three seconds (25 curl-ups per minute).

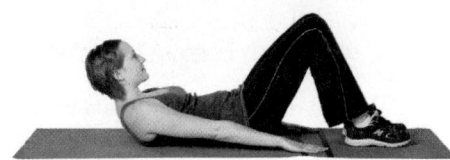

3. To start the test, curl your head and upper back upward, reaching your arms forward along the mat to touch the ending tape. Then curl back down so that your upper back and shoulders touch the floor. During the entire curl-up, your fingers, feet, and buttocks should stay on the mat. Your partner will count the number of correct repetitions you complete. Any curl-ups performed without touching the ending position tape will not be counted in the final results.

4. Perform as many curl-ups as you can without pausing, to a maximum of 25. Record your score below. Determine your muscular endurance rating for curl-ups using the chart below and record your results.

**Alternative: One-minute timed curl-ups. Your instructor may choose to have you complete as many curl-ups as you can within one minute (without the metronome pacing). Using the same start and end positions, perform controlled repetitions of curl-ups for one minute and record your results below.

Muscular Endurance Calisthenic Results

Push-Ups: Repetitions_____   Rating_____

Curl-Ups: Repetitions_____   Rating_____

**Alternative: One-minute timed curl-ups: Repetitions _____

SECTION III: REFLECTION

1. What was surprising about your muscular fitness results, if anything?

_____

_____

2. Based upon your assessment results, which aspect of muscular fitness will your program focus on, muscular strength or muscular endurance?

_____

_____

Muscular Endurance Rating

Push-ups						
Men	**Superior**	**Excellent**	**Good**	**Fair**	**Poor**	**Very Poor**
20–29 yrs	>36	31–36	24–30	21–23	16–20	<16
30–39 yrs	>30	24–30	19–23	16–18	11–15	<11
40–49 yrs	>25	19–25	15–18	12–14	9–11	<9
50–59 yrs	>21	15–21	12–14	9–11	6–8	<6
60–69 yrs	>18	13–18	10–12	7–9	4–6	<4
Women	**Superior**	**Excellent**	**Good**	**Fair**	**Poor**	**Very Poor**
20–29 yrs	>30	22–30	16–21	14–15	9–13	<9
30–39 yrs	>27	21–27	14–20	12–14	7–11	<7
40–49 yrs	>24	16–24	12–15	10–11	4–9	<4
50–59 yrs	>21	12–21	8–11	6–8	1–5	<1
60–69 yrs	>17	13–17	6–12	4–6	1–3	<1
Curl-ups						
Men	**Superior**	**Excellent**	**Good**	**Fair**	**Poor**	**Very Poor**
20–29 yrs	>25	22–25	16–21	13–15	10–12	<10
30–39 yrs	>25	19–25	15–18	13–14	10–12	<10
40–49 yrs	>25	19–25	13–18	8–12	5–7	<5
50–59 yrs	>25	18–25	11–17	9–10	7–8	<7
60–69 yrs	>25	17–25	11–16	8–10	5–7	<5
Women	**Superior**	**Excellent**	**Good**	**Fair**	**Poor**	**Very Poor**
20–29 yrs	>25	19–25	14–18	7–13	4–6	<4
30–39 yrs	>25	20–25	10–19	8–9	5–7	<5
40–49 yrs	>25	20–25	11–19	6–10	3–5	<3
50–59 yrs	>25	20–25	10–19	8–9	5–7	<5
60–69 yrs	>25	18–25	8–17	5–7	2–4	<2

Source: Adapted from Canadian Society for Exercise Physiology. *The Canadian Physical Activity, Fitness & Lifestyle Approach: CSEP-Health & Fitness Program's Health-Related Appraisal & Counseling Strategy*, 3rd ed. Canadian Society for Exercise Physiology: 2003.

LAB 4.3 • SETTING MUSCULAR FITNESS GOALS

Name: _____ Date: _____

Instructor: _____ Section: _____

Purpose: To learn how to set appropriate muscular fitness goals (short- and long-term).

SECTION I: SHORT- AND LONG-TERM GOALS

Create short- and long-term goals for muscular strength and muscular endurance. Be sure to use SMART (*Specific*, *Measurable*, *Action-Oriented*, *Realistic*, *Timed*) goal-setting guidelines. Apply information from the Chapter 4 text and use your results from Labs 4.1 and 4.2. Remember that aiming to improve your assessment scores is a measurable way to set goals. Select appropriate target dates and rewards for completing your goals.

Short-Term Goals (3–6 months)

1. Muscular Strength Goal:

_____

Target Date: _____

Reward: _____

2. Muscular Endurance Goal:

_____

Target Date: _____

Reward: _____

Long-Term Goals (12+ months)

1. Muscular Strength Goal:

_____

Target Date: _____

Reward: _____

2. Muscular Endurance Goal:

_____

Target Date: _____

Reward: _____

SECTION II: MUSCULAR FITNESS OBSTACLES AND STRATEGIES

What barriers or obstacles might hinder your plan to improve your muscular fitness? Indicate your top three obstacles below and list strategies for overcoming each obstacle.

a. _____

b. _____

c. _____

SECTION III: GETTING SUPPORT

1. List resources you will use to help change your muscular fitness:

Friend/partner/relative: _____   School-based resource: _____

Community-based resource: _____   Other: _____

SECTION IV: REFLECTION

1. How realistic are the short- and long-term target dates you have set for achieving your muscular fitness goals?

_____

_____

_____

_____

2. Are there any other strategies not listed above that could assist you in reaching your goals?

_____

_____

_____

_____

3. Think about all of the opportunities that present themselves in your daily life to work toward muscular fitness. List as many of these as you can think of:

_____

_____

_____

_____

LAB 4.4 • YOUR RESISTANCE-TRAINING WORKOUT PLAN

Name: _____ Date: _____

Instructor: _____ Section: _____

Purpose: To create a basic, personal resistance-training workout plan. Forms for following up and tracking your muscular fitness and your resistance-training program are included.

Directions: Complete the following sections.

SECTION I: MUSCULAR FITNESS PROGRAM QUESTIONS AND MOTIVATIONS

1. How many days per week are you planning to work on your muscular fitness program? _____

2. How experienced are you at resistance training? (select one below)

Novice　　　　　　**Intermediate (training 1 to 2 years)**　　　　　　**Advanced (training 3+ yrs)**

3. Which will you focus on first? (select one)　　**Muscular strength**　　**Muscular endurance**

4. The best muscular fitness programs are well rounded and work the entire body. However, some people want to focus more heavily on one area than another. Which muscle groups do you want to focus on?

_____

5. Which type of equipment do you plan to use and why? (check all that apply)

☐ **Weight machines**

☐ **Free weights**

☐ **No equipment (calisthenic exercises)**

6. How much time do you plan for your resistance-training program on each workout day? _____

7. Do you have a workout partner? Do you plan to work with a partner, trainer, or instructor to help you get started?

_____

*See **Activate, Motivate, Advance Your Fitness: A Resistance-Training Program** on page 169 for a sample resistance-training program that will match your preferences and goals outlined above.

SECTION II: RESISTANCE-TRAINING PROGRAM DESIGN

In the table on the following page, plan your resistance-training program using resources available to you (facility, instructor, text). Complete one line for each exercise you have chosen to do in your program.

Exercise	Muscle(s) Worked	Frequency (days/week)	Intensity (weight in lb)	Sets (number)	Reps (number per set)	Rest (time between sets)
LOWER BODY						
1.						
2.						
3.						
4.						
5.						
6.						
7.						
8.						
UPPER BODY						
1.						
2.						
3.						
4.						
5.						
6.						
7.						
8.						
9.						
10.						
11.						
12.						
TRUNK						
1.						
2.						
3.						
4.						
5.						

SECTION III: TRACKING YOUR PROGRAM AND FOLLOWING THROUGH

1. **Goal and program tracking:** Use a resistance-training chart (see next page) to monitor your progress. Change the amount of resistance, sets, or repetitions frequently to ensure continuing progress toward your goals.

2. **Goal and program follow-up:** At the end of the course or at your short-term goal target date, reevaluate your muscular fitness and answer the following questions:

   a. Did you meet your short-term goal or your goal for the course?

   b. If so, what positive behavioral changes contributed to your success? If not, which obstacles blocked your success?

   c. Was your short-term goal realistic? After evaluating your progress during the course, what would you change about your goals or resistance-training plan?

DATE																					
EXERCISE	Wt.	Sets	Reps	Wt.	Sets	Reps	Wt.	Sets	Reps	Wt.	Sets	Reps	Wt.	Sets	Reps	Wt.	Sets	Reps	Wt.	Sets	Reps
1.																					
2.																					
3.																					
4.																					
5.																					
6.																					
7.																					
8.																					
9.																					
10.																					
11.																					
12.																					
13.																					
14.																					

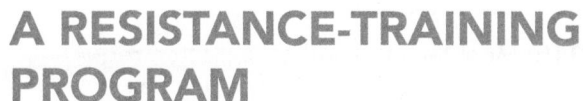

activate, motivate, & ADVANCE YOUR FITNESS

A RESISTANCE-TRAINING PROGRAM

ACTIVATE!

With the long list of health, wellness, and fitness benefits associated with resistance training, there is no doubt you want to get started now and give it all you've got! Just as with your cardiorespiratory program, don't make the mistake of trying to do too much, too soon. Doing too much too soon in a new resistance-training program is a leading cause of injury! Follow these programs to gradually increase the number of times you train each week, the number of exercises you incorporate into your weekly routine and, of course, the load (weight) and the volume (sets/repetitions).

What Do I Need for Resistance Training?

SHOES: For most resistance-training programs, you will want a pair of shoes with good traction and a non-slip sole. This gives you a stable base and prevents slipping when you lift.

CLOTHING: Wear comfortable, supportive clothing that allows for full range-of-motion movements. Choose materials that wick moisture away from your skin to help you regulate your body temperature and stay dry. In addition, you might find a pair of weight lifting gloves helpful for increasing your grip strength and preventing blisters and calluses.

How Do I Start a Resistance-Training Program?

TECHNIQUE: Safe and effective resistance training really depends on proper technique. Please be sure to read through each exercise description carefully and learn the proper technique for each exercise to ensure good form. If you need assistance with how to properly use or set up a weight machine or if you need an exercise demonstration, ask your instructor or the fitness specialist at your facility. In addition to maintaining good form, it is important to perform each exercise in a slow and controlled manner through the full range of motion, taking care to avoid "locking out" your joints. If you are unable to maintain good form, decrease the weight or even the number of repetitions. Keep the weight balanced and use collars on weight bars to keep weights stable and secure. When it comes to proper breathing technique, keep it simple.

In general, you will want to exhale during the exertion phase (when the exercise is hardest). Finally, when lifting free weights it is always advisable to have a spotter. This is especially important for heavier weight loads, for maximal efforts, and for exercises that require the weight to pass over your head, face, or chest and even when a weight actually rests on your shoulders.

ETIQUETTE: Most facilities will have posted regulations for all patrons, and there are a few basic guidelines to keep in mind when you are resistance training.

Remember, safety first. Place weights, collars, and other equipment back when you finish using them. The next user may not be as strong as you are and may not be able to move the weight plates. The last thing anyone in the gym needs is to be tripping over free weights, so put your weights back on the rack when you finish with them. Be sure to wipe down machines, equipment, and benches after use. Most gyms supply wipes or have spray bottles and rags spread out throughout the weight room, so you shouldn't use your personal sweat towel.

Another common courtesy is to let others use the machines or weights during your rest intervals between sets.

Resistance-Training Tips

AT THE GYM: One of the advantages of resistance training at a gym is access to the wide variety of equipment and the amount of actual weight: weight machines, barbells (long bars with weights attached or slots to add weight plates), dumbbells (smaller, hand-held weights), benches (flat, incline, decline), cable stations, the latest the industry has to offer. Utilizing essentials (machines and free weights) and the extras (balls, bands, etc.) provides exercise variety, which reduces boredom and increases exercise adherence. Another advantage to having a wide array of equipment and exercise options available relates to your specific muscular fitness goal and your progression. The exercise options included in the programs below and at the end of the chapter show options and modifications based on the equipment you have available. Feel free to mix up the mode you use for a basic exercise to challenge your body and increase your resistance or effort. Sometimes it is the little changes you make to an exercise that lead to the biggest progress.

AT HOME: You really have everything you need to get started. There are dozens of exercises that use your own bodyweight against gravity to increase your muscular endurance and strength. That being said, you can always add a few pieces of equipment to your home gym as you progress. Items you might consider include bands or tubing, a stability ball, medicine balls, suspension training systems, kettlebells, etc. These all store easily and most travel well. Each of these is simply one of many tools available to help you create a resistance to overcome. Training with different exercises and different exercise equipment allows you the opportunity to challenge your body with dynamic or functional exercises that mimic your movements in your activities of daily living (ADL) or your sport by introducing a fresh stimulus for physiological adaptation. For example, training with a medicine ball helps to develop total body power, muscular endurance, and flexibility. Bands can provide exercise options for beginning to advanced exercisers and athletes, an effective yet inexpensive way for your entire family to incorporate resistance training into their weekly routine. Stability balls can be used for everything from improving core stability, static and dynamic balance, strength, and flexibility and can enhance functional and sport performance. You can do an entire workout with a stability ball or use one as part of a well-rounded exercise program for greater variety and effective progression in your resistance-training program.

Resistance-Training Warm-Up and Cool-Down

A resistance-training warm-up and cool-down should include light cardiorespiratory exercises for 5 to 10 minutes. After breaking a light sweat in your warm-up, you will want to add dynamic exercises for increasing your range of motion and maybe a bit of foam rolling. Before you begin your lifts with full weight, you should complete a few repetitions with little or no weight to ensure proper form, posture, and body alignment. After you finish your cool-down, you can hold static stretches longer for improved flexibility.

Resistance-Training Programs

If you are new to resistance training or if you have taken a lay-off of more than three months, start slowly and build gradually. Start with Program A. This will help you increase overall muscular fitness (both muscular endurance and strength) and help to keep you injury free! If you are already resistance training two days a week (full body routine), then start with Program B. Adjust intensity, volume and training days to suit your personal fitness level and schedule; visit the companion website for more options.

PROGRAM A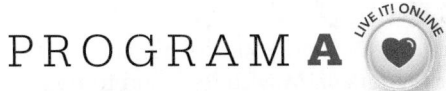

GOAL: Improve overall muscular fitness by performing 8 exercises twice a week.

Frequency	Intensity	Time			Number & Type of Exercises
		Reps	*Sets*	*Rest*	
2 non-consecutive days a week	60% 1RM	12	2	2 minutes between sets	8 multiple-joint exercises

Order of Exercises:

Leg Press
Heel Raises (can be performed through ankle plantar flexion while completing Leg Press)
Chest Press

Compound Row
Overhead Press
Lat Pull-Down
Abdominal Curl
Back Extension

PROGRAM B

GOAL: Continue to improve muscular fitness by performing a split resistance-training program (upper/lower) four days of the week.

Frequency	Intensity	Time			Number & Type of Exercises
		Reps	*Sets*	*Rest*	
4 days a week: Upper body M/W Lower body T/Th	70% 1RM	10	3	2.5 minutes between sets	Upper body: 7 multiple-joint exercises 1 single-joint exercise Lower body: 4 multiple-joint exercises 3 single-joint exercises

M/W Upper Body Order of Exercises:

Chest Press
Row
Chest Fly
Overhead Press
Lat Pull-Down
Upright Row
Biceps Curl
Triceps Extension

T/Th Lower Body Order of Exercises:

Squat
Lunge
Leg Extension
Leg Curl
Heel Raise
Abdominal Curl
Oblique Curl
Back Extension

MOTIVATE!

Create your own exercise log to track your resistance-training program—make note of days, actual exercises, sets, reps, load amounts, and rest intervals—or use the log available through the companion website. Here are a few other tips to keep you training strong.

ADJUST YOUR TRAINING ROUTINE: Boredom is a motivation killer. Regular changes to your training exercises, incorporating different equipment, and changing your training location from time to time are all ways to keep you engaged and ready for a new challenge.

MOTIVATION THROUGH MEDIA: Listen to music or podcasts during your rest intervals. In your downtime, try reading articles, blogs, or books about fitness, resistance training, healthy lifestyles, or your favorite sport. This helps to keep you interested and engaged to reach your goals.

STAY POSITIVE: Turn around your negative thoughts and self-talk and low energy days by surrounding yourself with positive affirmations and training partners. Stay focused and remember your goals. Take a moment to acknowledge how much you have already accomplished.

JOIN A FITNESS MESSAGE BOARD: Check out the message boards of fitness websites for inspiration from others who have accomplished their goals or who are working toward exercise goals similar to yours. Most message boards are designed to foster encouragement, discipline, and accountability.

MAKE A HEALTH CONTRACT WITH YOUR FAMILY MEMBERS: Everyone gets one private hour every day to exercise guilt-free. This will help establish your family's goal of a happy, healthy, and active lifestyle.

ADVANCE!

Now that you have established your resistance-training program, challenge yourself. Maybe it is time to try a few new exercises or new equipment. You may want to retake the estimated 1 RM and 20 RM tests and set new goals to take your training to the next level. Remember to follow the "10 percent rule" to safely progress to a new goal: do not increase frequency, intensity, or time more than 10 percent per week. Below are two more advanced resistance-training programs. You can follow these or log onto the companion website to find more options or to personalize this program or any of the programs in this book.

PROGRAM C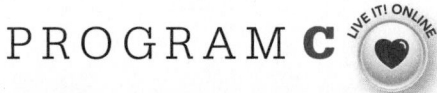

GOAL: Increase muscular endurance by performing 12 exercises three days a week.

Frequency	Intensity	Time			Number & Type of Exercises
		Reps	Sets	Rest	
3 non-consecutive days a week	50% 1RM	15	3	45–60 seconds between sets	10 multiple joint and 2 single joint

Order of Exercises:

Push-Up
Assisted Pull-Up
Squat
Lunge
Chest Fly
Row

Upright Row
Overhead Press
Biceps Curl
Pullover
Plank
Side Bridge (each side)

PROGRAM D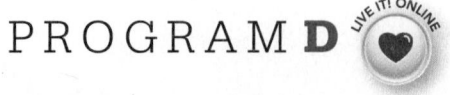

GOAL: Build muscular strength and mass by performing a high-intensity split resistance-training program (upper/lower) four days of the week.

Frequency	Intensity	Time			Number & Type of Exercises
		Reps	Sets	Rest	
4 days a week: Upper body M/W Lower body T/Th	80% 1RM	8	4	3 minutes between sets	Upper body: 7 multiple-joint exercises 1 single-joint exercise Lower body: 4 multiple-joint exercises 3 single-joint exercises

M/W Upper Body
Order of Exercises:

Chest Press
Row
Overhead Press
Lat Pull-Down
Lateral Raise
Biceps Curl
Tricep Extension
Back Extension

T/Th Lower Body
Order of Exercises:

Leg Press
Leg Extension
Leg Curl
Hip Abduction
Hip Adduction
Heel Raise
Abdominal Curl
Reverse Curl
Oblique Curl

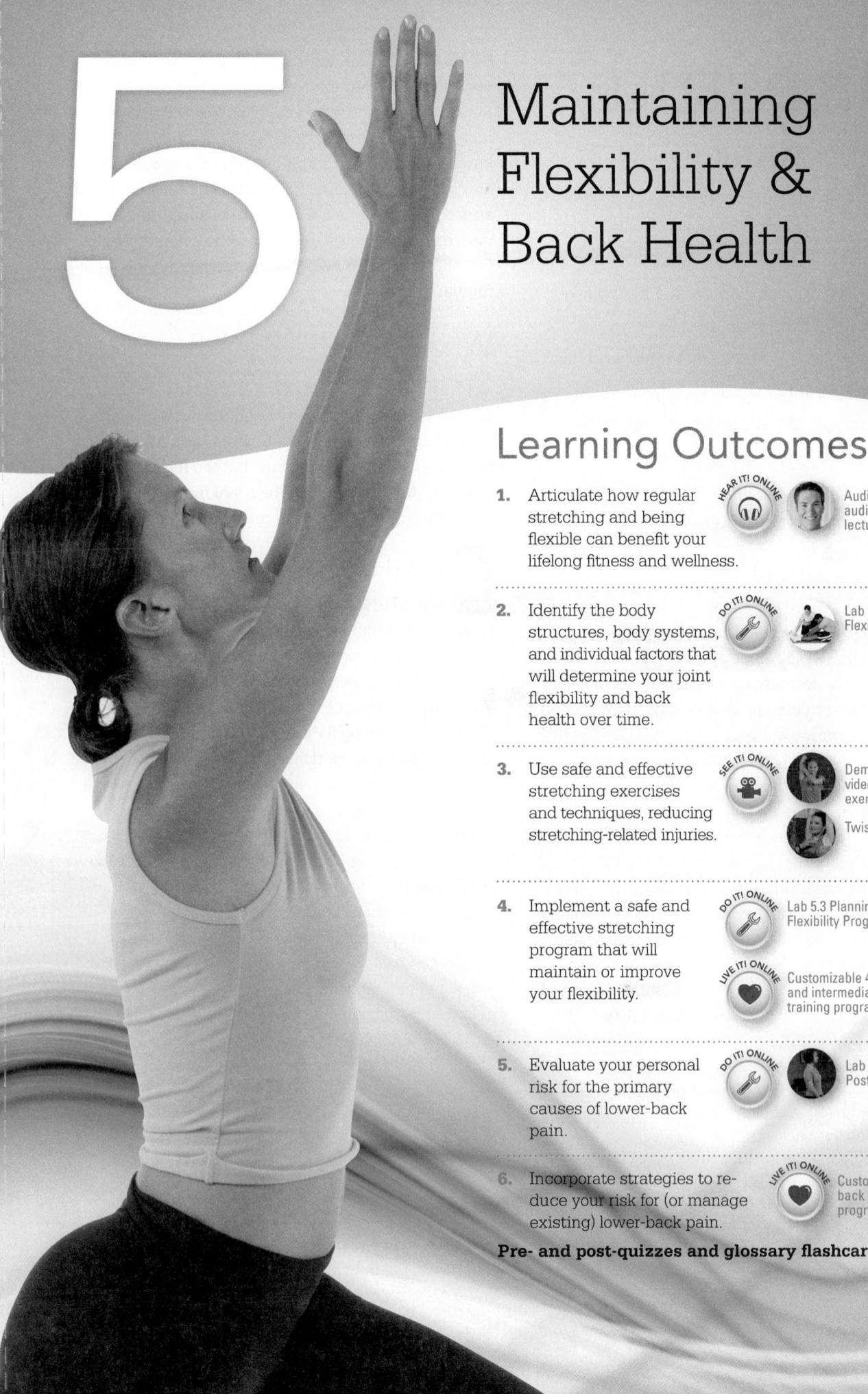

5

Maintaining Flexibility & Back Health

Learning Outcomes

1. Articulate how regular stretching and being flexible can benefit your lifelong fitness and wellness.

   HEAR IT! ONLINE — Audio case study and audio PowerPoint lecture

2. Identify the body structures, body systems, and individual factors that will determine your joint flexibility and back health over time.

   DO IT! ONLINE — Lab 5.1 Assess Your Flexibility

3. Use safe and effective stretching exercises and techniques, reducing stretching-related injuries.

   SEE IT! ONLINE — Demonstration videos of stretching exercises

   Twist to Get Fit

4. Implement a safe and effective stretching program that will maintain or improve your flexibility.

   DO IT! ONLINE — Lab 5.3 Planning a Flexibility Program

   LIVE IT! ONLINE — Customizable 4-week starter and intermediate flexibility training programs

5. Evaluate your personal risk for the primary causes of lower-back pain.

   DO IT! ONLINE — Lab 5.2 Assess Your Posture

6. Incorporate strategies to reduce your risk for (or manage existing) lower-back pain.

   LIVE IT! ONLINE — Customizable 4-week back health exercise programs

Pre- and post-quizzes and glossary flashcards *REVIEW IT! ONLINE*

casestudy

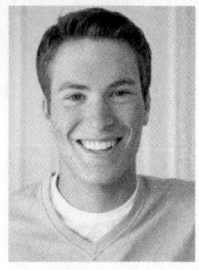

MARK

"Hi, I'm Mark. I live in Colorado Springs, at the foothills of the Rocky Mountains. I love the outdoors. I've been a backpacker, fisherman, and skier my whole life. My girlfriend is a fitness instructor and has been telling me that I should really stretch more, but I'm skeptical. What's so important about stretching? Will it help me be a better hiker or skier? How do I figure out what kind of stretches I should do? And when and how often should I stretch?"

HEAR IT! ONLINE

Flexibility is the ability of joints to move through a full **range of motion**. Flexibility tends to decrease as we get older,[1] so a good time to start a stretching program—if you don't stretch already—is when you are younger. Starting to stretch now will help you feel good and will increase your chances of staying flexible as you get older. A complete fitness program should include **stretching** and range-of-motion exercises to help you maintain flexibility and prevent joint problems.

Flexibility can be classified as static or dynamic. **Static (passive) flexibility** is a measure of the limits of a joint's overall range of motion.

Dynamic (active) flexibility is a measure of overall joint stiffness during movement (i.e., with muscular contraction). Active movement such as swinging a tennis racket or leaping over a hurdle on a track requires good dynamic flexibility.

> **flexibility** The ability of a joint (or joints) to move through a full range of motion
>
> **range of motion** The movement limits of a specific joint or group of joints
>
> **stretching** Exercises designed to improve or maintain flexibility
>
> **static (passive) flexibility** A joint's range-of-motion limits with an external force applied
>
> **dynamic (active) flexibility** A joint's range-of-motion limits with muscular contraction applied

In this chapter, we will cover how maintaining your flexibility can improve your mobility, keep your joints healthy, and help you relax. We will discuss the factors that determine how flexible a person is, present strategies for stretching safely and effectively, and provide guidelines for developing a personalized stretching program. We will also discuss the common problem of lower-back pain and offer strategies for incorporating a back-health component into your regular fitness plan.

What Are the Benefits of Stretching and Flexibility?

Like Mark, many people are not in the habit of stretching and are not sure why stretching is important. There are many benefits to stretching, but the most compelling is simple: Being flexible will help you move freely and complete activities you want to do with greater ease.

Improved Mobility, Posture, and Balance

A regular stretching program helps you maintain joint mobility throughout your body. Your joints allow you to *move*—whether you are bending your knees to tie a shoelace, riding a bicycle around campus, or reaching for a bowl on the top shelf of a cupboard. A reduction in your flexibility can result in a reduction in your ability to move about freely as you perform daily activities. Likewise, an improvement in your flexibility can result in greater freedom of movement. Keeping your body flexible and strong also helps you maintain your balance. Individuals who have better ankle strength and range of motion not only have better balance, but also a greater functional ability—which means fewer falls and injuries.[2]

Regular stretching can also help you maintain a balance of muscle strength and muscle flexibility, which is important for proper joint alignment and posture. For example, if the muscles on the front of your hips get too tight, your pelvis can get pulled forward and cause a larger sway in your lower back. This will alter your posture and could even affect your balance. Good flexibility, developed through stretching, helps you keep your joints and spine aligned and promotes overall body stability.

Healthy Joints and Pain Management

As many as 28 percent of all adults report pain or stiffness in joints. That number increases dramatically with age, and women are more likely to have those joint symptoms. Many adults also have or will develop **arthritis** at some point in their lives; 54 percent of people 75 years and older have been diagnosed with arthritis.[3] Regular exercise, including range-of-motion and flexibility exercises, is essential for people with arthritis to maintain function and manage joint pain.[4] Even in people without arthritis, stretching will increase joint flexibility, improve joint function, and decrease periodic joint pain.[5]

Possible Reduction of Future Lower-Back Pain

Having an adequate level of flexibility may reduce your risk of lower-back pain in the future; however, research on the subject is inconclusive. While poor flexibility has been linked to lower-back pain in adolescents, these relationships are less clear in adults.[6,7,8,9] Despite the mixed evidence, most experts agree that having a minimal level of joint mobility and flexibility through the hips and back is one of the strategies for reducing the risk of developing chronic lower-back pain.[10] We will discuss lower-back pain in more detail later in this chapter.

Muscle Relaxation and Stress Relief

After sitting at a computer for hours working on a term paper, doesn't it feel great to stand up and stretch? Staying in one position for too long, repetitive movement, and other stressors can result in stiff and "knotted" muscles. Gentle stretching and relaxation increases blood flow to tight muscles, stimulates the nervous system to decrease stress hormones, and ultimately helps relax areas of tension in your body.

What Determines My Flexibility?

What makes one person a human pretzel, while others can barely touch their toes? Is flexibility genetic, or can it be attributed entirely to the amount of stretching that you do? Many factors can affect your individual level of flexibility. Your joints, muscles, **tendons**, and nervous system—along with other characteristics such as age, gender, genetics, and activity level—can all influence your flexibility.

> **arthritis** An umbrella-term for more than 100 conditions characterized by inflammation of a joint
>
> **tendons** Connective tissues that attach muscle to bone
>
> **joint** The articulation or point of contact between two or more bones

Joint Structures, Muscles and Tendons, and the Nervous System

The range of motion possible in a particular **joint** is limited by the structures that comprise that joint, the muscles and tendons that cross over the joint, and the nervous system.

Joint Structures The individual components of a joint all affect the joint's mobility and stability (Figure 5.1). *Cartilage* is a strong, smooth tissue that cushions the ends of the bones, preventing them from rubbing directly against one another and providing impact protection. *Ligaments* are fibrous connective tissues that connect bone to bone. Some ligaments form the outer layer of the *joint capsule* to provide a reinforcing structure to the overall joint. Other ligaments, not part of the joint capsule, provide further stability to the joint. The *synovial membrane* forms the inner layer of the joint capsule and secretes *synovial fluid* into the *joint cavity.* Synovial fluid

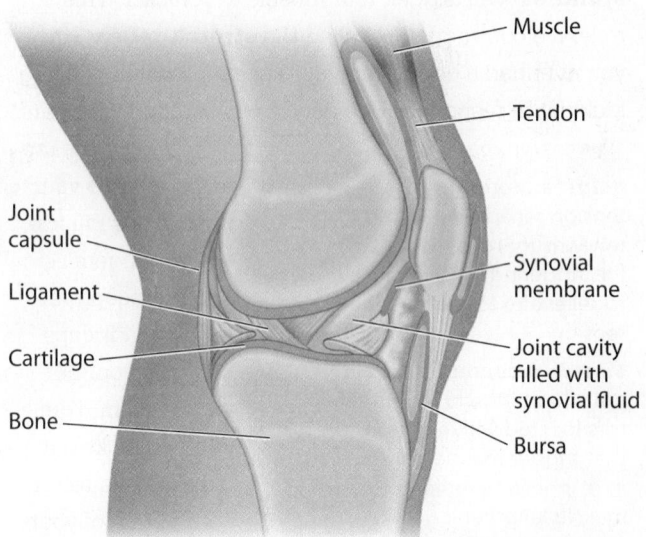

FIGURE **5.1** Joints are surrounded by a supportive joint capsule made of ligaments and synovial membranes. The joint cavity is filled with synovial fluid that (along with cartilage and bursa sacs) cushions and protects bones during movement. The stability of a joint is strengthened by muscle-tendon insertions surrounding the joint.

lubricates and protects the joint. *Bursae (singular, bursa)* are small fluid-filled sacs that lubricate the movement of muscles over one another or muscles over bone.

Muscles and Tendons Overall joint structure accounts for 47 percent of the resistance to movement around a joint (dynamic flexibility), while individual *soft tissues* (muscles, connective tissue, ligaments, tendons, and skin) account for 53 percent of the resistance to movement.[11] With regular activity and stretching, connective tissues within muscles remain supple and able to easily lengthen. With disuse and age, connective tissues become stiffer, limiting flexibility. Temperature can also affect the flexibility of soft tissues. When muscle temperature rises, connective tissues become softer and allow muscles to more easily lengthen.

The Nervous System Your nervous system is responsible for stimulating muscle contractions, and it also triggers muscle relaxation. Muscles and tendons contain nervous-system receptors that interpret information about the tension and length of muscles at any given moment. These receptors protect the muscle from damage caused by excessive amounts of tension or by stretching too far. If there is too much tension or force within a muscle, receptors in the tendon (called **golgi tendon organs**) will trigger your muscle to relax.

If your muscle is stretching too far, receptors in the muscle fibers (called **stretch receptors** or **muscle spindles**) will trigger your muscle to contract. This reflexive contraction is called the **stretch reflex**. Have you ever had a doctor tap your knee and watch your leg kick out in response? The doctor was striking your *patellar tendon*. This rapidly stretches your quadriceps muscle, which triggers stretch receptors in the quadriceps to signal your nervous system. Your leg then kicks out because of a reflex contraction of your quadriceps muscle stimulated by the nervous system.

Reducing the stretch reflex and activating the golgi tendon organs allows your muscles to relax, elongate, and gain improvements in flexibility.

golgi tendon organs Muscle tension receptors located in tendons that are responsible for triggering muscle relaxation to relieve excessive muscle tension

stretch receptors (muscle spindles) Muscle length receptors located within muscle fibers that trigger muscle contractions in response to rapid, excessive muscle lengthening

stretch reflex The reflex contraction of a muscle triggered by stretch receptors (muscle spindles) in response to a rapid overextension of that muscle

Individual Factors

Beyond the anatomical structures and physiological mechanisms that we all share, individual factors such as genetics, gender, age, body type, and activity level also affect flexibility.

Genetics Most people have a moderate level of flexibility. They have flexible and less-flexible areas of their bodies and need to work to maintain their present level of flexibility. However, some people are extremely flexible by nature, while others are exceptionally inflexible. Genetic differences in body structure and the elasticity of soft tissues help account for the wide variety of flexibility levels.

Gender Although it is widely assumed that females are more flexible than males, this may only be true for specific joints, as discussed in the box Men, Women, and Flexibility.

Age Flexibility changes throughout the lifespan. Flexible preschool children experience a decrease in joint range of motion until the preteen years, when flexibility increases again to its peak by 18 years of age.[12] In adulthood, flexibility decreases with age due to physical changes in muscles, joints, and connective tissues. These changes are joint specific and are primarily related to inactivity and disuse.

The good news is that with regular exercise, people of all ages can improve their current level of flexibility. In a study of men over 65 years of age, researchers observed flexibility improvements when the men participated in a regular resistance-training program.[13] These improvements disappeared when the men stopped training, reinforcing the notion that regular and sustained exercise is the key to maintaining and improving flexibility.

Body Type Body type can affect flexibility but typically only at the extremes of body shape and size. For example, body type may affect range of motion if an excessive amount of muscle or fat physically interferes with full joint movement. That said, genetics and training are far more influential factors in determining flexibility than is body type. There are people with long, lean bodies whom you might expect to be flexible but who actually are not due to genetics or inactivity.

DIVERSITY

Men, Women, and Flexibility

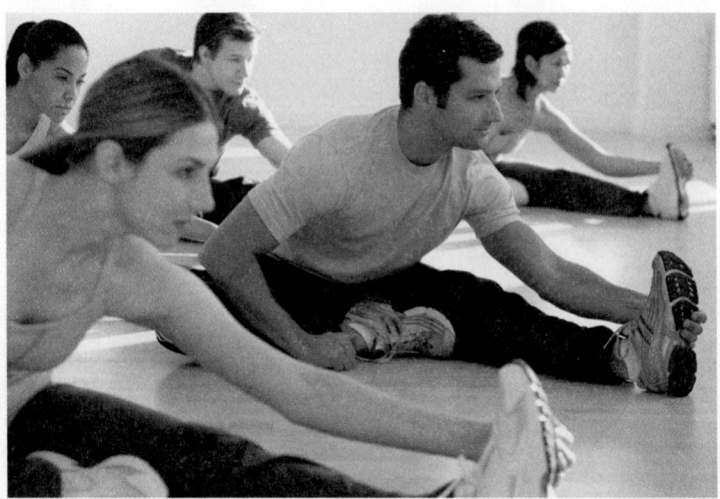

Women are more flexible than men, right? Not necessarily! This commonly held belief is not always true and may lull men into thinking that being inflexible is normal and okay. Women generally *are* more flexible in the hip joint and hamstrings, which are the most common sites for flexibility testing.[1] Women may have greater flexibility in these areas than males due to their wider hips, hormonal influences, and

tendency to participate in activities that develop greater flexibility. In other joints and areas of the body, however, there is not a large difference between males and females. In fact, males may have greater flexibility in other areas. For example, males may have greater trunk rotation capabilities.[2]

Interestingly, greater joint range of motion and flexibility may increase the chances of injury. Because women tend to have greater hip flexibility and internal rotation of the hip joint, they are more likely to have knee problems.[3] The bottom line is that adequate range of motion should be a goal for everyone, men and women. Being able to move your body without restriction opens up activity options and makes life easier!

Sources:
1. J. T. Manire and others, "Diurnal Variation of Hamstring and Lumbar Flexibility," *Journal of Strength and Conditioning Research* 24, no. 6 (2010): 1464–71.
2. J. T. Blackburn and others, "Sex Comparison of Hamstring Structural and Material Properties," *Clinical Biomechanics* 24, no. 1 (2009): 65–70.
3. R. H. Brophy and others, "The Core and Hip in Soccer Athletes Compared by Gender," *International Journal of Sports Medicine* 30, no. 9 (2009): 663–7.

Meanwhile, there are people with stocky, muscular builds who are exceptionally flexible, including many gymnasts.

Activity Level Inactivity can result in low levels of flexibility as muscles and connective tissues tighten and shorten with disuse. Overly repetitive physical activity can also result in muscle "stiffness." However, when done properly, stretching and regular physical activity can improve flexibility. We will introduce effective stretches and exercises later in this chapter.

Health Status Certain medical conditions can affect your joint health and range of motion. Diseases that affect your **collagen** and connective tissues can produce overly mobile or exceptionally inflexible joints. For example, arthritis speeds up the destruction of collagen and cartilage, leading to joint inflexibilty. In some genetic syndromes, reduced or ineffective collagen causes hypermobility. During pregnancy, many women will experience more flexible joints. Injuries or scar tissue can also affect your ability to move your

joints through their full range of motion.

collagen The primary protein of connective tissues throughout the body

casestudy

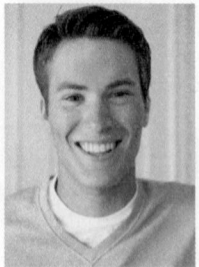

MARK

"I've heard that physical activity is supposed to improve your flexibility. If that's true, why do my muscles feel really stiff after a long day of skiing or hiking? I've noticed that this happens especially when I've gone for my first ski or hike of the season. Are my muscles just out of shape?"

THINK! What might explain Mark's muscle stiffness?

ACT! Make a list of at least five different factors that might play a role in Mark's flexibility.

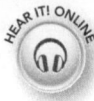

How Can I Assess My Flexibility?

Flexibility levels vary from joint to joint. As a result, most flexibility tests are designed to measure the flexibility of specific muscles and joints, not to measure your body's overall level of flexibility. However, if you take a variety of flexibility tests, you can get a sense of how your body's overall level of mobility is measuring up to recommended target ranges.

Perform the "Sit-and-Reach" Test

One of the most common measures of flexibility is the "sit-and-reach" test. This test measures the flexibility of your lower back, hip, and hamstring muscles. These areas are often tight in individuals who are inactive. This muscular imbalance can negatively influence posture, balance, and risk of back pain. **Lab 5.1** provides instructions for the sit-and-reach test.

Perform Range-of-Motion Tests

Having an adequate range of motion in your joints and maintaining that range over time should be the primary goal of a flexibility fitness program. Lab 5.1 provides instructions for performing range-of-motion tests on joints located in your neck, shoulders, trunk, hips, and ankles. By performing these tests, you can evaluate how the range of motion of your joints compares to those of the general population and determine whether your joints are more flexible or less flexible than average. This information will help you design a personalized program for developing flexibility. You can measure your progress over time by retaking the tests after months of training.

How Can I Plan a Good Stretching Program?

Regardless of whether you already stretch regularly, keep in mind the following guidelines to ensure a safe and effective program.

Set Appropriate Flexibility Goals

Decide up front what your goal is. Do you want to *maintain* your current level of flexibility (which is all that many people want to do), or do you want to *improve* your flexibility? Complete the sit-and-reach test and the range-of-motion tests described in Lab 5.1 before making this decision.

Once you've decided on your overall goal, follow the SMART guidelines for setting more specific goals. Recall that SMART stands for *specific, measurable, action-oriented, realistic,* and *time-oriented.* An example of a SMART goal designed to *maintain* your flexibility is, "My goal for the next year is to maintain the joint flexibility and range-of-motion levels recorded on my flexibility assessments by incorporating stretching into my workouts at least four times per week." An example of a SMART goal designed to *improve* your flexibility is, "My goal is to regularly stretch so that I can increase my lower-back, hip, and hamstring flexibility from 'poor' to 'good' on the sit-and-reach test by the end of the school semester." For most people, the primary goal should be the ability to move their joints through a normal range of motion. Achieving exceptionally high levels of flexibility may be desirable for some sports and activities but is not necessary for the average person.

Apply the FITT Program Design Principles

Recall that FITT stands for *frequency, intensity, time,* and *type.* Use the FITT principles to design your own personalized stretching program. Table 5.1 provides general guidelines from the American College of Sports Medicine. Refer to this table as a starting point for designing your own program.

Frequency Notice that the ACSM guidelines in Table 5.1 recommend stretching at least 2 to 3 days per week. If you've determined that your current level of flexibility is already within "normal" ranges and you

TABLE **5.1** ACSM's Flexibility Training Guidelines for Healthy Adults	
Frequency	2–3 days/week minimum
Intensity	Stretch to the point of feeling tightness or slight discomfort
Time	10–30 seconds per static stretch repetition 2–4 repetitions of each stretching exercise
Type	Static, dynamic, or PNF stretching of all major muscle groups*

*Ballistic stretching may be appropriate for some individuals in certain sports and recreational activities.

Source: C. E. Garner and others, "American College of Sports Medicine Position Stand: Quantity and Quality of Exercise for Developing and Maintaining Cardiorespiratory, Musculoskeletal, and Neuromotor Fitness in Apparently Healthy Adults: Guidance for Prescribing Exercise," *Medicine and Science in Sports and Exercise* 43, no. 7 (2011): 1334–59.

When Should I Stretch?

Many people incorrectly think that they have to stretch before a workout. In general, it is actually better to perform most of your static stretching *after* a workout, when your muscles are warm and your joint structures are more receptive to stretching.

For *most* individuals, light pre-exercise static stretches will not negatively affect exercise or recreational performance. If you are an athlete, though, you may want to avoid too much static stretching before a competition or high-intensity workout. Some studies have shown that extensive static stretching can result in a reduction in muscle strength and power that lasts 30 minutes or more.[1] The implications of this research are still unknown: A more recent study showed that stretching did not alter the 1 repetition maximum bench press performance in collegiate male athletes.[2]

It is also now generally accepted that pre-exercise stretching does not reduce over-use injuries.[3] This is a surprise to many people, but it doesn't mean that you have to give up your warm-up stretches. If you warm up properly first, you can stretch at any time of day and improve your flexibility.[4] More research must be done, but the recommendations now include stretching for maintaining joint mobility, but not as a primary means to reduce injury or enhance performance.

Key points:

- If you perform static stretches, stick to *light* static stretching (10 to 15 seconds)

- If you want to stretch before a workout, be sure to warm up beforehand. Stretching cold muscles can result in injury.

- Emphasize dynamic stretches in your warm-up and make sure the movements are similar to your exercise, sport, or recreational activity.

Sources:
1. T. Yamaguchi and K. Ishii, "Effects of Static Stretching for 30 Seconds and Dynamic Stretching on Leg Extension Power," *Journal of Strength and Conditioning Research* 19, no. 3 (2005): 677–83.
2. Z.D. Molacek, D. S. Conley, T. K. Evetovich, and K. R. Hinnerichs, "Effects of Low- and High-Volume Stretching on Bench Press Performance in Collegiate Football Players," *Journal of Strength and Conditioning Research* 24, no. 3 (2010): 711–16.
3. M. P. McHugh and C. H. Cosgrave, "To Stretch or Not to Stretch: the Role of Stretching in Injury Prevention and Performance," *Scandinavian Journal of Medicine & Science in Sports* 20, no. 2 (2010): 169–81.
4. G. G. Haff (ed.), "Round Table Discussion: Flexibility Training," *Strength and Conditioning Journal* 28, no. 2 (2006): 64–85.

merely want to maintain that level, you should stretch two days per week. If you've determined that your current level of flexibility needs improvement to reach a "normal" range, you should stretch three or more days per week. Should you stretch before a workout, after a workout, or both? The box When Should I Stretch? explores these questions and others.

Intensity The ACSM guidelines (see Table 5.1) state that you should stretch "to the point of feeling tightness or slight discomfort." If you are feeling pain, you are stretching too far and risking injury. Pay close attention to your body whenever you stretch; your flexibility level may vary slightly from day to day.

Time The ACSM guidelines state that you should perform your stretching program for at least 10 minutes at a time. In that time, stretch all major muscle groups, hold stretches for 10 to 30 seconds each, and repeat stretches two to four times. As soon as you start to stretch, your stretch reflex will activate: You can feel this as a slight increase in muscle tension when you move into a stretch position. By holding your stretches for at least 10 seconds, you are giving the stretch reflex time to lessen. You are also giving your golgi tendon organs time to activate and, thus, allow your muscles to lengthen farther.

By repeating stretches multiple times, you enable your muscles to relax and lengthen a little bit more each time. If you are beginning a stretching program for the first time and feel uncomfortable with multiple repetitions, you can perform one repetition of each stretch and still obtain benefits. After a few weeks of stretching consistently, gradually increase the number of repetitions to the recommended two to four times per session. Aim to have your total stretching time for each exercise add up to sixty seconds.

Type There are numerous kinds of stretching techniques. The most common are highlighted below.

- **Static stretching** involves moving slowly into a stretch and holding it for a prescribed amount of time. This is the simplest and safest method for individuals who are just starting a stretching program. Static stretching is effective, because the activity of slow stretching and holding reduces the activation of stretch receptors. After a workout, static stretching can help muscles recover and help you to maintain or improve your flexibility.

- **Dynamic stretching** involves stretching through movement. During dynamic stretching, you mimic the motions of your workout or

sports activity with slow, fluid movements. Dynamic stretching increases dynamic flexibility and can enhance muscle action during sports and recreational activities.[14] The warm-up phase of an exercise session is a good time to implement dynamic stretching, because it helps prepare the body for the more intense physical activity to come.

- **Ballistic stretching** is a stretching method characterized by bouncing, sometimes jerky, movements and high momentum. Ballistic stretching increases dynamic flexibility and can benefit trained athletes in sports requiring fast, explosive movements such as wrestling, gymnastics, tennis, and basketball. However, the bouncing movements in ballistic stretching rapidly activate the stretch receptors, making this method less effective at increasing static flexibility.

- **Proprioceptive neuromuscular facilitation (PNF)** uses the voluntary contraction of muscle

static stretching Stretching characterized by slow and sustained muscle lengthening

dynamic stretching Stretching characterized by controlled, full-range-of-motion movements that mimic exercise session movements

ballistic stretching Stretching characterized by bouncing, jerky movements and momentum to increase range of motion

proprioceptive neuromuscular facilitation (PNF) Stretching that is facilitated or enhanced by the voluntary contraction of the targeted muscle group or contraction of opposing muscles

casestudy

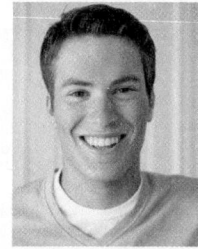

MARK

"The ski season just started. Out of curiosity, I asked a ski instructor for his opinions on stretching. He was surprised that I have been skiing my whole life but wasn't in the habit of stretching! He explained how stretching can help reduce muscle tension, improve my ability to make quick turns, and help prevent strains and stiffness. He recommended quadriceps and hamstrings stretches, for starters. He also suggested some stretching exercises that mimic the motion of skiing, in case I ever wanted to try skiing at a more advanced level."

THINK! Look at the quadriceps and hamstrings stretches in Figure 5.3. Are these static or dynamic stretches? What is the difference?

ACT! Assume that Mark wants to begin a general stretching program in the "off" season when he is not skiing, with the goal of improving his flexibility. Given the ACSM guidelines you have learned, write out a basic flexibility program for him.

HEAR IT! ONLINE

groups to help facilitate relaxation and stretching in target muscles. The most common method of PNF stretching is called *contract-relax PNF*. In contract-relax PNF, the exerciser experiences an isotonic or isometric contraction of the target muscle just prior to slow, passive stretching of that muscle. An example of contract-relax PNF in action is shown in Figure 5.2.

Table 5.2 lists some of the pros and cons of each stretching method. For most people starting a flexibility program on their own, static stretches are the safest option. Figure 5.3 illustrates some common stretching exercises you can select from, and Activate, Motivate, & Advance Your Fitness: A Flexibility Training Program located at the end of the chapter (page 210) offers options for sequencing and combining stretches. **Lab 5.3** walks you through the process of designing your own program.

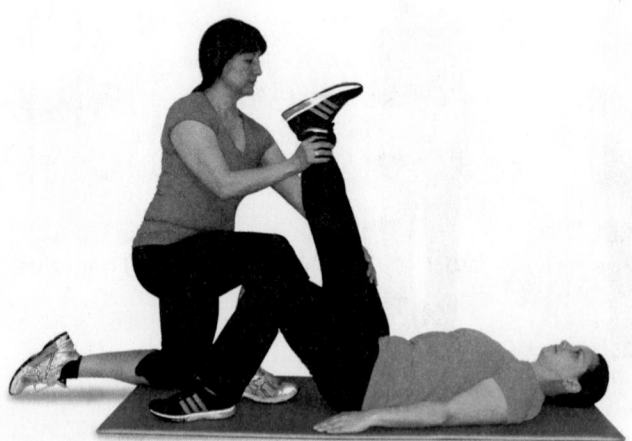 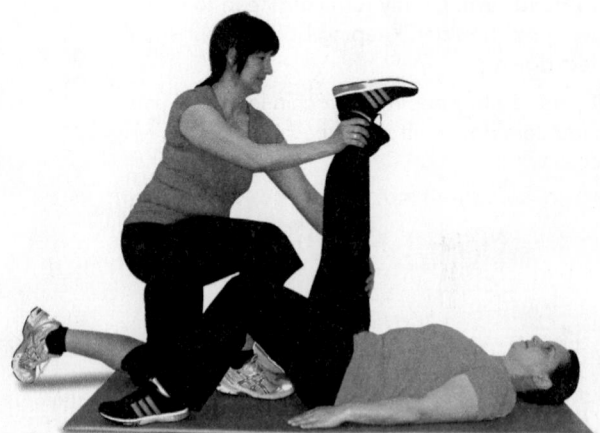

(a) Lie on your back with one leg bent and the other extended toward the ceiling. Have a partner hold your lifted leg as you try to press your leg to the ground for 6 seconds. Your partner can resist enough to allow no movement at all (isometric contraction) or just enough to allow gradual movement toward the ground (isotonic contraction). The contraction stimulates the golgi tendon organs to activate and promote muscle relaxation.

(b) Immediately following the 6-second contraction, relax your muscles and have your partner move your leg up and toward your chest into a passive stretch for the hips, hamstrings, and low back. Hold this stretch for 10–30 seconds and release.

FIGURE **5.2** An example of a contract-relax proprioceptive neuromuscular facilitation (PNF) partner exercise.

TABLE **5.2** Pros and Cons of Common Stretching Methods		
Stretching Method	Pro	Con
Static	Safe, simple to use, effective at increasing static flexibility	Can reduce muscle strength and power immediately after stretching, can be time consuming
Dynamic	Increases dynamic flexibility, functional movements	Takes time to learn correct movement patterns
Ballistic	Can be beneficial for ballistic sports, increases dynamic flexibility	Not as effective at increasing overall flexibility
PNF	Effective at increasing flexibility levels	Need a partner or equipment to perform, complicated method

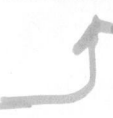

FIGURE **5.3**

STRETCHES TO MAINTAIN OR INCREASE FLEXIBILITY

All standing stretches should be started or performed from a good posture position (abs pulled in, feet facing forward, knees slightly bent). All one-arm or one-leg stretches should be performed on both sides.

Hold stretches for 10 to 30 seconds. (Refer to Figure 4.8 on page 132 for the full-body muscle diagram.)

Videos for these exercises and more are available online at www.pearsonhighered.com/hopson and on MyFitnessLab.

Upper-Body Stretches

1. Neck Stretches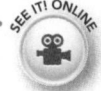

(a) **Head turn:** Gently turn your head to look over one shoulder, keeping both of your shoulders down.

(b) **Head tilt:** Keeping your chin level and your shoulders down, tilt your head to one side.

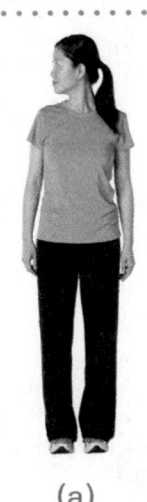 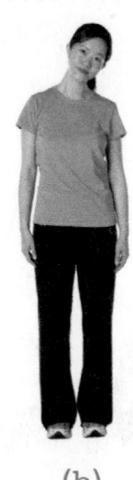

(a) (b)

Muscles targeted:

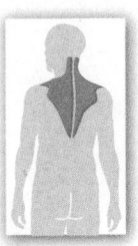

10 Trapezius

2. Pectoral and Biceps Stretch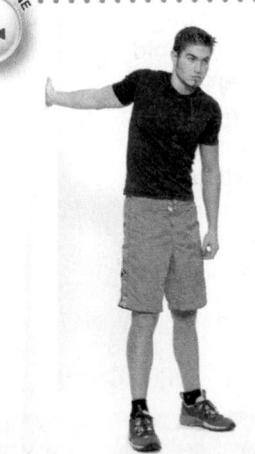

Stand arm's length away from a wall. Reach your arm out to the side and place your palm flat on the wall. Turn your body away from the wall until you feel a comfortable stretch.

Muscles targeted:

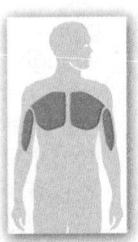

1 Pectoralis major
2 Biceps brachii

3. Upper-Back Stretch

Reach your arms out in front of you and clasp your hands while rounding out your back and lowering your head.

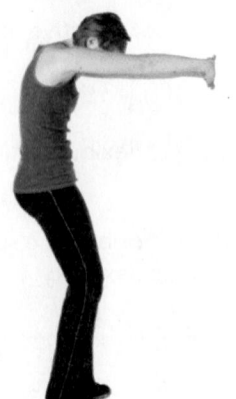

Muscles targeted:

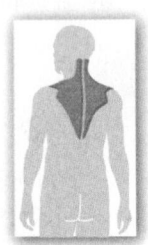 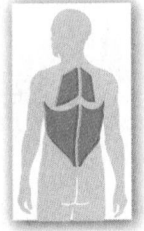

10 Trapezius   **11** Rhomboids
14 Latissimus dorsi

4. Side Stretch

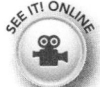
SEE IT! ONLINE

Reach one straight arm over your head and bend sideways at the waist. Focus on reaching up and over with your arm. The opposite hand can reach for the floor or be placed at your hip.

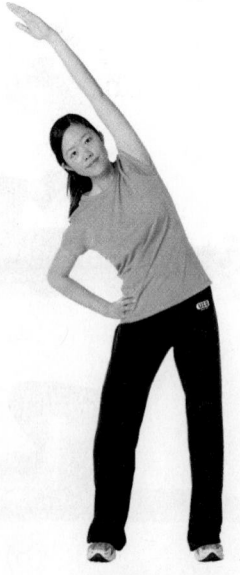

Muscles targeted:

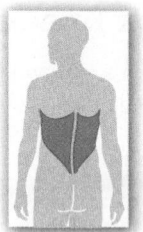
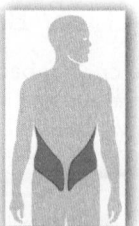

14 Latissimus dorsi   **4** External obliques

5. Shoulder Stretch

SEE IT! ONLINE

Reach one arm across the chest and hold it above or below the elbow with the other hand. Keep both shoulders pressed down.

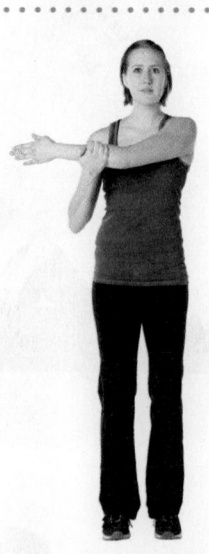

Muscles targeted:

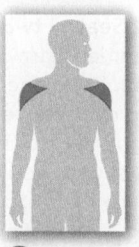

9 Deltoids

6. Triceps Stretch

SEE IT! ONLINE

Lift your arm overhead, reaching the elbow toward the ceiling and the hand down the back. Assist the stretch by using your other hand to either **(a)** press the arm back from the front or **(b)** reach over your head, grasp your arm just below the elbow, and pull back and toward your head.

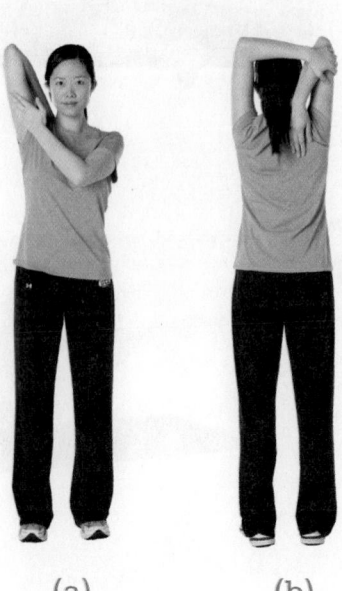

(a)   (b)

Muscles targeted:

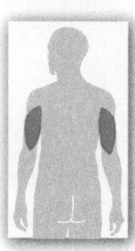

13 Triceps brachii

Lower-Body Stretches

7. Low-Back Knee-to-Chest Stretch

Lie on your back on a mat and lift either (a) one knee or (b) two knees toward the chest, grasping the leg(s) from behind for support.

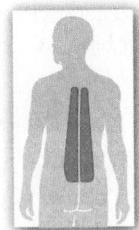

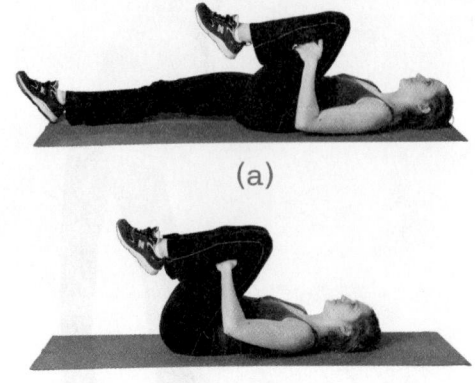

(a)

(b)

Muscles targeted:

12 Erector spinae

8. Torso Twist and Hip Stretch

(a) **Seated twist:** Sit on a mat with your legs straight out in front of you. Bend one knee and cross that leg over your other leg. Turn your body toward the bent knee and twist your body to look behind you. Place the opposite arm on the bent leg to gently press into the stretch further.

(b) **Lying cross-leg twist:** While lying on your back, bend the knee and hip of one leg to 90 degrees. Keep the other leg straight and slowly move the bent leg across your body toward the floor. Keep your arms wide for balance and both shoulders down.

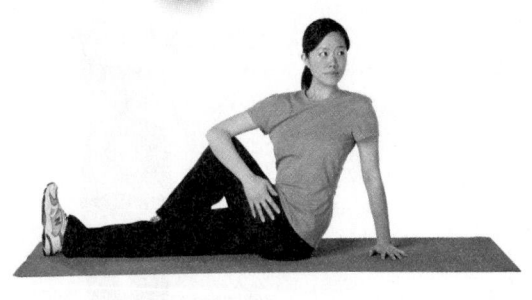

(a)

(b)

Muscles targeted:

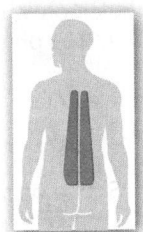 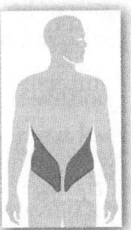

12 Erector spinae   **4** External obliques

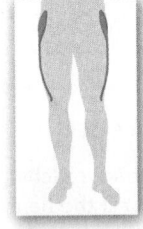 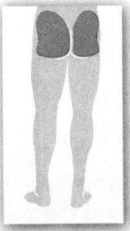

5 Tensor fasciae latae   **15** Gluteus maximus

9. Gluteal Stretch

Lie on your back with one leg bent and the foot on the floor. Place the ankle of the other leg on your thigh just below the knee. Lift both legs toward the chest and support them with your hands clasped behind your thigh.

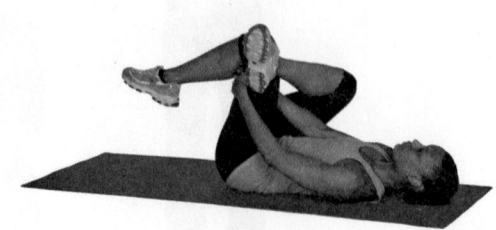

Muscles targeted:

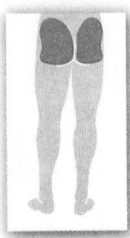

15 Gluteus maximus

10. Hip Flexor Stretch

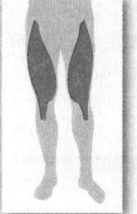

(a) **Standing stretch:** Stand tall with one foot forward and one foot back in a lunge position. Lift up the heel of the back leg and press your hips forward.

(b) **Low-lunge stretch:** Lunge forward and gently place your back knee on a mat and release your foot to point back. Lean forward into the hip and thigh stretch but make sure that your front ankle is directly under your front knee.

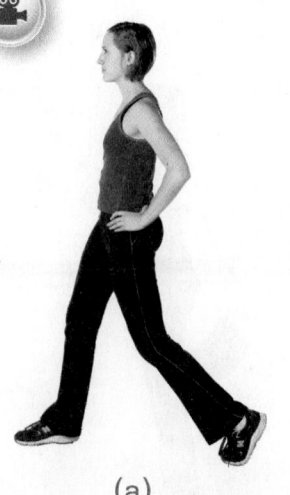
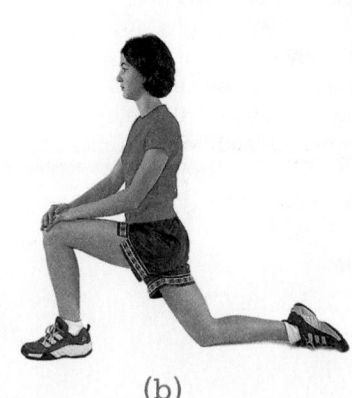

(a)   (b)

Muscles targeted:

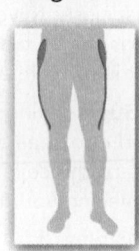

7 Quadriceps

11. Inner-Thigh Stretch

(a) **Side lunge stretch:** With a wide stance, shift your weight over onto one leg, bending that knee. Press your hips back to ensure that your bent knee does not extend beyond your ankle. Place your hands on your thigh, and keep your chest lifted and back straight.

(b) **Butterfly stretch:** Sitting on a mat, bring the bottoms of your feet together and pull your feet gently toward you. Actively contract your hip muscles to lower your knees closer to the ground. A slight lean forward will stretch the gluteal and low-back muscles as well.

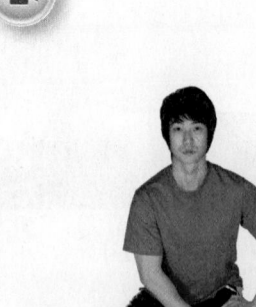
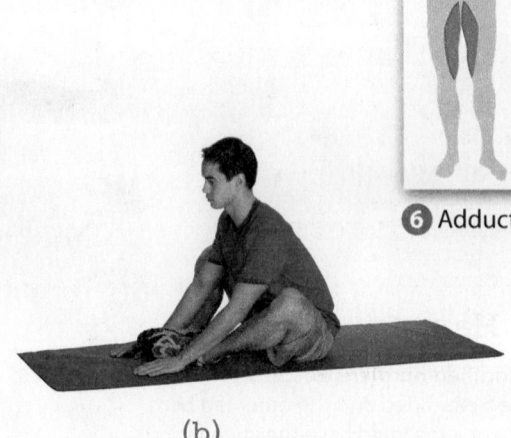

(a)   (b)

Muscles targeted:

6 Adductors

12. Outer-Thigh Stretch

Stand arm's length next to a wall. Place your outside foot on the floor closer to the wall, crossing over the inside leg. Lean your hip closer to the wall while you lean your upper body away from the wall for balance.

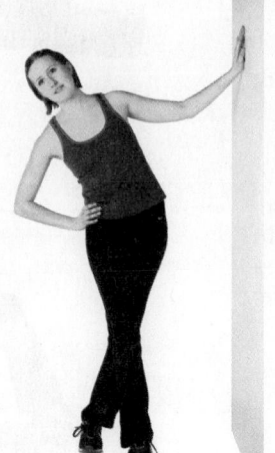

Muscles targeted:

5 Tensor fasciae latae

13. Quadriceps Stretch

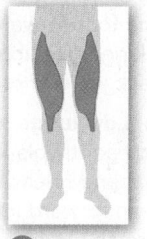

Grab your foot from behind and pull it back toward your rear until you feel a stretch in the front of your thighs. Maintain straight body alignment and keep your thighs parallel to one another. When **(a)** standing, assist your balance by holding a wall, a chair, or another form of support. The stretch can also be done from a **(b)** lying down position.

Muscles targeted:

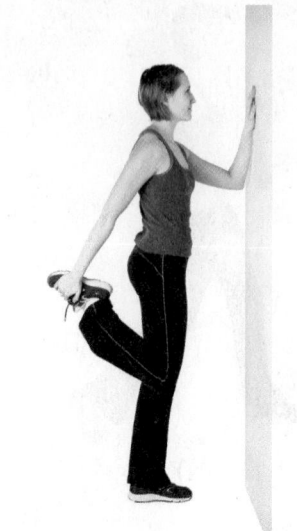

(a)

7 Quadriceps

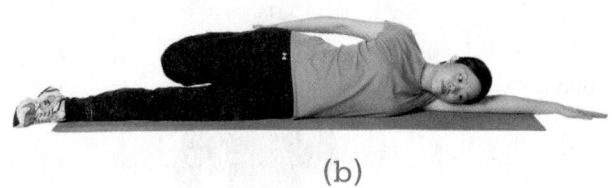

(b)

14. Hamstrings Stretch

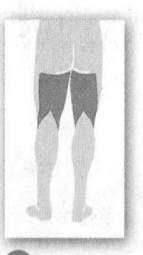

(a) Modified hurdler stretch: Sit with one leg extended and the other leg bent. The bent leg should have the knee facing sideways and the foot placed next to the extended leg near the calf, knee, or thigh. Keeping your back as straight as possible, lean your body forward, moving your chest closer to your extended leg. Your hands can be placed on the floor next to your knee, calf, or ankle for support.

(b) Supine lying: Lying on your back, bend one knee and extend the other toward the ceiling. Support the stretch by placing your hands or a towel above or below the knee. As you become more flexible, work at bringing your leg closer to your chest.

Muscles targeted:

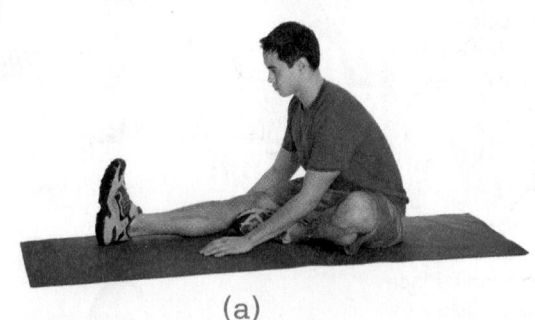

(a)

16 Hamstrings

(b)

15. Calf Stretches

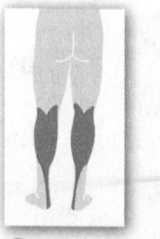 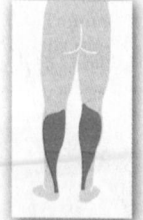

Muscles targeted:

17 Gastrocnemius   **18** Soleus

(a) Gastrocnemius lunge: Lean into a wall in a lunge position, extending one leg straight behind you. Press the heel of your straight leg into the floor as you lean your body and hips into the wall.

(b) Gastrocnemius heel drop: Stand tall and place your toes on a raised surface (mat or step) that will not tip over. Balance by holding on to a wall for support as you lower your heels toward the floor.

(c) Soleus stretch: Starting in a lunge position (a), bend the back knee until you feel a stretch in the soleus muscle.

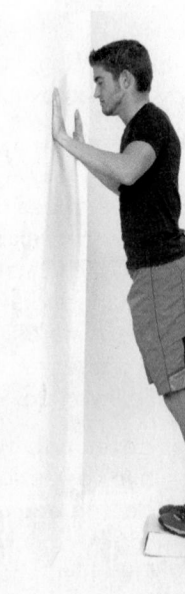

(a)   (b)   (c)

16. Shin Stretch

Reach one leg behind you and place the tips of your toes on the ground. Bend both knees and lower the body slightly as you press the top of your back foot toward the ground. You can use a wall for support if needed.

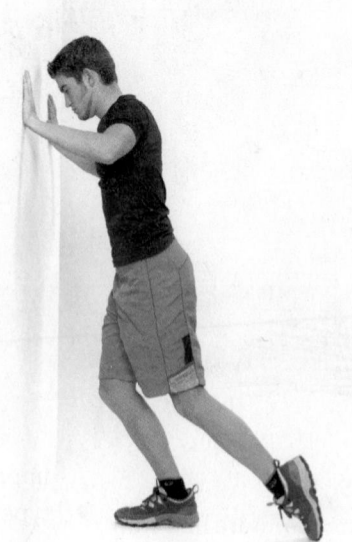

Muscles targeted:

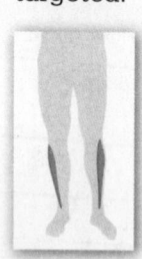

8 Tibialis anterior

Can I Become Flexible without Stretching?

If a regular stretching routine doesn't appeal to you, try one of these classes to help you reach your flexibility goals:

Yoga originated in India about 5,000 years ago and has become a popular activity in the United States. The forms of yoga most commonly practiced in the United States today require a combination of mental focus and physical effort while performing a variety of postures, or *asanas*. The physical aspect of yoga results in improvements in flexibility, posture, agility, balance, stamina, muscle endurance, and coordination. The mental aspect of yoga promotes attention, controlled breathing, relaxation, a union of mind and body, and an overall psychological sense of well-being.

Tai chi is a martial art that was developed in ancient China by monks wanting to defend themselves. Tai chi practice involves a slow-moving, smooth, and continuous series of positions or forms. These exercises increase balance, muscle endurance, flexibility, and coordination; they also reduce anxiety and stress.[1] Tai chi has become popular with many people, but older individuals in particular are drawn to this safe and effective way to exercise. There are other forms of martial arts that will develop flexibility, as well. You may want to look into classes for one of these popular martial arts: capoeira, karate, jujitsu, or tae kwon do.

Pilates was developed by Joseph Pilates in New York City in the 1920s. Pilates involves performing a sequence of exercises on a mat or specialized equipment designed to stretch and strengthen muscles. Specific breathing patterns are combined with stretching and resistance exercises to increase flexibility and muscle endurance, particularly in the core trunk-supporting muscles.

Dance is a fantastic and fun way to improve your flexibility and your overall fitness level. A group exercise class, such as aerobic dance, will usually give you a chance to work on your flexibility during the cool-down phase.

All of the activities described above require instruction by a trained professional, especially since some exercises can be risky for the untrained or novice participant.

Source:
1. C. Lan, S. Y. Chen, and J. S. Lai, "Changes of Aerobic Capacity, Fat Ratio, and Flexibility in Older TCC Practitioners: A Five-year Follow-up," *American Journal of Chinese Medicine* 36, no. 6 (2008): 1041–50; H. Liu and A. Frank, "Tai Chi as a Balance Improvement Exercise for Older Adults: a Systematic Review," *Journal of Geriatric Physical Therapy* 33, no. 3 (2010): 103–9.

Consider Taking a Class

LIVE IT! ONLINE

Twist to Get Fit

If you would like more structure and instruction in your stretching program, consider enrolling in a class. Yoga, tai chi, Pilates, dance, and martial arts classes can be fun, effective ways to maintain or improve your flexibility. For more information on these types of classes, see the box Can I Become Flexible without Stretching?. You may have heard of whole-body vibration or seen one of these machines in your college's gym. The box What Is Whole Body Vibration? gives more information about these machines.

What Is Whole Body Vibration?

In the 1960s, scientists who were looking for a way to help astronauts maintain or increase muscle and bone mass while in space started using whole body vibration (WBV) platforms as a solution. A motor under the whole body vibration platform transmits vibrations to the person using the platform. The vibrations occur quickly in one or more directions and stimulate muscle fiber contractions. The platforms are becoming more common in workout centers, and it makes sense: there is quite a bit of evidence to support the use of these vibration platforms for increased flexibility and muscle action. The evidence seems to be consistent for flexibility gains,[1] even over some of the other benefits such as bone density and muscle strength. Stretching during vibration on a WBV platform appears to be a good adjunct to static stretching and may help you retain the flexibility you gain.[2]

The down side with these machines is that they are expensive and they take up space. Given their cost, they probably aren't worth the investment for most people. If your gym has a WBV platform, talk with a fitness instructor or personal trainer about designing a program for you. Standing or lying muscle fitness exercises can be performed on the platform. Time on the platform should amount to 20 to 30 minutes a day, but work your way up to this. Use the platform a few times per week or every day to increase range of motion, muscle fitness, and bone density. If your gym doesn't have one, don't worry: just focus on incorporating well-balanced flexibility and muscle fitness routines into your schedule.

Sources:

1. D. G. Dolny and G. F. Reyes, "Whole Body Vibration Exercise: Training and Benefits," *Current Sports Medicine Reports* 7, no. 3 (2008): 152–7; R. Di Giminiani and others, "Effects of Individualized Whole-Body Vibration on Muscle Flexibility and Mechanical Power," *Journal of Sports Medicine Physical Fitness* 50, no. 2 (2010): 139–51; F. Fagnani and others, "The Effects of a Whole-Body Vibration Program on Muscle Performance and Flexibility in Female Athletes," *American Journal of Physical Medicine and Rehabilitation* 85, no. 12 (2006): 956–62.
2. J. B. Feland and others, "Whole Body Vibration as an Adjunct to Static Stretching," *International Journal of Sports Medicine* 31, no. 8 (2010): 584–9.

How Can I Avoid Stretching-Related Injuries?

We used to think of stretching as a way to avoid injury, but we now know that stretching can actually *cause* injury if done improperly. To avoid a stretching-related injury, adhere to the following guidelines.

Stretch Only Warm Muscles

An increase in body temperature prepares the joint fluid and structures for stretching and improves muscle elasticity. These changes allow you a greater range of motion while stretching. Static stretches, in particular, should be performed *after* a workout, when the muscles have been sufficiently warmed up.

Perform Stretches Safely

One of the keys to safe and effective stretching is to avoid activating stretch receptors when you want a muscle to relax. Stretch receptors are activated when muscles are lengthened rapidly. Muscle injury can occur from quick, bouncing movements, because the muscle is lengthening too far too quickly and the stretch reflex is creating tension at the same time. Avoid the stretch reflex by stretching carefully and slowly. Holding your stretches for at least 15 seconds will allow the stretch receptors and golgi tendon organs to make nervous system adjustments. These adjustments will allow further relaxation and lengthening of the muscles involved.

Know Which Exercises Can Cause Injury

Figure 5.4 shows common high-risk or **contraindicated** stretches with safer alternatives. Note that this figure

contraindicated Not recommended

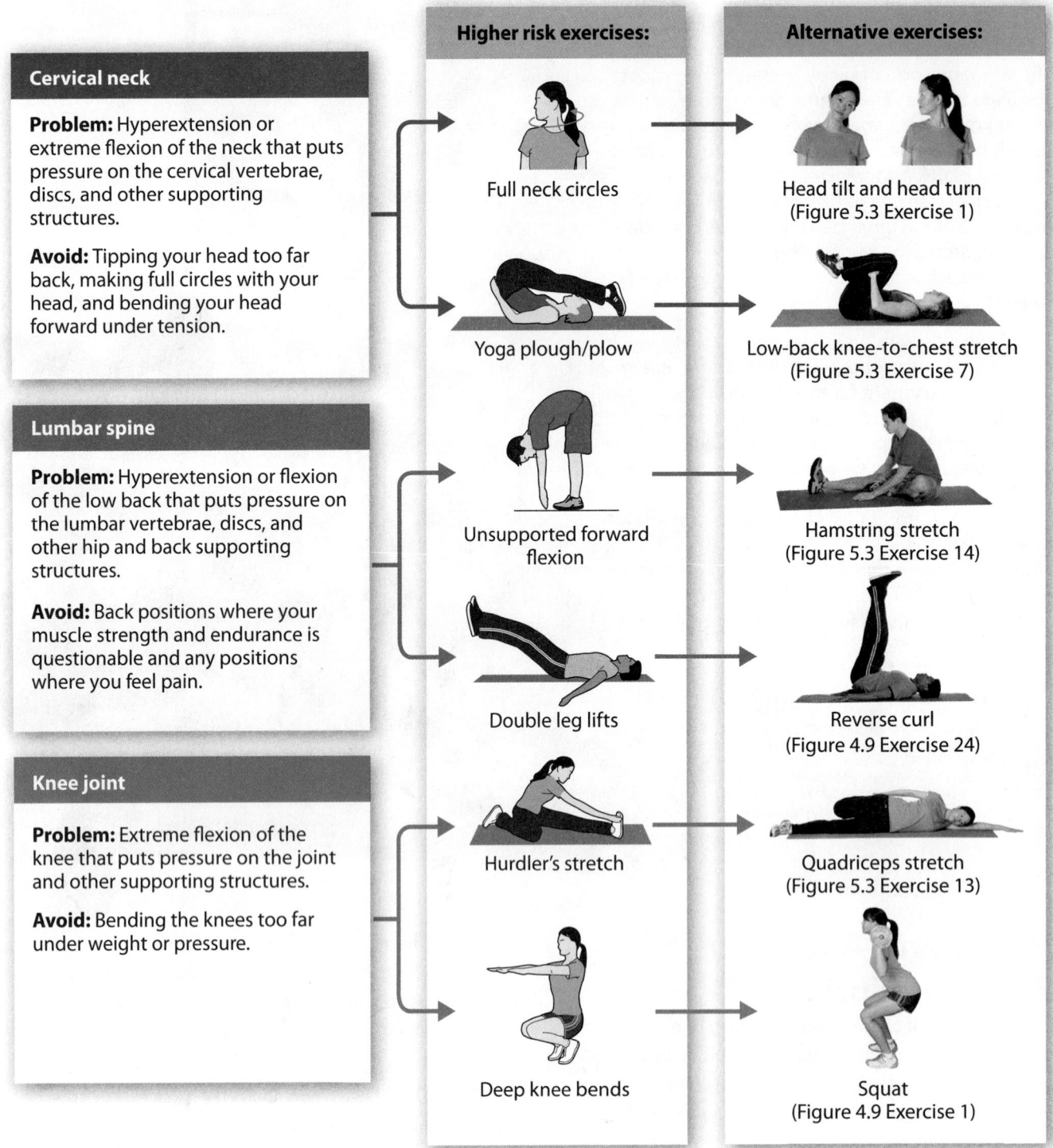

Cervical neck	Higher risk exercises:	Alternative exercises:
Problem: Hyperextension or extreme flexion of the neck that puts pressure on the cervical vertebrae, discs, and other supporting structures.	Full neck circles	Head tilt and head turn (Figure 5.3 Exercise 1)
Avoid: Tipping your head too far back, making full circles with your head, and bending your head forward under tension.	Yoga plough/plow	Low-back knee-to-chest stretch (Figure 5.3 Exercise 7)
Lumbar spine		
Problem: Hyperextension or flexion of the low back that puts pressure on the lumbar vertebrae, discs, and other hip and back supporting structures.	Unsupported forward flexion	Hamstring stretch (Figure 5.3 Exercise 14)
Avoid: Back positions where your muscle strength and endurance is questionable and any positions where you feel pain.	Double leg lifts	Reverse curl (Figure 4.9 Exercise 24)
Knee joint		
Problem: Extreme flexion of the knee that puts pressure on the joint and other supporting structures.	Hurdler's stretch	Quadriceps stretch (Figure 5.3 Exercise 13)
Avoid: Bending the knees too far under weight or pressure.	Deep knee bends	Squat (Figure 4.9 Exercise 1)

FIGURE **5.4** Choose safer alternatives to these common higher-risk exercises and stretches. Take into account your personal goals, experience, and limitations.

is *not* an all-inclusive list. Choosing safe exercises is a highly individual process. Consider your personal limitations and health issues when deciding which exercises are best for your body.

Be Especially Cautious If You Are a Hyperflexible or Inflexible Person

If you are really flexible, you may need to be more careful while stretching than the average exerciser. Excessive hypermobility increases joint laxity or looseness, decreases joint stability, and can lead to permanent changes in connective tissue. Take precautions to avoid overstretching, which may lead to injury or decreases in exercise performance. For example, if you are taking a yoga class, let your instructor know that you are hyperflexible and ask if there are any modified poses that would reduce your risk of overstretching.

Inflexibility is common in many people. If you have limited range of motion in one or more joints, avoid stretching beyond your abilities. Work gradually to improve your range of motion and overall flexibility. People with a very limited range of motion may be more susceptible to sudden acute injuries during sports, to activity-related injuries during daily-living tasks, and to lower-back injuries.

How Can I Prevent or Manage Back Pain?

While you are young, back pain is probably the furthest thing from your mind. However, lower-back pain affects at least 70 percent of the general U.S. population at some point in life, and about 28 percent of Americans at any given moment.[15] Some 31 percent of all Americans report limitations due to chronic back conditions.[16] In fact, back and spine problems are the self-reported cause of disability for 7.6 million Americans (16.8 percent), with women affected more often.[17] While Americans spend more than $86 billion each year treating back pain symptoms, the number and symptoms of sufferers continue to rise.[18]

Research has shown that college students are not immune to back-health issues. In recent studies, 29 to 43 percent of students reported regular lower-back pain, with higher numbers in students who were feeling sad, exhausted, or overwhelmed and those carrying heavy backpacks.[19,20] According to a recent American College Health Association survey of nearly 96,000 students, 12.5 percent reported having seen a physician in the last year for low back pain.[21]

Factors that increase your risk of lower-back pain include obesity, smoking, pregnancy, stress, inactivity, weak and inflexible muscles, and poor posture. In addition, a number of events can trigger back pain or cause a back injury, including accidents, sports injuries, repetitive movements, work trauma, and excessive sitting—especially if you already have other risk factors.

In the next sections, we will cover the causes of back pain, explain how the spine is structured and supported, and present strategies to reduce your risk of back pain. For those who already experience regular episodes of back pain, the next sections will also discuss ways to effectively manage, resolve, and prevent future recurrences of back pain.

Understand the Primary Causes of Back Pain

You experience back pain when your movement causes a sprain, strain, or spasm in one of the muscles, tendons, or ligaments in the back. You may also feel pain when your spine structures become misaligned or injured and the spinal nerves become compressed or irritated. Back pain can also result from age- or disease-related degeneration of the bones and joints of the spine. Ultimately, most back pain is caused by a *sedentary lifestyle,* which results in muscle weakness, inflexibility, and imbalance—all conditions that can lead to poor posture and body mechanics and to a higher risk of back pain and injury.

Muscular Weakness, Inflexibility, and Imbalance The supporting musculature of the spine is important for maintaining healthy posture, mobility, and spine structures. Weakness and inflexibility in key muscles can lead to muscular imbalances that affect the alignment of your spine. Weak abdominals, for instance, can cause your pelvis to rock forward and create a greater curvature in your lower back. This puts more pressure on spine structures and other spine-supporting muscles, potentially leading to back pain. Inflexible, tight hip flexor muscles can also cause a forward tilt of the pelvis and an increased curvature of the lower back.

Muscles become weak when they are not used on a regular basis. Repetitive movements or long hours of sitting can also cause muscles to shorten and tighten up. Some people have muscles of differing strength and flexibility levels around the spine and other joints. If your spine-supporting musculature does not have a muscle balance that promotes good posture and body mechanics, you may have back pain or injury in the future.

Improper Posture and Body Mechanics Improper posture can lead to increased forces within the spine structures and eventually to back pain. Altered body mechanics resulting from improper posture puts you at risk for injury during all of your daily activities, but especially during exercise and sports activities.

Acute Trauma, Risky Occupations, and Medical Issues Acute trauma to the back can happen to anyone at any age. Trauma could be the result of a car accident, a sports and recreation injury, or any other accident that affects the spine. Avoiding risky sports and recreational activities will reduce your chance of trauma.

Jobs that involve a lot of bending, twisting, and repeated lifting of heavy objects put workers at especially high risk of developing back pain. Jobs that involve a great deal of sitting every day are also considered high risk. Occupations with a high incidence of back pain include truck driving, nursing, firefighting, construction, and some professional sports (e.g., football, power lifting, golf, and wrestling). Occupations that are highly stressful and require long hours also increase the risk of back pain. Stress is a risk factor for back injury, and long hours at work can reduce the time you have to exercise and relax, further increasing the risk of developing back pain.

Medical issues and individual health factors can also significantly increase your chance of developing lower-back pain. For instance, smokers have an increased risk of low-back pain due to vascular damage, which facilitates disc degeneration.[22] Obesity and weight gain during pregnancy can increase lower-back pain due to greater loads on the spine, misalignment of the pelvis and low back, and muscular weakness. Pain can also result from degenerative conditions such as arthritis or disc disease, osteoporosis or other bone diseases, congenital abnormalities, viral infections, and general conditions that cause irritation to joints or discs.[23]

Understand How the Back Is Supported

The back comprises bones, muscles, and other tissues that form the back side of your trunk. The trunk contains most of your essential organs and bears the weight of your upper body. It is also responsible for transmitting forces and movements from the upper limbs to the lower limbs, and vice versa. If something is amiss with your back or your trunk overall, any upper- or lower-body movement can be difficult. Your back and trunk are supported by the bony structures of the spine and by the core trunk muscles.

The Structure of the Spine

The spine or *spinal column* (also called the *vertebral column*) is the series of bones called *vertebrae* that connect the upper-body and lower-body skeleton and protect the spinal cord. Figure 5.5 shows the basic structure of the spine. Note that the spine has four distinct regions and curvatures: *cervical*, *thoracic*, *lumbar*, and *sacral*. The curvatures are an essential part of the force-absorbing capabilities of the spine.

Intervertebral discs are round, spongy pads of cartilage that act as shock absorbers. The discs have fibrous outer rings that are filled with gel and water-like substances that will distend slightly when compressed. That distention acts to absorb shock. The discs also ensure that there is adequate space between the vertebrae. When a change in body mechanics or posture occurs—or when an acute injury occurs—the resulting change to spinal alignment can damage the disc structures.

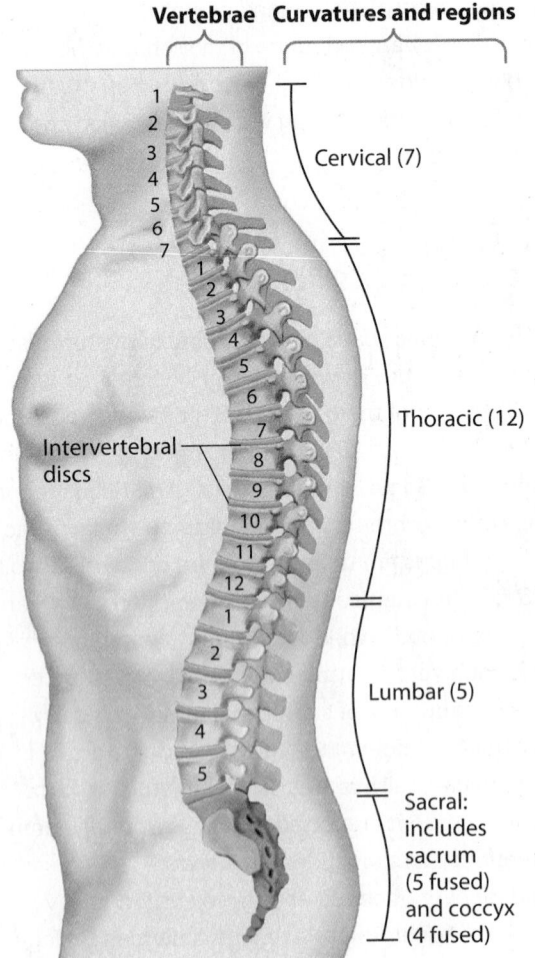

FIGURE 5.5 The spine has four distinct regions and curvatures (cervical, thoracic, lumbar, and sacral) made up of individual or fused vertebrae.

A permanent bulging of a disc out of the normal space is called a **disc herniation**. The disc can bulge toward the spinal column or nerves and cause pain or numbness in the back or other areas of the body. Disc herniations most often occur in the lower lumbar region, where most of the body weight and forces are applied.

Another problem that occurs with trauma or aging is dehydration, hardening, or degeneration of intervertebral discs. Without adequate fluid content and elasticity, discs cannot perform their shock-absorber role very well. The resulting smaller joint space between vertebrae applies pressure to the spinal nerves. This can cause back, hip, or leg pain and muscle weakness.

The Core Trunk Muscles The bones of the spinal column could not maintain their healthy curvatures and an upright posture without supporting muscles. Core trunk muscles support the trunk while you are standing, sitting, lying down, or moving. These muscles, located all around your body (Figure 5.6), are essential for supporting the spine and for performing sports, recreation, and everyday activities. **Core muscles** include back, abdominal, hip, gluteal, pelvis, pelvic floor, and lateral trunk muscles. Core muscles work together to effectively transmit forces between your upper and lower body. While weak core muscles can lead to back pain, strong core muscles can lead to increased performance levels in all of your activities.

Reduce Your Risk of Lower-Back Pain

You can reduce your risk of back pain by improving your body weight, muscle fitness, posture, and movement techniques. A review of multiple studies showed that exercise programs prevented back pain episodes in working-age adults, but other strategies, including shoe inserts and back supports, were not effective prevention measures.[24] Incorporating your new fitness knowledge from this course will help you gain strength and stability in your key spine-supporting muscles and reduce your risk of back pain.

Lose Weight The prevalence of lower-back pain rises with increases in body mass index or body weight and body fatness.[25] An increase in body weight puts extra strain and pressure on all the spinal structures. If the additional weight resides in the abdominal region, the pelvis may get pulled forward and result in a greater curvature of the lower back, causing back pain. Lowering your weight and body fat levels to within recommended ranges will reduce your risk of lower-back pain.

Strengthen and Stretch Key Muscles Most people's bodies have "weak" muscle areas, "tight" muscle areas, and areas that are both weak *and* tight.

- *Hip flexor muscles* tend to be tight in most people. This stems from extended sitting, resulting in shortened and inactive muscles. If you have tight hip flexor muscles, add hip flexor stretches (see Figure 5.3) to your weekly workout.

- *Hip extensor muscles* also tend to be tight and weak in many people and can benefit from stretching and strengthening.

- *Trunk flexor muscles* (abdominals) are often weak in individuals who are sedentary or overweight. Having a minimal level of strength in your abdominal muscles will help protect your spine and back and improve your exercise performance.

- *Trunk extensor muscles* are responsible for keeping your spine upright while sitting, standing, and moving.

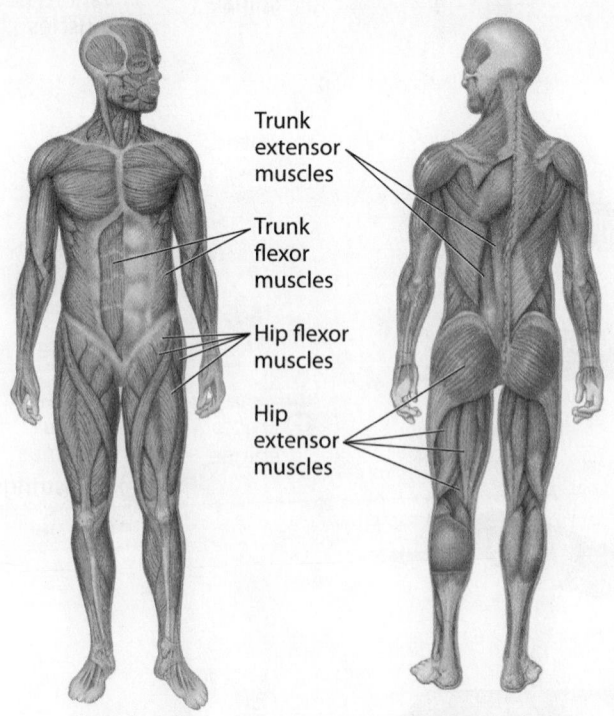

Trunk extensor muscles

Trunk flexor muscles

Hip flexor muscles

Hip extensor muscles

Anterior view　　　**Posterior view**

FIGURE **5.6** Strengthening and stretching of the spine-supporting core muscles is essential for a healthy back. The core muscles include extensors of the trunk and hip and flexors of the trunk and hip.

If you do a lot of hunched-over sitting, these muscles are probably weak, and you should add safe back extensor strengthening exercises to your program.

The simplest prescription for back health is to maintain a healthy weight and an active lifestyle. If you are predisposed to back pain due to other reasons (e.g., hyperflexibility, sport history, occupation), try to add some specific back health exercises to your current exercise routine. Figure 5.7 illustrates back health exercises that will help you stretch or strengthen the key areas of the trunk and hips; Activate, Motivate, & Advance Your Fitness: A Back-Health Exercise Program at the end of the chapter (page 213) will help you develop a plan to get started.

FIGURE **5.7**

EXERCISES FOR A HEALTHY BACK

Perform 3 to 10 repetitions of the back health exercises, holding where appropriate for 10 to 30 seconds. (See Figure 4.8 on page 132 for a full-body muscle diagram.)

Videos for these exercises and more are available online at www.pearsonhighered.com/hopson and on MyFitnessLab.

1. Cat Stretch

Start on your hands and knees with a flat back. Looking at the ground, align your head with your spine. Drop your head and look back toward your knees while lifting your upper back toward the ceiling.

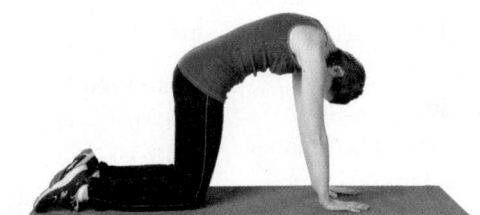

Muscles targeted:

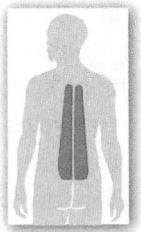 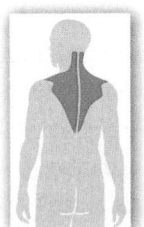

12 Erector spinae

10 Trapezius; various neck muscles

2. Arm/Leg Extensions

Start on your hands and knees with a flat back. Looking at the ground, align your head with your spine. Extend your arm straight out in front of you while extending the opposite leg straight out behind you. Keep your arm and leg in a straight line with your spine. Do not lift them too high, because this causes too much arch in your lower back.

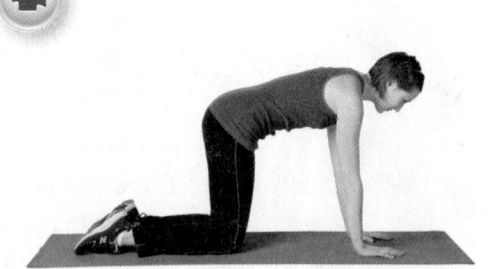

Muscles targeted:

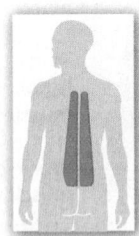 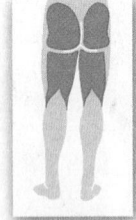

12 Erector spinae

15 Gluteus maximus

16 Hamstrings

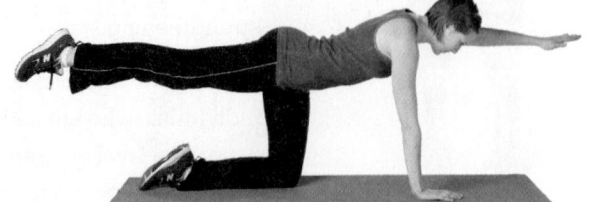

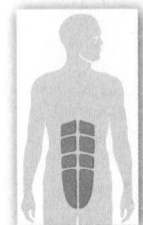

3 Rectus abdominis

(Continued)

3. Pelvic Tilt

Lie on your back with your knees bent and your feet flat on the floor. Relax in a comfortable posture, letting the natural curve of your spine bring your lower back off the mat. Breathe out as you tilt the bottom of your pelvis toward the ceiling, pulling your abdominals in and pressing your lower back flat against the floor.

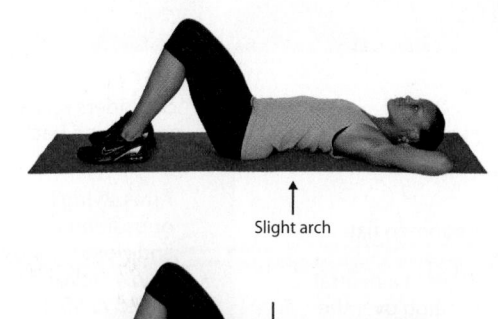

Slight arch

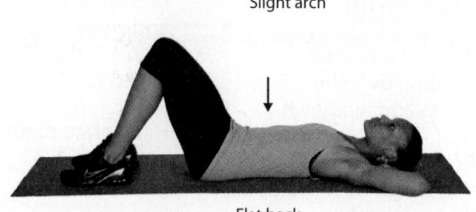

Flat back

Muscles targeted:

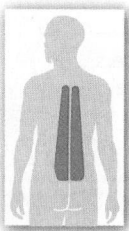

12 Erector spinae

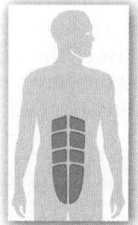

3 Rectus abdominis; various hip/ pelvis stabilizers

4. Back Bridge

Lie on your back with your knees bent, your feet flat on the floor, and your arms extended straight along your sides. Lift your hips off the ground and press your pelvis toward the ceiling until your thighs and back are in a straight line. Look at the ceiling and keep your neck extended throughout the exercise (do not tuck your chin to your chest).

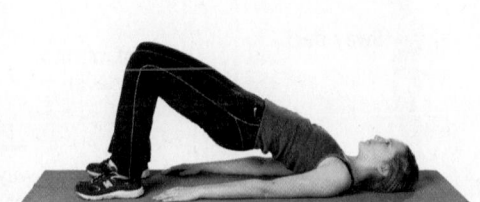

Muscles targeted:

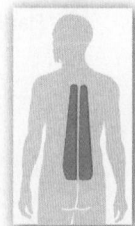

12 Erector spinae

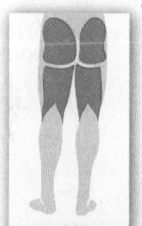

15 Gluteus maximus
16 Hamstrings

Other exercises that can help maintain back health include:

Plank (p. 145)
Side bridge (p. 145)
Knee-to-chest stretch (p. 184)
Hamstring stretch (p. 186)

Torso twist and hip stretch (p. 184)
Hip flexor stretch (p. 185)
Abdominal curl (p. 144)
Oblique curl (p. 145)

Maintain Good Posture and Proper Body Mechanics

If you have strong and flexible core trunk muscles, maintaining good posture and body mechanics is easier. The problem is that even with good muscular fitness, poor posture can become a habit. You might always hunch over at the computer and feel unnatural sitting up straight. Maybe you slouch back on the couch when you are watching TV. Over time, poor posture can create back problems.

Poor posture and poor muscle fitness can also lead to improper body mechanics while you perform everyday activities. Poor body mechanics put you at risk of muscle strain and back pain. **Lab 5.2** teaches you how to evaluate your posture, and Figure 5.8 illustrates proper postures for standing, walking, lifting, sitting, and lying down.

THINK! How long each day do you sit hunched over a pile of books, a laptop computer, or looking down at your smart phone?

ACT! Take a break every 20 minutes or so to do shoulder rolls, neck stretches, and dynamic hip and leg movements.

Properly Treat Lower-Back Pain

If you already experience regular back pain, you can do things to help manage your pain and prevent future recurrences. The box What Should I Do If I Already Have Back Pain? lists some strategies for back pain management.

Standing posture

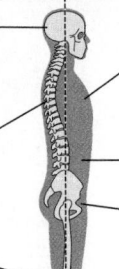

Head centered between the shoulders and the crown of the head extended

Shoulders over the pelvis, level and relaxed

Knees over the ankles and not hyperextended

Chest elevated

Abdomen flat

Pelvis in a neutral position over the knees and hips level

Feet facing forward and weight distributed through heels

Improper postures include:

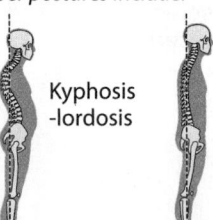

Kyphosis -lordosis

Flat-back

Sway-back

Walking posture

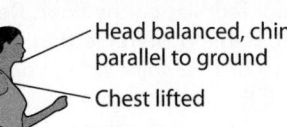

Shoulders relaxed, down, and back

Arms swing in opposition to legs and close to body; elbows relaxed or flexed to 90 degrees

Hips rotate naturally

Head balanced, chin parallel to ground

Chest lifted

Abdominals contracted and pelvis centered

Stride length is comfortable, not too short or long

Sitting posture

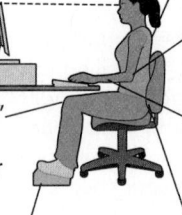

Top of monitor at eye level

If you have a "sway" back, elevate feet so knees are higher than hips; if you have a "flat" back, keep knees lower than hips

Feet flat on the floor or foot rest

Chest elevated and back extended tall, not slumping

Elbows bent at 90°; use armrest if available

Hands in line with forearms (wrists straight); use wrist supports if necessary

Low-back curvature supported by a back rest

Sleeping posture

Lying on one's back

Medium to firm mattress supports the spine

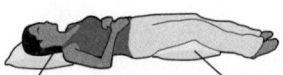

Head supported to maintain neck alignment, but avoiding a pillow that is too high

If needed, pillow or other lift placed under knees to reduce lumbar curvature and support the lower back

Lying on one's side

Hips and knees bent

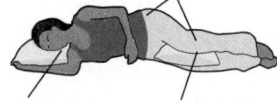

Head and neck supported enough to maintain a straight spine

If needed, pillow placed between knees for additional support of the lower back, hips, and pelvis

Lifting and carrying posture

Get help if the weight is too much for you

Bend at the knees and hips; don't bend over at the waist

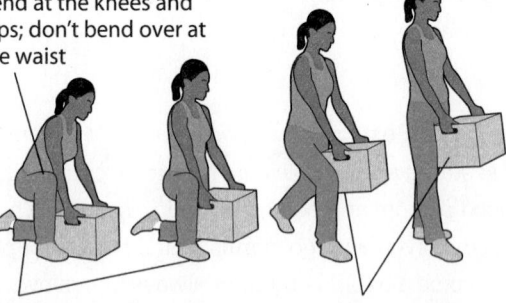

Use a wide straddle stance or a "stride" stance where one foot is forward and the other is back

Keep the weight close to your body when lifting and carrying

FIGURE **5.8** Proper posture is important for back health.

What Should I Do If I Already Have Back Pain?

While experiencing an acute episode of back pain, take the following treatment recommendations into account:

- Limit bed rest to 1 to 2 days at most. Bed rest alone may make back pain worse and may contribute to other problems such as muscle weakness and blood clots.

- Ice and heat may help with pain management, inflammation, and mobility. Apply cold treatments for 2 to 3 days after an acute event, and then add heat treatments as needed for increased muscle blood flow and relaxation.

- Engage in low-stress, back-healthy activities such as stretching, swimming, walking, and movement therapy as soon as you can.

- Check with a doctor before taking drugs for pain relief. Common medications include aspirin, ibuprofen, naproxen, topical muscle creams, and prescription muscle relaxers and pain medications.

- Spinal manipulation by a chiropractor or other qualified therapist can help some individuals with pain management and recovery.

- Nonconventional treatments (acupuncture, biofeedback, etc.) are considered by some patients when they are not responding to more traditional methods.

- Seek medical attention if you do not have a noticeable reduction in pain or if you experience continued inflammation after 72 hours of self–care.

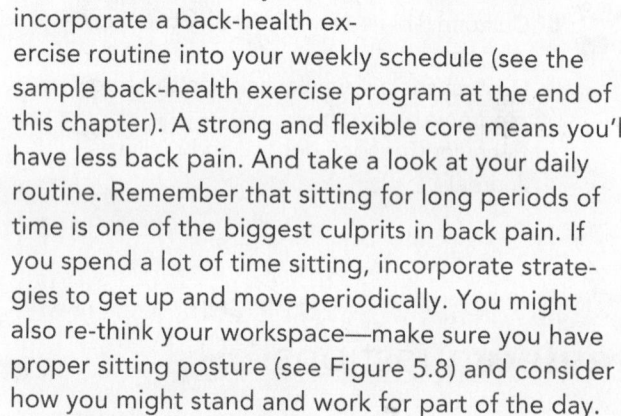

Once you have your current episode of back pain under control, try to incorporate a back-health exercise routine into your weekly schedule (see the sample back-health exercise program at the end of this chapter). A strong and flexible core means you'll have less back pain. And take a look at your daily routine. Remember that sitting for long periods of time is one of the biggest culprits in back pain. If you spend a lot of time sitting, incorporate strategies to get up and move periodically. You might also re-think your workspace—make sure you have proper sitting posture (see Figure 5.8) and consider how you might stand and work for part of the day.

Source: National Institute of Arthritis and Musculoskeletal and Skin Diseases, *Back Pain* NIH Publication No. 09-5282 (Information Clearinghouse, National Institutes of Health: Bethesda, MD, 2010).

• •

chapterin**review** ·······································

videos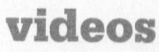

Log on to **www.pearsonhighered.com/hopson** or MyFitnessLab to view these chapter-related videos.

Flexibility Exercises
Calf Stretch
Cat Stretch
Gluteal Stretch
Hamstrings Stretch (Seated)
Head Turn and Head Tilt
Hip Flexor Stretch
Inner-Thigh Butterfly Stretch
Low-Back Knee-to-Chest Stretch

Modified Hurdler Stretch
Outer-Thigh Stretch
Pectoral and Biceps Stretch
Quadriceps Stretch
Shin Stretch
Shoulder Stretch
Side Stretch
Torso Twist and Hip Stretch
Triceps Stretch

Upper Back Stretch
Core Strength Exercises
Abdominal Curl (Stability Ball)
Abdominal Tuck (Stability Ball)
Arm/Leg Extensions
Back Bridge
Back Extension (Stability Ball)
Bridge Leg Curl (Stability Ball)
Bridge Up (Stability Ball)

Oblique Curl
Oblique Side Crunch (Stability Ball)
Pelvic Tilt
Pike-Up (Stability Ball)
Plank (Forearm Position)
Plank (Push-Up Position)
Plank (Stability Ball)

Reverse Curl
Side Bridge (Beginner)
Side Bridge (Intermediate)
Side Bridge (Advanced)
Assessments
Posture Evaluation
Range-of-Motion Assessment

Sit-and-Reach Assessment (Box)
Sit-and-Reach Assessment
  (Yardstick)
Shoulder Flexibility Assessment
Trunk Rotation Assessment

Twist to Get Fit

onlineresources

Log on to **www.pearsonhighered.com/hopson** or MyFitnessLab for access to these book-related resources, and for links to other useful websites.

 Audio case study
Audio PowerPoint lecture

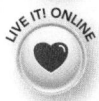 Customizable 4-week flexibility training programs
Customizable 4-week back-health exercise programs
Behavior Change Logbook and Wellness Journal

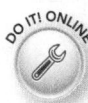 Lab 6.1 Assess Your Flexibility
Lab 6.2 Assess Your Posture
Lab 6.3 Planning a Flexibility Program
Alternate Lab: Modified Sit-and-Reach Test
Alternate Lab: Chair Sit-and-Reach Test
Alternate Lab: Assessing Shoulder Flexibility
Alternate Lab: Assessing Trunk Rotation

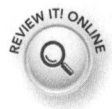 Pre- and post-quizzes
Glossary flashcards

reviewquestions

1. _____ is a measure of your overall joint stiffness during movement.
   a. Dynamic flexibility
   b. Static flexibility
   c. Passive flexibility
   d. Anatomical flexibility

2. Which of the following triggers a muscle to relax when there is too much force or tension in the muscle?
   a. Muscle spindle
   b. Baroreceptor
   c. Golgi tendon organ
   d. Reflex receptor

3. The intensity of each stretch should be stretching until you reach
   a. your toes.
   b. the point of tightness.
   c. moderate burning pain.
   d. your goal.

4. Stretching that involves voluntary muscle contractions to facilitate relaxation describes
   a. static stretching.
   b. dynamic stretching.
   c. ballistic stretching.
   d. PNF stretching.

5. Which of the following exercise styles uses a slow-moving series of forms to increase coordination, balance, and flexibility?
   a. Dance
   b. Pilates
   c. Yoga
   d. Tai chi

6. Which of the following is the primary underlying cause of low-back pain?
   a. Poor posture
   b. Sedentary living
   c. Muscle weakness
   d. Poor flexibility

7. The fluid of an intervertebral disc bulging outward and pressing on the nervous system structures in the spine is best described as disc
   a. dehydration.
   b. degeneration.
   c. herniation.
   d. hardening.

8. Which of the following sleep postures creates the most tension in your lower back and is not recommended?
   a. Lying on your side
   b. Lying on your stomach
   c. Lying on your back
   d. Sleeping in a chair

9. What approximate percentage of people will experience lower-back pain at some point in their lives?
   a. 25 percent
   b. 50 percent
   c. 70 percent
   d. 100 percent

10. Which of the following acute back pain self-care treatments is no longer recommended?
    a. Five days of bed rest
    b. Light exercise
    c. Pain relievers
    d. Cold and hot treatments

critical**thinking**questions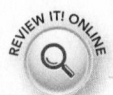

1. Explain how stretching can improve your posture and balance.
2. Describe how reducing the stretch reflex will enhance the effectiveness of your stretches.
3. Are the contraindicated stretches "off-limits" to everyone? Are there any sports, activities, or situations that would safely allow some of these movements and stretches? If so, which ones and which activities?
4. List three occupations that present high risk for low-back pain and explain why.

references

1. M. Nolan and others, "Age-related Changes in Musculoskeletal Function, Balance and Mobility Measures in Men aged 30–80 years," *Aging Male* 13, no. 3 (2010): 194–201.
2. M. J. Spink and others, "Foot and Ankle Strength, Range of Motion, Posture, and Deformity Are Associated with Balance and Functional Ability in Older Adults," *Archives of Physical Medicine and Rehabilitation* 92, no. 1 (2011): 68–75.
3. J. R. Pleis and others, National Center for Health Statistics, "Summary Health Statistics for U.S. Adults: National Health Interview Survey, 2009," *Vital Health Statistics* 10, no. 249 (2010).
4. H. B. Sun, "Mechanical Loading, Cartilage Degradation, and Arthritis," *Annals of the New York Academy of Science* 1211 (2010): 37–50; J. K. Cooney and others, "Benefits of Exercise in Rheumatoid Arthritis," *Journal of Aging Research* (2011): 681640; Y. Escalante, A. García- Hermoso, and J. M. Saavedra, "Effects of Exercise on Functional Aerobic Capacity in Lower Limb Osteoarthritis: A Systematic Review," *Journal of Science and Medicine in Sport* 14, no. 3 (2011): 190–8.
5. J. Peeler and J. E. Anderson, "Effectiveness of Static Quadriceps Stretching in Individuals with Patellofemoral Joint Pain," *Clinical Journal of Sport Medicine* 17, no. 4 (2007): 234–41.
6. F. Balagué and others, "The Association Between Isoinertial Trunk Muscle Performance and Low Back Pain in Male Adolescents," *European Spine Journal* 19, no. 4 (2010): 624–32 .

7. M. A. Jones and others, "Biological Risk Indicators for Recurrent Non-specific Low Back Pain in Adolescents," *British Journal of Sports Medicine* 39, no. 3 (2005): 137–40.
8. P. W. Marshall, J. Mannion, and B. A. Murphy, "Extensibility of the Hamstrings Is Best Explained by Mechanical Components of Muscle Contraction, Not Behavioral Measures in Individuals with Chronic Low Back Pain," *PM&R: The Journal of Injury, Function, and Rehabilitation* 1, no. 8 (2009): 709–18.
9. E. N. Johnson and J. S. Thomas, "Effect of Hamstring Flexibility on Hip and Lumbar Spine Joint Excursions during Forward-Reaching Tasks in Participants with and without Low Back Pain," *Archives of Physical Medicine and Rehabilitation* 91, no. 7 (2010): 1140–2.
10. N. Kofotolis and M. Sambanis, "The Influence of Exercise on Musculoskeletal Disorders of the Lumbar Spine," *Journal of Sports Medicine and Physical Fitness* 45, no. 1 (2005): 84–92.
11. R. J. Johns and V. Wright, "Relative Importance of Various Tissues in Joint Stiffness," *Journal of Applied Physiology* 17, no. 5 (1962): 824–8.
12. H. O. Kendall, F. P. Kendall, and G. E. Bennett, "Normal Flexibility According to Age Groups," *Journal of Bone and Joint Surgery* 30A, no. 3 (1948): 690–4; M. J. Alter, *The Science of Flexibility*, Human Kinetics, Champaign, IL, 2004.
13. I. G. Fatouros and others, "Resistance Training and Detraining Effects on Flexibility Performance in the Elderly Are

Intensity-Dependent," *Journal of Strength and Conditioning Research* 20, no. 3 (2006): 634–42.
14. M. Amiri-Khorasani, N. A. Abu Osman, and A. Yusof, "Acute Effect of Static and Dynamic Stretching on Hip Dynamic Range of Motion during Instep Kicking in Professional Soccer Players," *Journal of Strength Conditioning Research* 25, no. 6 (2011): 1647–52.
15. J. R. Pleis and others, "Summary Health Statistics for U.S. Adults: National Health Interview Survey, 2009," 2010.
16. National Center for Health Statistics, Health Promotion Statistics Branch, CDC Wonder. *DATA2010...the Healthy People 2010 Database.* (Hyattsville, MD; Centers for Disease Control, 2010), http://wonder.cdc.gov/data2010/focus.htm (accessed May 2011).
17. Centers for Disease Control and Prevention, "Prevalence and Most Common Causes of Disability among Adults—United States, 2005," *Morbidity and Mortality Weekly Report* 58, no. 16 (2009): 421–6.
18. B. I. Martin, and others, "Expenditures and Health Status among Adults With Back and Neck Problems," *JAMA* 299, no. 6 (2008): 656–64.
19. Z. Heuscher and others, "The Association of Self-Reported Backpack Use and Backpack Weight with Low Back Pain among College Students," *Journal of Manipulative Physiological Therapy* 33, no. 6 (2011): 432–7.

20. C. Kennedy and others, "Psychosocial Factors and Low Back Pain among College Students," *Journal of American College Health* 57, no. 2 (2008): 191–5.

21. American College Health Association, *American College Health Association–National College Health Assessment II (ACHA-NCHA II) Reference Group Executive Summary Spring 2010* (Linthicum, MD: American College Health Association, 2010).

22. M. Iwahashi and others, "Mechanism of Intervertebral Disc Degeneration Caused by Nicotine in Rabbits to Explicate Intervertebral Disc Disorders Caused by Smoking," *Spine* 27, no. 13 (2002): 1396–401.

23. National Institute of Neurological Disorders and Stroke, *Low Back Pain Fact Sheet* NIH Publication No. 03-5161 (Office of Communications and Public Liaison, National Institutes of Health: Bethesda, MD, 2003).

24. S. J. Bigos and others, "High-quality Controlled Trials on Preventing Episodes of Back Problems: Systematic Literature Review in Working-Age Adults," *The Spine Journal: Official Journal of the North American Spine Society* 9, no. 2 (2009): 147–68.

25. D.M. Urquhart and others, "Increased Fat Mass Is Associated with High Levels of Low Back Pain Intensity and Disability," *Spine (Philadelphia, PA 1976)* 36, no. 16 (2011): 1320–5.

LAB 5.1 • ASSESS YOUR FLEXIBILITY

Name: _____ Date: _____

Instructor: _____ Section: _____

Materials: Exercise mat, yardstick or sit-and-reach box, a partner

Purpose: To assess your current level of lower-back, hip, and hamstring flexibility and your current level of joint mobility or range of motion.

SECTION I: THE SIT-AND-REACH TEST

This test measures the general flexibility of your lower back, hips, and hamstrings. The results are specific to those regions of your body and do not reflect your flexibility in other body areas. Choose the **box** or the **yardstick** test based upon equipment availability and/or your instructor's preference. You **need not** perform both assessments.

1. **Warm-up.** Complete 3 to10 minutes of light cardiorespiratory activity to warm-up your body and then perform light range-of-motion exercises and stretches for the joints and muscles that you will be using.

2. **Prepare for the appropriate test.**

   SEE IT! ONLINE

   - **BOX Sit-and-Reach Test** – Place the sit-and-reach box against a wall to prevent it from moving during the test. Sit without shoes behind the box, place your feet flat against the box at the 26-cm mark (the "zero" or foot mark for this test), and put your hands on top of the box.

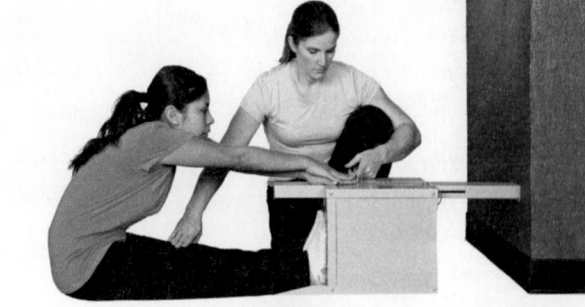

   SEE IT! ONLINE

   - **YARDSTICK Sit-and-Reach Test** – Sit straight legged on a mat with your shoes removed and your feet about 10 to 12 inches apart. Have your partner place a yardstick on the mat between your feet with the 15-inch mark at the edge of your heels. You can use a pre-placed and taped yardstick, tape the yardstick in place at the heels, or just have your partner hold the yardstick. Place your hands on top of the end of the yardstick.

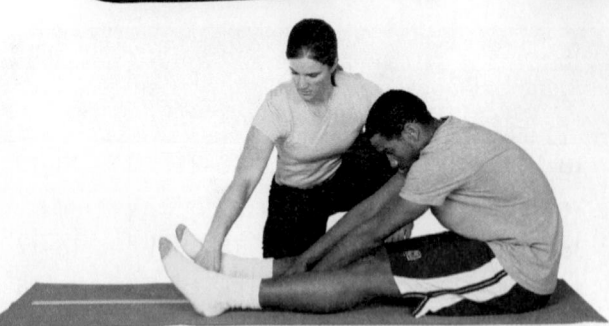

3. **Properly perform the test.** Keep one hand on top of the other. It is important that fingertips remain together and that your hands remain in contact with the yardstick or box ruler at all times. Reach forward as far as you can by slowly bending forward, reaching with your arms, and sliding your fingertips out along the yardstick or box. Keep your legs straight, drop your head between your arms, and breathe out as you perform the test. Hold your ending position for at least two seconds. Your partner will watch to ensure that you have proper hand position and straight legs during the test.

4. **Find your reach distance.** Your *reach distance* is the most distant point reached with both fingertips. If you cannot keep your hands from separating, the most distant point reached by the fingertips of the *hand that is farthest back* should be considered the reach distance. Record the reach distance in inches, as measured by the yardstick, or centimeters, as measured by the box. Perform the test twice. Have your partner point to your reach distance for each trial. Record your best reach distance of the two trials in the RESULTS section on the next page.

FLEXIBILITY RESULTS

Box Sit-and-Reach Test: Reach Distance (cm): _____   Rating:_____

OR

Yardstick Sit-and-Reach Test: Reach Distance (in): _____   Rating:_____

5. **Find your flexibility rating by using the charts provided below.** Your rating tells you how you compare to others who have completed this test in the past. Record your rating in the RESULTS section above.

BOX Sit-and-Reach Test (centimeters)					
Men	Excellent	Very Good	Good	Fair	Needs Improvement
15–19 yrs	≥39	34–38	29–33	24–28	≤23
20–29 yrs	≥40	34–39	30–33	25–29	≤24
30–39 yrs	≥38	33–37	28–32	23–27	≤22
40–49 yrs	≥35	29–34	24–28	18–23	≤17
50–59 yrs	≥35	28–34	24–27	16–23	≤15
60–69 yrs	≥33	25–32	20–24	15–19	≤14
Women	Excellent	Very Good	Good	Fair	Needs Improvement
15–19 yrs	≥43	38–42	34–37	29–33	≤28
20–29 yrs	≥41	37–40	33–36	28–32	≤27
30–39 yrs	≥41	36–40	32–35	27–31	≤26
40–49 yrs	≥38	34–37	30–33	25–29	≤24
50–59 yrs	≥39	33–38	30–32	25–29	≤24
60–69 yrs	≥35	31–34	27–30	23–26	≤22

Source: From *Canadian Physical Activity, Fitness & Lifestyle Approach: CSEP-Health & Fitness Program's Health-Related Appraisal & Counseling Strategy.* 3rd edition © 2003. Reprinted with permission from the Canadian Society for Exercise Physiology.

YARDSTICK Sit-and-Reach Test (inches)							
Men	Excellent	Good	Above Average	Average	Below Average	Poor	Very Poor
18–25 yrs	22–28	20–21	18–19	16–17	14–15	12–13	2–11
26–35 yrs	21–28	19	17	15–16	13–14	11–12	2–9
36–45 yrs	21–28	18–19	16–17	15	13	9–11	1–7
46–55 yrs	19–26	16–18	14–15	12–13	10–11	8–9	1–6
56–65 yrs	17–24	15–16	13	11	9	6–8	1–5
>65 yrs	17–24	14–16	12–13	10–11	8–9	6–7	0–4
Women	Excellent	Good	Above Average	Average	Below Average	Poor	Very Poor
18–25 yrs	24–29	22	20–21	19	17–18	16	7–14
26–35 yrs	23–28	21–22	20	18–19	16–17	14–15	5–13
36–45 yrs	22–28	20–21	18–19	17	15–16	13–14	4–12
46–55 yrs	21–27	19–20	17–18	16	14	12–13	3–10
56–65 yrs	20–26	18–19	16–17	15	13–14	10–12	2–9
>65 yrs	20–26	18–19	17	15–16	13–14	10–12	1–9

Source: Adapted with permission from *YMCA Fitness Testing and Assessment Manual,* 4th edition. Copyright © 2000 by YMCA of the USA, Chicago. All rights reserved.

SECTION II: JOINT MOBILITY—RANGE-OF-MOTION TESTS

SEE IT! ONLINE

Range-of-motion tests assess your joints' ability to move through a normal range of motion. Follow the instructions for each of the tests shown below. Perform each test on both your right and left sides. Stop each movement when you feel resistance. To avoid injury, do not try to push past your normal range. Have a partner observe your movements, "eyeball" your estimated joint angle, and record your range-of-motion results on page 204.

1. Neck Lateral Flexion— Sit or stand with your head neutral and looking forward. Tilt your head to the side and drop your ear toward your shoulder.

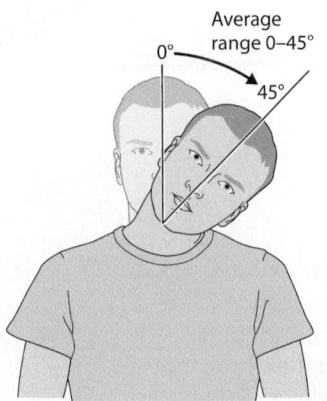

Average range 0–45°
0°
45°

2. Shoulder Flexion— Starting with your arms at your sides, reach a straight arm forward and up toward your head.

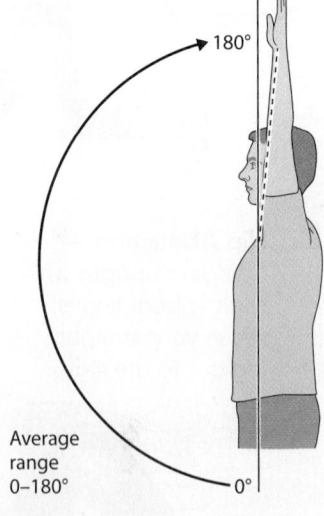

180°
Average range 0–180°
0°

3. Shoulder Extension— With your arms at your sides, reach a straight arm behind you and up.

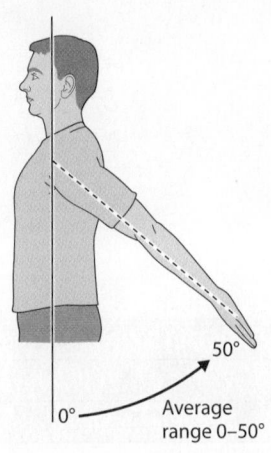

0°
50°
Average range 0–50°

4. Shoulder Abduction— Reach your straight arm out to the side and up to your head.

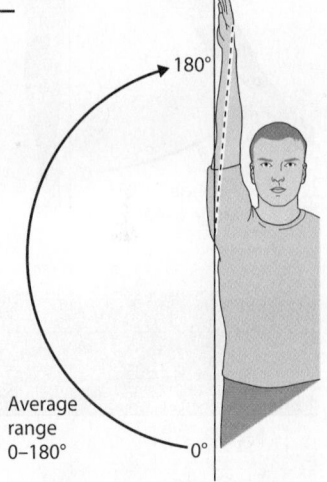

180°
Average range 0–180°
0°

5. Shoulder Adduction—Reach your straight arm down and across your body in front.

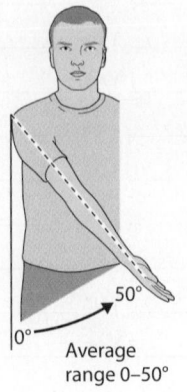

0°
50°
Average range 0–50°

6. Trunk Lateral Flexion— Standing upright with slightly bent knees and your arms at your sides, bend your torso sideways and reach your arm down your leg for support.

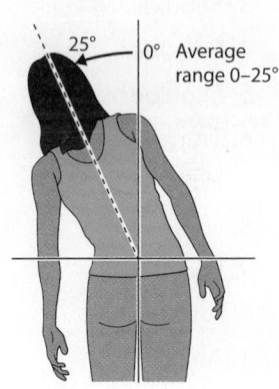

25°
0°
Average range 0–25°

7. Hip Flexion—Lying on your back, lift a straight leg up into the air while keeping the other leg bent with the foot flat on the ground.

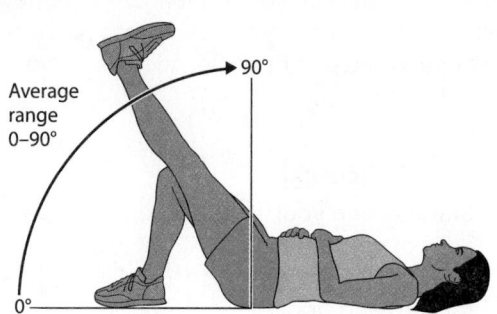

8. Hip Extension—Lying on your stomach with your head on the mat, reach your straight leg up behind you, keeping the other leg flat on the ground.

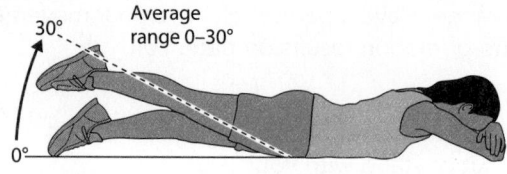

9. Hip Abduction—Standing upright with slightly bent knees, reach your straight leg out to the side.

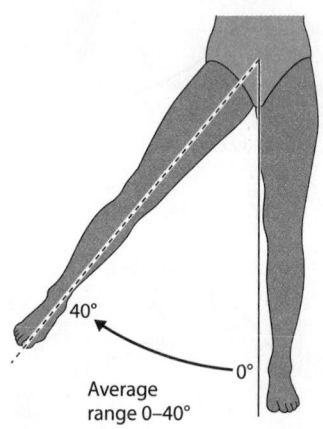

10. Ankle Dorsiflexion—Sitting without shoes and your legs extended in front of you, flex your foot back toward your knee.

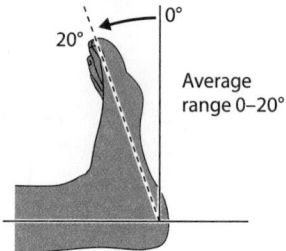

11. Ankle Plantar Flexion—Sitting without shoes and your legs extended in front of you, point your foot toward the floor.

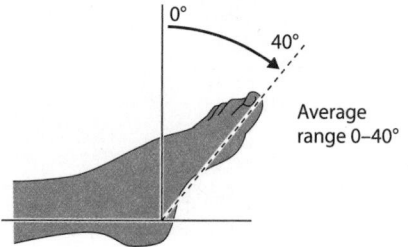

Joint Mobility RESULTS						
Joint	Movement and Average Range (degrees)	Full Average Joint Range?				
		Right Side			Left Side	
1. Neck	Lateral Flexion 0–45	_____ Yes	_____ No		_____ Yes	_____ No
2. Shoulder	Flexion 0–180	_____ Yes	_____ No		_____ Yes	_____ No
3. Shoulder	Extension 0–50	_____ Yes	_____ No		_____ Yes	_____ No
4. Shoulder	Abduction 0–180	_____ Yes	_____ No		_____ Yes	_____ No
5. Shoulder	Adduction 0–50	_____ Yes	_____ No		_____ Yes	_____ No
6. Trunk	Lateral Flexion 0–25	_____ Yes	_____ No		_____ Yes	_____ No
7. Hip	Flexion 0–90	_____ Yes	_____ No		_____ Yes	_____ No
8. Hip	Extension 0–30	_____ Yes	_____ No		_____ Yes	_____ No
9. Hip	Abduction 0–40	_____ Yes	_____ No		_____ Yes	_____ No
10. Ankle	Dorsiflexion 0–20	_____ Yes	_____ No		_____ Yes	_____ No
11. Ankle	Plantar Flexion 0–40	_____ Yes	_____ No		_____ Yes	_____ No

Sources: Adapted from American College of Sports Medicine, *ACSM's Health-Related Physical Fitness Assessment Manual.* 3rd ed. (Baltimore, MD: Lippincott Williams & Wilkins, 2009); American College of Sports Medicine, *ACSM's Resource Manual for Guidelines for Exercise Testing and Prescription.* 6th ed. (Baltimore, MD: Lippincott Williams & Wilkins, 2009).

LAB 5.2 • EVALUATE YOUR POSTURE

Name: _____ **Date:** _____

Instructor: _____ **Section:** _____

Purpose: To evaluate your posture.

Before you begin: Wear clothing that will not interfere with the assessment of your posture. If it is comfortable, men should wear shorts only, and women should wear shorts and a tank top. Remove your shoes. If you have long hair, pull it back into a ponytail for the assessment.

Stand against a wall and have a partner evaluate your posture using the chart on page 206. Your partner should assign you a score of between 1 and 5 for each of the 10 areas of your body shown on the next page.

SEE IT! ONLINE

Posture Results	
Posture Score	**Posture Rating**
45 or higher	Excellent
40–44	Good
30–39	Average
20–29	Fair
19 or less	Poor

Source: Adapted from *New York State Physical Fitness Test for Boys and Girls Grades 4–12. A Manual for Teachers of Physical Education*, Division of Physical Education and Research, State University of New York. Albany, NY: New York State Education Dept., 1972.

	Good—5	Fair—3	Poor—1	Score
Head	Head erect, gravity passes directly through center	Head twisted or turned to one side slightly	Head twisted or turned to one side markedly	
Shoulders	Shoulders level horizontally	One shoulder slightly higher	One shoulder markedly higher	
Spine	Spine straight	Spine slightly curved	Spine markedly curved laterally	
Hips	Hips level horizontally	One hip slightly higher	One hip markedly higher	
Knees and Ankles	Feet pointed straight ahead, legs vertical	Feet pointed out, legs deviating outward at the knee	Feet pointed out markedly, legs deviated markedly	
Neck and Upper back	Neck erect, head in line with shoulders, rounded upper back	Neck slightly foward, chin out, slightly more rounded upper back	Neck markedly forward, chin markedly out, markedly rounded upper back	
Trunk	Trunk erect	Trunk inclined to rear slightly	Trunk inclined to rear markedly	
Abdomen	Abdomen flat	Abdomen protruding	Abdomen protruding and sagging	
Lower back	Lower back normally curved	Lower back slightly hollow	Lower back markedly hollow	
Legs	Legs straight	Knees slightly hyperextended	Knees markedly hyperextended	
			Total score	

LAB 5.3 • PLANNING A FLEXIBILITY PROGRAM

Name: _____ Date: _____

Instructor: _____ Section: _____

Materials: Results from Lab 5.1

Purpose: To learn how to set appropriate flexibility goals and create a personal flexibility program.

SECTION I: SHORT- AND LONG-TERM GOALS

Create short- and long-term goals for flexibility and back health. Be sure to use SMART goal-setting guidelines (*s*pecific, *m*easurable, *a*ction-oriented, *r*ealistic, *t*ime-oriented). Select appropriate target dates and rewards for completing your goals.

Short-Term Goal for Flexibility (3 to 6 months)

_____

_____

Target Date: _____

Reward: _____

Optional: Short-Term Goal for Back Health (3 to 6 months)

_____

_____

Target Date: _____

Reward: _____

Long-Term Goal for Flexibility (12+ months)

_____

_____

Target Date: _____

Reward: _____

Optional: Long-Term Goal for Back Health (12+ months)

_____

_____

Target Date: _____

Reward: _____

SECTION II: FLEXIBILITY PROGRAM DESIGN

Complete one line for each exercise you have chosen to do in your program.

Stretching Exercises	Frequency (days/week)	Time (sec)	Reps (number)	Total Time (sec)
LOWER BODY				
1.				
2.				
3.				
4.				
5.				
6.				
7.				
8.				
UPPER BODY				
1.				
2.				
3.				
4.				
5.				
6.				
7.				
8.				

SECTION III: TRACKING YOUR PROGRAM AND FOLLOWING THROUGH

1. **Goal and Program Tracking:** Use the following chart to monitor your progress. Change the frequency, time, sets, and reps frequently to ensure continuing progress toward your goals.

2. **Goal and Program Follow-up:** At the end of the course or at your short-term goal target date, reevaluate your flexibility and answer the following questions:

   a. Did you meet your short-term goal or your goal for the course?

   b. If so, what positive behavioral changes contributed to your success? If not, which obstacles blocked your success?

   c. Was your short-term goal realistic? After evaluating your progress during the course, what would you change about your goals or training plan?

DATE	Stretches Completed (with time/reps)	COMMENTS (e.g., stretches modified, stretches held longer, how you felt, etc.)

Flexibility Training Log

activate, motivate, & ADVANCE YOUR FITNESS

A FLEXIBILITY TRAINING PROGRAM

LIVE IT! ONLINE

ACTIVATE!

Looking to improve your posture, circulation, and joint mobility? Follow these programs to gradually incorporate regular stretching into your weekly exercise routines.

What Do I Need for Flexibility Training?

GEAR: For flexibility training programs, you'll want a mat, towel, and something stable to hold onto for standing stretches. While you really don't need any other equipment for stretching, you may want to use a strap, foam roller, yoga block, or even a training partner.

CLOTHING: Wear comfortable clothing that allows for full range-of-motion movements.

How Do I Start a Flexibility Training Program?

TECHNIQUE: Safe and effective flexibility training depends on good body alignment and awareness. Read through each exercise description and take time to learn the proper form. If you need assistance, ask your instructor or a fitness specialist at your facility. Perform static stretches in a slow and controlled manner. Hold at the point of tightness but not pain. Exhale with the stretching exercise to help you relax and increase your flexibility.

ETIQUETTE: Most facilities will have mats, equipment, and a designated stretching area for you to use. Wipe down your mat or any other equipment after use.

STRETCHING BEFORE A WORKOUT: Dynamic stretching (stretching through movement) performed during your warm-up can prepare your body for the upcoming more intense activity. Incorporate slow and controlled movements that mimic the motions of your workout.

STRETCHING AFTER A WORKOUT: After your workout program your muscles are warm and ready to be stretched. Static or PNF stretching performed at this time will result in the biggest gains in flexibility, particularly after a cardiorespiratory workout.

Flexibility Training Warm-Up & Cool-Down

Warming up prior to stretching is crucial and should include gentle cardiorespiratory exercises for 5 to 10 minutes. After breaking a light sweat, add dynamic movements that increase your range of motion. Ease into the first repetition of each static or PNF stretching exercise. Ensure proper form, posture, and body alignment as you move into your full range of motion.

Flexibility Training Programs

If you are new to flexibility training or if you have not stretched for more than three months, start slowly and build gradually by beginning with Program A. If you already stretch two days a week, then start with Program B. Adjust intensity, volume and training days to suit your personal fitness level and schedule; visit the companion website for more options.

PROGRAM A  **GOAL:** Incorporate a full-body stretching routine into weekly schedule

Frequency	Intensity	Time	Number & Type of Stretches
2 non-consecutive days a week	Stretch to a point of mild tightness, not pain	Perform 2–3 repetitions of each stretch, holding for 10–20 seconds each time	8 static stretches

Order of Stretches

Side Stretch
Upper-Back Stretch
Pectoral and Biceps Stretch
Inner-Thigh Side Lunge

Quadriceps Stretch (Standing)
Hamstrings Stretch (Supine Lying)
Low-Back Knee-to-Chest Stretch (Two Knees)
Calf Stretch (Gastrocnemius Lunge)

PROGRAM B **GOAL:** Improve full body range of motion and overall physical function

Frequency	Intensity	Time	Number & Type of Stretches
3 non-consecutive days a week	Stretch to a point of mild tightness, not pain	Perform 2–4 repetitions of each stretch, holding for 20–30 seconds each time	12 static stretches

Order of Stretches

Neck Stretches (Head Turn)
Side Stretch
Upper-Back Stretch
Shoulder Stretch
Pectoral and Biceps Stretch
Inner-Thigh Side Lunge

Outer-Thigh Stretch
Quadriceps Stretch (Lying)
Hamstrings Stretch (Supine Lying)
Low-Back Knee-to-Chest Stretch (Two Knees)
Gluteal Stretch
Calf Stretch (Heel Drop)

MOTIVATE!

Create your own exercise log to track your flexibility training program—make note of days, actual stretches, type of stretch, repetitions, time—or use the log available through the companion website. Here are a few tips to keep you stretching.

FIND A PARTNER: With a stretching partner, you can keep each other accountable, help each other reach goals, and have greater options when incorporating PNF stretches, as well as a wider variety of both passive and active stretches. Bye-bye boredom!

TRY A NEW CLASS: Shorter classes specifically designed for stretching, foam rolling, core strength, and/or back health are popping up everywhere. You can also try a yoga or martial arts class and have exercises that increase flexibility built right in! Learn something new, meet new people, and keep "reaching" toward your goals.

STRESS? WHAT STRESS? Take a deep breath. Exhale. Slowly move into your stretch. Hold for at least 10 seconds. Repeat three more times. Before you know it you will feel refreshed and relaxed from head to toe. The simple act of performing your flexibility program can increase your circulation, decrease your blood pressure, and keep you calm and focused. Stretch more, stress less!

ADVANCE!

Now that you have established your flexibility program, you might find that you want more stretches that are specific to your sport or activity. Below are three more advanced flexibility programs specific for walkers/runners, cyclists, and swimmers. You can follow these or log onto the companion website to find more options or simply to personalize this program or any of the programs in this book.

PROGRAM C

GOAL: Add stretches of specific use for walkers and runners

Frequency	Intensity	Time	Number & Type of Stretches
3 non-consecutive days a week	Stretch to a point of mild tightness, not pain	Perform 2–4 repetitions of each stretch, holding for 20–30 seconds each time	5 additional static stretches*

*Perform following a walking/running cardiorespiratory workout, and in addition to Flexibility Program B.

Stretches to Add

Hip Flexor Stretch (Standing for walkers and Low Lunge for runners)
Torso Twist and Hip Stretch (Seated Twist)

Hamstrings Stretch (Modified Hurdler)
Calf Stretch (Soleus Stretch)
Shin Stretch

PROGRAM D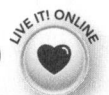

GOAL: Add stretches of specific use for cyclists

Frequency	Intensity	Time	Number & Type of Stretches
3 non-consecutive days a week	Stretch to a point of mild tightness, not pain	Perform 2–4 repetitions of each stretch, holding for 20–30 seconds each time	5 additional static stretches*

*Perform following a cycling cardiorespiratory workout, and in addition to Flexibility Program B.

Stretches to Add

Neck Stretches (Head Tilt)
Hip Flexor Stretch (Standing or Low Lunge)
Torso Twist and Hip Stretch (Seated Twist)

Calf Stretch (Soleus Stretch)
Shin Stretch

PROGRAM E

GOAL: Add stretches of specific use for swimmers

Frequency	Intensity	Time	Reps	Number & Type of Stretches
3 non-consecutive days a week	Stretch to a point of mild tightness, not pain	20–30 sec per stretch	2–4	5 additional static stretches

*Perform following a swimming cardiorespiratory workout, and in addition to Flexibility Program B.

Stretches to Add

Neck Stretches (Head Tilt)
Triceps Stretch
Hip Flexor Stretch (Standing)

Torso Twist and Hip Stretch (Seated Twist)
Shin Stretch

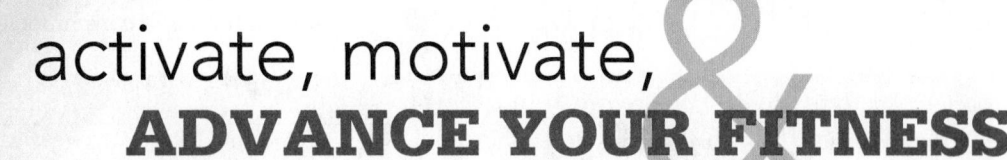

activate, motivate, & ADVANCE YOUR FITNESS

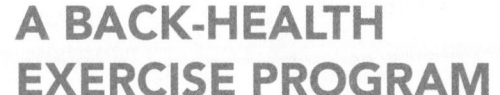

A BACK-HEALTH EXERCISE PROGRAM

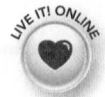

Want to avoid back pain or manage pain you may already have? Try the core stretching and strengthening exercise programs outlined on the next page. They are specifically designed to help you increase the strength of your core trunk muscles and decrease tightness. Combine programs A and B for a full-core back-health program. Together, these programs can stand alone; however, the exercises are designed to be incorporated into your current muscular fitness and flexibility programs. Visit the companion website to find more options or to personalize this or any of the programs in this book.

CORE PROGRAM A

GOAL: Increase core muscle endurance and strength

Frequency	Intensity	Time			Number & Type of Exercises
		Reps	Sets	Rest	
2 non-consecutive days a week	60% 1RM	12	2	2 minutes between sets	8 core muscle exercises

Core Strength Exercises

Arm/Leg Extensions
Plank (hold each plank for 15 to 30 seconds and complete 2 to 4 repetitions)
Back Extension
Abdominal Curl

Reverse Curl
Oblique Curl
Pelvic Tilt
Side Bridge (hold each side bridge for 15 seconds and complete 4 repetitions)

CORE PROGRAM B

GOAL: Decrease core muscle tightness

Frequency	Intensity	Time	Number & Type of Exercises
2 non-consecutive days a week	Stretch to a point of mild tightness, not pain	Perform 2–4 repetitions of each stretch, holding for 10–30 seconds each time	8 core stretch exercises

Core Stretches

Back Bridge
Low-Back Knee-to-Chest Stretch (Two Knees)
Gluteal Stretch
Hamstrings Stretch (Supine Lying)

Quadriceps Stretch (Lying)
Torso Twist and Hip Stretch (Seated Twist)
Cat Stretch
Hip Flexor Stretch (Low Lunge)

6

Understanding Body Composition

Learning Outcomes

1. Discuss how body composition is related to lifelong fitness and wellness.

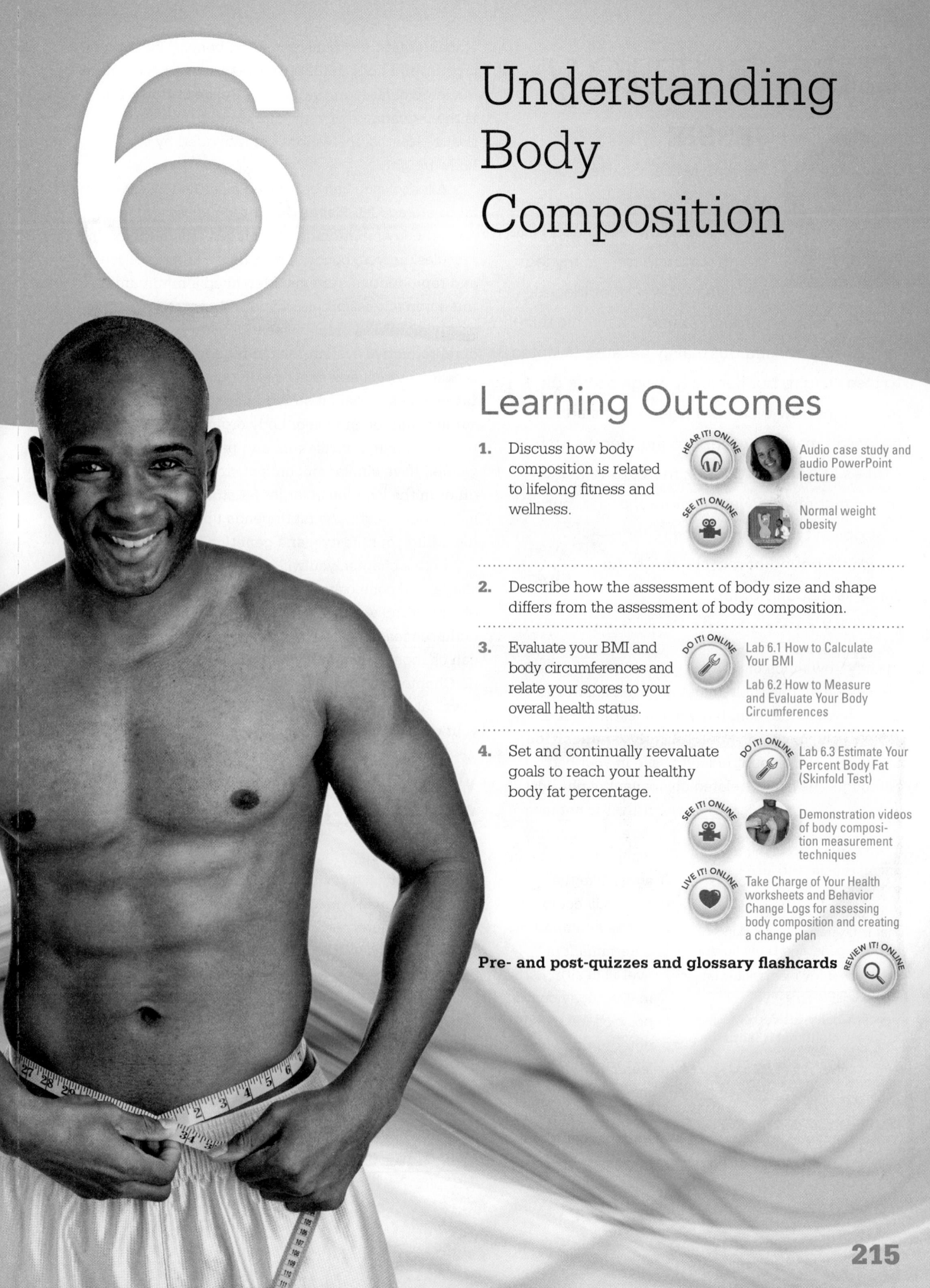 **HEAR IT! ONLINE** Audio case study and audio PowerPoint lecture

SEE IT! ONLINE Normal weight obesity

2. Describe how the assessment of body size and shape differs from the assessment of body composition.

3. Evaluate your BMI and body circumferences and relate your scores to your overall health status.

DO IT! ONLINE Lab 6.1 How to Calculate Your BMI

Lab 6.2 How to Measure and Evaluate Your Body Circumferences

4. Set and continually reevaluate goals to reach your healthy body fat percentage.

DO IT! ONLINE Lab 6.3 Estimate Your Percent Body Fat (Skinfold Test)

SEE IT! ONLINE Demonstration videos of body composition measurement techniques

LIVE IT! ONLINE Take Charge of Your Health worksheets and Behavior Change Logs for assessing body composition and creating a change plan

Pre- and post-quizzes and glossary flashcards REVIEW IT! ONLINE

casestudy

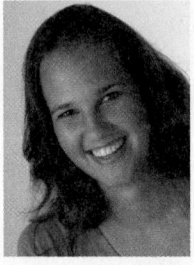

JESSIE

"Hi, I'm Jessie. I started running and resistance training two months ago and feel great! I like the new muscle tone in my legs, and I've made a lot of friends from the running group I joined. The ironic thing is, I started working out mainly because I wanted to lose weight, but I actually weigh a little bit more right now than I did when I first started. It doesn't make any sense to me, because my clothes fit better and I look more 'toned.' I've heard that muscle weighs more than fat, but that doesn't make any sense, either—doesn't a pound of muscle weigh the same as a pound of fat?"

HEAR IT! ONLINE

How much of your body is composed of fat? It's impossible to get an exact answer to that question, but you can estimate it. Body fat is a component of your total **body composition**, along with the amount of lean tissue in your body. Although this health-related component of physical fitness is not measured by your physical performance on a task like the others, body composition is an important determinant of overall health. Estimating body composition involves determining your lean body mass, fat mass, and percent body fat. Your **lean body mass** is your body's total amount of lean or fat-free tissue (muscles, bones, skin, other organs, and body fluids). Your **fat mass** is body mass made up of fat (adipose) tissue. **Percent body fat** is the percentage of your total weight that is fat tissue—that is, the weight of fat divided by total body weight.

All fat tissue can be labeled as either essential fat or storage fat. **Essential fat** is necessary for normal body functioning; it includes fats in the brain, muscles, nerves, bones, lungs, heart, and digestive and reproductive systems. Men need a minimum of three percent essential body fat. Women need significantly more (12 percent essential body fat) because of reproductive system-related fat deposits in their breasts, uterus, and elsewhere (Figure 6.1). **Storage fat** is nonessential fat stored in tissue near the body's surface and around major body organs. Storage fat provides energy, insulation, and padding. Men and women have similar amounts of storage fat but may differ in the location of larger fat stores. Your individual amount of storage fat depends upon many factors, including your lifestyle and genetics.

In this chapter, you will learn why body size, shape, and composition are useful measurements of fitness and wellness. You'll also learn how each of these measurements is determined and how you can change or maintain your body composition. (In Chapter 8, you will combine your knowledge of physical activity, body composition, and diet to create your own weight-management plan.)

Why Do My Body Size, Shape, and Composition Matter?

You might think of body size, shape, and composition mainly in terms of your physical appearance, but they encompass more than how you look. They are important components (as well as measurements) of your overall fitness and wellness.

Knowing Your Body Composition Can Help You Assess Your Health Risks

From the mid-1970s to 2008, the number of overweight children and adolescents increased from a mere 5 percent to 17 percent of the U.S. population![1]

---

body composition The relative amounts of fat and lean tissue in the body

lean body mass Body mass that is fat-free (muscle, skin, bone, organs, and body fluids)

fat mass Body mass that is fat tissue (adipose tissue)

percent body fat Percentage of total weight that is fat tissue

essential fat Body fat that is essential for normal physiological functioning

storage fat Body fat that is not essential but does provide energy, insulation, and padding

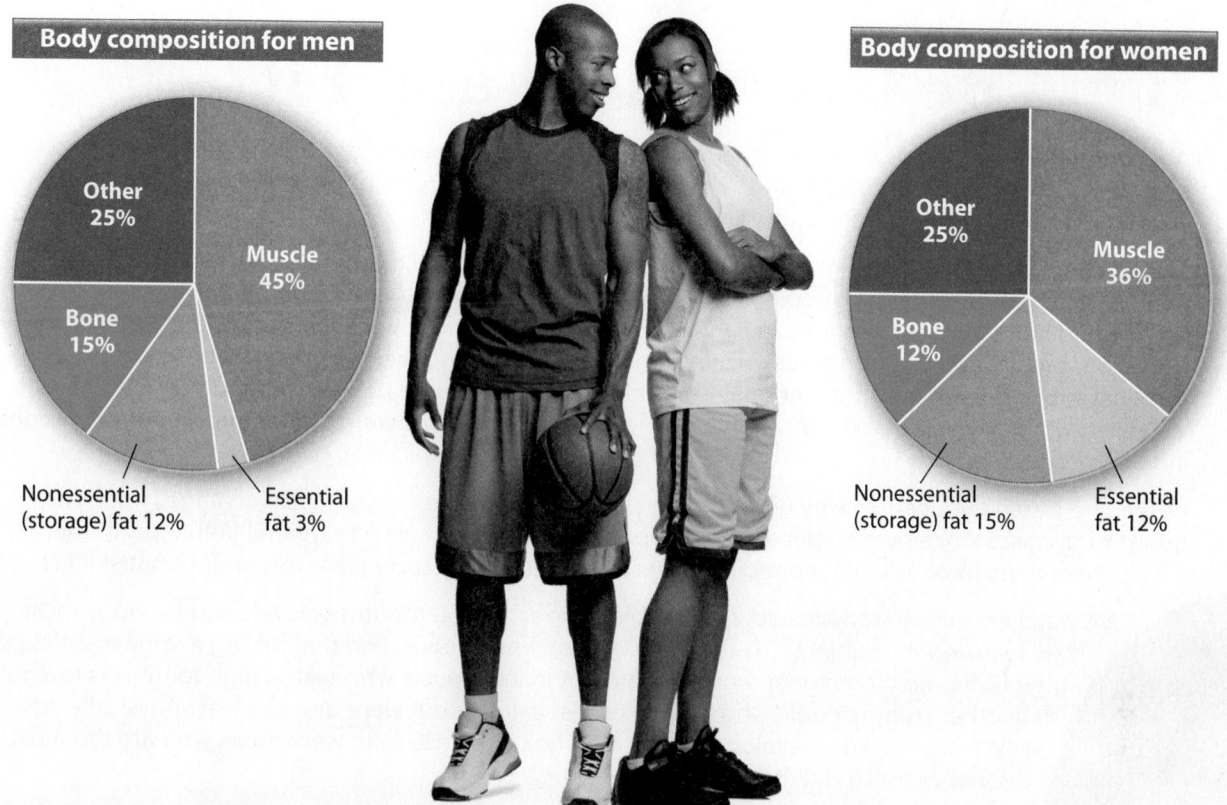

Body composition for men

Other 25%

Muscle 45%

Bone 15%

Nonessential (storage) fat 12%

Essential fat 3%

Body composition for women

Other 25%

Muscle 36%

Bone 12%

Nonessential (storage) fat 15%

Essential fat 12%

FIGURE **6.1** The body compositions of typical 20- to 24-year-old men and women vary primarily in the amounts of muscle and essential fat.

Data from McArdle and others, *Exercise Physiology: Energy, Nutrition, and Human Performance.* 7th ed. (Baltimore, MD: Lippincott Williams & Wilkins, 2010).

This is a problem because childhood obesity significantly increases your risk for heart disease and premature death and disability in adulthood.[2,3] Over a ten year period (1999–2008), the number of overweight or obese adults in the United States grew from 64 percent to 68 percent of the population. Of those, 38 percent are classified as obese![4]

Studies of obesity, however, often rely on measurements of total body weight rather than measurements of body composition. While measurements of total body weight can be useful in studying large populations, they are less useful in assessing an individual's health risks and body changes. For individuals, estimates of body composition—specifically, of lean and fat mass—provide additional important information. By knowing your percent body fat, you can more effectively determine your risks for chronic disease and decide just how much weight you should try to lose (or gain).

Evaluating Your Body Size and Shape Can Help Motivate Healthy Behavior Change

If you are just beginning an exercise program for fitness, it is often more useful to assess changes in body size and shape as a measurement of your progress, rather than weighing yourself daily on a bathroom scale. The reason: Healthy increases in muscle tissue (achieved by exercise) may cause you to temporarily gain weight, until the process of body fat loss catches up with muscle tissue gains. This is a *good* thing, but you would not know it if you relied solely on the scale to determine your progress. By monitoring improvements in your body size and shape instead, you can get a more realistic sense of your achievement and stay motivated to stick with an exercise program. The box Can I Be Overweight and Fit? discusses overweight, disease, and fitness in more detail.

Can I Be Overweight and Fit?

A recent federal study of 2.3 million American adults analyzed decades of mortality data from people over age 25.[1] The study divided all the subjects into standard BMI groupings: underweight, normal weight, overweight, and obese.

The study found that underweight people had higher-than-standard death rates for non-cancer and non-CVD causes. Overweight people had higher rates for cancer, diabetes, and heart disease. Obese people had higher death rates for CVD and slightly higher rates for the cancers associated with body fat: colon, breast, esophagus, uterus, ovary, kidney, and pancreas. Overweight and obese people may even have lower death rates than normal-weight individuals for some non-cancer and non-CVD causes. However, when all causes of death were combined, their death rates were higher than in normal-weight individuals.

Researchers aren't yet certain why underweight people tend to die in greater percentages from one group of diseases while overweight and obese people tend to succumb to others. In the meantime, other researchers have asked a more direct question: Can you be technically overweight but still fit?

Researchers in one study tested 2,600 subjects over age 60 for fitness levels and for body mass, then followed the subjects' health for 20 years.[2] The study found that having a large waistline or high BMI predicted higher mortality, but not in individuals who tested high for fitness levels. In another study, people who ate the fewest calories but were also the least physically active were more likely to develop and die from heart disease than were those who ate the most calories but also did the most exercise.[3]

Research says that fitness is important, particularly for boys who want to avoid adult diabetes, but cardiorespiratory fitness has benefits, independent of fatness, on disease markers in all adolescents.[4,5] The evidence is strong that muscular and cardiovascular fitness helps protect us from illness and disease as we grow older, too. One study found that elasticity in large arteries is altered by fitness level but not obesity level. So, being fit can help offset some of the risks associated with obesity and blood vessel health.[6] And while BMI, according to another study, had the greatest effect on blood pressure results, even a moderate level of fitness was associated with the lowest blood pressure grouping.[7] Finally, exercise can have a positive effect on depression, no matter what your BMI.[8]

Fitness allows us to stay healthier, to maintain mobility, and to experience a higher quality of life. Do you feel energetic, get plenty of exercise, and have a high fitness level? If so, you can probably worry less about current definitions of "overweight" and "high BMI" and instead focus on continuing to maintain or increase your fitness level.

Sources:
1. K. M. Flegal and others, "Cause-Specific Excess Deaths Associated with Underweight, Overweight, and Obesity," *Journal of the American Medical Association* 298, no. 17 (2007): 2028–37.
2. X. Sui and others, "Cardiorespiratory Fitness and Adiposity as Mortality Predictors in Older Adults," *Journal of the American Medical Association* 298, no. 21 (2007): 2507–16.
3. J. Fang and others, "Exercise, Body Mass Index, Caloric Intake, and Cardiovascular Mortality," *American Journal of Preventative Medicine* 25, no. 4 (2003): 283–89.
4. D. M. Cummings and others, "Fitness versus Fatness and Insulin Resistance in U.S. Adolescents," *Journal of Obesity* (2010): 195729.
5. S. Kwon, T. L. Burns, and K. Janz, "Associations of Cardiorespiratory Fitness and Fatness with Cardiovascular Risk Factors among Adolescents: The NHANES 1999-2002," *Journal of Physical Activity and Health* 7, no. 6 (2010): 746–53.
6. K. Davison and others, "Relationships between Obesity, Cardiorespiratory Fitness, and Cardiovascular Function," *Journal of Obesity* (2010): 191253.
7. J. Chen and others, "Fitness, Fatness, and Systolic Blood Pressure: Data from the Cooper Center Longitudinal Study," *American Heart Journal* 160, no. 1 (2010): 166–70.
8. L. G. Perraton, S. Kumar, and Z. Machotka, "Exercise Parameters in the Treatment of Clinical Depression: A Systematic Review of Randomized Controlled Trials," *Journal of Evaluation in Clinical Practice* 16, no. 3 (2010): 597–604.

How Can I Evaluate My Body Size and Shape?

How do you determine whether your body size and shape are "healthy"? This is a much-debated topic, but there are three common methods of doing so: calculating your body mass index, measuring your body circumferences, and identifying the patterns of fat distribution on your body. (Evaluating your body composition is a somewhat more complicated process, which we discuss later in this chapter.)

Calculate Your Body Mass Index (BMI) But Understand Its Limitations

Body mass index (BMI) is one of the most common measurements that doctors and researchers use to assess risk of weight-related disease, death, and disability. BMI is a measurement based on your weight and height. You can calculate your BMI now, using the chart in Figure 6.2.

Weight (pounds)

Height (feet and inches)	100	110	120	130	140	150	160	170	180	190	200	210	220	230	240	250	260
4'6"	24	27	29	31	34	36	39	41	43	46	48	51	53	55	58	60	63
4'8"	22	25	27	29	31	34	36	38	40	43	45	47	49	52	54	56	58
4'10"	21	23	25	27	29	31	33	36	38	40	42	44	46	48	50	52	54
5'0"	20	22	23	25	27	29	31	33	35	37	39	41	43	45	47	49	51
5'2"	18	20	22	24	26	27	29	31	33	35	37	38	40	42	44	46	48
5'4"	17	19	21	22	24	26	28	29	31	33	34	36	38	40	41	43	45
5'6"	16	18	19	21	23	24	26	27	29	31	32	34	36	37	39	40	42
5'8"	15	17	18	20	21	23	24	26	27	29	30	32	33	35	37	38	40
5'10"	14	16	17	19	20	22	23	24	26	27	29	30	32	33	34	36	37
6'0"	14	15	16	18	19	20	22	23	24	26	27	29	30	31	33	34	35
6'2"	13	14	15	17	18	19	21	22	23	24	26	27	28	30	31	32	33
6'4"	12	13	15	16	17	18	20	21	22	23	24	26	27	28	29	30	32
6'6"	12	13	14	15	16	17	19	20	21	22	23	24	25	27	28	29	30
6'8"	11	12	13	14	15	17	18	19	20	21	22	23	24	25	26	28	29
6'10"	11	12	13	14	15	16	17	18	19	20	21	22	23	24	25	26	27
7'0"	10	11	12	13	14	15	16	17	18	19	20	21	22	23	24	25	26

Key:
- Underweight
- Normal weight
- Overweight
- Obese

FIGURE **6.2** Estimate your BMI by finding where your weight and height intersect.

BMI scores place individuals in categories as follows:[5]

Underweight (BMI of <18.5)

Normal weight (BMI of 18.5 to 24.9)

Overweight (BMI of 25.0 to 29.9)

Obese—Class I (BMI of 30.0 to 34.9)

Class II (BMI of 35.0 to 39.9)

Class III (BMI of >40.0)

Figure 6.3 on page 220 illustrates that very low and very high BMI scores are correlated with greater risk of death and disability.

The limitation with using BMI scores to assess "fitness" or "fatness" is that they do not differentiate between fat mass and lean mass. BMI is solely determined by height and weight. While BMI measurements can be helpful for individuals of average muscle and bone density, they can be misleading for athletes, bodybuilders, and short or petite individuals. For instance, someone who has an exceptionally heavy skeleton and larger-than-average muscle mass may have a BMI score that classifies him or her as "overweight," even if his or her percent body fat is in the "healthy" range. Because of BMI's limitations, it helps to also consider other factors, such as percent body fat, when assessing the overall picture of a person's fitness. **Lab 6.1** walks you through how to calculate your own BMI.

> **body mass index (BMI)**
> A number calculated from a person's weight and height that is used to assess risk for health problems

THINK! Do you think BMI will be a good predictor of body fitness and/or fatness for you? Why or why not?

ACT! Look at the ranges above and guess which BMI category you fall into. Why do you think you are in that range? Use the chart in Figure 6.2 or go to www.cdc.gov/healthyweight/assessing/bmi/index.html to check your estimate.

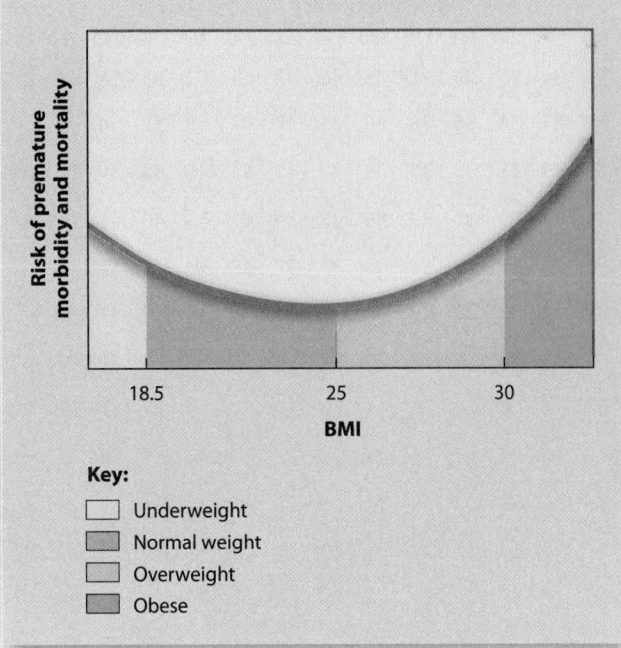

FIGURE 6.3 Extremely low or extremely high BMIs are associated with a greater risk of premature death and disability.

Data from Katherine Flegal and others, "Excess Deaths Associated with Underweight, Overweight, and Obesity," *Journal of the American Medical Association* 293, no. 15 (2005): 1861–67.

Measure Your Body Circumferences

You can measure circumferences of various parts of your body to monitor your body's changes over time and to further assess your risk of disease. If you want to gain or lose weight, you can measure the circumference of your waist, hips, neck, upper arm, chest, thigh, and calf and then monitor changes in your body over time. You can also use waist and hip circumferences to assess disease risk. As shown in Table 6.1, waist circumference (a marker of abdominal fat) can indicate greater risk of diabetes, high blood pressure, and heart disease if it is greater than 102 cm in males or 88 cm in females.[6] As the table also shows, the people at greatest risk

waist-to-hip ratio (WHR) Waist circumference divided by hip circumference

android Body shape described as "apple-shaped," with excess body fat distributed primarily on the upper body and trunk

gynoid Body shape described as "pear-shaped," where excess body fat is distributed primarily on the lower body (hips and thighs)

subcutaneous fat Adipose tissue that is located just below the surface of the skin

visceral fat Adipose tissue that surrounds organs in the abdomen

are those with high waist circumferences *and* high BMIs.

You can also use waist and hip circumferences to determine your waist-to-hip ratio (WHR). **Waist-to-hip ratio** is your waist circumference divided by your hip circumference. A higher WHR is associated with more health risks. Young men with a WHR of 0.94 or more and young women with a WHR of 0.82 or more fall into a high-risk category.[7] **Lab 6.2** will walk you through the process of measuring your body circumferences and determining your WHR. Although waist circumference and WHR are both measures of disease risk, waist circumference is generally preferred because it is simpler, because of its relationship with abdominal fat, and because of its strong association to disease risk factors.[8]

Identify Your Body's Patterns of Fat Distribution

Body fat distribution patterns are mostly genetically determined. You have probably noticed that people take after one parent in the way they "wear their fat." Some individuals tend to accumulate fat around their midsections; others collect it in the lower body or hips. These distributions contribute to an overall body shape that can be correlated to a higher or lower risk of disease.

The two most common body shapes are **android** ("apple-shaped") and **gynoid** ("pear-shaped") (Figure 6.4). A person with *android pattern obesity* has excess body fat on the upper body and trunk and has a greater risk of developing chronic disease than a person with *gynoid pattern obesity,* who carries excess body fat in the lower body. Higher waist circumferences due to excess abdominal fat are associated with higher levels of **subcutaneous fat** and **visceral fat**.[9] Although

TABLE 6.1 Waist Circumference, BMI, and Disease Risk

| Weight Classification | BMI (kg/m²) | Waist Circumference and Disease Risk* | |
		Smaller Waist Men ≤102 cm (40 in) Women ≤88 cm (35 in)	Larger Waist Men >102 cm (40 in) Women >88 cm (35 in)
Underweight	<18.5	—	—
Normal Weight	18.5–24.9	—	—
Overweight	25.0–29.9	Increased	High
Obese—I	30.0–34.9	High	Very High
Obese—II	35.0–39.9	Very High	Very High
Obese—III	>40.0	Extremely High	Extremely High

*Risk for type 2 diabetes, hypertension, and cardiovascular disease, relative to normal weight and waist circumference.

Source: Adapted from National Heart, Lung, and Blood Institute—Expert Panel on the Identification, Evaluation, and Treatment of Overweight in Adults, "Clinical Guidelines on the Identification, Evaluation, and Treatment of Overweight and Obesity in Adults: Executive Summary," *American Journal of Clinical Nutrition* 68 (1998): 899–917. Used with permission.

both are associated with metabolic diseases, fat in the abdominal cavity (visceral fat) has a stronger relationship to disease risk.[10] The good news is that a reduction in total body fat will result in reductions in subcutaneous fat, visceral fat, and disease risk.[11,12] While men tend to store fat in the abdomen and women tend to store it in the lower body, there are exceptions, and fat distribution is strongly influenced by genetics. If you have an "apple-shaped" body, understanding the health risks can help motivate you to keep your "apple" from getting too large and round!

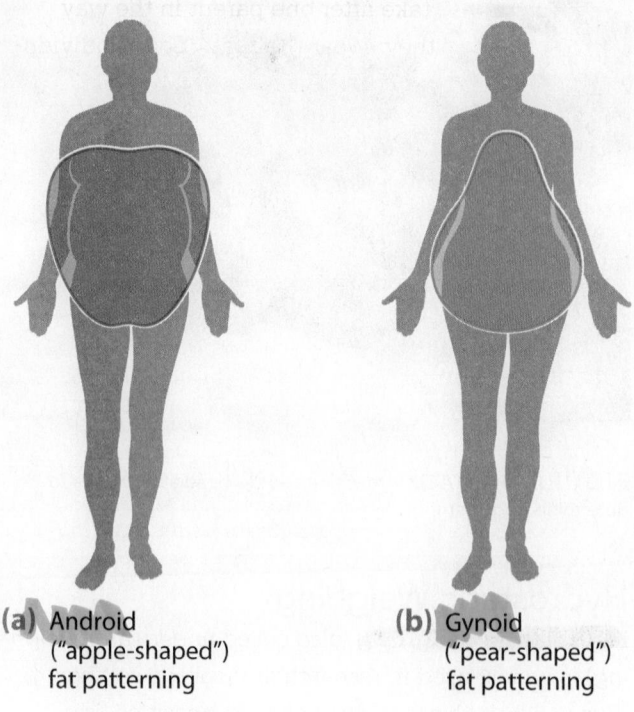

(a) Android ("apple-shaped") fat patterning

(b) Gynoid ("pear-shaped") fat patterning

FIGURE 6.4 (a) Android ("apple-shaped") fat distribution, associated with greater risk of heart disease and diabetes, is more common in men of all ages and postmenopausal women; (b) gynoid ("pear-shaped") fat distribution is more common in premenopausal women.

casestudy

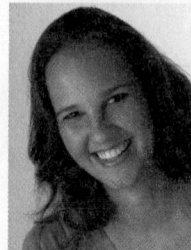

JESSIE

"My friend Emily explained to me that I probably gained weight after starting my exercise program because I was building muscle faster than I was losing fat and that I shouldn't worry about it. She suggested that I check my body measurements instead of getting on the scale. I like that idea, and she offered to help, but now I am not sure which ones to do. My problem areas have always been my hips and thighs. Should I measure those areas and call it good?"

THINK! Why would body measurements/circumferences be a better way for Jessie to measure her progress than body weight? What body shape, gynoid or android, does Jessie most likely have? Does her shape increase or decrease her risk for disease?

ACT! Write out three of your "problem" body areas. Next to each indicate whether you want to increase or decrease your size.

What Methods Are Used to Assess Body Composition?

Unlike BMI and body circumference measurements, body composition (lean mass vs. fat mass) can only be estimated indirectly. A true, direct assessment of body composition requires dissection after death; in fact, researchers judge the accuracy of the indirect measures by comparing them with dissection results from cadavers.

Methods of estimating body composition range from assessments that trained fitness instructors can easily administer, such as skinfold measurements and bioelectrical impedance analysis, to sophisticated tests that must be conducted by clinicians in a lab or hospital setting. The most accurate estimates of body composition are body scans such as an MRI (magnetic resonance imaging) or a CT (computed tomography) scan. These are used in medical settings to diagnose injury and illness but are not often used for body composition analysis alone. In the next section, we discuss methods that are commonly used to assess body composition.

Skinfold Measurements

Skinfold measurements are an easy, inexpensive way to estimate your percent body fat. **Calipers** (shown in Lab 6.3) are used to measure the thickness of a fold of skin and subcutaneous adipose tissue. Skinfold measurements at specific sites around the body are recorded and entered into an equation that predicts percent body fat. This prediction of percent body fat has an error range of 3 to 4 percent;[13] for example, if your body fat measurement is 16 percent, the true value could be anywhere from about 12 to 20 percent.

More recent research has shown that current equations to predict body fat from skinfolds will underestimate percent body fat levels by about 1.3% in men and 3.0% in women (compared to DXA measured body fat levels), and may result in additional over- or underestimates for ethnically and racially diverse populations.[14] If you use this method to estimate your body

fat, remember it is just that—an estimate! **Lab 6.3** provides instructions for skinfold measurements. Performing an accurate skinfold assessment takes education and practice, so be sure to ask a qualified fitness instructor to help you.

DO IT! ONLINE

Dual-Energy X-Ray Absorptiometry

Dual-energy X-ray absorptiometry (DXA) is the "gold-standard" reference method for body composition assessment in clinical and research settings (Figure 6.5). In a DXA scan, low-radiation X rays are used to distinguish fat, bone mineral, and bone-free lean components of the body. Measuring bone mineral (in addition to fat and lean mass) increases the accuracy of body fat estimates. In the medical setting, DXA scans are most often used to determine bone density for osteoporosis diagnosis. Body composition estimates can be obtained from whole body DXA scans that take less than 20 minutes. However, DXA tests are expensive, require a prescription for a medical X ray, and are not well designed to examine people who are extremely obese.

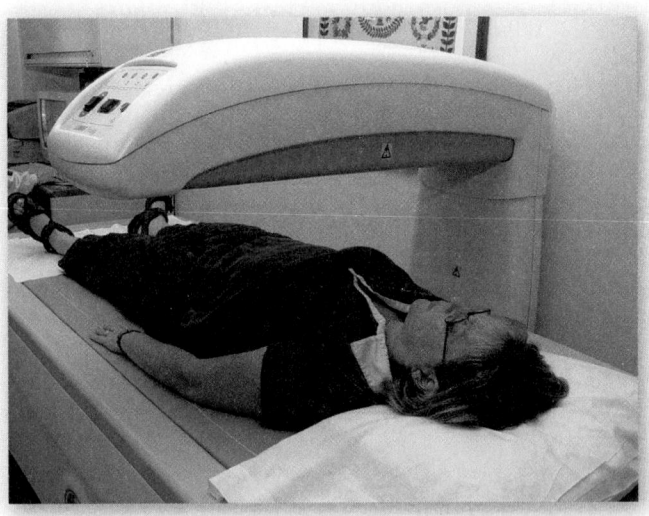

FIGURE **6.5** A DXA machine uses low-radiation X rays to determine body composition.

Hydrostatic Weighing

Hydrostatic weighing (also called *underwater weighing*) is widely used in research and college settings (Figure 6.6). In this method of body composition assessment, a person is first weighed outside a water tank and then weighed while completely submerged in the tank. Hydrostatic weighing is based on the concept that the more fat a person has, the more he or she will tend to float and the less weight he or she will exert against the bottom of the tank. From this process, a technician can assess total body volume and body density and use them to calculate

skinfold A fold of skin and subcutaneous fat that is measured with calipers to determine the fatness of a specific body area

calipers A handheld and spring-loaded instrument with calibrated jaws and a meter that reads skinfold thickness in millimeters

dual-energy X-ray absorptiometry (DXA) A technique using two low-radiation X rays to scan bone and soft tissue (muscle, fat) to determine bone density and to estimate percent body fat

hydrostatic weighing A technique that uses water to determine total body volume, total body density, and percent body fat

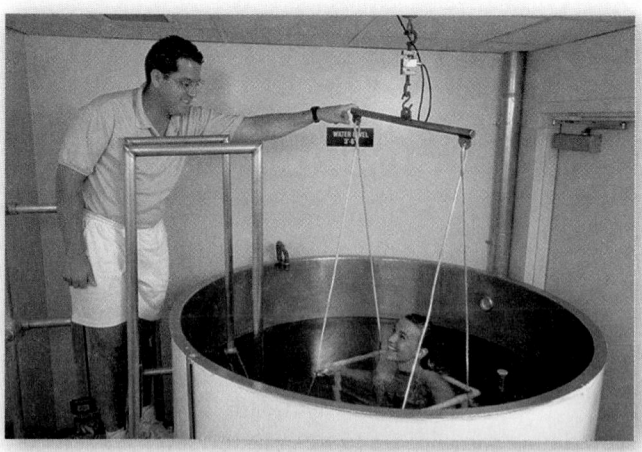

FIGURE **6.6** Hydrostatic (underwater) weighing uses total body water displacement to calculate estimated percent body fat.

an estimated percent body fat. The method is valid and reliable, but access to an equipped facility may be limited and not everyone is comfortable with being submerged.

Air Displacement (Bod Pod)

While hydrostatic weighing measures total body *water* displacement, the **Bod Pod** measures total body *air* displacement (Figure 6.7). The person being assessed puts on a swimsuit and then sits in the egg-shaped Bod Pod chamber while the air displacement is measured. The volume of air displaced is used together with other measures (such as weight) to determine total body volume and density and then to estimate percent body fat.

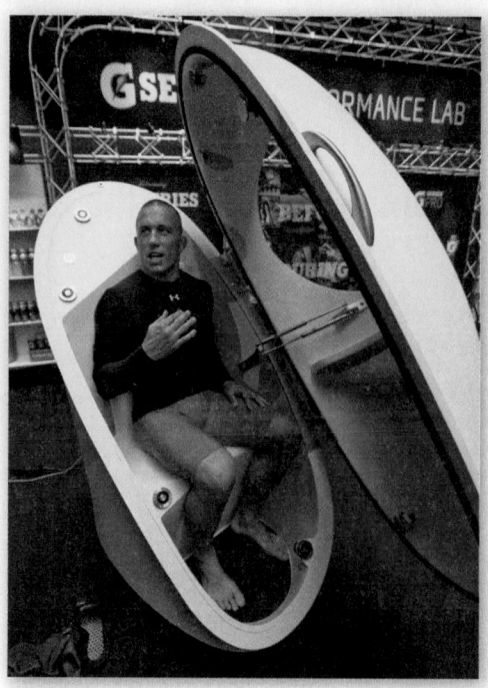

FIGURE **6.7** The Bod Pod uses total body air displacement to calculate estimated percent body fat.

Bod Pod percent body fat measurements are generally within 1–2% of hydrostatic weighing and DXA-measured levels of percent body fat.[15] Bod Pod measurements are available in many clinical and college settings, but availability in fitness settings is still somewhat limited.

> **Bod Pod** An egg-shaped chamber that uses air displacement to determine total body volume, total body density, and percent body fat
>
> **bioelectrical impedance analysis (BIA)** A technique that distinguishes lean and fat mass by measuring the resistance of various body tissues to electrical currents

Bioelectrical Impedance Analysis

In **bioelectrical impedance analysis (BIA)**, a machine measures the resistance of various body tissues to electrical currents. BIA machines send small electrical currents through the body via the hands, feet, or both (Figure 6.8). Fat does not conduct electricity very well, so fat tissues will demonstrate a resistance to the currents. Fat-free tissues have more body water and conduct electricity well; thus, fat-free tissues do not offer as much resistance to the currents. These resistance differences are used to estimate percent body fat. Higher resistance indicates higher levels of overall body fat. The error range of BIA is 3 to 4 percent, but accuracy depends upon the quality of the machine and upon the subject's following instructions, especially concerning his/her water intake.[16] Higher or lower levels of body water will significantly alter a BIA machine's results, so it is important to avoid drinking too much or too little prior to assessment.

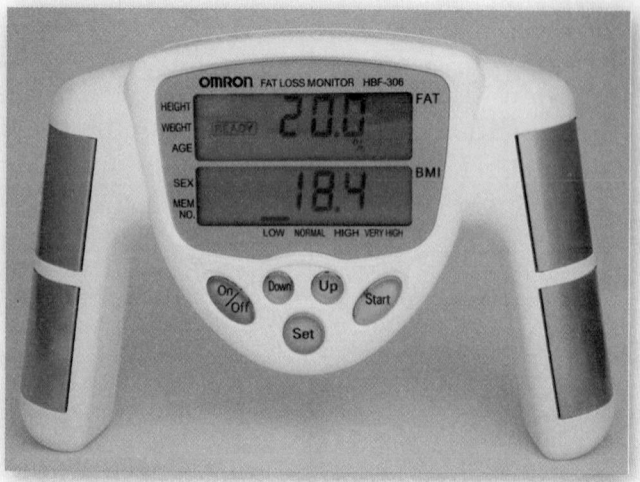

FIGURE **6.8** Bioelectrical impedance analysis (BIA) machines measure the resistance of different body tissues to electrical currents. These measurements are then used to estimate percent body fat. A handheld BIA machine is shown here.

How Can I Change My Body Composition?

After you assess your body size, shape, and composition, the next steps are evaluation, goal setting, and (if your results are not within healthy ranges) planning for change.

Determine Whether Your Percent Body Fat Is within a Healthy Range

Normal Weight Obesity

Because people accumulate fat very differently and not all fat is the same, it is difficult to specify the exact level of body fat that is "healthy" or "unhealthy" for an individual. For instance, abdominal fat increases your risk for disease much more than fat on your calves does. Because of these differences, researchers do not agree upon desired body fat percentages for people of all ages, and you will find that research articles, books, and websites differ in their recommendations. Table 6.2 provides percent body fat norms.

Set Reasonable Body Composition Goals

You have many choices in setting body composition goals. If you are already in the healthy ranges, you can set additional goals for increasing lean mass or decreasing fat mass (within the low limits). Keep in mind that real body composition changes take time. Quick weight

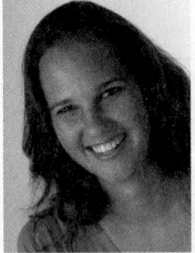
loss is easier for those with more weight to lose, but most weight that is lost quickly consists of water and muscle—the very things you *don't* want to lose. To lose fat only, you have to be committed to exercise and slow, consistent weight loss. Aim for a body composition goal

TABLE 6.2 Percent Body Fat Norms for Men and Women*

MEN

Age	Very Lean	Excellent	Good	Fair	Poor	Very Poor
20–29	≤6%	7–10%	11–15%	16–19%	20–23%	≥24%
30–39	≤10%	11–14%	15–18%	19–21%	22–25%	≥26%
40–49	≤13%	14–17%	18–20%	21–23%	24–27%	≥28%
50–59	≤14%	15–19%	20–22%	23–24%	25–28%	≥29%
60–69	≤15%	16–20%	21–22%	23–25%	26–28%	≥29%
70–79	≤15%	16–20%	21–23%	24–25%	26–28%	≥29%

WOMEN

Age	Very Lean	Excellent	Good	Fair	Poor	Very Poor
20–29	≤13%	14–16%	17–19%	20–23%	24–27%	≥28%
30–39	≤14%	15–17%	18–21%	22–25%	26–29%	≥30%
40–49	≤16%	17–20%	21–24%	25–28%	29–32%	≥33%
50–59	≤17%	18–22%	23–27%	28–30%	31–34%	≥35%
60–69	≤17%	18–23%	24–28%	29–31%	32–35%	≥36%
70–79	≤17%	18–24%	25–29%	30–32%	33–36%	≥37%

*Please note that there are no agreed-upon standards for recommended percent body fat; however, a range of 10–22% for men and 20–32% for women is considered healthy.

Adapted from American College of Sports Medicine, *ACSM's Guidelines for Exercise Testing and Prescription.* 8th ed. (Baltimore, MD: Lippincott Williams & Wilkins, 2010). Copyright © ACSM. Reprinted by permission of Wolters/Kluwer.

Will Spot Reduction Get Rid of My Belly Fat or Cellulite?

Have you ever thought, "I don't need to work on my whole body. I just need to lose some fat off my hips (or thighs or abdomen)!" Despite people's desire to spot-reduce and the multimillion-dollar industry it has spawned for ab-crunchers, thigh-slimmers, arm-toners, and cellulite creams, the answer is disappointingly simple: spot reduction doesn't work.

Researchers have punctured the spot-reduction myth with several carefully controlled studies and have verified that fat doesn't disappear through repeated exercise to one area. Instead, fat stores throughout the entire body dwindle when a negative caloric balance causes you to use up calories stored in fat tissue. In one study, researchers compared fat thickness in both arms of several tennis players. If anyone could work off fat selectively, it would be a tennis player, since he or she holds and swings a racquet thousands of times per week with the dominant hand and arm. The fat thickness, however, was identical in both arms.[1]

Research does show that laser therapy can spot-reduce fat and change body contours,[2] but in order to maintain such changes, the subject must make changes in diet and exercise. For most of us, it makes more sense to just go ahead and make the changes in diet and exercise and skip the time-consuming and expensive laser treatment!

You may be all too familiar with *cellulite*, a rippled appearance in the skin that typically appears around the buttocks and hips where fat deposits bulge. While no truly effective methods exist for getting rid of cellulite, tips for avoiding cellulite include:[3]

- Eating a healthy diet rich in fruits, vegetables, and fiber

- Staying hydrated with plenty of fluids

- Exercising regularly to keep muscles toned and bones strong

- Maintaining a healthy weight (no yo-yo dieting)

- Not smoking

The best strategy for reaching and maintaining a healthy body composition is still to exercise regularly—particularly with resistance training because you simultaneously strengthen and build lean tissue—and follow a structured diet.[4] If your calorie balance is also negative and you lose fat body-wide, your muscle definition will show more clearly, both in the offending spots and elsewhere as well!

Sources:
1. C. X. Bryant, "Why Is the Concept of Spot Reduction Considered a Myth?" *ACE FitnessMatters* 10, no. 1 (2004).
2. M. K. Caruso-Davis and others, "Efficacy of Low-Level Laser Therapy for Body Contouring and Spot Fat Reduction," *Obesity Surgery* 21, no. 6 (2010): 722–9.
3. National Library of Medicine, National Institutes of Health, Medline Plus, "Cellulite," www.nlm.nih.gov/medlineplus/ency/article/002033.htm, updated August 2011.
4. R. B. Kreider and others, "A Structured Diet and Exercise Program Promotes Favorable Changes in Weight Loss, Body Composition, and Weight Maintenance," *Journal of the American Dietetic Association* 111, no. 6 (2011): 828–43.

and a target weight that is healthy and that you can maintain for a lifetime. The box Will Spot Reduction Get Rid of My Belly Fat or Cellulite? discusses further the need for a whole-body approach to body composition.

Follow a Well-Designed Exercise and Nutrition Plan

Fad diets are just that: fads. Most of the time they do not work or only work for a short period of time. True body changes come from sticking with a carefully planned and executed nutrition and exercise program. This book will help you get started. For additional assistance, seek out qualified medical, nutrition, and fitness experts.

Monitor Your Body Size, Shape, and Composition Regularly

Stay motivated in your body change program by monitoring your progress regularly. Since body fat changes may take time, allow two to four months between body composition (percent body fat) assessments. Other types of assessments can be done more frequently. Here is a suggested schedule:

- Body size/shape (mirror and fit of clothes)—assess daily or weekly
- Weight—assess weekly
- Circumferences—measure monthly (or less frequently)
- BMI—measure monthly (or less frequently)
- Percent body fat—measure every other month (or less frequently)

In addition to tracking these measurements, log how you're feeling. Remember, improving your body composition should help you feel good about yourself! The box Self-Esteem and Unhealthy Body Composition Behaviors talks about some problems to be watchful for.

Keep a separate log, journal, or notebook of your progress, but do not feel burdened by it. Some people are more motivated by journaling than others—find the monitoring system that works best for you, and use it consistently.

DIVERSITY

Self-Esteem and Unhealthy Body Composition Behaviors

Body composition can become a major problem for athletes in certain sports—not because they are too fat, but because they are too thin. This is true for both sexes, though the problem is more common in females, who are at risk of developing the female athlete triad (described below). Men may also develop disordered eating habits, as well as a body composition disorder known as muscle dysmorphia, in which men who are of normal weight and even unusually muscular think that they are "puny." (Muscle dysmorphia is discussed further in Chapter 8.) Some sports—gymnastics, figure skating, wrestling, ballet dancing, body-building—place a huge emphasis on appearance and having a lean body. The pressure to look lean and to weigh less can push athletes to cut back on what they eat and increase their workouts to the point where they lose too much weight.

An athlete's self esteem can make a big difference. Lower self esteem can lead to believing that life events are out of your control (external locus of control) and vice versa. One study has shown that if a female athlete has an internal locus of control (or belief that she has power or control over her body and training), she will be more immune to coach and social pressures that can lead to disordered eating.[1] This can help her avoid the female athlete triad (see figure), a triangle of three interrelated problems: menstrual dysfunction, low bone density, and low energy availabilty as a result of disordered eating

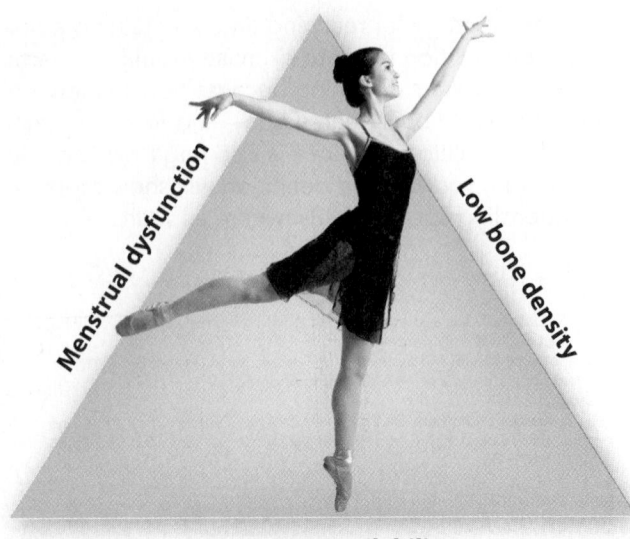

Menstrual dysfunction

Low bone density

Low energy availability

or eating disorders. In the triad, too little caloric intake coupled with too much exercise can lead to hormonal changes and the stopping of menstruation.[2] Improper nutrition, including too little calcium and vitamin D intake, can lead to altered hormones and to bone loss and a risk of fractures. Such changes taking place in adolescence or early adulthood can permanently reduce the size of a woman's skeleton and increase her lifelong risk for osteoporosis. In dancers, one study has shown that the triad negatively affects cardiovascular health.[3]

Athletes with low self-esteem and at high risk for the female athlete triad should carefully monitor their body composition, menstrual health, eating habits, and perhaps bone density. If the triad is suspected, the athlete should eat more nutritious food and/or exercise less, and may need to seek treatment for an eating disorder.

Sources:
1. S. Scoffier, Y. Paquet, and F. d'Arripe-Longueville, "Effect of Locus of Control on Disordered Eating in Athletes: The Mediational Role of Self-regulation of Eating Attitudes," *Eating Behaviors* 11, no. 3 (2010): 164–9.
2. A. M. McManus and N. Armstrong, "Physiology of Elite Young Female Athletes," *Medicine and Sport Science* 56 (2011): 23–46.
3. A. Z. Hoch and others, "Association between the Female Athlete Triad and Endothelial Dysfunction in Dancers," *Clinical Journal of Sport Medicine* 21, no. 2 (2011): 119–25.

chapterin**review**

videos

Log on to **www.pearsonhighered.com/hopson** or MyFitnessLab to view these chapter-related videos.

Measuring Hip-to-Waist Ratio   Skinfold Measurement   Normal Weight Obesity

onlineresources

Log on to **www.pearsonhighered.com/hopson** or MyFitnessLab for access to these book-related resources, and for links to other useful websites.

 Audio case study
Audio PowerPoint lecture

 Take Charge of Your Health! Worksheets
Behavior Change Log Book and Wellness Journal

 Lab 6.1 How to Calculate Your BMI
Lab 6.2 How to Measure and Evaluate Your Body Circumferences
Lab 6.3 Estimate Your Percent Body Fat (Skinfold Test)

 Pre- and post-quizzes
Glossary flashcards

reviewquestions

1. The proportion of your total weight that is fat is called
   a. body composition.
   b. lean mass.
   c. percent body fat.
   d. BMI.
2. Women have a greater amount of *essential fat* due to
   a. larger calves and thighs.
   b. their eating habits.
   c. less physical activity.
   d. reproduction-related fat deposits.

3. Which of the following statements about BMI is true?
   a. Your BMI is an estimate of your body fat percentage.
   b. BMI differentiates between lean mass and fat mass.
   c. Very low and very high BMI scores are associated with greater risk of mortality.
   d. BMI stands for "Basic Measure Indices."

4. Which of the following BMI ratings is considered "overweight"?
   a. 20   b. 25   c. 30   d. 35

5. Which of the following circumference measures indicates an increased risk of disease?
   a. A waist circumference over 100 cm for men and over 80 cm for women
   b. A waist circumference over 102 cm for men and over 88 cm for women
   c. A waist-to-hip ratio of 0.50 or higher
   d. A waist-to-hip ratio of 0.75 or higher

6. Which of the following body shapes or body fat distribution patterns is associated with an increased risk of heart disease and diabetes?
   a. Bell-shaped
   b. Android pattern obesity
   c. Pear-shaped
   d. Gynoid pattern obesity

7. Skinfold measurements are used to assess the amount of
   a. subcutaneous fat.
   b. visceral fat.
   c. essential fat.
   d. intramuscular fat.

8. Which of the following body composition measurement methods uses air displacement to estimate total body volume, density, and percent body fat?
   a. Bioelectrical impedance analysis
   b. Hydrostatic weighing
   c. The Bod Pod
   d. Skinfold measurement

9. Which body composition measurement method relies heavily on body water or hydration levels being normal (not too low or too high)?
   a. Bioelectrical impedance analysis
   b. Hydrostatic weighing
   c. The Bod Pod
   d. Skinfold measurement

10. The female athlete triad consists of the following interrelated issues:
   a. disordered eating, low bone density, and menstrual dysfunction.
   b. weak eyesight, poor nutrition, and brittle bones.
   c. low body weight, poor nutrition, and diabetes.
   d. excessive exercise, high blood pressure, and menstrual issues.

critical**thinking**questions  REVIEW IT! ONLINE

1. Explain the usefulness and limitations of using BMI to determine fitness goals.

2. What factors should you consider when determining a healthy percent body fat range for yourself?

references

1. C. Ogden and M. Carroll, National Center for Health Statistics, Health E-Stats: "Prevalence of Obesity Among Children and Adolescents: United States, Trends 1963–1965 Through 2007–2008." www.cdc.gov, June 2010.
2. J. J. Reilly and J. Kelly, "Long-term Impact of Overweight and Obesity in Childhood and Adolescence on Morbidity and Premature Mortality in Adulthood: Systematic Review." *International Journal of Obesity (London)*. 35, no. 7 (2011): 891–8.
3. J. L. Baker, L. W. Olsen, and T. I. Sorensen, "Childhood Body-Mass Index and the Risk of Coronary Heart Disease in Adulthood," *New England Journal of Medicine* 357, no. 23 (2007): 2329–37.
4. K. M. Flegal and others, "Prevalence and Trends in Obesity Among US Adults, 1999–2008," *Journal of the American Medical Association* 303, no. 3 (2010): 235–41.
5. National Heart, Lung, and Blood Institute—Expert Panel on the Identification, Evaluation, and Treatment of Overweight in Adults, "Clinical Guidelines on the Identification,

Evaluation, and Treatment of Overweight and Obesity in Adults: Executive Summary," *American Journal of Clinical Nutrition* 68, no. 4 (1998): 899–917.
6. Ibid.
7. V. H. Heyward, *Advanced Fitness Assessment and Exercise Prescription.* 6th ed. (Champaign, IL: Human Kinetics, 2010).
8. J. P. Reis and others, "The Relation of Leptin and Insulin with Obesity-Related Cardiovascular Risk Factors in U.S. Adults," *Atherosclerosis* 200, no. 1 (2008): 150–60.
9. A. Bosy-Westphal and others, "Measurement Site for Waist Circumference Affects Its Accuracy as an Index of Visceral and Abdominal Subcutaneous Fat in a Caucasian Population." *The Journal of Nutrition* 140, no. 5 (2010): 954–61.
10. C. S. Fox and others, "Abdominal Visceral and Subcutaneous Adipose Tissue Compartments: Association with Metabolic Risk Factors in the Framingham Heart Study." *Circulation* 116, no. 1 (2007): 39–48.
11. G. Fisher and others, "Effect of Diet with and without Exercise Training on Mark-

ers of Inflammation and Fat Distribution in Overweight Women." *Obesity (Silver Spring)* 19, no. 6 (2011): 1131–6.
12. B. H. Goodpaster and others, "Effects of Diet and Physical Activity Interventions on Weight Loss and Cardiometabolic Risk Factors in Severely Obese Adults: A Randomized Trial." *JAMA* 304, no. 16 (2010): 1795–802.
13. V. H. Heyward, *Advanced Fitness Assessment and Exercise Prescription* (2010).
14. A. S. Jackson and others, "Cross-validation of Generalised Body Composition Equations with Diverse Young Men and Women: The Training Intervention and Genetics of Exercise Response (TIGER) Study." *British Journal of Nutrition* 101, no. 6 (2009): 871–8.
15. D. A. Fields, M. I. Goran, and M. A. McCrory, "Body-composition Assessment via Air-displacement Plethysmography in Adults and Children: A Review." *American Journal of Clinical Nutrition* 75, no. 3 (2002): 453–67.
16. V. H. Heyward, *Advanced Fitness Assessment and Exercise Prescription* (2010).

LAB 6.1 • HOW TO CALCULATE YOUR BMI

Name: _____ **Date:** _____

Instructor: _____ **Section:** _____

Purpose: To learn how to calculate your BMI.

Materials: Weight scale, measuring tape, calculator

SECTION I: CALCULATE YOUR BMI

1. Record your weight and height below:

Weight _____ lb   Height _____ inches

2. Convert your weight and height to metric units:

Weight _____ lb ÷ 2.2 = _____ kg

Height _____ inches × 2.54 = _____ cm ÷ 100 = _____ meters (m)

3. Calculate your BMI:

BMI = _____ ÷ [_____ × _____]
       (weight in kg)   (height in m)   (height in m)

BMI = _____ kg/m²

Note: Square the height (multiply by itself) before dividing into weight.

4. Indicate your BMI rating in the table below:

Weight Classification	BMI (kg/m2)
Underweight	_____ <18.5
Normal Weight	_____ 18.5–24.9
Overweight	_____ 25.0–29.9
Obese—I	_____ 30.0–34.9
Obese—II	_____ 35.0–39.9
Obese—III	_____ >40.0

SECTION II: REFLECTION

1. Is your BMI category what you thought it would be?

_____

2. Remember that BMI categories can be misleading for individuals with above-average muscle mass. Do you

fall into this category? _____

3. Monitoring changes to your BMI over time is one way to assess your progress with a fitness program. Two
months after you begin a new exercise program, recalculate your BMI. Has it changed?

_____

LAB 6.2 • MEASURE AND EVALUATE YOUR BODY CIRCUMFERENCES

Name: _____ **Date:** _____

Instructor: _____ **Section:** _____

Purpose: To learn how to measure your body circumferences.

Materials: Measuring tape, partner

SECTION I: MEASURING CIRCUMFERENCES

Using a cloth or plastic tape measure, have a partner assist you with the following circumference measures. Be sure to mark your measurements (centimeters or inches) and record them to the nearest 0.5 cm or 0.25 inch.

Site	Description		Measurement
Waist	For those with a visible waist, measure at the narrowest part of the torso; for those with a larger torso, measure at the navel.		
Hip	Measure with the legs slightly apart. Measure where the hip/buttock circumference is the greatest.		
Upper Arm	Measure midway between the shoulder and elbow.		Right: Left:
Forearm	Measure at the greatest circumference between the wrist and elbow.		Right: Left:
Thigh	Measure with your leg on a bench or chair (knee at 90 degrees). Measure half way between the crease in your hip and your knee.		Right: Left:
Calf	Measure at the greatest circumference between the knee and ankle.		Right: Left:
Neck	Measure midway between the head and shoulders.		

Source: Adapted from American College of Sports Medicine, *ACSM's Guidelines for Exercise Testing and Prescription.* 8th Ed. (Baltimore, MD: Lippincott Williams & Wilkins, 2010).

SECTION II: EVALUATING CIRCUMFERENCES AND DISEASE RISK

1. Calculate your waist-to-hip ratio (WHR):

WHR = _____ ÷ _____

(waist circumference) (hip circumference)

WHR = _____

2. Evaluate your WHR using the table below:

Disease Risk and WHR				
Age (years)	Low	Moderate	High	Very High
Men: 20–29	<0.83	0.83–0.88	0.89–0.94	>0.94
30–39	<0.84	0.84–0.91	0.92–0.96	>0.96
40–49	<0.88	0.88–0.95	0.96–1.00	>1.00
50–59	<0.90	0.90–0.96	0.97–1.02	>1.02
60–69	<0.91	0.91–0.98	0.99–1.03	>1.03
Women: 20–29	<0.71	0.71–0.77	0.78–0.82	>0.82
30–39	<0.72	0.72–0.78	0.79–0.84	>0.84
40–49	<0.73	0.73–0.79	0.80–0.87	>0.87
50–59	<0.74	0.74–0.81	0.82–0.88	>0.88
60–69	<0.76	0.76–0.83	0.84–0.90	>0.90

Source: Reprinted with permission from V. H. Heywood, 2010, ADVANCED FITNESS ASSESSMENT AND EXERCISE PRESCRIPTION, 6th Edition. (Champaign: IL: Human Kinetics), 222.

Evaluate your waist circumference using the table below:

Waist Circumference (WC)		
Disease Risk Category	Women	Men
Very Low	<70 cm (<28.5 in)	<80 cm (<31.5 in)
Low	70–89 cm (28.5–35.0 in)	80–99 cm (31.5–39.0 in)
High	90–109 cm (35.5–43.0 in)	100–120 cm (39.5–47.0 in)
Very High	>110 cm (>43.5 in)	>120 cm (>47.0 in)

Source: From "Don't Throw the Baby Out with the Bath Water," George A. Bray, American Journal of Clinical Nutrition, 2004, Vol. 70, No. 3, pp. 347–349, by permission of the American Society for Nutrition.

3. Record your disease risk from WHR and waist circumference below:

Disease rating for WHR: _____

Disease rating for WC: _____

SECTION III: REFLECTION

1. Do your ratings for disease risk based upon circumferences surprise you? _____

2. Which of your circumference measures are you most interested in changing and why?

_____

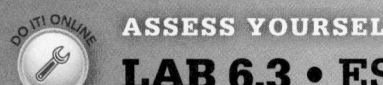
LAB 6.3 • ESTIMATE YOUR PERCENT BODY FAT (SKINFOLD TEST)

Name: _____ Date: _____

Instructor: _____ Section: _____

Materials: Skinfold calipers, appropriate clothing (shorts, tank top, sports bra for women)

Purpose: To assess your current percent body fat.

Directions: Complete the sections below with a trained instructor.

SECTION I: SKINFOLD MEASUREMENT

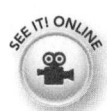

You will need an experienced, trained instructor to complete your measurements. Note the time of day of your measurements and perform any follow-up measurements at the same time of day.

1. Identify the correct skinfold locations. If you are male, locate the chest, abdomen, and thigh locations (see photos below). If you are female, locate the triceps, suprailiac, and thigh locations (see photos). Your instructor should mark these locations on the right side of the body with a pen before using the caliper.

Chest	A diagonal fold measured midway between the shoulder/armpit crease and the nipple.	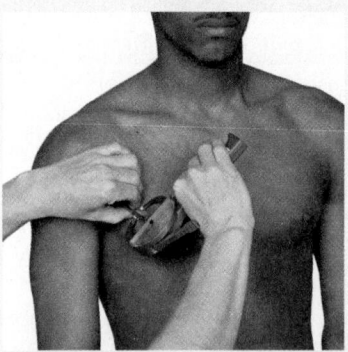
Abdomen	A vertical fold measured one inch to the right of the navel.	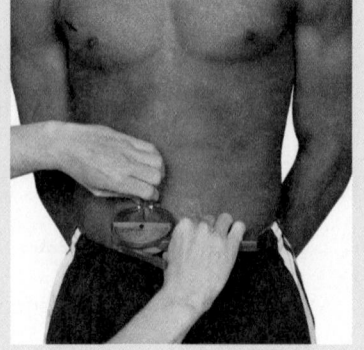

Thigh	A vertical fold measured midway between the crease in your hip and the top of your knee.	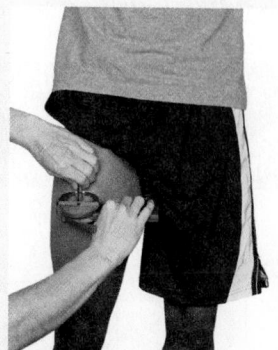
Triceps	A vertical fold on the back of the upper arm midway between the shoulder and elbow.	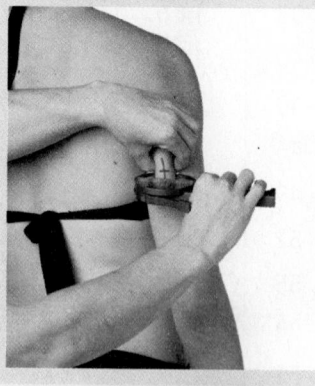
Suprailiac	A diagonal fold just above the hip bone, on the side of the body at the front edge of your relaxed arm.	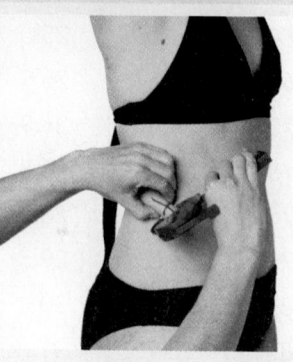

Source: Adapted from American College of Sports Medicine, *ACSM's Guidelines for Exercise Testing and Prescription.* 8th ed. (Baltimore, MD: Lippincott Williams & Wilkins, 2010).

2. Your instructor will measure each skinfold location using the technique below. Record the results below and then add up the numbers for the three skinfold sites to obtain your overall skinfold sum.

Skinfold measurement technique: After locating the correct sites, grab a double fold of skin on both sides of the skinfold location. Open your fingers about three inches when lifting the fold (> than three inches is required for larger individuals). Holding the fold in place, pick up the calipers with your other hand. While still holding the fold, place the caliper jaws on the skinfold location, measuring halfway between the crest and the base of the fold. You should measure perpendicular to the fold and about one cm away from your fingers. Read the measurement two to three seconds after placing the calipers and record the skinfold numbers to the nearest 0.5 mm. For accuracy, measure each site three times and average the two closest numbers.

MEN		WOMEN	
Chest	_____ mm	Triceps	_____ mm
Abdomen	_____ mm	Suprailiac	_____ mm
Thigh	_____ mm	Thigh	_____ mm
Sum of 3 =	_____ mm	Sum of 3 =	_____ mm

3. Using the sum of three skinfolds, find your estimated percent body fat in the tables for women and men.

Sum of Skinfolds (mm)	Percent Body Fat Estimates for WOMEN (from triceps, suprailiac, and thigh skinfolds) AGE (years)								
	Under 22	23–27	28–32	33–37	38–42	43–47	48–52	53–57	Over 57
23–25	9.7	9.9	10.2	10.4	10.7	10.9	11.2	11.4	11.7
26–28	11.0	11.2	11.5	11.7	12.0	12.3	12.5	12.7	13.0
29–31	12.3	12.5	12.8	13.0	13.3	13.5	13.8	14.0	14.3
32–34	13.6	13.8	14.0	14.3	14.5	14.8	15.0	15.3	15.5
35–37	14.8	15.0	15.3	15.5	15.8	16.0	16.3	16.5	16.8
38–40	16.0	16.3	16.5	16.7	17.0	17.2	17.5	17.7	18.0
41–43	17.2	17.4	17.7	17.9	18.2	18.4	18.7	18.9	19.2
44–46	18.3	18.6	18.8	19.1	19.3	19.6	19.8	20.1	20.3
47–49	19.5	19.7	20.0	20.2	20.5	20.7	21.0	21.2	21.5
50–52	20.6	20.8	21.1	21.3	21.6	21.8	22.1	22.3	22.6
53–55	21.7	21.9	22.1	22.4	22.6	22.9	23.1	23.4	23.6
56–58	22.7	23.0	23.2	23.4	23.7	23.9	24.2	24.4	24.7
59–61	23.7	24.0	24.2	24.5	24.7	25.0	25.2	25.5	25.7
62–64	24.7	25.0	25.2	25.5	25.7	26.0	26.2	26.4	26.7
65–67	25.7	25.9	26.2	26.4	26.7	26.9	27.2	27.4	27.7
68–70	26.6	26.9	27.1	27.4	27.6	27.9	28.1	28.4	28.6
71–73	27.5	27.8	28.0	28.3	28.5	28.8	29.0	29.3	29.5
74–76	28.4	28.7	28.9	29.2	29.4	29.7	29.9	30.2	30.4
77–79	29.3	29.5	29.8	30.0	30.3	30.5	30.8	31.0	31.3
80–82	30.1	30.4	30.6	30.9	31.1	31.4	31.6	31.9	32.1
83–85	30.9	31.2	31.4	31.7	31.9	32.2	32.4	32.7	32.9
86–88	31.7	32.0	32.2	32.5	32.7	32.9	33.2	33.4	33.7
89–91	32.5	32.7	33.0	33.2	33.5	33.7	33.9	34.2	34.4
92–94	33.2	33.4	33.7	33.9	34.2	34.4	34.7	34.9	35.2
95–97	33.9	34.1	34.4	34.6	34.9	35.1	35.4	35.6	35.9
98–100	34.6	34.8	35.1	35.3	35.5	35.8	36.0	36.3	36.5
101–103	35.3	35.4	35.7	35.9	36.2	36.4	36.7	36.9	37.2
104–106	35.8	36.1	36.3	36.6	36.8	37.1	37.3	37.5	37.8
107–109	36.4	36.7	36.9	37.1	37.4	37.6	37.9	38.1	38.4
110–112	37.0	37.2	37.5	37.7	38.0	38.2	38.5	38.7	38.9
113–115	37.5	37.8	38.0	38.2	38.5	38.7	39.0	39.2	39.5
116–118	38.0	38.3	38.5	38.8	39.0	39.3	39.5	39.7	40.0
119–121	38.5	38.7	39.0	39.2	39.5	39.7	40.0	40.2	40.5
122–124	39.0	39.2	39.4	39.7	39.9	40.2	40.4	40.7	40.9
125–127	39.4	39.6	39.9	40.1	40.4	40.6	40.9	41.1	41.4
128–130	39.8	40.0	40.3	40.5	40.8	41.0	41.3	41.5	41.8

Source: A. S. Jackson and M. L. Pollock, "Practical Assessment of Body Composition," *The Physician and Sportsmedicine* 13, no. 5 (1985): 76–90. Copyright © 1985 JTE Multimedia, LLC. Used with permission.

Sum of Skinfolds (mm)	Percent Body Fat Estimates for MEN (from chest, abdomen, and thigh skinfolds)								
	AGE (years)								
	Under 22	23–27	28–32	33–37	38–42	43–47	48–52	53–57	Over 57
8–10	1.3	1.8	2.3	2.9	3.4	3.9	4.5	5.0	5.5
11–13	2.2	2.8	3.3	3.9	4.4	4.9	5.5	6.0	6.5
14–16	3.2	3.8	4.3	4.8	5.4	5.9	6.4	7.0	7.5
17–19	4.2	4.7	5.3	5.8	6.3	6.9	7.4	8.0	8.5
20–22	5.1	5.7	6.2	6.8	7.3	7.9	8.4	8.9	9.5
23–25	6.1	6.6	7.2	7.7	8.3	8.8	9.4	9.9	10.5
26–28	7.0	7.6	8.1	8.7	9.2	9.8	10.3	10.9	11.4
29–31	8.0	8.5	9.1	9.6	10.2	10.7	11.3	11.8	12.4
32–34	8.9	9.4	10.0	10.5	11.1	11.6	12.2	12.8	13.3
35–37	9.8	10.4	10.9	11.5	12.0	12.6	13.1	13.7	14.3
38–40	10.7	11.3	11.8	12.4	12.9	13.5	14.1	14.6	15.2
41–43	11.6	12.2	12.7	13.3	13.8	14.4	15.0	15.5	16.1
44–46	12.5	13.1	13.6	14.2	14.7	15.3	15.9	16.4	17.0
47–49	13.4	13.9	14.5	15.1	15.6	16.2	16.8	17.3	17.9
50–52	14.3	14.8	15.4	15.9	16.5	17.1	17.6	18.2	18.8
53–55	15.1	15.7	16.2	16.8	17.4	17.9	18.5	19.1	19.7
56–58	16.0	16.5	17.1	17.7	18.2	18.8	19.4	20.0	20.5
59–61	16.9	17.4	17.9	18.5	19.1	19.7	20.2	20.8	21.4
62–64	17.6	18.2	18.8	19.4	19.9	20.5	21.1	21.7	22.2
65–67	18.5	19.0	19.6	20.2	20.8	21.3	21.9	22.5	23.1
68–70	19.3	19.9	20.4	21.0	21.6	22.2	22.7	23.3	23.9
71–73	20.1	20.7	21.2	21.8	22.4	23.0	23.6	24.1	24.7
74–76	20.9	21.5	22.0	22.6	23.2	23.8	24.4	25.0	25.5
77–79	21.7	22.2	22.8	23.4	24.0	24.6	25.2	25.8	26.3
80–82	22.4	23.0	23.6	24.2	24.8	25.4	25.9	26.5	27.1
83–85	23.2	23.8	24.4	25.0	25.5	26.1	26.7	27.3	27.9
86–88	24.0	24.5	25.1	25.7	26.3	26.9	27.5	28.1	28.7
89–91	24.7	25.3	25.9	26.5	27.1	27.6	28.2	28.8	29.4
92–94	25.4	26.0	26.6	27.2	27.8	28.4	29.0	29.6	30.2
95–97	26.1	26.7	27.3	27.9	28.5	29.1	29.7	30.3	30.9
98–100	26.9	27.4	28.0	28.6	29.2	29.8	30.4	31.0	31.6
101–103	27.5	28.1	28.7	29.3	29.9	30.5	31.1	31.7	32.3
104–106	28.2	28.8	29.4	30.0	30.6	31.2	31.8	32.4	33.0
107–109	28.9	29.5	30.1	30.7	31.3	31.9	32.5	33.1	33.7
110–112	29.6	30.2	30.8	31.4	32.0	32.6	33.2	33.8	34.4
113–115	30.2	30.8	31.4	32.0	32.6	33.2	33.8	34.5	35.1
116–118	30.9	31.5	32.1	32.7	33.3	33.9	34.5	35.1	35.7
119–121	31.5	32.1	32.7	33.3	33.9	34.5	35.1	35.7	36.4
122–124	32.1	32.7	33.3	33.9	34.5	35.1	35.8	36.4	37.0
125–127	32.7	33.3	33.9	34.5	35.1	35.8	36.4	37.0	37.6

Source: A. S. Jackson and M. L. Pollock, "Practical Assessment of Body Composition," *The Physician and Sportsmedicine* 13, no. 5 (1985): 76–90. Copyright © 1985 JTE Multimedia, LLC. Used with permission.

4. Record your estimated percent body fat and rating.

% body fat = _____

Indicate your body fat rating below:

Body Fat Rating	WOMEN	MEN
Athletic/Low	14–20%	6–13%
Fitness	21–24%	14–17%
Acceptable	25–31%	18–25%
Obese	>32%	>26%

Source: From "Percent Body Fat Norms for Men and Women" in ACE LIFESTYLE AND WEIGHT MANAGEMENT COACH MANUAL. Reprinted with permission from the American Council on Exercise® (ACE®), www.acefitness.org.

SECTION II: REFLECTION

1. Did your estimated percent body fat or rating surprise you? _____

2. How does your percent body fat rating compare with your other disease risk ratings from Lab 6.2?

_____

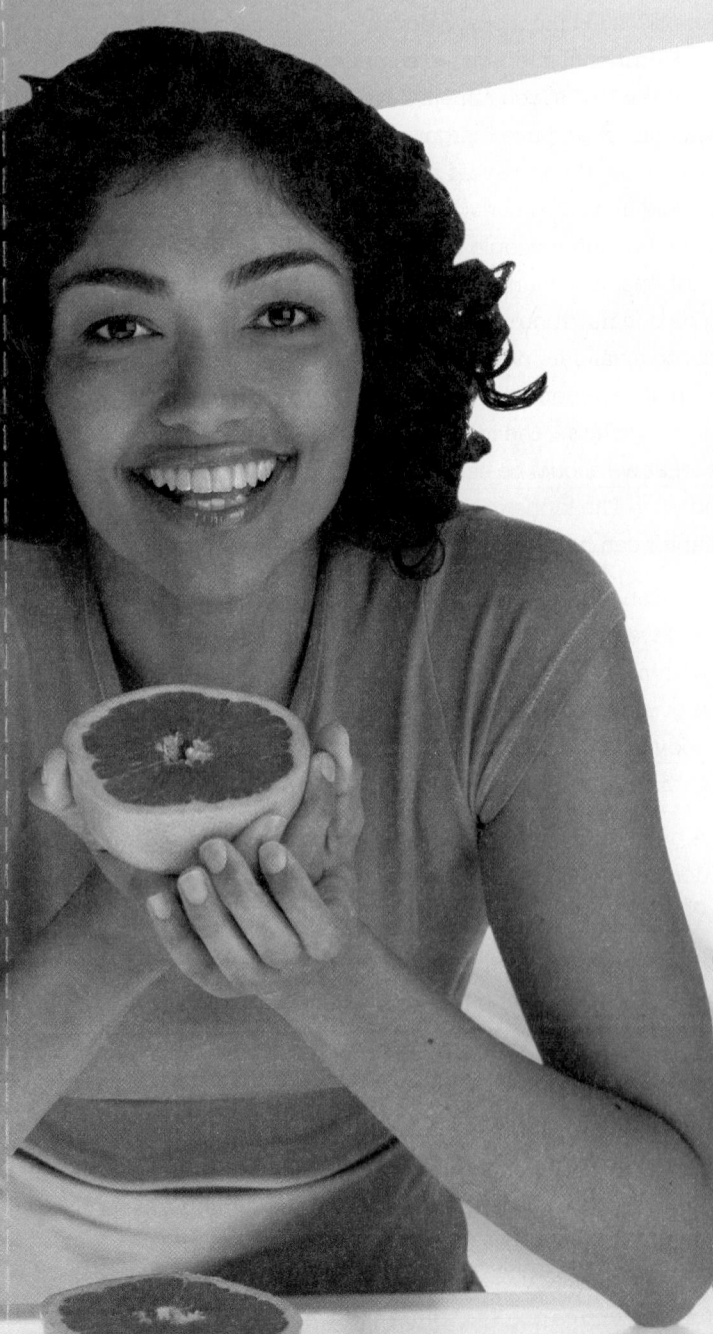

7

Improving Your Nutrition

Learning Outcomes

1. Describe ways to maintain a healthy diet during the college years and throughout your lifetime.

 HEAR IT! ONLINE

 Audio case study and audio Power-Point lecture

2. Identify the main nutrients in food and their roles in the body.

 SEE IT! ONLINE

 How Much Sugar?

3. Discuss the role of portion size, food labels, food groups, and whole foods in maintaining a balanced diet.

 DO IT! ONLINE

Lab 7.1 Reading a Food Label

 SEE IT! ONLINE

 Going Green

4. Describe the special dietary needs of elite athletes, women, children, adults over 50, and vegetarians.

5. Examine your own specific nutritional needs.

6. Assess your current diet.

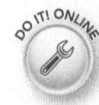 DO IT! ONLINE

Lab 7.2 Keeping a Food Diary and Analyzing Your Daily Nutrition

7. Create a plan for improved nutrition.

 DO IT! ONLINE

Lab 7.3 Improving Your Nutrition

 LIVE IT! ONLINE

Take Charge of Your Health! worksheets and Behavior Change Logs for logging eating habits and creating a change plan

 SEE IT! ONLINE

 You Are What You Eat?

Pre- and post-quizzes and glossary flashcards

 REVIEW IT! ONLINE

casestudy

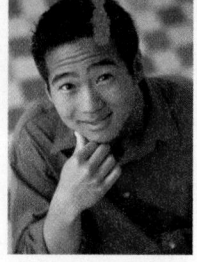

CHAU

"Hi, I'm Chau. I'm a freshman and I live on campus in a dorm with my roommate, Tom. I moved here to Connecticut from Chicago. Living away from home for the first time has been quite an experience! I've been studying hard, taking a full load of classes, and trying to figure out if I want to major in history or political science. Plus, I'm in a few clubs and I'm playing a lot of soccer. I'm not on the team, but I like to play for fun. I'll jump into just about any pick-up game if I have time. I'm always rushing, though, and then I realize I'm starving! When I lived at home, there was always food around. My meal plan at the cafeteria covers 60 meals a month. For the others, I'm often scrambling at the last minute to find something to eat."

HEAR IT! ONLINE

H unger is one of our basic motivators. Eating—seeing, smelling, and tasting foods—is one of life's great pleasures. Hunger compels us to seek and consume the food that will supply our bodies with energy and raw materials. The pleasure of eating compels us to find the foods we enjoy or even crave. Our challenge is to eat a healthy balance of foods we need and foods we want to eat.

Food contains **nutrients**, chemical compounds that supply the energy and raw materials for survival. Our cells break down food molecules and, in the process, change their shapes and release energy stored in their chemical bonds. The energy becomes available to drive the activities within our cells, tissues, and organs. The breakdown of nutrients also liberates raw materials that cells can take in, modify, and use in repair and growth.

Nutrition is the study of how people consume and use the nutrients in food. Nutrition researchers explore some of the basic questions about what we should be eating and how food affects our long-term health and disease. Is it better to eat butter or margarine? Should you drink tea, coffee, both, or neither? Should you take a daily vitamin pill? Is red meat okay? How much salt is too much?

Nutritional findings are sometimes contradictory. Since the 1970s, consumers have been advised to throw away butter and use margarine instead; then to do just the reverse; then to avoid almost all fats; then to avoid almost all carbohydrates, and so on. Understandably, some people have grown skeptical about nutritional information. As in every area of science, new studies in nutrition occasionally contain data that appear to invalidate older studies. Nevertheless, the field has made tremendous advances toward understanding our daily **diets**—the foods and drinks we select—as well as what we *should* be eating, what we should be *avoiding*, and why. The kinds of healthy diets we discuss in this chapter can help you stay fit and well. Keep in mind:

- A balanced diet helps sustain desirable body mass and weight and helps keep your fat-to-lean ratios within a recommended range. This, in turn, can improve appearance, make you more comfortable in your body, and reduce the risk of chronic illnesses related to excess weight and obesity.

- A good diet can help alleviate feelings of stress and depression, while a poor diet can contribute to them.

- A good diet can help prevent chronic diseases, frequent colds and infections, and the effects of vitamin deficiency. Conversely, poor diet is one of the biggest contributors to cardiovascular disease, diabetes, obesity, arthritis, osteoporosis, and several types of cancers.

If you are young and currently well, any of the above conditions may seem improbable and remote. However, the dietary habits you establish now either diminish or promote your later risk for all types of chronic illness. Optimal fitness and wellness—both now and in your future—requires good nutrition and good **eating habits**. This chapter shows you how to analyze and improve both.

nutrients Chemical compounds in food that are crucial to growth and function; include proteins, carbohydrates (starches and sugars), lipids (fats and oils), vitamins, and minerals

nutrition The study of how people consume and use the nutrients in food

diets The foods and drinks we select to consume

eating habits When, where, and how we eat; with whom we eat; what we choose to consume; and our reasons for choosing it

Why Are My College Years a Nutritional Challenge?

If you are like most college students, you often reach for cheap snacks and fast food to save time and money. You grab something tasty. You eat it quickly, maybe even while you walk or drive to the next class, job, study session, or social event. You may worry about calories and weight. But most students don't think much about vitamins, minerals, and other nutrients or worry much about the challenge of eating well during the college years.

The typical student's diet resembles the typical American diet: nearly one-third of Americans' total calories come from chips, cookies, donuts, desserts, French fries, candy bars, sugary drinks, beer, wine, and other alcoholic beverages.[1] The number-one takeout food is pizza, followed by Chinese food and fast food (burgers, fries, and so on). Other favorite "staples" of the American diet are coffee drinks, tacos, burritos, sandwiches, and salads. The most frequently eaten vegetables in America are iceberg lettuce and potatoes.[2]

Most Students Have Less-than-Optimal Eating Habits

Eating habits describe when, where, and how we eat; with whom we eat; what we choose to consume; and our reasons for choosing it. Like most Americans, college students, in general, have poor eating habits. Examples of poor eating habits are eating fast food and eating while driving or watching television. Good eating habits include sitting down to a relaxed meal and consuming fresh fruits and vegetables every day. How are your eating habits? Figure 7.1 can help you find out.

Less healthy eating habits	More healthy eating habits
Consuming sugary soft drinks with and between meals	Drinking water with and between meals
Skipping meals then gorging once or twice per day	Eating three meals plus one or two small, nutritious snacks at regular times
Eating large amounts of red meats, fatty meats, or fried meats	Choosing fish, lean poultry, tofu, or other proteins that are low in saturated fats
Choosing processed foods	Choosing whole foods such as fruits, vegetables, whole grains, nuts, seeds, and lean sources of protein
Hurriedly bolting down food on the run, in a car, on a bike	Sitting down to eat a relaxed meal with friends or family
Finishing the large portions served at restaurants	Eating half of a large restaurant portion and taking the rest home
Snacking before bed	Eating earlier in the evening
Eating heartily to be social, regardless of appetite	If you're not very hungry, drinking a low-cal beverage or eating a piece of fruit to be social
Eating out of habit or boredom, for example, while watching TV	Sitting down at a table to eat only when hungry, finding another outlet for boredom
Reaching for food when feeling stressed or angry	Learning stress reduction techniques

FIGURE **7.1** You can examine your own eating and snacking habits by comparing what, when, where, and how much you eat and drink to the sliding scale for each habit. You can also get ideas here for improving your daily diet.

Adapted from U.S. Department of Agriculture and U.S. Department of Health and Human Services, *Dietary Guidelines for Americans, 2010,* 7th Edition, "Chapter 5: Building Healthy Eating Patterns" (Washington, DC: U.S. Government Printing Office, 2010): 43–54.

Results of the American College Health Association's 2010 annual survey of nearly 96,000 students from colleges and universities throughout the United States highlighted the dietary deficiencies of today's students.[3] Taking produce as an example, only about 6 percent consumed the recommended five servings of fruits and vegetables each day. Fifty-eight percent reported eating only one to two servings each day, and 30 percent consumed three to four servings. Like their older counterparts, young adults report that they are interested in improving their health, yet they fall far short of the mark in meeting national dietary guidelines. It is no wonder that the term "Freshman 15" has become common language among students to describe the excess weight gain they often experience freshman year.

Good information and understanding can make a measurable difference in students' nutritional wellness, including the amount of weight they gain. The information throughout this book, especially in this chapter and in our discussion of weight management, can help you in the same ways.

THINK! How many servings of fruits and vegetables do you eat per day? One? Two? Five or more?

ACT! If you eat fewer than five servings a day, what specific things can you do to increase that number?

College Life Presents Obstacles to Good Nutrition

Food is easy to find in the many vending machines, cafeterias, bars, restaurants, and markets on campus and off. But nutritious foods—low in saturated fat, salt, and sugars, for instance, and high in fiber and vitamin content—are much harder to find on and near campus. Food choice is an important obstacle to student nutrition. There are other obstacles as well: time and money pressures, lack of home-cooking facilities, personal habits and attitudes, and the emotional stresses college can present.

Fast food and takeout appear to solve both time and money issues, but the food at these restaurants often provides poor nutrition. Even when students cook for themselves, however, nutritional misconceptions and a tight budget can still impede a good diet. If you do shop and cook, a few simple steps can help you achieve a healthy affordable diet: Buy fruits and vegetables that are in season. Watch for sales, use coupons, and shop at discount stores. Make a shopping list and stick to it. Buy

more plant proteins (e.g., beans and tofu) and less meat, fish, or poultry. And if possible, double your recipes and freeze portions for later.

Another obstacle to good nutrition is our natural human craving for sweet, fatty, salty, and high-protein foods. We love those treats! Students sometimes come to college with preexisting preferences and eating habits and then, away from parental influence for the first time, tip over into unhealthy dietary routines such as regularly eating junk food, skipping breakfast, snacking frequently, and limiting fruit and vegetable consumption.

Meal skipping or protein loading can also be an offshoot of body dissatisfaction at a time when social interaction and physical attractiveness are emphasized. Three-fifths of female college students and half of males are dissatisfied with their body size and

casestudy

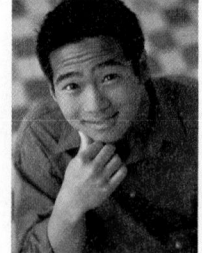

CHAU

"I like eating in the dorm cafeteria but I have to take care of about 30 meals on my own each month. The idea was that I'd eat two meals a day in the dorm—probably breakfast and dinner—and grab lunch somewhere between classes. So far, though, it's not quite working out that way. On days when I don't have an early class, I tend to sleep through breakfast. Then, I've got to rush to my 11:00, which means grabbing donuts and coffee in the campus store. Sometimes I manage to get back to the dorm for lunch, but if I don't, I usually eat something on the run at the food court. The good thing is that my dorm has a late night café that accepts my meal plan. So if I'm up late studying, I can grab a pizza or bowl of cereal. I don't pay much attention to my diet or how many calories I'm eating. I figure at my age, it's more about getting enough calories then eating a 'balanced meal.' Doesn't it all kind of balance out naturally?"

THINK! What aspects of college life are influencing Chau's dietary choices? How does your own living situation and schedule affect your efforts to eat right?

ACT! Make a list of small lifestyle changes you could make to improve your diet and try to incorporate at least one in the coming week, another the following week.

Tips for Ordering at Restaurants

No matter what type of cuisine you enjoy, there will always be healthier and less healthy options on the menu. To help you order wisely, here are lighter options and high-fat pitfalls. "Best" choices contain fewer than 30 grams of fat, a generous meal's worth for an active, medium-sized woman. "Worst" choices have up to 100 grams of fat.

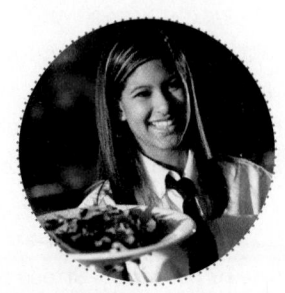

Cuisine	Best	Worst	Tips
Italian	Pasta with red or white clam sauce Spaghetti with marinara or tomato- and meat sauce	Eggplant parmigiana Fettucine Alfredo Fried calamari Lasagna	Stick with plain bread instead of garlic bread made with butter or oil. Avoid cream- or egg-based sauces. Try vegetarian pizza, and don't ask for extra cheese.
Mexican	Bean burrito (no cheese) Chicken fajitas with lots of vegetables	Beef chimichanga, deep fried Chile relleno, battered and fried	Choose soft tortillas (not fried) with fresh salsa, not guacamole. Order grilled shrimp, fish, or chicken. Ask for black or pinto beans made without lard or fat. Avoid cheeses and sour cream or ask for them on the side.
Chinese	Hot- and-sour soup Stir-fried vegetables Shrimp with garlic sauce Szechuan shrimp Wonton soup	Crispy chicken Kung pao chicken Moo shu pork Sweet-and-sour pork	Share a stir-fry. Request brown rice instead of white. Ask for vegetables steamed or stir-fried with less oil. Avoid fried rice, breaded dishes, egg rolls and spring rolls, and items loaded with peanuts or cashews. Avoid high-sodium sauces.
Japanese	Steamed rice and vegetables Tofu as a meat substitute Broiled or steamed chicken and fish	Fried rice dishes Miso Tempura	Avoid soy sauces. Avoid deep-fried dishes such as tempura. Eat sashimi and sushi (raw fish) only where the food is freshly made to avoid possible bacteria or parasites.
Thai	Clear broth soups Stir-fried chicken and vegetables Grilled meats	Coconut milk soup with chicken Peanut sauces for satay Deep-fried or batter-fried meats and vegetables	Avoid coconut-based soups and curries. Ask for steamed, not fried, rice. Try for brown rice rather than white. Avoid Thai iced tea, which is filled with sugar and high-fat evaporated milk.
American Breakfast	Hot or cold cereal with nonfat or one percent milk Pancakes or French toast with syrup Scrambled eggs with hash browns and plain toast	Belgian waffle with sausage Sausage and eggs with biscuits and gravy Ham-and-cheese omelet with hash browns and toast	Ask for whole-grain cereal or shredded wheat with two percent milk. Ask for whole wheat toast without butter or margarine. Order omelets without cheese. Order fried eggs without bacon or sausage.
Sandwiches	Veggies and tofu spread Roast beef Turkey	Tuna salad Reuben Submarine	Ask for mustard. Hold the mayonnaise and high-fat cheese.
Seafood	Broiled bass, halibut, or snapper Grilled scallops Steamed crab or lobster	Fried seafood platter Blackened catfish	Order fish broiled, baked, grilled, or steamed—not pan fried or sautéed. Ask for lemon instead of tartar sauce. Avoid creamy and buttery sauces.
Fast Food	Grilled chicken sandwich Lean roast beef sandwich Entrée salad, dressing on the side Water, nonfat or one percent milk, unsweetened iced tea Fresh fruit and yogurt	Extra-large or double-patty sandwiches Added cheese French fries and onion rings Fried chicken Fish fillets Chicken nuggets Apple pie Colas	Order sandwiches without mayo or special sauce. Avoid deep-fried items.

· ·

shape.[4] Most students want to lose weight, while a few want to gain weight or add muscle. Body dissatisfaction leads some students to skip meals; avoid particular classes of foods such as fats or carbohydrates; go on drastic very-low-calorie diets; or take other measures that can cause an imbalance of nutrients, vitamins, and minerals.

Stress and social eating are additional contributors to poor diet. Stress itself can cause people to eat more, especially high-calorie "comfort" foods. Stress can also reduce sleep, which can lead to using food, caffeine, sugar, and alcohol to alter mood and energy levels. People under stress also tend to seek out the relief of socializing for relaxation, and when people get together, they eat and drink. The box Tips for Ordering at Restaurants describes healthy and unhealthy food items on a wide variety of menus.

Research shows that when nutritious foods are readily available in a cafeteria setting, many students will choose them. For example, in one study male students chose more fruits and vegetables and leaner meats in dormitory dining halls than did males eating in apartments, in restaurants, and so on.[5] Female students eating in dining halls chose amounts of fruit closer to USDA recommendations. However, although free choice in cafeteria lines does seem to encourage better nutrition for many students, it can still lead to consuming too many calories. There are several keys to overcoming the food obstacles of college life:

- Learn about nutrition and what your body needs to maintain maximum wellness.

- Learn to distinguish good food choices from poor ones and good eating habits from bad ones.

- As often as possible, frequent those restaurants, stores, and cafeterias that offer a wide selection of healthy foods.

- Improve your eating habits and hang out with other students who care about nutritious eating.

What Are the Main Nutrients in Food?

We humans share the need to "refuel" with every other kind of animal, from soaring eagles to drifting sea cucumbers. Our bodies can't originate energy-containing raw materials for activity, growth, and repair. Like all animals, we must obtain these compounds from foods and liquids in sufficient quantities to supply our daily needs. Our required nutrients are water, proteins, carbohydrates (starches and sugars), lipids (fats and oils), vitamins, and minerals (Figure 7.2). Within each class of nutrients, the three-dimensional molecular shapes of the individual kinds of sugars, fats, and so on, determine the

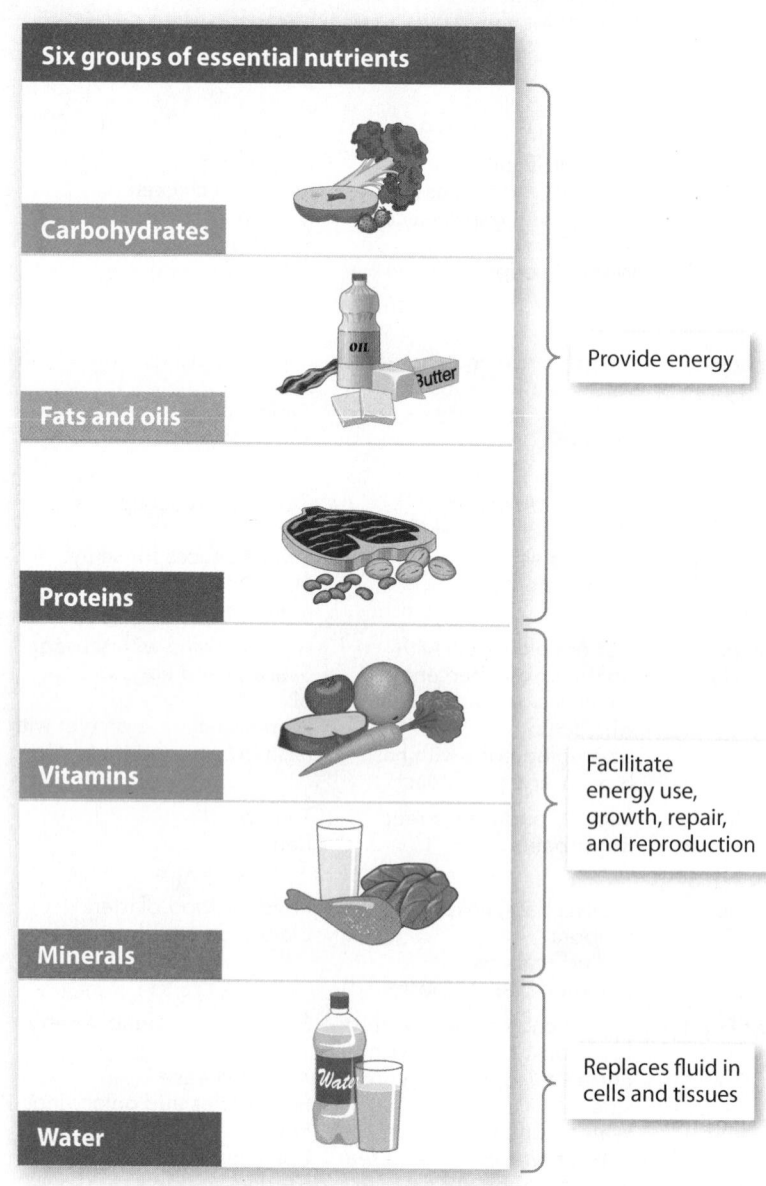

FIGURE **7.2** The six groups of essential nutrients in our foods provide energy, facilitate vital activities, and supply needed fluid for cells and tissues.

nutrients' unique chemical properties and in turn, their roles in the body.

Nutritionists use the term **essential nutrients** for those compounds we must get from foods in order to maintain normal body functioning. Our bodies chemically modify and use nutrients to build the thousands of components we need to allow our muscles to contract, our nerves to conduct, our cells to divide, and so on. Consuming nutrients keeps our internal "production line" efficiently manufacturing cell parts and usable energy compounds.

Nutritionists can measure the nutrients in individual foods—the natural sugars and starches in an apple, for example. They can measure the energy stored within those carbohydrates. And they can study the way our bodies release that stored energy during the digestion process. They measure the released energy in **calories**. One calorie (with a lowercase *c*) is the amount of energy required to raise the temperature of 1 gram of water 1 degree Celsius. When they refer to specific foods, nutritionists usually apply the larger measure **kilocalories (kcal)** or **Calories (C)**. One kilocalorie or Calorie (spelled with a capital *C*) equals 1,000 calories. A small-sized apple, for example, about the size of a tennis ball might have about 50 or 60 C.

To avoid confusion, this book will use "calories" when referring to food energy in general as well as when designating the energy in a specific food. Active adults need about 2,000 to 2,500 calories of food energy per day.

Proteins Are Building Blocks of Structure and Function

About 50 to 60 percent of your body weight is water; of the remainder, about half is protein. At 150 pounds, your body would contain about 75 pounds of water and about 37.5 pounds of protein, depending on your muscle mass. **Proteins** are major structural components of nearly every cell and are especially important to the building and repairing of bone, muscle, skin, and blood cells. Proteins are also critical to cell and body functioning: They make up the antibodies that protect us from disease, the enzymes that control all chemical reactions in the body, and many types of hormones that regulate body activities. Proteins also help transport oxygen, carbon dioxide, and various nutrients to body cells. When the body runs low on fats and carbohydrates as sources of ready energy, it can break down its own proteins as well. Protein supplies four calories of energy per gram.

Protein molecules are chains of subunits called *amino acids*. Sometimes called the "building blocks of life," amino acids contain carbon, hydrogen, oxygen, and nitrogen arrayed in particular ways. There are 20 different kinds of amino acids, each with a different three-dimensional shape. Your body uses the 20 types of amino acids to build tens of thousands of kinds of proteins. Many of these are *structural proteins* that make up parts of cells, tissues, and organs. Many kinds of structural proteins enable cells to move, to divide, and to transport materials around internally. Other structural proteins make up your hair strands, your fingernails and toenails, and the lenses of your eyes. A steady supply of amino acids in the diet allows your body to continuously build, repair, and replace its own structural proteins.

Proteins that perform crucial functions (rather than make up physical structures) are called *functional proteins* and include **enzymes**. Enzymes are proteins that enable thousands of kinds of chemical reactions to occur simultaneously within each body cell every second, including the enzyme reactions that break down food, absorb nutrients, and build new cell parts.

Proteins in the Diet Our bodies can manufacture only 11 of the 20 kinds of amino acids. Nutritionists call the other nine, which we must consume in food, the **essential amino acids**. Dietary protein that supplies all the essential amino acids is called *complete protein*, or *high-quality protein*. Typically, protein from animal products is complete. *Incomplete proteins* lack some of the essential amino acids and therefore some of the building blocks we need to produce the full spectrum of proteins for growth, repair, and activity.

essential nutrients Nutrients necessary for normal body functioning that must be obtained from food

calories A measure of the amount of chemical energy that foods provide. One calorie (lowercase *c*) can raise 1 gram of water 1 degree Celsius.

kilocalories (kcal) or **Calories (C)** A measure of energy equal to one thousand calories; also designated kilocalorie (kcal); nutritionists use kcal or C when they refer to specific foods.

proteins Biological molecules composed of amino acids. Proteins serve as crucial structural and functional compounds in living organisms.

enzymes Proteins that facilitate chemical reactions but are not permanently altered in the process; biological catalysts

essential amino acids Collectively, the nine of the 20 types of amino acids, or building blocks, that our bodies cannot manufacture and that we must consume in our foods

Proteins from plant sources are often incomplete, lacking one or two of the essential amino acids. Nevertheless, it is fairly easy for a vegetarian to combine plant foods to obtain *complementary proteins* from plant sources (Figure 7.3). Eating peanut butter on whole grain bread is one good example of combining plant foods to get all the essential amino acids. Eating corn and beans together is another.

Daily Protein Needs Nutritionists typically recommend that you get about 10 percent of your calories (or about 200 calories or more) from protein in a 2,000-calorie diet. Over a billion of the world's people face daily protein deficiency, but few Americans suffer it. The average American consumes between 60 and 100 grams (250 to 400 calories or more) of protein daily,

with as much as 70 percent of it coming from animal parts and products and dairy products high in saturated fats. Consuming too much protein, particularly animal protein, can place added stress on the liver and kidneys and can cause a painful disease called *gout.* An overload of protein may also increase calcium excretion in urine, which can increase your risk of bone loss and bone fractures.[6]

Use Figure 7.4 to calculate your daily protein needs. Here's an example: A healthy young woman weighing 132 pounds (60 kg) would need about 48 grams (60 × 0.8). One gram is equal to 0.035 ounce; therefore, she would need about 1.68 ounces of protein (0.035 × 48 = 1.68), which she could get, for example, by consuming 1 cup of skim milk, 3 ounces of chicken breast, and 3 ounces of salmon during the course of a day.

In recent years, millions of people have tried the Atkins diet and similar diets that nearly eliminate carbohydrates and prescribe large quantities of protein. While these diets *can* lead to weight loss, the dieter is losing weight due to total calorie reduction, not due to some magical property of dietary protein itself. Diets that are not nutritionally balanced are almost always flawed. People with fluid imbalances, kidney or liver problems, or cardiovascular disease should avoid these diets altogether, as they raise risk factors for various chronic diseases. Others who choose to try such unbalanced diets should limit the length of time they follow them.

Protein and Fitness It is fairly common for athletes and fitness buffs to load up on animal protein under the misguided notion that eating more protein will cause them to build bigger muscles. But muscles grow in response to being worked: you must use them to grow them! The many vegetarian Olympic athletes are proof that training and effort—not mountains of animal protein—are the crucial ingredients. Research has also shown that 1.0 gram/kg of protein is enough for all but the top athletes, most of whom can get all they need for heavy endurance and strength training in 1.5 to 1.6 g/kg/day.[7]

It's true that under some circumstances, you may need extra protein for cellular repair and replacement, such as when you are fighting off a serious infection, or if you are a pregnant woman. Most of us, though, need to be much more concerned with getting *low-fat* proteins than with meeting our daily protein needs.

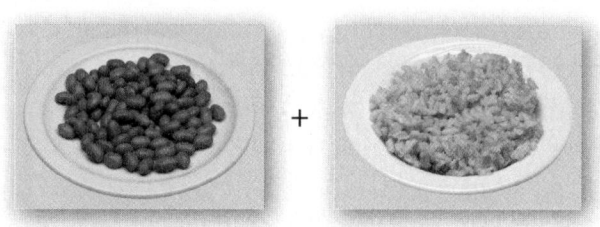

Legumes and grains

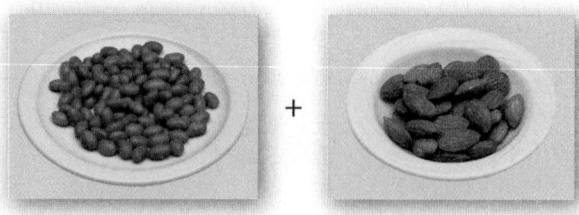

Legumes and nuts and seeds

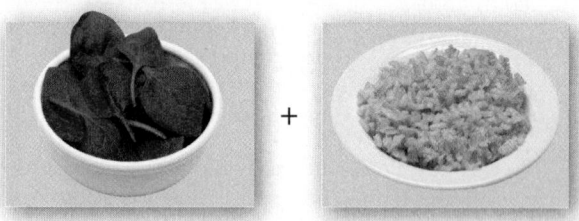

Green leafy vegetables and grains

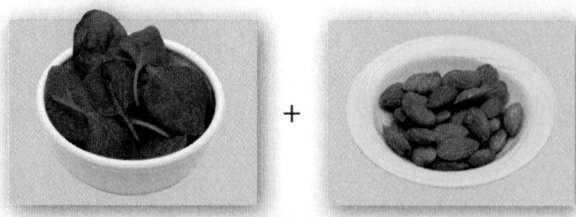

Green leafy vegetables and nuts and seeds

FIGURE **7.3** Combining plant foods from different groups (for example, grains and legumes) on the same day can provide complementary proteins and all the necessary amino acids, even without eating meat or other animal foods.

Group	Daily protein requirement (g/kg body weight)	Calculating your daily protein requirement	Example (for average adult)
Most adults	0.8 g/kg	① Determine your body weight	① Weight = 132 lb
Recreational athletes	1.0 –1.1 g/kg	② Convert pounds to kilograms: lb ÷ 2.21 lb/kg = kg	② 132 lb ÷ 2.21 lb/kg = about 60 kg
Elite athletes in training	1.2 –1.6 g/kg	③ Multiply by 0.8 g/kg for average adult to get requirement in grams per day	③ 60 kg × 0.8 g/kg = 48 g Result: a 132 lb adult would need 48 grams of protein a day

FIGURE **7.4**   Use these formulas to determine your daily protein requirements, depending on your activity level.

Carbohydrates Are Major Energy Suppliers

Carbohydrates, including the sugars and starches, have ring- and chain-like three-dimensional structures that allow them to store and supply much of the energy we need to sustain normal daily activity. The **simple carbohydrates** or **sugars** are common in whole, unprocessed foods such as beets, sugarcane, carrots, other vegetables, and fruits such as grapes (Figure 7.5a). The **complex carbohydrates** include the starches found abundantly in grains (such as rice and wheat); cereals (such as oats); some fruits and vegetables (such as bananas and squash); and many root vegetables (such as potatoes, yams, and turnips) (Figure 7.5b).

Our cells can rapidly break down sugar molecules and release energy stored in their chemical bonds. For this reason, sugars such as glucose, sucrose (table sugar), and lactose (milk sugar) are a source of immediate energy for the body. Your muscle cells and your brain and nerve cells are particularly dependent on a steady supply of glucose, whether from fruits and vegetables or from the starches in grains. This dependence is the reason low blood sugar, or *hypoglycemia*, can leave you feeling foggy-headed, weak, and shaky. According

carbohydrates A class of nutrients containing sugars and starches; supply most energy for daily activity

simple carbohydrates or sugars Carbohydrates made up of one or two sugar subunits that deliver energy in a quickly usable form

complex carbohydrates Energy-storing and structural compounds made up of long chains of sugar molecules; most deliver energy slowly

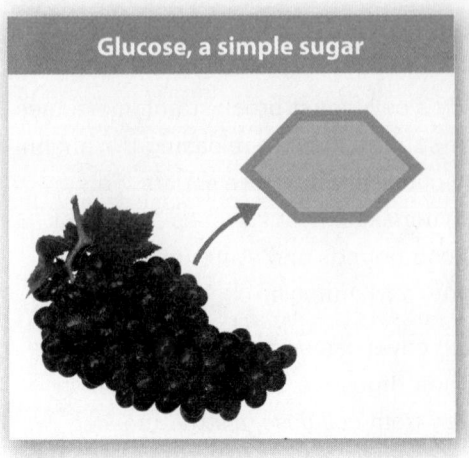

Glucose, a simple sugar

(a)

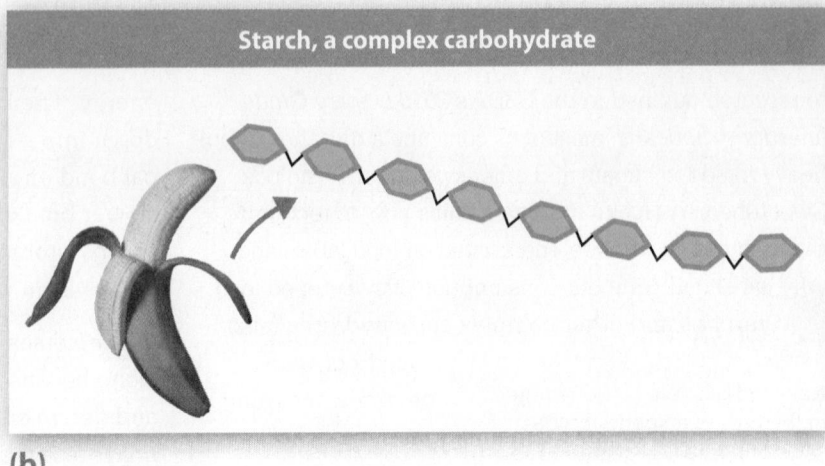

Starch, a complex carbohydrate

(b)

FIGURE **7.5**   (a) Grapes are rich in glucose, a simple sugar. (b) Bananas contain starch, a complex carbohydrate.

Sweeteners: A Health Primer

Full-Calorie Sweeteners

The average American consumes more than 355 calories (more than 22 teaspoons per day) of sugars such as honey, corn syrup, or sucrose (table sugar) added to their foods and beverages. Most of this is in processed foods. Sweeteners can boost flavor, texture, and bulk. However, added sugars have health consequences: they add calories but virtually no other nutrients. They promote tooth decay. They tend to replace more nutritious foods in the diet such as fruits, vegetables, seeds, nuts, and whole grains. And they raise triglyceride levels in the blood; this, in turn, can contribute to cardiovascular disease.[1] The American Heart Association recommends a maximum daily limit of 100 calories of added sugars (the equivalent of six teaspoons of sugar) for most women, and 150 calories (equivalent to nine teaspoons) for most men.[2]

Reduced-Calorie Sweeteners

Many products that claim to be "low in sugar" or "sugar free" include sugar alcohols: carbohydrates with a sweet flavor and a particular type of chemical structure. Examples of these ingredients include mannitol, sorbitol, xylitol, and hydrogenated starch hydrolysates. The products sometimes contain non-nutritive sweeteners, as well (see below). These "dietetic" foods do provide fewer calories—only about half of the calories in regular sweeteners—but can still be significant calorie and carbohydrate sources, depending on how much you consume.[3] They typically cost more, and to make them taste good, the manufacturers often add fat. Be sure to scan such food labels for these sweeteners as well as for *trans* fats and saturated fats.

SEE IT! ONLINE

How Much Sugar?

Non-nutritive Sweeteners

Artificial sweeteners contain synthetic compounds or chemicals derived from naturally occurring herbs or sugars. The products in this class are intensely sweet and provide essentially no calories. Most "sugar free" gums and beverages, for example, contain an artificial sweetener such as aspartame (Equal, NutraSweet); sucralose (Splenda); neotame; acesulfame potassium (Sunett, Sweet One), or saccharin (Sugar Twin, Sweet'N Low). A recently released product, Truvia, contains the sweet-tasting non-nutritive compound rebiana derived from the leaves of the stevia plant. In addition to rebiana, Truvia contains a sugar-alcohol (see above). Despite some concerns about the safety of nonnutritive sweeteners based on experiments feeding animals with saccharin, health agencies including the National Cancer Institute find no sound scientific evidence that artificial sweeteners raise cancer risk or promote other serious health problems. Some researchers, however, have suggested an association between weight gain and artificial sweetener use, for unknown reasons.[4]

Sources:
1. Mayo Clinic Staff, "Added Sugar: Don't Get Sabotaged by Sweeteners," MayoClinic Online, www.mayoclinic.com/health/added-sugar/MY00845 (November 2010).
2. American Heart Association, "Sugars and Carbohydrates," www.heart.org /HEARTORG/GettingHealthy/NutritionCenter/HealthyDietGoals/Sugars-and-Carbohydrates_UCM_303296_Article.jsp (updated October 2010).
3. American Diabetes Association, "Sugar Alcohols," www.diabetes.org/food-and-fitness/food/what-can-i-eat/sugar-alcohols.html (accessed September 2011).
4. Mayo Clinic Staff, "Artificial Sweeteners: Understanding These and Other Sugar Substitutes," Mayo Clinic Online, www.mayoclinic.com/health/artificial-sweeteners /MY00073 (October 2010).

• •

to research outlined in the USDA's *2010 Dietary Guidelines for Americans*, most of us consume a diet that is too heavy in added sugars and other sweeteners. The box Sweeteners: A Health Primer explains how to recognize the many kinds of sweeteners listed on food labels and why we should limit our consumption of sweetened food.

Starches and other complex carbohydrates (also called *polysaccharides*, meaning "many sugars") can be a source of "timed release"

fiber Indigestible carbohydrates in the diet that speed the passage of partially digested food through the digestive tract

energy. The body's cells must break starch molecules down into sugar subunits before releasing the chemical bond energy contained in those sugars. This slower breakdown makes most starches important energy-storage compounds and structural building materials in plants and animals.

Fiber Horses and cows can survive on grass and hay alone because their digestive systems break down and derive energy from *cellulose* (a structural carbohydrate that makes up the cell walls of plants). In humans, cellulose acts as indigestible **fiber** in one of two forms. *Insoluble fiber,* found in bran, whole grain breads and cereals, and in most fruits and vegetables, speeds the passage of foods and reduces bile acids and certain bacterial enzymes. *Soluble fiber,* which is in oat bran, dried beans, and some fruits and vegetables, attaches to water molecules. Soluble fiber appears to help lower blood cholesterol levels and the risk of cardiovascular disease. Both kinds of fiber assist the passage of partially digested food through the digestive tract. They also help control appetite and body weight by creating a feeling of fullness without adding extra calories.

While the evidence of a link between fiber consumption and reduced cancer risk is weak, eating fiber-rich foods is still recommended because they contain other nutrients that may help reduce cancer risk and have other health benefits.[8] Fiber also helps prevent constipation by absorbing moisture like a sponge and producing softer, bulkier stools that are easily passed. Fiber-induced gas may also initiate bowel movements. Reducing constipation helps protect against diverticulosis—the formation of tiny pouches in the colon that bulge out through the intestinal wall like bubbles protruding through holes in a tire. These pouches tend to get inflamed and can cause intestinal pain, bloating, bleeding, blockages, and other symptoms.

The USDA's *2010 Dietary Guidelines for Americans* recommends that we make at least half of our daily consumption of grains whole grain foods such as whole oats, whole wheat, and brown rice, and decrease our consumption of refined carbohydrates such as white flour, white bread and sandwich buns, and white rice. Table 7.1 lists many whole and refined grains. For tips on how to increase the fiber in your diet, see the box Tips for Eating More Fiber.

TABLE 7.1 Whole Grains and Refined Grains

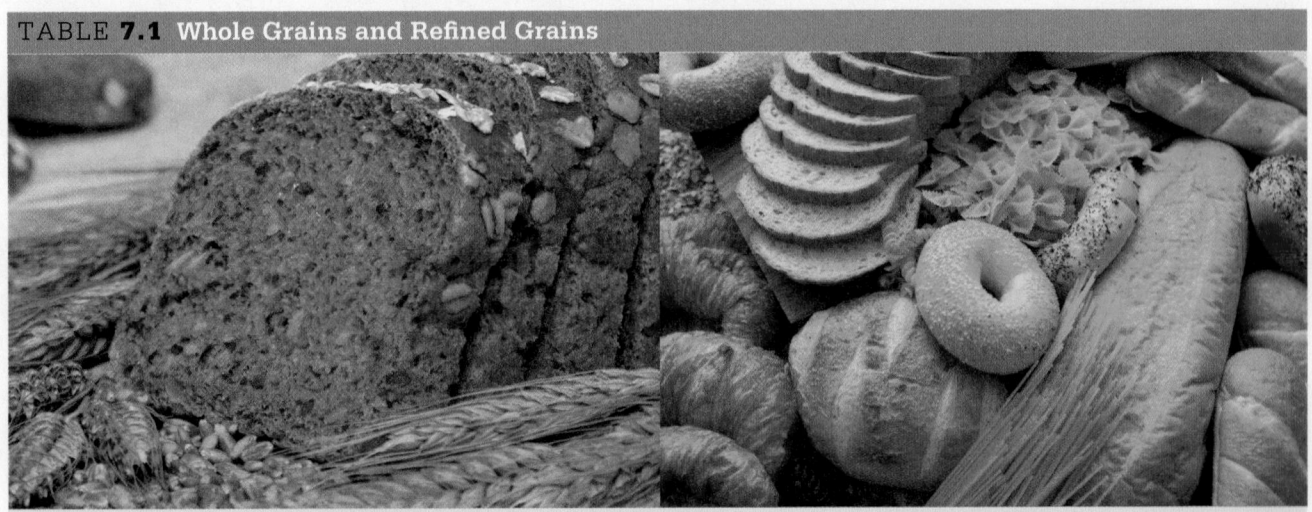

Whole grains		Refined grains	
brown rice	whole wheat bread	cornbread*	pitas*
buckwheat	whole wheat crackers	corn tortillas*	pretzels
bulgur (cracked wheat)	whole wheat pasta	couscous*	white bread
oatmeal	whole wheat sandwich	crackers*	white sandwich buns and
popcorn	buns and rolls	flour tortillas*	rolls
whole grain barley	whole wheat tortillas	grits	white rice
whole grain cornmeal	wild rice	noodles*	
whole rye		pasta*	*Ready-to-eat breakfast cereals*
	Less common whole grains:		corn flakes
Ready-to-eat breakfast cereals:	amaranth		
whole wheat cereal flakes	millet		
muesli	quinoa		
	sorghum		
	triticale		

*Most of these products are made from refined grains. Some are made from whole grains. Check the ingredient list for the words "whole grain" or "whole wheat" to decide whether they are made from a whole grain. Some foods are made from a mixture of whole and refined grains.

Source: USDA, "Food Groups: Grains," www.choosemyplate.gov/foodgroups/grains.html (modified June 2011).

Tips for Eating More Fiber

Most Americans should double their daily fiber intake. To increase the fiber in your diet, think "whole" and "traditional" foods instead of refined foods and choose more of these:

- Whole grains, including stone-ground wheat, bulgur wheat, wheat bran, wheat berries, whole barley, whole millet, whole quinoa, oatmeal, oat bran, popcorn, barley, cornmeal, whole rye, brown rice, and rice bran

- Peas, beans, nuts, and seeds

- Leafy greens such as baby spinach, endive, radicchio, arugula, mizuna, watercress, or dandelion greens

- Bran or flaxseed

- Fresh fruits and vegetables including, when edible, their cleanly scrubbed skins

- Plenty of liquids each day

At the same time, choose fewer of these:

- White bread, buns, or flour tortillas

- Cereals that list "enriched" flour as the main ingredient

- Cookies, pastries, desserts, candies

The daily recommended amount of fiber for an adult is 25 to 30 grams, but most Americans get less than that amount.[9] Some professional groups believe the requirements should be higher, perhaps even double the recommended amount. Food labels must list the fiber contents of foods and often break that number down into insoluble and soluble fiber.

The Glycemic Index of Foods Nutritionists use a tool called the **glycemic index** to measure the rate at which foods raise levels of glucose in the blood. If you eat food with a high glycemic index, especially in large portions, your bloodstream becomes flooded with glucose, and this, in turn, leads to an upsurge of the hormone insulin. The combination of glycemic index plus portion size is called *glycemic load*. Over time, this flooding and surging can contribute to being overweight and to type 2 diabetes, heart disease, and obesity.[10]

Using the glycemic index of foods to control the amount of sugar in your bloodstream requires some practice. A glycemic index chart can help you predict the effect a given food will have on your blood sugar levels. Note that not all sweet foods have a high index and many starchy or fatty foods do. See this book's website for links to these charts. The glycemic index of foods can help you plan a healthy diet, but it is just one factor to consider because some low–glycemic index foods are poor nutritional choices overall (i.e., premium ice cream, sausages) and some high–glycemic index foods are good choices overall (i.e., bran flakes, watermelon). The best approach to control your sugar intake is to develop a habit of reading food labels before you buy or eat something to discover the amount of dietary sugars in foods. Then, use glycemic index and glycemic load charts to help you get a feel for which foods raise your blood sugar levels quickly and which do not.

"Low-Carb" Foods In recent years, food manufacturers have introduced thousands of "low-carb" foods, influenced, in part, by the popularity of high-protein weight loss diets. As we've seen, however, whole grain foods are packed with healthful nutrients and fiber. The culprit is not the "carbs" themselves but the quantity most people eat and the refining of the carbohydrates. Whole fruits and vegetables, and foods made with whole grains, seeds, and nuts, are nutrient-dense and retain the fibrous cellulose in their skins and husks. Most "low-carb" foods are highly processed and contain substitute sugars such as mannitol, sorbitol, and dextrose. There is no solid evidence that "low-carb" products made with sweeteners protect you from diseases, and they cost much more than simple fruits, vegetables, whole grains, nuts, seeds, and beans.

glycemic index A measurement of the rate at which foods raise levels of glucose in the blood and, in turn, trigger the release of insulin and other blood-sugar regulators

Fats Are Concentrated Energy Storage

The "low-carb" diet craze was preceded by a "low-fat" craze that labeled all fats and oils as harmful. In fact, fats play vital roles in maintaining healthy skin and hair, padding the body organs against shock, insulating us against temperature extremes, storing energy to fuel muscle activity, and promoting healthy cell function. Although they are widely misunderstood nutrients, fats make foods taste better, carry the fat-soluble vitamins A, D, E, and K to cells, and provide certain essential compounds we can't get from other foods or manufacture in our own cells. They also provide a concentrated form of energy and raw materials that can stand in whenever carbohydrates are in short supply.

Types of Fats *Fat* is a common term for **lipids**, a class of molecules that includes fats and oils. **Fats**, such as butter, lard, and bacon grease, are solid at room temperature. **Oils** are usually liquid at room temperature; examples are corn and olive oils. Lipids also include *waxes,* such as beeswax, and *steroids,* such as steroid hormones, cholesterol, and certain vitamins.

Structurally, fats and oils are made up of long chains of carbon atoms, usually an even number between 4 and 28 linked in a chain. These chains are called **fatty acids**. The fatty acids in most foods and in the body occur in the form of **triglycerides**, molecules that have a "head," which contains the compound glycerol, and three tails (Figure 7.6a). The "tails" are made up of fatty acid chains of various lengths.

In lipid molecules of all types, the chemical bonding of carbon atoms is the key to whether the chains remain straight and form solid fats, or kink and form liquid oils. (Figure 7.6 b) Carbon atoms can form four bonds to other atoms. Where carbons are linked to each other in a chain (—C—C—), each carbon has two bonds left over,

$$C-C-C-C$$

and these often link to hydrogen atoms:

$$
\begin{array}{cccc}
& H & H & \\
& | & | & \\
C- & C- & C- & C \\
& | & | & \\
& H & H &
\end{array}
$$

In a fatty acid chain where every available carbon bond is *saturated* or filled with hydrogen atoms, the fat itself is called a **saturated fat**. Saturated chains remain straight and can pack solidly against each other. This explains why butter, beef fat, and lard—all saturated fats—occur as solids at room temperature (Figure 7.6c).

In an oil, there are also chains of carbon atoms, but at certain spots, the carbons have two bonds to other carbons (—C=C—). As a result, they have fewer bonds left over and can't be saturated or filled with hydrogen molecules at these points. The chains are said to be **unsaturated**. These double-bonded spots also cause the chains to kink and bend. Because the chains can't pack tightly together, they create a liquid oil rather than a solid fat. Fatty acid chains containing just one kinked (unsaturated) region are called **monounsaturated fatty acids (MUFAs)** (*mono* means "one"). Olive oil, canola oil, and cashew oil are all high in monounsaturated fatty acids. Chains containing two or more linked regions are called **polyunsaturated fatty acids (PUFAs;** *poly* means "many"). Corn oil, safflower oil, and cottonseed oil are all high in polyunsaturated fatty acids (Figure 7.6d).

Food manufacturers sometimes alter the properties of oils by adding hydrogen atoms to liquid oils, a process called hydrogenation. This results in partially hydrogenated oils that contain some *trans* fatty acids or **trans fats**. These have cooking properties of solid fats as well as their potentially negative effects on

lipids A category of compounds including fats, oils, and waxes that do not dissolve in water

fats Lipids, such as butter, lard, and bacon grease, which are usually solids at room temperature

oils Lipids, such as corn and olive oil, which are usually liquid at room temperature

fatty acids The most basic units of triglycerides

triglycerides Lipid molecules made up of three fatty acid chains or "tails" attached to one glycerol "head" containing a three-carbon backbone; common form of fats in foods and in organisms

saturated fat A lipid, usually a solid fat such as butter, in which most of the chains of carbon atoms are loaded (or "saturated") with as many hydrogen atoms as the chain can carry

unsaturated fat A lipid, usually a liquid oil, in which most carbon chains lack the maximum load of hydrogen atoms

monounsaturated fatty acids (MUFAs) Lipids whose fatty acid chains have just one kinked (unsaturated) region

polyunsaturated fatty acids (PUFAs) Lipids whose fatty acid chains have two or more kinked (unsaturated) regions

trans fats Unsaturated lipids or oils with hydrogen atoms added to cause more complete saturation and make the oil function as a solid

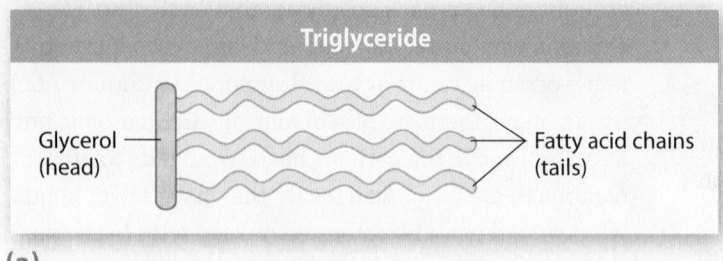

Triglyceride

Glycerol (head) — Fatty acid chains (tails)

(a)

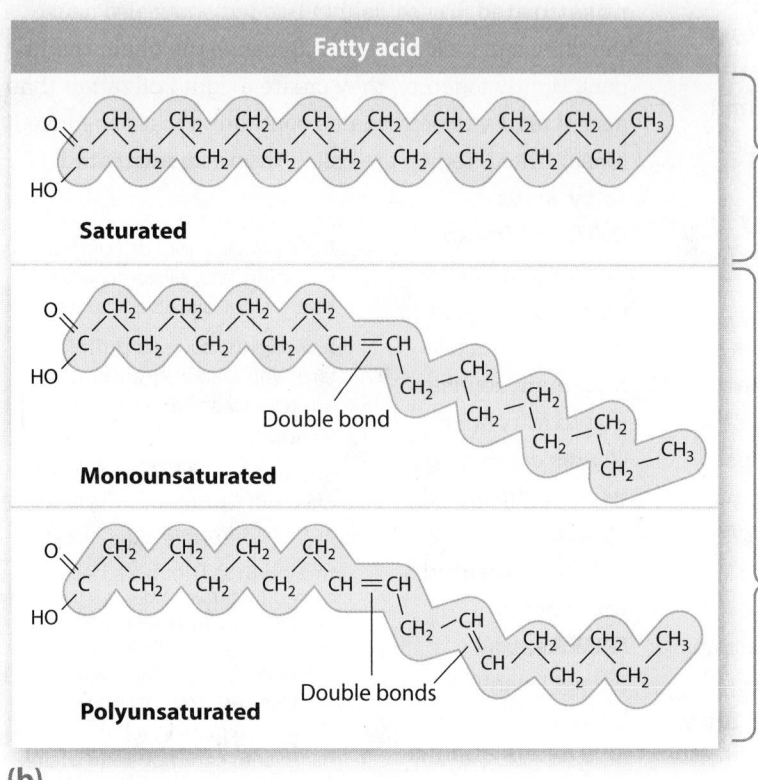

Fatty acid

Saturated

Double bond

Monounsaturated

Double bonds

Polyunsaturated

(b)

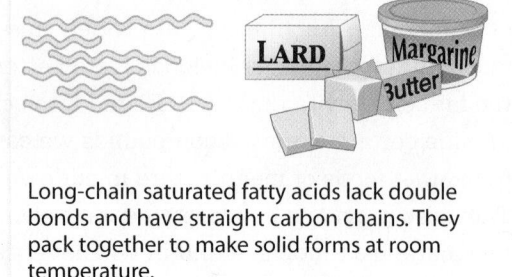

Long-chain saturated fatty acids lack double bonds and have straight carbon chains. They pack together to make solid forms at room temperature.

(c)

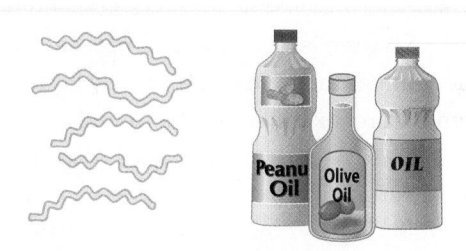

Mono- and polyunsaturated fatty acids can kink and bend at the double bond in the chain. Kinked chains slide past each other and act as liquid oils.

(d)

FIGURE **7.6** (a) Structure of triglyceride. (b) The chemical makeup of fatty acid chains in fats and oils helps explain why saturated fats (c) such as lard or butter are usually solid, and why mono- and polyunsaturated fats (d) such as olive and corn oil are usually liquids.

Adapted from NUTRITION: AN APPLIED APPROACH, 1st Edition, by Janice Thompson and Melinda Manore, © 2005. Reprinted by permission of Pearson Education, Inc., Upper Saddle River, NJ.

health. Margarines, shortenings, and many processed foods contain *trans* fats. Nutritionists often recommend that you eliminate or decrease foods containing *trans* fats from your diet. The *trans* fat content of foods is now indicated on food labels. We will discuss the health consequences of eating *trans* fats later.

All of our food sources of fats and oils contain both saturated and unsaturated fats, in different ratios (Figure 7.7). For example, a tablespoon of safflower oil contains 0.8 gram saturated fat, 10.2 grams of monounsaturated fat, and 2 grams polyunsaturated fat. A tablespoon of butter typically contains 7.2 grams saturated fat, 3.3 grams monounsaturated fat, and a trace of polyunsaturated fat. In general, lipids high in saturated fats are unhealthy for you, especially if you eat them frequently. While animals tend

to make saturated fats and plants tend to make unsaturated fats, some plants generate oils that are very high in saturated fats. Cocoa butter, palm kernel oil, and coconut oil contain more saturated fat per tablespoon than butter, beef fat, or lard! Since lipids high in mono- and polyunsaturated fats are much healthier for you than those high in saturated fat, it pays to learn about the types of oils so you can choose wisely. Figure 7.7 shows the oils containing the widest purple and red bands (which designate mono- and polyunsaturated fatty acids) are the healthiest. The fats and oils with the widest blue bands (designating saturated fatty acids) are the least healthy.

Omega-3 and Omega-6 Fatty Acids There are some types of fatty acids that our cells cannot construct and therefore we must consume in our diet. These fatty

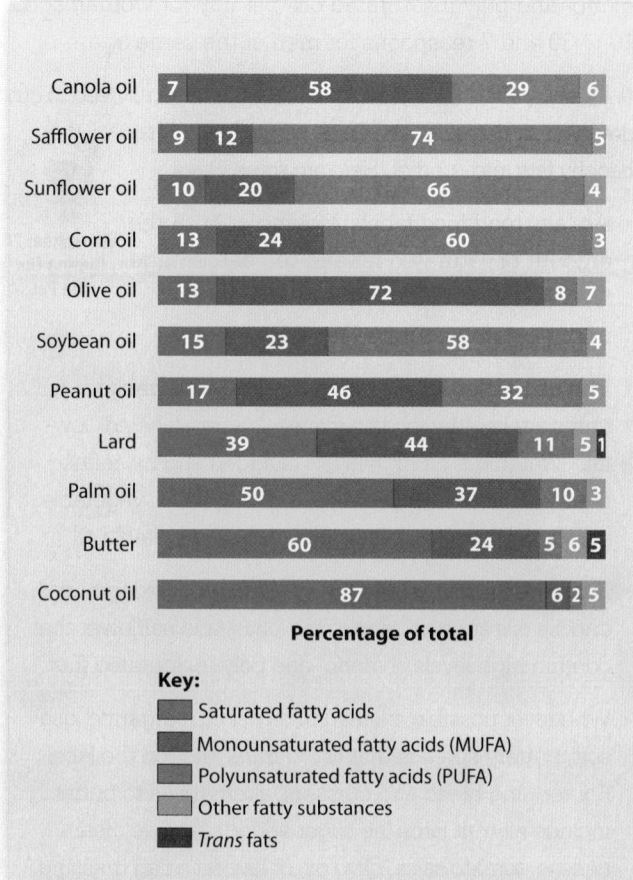

Percentage of total

Key:
- Saturated fatty acids
- Monounsaturated fatty acids (MUFA)
- Polyunsaturated fatty acids (PUFA)
- Other fatty substances
- *Trans* fats

FIGURE 7.7 Common fats and oils have varying percentages of saturated and unsaturated fats, making them more or less healthful in the diet.

acids are called **essential fatty acids**. They include *linoleic acid,* an omega-6 fatty acid, and *linolenic acid,* an omega-3 fatty acid. An **omega-6 fatty acid** is polyunsaturated and has double-bonded carbons at two sites, including one at the sixth carbon along the carbon chain. An **omega-3 fatty acid** has double-bonded carbons at three sites, including one at the third carbon along the chain. Other omega-3 fatty acids include EPA and DHA, which the human body can modify into linolenic acid. Polyunsaturated oils such as canola oil, corn oil, soybean oil, and sunflower oil all contain high levels of omega-6 fatty acids. Polyunsaturated oils such as flaxseed oil, walnut oil, and, to a lesser degree, certain fish oils, canola oil, and soybean oil contain relatively high percentages of omega-3 fatty acids. The body can modify both types of essential fatty acids into various fats we need for blood clotting, building cell membranes in the brain, protecting against heart disease by contributing to healthy blood vessel walls, and by helping to prevent inflammatory bowel disease and other autoimmune diseases.[11]

Dietary Fats and Your Health As your body breaks down the fats and oils in the food you eat, it packages the lipids into particles called **lipoproteins** that can move along easily in the bloodstream. Lipoproteins contain lipid and protein portions, and carry both triglycerides and **cholesterol**, the most common steroid in the body (recall that steroids are one structural class of fats). Our cells need and make cholesterol to keep membranes pliable and use it as a building block for making steroid hormones and other substances. In common usage, lipoproteins carrying cholesterol are simply called *cholesterol.*

Eating saturated fat and *trans* fat raises the level of **low-density lipoproteins** (also called **LDLs** or "bad cholesterol") in your bloodstream. Over time, elevated levels of LDLs can lead to plaque deposits inside the blood vessels. These plaques can constrict blood flow, raise blood pressure, and lead to heart disease, heart attacks, and strokes. Eating saturated fat also raises the level of **high-density lipoproteins** (**HDLs** or "good cholesterol") in the blood, but to a lesser degree. HDLs prevent and reduce plaque deposits in the blood vessels and therefore help protect against cardiovascular disease, strokes, and heart attacks.

You may be wondering how something the human body makes

essential fatty acids Lipid components, including linolenic acid, EPA, DHA, and linoleic acid, which the body cannot manufacture and which we must obtain in polyunsaturated oils

omega-6 fatty acid A polyunsaturated fatty acid that has double-bonded carbons at two sites, including one at the sixth carbon along the chain

omega-3 fatty acid A polyunsaturated fatty acid that has double-bonded carbons at three sites, including one at the third carbon along the chain

lipoproteins Lipid-plus-protein transport particles that can move along easily in the bloodstream; carry triglycerides or cholesterol

cholesterol A waxy lipid in the steroid class that is an important component of cell membranes and is transported in the blood by carriers called *LDL* and *HDL*

low-density lipoproteins (LDLs) A form of lipoprotein sometimes called "bad cholesterol;" LDL levels rise in response to saturated fats in the diet and can contribute to plaque deposits inside blood vessels

high-density lipoproteins (HDLs) A form of lipoprotein sometimes called "good cholesterol;" HDL levels rise in response to polyunsaturated fats and prevent and reduce plaque deposits in the blood vessels

and needs for its own cell membranes and hormones can be harmful in the diet. When some people consume cholesterol, their body cells make less cholesterol and their overall level stays constant. In other people, however, that "leveling mechanism" works inefficiently, and they tend to accumulate the extra dietary cholesterol in blood-vessel-narrowing plaques.[12] To be safe, the USDA recommends that you consume less cholesterol in the diet by cutting back on fatty meats, egg yolks, high-fat dairy products, and all sources of saturated or trans fats.

Research shows that *trans* fatty acids can be even more damaging than saturated fats. *Trans* fats increase LDLs and simultaneously lower HDLs, a doubly negative effect. A person who gets just two percent of his or her calories from *trans* fats would be raising his or her risk for heart disease by 23 percent and for sudden cardiac death by 47 percent.[13] The USDA recommends choosing products with little or no *trans* fats.[14] In fact, the USDA's ChooseMyPlate.gov website—which provides specific daily food recommendations based on your sex, size, age, and activity level—now classifies *trans* fats along with saturated fats and sugars as "empty calories." The site suggests you restrict your overall daily consumption of such empty calories to 260 per day (if you are a woman between 19 and 30) and to 330 per day (if you are a man in that same age group).

Trans fats also raise triglyceride levels. After a meal, the liver takes cholesterol and triglycerides that we don't use immediately in our tissues, packages them into HDLs and LDLs, and sends them through the blood to be stored in fat cells.[15] Coincidentally, consuming large quantities of refined starches, sugars, and/or alcohol also raises blood triglycerides. This helps explain why eating big helpings of such starches and sugars, as so many Americans do, can lead to obesity, diabetes, and heart disease.

Eating mono- and polyunsaturated fats lowers LDLs and raises HDLs, a doubly positive effect. As Figure 7.7 showed, most kinds of cooking oil are high in mono- and polyunsaturated fats and low in saturated fats, but there are exceptions, such as palm kernel oil and coconut oil. That's one reason it is important to read food labels rather than make assumptions about the fats in particular foods.

Some nutritionists encourage people to consume more oils. A popular plan called the Mediterranean diet encourages people to use olive oil liberally in cooking and at the table. Nutritionists from Harvard Medical School also encourage people to eat healthful plant oils at most meals.[16] The USDA ChooseMyPlate.gov website recommends a daily consumption of 6 teaspoons of

mono- and polyunsaturated oils per day for women aged 19 to 30 and 7 teaspoons for men of the same age.

A Healthy Plan for Fats in Your Diet Most of us need to cut down on saturated fats while getting more heart-healthy fats into our diet. Here are some ideas:

- Always read food labels, looking at both the amount of saturated fat and the percentage it represents of your daily recommended maximum for saturated fat and total fat.

- Don't be fooled into thinking that cookies, crackers, or chips are healthy foods because they are labeled "low-fat." Watch out for high levels of added sugars, refined flour, salt, and *trans* fats (the label may read "vegetable shortening" or "partially hydrogenated vegetable oil").

- For salad dressings, sautéing, and other cooking needs, choose oils such as canola, soy, olive, and safflower that contain high levels of mono- and polyunsaturated fats.

- Whenever possible, instead of butter or margarine, use soft, buttery spreads that list "0 *trans* fats" on the label. For topping bread and crackers, alternatives to butter include all-fruit jams (no sugar added), fat-free cream cheese, tomato salsa, olive oil, or low-fat salad dressing.

- For protein, choose beans, nuts, seeds, tofu, lean meats, fish, or poultry instead of fatty meats such as bacon, sausages, hot dogs, bologna, pepperoni, or organ meats. Remove skin. Avoid frying. Drain off fat after cooking.

- Choose dairy products that have zero or one percent fat, such as skim milk, nonfat yogurt, and fat-free cottage cheese. Avoid reduced-fat dairy products (two percent fat) and whole-milk dairy products (four percent fat) whenever possible. Choose nonfat or low-fat frozen yogurt or sorbet rather than ice cream.

- Cook with chicken broth, wine, vinegar, low-calorie salad dressings, or unsaturated oils (mono- and polyunsaturated) rather than butter, margarine, sour cream, mayonnaise, and creamy salad dressings.

- Eat fatty fish (i.e., salmon, tuna, bluefish, herring, or sardines) one or two times per week. However, be aware of high mercury levels in some types of fish (see the box Is It Safe to Eat Fish?).

- Add green, leafy vegetables, walnuts, walnut oil, and milled flaxseed to your diet.

- Limit processed and convenience foods. These often contain refined carbohydrates in addition to *trans* fats.

Is It Safe to Eat Fish?

You may have heard that eating too much of certain kinds of fish can pose health hazards, especially to women of childbearing age and to children. At the same time, there are many nutritional benefits to eating fish, including high levels of healthy omega-3 fatty acids. So what's safe and what's not?

The problem is that mercury (either released in the air due to industrial pollution, or naturally occurring) can accumulate in bodies of water, where it becomes methylmercury and contaminates fish. People who eat fish containing high amounts of methylmercury can, in turn, accumulate mercury in their bloodstream. Women of reproductive age and children should be careful about their fish consumption because mercury can damage the brain and nervous systems in developing fetuses and young children.

The EPA advises women and children to avoid four types of fish altogether: tilefish, swordfish, shark, and King mackerel,[1] as these fish tend to contain exceptionally high levels of mercury. They also advise the two groups to limit consumption of fish containing low-levels of mercury—such as salmon, canned light tuna, and catfish—to 12 ounces (two average meals) per week. Other seafood containing low levels of mercury include anchovies, clams, codfish, crab, herring, lobster, and North Atlantic mackerel.[2]

Sources:

1. Environmental Protection Agency, "What You Need to Know about Mercury in Fish and Shellfish," www.epa.gov/waterscience/fishadvice/advice.html (accessed July 2011).
2. U.S. Food and Drug Administration, "Mercury Levels in Commercial Fish and Shellfish, 1990–2010," www.fda.gov/Food/FoodSafety/Product-SpecificInformation/Seafood/FoodbornePathogensContaminants/Methylmercury/ucm115644.htm (updated May 2011).

Don't demand daily nutritional perfection from yourself. Try to balance your intake of different foods over a few meals and a couple of days at a time. If you have a high-fat breakfast or lunch, balance it with a low-fat dinner. If you forget to eat at least five servings of fruits and vegetables today, eat extra servings tomorrow. And closely monitor your diet to avoid consuming more than the small daily allotment the USDA recommends for empty calories such as sugars and saturated fats (no more than about 10 percent of daily calories).

Vitamins Are Vital Micronutrients

Vitamins are organic compounds that we need in tiny amounts to promote growth and help maintain life and health. Vitamins take part in the minute-by-minute cellular reactions that help maintain our nerves and skin, contribute to the production of blood cells, help us build bones and teeth, assist in wound healing, and help convert food energy to accessible fuel for cellular activities. Some vitamins are toxic in high doses, and for many vitamins, time spent on the shelf, the heat from cooking, and certain other environmental conditions can diminish their potency in foods.

Some vitamins can dissolve only in water and some only in fat. *Water-soluble vitamins,* including vitamin C and the B vitamins, dissolve easily in water and can be absorbed directly into the bloodstream.[17] Excess water-soluble vitamins are usually excreted in the urine and cause few toxicity problems. Because they are not stored in the liver, body fat, or other tissues, we must consume water-soluble vitamins on a regular basis in our foods. *Fat-soluble vitamins,* including vitamins A, D, E, and K, must associate with fat molecules in order to be absorbed through the intestinal tract. Excess, unused quantities of the fat-soluble vitamins tend to be stored in the body. High levels can accumulate in the liver

> **vitamins** Organic compounds in foods that we need in tiny amounts to promote growth and help maintain life and health

and cause damage. Table 7.2 lists 13 vitamins, their food sources, their chief functions in the body, and the symptoms caused by consuming too little or too much of each.

Vitamin vendors often make various claims about the benefits of taking vitamin supplements to augment what we consume in foods. For the most part, a careful diet will provide your vitamin needs, but because many people eat too few fruits and vegetables, they don't get optimal levels. In addition, certain groups of people, and all of us at certain life stages, do have special vitamin needs. People over 50, for example, must be careful to get enough vitamin B_{12} since absorption of certain nutrients,

TABLE **7.2** Guide to Vitamins				
Vitamin *RDI*	Best Food Sources	Main Functions in Body	Deficiency Symptoms	Toxicity Symptoms
Water-Soluble Vitamins				
B_1 (Thiamin) *1.5 milligrams (mg)*	Meat, pork, liver, fish, poultry, whole grain and enriched breads and cereals, pasta, nuts, legumes	Energy harvest and use from nutrients; normal appetite; nervous system function	Poor appetite, heart irregularities, mental confusion, muscle weakness, poor growth	None known
B_2 (Riboflavin) *1.7 mg*	Dairy products, dark green vegetables, liver, meat, whole grain and enriched breads and cereals	Energy harvest and use from nutrients; healthy skin, normal vision, normal growth	Eye problems, skin cracking around nose and mouth	None known
Niacin *20 mg*	Meat, eggs, poultry, fish, milk, whole grain and enriched breads and cereals, nuts, legumes, yeast, all protein foods	Energy harvest and use from nutrients; healthy skin, nervous system function, digestion	Skin rash, loss of appetite, dizziness, weakness, irritability, fatigue, mental confusion, indigestion	Flushing, blurred vision, glucose intolerance, abnormal liver function
B_6 (Pyridoxine) *2.0 mg*	Meat, poultry, fish, shellfish, legumes, whole grain foods, leafy greens, bananas	Breakdown of proteins and fats, formation of red blood cells and antibodies, conversion of niacin	Nervous disorders, skin rash, muscle weakness, anemia, convulsions, kidney stones	Sensory nerve damage, skin lesions
Folate *0.4 mg*	Leafy greens, liver, legumes, seeds	Forming red blood cells, breakdown of proteins, cell division, proper formation of neural tube in embryo	Anemia, heartburn, diarrhea, smooth tongue, poor growth and development	Nerve damage; high levels may mask a vitamin B_{12} deficiency
B_{12} *6 micrograms (mcg)*	Meat, fish, poultry, shellfish, milk, cheese, eggs, yeast	Nerve cell maintenance, red blood cell formation, building of new genetic material	Anemia, smooth tongue, fatigue, nerve degeneration progressing to paralysis	None known

TABLE **7.2** (*Continued*)

Vitamin RDI	Best Food Sources	Main Functions in Body	Deficiency Symptoms	Toxicity Symptoms
Pantothenic acid 10 mg	Widespread in foods	Crucial factor in energy harvest and use	Rare; sleep disturbances, nausea, fatigue	None known
Biotin 0.3 mg	Widespread in foods	Crucial factor in energy harvest and use, building fat molecules, energy storage in muscles	Loss of appetite, nausea, depression, muscle pain, weakness, fatigue, rash	None known
C (Ascorbic acid) 60 mg	Citrus fruits, cabbage-type vegetables, tomatoes, potatoes, dark green vegetables, peppers, cantaloupe, strawberries, mangos, papayas	Helps heal wounds; maintains connective tissue, bones, and teeth; strengthens blood vessels; antioxidant; boosts immunity; aids absorption of iron	Scurvy, anemia, blood vessel damage, depression, frequent infections, loose teeth, bleeding gums, bleeding, muscle wasting, rough skin, weak bones, poor wound healing	Nausea, abdominal cramps, diarrhea, red blood cell breakdown in some people, kidney stones in people with kidney disease. Upon withdrawing from high doses, deficiency symptoms may appear

Fat-Soluble Vitamins

Vitamin RDI	Best Food Sources	Main Functions in Body	Deficiency Symptoms	Toxicity Symptoms
A 5000 international units (IU)	Milk, cream, cheese, butter, eggs, liver, dark leafy greens, broccoli, deep orange fruits and vegetables	Healthy vision, growth and repair of tissues, formation of bones and teeth, immunity, building hormones, cancer protection	Night blindness; rough skin; frequent infections; impaired growth, especially of bones and teeth; eye problems leading to blindness	Miscarriage, birth defects, red blood cell breakage, nosebleeds, abdominal cramps, nausea, blurred vision, bone pain, dry skin, rashes, hair loss
D 200 IU	Sunlight on skin; fortified milk and margarine, eggs, liver, fish	Healthy bones and teeth; aids absorption of calcium and phosphorus	Rickets in children, weakened bones and bone problems in adults, abnormal growth, joint pain, soft bones	Raised blood calcium, constipation, weight loss, irritability, weakness, nausea, kidney stones, mental and physical retardation, calcium deposits
E 30 IU	Vegetable oils, leafy greens, wheat germ, whole grains, butter, liver, egg yolk, milk, nuts, seeds, fortified cereals, soybeans, avocado	Healthy red and white blood cells, healthy cell membranes in lungs and elsewhere, antioxidant activity	Muscle wasting, weakness, damage to red blood cells, anemia, bleeding, fibrocystic breast disease	Interference with anticlotting medication, intestinal discomfort, increased risk of stroke
K	Liver, milk, leafy greens, cabbage-type vegetables, vegetable oils	Aids digestion, blood clotting, regulation of calcium in blood, builds bone tissue	Bleeding	None known

Do I Have Special Vitamin and Mineral Needs?

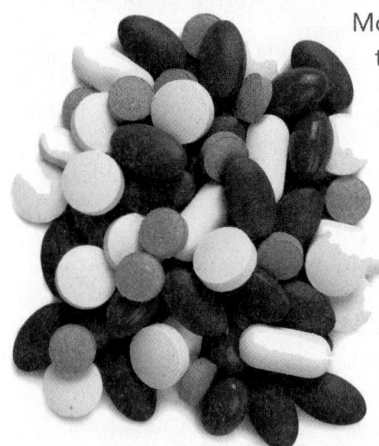

Most nutritionists agree that you should try to get your daily vitamins and minerals from a healthful diet rather than eating carelessly and relying on supplements. People in a number of population groups, however, are at risk for vitamin deficiencies. If you belong to one of these groups, you should pay extra attention to your diet and perhaps consider taking a multivitamin.[1]

- Women of reproductive age who could become pregnant need 400 micrograms of folate per day to prevent potential neurological defects in a developing fetus. Pregnant women need 600 micrograms per day.

- Premenopausal women, especially those with heavy menstrual bleeding, need 18 milligrams of iron per day in foods or in total from foods and a multivitamin. They must also get enough vitamin C to help them absorb iron from foods. Men and postmenopausal women need 10 milligrams per day and should be careful not to get too much.

- Everyone needs a good supply of calcium each day from low-fat dairy products, fortified juices, and other sources. The daily value for people under 50 is 1,000 milligrams. Pregnant women, nursing mothers, teens, and older adults need extra calcium (1,200 to 1,500 milligrams per day) for the development and maintenance of bones and to lower the risk of osteoporosis.

- Older adults need sufficient potassium for normal muscle contraction and nerve transmission and sodium within a healthy range to supply cellular needs but lower the risk of high blood pressure.

- Older adults, dark-skinned individuals, and people who do not get regular exposure to sunlight have a special need for vitamin D. The government currently recommends that people under 50 consume 200 IU (International Units) of vitamin D per day, people between 50 and 70 consume 400 I.U. per day, and people over 70 consume 600 I.U. per day.

- People over 50 naturally produce less stomach acid and absorb less vitamin B_{12} from foods. Older adults should be careful to get at least 2.4 micrograms of B_{12} per day or more, especially if they take stomach acid blockers.

- Cigarette smoking decreases bone density and interferes with the body's normal use of vitamin C. Smokers therefore need to consume higher levels of calcium (1,200 mg per day) and of vitamin C (110 mg in women, 125 mg per day in men) compared to 90 mg for nonsmoking adults.

- People with diseases that disrupt normal metabolism or nutrient absorption (diabetes and certain cancers, for example) can develop vitamin or mineral deficiencies. Physicians often recommend special diets or multivitamins as part of their treatment.[2]

- The USDA dietary guidelines provide specific pointers for parents and guardians to help kids and teens get the balance of nutrients they need to support their growth and development.

- Details about the special nutritional needs of vegetarians and diabetics are covered on pages 272–273.

If you plan to take a multivitamin, apply common sense. There is no need to get more than the RDI for vitamins and minerals. Doses exceeding 100 percent can lead to serious side effects. Since fat-soluble vitamins and certain minerals can build up in the body, be sure a multivitamin has less than the RDI for vitamins A, D, E, and K and for magnesium, chromium, selenium, and zinc.[3] To be safe, people in high-risk groups should consult a doctor before taking supplements regularly.

Sources:
1. Center for Science in the Public Interest, "The Multivitamin Maze" and "How to Read a Multi Label," *Nutrition Action Healthletter* (March 2006): 6–7.
2. U.S. Department of Agriculture and U.S. Department of Health and Human Services, *Dietary Guidelines for Americans, 2010*, 7th Edition (Washington, DC: U.S. Government Printing Office, 2010).
3. National Institutes of Health, "NIH State of the Science Panel Urges More Informed Approach to Multivitamin/Mineral Use for Chronic Disease Prevention," www.nih.gov/news/pr/may2006/od-17.htm (May 2006).

including B_{12}, declines naturally with age. The box Do I Have Special Vitamin and Mineral Needs? discusses both the vitamin needs of specific groups and the issue of taking vitamin supplements versus getting vitamins from food alone. Few Americans suffer from true vitamin deficiencies if they eat a fairly balanced diet. Taking very high levels of certain vitamins can even lead to a toxic condition know as *hypervitaminosis*.

Minerals Are Elemental Micronutrients

The micronutrients called **minerals** allow our nerves to transmit impulses, our hearts to beat, oxygen to reach our tissue cells, and our digestive tracts to absorb vitamins from food. They are usually not toxic, and we excrete excess quantities of most minerals from the body. The **major minerals** (also called *macrominerals*) are elements that the body needs in relatively large amounts. We need smaller amounts of the **trace minerals** (also called *microminerals*). Table 7.3 lists most of the major and trace minerals, their functions, food sources, and symptoms of deficiency and/or toxicity. We discuss three minerals—sodium, calcium, and iron—in more detail because of their crucial roles in the body and their excesses or deficiencies in many students' diets.

Sodium We need sodium, the Na in sodium chloride (NaCl), or table salt, for regulating the water contents of blood and body fluids; for the transmission of nerve impulses; for muscle contraction, including the heartbeat; and for several metabolic functions inside cells. However, most of us consume much more than we need.[18] The average adult at rest and not sweating profusely needs only 500 mg of sodium (about one-quarter teaspoon) per day. Nutritionists estimate, however, that the average American man consumes 3,100 to 4,700 mg per day and the average woman 2,300 to 3,100 mg per day in salted snacks and processed foods! The *2010 Dietary Guidelines for Americans* recommends that everyone restrict sodium to less than 2,300 mg per day, and that certain groups (those over 51 years old, African Americans, and people with hypertension, diabetes, or chronic kidney disease) reduce their sodium consumption to under 1,500 mg per day. Pickles, salty snack foods, processed cheeses, many breads and bakery products, and smoked meats and sausages often contain several hundred milligrams of sodium per serving. Many fast-food entrées and convenience entrées pack 500 to 1,000 mg of sodium per serving.

Many experts believe that there is a link between excessive sodium intake and hypertension (high blood pressure).[19] Researchers began recommending several years ago that people with hypertension cut back on sodium to reduce their risk of cardiovascular disorders.[20]

You can shake your own salt habit by choosing low-sodium or salt-free food products. For example, order popcorn without salt. Switch to kosher salt—it has 25% less sodium than regular table salt. Instead of adding salt to food you prepare, try using fresh or prepackaged herb blends to season foods. These small changes can add up to a significant reduction in unneeded sodium.

Calcium High sodium intake may also increase calcium loss in urine, which increases your risk for debilitating fractures as you age.[21] The element calcium (Ca) is crucial for the development and maintenance of bones and teeth, for blood clotting, muscle contraction, nerve transmission, and fluid balance between the cell's interior and its environment. Nevertheless, most Americans consume less than the 1,000 mg to 1,300 mg of calcium per day recommended by government guidelines.[22]

Osteoporosis is a disease of thinning, weakened, porous bones that affects more than 44 million Americans (women and men) over age 50. The risk for it climbs if you consume too little calcium during childhood and adolescence when bones are developing, if you have a small skeleton (or "frame"), and/or if you consume too little calcium during adulthood. Bone weakness can lead to pain, stooped posture, and fractures, and can diminish mobility and independence. Forty to 50 percent of women and 13 to 22 percent of men will break a bone as a result of osteoporosis.[23]

Dairy products are among the richest dietary sources of calcium, but calcium-fortified orange juice and soy milk are also good sources, as are leafy green vegetables and many other foods (see Table 7.3). Be aware that the added phosphoric acid (phosphate) in carbonated colas and possibly other soft drinks can cause you to excrete calcium

minerals Elements such as calcium or sodium that allow vital physiological processes including nerve transmission, heartbeat, oxygen delivery, and absorption of vitamins

major minerals Elements needed in relatively large amounts, including sodium, calcium, phosphorus, magnesium, potassium, and chloride

trace minerals Elements the body needs in very tiny amounts; includes iron, zinc, copper, iodine, selenium, fluoride, and chromium

osteoporosis A disease of thinning, weakened, porous bones during which too little calcium is deposited or retained in the bones

TABLE 7.3 Guide to Selected Minerals

Mineral RDI	Best Food Sources	Main Functions in Body	Deficiency Symptoms	Toxicity Symptoms
Calcium 1.0 g	Milk and dairy products, small fish with bones, tofu, leafy greens, legumes	Building bones and teeth, muscle contraction and relaxation, nerve function, blood clotting, blood pressure	Stunted growth in children, bone weakness and thinning in adults	Mineral imbalances, shock, kidney failure, fatigue, mental confusion
Phosphorus 1.0 g	All animal tissues	Component of every cell, helps regulate pH balance	Unknown	Can unbalance calcium; can lead to calcium deficiency, spasms, convulsions
Magnesium 400 mg	Nuts, legumes, whole grains, deep leafy greens, seafood, chocolate	Bone hardening, protein synthesis, enzyme activity, normal function of muscles and nerves	Weakness, confusion, poor growth, impaired hormone production, muscle spasms, disturbed behavior	Mega-doses can lead to nausea, cramps, dehydration, death
Sodium 2400 mg	Salt, soy sauce, processed foods, cured, canned, pickled foods	Helps maintain normal fluid balance and pH within body	Muscle cramps, mental apathy, loss of appetite	Hypertension, water retention, increased calcium loss
Chloride 2300 mg	Salt, soy sauce, processed foods, cured, canned, pickled foods	Component of stomach acid and needed for digestion, helps maintain normal fluid balance	Dangerous changes in pH, irregular heartbeat	Vomiting
Potassium 3500 mg	Meats, fruits, milk, vegetables, grains, legumes	Involved in biochemical reactions that help build protein, maintain fluid balance, transmit nerve impulses, contract muscles	Muscle weakness, paralysis, confusion; accompanies dehydration; can cause death	Muscular weakness, vomiting, irregular heartbeat; can stop heart
Iodine 150 mcg	Iodized salt, seafood	Component of thyroid hormone, helps regulate metabolism	Goiter; mental and physical retardation due to thyroid deficiency	Goiter or enlargement of thyroid gland
Iron 18 mg	Beef, fish, poultry, shellfish, eggs, legumes, dried fruits	Crucial component of hemoglobin in red blood cells, myoglobin in muscles; takes part in oxygen transfer, energy use	Anemia, weakness, pallor, headaches, frequent infections, difficulty concentrating	Nausea, vomiting, dizziness, rapid heartbeat, damage to organs, death
Zinc 15 mg	Meats, fish, poultry, grains, vegetables	Component of insulin and many enzymes; takes part in DNA, protein synthesis, immune response, taste, wound healing, normal development, sperm production, vitamin A transport	Growth failure in children, delayed sexual development, loss of taste, poor wound healing	Fever, nausea, vomiting, diarrhea, headaches, depressed immune function

TABLE **7.3** (*Continued*)

Mineral *RDI*	Best Food Sources	Main Functions in Body	Deficiency Symptoms	Toxicity Symptoms
Copper *2 mg*	Meats, drinking water	Absorption of iron, component of several enzymes	Anemia, bone changes (rare)	Liver damage if toxicity is due to certain diseases; nausea, diarrhea, vomiting
Fluoride *10 mg*	Drinking water (natural or fluoridated), tea, seafood	Formation and maintenance of bones and teeth	Susceptibility to tooth decay and bone loss	Discoloration of teeth, joint pain, stiffness
Selenium *400 mcg*	Seafood, meats, grains	Helps protect body compounds from oxidation	Muscle pain and possible deterioration, possible damage to nails and hair	Vomiting, nausea, rash, brittle hair and nails, cirrhosis of liver
Chromium *30 mcg*	Meats, whole foods, fats, vegetable oils	Associated with insulin, needed for breakdown and use of glucose	Diabetes-like condition with poor glucose utilization	Unknown. Occupational overexposure damages skin and kidneys

and thus deplete needed calcium from your bones.[24] Calcium/phosphorus imbalance may lead to kidney stones and bone spurs and to the deposits or plaques inside blood vessels that contribute to cardiovascular diseases.

Vitamin D improves absorption of calcium; that's why dairies are required by law to add it to milk. Sunlight shining on your skin also increases your body's own manufacture of vitamin D, so a moderate amount of sunlight helps improve calcium absorption. The best way to obtain calcium, like all nutrients, is to consume it as part of a balanced diet, but certain people do need calcium supplements (see the Diversity box on page 256).

Iron Each of us needs the element iron (Fe) for producing healthy blood, for muscle function, and for normal cell division. Females aged 15 to 50 need about 18 mg/day; males aged 19 to 50 need about 10 mg/day. Worldwide, iron deficiency is the most common nutrient deficiency, affecting more than one billion people. In developing countries, more than one-third of the children and women of childbearing age suffer from **iron-deficiency anemia**, in which the body fails to produce enough of the red hemoglobin pigment in the blood, leading to unusually low oxygen levels and unusually high carbon dioxide levels and resulting in mental and physical fatigue. About five percent of all Americans get too little iron in their food.[25] Among toddlers, adolescent girls, and women of childbearing age, about 10 percent show iron-deficiency anemia. Table 7.3 lists good dietary sources of iron.

Getting the right amount of iron is important. Researchers have linked iron deficiency to a host of problems, including poor immune system functioning

and a propensity toward certain cancers. Some research has also suggested a link between too much iron in the diet and/or stored in the body and a higher risk for cardiovascular disease.

Acute iron toxicity due to ingesting too many iron-containing supplements remains the leading cause of accidental poisoning in small children in the United States. Dozens of children have died from overdoses of as few as five iron tablets.[26]

Water Is Our Most Fundamental Nutrient

Imagine you are stranded on a desert island for a reality TV show and you can take along just one provision. Would you choose food, water, or a cell phone? We hope you said water!

Humans are mostly water—close to 60 percent. Watery fluids bathe each of our internal cells. They help maintain a proper balance of salts within our blood and tissues, help maintain pH balance, and help facilitate the transport of substances throughout the body. Human blood plasma (the fluid portion of blood exclusive of red and white blood cells and other solid components) is approximately 91.5 percent water.[27] This proportion must remain fairly constant for blood to efficiently carry oxygen and nutrients to the cells and carry away carbon dioxide and other wastes.

iron-deficiency anemia A disease in which the body takes in too little iron and makes too little oxygen-carrying hemoglobin

dehydrated Depleted of normal, necessary levels of body fluids

Even under the most severe conditions, the average person can live for weeks on the energy stored in body fat. You can also get along without certain vitamins and minerals from foods for an equal amount of time before experiencing serious deficiency symptoms. Without water, however, you would become **dehydrated**, or depleted of normal levels of body fluids, within hours. Within one day without drinking water, you would probably begin to feel sluggish, dizzy, and nauseated, and would experience headaches, muscle cramps, or weakness. After a few days without water, your tongue would be parched and swollen, your heart would be racing, and you'd very likely go into shock and die.

A person's need for water varies dramatically based on age, size, diet, exercise, overall health, and environmental temperature and humidity levels. Most of us get enough water through foods and beverages just by satisfying our thirst.[28] People with certain diseases such as diabetes or cystic fibrosis, however, excrete extra fluid and must generally take in a higher-volume. On a hot day, especially if exercising, you need to consciously replace fluids lost to sweat and exhalation. It is possible, though,

to take in too much water and become nauseated, confused, or weak or even to lose consciousness from excess hydration leading to *hyponatremia* (sometimes called water intoxication). This condition results from too much water in the blood and therefore a salt concentration that is too low due to dilution. It often occurs in conjunction with heavy perspiration. If your intake is high enough that you gain water weight during an active exercise session, you are probably imbibing too much.

Commercial energy drinks can help exercisers replenish water lost through sweat and to restore salt and sugar. Some energy drinks, however, include ingredients that are ineffectual or that can be harmful in large quantities. For example, researchers have failed to confirm any health benefit for ingredients such as taurine, bee pollen, and ginkgo biloba.[29] High concentrations of added sugars can boost energy in the short term but can create sluggishness later. Added vitamins C and B are unnecessary in a balanced diet. If overused, energy drinks containing the stimulants caffeine and/or ginseng can speed bone loss, raise blood pressure, and increase the risk of cardiovascular diseases.

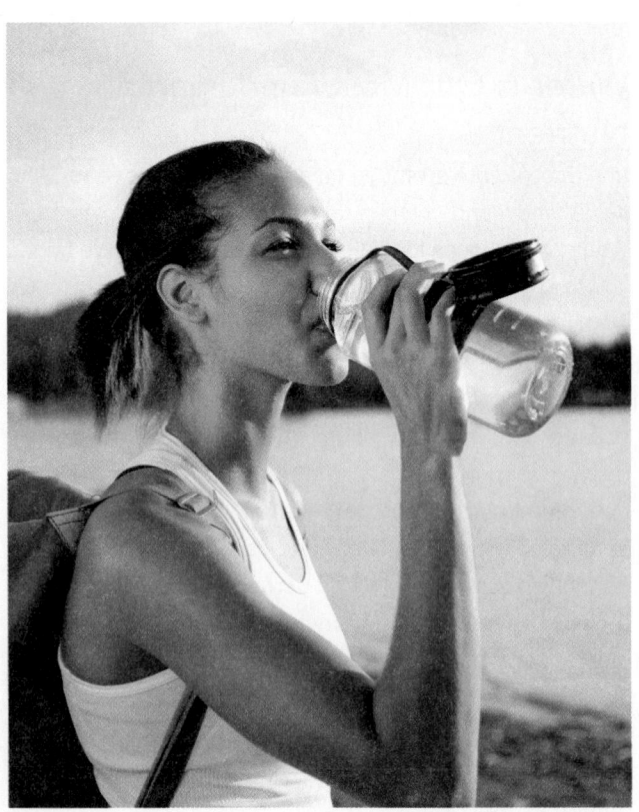

casestudy

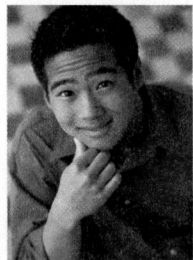

CHAU

"I kind of understand that your body uses different nutrients for different things. But I've never had a weight problem, so I've been more concerned with quantity than quality. I realize I'm eating a lot more carbs than I used to, mostly cereal and white bread. And Tom's girlfriend is always baking him cookies, so I load up on those. I also eat cheese and pepperoni pizzas in the cafeteria. Still, I don't worry about eating fat or being fat. Everyone in my family is thin!"

THINK! Chau often eats meals prepared on campus, where he has no access to nutrition labels. How could Chau estimate the amount of protein, carbohydrate, and fat in his diet? Given what you know about Chau's diet, which nutrients might he be deficient in? Which nutrients might he be consuming too much of?

ACT! Analyze your own diet. What nutrients, if any, are you deficient in? Calculate how much protein you need each day. Are you taking in more protein than you really need?

HEAR IT! ONLINE

How Can I Achieve a Balanced Diet?

The average American adult consumes about 1,000 calories more per day than the average citizen worldwide and yet still gets unbalanced nutrition. To counter these trends toward overeating and substandard nutrition, the U.S. government:

- Sets guidelines for minimum and recommended levels of nutrients, vitamins, and minerals

- Publishes an interactive website called ChooseMyPlate. gov to help individuals manage their daily nutrition, including calorie counting and energy expenditure through exercise

- Requires standardized nutrition labels on most packaged and processed foods

- Determines appropriate portion sizes, and

- Regulates the safety of our food supply

This massive effort is designed to improve our national wellness, and the many tools the USDA, FDA, National Academy of Sciences, and other governmental agencies provide can help you achieve a better diet, maintain a healthy weight, and help prevent several chronic diseases.

Follow Guidelines for Good Nutrition

There are so many parts to the government's nutritional advice to the public that they publish an overview—think of it as a cheat sheet for nutrition—called the *Dietary Guidelines for Americans*. The latest version came out in 2010 from the USDA and U.S. Department of Health and Human Services. We discuss the government's nutritional guidelines for specific sex, age, and ethnic groups later in the chapter. Here, we summarize the major recommendations in the 2010 version:

- *Balance calories to maintain weight.*
  - Balance the calories you take in from food with the calories your burn through activity and exercise. For most people, this means eating less and exercising more.
  - Learn about standard portion sizes so you can avoid oversized portions.

- *Increase certain foods and nutrients in your diet.*
  - Make at least half of your plate fruits and vegetables and eat a variety of produce types.
  - Consume at least half of your daily grains as whole grains and reduce refined grains.
  - Switch to fat-free or low-fat (one percent) dairy products.
  - Eat proteins low in solid (saturated) fats such as eggs, beans, seeds, soy, fish, lean meats, and poultry.
  - Eat more vegetables, whole grains, and fat-free or low-fat dairy products to increase potassium, dietary fiber, calcium, and vitamin D.

- *Decrease consumption of certain foods and components.*
  - Compare sodium in foods such as soup, bread, and frozen meals—and choose the foods with the lower numbers.
  - Drink water instead of sugary drinks.
  - Avoid *trans* fats and reduce saturated fat. Increase mono- and polyunsaturated oils to recommended levels for your sex, age, size, and activity level.
  - Reduce cholesterol.
  - Reduce added sugars and count the calories as "empty."
  - Reduce refined grains to less than half of your daily grains.
  - Limit alcohol consumption.

- *Build healthy eating patterns.*
  - Eat so that you can balance your nutrient and caloric needs over time.
  - Keep track of what you eat and drink and make sure they fit your long-term pattern.
  - Follow safety rules for food preparation and eating to avoid foodborne illnesses.

Several government scientific advisory boards serve up an "alphabet soup" of specific recommended daily minimum and maximum intakes for each type of nutrient (fat, carbohydrates, proteins), and for the various types of vitamins and minerals. The box What Do All Those Acronyms on the Food Label Mean? offers a short introduction to these **RDAs (Recommended Daily Allowances), DRVs (Daily Reference Values)**, and other daily intake recommendations. Sorting them out can be challenging, but it's easier if you keep in mind the simplified general guidelines just listed and concentrate on the **DVs (Daily Values)** listed on food labels.

RDAs (Recommended Dietary Allowances) A listing of the average daily nutrient intake level for a list of vitamins and minerals that meets most people's daily needs

DRVs (Daily Reference Values) Set of general intake guidelines of total fat, saturated fat, cholesterol, carbohydrates, protein, fiber, sodium, and potassium

DVs (Daily Values) A listing of all the important nutrients from two less inclusive government lists—the RDIs (Reference Daily Intakes) and the DRVs (Daily Reference Values); DVs are printed on all nutrition labels

What Do All Those Acronyms on Food Labels Mean?

- *DRI (Dietary Reference Intake)* is a listing of 26 nutrients essential to maintaining health. The DRI listing identifies recommended and maximum safe intake levels of the nutrients for healthy people, and identifies minimum levels needed to prevent deficiencies and diseases. DRIs are an umbrella category for several older classifications. The National Academy of Sciences Food and Nutrition Board publishes DRIs.

- *RDAs (Recommended Dietary Allowances)* are a listing of the average daily nutrient intake levels of vitamins and minerals that meet most people's daily needs. The National Academy of Sciences introduced RDAs in 1941 and updates the list periodically.

- *RDIs (Reference Daily Intakes)* are a listing of needed daily nutrients based on the National Academy of Science's RDAs. Tables 7.2 and 7.3 list the current RDIs for various vitamins and minerals.

- *DRVs (Daily Reference Values)* cover some nutrients the RDIs left out that proved to be important for daily dietary monitoring. They cover fat (including saturated fat and cholesterol), carbohydrates (including fiber), protein, sodium, and potassium. Table 7.4 lists the current DRVs for these nutrients.

- *DVs (Daily Values)* are the RDIs and the DRVs as printed on food labels. American consumers need to know what's in their food and what they should be eating without sorting through a bunch of confusing acronyms. Therefore, the U.S. Food and Drug Administration (FDA) invented a simpler term, DV, for all the important nutrients from the RDI and DRV lists to include on food labels. If you look on any food label, you will see a column labeled "% Daily Value."

You will probably come across the above-mentioned listings the most often. However, when looking into calorie requirements and safe levels of vitamins and minerals, you may also see references to a few other daily intakes:

- *EAR (Estimated Average Requirement)* is a listing of the intake that meets the requirement of half the healthy people of a certain gender at a certain life stage, such as adolescence, young adulthood, and so on.

- *AIs (Adequate Intakes)* are recommendations for daily nutrient intake where actual RDIs aren't known. Some of the values for vitamins and minerals are AIs because scientists have yet to discover exact daily requirements for those nutrients.

- *ULs (Tolerable Upper Intake Levels)* are recommendations for the highest levels that pose no risk when too much of a particular vitamin or mineral could be harmful.

- *EERs (Estimated Energy Requirements)* are calorie intake levels based on age, gender, height, weight, and activity level.

- *AMDRs (Acceptable Macronutrient Distribution Ranges)* are ranges of percentages for carbohydrate, fat, and protein consumption that provide adequate nutrition and reduces the risk of chronic diseases. For example, the AMDR for fat is 20 to 35 percent of total calories. For carbohydrate, it is 45 to 65 percent of total calories. For protein, it is 10 to 35 percent.

Reading Food Labels The U.S. government requires nutrition labels on the packages of most food products, including the familiar panel entitled "Nutrition Facts" (Figure 7.8). Reading and understanding these labels can help you judge both appropriate portion sizes and the nutritional merits of the foods you eat. By law, every food package must

- prominently identify the product, such as "multigrain cereal" or "fat-free milk";

- state the quantity of food product in the package by weight, volume, or number of pieces so you can judge the value of what you are buying;

- list all the ingredients by common name in order of amount from most to least by weight;

- give contact information for the food company in case you want more information;

- supply nutritional information in a standardized panel so you can compare and judge the dietary merits of the product before you buy it.

The Nutrition Facts panel provides the greatest concentration of information; it identifies a serving size and how many servings you'll get in a package. For example, the serving size of the soup in Figure 7.8 is 1 cup. The panel tells you how many calories each serving provides and how many of those calories come from fat. It lists daily recommended values (DVs) for nutrients that people should limit in their diets, including total fat, saturated fat, cholesterol, carbohydrates, and sodium. It also lists nutrients that many people should increase in their diets, such as vitamins A and C, calcium, and iron, giving the % Daily Value for each nutrient.

In 2010, First Lady Michelle Obama launched the "Nutrition Keys" front-of-package nutrition labeling initiative. She requested that the U.S. food industry create a new system of simplified front-of-package food labels that would act as a kind of "CliffsNotes" for quickly scanning and judging a food's nutrient content. In early 2011, some manufacturers responded by using streamlined front labels that highlight calories-per-serving information and the values per serving for three nutrients of interest for that type of food (Figure 7.9). A package of cookies, for example, might include calories, grams of saturated fat and sugar, and milligrams of sodium per serving. Other foods might highlight calories per serving

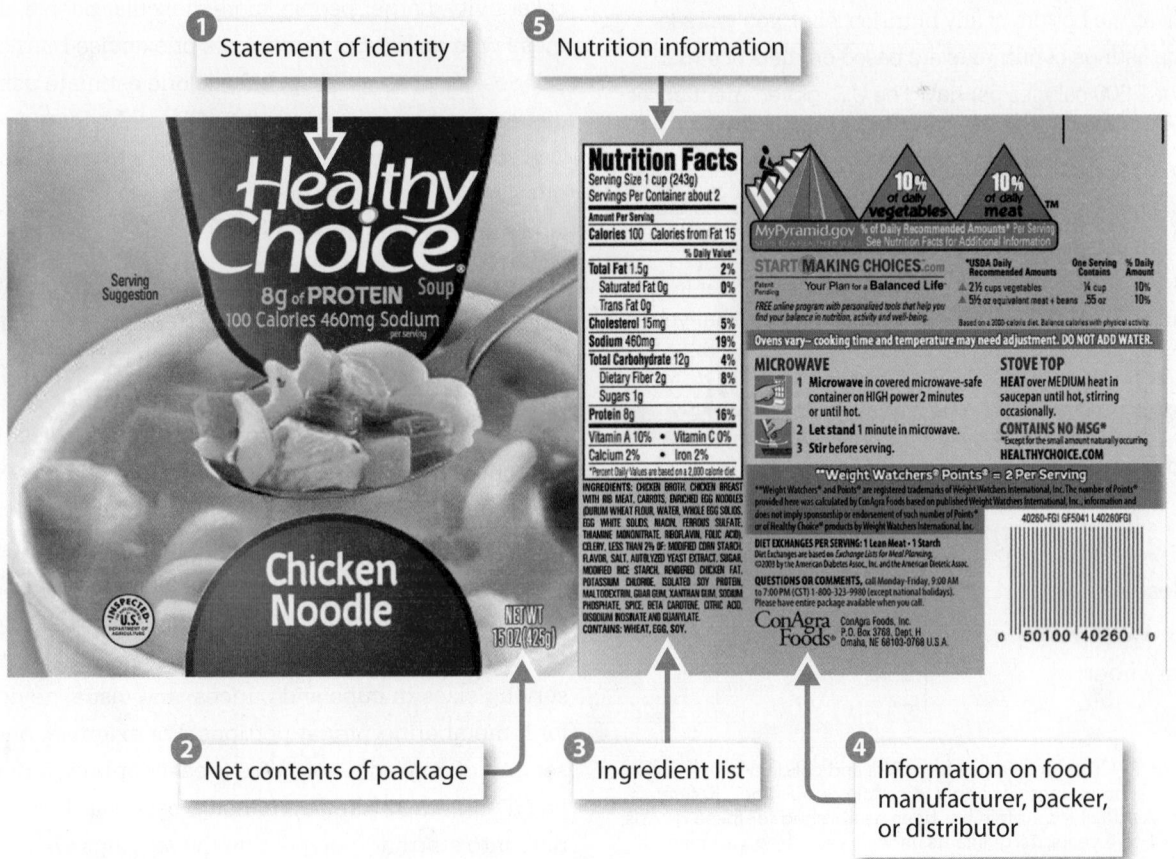

FIGURE 7.8 An important part of improving personal nutrition is reading food labels and understanding the information they provide.

Image © ConAgra Foods, Inc. Used with permission.

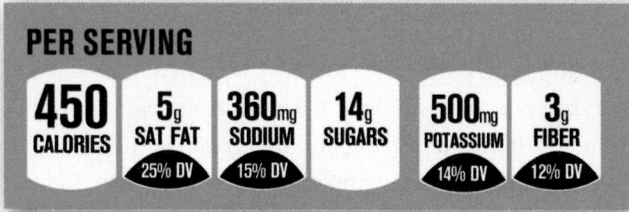

PER SERVING

| 450 CALORIES | 5g SAT FAT 25% DV | 360mg SODIUM 15% DV | 14g SUGARS | 500mg POTASSIUM 14% DV | 3g FIBER 12% DV |

FIGURE **7.9** One serving of this imaginary product has a whopping 450 calories, contains one-quarter of a day's saturated fat, one-sixth of a day's sodium, and the gram equivalent of three teaspoons of sugar. It does, however, also provide some potassium and fiber.

and three other types of nutrients such as vitamins A, C, or D; calcium; fiber; or protein content.

Without simplified front "keys" and more detailed side label panels, it would be easy for a consumer to eat half of a large bag of potato chips and think of that as one serving. Or to pick out a box of sweetened granola with 250 calories in one-half cup and mistakenly consider that food to be the nutritional equivalent of high-fiber, low-sugar multigrain flakes with only 100 calories in three-quarters of a cup. Individual consumers then must then provide the effort to read those labels, understand the issues behind the various values, and make intelligent choices.

Determining Your Calorie Needs If you read the fine print near the bottom of any nutrition label, you will see that the listings of nutrients are based on diets of either 2,000 or 2,500 calories per day. The U.S. government chose a 2,000 calorie-per-day diet as the basis for recommending the daily values of 65 grams of fat, 300 grams of carbohydrates, and 50 grams of protein (see Table 7.4). Does that mean you should be eating 2,000 calories per day regardless of whether you are 4' 9" tall and weigh 90 pounds, or 6' 9" and weigh 230 pounds? And does it mean that you

should adhere to those daily values regardless of your activity level? No, on both counts.

A round number like 2,000 calories makes it easy to extrapolate your actual calorie needs and serving sizes. It is also a maintenance level of energy input for a medium-sized person—about 150 pounds—who expends a medium amount of energy such as 30 minutes of moderate activity a few times per week. Food labels usually also provide a second level, 2,500 calories, as a calculation base for larger or more active people. Your actual calorie needs are determined by your size, age, gender, activity level, and medical conditions and your basal metabolic rate (BMR), which is partly inborn and partly activity-based.

Your BMR, the amount of energy your body uses in a given time period while resting or sleeping, accounts for 50 to 70 percent of your calorie consumption each day and allows you to maintain a steady heartbeat, a temperature of about 98.6°F, and so on. You use another 20 percent of your calories moving around and doing physical work such as walking, talking, carrying things, running, or sweeping the floor. Finally, eating and digesting food itself uses up about 5 to 10 percent of the calories you burn each day.

In determining calorie needs, the big variables are body size, BMR, and energy expenditure through physical activity. Larger people, more muscular people, and those who do hard physical work or exercise burn extra calories. You can get a specific calorie estimate using diet analysis tools such as www.ChooseMyPlate.gov. Use your own personal calorie estimate to calculate appropriate serving sizes and numbers when reading food labels and planning your diet.

Understanding Portion Sizes One reason that Americans eat an average of nearly 3,500 calories per day rather than the world average of 2,400 to 2,600 is that our typical food portions are too big. The U.S. government recommends that each of us eat a certain number of servings each day from each food group based on standard serving sizes. Most Americans, however, don't know how to recognize standard portions. It helps to have some visual aids for estimating proper serving sizes and recognizing the right amount of food. Figure 7.10 illustrates various foods, healthy serving sizes in cups and ounces, and visual devices for remembering proper portions. For example, one serving of cooked whole-wheat pasta or brown rice is half a cup, about the size of half a baseball. This figure puts into startling perspective the servings we receive at most restaurants: the mountains of pasta, the big wedges of pie, the stacks of plate-sized pancakes, the

TABLE **7.4** Daily Reference Values (DRVs)	
Food Component	DRV
Fat	65 grams (g)
Saturated fatty acids	20 g
Cholesterol	300 milligrams (mg)
Total carbohydrate	300 g
Dietary fiber	25 g
Protein*	50 g

(Based on 2,000 calories a day for adults and children over 4 only)
* DRV for protein does not apply to certain populations; Reference Daily Intake (RDI) for protein has been established for these groups: children 1 to 4 years: 16 g; infants under 1 year: 14 g; pregnant women: 60 g; nursing mothers: 65 g.

Adapted from U.S. FDA Food Labeling Guide, www.fda.gov/FoodLabelingGuide; (revised October 2009).

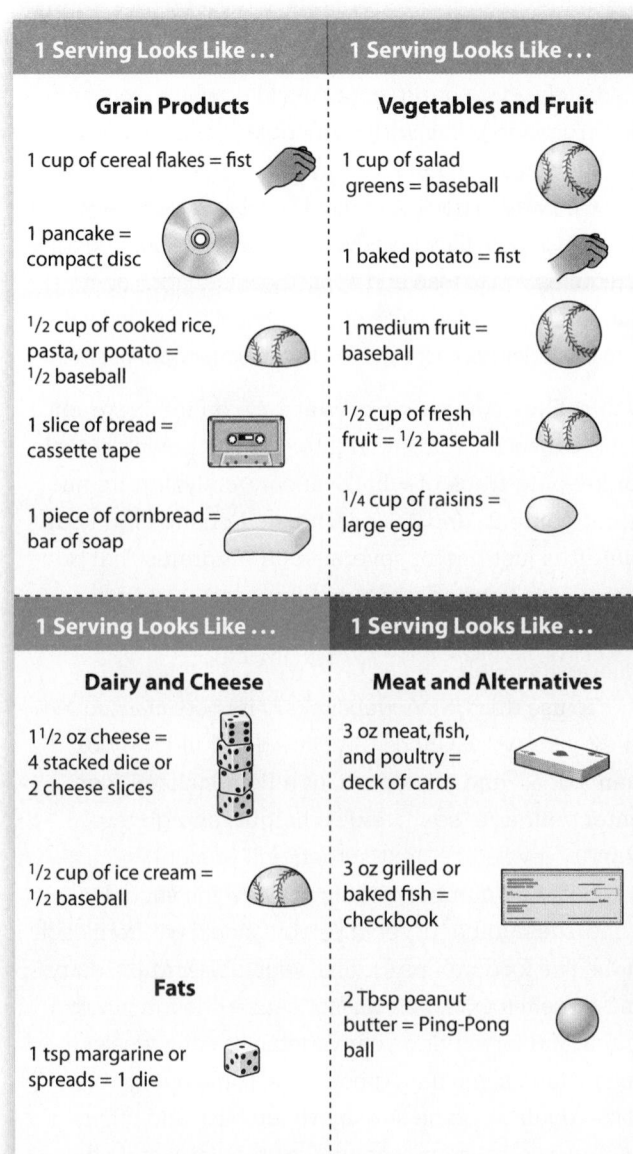

1 Serving Looks Like ...	1 Serving Looks Like ...
Grain Products	**Vegetables and Fruit**
1 cup of cereal flakes = fist	1 cup of salad greens = baseball
1 pancake = compact disc	1 baked potato = fist
1/2 cup of cooked rice, pasta, or potato = 1/2 baseball	1 medium fruit = baseball
1 slice of bread = cassette tape	1/2 cup of fresh fruit = 1/2 baseball
1 piece of cornbread = bar of soap	1/4 cup of raisins = large egg

1 Serving Looks Like ...	1 Serving Looks Like ...
Dairy and Cheese	**Meat and Alternatives**
1 1/2 oz cheese = 4 stacked dice or 2 cheese slices	3 oz meat, fish, and poultry = deck of cards
1/2 cup of ice cream = 1/2 baseball	3 oz grilled or baked fish = checkbook
Fats	2 Tbsp peanut butter = Ping-Pong ball
1 tsp margarine or spreads = 1 die	

FIGURE **7.10** One of the challenges of following a healthy diet is judging how big a portion size should be and how many servings you are really eating. The comparisons on this card can help you recall what a standard food serving looks like. For easy reference, photocopy or cut out this card, fold on the dotted line, and keep it in your wallet. You can even laminate it for long-term use.

Source: National Heart, Lung and Blood Institute, "Serving Size Card," http://hp2010.nhlbihin.net/portion/servingcard7.pdf (accessed April 2010).

bucket-sized soft drinks, and the other servings we accept and expect as normal.

Using Food Guides The USDA has issued Food Guides since the 1940s to help Americans select healthy diets as defined by contemporary nutritionists. They have used wheels, rectangles, pyramids, and most recently a divided plate to summarize and illustrate their recommendations simply for the public.[30] The plate icon introduced in 2011 uses segments of certain colors and sizes to symbolize the kinds and relative amounts of foods

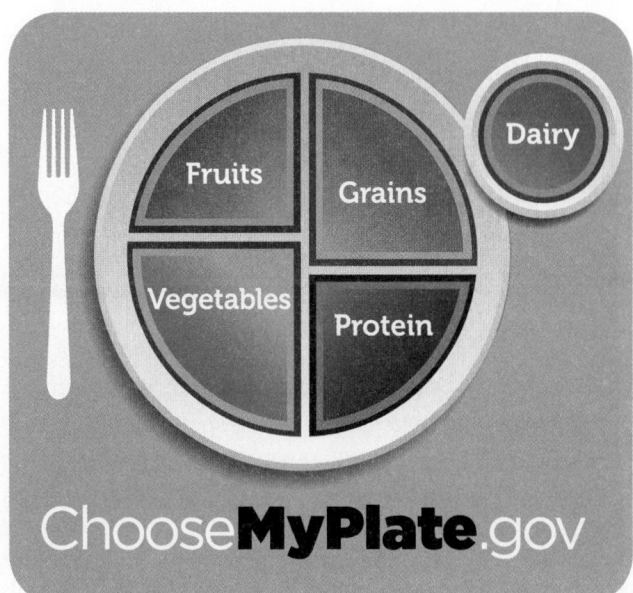

FIGURE **7.11** The ChooseMyPlate.gov icon shows the proper proportion of each food group in a healthy diet. The supporting website provides each visitor with an individualized recommendation for daily servings and portion sizes of each food type.

and nutrients (fruits, vegetables, grains, dairy, protein) consumers should select each day (Figure 7.11). The supporting website (www.ChooseMyPlate.gov) provides specific personalized diet analysis and recommendations based on your sex, age, size, and activity level.

Nongovernment nutritionists have published several alternative food plans. A pyramid published by Harvard Medical School's Department of Nutrition recommends that you minimize all sugars and refined or low-fiber carbohydrates such as white flour, white rice, pasta, and peeled potatoes. It also discourages the consumption of red meat, butter, cheese, and other sources of saturated fat. At the same time, it encourages consumption of vegetables, whole grains, nuts, beans, and unsaturated fats from plant oils. On the Internet, you can find alternative pyramids for Mediterranean, Asian, Latin American, and vegetarian eating patterns.

Acquire Skills to Improve Your Nutrition

Do you know the nutritional value of your diet? Do you know how to find out? A few simple skills will help you analyze and improve your diet. Developing a habit of quickly checking seven items from the typical food label can greatly improve your daily nutrition. **Lab 7.1** will encourage this habit. Here are the seven you should look for on a regular basis:

- *What is the normal serving size?* Let's say you bought a bag of corn chips and were planning to eat the whole thing. The label, however, says it contains 8.5 servings. That provides a valuable hint about the calorie density of that food, not to mention the amount of fat and sodium in the whole bag. If you decide to eat just one serving, you can count out your seven or eight chips and enjoy them—slowly!

- *What is the main ingredient?* If it is water, corn syrup, or enriched (translation, "white") flour, are you getting your money's worth—and good nutrition?

- *How do the total fats and saturated fats compare to the listed daily values?* Just 1 tablespoon of butter, for example, will provide one-third of your DV for saturated fat. Do you really want to consume that much fat in one pat?

- *What is the* trans *fat content?* Reduce or eliminate *trans* fats because of their potentially negative health consequences.

- *How does the sodium compare to % Daily Value?* People diagnosed with high blood pressure, diabetes, kidney disease, and certain other conditions must limit sodium levels. Others should limit sodium to within recommended levels.

- *Does the food provide any fiber?* If not, could you substitute something that does—for example, baby spinach leaves instead of iceberg lettuce in a salad, or a fresh apple instead of canned pineapple, or brown rice instead of white?

- *Finally, what is the % Daily Value of sugars?* Technically, there is no DV for sugars or other sweeteners, but you can see the content in grams listed on food labels. Sugars are common in cereals, sauces, and other processed foods and add empty calories that you could devote to more filling and nutritious foods. For example, instead of eating a cup of raisin bran with 19 grams of sugar and 188 calories of food energy, try choosing one cup of bran flakes with only 5 grams of sugar and 122 calories, and then adding a cup of sliced, fresh strawberries (high in volume, flavor, vitamin C, and fiber and containing only 55 calories).

Keeping a Food Diary Did you have three servings of fruit yesterday or two? 200 calories of fats and sugars or 600? If you are like most people, you can only remember a highlight or two from yesterday's meals, and not much of what you ate the other days of the week. To get an accurate idea of whether your diet is nutrient rich or

Worksheet 19
Food Log

poor and whether it provides enough fiber, try to record snacks and meals for a few days. This is best done immediately after eating, not hours later when you have discarded wrappers with nutrient labels or lost count of serving sizes.

One way to track your diet is to fill in a food diary. Keeping a food diary helps you learn to judge serving sizes. It requires you to read and apply the information on nutrition labels, learn the value of your typical foods, and substitute healthier items for the foods you usually choose.

Using Diet Analysis Software An online program such as www.ChooseMyPlate.gov is a powerful tool for keeping track of what you eat, analyzing its nutrient content, and making needed changes in your diet. It is just one of several such programs that can streamline your efforts to achieve better nutrition. Many smart phone "apps" help you keep track of calories, as well.

To use this USDA website and its personalized features, visit www.ChooseMyPlate.gov. Find the box "I want to…," and click on "Get a Personalized Plan." Enter your age, sex, weight, height, and general activity level. The next screen will present you with the number of daily calories you should consume; the number of servings you should eat from each of the five food groups (grains, vegetables, fruits, dairy, and protein foods); pointers for eating enough whole grains and for varying your vegetables each week so you include some dark green ones, some orange ones, some legumes, some starchy vegetables, and others; a reminder to consume enough healthful oils; and advice on limiting the calories in fats and sugars. You can then print out a personalized food plan based on your individual information. Beyond the personalized plan, the site also provides these features:

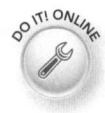

- You can use a meal tracking worksheet to keep tabs on each food you ate on a given day and save this for comparison with additional days.

- You can use the ChooseMyPlate Tracker to assess the nutrients—calories, fats, carbohydrates, vitamins, and so on—in specific foods such as a tuna fish sandwich or a slice of pizza (see **Lab 7.2**).

- You can make a data bank of nutritional information for foods or meals you eat routinely—say, your typical breakfast of cereal, juice, and toast—so you don't have to enter them individually each time.

- You can do a more detailed analysis of your physical activities to get an estimate of calories burned as you do a particular exercise for a certain period of time.

- Finally, you can keep track of trends in your diet and physical activity over time if you are making changes to benefit your fitness and wellness.

Choose the method—online or on paper—that works best for you, as that's the one you'll stick with.

Adopt the Whole Foods Habit

Analyzing your daily foods for calories and nutrients can help you achieve nutritional wellness. So can a simpler approach: making each bite you take more nutritious by choosing primarily **whole foods**, or dietary items produced with the minimum of refining, preservatives, or processing for quick preparation.

Going Green

Worksheet 18
Grocery
Shopping List

Decades ago, virtually all food was "whole," or real and unchanged. Many packaged foods today, however, have long lists of ingredients and additives that reduce the cost of ingredients, extend shelf life, intensify flavor, and make food preparation easier. People have learned to like the taste and convenience of processed foods, but these products tend to contain hidden fats and sugars, relatively large amounts of sodium, and various additives and preservatives. They also tend to have less naturally occurring fiber and fewer vitamins. Let's compare a medium-sized fresh apple, for example, with one cup of processed, preserved, and dried apple slices. The fresh apple contains about 95 calories, 17 grams of carbohydrates, 3 grams of fiber, and 13 grams of sugars. The cup of dried apple slices (derived from two or more whole apples) contain 209 calories, 51 grams of carbohydrates, 7 grams of fiber, and 49 grams of sugars, and may contain added sucrose or corn syrup and preservatives such as sulfur.

Shifting from a diet heavy in processed foods to one rich in whole foods doesn't mean you have to sacrifice good taste or feel hungry or dissatisfied. In fact, you will probably find snacks and meals very filling and delicious if you choose as many foods as possible that are nutrient-dense, high in volume but low in calories, high in fiber, and rich in antioxidants.

Nutrient-Dense Foods You may have heard people talk about foods—sugar, for example—that provide only "empty calories." What they mean is that such foods provide calories for energy without supplying other healthful nutrients. By contrast, **nutrient-dense foods** provide rich sources of vitamins, minerals, antioxidants, and fiber and minimize saturated fat, added sugars, sodium, and refined carbohydrates. Choosing nutrient-dense foods means striving to maximize the food value of each and every meal and snack you consume.

To see what this means in a practical way, compare two small meals—a glass of cola and a hot dog versus a glass of low-fat milk and a small serving of salmon. The cola provides 105 calories, all from refined carbohydrates. In about the same number of calories, the milk provides 8 grams

whole foods Dietary items produced and consumed with the minimum of processing (refining, adding preservatives, or altering form for quick preparation)

nutrient-dense foods Foods or beverages that provide a high level of nutrients and thus maximize the nutritional value of each meal and snack consumed

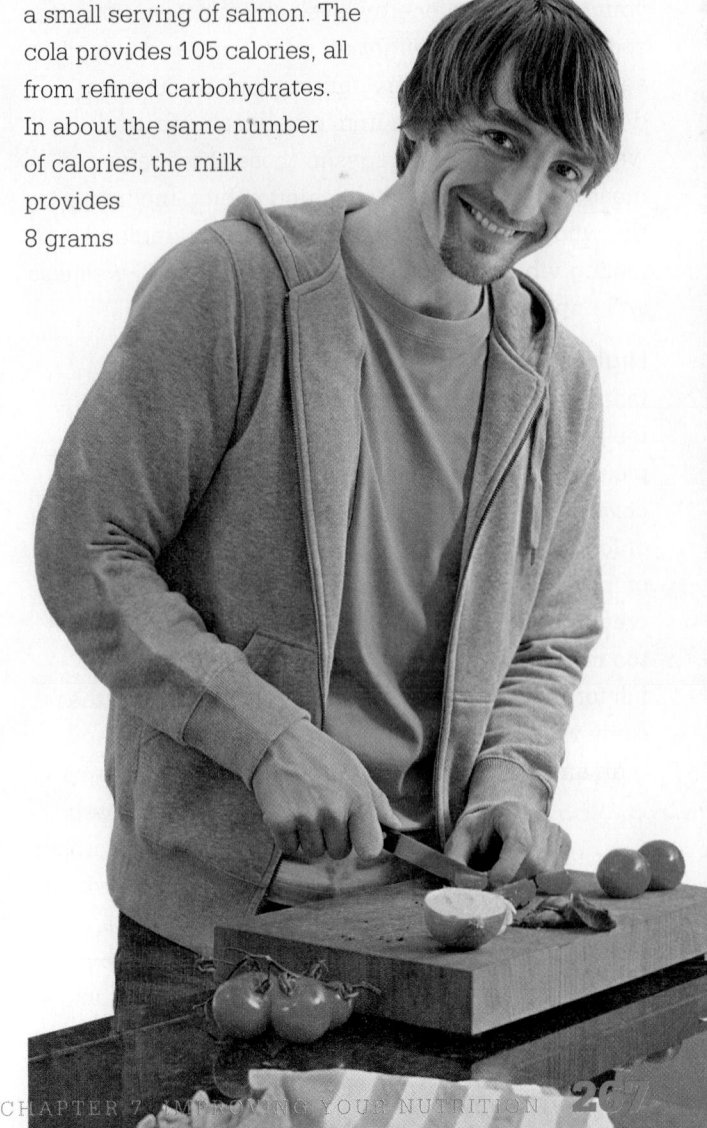

of protein along with vitamin D and calcium. The cola is nutrient-poor; the milk is nutrient-dense.

Now compare the hot dog and salmon. A hot dog on a white-bread bun supplies 420 calories. It contains more than a whole day's recommended amount of saturated fat, 9 grams of protein, most of a day's allotted sodium, and refined white flour lacking much fiber. In contrast, a serving of salmon provides fewer than 200 calories, 10 grams of heart-healthy omega-3 fatty acids, twice as much protein, and a small fraction of the sodium. The hot dog has fewer healthful nutrients while the salmon is nutrient-dense.

Learning to reach for nutrient-dense foods every time you get hungry will greatly benefit your lifelong fitness and wellness. If your diet consists primarily of processed foods such as pastries, coffee drinks, pizza, hamburgers, and cola, you may not even know what wellness feels like! Why should you care about eating too many calories, too much saturated fat, too many refined carbohydrates, and too much sodium? Because dietary excesses can affect your appearance, energy level, athletic performance, social life, ability to fight off infections, and overall sense of well-being. Try shifting toward nutrient-dense foods and away from empty calories, and watch for positive changes in those short-term measures. Focus on establishing habits, including the whole foods habit, that keep you looking and feeling vibrantly well today and your lifelong wellness will improve, too.

High-Volume, Low-Calorie Foods We eat for many reasons, but the primary one is *satiety*: a feeling of fullness and the physical and emotional pleasure it brings. Nutrition researchers have discovered that each of us has a characteristic weight of food that we eat in a day. You can eat that weight of food in candy bars, potato chips, steak, and ice cream, but you will be getting too few nutrients and too many calories and you probably wouldn't feel full for very long between meals. You could eat that same weight of food in celery, iceberg lettuce, and bran and still get too few nutrients, but the volume would help keep you full. The proper goal is somewhere in between: a filling, calorie-appropriate diet

that also emphasizes nutrient density. Relatively recent nutritional research has shown that eating nutritious foods with more volume due to higher air or water content can help people feel full and satisfied longer.[31] This is especially helpful for dieters or for people who want to maintain their weight and not gain more.

Foods with high contents of water, fiber, or protein tend to keep you full and satisfied longer, while those with high contents of fat, sugar, or refined carbohydrates leave you feeling hungry sooner. However, the water must be in the food (as in soups, fruits, and vegetables) and not just in a glass accompanying your meal. Apparently, your brain's satiety center knows the difference and isn't fooled by drinking water. Figure 7.12 compares two sandwiches with approximately the same number of calories, but very different ingredients. Table 7.5 lists familiar foods by calorie density.

High-Fiber Foods Fiber adds bulk and, often, a chewy quality to food. Both help satisfy hunger better and for longer periods. Soluble fiber such as that in oats, barley, and apples, for example, lowers LDL cholesterol. Grains that are intact (like brown rice or bulgur wheat) instead of finely ground (as in whole wheat flour) have a lower glycemic index. High-fiber foods also improve the passage of digested material through the digestive tract.

Antioxidant-Rich Foods *Free radicals* are molecules with unpaired electrons that the body produces in excess when it is overly stressed. Free radicals can damage or kill healthy cells, cell proteins, or genetic material in cells. **Antioxidants** produce enzymes that scavenge free radicals, slow their formation, and actually repair oxidative stress damage. Thus, the theory goes that if you

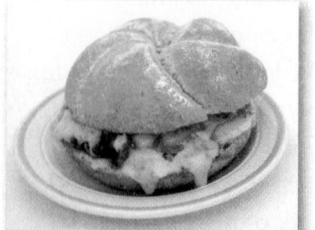 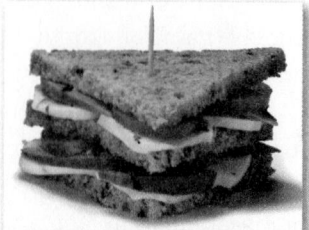

(a)   **(b)**

FIGURE **7.12** These two sandwiches have approximately the same number of calories (300), but one (a) is small and filled with saturated fat. It contains mayonnaise, butter, cheese, and bacon on a white roll. The other sandwich (b) is large, high-volume, and rich in fiber and vitamins. It contains whole wheat bread, tomato, lettuce, green and red peppers, and cheese.

antioxidants Compounds in foods that help protect the body against the damaging effects of oxygen derivatives called *free radicals*

TABLE **7.5** Comparing Calorie Density in Common Foods

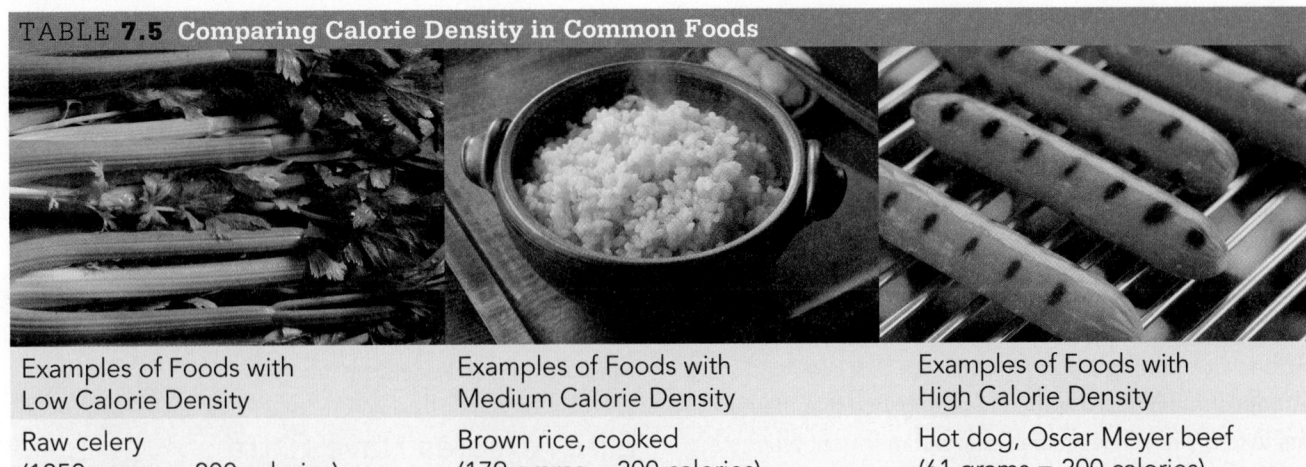

Examples of Foods with Low Calorie Density	Examples of Foods with Medium Calorie Density	Examples of Foods with High Calorie Density
Raw celery (1250 grams = 200 calories)	Brown rice, cooked (179 grams = 200 calories)	Hot dog, Oscar Meyer beef (61 grams = 200 calories)
Watermelon (666 grams = 200 calories)	Enriched spaghetti, cooked (126 grams = 200 calories)	French fries, McDonald's (59 grams = 200 calories)
Raw broccoli (588 grams = 200 calories)	Chicken breast, roasted (121 grams = 200 calories)	Potato chips, plain salted (37 grams = 200 calories)
Red or green grapes (290 grams = 200 calories)	Salmon, cooked, Alaskan wild (110 grams = 200 calories)	Peanut butter, smooth salted (34 grams = 200 calories)

Data from U.S. Department of Agriculture, Agricultural Research Service. 2007. USDA National Nutrient Database for Standard Reference, Release 20. Nutrient Data Laboratory Home Page, http://www.ars.usda.gov/ba/bhnrc/ndl

consume lots of antioxidants, you will nullify or greatly reduce the negative effects of oxidative stress. Among the more commonly cited nutrients touted as providing a protective effect are vitamin C, vitamin E, beta-carotene and other carotenoids, and the mineral selenium.

How valid is the theory? To date, many claims about the benefits of antioxidants in reducing the risk of heart disease, improving vision, and slowing the aging process have not been fully investigated; conclusive statements about their true benefits are difficult to make. Large, longitudinal epidemiological studies support the hypothesis that antioxidants in foods, mostly fruits and vegetables (Figure 7.13), help protect against cognitive decline and risk of Parkinson's disease. However, because of problems with study design and difficulties in isolating dietary effects from supplement effects, it is difficult to assess overall benefits of antioxidants.[32]

Some studies indicate that when people's diets include foods rich in vitamin C, they seem to develop fewer cancers, but other studies detect no effect from dietary vitamin C.[33] Recent studies indicate that high-dose vitamin C given intravenously, rather than orally, may be effective in treating cancer and providing protection from diseases affecting the central nervous system.[34] Early studies seemed to show that vitamin E had antioxidant effects that could help prevent heart disease and cancer. Large trials involving hundreds of people

taking vitamin E supplements, however, have shown very mixed results, with some indicating no benefit.[35] The vitamin E in foods does seem to help protect the cell membranes of red blood cells and the delicate surface lining our lungs.

Phytochemicals Plants make thousands of compounds collectively called *phytochemicals* (meaning literally "plant chemicals"), many of which have antioxidant properties. Fruit, flowers, and plant leaves form a bright palette of colors, in part because plants can generate pigments with antioxidant properties such as *beta-carotene* (yellow and orange pigments), *lycopene* (red

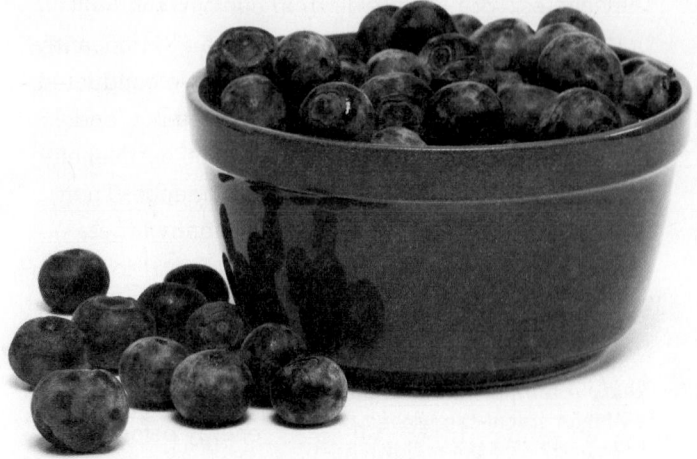

FIGURE **7.13** Fruits and vegetables such as blueberries and kale are high in antioxidants.

pigments), and *lutein,* found in various green, red, yellow, and orange foods.[36]

Most people love the idea of "magic bullets"—pills that will quickly solve their health problems with no other effort. Many people have begun taking antioxidant supplements despite a lack of evidence for their effectiveness in supplement form. Most nutrition researchers recommend getting your antioxidants from nutrient-dense foods or from multivitamin supplements.[37]

Foods Containing Folate In 1998, the U.S. Food and Drug Administration (FDA) started requiring food manufacturers to fortify all bread, cereal, rice, and macaroni products sold in the United States with **folate** (also called *folic acid*). Folate is a form of vitamin B that participates in the development of the spinal cord. Folate also helps break down the compound homocysteine, which is produced as the body digests meat and other high-protein foods. By helping break down homocysteine, folate may also protect against cardiovascular disease, heart attacks, and strokes.[38]

Do I Need Special Nutrition for Exercise?

Fitness requires physical activity, but does it also require a special diet? Active people may need some extra nutrients—a little more protein, perhaps, and some extra carbohydrates for fast energy and endurance. But big imbalances in the major nutrients, such as those caused by a high-protein diet or a low-carbohydrate regimen, cannot support improved fitness.

Most Exercisers Can Follow General Nutritional Guidelines

Exercisers often look for an "edge" and wonder what they can eat, drink, or swallow in pill form that will help them get into shape faster or better. Significantly, sports physiologists and nutritionists have conducted hundreds of studies of recreational, collegiate, and professional athletes, trying to determine optimal energy and nutrient levels for peak performance. Their findings may surprise and disappoint many fitness enthusiasts: they closely follow general nutritional guidelines with only a few minor adjustments.

folate A form of vitamin B that is vital for spinal cord development and helps break down homocysteine as the body digests proteins

should provide up to about 55 to 65 percent of daily calories.[39] Restricting carbohydrates can impede your fitness efforts by leaving you energy-deprived. Sugars can give a little energy boost but can also cause a rise in insulin and a drop in blood sugar that produces fatigue.

Proteins For moderate strengthening and endurance exercise, most of us need about 0.75 to 0.8 gram of protein per kilogram of body weight per day. Protein does not in itself help build muscle. Only activity, including weight training, adds new muscle.

Elite Athletes Have Extra Nutritional Needs

While most exercisers can get complete nutrition from a balanced diet of nutrient-dense foods, some elite athletes—those with the potential for intercollegiate, Olympic, or professional sports—do need to modify their eating patterns for better training and performance.

Calories People in regular training for competitive sports need extra calories. Athletes often have greater muscle mass than the average person, and muscle tissue consumes more calories than fat tissue, even at rest. A tall young man training with a football or basketball team, for example, could require 5,000 calories or more daily. High activity levels sustained for long periods—the running during a soccer match, for example—also require extra fuel. About 55 to 65 percent of that extra athletic fuel should come from complex carbohydrates—bread, pasta, cereals, grains, vegetables, and fruits.[40] Some nutritionists recommend up to 70 percent carbohydrates for sustained high-level activities.

Endurance events requiring heavy exertion for more than 90 minutes use two types of internal body fuels, glycogen and fat. Your muscles can store about 90 minutes' worth of glycogen, and additional storage in your liver can fuel a few more minutes of exercise. After that, your body uses its own fat to fuel activity (Figure 7.14). Endurance athletes such as marathon runners, swimmers, and soccer players often consume 60 or 70 percent of their diet in complex carbohydrates starting two to three days before an athletic event to store sufficient glycogen and fat. Consuming five to seven grams of carbohydrates per kilogram of body weight per day is usually enough for general training, while seven to 10 grams/kilogram/day will fuel endurance training and strenuous one-time events.

Pre- and Post-event Meals Trainers usually instruct athletes to drink plenty of water, to eat complex carbohydrates three or four hours before an event, and to avoid

Carbohydrates The best source of energy before and during exercise is carbohydrates; they

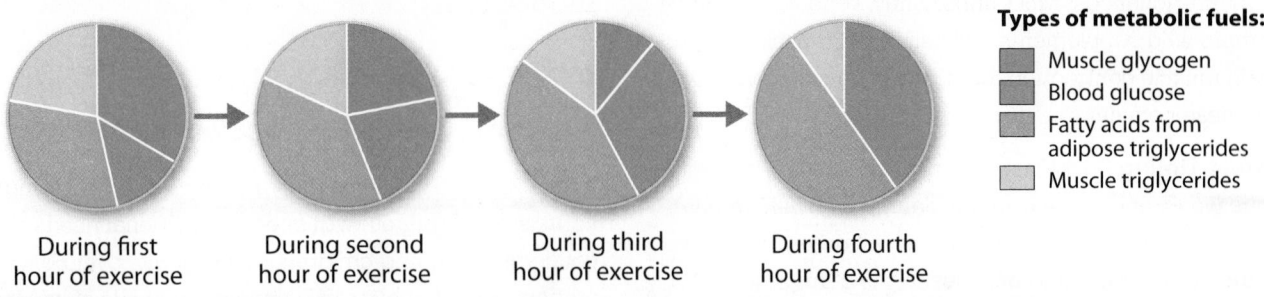

Types of metabolic fuels:

- Muscle glycogen
- Blood glucose
- Fatty acids from adipose triglycerides
- Muscle triglycerides

During first hour of exercise → During second hour of exercise → During third hour of exercise → During fourth hour of exercise

FIGURE **7.14** If you exercise for less than one hour, your body uses mostly glycogen and fatty acids (triglycerides) stored in your muscles. If you exercise for four hours, the fuel ratios shift dramatically and your activity is mainly powered by blood sugar and the breakdown of fat (adipose) tissue.

proteins, fats, refined sugars, caffeine, and gas-producing foods in the pregame meal. They recommend avoiding protein, because protein takes more time to digest and can lead to increased urination and dehydration. Likewise, fats and oils are slow to digest. Sugar is on the list because it induces a surge of insulin in the blood and later, during the event, can cause an energy dip. Caffeine can lead to increased urination and dehydration and to an accelerated heartbeat. Gas-producing foods can upset digestion.

Most athletes need water and additional carbohydrates during the event, and many choose sports drinks diluted with water to sustain energy and provide sufficient hydration. You can learn more about this by visiting the American College of Sports Medicine's website (www.acsm.org) to view their guidelines on exercise and fluid replacement.[41]

Selecting foods for post-performance meals is also important to help restore the muscles' energy supply. After a training or performance session you should eat simple and complex carbohydrates as soon as possible.

Is the popular practice of carbo-loading necessary? If you define *carbo-loading* as eating one huge starch meal the night before an athletic event, then no, it is not necessary or desirable. This kind of consumption can cause the body to retain water, the muscles to feel stiff the next day, and the athlete to feel slow and sluggish when the event starts.

If you define *carbo-loading* as eating 55 to 65 percent of your calories as complex carbohydrates at every meal for two to three days before an event, then it is desirable because it can load the muscles with glycogen for sustained activity if previous carbohydrate intake was low. Manipulating the pre-exercise diet with more or less sugar, fat, or protein seems to have little effect on most people's performance.[42]

Vitamins and Minerals The body's energy production and use requires B vitamins; bone- and blood-building require iron and calcium; sweating causes the loss of sodium and potassium that must be replenished during or after events. A balanced diet provides most athletes with enough vitamins and minerals to meet recommended intakes.

Supplements Optimal muscle growth and strength gain do not require nutritional supplements. Most competitive athletes in high school and college do take various kinds of supplements, including megadoses of certain vitamins and minerals as well as purported muscle builders.[43] Where there is no deficiency to start with, these mega-doses provide little or no benefit to performance.[44] The popular creatine monohydrate is chemically related to a natural substance called *creatine phosphate,* which helps fuel muscle contraction. Vendors claim creatine monohydrate helps build muscle, increases energy to improve performance, and delays muscle fatigue. Objective scientific studies suggest that taking creatine orally may cause muscles to temporarily retain more water, and this may boost short-term performance under anaerobic conditions. Thus, it may pump up the muscles a bit so they feel bigger, but it is not helpful for endurance events. And it does not do what many athletes are hoping for: build permanently bigger muscles. This requires regular physical strength training.

Also popular are individual, concentrated amino acid supplements such as taurine, arginine, glutamine, and leucine. Eating protein-rich foods provides these very same building blocks but in safe concentrations and in naturally occurring mixtures of multiple amino acids. In contrast, supplements provide artificially high concentrations of individual amino acids that may block your body's absorption of the full amino acid spectrum.

What's more, amino acid supplements can become contaminated and are far more expensive than eating protein-rich foods. Most importantly, vendors claim that amino acid supplements will help build muscle and sustain muscle contraction, but there is no good evidence of these benefits.

Meal Timing People use the term *meal timing* in various ways, and some trainers claim that *when* you eat fats, proteins, and carbohydrates will determine how quickly you can build muscles in the gym or how well you can sustain activity during a long bike ride. Carbo-loading and pre- and post-event meals are all forms of meal timing. So are regimens that instruct you to eat proteins early in the day, carbohydrates at lunch, and so on.

Research shows that the most significant thing about meal timing is the effect on your appetite. Skipping meals, getting ravenously hungry, then "gorging" most of your day's calories at dinner is far more likely to cause fat accumulation than "grazing" on five or six small meals throughout the day. Sumo wrestlers deliberately apply this principle to put on hundreds of pounds

• •

casestudy

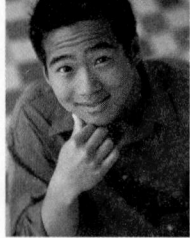

CHAU

"I'm not an 'athlete,' but I do like sports. I've never worried too much about supplementing my diet with extras. I figure as long as I eat enough to feel satisfied, my body's getting what it needs. Some of my friends—like Tom, who's a cross-country runner—are always drinking sports drinks and eating energy bars. I've also noticed Tom often has a pasta dinner two days before a big run, and then he will eat a lighter meal the night before the race. He's also pretty strict about taking a multivitamin every day. It makes me wonder if I should start taking vitamins too."

THINK! How do Chau's and Tom's nutritional needs differ? Should Chau begin taking vitamin supplements? Why would Tom eat pasta two nights before a big run, instead of the night before the race?

ACT! Analyze your own physical activity. Could you benefit from consuming more or fewer calories? Do you need to add nutrients to your diet, and if so which ones?

of fat. If they spread their daily 6,000 calories into five or six meals instead of two, they would weigh up to 25 percent less![45]

Do I Have Special Nutritional Needs?

In its *Dietary Guidelines for Americans*, the USDA highlights several groups with special nutritional needs and concerns, including children, teens, adults over 50, vegetarians, and diabetics. We review the needs of vegetarians and diabetics here.

Vegetarians Must Monitor Their Nutrient Intake

More and more people today are choosing partial or strict vegetarian diets. Between five and 15 percent of all Americans claim to be one of the following, arranged in order from the strictest and most exclusive of animal products to the least: Strict *vegetarians* (also called *vegans*) avoid all foods of animal origin, including dairy products and eggs; *lacto-vegetarians* avoid animal flesh but eat dairy products; *ovo-vegetarians* avoid animal flesh and dairy products but eat eggs; *lacto-ovo-vegetarians* consume both dairy products and eggs; or *semi-vegetarians,* consume fish and/or poultry but no red meat.

Vegetarian diets have certain benefits.[46] Most people who follow a balanced vegetarian diet weigh less than non-vegetarians of similar height. Most also have healthier cholesterol levels, less constipation and diarrhea, and a lower risk of heart disease. Research indicates that vegetarians may also have a lower risk for colon and breast cancers.[47] It is not clear whether these lower risks are due to their vegetarian diets per se or to some combination of lifestyle factors such as eating less saturated fat, avoiding smoking, and exercising more.

Despite their benefits, vegetarian diets can have deficiencies; with careful food choices, however, vegetarians can avoid deficiencies. Lacto-ovo vegetarians who eat dairy products and small amounts of chicken or fish are seldom nutrient-deficient. Vegans can get enough essential amino acids through complementary combinations of plant products (review Figure 7.3 on page 244). Lacto-vegetarians usually get enough vitamins D and B_{12} from dairy products, while strict vegans can develop deficiencies. Fortified products such as soy milk can usually provide enough of these vitamins. Vegans are sometimes deficient in vitamin B_2 (riboflavin) since

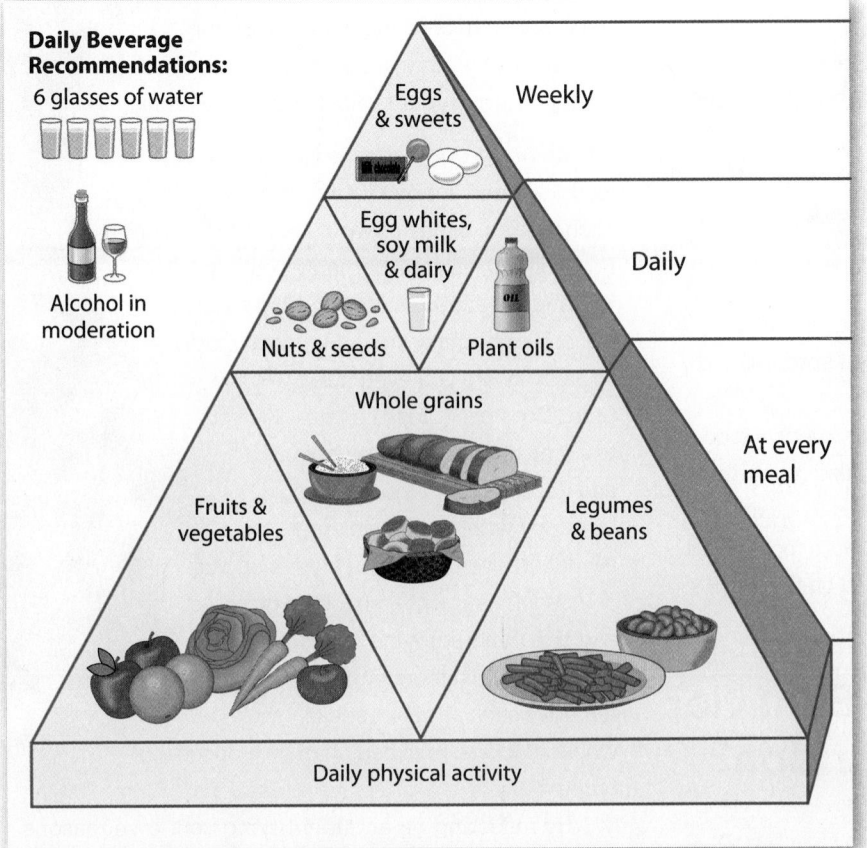

Daily Beverage Recommendations:

6 glasses of water

Alcohol in moderation

Eggs & sweets — Weekly

Egg whites, soy milk & dairy — Daily

Nuts & seeds / Plant oils

Whole grains

Fruits & vegetables / Legumes & beans — At every meal

Daily physical activity

FIGURE **7.15** Vegetarians must be careful to get enough protein, calcium, B vitamins, and other nutrients; they can do this by following this pyramid as a food guide.

Source: Oldways' Vegetarian Diet Pyramid. Copyright © 2000 Oldways Preservation and Exchange Trust. Used by permission, www.oldwayspt.org.

it is found mainly in meat, eggs, and dairy products. They can get enough B_2, however, by eating generous amounts of broccoli, asparagus, almonds, and fortified cereals. Because meat is rich in iron and dairy products are rich in calcium, vegans who avoid both can develop deficiencies of these minerals. Solutions include choosing mineral-rich plant foods (see Table 7.3) and/or taking multivitamin/mineral supplements.

In general, vegans can stay in excellent health by eating a wide variety of grains, legumes, fruits, vegetables, and seeds each day. Figure 7.15 shows a vegetarian food pyramid.

Those with Diabetes Must Reduce Carbohydrates

Anyone diagnosed with type 1 or type 2 diabetes will receive specific information from medical providers about both necessary drug treatments and dietary changes. Because diabetes is a disorder of blood-sugar regulation, patients usually must cut back on sweets

and desserts, both to reduce surges of sugar in the blood and to control obesity, which can lead to and intensify diabetes. Choosing foods with a lower rather than higher glycemic index (see page 248) is also beneficial, and this usually means less-processed foods and reduced fat content. The American Diabetes Association advises diabetics to eats lots of non-starchy vegetables and fruits, to choose whole grains over processed grain products, to include beans and lentils in the diet, to eat fish two to three times per week, to choose lean meats and nonfat dairy products, to drink water and diet drinks instead of sugary drinks, to avoid saturated fats and *trans* fats during cooking, and to watch portion sizes.[48]

Good Food Safety Practices Are for Everyone

Sometimes people think they have the flu when it is actually "food poisoning." Food-borne illnesses usually cause diarrhea, nausea, cramping, and vomiting. They usually occur five to eight hours after eating and last only a day or two. For many of us, food poisoning is unpleasant and inconvenient. For the very young, the elderly, or people with cancer, diabetes, AIDS, or other severe illnesses, it can be fatal.

Every year, millions of Americans become sick from unclean or poorly handled foods, sometimes with life-threatening consequences. The CDC estimates that every year 48 million Americans are sickened, 128,000 are hospitalized, and 3,000 die from food-borne illnesses.[49]

A rise in imports of fresh fruits and vegetables from developing countries, as well as increased urbanization, industrialization, travel, and restaurant dining raise the risk of unsafe food handling and resulting illness. Here are some tips for avoiding foodborne illness:

• Be aware of cleanliness in stores and restaurants. When purchasing food, be aware of the expiration dates on perishable foods.

- Use proper at-home techniques for storing and handling food.
  - Keep hands and cooking surfaces clean.
  - Separate raw foods from cooked foods during storage and cooking.
  - Scrub and thoroughly rinse produce before eating it.
  - Heat foods to high enough temperatures to kill germs.
  - Refrigerate perishable foods.
  - Safely handle the most common sources of food-borne illness: raw eggs, meat, poultry, and fish; unwashed or outdated bean or alfalfa sprouts; and unpasteurized milk and juices.

Some people have concerns about the safety of foods produced with the use of genetically modified organisms or their products, or foods that are irradiated to kill microorganisms and prolong shelf life. You can learn more about these issues by visiting the web links listed on this book's website.

How Can I Create a Behavior Change Plan for Nutrition?

You've no doubt heard the famous phrase, "You are what you eat." But did you know that its origin was a book written in 1825 by Anthelme Brillat-Savain—a French lawyer who loved the pleasures of the table above all else? What he actually wrote was, "Tell me what you eat and I shall tell you what you are." We could modify that slightly to make it perfectly relevant to this book and to you, the reader: tell us what you eat and we'll tell you how fit and well you're likely to be now and in the future!

SEE IT! ONLINE

You Are What You Eat?

Assess Your Current Diet

Would you benefit from changes to your current diet? The most successful way to change long-ingrained eating habits is to break the task into steps and keep track of your progress.

LIVE IT! ONLINE

Worksheet 20 Your Eating Habits

Recording What You Eat If you filled in Lab 7.2 using either a manual food diary or the food tracker found at www.ChooseMyPlate.gov, then you are on your way to a better diet. Self-awareness is the necessary starting point for change, followed by your own actions for self-improvement.[50]

You should get a pretty clear idea of how many calories your daily diet provides and whether your diet meets, exceeds, or falls short of the daily values for carbohydrates, fats, proteins, fiber, vitamins, and minerals. If there

are gaps in your food diary, keep track of your hour-by-hour food consumption for another day or two so you have a clear picture of your typical nutritional profile.

Identifying Your Patterns Go through your food diary and analyze your reasons for eating each meal and snack. Was it primarily hunger? Primarily socializing? Primarily boredom? If it is hunger, are you satisfying that need with nutrient-dense foods? If it is primarily socializing, are you even hungry at the time? Does peer pressure persuade you to eat an after-dinner snack of pizza and frozen yogurt when you could be happy with a salad, an apple, or a low-cal beverage? If you are eating out of boredom or stress—snacking on chips and cola while studying, for example—could you find a more nutritious alternative such as carrot sticks, whole wheat crackers, unsalted peanuts, popcorn, or grapes?

By reflecting on and identifying your own reasons for food preferences and eating habits, you can start to understand your patterns and perhaps change them for the better. It is seldom easy or automatic to improve your diet because it means breaking long-standing habits. But new behaviors become somewhat simpler if you realize when and why you reach for certain foods and that the resistance to change may come from within yourself or your family and friends.

Review Your Behavior Change Skills

Examining your current eating patterns is just one part of applying behavior change skills to improve your nutrition. Here are some other ways you can incorporate the behavior change model:

- *Look at your motivation.* Do you really want a different and better diet? What do you see as the immediate benefits of improved nutrition? What do you expect over the long term? Solidifying your motivation can help you get ready for change.

- *Identify barriers to a better diet.* What are some of the difficulties you foresee in achieving better nutrition? Time? Money? Eating in less-than-optimal ways with friends and family? Naming some of those barriers and coming up with alternatives can help you on the path to change. If you have trouble brainstorming solutions, the student health service or counseling center may be able to help you.

- *Make a commitment to learning about better nutrition.* Based on what you learn, list ways in which an improved diet will benefit your life. What could eating more whole grain fiber do for you? How about consuming more fruits and vegetables? Listing these will help you stick with your plan for change.

- *Choose a target behavior by identifying your biggest nutritional concern.* What is the most pressing issue with your current diet? Review your food diary. If you see that you're getting too much saturated fat every day, outline an approach for getting less saturated fat in your meals and snacks. If you discover that fried meats and cheese (on hamburgers, nachos, pizzas, etc.) are pushing up your daily total, think of lower-fat alternatives from those same menus, or try new places to eat.

- *Note where you stand in the typical stages of change.* Are you contemplating change? If so, gathering more information or talking more with friends and family might help. Are you planning for change and getting ready to take action?

- *Have you noticed any helpful role models?* Do you know people with good eating habits and a nutritious diet? Observing their food choices and talking to them about your nutritional issues may help you learn to counter your current habits with others based on better food choices, more successful eating patterns, and solid nutritional information.

Get Set to Apply Nutritional Skills

With this chapter, you've already begun to learn and apply nutritional skills. Review your use of them and look for ways to improve those skills and call upon them daily.

Examine food guides to compare your daily servings of various food groups with the amounts that nutritionists recommend from governmental agencies or from academic institutions. Read food labels more often and watch for those nutrients you've identified as problematic in your own diet. For example, watch for hidden fats and sugars and look for opportunities to increase fiber.

Recognize proper portion sizes and note when the helping you are served in a restaurant or cafeteria is way too big (three cups of pasta instead of half

a cup, for example) or way too small (a side salad the size of a golf ball, for example, instead of a softball). Use www.ChooseMyPlate.gov or other kinds of diet software to get an individual analysis of the daily calories and nutrients you consume and how they compare with the recommended daily intakes of each.

Both behavior-change skills and nutritional tools can help you plan your own program for improved nutrition. Working this plan can give you practice at recognizing nutrient-dense foods. You can start to choose high-volume, low-density alternatives to high-density, high-calorie foods. You may find that you now prefer whole grains to refined ones. And you may start to savor the colors, flavors, and textures of fruits and/or vegetables with every snack and meal.

Your plan may be your first deliberate application of nutritional tools and behavioral-change skills for nutrition. In time, however, it should become a continual and automatic part of each day. The goal is to balance nutrients and control calories naturally as part of your long-term efforts for fitness and wellness and your ongoing management of body mass and weight.

Create a Nutrition Plan

Begin planning your own program using **Lab 7.3**. As you work through the lab, write down your own notes and observations and swap them with others in your class, perhaps during a class discussion or in a small discussion group.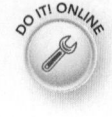

Keep track of calories for your new plan. Are you on track? Where could you cut or add without increasing saturated fats or sugars?

After two weeks, discuss the plan and your results with your fitness/health instructor, and revise if necessary. Again, if possible, discuss your experiences with others in your class to exchange successful ideas and get support for your efforts.

For several weeks, continue tracking your daily diet, either manually or using www.ChooseMyPlate.gov—at least for the number of servings of the main food groups. This helps you eat sufficient amounts of the foods you needed to increase (for example, whole grains, fruits, vegetables, beans, nuts) and helps you cut back on those that are already overrepresented (for example, saturated fat or refined carbohydrates). Be sure to continue applying nutritional skills such as reading labels and comparing serving sizes to the portions in Figure 7.10 (on page 265).

Don't try for perfection! Approach your diet in sets of two or three days at a time. When you have a day with too few fruits and vegetables, increase them the next day. When you have a day with too little protein, have more the next day. If you get too much protein one day, eat less the next or eat less-concentrated protein foods such as tofu, beans, or skim milk.

chapterin**review**

videos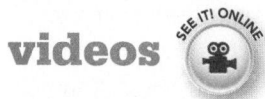

Log on to **www.pearsonhighered.com/hopson** or MyFitnessLab to view these chapter-related videos.

How Much Sugar?   Going Green   You Are What You Eat?
Which Fish Is Safest to Eat?

onlineresources

Log on to **www.pearsonhighered.com/hopson** or MyFitnessLab for access to these book-related resources, and for links to other useful websites.

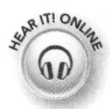 Audio case study
Audio PowerPoint lecture

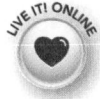 Take Charge of Your Health! Worksheets:
    Worksheet 18 Grocery Shopping List
    Worksheet 19 Food Log
    Worksheet 20 Your Eating Habits and
       Extra Calories
    Worksheet 24 Cutting out the Fat
Behavior Change Log Book and Wellness
Journal

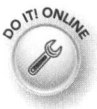 Lab 7.1 Reading a Food Label
Lab 7.2 Keeping a Food Diary and
Analyzing Your Daily Nutrition
Lab 7.3 Improving Your Nutrition

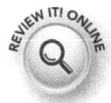 Pre- and post-quizzes
Glossary flashcards

reviewquestions

1. Which of the following would be considered a healthy, nutrient-dense food?
   a. Cheddar cheese
   b. Soft drink
   c. Potato chips
   d. Fat-free milk
2. Essential amino acids are
   a. found only in animal proteins.
   b. found only in plant proteins.
   c. best taken as supplements.
   d. protein building blocks your body can't produce.
3. Simple carbohydrates
   a. are important amino acid compounds.
   b. act as structural compounds in plants.
   c. provide fiber in the diet.
   d. deliver energy in a quickly usable form.

4. Using the glycemic index, one can determine
   a. the percentage of glucose in a food.
   b. the percentage of glycine in a food.
   c. how quickly a food will boost your blood sugar levels.
   d. the caloric content of a food.
5. What do nutritionists sometimes call "bad cholesterol"?
   a. Saturated fat
   b. Butter
   c. HDLs
   d. LDLs

6. Which of these is a poor source of essential fatty acids?
   a. Omega-3 fatty acids
   b. Omega-6 fatty acids
   c. Polyunsaturated oils
   d. Saturated oils such as palm kernel or coconut

7. Vitamins can
   a. act as structural components of bones and teeth.
   b. act as hormones that help regulate the body's use of glucose.
   c. help us convert food molecules into cellular fuel.
   d. delay wound healing.

8. Calcium can
   a. cause osteoporosis (brittle bones).
   b. delay blood clotting.
   c. prevent proper nerve impulse transmission.
   d. play an important role in muscle contraction.

9. An example of an antioxidant would be
   a. vitamin C.
   b. vitamin B 12.
   c. selenium.
   d. iron.

10. For proper food handling and safety
    a. use all produce straight from the garden or market without washing.
    b. avoid pasteurized milk and juices.
    c. observe expiration dates on food packaging.
    d. store raw and cooked foods together in airtight containers.

11. By law, a food label must
    a. tell the exact number of items in the package.
    b. give the manufacturer's business address.
    c. calculate the percentage of calories from fat.
    d. provide a recommended serving size.

critical**thinking**questions  REVIEW IT! ONLINE

1. Write out a healthy menu for yourself for one breakfast, one lunch, and one dinner, including portion sizes for each type of food you select.
2. Excluding water, what are the major types of nutrients in food? What are the main roles of each?
3. Name several protective functions of dietary fiber.
4. Differentiate *trans* fat and saturated fat. Name two dietary sources of each. Which is worse, and why?
5. How do antioxidants protect the body against the damaging effects of free radicals?
6. Describe the requirements for calcium and vitamin D in children, women of childbearing age, and people over 50.

references

1. U.S. Department of Agriculture, Agriculture Research Service, "What We Eat in America, NHANES 2003–2004," 2006.
2. U.S. Department of Agriculture, Agricultural Marketing Service, *How to Buy Fresh Vegetables*, Home and Garden Bulletin No. 258, 1994.
3. American College Health Association, *ACHA-National College Health Assessment Survey II: Reference Group Data Report Spring 2010* (Linthicum, MD: American College Health Association, 2010).
4. W. D. Hoyt, S. B. Hamilton, and K. M. Rickard, "The Effects of Dietary Fat and Caloric Content on the Body-Size Estimates of Anorexic Profile and Normal College Students," *Journal of Clinical Psychology* 59, no. 1 (2003): 85–91.
5. L. B. Brown, R. K. Dresen, and D. L. Eggett, "College Students Can Benefit by Participating in a Prepaid Meal Plan," *Journal of the American Dietetic Association* 105, no. 3 (2005): 445–8.
6. P. W. Lemon, "Is Increased Dietary Protein Necessary or Beneficial for Individuals with a Physically Active Lifestyle?" *Nutrition Review* 54, no. 4 pt. 2 (1996): S 169–75.
7. S. M. Phillips, "Protein Requirements and Supplementation in Strength Sports," *Nutrition* 20, nos. 7–8 (2004): 689–95.

8. American Cancer Society, "ACS Guidelines on Nutrition and Physical Activity for Cancer Prevention: Common Questions about Diet and Cancer," www.cancer.org /Healthy/EatHealthyGetActive /ACSGuidelinesonNutritionPhysical ActivityforCancerPrevention /acs-guidelines-on-nutrition-and-physical-activity-for-cancer-prevention-diet-cancer-questions (revised May 2011).
9. U.S. Food and Drug Administration, "How to Understand and Use the Nutrition Facts Label," www.fda.gov/food/labelingnutrition /consumerinformation/ucm078889.htm (updated March 2011).
10. J. Higdon, "Micronutrient Information Center: Glycemic Index and Glycemic Load," Linus Pauling Institute, Oregon State University, http://lpi.oregonstate.edu /infocenter/foods/grains/gigl.html (updated April 2010).
11. F. Sacks, "Ask the Expert: Omega-3 Fatty Acids," The Nutrition Source, Harvard School of Public Health, www.hsph .harvard.edu/nutritionsource/questions /omega-3/index.html (accessed February 2011); N. D. Riediger and others, "A Systemic Review of the Roles of n-3 Fatty Acids in Health and Disease," *Journal of the American Dietetic Association* 109, no. 4 (2009): 668–79.

12. J. Thompson and M. Manore, *Nutrition: An Applied Approach* 3rd Edition (San Francisco: Pearson, 2012).
13. W. Willett and D. Mozaffarian, "*Trans* Fats in Cardiac and Diabetes Risk: An Overview," *Current Cardiovascular Risk Reports* 1, no. 1 (2007): 16–23.
14. United States Department of Agriculture, "Empty Calories: What Are 'Solid Fats'?" www.choosemyplate.gov/foodgroups /emptycalories_fats.html (modified June 2011).
15. American Heart Association, "What Are Triglycerides?," American Heart Association internet publication, www.americanheart .org.
16. F. B. Hu and W. C. Willett, "Optimal Diets for Prevention of Coronary Heart Disease," *Journal of the American Medical Association* 288, no. 20 (November 2002): 2569–78.
17. J. May, "Ascorbic Acid Transporters in Health and Disease," paper given at Linus Pauling Diet and Optimum Health Annual Conference, Portland, OR, May, 2007.
18. L. J. Appel and C. A. M. Anderson, "Compelling Evidence for Public Health Action to Reduce Salt Intake," *New England Journal of Medicine* 362, no. 7 (2010): 650–2.
19. H. W. Cohen and others, "Sodium Intake and Mortality in the NHANES II Follow-Up Study," *American Journal of Medicine* 119, no. 3 (2006): 275.e7–14; J. Feng and others,

"Salt Intake and Cardiovascular Mortality," *American Journal of Medicine* 120, no. 1 (2007): e5–e7; H. Karppanen and E. Mervaala, "Sodium Intake and Hypertension," *Progress in Cardiovascular Diseases* 49, no. 2 (2006): 59–75.

20. J. Midgley and others, "Effects of Reduced Dietary Sodium on Blood Pressure: A Meta-Analysis of Randomized Controlled Trials," *The Journal of the American Medical Association* 275, no. 20 (1996): 1590–7.

21. Robert P. Heaney, "Role of Dietary Sodium in Osteoporosis," *Journal of the American College of Nutrition* 25, no. 3 suppl (2006): 271S–276S.

22. J. Ma, R. Johns, and R. Stafford, "Americans Are Not Meeting Current Calcium Recommendations," *American Journal of Clinical Nutrition* 85, no. 5 (2007): 1361–6.

23. I. A. Dontas and C.K. Yiannakopoulos, "Risk Factors and Prevention of Osteoporosis-Related Fractures," *Journal of Musculoskeletal and Neuronal Interactions* 7, no. 3 (2007): 268–272.

24. K. Tucker and others, "Colas, but Not Other Carbonated Beverages, Are Associated with Low Bone Mineral Density in Older Women: The Framingham Osteoporosis Study," *American Journal of Clinical Nutrition* 84, no. 4 (2006): 936–42.

25. World Health Organization, "Micronutrient Deficiencies: Iron Deficiency Anaemia," www.who.int/nutrition/topics/ida/en/index.html (accessed February 2011).

26. Office of Dietary Supplements, National Institutes of Health, "Dietary Supplement Fact Sheet: Iron," (Reviewed August 2007).

27. J. Postlethwait and J. Hopson, *Explore Life* (Pacific Grove, CA: Brooks/Cole, 2003): 400–1 .

28. Institute of Medicine of the National Academies, Food and Nutrition Board, *Dietary Reference Intakes for Water, Potassium, Sodium, Chloride, and Sulfate* (Washington, DC: The National Academies Press, 2004).

29. Consumers Union, "A Guide to the Best and Worst Drinks," *Consumer Reports on Health* (July 2006): 8–9.

30. USDA, Center for Nutrition Policy and Promotion, "A Brief History of USDA Food Guides," www.choosemyplate.gov/downloads/MyPlate/ABriefHistoryOf USDAFoodGuides.pdf (June 2011).

31. B. J. Rolls, E. A. Bell, and B. A. Waugh, "Increasing the Volume of a Food by Incorporating Air Affects Satiety in Men," *American Journal of Clinical Nutrition* 72, no. 2 (2000): 361–8.

32. A. Asherio, "Dietary Antioxidant Intakes and Neurological Disease Risks," Paper presented at the Linus Pauling Diet and Optimum Health Annual Conference (Portland, OR: May 2007).

33. J. Thompson and M. Manore, *Nutrition: An Applied Approach* 3rd Edition, 2012.

34. J. May, "Ascorbic Acid Transporters in Health and Disease," 2007.

35. E. R. Miller III and others, "Meta-Analysis: High-Dosage Vitamin E Supplementation May Increase All-Cause Mortality," *Annals of Internal Medicine* 142, no. 1 (2005): 37–46.

36. W. Willett, *Eat, Drink, and Be Healthy: The Harvard Medical School Guide to Healthy Eating* (New York: Free Press, 2003).

37. B. Frei, "Closing Remarks Summary, 2001," Paper presented at the Linus Pauling Institute International Conference on Diet and Optimum Health (Portland, OR: May, 2001).

38. Ibid.

39. M. Gonzalez-Gross and others, "Nutrition in the Sport Practice: Adaptation of the Food Guide Pyramid to the Characteristics of Athletes Diet," *Archives of Latino American Nutrition* 51, no. 4 (2001): 321–31.

40. L. M. Burke and others, "Carbohydrates and Fat for Training and Recovery," *Journal of Sports Science* 22, no. 1 (2004): 15–30.

41. M. N. Sawka, "American College of Sports Medicine Position Stand: Exercise and Fluid Replacement," *Medicine and Science in Sports and Exercise* 39, no. 2 (2007): 377–90.

42. W. H. Saris and L. J. van Loon, "Nutrition and Health: Nutrition and Performance in Sports," [article in Dutch] *Nederlands Tijdschrift voor Geneeskunde* 148, no. 15 (2004): 708–12.

43. J. J. Crowley and C. Wall, "The Use of Dietary Supplements in a Group of Potentially Elite Secondary School Athletes," *Asia-Pacific Journal of Clinical Nutrition* 13, suppl. (2004): S39.

44. R. Maughan, "The Athlete's Diet: Nutritional Goals and Dietary Strategies," *Proceedings of the Nutritional Society* 61, no. 1 (2002): 87–96.

45. J. B. Anderson and others, *Eat Right! Healthy Eating in College and Beyond* (San Francisco: Benjamin Cummings, 2007).

46. American Dietetic Association, "Position of the American Dietetic Association: Vegetarian Diets," *Journal of the American Dietetic Association* 109, no. 7 (2009): 1266–82.

47. S. Loft, "Diet, Oxidative DNA Damage, and Cancer," Paper presented at the Linus Pauling Institute International Conference on Diet and Optimum Health (Portland, OR: May, 2001).

48. American Diabetes Association, "Making Healthy Food Choices," www.diabetes.org/food-and-fitness/food/what-can-i-eat/making-healthy-food-choices.html (accessed September 2011).

49. Centers for Disease Control and Prevention, "CDC Estimates of Foodborne Illness in the United States: CDC 2011 Estimates: Findings," www.cdc.gov/foodborneburden/2011-foodborne-estimates.html (updated April 2011).

50. J. Kurman, "Self-Enhancement, Self-Regulation, and Self-Improvement Following Failures," *British Journal of Social Psychology* 45, pt 2. (2006): 339–56.

LAB 7.1 • READING A FOOD LABEL

Name: _____ **Date:** _____

Instructor: _____ **Section:** _____

Purpose: To learn how to read food labels and analyze the nutritional content of a packaged food.

Directions: Select any packaged food item from your kitchen or from a grocery store. Find the "Nutrition Facts" panel on the package and answer the following questions.

1. What is the name of the packaged food you are examining?

_____

2. What is the "serving size" stated on the Nutrition Facts panel?

_____

Does this "serving size" match the portion you typically consume of this food in one sitting? Is it bigger or smaller than the amount that you typically consume?

_____

3. Examine the ingredients. What are the main ingredients (i.e., which items are listed first)?

_____

Does this list of main ingredients surprise you? How nutritious are the main ingredients?

_____

4. Complete the following table for your chosen food, listing amounts and % Daily Value (% DV) for various nutrients:

Calories (per serving)	Total Fat	Saturated Fat	Trans Fat	Sodium	Dietary Fiber	Sugars	Vitamins/ Minerals
	Amount:	Amount:	Amount:	Amount:	Amount:	Amount:	Amount:
	% DV:	% DV:	% DV:	% DV:	% DV:	% DV:	% DV:

Examine your data. Is this food excessively high in fat, saturated fat, trans fat, or sodium? Does it provide any dietary fiber? How much sugar is in this food? Does this food supply any vitamins and minerals?

_____

_____

_____

5. What is your overall assessment of the nutritional value of the packaged food you have examined?

_____

_____

_____

LAB 7.2 • KEEPING A FOOD DIARY AND ANALYZING YOUR DAILY NUTRITION

Name: _____ Date: _____

Instructor: _____ Section: _____

Purpose: To get an initial assessment of your current nutrition and identify areas to be improved.

Directions: Follow the instructions below. You will need Internet access to complete this lab.

1. Log on to www.mypyramidtracker.gov.

2. Click "Assess Your Food Intake."

3. If you are accessing this site for the first time, click the link for New Users to set up your personalized login and password. When prompted, enter your age, gender, height, and weight. Then click "Proceed to Food Intake."

4. Enter all of the food items you have eaten today. (It's best to complete this at the end of the day, when you have finished all of your meals.) Enter each food individually by entering the name of the food in the search field, clicking "Search," and then clicking "Add." If you cannot find the exact food you are looking for, select the food that is the most similar. After you have "added" a food, it should pop up on the right side of the screen. Click "Select Quantity" and select a serving size from the drop-down menu. Enter the number of servings you consumed. Click "Enter Foods" to enter additional foods. Repeat until you have entered all of the foods you consumed today. (Don't forget to include any snacks and beverages!)

5. When your list of foods consumed is complete, click "Save and Analyze" or "Analyze Your Food Intake."

6. You will see a screen with several links to analyzed data. Click on "Calculate Nutrient Intakes from Foods." This screen will illustrate how your nutrient intake compares to the "recommended or acceptable range." Print this page.

   a. Does your intake of any nutrient fall short of the "recommended or acceptable" range? If so, which nutrient(s)?

   _____

   _____

   b. Does your intake of any nutrient exceed the "recommended or acceptable" range? If so, which nutrient(s)?

   _____

   _____

7. Click "Analyze Your Food Intake" to return to the main screen containing links to analyzed data. This time, click on "MyPyramid Recommendation." Print this page.

   How does your food intake compare to the recommendations?

   _____

   _____

Note: For more accurate results, record your intake for at least three consecutive days, and then analyze your data again.

Name: _____   **Date:** _____

Instructor: _____   **Section:** _____

Purpose: To create a detailed plan for improving your personal nutrition.

Materials: Results from Lab 7.2.

SECTION I: PLANNING CHANGES TO YOUR DIET

1. Look back at your results for Lab 7.2. Which nutrients do you consume too little of?

_____

_____

List at least three foods you could add to your diet in order to increase your consumption of these nutrients:

Food:_____   Rich in: _____

Food: _____   Rich in: _____

Food: _____   Rich in: _____

2. Do you consume too much protein, fat, saturated fat, cholesterol, or sodium? If so, what foods high in these substances could you reduce or eliminate from your diet? List at least 3:

Food: _____   High in: _____

Food: _____   High in: _____

Food: _____   High in: _____

3. How closely did your diet match up with the USDA recommendations? Fill in the blanks below.

Current Milk Intake: _____ cups   Recommended Milk Intake: _____ cups

Current Meat and Beans Intake: _____ oz.   Recommended Meat and Beans Intake: _____ oz.

Current Vegetables Intake: _____ cups   Recommended Vegetables Intake: _____ cups

Current Fruits Intake: _____ cups   Recommended Fruits Intake: _____ cups

Current Grains Intake: _____ oz.   Recommended Grains Intake: _____ oz.

How can you adjust your diet to more closely meet recommended intake levels for each food group?

- I would like to increase/decrease my milk intake by _____ cups.
- I would like to increase/decrease my meat and beans intake by _____ oz.
- I would like to increase/decrease my vegetables intake by _____ oz.
- I would like to increase/decrease my fruits intake by _____ cups.
- I would like to increase/decrease my grains intake by _____ oz.

SECTION II: SHORT- AND LONG-TERM GOALS

Create short- and long-term goals for your healthy eating plan. Be sure to use SMART (specific, measurable, action-oriented, realistic, time-limited) goal-setting guidelines and the information obtained from Section I of this lab and all of your Lab 7.2 materials. Choose appropriate target dates and rewards for completing your goals.

1. Short-Term Goal (3–6 Months)

   a. Goal:_____

   _____

   b. Target Date:_____

   c. Reward:_____

2. Long-Term Goal (12+ Months)

   a. Goal: _____

   _____

   b. Target Date:_____

   c. Reward: _____

SECTION III: BARRIERS TO GOOD NUTRITION; STRATEGIES FOR OVERCOMING THEM

1. What barriers or obstacles might hinder your plan for nutrition changes? Indicate your top three nutritional barriers here:

   a. _____

   b. _____

   c. _____

2. Overcoming these barriers to change will be an important step in reaching your goals. List three strategies for overcoming the obstacles listed:

   a. _____

   b. _____

   c. _____

SECTION IV: GETTING SUPPORT

List resources you will use to help you change your nutritional behavior and how each of these resources will support your goals:

Friend/partner/relative: _____

School-based resource: _____

Community-based resource: _____

Other: _____

8

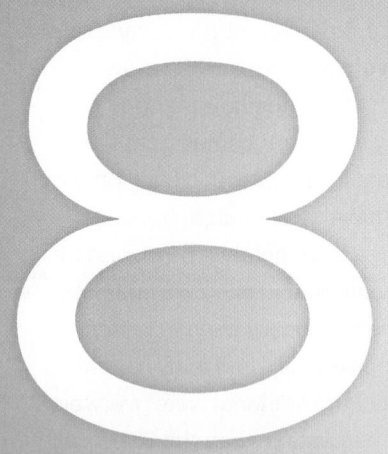

Managing Your Weight

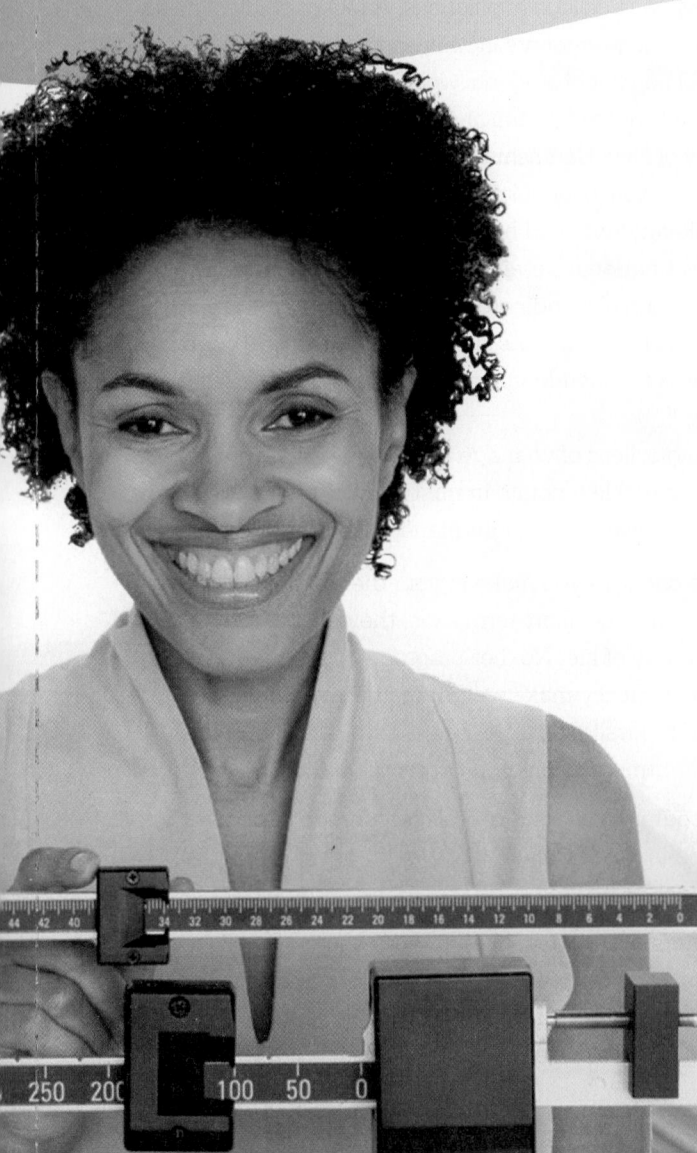

Learning Outcomes

1. Explain why obesity is both a worldwide trend and a serious concern in America.

 HEAR IT! ONLINE Audio case study and audio PowerPoint lecture

....

2. Discuss the effects of body weight on wellness.

....

3. Identify several effective tools for successful weight management.

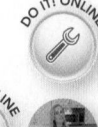 DO IT! ONLINE Lab 8.1 Calculating Energy Balance and Setting Energy Balance Goals

 SEE IT! ONLINE Miscounting Calories

....

4. List reasons why some diets work but most fail.

 SEE IT! ONLINE Food Diary Diet Writing

 Diet Dream Drug

....

5. Describe the major eating disorders.

 SEE IT! ONLINE Extreme Healthy Eating

....

6. Choose a realistic target weight based on your metabolic rate, activity level, eating habits, and environment.

....

7. Create a behavior change plan for long-term weight management.

 DO IT! ONLINE Lab 8.2 Your Diet IQ
Lab 8.3 Your Weight Management Plan

 LIVE IT! ONLINE Customizable 4-week starter weight loss fitness programs

Pre- and post-quizzes and glossary flashcards REVIEW IT! ONLINE

casestudy

MARIA

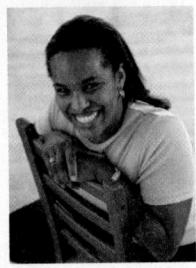

"My name is Maria. I'm 25 and a full-time student in southern Florida, finishing a BA in child development. I was halfway through college when my daughter, Anna, was born. Now that she's in preschool, I'm back to taking a full load of classes and hope to finish college in two more years. I love being a mom. The only thing I'd like to change is my weight! Ever since Anna was born, I've been trying to get back into my pre-pregnancy clothes. I've tried lots of ways to lose the extra pounds—diet pills, liquid diets, Atkins, South Beach—you name it, I've tried it! Sometimes it works for a while, but eventually the weight always comes back. I'm willing to try again, but how do I find a plan that will stick?"

HEAR IT! ONLINE

. . . .

overweight In an adult, a BMI of 25 to 29 or a body weight more than 10 percent above recommended levels

obese In an adult, a BMI of 30 or more or a body weight more than 20 percent above recommended levels

underweight In an adult, a BMI below 18.5 or a body weight more than 10 percent below recommended levels

energy balance The relationship between the amount of calories consumed in food and the amount of calories expended through metabolism and physical activity

Weight is a serious and growing health issue in America. While introducing a new campaign to combat obesity, First Lady Michelle Obama warned, "The surge in obesity in this country is nothing short of a public health crisis that is threatening our children, our families, and our future."[1] Over one-third of American adults (34.2 percent) are **overweight** (see Figure 8.1), meaning that their body weight is more than 10 percent over the recommended range and their body mass index, or BMI, is over 25.[2] Another one-third of adults (33.8 percent) are **obese**, with a BMI of 30 or above.[3] Only about 1.6 percent of Americans older than age 20 are **underweight**, with a BMI below 18.5 or a weight 10 percent below recommended range.[4]

Part of the First Lady's concern comes from the alarming trend in children: In the past 25 years, obesity rates for young children have more than doubled; for kids aged 6 to 11, the rates have nearly tripled; and for adolescents, they have more than tripled (Figure 8.2).[5]

College students have historically been in better shape than other adult populations. Until fairly recently, only about 25 percent of college students were overweight or obese, a much smaller percentage than the 66 percent of overweight and obese people in the population as a whole.[6,7] However, there is evidence that overweight is increasing in college populations. A recent study of nearly 10,000 college students in Minnesota indicated that over 39 percent of students were overweight, obese, or extremely obese.[8] A similar study of students at the University of New Hampshire indicated that over one-third of students were overweight or obese, and nearly 60 percent of male students had high blood pressure.[9] Results from a recent national survey by the National College Health Association also indicate a rise in overweight to 21.9 percent of the students surveyed; in obesity (to 11.6 percent of respondents); and in self-reports of disordered eating.[10]

Regardless of your age and stage of life, you should keep several key points in mind as you assess your own diet, exercise, and weight management strategies:

- The changes you make in your diet and exercise habits cannot be short-term fixes; they must become a new way of life. No diet program, product, or service will magically make weight melt away. Successful weight loss takes time, effort, motivation, and the commitment to change habits permanently.

- Recognize that your overall percentage of body fat is more important than your weight or the amount of weight you lose.

- Understand that fast weight loss usually involves a temporary decrease in tissue fluids and often a loss in lean muscle mass, as well. "Healthy weight loss" means the slow, sustained loss of fat, coupled with increases in muscle mass and the preservation and maintenance of lean body mass.

- Learn how long-term weight management balances calories consumed in foods with calories expended through metabolism, activity, and exercise—an equation called **energy balance**.

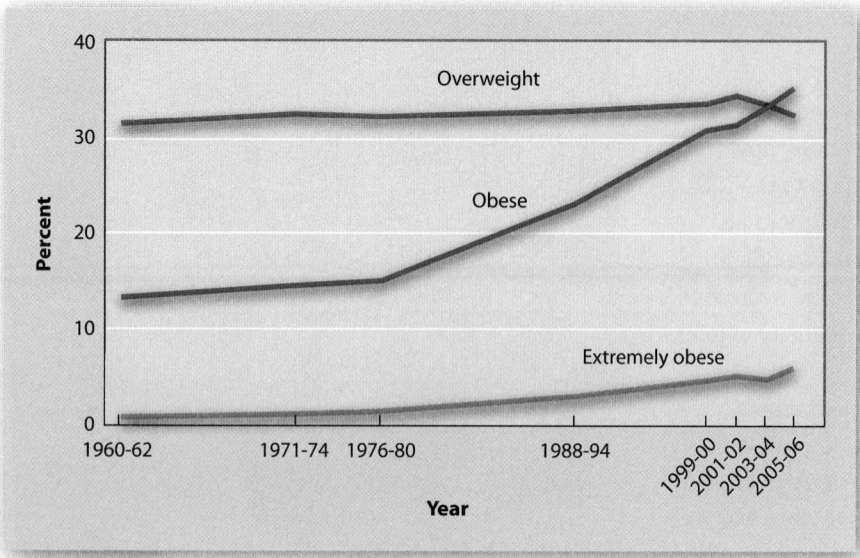

FIGURE **8.1** For the past half century, one-third of Americans have been overweight despite massive government campaigns and personal efforts at weight reduction. During that same period, the percentages of obese Americans have more than doubled.

Source: NCHS E-Stat: Prevalence of Overweight, Obesity and Extreme Obesity among Adults: United States, Trends 1960–1962 through 2007–2008, National Health and Nutrition Examination Survey (2010).

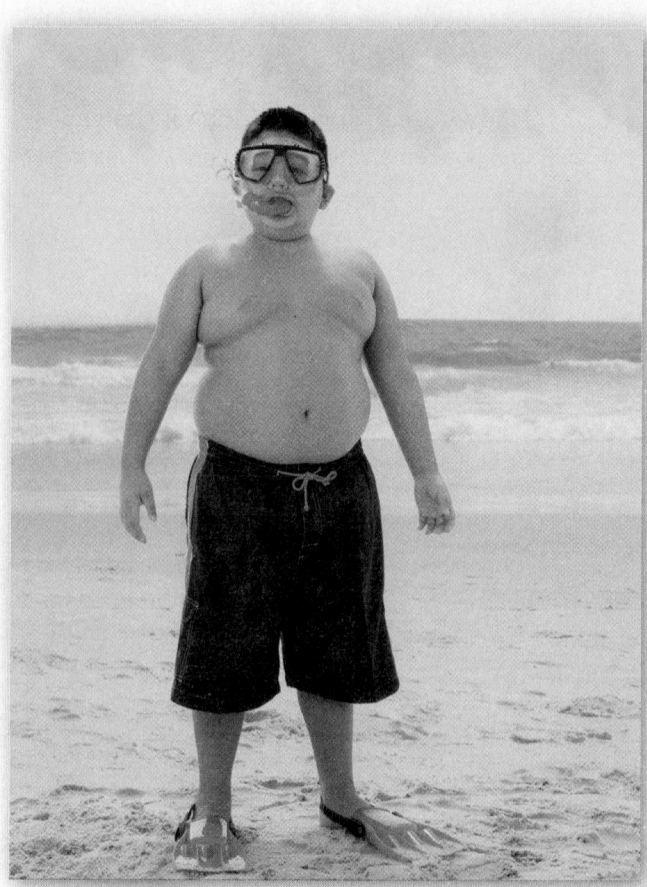

FIGURE **8.2** In the past 30 years, obesity rates for children aged 2 to 5 years have more than doubled, going from 5% to 10.4%, while rates for those aged 6 to 11 years went from 6.5% to 19.6%. The biggest increase was in adolescents aged 12 to 19 years, whose obesity rates more than tripled from 5% to 18.1%!

Data from NCHS E-Stat: Prevalence of Obesity among Children and Adolescents: United States, Trends 1963–1965 through 2007–2008, National Health and Nutrition Examination Survey (2010).

This chapter presents the tools and techniques you need to determine a healthy target weight and create a sound plan for reaching and maintaining it. Incorporating **weight management** into your ongoing wellness program will allow you to realize the significant benefits—physiological, social, and emotional—of sustaining your body mass and body composition within recommended ranges throughout adult life.

Why Is Obesity on the Rise?

In 2011, the World Health Organization (WHO) estimated that 1.6 billion of the world's people were overweight and that the number could increase to 2.3 billion by 2015. Obese adults number over 400 million worldwide and this number could grow to 900 million by 2015. The WHO coined the new term "globesity" to describe this trend. Obesity is a problem in high-income industrialized countries as well as in low- and middle-income developing countries.[11] Diets high in processed fats, meats, sugars, and refined starches provide excess calories while labor-saving devices and sedentary lifestyles reduce energy expenditure. In developing countries, entire cultures are moving away from traditional diets—rich in fruits, vegetables, grains, and low-fat proteins—as well as from manual labor. As a result, they are experiencing the same gain in body fat percentages and weight that Americans did three decades ago. Only the poorest countries of sub-Saharan Africa do not reflect this worldwide trend.[12]

Several Factors Contribute to Overweight and Obesity in America

In the last quarter century, the number of overweight Americans has risen slowly while the number of obese adults has more than doubled.[13] The maps in Figure 8.3 reveal that the rapid increase is distributed unevenly: the southern and upper Midwestern states show the highest

weight management A lifelong balancing of calories consumed and calories expended through exercise and activity to control body fat and weight

rates of obesity in the nation. Several factors contribute to the rapid increase.

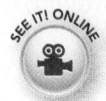

SEE IT! ONLINE

Miscounting Calories

Overconsumption Americans consume an average of 523 calories more per day now than they did in 1970 according to the U.S. Department of Agriculture.[14] Without additional exercise, this imbalance leads to weight gain. Many societal factors encourage overeating: "portion distortion," the constant availability of food, advertising, and price.

Food portions in restaurants and supermarkets have grown steadily over the past half-century (Figure 8.4). Researchers have also found that people don't read their own "fullness signals," or feelings of *satiety,* very well. So, the bigger the portions, the more they will eat overall.[15]

Easy access to food and food choices also encourages overeating.[16] Today, most drugstores, gas stations, schools, and public buildings sell packaged food. People eat more treats if they are available in plain sight than if the same food is less accessible.[17] Too, the more food choices people have, the more they tend to eat. People will eat more total food at a four-course meal than at a two-course meal—and even more at a buffet.[18]

Advertising also contributes to overeating. Amazingly, one third of our daily calories come from just a few categories of highly-advertised, empty-calorie foods: sweets, sodas and fruit drinks, alcoholic beverages, and salty snacks.[19] Food price also influences consumption: When experimenters lowered the price of snacks in vending machines, the sales grew immediately.[20]

Too Little Exercise The ease of our modern life is an improvement over the hard physical labor of past generations. Yet the exertion we are spared amounts to hundreds of calories per day that we *don't* burn off as we sit at our desks or change channels with a remote control.[21] Even the layout of modern towns and cities contributes to reduced energy expenditure. The majority of Americans live in suburbs—environments that encourage driving. The greater the urban or suburban sprawl, the less people walk, the more they weigh, and the more likely they are to have high blood pressure, heart disease, cancer, diabetes, and other diseases.[22]

Hereditary Factors With all these overconsumption factors in play, why isn't *everyone* overweight or obese? Part of the answer lies in heredity. If most of your relatives are overweight or obese, you are more likely to gain weight during adulthood yourself. If most of your relatives are thin, you are more likely to be thin as well.

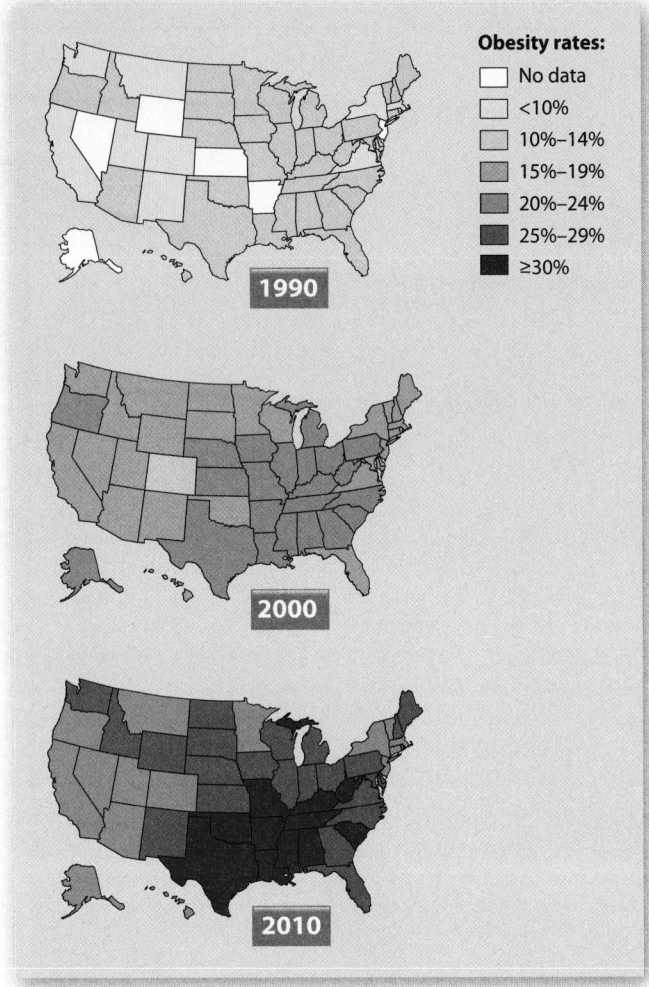

FIGURE 8.3 Obesity rates have risen dramatically over recent decades. Rates are highest in the upper Midwest and in the South.

Source: Centers for Disease Control, "U.S. Obesity Trends," www.cdc.gov/obesity/data/trends.html (updated July 2011).

Researchers have learned that dozens—perhaps hundreds—of genes help determine your weight.[23] Genes control whether our metabolism is fast, burning off most of our excess calories, or "thrifty," tending to conserve food energy.

"Non-Exercise" Activity Uses Energy In recent years, researchers have discovered another factor with hereditary underpinnings: our tendencies to save or use energy during rest and activity. Some people tend to conserve energy by sitting quietly for long stretches and being generally less active all day. Others tend to use energy by being fidgety, jiggling their head, hands, and feet, and getting up to walk around every few minutes. James Levine and colleagues at the Mayo Clinic have demonstrated that lean people burn 279 to 477

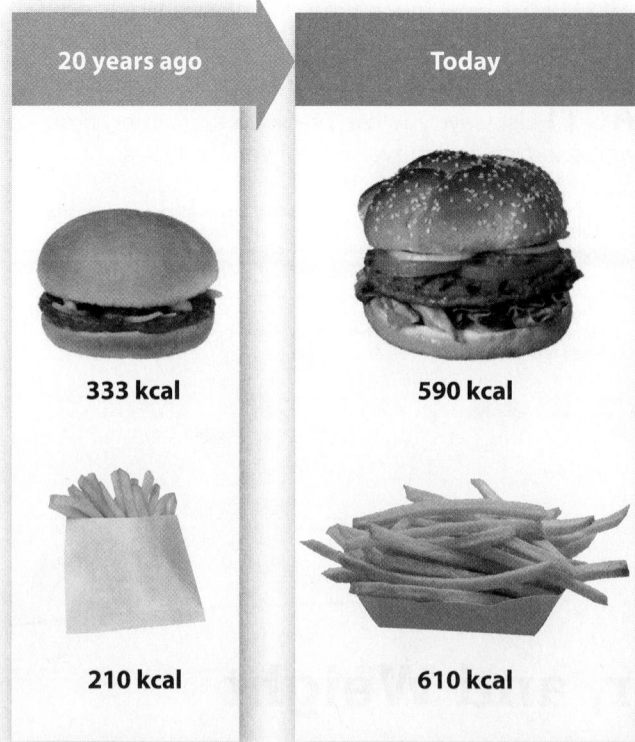

20 years ago	Today
333 kcal	590 kcal
210 kcal	610 kcal

FIGURE **8.4** Today's serving portions are significantly larger than those of past decades. A 25-ounce prime-rib dinner served at one local steak chain contains nearly 3,000 calories and 150 grams of fat. That's twice as many calories and more than three times the fat that most adults need in a whole day, and it's just the meat part of the meal!

Data are from National Heart, Lung, and Blood Institute, "Portion Distortion," http://hp2010.nhlbihin.net/portion (accessed September 2011).

more calories per day than obese people through this type of **non-exercise activity**—an expenditure that can significantly affect fat storage and body weight.[24]

The box Get Up from Your Chair! explores how even small, deliberate breaks from sitting can assist in weight management.

non-exercise activity Routine daily activities such as standing up and walking around that use energy but are not part of deliberate exercise

Demographic and Lifestyle Factors A mix of demographic factors both biological and non-biological—including sex, race/ethnicity, culture, education, and economic level—all influence weight. As the box Race/Ethnicity, Gender, and Weight explains, your body weight and likelihood of overweight or obesity vary by race/ethnic group as well as by sex. Biological and cultural factors interact, of course: Our family and ethnic group influences what, when, and how much we eat, as well as how much we exercise and participate in other activity. The choice of high-fat, high-calorie foods, for instance, is partly based on family upbringing, habit, and preference. And 25 percent of Americans engage in no exercise, sports, or other physical activity at all during their leisure time.[25] Education and income make a difference: The higher a person's education level, and the more money he or she makes, the more likely the individual is to be physically active and make healthy food choices. Tough economic times inspire many to choose less expensive foods which, in turn, tend to have more calories and be more highly processed.[26]

LIVE IT! ONLINE

Worksheet 23 Why Do You Eat?

TOOLS FOR **CHANGE** •

Get Up from Your Chair!

Researchers have discovered that sitting for long periods day after day can negatively impact your health—even if you exercise on those same days. Several studies have shown that people who spend the most time sitting also have the highest mortality rates from cardiovascular disease and other illnesses.[1]

Conversely, recent research shows that people who interrupt sedentary time with movement "breaks" have narrower waistlines and lower risk of cardiovascular disease. Scientists in Australia interpreted data from a large American study sponsored by the Centers for Disease Control and Prevention. They found

correlations with a trimmer waistline and less risk for cardiovascular diseases in 4,750 participants who wore devices that monitored movement and recorded breaks in sedentary time.[2]

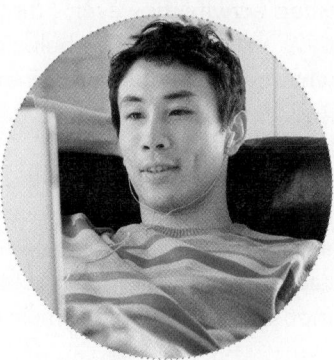

The team recommends that people take a "whole day approach" to increasing physical

(Continued)

activity, adding physical exercise but also breaking up sedentary time to benefit wellness.

First Lady Michelle Obama's "Let's Move!" campaign shares a similar goal, encouraging parents to walk with their families after dinner and kids to "Move everyday!" by getting one hour or more of active play time plus breaking up TV viewing with jumping jacks and other non-sitting activities.[3]

THINK! How much time do you spend sitting each day as you study, attend class, drive your car, and so on?

ACT! List ways you can break up that sitting time with exercise and movement of various types.

Sources:
1. N. Owen, A. Bauman, and W. Brown, "Too Much Sitting: A Novel and Important Predictor of Chronic Disease Risk?" *British Journal of Sports Medicine* 43, no. 2 (2009): 81–83
2. G. Healy, and others, "Sedentary Time and Cardio-Metabolic Biomarkers in U.S. Adults; NHANES 2003–06," *European Heart Journal* (2011) DOI: 10.1093/eurheartj/ehq451.
3. Let's Move!, "Move Everyday!" www.letsmove.gov/move-everyday (accessed September 2011).

DIVERSITY

Race/Ethnicity, Gender, and Weight

Body weight varies by racial/ethnic groups to some degree, based on genes as well as on cultural preferences for food and exercise. Hispanic males, African American males and females, Native American males and females, Pacific Islander males, and white males have the highest percentages of overweight (68 to 72 percent of adults in these groups). Hispanic females, Pacific Islander females, and white females have somewhat lower rates of overweight (51 to 62 percent). Asian Americans have the lowest percentages of overweight (men 46 percent, women 28 percent).

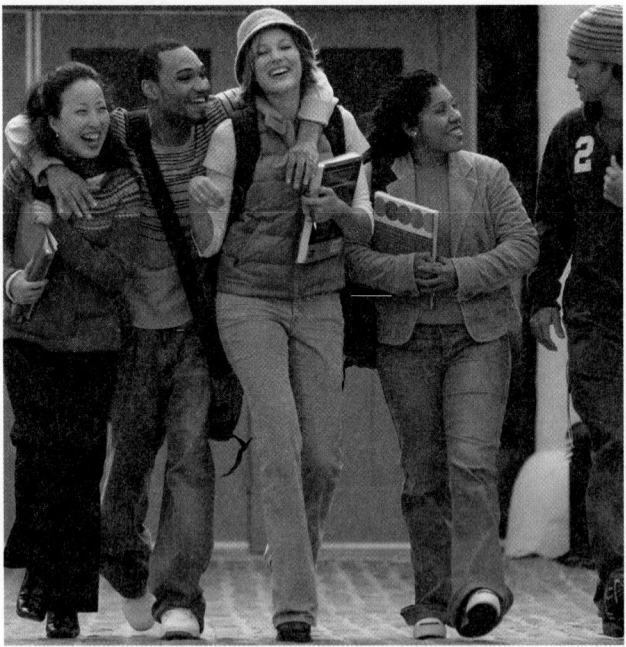

Some ethnic groups appear to have "thrifty genes" that helped their ancestors survive during extended periods of famine by slowing down metabolism to conserve food energy. In a modern environment of plentiful food, widespread mechanization, and diminished activity, however, "thrifty genes" can lead to easy weight gain. This helps explain, for example, why today, 90 percent of Pima Indians are overweight and 75 percent are obese.

Women have a tendency to burn fewer calories than men due to their higher level of essential body fat and lower ratio of lean body mass to fat mass. Because muscle cells burn more energy, and because men usually have more muscle tissue than women,

men burn 10 to 20 percent more calories than women do, even at rest. Monthly hormonal cycles and pregnancy also increase the likelihood of weight fluctuation and gain. Significantly, though, adult men are more likely to be overweight than adult women.

Sources: C. A. Schoenborn and P. F. Adams, National Center for Health Statistics, "Health Behaviors of Adults: United States, 2005–2007," *Vital and Health Statistics* 10, no. 245 (2010).

casestudy

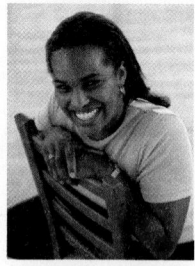

MARIA

"I was never overweight as a kid, and I gained a normal amount of weight during my pregnancy, but now I'm considered overweight. My parents, grandparents, and two older sisters are all on the heavy side, so I wonder if my "heavy" gene just decided to kick in! While I was pregnant, I got used to eating more food than before, and after giving birth to Anna, I guess I just didn't cut back. I spend a lot of time running around after Anna, but otherwise, I drive everywhere and don't set aside special time to exercise. Anna is a picky eater right now—she'll only eat macaroni and cheese, chicken strips, and pizza—so we end up eating those most of the time. That makes it really hard to diet!"

THINK! Do you share any of Maria's eating and exercise habits? Is she like any of your friends?

ACT! Write down your current BMI. Does it represent underweight, healthy weight, overweight, or obesity? List aspects of your lifestyle that may have contributed to your current BMI.

HEAR IT! ONLINE

How Does My Body Weight Affect My Wellness?

A leading nutritionist has written that body weight sits at the center of an intricate web of health and disease.[27] Indeed, research shows: You are more likely to remain healthy throughout life if (1) your BMI is between 21 and 23 for women and 22 and 24 for men; (2) you maintain approximately the same BMI and the same waist size throughout your adult life; and (3) your body's fat deposits tend to occur around the hips and thighs rather than the abdomen. High BMIs and abdominal fat (indicated by a large waist size) are associated with higher risk for several chronic diseases.[28]

Being underweight is an important but far less common problem. Fewer than five percent of Americans have a BMI under 18.5.[29] Underweight carries its own significant health risks and can be the result of an unusually fast metabolism, excessive dieting, extreme levels of exercise, eating disorders, smoking, or illness.

Body Weight Can Promote or Diminish Your Fitness

A stable, healthy-range BMI goes hand in hand with regular exercise. Maintaining weight and BMI within recommended ranges leads to increased energy and reduced likelihood of injury during fitness activities.

Overweight and under-weight can contribute to poor fitness. Overweight can lead to a downward fitness spiral: An over-accumulation of body fat can strain bones, joints, and muscles and make exercising harder and injury more likely. Resulting stiffness and pain in the hands, feet, knees, and back, in turn, make exercising even more difficult. They also make work, employment, and activities of daily living—walking up stairs, carrying books or grocery bags, shoveling snow, getting in and out of automobiles, and so on—harder.

Underweight can lead to muscle wasting as the body breaks down muscle tissue for energy when fat stores are low. Muscle wasting, in turn, can lead to weakness and declining ability to exercise and accomplish daily tasks. These inevitably reduce both fitness and wellness.

Body Weight Can Have Social Consequences

Being overweight can subject a person to significant discrimination in education, employment, health care, and social interactions, starting in childhood.[30] "Weight stigma," or prejudice against overweight and obese people, is widespread in society and often starts with parents and teachers of overweight youngsters. Researchers have discovered, for example, that parents spend less money sending their overweight children to college than they do their thinner children, even when money isn't a limiting factor and the children have equivalent grades.[31] Adoption agencies and prospective parents are less likely to choose an overweight child for adoption than a thin one.[32] And adult attitudes rub off on children. Preschoolers are more likely to describe overweight kids their own age as "mean, ugly, or stupid."[33]

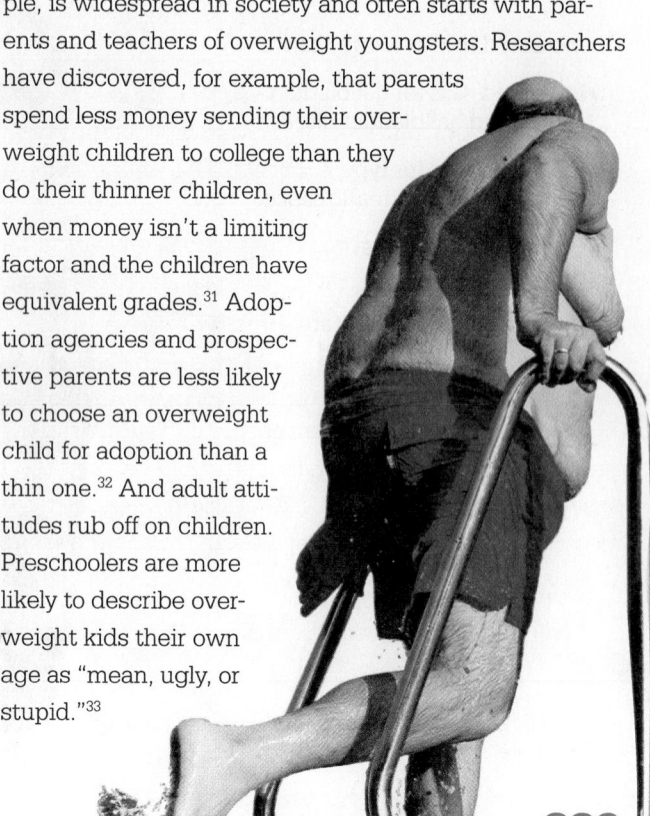

Weight stigma is also quite common among employers. Overweight job applicants suffer discrimination, get hired less often, and get fired more often than thinner individuals with similar qualifications.[34] In one study, job applicants standing near obese people were less likely to get hired, even if they were strangers![35] Weight stigma is even pronounced among health professionals, including specialists who treat the obese.[36]

Negative self-images and beliefs can lead to discouragement, shame, hopelessness, and in many, to eating "comfort foods" that temporarily boost mood but cause more weight gain.[37] Weight stigma scholars consider anti-fat bias to be a serious societal issue in need of more study and creative solutions. Awareness is a good starting place.

THINK! Do you say or do things that reveal weight stigma?

ACT! If so, think of substitute thoughts and actions that you could choose and have them ready.

Body Weight Can Influence Your Risk for Chronic Disease

Researchers have confirmed that people with excess body fat have higher levels of several serious chronic diseases (Figure 8.5).[38] Specific cancers linked to high BMI include cancers of the prostate, colon, rectum, esophagus, pancreas, kidney, gallbladder, ovary, cervix, liver, breast, uterus, and stomach.[39]

Fat accumulation around the waist (a 40-inch waistline or higher for a man, or a 35-inch waistline or higher for a woman) increases the risk for developing *metabolic syndrome*. This serious medical condition is a combination of high blood cholesterol, high blood pressure, abdominal fat deposits, and insulin resistance or full-fledged type 2 diabetes.[40] A weight loss of just 10 pounds can bring measurable health benefits, even to an obese individual.[41]

Body Weight Can Affect Your Life Expectancy

You can expect to live longer if your body weight and BMI are within recommended ranges than you can if they fall under the categories for obesity or underweight.

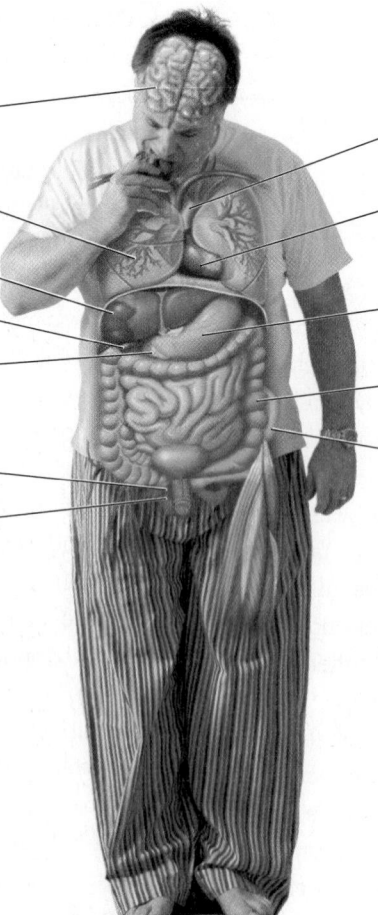

Negative health effects

- Increased risk of stroke
- Increased risk of sleep apnea and asthma
- Increased risk for kidney cancer
- Increased risks for gallbladder cancer and gallbladder disease
- Increased risks for type 2 diabetes and pancreatic cancer
- Higher rates of sexual dysfunction
- Increased risks for prostate, endometrial, ovarian and cervical cancer
- Increased risk of breast cancer in women

Negative health effects

- Higher triglyceride levels and decreased HDL levels
- High blood pressure and increased risk for all forms of heart disease
- Increased risks for stomach and esophageal cancer
- Increased risks for colon and rectal cancer
- Increased risk of osteoarthritis, especially in weight-bearing joints, such as knees and hips
- In pregnant women, increased risks of fetal and maternal death, labor and delivery complications, and birth defects

FIGURE **8.5** Body weight can influence the risks for chronic disease.

As Figure 8.6 shows, being fit significantly reduces mortality risk, especially when combined with healthy weight. Being obese (having a BMI of 30 or above) cuts an average of six to seven years from the life of a non-smoker and 13 to 14 years from a smoker.[42] Research indicates that Americans' average life expectancy may begin to decline because obesity is so prevalent and can shorten life so dramatically.[43]

Underweight people have a shorter life expectancy than normal-weight or overweight people.[44] In fact, some studies indicate that underweight people may have more than 18 times the risk of dying of cancer, and four times the risk of CVD death.[45] Only obese people have a shorter life expectancy. The statistics for early deaths among the underweight reflect the fact that a low BMI is characteristic of patients with illnesses such as cancer, uncontrolled diabetes, and disordered eating. People who are underweight but *not* ill and who are careful to get complete daily nutrition may actually realize greater longevity.[46] Underweight associated with poor nutrition, however, can lead to life-shortening conditions such as anemia, susceptibility to disease and infection, slower recovery from illness, muscle wasting and weakness, and osteoporosis and bone fractures.

Why Don't Most Diets Succeed?

Food Diary
Diet Writing

Overweight or obese Americans face a discouraging cultural phenomenon. Most media images, such as television and magazines, show slim people or buffed up athletes. This leads to high levels of body dissatisfaction and in turn, fuels a $30 billion per year diet industry. Many people are convinced that they will successfully lose weight if they can simply find the right diet. They bounce from one highly publicized diet to another: low-fat, high carbohydrate; low carbohydrate, high protein and so on. Experts tend to agree that any calorie-cutting diet can produce weight loss in the short-term, often through water-weight loss. They also acknowledge that most diets are ineffective and that most people's attempts at weight loss will fail over the long run unless they change their eating habits permanently and make sustained exercise and activity part of their daily lives. Let's look more closely at dieting and why most diets fail.

Diets Often Lead to Weight Cycling

Do you know someone who is dieting? The Centers for Disease Control and Prevention estimates that about one-quarter of women aged 18 to 45 dieted in a recent six-month period.[47] Dismayingly, three-quarters of dieters will regain their weight within two years (or sooner) after a major diet. Most will wind up in a process called **weight cycling**—a pattern of repeatedly losing and regaining weight.

Weight experts refer to this pattern as **yo-yo dieting** (Figure 8.7). Yo-yo dieting may have significant health consequences. Some studies show a link to high blood pressure and other chronic diseases, but experts are not sure whether weight cycling in itself leads to physical health problems.[48] It is a common misconception that yo-yo dieting slows your metabolism and makes each new diet harder and less likely to succeed.[49] Studies of weight cycling do not reveal increases in fat

weight cycling The pattern of repeatedly losing and gaining weight, from illness or dieting

yo-yo dieting A series of diets followed by eventual weight gain

FIGURE **8.6** Being fit significantly reduces your mortality risk in any given year, regardless of your degree of body fat.

From "Cardiorespiratory fitness, body composition and all-cause and cardiovascular disease mortality in men," Chong Do Lee, et al., American Journal of Clinical Nutrition, 1999, Vol. 69, No. 3, pp. 373-380, by permission of the American Society for Nutrition.

Lean, fit body
Lean, unfit body

Normal, fit body
Normal, unfit body

Obese, fit body
Obese, unfit body

0   0.5   1.0   1.5   2.0   2.5   3.0
Relative risk of all-cause mortality

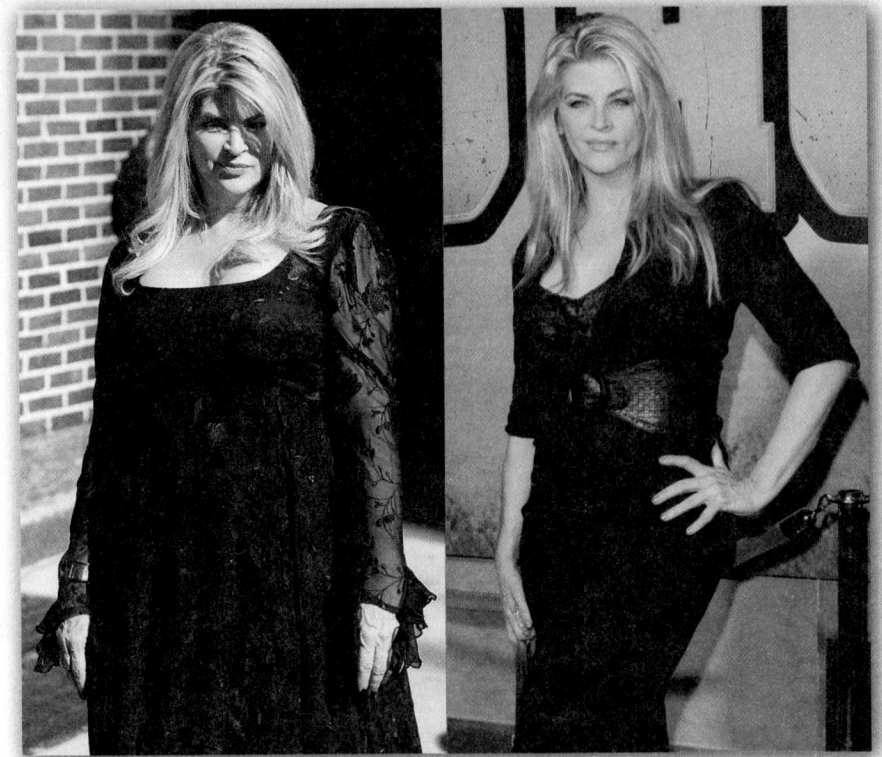

FIGURE **8.7** Actress Kirstie Alley, who was recently a contestant on *Dancing with the Stars,* has long struggled with "yo-yo dieting" or weight cycling.

calories tomorrow and increase your exercise regimen to compensate. As a result, people tend to stay on flexible diets longer and in the process, learn better long-term eating habits.

Everyone who diets will experience some degree of lowered metabolism during a period of calorie restriction as the body "defends" its fat stores. That's why even in a sensible diet, weight loss tends to slow down after an initial quick drop. It's also part of the reason why successful weight maintenance requires permanent changes to your old eating habits.

Our Built-In Appetite Controls Make Diets Less Effective

Our bodies have a complicated set of internal chemical signals and control mechanisms that tell us when to eat, how much to eat, how much fat our bodies should store, and how we should respond when those fat stores start to shrink.[51] Researchers have learned, for example, that we produce powerful appetite stimulants such as leptin and ghrelin. Fat cells make the hormone leptin. The levels of this hormone fall when your body uses stored fat. This stimulates your appetite—and contributes to the difficulty of dieting. Before a meal, your stomach and small intestines make more of a hormone called ghrelin that stimulates food consumption. When leptin levels fall or ghrelin levels climb, your nervous system stimulates food seeking and eating behaviors.

Our bodies do make natural compounds that suppress appetite and signal a feeling of fullness. These compounds help diminish our appetites and get us to stop eating when full. They are less powerful than the factors that increase appetite, though, so they are much easier for most people to tolerate or ignore.[52] Thus, the biology of appetite control works against dieting.

tissue, decreases in muscle tissue, or decreased metabolic rate as a result of weight cycling. Weight cycling can, however, lead to feelings of depression or failure.

Marketers of diet plans, books, and foods often promise quick weight loss with no hunger and very little effort. These diets usually backfire. One major reason they do is that they are rigid. **Rigid diets** specify rules like "eat only cabbage soup and grapefruit," or "never eat after 6:00 PM." Because rigid diets are unpleasant and restrictive, people seldom stick with them. People on rigid diets tend to have a higher percentage of body fat than people on more flexible plans.[50] The followers of rigid diets tend to exhibit more depression, anxiety, and binge eating as well.

In contrast to rigid diets, **flexible diets** are based on energy balancing of calories eaten and burned. They focus on portion size and make allowances for variations in daily routine, appetite, and food availability. For example, if you go to a party and overeat, a flexible diet allows you to cut extra

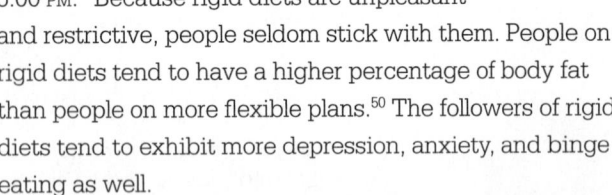

LIVE IT! ONLINE

Worksheet 21
All-or-Nothing
Thinking

rigid diets Weight-loss regimens that specify strict rules on calorie consumption, types of foods, and eating patterns

flexible diets Weight-loss regimens that focus on portion size and make allowances for variations in daily routine, appetite, and food availability

Most Diet Products and Plans Are Ineffective

Most over-the-counter products—"fat burners," "starch blockers," muscle stimulators, diet books, diet supplements, weight-loss

SEE IT! ONLINE

Diet Dream
Drug

program memberships, meal replacements, and other diet aids—are ineffective, and some are even dangerous. In 2004, the U.S. Food and Drug Administration banned the popular supplement ephedra (also called *ma huang*) after it caused heart attacks, seizures, and strokes in more than 16,000 people and precipitated more than 100 deaths. Even prescription diet drugs are only modestly effective and can have serious side effects.[53] As the box Do Drastic Weight Loss Methods Work? explains, prescription diet drugs and surgery are a viable option for only a small minority of overweight and obese people.

What about commercial diet plans and programs? One comprehensive study revealed that none of the nationally known programs—Weight Watchers, Jenny Craig, Optifast, eDiets.com, and Overeaters Anonymous—really deliver.[54] For example, after two years, people who joined Weight Watchers had lost an average of just 6.4 pounds. Equally ineffective are diet books that promise easy, permanent weight loss; invoke spurious factors such as your blood type or food allergies; or prescribe extreme diets (very low-calorie or based on eliminating whole categories of nutrients such as carbohydrates or fats).

What, then, should a would-be dieter do? If you are buying a book, look for one that advocates balanced nutrients and regular exercise. If you are joining a program, low-cost support groups are probably the best alternative for most people. They provide one important component: encouragement and support, either in person, through weekly groups, or online. Campus health centers can usually help students find group support for dieting. It's also important to enlist the personal encouragement of friends, roommates, and family members. If people undermine your diet efforts, tell them firmly that you need a different approach. We consider more tools for effective weight loss and management later in the chapter.

What Are Eating Disorders?

Skipping meals, going on diet after diet, and binging on junk food are all forms of **disordered eating**: atypical, abnormal food consumption that is common in the general public. Disordered eating diminishes your wellness but is usually neither long-lived nor disruptive to everyday life. **Eating disorders** are long-lasting, disturbed patterns of eating, dieting, and perceptions of body image that have psychological, environmental, and possibly genetic underpinnings.

Eating disorders can disrupt relationships, emotions, and concentration and can lead to physical injury, hospitalization, and even death. They require diagnosis and treatment from a psychiatrist or other physician.

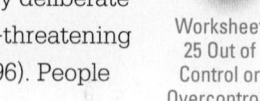

SEE IT! ONLINE

Extreme Healthy Eating?

Recognizing an eating disorder in yourself or a loved one can lead to treatment that improves or stops the behavior. The statements in Figure 8.8 can help you recognize abnormal or disordered thoughts about food and body image. People with eating disorders often believe they look fat even when they are rail thin. This unrealistic and negative self-perception can be part of a related syndrome called **body dysmorphic disorder** (BDD), in which a person becomes obsessed with a physical "defect" such as nose size or body shape.

The three most common types of eating disorders are anorexia nervosa, bulimia nervosa, and binge eating disorder. About eleven million Americans—ten million of whom are young women—meet the criteria for one of these disorders.[55]

Eating Disorders Have Distinctive Symptoms

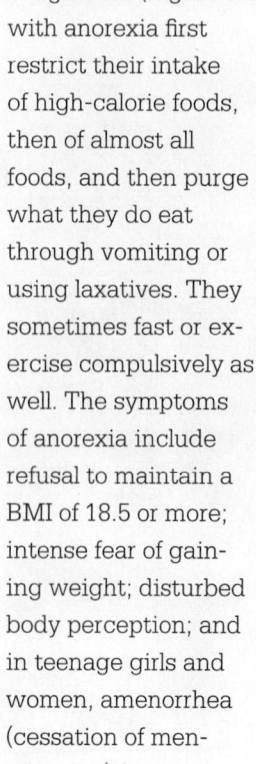

LIVE IT! ONLINE

Worksheet 25 Out of Control or Overcontrol?

Anorexia nervosa is a persistent, chronic eating disorder characterized by deliberate food restriction and severe, life-threatening weight loss (Figure 8.9, page 296). People with anorexia first restrict their intake of high-calorie foods, then of almost all foods, and then purge what they do eat through vomiting or using laxatives. They sometimes fast or exercise compulsively as well. The symptoms of anorexia include refusal to maintain a BMI of 18.5 or more; intense fear of gaining weight; disturbed body perception; and in teenage girls and women, amenorrhea (cessation of menstruation) for three

disordered eating Atypical, abnormal food consumption that diminishes wellness but is usually neither long-lived nor disruptive to everyday life

eating disorders Disturbed patterns of eating, dieting, and perceptions of body image that have psychological, environmental, and possibly genetic underpinnings and that lead to consequent medical issues

body dysmorphic disorder A psychological syndrome characterized by unrealistic and negative self-perception focusing on a perceived physical defect

anorexia nervosa A persistent, chronic eating disorder characterized by deliberate food restriction and severe, life-threatening weight loss

Do Drastic Weight Loss Methods Work?

Millions of people think to themselves, "I hate diets and exercise, and they don't work for me, anyway. Why can't I just take drugs or have surgery to get thin?" Unfortunately, prescription diet drugs are expensive, relatively ineffective, and have side effects. Over-the-counter diet drugs can be dangerous and are even less effective. And weight loss surgical procedures carry significant risks and are generally reserved for the severely obese or those with uncontrolled weight-related diseases like diabetes or high blood pressure.

Users of the prescription drug Xenical (orlistat), which partially blocks digestion of fats, lose an average of 13 pounds in a year (about 4 ounces per week), but side effects include oily stools and spotting, gas with fecal discharge, and urgent elimination. The prescription drugs Phentride (phentermine) and Tenuate (diethylpropion) suppress appetite.[1] However, these drugs are addictive and are prescribed only for short periods. For long-term success, people who take prescription diet drugs must still change their eating and exercise habits permanently. Without these changes, virtually all will regain the weight after the prescription ends.

The FDA has banned many other drugs and supplements (for example, drugs containing ephedra or phenylpropanolamine, also called *fen-phen*) and discouraged the use of others (such as Meridia) because of harmful side effects.[2] Over-the-counter diet remedies have not proven to be effective and can be harmful as well. *Hoodia gordonii* is widely advertised and sold but lacks convincing evidence for effectiveness. Other unproven supplements include St. John's wort, herbal laxatives, bitter orange, ginseng and ginkgo, and green tea extracts.

Surgery for weight loss (known as bariatric surgery) has grown more than ten-fold, from about 16,000 procedures per year in the 1990s to an estimated 220,000 in 2008. During gastric banding, the surgeon partitions the stomach into two parts using an inflatable band that acts like a belt. The patient then eats far less before feeling full and stays full longer. This procedure is surgically reversible. In gastric bypass, the surgeon creates a permanent small stomach pouch that connects to the small intestine. This drastically reduces the amount a person can eat as well as the nutrients he or she can absorb—vitamins and minerals as well as calories. This irreversible surgery poses many medical risks but it has been shown to improve type 2 diabetes in obese patients and can lead to significant weight loss.[3] The high cost of bariatric surgery ($15,000 and up) and its on-going medical risks restrict access for most people. Fifteen percent of those who have had bariatric surgery regain all of their original weight.[4] About half experience medical complications or nutrient deficiencies.[5] This discouraging picture could change with future medical research and development.

Sources:
1. D. Rucker and others, "Long-Term Pharmacotherapy for Obesity and Overweight: Updated Meta-Analysis," *British Medical Journal* 335, no. 7631 (2007): 1194–99.
2. A. Pollack, "Abbot Lab Withdraws Meridia, It's Diet Drug, From the Market," *New York Times*, October 9, 2010.
3. F. Rubino and others, "Metabolic Surgery to Treat Type 2 Diabetes: Clinical Outcomes and Mechanisms of Action," *Annual Review of Medicine* 61 (2010): 393–411.
4. D. Grady, "Operation for Obesity Leaves Some in Misery," *New York Times*, May 4, 2004.
5. G.J. Service and others, "Hyperinsulinemia Hypoglycemia with Nesidioblastosis after Gastric-Bypass Surgery," *New England Journal of Medicine* 353, no. 3 (2005): 249–54.

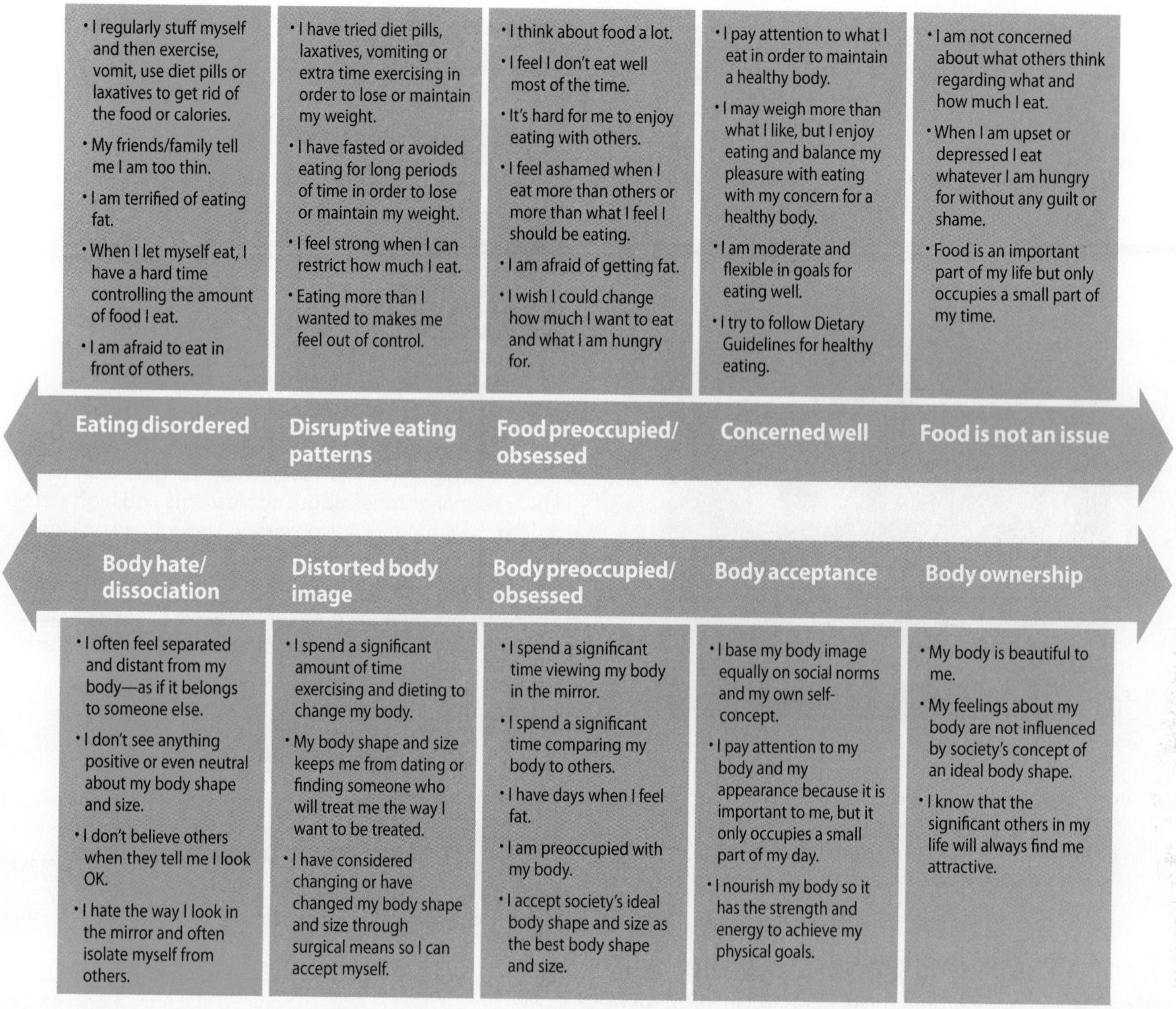

Eating disordered
- I regularly stuff myself and then exercise, vomit, use diet pills or laxatives to get rid of the food or calories.
- My friends/family tell me I am too thin.
- I am terrified of eating fat.
- When I let myself eat, I have a hard time controlling the amount of food I eat.
- I am afraid to eat in front of others.

Disruptive eating patterns
- I have tried diet pills, laxatives, vomiting or extra time exercising in order to lose or maintain my weight.
- I have fasted or avoided eating for long periods of time in order to lose or maintain my weight.
- I feel strong when I can restrict how much I eat.
- Eating more than I wanted to makes me feel out of control.

Food preoccupied/obsessed
- I think about food a lot.
- I feel I don't eat well most of the time.
- It's hard for me to enjoy eating with others.
- I feel ashamed when I eat more than others or more than what I feel I should be eating.
- I am afraid of getting fat.
- I wish I could change how much I want to eat and what I am hungry for.

Concerned well
- I pay attention to what I eat in order to maintain a healthy body.
- I may weigh more than what I like, but I enjoy eating and balance my pleasure with eating with my concern for a healthy body.
- I am moderate and flexible in goals for eating well.
- I try to follow Dietary Guidelines for healthy eating.

Food is not an issue
- I am not concerned about what others think regarding what and how much I eat.
- When I am upset or depressed I eat whatever I am hungry for without any guilt or shame.
- Food is an important part of my life but only occupies a small part of my time.

Body hate/dissociation
- I often feel separated and distant from my body—as if it belongs to someone else.
- I don't see anything positive or even neutral about my body shape and size.
- I don't believe others when they tell me I look OK.
- I hate the way I look in the mirror and often isolate myself from others.

Distorted body image
- I spend a significant amount of time exercising and dieting to change my body.
- My body shape and size keeps me from dating or finding someone who will treat me the way I want to be treated.
- I have considered changing or have changed my body shape and size through surgical means so I can accept myself.

Body preoccupied/obsessed
- I spend a significant time viewing my body in the mirror.
- I spend a significant time comparing my body to others.
- I have days when I feel fat.
- I am preoccupied with my body.
- I accept society's ideal body shape and size as the best body shape and size.

Body acceptance
- I base my body image equally on social norms and my own self-concept.
- I pay attention to my body and my appearance because it is important to me, but it only occupies a small part of my day.
- I nourish my body so it has the strength and energy to achieve my physical goals.

Body ownership
- My body is beautiful to me.
- My feelings about my body are not influenced by society's concept of an ideal body shape.
- I know that the significant others in my life will always find me attractive.

FIGURE 8.8 Thought patterns associated with healthy and disordered eating habits exist on a continuum, as do thought patterns associated with positive and negative body image.

Adapted from Smiley/King/Avery: Campus Health Service. Original continuum, C. Schislak: *Preventive Medicine and Public Health*. Copyright 1997 Arizona Board of Regents. Used with permission.

months or more. Five to twenty percent of anorexics eventually die from medical conditions brought on by vitamin or mineral deficiencies or physiological results of starvation. This gives anorexia the highest death rate of any psychological illness.[56]

Bulimia nervosa is characterized by frequent bouts of binge eating followed by purging (self-induced vomiting), laxative abuse, or excessive exercise. Bulimics tend to consume much more food than most people would during a given time period and feel a loss of control over it. Binging and purging are often done secretly. A medical diagnosis includes binging and purging at least twice a week for three months. People with bulimia are also obsessed with their bodies, weight gain, and how they appear to others. Unlike those with anorexia, however, people with bulimia are often normal weight. Treatment appears to be more effective for bulimia than for anorexia.

Binge eating disorder, a variation of bulimia, involves binge eating but usually no purging, laxatives, exercise, or fasting. Individuals with BED often wind up significantly overweight or obese but tend to binge much more often than does the typical obese person.

bulimia nervosa An eating disorder characterized by frequent bouts of binge eating followed by purging (self-induced vomiting), laxative abuse, or excessive exercise

binge eating disorder A variation of bulimia that involves binge eating but usually no purging, laxatives, exercise, or fasting

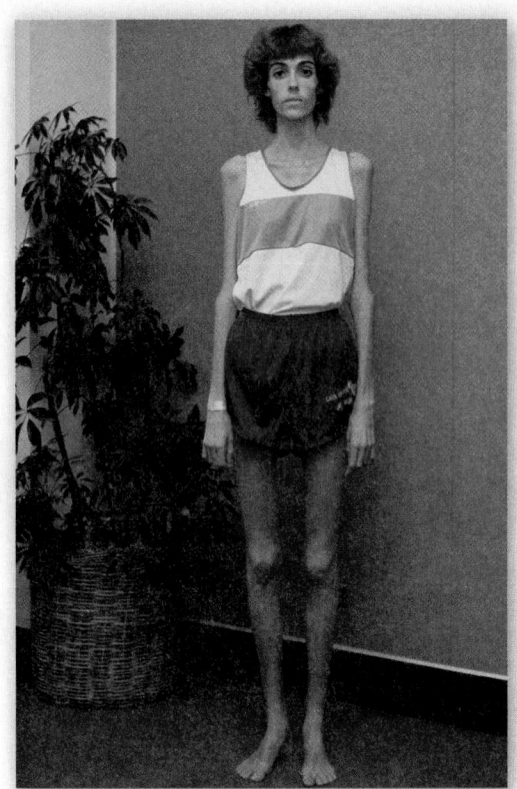

FIGURE 8.9 Anorexia nervosa is characterized by severe, life-threatening weight loss.

casestudy

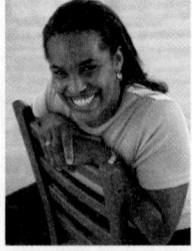

MARIA

"I've never had an eating disorder, but I admit that at times I've been tempted to binge and purge or take a laxative that I don't need. There's so much pressure from all sides. You go to a family party and everyone tells you to eat, eat, eat. At the same time, all you see on TV are super-thin people. How can you please everyone—and yourself?

"My daughter Anna is still a little kid, but I worry about the pressures she'll feel when she gets older. I hear so many stories about adolescents and high school students with eating disorders. Although I want—and need—to lose weight, I don't want Anna to get the message that being thin matters above everything else. There's a big difference between being overweight and wanting to lose excess weight to become healthier, and wanting to be stick-thin like a model or actress."

THINK! What signs of eating disorders or disordered eating should Maria watch for as Anna gets older?

ACT! If you suspect symptoms of an eating disorder in yourself or a friend, review the section in this chapter on eating disorders, look carefully at Figure 8.8, and if appropriate, consult a campus counselor or eating disorder support group.

HEAR IT! ONLINE

Eating Disorders Can Be Treated

Because eating disorders have complex physical, psychological, and social causes that unfold over many years, there are no quick or simple solutions for them. Still, eating disorders *are* treatable. The primary goal of treatment is usually to reduce the threat to the patient's life posed by his or her eating behaviors and the physical damage they can cause to the bones, teeth, throat, esophagus, stomach, intestines, heart, and other organs. Once the patient is stabilized medically, long-term therapy can begin. Often, the affected individual comes from a family that places undue emphasis on achievement, body weight, and appearance. Genetic susceptibility can also play a role.[57] Therapy focuses on the psychological, social, environmental, and physiological factors that have contributed. Therapy is aimed at helping the patient develop new eating behaviors, build self-confidence, deal with depression, and find constructive ways of dealing with life's problems. Eating disorder support groups can be pivotal as well.

What Concepts Must I Understand to Achieve My Weight Goals?

Understanding the role of metabolic rates, recognizing your body's set point, and understanding the energy balance equation are all important weight management tools. Taking lessons from successful weight maintainers can help you set and achieve realistic weight goals. And balancing your energy equation by keeping track of your calorie intake and by adding or continuing a regular exercise program can help you maintain a healthy weight over time.

Recognize the Role of Your Metabolic Rate

As much as 60 to 70 percent of your daily calorie intake—typically between 900 and 1,800 calories per day—is consumed as your body sustains functions such as heartbeat, breathing, and maintenance of body temperature.[58] The rate at which your body consumes food energy to sustain these basic functions is your **basal metabolic rate** (**BMR**). Your **resting metabolic rate** (**RMR**) is slightly higher, because it includes the energy you expend to digest food. BMR can be influenced by your activity level and your body composition. The more lean tissue you have, the greater your BMR; the more fat tissue you have, the lower your BMR. The higher your fitness level, the greater your ratio of lean tissue to fat mass is likely to be, and the more energy you will burn while exercising and at rest. Cardiovascular and strength-building exercises contribute most directly to speeding up BMR.

Recognize Your Body's Set Point

Perhaps you've noticed that your body is programmed around a certain weight or **set point** that it returns to fairly easily when you gain or lose a few pounds. Many dieters reach a plateau after a certain amount of weight loss and can't seem to trim off more pounds. This plateau is due, in part, to a downshifted metabolism balancing out lower calorie intake: the person's energy balance is now at a weight-maintenance, not a weight-loss, level. To "outsmart" and reset one's set point, a dieter must lose weight slowly and increase exercise.

Balance Your Energy Equation

Long-term weight management relies on balancing your energy equation—that is, reaching a balance where the calories you eat equal the calories you burn over time. To lose or gain weight, you must deliberately "unbalance" that equation for a while. If you expend more calories than you consume over time, you'll lose weight due to a **negative caloric balance** (Figure 8.10). Consume more calories than you expend

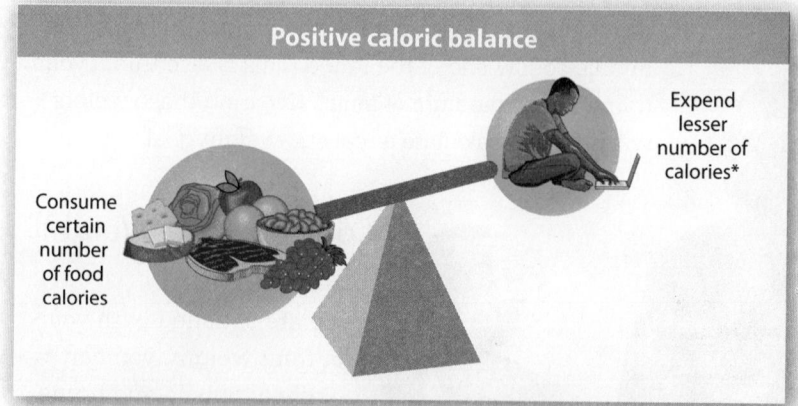

(a) Energy intake < Energy expenditure ⟶ Weight loss

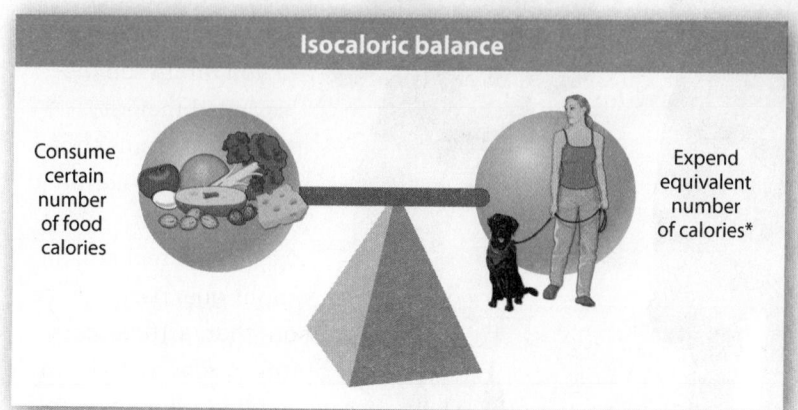

(b) Energy intake > Energy expenditure ⟶ Weight gain

(c) Energy intake = Energy expenditure ⟶ Weight maintenance

basal metabolic rate (BMR) Your baseline rate of energy use, dictated by your body's collective metabolic activities

resting metabolic rate (RMR) Basal metabolic rate plus the energy expended in digesting food

set point A pre-programmed weight that your body returns to easily when you gain or lose a few pounds

negative caloric balance A state in which the amount of calories consumed in food falls short of the amount of calories expended through metabolism and physical activity

FIGURE **8.10** On any given day, each of us has a personal energy equation with either a negative caloric balance, a positive caloric balance, or an isocaloric balance. Over time, this equation helps determine our body weight.

*Calories are expended through metabolism, activity, and exercise.

and you'll gain weight due to a **positive caloric balance**. Consume and expend approximately the same number of calories over a period of time and you'll reach an **isocaloric balance**—and with it, be able to maintain your weight.

There are several ways to approximate your daily calorie consumption and expenditure. You can calculate your current energy balance and set goals for a better balance in **Lab 8.1.** Another approach is logging on to the ChooseMyPlate website at www.ChooseMyPlate.gov to get a target number for calorie consumption based on your age, sex, and level of daily moderate or vigorous activity. This website provides calorie counts for specific foods and portions so you can keep track of how many calories you consume each day. You can also get calorie-counting programs for smart phones, or find them online at websites such as www.caloriecontrol.org.

positive caloric balance A state in which the amount of calories consumed in food exceeds the amount of calories expended through metabolism and physical activity

isocaloric balance A state in which the amount of calories consumed in food is approximately the same as the amount of calories expended through metabolism and physical activity

Height (feet and inches)	100	110	120	130	140	150	160	170	180	190	200	210	220	230	240	250	260
4'6"	24	27	29	31	34	36	39	41	43	46	48	51	53	55	58	60	63
4'8"	22	25	27	29	31	34	36	38	40	43	45	47	49	52	54	56	58
4'10"	21	23	25	27	29	31	33	36	38	40	42	44	46	48	50	52	54
5'0"	20	22	23	25	27	29	31	33	35	37	39	41	43	45	47	49	51
5'2"	18	20	22	24	26	27	29	31	33	35	37	38	40	42	44	46	48
5'4"	17	19	21	22	24	26	28	29	31	33	34	36	38	40	41	43	45
5'6"	16	18	19	21	23	24	26	27	29	31	32	34	36	37	39	40	42
5'8"	15	17	18	20	21	23	24	26	27	29	30	32	33	35	37	38	40
5'10"	14	16	17	19	20	22	23	24	26	27	29	30	32	33	34	36	37
6'0"	14	15	16	18	19	20	22	23	24	26	27	29	30	31	33	34	35
6'2"	13	14	15	17	18	19	21	22	23	24	26	27	28	30	31	32	33
6'4"	12	13	15	16	17	18	20	21	22	23	24	26	27	28	29	30	32
6'6"	12	13	14	15	16	17	19	20	21	22	23	24	25	27	28	29	30
6'8"	11	12	13	14	15	17	18	19	20	21	22	23	24	25	26	28	29
6'10"	11	12	13	14	15	16	17	18	19	20	21	22	23	24	25	26	27
7'0"	10	11	12	13	14	15	16	17	18	19	20	21	22	23	24	25	26

Weight (pounds)

Key:
- Underweight
- Normal weight
- Overweight
- Obese

FIGURE 8.11 Locate your height, read across to find your weight, and then read up to determine your BMI. Note that BMI values have been rounded to the nearest whole number.

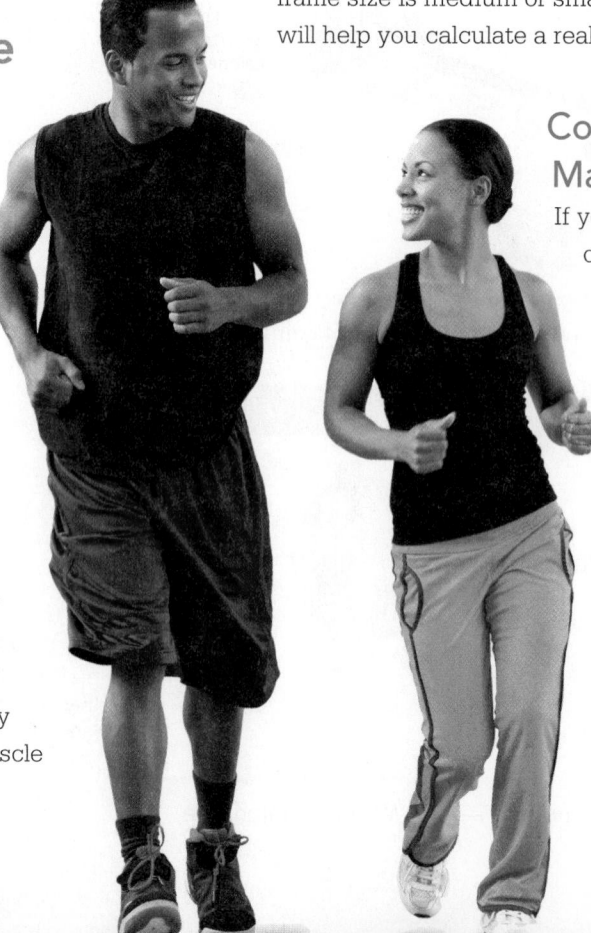

How Can I Create a Behavior Change Plan for Weight Management?

Let's look at the steps you can take to manage your weight.

Assess Your Current Weight and Choose a Realistic Goal

Figure 8.11 shows healthy weight and BMI ranges based on height. If your body fat percentage is low and your muscle development is high, your healthy weight and your BMI will be on the higher end of the range. The same is also true if your frame size is large. If your body fat percentage is high and your muscle development is low, your healthy weight will be in the middle-to-low end of the range. This is also true if your frame size is medium or small. Knowing these factors will help you calculate a realistic weight goal.

Contemplate Weight Management

If you are satisfied with your current weight, you can simply pursue and refine your application of good nutritional principles and regular exercise. If you are in the dissatisfied majority, use the assessment of your current weight and BMI from Figure 8.11 to choose a realistic weight goal based on no more than a 10 percent initial loss or gain. Even if you don't need weight change now, you can use the specifics in this section to stabilize your current weight and maintain it for the next few decades. Readiness requires motivation, commitment, goals, and a positive attitude. **Lab 8.2** at the end of this chapter helps you assess your readiness for weight change—your diet IQ.

Prepare for Better Weight Management

- *Think about your beliefs and attitudes.* Do you see yourself as a hopeless victim of "bad genes," overwork, or low budget? Think you are too young to worry about deliberate weight management? Believe that you can take effective control of your body composition and weight largely through eating intelligently, limiting your calorie intake, and establishing a program of regular exercise? Talk

with others or write in your journal to clarify your attitudes in preparation for making an effective weight management plan.

- *Consider your goals.* Motivating goals are usually personal and extended, such as looking good, feeling fit and capable, and staying well over a period of years. Avoid short-term goals that can lead to weight cycling. If one of your reasons is a specific upcoming event (a beach trip or a sports match, for example), find additional reasons with longer time frames. Long-term goals help you see beyond poorly designed quick-fix diet remedies. You can write out your specific goals in **Lab 8.3**.

- *Identify barriers to change.* What keeps you from changing or maintaining your weight? A lack of information about good weight management techniques? Poor nutrition and eating habits? Eating triggers that encourage overconsumption? Lack of social

TOOLS FOR **CHANGE** •

Tips for Weight Management

Try these ideas for reframing weight loss in your mind, rather than jumping right in to a diet regimen unprepared:

LIVE IT! ONLINE

Worksheet 22 It Doesn't Last If You Fast

- Think substitution. Instead of cookies or ice cream at snack time, substitute fresh fruit. Instead of chips or fries, substitute unbuttered popcorn, nuts, or vegetable sticks and low-fat dip.

- Consider yourself successful if you lose 1/2 to 1 pound per week. Faster weight loss stimulates too much hunger, slows metabolism, and loses lean tissue.

- Avoid feeling famished by choosing high-volume, nutrient-dense foods. Items such as clear soups, light salads, whole grains, fruits, vegetables, and beans fill you more quickly and control hunger longer.

- Avoid rigid dieting. Strictly limiting calorie counts or forbidding yourself certain foods can trigger binging and weight gain, not loss. Flexible dieting works better and emphasizes portion control and lower-calorie, higher-volume foods.

- Don't drink "empty" calories. Drinks sweetened with sugar or corn syrup contribute disproportionately to weight gain. Alcoholic drinks pack a lot of calories and stimulate the appetite.

- Sleep well. Get seven to nine hours of sleep each night. Sleep deprivation triggers greater levels of hunger and eating.

- Increase the physical activity in your life. Take the stairs instead of the elevator. Walk the last mile to class instead of riding in a car or bus. Turn off the TV and go play Frisbee with a friend.

- Join a support group. Support groups help most people lose at least a small amount of weight and keep it off.

- Use an online or smartphone application to track calories, keep food diaries, calculate body fat and fat grams in foods, log in your weight to a social site, and so on. These high tech tools can't substitute for your own motivation and adherence, but they can make tracking your information and getting support easier and more fun!

or emotional support? Lack of exercise? Identify your barriers and brainstorm solutions to them.

- *Visualize new behaviors.* What specific new behaviors will you adopt to improve your BMI and body composition? Here are some good choices: Choosing only nutritious foods. Avoiding foods filled with saturated fats, sweeteners, or sodium. Tracking the numbers of servings you eat from each food group. Planning for exercise most days of the week. Keeping a log of your daily and weekly exercise. Asking friends for support.

Take Action

- *Commit to your goals.* Behavior change requires commitment. Thinking and talking about your commitment with friends is helpful; so is writing it down and showing it to someone.

- *Set up support.* Solicit the help of people you can trust to support your efforts. Let's say it is 9:30 PM, you've finished studying and you're hungry, but you've already eaten the 1,800 calories on your day's food plan. A supportive friend might say, "Well, you can always have some raw vegetables to fill up. You'll be glad you stuck with your program. Just think, once you've lost weight, you can add back some extra calories each day—and that won't be so long from now!" The box Tips for Weight Management tells more.

Establish a Regular Exercise Program

Along with monitored and controlled eating, physical activity is crucial both to weight change (loss or gain) and to weight maintenance. In addition to following a healthy diet, you may need to be active for more than an hour per day in order to lose weight, while sixty minutes per day will sustain weight at current levels. These figures are cumulative: Add seven minutes of stair-climbing here, plus eleven minutes of brisk walking across campus there, plus twenty minutes of stationary biking, and so on. Aerobic exercise is the best calorie burner.

The greater the frequency, intensity, and time spent on an activity, the more energy you use and the more calories you burn. There are other considerations for choosing types of fitness exercise as well. The larger the muscle groups you use, the more you boost your metabolism and, in turn, your calorie expenditure. Kick boxing, for example, uses the thigh, calf, and gluteus muscles as well as those that move and support your torso. By contrast, lifting small hand weights works mainly the smaller muscles

of the hand, wrist, and lower arms. Table 8.1 lists the caloric expenditures for several popular activities, sports, and exercises for adults of different weight levels.

Achieve Weight Maintenance

Weight management and weight change are similar in principle. The tools are the same; your daily calorie goal for weight management will simply be isocaloric while your daily goal for weight loss or gain will have a negative or positive caloric balance. Some degree of

TABLE **8.1** Calories Burned through Activity			
Activity, Sport, or Exercise	Calories You Expend per Minute If You Weigh...		
	110 lb	150 lb	190 lb
Aerobics, 10" step	7.0	9.5	12.0
Basketball, pick-up	7.0	9.5	12.0
Biking, slow	5.3	7.1	9.0
Bowling	2.6	3.6	4.5
Dancing, moderate pace	4.2	5.7	9.0
Downhill skiing, moderate pace	5.5	7.5	9.5
Driving	1.8	2.4	3.0
Frisbee, casual	2.6	3.6	4.5
Golf, walking and pulling clubs	4.4	6.0	7.5
Grocery shopping	3.1	4.2	5.3
Hiking, hills	5.3	7.1	9.0
Jogging, moderate pace	5.3	7.1	9.0
Kickboxing	8.8	12.0	14.7
Office work	1.3	1.8	2.3
Ping-Pong	3.5	4.8	6.0
Reading	0.9	1.2	1.5
Soccer, noncompetitive	6.1	8.3	10.5
Softball	4.4	6.0	7.5
Stair climbing, 40 stairs/minute	6.1	8.3	10.2
Stretching	3.5	4.8	5.8
Swimming	~8	~10	~13
Tennis, singles, recreational	7.0	9.5	12.0
Watching TV	1.0	1.4	1.8

Source: Adapted from *Calorie Expenditure Charts*, by Frank I. Katch, Victor L. Katch, and William D. McArdle (Ann Arbor, Michigan: Fitness Technologies Press, 1996).

casestudy

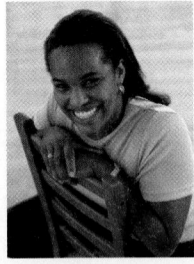

MARIA

"We moved to a new apartment recently, and after living there for a month, it's gotten easier to climb up and down the three flights of stairs. I guess I'm getting used to it! I know this isn't enough exercise to make me lose weight, but at least I'm a little more active. I can see that I need to change daily habits—eating and exercising—instead of just 'going on a diet.' Because I'll regain everything I lose as soon as I go off of it, right? So I need to figure out more ways to be active—ways that feel natural, like taking the stairs; not forced, like doing push ups!

"I weigh 155 right now. I need to lose 35 pounds to get back to my prepregnancy weight of 120. For now, I'm just going to try losing 10 pounds, at least to start off with. I've heard about weight-loss groups that help you plan meals, control how much you eat, and get regular exercise. I think a group might be a good approach for me."

THINK! You've just read about several tools for effective weight management. Which tools is Maria considering? Which tools do you already use? Which others could you use?

ACT! Write down some steps you can take to begin a regular exercise program, to improve the one you already have, or just to fit more physical activity into your day.

. . . .

calorie-tracking is usually involved in both maintenance and change, and a weekly weigh-in is important. If you have lost or gained ten percent of your body weight, you will need to maintain that level for a few months before resuming more weight change. The skills you employ during an interim phase of weight maintenance will be excellent practice for the rest of your life! Once weight management skills, good nutrition, and daily exercise and activity become second nature, both change and maintenance become relatively easy for most people.

Take Lessons from Successful Weight Maintainers

Most people who sustain a normal, healthy weight over years or decades engage in a physically active lifestyle, averaging an hour per day of moderate to vigorous physical activity.[59] They don't skip meals; they eat breakfast every day. They eat a nutritious diet that is low in fats and high in complex carbohydrates, has moderate levels of protein, and has a high volume but a low calorie density—even on weekends! They avoid sodas and juice drinks sweetened with sugar or corn syrup.

Successful weight maintainers also stay conscious of situations that trigger overeating and they apply strategies to prevent overeating. They are motivated to stay at a healthy weight, and they respond quickly by cutting back calories and increasing activity when their weight starts to creep up.[60]

People who are successful at maintaining a healthy weight typically have tools for coping with problems and handling life stresses. They assume responsibility for their lifestyle behaviors, know where to seek help, and tend to be self-reliant. They have a good social support system, both for their weight maintenance and their lives in general.[61]

Maintaining recommended weight and BMI confer so many benefits upon your appearance, energy level, and overall wellness that once you master the needed skill set, you'll rarely miss the junk food you used to eat, nor will you miss the few minutes it will take each day to track energy consumed and expended. The rewards in lifelong wellness are fully worth the trade-off!

chapterinreview

videos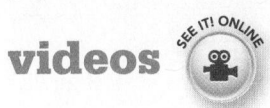

Log on to **www.pearsonhighered.com/hopson** or MyFitnessLab to view these chapter-related videos.

Diet Dream Drug   Food Diary Diet Writing   Extreme Healthy Eating
Miscounting Calories

onlineresources

Please visit this book's website at **www.pearsonhighered.com/hopson** to access links related to topics in this chapter.

 Audio case study
Audio PowerPoint lecture

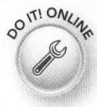 Lab 8.1 Calculating Energy Balance and Setting Energy Balance Goals
Lab 8.2 Your Diet IQ
Lab 8.3 Your Weight Management Plan

 Take Charge of Your Health! Worksheets:
Worksheet 21 All-or-Nothing Thinking and "Safe Foods" versus "Forbidden Foods"
Worksheet 22 It Doesn't Last If You Fast
Worksheet 23 Why Do You Eat?
Worksheet 25 Out of Control or Overcontrol?
Behavior Change Log Book and Wellness Journal

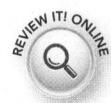 Pre- and post-quizzes
Glossary flashcards

reviewquestions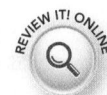

1. The World Health Organization coined the term "globesity" to promote an understanding of
   a. global hunger.
   b. rising obesity rates in underdeveloped countries.
   c. rising obesity rates in developed countries.
   d. the epidemic of obesity in the global population.

2. Excess body weight can affect body systems negatively. Indicate the one least likely to be affected negatively.
   a. Cardiovascular system (heart and lungs)
   b. Digestive system (gallbladder, kidneys, colon)
   c. Musculoskeletal system (bones and joints)
   d. Integumentary system (skin and hair)

3. At more than 20 percent above the recommended weight range, a person who is 5'8" tall is considered
   a. overweight.
   b. obese.
   c. at ideal weight.
   d. at his/her set point.

4. A BMI of 16 in a woman indicates
   a. overweight.
   b. underweight.
   c. normal weight.
   d. obesity.

5. Getting up, walking around, and jiggling your feet when seated are all examples of
   a. energy conservation.
   b. appetite control.
   c. non-exercise activity.
   d. depression.

6. To lose weight, you must establish a(n)
   a. negative caloric balance.
   b. isocaloric balance.
   c. positive caloric balance.
   d. set point.

7. Weight cycling is
   a. a pattern of repeatedly losing and regaining weight.
   b. characterized by rigid diets.
   c. characterized by flexible diets.
   d. uncommon.

8. Anorexia nervosa is characterized by
   a. frequent bouts of binge eating followed by self-induced vomiting.
   b. deliberate food restriction and severe, life-threatening weight loss.
   c. the use of laxatives.
   d. obesity.

9. The rate at which your body consumes food energy to sustain basic functions is your
   a. basal metabolic rate.
   b. resting metabolic rate.
   c. BMI.
   d. set point.

10. Successful weight maintainers are most likely to do which of the following?
    a. Indulge in junk food on weekends
    b. Skip meals
    c. Drink diet sodas
    d. Eat a nutritious diet that is low in fats, with high volume but low calorie density

critical**thinking**questions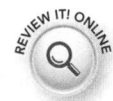

1. How do height, physical build, and musculature affect recommended weight and BMI?
2. What do you see as the greatest contributor to "globesity"? Defend your answer.
3. List several effective tools for successful weight management. Is one more important than the others? If so, discuss.
4. Why do most diets fail?

references

1. First Lady Michelle Obama, Introduction of New Plan to Combat Overweight and Obesity, Press Conference, Alexandria, Virginia, January 28, 2010.
2. K. M. Flegal and others, "Prevalence and Trends in Obesity among U.S. Adults, 1999–2008," *Journal of the American Medical Association* 303, no. 3 (2010): 235–41.
3. Ibid.
4. C. D. Fryar and C. L. Ogden, "NCHS Health E-Stat: Prevalence of Underweight Among Adults Aged 20 Years and Over: United States, 2007–2008." National Health and Nutrition Examination Survey, www.cdc.gov/nchs/data/hestat/underweight/underweight_adults.htm (updated May 2009).
5. M. Ogden and M. Carroll, "NCHS E-Stat: Prevalence of Obesity among Children and Adolescents: United States, Trends 1963–1965 through 2007–2008," National Health and Nutrition Examination Survey, www.cdc.gov/nchs/data/hestat/obesity_child_07_08/obesity_child_07_08.htm (updated June 2010).
6. American College Health Association, *American College Health Association–National College Health Assessment II (ACHA-NCHA II) Reference Group Executive Summary Spring 2010* (Linthicum, MD: American College Health Association, 2010).
7. Charlotte A. Schoenborn and others, "Body Weight Status of Adults: United States, 1997–1998." *Advance Data from Vital and Health Statistics* no. 330 (2002).
8. University of Minnesota, Boynton Health Service, "News Release: First Ever Comprehensive Report on the Health of Minnesota College Students Looks at Mental Health, Obesity, Financial Health, Sexual Health and More," www1.umn.edu/news/news-releases/2007/UR_RELEASE_MIG_4318.html (November 2007).
9. University of New Hampshire, "College Students Face Obesity, High Blood Pressure, Metabolic Syndrome." *ScienceDaily* www.sciencedaily.com/releases/2007/06/070614113310.htm (June 2007).
10. American College Health Association, *ACHA-NCHA II Reference Group Executive Summary Spring 2010,* 2010.
11. World Health Organization, "Fact sheet no. 311: Obesity and Overweight," www.who.int/mediacentre/factsheets/fs311/en/index.html (updated March 2011).
12. International Union of Nutritional Sciences, "The Global Challenge of Obesity and the International Obesity Task Force," September 2002, www.iuns.org/features/obesity/obesity.htm (accessed March 2011).
13. M. Ogden and M. Carroll, "NCHS E-Stat: Prevalence of Overweight, Obesity, and Extreme Obesity among Adults: United States, Trends 1960–1962 through 2007–2008," National Health and Nutrition Examination Survey, www.cdc.gov/nchs/data/hestat/obesity_adult_07_08/obesity_adult_07_08.htm (updated June 2011).
14. U.S. Department of Agriculture Economic Research Service, "U.S. Food Consumption Up 16 Percent Since 1970," *Amber Waves,* November 2005, www.ers.usda.gov/AmberWaves/November05/findings/usfoodconsumption.htm.
15. B. Wamsink, J. E. Painter, and J. North, "Bottomless Bowls: Why Visual Cues of Portion Size May Influence Intake," *Obesity Research* 13, no. 1 (2005): 93–100.
16. J. C. Spence and others, "Relation between Local Food Environments and Obesity among Adults," *BMC PublicHealth* 9 (2009): 192; M. Wang and others, "Changes in Neighbourhood Food Store Environment, Food Behaviour, and Body Mass Index, 1981–1990," *PublicHealth Nutrition* 11, no. 9 (2008): 963–70.
17. B. Wansink, "Environmental Factors that Increase the Food Intake and Consumption Volume of Unknowing Customers," *Annual Review of Nutrition* 24 (2004): 455–79.
18. B. Wansink, J. E. Painter, and J. North, "Bottomless Bowls: Why Visual Cues of Portion Size May Influence Intake," 2005.
19. G. Block and others, "Foods Contributing to Energy Intake in the U.S.: Data from NHANES III and NHANES 1999–2000," *Journal of Food Chemistry and Analysis* 17, no. 3–4 (2004): 439–47.
20. S. A. French, "Public Health Strategies for Dietary Change: Schools and Workplaces," *Journal of Nutrition* 135, no. 4 (2005): 91–92.
21. National Center for Health Statistics, "NCHS Health E-Stat: Prevalence of Sedentary Leisure-Time Behavior among Adults in the United States," www.cdc.gov/nchs/data/hestat/sedentary/sedentary.htm (updated February 2010); M. S. Treuth and others, "A Longitudinal Study of Sedentary Behavior and Overweight in Adolescent Girls," *Obesity* 17, no. 5 (2009): 1003–08.
22. M. Papas and others, "The Built Environment and Obesity," *Epidemiological Reviews* 29, no. 1 (2007): 129–43; M. Rao and others, "The Built Environment and Health," *The Lancet* 370, no. 9593 (2007): 1111–13.
23. I. S. Farooqi and S. O'Rahilly, "Genetic Factors in Human Obesity," *Obesity Reviews* 8, Suppl 1 (2007): 37–40.
24. J. A. Levine and others, "Interindividual Variation in Posture Allocation: Possible Role in Human Obesity," *Science* 307, no. 5709 (2005): 584–86.
25. Centers for Disease Control and Prevention, U.S. Physical Activity Statistics, "1988–2008 No Leisure-Time Physical Activity Trend Chart," www.cdc.gov/nccdphp/dnpa/physical/stats/leisure_time.htm (updated February 2010).
26. M. Beydoun, L. Powell, and Y. Yang, "The Association of Fast Food, Fruit, and Vegetable Prices with Dietary Intakes among U.S. Adults: Is There Modification by Family Income?" *Social Science and Medicine* 66, no. 11 (2008): 2218–29.
27. W. Willett, *Eat, Drink, and Be Healthy: The Harvard Medical School Guide to Healthy Eating* (New York: Free Press, 2003): 35.
28. D. Canoy and others, "Body Fat Distribution and Risk of Coronary Heart Disease in Men and Women in the European Prospective Investigation into Cancer and Nutrition in Norfolk Cohort: A Population-Based Prospective Study," *Circulation* 116, no. 25 (2007): 2933–43.
29. C. D. Fryar and C. L. Ogden, "Prevalence of Underweight among Adults Aged 20 Years and Over: United States, 2007–2008," 2009.
30. R. Puhl and K.D. Brownell, "Bias, Discrimination, and Obesity," *Obesity Research* 9, no. 12 (2001): 788–805.
31. D. R. Musher-Eizenman and others, "Body Size Stigmatization in Preschool Children: The Role of Control Attributions," *Journal of Pediatric Psychology* 29, no. 8 (2004): 613–20; S. H. Thompson and S. Digsby, "A Preliminary Survey of Dieting, Body Dissatisfaction, and Eating Problems among High School Cheerleaders," *Journal of School Health* 74, no. 3 (2004): 85–90.
32. R. Puhl and K.D. Brownell, "Bias, Discrimination, and Obesity," 2001.
33. D. R. Musher-Eizenman and others, "Body Size Stigmatization in Preschool Children," 2004.
34. R. Puhl and K.D. Brownell, "Bias, Discrimination, and Obesity," 2001; M. R. Hebl and L. M. Mannix, "The Weight of Obesity in Evaluating Others: A Mere Proximity Effect," *Perspectives in Social Psychology Bulletin* 29, no. 1 (2003): 28–38.
35. M. R. Hebl and L. M. Mannix, "The Weight of Obesity in Evaluating Others," 2003.
36. M. B. Schwartz and others, "Weight Bias among Health Professionals Specializing in Obesity," *Obesity Research* 11, no. 9): 1033–39.
37. S. S. Wang and others, "The Influence of the Stigma of Obesity on Overweight Individuals," *International Journal of Obesity* 28, no. 10 (2004): 1333–37.

38. C. O'Neil and T. Nicklas, "State of the Art Reviews: Relationship between Diet/Physical Activity and Health," *American Journal of Lifestyle Medicine* 1, no. 6 (2007): 457–81.

39. E. Calle and others, "Overweight, Obesity, and Mortality from Cancer in a Prospectively Studied Cohort of U.S. Adults," *New England Journal of Medicine* 348, no. 17 (2003): 1625–38.

40. N. Pandey and V. Gupta, "Trends in Diabetes," *Lancet* 369, no. 9569 (2007): 1256–57.

41. Mayo Clinic Staff, "Metabolic Syndrome," www.mayoclinic.com/health/metabolic%20syndrome/DS00522 (November 2009).

42. C. C. Mann, "Provocative Study Says Obesity May Reduce U.S. Life Expectancy," *Science* 307, no. 5716 (2005): 1716–17.

43. S. J. Olshansky and others, "A Potential Decline in Life Expectancy in the United States in the 21st Century," *New England Journal of Medicine* 352, no. 11 (2005): 1138–45.

44. K. Flegal and others, "Excess Deaths Associated with Underweight, Overweight, and Obesity," *Journal of the American Medical Association* 298, no. 17 (2007): 2028–37; K. M. Flegal and B. I. Graubard, "Estimates of Excess Deaths Associated with Body Mass Index and Other Anthropometric Variables," *American Journal of Clinical Nutrition* 89, no. 4 (2009): 1213–19.

45. Y. Takata and others, "Association between Body Mass Index and Mortality in an 80-Year-Old Population," *Journal of the American Geriatric Society* 55, no. 6 (2007): 913–17.

46. L. Fontana and others, "Long-Term Calorie Restriction Is Highly Effective in Reducing the Risk for Atherosclerosis in Humans," *Proceedings of the National Academy of Sciences* 101, no. 17 (2004): 6659–63.

47. S. L. Boulet and others, "Folate Status in Women of Childbearing Age, by Race/Ethnicity—United States, 1999–2000, 2001–2002, and 2003–2004," *Morbidity and Mortality Weekly Report*, 54, no. 38 (2005): 8.

48. U.S. Department of Health and Human Services, National Institute of Diabetes and Digestive and Kidney Diseases (NIDDK), "Weight Cycling," NIH Publication No. 01-3901, www.win.niddk.nih.gov/publications/PDFs/wtcycling2bw.pdf (May 2008).

49. NIDDK, "Weight Cycling," 2008.

50. C. F. Smith and others, "Flexible versus Rigid Dieting Strategies: Relationship with Adverse Behavioral Outcomes," *Appetite* 32, no. 3 (1999): 295–305.

51. S. Stock and others, "Ghrelin, Peptide YY, Glucose-Dependent Insulinotropic Polypeptide, and Hunger Responses to a Mixed Meal in Anorexic, Obese, and Control Female Adolescents," *Journal of Clinical Endocrinology and Metabolism* 90, no. 4 (2005); E. T. Poehlman, "Reduced Metabolic Rate after Caloric Restriction," *Journal of Clinical Endocrinology and Metabolism* 88, no. 1 (2003): 14–15.

52. D. Rucker and others, "Long-Term Pharmacotherapy for Obesity and Overweight: Updated Meta-Analysis," *British Medical Journal* 335, no. 7631 (2007): 1194–99; ConsumerSearch, "Diet Pills: Reviews," www.consumersearch.com/diet-pills (updated August 2009).

53. Ibid.

54. A. Tsai and T. Wadden, "Systematic Review: An Evaluation of Major Commercial Weight Loss Programs in the U.S.," *Annals of Internal Medicine* 142, no. 1 (J2005): 56–66.

55. National Eating Disorder Association, "Statistics: Eating Disorders and Their Precursors," www.nationaleatingdisorders.org/information-resources/general-information.php#facts-statistics (2005).

56. K. Beals and A. Hill, "The Prevalence of Disordered Eating, Menstrual Dysfunction, and Low Bone Mineral Density among US Collegiate Athletes," *International Journal of Sport Nutrition and Exercise Metabolism* 16, no. 1 (2006): 1–23; American Psychiatric Association, "DSM-5 Development: Proposed Revision: 307.1 Anorexia Nervosa," www.dsm5.org/ProposedRevisions/Pages/proposedrevision.aspx?rid=24 (updated October 2010).

57. C. M. Bulik and others, "The Genetics of Anorexia Nervosa," *Annual Review of Nutrition* 27 (2007): 263–75.

58. Mayo Clinic Staff, "Metabolism and Weight Loss: How You Burn Calories," www.mayoclinic.com/health/metabolism/WT00006 (October 2009).

59. R. R. Wing and S. Phelan, "Long-Term Weight Loss Maintenance," *American Journal of Clinical Nutrition* 82, no. 1 (2005): 222S–25S.

60. K. Elfhag and S. Rossner, "Who Succeeds in Maintaining Weight Loss?" *Obesity Review* 6, no. 1 (2005): 67–85.

61. Ibid.

LAB 8.1 • CALCULATING ENERGY BALANCE AND SETTING ENERGY BALANCE GOALS

Name: _____ **Date:** _____

Instructor: _____ **Section:** _____

Materials: Calculator, access to Internet (optional)

Purpose: To learn how to calculate energy balance and set realistic goals for calorie intake and energy expenditure.

Directions: Complete the following sections.

SECTION I: CALCULATING BMR AND ENERGY EXPENDITURE

Your **basal metabolic rate (BMR)** is the rate at which you burn calories to sustain life functions at rest at a normal room temperature. Your activities, fitness level, stress level, and many other things will affect your BMR.

1. Calculate your BMR (the method shown here uses the Harris-Benedict formula):

Men

1. BMR = 66 + (6.3 × weight in pounds) + (12.9 × height in inches) − (6.8 × age in years)

2. BMR = 66 + (   ) + (   ) − (   )

3. BMR = _____ calories

Women

1. BMR = 655 + (4.3 × weight in pounds) + (4.7 × height in inches) − (4.7 × age in years)

2. BMR = 655 + (   ) + (   ) − (   )

3. BMR = _____ calories

2. Estimate your total energy expenditure (EE):

Total energy expenditure takes into account your amount of activity within a 24-hour period. You can calculate your energy expenditure by keeping an activity log and adding up the calories expended during any nonsleep time. To do this, use the physical activity tracking tool on the ChooseMyPlate website (www.choosemyplate.gov). Another way to estimate total energy expenditure is to use the following calculations. Choose your level of activity on *average* and use that formula to calculate your energy expenditure (EE).

Multiply your BMR by the appropriate activity factor, completing ONE equation below:

- If you are **sedentary** (little or no exercise):

  EE = _____(BMR) × **1.2** = _____ calories

- If you are **lightly active** (light exercise/sports 1–3 days/week):

  EE = _____(BMR) × **1.375** = _____ calories

- If you are **moderately active** (moderate exercise/sports 3–5 days/week):

  EE = _____(BMR) × **1.55** = _____ calories

- If you are **very active** (hard exercise/sports 6–7 days/week):

  EE = _____(BMR) × **1.725** = _____ calories

- If you are **extra active** (very hard daily exercise/sports & physical job or 23-day training):

  EE = _____(BMR) × **1.9** = _____ calories

SECTION II: CALCULATING ENERGY BALANCE

1. Estimated **calorie INTAKE**

_____ calories

2. Estimated **calorie EXPENDITURE** (EE from Section I)

_____ calories

3. Subtract your EXPENDITURE (#2) from your INTAKE (#1) to get:

Out of balance calories = _____ calories

SECTION III: TOOLS FOR YOUR WEIGHT MANAGEMENT PLAN

1. What was your caloric intake from your dietary analysis? _____ What was your energy expenditure? _____ What was your overall energy balance? _____

- **Energy balance** (+/− 200 calories): You are supplying your body with its energy needs and maintaining current weight.
- **Negative energy balance** (−201 calories): You are expending more energy than you are eating and should be losing weight.
- **Positive energy balance** (+201 calories): You are eating more energy than you are expending and should be gaining weight.

2. Do you want or need to lose body fat? **YES or NO**

3. What is your **goal** for your body fat percentage? _____

4. Complete the following calculations to figure out how many **pounds of fat** you need to lose in order to reach this goal:

- Find your **current fat weight:**

  _____ (current weight, lb) × _____ (current % body fat, expressed as a decimal) = _____ current fat weight (lb)

- Find your **lean body mass**

  (LBM): _____ (weight, lb) − _____ (fat weight, lb) = _____ LBM (lb)

- Find your **target body weight:**

  _____ (LBM) ÷ (1 − goal % body fat expressed as a decimal) = _____ target body weight (lb)

- Find the **lb of fat loss** needed to reach your body fat percentage goal:

  _____ (current weight, lb) − _____ (target weight, lb) = _____ fat loss needed (lb)

5. If you lose 1 pound of fat per week (500 calorie deficits per day), how many weeks will it take you to lose your desired fat weight? _____

6. Brainstorm ways that you can get to a −500 calorie deficit per day through diet and exercise/activity changes.

DIET CHANGE (−250 calories)

_____

_____

_____

_____

ACTIVITY CHANGE (−250 calories)

_____

_____

_____

_____

LAB 8.2 • YOUR DIET IQ

Name: _____   **Date:** _____

Instructor: _____   **Section:** _____

Purpose: To encourage students to think critically about their dieting history, ways of controlling food consumption, and readiness for weight changes.

Directions: Complete the following sections to analyze your dieting patterns.

SECTION I: DIET HISTORY

1. **How many times have you been on a diet?**

_____0 times   _____1–3 times   _____4–10 times   _____11–20 times   _____more than 20

2. **How much weight did you lose?**

_____0 lb.   _____1–5 lb.   _____6–10 lb.   _____11–20 lb.   _____more than 20 lb.

3. **How long did you stay at the new lower weight?**

_____Under 1 mo.   _____2–3 mos.   _____4–6 mos.   _____6 to 12 mos.   _____Over 1 yr.

4. Put a check mark by each dieting method you have tried:

_____skipping breakfast   _____skipping lunch or dinner

_____cutting out all snacks   _____counting calories

_____cutting out most fats   _____cutting out most carbohydrates

_____increasing regular exercise   _____taking "weight loss" supplements

_____taking appetite suppressants   _____using meal replacements such as Slim Fast

_____taking laxatives   _____inducing vomiting

_____taking prescription appetite suppressants

_____other _____

SECTION II: READINESS TO START A WEIGHT-LOSS PROGRAM

If you are thinking about starting a weight-loss program, answer questions A–F:

A. **How motivated are you to lose weight?**

1	2	3	4	5
Not at all motivated	Slightly motivated	Somewhat motivated	Quite motivated	Extremely motivated

B. **How certain are you that you will stay committed to a weight-loss program long enough to reach your goal?**

1	2	3	4	5
Not at all certain	Slightly certain	Somewhat certain	Quite certain	Extremely certain

C. Taking into account other stresses in your life (school, work, and relationships), to what extent can you tolerate the effort required to stick to your diet plan?

1	2	3	4	5
Cannot tolerate	Can tolerate somewhat	Uncertain	Can tolerate well	Can tolerate easily

D. Assuming you should lose no more than 1 to 2 pounds per week, have you allotted a realistic amount of time for weight loss?

1	2	3	4	5
Very unrealistic	Somewhat unrealistic	Moderately realistic	Somewhat realistic	Realistic

E. While dieting, do you fantasize about eating your favorite foods?

1	2	3	4	5
Always	Frequently	Occasionally	Rarely	Never

F. While dieting, do you feel deprived, angry, upset?

1	2	3	4	5
Always	Frequently	Occasionally	Rarely	Never

Total your scores from questions A–F, circle your score category, and answer any questions below:
6 to 16: This may not be a good time for you to start a diet. Inadequate motivation and commitment and unrealistic goals could block your progress. Think about what contributes to your unreadiness. What are some of the factors? Consider changing these factors before undertaking a diet. How could you alter the most important ones?

17 to 23: You may be nearly ready to begin a program but should think about ways to boost your readiness. Regardless of readiness level, what are a few additional things you could do at this time to prepare?
24 to 30: The path is clear—you can decide how to lose weight in a safe, effective way.
Section II Comments:

SECTION III: HUNGER, APPETITE, AND EATING

Think about your hunger and the cues that stimulate your appetite or eating, and then answer parts A–C.

A. When food comes up in conversation or in something you read, do you want to eat, even if you are not hungry?

1	2	3	4	5
Never	Rarely	Occasionally	Frequently	Always

B. How often do you eat for a reason other than physical hunger?

1	2	3	4	5
Never	Rarely	Occasionally	Frequently	Always

C. When your favorite foods are around the house, do you succumb to eating them?

1	2	3	4	5
Never	Rarely	Occasionally	Frequently	Always

Total your scores from questions A–C, circle your score category, and answer any questions below:

3 to 6: You might occasionally eat more than you should, but it is due more to your own attitudes than to temptation and other environmental cues. Controlling your own attitudes toward hunger and eating may help you. What are some of these attitudes, and how could you control or change them?

7 to 9: You may have a moderate tendency to eat just because food is available. Losing weight may be easier for you if you try to resist external cues and eat only when you are physically hungry. What are some ways you could better resist external cues?

10 to 15: Some or much of your eating may be in response to thinking about food or exposing yourself to temptations to eat. Think of ways to minimize your exposure to temptations so you eat only in response to physical hunger.

Section III Comments:

SECTION IV: CONTROLLING EATING

How good are you at controlling overeating when you are on a diet? Answer parts A–C.

A. **A friend talks you into going out to a restaurant for a midday meal instead of eating a brown-bag lunch. As a result, you:**

1	2	3	4	5
Would eat much less	Would eat much less	Would make no difference	Would eat somewhat more	Would eat much more

B. **You "break" your diet by eating a fattening, "forbidden" food. As a result, for the day, you:**

1	2	3	4	5
Would eat much less	Would eat much less	Would make no difference	Would eat somewhat more	Would eat much more

C. **You have been following your diet faithfully and decide to test yourself by taking a bite of something you consider a treat.** As a result, for the day, you:

1	2	3	4	5
Would eat much less	Would eat much less	Would make no difference	Would eat somewhat more	Would eat much more

Sum your scores from questions A–C, circle your score category, and answer any questions below:

3 to 7: You recover rapidly from mistakes. However, if you frequently alternate between out-of-control eating and very strict dieting, you may have a serious eating problem and should get professional help. Does that kind of alternation describe your pattern? If so, where on your college campus could you turn for professional guidance?

8 to 11: You do not seem to let unplanned eating disrupt your program. This is a flexible, balanced approach. Do "flexible" and "balanced" describe your dieting? How could you achieve even more flexibility and balance?

12 to 15: You may be prone to overeating after an event breaks your control or throws you off track. Your reaction to these problem-causing events could use improvement. What are some ways you could try to more effectively control an overeating reaction?

Section IV Comments:

SECTION V: REFLECTION

1. Were your previous dieting patterns successful? Why or why not? Was it hard to be consistent with these dieting methods?

2. Which dieting methods were challenging or did not work for you at all? Why were these methods more difficult? What would be the ideal dieting method for you?

LAB 8.3 • YOUR WEIGHT MANAGEMENT PLAN

Name: _____ Date: _____

Instructor: _____ Section: _____

Materials: None

Purpose: To create an appropriate weight management goal, you must apply behavior change tools and make a plan to implement your goals.

Directions: Complete the following sections.

SECTION I: SHORT- AND LONG-TERM GOALS

1. **Short-Term Goals**

• My 3-month *or* 6-month (circle one) % body fat goal is _____%.

• My 3-month *or* 6-month (circle one) weight goal is _____ lb.

• My 3-month *or* 6-month (circle one) BMI goal is _____ kg/m².

2. **Long-Term Goals**

a. Based on my current weight, BMI, % body fat, and the tools gained in Lab 8.2:

• My 1-year % body fat goal is _____%.

• My 1-year weight goal is _____ lb.

• My 1-year BMI goal is _____ kg/m².

b. I plan to reach that goal by consuming about _____ calories per day and adding _____ activity calories per day.

SECTION II: DIET OBSTACLES AND STRATEGIES

1. **Negative Food and Eating Triggers**

Eating and food preferences can be triggered by emotions, social situations, and the sights and smells around you.

a. Fill out the following table exploring your negative food and eating triggers. For example, a situational trigger for you eating sugary foods may be "attending holiday parties."

Diet Behavior	Emotional Triggers	Social Triggers	Situational Triggers
Eating More Food			
Eating Late at Night			
Eating More Often			
Eating Sugary Foods			
Eating Fatty Foods			
Eating Fast Foods			
Eating Out			
Others:			

b. List three strategies to overcome or manage your food and eating triggers:

(1) _____

(2) _____

(3) _____

2. **Changing Food Patterns**

a. I will eat LESS of the following foods and beverages:

_____

_____

b. For good nutrition and weight management goals, I will replace the above foods and beverages with the following:

_____

_____

SECTION III: EXERCISE AND ACTIVITY OBSTACLES AND STRATEGIES

1. **Reducing Sedentary Behaviors**

a. Evaluate your sedentary activities in the space below. List your top three sedentary activities (not including time spent in class), the number of days per week you do them, and how many minutes per day.

	Sedentary Activity	Days/wk	Min/day
1			
2			
3			

b. Which sedentary activity could you replace with physical activity or even supplement with physical activity (such as exercising while you watch TV, or stretching while on your cell phone)? Write down three ideas for replacing sedentary activities with more active ones.

(1) _____

(2) _____

(3) _____

2. List a few of the obstacles to replacing sedentary activity with more energy-intensive physical activity, along with strategies for overcoming these obstacles.

Activity Obstacle	Strategy to Overcome
(1) _____	_____
(2) _____	_____
(3) _____	_____

SECTION IV: GETTING SUPPORT

1. **I feel supported in my weight goals by these people:**

_____

Here's what they do that assists me:

_____

2. **I need additional support from these people:**

_____

Here's what I need to ask for:

_____

3. **If I need group or medical support,** here are a few places to seek it: student health service, family physician, local hospital, local Weight Watchers chapter, online groups. If needed, I would be inclined to use _____ for support.

SECTION V: REWARDS

1. When I make the **short-term** behavior change described above, my reward will be:

_____

Target date _____

2. When I make the **long-term** behavior change described above, my reward will be:

_____

Target date _____

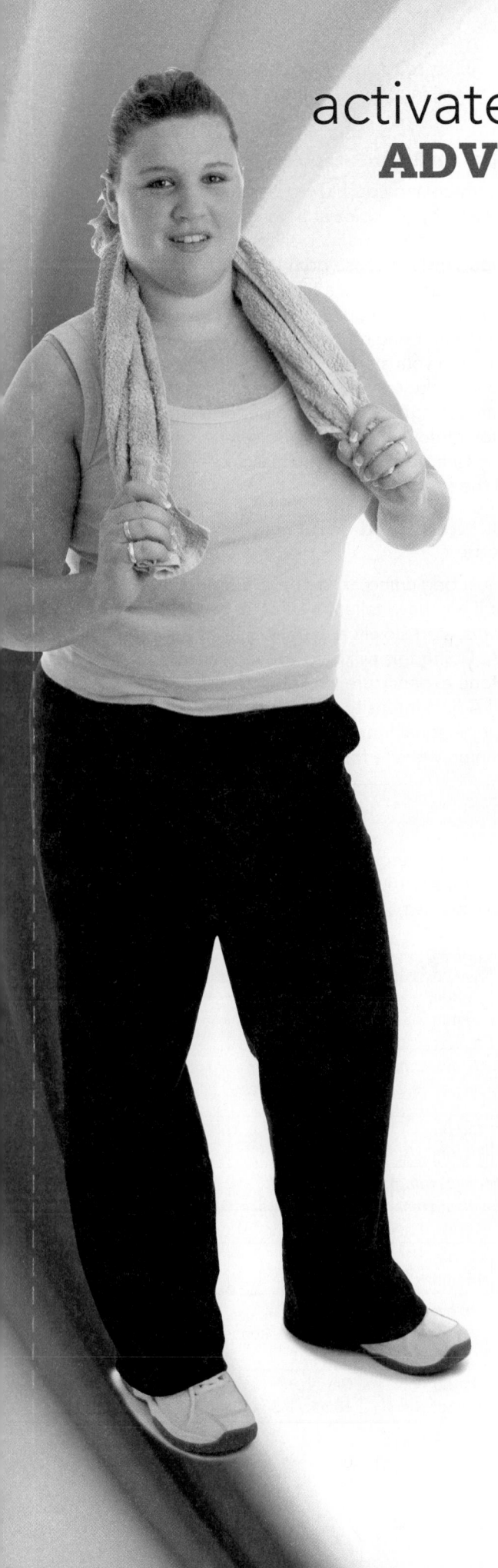

activate, motivate, & ADVANCE YOUR FITNESS

A WEIGHT MANAGEMENT EXERCISE PROGRAM

LIVE IT! ONLINE

ACTIVATE!

With weight management, progression is the key. Don't make the mistake of doing too much too soon. That is a leading cause of injury and will set you back even further from your goals. Start slowly and go at your own pace, building up stamina and strength; start where you are. Eventually, you will progress and increase the time or the intensity of your workouts (or both) as you become stronger and the sessions become easier. Follow these programs to gradually increase the number of minutes you train each week, the intensity of each session, and the calories you burn with each workout.

What Do I Need?

SHOES AND CLOTHING: The right shoes and clothes can go a long way toward keeping you comfortable and injury free as you begin a complete weight management program. Please refer to the cardiorespiratory programs in this book (Chapter 3) for details and tips to consider when choosing shoes and exercise clothing that are right for you.

How Do I Start?

TECHNIQUE: Safe and effective training really depends on proper technique. This is true whether you are just starting to become active or whether you are incorporating more vigorous activities into your program. Be sure to read through each of the previous chapters for detailed exercise descriptions and to learn proper technique and form. If you are unable to maintain good form, simply decrease the weight, the speed of the movement, the number of repetitions, or the length of your workout session.

Where Do I Start?

AT HOME: Walking is the best place to start. Whether it is a walk inside your home or around the campus or neighborhood, walking is the easiest way to add more activity to your day. Start with flat and forgiving surfaces and as you progress, add inclines or increase your pace or your overall minutes each week.

Although walking may be the best way to get started and increase your cardiorespiratory fitness, you will need to incorporate some resistance training to increase your muscular fitness, begin to change your body composition, and assist with increasing your overall weekly calorie expenditure. In the beginning weeks, you can complete your weight management resistance training program by using your own bodyweight against gravity to increase muscular endurance and strength. However, a few key items might help your motivation by keeping you comfortable and interested: a sturdy chair, a towel or mat, and maybe a few household items (books in your backpack, for instance). As you progress, you can add pieces of equipment to provide more resistance and increase your intensity (bands or tubing, a good stability ball, and even medicine balls).

AT THE GYM: Here, too, walking is the best way to start a weight management program. The treadmill is a great option and offers less impact than cement and asphalt. An elliptical machine is another good option that reduces the stress placed on hips, knees, ankles, and feet. If your gym has a pool, make use of it. Water walking (shallow or deep) is a great way to move your body without placing stress on your joints. Water also adds resistance to your workout and of course, the pool can help you to stay cool!

For resistance training sessions, a gym provides access to the wide variety of equipment. You will be able to incorporate the use of barbells (long bars with weights attached or slots to add weight plates), dumbbells (smaller, hand-held weights), benches (flat, incline, decline), plus cable stations and the latest the industry has to offer. All of these will help

you to progress, reducing your chances of boredom and increasing your likelihood of continued exercise.

Warm-Up and Cool-Down

A good warm-up and cool-down consists of simply doing your activity of choice at a slower pace and easing into and out of your training session. Break a light sweat as you slowly increase both your respiratory rate and your heart rate. Include a few dynamic range-of-motion exercises. After you finish your workout session, cool-down slowly, bringing your heart rate and respiratory rate back to your starting point. Once you have cooled down, include a few more dynamic moves or try a bit of foam rolling. Then begin to perform your static stretches for improved flexibility. (Be sure to review the programs in Chapter 5 for more ideas and descriptions of each of the stretches.)

Four-Week Weight Management Programs

If you are just beginning, if you have a BMI of 30 or greater, or if you have taken a lay-off of more than three months, start slowly and build gradually with Program A. Doing this will help you increase your overall calorie expenditure while helping to keep you injury free! Adjust intensity, volume, and training days to suit your personal fitness level and schedule; visit the companion website for more options.

PROGRAM A 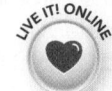 **GOAL:** Increase cardiorespiratory exercise frequency to 3 days a week and time to 15 minutes continuously, 100+ minutes/week; also incorporate resistance training 2 days a week.

	Mon	Tue	Wed	Thurs	Fri	Sat	Sun
Week 1	Cardio, 10 min ×3	Resistance, 1 circuit	Cardio, 10 min ×3	Resistance, 1 circuit	Cardio, 10 min ×3		
	Cardio workout: Walk 10 minutes continuously 3× (morning, afternoon, evening) *Resistance circuit workout: Do each exercise for 60 seconds with 15-second rests between exercises*						
Week 2	Cardio, 10 min ×3	Resistance, 2 circuits	Cardio, 10 min ×3	Resistance, 2 circuits	Cardio, 10 min ×3	Cardio, 10 min ×3	
	Cardio workout: Walk 10 minutes continuously, 3× (morning, afternoon, evening) *Resistance circuit workout: Do each exercise for 60 seconds with 15-second rests between exercises, 60-second rests between circuits*						
Week 3	Cardio, 15 min ×3	Resistance, 2 circuits	Cardio, 15 min ×3	Resistance, 2 circuits	Cardio, 15 min ×3		
	Cardio workout: Walk 15 minutes continuously, 3× (morning, afternoon, evening) *Resistance circuit workout: Do each exercise for 60 seconds with no rest between exercises, 60-second rests between circuits*						
Week 4	Cardio, 15 min ×3	Resistance, 3 circuits	Cardio, 15 min ×3	Resistance, 3 circuits	Cardio, 15 min ×3	Cardio, 15 min ×3	
	Cardio workout: Walk 15 minutes continuously, 3× (morning, afternoon, evening) *Resistance circuit workout: Do each exercise for 45 seconds with 10-second rests between exercises, 60-second rests between circuits*						

Order of Resistance Circuit Exercises for Home Workout

Squat
Push-Up or Modified Push-Up
Lunge
Plank or Modified Plank
Row with Resistance Band or dumbbell
Lat Pull-Down with Resistance Band
Side Bridge (each side)
Back Extension

Order of Resistance Circuit Exercises for Facility Workout

Chest Press
Squat or Leg Press Machine
Upright Row
Leg Extension
Rows
Overhead Press
Lat Pull-Down
Biceps Curl
Triceps Extension
Plank

MOTIVATE!

Create an exercise log to track your own weight management exercise program—make note of days, actual exercises, sets, reps, load amounts, rest intervals—or use the one on the companion website. Here are a few tips to get you moving:

MOTIVATING MEASUREMENTS: Whether you use a scale, a tape measure, or simply your favorite jeans, be sure to check your progress each week. This can encourage and motivate you, and it will serve as a good catch to help you get back on track if you are not maintaining your nutrition and exercise program.

BAN THE FAT TALK: Stop your negative self-talk and start anew! Surround yourself with only positive comments, upbeat training partners, and true supporters of your new healthy behaviors and lifestyle. Stay focused. Remember your goals. Be patient with yourself and be sure to acknowledge how much you have already accomplished!

TAKE A LITTLE "YOU" TIME: Make fitness and nutrition a priority. Take time for you—schedule your favor-

ite fitness activity (a stroll, your yoga DVD, pool time) and keep the appointment as you would for any other priority.

KEEP A DIGITAL PHOTO LOG: Take a "before" picture, and take a new picture each week. It may sound like the last thing you want to do at first. However, it can remind you of just how far you've come and keep you motivated to continue. This also works for your meals (especially when you eat out). Take pictures of your meals and gain a different perspective on what you are eating, how much, and when.

ADVANCE!

Now that you have established your exercise and weight management program, challenge yourself. Follow Program B if you already exercise at least two days a week, if you have a BMI of 25 to 29, or if you simply want to take your weight management program to the next level. Visit the companion website to find more options or to personalize this or any of the programs in this book.

PROGRAM B

 GOAL: Increase cardiorespiratory exercise frequency to 5 days a week and time to 30 minutes continuously, 300+ minutes/week; also incorporate resistance training 3 days a week.

	Mon	**Tue**	**Wed**	**Thurs**	**Fri**	**Sat**	**Sun**
Week 1	Walk/jog 15 min continuously, ×3 (morning, afternoon, evening)	Resistance, 2 circuits	Walk/jog 15 min continuously, ×3 (morning, afternoon, evening)	Resistance, 2 circuits	Walk/jog 15 min continuously, ×3 (morning, afternoon, evening)	Walk/jog 20 min continuously, ×2 (morning, evening)	
	Resistance circuit workout: Do each exercise for 60 seconds with 10-second rests between exercises, 60-second rests between circuits						

	Mon	Tue	Wed	Thurs	Fri	Sat	Sun
Week 2	Walk/jog 20 min continuously, ×3 (morning, afternoon, evening)	Walk/jog 15 min + Resistance, 2 circuits	Walk/jog 20 min continuously, ×3 (morning, afternoon, evening)	Walk/jog 15 min + Resistance, 2 circuits	Walk/jog 20 min continuously, ×3 (morning, afternoon, evening)	Walk/jog 25 min continuously, ×2 (morning, evening)	
	Resistance circuit workout: Do each exercise for 60 seconds with 10-second rests between exercises, 60-second rests between circuits						
Week 3	Walk/jog 25 min continuously, ×3 (morning, afternoon, evening)	Walk/jog 15 min + Resistance, 3 circuits	Walk/jog 25 min continuously, ×3 (morning, afternoon, evening)	Walk/jog 15 min + Resistance, 3 circuits	Walk/jog 25 min continuously, ×3 (morning, afternoon, evening)	Walk/jog 30 min continuously, ×2 (morning, evening)	
	Resistance circuit workout: Do each exercise for 60 seconds with 10-second rests between exercises, 60-second rests between circuits						
Week 4	Walk/jog 30 min continuously, ×3 (morning, afternoon, evening)	Walk/jog 15 min + Resistance, 3 circuits	Walk/jog 30 min continuously, ×3 (morning, afternoon, evening)	Walk/jog 15 min + Resistance, 3 circuits	Walk/jog 30 min continuously, ×3 (morning, afternoon, evening)	Walk/jog 15 min + Resistance, 3 circuits	
	Resistance circuit workout: Do each exercise for 60 seconds with 10-second rests between exercises, 60-second rests between circuits						

Order of Resistance Circuit Exercises for Home Workout

Squat + Overhead Press with Resistance Band or Dumbbells
Push-Up or Modified Push-Up
Lunge + Biceps Curl with Resistance Band or Dumbbells
Row with Resistance Band or Dumbbells
Lat Pull-Down with Resistance Band
Triceps Extension with Resistance Band or Dumbbells
Oblique Curl
Plank or Modified Plank
Back Extension

Order of Resistance Circuit Exercises for Facility Workout

Squats or Leg Press Machine
Chest Press
Leg Extension
Overhead Press
Leg Curl
Upright Row
Lunge + Biceps Curl with Resistance Band or Dumbbells
Rows
Lat Pull-Down
Pullover
Plank
Abdominal Curl
Back Extension

9 Managing Stress

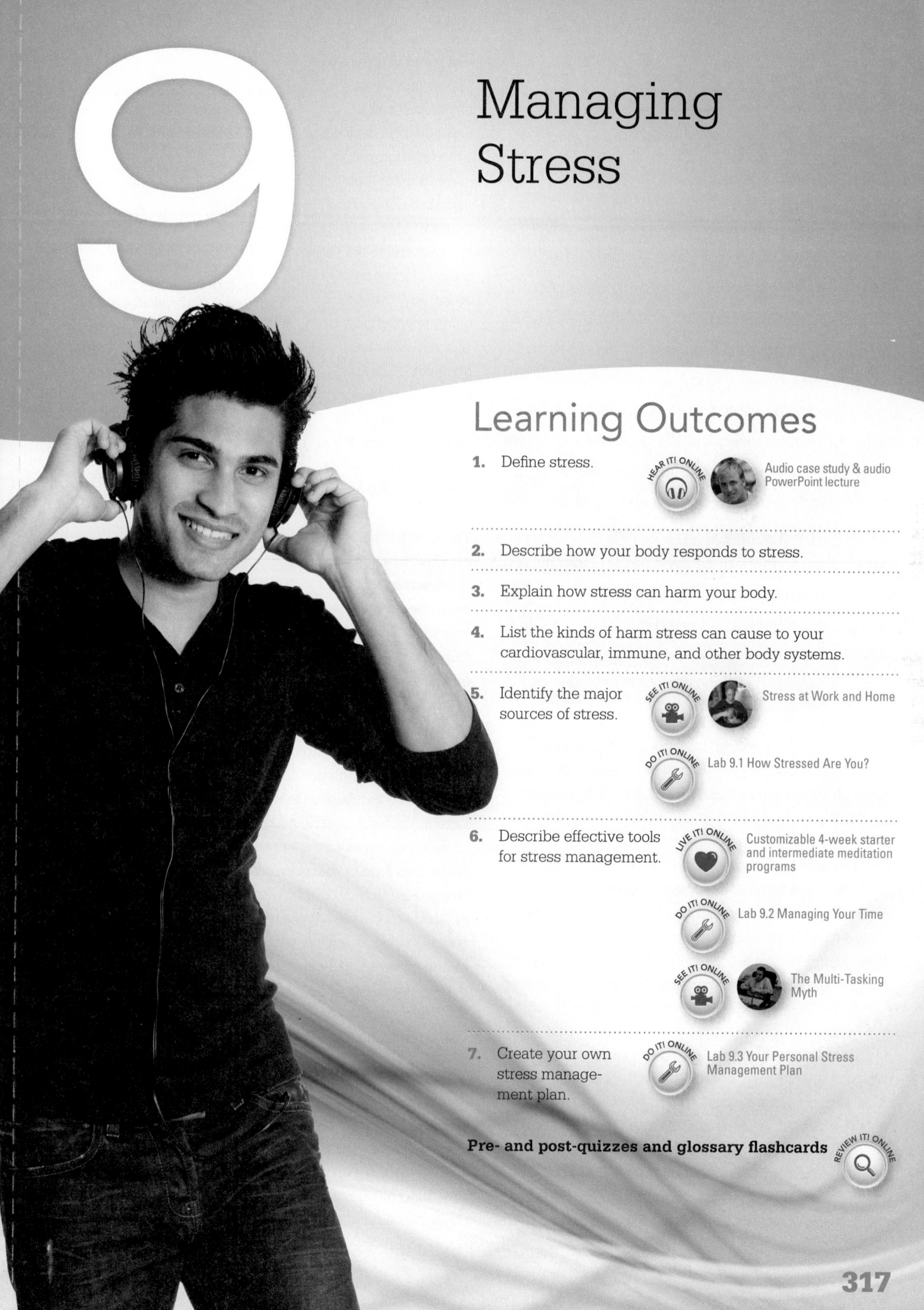

Learning Outcomes

1. Define stress.

   HEAR IT! ONLINE — Audio case study & audio PowerPoint lecture

2. Describe how your body responds to stress.

3. Explain how stress can harm your body.

4. List the kinds of harm stress can cause to your cardiovascular, immune, and other body systems.

5. Identify the major sources of stress.

   SEE IT! ONLINE — Stress at Work and Home

   DO IT! ONLINE — Lab 9.1 How Stressed Are You?

6. Describe effective tools for stress management.

   LIVE IT! ONLINE — Customizable 4-week starter and intermediate meditation programs

   DO IT! ONLINE — Lab 9.2 Managing Your Time

   SEE IT! ONLINE — The Multi-Tasking Myth

7. Create your own stress management plan.

   DO IT! ONLINE — Lab 9.3 Your Personal Stress Management Plan

Pre- and post-quizzes and glossary flashcards

REVIEW IT! ONLINE

317

casestudy

CORY

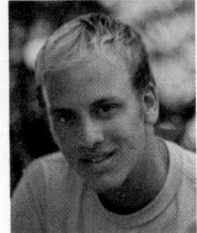

"Hi, I'm Cory. I'm a junior, majoring in biology. I'm from Denver, Colorado, and just transferred schools in August to be closer to my dad, who lives alone and has diabetes. I take five classes, I work part-time as a lab assistant, and I'm up late every night studying so that I can keep up my grades for applying to medical school. I've always been able to work under pressure, but I have to admit, these past few months have been rough. I am constantly worn out, worried about my dad, and I can barely stay awake in class sometimes. I know that medical school will be even harder, so maybe I should just get used to living like this! But I am so tired of feeling dragged out."

HEAR IT! ONLINE

Everyone feels stress at least some of the time, be it from traffic, competition for the courses you need, job hunting, fast-changing technology, or a hectic pace that seems to accelerate yearly. Over time, stress can diminish not just our enjoyment of life, but our health and well-being, too.[1] Thus, learning effective stress-management techniques is an important part of any complete wellness program.

This chapter explains the stress response, details the ways accumulated stress can affect your health, and proposes several helpful strategies you can use to counteract stress. Using the stress-management tools in this chapter, you can better face the pressures of college life and beyond.

What Is Stress?

In a recent national survey, college students reported stress as the biggest impediment to their academic success, with a greater impact on achievement than colds, flu, sleep difficulty, relationship issues, and all other concerns.[2] But what, exactly, *is* stress?

Stress is a term that is commonly used in many different ways. In this book, we'll define stress as the disturbed physical and/or emotional state that a person experiences as a result of an event. The event may be physical, social, or psychological, such as a threat, aggravation, or excitement that disturbs an individual's "normal" physiological state and to which the body must try to adapt. Any event that disrupts your body's "normal" state is a **stressor**. A stressor can be physical, such as an uncomfortably heavy backpack. It can also be emotional, like the anxiety you feel before a major exam. The term for the physical effect of a stressor is the **stress response**: the set of physiological changes initiated by your body's nervous and hormonal signals. The stress response prepares the brain, heart, muscles, and other organs to respond to a perceived threat or demand.

A more traditional view of stress includes the concepts of both positive stress and negative stress. Positive stress, or **eustress**, presents an opportunity for personal growth, satisfaction, and enhanced well-being. Eustress can invigorate us and motivate us to work harder and achieve more. Entering college, starting a job, and developing a new relationship are all challenges that can produce eustress. Negative stress, or **distress**, can result from negative stressors such as academic pressures, relationship discord, or money problems. It can even result from an overload of positive stressors such as graduating from college, getting married, moving to a new state, and starting a new job all in the same week. Distress can reduce wellness by promoting cardiovascular disease, impairing immunity, or causing mental and emotional dysfunction.

How Does My Body Respond to Stress?

As you sit down in the lecture hall to take your hardest midterm exam, you realize your heart is pounding, your breathing has quickened, your hands are sweating, you have "butterflies" in your stomach, and you feel a sense

stress The disturbed physical or emotional state experienced as a result of a physical, social, or psychological event or circumstance that disturbs the body's "normal" state and to which the body must try to adapt

stressor A physical, social, or psychological event or circumstance to which the body tries to adapt; stressors are often threatening, unfamiliar, disturbing, or exciting

stress response A set of physiological changes initiated by your body in response to a stressor

eustress Stress based on positive circumstances or events; can present an opportunity for personal growth

distress Stress based on negative circumstances or events, or those perceived as negative; can diminish wellness

of dread. You are experiencing a stress response: a reaction involving nervous and hormonal activities that prepare both body and mind to deal with the disturbance to your normal state.

The Stress Response

Here's what happens during the seconds that the body initiates a stress response and in the minutes and hours as the response continues (Figure 9.1):

1. Your senses perceive and your brain interprets something as a threat; in the example above, an exam that will determine half your grade.

2. The threat triggers a region of your brain called the *hypothalamus* to release a hormone that in turn triggers your pituitary gland to secrete **adrenocorticotropic hormone (ACTH)** into your blood.

3. ACTH travels through the bloodstream and reaches the outer zone of each adrenal gland (located on top of each kidney). ACTH causes the adrenal glands to secrete **cortisol**, your body's main stress hormone.

adrenocorticotropic hormone (ACTH) A hormone secreted by the pituitary gland that causes adrenal glands to secrete cortisol

cortisol The body's main stress hormone, secreted by the cortex or outer layer of the adrenal glands located on top of the kidneys; stimulates the sympathetic nervous system; can also damage or destroy neurons.

At the same time, nerve signals from your brain and spinal cord reach and stimulate the central zone of each adrenal gland. Both adrenals respond

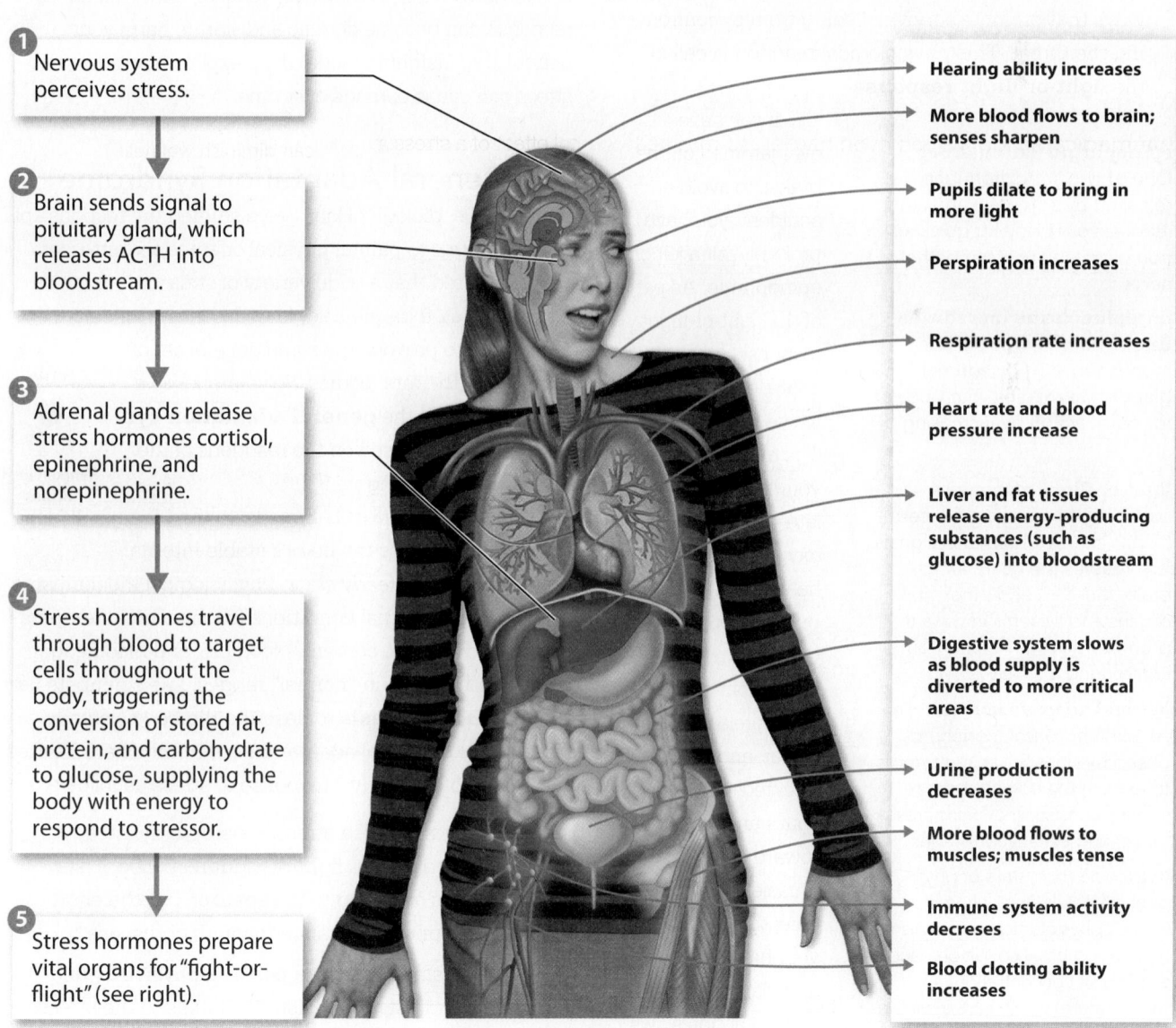

① Nervous system perceives stress.

② Brain sends signal to pituitary gland, which releases ACTH into bloodstream.

③ Adrenal glands release stress hormones cortisol, epinephrine, and norepinephrine.

④ Stress hormones travel through blood to target cells throughout the body, triggering the conversion of stored fat, protein, and carbohydrate to glucose, supplying the body with energy to respond to stressor.

⑤ Stress hormones prepare vital organs for "fight-or-flight" (see right).

Hearing ability increases

More blood flows to brain; senses sharpen

Pupils dilate to bring in more light

Perspiration increases

Respiration rate increases

Heart rate and blood pressure increase

Liver and fat tissues release energy-producing substances (such as glucose) into bloodstream

Digestive system slows as blood supply is diverted to more critical areas

Urine production decreases

More blood flows to muscles; muscles tense

Immune system activity decreses

Blood clotting ability increases

FIGURE **9.1**   The stress response.

by releasing two additional stress hormones that ready the body for quick action: **epinephrine** (also called **adrenaline**) and **norepinephrine** (or **noradrenaline**).

4. Traveling inside the bloodstream, cortisol reaches specific *target cells* within the body fat and within several organs, including the liver and intestines. Cortisol quickly triggers target cells to convert stored fat, protein, and carbohydrate molecules into glucose. Soon, more glucose is circulating in the blood, supplying the whole body—especially the brain and skeletal muscles—with the extra energy needed to respond to the stressor.

5. The epinephrine and norepinephrine released into the blood rapidly reach target cells in the heart, lungs, stomach, intestines, sense organs, and muscles. Along with signals from sympathetic nerves, these additional stress hormones ready the vital organs in ways that promote survival: fleeing from or confronting the threat. This physiological reaction is called the **fight-or-flight response**.

epinephrine (adrenaline) One of two stress hormones released by adrenal glands that readies your body for quick action by stimulating sympathetic nerves

norepinephrine (noradrenaline) One of two stress hormones secreted by adrenal glands that readies your body for quick action by increasing arousal

fight-or-flight response A physiological reaction induced by nervous and hormonal signals that readies the heart, lungs, brain, muscles, and other vital organs and systems in ways that promote survival: fleeing from or confronting a threat

general adaptation syndrome (GAS) A historical model proposed by Hans Selye; it attempts to explain the body's stress response consisting of alarm, resistance, and exhaustion stages.

homeostasis A state of physiological equilibrium wherein various physiological mechanisms maintain internal conditions (such as pH, salt concentration, and temperature) within certain viable ranges

If you have ever jammed on the brakes to avoid an accident, you have probably felt a jolt of epinephrine. As part of the fight-or-flight response, your pupils dilate, enabling you to see more clearly. The air passages in your lungs also dilate, allowing more oxygen to enter. Your heart beats faster and pumps more blood to your muscles and brain. Your sweat glands release more sweat, and blood is directed away from your hands and feet toward your large muscles and body core; this can make your hands feel cold and clammy. Your digestive action slows or stops, and your

bladder function slows, since neither process is crucial to short-term survival. Primed in all these ways, your body is ready to handle the stressor, at least in the short term.

After a perceived stressor subsides, your nervous system returns the body to its "normal" state with slower heartbeats, normal breathing rate, normal digestion, and so on. The stress-reduction techniques you will learn later deliberately encourage the body's return to this more relaxed state.

Why Does Stress Cause Harm?

Why is chronic stress harmful? After all, if a truck is speeding toward you, your fight-or-flight response could save your life. However, if you are faced with financial hardship or excessive work pressures for years on end, your stress response can become chronic and start to harm your health. Two insightful models help explain how *sustained* stress can cause damage over time.

The General Adaptation Syndrome

In the 1930s, biologist Hans Selye studied the response of laboratory rats to painful physical or emotional stressors. He discovered that a wide variety of stressors—such as extreme heat, extreme cold, forced exercise, or surgery—all seemed to provoke the same general set of changes in the rats' bodies. Selye proposed a model he called the **general adaptation syndrome (GAS)**, based on the reactions of the rats he observed (Figure 9.2).[3]

LIVE IT! ONLINE
Worksheet 8
Stress
Reaction

Central to Selye's GAS model is the idea that stress disrupts the body's stable internal environment, or *steady state*. Physiological mechanisms work to keep internal conditions (such as body temperature, blood-oxygen content, blood pH, and blood sugar levels) within certain "normal" ranges. Life scientists use the term **homeostasis** to describe the body's steady state. Selye's general adaptation syndrome characterizes the stages of the body's response to stress as follows:

1. In the *alarm stage*, a stressor disrupts the steady state and triggers a fight-or-flight response. The body starts adapting to the stressor, but the effort can lower one's resistance to injury or disease.[4]

2. In the *resistance stage*, a person's physiology and behavior adjust, and resistance builds to the stressor. The body establishes a new level of homeostasis, despite the continued presence of the stressor.

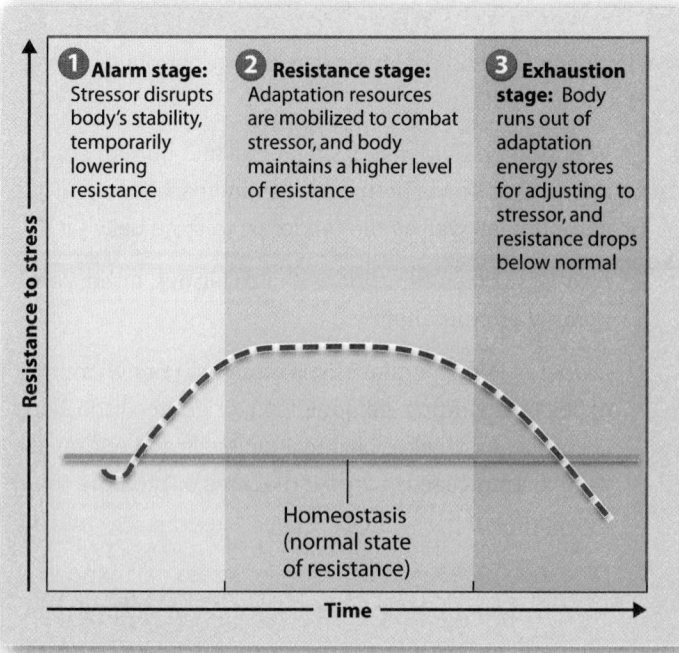

① **Alarm stage:** Stressor disrupts body's stability, temporarily lowering resistance

② **Resistance stage:** Adaptation resources are mobilized to combat stressor, and body maintains a higher level of resistance

③ **Exhaustion stage:** Body runs out of adaptation energy stores for adjusting to stressor, and resistance drops below normal

Resistance to stress

Homeostasis (normal state of resistance)

Time

FIGURE **9.2** Hans Seyle's general adaptation syndrome.

3. In the hypothetical *exhaustion stage,* the body runs out of resources to successfully adapt to the stressor, resulting in physiological harm in the form of reduced immunity and increased susceptibility to physical or mental illness.

The general adaptation syndrome recognized that sustained stress can take a toll on wellness. However, scientists have since modified Selye's concept of an "exhaustion stage" and the idea that illness results from running out of resources to adapt to a stressor. Rather, they now believe that over time, the stress response *itself* can damage the body and increase one's risk of developing illness, as we will see in the next section.

Allostatic Load

Today's stress researchers use the term **allostasis** to describe the many simultaneous changes that occur in the body to maintain homeostasis, and they use the term **allostatic load** to refer to the long-term wear and tear on the body that is caused by prolonged allostasis.[5]

Allostatic load can result if your body's ability to shut off the stress response (after a stressor has disappeared) is impaired, allowing high levels of stress hormones to remain in the bloodstream. It can also develop when your body releases too *few* stress hormones and cannot mount an adequate stress response.[6] And it can build up if you experience a sustained string of stressful events over a long period of time. A classic example of a consequence

of allostatic load is the development of stress-induced high blood pressure (hypertension.) As you will see shortly, chronically high blood pressure can damage arteries and increase one's risk of developing cardiovascular disease.[7]

A person's behavior and choices can also result in allostatic load. For example, some people respond to stress by exercising more, meditating, getting extra sleep, and avoiding drugs and alcohol—all behaviors that can help minimize allostatic load. Others respond by exercising less, staying up late, drinking more, or starting to smoke or take drugs. Such counterproductive measures can result in allostatic load and increase one's susceptibility to developing illness.

> **allostasis** The many simultaneous changes that occur in the body to maintain homeostasis
>
> **allostatic load** The long-term wear and tear on the body that is caused by prolonged allostasis

casestudy

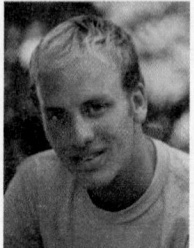

CORY

"I knew this year was going to be a challenge—transferring to a new school and taking upper-level classes. The first month actually went okay. I liked my classes, my dad seemed to be doing better, and I got used to getting by on five hours of sleep each night. Then sometime in September I caught a cold that didn't go away for four weeks! I was coughing all night, could barely pay attention in class, and did badly on one of my midterms. Now I have to work even harder to make up for the bad grade."

THINK! List Cory's main sources of stress. Which would you classify as *eustress* and which would you classify as *distress*? How might the allostatic load model explain what is happening with Cory?

ACT! Make a list of your own major sources of stress, organizing them into eustress and distress. How does stress affect your body and mind? What do you do when you feel stressed out? If you typically choose unhealthy responses to stress, list some alternative healthy responses you'd like to try.

HEAR IT! ONLINE

What Kinds of Harm Can Stress Cause?

Studies indicate that 40 percent of deaths and 70 percent of disease in the United States are related, in whole or in part, to stress.[8] The list of ailments related to chronic stress includes heart disease, diabetes, cancer, headaches, ulcers, low back pain, depression, and the common cold.

Stress and Cardiovascular Disease

Perhaps the most studied and documented health consequence of unresolved stress is cardiovascular disease (CVD). Research on this topic has demonstrated the impact of chronic stress on heart rate, blood pressure, heart attack, and stroke.[9] Historically, the increased risk of CVD from chronic stress has been linked to increased plaque buildup due to elevated cholesterol, hardening of the arteries, alterations in heart rhythm, and increased and fluctuating blood pressure. Recent research also points to metabolic abnormalities, insulin resistance, and inflammation in blood vessels as major contributors to heart disease.[10] In the past 15 to 20 years, researchers have identified direct links between the incidence and progression of CVD and stressors such as job strain, caregiving, bereavement, and natural disasters.[11] Whatever the mechanism, the evidence is clear that stress is a significant contributor to CVD morbidity and mortality.

Stress and the Immune System

A growing area of scientific investigation known as **psychoneuroimmunology (PNI)** explores the intricate relationship between the mind's response to stress and the immune system's ability to function effectively. Research suggests that too much stress over a long period can negatively regulate various aspects of the cellular immune response.[12] Whereas a short-term fight-or-flight response is usually protective, prolonged stress depresses the immune system. During prolonged stress, elevated levels of adrenal hormones (such as cortisol) destroy or reduce the ability of certain white blood cells, known as killer T cells, to aid the immune response.[13] When killer T cells aren't working correctly, the body becomes more susceptible to illness.

psychoneuroimmunology (PNI) Science of the interaction between the mind and the immune system

post-traumatic stress disorder (PTSD) An acute stress disorder caused by experiencing an extremely traumatic event

Stress and Other Physical Effects

Prolonged periods of stress can have other physical effects, as well:

- *Weight gain* Evidence from animal and human studies shows that stress hormones can increase food consumption as well as the tendency to store belly fat.[14]

- *Hair loss* Stress can trigger hair to fall out, either temporarily or permanently.[15]

- *Diabetes* People under stress often eat poorly, drink to excess, take drugs, eat junk food, or get too little sleep. All of these can alter blood sugar levels and aggravate pre-existing cases of type-2 diabetes or promote their development.[16]

- *Digestive problems* People under stress can experience nausea, vomiting, stomach pain, intestinal pain, or diarrhea. Stress hormones can cause existing digestive problems to flare. A classic example is irritable bowel syndrome.[17]

- *Loss of libido* Even in young people, stress can alter normal levels of sex hormones and this, in turn, can lead to erectile dysfunction, emotional swings, and loss of sex drive.[18]

If you experience any of these problems, a trip to the student health center may help you discover links to stress and solutions to the problems.

Stress and the Mind

Stress may be one of the single greatest contributors to mental impairment and disability and to emotional dysfunction in industrialized nations. One of the most common impairments is disrupted short-term memory, especially a person's ability to remember words as quickly as he or she could before the period of stress.[19] Animal studies show that stress hormones can actually shrink the brain's memory center (the *hippocampus*) and negatively impact verbal and other memory functions.[20] Stress can lead to mental disorders, as well. Studies have shown that environmental stressors, including divorce, marital conflict, and economic hardship can aggravate or affect the onset of mental disorders, particularly depression and anxiety (see the box Can Stress Cause Depression?).[21]

In severe cases, an individual's response to stress may develop into **post-traumatic stress disorder (PTSD)**. Traumas that can trigger PTSD include wartime experiences, rape, near-death experiences in accidents, witnessing a murder or death, being caught in a natural disaster, or a terrorist attack.

Can Stress Cause Depression?

Stress and depression have complicated interconnections based on emotional, physiological, and biochemical processes. Prolonged stress can trigger depression in susceptible people, and prior periods of depression can leave individuals more susceptible to stress.[1]

The physical links between stress and depression are strong. During the stress response, the body is flooded with cortisol and with chemicals called *cytokines*. These factors promote inflammation as part of the body's immune response. Researchers think that exposure to both kinds of chemicals can damage or kill neurons in a part of the brain called the *hippocampus* and can alter nerve transmission within the brain. One result of hippocampal damage is impaired learning and memory.[2] Another is the onset of depression symptoms in genetically susceptible individuals.[3] Research confirms that loss of hippocampal neurons is present in many who suffer depression.[4]

Realizing the important interconnections between stress and depression can help you take appropriate steps to handling one or both. Because stress and depression symptoms overlap, applying the stress-management techniques outlined in this chapter may help alleviate depression.

Physical activity is a particularly potent tool. A recent survey or more than 43,000 college students revealed that students who exercise or engage in physical activity each week have fewer feelings of depression, hopelessness, and suicidal behavior than do inactive students.[5]

If depression symptoms become severe enough to interfere with studying or other aspects of daily life, you should seek help. Potential sources for help are the student health service, the campus counseling center, a doctor or mental health professional in your community, and your local depression or suicide hotline.

Sources:
1. M. A. Ilgen and K. E. Hutchison, "A History of Major Depressive Disorder and the Response to Stress," *Journal of Affective Disorders* 86, no. 2 (2005): 143–50.
2. F. A. Scorza and others, "Neurogenesis and Depression: Etiology or New Illusion?" *Review of Brazilian Psychiatry* 27, no. 3 (2005): 249–53.
3. M. A. Ilgen and K. E. Hutchison, "A History of Major Depressive Disorder and the Response to Stress," 2005.
4. P. Price, "Stress and Depression," www.allaboutdepression.com/gen_05.html (updated June 2010).
5. L. Taliaferro and others, "Associations between Physical Activity and Reduced Rates of Hopelessness, Depression, and Suicidal Behavior among College Students," *Journal of American College Health* 57, no. 4 (2009): 427–36.

What Are the Major Sources of Stress?

College students can experience a flood of new stressors, and these can differ depending on age, sex, and year in school.[22] First-year students, for example, primarily feel academic pressure.[23] Fully 29 percent of freshman report feeling frequently overwhelmed by all they have to do.[24] Female freshmen also tend to report dieting and weight gain as stressful, while male students worry more about being underweight, relationship issues, and substance use (drugs, alcohol).[25] In addition, nontraditional and foreign students may experience other sources of stress, as described in the box International Student Stress.

Sources of Stress Can Be Internal or External

Interactions with others, expectations we and others have of ourselves, and the social and environmental conditions we live in force us to readjust constantly. Examining the causes of stress may help you identify your sources of stress and learn new ways to cope with them (Figure 9.3).

Change Alterations from your normal routine can cause stress. The greater the change and your necessary adjustments to it, the more stress and the greater the potential impact on your immune system.[26] Certain life events predict increased risk for stress-related illness. Knowing them can help, as you'll discover in **Lab 9.1**.

Performance Demands We experience stress when we must meet higher standards or unfamiliar de-

Stress at Work and Home

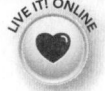

Worksheet 9
Stress
Tolerance Test

mands. In college, competition for grades, athletic positions, club memberships, internships, graduate school acceptance, and job interviews can exert considerable pressure. We can lessen the impact of such demands by setting priorities and realistic deadlines.

Inconsistent Goals and Behaviors The negative effects of stress can be magnified when we don't match our goals with our actions. For instance, you may want good grades. But if you party and procrastinate throughout the term, your goals and behaviors are inconsistent. Behaviors that are consistent with your goals—for example, studying harder and partying less to achieve good grades—can help alleviate stress.

Overload and Burnout Time pressure, responsibilities, course work, tuition, and high expectations for yourself and those around you—coupled with a lack of support—can lead to *overload:* a state of feeling overburdened, unable to keep up, and longing for

DIVERSITY

International Student Stress

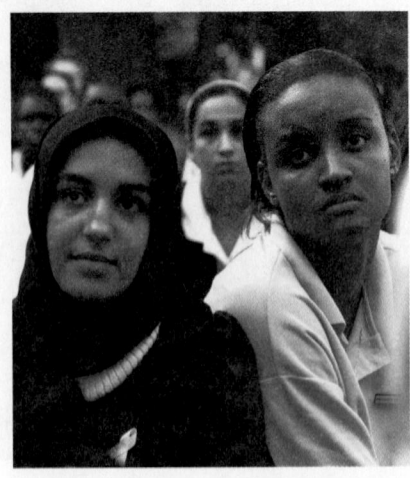

International students experience unique adjustment issues related to language barriers, cultural barriers, and a lack of social support, among other challenges. Academic stress may pose a particular problem for the more than 670,000 international students who have left support networks of family and friends in their native countries to study in the United States. Accumulating evidence suggests that seeking emotional support from others is among the most effective ways to cope with stressful and upsetting situations. Yet,

many international students refrain from doing so because of cultural norms, feelings of shame, and the belief that seeking support is a sign of weakness that calls inappropriate attention to both the individual and the respective ethnic group. This reluctance, coupled with the language barriers, cultural conflicts, and other stressors, can lead international students to suffer significantly more stress-related illnesses than their American counterparts. Even if we can't solve the many problems international students encounter, there are things we can do to make one person's life (or maybe two or three persons' lives) a little less stressful: share companionship and communication and lend a helping hand. To paraphrase a popular Hindu proverb: "Help thy neighbor's boat across and thine own boat will also reach the shore."

Sources: S. Sumer, "International Students' Psychological and Sociocultural Adaptation in the United States," Georgia State University, Doctoral Dissertation, http://digitalarchive.gsu.edu/cps_diss/34 (2009); Institute of International Education, "Record Numbers of International Students in U.S. Higher Education," Press Release, http://opendoors.iienetwork.org/?p=150649 (November 2009).

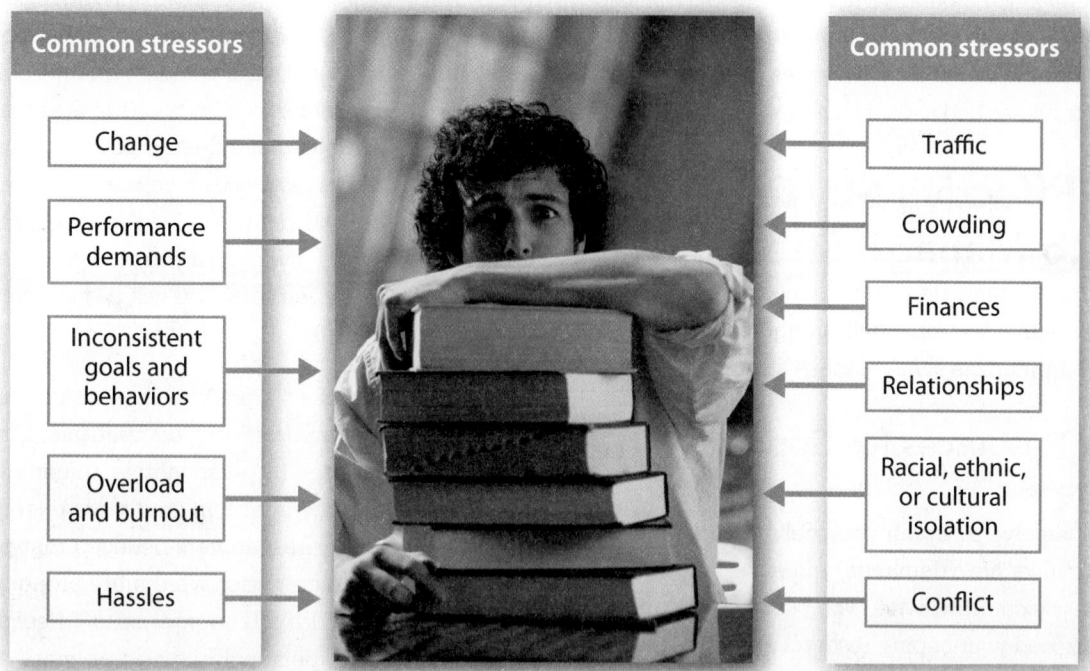

FIGURE **9.3** Which of these stressors impact you?

escape. Overload pushes some students toward depression or substance abuse; others respond by using stress-management tools to alleviate tension before it piles up. Unrelieved overload can lead to *burnout,* a state of stress-induced physical and mental exhaustion. Teachers, nurses, and law enforcement officers, for example, experience high levels of burnout, and highly pressured professionals often use stress-management techniques to avoid reaching this point.

Hassles Petty annoyances and frustrations may seem unimportant if taken one by one: getting stuck in a long line at the bookstore, for example, or finding out that a school administrator has misplaced your paperwork. However, minor hassles can build to major stress if you perceive them negatively and let the feelings mount.[27] Regular release through stress management can counter this buildup.

Environmental Sources of Stress Environmental stress results from events occurring in the physical environment. People living in crowded urban environments tend to experience stress from things such as traffic, housing density, and a high cost of living. Meanwhile, people living in rural areas may experience different stresses such as limited employment opportunities and decreased services.

Relationships Relationships with friends, partners, family members, and co-workers can be important sources of strength and support, but they can also exert stress in our lives. These relationships can inspire and encourage us to achieve our highest goals and give us hope for the future. Staying connected can improve our mental, emotional, and physical health. Sometimes, though, relationships can diminish our self-esteem and leave us reeling from a destructive interaction. This kind of stress can diminish our wellness.

Racial, Ethnic or Cultural Isolation Those who act, speak, or dress differently sometimes face additional pressures that do not affect more "typical" students. Students perceived as different—whether due to race, ethnicity, religious affiliation, age, physical handicap, or sexual orientation—may become victims of subtle and not-so-subtle forms of bigotry, insensitivity, harassment, or hostility and this can increase the other forms of stress inherent in going to college.

Conflict Conflict occurs when we have to choose between competing motives, behaviors, or impulses, or when we must face incompatible demands, opportunities, needs, or goals. For example, what if your best friend wanted you to help her cheat on an exam, but you didn't feel right about it? College students often experience stress because their own developing set of beliefs conflicts with the values they learned from their parents.

What stresses do you face, and how are they affecting you? Lab 9.1 charts many common sources of stress for college students and others. Completing this lab will help you measure your current stress level. Reading through the next section will then supply a series of helpful stress-reduction strategies and tools for using them.

What Effective Strategies Can I Use to Manage Stress?

Most college students are able to manage their stress and do best with a low-key, multipronged approach. Figure 9.4 summarizes some of these strategies.

Internal Resources for Coping with Stress

When you perceive that your personal resources are sufficient to meet life's demands, you experience little or no stress. By contrast, when you perceive that life's demands exceed your coping resources, you are likely to feel strain and distress.

appraisal The interpretation and evaluation of information provided to the brain by the senses

psychological hardiness Personal characteristics of control, commitment, and an embrace of challenge that help individuals cope with stress

Self-Esteem and Self-Efficacy Several coping resources influence your stress **appraisal**, how you appraise the stress in your life. Two of the most important are *self-esteem* and

self-efficacy. Self-esteem is a sense of positive self-regard, or how you feel about yourself. Self-efficacy is a belief or confidence in personal skills and performance abilities. Researchers consider self-efficacy one of the most important personality traits that influence psychological and physiological stress responses.[28] Low self-esteem or low self-efficacy can lead you to feel helpless to cope with the stress in your life. Conversely, if you work to build your self-esteem and self-efficacy, you will add the benefit of less stress in your life!

Hardiness So-called "Type A" personalities are characterized as hard-driving, competitive, time-driven perfectionists. "Type B" personalities, in contrast, are more relaxed, noncompetitive, and more tolerant of others. Historically, researchers believed that people with Type A characteristics were more prone to heart attacks than their Type B counterparts.[29] Researchers today believe that personality types are more complex than previously thought—most people are not one personality type all the time, and other variables must be explored.

Psychological hardiness may negate self-imposed stress associated with Type A behavior. Psychologically hardy people are characterized by control, commitment, and an embrace of challenge.[30] People with a sense of control are able to accept responsibility for their behaviors and change those that they discover to be debilitating. People with a sense

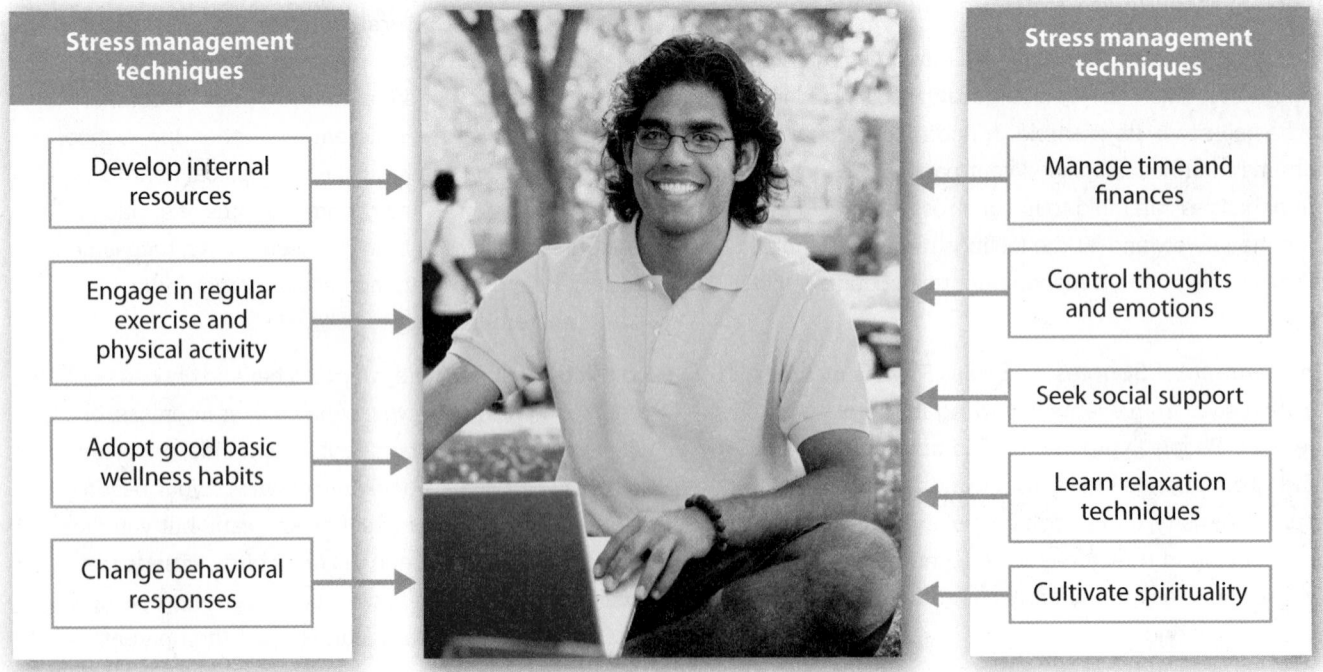

Stress management techniques		Stress management techniques
Develop internal resources		Manage time and finances
Engage in regular exercise and physical activity		Control thoughts and emotions
Adopt good basic wellness habits		Seek social support
Change behavioral responses		Learn relaxation techniques
		Cultivate spirituality

FIGURE **9.4** There are many effective techniques for helping you manage stress.

of commitment have good self-esteem and understand their purpose in life. People who embrace challenge see change as an opportunity for personal growth. The concept of hardiness has been studied extensively, and many researchers believe it is the foundation of an individual's ability to cope with stress and remain healthy.[31]

Exercise, Fun, and Recreational Activity

Improving your overall level of fitness may be the most helpful thing you can do to combat stress. Interestingly, research shows that exercise actually stimulates the stress response, but that a well-exercised body adapts to the *eustress* of exercise, and as a result is able to tolerate greater levels of *distress* of all kinds.[32] Compared to an unfit person, a fit individual develops a milder stress response to any given stressor.[33] Research also shows that exercise reduces both psychosocial stress and metabolic disturbances leading to belly fat, high blood pressure, high blood cholesterol, and vascular disease.[34]

Many physical activities relieve the feeling of stress and tension, while others—especially those that involve competition, high skill levels, or physical risk—may add to your stress load. Some activities are high in one value and low in the other, but many can build fitness and promote relaxation at the same time. The trick is to balance exercise, fun, and recreational activities in your free time so that you can stay fit and reduce chronic stress.

Basic Wellness Measures

Many of the habits you cultivate to improve your wellness can also fight the negative effects of stress.

Eating Well Eating nutrient-dense foods rather than fast foods and junk foods gives you more mental and physical energy, improves your immune responses, and helps you stay at a healthy weight. Undereating, overeating, or eating nutrient-poor foods can contribute to your stress levels by diminishing your overall wellness. Most claims about vitamins and supplements that reduce stress are unsupported. Vitamin and mineral supplementation beyond your daily requirements may only add to your stress—financial stress, that is!

Getting Enough Sleep Sleep is a central wellness component. As explained in the box How Does Sleep

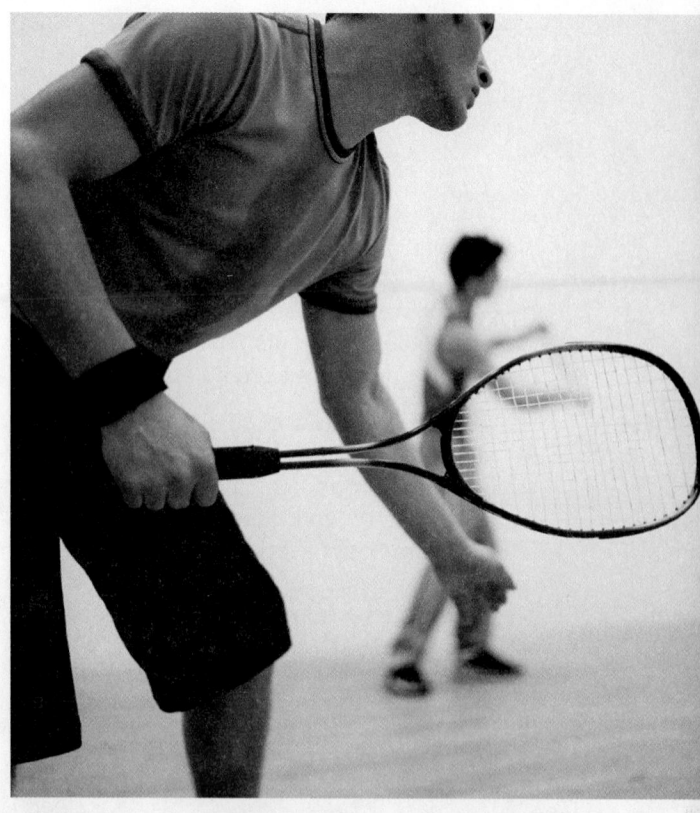

Affect My Performance and Mood?, sleep loss hinders learning, memory, academic work, and physical performance. It can also depress mood and prompt feelings of stress, anger, and sadness. *Sound* sleep is important, too. Some people find that inexpensive earplugs or eye masks from a drugstore block sleep-disturbing sound and light. Others require a quieter, darker room or more considerate roommates to solve their sleep problems.

Worksheet 4
Sleep
Inventory

Avoiding Alcohol and Tobacco Both drinking and smoking can disrupt sleep patterns during the night. Alcohol can disrupt the length of time it takes you to fall asleep as well as the sequence and duration of your sleep states.[35] The nicotine in tobacco is highly addictive and acts as a mild stimulant. Tobacco use also impairs normal breathing and diminishes your ability to fight off colds and other infections.

Change Your Behavioral Responses

Realizing that stress is harming your fitness, wellness, relationships, or productivity is often the first step toward making positive changes. Start by assessing all aspects of a stressor, examining your typical response, determining ways to change it, and learning to cope. Often, you cannot change the stressors you face: the

How Does Sleep Affect My Performance and Mood?

Sleep experts suggest that 18- to 20-year-olds need about 8.5 to 9.25 hours of sleep per night, while adults over 21 need about 7 to 9 hours of sleep (depending on individual physiology).[1] In the 1980s, college students got an average of 7 to 7.5 hours of sleep per night. Today, however, that has slid to between 6 and 6.9 hours. In addition, the typical student sleeps less at the end of a semester than at the beginning due to the accumulation of assignments and exams.

Losing an hour or two of sleep actually does matter, even to young, active, healthy college students. Research shows that sleep loss degrades learning and memory, physical performance, and mood in both young and older adults. One piece of evidence for this is a German study that presented students with a math puzzle to work out. Most of those who "slept on it" realized a shortcut to solving the problem by morning and could accomplish the task much more quickly. Three-quarters of those who didn't "sleep on it" failed to intuit the way to a faster, simpler solution.[2] This was the first scientific proof that sleep can promote insight and problem solving.

Sleep deprivation can also increase feelings of stress, anger, anxiety, and sadness.[3] These emotional states can, in turn, make sleeping even harder. Feeling extremely stressed out and having a negative emotional response to that stress is, in fact, the best predictor that a student will have sleep problems.[4]

Poor sleep is defined as getting fewer-than-recommended hours of sleep, having irregular bedtimes and rising times, and experiencing interrupted sleep. To improve your sleep and adopt better sleep habits,

- go to bed and wake up at as regular a time as possible;
- sleep in a room that is as quiet and dark as possible;
- get regular exercise such as brisk walking or resistance training, but not too close to bedtime;[5]
- avoid caffeine in the afternoon or evening;
- avoid taking naps;
- sleep where it is cool (not cold) and ventilated (but not drafty); and
- avoid excess alcohol.

Sources:
1. National Sleep Foundation, "How Much Sleep Do We Really Need?" www .sleepfoundation.org/article/how-sleep-works/how-much-sleep-do-we-really- need (accessed October 2011).
2. U. Wagner and others, "Sleep Inspires Insight," *Nature* 427, no. 6972 (2004): 352–5.
3. B. A. Marcks, "Co-Occurrence of Insomnia and Anxiety Disorder: A Review of the Literature," *American Journal of Lifestyle Medicine* 3, no. 4 (2009): 300–9.
4. L. A. Verlander, J. O. Benedict, and D. P. Hanson, "Stress and Sleep Patterns of College Students," *Perceptual Motor Skills* 88, no. 3 (1999): 893–8.
5. M. Burman and A. King, "Exercise as Treatment to Enhance Sleep," *American Journal of Lifestyle Medicine* 4, no. 6 (2010): 500–14.

death of a loved one, the stringent requirements of your major, stacked-up course assignments, and so on. You can, however, change your reactions to them and better manage your stress.

Assess the Stressor List and evaluate the stressors in your life. Can you change the stressor itself? If not, you can still change your behavior and reactions to reduce the levels of stress you experience. For example, if you have a heavy academic workload, such as five term papers due for five different courses during the same quarter or semester, make a plan to start the papers early and space your work evenly so you can avoid panic over deadlines and all-night sessions to finish papers on time.

Change Your Response If something causes you distress—a habitually messy roommate, for example—you can (1) express your anger by yelling; (2) pick up the mess yourself but then leave a nasty note; (3) use humor to get your point across; or (4) initiate an even-tempered, matter-of-fact conversation about the problem. Before you respond, think through the most effective choice. Humor and laughter are surprisingly good ways to deescalate tense situations and to benefit your wellness generally. Laughter can boost your immune response, not to mention lightening your mood and even bringing extra oxygen into your lungs![36] A calm, rational conversation can work well, too.

Cognitive Coping Strategies Thinking things through before acting may help you avoid destructive or ineffective responses to potentially stressful events. Forethought and planning can also help you tolerate increasingly higher stress levels while limiting physical and mental wear and tear.

Prepare Before Stressful Events Preparing yourself for an event that you know will be stressful can diminish its impact. For example, practicing in front of friends may help you find and correct rough spots, and in turn, lower your levels of stress during the actual speech.

Downshift You may experience stress because you want to "have it all": a college diploma, a successful career, a family, a wide circle of friends, possessions, status in the community, and so on. But many people are **downshifting**: stepping back to a simpler life by, for example, moving from a large urban area to a smaller town, changing from a hectic high-pressure career to a low-key one, or scaling back to fewer, less-expensive possessions.

Consider some immediate and longer-term steps for simplifying your life:

- Avoid unnecessary spending.

- Choose a career that you enjoy for itself, not primarily for the salary it commands. Some lower-paying jobs are less stressful and allow more free time for relaxation.

- Clear out clutter. Having fewer unnecessary, unused items means keeping track and taking care of that much less.

Managing Your Time and Finances

The world presents us with plenty of stressors. We create some of our own through ineffective time and finance management habits. Habits are learned behaviors, and you can *unlearn* bad habits or replace them with new habits that serve you better in managing stress. Here is what to aim for.

Manage Your Time Time—or our perceived lack of it—is one of our biggest stressors. If you learn to handle demands in a more streamlined, efficient way, you can leave more time for other things, such as studying and having fun. To get a handle on time management, try working through **Lab 9.2**. The following tips can also help:

DO IT! ONLINE

- *Use a calendar.* A calendar can help you keep track of due dates, events, commitments, and the like. Pick out a calendar that fits your life. Don't use a wall calendar if you are constantly on the go. Electronic calendars work well, especially because you can set reminders in them. Some people like the feel of paper and pen. Whatever works for you is fine, just get something you'll use.

- *Multitask only when it's truly appropriate.* Save multitasking for things that take less concentration, such as doing the laundry and paying bills.

SEE IT! ONLINE

The Multi-Tasking Myth

- *Break up big tasks.* Divide big tasks like finishing a term paper into smaller segments and then allocate a certain amount of time to each piece. If you find yourself floundering in a task, move on and come back to it when you are refreshed.

- *Clean your desk.* Periodically weed out unneeded papers and file the

downshifting Forging new values that include stepping back to a simpler life

useful ones in separate folders. Promptly read, respond to, file, or toss mail into the recycle bin.

- *Accommodate your natural rhythms.* If you are a morning person, study and write papers in the morning, and take breaks when you start to slow down.

- *Avoid overcommitment.* Set your school and personal priorities and don't be afraid to say no to things you cannot or should not agree to do.

- *Avoid interruptions.* When you have a project that requires total concentration, schedule uninterrupted time. Go to a quiet room in the library or student union where no one will find you. Shut off your cell phone.

- *Remember that time is precious.* Many people learn to value their time only when they face a terminal illness. Try to value each day. Time spent not enjoying life is a tremendous waste!

Manage Your Finances Higher education can impose a huge financial burden on parents, students, and communities. In recent studies, nearly two-thirds of students indicated that they have "some" or "major" concerns regarding their ability to pay for their education.[37] The economic downturn of the past few years is pushing already financially stressed students and their families further toward the breaking point. Many students must work part- or full-time in addition to carrying heavy class loads, and some have increasing levels of credit card debt.

Here are a few tips for easing your financial stress:

- Develop a realistic budget of monthly expenses and what you really need.

- Pay bills immediately and consider online banking to avoid late fees.

- Take money management seminars and courses.

- Avoid unsolicited credit card offers.

- Take on as little new debt as possible.

Managing Your Thoughts and Emotions

Just as we can manage our time and finances, we can learn to manage how we think and react to events and to our emotions.

Manage Your Thinking Our "negative scripts" about ourselves contribute to our stress. When we see ourselves as unable to cope (that is, when we have low

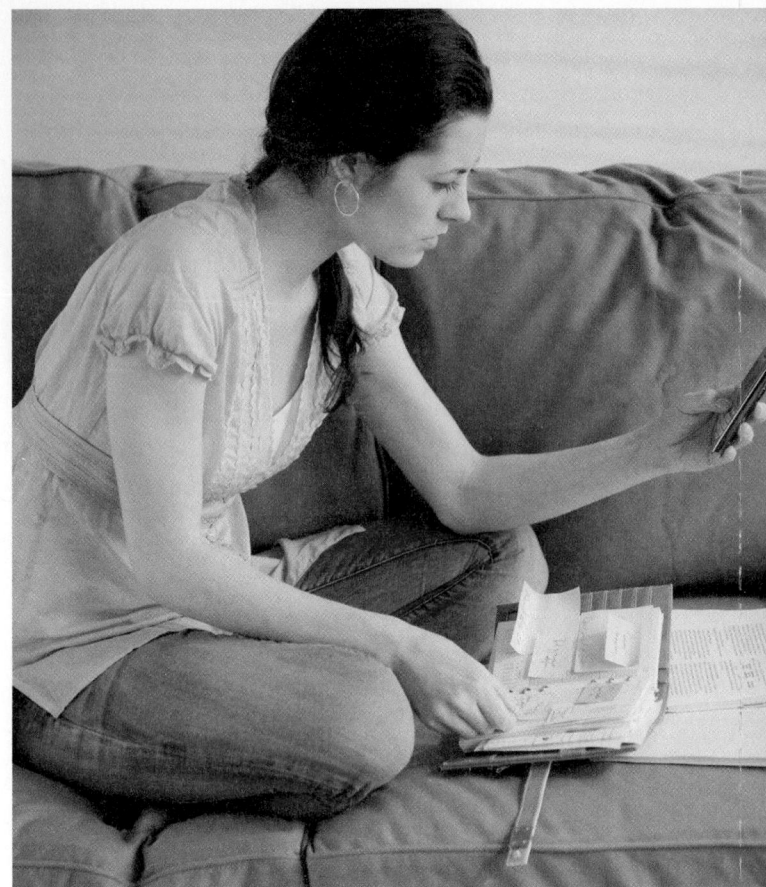

self-efficacy), we tend to handle life's problems and stresses more poorly. You can change negative scripts to more positive ones, however, and in the process reduce your stress responses. Successful stress management involves developing and practicing self-esteem skills, such as applying positive thinking and examining self-talk to reduce negative and irrational responses. Focus on your current capabilities rather than on past problems.

Here are specific actions you can take to develop better mental skills for stress management:

- *Worry constructively.* Don't waste time and energy worrying about things you can't change or events that may never happen.

- *Perceive life as changeable.* If you accept that change is a natural part of living and growing, the jolt of changes will become less stressful.

- *Consider alternatives.* Remember, there is seldom only one appropriate action. Anticipating options will help you plan for change and adjust more rapidly.

- *Moderate your expectations.* Aim high but be realistic about your circumstances and motivation.

- *Don't rush into action.* Think before you act. Tolerate mistakes by yourself and others. Rather than getting angry and stressed by mishaps, evaluate what happened, learn from them, and plan to avoid future occurrences.

- *Take things less seriously.* Try to keep the real importance of things in perspective. Ask yourself: How much will this matter in two weeks? Six months?

Manage Negative Emotions and Anger

Stress management involves learning to identify emotional reactions that are based on irrational beliefs and negative self-talk. Identifying those can allow you to deal with the belief or emotion in a healthy and appropriate way.[38]

LIVE IT! ONLINE

Worksheet 11
Anger Log

Learning how to manage anger is particularly important. Anger can be constructive if it mobilizes us to stand up for ourselves or to accomplish something others think we are incapable of. However, a habit of responding angrily when our wants or desires are thwarted can be destructive.

Hotheaded, short-fused people are at risk for health problems. Numerous studies show that anger can significantly increase the risk of heart disease. Stress hormones released during anger may constrict blood vessels in the heart or actually promote clot formation, which can trigger a heart attack.[39] Strategies for controlling and redirecting anger include practicing problem-solving techniques in place of complaining; seeking objective opinions and constructive advice from friends; anticipating situations that trigger your anger and brainstorming solutions in advance; learning to express your feelings constructively; learning to de-escalate from anger by taking deep breaths or counting to 10; and keeping a journal to observe your own reactions and progress in controlling anger.

Seeking Social Support

Making, keeping, and spending time with friends is a central stress-management tool that helps protect you against harmful stressors.[40] Social interactions are important buffers against the effects of stress: A person who is well-integrated socially is only half as likely to die from any cause at any age than is a person with few or no sources of social support.[41] This makes social connections a factor as large as being a nonsmoker versus a smoker! Social networking—through Facebook and Twitter, for example—has been an enormously popular way to stay connected. A few users do so obsessively, however, and this can become its own source of stress.[42] In addition, some recent research suggests that smoking, obesity, and other behaviors may tend to spread through networks of friends.[43] Clearly, social connectedness—pursued in moderation and with intelligent choices made toward eating, smoking, and other socially influenced behaviors—is important to wellness.

The flip side of social connectedness is social isolation, and it, too, has important health implications. Compared to students with a network of friends, isolated students experience more stress, poorer moods, and lower quality sleep.[44] Studies have found deleterious changes to the cardiovascular, immune, and nervous systems in chronically lonely people and these changes may help explain the increased risks for heart disease, infection, and depression in isolated individuals.[45] This research also suggests that a person's actual number of social contacts is less important to wellness than the subjective experience of being unpopular or lonely.[46]

While friends can be important stress reducers, people sometimes need the help of a counselor or support group. Most colleges and universities offer counseling services at no cost for short-term crises. Clergy, instructors, and dorm supervisors also may be helpful resources. Sometimes university services are unavailable and you may be concerned about confidentiality. Most communities offer low-cost counseling through mental health clinics. You may be able to find and join a stress-reduction program or stress support group through one of these professional resources. Many individual counselors and classes teach stress-reduction techniques to help you manage your stress.

> **relaxation breathing** Inhaling deeply and rhythmically, expanding and then relaxing the abdomen; this breathing technique can help relieve tension and increase oxygen intake.
>
> **progressive muscle relaxation (PMR)** A stress-management technique that identifies tension stored in the muscles and releases it, one muscle group at a time

Relaxation Techniques

Relaxation techniques tend to focus the mind and breathing while the body remains fairly stationary. Here are some of the most popular examples.

Relaxation Breathing When we're tense, we often breathe shallowly in the upper chest or even hold our breath, but this kind of breathing can increase anxiety.[47] **Relaxation breathing**—inhaling deeply and rhythmically and involving the abdominal muscles—can help relieve tension and increase oxygen levels in the blood. This, in turn, can boost energy and sharpen thinking. Relaxation breathing, also called *diaphragmatic breathing,* is easy and can be done sitting in a chair or lying down, alone or in a small group, and for a few minutes or longer. The object is to expand the lungs fully by drawing downward with the diaphragm and outward with the abdomen, then releasing fully.

Progressive Muscle Relaxation **Progressive muscle relaxation (PMR)** releases tension in the muscles, muscle group by muscle group. To do PMR, lie down in a quiet, comfortable place and devote 10 or 20 minutes to gradually letting go of accumulated stiffness and

TOOLS FOR CHANGE ●

Progressive Muscle Relaxation

Progressive muscle relaxation involves systematically contracting and relaxing different muscle groups in your body. The standard pattern is to begin with the feet and work your way up your body, contracting and releasing as you go. With practice, you can quickly identify tension in your body when you are facing stressful situations and consciously release that tension to calm yourself.

Sit or lie down in a comfortable position and follow the steps below: Start with one foot. Inhale to the count of five, contracting the muscle of your foot. Hold for three seconds and notice the feeling of tension. Exhale to the count of eight, slowly releasing the muscles. Notice the feeling of tension flowing away. Repeat the same steps contracting and releasing your foot and lower leg, then your entire leg.

Follow the same sequence with your other foot and leg. Starting with one hand, follow the same sequence for both arms. Continue these isolations as you progress up your body, contracting and then relaxing your abdomen, then chest, followed by neck and shoulders, and ending with your face.

Hint: when you isolate and tense a muscle group, be sure not to contract too tightly. This can cause cramping, especially in your toes, feet, calves and neck. You many want to record the steps of PMR on a tape recorder. Some prefer to memorize the sequence of muscle groups and repeat the instructions mentally. Alternatively, ask another person to read the instructions to you out loud.

● ●

tension in the affected muscles. The box Progressive Muscle Relaxation, shows you how. You can do this alone or in a group as a way to relax and refresh yourself fully. Some people also use it as a means of falling asleep.

Meditation There are dozens of forms of meditation. Most involve sitting quietly for 15 to 30 minutes and focusing on breathing. Researchers have confirmed that meditation reduces the stress response and boosts the immune response.[48] Meditation also shifts brain activity from the right prefrontal lobe, associated with unhappiness, anger, and distress, and toward the left prefrontal lobe, associated with happiness and enthusiasm. See Activate, Motivate, and Advance: A Meditation Program at the end of the chapter for guidance on beginning a meditation practice.

Biofeedback **Biofeedback** involves monitoring physical stress responses such as brain activity, blood pressure, muscle tension, and heart rate with a special machine and then learning to consciously alter these responses. Biofeedback is effective for several stress-related conditions, including high blood pressure, headaches, irritable bowel syndrome, and asthma.[49]

Hypnosis **Hypnosis** trains people to focus on one thought, object, or voice and to become unusually responsive to suggestion. A qualified hypnotherapist can implant a suggestion that directs a patient to resist habits such as smoking or overeating or to lessen phobias such as fear of snakes or air travel. The patient then learns to induce a state of selfhypnosis as a way to relax deeply and reinforce the behavioral changes.

People who exercise regularly and practice one or more of these relaxation methods—relaxation breathing, progressive muscle relaxation, meditation, biofeedback, and hypnosis—can achieve effective relief from stress symptoms.[50] Many will also see improvement in medical conditions that are worsened by stress.

Spiritual Practice

Several medical studies have discovered correlations between spirituality and wellness. Prayer, for example elicits the same relaxation response attained through other stress-management techniques: lowered blood pressure, heart rate, breathing and metabolism, and a more vigorous immune response.[51] Spirituality is also correlated with a reduced *perception* of stress in one's life.

Developing one's spirituality can be more than just an internal process. It can also be a social process that enhances your relationships with others. The abilities to give and take, speak and listen, and forgive and move on are integral to any process of spiritual development.

biofeedback A stress-management technique that teaches you to alter automatic physiological responses such as body temperature, heart rate, or sweating.

hypnosis A medical and psychiatric tool that trains people to focus on one thought, object, or voice and to become unusually responsive to suggestion

LIVE IT! ONLINE

Worksheet 7
Developing
Your Spirituality

casestudy

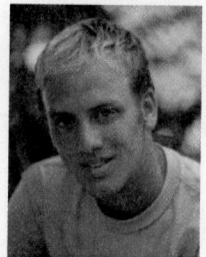

CORY

"This semester was getting out of control. I was exhausted but would have trouble falling asleep, so that was a vicious cycle. I stopped working out—which I used to do twice a week but just didn't have the time for anymore. And I caught another cold at the end of October. My dad started joking that he was healthier than I was! I had to cut out something so I dropped my only elective, Spanish, even though I liked it. I used the extra time to start going back to the gym, and that actually seemed to give me back some energy. I honestly think just those two things alone helped me to get through the rest of the semester. Now, I just need to ace my MCATs …"

THINK! What kinds of stress-related problems was Cory exhibiting? Review the section on stress-management tools. Which strategies did Cory employ?

ACT! Make a list of the stress-management strategies you use. Using that same list, put a check by the techniques that seem to be the most effective for you. How could you make the others work better?

HEAR IT! ONLINE

How Can I Create My Own Stress Management Plan?

You can use many of the fitness and wellness tools you read about in earlier chapters to help reduce your stress levels. These tools include self-assessment, drawing up a behavior change contract, and journaling. Lab 9.1 helps you assess situations that may leave you susceptible to stress. It also reveals signs of chronic stress. Using this information, target for change one or more behaviors that contribute to your increased stress.

Then, evaluate the behavior(s) you have chosen. Identify your stress-producing behavior patterns. What can you change now? What can you change in the near future? Select one stress-producing behavior pattern that you want to change. Devise an action plan and create a behavior change contract using **Lab 9.3**. As you learned earlier, your

behavior change contract should include your long-term goal for change, your short-term goals, the rewards you will give yourself for reaching these goals, potential obstacles along the way, and strategies for overcoming these obstacles.

Chart your progress in your journal. At the end of a week, evaluate how successful you were in following your plan. What helped you be successful? What obstacles to change did you encounter? What will you do differently next week? After you assess yourself, make a plan and revise it as needed. Are your short-term goals attainable? Are the rewards satisfying? Do you need to go beyond your own self-efforts and enlist the help of your peers or professionals? If you think you need professional support, start by consulting the student health service for advice and direction on finding suitable counselors, therapists, or stress-management support groups.

chapterin**review**

videos

Log on to **www.pearsonhighered.com/hopson** or MyFitnessLab to view these chapter-related videos.

Stress at Work and Home   The Multi-Tasking Myth

online**resources**

Log on to **www.pearsonhighered.com/hopson** or MyFitnessLab for access to these book-related resources, and for links to other useful websites.

Audio case study
Audio PowerPoint lecture

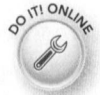
Lab 9.1 How Stressed Are You?
Lab 9.2 Managing Your Time
Lab 9.3 Your Personal Stress Management Plan

Customizable 4-week starter and intermediate meditation programs
Take Charge of Your Health! Worksheets:
  Worksheet 4 Sleep Inventory
  Worksheet 7 Developing Your Spirituality
  Worksheet 8 Stress Reaction
  Worksheet 9 Stress Tolerance Test
  Worksheet 11 Anger Log
Behavior Change Log Book and Wellness Journal

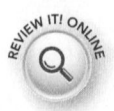
Pre- and post-quizzes
Glossary flashcards

reviewquestions

1. Graduating from college and moving to a new city can create stress as well as provide an opportunity for growth. This type of stress is called
   a. strain.
   b. distress.
   c. eustress.
   d. adaptive response.

2. The physiological instinct to flee from or confront a threat is called
   a. homeostasis.
   b. the fight-or-flight response.
   c. allostasis.
   d. allostatic load.

3. *Homeostasis* describes
   a. the body's "normal" or "steady state."
   b. long-term wear-and-tear on the body.
   c. sustained stress.
   d. the exhaustion stage of the general adaptation syndrome.

4. Contemporary researchers have modified one stage of Hans Selye's general adaptation syndrome. Which one is it?
   a. The alarm stage
   b. The resistance stage
   c. The allostasis stage
   d. The exhaustion stage

5. Find the true statement:
   a. Stress reduces the risk of cardiovascular disease.
   b. Stress improves immune system function.
   c. Stress alleviates depression and anxiety.
   d. Stress reduces overall health and wellness.

6. Change, hassles, performance demands, and burn-out are all examples of
   a. psychosocial sources of stress.
   b. environmental sources of stress.
   c. internal sources of stress.
   d. homeostasis.

7. *Allostatic load* refers to
   a. changes that occur in the body to maintain homeostasis.
   b. long-term wear-and-tear on the body caused by stress.
   c. the first stage of the general adaptation syndrome.
   d. eustress.

8. Find the true statement: Effective stress management includes
   a. getting by on little sleep.
   b. reducing exercise and physical activity to allow more time for studying.
   c. eating fast food and junk food to save money and provide comfort.
   d. avoiding alcohol and tobacco.

9. *Relaxation breathing* refers to
   a. inhaling deeply and rhythmically to relieve tension and increase oxygen levels in the blood.
   b. progressive muscle relaxation.
   c. monitoring physical stress responses and then consciously working to alter those responses.
   d. biofeedback.

10. What stress-fighting technique allows people to become unusually responsive to suggestion?
    a. Meditation
    b. Massage
    c. Biofeedback
    d. Hypnosis

critical**thinking**questions

1. Compare and contrast distress and eustress. In what ways are both types of stress potentially harmful?
2. Describe the body's physiological response to stress.
3. What are some of the health risks that result from chronic stress? Summarize the main points of the general adaptation syndrome and the allostatic load model.

4. What major factors seem to influence the nature and extent of a person's susceptibility to stress? Explain how social support, self-esteem, and personality may make a person more or less susceptible.

references

1. American Psychological Association, *Stress in America 2009, Executive Summary,* www.apa.org/news/press/releases /stress-exec-summary.pdf (2009).
2. American College Health Association, *American College Health Association– National College Health Assessment II (ACHA-NCHA II) Reference Group Executive Summary Spring 2010* (Linthicum, MD: American College Health Association, 2010).
3. H. Selye, "The General-Adaptation-Syndrome" *Annual Review of Medicine* 2 (1951): 327–42.
4. D. G. Myers, *Psychology* 5th ed. (New York: Worth Publishers, 1998): 518.
5. B. McEwen and T. Seeman, "Allostatic Load and Allostasis," John D. and Catherine T. MacArthur Research Network on Socio-economic Status and Health, University of California at San Francisco (revised 2009).

6. Ibid.
7. R. Sapolsky, *Why Zebras Don't Get Ulcers: An Updated Guide to Stress, Stress-Related Diseases, and Coping* (New York: Owl Books, 2004).
8. A. Mokdal and others, "Actual Causes of Death in the United States 2000," *Journal of the American Medical Association* 291, no. 10 (2004): 1238–45.
9. S. Cohen, D. Janicki-Deverts, and G. Miller, "Psychological Stress and Cardiovascular Disease," *Journal of the American Medical Association* 298, no. 14 (2007): 1685–7.
10. F. Sparrenberger and others, "Does Psychological Stress Cause Hypertension? A Systematic Review of Observational Studies," *Journal of Human Hypertension* 23, no 1 (2009): 12–9; J. Dimsdale, "Psychological Stress and Cardiovascular Disease," *Journal of the American College of Cardiology* 51, no. 13 (2008): 1237–46.
11. S. A. Everson-Rose and T. T. Lewis, "Psychosocial Factors and Cardiovascular Diseases," *Annual Review of Public Health* 26 (2005): 469–500.
12. S. C. Segerstrom and G. E. Miller, "Psychological Stress and the Human Immune System," *Psychological Bulletin* 130, no. 4 (2004): 601–30. R. M. Lucas and others, "Mid-life Stress Is Associated with Both Up- and Down-Regulation of Markers of Humoral and Cellular Immunity," *Stress* 10, no. 4 (2007): 351–61.
13. S. C. Segerstrom and G. E. Miller, "Psychological Stress and the Human Immune System," 2004.
14. V. Vicennati and others, "Stress-Related Development of Obesity and Cortisol in Women," *Obesity* 17, no 9 (2009): 1678–83.
15. D. K. Hall-Flavin, "Stress and Hair Loss: Are They Related?" MayoClinic.com, www.mayoclinic.com/health/stress-and-hair-loss/AN01442 (2008).
16. M. Scollan-Koliopoulos, "Managing Stress Response to Control Hypertension in Type 2 Diabetes," *The Nurse Practitioner* 30, no. 2 (2005): 46–9.
17. Johns Hopkins Health Alerts, "Four Relaxation Techniques to Soothe Your Digestive Discomfort," www.johnshopkinshealthalerts.com/reports/digestive_health/2683-1.html (2008).
18. V. Bitsika, C. Sharpley, and R. Bell, "The Contribution of Anxiety and Depression to Fatigue among a Sample of Australian University Students: Suggestions for University Counselors," *Counseling Psychology Quarterly* 22, no. 2 (2009): 243–53.
19. L. Schwabe, T. Wolf, and M. Oitzl, "Memory Formation under Stress: Quantity and Quality," *Neuroscience and Biobehavioral Reviews* 34, no. 4 (2009): 584–91.
20. E. Dias-Ferreira and others, "Chronic Stress Causes Frontostriatal Reorganization and Affects Decision-Making," *Science* 325, no. 5940 (2009): 621–5.
21. D. A. Katerndahl and M. Parchman, "The Ability of the Stress Process Model to Explain Mental Health Outcomes," *Comprehensive Psychiatry* 43, no. 5 (2002): 351–60.
22. J. Burris and others, "Factors Associated with the Psychological Well-Being and Distress of University Students," *Journal of American College Health* 57, no. 5 (2009): 536–43.
23. P. Jackson and M. Finney, "Negative Life Events and Psychological Distress among Young Adults," *Social Psychology Quarterly* 65, no. 2 (2002): 186–201.
24. J. H. Pryor and others, *The American Freshman: National Norms Fall 2010* (Los Angeles: Higher Education Research Institute at UCLA, 2011): 1–4.
25. Ibid.
26. T. Holmes and R. Rahe, "The Social Readjustment Rating Scale," *Journal of Psychosomatic Research* 11 (1967): 213–8.
27. D. J. Maybery and D. Graham, "Hassles and Uplifts: Including Interpersonal Events," *Stress and Health* 17, no 2 (2001): 91–104; R. Blonna, *Coping with Stress in a Changing World,* 4th ed. (New York: McGraw-Hill, 2006).
28. A. D. Von and others, "Predictors of Health Behaviors in College Students," *Journal of Advanced Nursing* 48, no. 5 (2004): 463–74.
29. M. Friedman and R. H. Rosenman, *Type A Behavior and Your Heart* (New York: Knopf, 1974).
30. S. Kobasa, "Stressful Life Events, Personality, and Health: An Inquiry into Hardiness," *Journal of Personality and Social Psychology* 37 (1979): 1–11.
31. B. J. Crowley and others, "Psychological Hardiness and Adjustment to Life Events in Adulthood," *Journal of Adult Development* 10 (2003): 237–48.
32. A. Leal-Cerro and others, "Mechanisms Underlying the Neuroendocrine Response to Physical Exercise," *Journal of Endocrinological Investigation* 26, no. 9 (2003): 879–85.
33. U. Rimmele and others, "Trained Men Show Lower Cortisol, Heart Rate, and Psychological Responses to Psychosocial Stress Compared with Untrained Men," *Psychoneuroendocrinology* 32, no. 6 (2007): 627–35.
34. A. Tsatsoulis and S. Fountoulakis, "The Protective Role of Exercise on Stress System Dysregulation and Comorbidities," *Annals of the New York Academy of Sciences* 1083 (2006): 196–213.
35. National Institute of Alcohol Abuse and Alcoholism, "Alcohol and Sleep," *Alcohol Alert* 41, http://pubs.niaaa.nih.gov/publications/aa41.htm (1998).
36. M. Bennett and C. Lengacher, "Humor and Laughter May Influence Health IV: Humor and Immune Function," *Evidence-Based Complementary and Alternative Medicine* 6, no. 2 (2009): 159–64.
37. J. H. Pryor and others, *The American Freshman: National Norms Fall 2010,* 2011.
38. B. L. Seward, *Managing Stress: Principles and Strategies for Health and Well-Being,* 6th ed. (Sudbury, MA: Jones and Bartlett, 2009): 8.
39. L. D. Kubzansky and others, "Shared and Unique Contributions of Anger, Anxiety, and Depression to Coronary Heart Disease: A Prospective Study in the Normative Aging Study," *Annals of Behavioral Medicine* 31, no. 1 (2006): 21–9.
40. P. A. Bovier, E. Chamot, and T. V. Perneger, "Perceived Stress, Internal Resources, and Social Support as Determinants of Mental Health among Young Adults," *Quality of Life Research* 13, no. 1 (2004): 161–70; A. M. McLaughlin and others, *Determinants of Minority Mental Health and Wellness* (New York: Springer, 2009); L. Crockett and others, "Acculturative Stress, Social Support and Coping: Relations to Psychological Adjustment among Mexican American College Students," *Cultural Diversity and Ethnic Minority Psychology* 13, no. 4 (2007): 347–55; J. Ruthig and others, "Perceived Academic Control: Mediating the Effects of Optimism and Social Support on College Students' Psychological Health," *Social Psychology of Education* 12, no. 7 (2009): 233–49.
41. S. Levine, D. M. Lyons, and A. F. Schatzberg, "Psychobiological Consequences of Social Relationships," *Annals of the New York Academy of Sciences* 89, no. 7 (1999): 210–8.
42. A. Lenhart and others, "Social Media and Young Adults," Pew Internet and American Life Project, www.pewinternet.org/Reports/2010/Social-Media-And-Young-Adults.aspx (2010).
43. J. Couzin, "Friendship as a Health Factor," *Science* 323, no. 5913 (2009): 454–7.
44. J. T. Cacioppo and L. C. Hawkley, "Social Isolation and Health, with an Emphasis on Underlying Mechanisms," *Perspectives in Biology and Medicine* 46, no. 3 Suppl (2003): S39–52.
45. G. Miller, "Why Loneliness Is Hazardous to Your Health," *Science* 331, no. 6014 (2011): 138–40.
46. Ibid.
47. A. Conrad and others, "Psychophysiological Effects of Breathing Instructions for Stress Management," *Applied Psychophysiology and Biofeedback* 32, no. 2 (2007): 89–98.
48. S. Jain and others, "A Randomized Controlled Trial of Mindfulness Meditation Versus Relaxation Training: Effects on Distress, Positive States of Mind, Rumination, and Distraction," *Annals of Behavioral Medicine* 33, no. 1 (2007): 11–21; R. J. Davidson and others, "Alterations in Brain and Immune Function Produced by Mindfulness Meditation," *Psychosomatic Medicine* 65, no. 4 (2003): 564–70.
49. Mayo Clinic Staff, "Biofeedback: Using Your Mind to Improve Your Health," www.mayoclinic.com/health/biofeedback/MY01072 (January 2010).
50. Mayo Clinic Staff, "Relaxation Techniques: Try These Steps to Reduce Stress," www.mayoclinic.com/health/relaxation-technique/SR00007 (May 2011); Mayo Clinic Staff, "Exercise and Stress: Get Moving to Combat Stress," www.mayoclinic.com/print/exercise-and-stress/SR00036 (July 2010).
51. D. K. Reibel and others, "Mindfulness-Based Stress Reduction and Health-Related Quality of Life in a Heterogeneous Patient Population," *General Hospital Psychiatry* 23, no. 4 (2001): 183–92, R. Sethness and others, "Cardiac Health: Relationships among Hostility, Spirituality, and Health Risk," *Journal of Nursing Care Quality* 20, no. 1 (2005): 81–9; L. E. Carlson and others, "Mindfulness-Based Stress Reduction in Relation to Quality of Life, Mood, Symptoms of Stress and Levels of Cortisol, Dehyroepiandrosterone Sulfate (DHEAS) and Melatonin in Breast and Prostate Cancer Outpatient," *Psychoneuroendocrinology* 29, no. 4 (2004): 448–74.

LAB 9.1 • HOW STRESSED ARE YOU?

Name: _____ **Date:** _____

Instructor: _____ **Section:** _____

Purpose: To uncover your major stressors and your stress levels during the last year.

Directions: The following Life Experiences Survey lists events that can cause a buildup of chronic stress. If you did not experience a listed event, circle the zero in front of a statement. If you experienced the event but feel that it had a positive impact on your life, also mark a zero. If you experienced an event and feel it had a *negative* impact, use the scale below and circle the number 1, 2, or 3.

Life Experience Survey

3 = Extremely negative impact
2 = Moderately negative impact
1 = Somewhat negative impact
0 = No impact or a positive impact

College

0 1 2 3   Beginning a new school experience at a higher academic level

0 1 2 3   Changing to a new school at same academic level

0 1 2 3   Academic probation

0 1 2 3   Failing an important exam

0 1 2 3   Changing a major

0 1 2 3   Failing a course

0 1 2 3   Dropping a course

0 1 2 3   Joining a fraternity/sorority

0 1 2 3   Ending formal college education

0 1 2 3   Financial problems concerning college

Family

0 1 2 3   Marriage

0 1 2 3   Death of spouse

Death of a close family member

     0 1 2 3   Mother

     0 1 2 3   Father

     0 1 2 3   Brother

     0 1 2 3   Sister

     0 1 2 3   Child

     0 1 2 3   Grandmother

     0 1 2 3   Grandfather

     0 1 2 3   Other _____

0 1 2 3   Male: Wife/girlfriend's pregnancy

0 1 2 3   Female: Pregnancy

Serious illness or injury of close family member:

     0 1 2 3   Father

     0 1 2 3   Mother

     0 1 2 3   Sister

     0 1 2 3   Brother

     0 1 2 3   Grandmother

     0 1 2 3   Grandfather

     0 1 2 3   Spouse

     0 1 2 3   Child

     0 1 2 3   Other _____

0 1 2 3   Trouble with in-laws

0 1 2 3   Major change in closeness of family members (decreased or increased)

0 1 2 3   Gaining a new family member (birth, adoption, marriage of a relative)

0 1 2 3   Separation from spouse due to work, travel, school, etc.

0 1 2 3   Marital separation from mate (due to conflict)

0 1 2 3   Marital reconciliation with mate

0 1 2 3   Major change in number of arguments with spouse (a lot more, a lot fewer)

0 1 2 3   Married person: Change in a spouse's work outside the home (beginning work, loss of job, changing job, retirement, etc.)

0 1 2 3   Male: Wife/girlfriend having abortion

0 1 2 3   Female: Having an abortion

0 1 2 3   Major change in living condition of family (new home, remodeling, damage to home, loss of home)

0 1 2 3   Divorce

0 1 2 3   Son or daughter leaving home

0 1 2 3   Leaving home for first time

Fitness/Wellness Issues

0 1 2 3   Major changes in sleeping habits (much more or much less sleep)

0 1 2 3   Major change in eating habits (much more or much less food intake)

0 1 2 3   Major personal illness or injury

0 1 2 3   Sexual difficulties

Social Issues

0 1 2 3   Detention in jail or comparable institution

0 1 2 3   Minor law violation (traffic ticket, disturbing the peace, etc.)

0 1 2 3   Death of a close friend

0 1 2 3   Change of residence (moving)

0 1 2 3   Major change in church activities (increased or decreased attendance)

0 1 2 3   Major change in usual type or amount of recreation

0 1 2 3   Major change in social activities such as parties, movies, visiting (increased or decreased participation)

0 1 2 3   Serious injury or illness of close friend

0 1 2 3   Breaking up with boyfriend/girlfriend

0 1 2 3   Engagement

0 1 2 3   Reconciliation with boyfriend/girlfriend

Money Matters

0 1 2 3   Foreclosure on mortgage or loan

0 1 2 3   Major change in financial status (a lot better off, a lot worse off)

0 1 2 3   Borrowing more than $10,000 (buying a home, business, etc.)

0 1 2 3   Borrowing less than $10,000 (buying a car or TV, getting a school loan)

Work

0 1 2 3   New job

0 1 2 3   Changed work situation (different working conditions, working hours, etc.)

0 1 2 3   Trouble with employer (in danger of losing job, being suspended, demoted, etc.)

0 1 2 3   Being fired from job

0 1 2 3   Retirement from work

Additional Factors

Other experiences that have had a negative impact on your life in the past year.

_____

_____

_____

_____

RESULTS

Sum of negative scores: _____

Use the table below to find the rating of your score and write it here: _____

Life Experience Survey Scores		
Sum of Negative Score	Interpretation	Action
<6	Below-normal stress	None needed
6–9	Average stress	Consider improving your fitness and wellness
9–13	Above-average stress	Consider improving fitness and applying stress-reduction techniques
14+	Much-above-average stress	Consider improving fitness, reducing stress, and seeking counseling or group support

Source: Adapted from I.G. Sarason and others, "Assessing the Impact of Life Changes: Development of the Life Experiences Survey," *Journal of Consulting and Clinical Psychology* 46, no. 5 (1978): 932–46. Copyright 1978 by the American Psychological Association.

LAB 9.2 • MANAGING YOUR TIME

Name: _____ **Date:** _____

Instructor: _____ **Section:** _____

Purpose: Learn a concrete way to manage your time so you can accomplish the things you want to.

SECTION I: ANALYZING YOUR TIME

Every evening for a week fill out the following table, listing how much time you spent doing each activity that day.

Activity	Monday	Tuesday	Wednesday	Thursday	Friday	Saturday	Sunday	Total Hours
Getting ready								
On the road								
In class								
Working for pay								
Exercising								
Eating								
Studying								
Watching TV or videos								
Using computer (school)								
Using computer (recreational)								
Spending time with friends								
Leisure activities								
Sleeping								
Other (specify)								

At the end of the week, total the hours for each activity. Are there any activities that you would like to do more or less frequently? You can use the rest of this lab to clarify your goals and set up your calendar so that you accomplish the things that you want to accomplish.

SECTION II: CLARIFY YOUR GOALS AND CREATE YOUR TASK LIST

1. On a piece of paper or in a journal, list your goals down the left side. Goals can be anything from "go to nursing school" to "learn to play racquetball." Make the goals specific. Instead of "be more musical," come up with a concrete goal such as "learn to play guitar."

2. On the right side of the paper, break each of your goals down into specific tasks. For example, as part of the nursing school goal, you might add "make a list of possible schools" to the task list.

3. Next, prioritize the tasks by numbering them in order of importance.

SECTION III: ENTER YOUR TASKS ONTO YOUR CALENDAR

In your calendar, write the commitments you have already—classes, job, exercise, rehearsals, and so on. Be sure to look at the schedule you filled out in section one. Now is your chance to think about what activities you want to continue and which you would like to curb.

When you have all of your commitments written in, you'll be able to see where your free time is. Now review your task list from section two above and choose the most important tasks to put in your free time. Make sure these tasks are things that are really important to you to accomplish.

SECTION IV: MAKE IT HAPPEN

Go over your schedule at the start of each day. This gives you a chance to prepare for the day and remember things that you need to take with you. At the end of the day, cross off tasks you were able to accomplish and re-arrange (or delete) tasks that you didn't do.

SECTION IV: REFLECTION AND EVALUATION

1. Describe any times you found yourself procrastinating. What do you think caused that? Were you bored? Were you overwhelmed? What specific thing could you do next time to get back on track quicker? For example, if you were overwhelmed, is there an advisor you could talk to who could help you prioritize?

_____

_____

2. Did you check your planner each morning, writing in tasks, checking them off, doing weekly planning? If not, what got in the way? What could you do differently next time?

_____

_____

3. Did you find other people encroaching on your time? What happened? How could you handle that differently next time?

_____

_____

4. Review your goals and tasks for the next week, adjust the list to reflect things you've accomplished or any other changes, and then block off time on your calendar for the most important things. Remember that time management is an ongoing exercise. Spend at least 20 minutes at the start of your week planning for the upcoming week, then stay focused on the things you want to accomplish!

LAB 9.3 • YOUR PERSONAL STRESS-MANAGEMENT PLAN

Name: _____ Date: _____

Instructor: _____ Section: _____

Purpose: To develop a stress-management plan that targets the key sources of stress in your life.

SECTION I: EXAMINE YOUR BEHAVIOR AND ATTITUDES

1. Enter your results from Lab 9.1 here:

Score: _____ Interpretation: _____

Action: _____

2. Do you feel that stress is a problem in your life right now?   ☐ Yes   ☐ No

If you scored above average in Lab 9.1, indicating relatively high exposure to stressors and fairly high stress levels, and yet you don't see stress as an issue to address, consider your readiness for change.

SECTION II: IDENTIFY MAJOR SOURCES OF STRESS

After reviewing your entries in the Life Experiences Survey in Lab 9.1, describe your main sources of stress, grouping them into the following categories:

College

_____

_____

Family

_____

_____

Fitness/Wellness Issues

_____

_____

Social Issues

_____

_____

Money Matters

_____

_____

Time-Management Issues

_____

_____

SECTION III: SET REALISTIC GOALS

Use this chart to rank your top five stressors from Section II, in order of urgency. Note ways to modify or eliminate each stressor. Note stress-reduction techniques that you can apply when the stressor arises.

	Stressors	Can I Modify or Eliminate the Stressor? Y/N	Can I Reduce Stress Symptoms? Y/N
Most urgent	1.		
⇓	2.		
⇓	3.		
⇓	4.		
Least urgent	5.		

SECTION IV: DEVISE A STRATEGY AND AN ACTION PLAN

Use this section to target the most urgent source of stress in your life first, and then address additional stressors as you feel ready to work on them.

1. Stressor: _____

2. Is it possible that I will need help from others? ☐ Y   ☐ N

If yes, ask yourself the following:

What professional resources are available where I live, work, or go to school? _____

_____

_____

How can I get my friends or family involved? _____

_____

3. List general strategies for modifying or eliminating environmental stressors that apply to more than one of your most urgent examples: _____

_____

4. What stress-management techniques can I use to relieve my own ongoing or recurrent symptoms of stress? (Consider relaxation breathing, progressive muscle relaxation, visual imagery, meditation, yoga, improved fitness, improved diet, better time-management skills, and enhanced spiritual connectedness.)

_____

_____

5. How can I plan ahead to avoid this stressor in the future?

_____

_____

6. How will I reward myself for sticking to my plan? _____

_____

SECTION V: CREATE A BEHAVIOR CHANGE CONTRACT

Use the information from Part IV to develop a behavior change contract that targets the stressor(s) you selected. A basic behavior change contract is included at the front of this book.

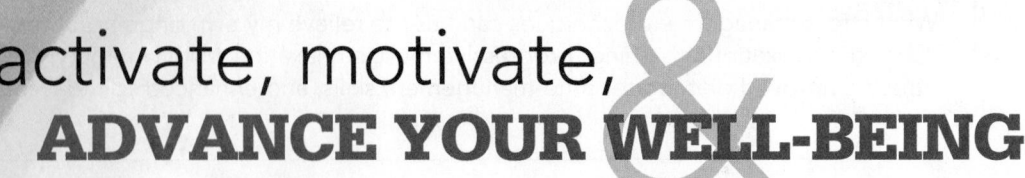

activate, motivate, & ADVANCE YOUR WELL-BEING

A MEDITATION PROGRAM

LIVE IT! ONLINE

ACTIVATE!

Meditation is a popular relaxation and centering activity. We all experience tension from worrying about or anticipating our problems. Meditation can help us relax and compose ourselves. It instills a sense of well-being that improves many aspects of our life. People who meditate regularly often enjoy a realistic optimism, enhanced intimacy, more satisfying social relations and a stronger ability to pay attention. In short, meditation brings physical, emotional, and intellectual enhancement.

What Do I Need?

LOCATION: You may meditate in your own living space, but be on the lookout for quiet places to meditate on campus, indoors or out. If you meditate at home, be sure to put your living space in order before you start. A clean, tidy place in which to meditate invites the mind to settle down.

TIME: If you live with others, plan to sit at a quiet time of the day, perhaps before your roommates get up or after they leave for the morning. Turn off your cell phone. For the period of time that you meditate you are not available. Place a silent timer, such as a watch or digital alarm clock, in your meditation area so that you can set it and not have to be concerned with keeping track of time while you meditate.

POSTURE: Sitting on the floor with crossed legs is by far the best posture for meditation. Place your hands in your lap or on your thighs, whichever is comfortable for you. Sit on a firm cushion that supports your spine and lifts your buttocks higher than your knees. The height of the cushion is a very individual matter based on comfort.

The first advantage of this posture is its stability. The broad base supports you, inviting relaxation at the physical and mental level. Second, the spine is self-supporting, not resting against anything. This discourages sleepiness and promotes balanced energy. Meditation is very much a physical activity.

If sitting on the floor is too uncomfortable, use a kneeling bench or sit on a firm chair such as a folding chair or a dining room chair. Sit toward the forward edge of the chair—don't lean against the backrest.

CLOTHING: Loose-fitting pants allow the abdomen to relax and they give room for the thighs to rotate out. Bare feet are most comfortable for sitting cross-legged. It's a good idea to wear a long-sleeved shirt for warmth.

How Do I Start?

BEGIN BY FOCUSING YOUR ATTENTION ON YOUR BREATH: Close your eyes and draw your attention to the area of your abdomen where you find the sensations of breathing most obvious; Follow the sequence of sensations occurring as you inhale and exhale. As you mindfully observe the rising and falling of the abdomen, make soft mental notes, "rising" and "falling." Noticing the breath is the primary activity of meditation, and it helps to sharpen and strengthen your attention.

Don't exaggerate the breath, let it be natural. Don't use your imagination to create an image of the breath, just attend to the sensations that are actually occurring.

You may find that your mind wanders off. Gently re-apply your attention to your breath. Your mind may wander, and you cannot control it with your will power. Relax! Make a mental note, "wandering, wandering," and aim your focus on the breath again. Already you are learning about stress and how to let go. Try to notice every breath. Watch each breath from the beginning, through the middle, to the end. As a beginner you won't be able to be present with every breath, but you must try. To be patient about this wandering, appreciate how passive your attention is generally. Your attention is drawn to stimulating things and is held there by the excitement. Think about the opening moments of a movie. Does it excite your interest? Must you make a special effort to stay with it, or are you swept along?

By contrast, in meditation you focus inward, on your breath. To avoid boredom, sleepiness, and wandering thoughts you attend to your breath. Through noticing the breath and the sensations of the rising and falling of the abdomen—stretching, tightness, swelling; and softness, cascading, and deflation—you will feel stress leave you.

As you become more skilled, your attention will become sustained and steadier for longer periods of time. Gradually your mind will settle down and your body will relax. This composure of mind and body is energizing, bright, and pleasant.

FOCUSING ATTENTION ON THE FELT SENSE OF DISCOMFORT: Physical pain or mental pain can be difficult for the body and mind. In trying to push them away, you may experience tension and stress. Try to turn toward what you have been avoiding. The rewards will be immediate.

When physical pain or mental displeasure arises for you, track and scrutinize the sensation, applying a soft mental label "pain" or "disliking" three or so times. As best you can, track the changing sensations of pressure, hardness, and heat, for example. The fear of pain will start to lose its grip as you see that pain is a collection of intense sensations.

When you are disturbed by thinking about someone you dislike, try saying this mantra: "If I have hurt, harmed, or offended anyone knowingly or unknowingly, may I be forgiven." Repeat that several times and then continue with this: "And anyone who may have hurt, harmed, or offended me knowingly or unknowingly, I freely forgive them."

When the strength of attention on the discomfort weakens, turn back to the breath to make a fresh start, setting aside the negativity. Your composure will grow as you focus on the breath.

ENDING THE SESSION: When it is time to stop meditating, move slowly. Take a little time to stretch and rest, write in your journal, and transition from quiet and stillness into activity. Wait for 20 minutes or so before making phone calls, texting, or getting into conversations.

Four-Week Beginning Meditation Program

After you sit, take a few minutes to record notes. Write down what you observed of the breath. The purpose of this exercise is to enhance your ability to pay attention to the breath as it is, in the same spirit as if you were an artist who kept a sketchbook in which to record things seen during the day.

PROGRAM **A** **GOAL:** Sit for 15 minutes every other day for four weeks.

	Mon	Tue	Wed	Thurs	Fri	Sat	Sun
Week 1	15 min		15 min		15 min		15 min
Week 2		15 min		15 min		15 min	
Week 3	15 min		15 min		15 min		15 min
Week 4		15 min		15 min		15 min	

MOTIVATE!

Create a journal—or use the log on the companion website—to keep track of your meditation sessions and become aware of the changing quality of your meditation experiences. Here are some other things to bear in mind and potential motivators to consider as you progress in your meditation practice:

ACCEPT THE CHALLENGE: Meditation can bring the benefits of centeredness, relaxation, and brightness of mind. Learning to meditate is a lifelong endeavor. To sit still, watch the breath, focus attention and calm down sounds simple, but it's a challenge! To do it, one must meet and overcome doubt, boredom, desire, irritability, and restlessness in turn.

FACE DISTRACTIONS: When you find yourself stopped by doubt, remember that being able to meet life's challenges with a calm mind is a valuable thing—worth working for. If you keep wanting to get up and eat something or check for text messages, then observe each mental interruption, acknowledge it, and let it go.

ENJOY THE FREEDOM: It is usually a great relief to detach from discomfort and from taking things personally. It is uplifting to be able to relax in the face of annoyances that previously would have provoked resistance and retaliation. When you truly attend to displeasure, annoyances don't dominate or push you around as they used to. Introspection gives rise to insight and inner freedom.

JOIN A GROUP: Beginners can find it motivating to join a meditation class with a teacher. You may be able to find such a meditation class through a yoga center, through your fitness instructor, or in a local alternative newspaper. If you sit with a group you will enjoy the inspiration and support of the group energy and can begin to feel confident about the benefits of daily practice. If you can't find an established group, you may form your own group of people with similar goals. In a quiet setting, you may want to read a book together, selecting an interesting passage to precede the sitting, or listen to a recorded talk from the Internet before you sit.

ATTEND A RETREAT: In addition to a weekly sitting group, you may want to deepen your learning by going on a silent retreat. Retreats may be for a weekend or for as long as three months! Some retreats are specifically for young people.

ADVANCE!

Meditation is a lifelong affair. When you learn how to meditate you learn how to be attentive and reflective all the time. You will want to sit every day. People often find that 45 minutes to an hour daily is enough to see real effects in personality, friendships, and ability to concentrate on work.

PROGRAM B **GOAL:** Sit for 20 minutes five days a week, working up to sitting daily for a minimum of 20 minutes.

	Mon	Tue	Wed	Thurs	Fri	Sat	Sun
Week 1	20 min	20 min	20 min	20 min	20 min		
Week 2	20 min	20 min	20 min	20 min	20 min		
Week 3	20 min	20 min	20 min	20 min	20 min	20 min	
Week 4	20 min	20 min	20 min	20 min	20 min	20 min	20 min

10 Reducing Your Risk of Cardiovascular Disease

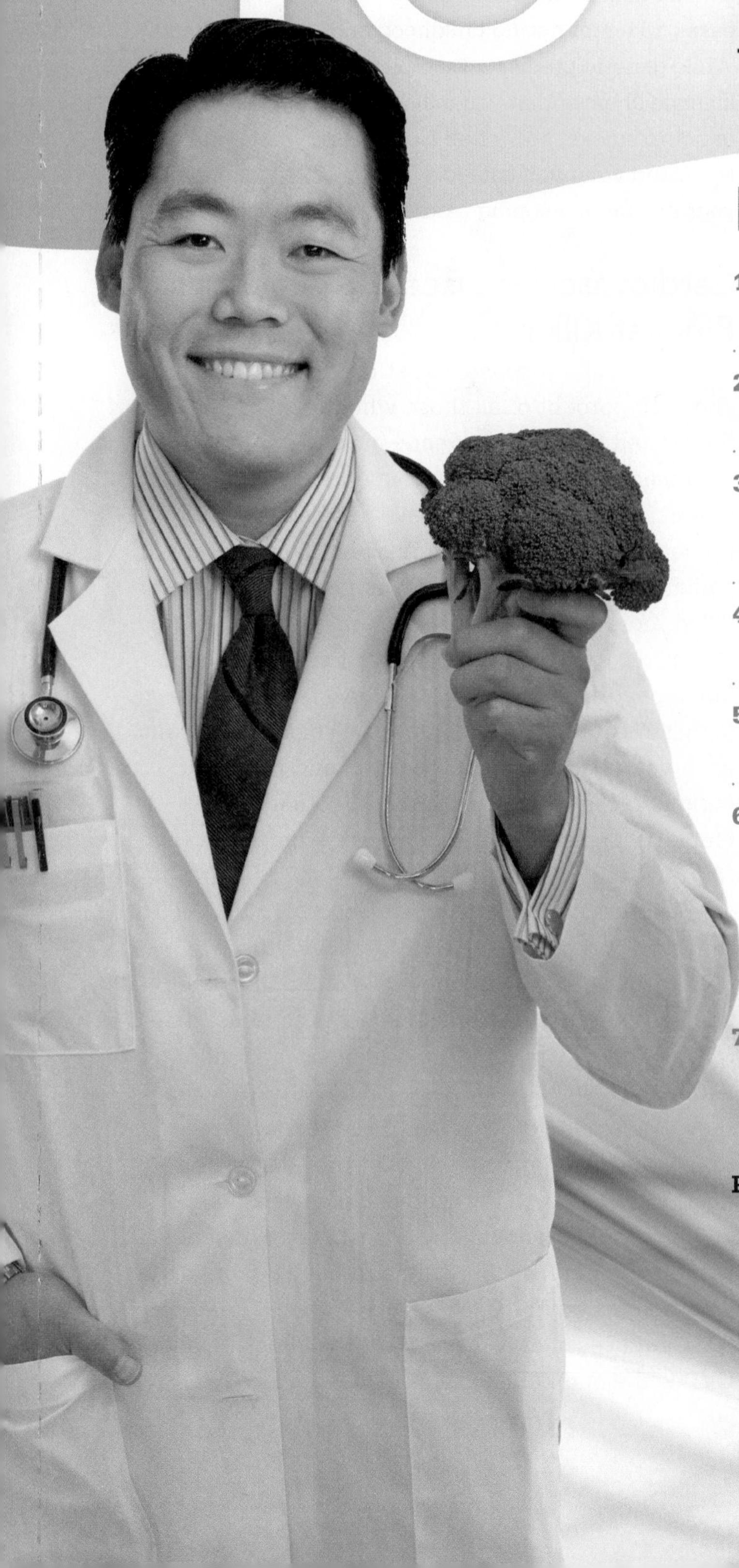

Learning Outcomes

1. Define cardiovascular disease (CVD).

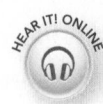 HEAR IT! ONLINE — Audio case study and audio PowerPoint lecture

2. Explain why a college student should be concerned about CVD.

3. List the human and economic impacts of CVD.

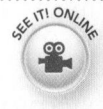 SEE IT! ONLINE — Heart Disease in America — TIM RUSSERT 1950-2008

4. Explain how CVD affects the heart and blood vessels, and the symptoms it produces.

5. Describe various forms of CVD, including hypertension, atherosclerosis, stroke, heart disease, and others.

6. Outline the main risk factors for CVD, including those you can and cannot control.

 DO IT! ONLINE — Lab 10.1 Understand Your CVD Risk

  SEE IT! ONLINE — Tips to Raise Good Cholesterol

7. Create a plan and apply behavior-change skills to lower your own risk of CVD.

 LIVE IT! ONLINE — Take Charge of Your Health worksheets and Behavior Change Logs for assessing your CVD risk and creating a change plan

Pre- and post-quizzes and glossary flashcards  REVIEW IT! ONLINE

casestudy

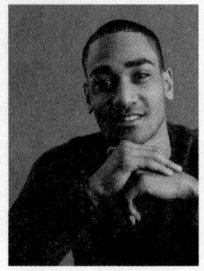

DARYL

"Hi, I'm Daryl. I'm a junior, majoring in education. I'm also a jazz pianist and I play at clubs around town about three times a week. I love jazz, and the gigs help me pay my college tuition.

"I think I'm pretty healthy—I've never been hospitalized for anything in my life—but I do have a family history of heart disease. Both of my grandfathers died from heart attacks when they were in their 40s. My dad died of a stroke when I was 10, and my mom is currently getting treatment for high blood pressure and high cholesterol. I know I'm still young, but given the family history, I'm worried. Are there things I can be doing to protect myself? And how can I help my mom?"

C ardiovascular disease (CVD) is the term commonly used to describe diseases of the heart and the blood vessels brought on by a build-up of fatty, waxy accumulations that restrict or block blood flow. CVD can bring on potentially devastating consequences such as a heart attack and stroke, which are the number one and number three leading causes of death in America (cancer being number two).[1] You may think that cardiovascular problems strike only older people but in fact, 9 to 15 percent of women and men under age 40 have some form of CVD.[2] The prevalence rises to about 40 percent in middle-aged adults of both sexes and then climbs sharply after age 60, involving about three-quarters or more of older Americans.[3] Among Americans of all age groups, approximately one out of every three has some form of cardiovascular disease.[4]

cardiovascular disease (CVD) A disease of the heart and/or blood vessels

Why Should I Worry about Cardiovascular Disease?

As a college student, your most pressing concerns are probably things like getting good grades, paying tuition, and landing a job. Cardiovascular disease could be the furthest thing from your mind. However, it is not too early to start learning about CVD. For many people, the earliest manifestations of heart and blood vessel diseases take root during childhood and early adulthood.[5] While genetic predisposition plays an important role, lifestyle choices that you make now—such as whether or not to smoke, how often to exercise, your stress level, and what you eat—can also greatly influence your risk for developing cardiovascular disease later.

LIVE IT! ONLINE

Worksheet 39 Healthy Heart I.Q.

Cardiovascular Disease Is America's Biggest Killer

Cardiovascular disease and stroke kill about 30 percent of all those who die in the United States each year—more than any other single cause of death in America.[6] In fact, cardiovascular disease has been the leading cause of death in the U.S. every year since 1900, except in 1918, when pandemic flu killed more Americans. If we completely eliminated CVD in the United States, experts estimate our average life expectancy would rise by almost 7 years.[7] Together, heart disease and strokes kill more Americans each year—both men and women and people of various races—than cancer or any other cause (Table 10.1; also, see the box Men, Women, and Cardiovascular Disease).

SEE IT! ONLINE

Heart Disease in America

Figure 10.1 shows the prevalence of CVD throughout the country. Cardiovascular disease costs Americans an estimated $475.3 billion each year, a figure that includes the costs of actual care (physicians, hospitals, nursing homes, and medications) as well as lost productivity.[8] By 2030, the prevalence of cardiovascular disease is expected to increase 9.9 percent, with the prevalence of heart failure and stroke increasing approximately 25 percent, and annual direct costs are expected to increase to $818 billion, with another $276 billion in lost productivity.[9]

Cardiovascular disease is a global problem, and CVD is the number one cause of death globally.

TABLE 10.1 Five Leading Causes of Death in the U.S.	
Cause	Number of deaths
Heart disease and Stroke	727,210
Cancer	568,668
Chronic lower respiratory diseases	137,082
Accidents (unintentional injuries)	117,176
Alzheimer's disease	78,889

Source: K. D. Kochanek, "Deaths: Preliminary Data for 2009," *National Vital Statistics Reports* 59, no. 4 (Hyattsville, MD: National Center for Health Statistics, 2011).

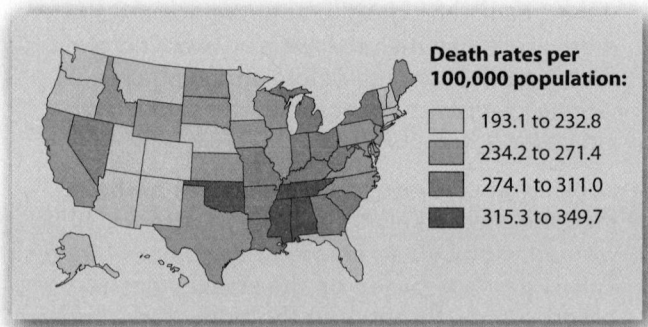

FIGURE 10.1 Cardiovascular disease age-adjusted death rates by state.

Reprinted with permission from CIRCULATION 2011; 123:e18-e209. © 2010, American Heart Association, Inc.

Of an estimated 17.3 million global deaths from CVD in 2008, about 7.3 million were due to coronary heart disease and 6.2 million were due to stroke.[10] The World Health Organization predicts that by 2030, CVD will still be the single leading cause of death and will claim almost 23.6 million lives each year, mainly from heart disease and stroke.[11]

Among developed nations, eastern European countries such as Russia, Bulgaria, and Romania have the highest incidence of deaths attributed to CVD, with over 500 deaths per 100,000 population per year.[12] France, Japan, Switzerland, Spain, and Italy are at the bottom of the list, with about 200 deaths or fewer per 100,000 population. The United States is in the middle—along with countries such as England, Denmark, New Zealand, and Germany—with 300 to 400 deaths per 100,000 population per year, depending on demographic groups within the populations.[13]

Cardiovascular Disease Can Greatly Decrease Your Quality of Life

The potential of cardiovascular disease to cause death is obviously its most serious consequence, but even when it is not fatal, it can seriously impact daily life. Heart attack and stroke survivors may lose their ability to walk, talk, read, exercise, or carry out other daily activities normally. Cardiovascular disease can cause chest pain, shortness of breath, and damage to internal organs. It can also require expensive drugs, which have their own negative side effects.

Cardiovascular Disease Can Begin Early in Life

Childhood and early adolescence are often the time when people first start experiencing the risk factors for cardiovascular disease—poor diet, lack of exercise, BMI above 25, and smoking.[14] These, in turn, can trigger physical processes that initiate the start of cardiovascular disease itself surprisingly early in life. In a classic study of blood vessel tissue from 3,000 young people between the ages of 15 and 34 who had died of accidents, homicides, or suicides, researchers found glistening streaks of fat and fatty, waxy buildup in some of the vessel specimens— deposits that marked the unmistakable beginnings of cardiovascular disease. The researchers found early signs of CVD in 2 percent of males aged 15 to 19. They also observed advanced markers of CVD in 20 percent of 30- to 34-year-old males, and 8 percent of females in the same age group. In examining the individual health records of those young people with blood vessel deposits, the researchers found a higher incidence of poor diet, lack of exercise, high BMI, and smoking than in healthier young people lacking those deposits.[15] These same habits continue to contribute to cardiovascular disease in middle-aged and older adults. More recent studies reflect the result of those early risk factors and blood vessel deposits: A 2011 CDC study revealed that stroke-related hospitalizations rose dramatically in 15- to 44-year-olds between the years 1994 and 2007.[16] Among 15- to 34-year-old men, they found a 51 percent jump in stroke hospitalizations, and among boys and girls aged 5 to 14, a 30 percent rise. The actual numbers of young people who suffer strokes are small but the trend is clear; CVD prevention must begin in childhood.

Men, Women, and Cardiovascular Disease

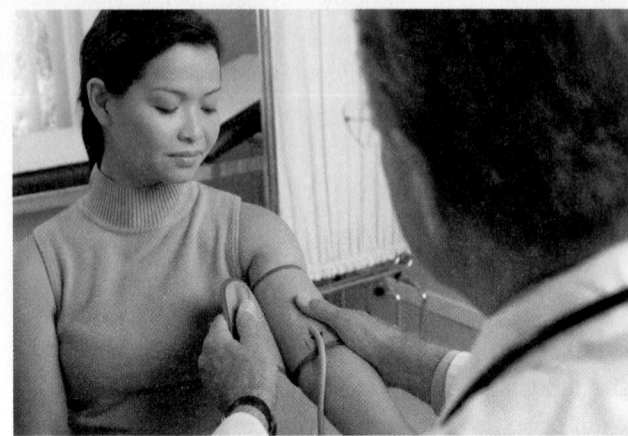

Many people are aware that cardiovascular disease is the leading cause of death in men in the United States, claiming 388,049 male victims in 2007.[1] Few realize, however, that cardiovascular disease is the leading cause of death in American women as well—and in fact kills more women than men each year; in 2007, CVD claimed 418,107 female victims. This figure is higher than the number of female lives lost in 2007 due to cancer, Alzheimer's, diabetes, and accidents *combined*.

Even physicians can harbor misconceptions about women and cardiovascular disease. In one study, fewer than one doctor in five knew that CVD kills more women than men annually.[2] Another study has shown that doctors are more likely to screen male patients for heart disease and make recommendations for intervention than they are to screen or treat female patients for the same.[3]

Researchers have also found significant differences in the ways men and women tend to express patterns and symptoms of cardiovascular disease. For example:

- Men tend to develop heart disease 10 to 15 years earlier than women. Women rarely have heart attacks before menopause (early 50s); they show rates of CVD two or three times higher after menopause than before.

- While having a heart attack, men tend to experience the classic "squeezing" sensation in the chest, pain in the chest or arm, and/or shortness of breath. Women, however, are less likely to feel these symptoms. Instead, they are more likely to experience shortness of breath, weakness or fatigue, a cold sweat, or dizziness. If they feel any localized pressure, it tends to be between the shoulder blades rather than in the chest or arm. Women are also more likely than men to have early warning symptoms up to one month before, including unusual fatigue, sleep disturbances, shortness of breath, indigestion, and anxiety.[4]

- Looking at cardiovascular disease as a whole, men are more likely to have heart attacks, while women with CVD are more likely to have strokes. This is perhaps based on the smaller size of blood vessels throughout the body, including the brain.[5]

- Doctors have long prescribed daily aspirin to both sexes as a way to prevent heart attacks. Recent studies, however, have shown that aspirin seems to prevent some heart attack deaths in men and some stroke deaths in women but does not seem to prevent stroke deaths in men or heart attack deaths in women.[6]

Sources:
1. J. Xu and others, "Deaths: Final Data for 2007," *National Vital Statistics Reports* 58, no. 19 (Hyattsville, MD: National Center for Health Statistics, 2010).
2. L. Mosca and others, "National Study of Physician Awareness and Adherence to Cardiovascular Disease Prevention Guidelines," *Circulation* 111, no. 4 (2005): 499–510.
3. J. H. Mieres, "Review of the American Heart Association's Guidelines for Cardiovascular Disease Prevention in Women," *Heart* 92, Suppl 3 (2006): iii10–3.
4. J. C. McSweeney and others, "Women's Early Warning Symptoms of Acute Myocardial Infarction," *Circulation* 108 (2003): 2619–23.
5. T. Kurth and others, "Healthy Lifestyle and the Risk of Stroke in Women," *Archives of Internal Medicine* 166, no. 13 (2006): 1403–9.
6. J. S. Berger and others, "Aspirin for the Primary Prevention of Cardiovascular Events in Women and Men: A Sex-Specific Meta-analysis of Randomized Controlled Trials," *Journal of the American Medical Association* 295, no. 3 (2006): 306–13.

How Does Cardiovascular Disease Affect the Body?

Learning about how cardiovascular disease affects your body is useful for understanding why it causes the symptoms it does and what you can do to keep your cardiovascular system healthy.

Cardiovascular Disease Affects the Heart and Blood Vessels

Your body contains trillions of living cells, all needing a continuous supply of oxygen and energy compounds. The cardiovascular system—the heart and blood vessels—does the critical work of delivering that oxygen and energy *to* your cells. It also removes carbon dioxide and other wastes *from* your cells. (To review the anatomy of the cardiovascular, or circulatory, system, see Chapter 3.)

In a healthy 10-year-old, the heart is almost adult size. The blood vessel walls are smooth inside and out. The walls of the arteries are strong and elastic, while the walls of the veins are thinner and more fixed in diameter. Blood can flow freely down the long narrow opening in the middle of each vessel. The ventricles fill smoothly and forcibly push blood out. Tight-closing valves help prevent blood from flowing backward. The circulating blood reaches all the distant capillary beds in the brain, limbs, kidneys, skin, and other organs, then returns quickly through the venous system.

Atherosclerosis Starting at age 10 or even earlier, abnormal accumulations inside the blood vessels can begin to restrict blood flow. The process of accumulation and restriction in blood vessels is known as **atherosclerosis** (from the Greek words "athero," meaning gruel, and "sclerosis," meaning hardness.) Atherosclerosis is a major factor in many forms of cardiovascular disease. Both lifestyle and genetic factors can cause deposits of fatty, waxy, yellowish, sludgelike debris called *atheromas* to accumulate inside arteries and smaller arterioles. Other substances such as calcium salts, cholesterol, cellular waste, blood clotting proteins, and white blood cells can accumulate around the atheromas, enlarging and solidifying the yellowish deposits into hardened blockages called **plaques**. These plaques, in turn, tend to bulge inward and cause a narrowing of the vessels' inner channels. This narrowing is called **arterial stenosis**. Plaques can eventually grow large enough to block blood passage through the vessel (see Figure 10.2) or even cause the vessel to rupture. The buildup process can take decades, but atherosclerosis can start in childhood, especially in the overweight and obese.[17]

Arteries with plaques that cause a narrowed channel or inward-bulging side walls transport less blood and are stiffer and less flexible. Just as the pressure builds up in a hose if you prevent normal water flow with your thumb, channel narrowing and plaque buildup can increase pressure within the blood vessels. Unhealthy lifestyle characteristics including smoking, chronic stress, inactivity, high alcohol consumption, high blood sugar, high blood pressure, obesity, and unfavorable levels of certain fats and cholesterol in the blood can all increase the speed and severity of atherosclerosis and, in turn, contribute to CVD.[18] Atherosclerotic cardiovascular disease is America's leading cause of death and disability.[19]

In recent years, medical researchers have studied the role of *inflammation* in atherosclerosis. Inflammation is an immune response that causes redness and swelling in response to injury. Researchers think that LDL (low-density lipoprotein) cholesterol, cigarette smoking, hypertension, diabetes mellitus, and disease-causing bacteria may all promote inflammation. The most likely disease-causing bacteria are *Chlamydia pneumoniae* (a common cause of respiratory infections), *Helicobacter pylori* (which causes ulcers), herpes simplex virus (to which the majority of Americans are exposed by the age of 5), and cytomegalovirus (another herpes virus transmitted through body fluids and infecting most Americans before the age of 40).

During an inflammatory reaction, researchers can often detect high levels of two or more substances. One is a set of proteins called *C-reactive proteins* (CRPs), the other is an amino acid called *homocysteine*. These substances may inflame the inner linings of arteries and promote plaque deposits and blood-clot formation. At the very least, their presence is an indicator of inflammation. In the near future, physicians may be able to order sensitive tests that detect CRPs and homocysteine as markers of atherosclerosis.[20] Lifestyle changes such as regular exercise, weight management, smoking

atherosclerosis Hardening or stiffening of the arteries as plaque accumulates, often at injury sites, in the inner linings of arteries

plaques A pinpoint area of fatty, waxy debris that accumulates at a site along the inner wall of an artery or arteriole

arterial stenosis A narrowing of the inner channel of arteries and smaller arterioles due to the buildup of a sludge-like layer of fatty, waxy debris

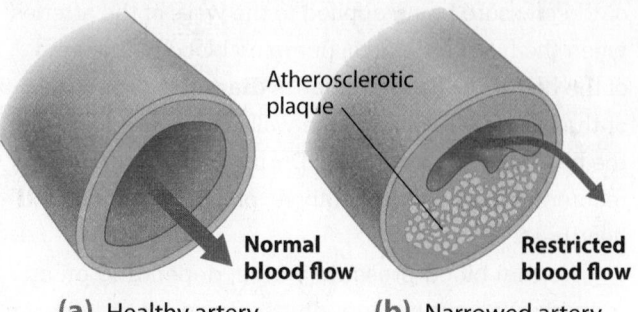

Atherosclerotic plaque

Normal blood flow

Restricted blood flow

(a) Healthy artery   **(b)** Narrowed artery

FIGURE **10.2** (a) Cross-section of a healthy artery, allowing normal blood flow. (b) Cross-section of an artery with plaque buildup narrowing the channel and restricting blood flow.

cessation, moderation of alcohol intake, and eating less saturated fat and cholesterol appear to reduce inflammation and its markers in the blood.

Cardiovascular Disease Takes Many Forms

Table 10.2 identifies the most common forms of cardiovascular disease and their prevalence in American adults. Let's look at each of these forms of CVD in more detail.

Hypertension **Hypertension**, or sustained high blood pressure, is the most common form of cardiovascular disease. It is also considered a risk factor for other forms of CVD. About 30 percent of all Americans have hypertension.[21] Because it has no initial symptoms,[22] many are unaware they have the condition, causing experts to refer to it as a "silent killer." Hypertension causes blood vessel damage and promotes plaque development.[23] As mentioned earlier, plaque deposits and vessel-channel narrowing can in turn increase resistance to blood flow throughout the circulatory system and can cause blood pressure to rise further, creating a damaging vicious cycle. In

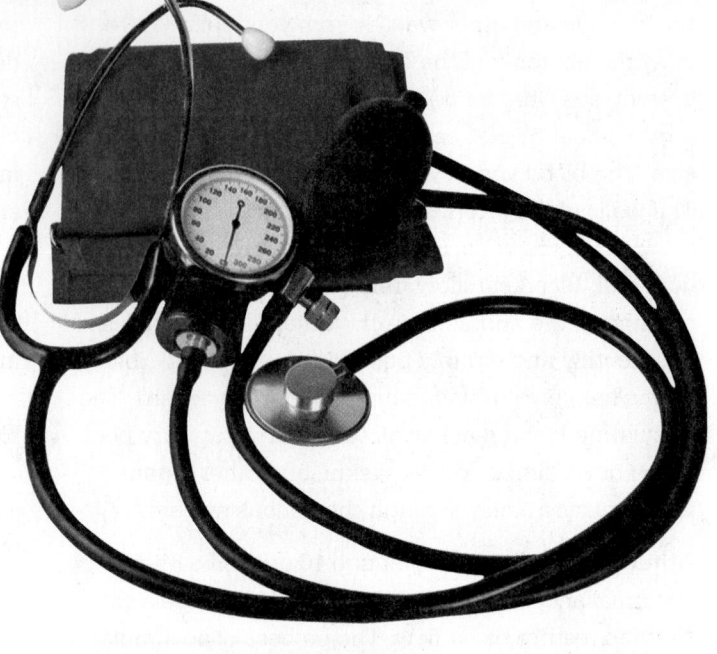

addition to leading to other forms of CVD, hypertension can cause your thinking to slow down or make you more susceptible to dementia later in life.[24] You may think of high blood pressure as an older person's disease, but it can begin in your college years and is common by middle age.[25] The condition can result from consuming too much sodium in the diet, leading to water retention and increased blood volume. Other causes of hypertension include kidney or heart abnormalities, aging, inherited tendencies, obesity, sleep apnea, stress, or certain kinds of tumors. Could hypertension impact you? See the box College Students and Hypertension to find out more.

A blood pressure device can help diagnose hypertension. Such devices measure your blood pressure in two parts, expressed as a fraction—for example, 120/80. Both values are measured in millimeters of mercury (mm Hg). The first number refers to **systolic pressure**, or the pressure being applied to the walls of the arteries when the heart contracts, pumping blood to the rest of the body. The second value is **diastolic pressure**, or the pressure applied to the walls of the arteries during the heart's relaxation phase. During this phase, blood is reentering the heart's chambers, preparing for the next heartbeat.

Normal blood pressure varies, depending on an individual's weight, age, physical condition, gender, and ethnic background. Systolic blood pressure tends to increase with age, while diastolic blood pressure tends to increase until age 55, and then decline. Generally, men have a greater risk for high

hypertension Sustained blood pressure over 130/85 mm Hg

systolic pressure The pressure applied to the walls of the arteries when the heart contracts

diastolic pressure The pressure applied to the walls of the arteries during the heart's relaxation phase

TABLE **10.2** Major Types of Cardiovascular Disease and Prevalence of Each	
Type of Cardiovascular Disease	Prevalence in the United States
Hypertension	76.4 million
Coronary heart disease (including heart attack)	16.3 million
Angina pectoris	9.0 million
Arrhythmia	2.2 million
Congestive heart failure	5.7 million
Congenital cardiovascular defects	Eight defects per 1,000 live births
Stroke	7.0 million; 795,000 new or recurrent cases of stroke each year

Data from American Heart Association *Heart Disease and Stroke Statistics 2011 Update* (2011).

DIVERSITY

College Students and Hypertension

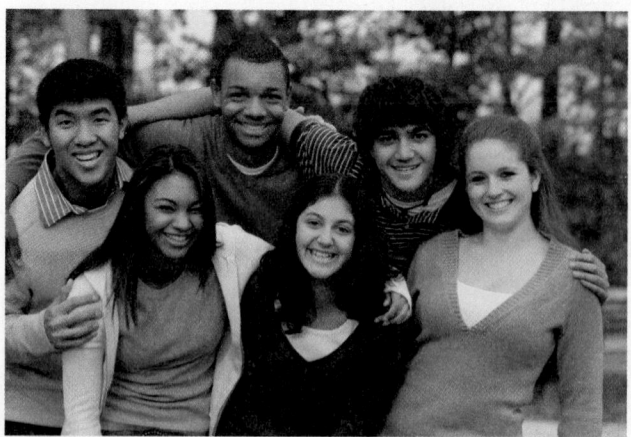

Our discussion of increased hospitalizations for stroke among young people is part of a bigger trend: increased hypertension in people from 20 to 44. A revealing study of 800 students at the University of New Hampshire, for example, showed that one-third were overweight or obese and that fully 60 percent of male students had high blood pressure.[1] Other reports have shown that more than four million young adults (about 4 percent) are now taking anti-cholesterol medications, while 8.5 million (8 percent) are now taking medications to combat high blood pressure (hypertension).[2]

As with the general U.S. adult population, college students of both sexes are at risk of hypertension based on the prevalence of obesity, poor diet, and sedentary lifestyles in our culture. But young men, particularly young African American men, seem to be at highest risk.[3] This may be partly because men under age 35 are more likely to ignore early symptoms and delay return visits to doctors after a preliminary discussion about their high blood pressure. Depression and high alcohol consumption can also increase the risk for hypertension, and both are common among college students of both sexes.[4]

Hypertension can have devastating long-term effects on nearly every organ of the body. Among the many health problems that they may encounter, men with prehypertension and hypertension are nearly three times as likely to experience erectile dysfunction as men without these cardiac problems. Reducing sodium consumption, losing weight, and exercising, among other measures, can make a huge difference in risk reduction and help you avoid the need for medical intervention.

Sources:
1. University of New Hampshire, "College Students Face Obesity, High Blood Pressure, Metabolic Syndrome," *ScienceDaily*, www.sciencedaily.com /releases/2007/06/070614113310.htm (June 18, 2007).
2. J. T. Flynn, "Pediatric Hypertension Update," *Current Opinion in Nephrology and Hypertension* 19, no. 3 (2010): 292–7; *Washington Times*, "Heart Patients Getting Younger," www.washingtontimes.com/news/2007/oct /30/heart-patients-getting-younger (October 30, 2007).
3. B. Rosner, "Blood Pressure Differences by Ethnic Group among United States Children and Adolescents," *Hypertension* 54, no. 3 (2009): 502–8; D. T. Lackland, "High Blood Pressure: A Lifetime Issue," *Hypertension* 54, no. 3 (2009): 457–8.
4. S. B. Patten and others, "Major Depression as a Risk Factor for High Blood Pressure: Epidemiologic Evidence from a National Longitudinal Study," *Psychosomatic Medicine* 71, no. 3 (2009): 273–9.

blood pressure than women until age 55; at that point, the risks become about equal. After age 75, women are more likely to have high blood pressure than men.[26]

For a healthy adult, normal systolic blood pressure is less than 120, and normal diastolic blood pressure is less than 80.[27] A physician may diagnose *prehypertension* or the potential beginnings of hypertension when systolic pressure is between 120 and 139 and diastolic pressure is between 80 and 89. *High blood pressure* (HBP) is usually diagnosed when systolic pressure is 140 or above and diastolic pressure is 90 or above (although the latter reading may not necessarily be elevated). When only systolic pressure is high, the condition is known as *isolated systolic hypertension* (ISH), the most common form of high blood pressure in older Americans. If your blood pressure exceeds 140/90, you need to work with your physician to lower it through diet, exercise, stress reduction, and prescription drugs. Table 10.3 presents a summary of blood pressure values.

If you are diagnosed with high blood pressure in college, you can do something about it. Lifestyle modifications are helpful in reducing or preventing hypertension in early adulthood. These include losing weight, exercising, reducing stress, and reducing dietary salt and sugar (see the box Do Salt and Sugar Increase My Risk of Cardiovascular Disease?).[28]

TABLE 10.3 Blood Pressure Readings

Classification	Systolic Reading (mm Hg)	Diastolic Reading (mm Hg)
Normal	Less than 120	Less than 80
Prehypertension	120–139	80–89
Hypertension		
Stage 1	140–159	90–99
Stage 2	160 or higher	100 or higher

Note: If systolic and diastolic readings fall into different categories, treatment is determined by the highest category. Readings are based on the average of two or more properly measured, seated readings on each of two or more health care provider visits.

Source: National Heart, Lung, and Blood Institute, *Seventh Report of the Joint National Committee on Prevention, Detection, Evaluation, and Treatment of High Blood Pressure* (NIH Publication No. 03-5233) (Bethesda, MD: National Institutes of Health, May 2003).

Coronary Heart Disease When atherosclerosis occurs in the heart's main blood vessels, it is called **coronary artery disease (CAD)** or **coronary heart disease (CHD)**. When it occurs in the feet, ankles, calves, hands, or forearms, it is called *peripheral artery disease*. Of all the types of cardiovascular disease, CHD is the greatest killer. Each year, an estimated 1.25 million Americans will suffer a *coronary attack* or heart attack: 785,000 will have their first heart attack and 470,000 will have a recurrent attack.[29] The American Heart Association calculates that approximately every *minute*, somewhere in the U.S., someone dies of a first or subsequent heart.

A heart attack, also called a **myocardial infarction (MI)**, occurs when an area of the heart suffers permanent damage after its normal blood supply has been blocked. The blockage can be caused by a blood clot in a coronary artery or by atherosclerotic narrowing. When blood flow slows dramatically or stops, the surrounding tissue is deprived of oxygen. If the blockage is extremely minor, an otherwise healthy heart will adapt over time as small blood vessels reroute needed blood through other areas.

When heart blockage is more severe, a person can experience the symptoms of a heart attack and will require life-saving support. The box In the Event of a Heart Attack, Stroke, or Cardiac Arrest (on page 357) describes how you should respond if you recognize such symptoms in someone else or yourself.

Angina Pectoris Atherosclerosis and other circulatory impairments may reduce the heart's blood and oxygen supply and cause a condition called **ischemia**. People with ischemia often suffer from varying degrees of chest pain, also called **angina pectoris**. The American Heart Association estimates that more than nine million Americans suffer from angina.[30] Many people experience short episodes of angina whenever they exert themselves physically. Symptoms may range from slight indigestion to a feeling that the heart is being crushed. Generally, the more serious the oxygen deprivation, the more severe the pain.

Doctors currently use several methods of treating angina. In mild cases, they prescribe rest. To treat more serious chest pain, they may recommend nitroglycerin tablets to relax veins and lessen the heart's workload. Calcium channel blockers can also relieve angina caused by spasms of the coronary arteries. Drugs called *beta blockers* can control potential overactivity of the heart muscle.[31]

Arrhythmias An **arrhythmia**, or irregular heartbeat, is relatively common: More than 2.2 million Americans experience it each year.[32] The disturbance of heartbeat rhythm can take several forms: a racing heart in the absence of exercise or anxiety (called *tachycardia*); an abnormally slow heartbeat (called *bradycardia*); or a sporadic, quivering pattern called *fibrillation*. **Fibrillation** renders the heart extremely inefficient at pumping blood

coronary artery disease (CAD) or **coronary heart disease (CHD)** Atherosclerosis (the buildup of plaque deposits) in the main arteries that supply oxygen and other materials to the heart muscle.

myocardial infarction (MI) Medical term for a heart attack; involves permanent damage to an area of the heart muscle brought on by a cessation of normal blood supply

ischemia A damaging reduction in the blood (and therefore the oxygen supply) to a region of the heart, brain, or other organ

angina pectoris Chest pain due to ischemia, or reduction in blood flow to the heart muscle and surrounding tissues

arrhythmia Irregular heartbeat; can involve abnormally fast or slow heartbeat or the disorganized, sporadic beat of fibrillation

fibrillation A sporadic, quivering heartbeat pattern that results in inefficient pumping of blood

Do Salt and Sugar Increase My Risk of Cardiovascular Disease?

The average American adult consumes 3,466 mg of sodium per day in salt (NaCl)[1]—more than twice the USDA-recommended level of 1500 mg for those over 50, African Americans, and those who have high blood pressure. The 2010 Federal Dietary Guidelines recommend that all other adults consume below 2300 mg per day (the American Heart Association recommends a more conservative limit of 1500 mg per day for adults and children of all ages). These health organizations advocate limiting salt because excess sodium induces fluid retention. This, in turn, elevates blood pressure and contributes to hypertension and CVD. To get below 2300 mg, most adults would have to cut overall salt consumption by about half a teaspoon.

Most of the salt in our national diet comes from foods high in processed grains (such as pizza and cookies) and from meats, poultry, and lunch meats.[2] Researchers estimate that a population-wide average drop in dietary salt by 1200 mg/day would annually cut new cases of cardiovascular disease by 60,000 to 120,000 and prevent 32,000 to 66,000 new strokes, 54,000 to 99,000 new heart attacks, and 44,000 to 92,000 deaths. They also projected this trend would save $10 to $24 billion in annual health care costs.[3] Some medical researchers have criticized a few of the team's assumptions and thus disagree with their specific figures.[4] However, few, if any, disagree with the major premise that dietary salt causes hypertension and cutting consumption would help improve and prevent CVD.

What about sugar? The average American consumes more than 150 pounds of caloric sweeteners (sugar, corn syrup, brown sugar, honey, agave syrup, concentrated fruit juice, and so on) each year. That's almost three pounds per week![5] Most of this extra sugar comes from sweetened sodas, sports drinks, energy drinks, coffee drinks, and tea drinks. Like salt, sugar takes a toll on our cardiovascular health by increasing weight gain and by raising both glucose and triglyceride levels in the blood. Consuming an extra 2.6 ounces per day of corn syrup (the amount in two or three sweetened drinks) doubles a person's risk for high systolic blood pressure.[6] In one large study, women who consumed two sweetened drinks per day had a 20 percent greater risk of heart disease over those who drank sugary drinks only about once per month.[7] In another large study, drinking one sugary drink per day increased the risk of metabolic syndrome by 44 percent.[8] Dietary sugar, in other words, increases the risks of CVD, just as salt does.

Sources:
1. Centers for Disease Control and Prevention, "CDC Survey Find Nine in Ten U.S. Adults Consume Too Much Sodium," Press Release www.cdc.gov/media/pressrel/2010/r100624.htm (2010).
2. Ibid.
3. K. Bibbins-Domingo and others, "Projected Effect of Dietary Salt Reductions on Future Cardiovascular Disease," The New England Journal of Medicine 362, no. 7 (2010): 590–9.
4. P. Belluck, "Big Benefits Are Seen from Eating Less Salt," New York Times, www.nytimes.com/2010/01/21/health/nutrition/21salt.html (January 20, 2010).
5. USDA, "Chapter 2: Profiling Food Consumption in America," Agricultural Fact Book 2001–2002, www.usda.gov/factbook/chapter2.htm (2002).
6. D. I. Jalal and others, "Increased Fructose Associates with Elevated Blood Pressure," Journal of the American Society of Nephrology 21, no. 9 (2010): 1543–9.
7. T. T. Fung and others, "Sweetened Beverage Consumption and Risk of Coronary Heart Disease in Women," American Journal of Clinical Nutrition 89, no. 4 (2009): 1037–42.
8. R. Dhingra and others, "Soft Drink Consumption and Risk of Developing Cardiometabolic Risk Factors and the Metabolic Syndrome in Middle-Aged Adults in the Community," Circulation 116, no. 5 (2007): 480–8.

through the vessels. If a fibrillation incident or series of incidents go untreated, the condition may be fatal. Even without cardiovascular disease, you may feel heart arrhythmias from drinking too much caffeine or from the nicotine in tobacco. Mild cases like this are seldom life-threatening. If you develop a severe case due to disease, you may require drug therapy or a pacemaker.

Congestive Heart Failure More than five million Americans suffer from **congestive heart failure (CHF)** each year.[33] Causes include past heart attack, high blood pressure, heart valve defects or damage, birth defects, or damage to the heart from infection or inherited disease. In CHF, the heart muscle is damaged or overworked, the pumping chambers are often taxed to the limit, and the heart lacks the strength to keep blood circulating normally through the body. Heart muscle damage can result from viral or bacterial pneumonia, heart attack, other cardiovascular problems, or even treatments for cancer. The weakened heart pumps less blood out through the arteries. As a result, the "return" blood can't flow back through the veins to the heart in normal amounts. As the blood begins to back up, it causes congestion in body tissues. Blood pooling enlarges the heart, making it even less efficient, and fluid accumulates in the legs, ankles, or lungs, where it can cause swelling or difficulty in breathing.

Congestive heart failure can be fatal if untreated, but most cases respond well to drug treatment. Diuretics (water pills) increase urination and reduce fluid accumulation, drugs such as digitalis increase the heart's pumping action, and vasodilators expand blood vessels so blood can flow through more easily and reduce the heart's workload.

Congenital Heart Disease **Congenital heart disease**, meaning heart disease present at birth, affects nine out of every 1,000 live births.[34] A baby may be born with a slight *heart murmur,* an audible sound based on an irregular heart valve that allows turbulent blood flow through the heart. Some children outgrow such heart murmurs and have no further problems. Others, however, can have more serious congenital irregularities with heart anatomy or function that require surgical repair. Causes may include hereditary factors, a mother's case of rubella or certain other infections during pregnancy, or the mother's use of alcohol or drugs during fetal development. Advances in treatment continually improve the prospects for children with congenital heart defects.

Stroke The American Heart Association's most recent statistics show that approximately seven million Americans alive today have suffered a stroke at some point in their lives. Each year more than 795,000 people experience a new or recurrent stroke, and 136,000 of them die, making stroke the third leading cause of death after heart disease and cancer.[35] In recent years, the incidence of stroke has been rising in adults aged 15 to 44.

We saw that a heart attack can occur when a blocked vessel prevents a region of the heart from getting enough oxygenated blood. In a similar way, a **stroke** is a sudden loss of function in a region of the brain caused by blockage in or rupture of a blood vessel, leading to oxygen deprivation and cell damage or death. *Ischemic* strokes are the result of a plaque-blocked vessel or a floating blood clot that lodges in a vessel and cuts off blood supply to a brain region. *Hemorrhagic* strokes occur when a blood vessel bursts, spilling oxygenated blood rather than transporting it to a distal brain region, allowing that unsupplied area to become damaged through oxygen deprivation. Family history, advancing age, atherosclerosis, heart disease, congestive heart failure, hypertension, smoking, diabetes, inactivity, overweight, heavy drinking, stimulant drug use, and other factors can all contribute to triggering strokes.[36]

Some strokes are mild and cause only temporary dizziness or slight weakness or numbness. If an affected area is large or in a crucial part of the brain, stroke may cause speech impairments, memory problems, loss of motor control, or death. About 1 in 10 major strokes is preceded days, weeks, or months earlier by *transient ischemic attacks (TIAs)*, brief interruptions of the blood supply to the brain that cause only temporary dizziness, weakness, paralysis, numbness, or other symptoms.[37] Deaths due to strokes have decreased in recent years thanks to better diagnosis, better surgical options, new clot-busting drugs that can be injected immediately after a stroke has occurred, and better aftercare for stroke patients. Campaigns to teach awareness and avoidance of risk factors could prevent up to half of annual strokes if people followed them carefully.

congestive heart failure (CHF) A cardiovascular disease in which the heart muscle is damaged or overworked, and the heart lacks the strength to keep blood circulating normally through the body

congenital heart disease Heart disease present at birth

stroke A sudden loss of function in a region of the brain caused by blockage in or rupture of a blood vessel, leading to oxygen deprivation, cell damage, or death

In the Event of a Heart Attack, Stroke, or Cardiac Arrest

Knowing what to do in a cardiovascular emergency could save a friend's life—or your own.

Warning Signs of a Heart Attack

- Uncomfortable pressure, fullness, squeezing, or pain in the center of the chest (more likely in men) or between the shoulder blades (more likely in women), lasting two minutes or longer

- Jaw pain and/or shortness of breath

- Pain spreading to the shoulders, neck, or arms

- Dizziness, fatigue, fainting, sweating, and/or nausea

Not all of these warning signs occur in every heart attack. For instance, a woman's heart attack may show up as shortness of breath, fatigue, and jaw or shoulder blade pain or pressure, stretched out over hours rather than minutes. If any of these symptoms appear, don't wait. Get help immediately!

Warning Signs of a Stroke

- Sudden numbness or weakness, especially on one side of the body, affecting face, arm, and/or leg

- Sudden mental confusion, especially trouble speaking or understanding words

- Sudden vision problems in one or both eyes

- Sudden dizziness, loss of balance, lack of coordination, or trouble walking

- Sudden severe headache without apparent cause

Warning Signs of a Cardiac Arrest

- Sudden loss of responsiveness (won't respond if tapped on either shoulder)

- Cessation of normal breathing (tilt head up; check for breathing for 5 seconds)

Know What to Do before an Emergency Strikes

- Find out which hospitals in your area have 24-hour emergency cardiac care.

- Determine (in advance) the hospital or medical facility that is nearest your home and office and tell your family and friends to call this facility in an emergency.

- Keep a list of emergency rescue service numbers next to your telephone and in your pocket, wallet, or purse. Remember 911 if you don't have time to call emergency rescue numbers.

- If you have chest or jaw discomfort that lasts more than two minutes, call the emergency rescue service or 911. Do not drive yourself to the hospital unless there is no other alternative.

Be a Lifesaver during a Crisis

- If you are with someone who is showing signs of a heart attack or stroke and the warning signs last for two minutes or longer, act immediately.

- Expect a denial. It is normal for a person with chest discomfort to deny the possibility of anything as serious as a heart attack. Don't take no for an answer. Insist on taking prompt action.

- Call 911 or an emergency rescue service, or get to the nearest hospital emergency room that offers 24-hour emergency cardiac care.

- If you are with someone in cardiac arrest and if you are properly trained, give chest compressions and mouth-to-mouth breathing. Continual chest compressions appear to be more important for adult heart attack victims; combined compressions and breathing (CPR or cardiopulmonary resuscitation) seem to be more important for children having a heart, stroke, or breathing-related emergency. Get instructions on which to use from a 911 operator, emergency medical technician, or other rescue personnel if possible.

- An automated external defibrillator (AED) may save a person during cardiac arrest. These devices are increasingly common in public places—workplaces, restaurants, health clubs, sports stadiums, schools, shopping centers, airports, hotels, and so on. Try to cultivate the habit of noticing their location in case of emergency.

Source: Adapted from American Heart Association, "Heart Attack, Stroke, and Cardiac Arrest Warning Signs," www.americanheart.org, March 18, 2011.

What Are the Main Risk Factors for Cardiovascular Disease?

The prevalence of cardiovascular disease is an unfortunate reality. However, we can modify many of our individual risk factors. By identifying your risks and understanding which are controllable, (see **Lab 10.1**), you can learn to modify risk-promoting behaviors and lower your chances of developing CVD.

Risks You Can Control

Experts have identified at least 10 significant risk factors for CVD: tobacco use, hypertension, high blood fats, obesity/overweight, physical inactivity, type 2 diabetes, metabolic syndrome, heavy alcohol consumption, poor diet, and uncontrolled stress. Since lifestyle choices underlie many of these risk factors, changes to daily habits can often reduce the chances of developing cardiovascular disease. Many people have multiple risk factors for CVD; the more risk factors they have, the greater their chances of experiencing a heart attack, stroke, angina, atherosclerosis, and other specific forms of CVD.[38] Let's look at each of these risk factors more closely.

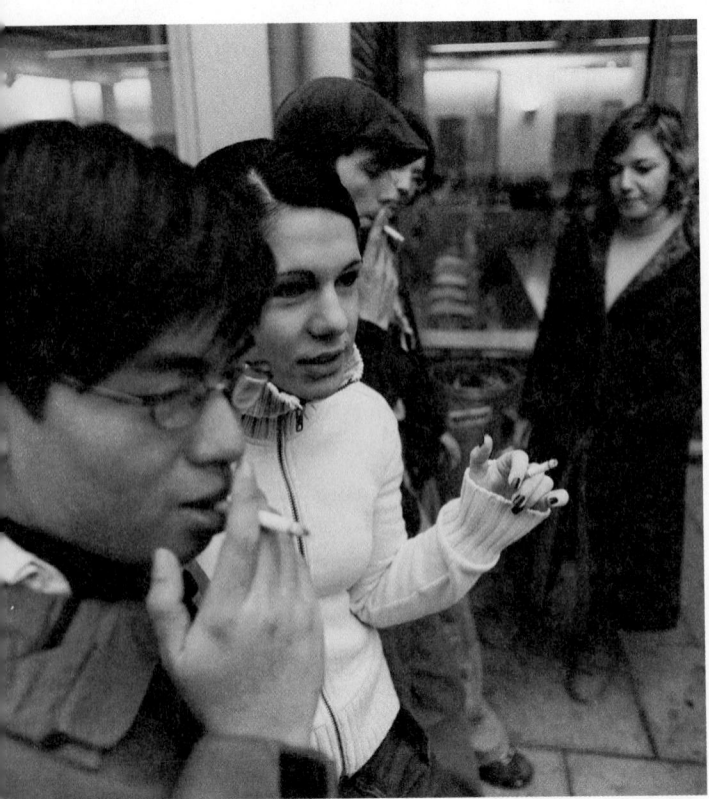

Tobacco Use In 1964, the Surgeon General of the United States asserted that smoking was the greatest risk factor for heart disease. Today, more than 20 percent of deaths from CVD are directly related to smoking. The risk for cardiovascular disease is 70 percent greater for smokers than for nonsmokers. Smokers who have a heart attack are more likely to die suddenly (within one hour) than are nonsmokers.[39] Evidence also indicates that an estimated 46,000 *non*smokers die from cardiovascular disease each year as a result of chronic exposure to environmental tobacco smoke.[40]

How does tobacco use damage the cardiovascular system? Researchers have several plausible explanations. One is that the nicotine in all forms of tobacco (cigarettes, cigars, chewing tobacco, etc.) increases heart rate, heart output, blood pressure, and oxygen use by the heart muscle. Another is that cigarette smoke is filled with carbon monoxide, which displaces oxygen in heart tissue and requires a smoker's heart to work harder to obtain enough oxygen. Chemicals in smoke can cause injuries to arteries that lead to both plaque formation and inflammation. Finally, smokers have a higher level of a natural blood-clotting factor, and these increased levels may contribute to the blood clots that trigger heart attacks and strokes.[41]

Hypertension We have seen that hypertension can damage artery walls and lead to atherosclerosis. It can also weaken artery walls and lead to an *aneurysm,* an abnormal, blood-filled bulge in a blood vessel that has the potential to rupture. Hypertension can damage coronary arteries, enlarge the heart, or weaken the heart muscle. By affecting blood vessels in the brain, hypertension can cause strokes and TIAs, promote dementia, and impair cognitive functioning. By damaging delicate blood vessels in the kidneys and eyes, hypertension can lead to kidney damage or failure and to impaired vision or vision loss. In addition, hypertension can reduce sexual function, disrupt sleep, and magnify the bone loss of osteoporosis.[42] Reducing dietary sodium, blood fats, and excess weight can help lower blood pressure, as can managing stress and taking certain prescription drugs.

High Levels of Fats in Your Blood *Hyperlipidemia*—or high levels of cholesterol, triglycerides, and other fats in the blood—is correlated with increased risk of several cardiovascular diseases. According to a recent report, more than 50 percent of American men aged 65 and older and 40 percent of American women aged 65 or older are on some type of anti-hyperlipidemia prescription drug, including such medications as the "statins"

(Lipitor, Crestor, Zocor) and others drugs designed to reduce blood fats.[43] Unfortunately, many of these medications carry significant risks of their own. Additionally, many people use these medications as "crutches" and continue to eat high fat-foods, assuming that the medications will keep any risks from CVD at bay.

Diets high in saturated fats and/or *trans* fats can raise blood cholesterol levels and contribute to atherosclerosis. They can also switch on the body's blood-clotting system, making the blood thicker and stickier. All of these blood changes increase the risk of heart attack or stroke.

Increases in blood cholesterol can also contribute to hardening of the arteries, or atherosclerosis, with its long-term effects on CVD. Table 10.4 shows recommended levels for blood cholesterol. People with several risk factors for CVD should follow the most stringent range of the guidelines.

Total cholesterol levels are just one measure of cardiovascular disease risks. Another is the ratio of "bad" to "good" cholesterol. Low-density lipoprotein (LDL), often referred to as "bad" cholesterol, is believed

SEE IT! ONLINE

Tips to Raise Good Cholesterol

to contribute to plaque buildup on artery walls. High-density lipoprotein (HDL), or "good" cholesterol, appears to remove plaque from artery walls, thus serving as a protector. In theory, if LDL levels get too high relative to HDL levels, plaque will tend to accumulate inside arteries and lead to cardiovascular problems. The LDL/HDL ratio can increase because of too much saturated fat in the diet, lack of exercise, high stress levels, or genetic predisposition.

It can be useful to obtain an accurate assessment of your total cholesterol and LDL and HDL levels. This analysis requires a fasting blood test (no eating or drinking for 12 hours prior to the test) administered by a reputable health provider. You can compare your numbers to Table 10.4 and discuss their significance with your physician.

A second type of blood fat called *triglycerides* also appears to promote atherosclerosis. As people get older, heavier, or both, their triglyceride and cholesterol levels tend to rise. No one has yet proved that high triglyceride levels cause atherosclerosis and thus underlie CVD. However, these blood fats may contribute to faster plaque development.

Overweight and Obesity Being overweight or obese can strain the heart, forcing it to push blood through "extra" miles of capillaries that supply each pound of fat. A heart that must continuously move blood through an overabundance of vessels has to work harder and may become weakened or damaged. The same high-fat, high-sugar, and high-calorie diets that lead to overweight and obesity can also contribute to plaque formation.

Overweight people are more likely to develop heart disease and stroke even if they have no other CVD risk factors.[44] Losing even 5 to 10 pounds can make a significant difference to CVD risk.[45] This is especially true for people who tend to store fat around the upper body and waist (an "apple" shape) as opposed to those who tend to store fat around the hips and thighs (a "pear" shape.)

Physical Inactivity A sedentary lifestyle is one of the most significant risk factors for CVD. Elevating the heart rate and blood flow through moderate to vigorous activity benefits the heart muscle and helps prevent plaque deposits on artery walls. Conversely, inactivity decreases the efficiency of the heart muscle and allows plaque buildup to occur more easily. Even modest levels of low-intensity physical activity—walking, gardening, housework, dancing—are beneficial if done regularly and over the long term. Despite the clear

TABLE 10.4 LDL, Total, and HDL Cholesterol and Triglycerides (mg/dL) Levels for Adults	
LDL Cholesterol	
Less than 100	Optimal
100–129	Near optimal/above optimal
130–159	Borderline high
160–189	High
190 or higher	Very high
Total Cholesterol	
Less than 200	Desirable
200–239	Borderline high
240 or higher	High
HDL Cholesterol	
Less than 40	Low
60 or higher	Desirable
Triglycerides	
Less than 150	Normal
150–199	Borderline high
200–499	High
500 or higher	Very high

Source: National Heart, Lung, And Blood Institute, "Detection, Evaluation, and Treatment of High Blood Cholesterol in Adults" (NIH Publication No. 02-5215), 2002.

benefits of regular exercise, only 34.4 percent of Americans over age 18 engage in any regular physical activity.[46]

Diabetes Mellitus Chronic diseases are interrelated: people who have one tend to have others. This connection is especially clear when it comes to diabetes and cardiovascular disease. Having diabetes significantly increases one's risk for CVD even if blood sugar levels are well controlled. When they're uncontrolled, the risks are even higher. People with diabetes have death rates from CVD that are 2–4 times higher than those of people without diabetes.[47] Some experts estimate that as many as 50 percent of people with diabetes eventually die of CVD.[48] In fact, the risk is so great, many physicians consider someone with pre-diabetes or with the early stages of diabetes to have the same risks as someone who has already had their first heart attack. Diabetics also tend to have elevated blood fat levels, increased atherosclerosis, and a tendency toward deterioration of small blood vessels, particularly in the eyes and extremities.

Metabolic Syndrome **Metabolic syndrome** refers to a cluster of obesity-related risk factors associated with CVD and type 2 diabetes.[49] People with metabolic syndrome have several characteristics in common (see Figure 10.3):

metabolic syndrome A group of metabolic conditions occurring together that increase a person's risk of heart disease, stroke, and diabetes

- Abdominal obesity, meaning a large waistline (more than 40 inches in men or 35 inches in women).

- Elevated levels of triglycerides in the blood (more than 150 mg/dL).

- Low levels of "good cholesterol" (HDLs below 40 mg/dL in men or 50 mg/dL in women)

- High blood pressure (greater than 130/85 mm Hg)

- High levels of the sugar glucose in the blood (more than 100 mg/dL after fasting)

- High levels of C-reactive protein (more than 10 mg/L), indicating inflammation

The National Heart, Lung, and Blood Institute estimates that 47 million American adults—fully one quarter of our adult population—have metabolic syndrome.[50] By definition, they have multiple risk factors for CVD, and thus their overall risk of developing cardiovascular illness is high.

The prevalence of metabolic syndrome in adolescents and young adults is causing concern among many health professionals. A recent study of nearly 2,000 teenagers revealed that one-third of overweight or obese teens had metabolic syndrome, as did 10 percent of all the adolescents tested.[51] Nutrition—specifically low intake of fruits and vegetables and high intake of sweetened beverages—can play an important role in this early onset.[52]

Studies of college students have found similar rates of metabolic syndrome, with both low levels of fitness and overweight status correlating with higher risk for metabolic syndrome.[53] As with adolescents, only 10 percent of college students in one study had several of the measurable parameters that define metabolic syndrome; however, 43 percent had at least one of the indicators.[54] The message here is clear: Being young does not make you immune to metabolic syndrome and its multiple risk factors for cardiovascular disease.

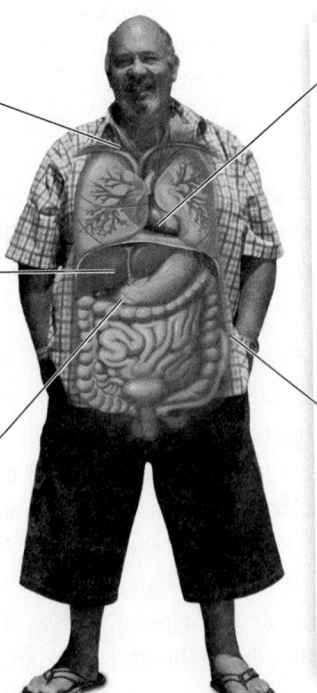

ELEVATED BLOOD TRIGLYCERIDES
- Greater than or equal to 150 mg/dL

REDUCED BLOOD HDL CHOLESTEROL
- *Men:* Less than 40 mg/dL
- *Women:* Less than 50 mg/dL

ELEVATED FASTING BLOOD GLUCOSE
- Greater than or equal to 100 mg/dL

ELEVATED BLOOD PRESSURE
- *Systolic* blood pressure greater than or equal to 130 mm Hg
- *Diastolic* blood pressure greater than or equal to 85 mm Hg

INCREASED WAIST CIRCUMFERENCE
- *Men:* Greater than or equal to 40 inches
- *Women:* Greater than or equal to 35 inches

FIGURE **10.3** Risk factors associated with metabolic syndrome.

Other Controllable Factors Stress can act as a risk factor for CVD. Your body's stress response can cause blood pressure to rise and can trigger blood-clotting and heart rhythm abnormalities.[55] Stress can also foster habits that promote CVD, such as overeating or smoking.

Poor nutrition also increases CVD risk. Too much saturated fat, salt, and refined carbohydrates and too little fiber and too few fruits and vegetables all heighten risk, while improved nutrition lowers risk.

Although some studies have suggested that *moderate* amounts of alcohol may help lower the risk of cardiovascular disease, excessive alcohol consumption can raise blood triglycerides, trigger arrhythmias, raise blood pressure, promote obesity, and contribute to heart failure and strokes. Stimulant drugs, such as amphetamines or cocaine, can also trigger strokes—even in young people.[56]

Risks You Cannot Control

Unfortunately, there are risk factors for cardiovascular disease that you cannot control, including the following:

Heredity A family history of cardiovascular disease—that is, CVD in several generations of an extended family—appears to increase risk significantly. Researchers are unsure whether the increase is due to genetics, to the environment in which you were raised (including diet, exercise, and stress levels), or both.

Age Seventy-five percent of all heart attacks occur in people over age 65. The risk for CVD increases with age for both sexes.[57]

Gender Men are at greater risk for CVD until about age 60.[58] Women under 35 have a fairly low risk unless they have high blood pressure, kidney problems, or diabetes. Being a smoker while using oral contraceptives also increases a woman's risk. Hormonal factors appear to protect women before menopause; after menopause or after estrogen levels decline due to hysterectomy or ovary disease, a woman's LDL levels tend to rise and with them, the chances of developing cardiovascular disease.[59]

Race Members of certain racial/ethnic groups may face increased cardiovascular disease risk (see Figure 10.4).[60] African Americans have the highest rates of cardiovascular disease, followed by Caucasian Americans and Mexican Americans. Rates for Asian Americans are below 25 percent.[61]

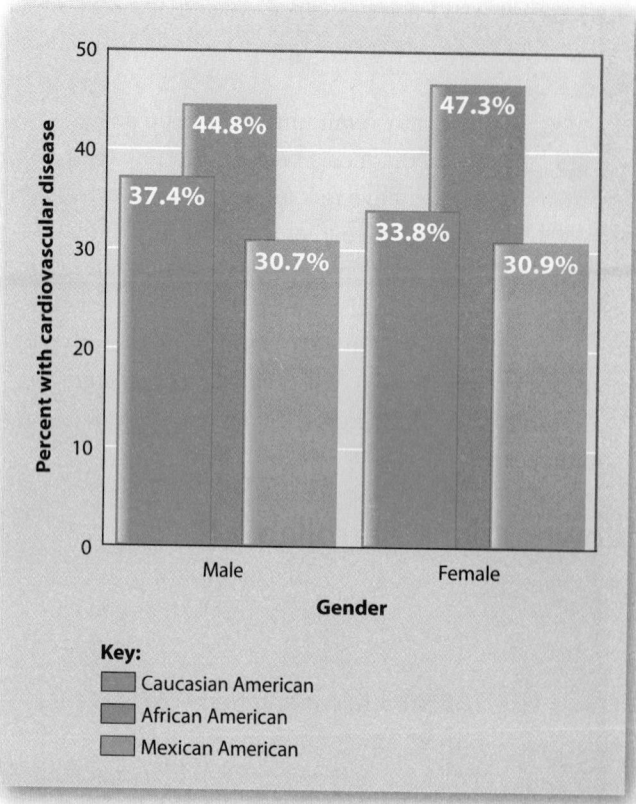

FIGURE **10.4** Cardiovascular disease affects a disproportionate percentage of African Americans.

Data from American Heart Association, *Heart Disease and Stroke Statistics 2010 Update-at-a-Glance*. Comparable data on Hispanic American and Asian American populations were not available in this report.

casestudy

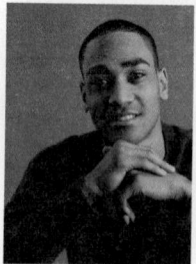

DARYL

"I took my mom in for a check-up the other day. The good news is that her blood pressure and cholesterol have both come down since her last visit. While I was sitting in the waiting room, though, I read a brochure about risk factors for heart disease. I knew genetics was a factor, but I was surprised at how many other risk factors I had: not being very active (unless you count playing the piano!), breathing in other people's smoke at jazz clubs, too much fast food, and stress."

THINK! What else could Daryl do to assess his risk for cardiovascular disease? What risk factors for cardiovascular disease do you have?

ACT! Sort your risk factors by "controllable" and "non-controllable." For each controllable risk factor, list ways you could change your lifestyle to reduce your vulnerability.

How Can I Avoid Cardiovascular Disease?

Worksheet 38 Cardiovascular Risk Assessment

People often wait until they get a scary medical diagnosis before changing their habits. If you have risk factors for cardiovascular disease, the earlier you confront them, the better your chances of avoiding CVD later. Identifying the controllable risk factors for cardiovascular disease in your life, and making simple changes to reduce them, will give you a head start toward protecting your cardiovascular health throughout adulthood!

Lower Your Controllable Risks

Here are specific behavioral tips for avoiding cardiovascular disease by reducing the risk factors you can control.

Don't Use Tobacco According to the American Heart Association, smoking is the greatest preventable cause of disease and death. Even light smoking—just two cigarettes per day—increases your CVD risk. When people stop smoking, regardless of how long or how much they have smoked, their risk of heart disease declines rapidly. Three years after quitting, the risk of death from heart disease and stroke for people who smoked a pack a day or less is almost the same as for people who never smoked. Women appear to recover lung function more fully than men.[62] Since secondhand smoke is a potent risk factor, avoid smoky places when possible. Avoid all forms of tobacco, since nicotine increases blood pressure, heart rate, blood clotting, and plaque buildup.

Eat Well There are numerous ways you can promote cardiovascular health through better nutrition. The American Heart Association recommends the following:[63]

- Aim to use up at least as many calories as you consume.

- Eat a wide variety of foods from all the basic food groups.

- Aim to have a diet that consists of mainly nutrient-rich foods such as vegetables, fruits, and whole-grain products. Fruits and vegetables are high in vitamins, minerals, and fiber, and are low in calories. Meanwhile, the fiber in unrefined whole-grain foods can help lower cholesterol and help you feel full (which can help with weight management).

- Eat fish at least twice a week. The omega-3 fatty acids in fish such as salmon and trout may help lower the risk of death from coronary artery disease.

- Consume lean meats without skin, and cook them without added saturated and *trans* fat. Or substitute beans and legumes as a protein source instead of meats.

- Avoid high-fat dairy products, and instead consume fat-free, 1 percent fat, or low-fat dairy products.

- Reduce your consumption of foods containing partially hydrogenated vegetable oils to lower the amount of *trans* fat in your diet.

- Cut back on foods high in dietary cholesterol. Aim to eat less than 300 milligrams of cholesterol each day.

- Cut back on beverages and foods with added sugars.

- Reduce your intake of sodium to 1,500 milligrams or less per day.

- Drink alcohol in moderation.

- Be aware of portion sizes, especially while dining out.

If you have (or are at risk of developing) hypertension, your physician may suggest that you adopt the DASH (Dietary Approaches to Stop Hypertension) diet. Following this diet can help lessen your risk of hypertension and other forms of cardiovascular disease. The box on the DASH Diet discusses the diet's specific recommendations.

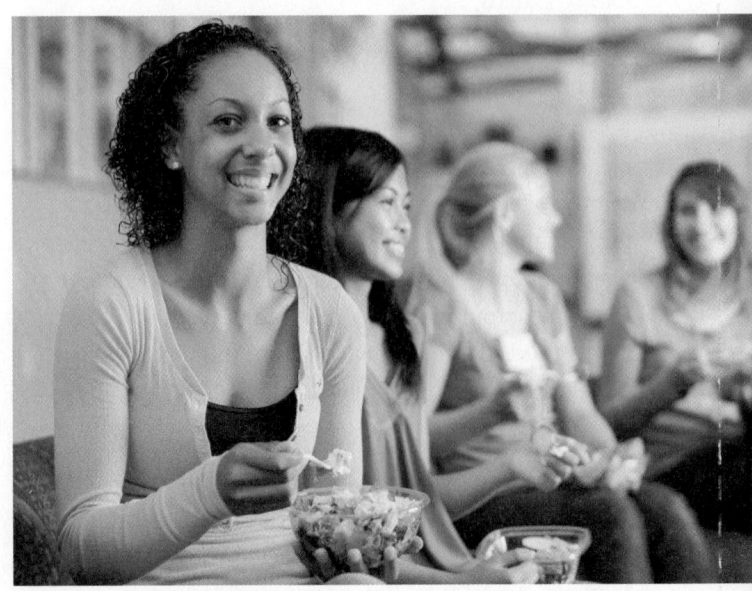

Exercise Regularly Regular cardiovascular exercise strengthens the heart muscles and helps keep the blood vessels resilient. Performing 30 to 60 minutes or more of moderate activity most days of the week will help prevent cardiovascular disease, especially if you reach your target heart rate. Strength training and flexibility are also important components of your exercise plan for cardiovascular wellness, helping you to maintain muscle mass, speed metabolism, control weight, and prevent injury.

Manage Your Stress The physiological stress response raises blood pressure, speeds the heart rate, and floods the bloodstream with glucose. All of these, in turn, can promote cardiovascular disease by damaging the blood vessels and directly contributing to atherosclerosis, and by weakening the heart through electrical and hormonal overstimulation. Learning specific techniques for stress reduction, relaxation, and anger management can give you important tools for lowering your risk of cardiovascular disease.

Control Diabetes Because elevated sugar levels in the blood greatly increase the risk for heart disease, stroke, and artery disease, people with diabetes are at tremendous risk. The very factors that contribute to the development of diabetes (obesity, hypertension, elevated blood cholesterol and triglycerides, inactivity) are additional risks for CVD. Careful diet, increased exercise, and medication help most diabetics control their condition and lower their CVD risk.

Avoid Alcohol and Drug Abuse If you drink, keep your consumption below one drink per day for women and two per day for men. Greater consumption raises blood sugar and triglyceride levels. Avoid recreational drugs, especially stimulants.

TOOLS FOR CHANGE •

The DASH Diet

The DASH (Dietary Approaches to Stop Hypertension) diet is a set of nutritional guidelines designed to reduce blood pressure. Recommended by the National Heart, Lung, and Blood Institute and the American Heart Association, it is characterized by the following:

- Reduced consumption of saturated fat, total fat, red meats, sodium, sweets, added sugars, and sugar-containing beverages

- Increased consumption of fruits, vegetables, fat-free or low-fat dairy products, whole-grain foods, fish, poultry, and nuts

- Special care to consume recommended levels of potassium, magnesium, calcium, protein, and fiber

You can find the entire DASH eating plan—including nutrient goals and serving recommendations at different calorie levels for various food groups—online at www.nhlbi.nih.gov/health/public/heart/hbp/dash/new_dash.pdf.

In addition to these guidelines, the DASH diet provides tips for reducing sodium—often hidden in processed foods—that can benefit virtually everyone:

- Buy the low- or reduced-sodium versions of soups, condiments, crackers, and other packaged foods. Read labels carefully and watch for sodium in such items as breakfast cereals and salad dressings.

- Choose fresh or frozen vegetables. If buying canned, look for no-sodium or low-sodium versions.

- Watch out for canned, smoked, cured, or processed meats and brined foods such as pickles and olives, which are usually very high in sodium. Rinse when practical to wash away some of the salt.

- Some processed foods have so much sodium you may simply have to avoid them; examples include packaged cake and sauce mixes, pizzas, and frozen dinners.

Source: U.S. Department of Health and Human Services, National Institutes of Health, National Heart, Lung, and Blood Institute, *DASH Eating Plan: Lower Your Blood Pressure* (NIH Publication #06-4082, Revised April, 2006).

• •

chapterin**review**

videos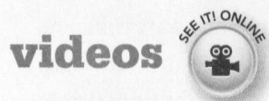

Log on to **www.pearsonhighered.com/hopson** or MyFitnessLab to view these chapter-related videos.

Heart Disease in America   Tips to Raise Good Cholesterol

online resources

Log on to **www.pearsonhighered.com/hopson** or MyFitnessLab for access to these book-related resources, and for links to other useful websites.

 Audio case study
Audio PowerPoint lecture

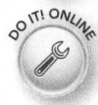 Lab 10.1 Understand Your CVD Risk

 Take Charge of Your Health! Worksheets:
    Worksheet 38 Cardiovascular Risk
       Assessment
    Worksheet 39 Healthy Heart I.Q.
Behavior Change Log Book and Wellness
Journal

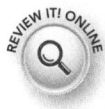 Pre- and post-quizzes
Glossary flashcards

review questions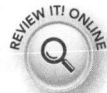

1. Cardiovascular disease and stroke are responsible for about _____ of deaths in the United States each year.
   a. one-half
   b. one-tenth
   c. one-sixth
   d. one-third

2. In annual medical care costs and lost productivity, CVD collectively costs Americans
   a. about $475,000.
   b. about $47.5 million.
   c. about $475 million.
   d. about $475 billion.

3. Which of the following is an example of cardiovascular disease (CVD)?
   a. Diabetes
   b. Low blood pressure
   c. Coronary heart disease
   d. Systolic pressure

4. Which of the following accurately describes *hypertension*?
   a. Sustained high blood pressure
   b. A thickening or hardening of the arteries
   c. Heart blockage
   d. Irregular heartbeat

5. Which of the following is characteristic of cardiovascular disease?
   a. Joint pain
   b. Feeling energized
   c. Having no symptoms at all
   d. Dry skin

6. When atherosclerosis occurs in the heart's main blood vessels, it is called
   a. peripheral artery disease.
   b. coronary artery disease.
   c. inflammation.
   d. homocysteine.

7. Which of the following is a significant risk factor for CVD?
   a. Regular exercise
   b. Managed stress
   c. Underweight
   d. Tobacco use

8. A person with metabolic syndrome is likely to have which one of the following?
   a. Abdominal obesity or a large waistline
   b. Depressed levels of triglycerides in the blood
   c. High levels of "good" cholesterol (HDLs)
   d. Hypoglycemia or low blood sugar

9. Which of the following statements is true?
    a. The earliest manifestations of cardiovascular disease often take root during childhood.
    b. Only seniors need to worry about cardiovascular disease.
    c. Heavy alcohol consumption is unrelated to your risks for developing cardiovascular disease.
    d. People who are skinny are protected against cardiovascular disease.

10. Low-density lipoprotein (LDL) is often referred to as
    a. "good" cholesterol.
    b. "bad" cholesterol.
    c. diabetes mellitus.
    d. metabolic syndrome.

critical**thinking**questions

 REVIEW IT! ONLINE

1. List six different forms of CVD. Compare and contrast their risk factors, symptoms, and prevention.
2. Describe the atherosclerosis process and explain the medical term "atherosclerotic cardiovascular disease."
3. Discuss the evidence that people in your age group are at risk for developing CVD.
4. Discuss specific ways that exercise and dietary changes can help prevent CVD.

references

1. National Center for Health Statistics (NCHS), "FastStats: Leading Causes of Death," www.cdc.gov/nchs/fastats/lcod.htm (updated September 2011).
2. American Heart Association, "Heart Disease and Stroke Statistics 2011 Update: A Report from the American Heart Association," *Circulation* 123, no. 4 (2011): e18–209.
3. Ibid.
4. Ibid.
5. L. L. Hayman, "Starting Young: Promoting a Healthy Lifestyle with Children," *Journal of Cardiovascular Nursing* 25, no. 3 (2010): 228–32; American Heart Association, "Heart Disease and Stroke Statistics 2011 Update," 2011.
6. J. Xu and others, "Deaths: Final Data for 2007," *National Vital Statistics Reports* 58, no. 19 (Hyattsville, MD: National Center for Health Statistics, 2011); M. Heron, "Deaths: Leading Causes for 2006," *National Vital Statistics Reports* 58, no. 14 (Hyattsville, MD: National Center for Health Statistics, 2010); K. D. Kochank and others, "Deaths: Preliminary Data for 2009," *National Vital Statistics Reports* 59, no. 4 (Hyattsville, MD: National Center for Health Statistics, 2011).
7. American Heart Association, "American Heart Association Scientific Statement: Combined Behavioral Interventions Best Way to Reduce Heart Disease Risk," http://newsroom.heart.org/pr/aha/1073.aspx (July 12, 2010).
8. American Heart Association, "Cardiovascular Disease Cost," www.americanheart.org/presenter.jhtml?identifier=4475 (2011).
9. P. A. Heidenreich and others, "Forecasting the Future of Cardiovascular Disease in the United States: A Policy Statement from the American Heart Association," *Circulation* 123, no. 8 (2011): 933–44.
10. World Health Organization, "Cardiovascular Diseases (CVDs)," Fact sheet no. 317, www.who.int/mediacentre/factsheets/fs317/en/index.html (September 2011).
11. Ibid.
12. World Health Organization, "Cardiovascular Disease: Prevention and Control," Global Strategy on Diet, Physical Activity, and Health, www.who.int/dietphysicalactivity/publications/facts/cvd/en/index.htm (accessed August 2007).
13. World Health Organization, "Cardiovascular Diseases (CVDs)," 2011.
14. H. C. McGill and others, "Origin of Atherosclerosis in Childhood and Adolescence," *American Journal of Clinical Nutrition* 72, no. 5 (2000): 1307S–15S.
15. H. C. McGill and others, "Association of Coronary Heart Disease Risk Factors with Microscopic Qualities of Coronary Atherosclerosis in Youth," *Circulation* 102, no. 4 (2000): 374–9.
16. T. Parker-Pope, "Stroke Rising among Young People," *New York Times* http://well.blogs.nytimes.com/2011/02/10/stroke-rising-among-young-people (February 10, 2011).
17. P. Franks and others, "Childhood Obesity, Other Cardiovascular Risks, and Premature Death," *New England Journal of Medicine* 362, no. 6 (2010): 485–93; D. H. Whincup and J. E. Deanfield, "Childhood Obesity and Cardiovascular Disease: The Challenge Ahead," *Nature Clinical Practice Cardiovascular Medicine* 2, no. 9 (2005): 432–3; R. E. Kavey and others, "American Heart Association Guidelines for Primary Prevention of Atherosclerotic Cardiovascular Disease Beginning in Childhood," *Circulation* 107, no. 11 (2003): 1562–6.
18. A. G. Mainous III and others, "Life Stress and Atherosclerosis: A Pathway through Unhealthy Lifestyle," *International Journal of Psychiatry in Medicine* 40, no. 2 (2010): 147–61; Mayo Clinic Staff, "Arteriosclerosis/Atherosclerosis: Causes," www.mayoclinic.com/health/arteriosclerosisatherosclerosis/DS00525 (June 2010).
19. R. E. Kavey, "American Heart Association Guidelines for Primary Prevention of Atherosclerotic Cardiovascular Disease," 2003.
20. "Inflammation, Heart Disease, and Stroke: The Role of C-Reactive Protein," American Heart Association, www.americanheart.org/presenter.jhtml?identifier=4648 (March 2011).
21. B. M. Egan, Y. Zhao, and R. N. Axon, "US Trends in Prevalence, Awareness, Treatment, and Control of Hypertension, 1988–2008," *Journal of the American Medical Association* 303, no. 20 (2010): 2043–50.
22. Mayo Clinic Staff, "High Blood Pressure (Hypertension)," www.mayoclinic.com/health/high-blood-pressure/DS00100 (March 2011).
23. S. I. Sharp and others, "Hypertension Is a Potential Risk Factor for Vascular Dementia: Systematic Review," *International Journal of Geriatric Psychiatry* 26, no. 7 (2011): 661–9; F. D. Testai and P. B. Gorelick, "Vascular Cognitive Impairment and Alzheimer's Disease: Are These Disorders Linked to Hypertension and other Cardiovascular Risk Factors?" in V. Aiyagari and P. B. Gorelick (eds.) *Hypertension and Stroke: Pathophysiology and Management* (New York: Humana Press, 2011): 195–210.
24. Ibid.
25. C. L. Williams and B. A. Strobino, "Childhood Diet, Overweight, and CVD Risk Factors: The Healthy Start Project," *Preventive Cardiology* 11, no. 1 (2008): 11–20; P. K. Elias and others, "Blood Pressure-Related Cognitive Decline: Does Age Make a Difference?" *Hypertension* 44, no. 5 (2004): 631–6.
26. American Heart Association, "About High Blood Pressure," www.heart.org/HEARTORG/Conditions/HighBloodPressure/AboutHighBloodPressure/About-High-Blood-Pressure_UCM_002050_Article.jsp (updated June 2011).
27. Ibid.
28. J. Flynn, "Hypertension in the Young: Epidemiology, Sequelae, and Therapy," *Nephrology, Dialysis, Transplantation* 24, no. 2 (2009): 370–75.
29. American Heart Association, "Heart Disease and Stroke Statistics 2011 Update," 2011.
30. Ibid.

31. Mayo Clinic Staff, "Angina," www .mayoclinic.com/health/angina/DS00994 (June 2011).

32. American Heart Association, "About Arrhythmia," www.heart.org/HEARTORG /Conditions/Arrhythmia/AboutArrhythmia /About-Arrhythmia_UCM_002010_Article .jsp (updated June 2011).

33. American Heart Association, "About Heart Failure," www.heart.org/HEARTORG /Conditions/HeartFailure/AboutHeartFailure /About-Heart-Failure_UCM_002044_Article .jsp (updated September 2011).

34. American Heart Association, "About Congenital Heart Defects," www.heart.org /HEARTORG/Conditions/Congenital HeartDefects/AboutCongenitalHeart Defects/About-Congenital-Heart-Defects _UCM_001217_Article.jsp (updated January 2011).

35. American Heart Association, "Heart Disease and Stroke Statistics 2011 Update," 2011.

36. Mayo Clinic Staff, "Stroke: Risk Factors," www.mayoclinic.com/health/stroke /DS00150 (July 2011).

37. Mayo Clinic Staff, "Transient Ischemic Attack (TIA)," www.mayoclinic.com /health/transient-ischemic-attack/DS00220 (March 2011).

38. National Heart, Lung, and Blood Institute, "What Are Coronary Heart Disease Risk Factors?" www.nhlbi.nih.gov/health/dci /Diseases/hd/hd_prevention.html (February 2011).

39. U.S. Department of Health and Human Services, The Health Consequences of Smoking: A Report of the Surgeon General (Atlanta: U.S. Department of Health and Human Services, Centers for Disease Control and Prevention, National Center for Chronic Disease Prevention and Health Promotion, Office on Smoking and Health, 2004), available at www.surgeongeneral .gov/library/smokingconsequences/index .html.

40. American Cancer Society, "Secondhand Smoke," www.cancer.org/cancer/cancer causes/tobaccocancer/secondhand-smoke (revised June 2011).

41. American Heart Association, "Why Quit Smoking?" www.heart.org/HEARTORG /GettingHealthy/QuitSmoking /QuittingSmoking/Why-Quit-Smoking _UCM_307847_Article.jsp (updated August 2011); V. F. Tapson, "The Role of Smoking in Coagulation and Thromboembolism in Chronic Obstructive Pulmonary Disease," Proceedings of the American Thoracic Society 2, no. 1 (2005): 71–7.

42. Mayo Clinic Staff, "High Blood Pressure Dangers: Hypertension's Effects on Your Body," www.mayoclinic.com/health /high-blood-pressure/HI00062 (January 2011).

43. National Center for Health Statistics, Health, United States, 2010: With Special Feature on Death and Dying (Hyattsville, MD: U.S. Department of Health and Human Services, 2011) Table 95.

44. American Heart Association, "Heart Disease and Stroke Statistics 2011 Update," 2011.

45. Mayo Clinic Staff, "Top 5 Lifestyle Changes to Reduce Cholesterol," www.mayoclinic .com/health/reduce-cholesterol/CL00012 (May 2010).

46. National Center for Health Statistics, "National Health Interview Survey, 1997–2010, Leisure-Time Physical Activity," www.cdc.gov/nchs/data/nhis/earlyrelease /201106_07.pdf (June 2011).

47. American Diabetes Association, "Diabetes Statistics: 2011 National Diabetes Fact Sheet," www.diabetes.org/diabetes-basics/diabetes-statistics (January 2011).

48. World Heart Federation, "Diabetes and Cardiovascular Disease," www.world-heart-federation.org/press/fact-sheets /diabetes-and-cvd (January 2011).

49. American Heart Association, "Heart Disease and Stroke Statistics 2011 Update," 2011.

50. National Heart, Lung, and Blood Institute, "What Is Metabolic Syndrome?" www .nhlbi.nih.gov/health/dci/Diseases/ms /ms_whatis.html (April 2011).

51. S. D. de Ferranti and others, "Prevalence of the Metabolic Syndrome in American Adolescents: Findings from the Third National Health and Nutrition Examination Survey," Circulation 110, no. 16 (2004): 2494–7.

52. American Diabetes Association, "Metabolic Syndrome Risk Factors in Young Adults," DOC NEWS 2, no. 1 (2005): 23.

53. J. Schilter and L. Dalleck, "Fitness and Fatness: Indicators of Metabolic Syndrome and Cardiovascular Disease Risk Factors in College Students?" Journal of Exercise Physiology 13, no. 4 (2010): 29–39.

54. T. L. Keown, C. B. Smith, and M. S. Harris, "Metabolic Syndrome among College Students," The Journal for Nurse Practitioners 5, no. 10 (2009): 754–9.

55. M. Esler and others, "Chronic Mental Stress Is a Cause of Essential Hypertension: Presence of Biological Markers of Stress," Clinical and Experimental Pharmacology and Physiology 35, no. 4 (2008): 498–502; A. Flaa and others, "Sympatho-adrenal Stress Reactivity Is a Predictor of Future Blood Pressure: An 18-Year Follow-Up Study," Hypertension 52, no. 2 (2008): 336–41; T. Chandola et al., "Work Stress and Coronary Heart Disease: What Are the Mechanisms?" European Heart Journal 29, no. 5 (2008): 640–8.

56. A. N. Westover, S. McBride, and R. W. Haley, "Stroke in Young Adults Who Abuse Amphetamines or Cocaine," Archives of General Psychiatry 64 (2007): 495–502.

57. American Heart Association, "Heart Disease and Stroke Statistics 2011 Update," 2011.

58. Ibid.

59. National Heart, Lung, and Blood Institute, National Cholesterol Education Program, "High Blood Cholesterol: What You Need to Know," NIH Publication No. 05-3290, www.nhlbi.nih.gov/health /public/heart/chol/wyntk.htm (revised June 2005).

60. American Heart Association, "Heart Disease and Stroke Statistics 2011 Update," 2011.

61. Ibid.

62. Centers for Disease Control and Prevention, "Tobacco Use: Targeting the Nation's Leading Killer—At A Glance 2011," www .cdc.gov/chronicdisease/resources /publications/AAG/osh.htm (updated February 2011).

63. American Heart Association, "American Heart Association Supports New USDA /HHS Dietary Guidelines and Encourages Adherence: AHA Also Expresses Disappointment That Sodium, Saturated Fat Guidance Is Weak." Press Release http://newsroom.heart.org/pr/aha/1243 .aspx (January 2011).

LAB 10.1 • UNDERSTAND YOUR CVD RISK

Name: _____ Date: _____

Instructor: _____ Section: _____

Purpose: To engage students in critical thinking about their own risk factors for CVD.

Directions: Complete each of the following questions about CVD risk and total your points in each section—the higher the score, the greater your risk. If you answered "don't know" for any question, talk to your parents or other family members as soon as possible to find out whether you have any unknown risks.

SECTION I: ASSESS YOUR FAMILY RISK FOR CVD

	Yes	No	Don't Know
1. Do any of your primary relatives (mother, father, grandparents, siblings) have a history of heart disease or stroke?	1	0	
2. Do any of your primary relatives (mother, father, grandparents, siblings) have diabetes?	1	0	
3. Do any of your primary relatives (mother, father, grandparents, siblings) have high blood pressure?	1	0	
4. Do any of your primary relatives (mother, father, grandparents, siblings) have a history of high cholesterol?	1	0	
5. During the time you lived at home, did your family consume red meat and high-fat dairy products several times per week?	1	0	
Total for Section I = _____			

SECTION II: ASSESS YOUR LIFESTYLE RISK FOR CVD

	Yes	No	Don't Know
1. Do you have high blood pressure?	1	0	
2. Is your total cholesterol level higher than recommended? (See Table 10.4)	1	0	
3. Have you been diagnosed as pre-diabetic or diabetic?	1	0	
4. Do you smoke three or more cigarettes per day?	1	0	
5. Would you describe your life as being highly stressful?	1	0	
Total for Section II = _____			

SECTION III: ASSESS YOUR ADDITIONAL RISKS FOR CVD

1. How would you best describe your current BMI?

<18.5 (1 point)	25–29.9 (1 point)
18.5–24.9 (0 point)	≥30 (2 points)

2. How would you describe your level of exercise?

Moderate activity for 30 to 60 minutes on fewer than 3 days per week, plus fewer than three cardio workouts per week and fewer than two strength-training workouts per week	1 point
Moderate activity for 30 to 60 minutes most days of the week, plus three cardio workouts and two strength-training workouts per week	0 points
Moderate activity for 60 minutes or more most days of the week, plus more than three cardio workouts and two strength-training workouts per week	0 points

3. How would you describe your dietary behaviors?

I eat more than the recommended number of calories each day.	1 point
I eat about the recommended number of calories/day for my age, BMI, and activity level.	0 points
I eat fewer than the recommended number of calories each day.	0 points

4. Which of the following best describes your typical dietary behavior?

I eat several servings of red meat per week and consume saturated fat from other meats and high-fat dairy products most days.	1 point
I eat from the major food groups, trying hard to get the recommended fruits and vegetables.	0 points
Whenever possible, I try to substitute olive oil or canola oil for other forms of dietary fat.	0 points

Total for Section III = _____

Scoring: Look at each section. If your total score for that section is 0, your CVD risk is minimal. Keep up the good work! If your score is between 1 and 3, your risk is moderate and you should initiate some change to lower it. If you score a 4 or 5, you should make substantial changes in those factors that you can control. Your behavior change plan for the chapter will help, and you can get additional advice from your instructor.

SECTION IV: REFLECTION

1. What are your risk factors for CVD? Identify any behaviors that put you at risk for CVD. What can you change right now? What can you change in the future to reduce your risk?

_____

_____

2. Which risk factors for CVD are outside of your control? What can you do to reduce your risk of CVD, even though you have some uncontrollable risk factors?

_____

_____

Appendix

Answers to End-of-Chapter Questions

Chapter 1
1.b; 2.b; 3.d; 4.a; 5.a; 6.b; 7.b; 8.d; 9.a; 10.d

Chapter 2
1.b; 2.c; 3.d; 4.a; 5.b; 6.d; 7.d; 8.b; 9.d; 10.a

Chapter 3
1.c; 2.a; 3.a; 4.d; 5.c; 6.b; 7.d; 8.c; 9.a; 10.c

Chapter 4
1.d; 2.c; 3.a; 4.d; 5.a; 6.b; 7.c; 8.b; 9.a; 10.c

Chapter 5
1.a; 2.c; 3.b; 4.d; 5.d; 6.b; 7.c; 8.b; 9.c; 10.a

Chapter 6
1.c; 2.d; 3.c; 4.b; 5.b; 6.b; 7.a; 8.c; 9.a; 10.a

Chapter 7
1.d; 2.d; 3.d; 4.c; 5.d; 6.d; 7.d; 8.a; 9.c; 10.d

Chapter 8
1.d; 2.d; 3.b; 4.b; 5.c; 6.a; 7.a; 8.b; 9.a; 10.d

Chapter 9
1.c; 2.b; 3.a; 4.d; 5.d; 6.a; 7.b; 8.d; 9.a; 10.d

Chapter 10
1.d; 2.d; 3.c; 4.a; 5.c; 6.b; 7.d; 8.a; 9.a; 10.b

Photo Credits

Chapter 1

Chapter Opener p. 1 moodboard/Alamy; 1.1 Ale Ventura/Jupiter Images; p. 2 Image Source/Jupiter Images Royalty Free; 1.2 Irreversible damage: ImageState Royalty Free/Alamy; Chronic illness: MBI/Alamy; Signs of illness: Ariel Skelley/Alamy; Average wellness: Fancy/Alamy; Increased wellness: Tetra Images/Alamy; Optimum wellness: Blend Images/Alamy; 1.3 Alamy; p. 4 Corbis RF; p. 6 Thinkstock; 1.4 iStock; 1.7 Goodshoot/Jupiter Images Royalty Free; p. 9 Masterfile Royalty Free Division; p. 11 Corbis RF; p. 12 Masterfile Royalty Free Division; p. 13 Alamy; p. 15 Andrew Manley/iStockphoto.com; p. 17 Edyta Pawlowska/Shutterstock.

Chapter 2

Chapter Opener p. 31: Nicole Hill/RubberBall/Alamy; p. 32 Ryan McVay/Getty Images Inc. - PhotoDisc; 2.1a Light physical activity: Ken Gillespie Photography/Alamy; 2.1b Moderate physical activity: Doug Menuez/Getty Images Inc.-PhotoDisc; 2.1c Vigorous physical activity: Getty Images - Stockbyte; p. 34 Denkou Images/AGE Fotostock America, Inc - Royalty-free; p. 37 George Doyle/Getty Images, Inc - Stockbyte Royalty Free; 2.4a cardiorespiratory endurance: Dan Dalton/Getty Images/Digital Vision; 2.4b muscular fitness: MIXA/Getty Images Inc. RF; 2.4c flexibility: Daniel Grill/Alamy; p. 41 Alamy; p. 43 Dreamstime; p. 44 Alamy; p. 45 Shutterstock; p. 46 Paul Burns/Jupiter Images Royalty Free; p. 48 Alamy; p. 50 Dreamstime.

Chapter 3

Chapter Opener p. 67: Franck Camhi/Alamy; 3.1 rubberball/Getty Images Inc - Rubberball Royalty Free; p. 68 Jupiter Images - Thinkstock Images Royalty Free; 3.2 Radius Images/Jupiter Images Royalty Free; p. 73 Alamy Images Royalty Free; 3.5 Andres Rodriguez/Alamy; p. 75 Dennis Welsh/AGE Fotostock America, Inc - Royalty-free; 3.6a Elena Dorfman/Elena Dorfman; 3.6b Elena Dorfman/Elena Dorfman; 3.7 Thinkstock; p. 78 PhotoLibrary; p. 82 Eric Fowke/PhotoEdit Inc.; p. 85 iStock; p. 86 Thinkstock; p. 87 iStock; p. 89 Rob Melnychuk/Getty Images/Digital Vision; Table 3.4 Alamy; p. 97 Elena Dorfman/Pearson Education/Pearson Science; p. 112 Asia Images Group/PhotoLibrary.

Chapter 4

Chapter Opener p. 115 Tero Sivula/Alamy; p. 116 Comstock Images/Jupiter Images PictureArts Corporation/Brand X Royalty Free; 4.4 Alamy; p. 122 Masterfile Royalty Free Division; 4.5a, b U.S. Department of Agriculture; Table 4.1 p. (both) Elena Dorfman/Pearson Education/Pearson Science; p. 128 Alamy; p. 130 Masterfile Royalty Free Division; 4.9.1-4.9.3 (all) Elena Dorfman/Pearson Education/Pearson Science; 4.9.4-4.9.5 (all) Rolland Renaud/Pearson Education/Pearson Science; 4.9.5a Rolland Renaud/Pearson Education/Pearson Science; 4.9.5b Jac Mat/Pearson Education/Pearson Science; 4.9.6a (both) Rolland Renaud/Pearson Education/Pearson Science; 4.9.6b (both) Elena Dorfman/Pearson Education/Pearson Science; 4.9.7a (both) Rolland Renaud/Pearson Education/Pearson Science; 4.9.7b (both) Elena Dorfman/Pearson Education/Pearson Science; 4.9.7c hip adduction with ball: Jac Mat/Pearson Education/Pearson Science; 4.9.8a, b (both) Elena Dorfman/Pearson Education/Pearson Science; 4.9.9 (both) Jac Mat/Pearson Education/Pearson Science; 4.9.10 (both) Rolland Renaud/Pearson Education/Pearson Science; 4.9.11a (both) Elena Dorfman/Pearson Education/Pearson Science; 4.9.11b (both) Creative Digital Visions/Pearson Education/Pearson Science; 4.9.12a, b (both) Elena Dorfman/Pearson Education/Pearson Science; 4.9.13a (both) Elena Dorfman/Pearson Education/Pearson Science; 4.9.13b (both) Jac Mat/Pearson Education/Pearson Science; 4.9.14-4.9.18 (all) Elena Dorfman/Pearson Education/Pearson Science; 4.9.19a (both) Rolland Renaud/Pearson Education/Pearson Science; 4.9.19b (both) Elena Dorfman/Pearson Education/Pearson Science; 4.9.20a, b Elena Dorfman/Pearson Education/Pearson Science; 4.9.20c (both) Jac Mat/Pearson Education/Pearson Science; 4.9.20d Elena Dorfman/Pearson Education/Pearson Science; 4.9.20e Jac Mat/Pearson Education/Pearson Science; 4.9.21a (both) Elena Dorfman/Pearson Education/Pearson Science; 4.9.21b (both) Creative Digital Solutions/Pearson Education/Pearson Science; 4.9.22a, b Elena Dorfman/Pearson Education/Pearson Science; 4.9.22c p. 143 triceps extension with resistance band: Jac Mat/Pearson Education/Pearson Science; 4.9.23a, b Elena Dorfman/Pearson Education/Pearson Science; 4.9.23c (both) Jac Mat/Pearson Education/Pearson Science; 4.9.24a (both) Elena Dorfman/Pearson Education/Pearson Science; 4.9.24b (both) Jac Mat/Pearson Education/Pearson Science; 4.9.25-4.9.28 (both) Elena Dorfman/Pearson Education/Pearson Science; p. 150 (left) Shutterstock; p. 150 (right) Superstock; p. 150 (bottom) Ralph Kerpa/PhotoLibrary; p. 152 Shutterstock; p. 161 (all) Elena Dorfman/Pearson Education/Pearson Science; p. 162 (both) Elena Dorfman/Pearson Education/Pearson Science; p. 169: GoGo Images Corporation/Alamy.

Chapter 5

Chapter Opener p. 173 Superstock Royalty Free; p. 174 Alamy; p. 174 Plush Studios/Getty Images Inc. - PhotoDisc; p. 177 Tetra Images/Getty Images, Inc/Tetra Images Royalty Free; p. 179 John Cumming/Getty Images/Digital Vision; 5.2a, b Elena Dorfman/Pearson Education/Pearson Science; 5.3.2 Jac Mat/Pearson Education/Pearson Science; 5.3.3-5.312 (all) Elena Dorfman/Pearson Education/Pearson Science; 5.3.10a Elena Dorfman/Pearson Education/Pearson Science; 5.3.10b Rolland Renaud/Pearson Education/Pearson Science; 5.3.11-5.3.14 Elena Dorfman/Pearson Education/Pearson Science; 5.3.16 Jac Mat/Pearson

Index

F

G

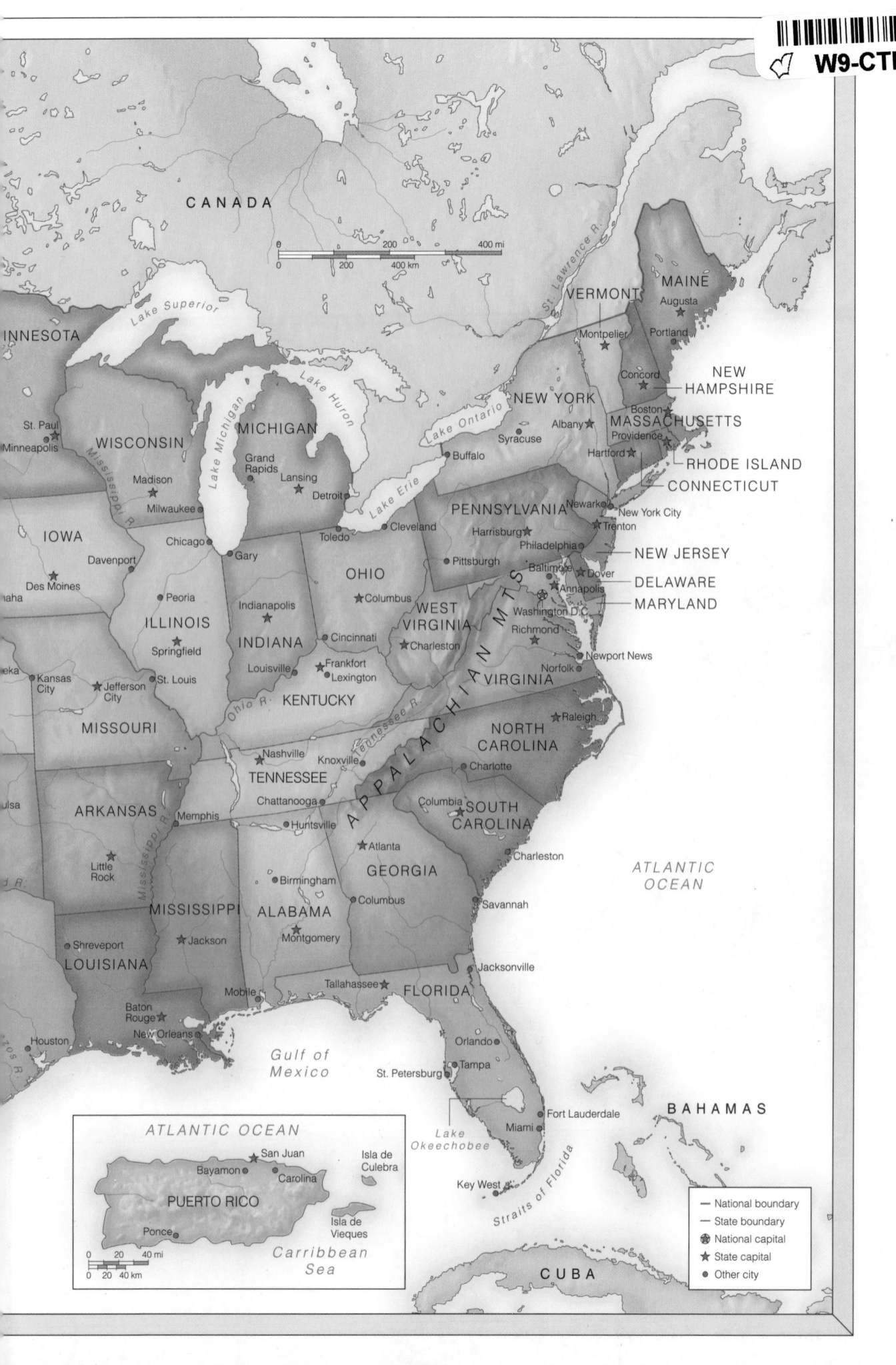

W9-CTI-035

CANADA

200   400 mi

200   400 km

Lake Superior

MINNESOTA

St. Paul ★
Minneapolis

WISCONSIN

Lake Michigan

Lake Huron

MICHIGAN

Grand Rapids
Lansing ★
Detroit

VERMONT

Montpelier ★

MAINE

Augusta ★

Portland

NEW HAMPSHIRE

Concord ★

St. Lawrence R.

Lake Ontario

Syracuse

Buffalo

NEW YORK

Albany ★

Boston ★
MASSACHUSETTS
Providence ★
Hartford ★

——— RHODE ISLAND
——— CONNECTICUT

Madison ★
Milwaukee

IOWA

Davenport
Des Moines ★

maha

Chicago
Gary

Peoria

ILLINOIS
Springfield ★

Toledo

OHIO

Columbus ★

Cleveland

Indianapolis ★

INDIANA

Cincinnati

PENNSYLVANIA

Harrisburg ★
Pittsburgh

WEST VIRGINIA

Charleston ★

Newark
New York City
Trenton ★

Philadelphia

Baltimore
Washington D.C. ⊛
Annapolis ★

——— NEW JERSEY
——— DELAWARE
——— MARYLAND

Dover

Mississippi R.

Kansas City
Jefferson City ★

St. Louis

Louisville
Frankfort ★
Lexington

KENTUCKY

Ohio R.

Richmond ★

VIRGINIA

Norfolk

Newport News

MISSOURI

TENNESSEE

Nashville ★
Knoxville

Chattanooga

Tennessee R.

A
P
P
A
L
A
C
H
I
A
N
   M
T
S
.

NORTH CAROLINA

Raleigh ★

Charlotte

Tulsa

ARKANSAS

Memphis

Huntsville

Little Rock ★

MISSISSIPPI

Jackson ★

ALABAMA

Birmingham

Columbus

GEORGIA

Atlanta ★

Columbia ★
SOUTH CAROLINA

Charleston

Savannah

ATLANTIC OCEAN

R.

Shreveport

LOUISIANA

Montgomery ★

Mobile

Tallahassee ★

FLORIDA

Jacksonville

Houston

Baton Rouge ★
New Orleans

Gulf of Mexico

St. Petersburg

Orlando

Tampa

Lake Okeechobee

Fort Lauderdale
Miami

BAHAMAS

zos R.

Key West

Straits of Florida

CUBA

ATLANTIC OCEAN

San Juan ★
Bayamon
Carolina

Isla de Culebra

PUERTO RICO

Ponce

Isla de Vieques

Carribbean Sea

0   20   40 mi
0   20   40 km

——— National boundary
——— State boundary
⊛ National capital
★ State capital
● Other city

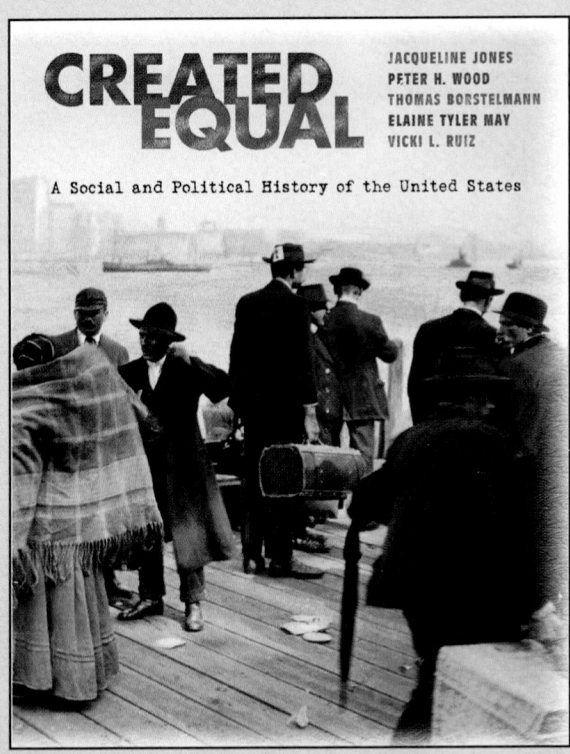

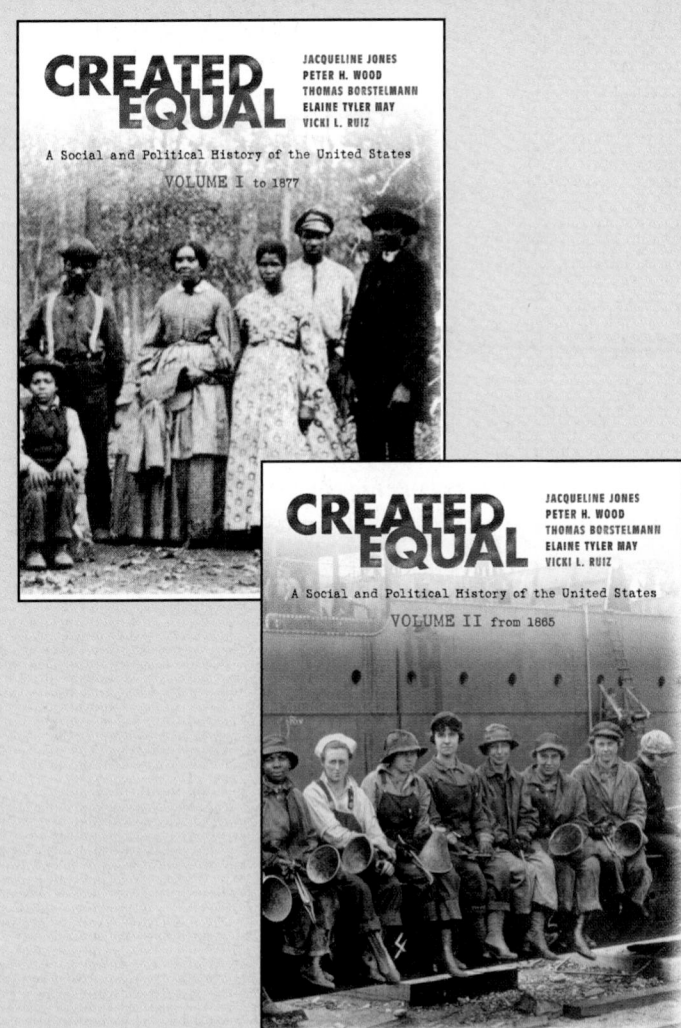

Jacqueline Jones, *Brandeis University*
Peter H. Wood, *Duke University*
Thomas Borstelmann, *Cornell University*
Elaine Tyler May, *University of Minnesota*
Vicki L. Ruiz, *University of California, Irvine*

With its sweeping inclusive view of American history, *Created Equal* emphasizes social history — including the lives and labors of women, immigrants, working people, and persons of color in all regions of the country — in the context of political and economic history. This new text from Longman Publishers acknowledges and reflects the diversity of class, race, culture, region, and gender that has always been part of the American story, and pays unique attention to the large middle class that has been central to the development of American society.

SVE • ©2003 • 1168 pages • Hardcover • ISBN 0-321-05296-X
Volume I • ©2003 • 656 pages • Paper • ISBN 0-321-05298-6
Volume II • ©2003 • 640 pages • Paper • ISBN 0-321-05300-1

Outstanding Features in *Created Equal*

▶ **Part Openers and Timelines.**
Part Openers preview the key issues and the political, cultural, ethnic, and regional diversity characteristic of the distinctive historical period covered in each three-chapter part. **Illustrated timelines** highlight significant events and trends and serve as a convenient preview/review for students. Each part covers approximately the era of a single generation of Americans.

1900	U.S. troops sent to China to crush Boxer Rebellion
1901	McKinley is assassinated; Vice President Theodore Roosevelt becomes President
1902	Newlands Act spurs dam building and irrigation in the Southwest
1903	First motorized flight by Orville and Wilbur Wright
	Henry Ford founds Ford Motor Company
1904	Roosevelt Corollary to the Monroe Doctrine
1905	Industrial Workers of the World founded
	Japan defeats Russia
1906	San Francisco Earthquake
	Sinclair Lewis, The Jungle
	Pure Food and Drug Act
	Indiana becomes first state to pass compulsory sterilization law
1907	"Gentlemen's Agreement" with Japan
	Oklahoma (former Indian Territory) becomes a state
1908	Muller v. Oregon upholds maximum hours for working women
1909	New York City garment workers' "Uprising of the 20,000"
	Peary/Henson Expedition reaches North Pole with four Greenland Inuit
1910	Mexican Revolution begins
	National Association for the Advancement of Colored People (NAACP) founded
1911	Triangle Shirtwaist fire, New York City
	Society of American Indians founded
1912	Theodore Roosevelt helps form Progressive Party
1913	Federal Reserve Act
	Sixteenth Amendment (federal personal

PART SEVEN

Reform at Home, Revolution Abroad, 1900-1929

MANY AMERICANS GREETED THE FIRST YEARS OF THE TWENTIETH century with optimism. Developments at home and abroad seemed to promise a new era of prosperity and progress. The mass manufacturing of automobiles proved a boon to the economy and transformed patterns of travel, leisure, and consumption. The beginning of commercial air flights heralded a revolution in communication and transportation. Moving pictures and new musical forms such as jazz delighted millions.

Focused on the new challenges of urbanization and industrialization, Progressive reformers sought to use science to solve a wide range of problems related to public health and welfare. Some advocated overhauling the system of public education; others pressed for legislation affecting the sale and distribution of alcohol. Some lobbied for worker health and safety legislation, while still others sought to exercise social control through eugenics and state-mandated sterilization.

A variety of social groups challenged white men's exclusive claim to civil rights. African Americans took the national stage to argue for equality under the law and for freedom from state-sanctioned violence in the form of lynching and debt peonage. Beginning with the "Great Migration" of World War I, southern blacks abandoned the southern cotton fields to seek jobs in northern cities.

The changing roles of women bolstered the women's suffrage movement. Growing numbers of women were becoming labor organizers, reformers, and college professors. Rising divorce rates and the emergence of birth control as a political as well as medical issue signaled challenges

---

CONNECTING HISTORY

Systems of Unfree Labor

The controversy over slavery ultimately precipitated the Civil War, the bloodiest conflict in the nation's history. Yet the abolition of slavery (with the ratification of the Thirteenth Amendment in 1865) did not eradicate forms of coerced labor. Indeed, systems of unfree labor—in which individuals are forced to work without compensation and for the benefit of someone else—have characterized the whole sweep of American history.

In the seventeenth century, most tobacco field workers in the Chesapeake region were indentured servants. These young men and women received passage from Europe to the colonies. In return, they bound themselves to a master for a stipulated amount of time (usually 7 years). Apprentices, children and young people, labored for a master artisan until they reached age 21.

Beginning in the late seventeenth century, the institution of slavery spread throughout the colonies. This system, which depended on the labor of Africans and their descendants, differed in crucial ways from indentured servitude and apprenticeship. Slaves remained slaves for life, and they had no rights under law. Children took the status of their enslaved mother.

States outside the South had emancipated their slaves by the mid-

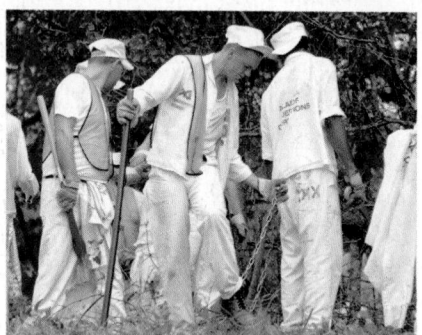

Shackled inmates work to clear brush along a highway near Prattville, Alabama. A 1996 settlement prevented the state from shackling prisoners together on a "chain gang" but shackling of individual convict laborers was still permissible.

such as growing crops, spinning thread, weaving cloth, and producing handicrafts. In some cases, ship captains kidnapped sailors and forced them to work for no pay on long voyages. Indian and African American children remained at risk as labor-hungry whites forcibly "apprenticed" them with the aid of the courts.

By the late nineteenth century, peonage characterized the southern staple crop economy as well as the rural extractive sector (logging, sawmills, turpentine production, and

men) into the rough and dangerous work of building roads through swamps and digging coal out of the earth. Convict labor officials often demonstrated a reckless disregard for human life. Unlike slave owners, prison officials and the private individuals who leased convicts had few incentives to treat these workers in a humane way.

In the early twenty-first century, coerced labor persists. Some illegal immigrants continue to indenture themselves to smugglers and remain indebted to these smugglers for many

▶ **"Connecting History"** features demonstrate the relationship between the ways we experience and the ways we remember history. These short essays examine a specific topic related to the chapter content tracing it both forward and backward in time, showing students how the issues and concerns relevant to one period of American history reverberate in other eras.

U.S. History Readers

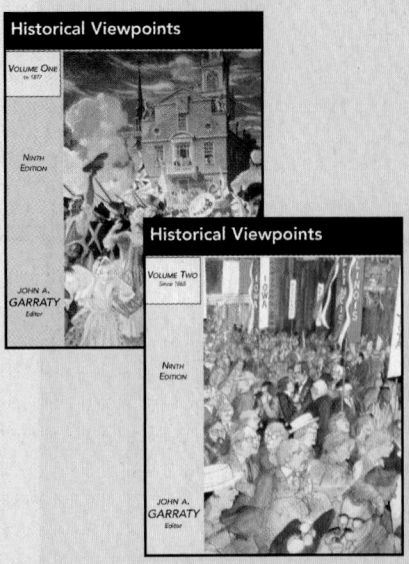

Historical Viewpoints, 9/e

John A. Garraty

Volume One — ISBN 0-321-10299-1
Volume Two — ISBN 0-321-10211-8

This collection of secondary source readings features articles adapted from the popular magazine *American Heritage*. Accessible, interesting, and significant, *Historical Viewpoints*, introduces students to a broad spectrum of historical issues and opinions from many of the world's foremost historians.

The Social Fabric, 9/e

Thomas L. Hartshorne
Robert A. Wheeler
John H. Cary
Julius Weinberg

Volume One — ISBN 0-321-10139-1
Volume Two — ISBN 0-321-10140-5

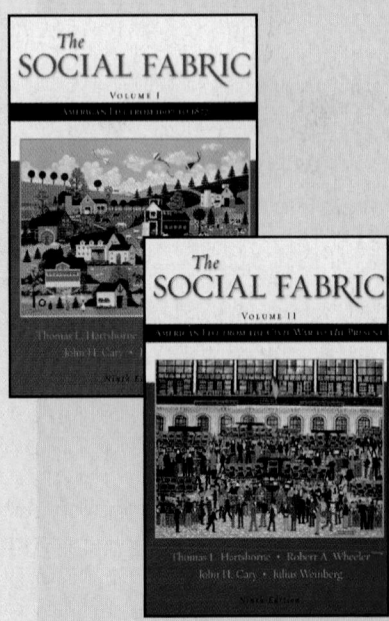

An engaging collection of secondary sources oriented to social history, this reader leads students to consider the role of women, ethnic groups, and laboring Americans in the weaving of the nation's social fabric.

Retracing the Past, 5/e

Gary B. Nash
Ronald Schultz

Volume One — ISBN 0-321-10137-5
Volume Two — ISBN 0-321-10138-3

This anthology of readings — both secondary and primary ("Past Traces") — describes the lives of ordinary Americans and examines the diversity of the American people, from the earliest settlement of America to the present day.

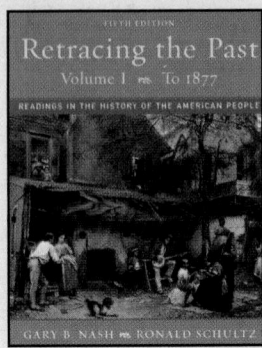
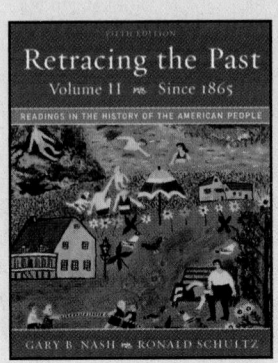

U.S. History Readers continued

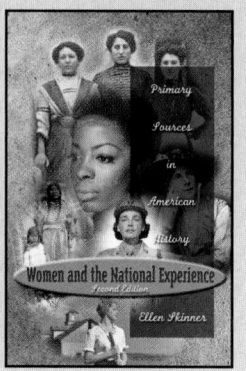

Women and the National Experience, 2/e

Ellen Skinner, *Pace University*

ISBN 0-321-00555-4

This brief, affordable primary source reader contains over one hundred different sources that describe the history of women in the United States. Combining classic and unusual sources, this anthology explores the private voices and public lives of women throughout U.S. history.

20th Century U.S. Foreign Policy

Gary A. Donaldson, *Xavier University*

ISBN 0-321-10506-0

With full-length primary source documents, including several contemporary opposing viewpoints, this collection is intended as a supplement to a U.S. Foreign Policy course that covers the 20th Century.

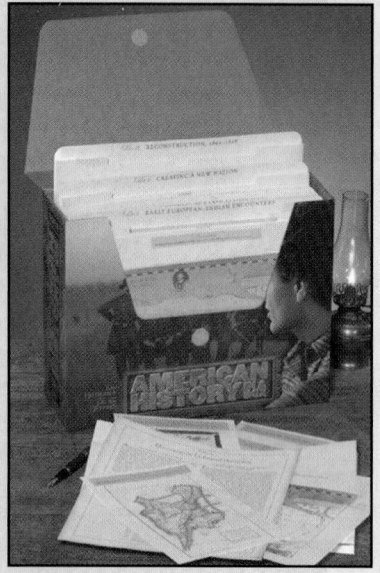

American History in a Box

Julie Roy Jeffrey, *Goucher College*
Peter J. Frederick, *Wabash College*

Volume One — ©2002 • Boxed Set • 12 folders • ISBN 0-321-03005-2
Volume Two — ©2002 • Boxed Set • 13 folders • ISBN 0-321-03006-0

American History in a Box takes your students on a fascinating journey through our nation's past. Containing a wealth of facsimiles of original documents – poems, photographs, speeches, cartoons, advertisements, sheet music, letters, and much more – these two volumes allow your students to learn first-hand what history is and what historians actually do.

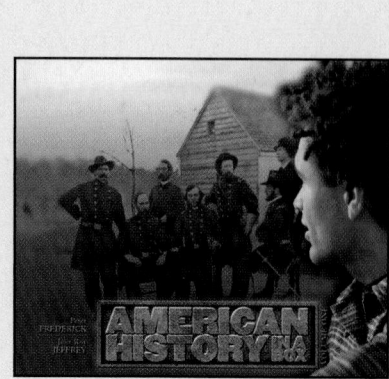

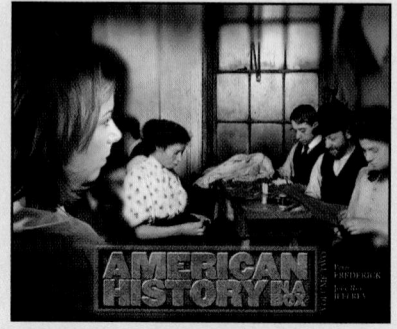

CREATED EQUAL

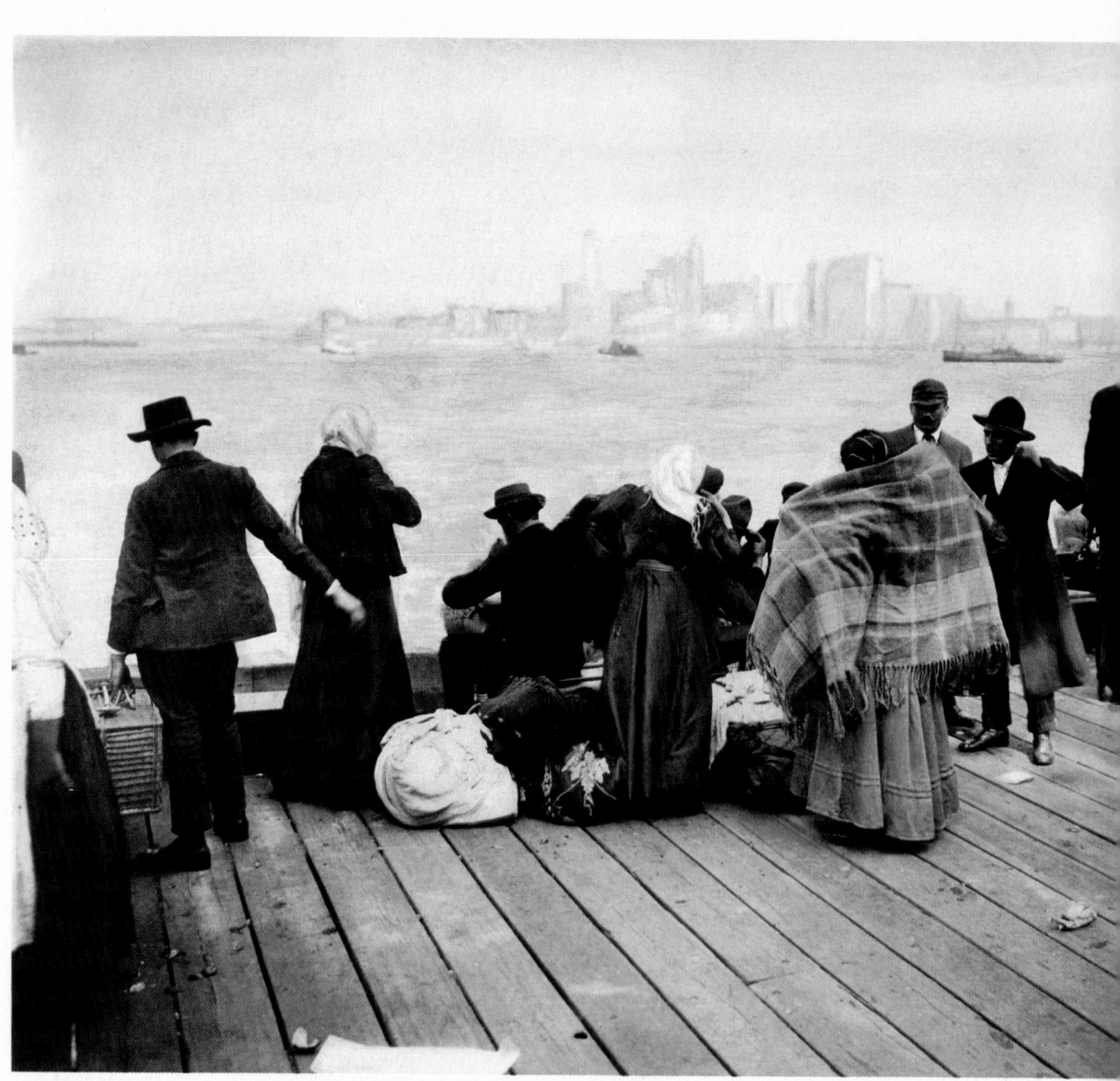

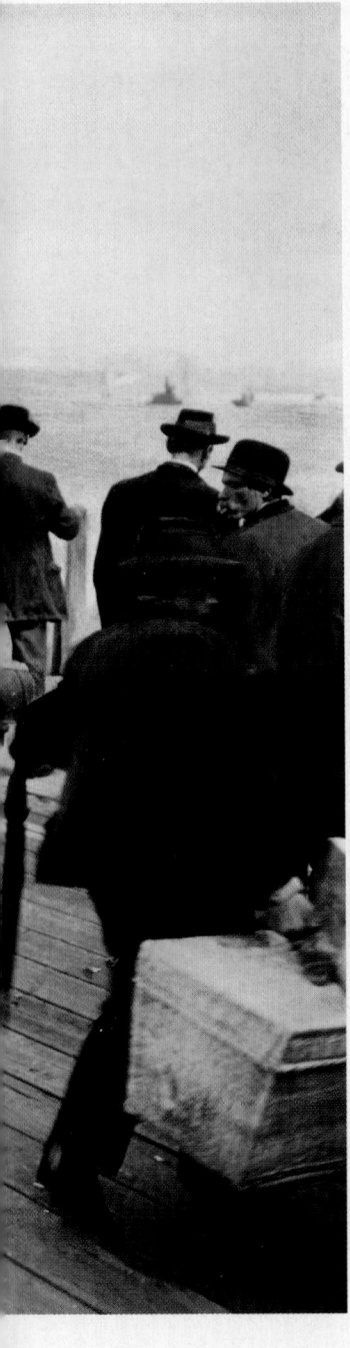

CREATED EQUAL

A SOCIAL AND POLITICAL
HISTORY OF THE UNITED STATES

Jacqueline Jones
Brandeis University

Peter H. Wood
Duke University

Elaine Tyler May
University of Minnesota

Thomas Borstelmann
Cornell University

Vicki L. Ruiz
University of California, Irvine

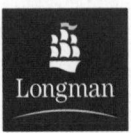

Longman

New York San Francisco Boston
London Toronto Sydney Tokyo Singapore Madrid
Mexico City Munich Paris Cape Town Hong Kong Montreal

Vice President and Publisher: Priscilla McGeehon
Acquisitions Editor: Ashley Dodge
Director of Development: Lisa Pinto
Development Manager: Betty Slack
Executive Marketing Manager: Sue Westmoreland
Media Editor: Patrick McCarthy
Supplements Editor: Kristi Olson
Director of Market Research: Laura Coaty
Production Manager: Ellen MacElree
Project Coordination, Electronic Page Makeup, and Cartography: Electronic Publishing Services Inc., NYC
Interior Design: Pearson Education Development
Cover Designer/Manager: Wendy Ann Fredericks
Photo Researcher: Photosearch, Inc.
Manufacturing Buyer: Lucy Hebard
Printer and Binder: Webcrafters
Cover Printer: Phoenix Color Corps.
Cover/Frontispiece Photo: Newly landed European immigrants on the dock at Ellis Island, New York City; oil over
    a photograph, 1900 © The Granger Collection, New York

Credits for literary selections, selected maps and figures, and timeline photos appear on pages C-1–C-3.

Library of Congress Cataloging-in-Publication Data
Created equal : a social and political history of the United States / Jacqueline Jones ... [et al.].
    p. cm.
    Includes bibliographical references and index.
    ISBN 0-321-05296-X
    1. United States—History. 2. United States—Social conditions. 3. United States—Politics
and government. 4. Pluralism (Social sciences)—United States—History. 5.
Minorities—United States—History. 6. Pluralism (Social sciences)—United
States—History—Sources. 7. Minorities—United States—History—Sources. I. Jones,
Jacqueline, 1948–
E178 .C86 2003
973—dc21

                                                            2002069476

Please visit our website at www.ablongman.com

ISBN: 0-321-05296-X (Complete Edition)
ISBN: 0-321-05298-6 (Volume I)
ISBN: 0-321-05300-1 (Volume II)

1 2 3 4 5 6 7 8 9 10—WC—05 04 03 02

To our own teachers, who helped set us on the historian's path, and to our students, who help keep us there. You have touched our intellects, our hearts, and our lives.

A nuestros propios maestros, quienes nos ayudaron a seguir en el sendero de historiador, y a nuestros estudiantes que ayudan a mantenernos alli. Usted ha tocado nuestros intelectos, nuestros corazones, y nuestras vidas.

Brief Contents

Detailed Contents

■ **CONNECTING HISTORY**
Homeland Security and Deep Fears of the Enemy Within   *98*

■ **INTERPRETING HISTORY**
"They Are Really Better to Us Than We Are to Them": Tension on North Carolina Coast   *108*

■ **CONNECTING HISTORY**
Reparations for Slavery?   *120*

■ **INTERPRETING HISTORY**
"Releese Us out of This Cruell Bondegg"   *139*

■ **INTERPRETING HISTORY**
"Pastures Can Be Found Almost Everywhere": Joshua von Kocherthal Recruits Germans to Carolina   *160*

■ **CONNECTING HISTORY**
Sounds Around Us: The Lost World of High Fidelity   *172*

■ CONNECTING HISTORY
Civil Liberties Under Siege During Wartime and Other National
Crises   *300*

■ INTERPRETING HISTORY
A Sailmaker Discusses "Means for the Preservation of Public
Liberty" on the Fourth of July, 1797   *314*

■ INTERPRETING HISTORY
Cherokee Women Petition Against Further Land Sales to Whites
in 1817   *343*

■ CONNECTING HISTORY
Revolutions in Transportation   *346*

■ CONNECTING HISTORY
The Strange Career of the Monroe Doctrine   *368*

■ INTERPRETING HISTORY
José Agustin de Escudero Describes New Mexico as a Land
of Opportunity, 1827   *375*

■ INTERPRETING HISTORY
Songs of the Great Depression   742

■ CONNECTING HISTORY
Presidents and the Media   750

CHAPTER 23
Global Conflict: World War II, 1937–1945   768

■ INTERPRETING HISTORY
Zelda Webb Anderson, "You Just Met One Who Does Not Know How to Cook"   789

■ CONNECTING HISTORY
The Atomic Bomb: Political and Cultural Fallout   796

CHAPTER 24
Cold War and Hot War, 1945–1953   800

■ CONNECTING HISTORY
The Origins of the Cold War   814

■ INTERPRETING HISTORY
NSC-68   825

PART NINE
The Cold War at Full Tide, 1953–1979   832

CHAPTER 25
Domestic Dreams and Atomic Nightmares, 1953–1963   834

List of Maps

List of Figures and Tables

Figures

Tables

List of Features

Connecting History

Interpreting History

Preface

> *"We hold these truths to be self-evident: That all men are created equal; that they are endowed by their Creator with certain unalienable rights; that among these are life, liberty, and the pursuit of happiness. . . . "*

Ever since the Continental Congress approved the Declaration of Independence on July 4, 1776, the noble sentiments expressed in the document have inspired people in the United States and around the world. The Founding Fathers conceived of the new nation in what we today would consider narrow terms—as a political community of white men of property. Gradually, as the generations unfolded, diverse racial and ethnic groups, as well as women of all backgrounds, cited the Declaration in their struggle to achieve a more inclusive definition of American citizenship. American history is the story of various groups of men and women, all "created equal" in their common humanity, claiming an American identity for themselves.

In fact American history consists of many stories—the story of territorial growth and expansion, the story of the rise of the middle class, the story of technological innovation and economic development, and the story of U.S. engagement with the wider world. *Created Equal* incorporates these traditional narratives into a new and fresh interpretation of American history, one that includes the stories of diverse groups of people and explores expanding notions of American identity.

The book's basic framework focuses on the political events and economic structures discussed in most American history textbooks. *Created Equal* aims not to overturn the familiar chronology of American history, but to incorporate into it a variety of groups and individuals whose stories help us to provide an accurate, comprehensive, and compelling view of the past.

Four Themes

We have chosen to highlight four significant themes that run throughout American history.

- **Diversity.** In considering the theme of diversity, we acknowledge that the formation of social identity is a central element of the American story. We examine how individual Americans have understood and identified themselves by gender, religion, region, income, race, and ethnicity, among other factors. Native Americans, African Americans, Spanish-speaking inhabitants of the Southwest, Chinese immigrants, members of the laboring classes, women of all groups—all of these people have played a major role in defining what it means to be an American. At the same time, diverse forms of identity are by no means fixed or static. For example, in the early twentieth century, a Russian immigrant garment worker on New York's Lower East Side might think of herself in any number of ways—as a Jew, an employee, a union member, a single woman, a resident of a thriving city—and these forms of identity might change over time, depending on the woman's circumstances.

- **Class and systems of power.** These have also shaped American society in profound ways and an understanding of them is fundamental to understanding events in American history. Those systems take many forms. The institution of slavery denied people of African descent basic human freedoms. Class differences based on income and formal education mocked broader ideals of social equality. Some groups used the law to deny other groups the right to participate in the political system. Popular ideas related to alleged social differences and innate inferiority served to justify the treatment of certain groups as second-class citizens. U.S. military leaders launched military campaigns against vulnerable peoples within and outside the nation's borders. By the end of the nineteenth century, the United States boasted the largest and most comfortable middle class in the world—and yet the most substantial political and economic power was distributed among a relatively small contingent of white men. During the twentieth century, Americans dismantled the legal system of inequality that reduced blacks, women, and other groups to second-class citizenship. Nevertheless, a growing gap between the rich and poor continued to mock the notion of true equality.

- **Environment.** The role of the environment in American history has been significant. The physical landscape has profoundly shaped American society, and has in turn been shaped by it. The theme of the environment is key to understanding cultural, political, and economic developments. Many Native American groups shared a sense of oneness with the land; for them, the material and spiritual worlds were intimately related. In contrast, many European Americans saw the land as a means of making a living or making money, or as the source of valuable raw materials—in other words, as a thing to be bought, sold, and used. The vast richness of the American landscape has provoked violent conflict over the years, even as it has formed a key component in American wealth and power. We examine regional differences in all geographical areas—not just the eastern seaboard.

- **Globalization.** Finally, the increasing globalization of the United States' economy and society in recent decades reminds us of how deeply the country has always been engaged with the rest of the world. Since the earliest days of colonial settlement, Americans have traded goods, cultural practices, and ideas with peoples outside their borders. As an immigrant nation and the modern world's superpower, America's foreign and domestic relations have always been intertwined. After World War II, Americans' fears of Communism and the Soviet Union exerted a profound effect upon the country's politics and society. In the wake of the attacks of September 11, 2001, all Americans were forced to confront the role of the United States in the larger world, with all the opportunities and dangers that role entailed.

These four themes serve as the lenses through which we view the traditional narrative framework of American history. Readers of *Created Equal* will understand the major political developments that shaped the country's past, as well as the role of diverse groups in initiating and reacting to those developments. Chapter 13, for example, which focuses on the 1850s, includes a detailed account of the effects of the slavery crisis on Congress and the political party system, as well as a discussion of shifting group identities affecting Indians, Latinos, northern women, and enslaved and free blacks. Chapter 18, focusing on the 1890s, covers the rise of the Populist Party and stirrings of American imperialism, as well as a discussion of barriers to a U.S. workers' political party and challenges to traditional gender roles. Thus *Created Equal* builds upon the basic history that forms the foundation of most major textbooks and offers a rich and comprehensive look at the past by including the stories of all Americans, in addition.

Chronological Organization

One of the challenges in writing *Created Equal* has been to emphasize the way in which the four major themes come together and influence each other, affecting specific generations of Americans. Thus, the text is organized into ten parts, most of these covering a generation. Many textbooks organize discussions of immigrants, cities, the West, and foreign diplomacy (to name a few topics) into separate chapters that cover large time periods. In contrast, *Created Equal* integrates material related to a variety of topics within individual chapters. Although the text adheres to a chronological organization, it stresses coherent discussions of specific topics within that framework. This provides students with a richer understanding of events. Chapter 15, for example, which covers the dozen or so years after the end of the Civil War, deals with Reconstruction in the South, Indian wars on the High Plains, and the rise of the women's and labor movements, stressing the relationships among all these developments. To cite another example: Many texts devote a chapter exclusively to America's post–World War II rise to global power; *Created Equal* integrates material related to that development in a series of six chapters that cover the period of 1945 to 2000. Each of these chapters illustrates the effects of dramatic world developments on American social relations and domestic policy on a decade-by-decade basis. This approach allows readers to appreciate the rich complexity of any particular time period and to understand that major events occur not in a vacuum, but in a larger social context.

Special Features

The book includes a number of features designed to make American history clear and engaging to the reader, and to encourage students to "do" history on their own. These features include:

- **Parts and timelines.** *Created Equal* consists of ten parts covering three chapters each. An opening section that lays out the basic themes of the period introduces each part. Each part opener also includes an illustrated timeline highlighting major events covered in the three chapters that follow.

- **Chapter introductory vignettes and conclusions.** Each chapter begins with a story that introduces the reader to groups and individuals representative of the themes developed in the chapter. Among the chapter introductory vignettes are the stories of a Norwegian immigrant woman in Wisconsin (Chapter 12), a group of runaway slaves accused of treason by Confederate authorities in wartime (Chapter 14), Spanish-speaking inhabitants of Northern New Mexico struggling to retain their culture in the face of an onslaught of European American settlers (Chapter 17), and a Sioux Indian boy at a government boarding school (Chapter 18). At the end of each chapter, a concluding section sums up the chapter's themes and points the reader toward the next chapter.

- **"Connecting History."** *Created Equal* encourages students to think outside the boundaries of specific periods by including in each chapter a boxed feature called "Connecting History." A topic is examined at two different periods, or as it evolved over time. Several of these mini-essays span the entire sweep of American history. Topics include the history of naval navigation, civil liberties, education, advertising, the Ku Klux Klan, and the Internet.

- **"Interpreting History."** This feature consists of a primary document on a topic relevant to the chapter's themes. Through this feature we hear the voices of a variety of Americans—a seventeenth-century slave, a sail maker in post-Revolutionary New York City, a Mexican lawyer visiting New Mexico in the early nineteenth century, a group of Cherokee women in early nineteenth-century Georgia, an antebellum southern professor, industrial titan Andrew Carnegie, and the environmental activist Rachel Carson. The "Interpreting History" feature takes many different forms—letters, sermons, court decisions, labor contracts, Congressional hearings, and songs. Students thus have an opportunity to analyze primary documents and to better appreciate the historian's task—to read materials critically and to place them in their larger socio-historical context.

- **Maps, charts, pullout quotes, and artifacts.** Illustrations—photographs, tables, pictures of objects from the time period, and figures—enhance the narrative. Large maps offer greater geographical detail and invite students to see the relationship between geography and history. Highlighted quotes help the reader grasp the chapter's major themes.

- **"Sites to Visit" and "For Further Reading."** At the end of each chapter is a list of "Sites to Visit," identifying sites on the World Wide Web relevant to the chapter and occasionally listing the location of important historical sites and landmarks as well. There is also a list of suggested works related to each section of the chapter. These features encourage students to follow up on major topics on their own—either on the computer or in the library.

Created Equal introduces students to recent scholarship in social history as well as providing a firm grounding in the traditional political narrative. In recent decades social identity has emerged as a central theme of American history. However, exclusive attention to cultural and social diversity can overshadow the political and economic structures of American society. Students should gain an understanding of our nation's social diversity but also learn about the power relations that have shaped that past—which groups have had influence and how they have maintained and wielded that influence. Placing these issues at the forefront, *Created Equal* tells the dramatic, evolving story of America in all its complexity—a story of a diverse people "created equal" yet struggling to achieve equality.

The Authors

Meet the Authors

Jacqueline Jones was born in Christiana, Delaware, a small town of 400 people in the northern part of the state. The local public school was desegregated in 1955, when she was a third grader. That event, combined with the peculiar social etiquette of relations between blacks and whites in the town, sparked her interest in American history. She attended the University of Delaware in nearby Newark and went on to graduate school at the University of Wisconsin, Madison, where she received her Ph.D. in history. Her scholarly interests have evolved over time, focusing on American labor, and women's, African American, and southern history.

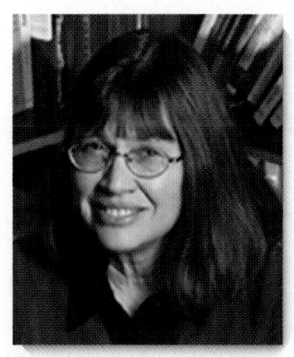

One of her biggest challenges has been to balance her responsibilities as teacher, historian, wife, and mother (of two daughters). One of her proudest achievements is the fact that she has been able to teach full-time and still pick up her daughters at school every day at 2:30 in the afternoon (thanks to a flexible professor's schedule). She is the author of several books, including *Soldiers of Light and Love: Northern Teachers and Georgia Blacks* (1980); *Labor of Love, Labor of Sorrow: Black Women, Work, and Family Since Slavery* (1985), which won the Bancroft Prize and was a finalist for a Pulitzer Prize; *The Dispossessed: America's Underclasses Since the Civil War* (1992); and *American Work: Four Centuries of Black and White Labor* (1998). In 2001, she completed a memoir that recounts her childhood in Christiana: *Creek Walking: Growing Up in Delaware in the 1950s.*

She teaches American history at Brandeis University, where she is Harry S. Truman Professor. In 1999, she received a MacArthur Fellowship.

Peter H. Wood was born in St. Louis (before the famous arch was built). He recalls seeing Jackie Robinson play against the Cardinals, visiting the courthouse where the Dred Scott case originated, and traveling up the Mississippi to Hannibal, birthplace of Mark Twain. Summer work on the northern Great Lakes aroused his interest in Native American cultures, past and present. He studied at Harvard (B.A., 1964; Ph.D., 1972) and at Oxford, where he was a Rhodes Scholar (1964–1966). His pioneering book, *Black Majority* (1974), concerning slavery in colonial South Carolina, won the Beveridge Prize of the American Historical Association. Since 1975, he has taught early American history at Duke University, where he also coached the women's lacrosse club for three years. The topics of his articles range from the French explorer LaSalle to Gerald Ford's pardon of Richard Nixon. He coauthored *Winslow Homer's Images of Blacks,* and he has written *Strange New Land,* a book about early African Americans. In 1989 he coedited *Powhatan's Mantle: Indians in the Colonial Southeast.* His demographic essay in that volume provided the first clear picture of population change in the eighteenth-century South. Dr. Wood has served on the boards of the Highlander Center, Harvard University, Houston's Rothko Chapel, the Menil Foundation, and the Institute of Early American History and Culture in Williamsburg. He is married to colonial historian Elizabeth Fenn; his varied interests include archaeology, documentary film, and growing gourds. He keeps a baseball bat used by Ted Williams beside his desk.

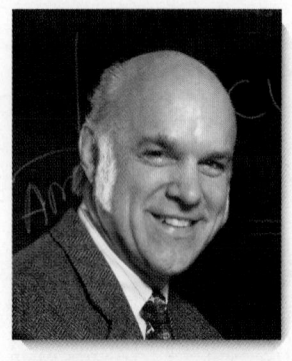

Thomas Borstelmann, the son of a university psychologist, has taught at the elementary, high school, and college levels. He taught second-grade physical education, taught and coached high school lacrosse, soccer, and basketball, and since 1991 has taught American history at Cornell University. In addition to his teaching experience, he also served as "Head Maid" of a conference center near Lake Tahoe. He lives with his wife and two sons in Syracuse, New York, where his greatest challenge—and delight—is doing the bulk of childcare while commuting 60 miles to Cornell. An avid bicyclist, runner, and cross-country skier, he earned his B.A. from Stanford University in 1980 and Ph.D. from Duke University in 1990.

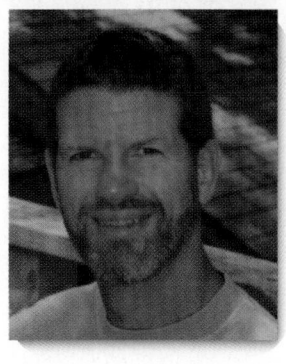

He became a historian to figure out the Cold War and American race relations, in part because he had grown up in the South. His first book, concerning American relations with southern Africa in the mid-twentieth century, won the Stuart L. Bernath Book Prize of the Society for Historians of Foreign Relations. His second book, *The Cold War and the Color Line*, appeared in 2002. His commitment to the classroom remains clear at Cornell University, where he has won a major teaching award: the Robert and Helen Appel Fellowship. He found writing *Created Equal* a natural complement to what he does in the classroom, trying to provide both telling details of the American past and the broad picture of how the United States has developed as it has. A specialist in U.S. foreign relations, he is equally fascinated with domestic politics and social change. He is currently working on a book about the 1970s.

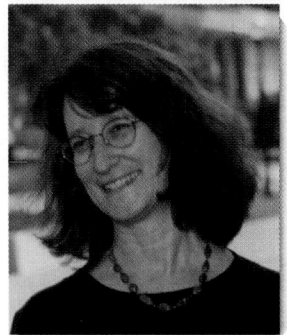

Elaine Tyler May grew up in the shadow of Hollywood, performing in neighborhood circuses with her friends. She went to high school before girls could play on sports teams, so she spent her after-school hours as a cheerleader and her summer days as a bodysurfing beach bum. Her passion for American history developed in college when she spent her junior year in Japan. The year was 1968. The Vietnam War was raging, along with turmoil at home. As an American in Asia, often called on to explain her nation's actions, she yearned for a deeper understanding of America's past and its place in the world. She returned home to study history at UCLA, where she earned her B.A., M.A., and Ph.D. She has taught at Princeton and Harvard Universities and since 1978 at the University of Minnesota. She has written four books examining the relationship between politics, public policy, and private life. Her widely acclaimed *Homeward Bound: American Families in the Cold War Era* was the first study to link the baby boom and suburbia to the politics of the Cold War. The *Chronicle of Higher Education* featured *Barren in the Promised Land: Childless Americans and the Pursuit of Happiness* as a pioneering study of the history of reproduction. *Lingua Franca* named her coedited volume *Here, There, and Everywhere: The Foreign Politics of American Popular Culture* a "Breakthrough Book." She served as president of the American Studies Association in 1996 and as Distinguished Fulbright Professor of American History in Dublin, Ireland, in 1997. She is married to historian Lary May and has three children who have inherited their parents' passion for history.

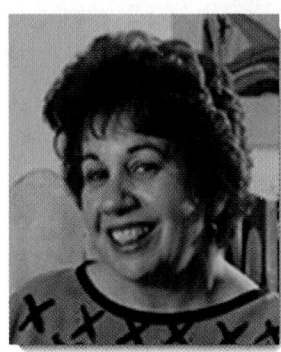

Vicki L. Ruiz is a professor of history and Chicano/Latino studies at the University of California, Irvine. For her, history remains a grand adventure, one that she began at the kitchen table listening to the stories of her mother and grandmother and continued with the help of the local bookmobile. She read constantly as she sat on the dock catching small fish ("grunts") to be used as bait on her father's fishing boat. As she grew older, she was promoted to working with her mother selling tickets for the *Blue Sea II*. The first in her family to receive an advanced degree, she graduated from Gulf Coast Community College and Florida State University, then went on to earn a Ph.D. in history at Stanford in 1982, the fourth Mexican American woman to receive a doctorate in history. Her first book, *Cannery Women, Cannery Lives*, received an award from the National Women's Political Caucus, and her second, *From Out of the Shadows: Mexican Women in 20th-Century America*, was named a *Choice* Outstanding Academic Book of 1998 by the American Library Association. She is coeditor with Ellen Carol Dubois of *Unequal Sisters: A Multicultural Reader in U.S. Women's History.* She and Virginia Sánchez Korrol coedit *Latinas in the United States: A Historical Encyclopedia,* and both were recognized by *Latina Magazine* as Latinas of the Year in Education for 2000. Active in student mentorship projects, summer institutes for teachers, and public humanities programs, Dr. Ruiz served as an appointee to the National Council of the Humanities. She has also served on the national governing bodies of the American Historical Association, the Organization of American Histories, and the American Studies Association. The mother of two grown sons, she is married to Victor Becerra, urban planner and gourmet cook extraordinaire.

A Conversation with the Authors

> Created Equal *tells stories across generations, regions, and cultures, integrating the lives of individuals within the economic, political, cultural, global, and environmental vectors shaping their lives. These tales of simple courage breathe life into history, bringing an immediacy and vibrancy to the past. We cherish the telling of stories for it is within these tales that we remember the* ánimo y sueños *(spirit and dreams) of the American people.*
>
> VICKI RUIZ

How Did This Project Begin?

PETER: It started with a videocassette. The Longman history editor taped a lively conversation with a dozen exceptional history teachers from very different backgrounds. They were all energized about teaching U.S. history in new ways, but they felt frustrated by their current texts. Then Longman sent the video to me. The video was not great cinematography, just talking heads. But their voices were so articulate, and I shared so many of their concerns. I remember watching the cassette on a Sunday night, and it set my mind spinning. I couldn't get much sleep. Here were real teachers like me who wanted a dramatically different text. And here was a major publisher, Longman, saying, "What do you think?"

At the time, I was teaching one of those special classes, a group of history majors that really clicked. Four of the best students had parents from other countries—South Africa, Mexico, Haiti, Vietnam—and all four were fascinated by American history. I remember thinking, "I'd love to be part of a team of historians who developed a text that would excite Darlene Aquino from Texas and Minh-Thu Pham from North Carolina." I called Longman and said, "Let's find a way to do it."

How Did You Come to the Decision to Write This Book?

JACKIE: I thought that writing a new kind of text would be a real intellectual challenge. We have the opportunity to rethink and reconfigure the traditional American history narrative, and that's exciting.

PETER: I was not eager to write a "feel good" text. American history has not been a big happy rainbow. I was convinced that we could be much more open and inclusive than most current texts. We could also be more direct and matter-of-fact in many areas. It is important to be frank about differences and contradictions in the American story in a way that actually helps explain things.

THOMAS: Writing a textbook was attractive because it's so complementary to what I do in the classroom, particularly teaching the introductory American history survey. Having the chance to try to tell the entire story of the American past was exciting as a balance to the other work we do.

How Did the Author Team Come Together, Work Together?

PETER: The Longman videotape circulated. Eventually, we had a team of people who felt that they could answer, collectively, the challenge presented by those articulate teachers. Obviously, no one could do it alone, but the right combination might be able to pull it off.

Having watched the Duke basketball team for two decades, I know what five very different people can do if they pay attention to each other, and if they all have the same goal in mind. An author team is like a basketball team: The players have to complement one another. (Sometimes we *compliment* each other, too!) And each person gets better and contributes more through practice and hard work. This team works hard.

VICKI: I joined the *Created Equal* team out of the profound respect I have for the scholarship of my colleagues. I had met Elaine and Jackie previously at conferences and knew Peter and Thomas only from their scholarship. The first brainstorming meeting I attended in New York City was intellectual magic, pure and simple. From the first hour onward, we exchanged our separate visions and expectations, debated periodization and conceptual frames, and began the process of intellectual coalescence that marks this truly collaborative enterprise. I left New York exhilarated and exhausted.

> *I joined the* Created Equal *team out of the profound respect I have for the scholarship of my colleagues.*
>
> VICKI RUIZ

ELAINE: I joined this project because I was excited about the challenge of writing a textbook that would convey the drama and excitement of the nation's history. It offered an opportunity to work with a team of scholars who I have long admired, and it has been a joy and a privilege to collaborate with them. We have become a close group of friends and colleagues, and our text reflects the lively exchanges, debates, and brainstorming sessions we've had over email, phone calls, and gatherings when we have come together to work on the project.

Tell Us About the Title—*Created Equal*.

JACKIE: The title reflects our commitment to be inclusive in our coverage of different groups and the part they played in shaping American history. Of course, we are invoking the Declaration of Independence: "We hold these truths to be self-evident, that all men are created equal." That document, and those words, have inspired countless individuals, groups, and nations around the world.

PETER: We all recognize the phrase, "Created Equal" from the Declaration of Independence, but we rarely ponder it. For me, it represents an affirmation of humanity, the family of mankind. But it also raises the deepest American theme—the endless struggles over defining whose equality will be recognized. I suppose you could say that there is equality in birth and death, but a great deal of inequality in between.

Many of those inequities—and their partial removal—drive the story of American History. Tom Paine understood this in 1776 when he published *Common Sense*. Months before the Declaration of Independence appeared, Paine put it this way: "Mankind being originally equal in the order of creation, the equality could only be destroyed by some subsequent circumstance."

How and Why Did You Choose the Themes that Structure the Text?

THOMAS: The themes that we chose to highlight in *Created Equal* reflect what we see as the current and future state of the field of U.S. history, as well as the needs of future generations of students.

The prominence of multiculturalism in recent decades made clear that identity remains a central piece of the American story: how individual Americans understand and identify themselves (by religion, class, region, sex, race, ethnicity, etc.). But too much attention to cultural issues has often led to a discounting of the political and economic structure of American society: Who has material wealth and power, and how they use it, is fundamental for determining the course of the past and present. The increasing globalization of the U.S. economy and American society (e.g., through rising immigration) in recent decades has reminded us of how deeply the United States has always been engaged with the rest of the world—as an immigrant nation and the modern world's superpower, America's foreign and domestic affairs have always been intertwined. And the deepening awareness in recent decades of the fragility of the earth's environment has stimulated a whole subfield of American environmental history, which we try to tap into—in a sense, the environment represents the clearest example of the interconnectedness of American and international history.

JACKIE: It was time to integrate recent scholarship related to the many different groups that have been part of the American story, and to open up that story to include all geographical areas (and not just the eastern seaboard). The theme of the environment is key to understanding American history; we explore the ways American cultural, political, and economic developments influence and are shaped by the nation's natural resources and landscape. The theme of power relations helps students to understand that differences of class, and differences in political and material resources, are significant aspects of the country's history. We balance this perspective by showing how America emerged as a uniquely open and middle-class nation—one that has attracted immigrants from all over the world throughout its history.

ELAINE: *Created Equal* brings together aspects of the nation's story that are usually examined separately. It demonstrates that the people who make change are not only those in major positions of power—they are also ordinary Americans from all backgrounds. We illuminate ways that ordinary Americans have seized opportunities to improve their lives and their nation. In *Created Equal*, the land itself is a major player in the story—the environment, the different regions, and the ways in which people, businesses, public policies, and the forces of nature have shaped it. We also address the ongoing interaction between the United States and the rest of the world, examining the nation in a truly global context.

> **Created Equal** *brings together aspects of the nation's story that are usually examined separately.*
>
> ELAINE TYLER MAY

How Is the Book Organized?

PETER: History is the study of change over time, so chronology becomes extremely important. We wanted to emphasize central themes, but we wanted to explore and explain how they related to one another at any given moment. So we made a conscious decision to be more chronological than many recent texts in our presentation. It makes for less confusion, less jumping back and forth in time, than when broad themes are played out separately. After all, this is the way we lead our own lives—sequentially.

JACKIE: Most of the 10 separate parts in the book each cover about a generation. The parts give students a sense of the big picture over a longer period—the way our themes fit together and the impact of major developments on a particular generation of Americans. The chronological organization of the book forces us to understand the "wholeness" of any particular period—to consider links among political, social, economic, and cultural developments. By maintaining a strictly chronological focus, we hope to show students how the events and developments of any one period are intertwined with each other. For example, for coverage of the period after the end of the Civil War, it is important to show links between the Indian wars in the West and the process of Reconstruction in the South. In most texts, those regional perspectives are separated into different chapters, but, in *Created Equal*, these connections are presented together in Chapter 15.

Each of the Chapters Has Two Feature Essays: "Interpreting History" and "Connecting History." What are the Benefits of These Features?

JACKIE: The "Interpreting History" feature provides students with an opportunity to "do history" on their own. These are brief primary documents related to the issues presented in a particular chapter. We have chosen documents that are particularly rich in terms of providing material for discussion and analysis. By working with this material, students will learn how to balance the close reading of a text with an understanding of the larger historical context of the document.

The "Connecting History" feature follows a particular subject backward and forward in time, suggesting ways that a topic discussed in a particular chapter has evolved through American history. These mini-essays encourage students to consider change over long periods of time.

What Did You Enjoy Most About Writing this Text?

JACKIE: The intellectual stimulation and the opportunity to work with a wonderful group of people.

PETER: Three things. My teammates and their different energies, for sure. Also, the staff at Longman. I had never worked on a big collective effort like this, and I still marvel at the intricacies and coordination of the whole operation.

But most of all, writing this text has reinforced my sense of the intense relevance of history. We were hard at work when the World Trade Center attack occurred, and our editor lived only a few blocks from the destruction. I saw the hole in the Pentagon first-hand.

> *Writing this text has reinforced my sense of the intense relevance of history.*
> PETER WOOD

Suddenly, our entire society was on a new footing. A culture oriented to the present and the future had to re-examine the past, both locally and globally, recent and distant. In reconnecting to our history in new ways—examining it openly and fearlessly and critically—we find a story that is more relevant than most of us imagined. It is complex, dramatic, sobering, and uplifting all at once. . .like life itself.

THOMAS: It's been a pleasure to work as a team. When I first joined the project in its early phases, I was lured by the prospect of working with Peter—and then I got that much more excited as the rest of the team was filled in. I've been deeply impressed by how well we communicate, especially the combination of serious intellectual challenges to each other and our great personal support for each other. I simply learn a lot every time we communicate, and I'm grateful for the friendships that have emerged out of our joint endeavor.

What Do You Hope Students Will Get Out of the Book?

PETER: I want readers to connect. As a child, you connect to your family, your neighbors, your schoolmates. As you get older, that circle expands; you begin to relate to people in other places and other times. In a good history class, or a strong history book, that relationship becomes close. You start to care about, argue with, and connect to the persons you are studying. Pretty soon, their tough choices and surprising experiences in life start to resemble our own in ways we never expected, even though their worlds are dramatically different from ours.

JACKIE: By presenting an inclusive view of the past, we give students a more accurate account of American history. Many texts only pay lip service to diversity. Non-elite groups are tacked on, marginalized, or segregated from the "real" story of America. In contrast, we believe that the history of all groups constitutes the real story of America.

Acknowledgments

As authors, we could not have completed this project without the loving support of our families. We wish to thank Jeffrey Abramson, Lil Fenn, Lynn Borstelmann, Lary May, and Victor Becerra for their interest, forbearance, and encouragement over the course of many drafts. Our children, now ranging in age from 6 to 32, have been a source of inspiration, as have our many students, past and present. We are grateful to scores of colleagues and friends who have helped shape this book, both directly and indirectly, in more ways than they know.

Special thanks are due to Pam Gordon for pulling this team together and launching the project, to Dan Usner and Jay O'Callaghan for their useful involvement in the early stages, and to Steve Fraser for his insightful midcourse corrections, which came at a crucial time in the process. Along the way, Matt Basso, Chad Cover, Eben Miller, Andrea Sachs, Mary Strunk, and Melissa Williams provided useful research and administrative assistance; their help was invaluable. Louis Balizet provided careful reading of several chapter drafts. Thanks to Deborah Anderson for a stellar job in locating images, and to Jennifer Mazurkie for all her terrific work in overseeing the layout.

Our friends at Longman have shown their belief in this project from the beginning. They supported an invaluable two-day retreat at Truro, on Cape Cod, and they worked hard to smooth out numerous bumps along this long road. We thank all the creative people at Longman (and there are many) who have had a hand in bringing this book to life. We are especially grateful to Priscilla McGeehon, Lisa Pinto, Betty Slack, and Sue Westmoreland for their enthusiastic devotion to this project and their expertise and friendship from start to finish. Ashley Dodge, joining the Longman team recently, has embraced *Created Equal* and given it her full and timely support.

From the beginning, we knew that we wanted a unique and distinctive look for this book. For their comments and feedback on sample design material, we thank the following reviewers:

Scott Barton
East Central University

Constance M. McGovern
Frostburg State University

Keith Pacholl
*California State
  University–Fullerton*

Robert E. Rook
Fort Hays State University

Rachel Standish
Foothill College

Michael M. Topp
University of Texas–El Paso

Finally, we wish to express our deep gratitude to the following people who read and commented on the manuscript as it went through its several drafts. Collectively, they pushed us hard with their high standards, tough questions, and shrewd advice. The thoughtful criticisms and generous suggestions from these colleagues have helped improve the book.

Ken Adderley
Upper Iowa University

Leslie Alexander
Ohio State University

John Andrew
Franklin and Marshall College

Abel Bartley
University of Akron

Donald Scott Barton
*Central Carolina Technical
  College*

Mia Bay
Rutgers University

Chris Bierwith
*Treasure Valley Community
  College*

Charles Bolton
*University of Arkansas at Little
  Rock*

Susan Burch
Gallaudet University

Tommy Bynum
Georgia Perimeter College

Robert B. Carey
Empire State College–SUNY

Todd Carney
Southern Oregon University

Kathleen Carter
Highpoint University

Jonathan Chu
University of Massachusetts

Amy E. Davis
University of California–Los Angeles

Judy DeMark
Northern Michigan University

James A. Denton
University of Colorado

Joseph A. Devine
Stephen F. Austin University

Margaret Dwight
North Carolina Agricultural and Technical University

Nancy Gabin
Purdue University

Lori Ginzberg
Pennsylvania State University

Gregory Goodwin
Bakersfield College

Amy S. Greenberg
Pennsylvania State University

Nadine Isitani Hata
El Camino College

James Hedtke
Cabrini College

Fred Hoxie
University of Illinois

Tera Hunter
Carnegie Mellon University

David Jaffe
City College of New York

Jeremy Johnson
Northwest College

Yvonne Johnson
Central Missouri State University

Kurt Keichtle
University of Wisconsin

Anne Klejment
University of St. Thomas

Dennis Kortheuer
California State University–Long Beach

Joel Kunze
Upper Iowa University

Joseph Laythe
Edinboro College of Pennsylvania

Chana Kai Lee
Indiana University

Dan Letwin
Pennsylvania State University

Gaylen Lewis
Bakersfield College

Kenneth Lipartito
Florida International University

Kyle Longley
Arizona State University

Edith L. Macdonald
University of Central Florida

Lorie Maltby
Henderson Community College

Sandra Mathews-Lamb
Nebraska Wesleyan University

Constance M. McGovern
Frostburg State University

Henry McKiven
University of South Alabama

James H. Merrell
Vassar College

Earl Mulderink
Southern Utah State University

Steven Noll
University of Florida

Jim Norris
North Dakota State University

Elsa Nystrom
Kennesaw State University

Keith Pacholl
California State University–Fullerton

William Pelz
Elgin Community College

Melanie Perrault
University of Central Arkansas

Delores D. Petersen
Foothill College

Robert Pierce
Foothill College

Louis Potts
University of Missouri–Kansas City

Sarah Purcell
Central Michigan University

Niler Pyeatt
Wayland Baptist University

Steven Reschly
Truman State University

Arthur Robinson
Santa Rosa Junior College

Robert E. Rook
Fort Hays State University

Steven Ruggles
University of Minnesota

Christine Sears
University of Delaware

Rebecca Shoemaker
Indiana State University

Howard Shore
Columbia River High School

James Sidbury
University of Texas

Arwin D. Smallwood
Bradley University

Margaret Spratt
California University of Pennsylvania

Rachel Standish
Foothill College

Jon Stauff
St. Ambrose University

David Steigerwald
Ohio State University–Marion

Kay Stockbridge
Central Carolina Technical College

Daniel Thorp
Virginia Tech University

Michael M. Topp
University of Texas–El Paso

Clifford Trafzer
University of California–Riverside

Deborah Gray White
Rutgers University

Scott Wong
Williams College

Bill Woodward
Seattle Pacific University

Nancy Zens
Central Oregon Community College

David Zonderman
North Carolina State University

CREATED
EQUAL

25,000 to 11,000 years ago
Low ocean levels expose land bridge linking Siberia to Alaska.

14,000 years ago
Early Paleo-Indians in Florida and Pennsylvania regions, and also in Monte Verde, Chile.

13,900 to 12,900 years ago
Clovis hunters spread across North America.

10,000 to 3000 years ago
Archaic Indians flourish in diverse settings.

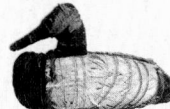

4200 to 2700 years ago
Poverty Point culture existing in Louisiana.

300 to 900 A.D.
Mayan culture flourishes in Mesoamerica.

400
Polynesian explorers reach the Hawaiian Islands.

500 to 600
Teotihuacan in central Mexico becomes one of the world's largest cities.

900 to 1100
Anasazi culture centered in Chaco Canyon in Southwest.

1000
Norse explorers establish a Vinland colony in Newfoundland.

1100
Cahokia in Illinois becomes one focus of Mississippian culture.

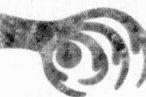

1250 to 1400
Mississippian culture reflected at Moundville in Alabama.

1400
Aztecs build capital at Tenochtitlán (site of modern Mexico City).

1405 to 1433
Chinese fleet of Admiral Zheng He reaches Indian Ocean and Africa's east coast.

1420 to 1460
Prince Henry of Portugal sends ships to explore Africa's west coast.

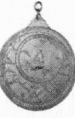

1492
First voyage of Columbus.

1494
Treaty of Tordesillas arranges division between overseas claims of Spain and Portugal.

1497 to 1499
Vasco da Gama completes trading voyage from Portugal to India.

1517
Martin Luther launches Protestant Reformation.

1519
Cortés invades Mexico.

PART ONE

North American Founders

WE SOMETIMES CALL THE FRAMERS OF THE U.S. CONSTITUTION America's Founding Fathers, using capital letters for emphasis. The men who met in Philadelphia in 1787 were indeed founders in a political sense, having drafted our enduring frame of government. But the 1780s seem recent in relation to most of North America's long human history. We must explore far back in time, long before the eighteenth century, to find the varied men and women who were the continent's first founders.

Two kinds of foundation builders emerge: the distant ancestors of today's Native Americans and newcomers from abroad who colonized North America in the sixteenth and seventeenth centuries.

Our earliest human ancestors evolved in Africa and then spread across the landmass of Eurasia. In the Southern Hemisphere, they managed to cross to Australia some 40,000 years ago, but evidence suggests that they reached the Americas from Asia much later, probably less than 20,000 years ago. These first human arrivals took advantage of the land bridge that joined Siberia to Alaska when Ice Age glaciers prompted a dramatic decline in sea levels. Roughly 14,000 years ago, these hunters apparently bypassed melting glaciers to reach the North American interior. They came on foot, but additional newcomers may have skirted the Pacific coast in small boats or even drifted across the South Pacific.

We still understand very little about these earliest Americans. What we do know is that they spread rapidly across North America over the next thousand years, and they continued to hunt mammoths and other large animals until these ancient species became extinct. Later, their descendants adapted to a wide range of different environments, learning to fish, hunt for smaller game, and gather berries. It has been 10,000 years since the extinction of the mammoths and 3000 years since the early signs of agriculture in the Americas. By 500 A.D. complex societies were beginning to appear in equatorial America, and a succession of diverse and rich societies had arisen in the Americas by the time a second set of founders appeared around 1500 A.D.

Although Vikings from Scandinavia had preceded Christopher Columbus by five centuries, their small outpost on the coast of Newfoundland lasted only a few years. In contrast, when Columbus reached the West Indies and returned to Spain in 1492, his voyage launched a human and biological exchange between the Eastern and Western Hemispheres that has never ceased. Spanish and Portuguese ships initiated this exchange, but they were soon followed by vessels from England, France, and Holland. Half a century after Columbus's first voyage, Spanish overland expeditions had already pushed from Florida to Arkansas and from Mexico to Kansas. French explorers, hoping to find a Northwest Passage to Asia, had penetrated far up the St. Lawrence River in Canada.

Europeans brought new materials such as iron and new animals such as horses, cattle, and pigs. They also brought deadly diseases previously unknown in the Americas, such as measles and smallpox, which had a catastrophic impact on Native American societies. By 1565 Europeans had established their first lasting outpost in the North American continent, the town of St. Augustine in Spanish Florida. Two decades later the English tried, unsuccessfully, to plant a similar colony at Roanoke Island along the coast of what is now North Carolina.

In the first decades of the seventeenth century, permanent European settlements took hold at Quebec on the St. Lawrence River and at Santa Fe near the Rio Grande. A trans-Atlantic outpost of English society appeared at Jamestown on Chesapeake Bay in 1607. Farther north, behind the sheltering hook of Cape Cod, other settlers formed additional coastal outposts and renamed the region New England.

Numbers were small at first, but these communities and others endured and expanded, often with crucial help from Native Americans who knew the keys to survival in their own domains. The gradual success of these European footholds prompted imitation and competition; colonizers clashed with each other and with long-time Indian inhabitants over control of the land and its resources. Disappointed in their early searches for easy mineral wealth, the new arrivals made do in various ways: cutting timber, catching fish, raising tobacco, or trading for furs. The French in particular, with aid once again from Native Americans, explored the interior of the continent. By 1700, they had laid claim to the entire Mississippi River valley and established a colony on the Gulf of Mexico.

Each new colonizing enterprise in the seventeenth century took on a distinctive life of its own—or, rather, numerous lives. First of all, there was the internal life of the community: Who would be allowed to take part, how would participants govern themselves, and how would they subsist? In each instance, relations with the region's native inhabitants constituted a second unfolding story. Complicated ties to Europe—economic, religious, social, and political—made a third crucial narrative. Furthermore, relations between colonies and between the distant European powers that backed them had a determining influence, as when England took over the Dutch colony at New Netherland in the third quarter of the seventeenth century. Finally, there was the compelling drama of the newcomers' relationship to the environment itself. These founding generations labored to understand—or to subdue and exploit without fully understanding—the continent they had started to colonize.

1519 to 1522
Magellan's ship circumnavigates the globe and returns to Spain.

1533 Pizarro overthrows Inca Empire in Peru.

1534 to 1543
Expeditions of Cartier (Canada), De Soto (Southeast), and Coronado (Southwest) probe North America.

1565 Spanish establish St. Augustine.

1577 to 1580
Voyage of Drake challenges Spanish dominance in the Pacific.

1585 to 1590
English attempt to establish Roanoke colony fails.

1588 Spanish Armada fails in an effort to invade England.

1599 Spanish colonize New Mexico.

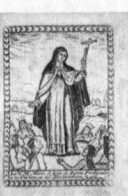

1607 England's Virginia Company launches colony at Jamestown.

1620 *Mayflower* passengers establish Plymouth Colony.

1630 English Puritans found Massachusetts Bay Colony.

1637 Pequot War in New England.

1660 Restoration of monarchy in England under Charles II.

1664 Charles II grants a charter to his brother James, Duke of York, sanctioning the takeover of the Dutch New Netherland colony and the creation of New York.

1675 to 1676
Metacom's War in New England.

1676 Bacon's Rebellion in Virginia.

1680 Pueblo Revolt in New Mexico.

1681 Quaker William Penn receives charter for Pennsylvania.

1682 La Salle explores the Mississippi River and claims Louisiana for France.

1689 Dutch leader William of Orange and his wife Mary become joint English sovereigns in the Glorious Revolution, replacing King James II.

1691 Witchcraft trials in Salem, Massachusetts.

1699 Iberville begins colony in French Louisiana.

1711 to 1715
Tuscarora Indians in North Carolina, and then the Yamasee in South Carolina, resist English colonial expansion.

CHAPTER

1

First Founders

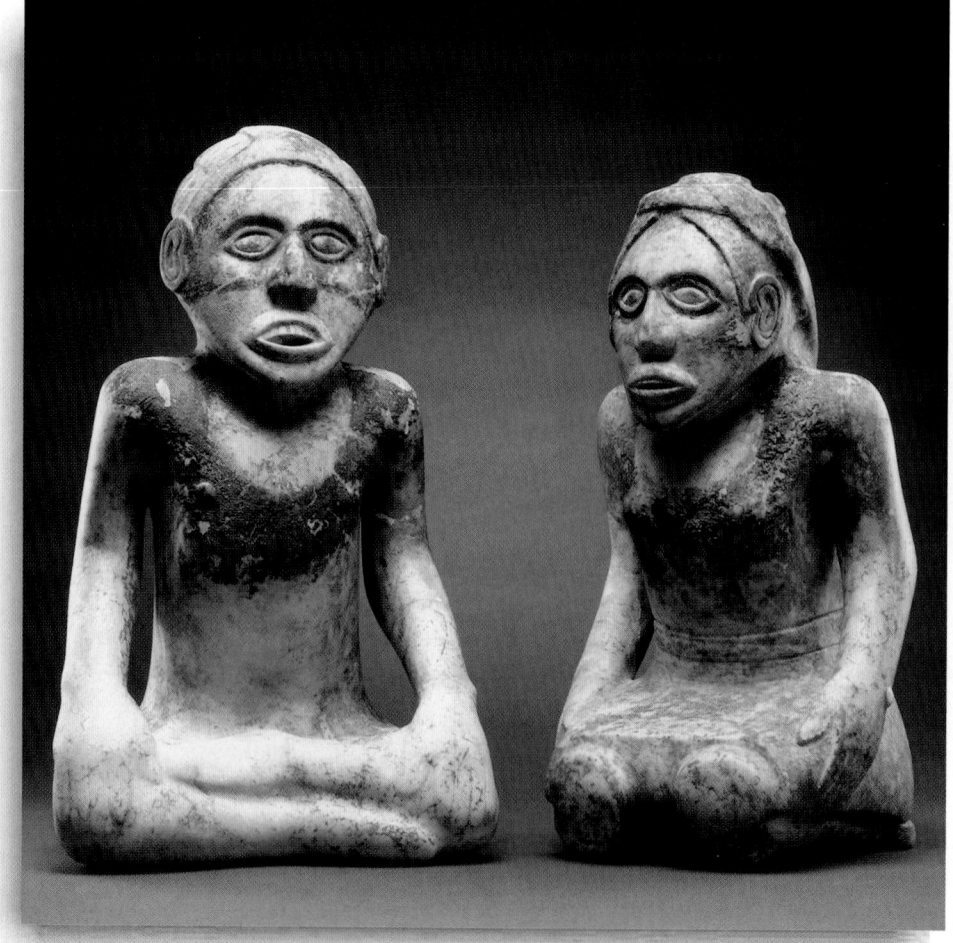

CHAPTER OUTLINE

Georgia Department of Natural Resources. Photograph ©1985 The Detroit Institute of Arts

■ Carved stone figures created nearly 1000 years ago at Etowah in Georgia.

ONE DAY IN 1908, A COWBOY NAMED GEORGE MCJUNKIN WAS CHECKING FENCES ON A cattle ranch near Folsom, New Mexico, when something strange caught his eye. McJunkin noticed several large bones protruding from the earth. Dismounting from his horse, he also spotted an old arrowhead, something common in these parts. But it was the bones beside it that seemed unusual. They were larger than cattle bones and buried under layers of dirt, so McJunkin decided to show them to others. Nearly 20 years later, ancient-bones expert Jesse Figgins came to Folsom after seeing McJunkin's evidence. Soon Figgins unearthed an extensive bone bed containing the remains of 23 large Ice Age bison of a species that had been extinct for 10,000 years. He also uncovered a spear point, clearly fashioned by human hands, embedded between two bison ribs. Figgins's finds confirmed McJunkin's earlier discovery. The objects stirred first disbelief and then excitement, for they proved that human hunters had existed in North America 7000 years earlier than scientists had supposed. The discovery of the thin projectile tips, named Folsom points after the site, sparked a revolution in North American archaeology.

In 1908, the year of McJunkin's discovery, the nation still had a great deal to learn about the oldest chapters in American history. The United States had just commemorated the 300th anniversary of England's Jamestown settlement in Virginia, and across the country, U.S. citizens memorialized Anglo-American beginnings. They expected newly arrived immigrants to learn English quickly and leave their Old World cultures behind. Textbooks of the era shared in the celebration of English colonization. They paid scant attention to the earlier Spanish and French arrivals in North America and none at all to the Native American inhabitants who had preceded them by thousands of years. *The Beginner's American History,* like most popular texts of the time, opened by relating the voyages of Christopher Columbus, the Italian explorer who encountered America while sailing for the Indies in 1492.

Even as far back as the sixteenth century, European newcomers to North America showed only occasional interest in the origins of the people who already lived there. Columbus, thinking he had reached the Asian islands close to India and China ("the Indies"), mistakenly lumped America's peoples together as "Indians." Euro-peans who were curious about Native Americans had little but the Bible to guide their inquiries. Christians speculated that North America's original residents were descendants of the Lost Tribe of Israel who had somehow wandered to these lands in Old Testament times. Whatever their origin, these inhabitants could hardly have been here more than 3000 years, the Europeans reasoned, for the world itself was thought to be scarcely 6000 years old.

Such views had changed little by the nineteenth century when American settlers swarmed westward in search of farmsteads. The newcomers speculated on the origin of

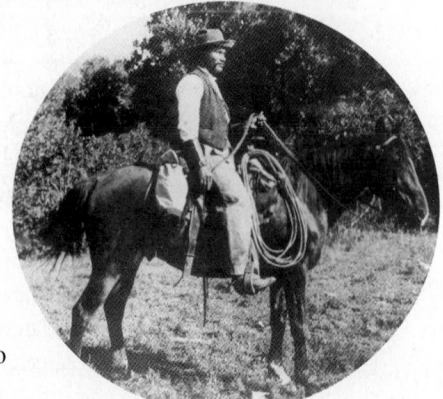

In 1908 a discovery by African American cowboy George McJunkin started a revolution in American archaeology.

mysterious burial mounds they saw throughout much of the Mississippi valley. Impressed by the size of these structures but convinced that Indians could not have built them, these new settlers suggested that the hills had to be the work of another race. Perhaps the ancient builders were European in origin and had somehow fallen victim to ancestors of the Native Americans. By 1890, as decades of Indian wars on the Great Plains drew to a close, only a few scientists took an interest in who the earliest North Americans really were, where they came from, when they arrived on the continent, and how they lived.

In the century since George McJunkin picked up a prehistoric bison bone, all of that has changed. Scholars who explore and debate the long history of early North America have steadily learned more about the continent's first inhabitants. An expanding American history now stretches back in time far before the Jamestown settlement and reaches broadly from coast to coast. Its earliest roots lie with the indigenous inhabitants of the continent over many millennia. In addition, the foreigners who suddenly intruded into portions of the Native American world in the sixteenth century—speaking Spanish, French, and occasionally English—also represent a significant beginning. All these people now number, in different ways, among America's first founders.

Ancient America

The discoveries at Folsom more than doubled archaeologists' estimates of the time span that humans had lived in North America. Clearly, they had resided on the continent for at least 10,000 years. After the Folsom find, collectors immediately began combing the Southwest for additional evidence. They soon found it at nearby Clovis, New Mexico, 170 miles south of Folsom and close to the Texas border.

In 1929 a teenager reported spotting large, well-chipped spear heads near Clovis. Three years later, amateur collectors located more in the same vicinity, this time beside the tooth of an extinct mammoth. These so-called Clovis points lay beneath a soil layer containing Folsom points, so they were clearly older than McJunkin's and Figgins's finds. Ever since, scientists have unearthed Clovis-like points throughout much of North America. According to the latest calculations, humans started creating these weapons roughly 13,900 years ago and ceased about 12,900 years ago. This means that people were hunting widely on the continent nearly 14,000 years ago. Archaeologists continue to push back and refine the estimated date for the appearance of the first people in the Americas. Recently, they have unearthed evidence suggesting the possible presence of pre-Clovis inhabitants.

The Question of Origins

Like all other peoples, the Indian societies whose ancestors have lived in America for at least 14,000 years retain rich and varied accounts of their own origins. No amount of scientific data can diminish or replace the powerful creation stories, in the Americas or elsewhere throughout the world, that have been passed down from distant ancestors and continue to serve an important cultural purpose. Nevertheless, modern researchers continue to compile evidence about the origin and migration of humans, very recent newcomers on a planet estimated to be 4.5 billion years old.

Scientists have determined that multicelled organisms began to evolve less than 600 million years ago. The higher primates who were humans' direct ancestors (that is, in the genus *Homo,* like today's humans) first emerged in Africa some 2.5 million years ago. Some ancient members of the *Homo* family tree may have migrated out of Africa as far as the Black Sea region by 1.7 million years ago. But it was scarcely 70,000 years ago when the most recent

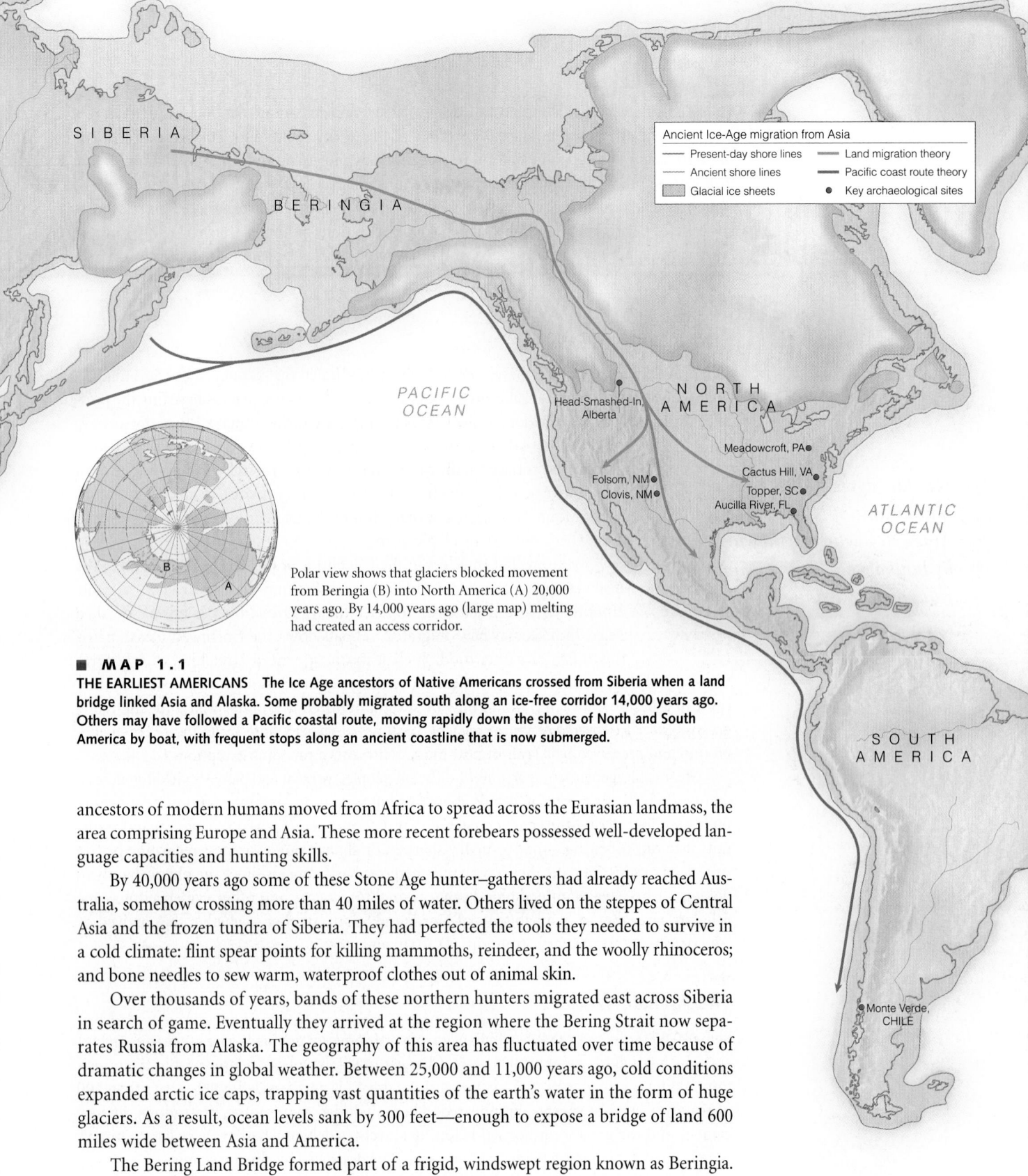

SIBERIA

BERINGIA

PACIFIC
OCEAN

NORTH
AMERICA

ATLANTIC
OCEAN

SOUTH
AMERICA

Head-Smashed-In,
Alberta

Meadowcroft, PA●
Cactus Hill, VA●
Folsom, NM●
Clovis, NM●
Topper, SC●
Aucilla River, FL●

Monte Verde,
CHILE

Ancient Ice-Age migration from Asia

— Present-day shore lines	— Land migration theory
— Ancient shore lines	— Pacific coast route theory
▨ Glacial ice sheets	● Key archaeological sites

Polar view shows that glaciers blocked movement
from Beringia (B) into North America (A) 20,000
years ago. By 14,000 years ago (large map) melting
had created an access corridor.

■ **MAP 1.1**

THE EARLIEST AMERICANS   The Ice Age ancestors of Native Americans crossed from Siberia when a land
bridge linked Asia and Alaska. Some probably migrated south along an ice-free corridor 14,000 years ago.
Others may have followed a Pacific coastal route, moving rapidly down the shores of North and South
America by boat, with frequent stops along an ancient coastline that is now submerged.

ancestors of modern humans moved from Africa to spread across the Eurasian landmass, the
area comprising Europe and Asia. These more recent forebears possessed well-developed language capacities and hunting skills.

By 40,000 years ago some of these Stone Age hunter–gatherers had already reached Australia, somehow crossing more than 40 miles of water. Others lived on the steppes of Central
Asia and the frozen tundra of Siberia. They had perfected the tools they needed to survive in
a cold climate: flint spear points for killing mammoths, reindeer, and the woolly rhinoceros;
and bone needles to sew warm, waterproof clothes out of animal skin.

Over thousands of years, bands of these northern hunters migrated east across Siberia
in search of game. Eventually they arrived at the region where the Bering Strait now sepa-
rates Russia from Alaska. The geography of this area has fluctuated over time because of
dramatic changes in global weather. Between 25,000 and 11,000 years ago, cold conditions
expanded arctic ice caps, trapping vast quantities of the earth's water in the form of huge
glaciers. As a result, ocean levels sank by 300 feet—enough to expose a bridge of land 600
miles wide between Asia and America.

The Bering Land Bridge formed part of a frigid, windswept region known as Beringia.
Small groups of people could have subsisted in this cold landscape by hunting mammoths
and musk oxen. As the climate warmed and the ocean rose again, some might have headed farther east onto higher ground in Alaska. If so, these newcomers would have been cut off permanently from Siberia as water once more submerged the land bridge. But the same warming
process also eventually opened a pathway through the glaciers blanketing northern America.
This opening could account for the sudden appearance of Clovis hunters across much of North
America nearly 14,000 years ago.

Geologists have shown that as Ice Age glaciers receded about 14,000 years ago, an ice-free corridor opened along the eastern slope of the Rocky Mountains. For decades, scholars have conjectured that small bands of people probably moved south from Alaska through that route. Presumably these hunters, armed with razor-sharp Clovis points, spread rapidly across the continent, destroying successive herds of large animals that had never faced human predators before. Perhaps, according to this theory, generations of hunters moved swiftly south as local game supplies dwindled. They would have migrated as far as the tip of South America within several thousand years.

The Newest Approaches

In recent decades, intriguing developments have complicated the picture. At Cactus Hill, Virginia, and Topper, South Carolina, archaeologists have uncovered artifacts suggesting the presence of immediate predecessors to the Clovis people. At Florida's Aucilla River, divers have recovered a 14,000-year-old cache of ivory and bone tools. Other pre-Clovis objects have surfaced at the Meadowcroft site southwest of Pittsburgh. The most provocative new discovery has come from South America. In an ancient campsite at Monte Verde, Chile, experts found knotted cords, and even a footprint, dating back more than 14,000 years.

Scholars agree that early inhabitants of North and South America—whether they arrived by land or sea—came primarily from distant Asian ancestry.

We know that travelers in the Paleolithic era reached Australia from the Asian landmass by water. Could other small groups have used a coastal route around the North Pacific rim to reach the Americas? If so, bands of so-called Paleo-Indians may have migrated in boats down the Northwest Coast, pausing to fish or gather food. Such seaborne journeys, stretching over generations, could help explain the rapid diffusion of humans into South America. Most of their campsites beside the Pacific would now be several hundred feet under water, for the rising oceans have since covered America's ancient coastlines. Perhaps Monte Verde, located on higher ground and preserved by a layer of peat moss, represents a revealing exception.

Meanwhile, genetic comparisons of different peoples, present and past, are yielding increasingly specific, if controversial, details about ancient migrations and interactions. Advances in understanding DNA—the genetic material that determines our physical make-up and transmits it to our offspring—may someday sharpen or change our awareness regarding Native American origins. To date, they have confirmed one basic conclusion of the physical anthropologists who have examined blood types, dental formation, and other evidence for years. Scholars agree that early inhabitants of North and South America—whether they arrived by land or sea—came primarily from distant Asian ancestry.

The Archaic World

Some 10,000 years ago, the Paleo-Indian era in North America gradually gave way to the Archaic era, which lasted for roughly 7000 years. Changes in wildlife played a large part in the transition. As the continent warmed further and the great glaciers receded north, more than 100 of America's largest species disappeared. These included mammoths, mastodons, horses, camels, and the great long-horned bison. Researchers debate whether these large animals were hunted to extinction, wiped out by disease, or destroyed by climate change.

Whatever the causes—and probably there were many—human groups had to adapt to the shifting conditions. They developed new methods of survival. Inhabitants turned to the smaller bison, similar to modern-day ones, that had managed to survive and flourish on the northern plains. Hunters learned to drive herds over cliffs and use the remains for food, clothing, and tools. One such bison jump is located in eastern Colorado. Another mass kill site, known as Head-Smashed-In, is in western Alberta; native peoples used it for 7000 years.

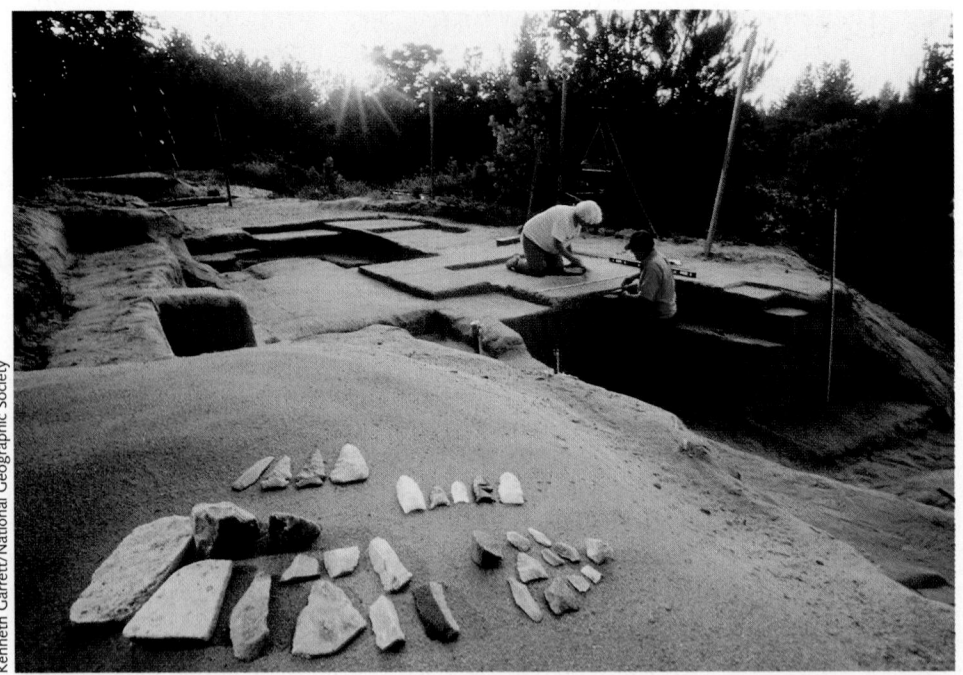

Kenneth Garrett/National Geographic Society

■ Archaeologists digging at Cactus Hill, Virginia, and several other sites have unearthed artifacts that suggest human habitation before the arrival of hunters using Clovis points. The foreground objects are laid out clockwise by apparent age, with the most recent at the top. Clovis-like spearheads appear in the second group. The third and fourth groups, taken from lower layers of soil, are thought to be older items, some reaching back well beyond 14,000 years. With the most primitive tools, it becomes difficult to separate implements made by humans from natural rock fragments.

A weighted spear-throwing device, called an atlatl, let hunters bring down medium-sized game. Archaic peoples also devised nets, hooks, and snares for catching birds, fish, and small animals. By 4000 years ago, they were even using duck decoys in the Great Basin of Utah and Nevada.

Though genetically similar, these far-flung bands of Archaic Indians developed diverse cultures as they adapted to very different landscapes and environments. Nothing illustrates this diversity more clearly than speech. A few early languages branched into numerous language families, then divided further into hundreds of separate languages. The Algonkian family of North American languages, which includes Wampanoag in the east and Cheyenne in the west, in turn has links to Choctaw, Chickasaw, and other southeastern languages of the Muskogean family. Similar cultural variations emerged in everything from diet and shelter to folklore and spiritual beliefs.

All of these variations reflected local conditions, and each represented an experiment that might potentially lead to more elaborate social arrangements. Among hunting and gathering societies, subsistence was a way of life, and people lived in small and widely dispersed groups, moving regularly to take advantage of seasonal food sources. As a result, their social structure remained very simple. Eventually in the Americas, as elsewhere, the cultivation of domesticated plants led to settled horticultural societies. A more stable food supply allowed the creation of surpluses, prompting larger permanent villages, wider trade, and a greater accumulation of goods. With this settled lifestyle came greater social stratification and the emergence of hereditary chiefdoms.

Frequently, a class of priests appeared near the top of the expanding hierarchy, mediating between the people and a god or gods who were intimately involved in human affairs. And slaves, unknown in hunting and gathering societies, appeared at the bottom of the hierarchy, since captives could be put to work for their conquerors, and an expanded population meant an increased labor force, not only to produce more food but also to create the public works that demonstrated, and enhanced, the power of the chiefs and priests. As the social structures became more complex, greater specialization ensued, allowing the development of more extensive communities with more elaborate political and religious activities and greater concentrations of power. But such developments were slow and uneven, depending on local conditions.

The Rise of Maize Agriculture

One condition remained common to all the various Archaic American groups, despite their emerging regional differences: they all shared a lack of domesticated animals. Diverse peoples living in the Eurasian landmass had managed to domesticate five important species—sheep, goats, pigs, cows, and horses—by 6000 years ago, leading to the creation of stable pastoral societies. But none of these mammals existed in the Americas, nor did camels, donkeys, or water buffalo. Archaic Indians, like their Asian forebears, did possess dogs, and settlers in the Andes domesticated the llama over 5000 years ago. Herds of buffalo and deer could be followed, and even managed and exploited in various ways. But no mammal remaining in the Americas could readily be made to provide humans with milk, meat, hides, and hauling power.

Although their prospects for domesticating animals were severely limited, early Americans had many more options when it came to the domestication of plants. Humans managed to domesticate plants independently in five different areas around the world, and three of those regions were located in the Americas. First, across parts of South America, inhabitants learned to cultivate root crops of potatoes and manioc (also known as cassava, which yields a nutritious starch). Second, in Mesoamerica (modern-day Mexico and Central America), people gradually brought squash, beans, and maize (corn) under cultivation—three foods that complement one another effectively in dietary terms.

Maize agriculture became a crucial ingredient for the growth of complex societies in the Americas, but its development and diffusion took time. Unlike wheat, the Eurasian cereal crop which offered a high yield from the start, maize took thousands of years of cultivation in the Americas to evolve into an extremely productive food source. Moreover, most of Eurasia stretches east-west through a temperate climate that fosters the spread of similar agriculture. Because of this similarity of climate, a crop that succeeds in one place can readily be grown in another. The western hemisphere, in contrast, lies on a north-south axis; the Americas stretch through numerous different climate zones. Some experts speculate that this geographical fact of life made crop diffusion more difficult. For example, the differences between Mesoamerica and North America proved substantial when it came to mastering maize agriculture. Southwestern Indians in North America began growing thumb-sized ears of maize only about three thousand years ago (at a time of increasing rainfall), well after the crop had taken hold in Mesoamerica. More than a thousand years later, maize reached eastern North America, where it adapted slowly to the cooler climate and shorter growing season.

Southwestern Indians in North America began growing thumb-sized ears of maize only about three thousand years ago.

In the east, a different agriculture had already taken hold, centered on other once-wild plants. This was the third zone where the independent domestication of plants occurred in the Americas. As early as 4000 years ago, eastern Indians at dozens of Archaic sites were cultivating domesticated squash and sunflowers. The latter yielded edible seeds, as did several less familiar plants. Sumpweed, or marsh elder, flourished near lakes and rivers and produced an oily seed. Goosefoot, knotweed, and maygrass all produced starchy seeds that have been found near Archaic sites in Kentucky, Illinois, and elsewhere. These domesticated plants provided supplemental food sources for eastern communities that continued to subsist primarily by hunting and gathering until the arrival introduction of maize agriculture into the eastern woodlands during the first millennium A.D.

About 3000 years ago, as maize cultivation began in the Southwest and gardens of squash and sunflowers appeared in the Northeast, the first of several powerful Mesoamerican cultures—the Olmecs—emerged in the lowlands along the southwestern edge of the Gulf of Mexico. Their name meant "those who live in the land of rubber," for they had learned how to turn the milky juice of several plants into an unusual elastic substance. The Olmecs grew maize and manioc in abundance, and their surplus of food supported a hierarchical society. Its leaders built large burial mounds and pyramids, and they erected distinctive stone monuments—huge heads standing five to nine feet high. The Olmecs, who revered the jaguar in their religion, developed a complex calendar and played a distinctive game with a large ball of solid rubber. Since they traded widely with people across Mesoamerica, they passed on these cultural traits, which reappeared later in other societies in the region.

Olmec traders, traveling by coastal canoe, may even have encountered and influenced the Poverty Point culture that existed near the lower Mississippi River 4,200 to 2,700 years ago. Numerous late Archaic locations near the Gulf Coast shed light on Poverty Point culture. It takes its name from the largest of these sites—a 500-acre complex in northeast Louisiana first rediscovered through aerial photography in the mid-twentieth century. Since then, archaeologists have determined that workers constructed Poverty Point between 3,500 and 2,700 years ago. This religious and political center consists of a vast semicircle of six concentric earthen ridges that span four-fifths of a mile. Researchers estimate that the complex required three million worker-hours to build. Each ridge, more than 80 feet wide and 8 feet high, may have served to raise human dwellings above the flood plain.

The Poverty Point culture, with its trade network on the lower Mississippi and its tributaries, stands as a mysterious precursor to the mound-building societies of the Mississippi Valley that emerged much later. (In a similar way, the Olmecs prefigured the later Mayan, Toltec, and Aztec cultures in Mesoamerica.) Remnants of these more extensive Mississippian cultures still existed when newcomers from Europe arrived to stay, around A.D. 1500. But in many parts of North America, smaller and less stratified Archaic cultures, that combined hunting for a variety of animals with gathering and processing local plant foods, remained intact well into the era of European colonization.

A Thousand Years of Change: A.D. 500 to 1500

The millennium stretching from the fifth century to the explorations of Columbus in the fifteenth century witnessed dramatic and far-reaching changes in the separate world of the Americas. In the warm and temperate regions on both sides of the equator, empires rose and fell as maize agriculture and elaborate irrigation systems provided food surpluses, allowing the creation of cities and the emergence of hierarchical societies.

On the coast of Peru, for example, the Moche people excelled in delicate gold work, intricate pottery, and bright weavings made from domesticated cotton. The Moches built huge pyramids to honor the sun, and their realm prospered for centuries. But around A.D. 800 it collapsed suddenly, perhaps a victim of the periodic disturbance in Pacific weather known as El Niño.

In the 1400s, centuries after the Moches and their neighbors disappeared, the expansive Inca empire emerged in their place. Inca emperors, ruling from the capital at Cuzco, prompted the construction of a vast road system throughout the Peruvian Andes. Stonemasons built large storage facilities at provincial centers to hold food for garrisons of soldiers and to store tribute items such as gold and feathers destined for the capital. Until the empire's fall in the 1530s, officials leading pack trains of llamas ferried goods to and from Cuzco along mountainous roadways.

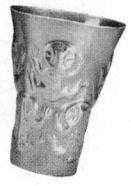

Similarly, Mesoamerica also saw a series of impressive civilizations—from the Mayans to the Aztecs—in the millennium spanning A.D. 500 to 1500 in the western calendar. Developments in North America in the same millennium were very different but bear enough resemblance to patterns in Mesoamerica to raise intriguing and still unanswerable questions. Did significant migrations northward from Mesoamerica ever take place? And if not, were there substantial trade links at times, allowing distinctive materials, techniques, ideas, and seeds to reach North American peoples? Or did the continent's distinctive societies, such as the Anasazi in the Southwest and the Cahokia mound builders on the Mississippi River, develop almost entirely independently? Not surprisingly, North American archaeologists continue to debate the extent of possible links to Mesoamerica in the centuries before Columbus.

Valleys of the Sun: The Mesoamerican Empires

In Mesoamerica, the Mayans and the Aztecs established rich empires where worship of the sun was central to their religious beliefs. Mayan culture flourished between A.D. 300 and 900. The Mayans controlled a domain stretching from the lowlands of the Yucatan peninsula to the highlands of what is now southern Mexico, Guatemala, Honduras, and El Salvador—an area half the size of Texas. They derived their elaborate calendar—a 52-year cycle made up of 20-day months—and many other aspects of their culture from the earlier Olmecs, but they devised their own distinctive civilization.

The Mayan people built huge stone temples and held ritual bloodletting ceremonies to appease their gods. They also constructed narrow courts for a ball game—which some Mexicans still play—where opposing players hit a rubber ball with their hips. Recently, researchers have deciphered the complex glyphs that appear throughout Mayan art. These pictographs are yielding detailed information and precise dates for individual rulers. The Mayans, like the Moches in Peru, declined mysteriously, and dominance in Mesoamerica moved farther west, where great cities arose in the highlands of Central Mexico, first at Teotihuacan and then nearby at Tenochtitlán, the capital of the powerful but short-lived Aztec empire.

The people who constructed the metropolis of Teotihuacan in the Mexican highlands remain an enigma. They appear to have traded with the Mayans and perhaps with the Olmecs before that. They laid out their immense city in a grid, dominated by the 200-foot Pyramid of the Sun. By A.D. 500, the city held more than 100,000 inhabitants, making it one of the largest in the world. But Teotihuacan's society declined fast, for unknown reasons, succeeded first by the Toltecs and then by the Aztecs.

Eager to expand their empire and to extend their rule, the Aztecs launched fierce wars against neighboring lands.

The Aztecs (or Mexicas) had migrated to the central Valley of Mexico from the north in the twelfth century. Looked down upon at first by the local people, they swiftly rose to power through strategic alliances and military skill. According to legend, the Aztecs' war god instructed their priests to locate the place where a great eagle perched on a cactus. They found such a spot, on a swampy island in Lake Texcoco. By the 1400s the Aztecs had transformed the island into Tenochtitlán, an imposing urban center, located on the site of modern Mexico City.

The impressive city of Tenochtitlán, surrounded by Lake Texcoco and linked to shore by causeways, became the Aztec capital. Its architecture imitated the ruined temple city of Teotihuacan, which lay 35 miles to the north, and exceeded it in grandeur. The Aztecs also adopted many other features of the cultures they had displaced. They used the cyclical 52-year Mesoamerican calendar, and they worshipped the great god Quetzalcoatl, the plumed serpent associated with wind and revered by the Toltecs, their predecessors in the Valley of Mexico.

Schooled in hardship, pessimism, and violence, the Aztecs saw themselves as living in the World of the Fifth Sun, a final human era destined to end in cataclysm just as earlier epochs had. Eager to expand their empire and to extend their rule as long as possible, they launched fierce wars against neighboring lands. But their primary objective was not to kill enemies or gain more territory. Instead, Aztec warriors demanded tribute and took prisoners from the people they subdued. They then sacrificed numerous captives at pyramid temples to placate the gods. These deities, they believed, would in turn protect them as they conducted further wars of capture, leading to more tribute and sacrifices.

The Aztecs' grim cycle of conflict helped them ward off deep fears of extended drought and lasting destruction. But it also weakened their expanding realm. Like the Incas of Peru, the Aztecs imposed harsh treatment on the peoples they conquered, extracting heavy annual tributes. This harsh policy alienated the provinces from the Aztecs and made their centralized empire vulnerable to external attack. When a foreign assault prompted their downfall in the early sixteenth century, it came from a direction the Aztec priests and generals could not predict.

The Anasazi: Chaco Canyon and Mesa Verde

The great urban centers of Peru and Mesoamerica had no counterparts farther north. The peoples inhabiting North America in the millennium before Columbus never developed the levels of social stratification, urban dynamism, architectural grandeur, astronomical study, or intensive corn agriculture that characterized the Mayans, Incas, or Aztecs. Yet elements of all these traits appeared in North America, especially in the Southwest and the Mississippi valley, with the emergence of increasingly settled societies and widening circles of exchange.

Modern scholars wonder whether the maize, squash, and bean agriculture, sun worship, and astronomical knowledge found among North America's southwestern peoples had roots farther south. After all, the Aztecs' ancestors had apparently migrated down from this dry region to the interior of Mexico after A.D. 1100. Could other north–south movements back and forth have occurred, earlier or later, between Central Mexico and the American Southwest? Links of migration or trade would help to explain the dozens of ancient ball courts, similar to those in Mesoamerica, that archaeologists have excavated in Arizona. Recently, researchers have identified a north–south traffic in turquoise, highly prized in both Mexico and the Southwest.

Three identifiably different cultures were already well established in the North American Southwest by A.D. 500. The Mogollons occupied the dry, mountainous regions of eastern Arizona and southern New Mexico. Mogollon women were expert potters who crafted delicate bowls from the fine clay of the Mimbres River. Families lived in sunken pit houses that were cool in summer and warm in winter. The Hohokams, their neighbors to the west in south-central Arizona, did the same. The Hohokams also constructed extensive canal and floodgate systems to irrigate their fields from the Gila and Salt rivers. According to their Native American successors, who still dwell in the Phoenix area, the name *Hohokam* means "those who have gone."

Farther north, in what is now the Four Corners Region, where Utah and Colorado meet Arizona and New Mexico, lived the people remembered as the Anasazi, or "ancient ones." By A.D. 750 the Anasazi inhabited aboveground houses clustered around a central ceremonial room dug into the earth. They entered this circular space by descending a ladder through the roof. The climb back up from this sunken chamber, known as a kiva, symbolized the initial ascent of humans into the Upper World from below. European explorers used the Spanish word for town, *pueblo,* to describe the Anasazis' multiroom and multistory dwellings of masonry or adobe.

Beginning in the 850s, Chaco Canyon in the San Juan River basin of northwest New Mexico emerged as the hub of the Anasazi world. Wide, straight roads radiating out from Chaco let builders haul hundreds of thousands of logs for use as roof beams in the nine great pueblos that still dot the canyon. The largest of them, Pueblo Bonito, rises five stories high in places and has 600 rooms arranged in a vast semicircle. Yet the canyon's population remained small,

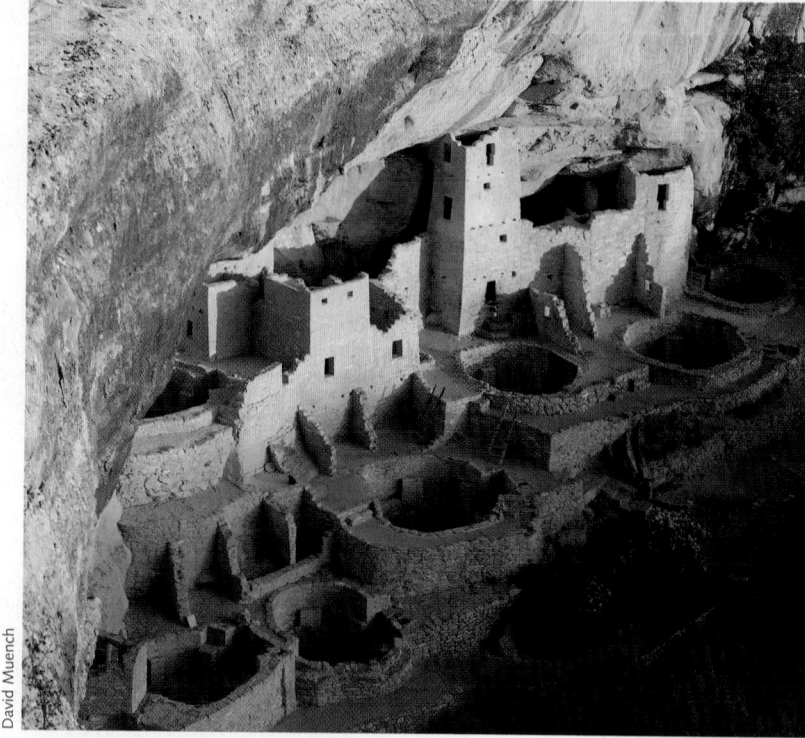

David Muench

■ Cliff Palace, at Mesa Verde National Park in southwest Colorado, was created 900 years ago, when the Anasazi left the mesa tops and moved into more secure and inaccessible cliff dwellings. Facing southwest, the building gained heat from the rays of the low afternoon sun in winter, and overhanging rock protected the structure from rain, snow, and the hot midday summer sun. The numerous round kivas, each covered with a flat roof originally, suggest that Cliff Palace may have had a ceremonial importance.

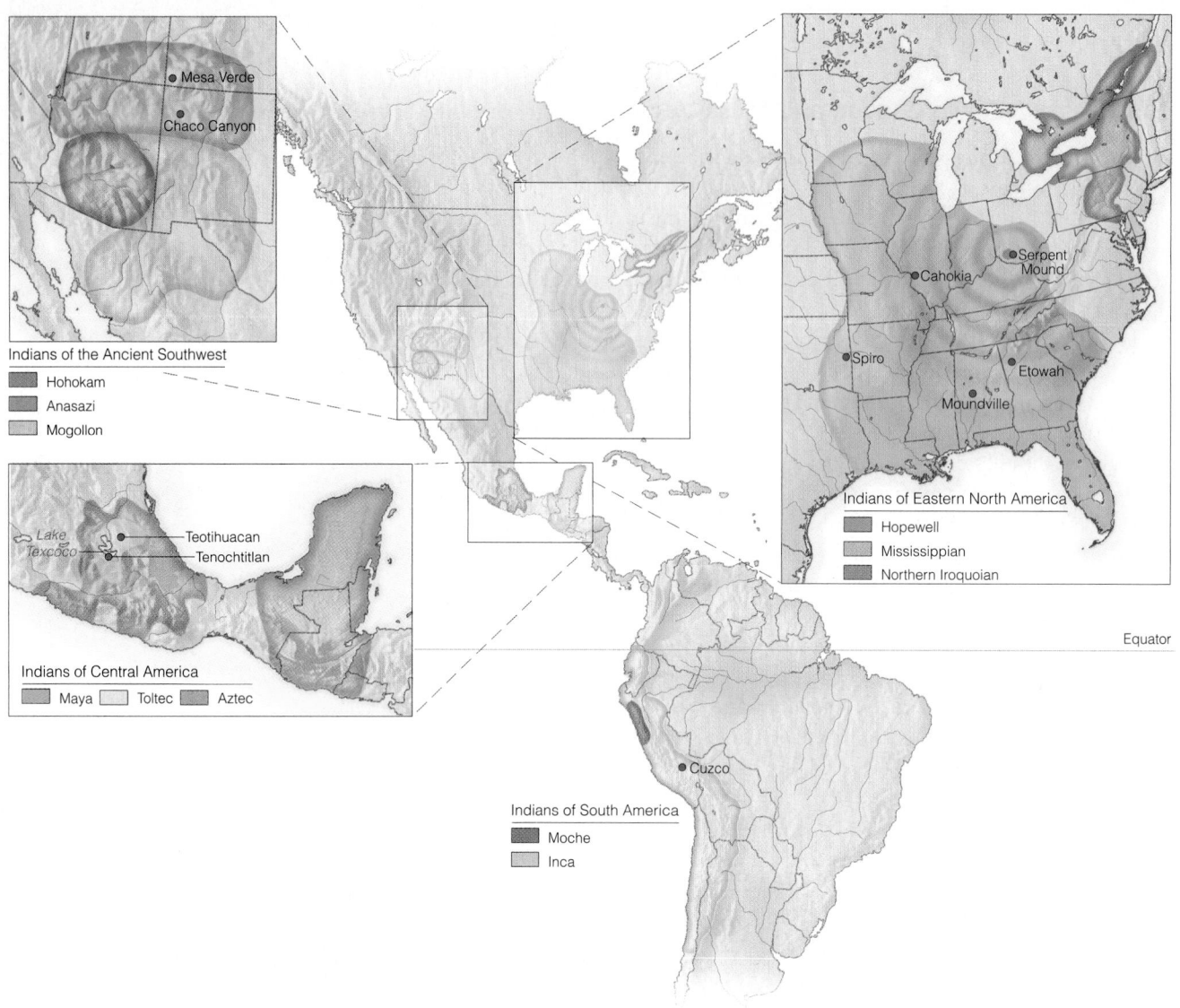

■ MAP 1.2

AMERICA IN THE MILLENNIUM BEFORE COLUMBUS, A.D. 500–1500   A number of distinctive cultures emerged in the Americas during the ten centuries before 1500. Most learned from their predecessors—Mississippians from Hopewells and Aztecs from Mayans, for example—but debate continues over the full extent of trade and travel networks at any given time.

perhaps dominated by priestly rulers who used violence to extract labor, food, and tribute from the region's inhabitants.

Violence and warfare played a significant part in Anasazi life, as they did in the Mesoamerican world of the same era. But in the end, environmental change exerted the greatest destructive force. Tree rings show that after 1130, a drought gripped the Colorado Plateau for half a century. The turquoise workshops of Chaco Canyon fell silent. Most of the inhabitants moved away. Some no doubt headed north, where dozens of Anasazi communities with access to better farming conditions dotted the landscape. Earlier, they had resided atop mesas (from the Spanish word meaning "table," for the region's distinctive hills with steep sides and level tops). But gradually—with populations growing, the climate worsening, and competition for resources stiffening—they moved into sheltered cliff dwellings built into the mesa walls. Cliff Palace at Mesa Verde in southwestern Colorado, with its 220 rooms and 23 kivas, remains the most famous today because of its ready access and careful preservation. Yet other sites were even larger. Reached only by ladders and steep trails, these pueblos offered protection from enemies and shelter from the scorching summer sun. Still, another prolonged drought (1276–1299) forced the Anasazi to move once again by 1300. Survivors dispersed south into lands later occupied by the Hopi, Zuni, and Rio Grande peoples.

The Mississippians: Cahokia and Moundville

Earlier, in the Mississippi Valley, the Hopewell people had prospered for half a millennium before A.D. 500 (in the era of the Roman Empire in Europe). The Hopewell lived primarily in southern Ohio and western Illinois. But their network of trade extended over much of the continent. Archaeologists excavating ornate Hopewell burial sites have found a wide array of objects, including pipestone and flint from the Missouri River Valley, copper and silver from Lake Superior, mica and quartz from Appalachia, sea shells and shark teeth from Florida, and artwork made from Rocky Mountain obsidian and grizzly-bear teeth. Hopewell trading laid the groundwork for larger mound-building societies, known as the Mississippian cultures that emerged in the Mississippi Valley and the Southeast in roughly the same centuries as the great Mesoamerican civilizations and the Anasazi in the Southwest.

The more elaborate and widespread Mississippian tradition developed gradually after A.D. 500. Then after A.D. 900, it flourished broadly for six centuries. Shifts in technology and agriculture facilitated the rise of the Mississippians.

Bows and arrows, long used in arctic regions of North America but little known elsewhere, began to see widespread use in the eastern woodlands around A.D. 700. At the same time, maize underwent a transformation from a marginal oddity to a central staple crop. Growers as far east as northern Florida were producing it by the eighth century, and it soon appeared farther north with the spread of a more hardy variety. By 1300, maize and bean agriculture reached all the way to the Iroquoian peoples around Lake Ontario and in the St. Lawrence River valley. Across the east, food supplies expanded as Native American communities planted corn in the rich bottomland soil along the region's many rivers. More and more people began settling in these fertile areas. Maize agriculture also spurred bureaucracy and hierarchy. With greater productivity, commercial and religious elites asserted greater control over farmers to take advantage of the community's expanding resources.

The extent of contacts, rivalries, and exchanges between separate Mississippian mound-building centers remains uncertain. Mississippian sites have been found as far apart as Spiro, in eastern Oklahoma, and Etowah, in northern Georgia. The largest complex was at Cahokia in American Bottom, the 25-mile floodplain below where the Illinois and Missouri rivers flow into the Mississippi. We will never know Cahokia's full extent, for city planners expanding St. Louis in the nineteenth century flattened more than two dozen mounds on the Mississippi's west bank, leaving little record of their work. Across the river, builders in East St. Louis, Illinois, and farmers eager to increase their acreage leveled more mounds. But nearby, on Cahokia Creek, dozens of rectangular, flat-topped temple mounds still remain after almost a thousand years. The largest mound at Cahokia—indeed, the largest ancient earthwork in North America—rises 100 feet in four separate levels, covering 16 acres and using nearly 22 million cubic feet of earth. A log palisade with gates and watchtowers once enclosed this temple mound and its adjacent plaza in a 200-acre central compound. In a separate construction nearby, residents used engineering and astronomy skills to erect 48 posts in a huge circle, 410 feet in diameter. This creation, now called Woodhenge after England's Stonehenge, functioned as a calendar to mark the daily progression of the sun throughout each year.

The largest mound at Cahokia—indeed, the largest ancient earthwork in North America—rises 100 feet in four separate levels.

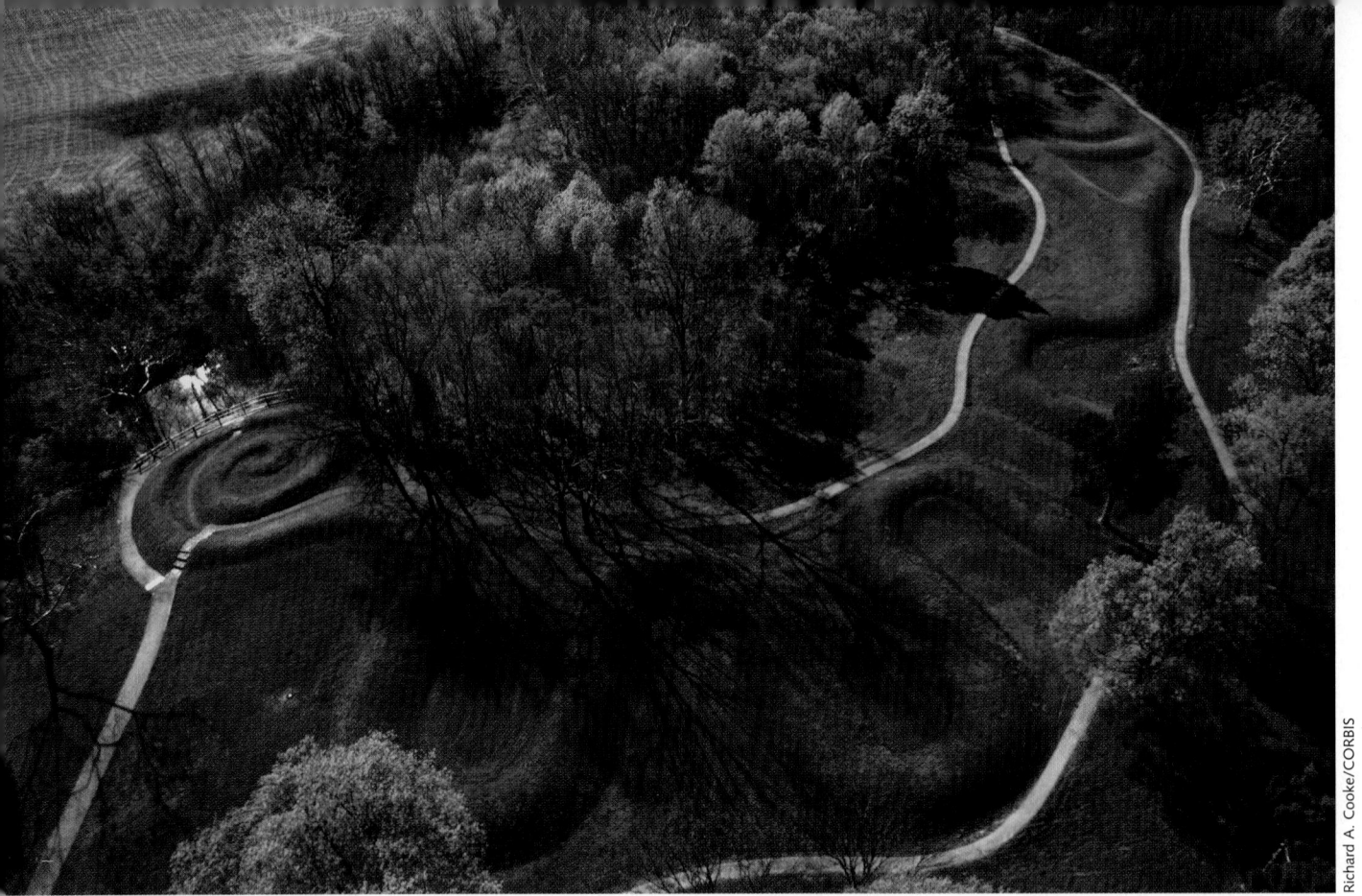

■ The most striking Mississippian earthwork to survive is the enigmatic Serpent Mound, built in the eleventh century by the Fort Ancient people in southern Ohio. The snake (holding an egg in its mouth) has links to astronomy because its curves are aligned toward key positions of the sun. The serpent may even represent Halley's Comet, which blazed in the heavens in A.D. 1066. Completely uncoiled, the earthwork would measure more than a quarter mile in length.

Cahokia's mounds rose quickly in the decades after A.D. 1050, as the local population expanded beyond 10,000. A succession of powerful leaders reorganized the vicinity's small, isolated villages into a strong regional chiefdom that controlled towns on both sides of the river. These towns provided the chiefdom's centralized elite with food, labor, and goods for trading. The elaborate religious rituals and the wealth and power of the leaders are seen in a burial site opened by archaeologists in the 1970s. The body of one prominent figure, presumably a chief, was laid out on a surface of 20,000 shell beads. Near him lay six young adults who must have been relatives or servants sacrificed at the ruler's funeral. They were supplied with hundreds of stone arrowheads—finely chipped and neatly sorted—plus antler projectile points, a rolled tube of sheet copper, bushels of glistening mica (a transparent mineral crystallized into very thin sheets), and 15 stone disks used in the popular spear-throwing game known as chunkey. Archaeologists found further evidence of sacrifice nearby. They uncovered the remains of four men, whose heads and hands had been cut off, and a pit filled with nearly four dozen young women who apparently had been strangled.

The population of Cahokia perhaps exceeded 15,000 people around A.D. 1100. It then waned steadily over the next two centuries as the unstable hierarchy lost its sway over nearby villages. As Cahokia declined, other regional chiefdoms rose along other rivers. The most notable appeared at Moundville in west-central Alabama, 15 miles south of modern Tuscaloosa. A century of archaeological work at this site has revealed clear phases of development after A.D. 900. First, the inhabitants adopted corn agriculture. This in turn allowed them to intensify craft production, and a budding elite emerged. Before long, the leaders directed the creation of mounds in several small villages. Shortly before 1250, workers laid out an 80-acre rectangular plaza at the Moundville site. They began construction on more than 20 flat-topped mounds (some larger than football fields), which provided dwelling sites and burial locations for the small ruling class. Excavated burial objects—ceremonial axes, beads carved from conch shells, and distinctive copper spools worn as giant earrings—reveal evidence of long-distance trade and elaborate rituals. But by 1400, Moundville had started to lose its grip as a dominant ceremonial center. The causes of this decline remain unclear, but once again small villages became the norm.

Linking the Continents

Estimates vary widely, but probably around one-sixth of the world's population—as many as 60 to 70 million people—resided in the Americas when Columbus arrived in 1492. Most of them lived near the equator, where their ancient ancestors had developed efficient forms of tropical agriculture. But roughly one-tenth of the hemisphere's population (6 to 7 million people) was spread across North America from coast to coast.

We cannot rule out the appearance in America of ancient ocean travelers on occasion. Around A.D. 400, Polynesian mariners sailed their double-hulled canoes from the Marquesas Islands in the South Pacific to the Hawaiian archipelago. Conceivably, in the millennium before 1500, one or two boats from Africa, Ireland, Polynesia, China, or Japan sailed—or were blown—to the American mainland. But any survivors of such a journey would have had little genetic or cultural impact, for no sustained back-and-forth contact between the societies occurred. Even the seafaring Norse from Scandinavia, known as Vikings, whose brief settlement on Canadian soil a thousand years ago is now well documented, remained for only a few years and never established a lasting colony. Native American societies, therefore, knew nothing of the people, plants, animals, and viruses of the Eastern Hemisphere.

America's near isolation ended dramatically, beginning in the late fifteenth century, after innovations in deep-sea sailing opened the world's oceans as a new frontier for human exploration. Chinese sailors in the North Pacific or Portuguese mariners in the South Atlantic could well have been the first outsiders to establish ongoing contact with the peoples of the Western Hemisphere. But instead, it was Christopher Columbus, an Italian navigator in the service of Spain, who became the agent of this sweeping change. He encountered the Americas by accident and misinterpreted what he had found. But his chance encounter with a separate realm would spark new patterns of human migration, cultural transfer, and ecological exchange, which would reshape the modern world.

The Vikings Reach Newfoundland and Beyond

Scandinavian settlers had colonized Ireland in the 830s and Iceland in the 870s. A century later, these Norse seafarers—led by Erik the Red—reached Greenland in the 980s. When Erik's son, Leif, learned that Vikings blown off course had sighted land farther west, he sailed from Greenland to the North American coast. Here he explored a region near the Gulf of St. Lawrence that he named Vinland. Around A.D. 1000, Leif Eriksson's relatives directed several return voyages to Vinland, where the Vikings built an outpost called Straumfjord. The tiny colony of 160 people, including women and children, lived and grazed livestock in Vinland for several years until native peoples drove them away.

For centuries, this Norse contact was known only through epic Icelandic tales called the Vinland Sagas—medieval transcriptions of oral traditions. But in the 1960s archaeologists found Viking artifacts at L'Anse aux Meadows, a coastal site in northern Newfoundland. Perhaps this secure base, today reconstructed with Viking-style sod houses, was Straumfjord. Researchers believe that Norsemen returned occasionally to cut timber and that they traded with inhabitants of northeastern Canada for generations.

For three centuries, the Viking community in Greenland endured. The Norse settlers shipped walrus tusks and hunting falcons to Europe in return for farm tools and livestock. But trade slumped in Europe after the plague known as the Black Death swept away a third of the continent's population around 1350. Other factors made the settlement less viable as well. Climate changes brought colder, wetter weather, and conflict increased with Inuit natives. Soil erosion, caused by tree-cutting and overgrazing of sheep, goats, and cattle, also took a toll. By 1450 Viking settlements in Greenland had died out completely. Whether sailors elsewhere in Europe knew much about Norse exploits in the North Atlantic remains shrouded in mystery.

Oceanic Travel and the Beginnings of Globalization

What Europeans did know, vaguely, was the existence of the distant Chinese Empire. They called the realm Cathay, a term used by Italian merchant Marco Polo, who journeyed from Venice across Asia along the fabled Silk Road in the 1270s. Polo returned to Italy in 1292 to publish his *Travels*, an account of adventures in China during the reign of Kublai Khan. He told of many things unknown to Europeans, including rocks that burned like wood (coal) and spices that preserved meat. Lacking winter fodder for their herds, Europe's farmers regularly slaughtered numerous cattle in the fall and pickled or salted the beef to preserve it. Asian spices such as nutmeg, cinnamon, pepper, ginger, and cloves, if they could be obtained, would offer new preservatives. When renewed Islamic power in the Middle East cut off the Silk Road to Cathay, Europeans searched for other ways to reach that far-off region.

The desire to obtain oriental spices at their source fueled European oceanic exploration, leading eventually to the transformation of the Americas, yet it was China, not Europe, that first mastered ocean sailing. In 1281, during Marco Polo's sojourn in Beijing, Kublai Khan's formidable navy sailed with 4500 ships to invade Japan, only to fall victim to a huge typhoon en route. Still, China increased its deep-sea commerce with Southeast Asia, India, and the Persian Gulf. Chinese strength in overseas exploration and trade reached its height in the early fifteenth century under Admiral Zheng He (pronounced "Jung Huh"). Between 1405 and 1433, this brilliant officer led seven large fleets to the Indian Ocean, sailing as far as east Africa. His squadron included immense treasure ships 400 feet long and equipped with 24 cannon.

Then, abruptly, China turned away from the sea, losing its opportunity to become the first global maritime power and to play a leading role in shaping oceanic trade and the destiny of North America. Within a century of Zheng He's accomplishments, the empire grew dismissive of foreign trade and turned inward. Chinese officials destroyed the log books of earlier voyages and curtailed production of oceangoing vessels. Instead of powerful China on the Pacific, it was tiny Portugal, overlooking the Atlantic from the Iberian peninsula, that emerged as the leader in maritime innovation and exploration in the fifteenth century.

Geography and religious zeal helped to spur Portugal's unlikely rise to world prominence. The tiny country faced the sea at the crossroads between Mediterranean commerce and the coastal traffic of Northern Europe. This strategic location also exposed Portugal to the ongoing conflict between Christianity and Islam. The religion founded by Muhammad (born at Mecca in 570) had spread rapidly across North Africa from Arabia. By the eighth century, followers of Islam (known as Muslims, Moslems, or Moors) had crossed the Straits of Gibraltar to establish a kingdom in southern Spain. Centuries later, Spanish and Portuguese Christians rallied to force Islam out of the Iberian peninsula—a campaign that concluded in 1492—and to join other militant Europeans in fighting against Islamic power in the Middle East.

When Christian crusades to the holy land failed to defeat Islam and reopen overland trade routes to China, European strategists dreamed of skirting Africa by sea to reach Asia. The Portuguese were well positioned to lead this flanking movement around Islam. And if no such oceanic route to Asia existed, some speculated that Portuguese exploration south beyond the Sahara Desert, along the coast of sub-Saharan Africa, still might yield contact with strong Chris-

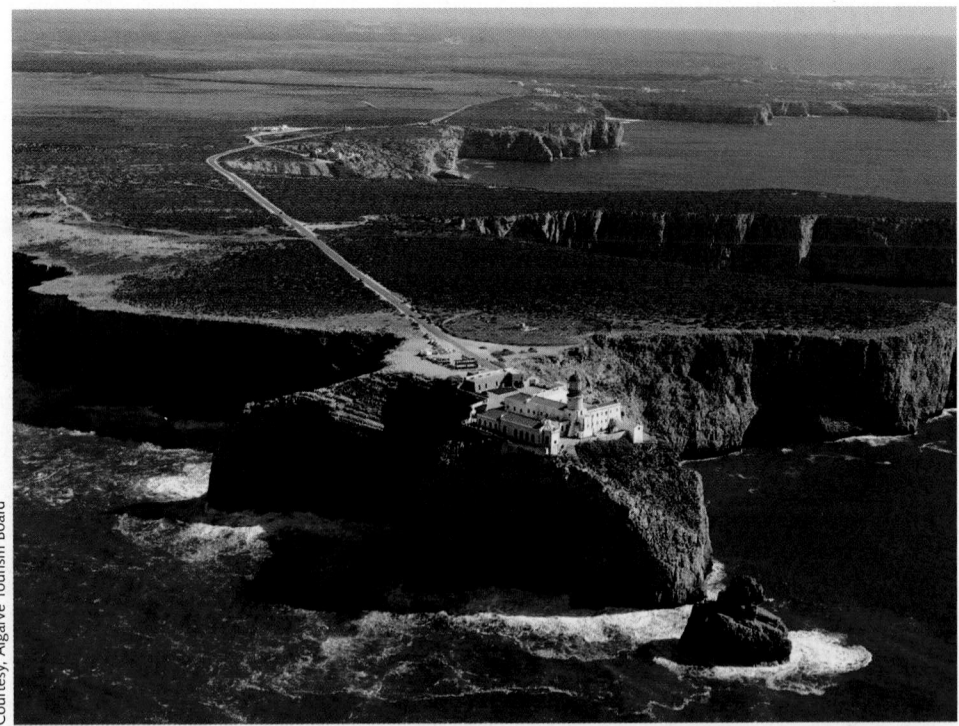

Courtesy, Algarve Tourism Board

■ **Prince Henry of Portugal rarely went to sea himself. Instead, he established a base at Sagres, overlooking the Atlantic Ocean. From here, beginning in 1418, he sent mariners south along the African coast. They quickly laid claim to the islands of the eastern Atlantic, and by the 1440s they had initiated trade along the west African coast, carrying gold and slaves back to Portugal.**

tian allies. For generations, Europeans had fostered legends of a wealthy kingdom somewhere in Africa, said to be ruled by a black Christian known as Prester John. Even if Prester John's imaginary realm could not be found, probes south from the Iberian Peninsula in ships might explore the full extent of Islamic influence in Africa and seek out fresh converts to Christianity.

Intellectual and economic motives also existed for these ventures. Such journeys could boost European knowledge of the unknown, based upon observations of the real world, and they might well open new markets for trade if technical difficulties could be overcome. The Portuguese had fished and traded in Atlantic coastal waters and the Mediterranean for ages, but long voyages far from land presented new challenges in shipbuilding and navigation. The first step involved an investment of leadership and resources, before early efforts could bear fruit and give the exploration process a momentum of it own.

Prince Henry of Portugal (1394–1460) provided these initial ingredients. The young prince—later honored as "Henry the Navigator"—had been appointed by the pope to head Portugal's military Order of Christ, an elite and wealthy organization of knights committed to the campaign against Islam. In 1415, at age 22, he crossed the Straits of Gibraltar to fight Muslims at Ceuta in North Africa. For the next 45 years, Henry waged a religiously inspired crusade-at-sea. He built his headquarters at Sagres in southwest Portugal. The center overlooked the ocean near Cape St. Vincent, the western tip of Europe. From there, his sailors launched a far-reaching revolution in human communication and trade, perhaps the most momentous single step in a globalization process that continues to the present day.

Henry's small ships, known as caravels, pushed south along the African coast. Innovative in design, caravels boasted narrow hulls, deep keels, and high gunwales for ocean sailing. Most importantly, they used triangular lateen sails, an idea that Mediterranean sailors had borrowed from Arab boats on the Red Sea. The lateen sail let a vessel travel into the breeze, tacking back and forth on a zigzag course against a prevailing wind; traditional square sails could not do this. Henry's experts at Sagres also drew on the work of Jewish cartographers from the island of Majorca to develop state-of-the-art charts, astronomical tables, and navigational instruments. His captains mastered the winds and currents off western Africa, but when he died in 1460, they

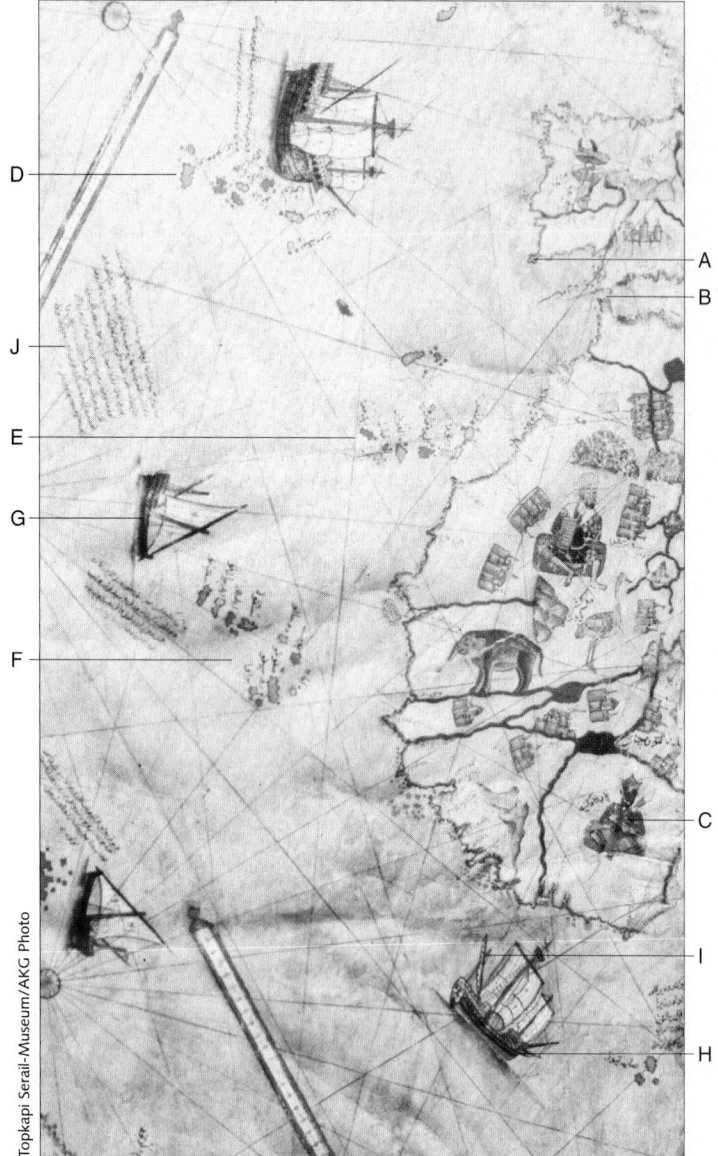

Topkapi Serail-Museum/AKG Photo

■ **This Atlantic chart illustrates key aspects of Portuguese success in overseas exploration.** Cape St. Vincent (A) where Prince Henry built his headquarters at Sagres, lies near the Strait of Gibraltar (B), the narrow entrance to the Mediterranean Sea. As Henry's mariners explored along the African coast for a sea passage to Asia, they also looked for possible allies such as Prester John, a mythical black king (C). They used the island groups of the eastern Atlantic to check their position: Azores (D), Madeiras (E), Canaries (F). Their small caravels (G) adopted the triangular lateen sail seen on traditional Arab boats in the Red Sea. Larger square-rigged ships that later sailed from Portugal to India (H) also incorporated lateen sails on a mast at the stern (I). A skilled Turkish navigator—who had never sailed on the Atlantic—made this unusual map in 1513. Piri Re'is used charts captured from a Christian ship in the Mediterranean; his inscriptions (J) are in Turkish.

had only sailed as far as what is now Sierra Leone. While skeptics wondered when the expensive ventures would see a tangible payoff, optimists noted that the African coast near Sierra Leone trended to the east and might eventually lead to Asia, despite the teaching of ancient scholars that no such route existed.

The early voyages during Henry's lifetime launched two developments that would have a lasting impact on the world. First, the Portuguese pioneered the course of European overseas colonization that would continue unabated for centuries. The harsh process began with the European discovery of three island groups off Northwest Africa— the Canaries, the Madeiras, and the Azores. Settlers sent to these islands from Portugal killed the native peoples; introduced crops such as sugar for export; and imported thousands of laborers to plant and process the sugar cane.

Second, in the 1440s Portuguese mariners initiated the Atlantic slave trade. They began by seizing people who lived on the coast of West Africa and deporting them to the new Atlantic sugar islands. Portuguese captains also carried slaves back to Europe and sold them there to supplement the growing sub-Saharan trade in ivory and gold. Africans themselves already had their own domestic slave trade. But this new Atlantic traffic, which grew relentlessly, eventually proved far more elaborate and devastating.

Looking for the Indies: da Gama and Columbus

During the 1480s, following a war with Spain, the Portuguese continued their African designs. In 1482 they erected a trading fort called Elmina Castle on the Gold Coast (modern Ghana) to guard against Spanish competition and to support exploration toward the east. But they soon encountered a new obstacle: Africa's long coastline turned abruptly south and continued in that direction for a vast distance. This led Portuguese captains below the equator, where they observed strange new constellations of stars in the night sky. Rather than sailing directly east toward China, as they had hoped, they had entered the unfamiliar Southern Hemisphere for the first time. Several years later, they reached the vast Congo River.

Finally, in 1487, Bartolomeu Dias rounded the southernmost tip of Africa, around the Cape of Good Hope, proving that a link existed between the Atlantic and Indian oceans. The Portuguese rejoiced: It now seemed possible to sail from Lisbon to India and tap into the rich spice trade flowing from the islands of Southeast Asia that Europeans vaguely called the Indies. Success came a decade later with the voyage of Vasco da Gama (1497–1499). When his ship returned to Portugal from India laden with pepper and cinnamon, Europeans realized they had finally opened a southeastern sea route to the silk and spice markets of the East.

Meanwhile, the rulers of rival Spain, who were reconquering their realm from Muslim control at great expense, gambled on finding a profitable *westward* route to the Indies. In 1492, King Ferdinand and Queen Isabella finally succeeded in driving Islam from their realm by military means. The monarchs imposed Christian orthodoxy and forced Jews into exile. That same year, they agreed to sponsor an Atlantic voyage by Christopher Columbus. Leaving Spain with 90 men aboard three small vessels, the Italian-born navigator headed for the Canary Islands, eluding Portuguese caravels sent to stop him. From the Canaries, he sailed due west on September 6. After a voyage of three or four weeks, he expected to encounter the island of Cipangu (Japan), which Marco Polo had mentioned, or to reach the coast of Asia. After weeks without sight of any land, his crewmen worried that they might not have enough supplies for the long return home. So Columbus gave out a false, reduced estimate of each day's headway, leading his sailors to believe they were still close to Europe. He recorded the much longer, more accurate distance in his own private log.

Early on October 12, the distressed seamen finally sighted a small island, naming it San Salvador after their Christian savior. The inhabitants proved welcoming, and Columbus recorded pleasure over the "gold which they wear hanging from their noses. But I wish to go and see if I can find the island of Cipangu." Within several weeks he located an impressively large island and found reason to hope that the mainland of the Great Khan was only "a 10 days' journey" further west. He claimed a nearby island as La Isla Española, the Spanish island, or Hispaniola (current-day Haiti and the Domican Republic). He noted stories of hostile islanders further south called Caribs, or Caniba, who were said to devour their enemies. "I repeat," he asserted, "the Caniba are no other than the people of the Grand Khan." (Upon hearing of these fierce Caribs, Europeans soon fashioned the word *cannibal* and named the region the Caribbean.)

Bolstered by these encounters, the explorers returned hastily across the Atlantic on a more northerly route. They weathered a horrendous winter storm to reach Spain in March 1493. Columbus told the Spanish court that he had reached the Indies off the Asian coast, and he displayed several natives he called "Indians" to prove it. His three later voyages did not shake this belief, which he clung to until his death in 1506. But in fact San Salvador, the tiny islet where Europeans had waded ashore on October 12, 1492, was not close to Asia but rather a

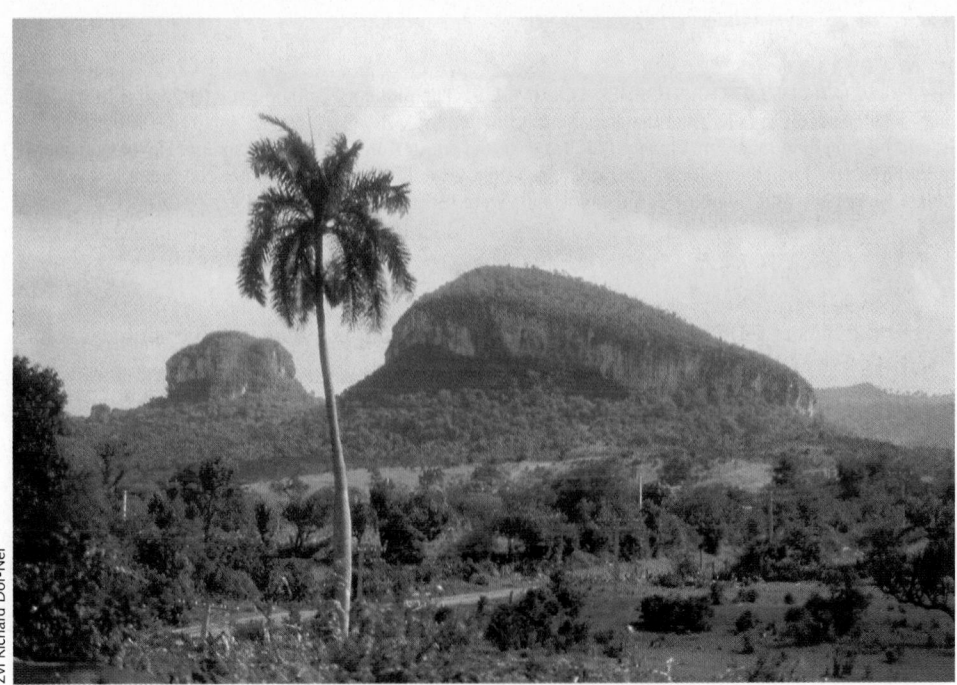

Zvi Richard Dor-Ner

■ Two weeks after his initial landfall in the Bahamas, Columbus approached the island of Cuba. "I have never seen anything so beautiful," he wrote in his diary. "There are many birds of all sizes that sing very sweetly, and there are many palms different from those in Guinea or Spain." The Indians he brought with him from the Bahamas told him the huge island contained many rivers and rich gold mines and that other lands lay farther west.

On Cuba's northeast coast, Columbus noted these "two very round mountains," one of them shaped "like a beautiful little mosque."

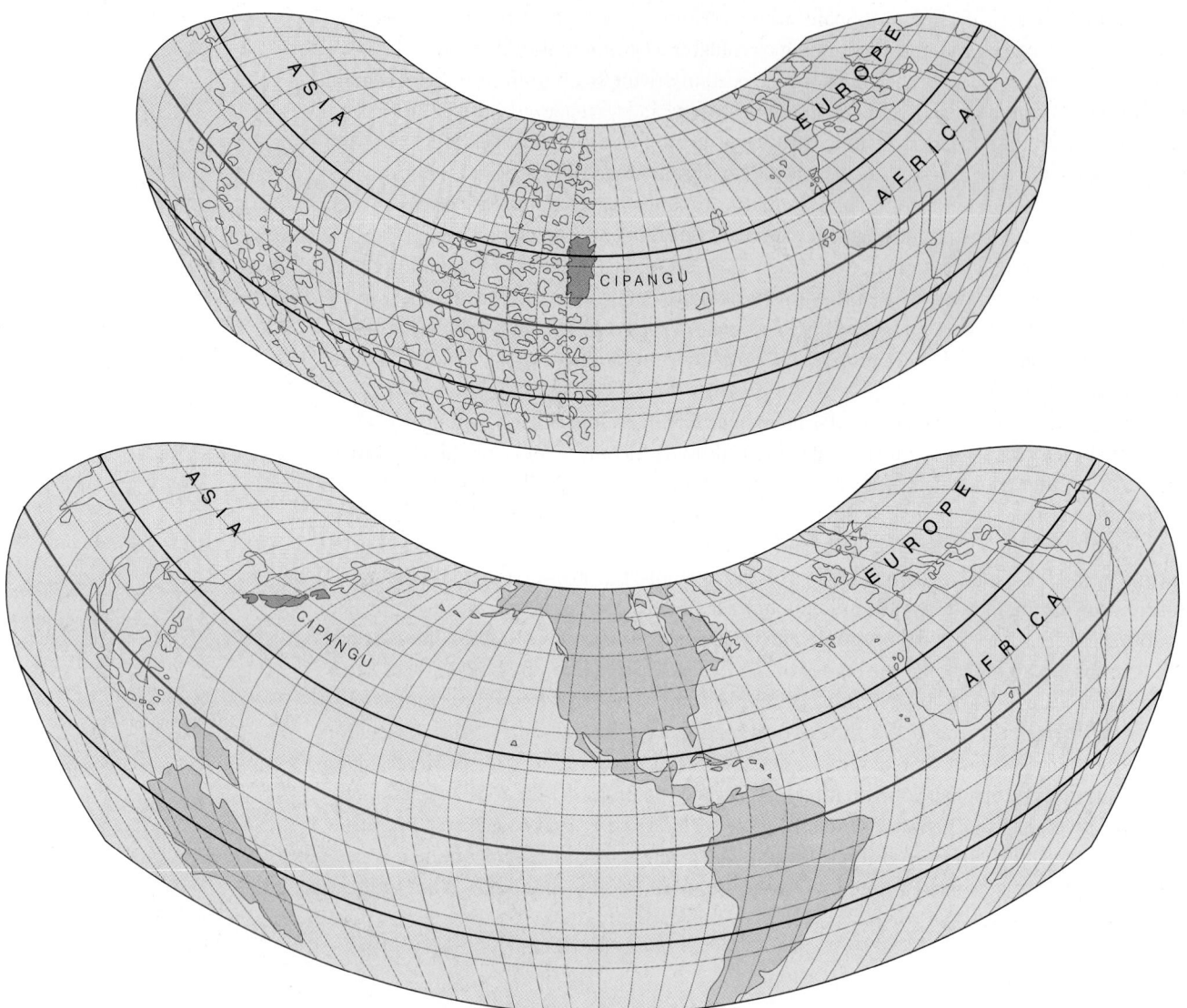

■ **MAP 1.3**

THE EXPECTATIONS OF CHRISTOPHER COLUMBUS   The globe as Columbus understood it (upper map) was decidedly smaller than the actual earth (lower map). He also believed Asia to be wider than it is, and he imagined Japan, or Cipangu, too far east and south from the Asian coastline. He was unaware of the Western Hemisphere. Therefore, when he sailed west and encountered Cuba, he thought it was Japan. He believed the adjacent Caribbean islands were the spice-rich Asian Indies.

part of the Bahamas (now called Watling's Island). Columbus's island of Hispaniola was half a world away from Cathay. The people who inhabited the region, Tainos and Caribs, were not subjects of the Great Khan. Nor was Cuba the land of Cipangu (Japan), which Marco Polo had mentioned.

Why these huge misunderstandings? The mariner made several crucial mistakes. Columbus, born in Genoa, had grown up in a European generation eager to find access to the East. Like others, he knew the world was round, not flat. He also accepted the idea of ancient geographer Ptolemy that by using north–south lines, one could divide the globe into 360 degrees of longitude. But he questioned Ptolemy's estimate that each degree measures 50 nautical miles at the equator. (Each actually measures 60 miles.) Instead, Columbus accepted an alternative figure of 45 miles, which made the circumference of his theoretical globe 25 percent smaller than the real distance around the earth. Although he underestimated the world's circumference, he also compounded his error by overestimating two other crucial distances: the breadth of the Eurasian landmass and the extent of Japan's separation from China. The first distance is actually 130 degrees of longitude, and the second is 20. Columbus used authorities who suggested 225 and 30 degrees, respectively. His estimates placed Japan 105 degrees closer to Europe, at the longitude that runs through eastern Lake Superior and western Cuba.

Columbus's errors came from relying on obscure passages in Christian scripture and dwelling on conflicting ancient geography treatises. But the navigator had practical familiarity with the Atlantic world. He visited the Madeiras, West Africa (Guinea), and perhaps even Iceland. He also benefited from the knowledge of his brother Bartolomew, a mapmaker. Both men heard stories from English and Portuguese fishermen about islands, real and imagined, that dotted the Atlantic. And they presented their unusual ideas in Portugal, England, and France before finding support. It was Columbus's experience and knowledge that gained him the trust of Spain's king and queen. The captain, one observer wrote in 1493, "has sailed. . ., as he believes, to the very shores of India, . . .even though the size of the earth's sphere seems to indicate otherwise." Columbus had not reached the lands he sought, but his exploits would have immediate and extraordinary consequences.

In the Wake of Columbus: Competition and Exchange

Within months of Columbus's return, the pope in Rome issued a papal bull, or decree. This pronouncement, titled *Inter Caetera*, viewed the world as the rightful inheritance of Christianity, ignoring the rights of non-Christians in all lands, whether known or unknown to Europeans. It brashly divided the entire world between two Christian powers, Spain and Portugal, by drawing a line down through the western Atlantic Ocean from the North Pole to the South Pole. For 180 degrees west of the line, the Spanish alone could continue to seek access to Asia. East of the line, on the other half of the globe, Portugal would have a monopoly in developing the route that Dias had opened around the Cape of Good Hope.

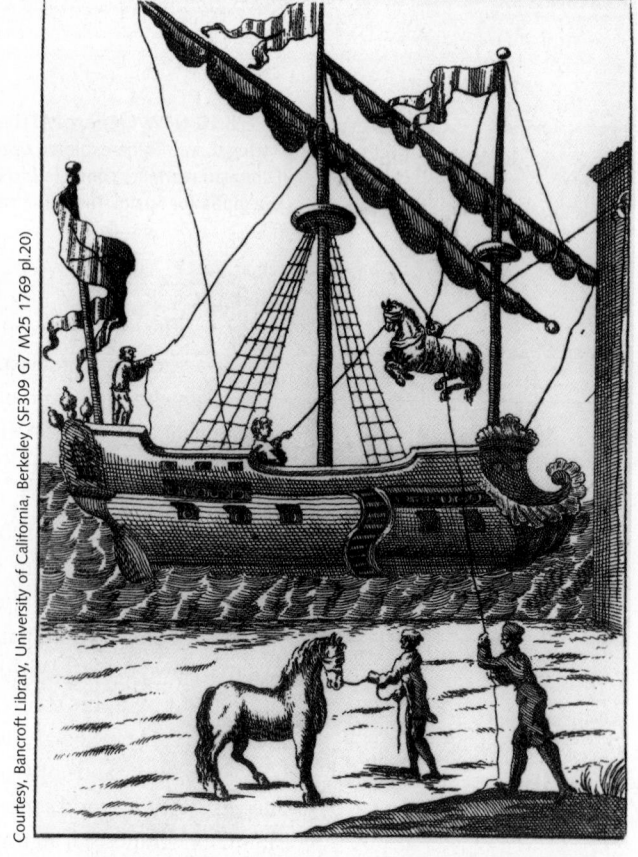

The two Iberian powers affirmed this division of the earth in the Treaty of Tordesillas (1494), which put the line 370 leagues west of the Cape Verde Islands. Within years, both parties realized that this agreement placed Brazil on the Portuguese side of the demarcation line, so Portugal quickly claimed the region. But by then, the Portuguese had already focused their attention on the African route to Asia, following da Gama's successful voyage to India in 1497. Despite their new foothold in the Americas, they left further Atlantic exploration to other European countries.

Spain and England acted swiftly. In 1494, Columbus led a huge venture back to Hispaniola, taking 1200 men aboard 17 ships. By employing only men at first to launch Spain's overseas empire, the expedition initiated a pattern of warfare against native Caribbean men and intermarriage with indigenous women. A mestizo, or mixed-race, population emerged swiftly in Spanish settlements there. On his third Atlantic crossing (1498), Columbus glimpsed the wide mouth of Venezuela's Orinoco River. Given the huge volume of fresh water entering the sea, he knew he had reached a large landmass, perhaps a part of Asia. When Amerigo Vespucci, another Italian in the service

Courtesy, Bancroft Library, University of California, Berkeley (SF309 G7 M25 1769 pl.20)

■ Horses, absent from the Americas for nearly 10,000 years, returned aboard Spanish ships. They awed Native Americans at first and played a crucial role in European conquests. "After God," the Spanish wrote, "we owe victory to the horses."

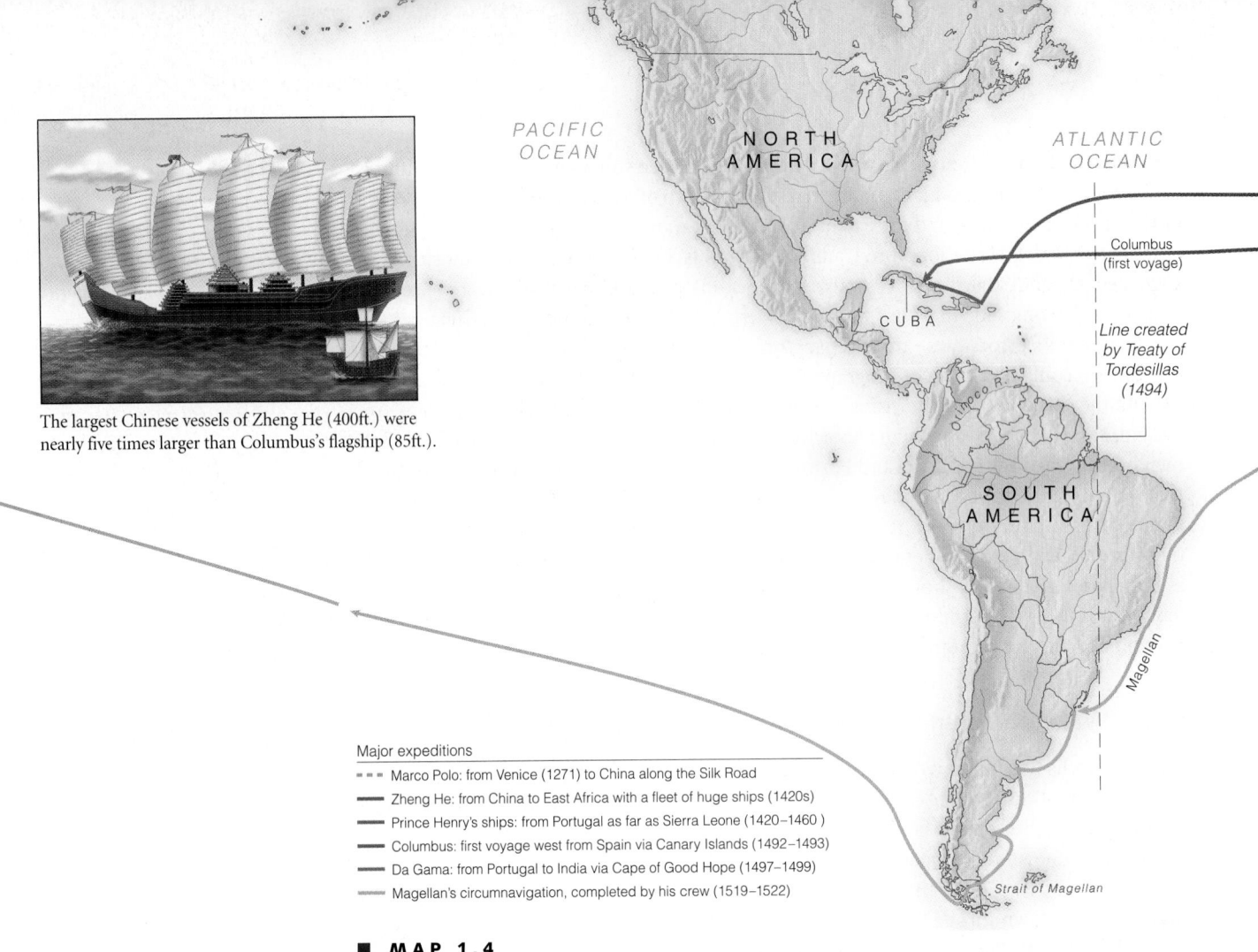

The largest Chinese vessels of Zheng He (400ft.) were nearly five times larger than Columbus's flagship (85ft.).

Major expeditions

- - - Marco Polo: from Venice (1271) to China along the Silk Road
— Zheng He: from China to East Africa with a fleet of huge ships (1420s)
— Prince Henry's ships: from Portugal as far as Sierra Leone (1420–1460)
— Columbus: first voyage west from Spain via Canary Islands (1492–1493)
— Da Gama: from Portugal to India via Cape of Good Hope (1497–1499)
— Magellan's circumnavigation, completed by his crew (1519–1522)

■ **MAP 1.4**

OPENING NEW OCEAN PATHWAYS AROUND THE GLOBE, 1420–1520   In the 1420s, ships from Portugal and China explored opposite coasts of Africa. But China withdrew from oceanic trade, and European mariners competed to explore the earth by sea. Within a century, Magellan's ship had circled the globe for Spain. The colonization in North America is a chapter in this larger saga of exploration.

of Spain, saw the same continent in 1499, he described it as a *Mundus Novus,* or New World. European geographers wrote his name, *America,* across their maps.

Meanwhile, a third Italian navigator—John Cabot (or Caboto)—obtained a license from the English king, Henry VII, to probe the North Atlantic for access to Cathay. Cabot knew that English mariners from the port of Bristol had been fishing in the waters off Newfoundland for decades. In 1497, Cabot sailed west from Bristol across the Atlantic to Newfoundland and perhaps Nova Scotia, thinking he was viewing the coast of Asia. When Cabot died at sea during a follow-up voyage the next year, Henry VII, the founder of England's new Tudor monarchy, lacked the resources to pursue the explorer's claims. Nevertheless, the ventures of Columbus had sparked widespread excitement and curiosity in European ports about what lay to the west. Within a generation, navigators and cartographers began to comprehend the geographic reality that Columbus had so thoroughly misunderstood. Their increasing knowledge fueled greater contact.

After thousands of years, the long separation of the hemispheres had been broken. The destinies of the world's most divergent continents swiftly became linked. Those links fostered human migrations of an unprecedented scale. With European ships came transfers of seeds and viruses, bugs and birds, plants and animals that forever reshaped the world. Scholars call this phenomenon the Columbian Exchange. The term also underscores the two-way nature of the flow. West across the Atlantic went horses, cows, sheep, pigs, chickens, and honeybees

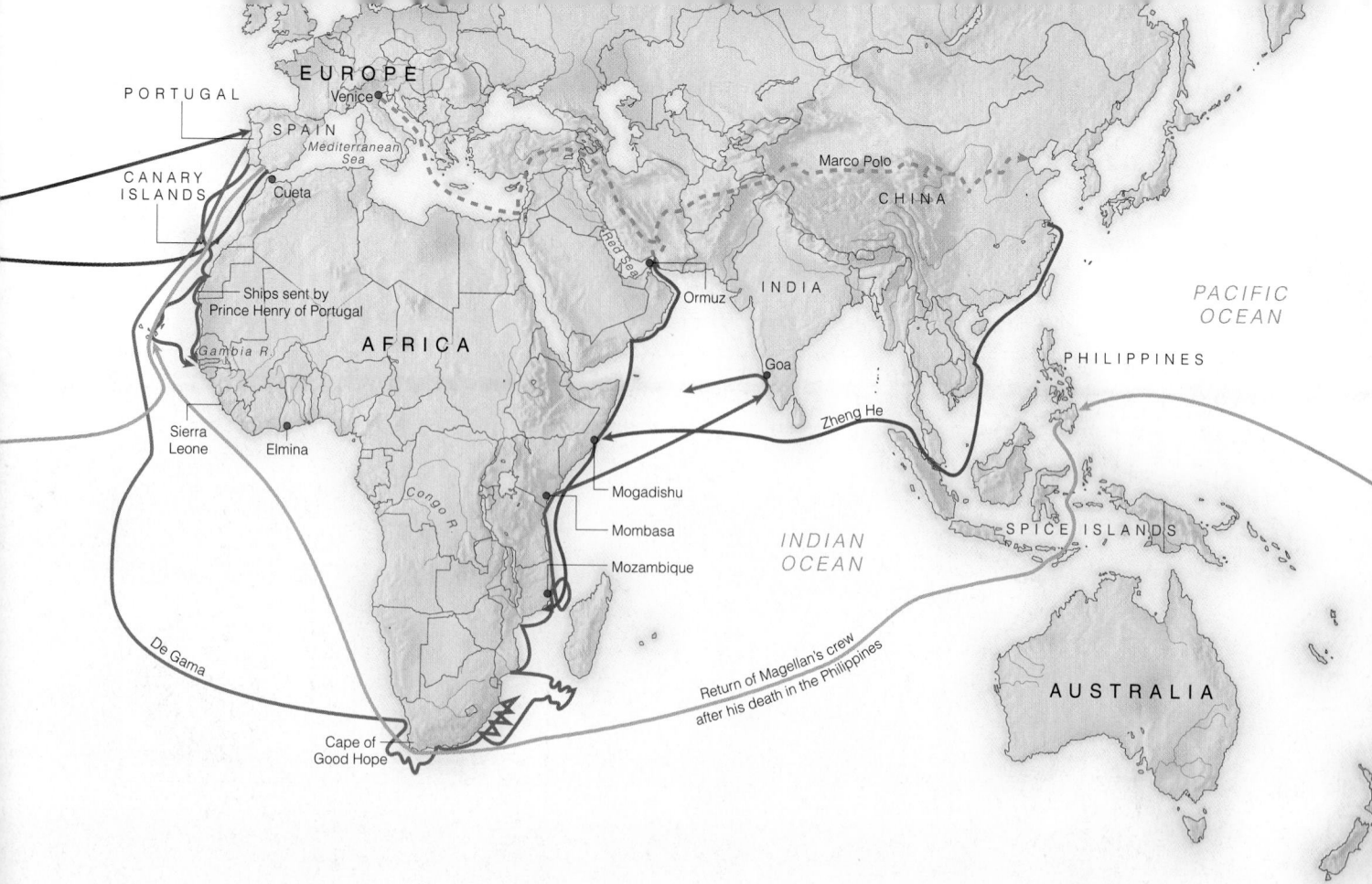

and important foods such as sugar cane, coffee, bananas, peaches, lemons, and oranges. But Europeans' westbound ships also carried devastating diseases unknown in the Americas such as smallpox, measles, malaria, and whooping cough. East in the opposite direction traveled corn, potatoes, pumpkins, chili peppers, tobacco, cacao, pineapples, sunflowers, turkeys— and perhaps syphilis. The planet and all its inhabitants would never be the same again.

Spain Enters the Americas

Throughout the sixteenth century, European mariners, inspired by the feats of Columbus and da Gama, risked ocean voyaging in hopes of scoring similar successes. Those who survived brought back novelties for consumers, information for geographers, and profits for ship owners. New wealth prompted further investment in exploration, and expanding knowledge awakened cultural changes for both explorers and the people they met. The dynamic European era known as the Renaissance owed much to overseas exploration. Returning mariners brought reports of suprising places and people. Their experiences challenged the inherited wisdom of traditional authorities and put a new premium on rational thought, scientific calculation, and careful observation of the natural world.

In turn, Europe's Renaissance, or rebirth, stimulated ever wider exploration as breakthroughs in technology and navigation yielded practical results. Sailing south around Africa and then east, Portuguese caravels reached China by 1514 and Japan by 1543. Sailing west, Spanish vessels learned first that the Caribbean did not offer a passage to Asia and then later— through the voyage of Magellan (1519–1522)—that the ocean beyond America was enormous. In the West Indies, and then elsewhere in the Western Hemisphere, Native Americans began to pay dearly for the exchange that ships from Spain had initiated.

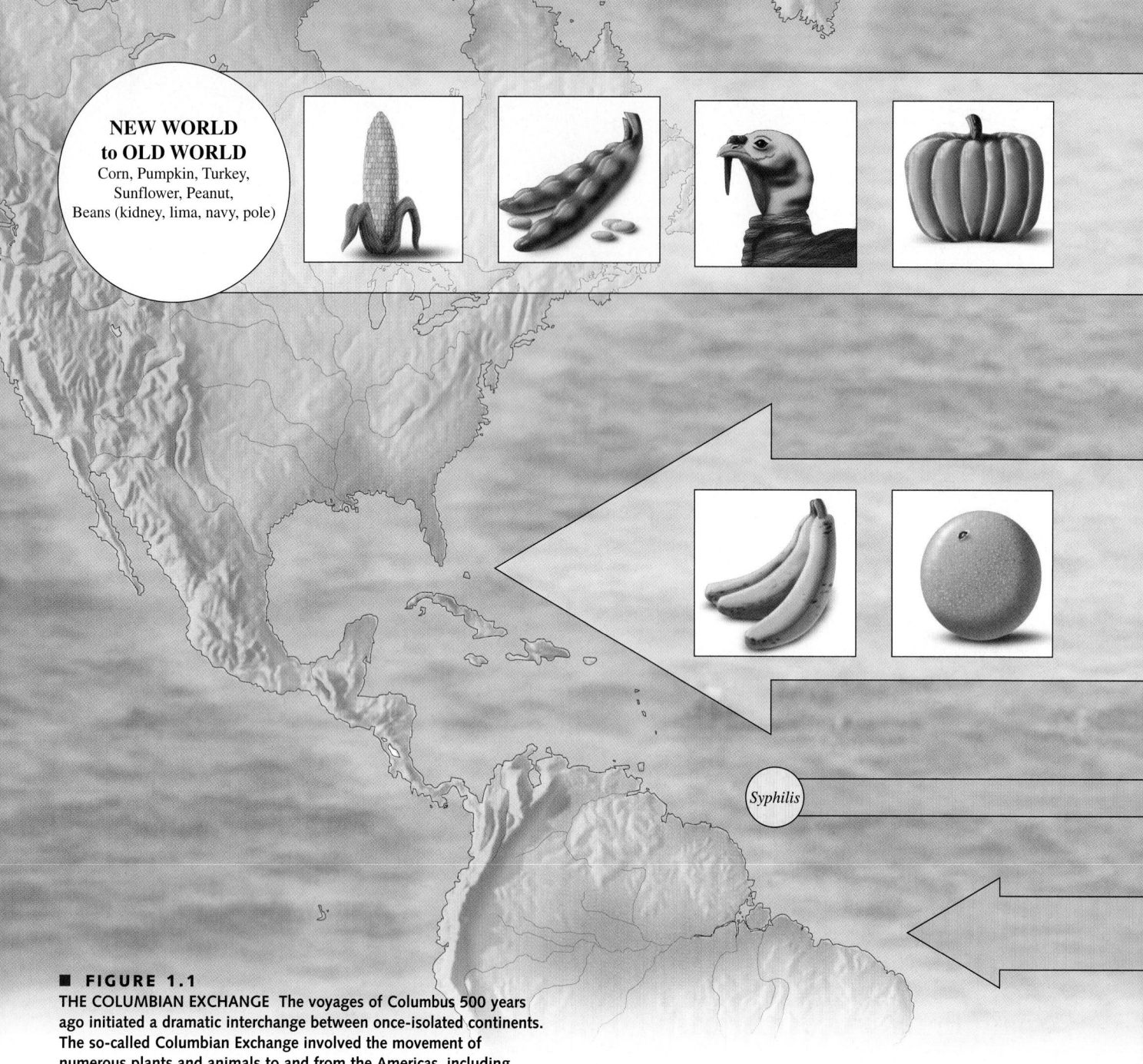

Syphilis

■ **FIGURE 1.1**
THE COLUMBIAN EXCHANGE The voyages of Columbus 500 years ago initiated a dramatic interchange between once-isolated continents. The so-called Columbian Exchange involved the movement of numerous plants and animals to and from the Americas, including those shown here. Seeds and microorganisms have been a crucial part of this process, which continues at an ever-increasing rate.

The Devastation of the Indies

Spanish arrival in the West Indies in 1492 triggered widespread ecological and human disaster within decades. Well-armed and eager for quick wealth, the early colonizers brought havoc to the Taino Indians and Caribs who inhabited the islands. The strange newcomers killed and enslaved native peoples and extracted tribute from the survivors in the form of gold panned from streams. Spanish livestock trampled or consumed native gardens, prompting severe food shortages. Worse, European diseases ravaged countless villages. The West Indian population plummeted as island societies totaling more than 1 million lost 19 of every 20 people within a generation.

This near-extinction had three consequences. First, devout Catholics back in Spain protested the loss of potential American converts. When Dominican friars reached Cuba in

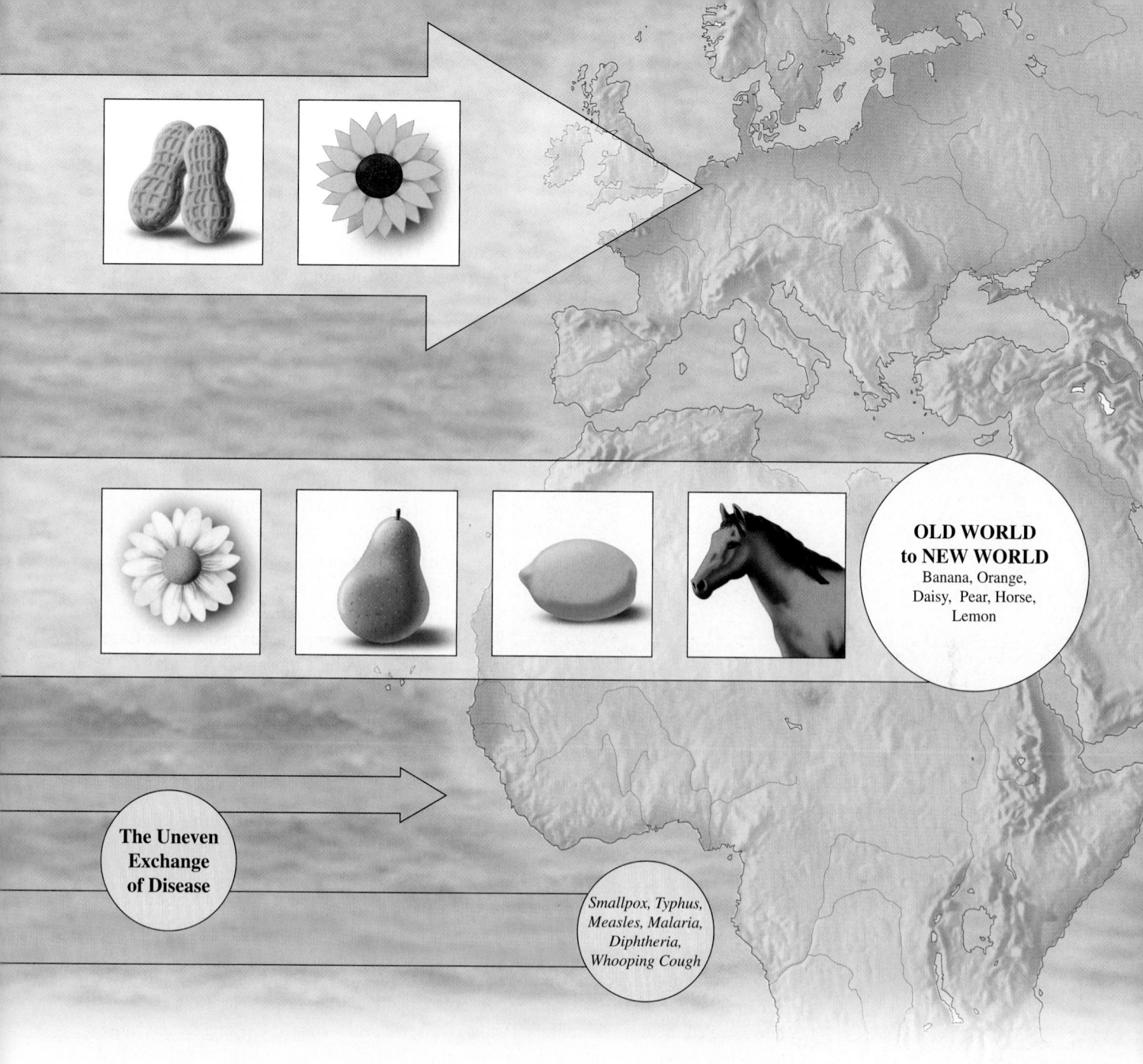

OLD WORLD to NEW WORLD
Banana, Orange, Daisy, Pear, Horse, Lemon

The Uneven Exchange of Disease

Smallpox, Typhus, Measles, Malaria, Diphtheria, Whooping Cough

1510, they denounced Spanish brutality as sinful. The Indians, they argued, possessed souls that only Christian baptism could save. A Spanish soldier named Bartholomé de Las Casas, who repented and joined the Dominican order, led the outcry for reform. He published a scathing exposé titled *The Devastation of the Indies.*

Second, in response to the steep drop in population, Spanish colonizers began importing slaves from Africa to replace the decimated Indian workforce. The same Christians who bemoaned Native American enslavement (including Las Casas) justified this initiative and overlooked the contradictions. The first importation of Africans came in 1502, following the Portuguese precedent in the Azores. Over the coming centuries, the African slave trade to the Americas slowly evolved into an enormous system of human exploitation.

Third, decimation in the islands prompted the Spanish to intensify their explorations. They sought new sources of Indian labor close at hand, fresh lands to exploit, and easy

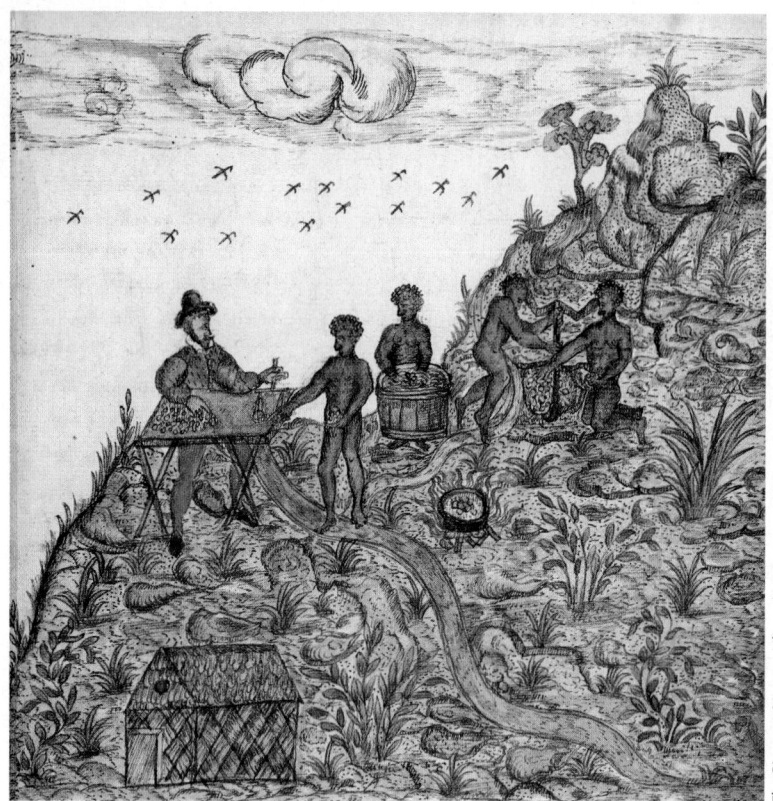

The Pierpont Morgan Library/Art Resource, NY

■ As the Indian population of the Caribbean plummeted in the face of new diseases and exploitation, the Spanish began importing Africans to the New World as slaves. Many were put to work mining precious metals. Here men are forced to dig for gold nuggets beside a mountain stream, then wash them in a tub and dry them over a fire, before handing them to their Spanish master to weigh in his hand-held scale.

passageways to the Pacific. They pushed out from the Caribbean in several directions. In 1510, they established a mainland outpost at Darien on the Atlantic coast of Panama. From there, Vasco Núñez de Balboa pressed south over the mountainous isthmus to glimpse the Pacific in 1513. That same year, Juan Ponce de León sailed northwest from Puerto Rico, where he had amassed a fortune as governor. Despite later tales that he sought a fountain of youth, he actually hoped the nearby land would yield new gold and slaves. "He named it Florida, because he discovered it on the Feast of the Resurrection, which is called *Pasqua Florida*" in Latin, explained Peter Martyr, an Italian humanist of the day who chronicled early European explorations of America in *Decades of the New World*. "They got a bad reception," Martyr reported, for the peninsula's Indians already were familiar with Spanish raiders. The Ais people near Cape Canaveral and the Calusas on Florida's west coast turned Ponce de León away after he claimed the region for Spain.

The Spanish Conquest of the Aztecs

By 1519, the Spanish had determined that the Gulf of Mexico offered no easy passage to Asia. They needed fresh alternatives. In Spain, crown officials sought someone to sail southwest, around the South American continent that Columbus and Vespucci had encountered. For this perilous task, they recruited a Portuguese navigator named Ferdinand Magellan, who had sailed in the Indian Ocean. On his epic voyage (1519–1522), Magellan located a difficult passage through the tip of South America—now called the Strait of Magellan. But the journey also revealed the vast width of the Pacific. The crew nearly starved crossing its enormous expanse, which covers one-third of the earth's surface. Warring factions in the Philippines killed Magellan and 27 of his men shortly after they reached the islands. However, one of his ships, the *Victoria*, made it back to Spain via Africa's Cape of Good Hope, becoming the first vessel to circumnavigate the globe.

If the western route to Asia was far longer than Columbus had estimated, the New World itself soon proved more enticing than Europeans had first imagined. As news of Magellan's voyage raced through Spain in 1522, word also arrived that a Spanish soldier, or *conquistador*, named Hernán Cortés had toppled the gold-rich empire of the Aztecs in Central Mexico. Like other ambitious conquistadores, Cortés had followed Columbus to the Caribbean. In 1519, hoping to march overland to the Pacific as Balboa had done, Cortés sailed along Mexico's east coast and established a base camp at Vera Cruz. He quickly realized he had reached the edge of a powerful empire.

At Tenochtitlán the Aztec emperor, Moctezuma, reacted with uncertainty to news that bearded strangers aboard "floating islands" had appeared off his coast. Ominous signs—shooting stars, fierce storms, unknown birds—had foretold an extraordinary arrival. If the newcomers' leader was the returning god Quetzalcoatl, the court had to welcome him with the utmost care. The emperor sent basketloads of precious objects encrusted with gold to Cortés's camp. But the elaborate gifts only alerted Cortés and his men to the Aztecs' wealth.

Although the Spanish numbered scarcely 600, they had several key advantages over the Aztecs. Their guns and horses, unknown in America, terrified the Indians. So did their ruthless European style of warfare, for the Spanish gained victory by killing enemies, whereas the Aztecs measured military success by taking captives. If European war making surprised the Aztecs, the Indians' rituals of human sacrifice shocked the Spanish. The Europeans could now add moral indignation to their lust for gold as reasons to vanquish the Aztecs. When Cortés found coastal peoples staggering under heavy Aztec taxes, he recruited them as willing allies. Where Aztec leadership proved weak and divided, Cortés acted aggressively. He marched directly to the capital and seized Moctezuma as his hostage. An Indian woman (christened Doña Marina, or La Malinche) acted as his translator and companion.

To be sure, the Spanish still faced daunting obstacles. But sickness worked decisively to their advantage. Smallpox was a disease the Aztecs had never encountered before, so they lacked any immunity. The European illness reached the mainland with the invading army, and a crushing epidemic swept the Aztec capital in 1521. The disaster let Cortés conquer Tenochtitlán (which he renamed Mexico City) and claim the entire region as New Spain. He expanded his control by introducing the encomienda system, which became central to Spanish colonization. Cortés granted encomiendas to his restless lieutenants, expanding their power and control. Each grant "commended" a group of villages to an officer. The newcomers received payments of tribute and

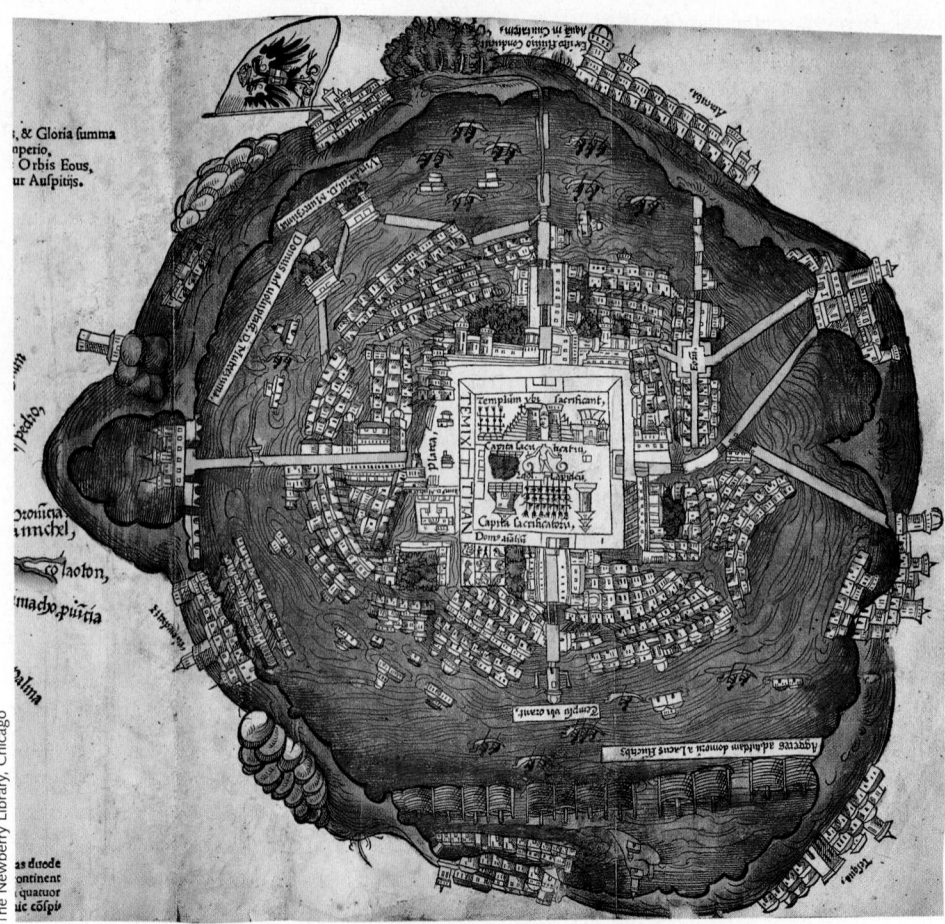

■ Cortés enclosed this map of Tenochtitlán in a letter to King Charles V (the Holy Roman Emperor and grandson of Ferdinand and Isabella). The map remained secret in Spain, but it was published in a 1524 Nuremberg edition of the letter, giving many Europeans their first glimpse of the defeated Aztec capital that was later rebuilt as Mexico City. The city plan shows the causeways over Lake Texcoco and the central square, with high temples where Aztec priests conducted human sacrifices. The flag with the double-headed eagle of Charles V's Hapsburg dynasty may mark Cortés's headquarters.

labor similar to those the Aztec overlords once demanded. In return, the Spanish agreed, at least in theory, to protect their villagers and convert them to Christianty. More often they exploited them as workers.

Magellan and Cortés Prompt New Searches

Cortés's conquest of Mexico raised Spain's hopes of additional windfalls in the Americas. Moreover, the length of Magellan's voyage spurred European interest in finding a shorter route to Asia. By 1524, the Spanish controlled the Pacific coast of Mexico, Guatemala, and the Isthmus of Panama, and they were building ships for further expansion. They explored the Pacific coastline north and south, and in 1531 Spanish raiders under Francisco Pizarro set sail from Panama for Peru, with plans to overthrow the Inca empire.

Pizarro had limited resources (180 men and 37 horses), but smallpox assisted him, as it had helped Cortés, and his invaders accomplished their mission. Marching overland to Cuzco in 1533, they killed the emperor, Atahualpa, and sacked the mountain capital for the gold it contained. The Spanish also pressed west across the Pacific, emboldened by Magellan's success. One of three ships dispatched by Cortés from Mexico for the Philippines actually reached its destination. Still, not until the 1560s did Spanish cargo ships, known as galleons, accomplish the arduous round trip from Acapulco to the Philippines and back across the Pacific.

In 1524, Italian navigator Giovanni da Verrazzano, sailing for the French, reached North America near modern Cape Fear, North Carolina, later cruising north to enter New York harbor and explore further along the coast. In 1526, Lucas Vásquez de Ayllón led 500 men and women from the Spanish Caribbean to the Santee River region (near present-day Georgetown, South Carolina) to settle and explore. But Ayllón fell sick and died, and the colony proved short-lived. Two years later, Pánfilo de Narváez directed an even greater disaster.

A rival of both Cortés and Ayllón, Narváez launched his expedition from Cuba in 1528. He landed near Florida's Tampa Bay, intending to bring wealth and glory to his 400 soldiers. But disease, hunger, and Indian hostilities plagued the party's journey along the Gulf Coast. Only four men—three Spanish and one north African black named Esteban—survived to make an extended trek on foot across the Southwest from Galveston Bay to Mexico City. Their leader, Álvar Núñez Cabeza de Vaca, wrote about the odyssey after he returned to Spain in 1537. Scholars now recognize Cabeza de Vaca's *Relation* (1542) as an early classic in North American literature.

Three New Views of North America

Even before Cabeza de Vaca published his narrative, Europeans initiated three more expeditions into North America. Each probed from a different direction, hoping to gauge the land's dimensions, assess its peoples, and claim its resources. Competing with one another, the three parties entered separate regions of the continent. But together, the enterprises led by Jacques Cartier, Hernando de Soto, and Francisco Vásquez de Coronado made the brief span between 1534 and 1543 the most extraordinary decade in the early European exploration of North America, for Native Americans and newcomers alike.

In the Northeast, Frenchman Jacques Cartier visited the Gulf of St. Lawrence in 1534 and bartered for furs with the Micmac Indians. He returned the next year and penetrated southwest up the St. Lawrence River into Canada. (The name comes from *kanata*, the Huron–Iroquois word for "village.") After a friendly reception at the large Indian town of Hochelaga near modern Montreal, the French returned downriver to camp at Stadacona, the future site of Quebec. Following a hard winter, in which he lost 25 men to scurvy, the explorer and his remaining crew sailed for France.

Cartier came back to Quebec in 1541, seeking precious minerals and signs of a water passage farther west to the Pacific Ocean. He found neither. When he returned to France,

"These Gods That We Worship Give Us Everything We Need"

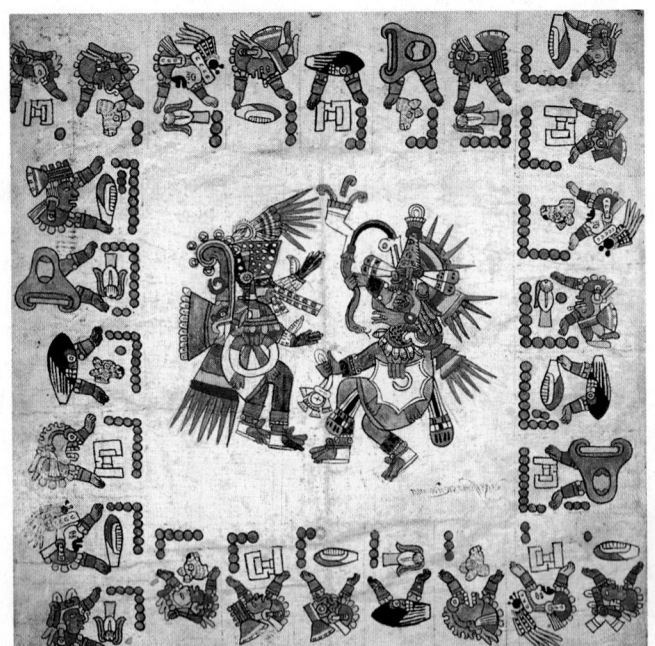

The Bibliothèque Nationale, Paris

Three years after the army of Cortés captured the city of Tenochtitlán, a dozen missionaries from the Franciscan Order arrived in Mexico to preach Christianity to the conquered Aztecs. In several meetings with principal elders and priests from the city, they explained their beliefs and laid out their plans through a translator. Similar talks would take place throughout America in later generations.

No transcript of the 1524 conversations exists, but another Franciscan, the famous preserver of Aztec culture Bernardino de Sahagún, gathered recollections of the encounter from both sides and reconstructed the dialogue. He published his version in 1564, creating parallel texts in Spanish and Nahuatl, the Aztec language. "Having understood the reasoning and speech of the twelve," Sahagún reports, the city leaders "became greatly agitated and fell into a great sadness and fear, offering no response." The next morning, they requested a complete repetition of the unsettling message. "Having heard this, one of the principal lords arose, asked the indulgence of the twelve, . . . and made the following long speech."

> Our lords, leading personages of much esteem, you are very welcome to our lands and towns. . . . We have heard the words that you have brought us of the One who gives us life and being. And we have heard with admiration the words of the Lord of the World which he has sent here for love of us, and also you have brought us the book of celestial and divine words.
>
> You have told us that we do not know the One who gives us life and being, who is Lord of the heavens and of the earth. You also say

that those we worship are not gods. This way of speaking is entirely new to us, and very scandalous. We are frightened by this way of speaking because our forebears who engendered and governed us never said anything like this.

> On the contrary, they left us this our custom of worshiping our gods. . . . They taught us how to honor them. And they taught us all the ceremonies and sacrifices that we make. They told us that . . . we were beholden to them, to be theirs and to serve countless centuries before the sun began to shine and before there was daytime. They said that these gods that we worship give us everything we need for our physical existence: maize, beans, chia seeds, etc. We appeal to them for the rain to make the things of the earth grow.
>
> These our gods are the source of great riches and delights, all of which belong to them. . . . They live in very delightful places where there are always flowers, vegetation, and great freshness, a place . . . where there is never hunger, poverty, or illness. . . . There has never been a time remembered when they were not worshiped, honored, and esteemed. . . .

It would be a fickle, foolish thing for us to destroy the most ancient laws and customs left by the first inhabitants of this land. . . . We are accustomed to them and we have them impressed on our hearts. . . . How could you leave the poor elderly among us bereft of that in which they have been raised throughout their lives? Watch out that we do not incur the wrath of our gods. Watch out that the common people do not rise up against us if we were to tell them that the gods they have always understood to be such are not gods at all.

> It is best, our lords, to act on this matter very slowly, with great deliberation. We are not satisfied or convinced by what you have told us, nor do we understand or give credit to what has been said of our gods. . . . All of us together feel that it is enough to have lost, enough that the power and royal jurisdiction have been taken from us. As for our gods, we will die before giving up serving and worshiping them. This is our determination; do what you will. ∎

Source: Kenneth Mills and William B. Taylor, *Colonial Spanish America: A Documentary History* (Wilmington: Scholarly Resources, 1998), 21–22.

Parisians ridiculed his rock crystals as "Canada diamonds." In Cartier's wake came a colonizing party of several hundred in 1542, led by a nobleman named Roberval. This was the first French expedition to include women. But again, scurvy and cold took a heavy toll at the Quebec campsite, and the weakening colony withdrew after a single winter. Despite a decade of effort, the French still had not established a beachhead in the New World. Nevertheless, they had demonstrated their resolve to challenge Spain's exclusive claim to American lands, sanctioned by the pope 50 years earlier.

In the Southeast, news of Pizarro's 1533 triumph over the Incas in Peru renewed the Spanish search for wealthy kingdoms to conquer. In 1537, Emperor Charles V of Spain granted one hardened veteran of the Peruvian campaign—Hernando de Soto—the right to explore and conquer in Florida. De Soto could divide all gold and jewels with the crown while establishing a hereditary domain for himself and his descendants. The conquistador spent most of his fortune assembling a force of more than 600 soldiers that reached Tampa Bay in 1539. The enterprise included several women and priests, along with scores of servants and African

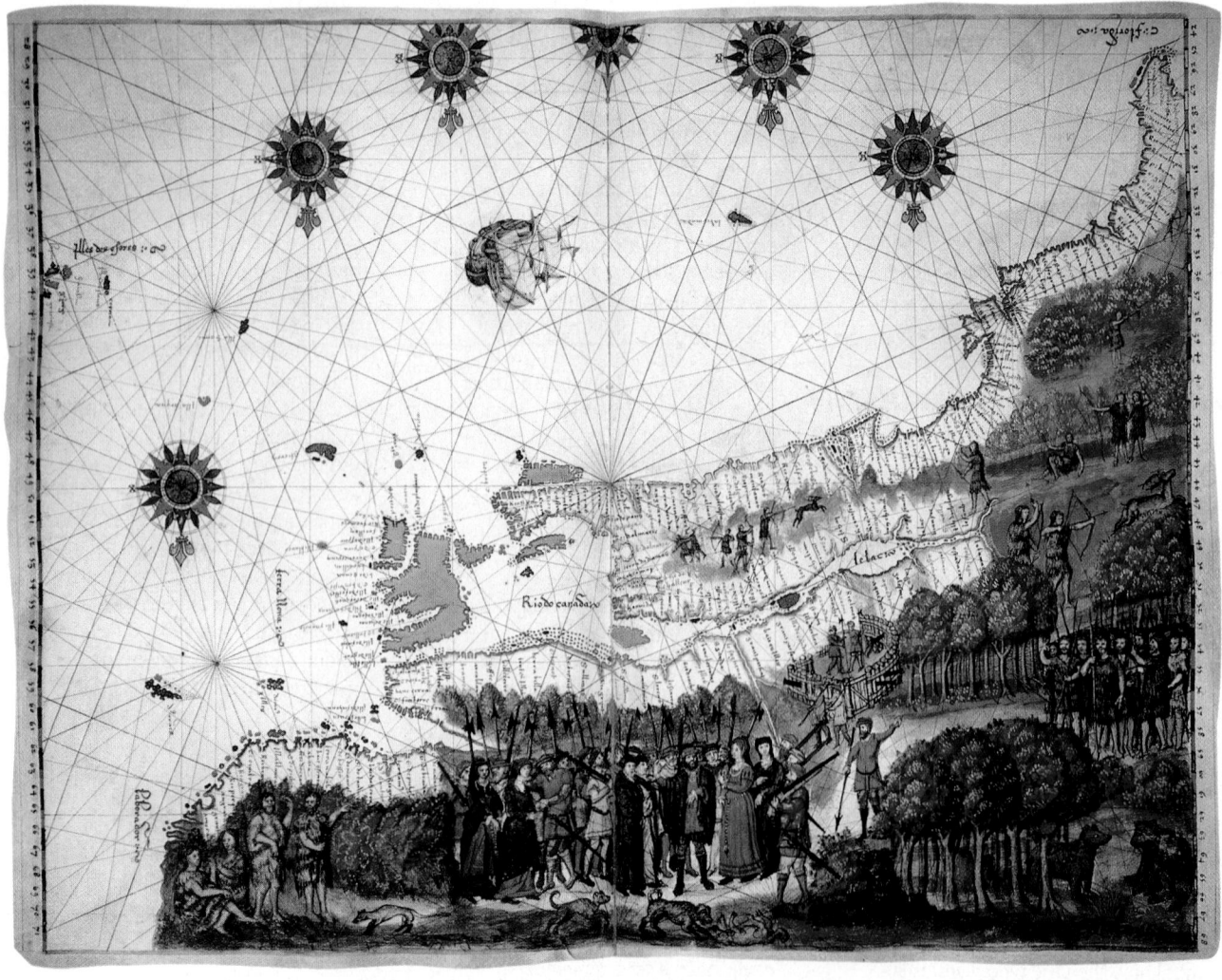

■ In 1547, a mapmaker prepared this elegant chart of North America's Atlantic coast to document the early explorations and claims of France. (South is at the top; Florida is at the upper right.) It shows the men and women of Roberval's short-lived colonizing expedition as they disembarked in Canada in 1542, watched by Native Americans.

slaves, plus 200 horses. De Soto had also brought along a herd of 300 pigs that multiplied rapidly and provided food during the long march through the interior.

During the next four years, de Soto's party traversed a wide region, eventually traveling through ten modern southern states. They hoped to find a city as wealthy as Cuzco in Peru or Tenochtitlán in Mexico. Instead, they found scattered towns inhabited by surprised and frightened villagers. At Cofitachequi, in what is now central South Carolina, the invaders also found something else: evidence of Ayllón's coastal visit in the form of Spanish axeheads, Catholic rosaries, and villages decimated by disease. Cofitachequi's woman leader welcomed de Soto warmly but then watched in horror as the Spanish pillaged her town for pearls. Settlements that refused to provide the intruders with porters or guides met with brutal reprisals that included the use of attack dogs. After passing through Cherokee Indian country in the southern mountains, de Soto's army descended into lands once dominated by Mississippian chiefdoms.

Here, tensions between the foreigners and the North American inhabitants intensified. Violence escalated. On October 18, 1540, a native leader named Tuscaluza attacked the Spanish at the village of Mabila near modern-day Selma, Alabama. Tuscaluza's bowmen proved no match for the mounted, armored riders brandishing swords and lances. Spanish accounts put Indian deaths at 2500 and de Soto's losses at only 22 men. Still, the conquistador's elaborate enterprise slowly unraveled as frustrations grew stemming from the difficult terrain, stiff Indian resistance, and failure to find riches. Exhausted and depressed, de Soto died of a fever in 1542 after exploring beyond the Mississippi River. His disheartened followers escaped downstream to the Gulf of Mexico the next year, leaving epidemic sickness in their wake.

At the same time, an equally complex encounter was unfolding in the Southwest. By 1539, Spanish sailors voyaging up Mexico's West Coast had explored the Gulf of California and skirted the Baja Peninsula. Over the next four years, similar expeditions cruised the coast of California and southern Oregon. Once again, they found no signs of a passage linking the Pacific and Atlantic oceans. In Mexico, speculation about gold in the north intensified with the return of Cabeza de Vaca. His African companion, Esteban, guided a reconnaissance party north in 1539. Esteban was killed by the Zuni Indians, but exaggerated accounts of the region's pueblos prompted rumors about the seven golden cities known as Cibola.

Desperate to get rid of Coronado, the Pueblos told him stories of a far-off, wealthy land called Quivira.

The next year, aspiring conquistador Francisco Vásquez de Coronado set out from northern Mexico to reach these wealthy towns before de Soto could. He left his post as a frontier governor to lead a huge expedition. Only 30 years old, Coronado assembled more than 300 Spanish adventurers and a thousand Indian allies. However, his grandiose expectations were quickly dashed. The pueblos of the Zunis, he reported, "are very good houses, three and four and five stories high," but the fabled "Seven Cities are seven little villages." Hoping to gauge his distance from the Pacific, Coronado sent explorers northwest. They returned after reaching the impassable Grand Canyon and realizing they could go no farther.

The presence of Spanish forces soon imposed a heavy burden on the Pueblo Indians, as the newcomers demanded food and burned helpless towns. Desperate to get rid of Coronado, the Pueblos told him stories of a far-off, wealthy land called Quivira. They secretly recruited a Plains Indian to lead the Spaniards to some place where men and horses "would starve to death." In the spring of 1541, Coronado's seemingly earnest guide led his party far out onto the Great Plains, repeating tantalizing tales of gold and silver. Coronado's soldiers became the first Europeans to see this rolling ocean of grass and its endless herds of buffalo. But when Quivira proved to be a Wichita Indian village in what is now central Kansas, the Spanish strangled their deceitful guide and made their way back south to New Spain. They left several Indians and Africans behind in the Rio Grande valley. At one point, as they crossed northern Texas, they even came within 300 miles of de Soto's ill-fated party in eastern Arkansas. But neither de Soto nor Coronado—nor Cartier in the north—ever discovered the wealthy cities or the passage to the Far East that had seemed such real and alluring possibilities.

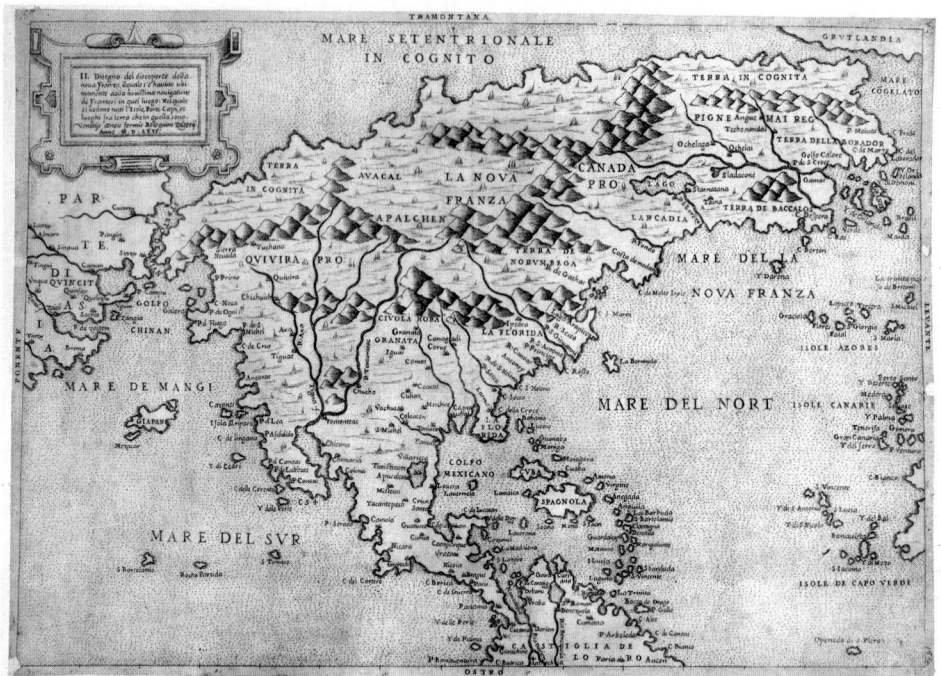

■ European mapmakers learned quickly about the expeditions into the North American interior led by Cartier, de Soto, and Coronado. This 1566 Italian chart places New France, or Canada, in the North, and shows the Indian town of "Ochelaga" visited by Cartier. "La Florida," labeled twice, includes not only the crudely drawn peninsula but also all of the Southeast explored by de Soto. The imagined regions of Cibola and Quivira, sought by Coronado, appear in the Southwest. European hope of a Northwest Passage from the Atlantic to Asia continues, and the size of the North Pacific remains uncertain, so Japan (Giapan) is shown near the coast of California.

The Protestant Reformation Plays Out in America

In 1520, while Cortés vied with the Aztecs for control in Mexico and Magellan maneuvered around South America, the pope excommunicated a German monk named Martin Luther. Three years earlier, Luther had nailed to Wittenberg's cathedral door a list of 95 theses, statements challenging long-standing church practices and papal authority. Luther's followers questioned lavish church spending—construction of the ornate St. Peter's Basilica was under way in Rome at the time—and the practice of selling religious pardons to raise money. They also rejected the church's elaborate hierarchy and criticized its refusal to translate the Latin Bible into modern languages. Luther's reform movement triggered sharp doctrinal disputes and the division of western Christianity into competing faiths. For their written protestations against the papacy, Luther and his fellow insurgents received the enduring name *Protestants*. Their movement became known broadly as the Reformation. Those who opposed it, siding with Rome, launched a Counter-Reformation to defend and revitalize the Roman Catholic church.

For the first time in history, a controversy in Europe made waves that washed onto American shores. Throughout the remainder of the sixteenth century, European national and religious conflict played out in part overseas, a pattern that repeated itself in future centuries. France and Spain, competing in Europe, wrestled to claim control of Florida. And England, an upstart island nation with a rising population and an expanding navy, seized control of Ireland and launched its first attempt to plant a colony in North America.

Reformation and Counter-Reformation in Europe

As zeal for Luther's religious reforms spread across Europe, it split communities and even sparked armed conflict. In Switzerland, a priest named Ulrich Zwingli led the revolt. He abolished the practice of confession, condemned the church calendar full of fasts and saints' days, and defied the tradition of a celibate clergy by marrying. Zwingli was killed in battle in 1531, but the Swiss Reformation soon found a new leader in John Calvin. A French Protestant, Calvin settled in Geneva and ruled the city as a church-centered state for more than two decades (1541–1564).

Calvin imposed his own strict interpretation on Lutheranism and drew dedicated followers to his church. Offended by expensive vestments and elaborate rituals, he donned a simple black "Geneva" robe. He argued that faith alone, not "good works," would lead Christians to be saved. Salvation, he preached, was determined by God, not bought by giving tithes to the church. Only a select few people, Calvin explained, were destined to be members of God's chosen elect. Moreover, only an informed clergy and the careful study of scripture could reveal signs of a person's status. Soon Calvinist doctrine helped shape Protestant communities across northern Europe: Huguenots in France, Puritans in England, Presbyterians in Scotland, and the Dutch Reformed Church in the Netherlands.

The Protestant Reformation that Luther had ignited coincided roughly with another important change in Europe, the emergence of the modern nation-state. Kings and queens gradually expanded court bureaucracies and asserted greater control over their subjects and economies. They strengthened their armies, gaining a near-monopoly on the use of force, and they took full advantage of the new medium of printing. Monarchs also surveyed the boundaries of their kingdoms, claiming control over persons because they inhabited a particular territory, rather than because they held an established relationship to the ruler. As religious ferment spread and local allegiances gave way to a broader sense of national identity, strong sovereigns moved to distance themselves from papal authority in Rome.

In 1542, Catholic authorities established a new religious-judicial proceeding, known as the Inquisition, to help resist the spread of Protestantism.

The emergence of England as a nation-state under the Tudor dynasty (founded by Henry VII in 1485) illustrates this shift in power away from Rome. In 1533, when the pope refused to grant Henry VIII an annulment of his first marriage, the king wrested control of the English church from papal hands and had Parliament approve his divorce and remarriage. The new Church of England, or Anglican Church, continued to follow much of the Catholic Church's doctrine. However, its "Protector and only Supreme Head" would now be the English monarch. During her long reign from 1558 to 1603, Henry VIII's daughter Queen Elizabeth I managed to steer the Church of England on a middle course between advocates of Catholicism and extreme Protestants.

Throughout Europe, as zealous believers on both sides of the debate staked out their positions, attempts to heal religious divisions gave way to confrontation. Challenges to the pope in Rome, whether from Christian parishes or powerful monarchs, met with stiff resistance as Catholic leaders mobilized opposition. Their followers rallied to defend Roman Catholicism in a variety of ways. Taken together, these efforts are known as the Counter-Reformation.

One dimension of the Counter-Reformation is represented in the Jesuit order, founded by Ignatius Loyola. This Spanish soldier had studied alongside Calvin at a Paris college in the 1530s, but he took an opposite path from that of the Geneva preacher. By 1540, Loyola had organized a militant new Catholic religious community called the Society of Jesus, or the Jesuits. Willing to give their lives for their beliefs, these dedicated missionaries and teachers helped to reenergize the Catholic faith and spread it to distant parts of the world.

Another institution, the Inquisition, reflects a different side of the Counter-Reformation. In 1542, Catholic authorities established a new religious-judicial proceeding, known as the

Inquisition, to help resist the spread of Protestantism. Heretics—persons accused of deny-ing or defying church doctrine—were brought before the Inquisition's religious courts. Any-one who refused to renounce heretical beliefs suffered severe punishment. These heresy trials made clear to Inquisition leaders that the advent of printing was helping to spread the works of Luther and his Protestant allies. In 1557, therefore, the Vatican issued an "Index" of pro-hibited books.

Royalty also played a part in the Counter-Reformation. In France, where religious wars raged until the end of the century, struggles for control between competing dynasties became entwined with disputes over church doctrine. In Spain, King Philip II, who ruled from 1556 to 1598, led an Inquisition to root out Protestant heresy. His harsh policies sparked a lengthy revolt in the Spanish Netherlands that resulted in the creation of the United Provinces, Europe's first Protestant republic. Philip expanded Spain's power in 1581, when he acquired Portugal. The move combined Europe's two great overseas empires until their separation in 1640.

The Spanish monarch came close to acquiring England as well. In 1588 he sent a fleet of warships—the Spanish Armada—to England in hopes of reconquering it for the Catholic church. A timely storm and hasty mobilization by the island nation foiled the Spanish king's invasion. But Philip II's confrontation with the navy of Queen Elizabeth epitomized the sharp new division between Catholic and Protestant power in Europe. This deepened antagonism—religious, ideological, and economic—shaped events overseas in the second half of the sixteenth century. The struggle became especially clear in Florida, the vague region claimed by Spain that encompassed Indian lands from Chesapeake Bay to the Gulf of Mexico.

Competing Powers Lay Claim to Florida

As Spain used force to obtain the dazzling wealth of New World societies, its European rivals looked on jealously. As early as 1523, French sea raiders had captured Spanish ships return-ing from Mexico with Cortés's Aztec bounty: coffers of jewels and pearls, ingots of silver, and bags filled with 500 pounds of gold dust. Ten years later, French pirates made a similar haul. To protect the flow of riches from America, the Spanish soon initiated a well-armed annual convoy to escort their wealth from Havana to Seville. Each year, Spain's huge West Indies treasure fleet made an enticing target as it followed the Gulf Stream along the Florida coast. "Thus it is a matter of great moment in the preservation of the Indies, and for its trade and commerce," Spanish officials realized, "that Florida remain Spanish and be strongly guarded."

Each year, Spain's huge West Indies treasure fleet made an enticing target as it followed the Gulf Stream along the Florida coast.

But France had its own designs, furthered by the special concerns of French Huguenots. Unsure of their future in a religiously divided country, these Protestants took a leading role in the colonization efforts of France. When Gaspard de Coligny became admiral of the French Navy in 1552, he saw a way to help fellow Huguenots and the realm by encouraging the formation of anti-Catholic colonies in the New World. French Huguenots established a settlement in Brazil in 1555. But after the Portuguese uprooted it, Coligny turned his attention to the Florida region. In 1562 he supported a Protestant colony at Port Royal Sound (Parris Island, South Carolina), close to the route of Spain's annual treasure fleet. The effort lasted only two years and aroused Spanish suspicions of "Lutheran" intruders.

Undaunted, Admiral Coligny backed a larger colonizing effort to Florida in 1564. French Protestants erected Fort Caroline on the St. John's River at present-day Jacksonville. This time, the Spanish crown took swift action against the Huguenots. In 1565 Philip II sent 300 sol-diers and 700 colonists under Pedro Menéndez de Avilés to oust the French and secure Florida. Menéndez carried out his assignment with zeal. He captured Fort Caroline and massacred hun-dreds of French settlers. The heretics, he feared, might attack the treasure fleet, forge alliances with Florida's Indians, or provoke revolt among slaves in the Spanish Caribbean.

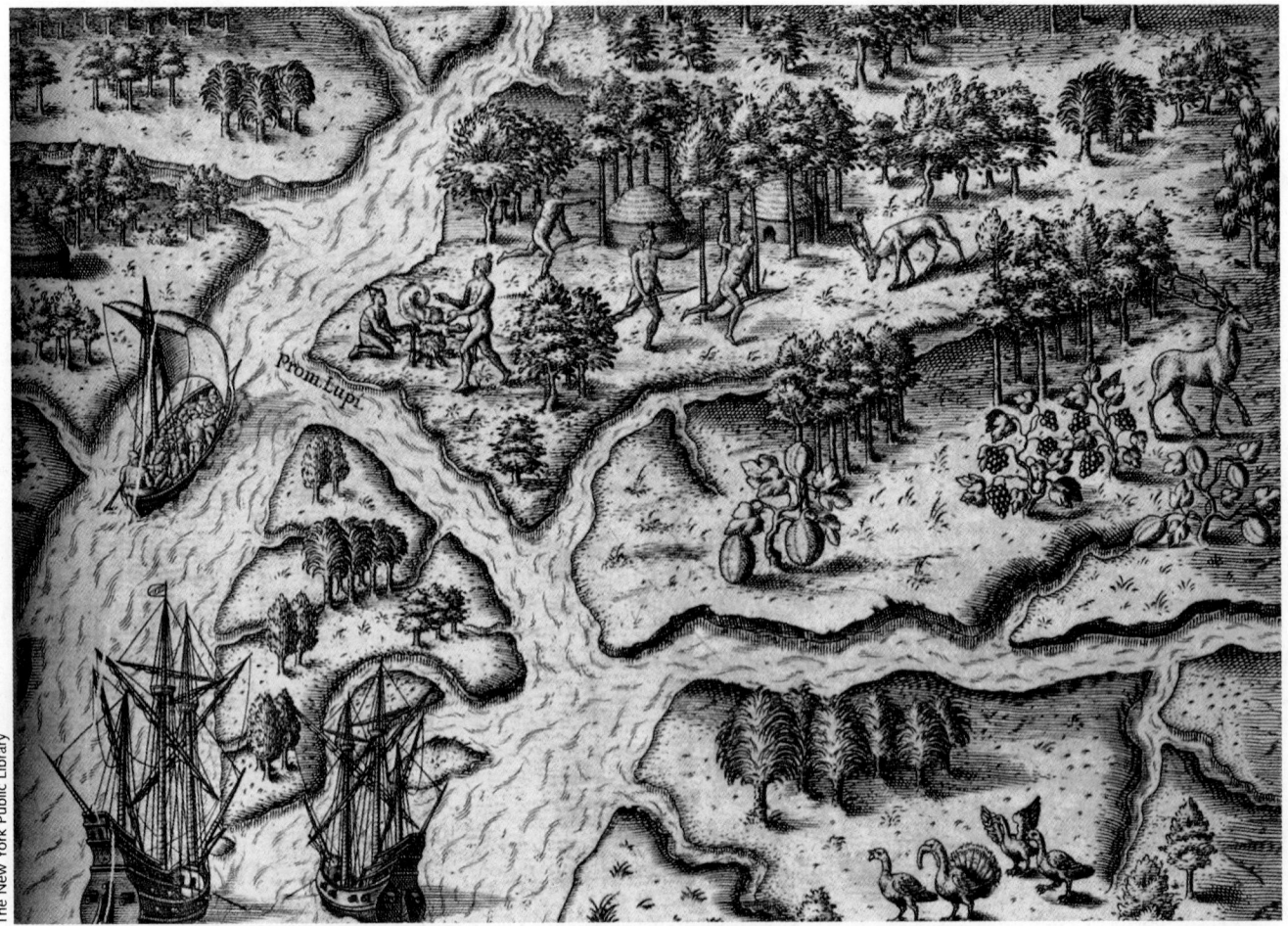

The New York Public Library

■ In 1562, French Protestants established a short-lived colony at Port Royal Sound on the South Carolina coast. "The commander, on landing with some soldiers, found the country very beautiful, as it was well wooded with oak, cedar, and other trees. As they went through the woods, they saw Indian peacocks, or turkeys, flying past, and deer going by." Traveling upstream beyond Parris Island, they surprised an encampment of Indians, "who, on perceiving the boats, immediately took flight," leaving behind the meat "they were roasting."

To prevent further French incursions on Florida's Atlantic coast, Menéndez established a new outpost at nearby St. Augustine. He also laid out ambitious plans to discover precious resources from Chesapeake Bay to the Mississippi. As part of this design, explorer Juan Pardo led several parties inland from the Carolina coast in the 1560s, establishing a post far up the Savannah River and crossing the southern Appalachian Mountains, as de Soto had done, but to no avail. Because the Spanish did not yet understand the magnitude of the distance between Florida and New Spain, they even discussed building a road for transporting silver from mines in northern Mexico to their posts on the Atlantic shoreline.

With French threats defeated, the Spanish at St. Augustine attempted to plant strategic missions farther north to convert Native Americans to Christianity and secure Spain's land claims. In 1570, eight missionaries from Loyola's Society of Jesus sailed north from Florida to Chesapeake Bay. There, the Jesuits established a mission to convert local Indians and looked for "an entrance into the mountains and on to China." But the friars' rules and beliefs antagonized the Native Americans. All the missionaries had been killed by the time Menéndez visited the region in 1572. Spain's failure to secure a foothold on Chesapeake Bay soon proved costly as a new European rival appeared on the scene. Almost

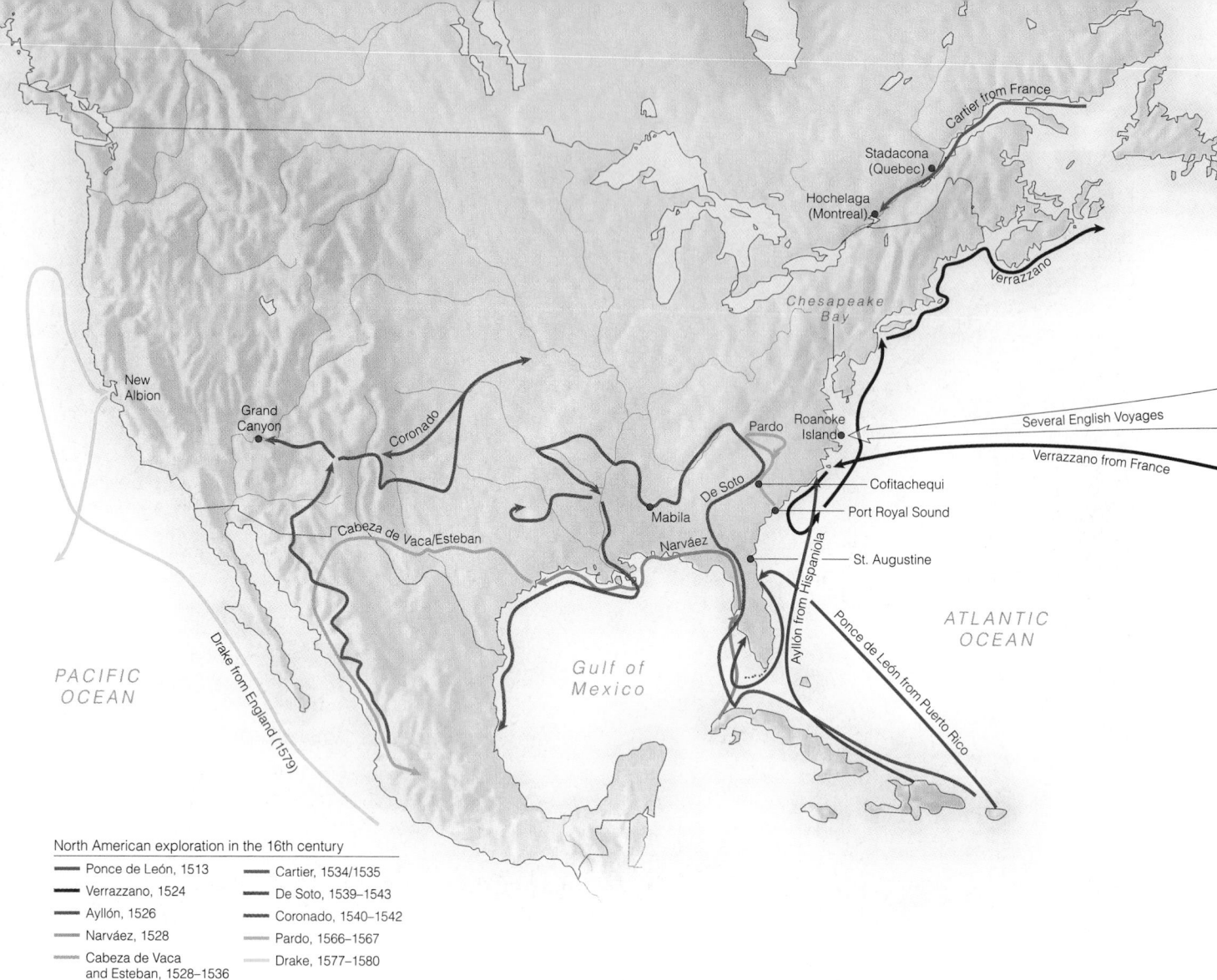

■ MAP 1.5

THE EXTENT OF NORTH AMERICAN EXPLORATION BY 1592 By 1592, a century after Columbus's initial voyage, European explorers and colonists had touched the edges of North America, and a few had ventured far inland. But they had not found riches or a passageway to the Pacific, and only the Spanish had managed to establish a lasting foothold along the Florida Coast.

overnight, Protestant England emerged as a contending force in the Atlantic world. Now English adventurers began challenging Spanish dominance in the Caribbean and along North America's southeastern coast.

The Background of English Expansion

The voyages of John Cabot and the visits of Bristol fishing vessels to Newfoundland's Grand Banks had stimulated an early English interest in the Atlantic. But for several reasons this curiosity intensified after 1550. Henry VIII had used his power, plus the wealth he had seized from the Catholic Church, to begin a fleet that would one day dominate the world's oceans. Inheriting a navy of only 5 ships in 1509, the monarch added 85 vessels before he died in 1547. The merchant fleet grew as well, carrying English wool and cloth to Antwerp and other European ports. In addition, the English population, which had declined in the previous 150 years, grew steadily after 1500. Overall numbers more than doubled during the sixteenth century, cre-

Legend for map:

North American exploration in the 16th century

- Ponce de León, 1513
- Verrazzano, 1524
- Ayllón, 1526
- Narváez, 1528
- Cabeza de Vaca and Esteban, 1528–1536
- Cartier, 1534/1535
- De Soto, 1539–1543
- Coronado, 1540–1542
- Pardo, 1566–1567
- Drake, 1577–1580

Lost at Sea

Lost at sea? Nowadays you can hold in your palm a marine global positioning system (GPS) receiver. It lets you know exactly where you are, which direction you are heading, what course you have traveled, and how fast you are moving. To increase your confidence, one maker of GPS devices uses the name of one of the world's greatest navigators: Magellan.

Thanks to GPS, we are getting used to knowing our precise location on the globe at any moment. Originally developed and operated by the U.S. Department of Defense for military purposes, GPS uses signals from satellites to determine an object's latitude and longitude within a matter of inches. But it hasn't always been that way.

Before the 1400s, countless generations of sailors navigated only within sight of land, where they could take their bearings from familiar landmarks such as mountains and rivers. Captains on the Mediterranean Sea carried charts listing the visible guideposts along every coast. If fog surrounded them, a piece of lead lowered over the bow until it touched bottom told them whether they were in dangerously shallow water. Norse seafarers in the Atlantic and some ancient mariners in the Pacific learned to read ocean swells and follow the stars well enough to undertake long ocean voyages. But most Europeans avoided sailing out of sight of land until the fifteenth century.

It took centuries for navigators to experience, and overcome, the numerous dilemmas associated with deep sea sailing. For one thing, a compass needle does not point to true north but to a slightly different magnetic north. And that difference varies from one place to another. Also, winds and currents imperceptibly nudge a boat off course, making it harder to estimate exact location. Position is relative and concerns relationships to known places. So it was important for mariners at sea to have a grid on which to fix their position. Ancient geographer Ptolemy had suggested that horizontal lines of latitude running parallel to the equator and meridians of longitude circling the earth vertically could provide that grid.

Locating your position on such a grid proved simple in one way and impossibly hard in another. Latitude was the easy part, finding one's north–south location between the pole and the equator. Sailors in the Northern Hemisphere could determine their latitude by measuring the angle of the North Star (or Pole Star) above the horizon at night. By keeping the Pole Star at the same height in the sky, they could steer along the same latitude, parallel to the equator.

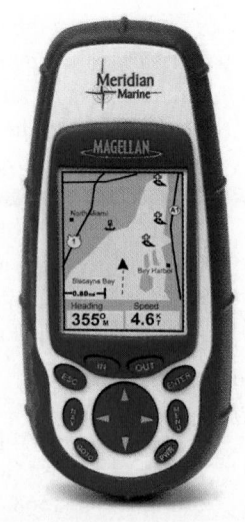

Magellan Handheld Marine GPS Receiver

Columbus used this technique in sailing due west across the Atlantic from the Canary Islands.

But finding east–west location, or longitude, at sea was a more difficult matter. Mariners had to guess at longitude, and often over the years those guesses proved fatal. A notorious example occurred in October 1707 when fog enveloped a British fleet returning home. Officers estimated that they were a safe distance west of the English coast. They were wrong, and nearly 2000 men drowned when the ships crashed ashore at night. The British Parliament responded in 1714 by offering a huge reward to anyone who could finally solve the vexing "longitude problem." The solution came half a century later from English clockmaker John Harrison. He revolutionized navigation by creating a clock (using a spring instead of a pendulum) that could keep time at sea.

From the late eighteenth century to the late twentieth century, timepieces grew increasingly portable, durable, and accurate, helping sailors determine their positions. Now GPS has created yet another revolution, bringing a new technology to bear on the mariner's ancient question: "Where am I?" Ferdinand Magellan would be amazed. ■

ating pressure for limited resources, especially land. Adding to the squeeze, property owners, eager to enclose pastures for sheep grazing, pushed tenants off their land. This "enclosure movement" set even more people adrift to seek work in towns and cities. London's population soared from 50,000 in 1500 to 200,000 a century later. And when Europe's saturated woolen textile market collapsed suddenly, English cloth exports fell 35 percent in 1551. Merchants searched hastily for new avenues of foreign commerce.

Starting in the 1550s, therefore, England's overseas exploration pushed in all directions. Investors in the new Muscovy Company sent ships north around Scandinavia through the Arctic Ocean as far as Archangel on the White Sea. They established contact with Czar Ivan the Terrible in Moscow and opened trade with Russia, but they failed to find a northeastern route above the Asian landmass to China. Other English vessels sailed south to Morocco and the Gold Coast, challenging the Portuguese monopoly of the African trade. English mariner John Hawkins conducted three voyages to west Africa during the 1560s. Horning in on the growing transatlantic slave traffic, he purchased Africans and then sold them in Caribbean ports to Spanish buyers. In doing so, he marked out a grim "triangular trade" linking England, west Africa, and the Americas. In later centuries this inhuman trade yielded untold profits for the owners and investors who funded thousands of slaving voyages.

Philip II, having driven the French out of Florida, had had enough of Protestant interlopers. A Spanish fleet forced Hawkins and his young kinsman Francis Drake out of Mexican waters in 1568. But thereafter, English sea rovers stepped up their challenges to Spain on the high seas, with quiet support from Queen Elizabeth. Drake proved the most wide-ranging and successful. On a voyage to the Pacific (1577–1580) he plundered Spanish ports in Peru and landed near San Francisco Bay. He claimed California for England as New Albion and then sailed around the globe. In the 1580s, Drake continued, in his words, "to singe the Spaniard's beard." He sacked ports in the West Indies, encouraged slave uprisings against the Spanish, and attacked the settlement at St. Augustine. He also captured numerous treasure ships, sank two dozen enemy vessels in their home port at Cadiz, and helped to defeat Philip's Spanish Armada in 1588.

England's anti-Catholic propagandists made Drake a national hero. Moreover, they painted Spanish cruelties toward Indians in the New World in the worst possible terms. To bolster their case, they translated the vivid writings of Las Casas into English. But the English were not blameless themselves. In their brutal conquest of Ireland, they established their own pattern of violence during the Elizabethan years. Sir Humphrey Gilbert and others who played leading roles in this bloody takeover came to view a colony in America as the next logical step in England's aggressive overseas expansion.

In 1576 Gilbert published his *Discourse for a Discovery for a New Passage to Cathay*. In it, he speculated on a short northwestern route to China. Martin Frobisher, another veteran of the Irish campaign, undertook voyages to locate such a route. He mistakenly thought he had found the passage, or strait, to Asia. As evidence, he brought back an Eskimo family he believed to be Chinese, and English artist John White drew their pictures. The next year, writing an essay on "How Her Majesty May Annoy the King of Spain," Gilbert proposed a colony in Newfoundland. The queen granted him a patent—a license giving him exclusive rights—for such a project. But the venture failed because of shipwrecks and desertions. When Gilbert died at sea on the homeward voyage, his half-brother, Walter Raleigh, obtained a similar patent to plant a colony in North American lands "not actually possessed by any Christian prince."

Lost Colony: The Roanoke Experience

In 1584 Raleigh sent explorers to the Outer Banks, the string of barrier islands below Chesapeake Bay that Verrazzano had glimpsed 60 years earlier. The men visited Roanoke Island and then returned to England in September. They brought back positive reports about the land and two Indian informants. The next month, Richard Hakluyt, England's foremost advocate and chronicler of overseas expansion, handed Queen Elizabeth an advisory paper entitled "Western Planting." The document called for the establishment of a strategic outpost on the North American coast, where the English could launch attacks against Spanish shipping, hunt for useful commodities, and convert Indians to Protestant Christianity.

Raleigh's three efforts to establish such an outpost failed in rapid succession. In 1585, he first sent Ralph Lane, a hardened veteran of the Irish campaigns, to build a fort at Roanoke Island. Like other Europeans who had preceded him to America, Lane anticipated "the discovery of a good mine, or a passage to the South Sea." But storms at sea scattered his ships, and most of Lane's initial force never arrived. Those who did, including artist John White, fared badly because of scarce food, bad discipline, and hostile relations with the Indians. Francis Drake, arriving in 1586 after harassing the Spanish in the West Indies and Florida, expected to find a thriving enterprise. Instead, he carried the disheartened soldiers back to England. They had paid a price, Hakluyt commented, "for the cruelty and outrages committed by some of them against the native inhabitants of that country." A second expedition diverted to the Caribbean to prey on enemy shipping, after leaving a few men at Roanoke, who did not survive.

In May 1587 John White led a third English venture to America, with 110 people, including women and children. They planned to settle on Chesapeake Bay, but a contentious captain refused to carry them farther north after an initial stop at Roanoke Island. So the settlers remained huddled at Roanoke, unseen by a Spanish ship from Florida sent north to check on rumors of English activity. In August they agreed to send White back to England for more supplies and to leave a message for him if they moved. When he finally returned in 1590—delayed by England's clash with the Spanish Armada—he found the site deserted. The word *Croatoan* carved on a post suggested that survivors had joined the nearby Croatan Indians, but the Lost Colony's fate remains a source of endless speculation. The Spanish, worried by the English foray, drew up plans for a fortification at Chesapeake Bay, but warfare between Spain and England kept both countries preoccupied elsewhere until Philip II and Elizabeth I had died.

Conclusion

Over approximately 150 centuries, people of distant Asian ancestry had explored and settled the bountiful Western Hemisphere. In every region of North America, from the arctic North to the semitropical Florida Keys, they had adapted and prospered over countless generations. Then suddenly, in a single century, unprecedented intrusions brought newcomers from foreign lands to the coasts of the Americas, in wooden castles that floated on the sea. Their numbers only increased with time. In the next century, the contest for European control of the Atlantic seaboard began in earnest.

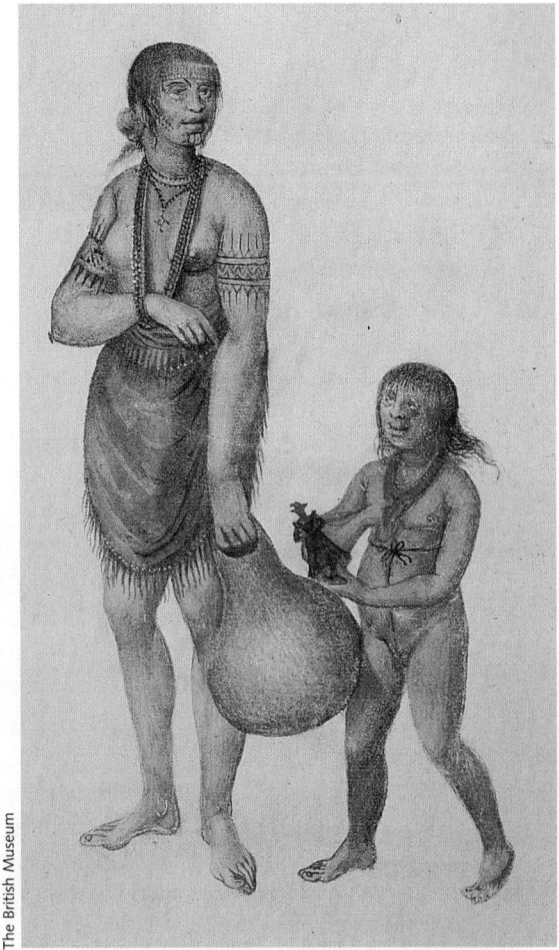

The British Museum

■ John White took part in several voyages to Roanoke Island in the 1580s. A skilled artist, the Englishman made valuable first-hand drawings of Native Americans living in what is now coastal North Carolina, including the wife and daughter of a local leader. The woman kept her "haire trussed opp in a knott," had tattoos on her arms, wore "a chaine of great pearles," and often carried "a gourde full of some kinde of pleasant liquor." The girl holds an English doll, for Indian children "are greatly Deligted with puppetts . . . brought oute of England."

Sites to Visit

Cahokia Mounds State Historic Site

Covering 2200 acres just south of Highway 40 near Collinsville, in East St. Louis, Illinois, Mississippian earthworks dot this World Heritage Site. The Cahokia Mounds Museum Society conducts an archaeological field school each summer.

Chaco Culture National Historical Park

The most striking structure in this park is Pueblo Bonito, the largest building in North America until 1882. Lying in Chaco Canyon northwest of Albuquerque, New Mexico, these Anasazi ruins can be reached by driving south from Aztec (where there are several important museums) or north from Thoreau.

Makah Cultural and Research Center

This site, in Neah Bay, Washington, at the tip of Olympic Peninsula, houses thousands of artifacts from an ancestral Macah Indian village, at nearby Ozette, that was covered in a mudslide shortly before European contact and revealed by a 1970 winter storm.

Mesa Verde National Park

Located near Cortez, Colorado, this is the oldest archaeological national park in the United States. It covers 80 square miles in southwest Colorado, adjoining the Ute Mountain Indian Reservation. The park contains impressive Anasazi ruins, the most famous of which is Cliff Palace.

Moundville Archaeological Park

Located half a mile west of State Route 69, on the Black Warrior River outside Moundville, Alabama, just south of Tuscaloosa, this well-preserved Mississippian mound complex also contains an archaeological museum.

Poverty Point State Commemorative Area

A visitors' center is located near the center of the geometric earthworks from the late Archaic era on this 400-acre site on State Route 577 near Epps, Louisiana.

Pueblo Grande Museum

This downtown Phoenix, Arizona, museum, just off State Route 143, contains artifacts of the Hohokam culture. A large platform mound, a ball court, and ancient irrigation canals are preserved within the park.

Fort Raleigh National Historical Site

This site is on Route 64 at the north end of Roanoke Island, in eastern North Carolina. A reconstructed Elizabethan ship at nearby Manteo suggests the experience of England's sixteenth-century "lost colony." A drive or walk on the sandy Outer Banks (Route 12) recalls the coastline seen by Verrazzano in 1524.

Serpent Mound State Memorial

Four miles northwest of Locust Grove, Ohio, on State Route 73, this site includes a small museum and a viewing tower that allows visitors to look down on the winding effigy mound, now thought to be roughly 1000 years old.

L'Anse aux Meadows National Historic Site

parkscanada.pch.gc.ca/parks/newfoundland/
anse_meadows/anse_meadows_e.htm

Take a tour of the reconstructed Viking settlement at this Web site.

www.acs.ucalgary.ca/applied_history/tutor/eurvoya/
index.html

The University of Calgary has developed a course around this Web site titled "The European Voyages of Exploration: The Fifteenth and Sixteenth Centuries."

www.pbs.org/weta/thewest/resources/archives/one/
cabeza.htm

Read the narrative by Cabeza de Vaca of his journey across the Southwest in the 1530s.

www.win.tue.nl/cs/fm/engels/discovery/

See the "Discoverers Web" for numerous links concerning the era of European exploration.

For Further Reading

General

John Logan Allen, *North American Exploration, Volume 1, A New World Disclosed* (1997).

Alfred W. Crosby, *Ecological Imperialism: The Biological Expansion of Europe, 900–1900* (1986; Canto edition, 1993).

Jared Diamond, *Guns, Germs, and Steel: The Fates of Human Societies* (1997).

Henry F. Dobyns, *Their Number Become Thinned: Native American Population Dynamics in Eastern North America* (1983).

Brian M. Fagan, *Ancient North America* 3rd ed. (2000).

William H. Goetzmann and Glyndwr Williams, *The Atlas of North American Exploration: From the Norse Voyages to the Race to the Pole* (1992).

J.C.H. King, *First Peoples, First Contacts: Native Peoples of North America* (1999).

David B. Quinn, *North America from Earliest Discovery to First Settlements: The Norse Voyages to 1612* (1977).

David Hurst Thomas, *Exploring Native North America* (2000).

Ancient America

Brian M. Fagan, *The Great Journey: The Peopling of Ancient America* (1987).

Brian M. Fagan, *The Journey from Eden: the Peopling of Our World* (1990).

Stuart J. Fiedel, *Prehistory of the Americas* (1987).

Francis Jennings, *The Founders of America* (1993).

Helen Roney Sattler, *The Earliest Americans* (1993).

Robert Silverberg, *Mound Builders of Ancient America: The Archaeology of a Myth* (1968).

A Thousand Years of Change: A.D. 500 to 1500

Sally A. Kitt Chappell, *Cahokia: Mirror of the Cosmos* (2002).

Brian M. Fagan, *Kingdoms of Gold, Kingdoms of Jade: The Americas Before Columbus* (1991).

Alvin M. Josephy, Jr., ed., *America in 1492: The World of the Indian Peoples Before the Arrival of Columbus* (1992).

Thomas C. Patterson, *The Inca Empire: The Formation and Disintegration of a Pre-Capitalist State* (1991).

Linda Schele and David Freidel, *A Forest of Kings: The Untold Story of the Ancient Maya* (1990).

David Hurst Thomas, *Exploring Native North America* (2000).

Linking the Continents

Alfred W. Crosby, Jr., *The Columbian Exchange: Biological and Cultural Consequences of 1492* (1972).

Zvi Dor-Ner, *Columbus and the Age of Discovery* (1991).

William W. Fitzhugh and Elisabeth I. Ward, eds., *Vikings: The North Atlantic Saga* (2000).

Louise Levathes, *When China Ruled the Sea: The Treasure Fleet of the Dragon Throne* (1994).

Samuel Eliot Morison, *The European Discovery of America: The Northern Voyages, A.D. 500–1600* (1971).

J. H. Parry, *The Age of Reconnaissance: Discovery, Exploration, and Settlement, 1450–1650* (1963).

Peter Russell, *Prince Henry "The Navigator": A Life* (2000).

Carl Ortwin Sauer, *The Early Spanish Main* (1969).

Spain Enters the Americas

Herbert E. Bolton, *Coronado: Knight of Pueblos and Plains* (1990).

Hernán Cortés, *Letters from Mexico,* translated and edited by Anthony Pagden (1986).

Cyclone Covey, trans. and ed., *Cabeza de Vaca's Adventures in the Unknown Interior of America* (1961).

W. J. Eccles, *France in America* (1972).

Charles Hudson, *Knights of Spain, Warriors of the Sun: Hernando de Soto and the South's Ancient Kingdoms* (1997).

Miguel Leon-Portilla, *The Broken Spears: The Aztec Account of the Conquest of Mexico* (1962).

Jerald T. Milanich, *Florida Indians and the Invasion from Europe* (1995).

The Protestant Reformation Plays Out in America

Karen Ordahl Kupperman, *Roanoke: The Abandoned Colony* (1984).

Eugene Lyon, *The Enterprise of Florida: Pedro Menéndez de Avilés and the Spanish Conquest of 1565–1568* (1976).

John T. McGrath, *The French in Early Florida: In the Eye of the Hurricane* (2000).

David Beers Quinn, *Raleigh and the British Empire* (1962).

David Beers Quinn, *England and the Discovery of America, 1481–1620* (1974).

Carl Ortwin Sauer, *Sixteenth Century America: The Land and the People as Seen by the Europeans* (1971).

Online Practice Test

Test your understanding of this chapter with interactive review quizzes at

www.ablongman.com/jonescreatedequal/chapter1

Additional Photo Credits

Page 5: Courtesy, Museum of New Mexico (#50884)
Page 8: Lee Boltin Picture Library
Page 11: Collection of Duke University Museum of Art; DUMA Acquisiton Fund (1993.7.1-2)
Page 15: The Ohio Historical Society
Page 18: Sheldon Jackson Museum, Sitka. Photograph by Randy Miller
Page 19: Museum of the History of Science, Oxford, Oxfordshire, UK/Bridgeman Art Library
Page 39: Used by permission, Thales Navigation 2

CHAPTER

2

European Footholds on the Fringes of North America, 1600–1660

CHAPTER OUTLINE

Spain's Ocean-Spanning Reach

France and Holland:
Overseas Competition
for Spain

English Beginnings
on the Atlantic Coast

The Puritan Experiment

The Chesapeake Bay Colonies

Conclusion

Sites to Visit

For Further Reading

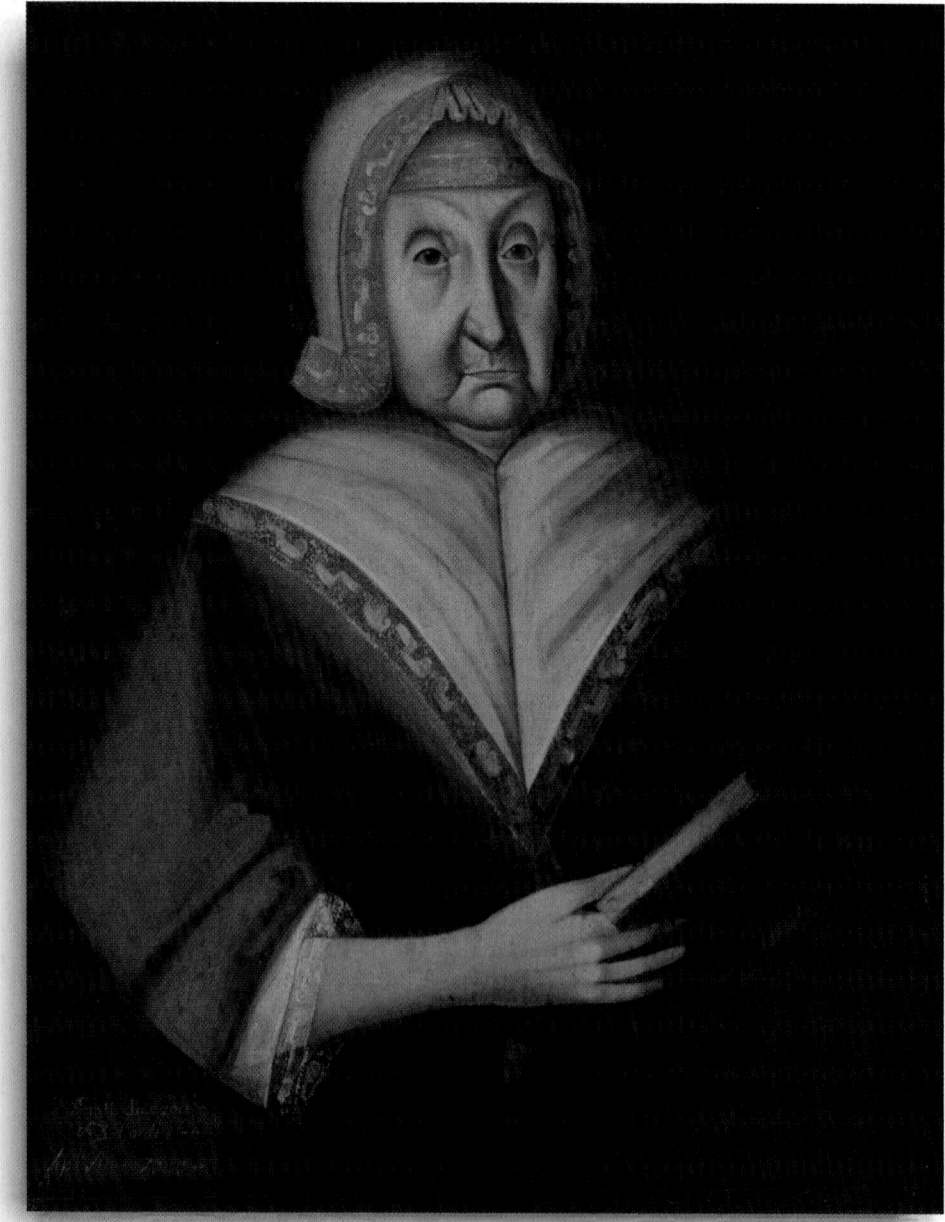

Unknown Artist, *Mrs. William Pollard*, 1721. Courtesy of the Massachusetts Historical Society, MHS #1495

■ Mrs. William Pollard, 1721. Anne Pollard migrated to New England as a young woman.

IN THE SUMMER OF 1621, AN ENGLISHMAN AND AN INDIAN LEFT PLYMOUTH VILLAGE ON foot to visit a Native American leader named Massasoit. Stephen Hopkins and Squanto had a threefold purpose: to "view the country," to assess Massasoit's military strength, and to secure his support for the struggling English colony. During their 40-mile journey, the two men saw numerous signs of a wave of disease that had swept the New England coast four years earlier, killing thousands of Indians. Weakened survivors had lacked the energy to bury the dead, whose skulls and bones still lay aboveground in many places.

The two men who encountered these grim scenes had come together from strikingly different backgrounds. Back in 1609, Hopkins had boarded the *Sea Adventure* and left England in a fleet of nine vessels, all heading for Jamestown in Virginia. When a storm wrecked his ship on the uncharted island of Bermuda, Hopkins and others rebelled against their official leader. They refused to go further under his command. Accused of mutiny and sentenced to hang, Hopkins pleaded his case and narrowly escaped the noose. When the rest of the company finally managed to build two small boats and sail safely to Virginia, he went along. Soon after that, he managed to return to England and start a family, but he could not shake off the lure of America.

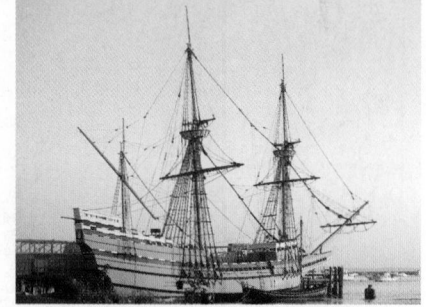

A Mayflower replica is now part of the restored Plymouth Colony site.

In 1620 Hopkins decided to return. At the English port of Plymouth, Hopkins, his pregnant wife, Elizabeth, and several children and servants boarded another vessel: the *Mayflower*. Headed for Virginia, the *Mayflower* had been chartered to carry a group of English Protestants to America from their exile in Holland. Paying passengers such as the Hopkins family also joined the journey. Tensions mounted when a midpassage decision changed the *Mayflower*'s destination from Virginia to New England. Hopkins, remembering his experiences in Bermuda, was among those who muttered "mutinous speeches" and argued that "when they came ashore, they should use their own libertie, for none had power to command them." But after Elizabeth gave birth, Hopkins joined the other 40 men aboard in signing the *Mayflower* Compact. The agreement bound all the passengers together in a "Civil Body Politic" to be governed by laws "most meet and convenient for the general good." They reached New England in early winter, and Hopkins and others laid out the village of Plymouth in the snow. There, the newcomers met Squanto, a Native American with a command of English who helped them negotiate with local Indians.

Squanto had also endured great hardship and Atlantic travel. He remembered the first French and English fishing vessels, which had appeared when he was a small boy. The sailors mapped the coast, traded with local tribes for beaver pelts or corn, and occasionally took Indian hostages back to Europe. In 1614 Squanto was among 27 Indians seized by an Englishman departing with a cargo of fish for the Mediterranean port of Malaga. Rescued from certain slavery by Spanish friars, Squanto somehow reached England, voyaged to Newfoundland, and returned to his homeland in 1619, only to find his entire village swept away by disease.

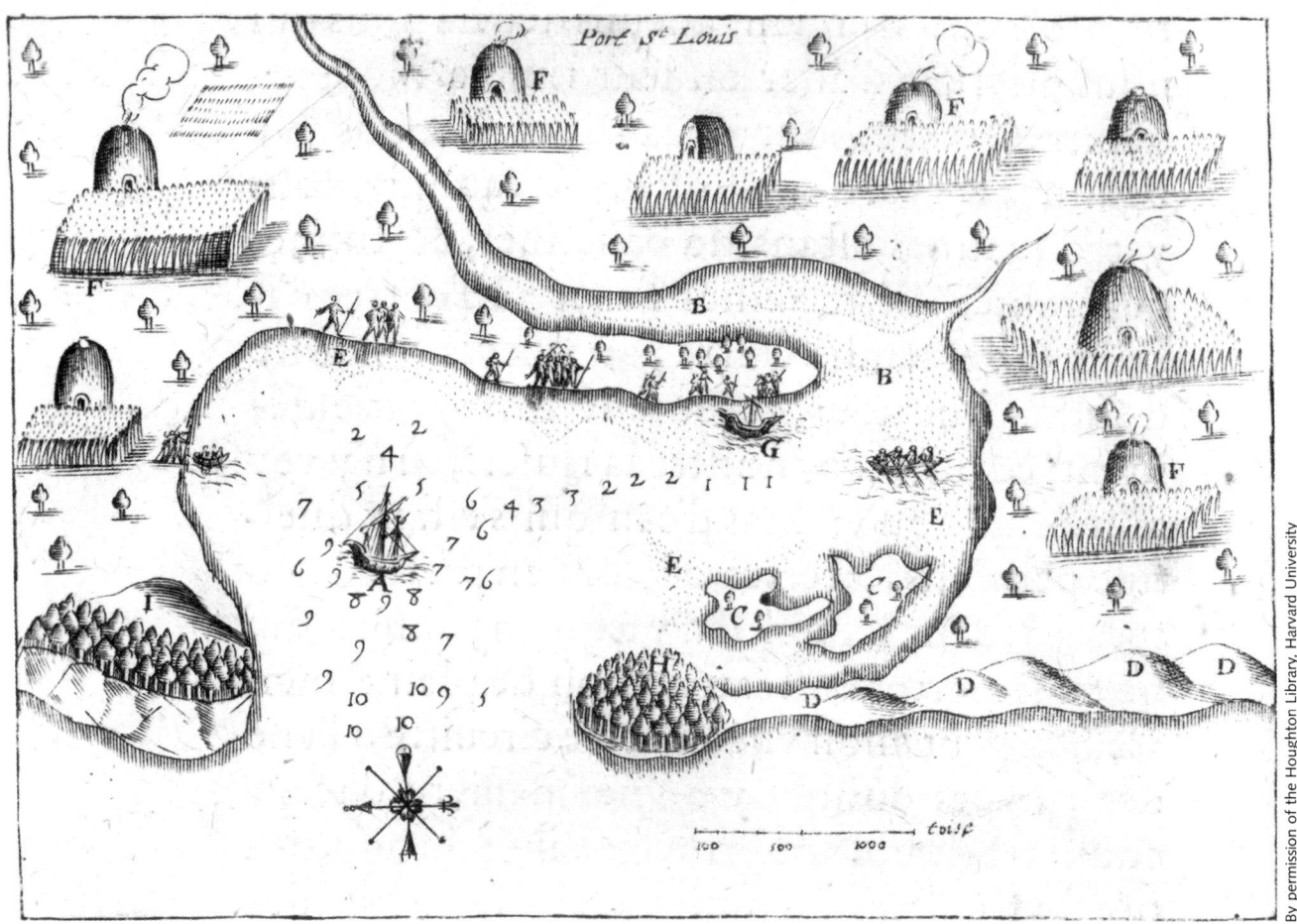

■ As a boy, Squanto probably saw Samuel de Champlain's vessel enter this bay in July 1605. The French dropped anchor (A) and took soundings until they ran aground (G). Champlain climbed a sand dune (D) to sketch this map, noting numerous Indian dwellings and gardens (F). These settlements had been devastated by disease when the *Mayflower* colonists arrived in December 1620. They renamed the harbor Plymouth and spent their first night ashore on Clark's Island (C).

The *Mayflower* pilgrims, arriving a year after Squanto's return, would also suffer heavy losses. Of the 102 settlers who had begun the voyage, half of them died in Plymouth colony by the next spring. But in New England, as elsewhere in America, death seemed to play favorites in the following years. As colonization continued, recurrent epidemics took a particularly heavy toll on Native Americans, who lacked immunity when exposed to foreign diseases for the first time. In 1622 Squanto fell sick and died of a fever, leaving no relatives behind. In contrast, Stephen and Elizabeth Hopkins lived on to see numerous children and grandchildren thrive.

By the middle of the seventeenth century, English settlements had taken root in both Virginia and Massachusetts. The success of these colonies would exert a lasting influence on the future direction of American society. But their stories unfolded as part of a far wider North American drama. It embraced both the Atlantic and the Pacific shores, and it included a diversity of European groups besides the English settlements near Cape Cod and Chesapeake Bay. The French founded towns at Quebec and Montreal, while the Spanish held onto St. Augustine and established Santa Fe in the Southwest. Dutch traders built New Amsterdam on Manhattan Island, overlooking the Hudson River, and Swedish colonists erected a fort near the mouth of the Delaware.

Nor was the drama confined to the tiny colonies, struggling against steep odds to establish lasting footholds on the fringes of the continent. In each outpost the lives of the new arrivals remained linked to the broad religious struggles, economic ambitions, and imperial contests that absorbed the Atlantic powers in far-off Europe. And closer at hand, the wellbeing of Indian groups, near and far, proved to be linked with the lives of colonists such as the Hopkins family. As the story of Squanto illustrates, Native American communities faced their own set of new challenges that altered traditional ways of living and threatened their very survival.

Spain's Ocean-Spanning Reach

In 1580 Spain's Philip II had laid claim to the throne of Portugal. This consolidation, (which endured until 1640) unified Europe's two great richest seaborne empires, for Spain and Portugal had each been sanctioned by the pope nearly a century earlier to explore opposite sides of the globe.

Both kingdoms had had remarkable success in these overseas endeavors. The Portuguese had established trade with India and Southeast Asia, and their traders and Catholic missionaries had even created a foothold in Japan. The Spanish, sailing in the opposite direction, had staked out huge claims in the Americas and had founded Manila in the Philippines as a Pacific port of trade. By the turn of the century, however, Spain faced two fresh problems. First, combining with Portugal put huge additional burdens on the overstretched Spanish bureaucracy. Second, the global success of the combined Iberian empires invited challenges from envious rivals in northern Europe. The new international competition came from the French, the Dutch, and the English. Each of these realms constituted an aspiring naval power with imperial ambitions of its own.

In 1598, for example, ten Dutch ships found their way to the Pacific, defying Spanish claims for control of that ocean. One of these vessels, piloted by Englishman Will Adams, ended up in Japan, where the new Tokugawa dynasty (1600–1868) was consolidating its control. Adams visited Edo—the rising military town that would grow into modern Tokyo. He even built a ship for the *shogun* (ruler) and trained Japanese carpenters to become shipwrights. Adams's experience in Japan serves as a reminder that in the decades before the *Mayflower* sailed the Atlantic, the issue of who would dominate Pacific sea lanes to America was anything but clear.

Vizcaíno in California and Japan

In April 1607, a letter from the king of Spain reached Mexico City. The king commanded his viceroy in charge of affairs in Mexico (New Spain) to create an outpost on California's Monterey Bay in order to aid Spanish galleons crossing the Pacific from Manila. The logical person to execute the plan for the viceroy was Sebastián Vizcaíno, a seasoned navigator who had already explored Monterey Bay on the California coast four years earlier.

Vizcaíno understood the Pacific trade, having sailed between Acapulco on Mexico's west coast and the new Spanish stronghold at Manila. His ships had carried American chocolate to the Philippines and brought back silks and spices from Asia. Vizcaíno knew that galleons returning through the North Pacific to the west coast of Mexico desperately needed a haven along the route, after crossing the immense ocean. As he had seen, Monterey Bay was well supplied with water, food, and timber. The sheltering harbor would provide a perfect way station, where ships could take on supplies and make repairs before heading south. The royal plan directed Vizcaíno to sail to Manila and then establish a new colony at Monterey during his return voyage.

But the viceroy in Mexico City had other ideas. He diverted the necessary funds into a search for the fabled North Pacific isles of Rica de Oro ("Rich in Gold") and Rica de Plata ("Rich in Silver"). In 1611, the viceroy authorized Vizcaíno to search for the mysterious islands. The venture took Vizcaíno to Japan. When he finally returned east in 1613 aboard a vessel built

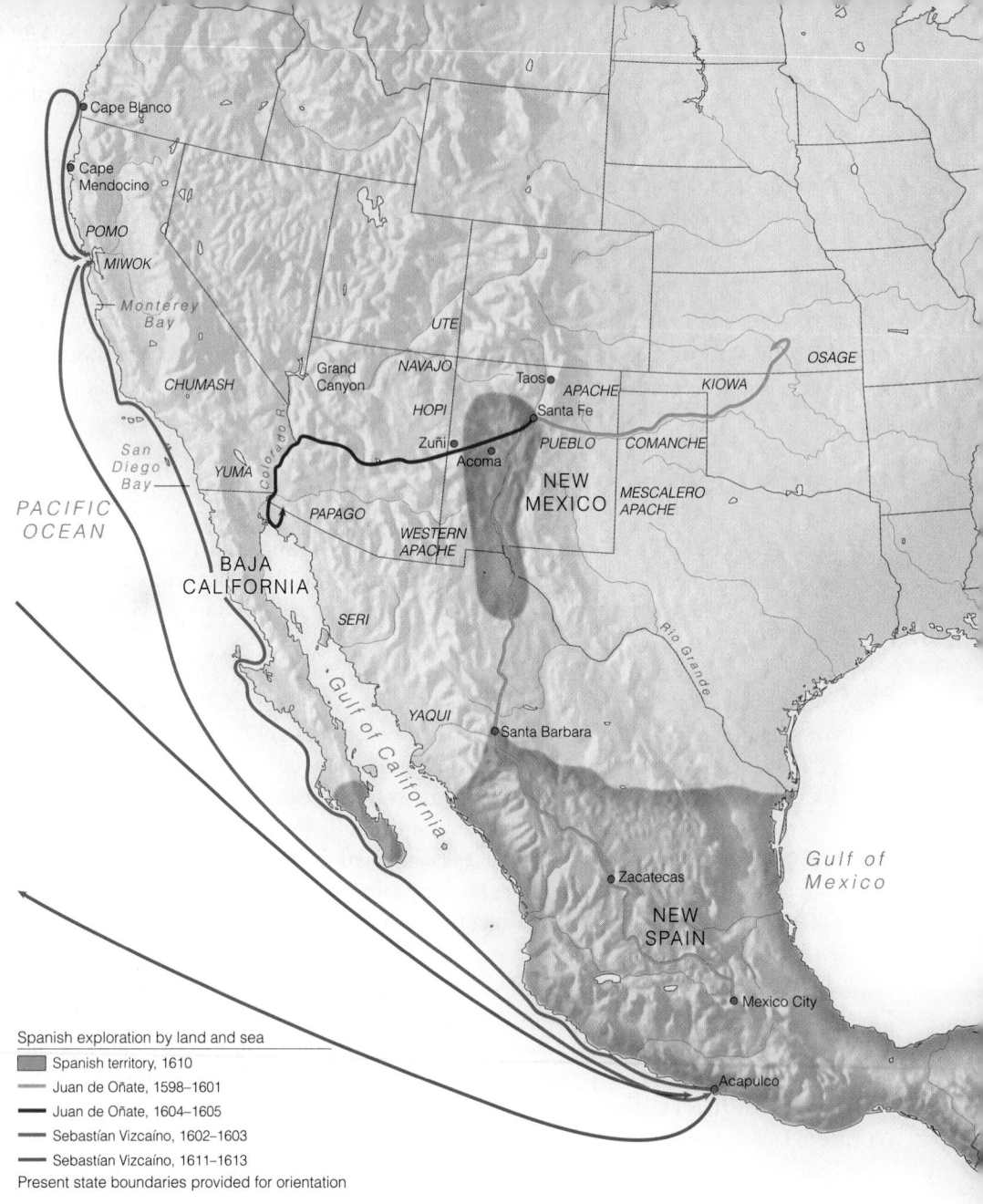

Spanish exploration by land and sea

▮ Spanish territory, 1610
— Juan de Oñate, 1598–1601
— Juan de Oñate, 1604–1605
— Sebastían Vizcaíno, 1602–1603
— Sebastían Vizcaíno, 1611–1613
Present state boundaries provided for orientation

■ **MAP 2.1**
THE SPANISH SOUTHWEST IN THE EARLY SEVENTEENTH CENTURY

in Japan, he brought 180 Japanese with him to Mexico. This unique delegation was bound for Spain and Italy to open doors between East and West. However, the Tokugawas soon began to persecute the European traders and Christian missionaries who had been allowed in the Japanese islands for a generation. Because of this persecution, the frail link between Europe and Japan through Mexico never developed further.

Tokugawa officials, it seems, feared that tolerating foreigners in Japan's ports might foster the spread of Christianity and undermine their supremacy. Moreover, developing Japanese fleets might bring guns to warlords and disrupt hard-won peace. So Japan passed up an opportunity for naval expansion, just as Ming China had done two centuries earlier after the voyages of Cheng Ho. Instead, the new dynasty adopted a policy of commercial and cultural isolation that would last for more than two hundred years. Had Japanese society followed another route, co-opting Western technologies and aggressively exploring and colonizing the Pacific, the subsequent history of North America and the world would almost certainly have taken a very different path.

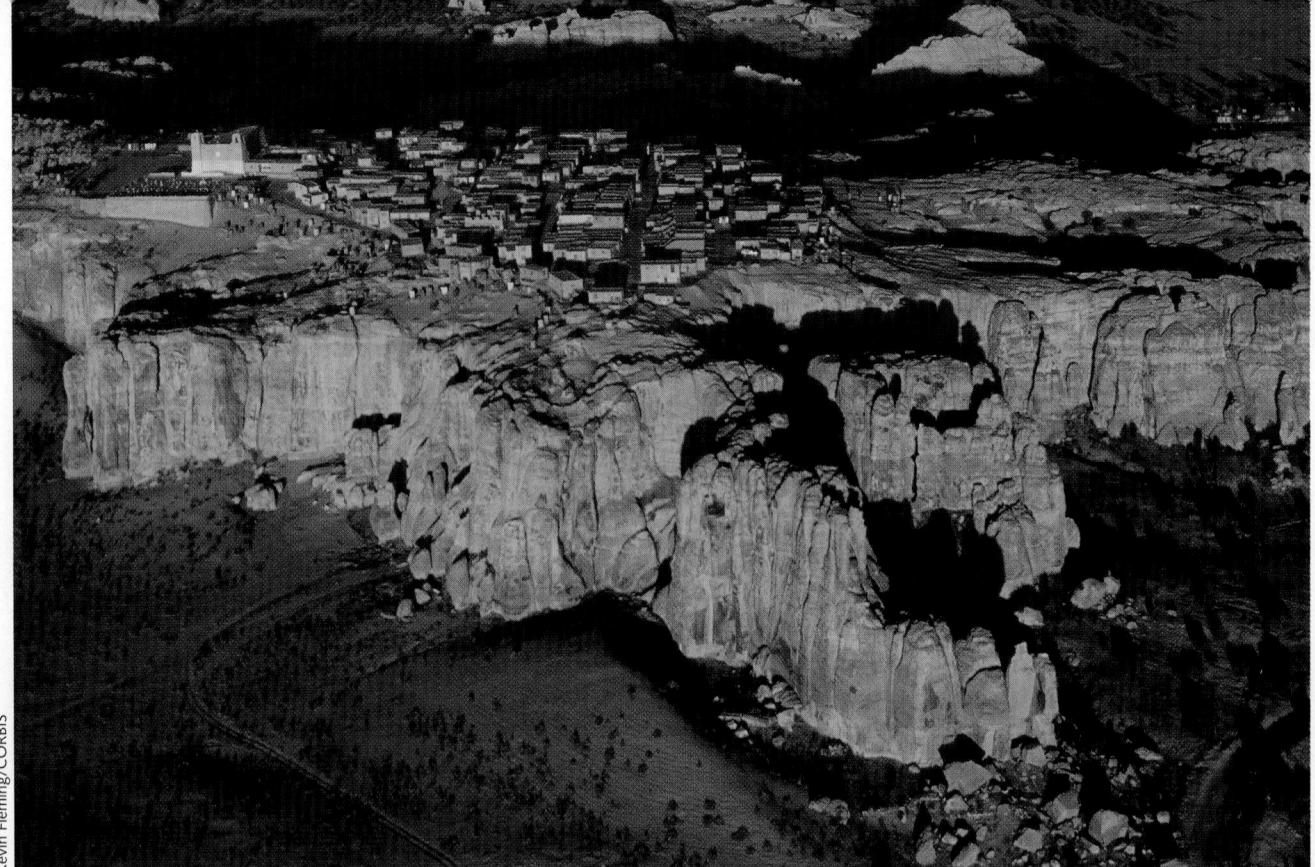

■ Acoma, often called Sky City, sits atop a high sandstone mesa west of Albuquerque, New Mexico. The name means "place that always was," and the pueblo has been continuously inhabited for roughly 1000 years. Acoma's Native American community survived a devastating attack by Spanish colonizers in 1599.

For the Spanish, Vizcaíno's Pacific adventure also failed to open new prospects. His fruitless search for gold and silver consumed crucial funds, and the possibility of a Spanish settlement at Monterey quickly disappeared. Spanish mariners knew California's rugged coastline only from the sea, and the steep cliffs discouraged them from approaching the mainland too closely. Moreover, fresh probes by ships sailing to the north along California's coast might reveal the "Straits of Anian"—the mythic Northwest Passage from the Atlantic to the Pacific that Spain's rivals had been seeking. Concerned that their empire had already become overextended, Spanish officials postponed plans to colonize California's coast. In addition, Spain wondered whether to maintain its existing North American colony in Florida and its newest frontier province: New Mexico.

Oñate Creates a Spanish Foothold in the Southwest

In 1598 Juan de Oñate renewed the northern efforts of Coronado's expedition several generations earlier. Setting out from New Spain, he led 500 men, women, and children north into the upper Rio Grande valley to create the province of New Mexico. Oñate was a wealthy man—his father had discovered a major silver mine at Zacatecas—and he had bold ambitions. Aided by Franciscan friars (organized followers of St. Francis loyal to the Roman Catholic pope), Oñate and his colonists expected to convert the Indians to Christianity. (The newcomers called these local inhabitants the Pueblo people, using the Spanish word for *town*, since they lived in compact apartment-like villages.) Expanding outward from the native towns, or pueblos, the intruders hoped to open a vast new colonial realm. It would be a "new world," they proclaimed, "greater than New Spain."

But Oñate drastically underestimated the difficulties. When embittered Indians at Acoma pueblo killed 11 of his soldiers in 1599, he retaliated by bombarding the mesa-top citadel, killing 800 inhabitants and enslaving nearly 600 others. Hearing of the brutal repression of the

49

residents of Acoma, neighboring pueblos reluctantly submitted to Spanish demands for labor and food. Oñate had expended his entire personal fortune to establish a fragile toehold in the region. But reinforcements arriving in 1600 were dismayed by the harsh conditions; Oñate needed new discoveries if the colony were to prosper. In 1601, he launched an expedition east onto the Great Plains, mistakenly believing that the Atlantic Ocean was not far away. The venture proved as futile as Coronado's earlier march had been.

To make matters worse, 1601 proved to be a year of drought. When Oñate returned to the Rio Grande, he found that two-thirds of his tiny colony—including many of the recent reinforcements—had given up and departed. Instead of silver, they had found sand. The disillusioned settlers returned to Mexico in a pitiful condition. Asked why they had deserted the colony, they said that the region lacked woods, pastures, water, and suitable land.

Foiled on the east and weakened along the Rio Grande, Oñate next pressed west to seek a link to the Pacific. When he reached the Gulf of California in 1605, he mistook it for the great ocean. He even inscribed a notice of his feat (still visible) on the great sandstone rock, El Morro, between Acoma and Zuni pueblos. But his new "Mexico" remained isolated and impoverished, with the remaining colonists strapped for clothing and food. The newcomers, desperate to survive, pressed hard on the native peoples they had harried into submission. They demanded tribute in the form of cotton blankets, buffalo hides, and baskets of scarce maize. In winter, ill-equipped Spanish soldiers stripped warm robes off the backs of shivering women and children; in summer, they scoured each pueblo for corn. Sometimes they tortured residents to find out where food was hidden.

Meanwhile, a few hundred Pueblo Indians—intimidated by the Spanish, desperate for a share of the food they had grown, and fearful of attacks by neighboring Apaches—began to accept Christian baptism and seek Spanish protection. By 1608, when the crown threatened to withdraw support from the struggling province, the colony's Franciscan missionaries appealed that their converts had grown too numerous to resettle and too dependent to abandon. Their argument may have been exaggerated, but it caught the attention of authorities.

Besides, England and France were launching new colonies in Virginia and Canada. Since mapmakers still could not accurately calculate longitude (east-west distance on the globe), no one was sure whether these bases created by international rivals posed a threat that was dangerously close at hand. England's failed Roanoke colony, after all, had the same latitude (or north-south position) as Santa Fe, and many Europeans still estimated the two points were not far apart. Worried Spanish officials finally agreed with the Franciscan friars that New Mexico must carry on. But, they replaced Oñate with a new governor and asserted royal control over the few dozen settlers who remained in the colony.

New Mexico Survives: New Flocks Among Old Pueblos

The Spanish decision to hold on in New Mexico reshaped life for everyone in the region. At least 60,000 Indians living in nearly separate pueblos found their world transformed and their survival threatened over the next half-century. In 1610 the new governor, ruling over scarcely 50 colonists, created a capital at the village of Sante Fe. Every three years, a government supply train of 30 wagons made the long trip to the new capital from Mexico City. Within two decades, roughly 750 colonists inhabited the remote province, including Spanish, Mexican Indians, Africans, and mixed-race children.

The racial and ethnic diversity of New Mexico repeated the colonial pattern established in New Spain. Similarly, labor practices and

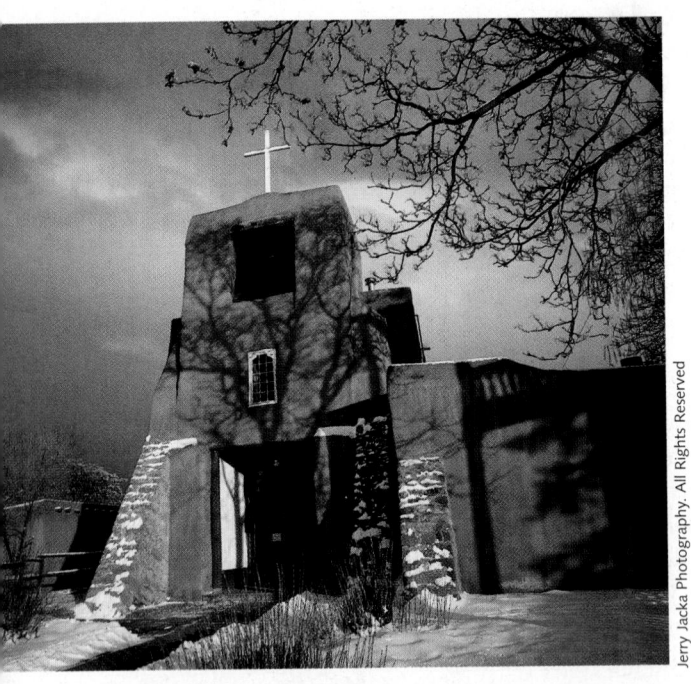

■ The Spanish made Santa Fe the capital of their New Mexico colony in 1610 and built the church of San Miguel there in 1626. Though destroyed in the Pueblo Revolt of 1680, it was rebuilt and has remained in use. "The floor is bare earth," wrote an eighteenth-century observer, "the usual floor throughout these regions."

religious changes also followed models established after the conquest of the Aztecs in Mexico. As in New Spain, certain privileged people in the new colony received *encomiendas*; such grants entitled the holders (known as an *encomenderos*), to the labor of a set number of Native American workers. With labor in short supply throughout the Spanish colonies, other settlers led occasional raids against nomadic Plains Indians, keeping some captives and shipping others south to toil as slaves in the Mexican silver mines.

Meanwhile, the number of missionaries rose rapidly, just as it had throughout Spain's American empire. By the 1630s, 46 Franciscan friars staffed missions in 35 pueblos. They preached a mix of Christian religion and Hispanic cultural values. They forbade traditional Pueblo celebrations, known as kachina dances, and destroyed sacred kachina masks. Their combination of intense zeal and harsh punishments prompted many Indians to learn Spanish and become obedient converts. However, it also drove the Indians' own religious practices underground—literally, into the hidden, circular kivas that had long been a focal point for Native American spiritual activities in the region. There, people kept their traditional faith alive in secret and passed sacred rituals along to the next generation.

The Spanish brought more than Christianity to New Mexico. The newcomers also transferred novel crops (wheat, onions, chilies, peas) and planted new fruits (peaches, plums, cherries). Settlers introduced metal hoes and axes to the area as well, along with donkeys, chickens, and other domesticated animals previously unknown to the native inhabitants. Horses and cattle, led north from New Spain in small herds, eventually revolutionized life across the North American West. But Spanish sheep, well suited to the semi-desert conditions, exerted the most immediate impact. Each friar soon possessed a flock of several thousand. Pueblo artisans, skilled at spinning cotton, now wove woolen cloth for their own use and for export.

But the Pueblo world, like Squanto's world, was eroding under the onslaught of new European diseases. The large Pueblo population, cut in half in the 60 years after Coronado's appearance, still numbered more than 60,000 in 1600, after the arrival of Oñate's colonizing expedition. Yet sickness, along with warfare and famine, cut this number in half again by 1650 and in half once more by 1680.

Conversion and Rebellion in Spanish Florida

The flat, lush environment of the Florida peninsula contrasts sharply with the dry, rugged landscape of New Mexico. Yet by 1600, Spain's Florida colony had also disappointed imperial officials. Dreams of gold-filled kingdoms and a strategic passage from the Southeast to the Orient had never materialized. The 500 needy soldiers, settlers, and slaves who resided in thatched huts at St. Augustine struck Spanish officials at home as an undue burden. The government planned to disband the colony and end its annual subsidy. But Franciscan missionaries won the day, as in New Mexico. They argued that scores of Indian towns appeared ready to receive Christianity. By 1608, the crown had decided to let the colony continue. A handful of missionaries fanned out among the Indians of northern Florida, erecting small churches, celebrating mass, and explaining the rudiments of the Catholic faith.

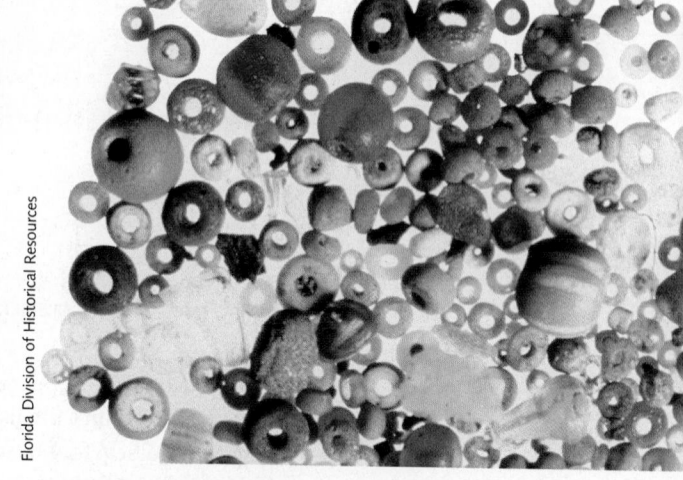

■ The Spanish found that glass beads, colorful and easy to transport, made fine gifts and trade items in their contacts with Florida Indians. Chiefs often received special quartz crystal beads and pendants to retain their loyalty.

Florida Division of Historical Resources

However, the Franciscans soon realized that literacy itself held a more powerful appeal among Florida Indians than the Christian word. The friars therefore set up schools "for imprinting the Christian discipline and doctrine in those hearts and lands with letters." At missions (known as *doctrinas*), where a resident friar taught church doctrine, they recruited Indian students aggressively without regard to age or sex. In 1612 Francisco de Pareja published an illustrated, bilingual confessional in Castilian and Timucuan, the earliest text in any North American Indian language. The book enabled wary friars to ask villagers, "Have you said suggestive words?" and "Have you desired to do some lewd act with some man or woman or kin?"

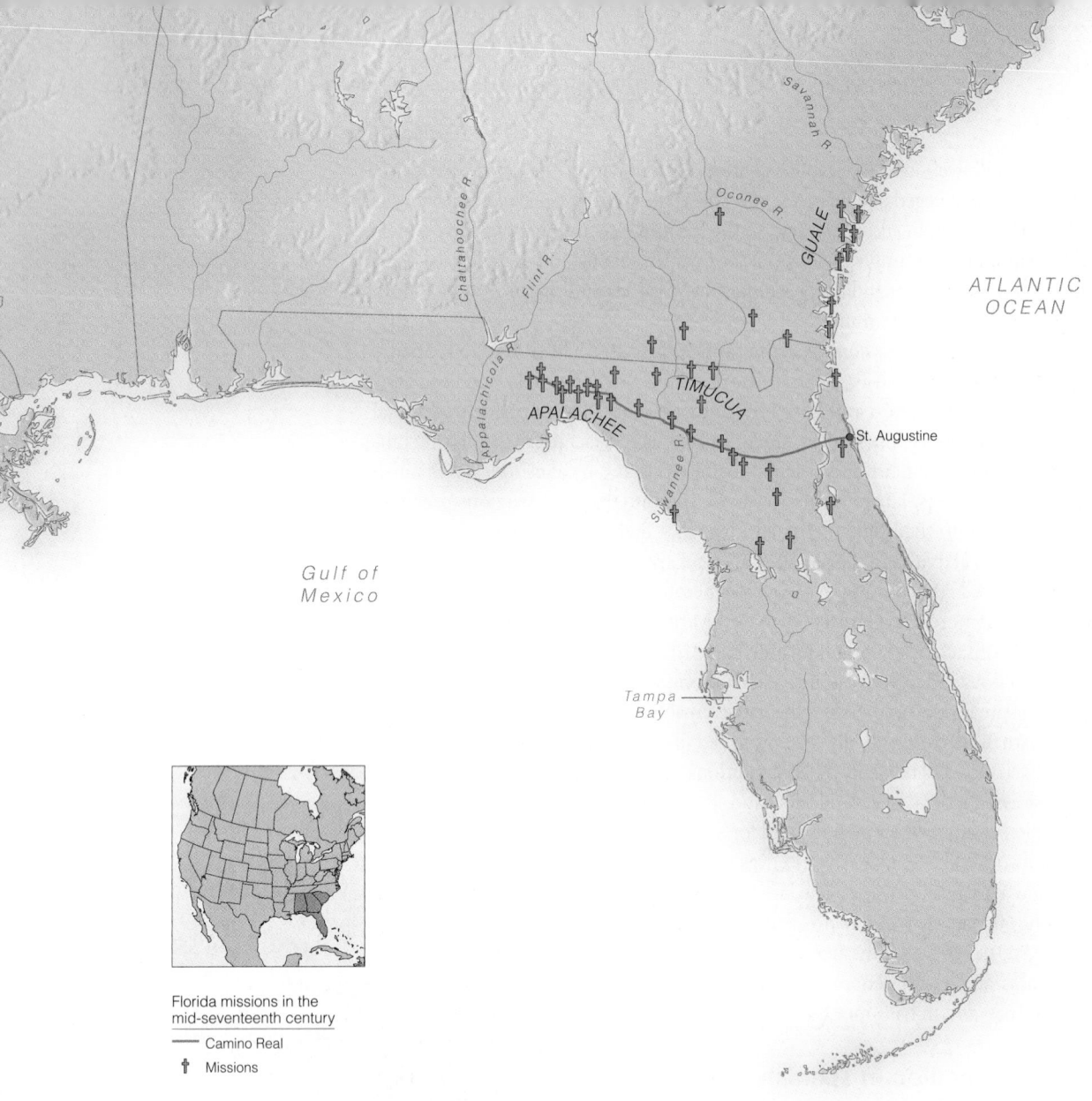

ATLANTIC
OCEAN

GUALE

TIMUCUA

APALACHEE

St. Augustine

Gulf of
Mexico

Tampa
Bay

Florida missions in the
mid-seventeenth century
—— Camino Real
† Missions

■ **MAP 2.2**
SITES OF CATHOLIC MISSIONS IN SPANISH FLORIDA IN THE MID-SEVENTEENTH CENTURY

Contact with Christian beliefs and books came at a steep price, for each inland village was expected to help feed the colonial garrison at St. Augustine. Local women neglected their own household crops to grow additional maize and grind it into meal. Annually, the crown requisitioned the labor of Indian men from each village. Spanish officials compelled them to transport the cornmeal overland to the Atlantic coast and return to the mission bringing supplies back to the Franciscans. Imported candles, communion wine, and mission bells all had to be hauled inland from St. Augustine. The trip to and from the coast took several weeks, and each bearer shouldered a 75-pound load. When missions appeared in the western province of Apalachee (around modern-day Tallahassee) after 1633, the treks from the coast needed to cover even greater distances.

Friars and Indian bearers traveling to the interior also carried sicknesses from St. Augustine. Epidemics of measles, bubonic plague, malaria, typhus, smallpox, and influenza took a devastating toll on the Native Americans. Harsh work conditions and poor diets lowered people's resistance to illness. Indians expired more rapidly than the Spanish could convert them, and friars hastened to baptize the dying and claim their souls for Christ. In a letter to the Spanish king in 1617, a Franciscan reported that the local population had been cut in half in the five years since his arrival "on account of the great plagues and contagious diseases that the Indians have suffered." But he reassured his majesty that "a very rich harvest of souls for heaven has been made in the midst of great numbers of deaths."

Even though the small cadre of friars grew, reaching a high of 70 after midcentury, the region's overall population plummeted. A report from 1635, shortly after Spanish expansion into Apalachee, claimed 30,000 baptisms at 44 missions. But within a generation, the number of native Floridians, whether baptized or not, had plunged by nearly half. In 1655 the governor noted "high mortality" throughout Timucua caused by a "series of small-pox plagues which have affected the country for the last ten months" and by "the trials and hunger which these unfortunate people have suffered." Two years later, he reported that the people of Timucua and Guale had been almost "wiped out with the sickness of the plague and small-pox which has overtaken them."

As whole villages disappeared, Spanish entrepreneurs began to expand cattle ranching across the newly vacated lands of northern Florida. Faced with encroaching farms, crushing labor demands, and frightful mortality, local native leaders saw their power reduced and their communities depleted. When the Spanish established a cattle ranch in Apalachee in 1645, a local chief protested that they drew in "all the men and the women, boys and girls," to provide labor, and "what we gained from all this work was solely fatigue and nothing else."

Two years later, in 1647, Indians at Apalachee staged a revolt. They burned down seven of the area's mission compounds, killing three friars, the deputy governor and his family, and a number of recent converts. But the garrison at St. Augustine reacted quickly, and when its soldiers arrived, they tried and executed 12 of the rebel leaders. In 1656 a wider Native American uprising shook Timucua in north central Florida. The rebellion occurred because the governor of Florida feared a possible attack by English ships on the garrison at St. Augustine. He therefore requisitioned 500 Indian warriors from the Timucua region to help fend off the rumored invasion, and he required each man to bring along 75 pounds of corn for the campaign. Insulted by the demand, Timucuan leaders staged a revolt that took months to suppress.

In the end, the English threat to Spanish Florida did not materialize, but the rumor in 1656 underscored how much had changed in the preceding half-century. Two generations earlier, in 1600, no European power besides Spain had possessed a solid foothold in any portion of the Americas.

Even Portuguese Brazil had recently come under the rule of Spain. But over the next six decades, France, Holland, and England all asserted claims on the American mainland. These rivals challenged Spain not only in the Atlantic but in the Pacific as well.

France and Holland: Overseas Competition for Spain

At the turn of the seventeenth century, interlopers from Holland had challenged Spanish colonizers in the Philippines and Portuguese traders in Japan. These Dutch efforts illustrated the growing competition between European powers for control of the world's oceans. In London, commercial leaders received a royal charter to create the English East India Company in 1600, and merchants in Amsterdam took a similar step. Hoping to capture Portugal's lucrative Asian trade, they established the Dutch East India Company in 1602. Four years later, Dutchman Willem Jansz became the first European to glimpse Australia. Within a generation (as the Ming dynasty ended in China during the 1640s), Dutch sailors expanded their Asian reach still farther. They took Malacca (near Singapore) from the Portuguese in 1641, reached Tasmania and New Zealand in 1642, and charted the coast of northern Japan in 1643. By 1652 they had also founded a Dutch colony at Cape Town, on the southern tip of Africa.

The united powers of Spain and Portugal proved even more vulnerable in the Atlantic. To be sure, Spanish convoys continued to transport Mexican gold and silver to Europe annually, along with Asian silks and spices shipped to Mexico via the Pacific trade. Portuguese vessels carried Africans to the New World at a profit. But ships from rival European nations preyed on these seaborne cargoes with increasing success. Defiantly, they also laid claim to numerous islands in the Caribbean.

By 1660, the English had taken control of Barbados, Providence Island, Antigua, and Jamaica; the Dutch had acquired St. Maarten, St. Eustacius, Saba, and Curaçao; and the French had claimed Guadeloupe, Martinique, Grenada, and St. Lucia. For France, however, the most promising Atlantic prospects lay farther north in Canada. There, Spanish power was absent, hopes for a Northwest Passage persisted, and French imperial claims stretched back generations.

The Founding of New France

Since the time of Jacques Cartier, fishing boats from the coast of France had crisscrossed New-foundland's Grand Banks. One old French salt claimed to have made the voyage for 42 consecutive years. The trade increased after 1580 as crews built seasonal stations along the American coast for drying codfish. These stations brought them into greater contact with Indians; soon both parties were exchanging metal goods for furs on terms that pleased all. A Native American could trade a worn-out robe made from beaver skins for a highly valued iron kettle. For a European, the older the robe the better, for its Indian owner wore it with the fur side in. Steady wear rubbed away the long guard hairs and left the soft underlayer of fur. Back home in Europe, workers removed these greasy short hairs and matted them into felt for the manufacture of beaver hats. (They used mercury in the process, not knowing that its poison made some of them insane, hence the phrase "mad as a hatter.") The finished product proved warm, waterproof, and fashionable. Because one robe yielded felt for six to eight hats (each worth a steep three pounds), its high sale price let dealers purchase scores of kettles and knives for the next year's exchange.

As North Atlantic fishing and trading expanded, the domestic situation in France improved after 1600. In 1598, a generation of religious war between Catholics and Protestants in France ended when King Henry IV issued the Edict of Nantes. The decree granted political rights and limited toleration to French Protestants, or Huguenots. With peace restored, the king could now afford to look favorably on new colonization initiatives in America. An experienced French soldier and sailor named Samuel de Champlain emerged as a key leader in this effort. Between 1599 and 1601, Champlain scouted Spain's New World empire and brought back suggestions to Paris for overseas advancement of French interests. He even offered a proposal to create a canal across the Isthmus of Panama. But from 1602 until his death in 1635, Champlain devoted himself to the St. Lawrence River region, where Acadia on the Atlantic coast and Canada along the extensive river valley made up the anticipated realm of New France.

Year-round French settlements in Acadia could support the Atlantic fisheries, extend the fur trade, and preempt the English, who were eyeing the same coast. Spurred by rumors of precious metals and western passages to Asia, Champlain explored and mapped the coast from Cape Breton to Cape Cod. But settlement efforts came to nothing, so the French directed their attention inland. In 1608 Champlain and several dozen other men established the outpost of Quebec at a narrow spot in the St. Lawrence River, where Cartier and Rober-val had wintered generations earlier.

In June 1609 Champlain joined a band of Algonquin and Huron Indians in a raid on the Iroquois. They journeyed south to a large lake in modern New York, which he proudly renamed as Lake Champlain. When they engaged their Iroquois enemies in battle, Champlain fired his gun to kill several war chiefs. A novelty in the region, the gun sparked a rout. For the powerful Iroquois League south of the St. Lawrence (the Five Nation confederation composed of the Seneca, Cayuga, Onondaga, Oneida, and Mohawk Indians), the defeat spawned lasting bitterness. But the victory sealed good relations for the French with the Algonquins and Hurons, ensuring the survival of Quebec and spurring unprecedented commerce. Within 15 years, Native Americans were trading 12,000 to 15,000 beaver pelts annually via the St. Lawrence River valley.

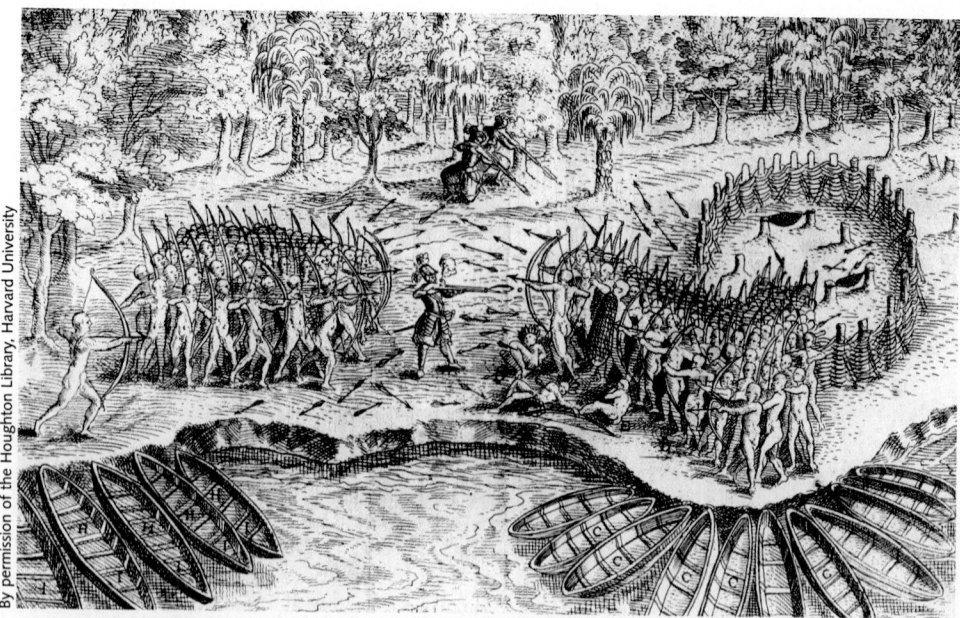

By permission of the Houghton Library, Harvard University

■ **Champlain's drawing of the battle on Lake Champlain, 1609**

In 1627, the powerful first minister in France, Cardinal Richelieu, pressed for greater French settlement in Canada through a new private company. He banned Huguenots from participating and pushed to make sure that only Roman Catholics were allowed to migrate to Canada. But his expansive policies alarmed England, which began aggressive efforts to force out the French colonists. In 1628 English privateers (privately owned ships commissioned to seize enemy vessels for profit) captured an arriving convoy of 400 French Catholic settlers. The next year, they forced the surrender of Quebec. When restored to French control several years later, the tiny outpost contained fewer than a hundred people. In an effort to expand the meager settlement and populate the fertile valley upriver from Quebec, French authorities began granting narrow strips of land with river frontage to any Catholic lord who would take up residence there and bring French tenants to his estate.

Competing for the Beaver Trade

Cardinal Richelieu's power in France epitomized the ongoing Counter-Reformation. Indeed, the effects of this outpouring of Catholic zeal reached as far as North America. In 1635 Jesuits from the Society of Jesus, created a century earlier by Ignatius Loyola to defend and spread the Catholic faith, founded a college in Quebec to educate the sons of colonists, and in 1639 six nuns arrived to begin a school and a hospital for Indian girls. Other religious workers established a station farther west in 1641. Their outpost where the Ottawa River joined the St. Lawrence, in territory recently dominated by the Iroquois, marked the beginnings of Montreal. This move upstream had strategic as well as religious significance. The French wanted to control the beaver trade as it expanded west. They also hoped to prevent the Iroquois League from diverting furs south to Holland's new colony on the Hudson River.

But the desperate Iroquois nations, facing collapse, took a stand. Increasing contact with Europeans and their contagious diseases had brought catastrophic epidemics to the Iroquois homelands below Lake Ontario. Beginning in 1633, sicknesses that were new to the region swept away some 10,000 people and cut the Five Nations' population in half within a decade. The Mohawks—farthest east and most exposed to French, Dutch, and English newcomers—suffered the most, losing as many as three out of four people from the distinctive longhouses

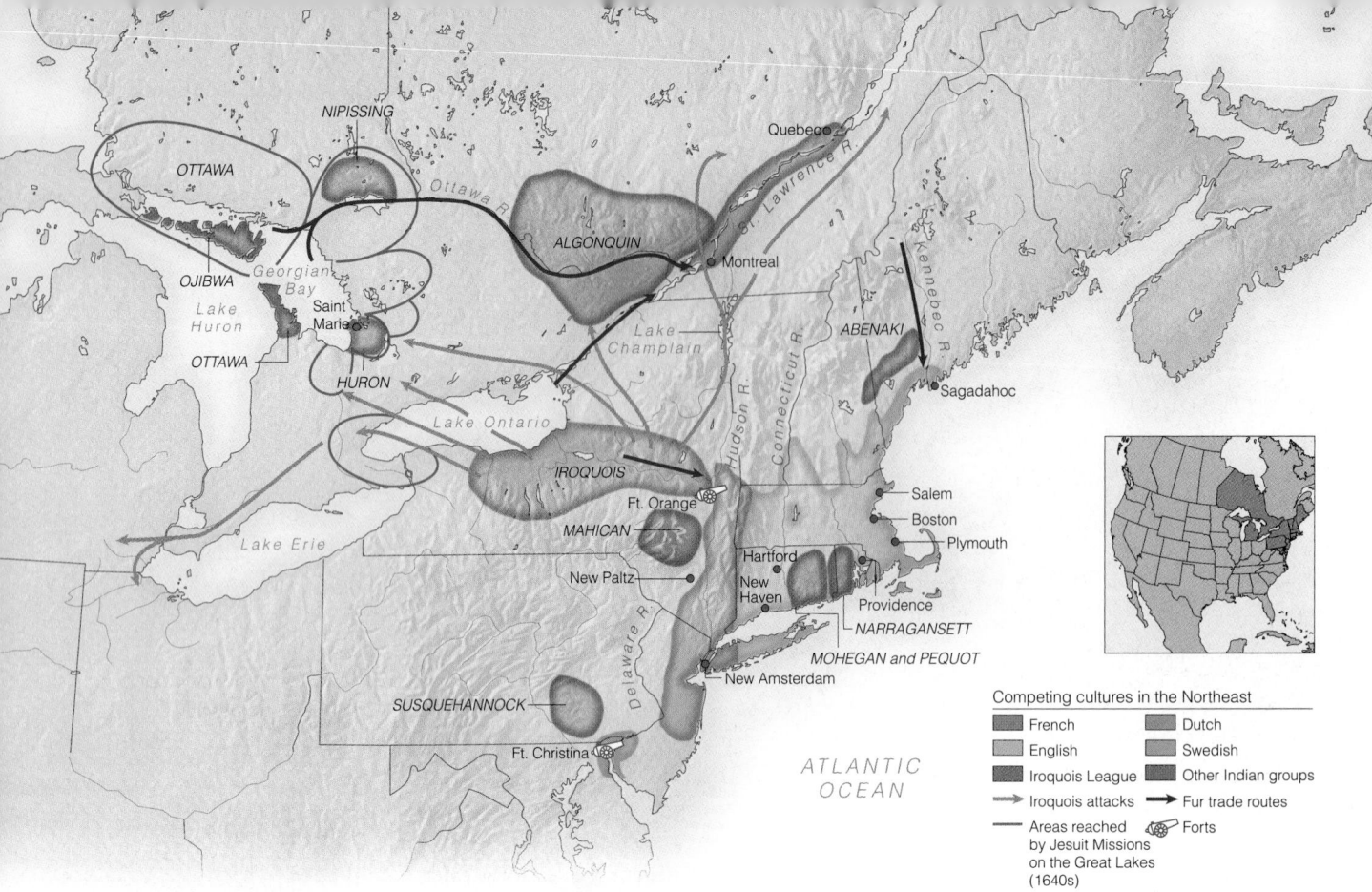

■ **MAP 2.3**
EUROPEAN AND NATIVE AMERICAN CONTACT IN THE NORTHEAST, 1600–1660 French and English colonization efforts brought devastating diseases to the Five Nations of the Iroquois League. Eager to take captives and profit from the growing trade in furs, the Iroquois ranged north and west to make war on the French and their Huron Indian allies.

that made up Iroquois villages. According to Iroquois tradition, survivors must replace deceased individuals swiftly with captives to maintain the community's strength and continuity. Pressed by grieving families, Iroquois warriors initiated a generation of violent campaigns intended to capture and absorb neighboring groups. These so-called mourning wars are also remembered as the Beaver Wars because they included a clear economic as well as cultural motive. Besides captives, the Iroquois aggressors sought furs. If they could seize pelts before the valuable items reached the French, they could trade them to the Dutch for guns and powder. Well armed, they could then engage in further wars for captives and furs.

This spiral of aggression put the Iroquois on a collision course with the Hurons and their Catholic allies, a small band of Jesuit missionaries from France. These members of the militant Society of Jesus were willing to risk martyrdom to win converts in New France. But the seasonal mobility of most local Indians frustrated them. According to one discouraged priest, "Not much ought to be hoped for from the savages as long as they are wanderers." Eager to find "a stable nation" for potential converts, the Jesuits focused their attention on Huronia, the region east of Lake Huron and Georgian Bay. There, 30,000 Huron Indians lived in large, settled villages. The Jesuits erected chapels at four of these towns. And in 1639, they constructed a central base at St. Marie on the Wye River, part fort and part mission. Having volunteered for hardship, they witnessed far more of it than they ever imagined.

First came the same foreign epidemics that had wasted the Iroquois; smallpox cut down roughly two-thirds of the Huron population, or 20,000 people, between 1635 and 1640. Then came the Iroquois themselves, bent on capturing Huron women and children to revitalize their longhouses, swept empty by disease in the 1630s. Armed by Dutch traders eager for furs, 1000 warriors descended on the weakened Hurons in March 1649. They burned villages, secured captives, tortured several priests to death, and seized large stocks of pelts. Some lucky survivors dispersed to neighboring tribes, and the 500 who remained behind took refuge near Quebec. The Iroquois then launched raids on the St. Lawrence valley, disrupting the fur trade and frightening the several thousand French inhabitants. By 1660, it seemed that New France—thinly settled, weakly defended, and poorly supplied—might face the same extinction that the much older and larger Huronia community had suffered.

A Dutch Colony on the Hudson River

The Dutch traders who supplied firearms to the Iroquois in exchange for furs owed their start to English-born navigator and arctic explorer Henry Hudson. In 1608 the Dutch East India Company, eager to locate a northeastern route to China, hired Hudson and his crew to probe above Scandinavia. But when snowstorms blocked their way, Hudson sailed his vessel, the *Half Moon,* across the Atlantic in search of a western passage to the Orient. During the summer of 1609, the *Half Moon* visited Chesapeake Bay and Delaware Bay, then rediscovered modern-day New York harbor, the bay that Verrazzano had entered in 1524. Flying the Dutch flag, Hudson sailed north up the broad river that now bears his name. Along the way, he obtained food and furs from Algonkian Indians in exchange for knives and beads. He noted that saltwater and ocean tides pushed 60 miles upstream—Indians called the river "the water that flows two ways." But no channel to the Pacific materialized.

The Dutch moved quickly to gain a foothold in the region. Ships from Amsterdam soon appeared far up the Hudson, exchanging metal goods for beaver pelts and occasionally leaving men behind to engage in trading with the Indians. One Dutch captain arriving in 1613 encountered Juan Rodrigues, a mulatto from the West Indies who had jumped ship the previous year with 80 hatchets and other trade goods. The captain, in turn, left behind a young Amsterdam clerk and took away two sons of the principal Indian leader, or *sachem*. Soon the Dutch clerk had established a year-round trading post at Fort Orange (near present-day Albany). Mohawk traditions recall how the Indians "Planted the Tree of Good Understanding" with the Dutch newcomers, whom they called *Kristoni,* for "I am a metal maker."

In 1621, responsibility for New Netherland—the region claimed between the Delaware and Connecticut rivers—fell to the newly chartered Dutch West India Company (DWIC).

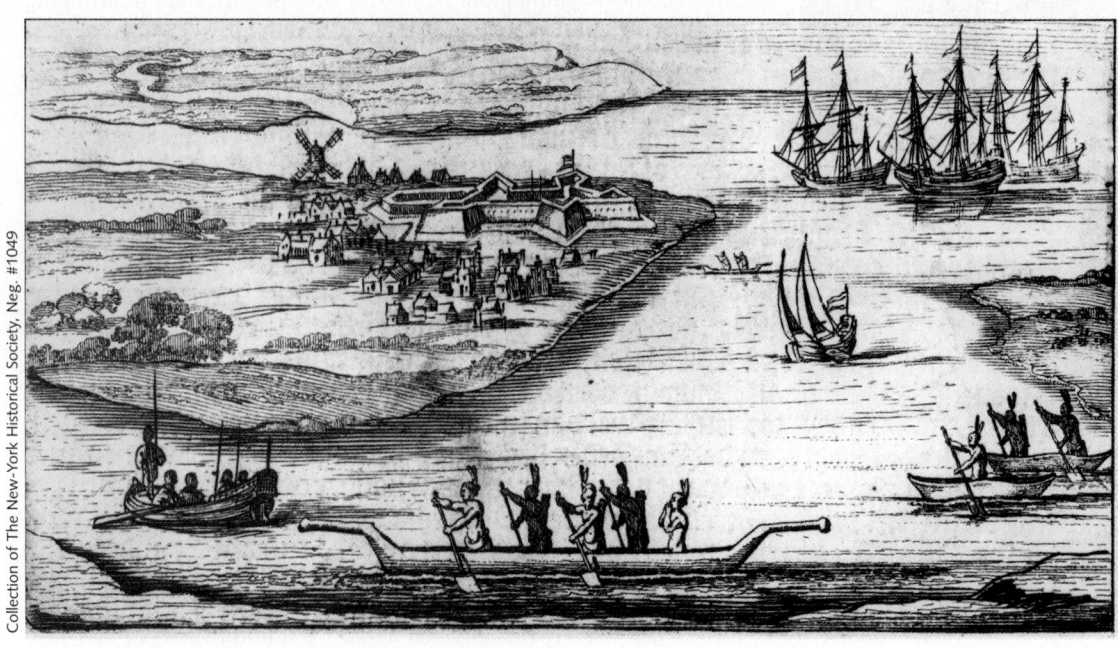

Collection of The New-York Historical Society, Neg. #1049

■ **New Amsterdam Fort on Manhattan Island**

Modeled on the Dutch East India Company, this enterprise made Holland a formidable force in the Atlantic, especially after the spectacular Dutch capture of the Spanish silver fleet off Cuba in 1628. The DWIC concentrated on piecing together an empire in the South Atlantic. Dutch ships seized part of sugar-rich Brazil (1632), the island of Curaçao near Venezuela (1634), and Portugal's African outpost at Elmina, on the coast of modern-day Ghana (1637). But the DWIC also laid plans for a North American colony.

To begin, company officials recruited a group of Walloon refugees, French-speaking Belgians who had hoped to found a community in English Virginia. They transported these people to New Netherland in 1624. To secure the boundaries of the province, they deposited farm families far up the Hudson at Fort Orange and along the Connecticut and Delaware rivers. However, Peter Minuit, the colony's director from 1626 to 1631, saw danger in this dispersal. He worried that the widely scattered newcomers lacked defenses, trade, and community ties. To consolidate Dutch settlement, he purchased Manhattan Island at the mouth of the Hudson from the local Indians. By 1630, the village of New Amsterdam boasted 270 settlers clustered in cottages around a waterfront fort at the southern tip of Manhattan. (When the inhabitants built a wall around the village to protect against Indian attacks, the road inside this palisade became known as Wall Street.)

Next, the DWIC began granting land along the Hudson to wealthy *patroons* (patrons), similar to the French seigneurs along the St. Lawrence. Hoping that private investment would strengthen their colony, the company gave a huge tract with 18 miles of river frontage to any wealthy investor who could send 50 people to farm there as tenants. An Amsterdam merchant named Kiliaen van Rensselaer formed the first and most lucrative of these patroonships near Fort Orange. But this effort to promote migration faltered, and new conflicts began to appear on several fronts.

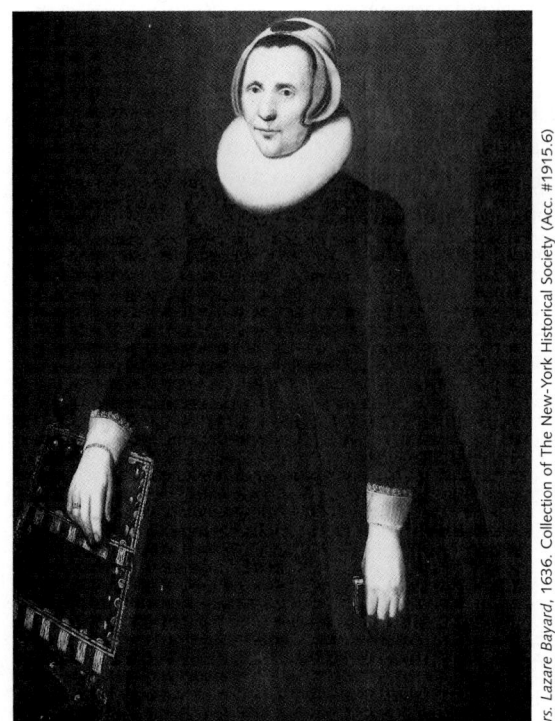

■ When Judith Bayard Stuyvesant arrived in New Amsterdam with her husband in 1647, she carried this portrait of her mother, Judith de Vos Bayard, painted in Holland in 1636. Dutch painting flourished at the time, led by Rembrandt and Hals.

Mrs. Lazare Bayard, 1636. Collection of The New-York Historical Society (Acc. #1915.6)

When the company threw open the Indian trade to others besides its own agents, the careless and greedy actions of unregulated traders sparked a series of violent wars with coastal tribes. Settlers also squabbled with neighboring English settlers over fur-trading rights and other matters. The small colony of New Sweden, which materialized on the west side of the Delaware River in 1637, posed yet another problem. That short-lived venture was sponsored partly by Dutch capital, and Peter Minuit was put in charge. But the settlers who actually built Fort Christina (now Wilmington, Delaware) were Swedes and Finns hoping to establish their own trade with the Indians. But in 1655, these several hundred Scandinavian settlers were obliged to surrender to Dutch power.

"All Sorts of Nationalities": Diverse New Amsterdam

The symbol of Dutch power in the region, and the commander of the fleet that seized New Sweden, was Peter Stuyvesant. He ruled New Netherland aggressively for several decades before England seized the colony in 1664. His career reveals the close ties among the DWIC's Atlantic ventures. Stuyvesant had served as governor of Dutch Curaçao (losing his right leg in an attack on the Spanish at St. Maarten). His next commission made him director general of several DWIC dependencies, including New Netherland and Curaçao. He married Judith Bayard in Holland, and the couple sailed from Amsterdam for New Netherland in 1647.

Stuyvesant, age 37, moved swiftly to assert control. He limited beer and rum sales, fined settlers for promiscuity and knife fighting, and established a nine-member night watch. If disobeyed, he turned to whippings. "He proceeds no longer by words or writings," a resident complained in 1651, "but by arrests and stripes." When a group of English Quakers, members of the newly formed Society of Friends, arrived aboard a trading vessel in 1657, he attempted to expel the radical Protestants and fine any who gave them shelter. However, Dutch residents of Flushing, on Long Island, defied his ban and signed a public letter of objection stressing religious toleration. "Whether Presbyterian, Independent, Baptist or Quaker," they protested, "let every man stand and fall to his own."

To address the colony's chronic labor shortage, Stuyvesant endorsed trade in African slaves, by now a mainstay in Holland's South Atlantic commerce. He also used his Caribbean connections to expand this traffic. When the Portuguese forced Holland out of Brazil in 1654 and closed that sugar colony to Dutch slave vessels, some of the ships brought their cargoes to New Amsterdam instead. Like the Dutch-speaking blacks who already lived in the colony, most of these newcomers were enslaved for life. But the DWIC, the largest importer and owner of slaves in New Netherland, granted "half-freedom" to some people whom it could not employ year-round. These people, in return for an annual fee, could travel and marry freely, acquire property, and hire out their labor. By 1664, African arrivals made up more than 10 percent of New Netherland's population, and at least half of them lived in Lower Manhattan. These 375 black New Amsterdam residents—most enslaved, some half-free, and at least 75 entirely free—made up 20 percent of the town's populace.

> *Compared with New France, New Netherland seemed far more populous, prosperous, and ethnically diverse.*

New Amsterdam, home to fewer than 2000 people, also had a small Jewish contingent, the first in mainland North America. In 1654, 23 Sephardic Jews (forced out of Brazil when the Portuguese took over) reached New Amsterdam aboard the French frigate *Sainte Catherine*. But Stuyvesant promptly asked the DWIC for permission to expel the refugees. Strident in his anti-Semitism, he claimed such "blasphemers of the name of Christ" would "infect and trouble this new colony." The DWIC, which included Jewish stockholders and was eager for newcomers of all kinds, overruled the governor's request. In the end, colony officials authorized a Jewish ghetto, or segregated neighborhood. They instructed the newcomers to build homes "close together in a convenient place on one or the other side of New Amsterdam." Here, they could pray together freely in private. At first, however, they were not allowed to construct a synagogue for public worship.

In the early 1660s, the colony continued to grow, "slowly peopled by the scrapings of all sorts of nationalities," as Stuyvesant complained. Huguenots occupied New Paltz near the Hudson; farther north, other newcomers founded Schenectady in 1661. Swedes and Finns continued to prosper along the Delaware, and numerous English had settled on Long Island. Compared with New France, New Netherland seemed far more populous, prosperous, and ethnically diverse. But whereas the French colony to the north endured for another century, the Dutch enterprise soon was absorbed by England. For, despite a slow start and innumerable setbacks, the English managed to outdistance all their European rivals and establish thriving North American colonies in the first half of the seventeenth century.

English Beginnings on the Atlantic Coast

When Queen Elizabeth I passed away in 1603, several important elements were already in place to help England compete for colonial outposts. The so-called enclosure movement, where large landholders had fenced in their fields and turned to raising sheep, had pushed thousands of tenants off rural farms. These people, who roamed the countryside and flocked to urban centers in search of work, formed a restless supply of potential colonists. Also, the country had an expanding fleet of English-built ships, sailed by experienced mariners who had accumulated extensive knowledge of the North Atlantic. In addition, England had a group of seasoned and ambitious leaders. A generation of soldiers (many of them younger sons of the property-holding elite known as the gentry) had participated in the brutal colonization of Ireland or sailed as privateers in the conflict with Spain. Some, including John Smith, who later became a leader of the Jamestown Colony, had skipped school and fought Spanish forces in the Netherlands. Smith himself had even survived battles and enslavement in Hungary, Turkey, and Russia.

Because Elizabeth died without heirs, the king of Scotland, James Stuart, succeeded her as ruler. During the reigns of James I (1603–1625) and his son Charles I (1625–1649), religious and economic forces in England prompted an increasing number of people to consider migrating overseas. With the expansion of the country's Protestant Reformation, religious strife escalated toward civil war, which erupted in 1642. During the tumultuous 1630s, English public officials were glad to transplant Puritans and Catholics alike to foreign shores. In turn, many ardent believers—weary of conflict or losing hope for their cause at home—welcomed the prospect of a safe haven abroad. Others, eager to support their faith, saw an opportunity to spread their beliefs more widely. Economically, the development of joint stock organizations enabled merchants to raise capital and spread the high risk of colonial ventures by selling numerous shares to small investors. At the same time, the fluctuating domestic economy prompted many people to consider seeking their fortunes elsewhere.

Nor had English geographers given up on finding a sea route somewhere in the Northern Hemisphere leading to the riches of Asia. Perhaps Virginia would prove no wider than the Isthmus of Panama, or a short passage to China would reveal itself farther north. With this latter prospect in mind, England pressed Henry Hudson into service in 1610, shortly after his promising voyage for the Dutch. The experienced explorer ventured far to the northwest, navigating the strait and bay in northern Canada that still bear his name. Mutinous crewmen set the captain adrift in a small boat—resulting in his death—and returned to England claiming they had found the Northwest Passage. But efforts to discover a northern "Passage into the South Sea" proved futile, and English attention moved elsewhere.

The Virginia Company and Jamestown

For Richard Hakluyt, England's leading publicist for overseas expansion, the proper focus seemed clear: "There is under our noses," he wrote in 1599, "the great & ample countrey of Virginia." Great and ample, indeed, especially before the rival Dutch established New Netherland. On paper, the enormous zone that England claimed as Virginia stretched north to south from the top of modern-day Vermont to Cape Fear on Carolina's Outer Banks. From east to west, it spanned North America from the Atlantic to the Pacific, however narrow or wide the continent might prove to be.

In 1606 James I chartered the Virginia Company as a two-pronged operation to exploit the sweeping Virginia claim. Under the charter, a group of London-based merchants took responsibility for colonizing the Chesapeake Bay region. Meanwhile, merchants from England's West Country, based in the seaports of Plymouth, Exeter, and Bristol, took charge of developing the northern latitudes of the American coast. In 1607, two ships from Plymouth deposited roughly a hundred colonists at the Sagadahoc (Kennebec) River in Maine. The Sagadahoc settlers erected a fort and buildings; they even constructed a small sailing vessel called the *Virginia*, the first of hundreds of ships that the English built from American forests. But frostbite, scurvy, and dwindling supplies prompted a retreat home in 1608, two decades after the Roanoke failures.

A parallel effort by the Londoners proved more enduring—but just barely. In April 1607, three ships from the Thames sailed into Chesapeake Bay carrying 105 men. They disembarked on what appeared to be a secluded island near a broad river. In fact, they had entered the territory of a large Indian confederation. The confederacy numbered more than 13,000 people living in dozens of villages spread across the Tidewater area. The paramount chief, Powhatan, had been steadily expanding his power in the region. Initially, his councilors wondered whether to view the new arrivals as dangerous intruders or as potential trading partners, military allies, and members of the confederacy. The isolated English proved equally unsure whether to offer friendship or defiance. Within months, these subjects of James I had named the waterway the James River and established a fortified village beside it called Jamestown. In June, hoping for quick rewards, they shipped to London various stones that they thought contained precious gems and gold ore.

When the rocks proved worthless, the colonists' dreams of easy wealth evaporated. So did ideas about pushing west beyond the watershed. During the outpost's first winter, a fire destroyed the tiny settlement, and death from hunger, exposure, and sickness cut the garrison's population in half. The governor and council appointed by the Virginia Company to oversee the enterprise bickered among themselves, providing poor leadership in the face of hardship. Fully one-third of the early arrivals claimed to be gentlemen, from England's leisure class—a proportion six times higher than in England—and most proved unaccustomed to hard manual labor. Moreover, all the colonists were employees of the company, so any profits from their labor went to repay London investors.

Despite the unsuitable make-up of the garrison and the stiff rules governing work, conditions improved briefly with the emergence of John Smith as an artful and vigorous leader who dealt forcefully with the Indians. (Later, he claimed to have been assisted and protected by Powhatan's young daughter, Pocahontas.) Fears of Spanish attacks on the infant outpost came to nothing. Still, the poorly supported enterprise limped along.

With hopes of a swift bonanza dashed, the London merchants decided to alter their strategy. They would salvage the venture by attracting fresh capital; then they would recoup their high initial costs by recruiting new settlers who could produce staple products suited for export—perhaps grapes, sugar, cotton, or tobacco. In 1609, amid much fanfare, the company began to sell seven-year joint stock options to the English public. Subscribers could invest money or, as "adventurers of person," they could sign on for service in Virginia according to their needed skills. Company officials promised them at least a hundred acres of land when their investment matured in 1616. Surprising numbers responded, including Stephen Hopkins. In June 1609, he joined another 500 men and 100 women departing for the Chesapeake.

"Starving Time" and the Lure of Tobacco

In retrospect, Hopkins and the other passengers of the *Sea Adventure* who were shipwrecked on Bermuda appear to have been the lucky ones. When the fleet's remaining vessels arrived at Jamestown, they found insufficient supplies to feed the hundreds of additional colonists. Moreover, the first round of settlers had failed to discover a profitable staple crop. Even the local tobacco proved "poor and weake, and of a byting tast." The settlers, now numbering 500, depended heavily on the Native Americans for food, and Powhatan's Confederacy proved increasingly unwilling and unable to supply it. As one Indian told them, "We know that you cannot live" without "our harvest" and the "reliefe we bring you." Indeed, most of the settlers did not live. In a grim "starving time," caused in large part by drought conditions, the ill-equipped newcomers scavenged for berries and bark. Extreme hunger drove a few to cannibalize the dead before dying themselves. By the spring of 1610, seven of every eight people had died; scarcely 60 remained alive.

In June, these survivors abandoned their ghost town altogether. But they had scarcely set sail for England when they encountered three long-overdue ships entering Chesapeake Bay with fresh supplies and 300 new settlers. Reluctantly, they agreed to try again. More years of harsh discipline, Indian warfare, and scarce resources followed. The beleaguered colony continued to face mismanagement and factionalism, underfunding and misinformation, inexperience, and poor communication. But another force—a severe dry spell—also conspired against the hapless newcomers. Indian and English crops alike shriveled from 1607 through 1612.

Relief came from an unexpected quarter: *Nicotiana tabacum,* or Orinoco tobacco, a variety of tobacco grown in parts of the West Indies and South America. John Rolfe and his pregnant wife had endured the wreck of the *Sea Adventure* with Stephen Hopkins in 1609. Their child died in infancy, and Mrs. Rolfe perished shortly after reaching Jamestown in 1610. But her husband survived and promptly joined in the colonists' search for a viable staple. He found

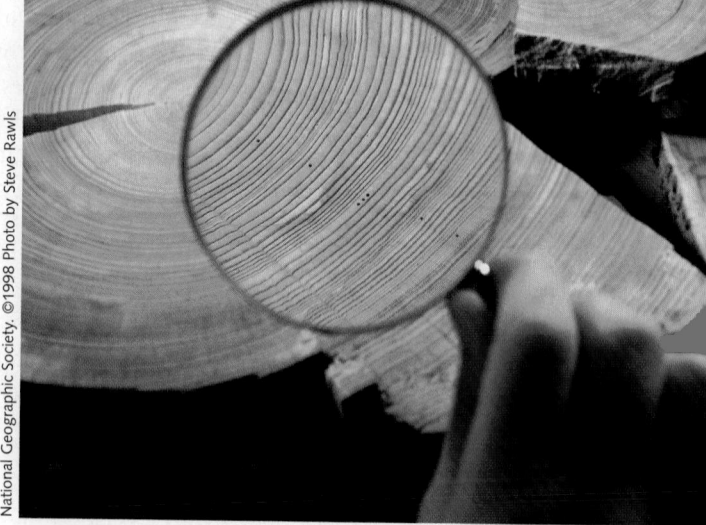

National Geographic Society. ©1998 Photo by Steve Rawls

■ Inexperience prompted initial English difficulties at Roanoke and Jamestown, but so did poor weather. Scientists studying the region's bald cypress trees have recently shown (from certain narrow rings) that terrible droughts struck the coastal area in the late 1580s and again from 1606 through 1612. These two sequences of narrow annual rings are visible under the magnifying glass.

that local Indians cultivated an indigenous tobacco plant, *Nicotiana rustica*. Rolfe, a smoker himself, wondered whether better-tasting varieties might also prosper in Virginia soil.

Within a year, Rolfe had somehow managed to obtain seeds for the sweet-flavored Orinoco tobacco. This "bewitching vegetable" had captured English taste in the previous generation. Sales of this New World product in England sent profits to the Spanish crown and prompted James I to launch a vigorous antismoking campaign in 1604. In his tract titled *Counterblaste to Tobacco,* the king condemned inhaling the noxious weed as a dangerous, sinful, and enfeebling custom, "lothsome to the eye, hatefull to the Nose, harmefull to the braine, daungerous to the Lungs." But by 1612, Rolfe's patch of West Indian tobacco was flourishing. The next year, he grew a sample for export. Desperate settlers and impatient London investors were delighted by Rolfe's successful experiment with tobacco. Production of the leaf soared at Jamestown, to the neglect of all other pursuits.

The colony's tobacco exports rose exponentially from 2000 pounds in 1615 to 20,000 in 1617, 40,000 in 1620, 60,000 in 1622, 500,000 in 1626, and an astounding 1,500,000 pounds in 1629. That year, saturated markets and stiff taxes led to slumping prices. Profits declined in ensuing decades. A dubious luxury good rather than a crucial resource, tobacco nevertheless could yield a profit. Thus authorities in England began to regulate its sale to raise customs revenues and reduce foreign competition. The island of Bermuda also became a tobacco colony after 1613. A decade later, the crown gave Virginia and Bermuda a virtual monopoly on English tobacco sales, lowering import duties for the two colonies when they shipped tobacco to England and aiding them further by imposing limits on the same product from Spanish America.

> *The Virginia Company went out of its way to assure its colonists access to established English freedoms.*

During Virginia's initial tobacco boom, recently starving settlers saw handsome profits within reach. Because land was plentiful at first (a novelty for the English), the only limitations to riches were the scarcity of workers and the related high cost of labor. Any farmer who could hire half a dozen field hands could increase his profits fivefold, quickly earning enough to obtain more land and import more servants. The company transported several shiploads of apprentices, servants, and London street children to the labor-hungry colony. When a Dutch captain delivered 20 enslaved blacks in 1619, settlers eagerly purchased these first Africans to arrive in English Virginia. They also bid on the 100 women who disembarked the same year, shipped from England by the company to be sold as wives and workers. Still, men continued to outnumber women more than three to one for decades to come.

To encourage English migration further, the Virginia Company offered transportation and 50 acres to tenants, promising them ownership of the land after seven years of work. Men who paid their own way received 50 acres and an additional "headright" of 50 acres for each household member or laborer they transported. The Virginia Company went out of its way to assure its colonists access to such established English freedoms as the right to trial by jury and to a representative form of government. The company established civil courts controlled by English common law. It also instructed its appointed governor to summon an annual assembly of elected burgesses—the earliest representative legislature in North America. First convened in 1619, the House of Burgesses wasted no time in affirming its commitment to fundamental English rights. The governor, the house said, could no longer impose taxes without the assembly's consent.

Launching the Plymouth Colony

To attract additional capital and people, the Virginia Company also began awarding patents (legal charters) to private groups of adventurers "to erect and build a town and settle and plant dyvers inhabitants there for the advancement of the general plantation of the country." The newcomers would live independently on a large tract, with only minimal control from the governor and his council. Between 1619 and 1623, the company granted more than 40 such patents, with the exact location of each settlement to be determined on the colonists' arrival. Two such small colonies originated among English Protestants who were living in exile in Holland because their separatist beliefs did not allow them to profess loyalty to the Church of England. The first group of 180, based in Amsterdam, obtained a patent late in 1618 and departed for America on a crowded ship. Winter storms, sickness, and a shortage of fresh water destroyed the venture; scarcely 50 survivors straggled ashore in Virginia.

A second group of English Separatists, residing in the smaller Dutch city of Leiden, fared better. Most had migrated to Holland from northeast England in 1608, led by William Brewster, who had often hosted their prayer meetings at his home in Nottinghamshire. This group openly opposed the hierarchy, pomp, and inclusiveness of the Church of England. Instead, they wanted to return to early Christianity, where small groups of worthy (and often persecuted) believers formed their own communities of worship. After a decade in Holland, many of them had wearied of the foreign culture. Dismayed by the effect of worldly Leiden on their children, they also sensed, correctly, that warfare would soon break out in Europe. A few families pushed for a further removal to America, despite the obvious dangers of such a journey.

Possible destinations ranged from Guiana in South America to the Gulf of St. Lawrence in Canada. Dutch entrepreneurs suggested the Hudson River. But in the end, still loyal to England, the Separatists decided to use a patent granted by the Virginia Company to a group of English capitalists. On the negative side, they had to work for these investors for seven years. They also had to take along outsiders who did not share their beliefs: paying passengers, as well as artisans assigned to the venture. On the positive side, they received financial support from backers who paid to rent a ship. Moreover, instead of having their daily affairs controlled from London, they could elect their own leader and establish civil authority as they saw fit. In short, they had the power to govern themselves.

In September 1620, after costly delays, 35 members of the Leiden congregation and additional Separatists from England departed from Plymouth, along with other passengers (including the family of Stephen and Elizabeth Hopkins). They were crowded aboard the *Mayflower*, a 160-ton vessel converted from the wine trade, and bound for Virginia. But a stormy two-month crossing brought them to Cape Cod, in modern-day Massachusetts, no longer considered part of the Virginia Company's jurisdiction. Already sickly from their long journey, they feared pressing south with winter closing in. They decided to disembark and establish their Plymouth Plantation, having signed a compact aboard the *Mayflower* binding them together in a civil community.

William Bradford, the chronicler and longtime governor of the Plymouth Colony, later recalled their plight:

> They had now no friends to welcome them nor inns to entertain or refresh their weatherbeaten bodies; no houses or much less towns to repair to. . . . And for the season it was winter, and they that know the winters of that country know them to be sharp and violent. . . . Besides, what could they see but a hideous and desolate wilderness. . . . If they looked behind them, there was the mighty ocean which they had passed and was now as a main bar and gulf to separate them from all the civil parts of the world. . . . What could now sustain them but the Spirit of God and His grace?

Bradford could scarcely exaggerate the challenge. His own wife drowned (an apparent suicide) shortly after the *Mayflower* dropped anchor. And by the time the ship departed for its return voyage in April, an illness had swept away half the colonists. When those remaining planted barley and peas, the English seeds failed to take hold. But settlers had abundant fish and wildlife, along with ample Indian corn, and soon reinforcements arrived from England bringing needed supplies. The newcomers also brought a legal patent for the Plymouth colony's land. With Squanto's aid, the settlers secured peaceful relations with Massasoit's villages. When survival for another winter seemed assured, they invited Massasoit and his followers to join in a three-day celebration of thanksgiving so that, according to one account, all might "rejoice together after we had gathered the fruit of our labors."

Colonization Then and Now

You may not be set to blast off yet, but lots of people are ready. Before the first space shuttle lifted off a generation ago, a Tucson engineer named Keith Henson had formed the L–5 Society for people eager to live beyond the earth. By 2000 the Hilton Hotel chain was beginning to plan stays in space. Scientists talk hopefully of launching settlers on an eight-month voyage to Mars by October 2007, when Earth comes closest to the Red Planet's orbit. A private advocacy group called the Mars Society is already conducting practice expeditions in the Arctic.

Space attracts Americans in part because colonization played such a large part in our own beginnings. The "ships" look different, but basic issues remain the same. Motivation, for instance, may spring from scientific fascination, social necessity, or a desire for material success. "It's raining gold," Henson observed about space opportunities back in 1978, "and we're trying to figure out how to get a bucket." And what of saving souls? Because strange encounters between human beings proved a crucial aspect of earthbound colonization, our *Star Trek* imaginings often turn on confrontations with life forms like our own. Will we be the colonizers or the colonized? Will we save the extraterrestrials or be saved by them?

Financing remains crucial too. European governments once debated the proper mix of public and private funds to support colonization and argued the costs and benefits of each successive venture. They also developed new ways, such as joint stock companies, for mobilizing the capital to cover huge start-up costs and to spread enormous risks. U.S.–Russian competition fueled the initial space race, but resources dried up with the end of the Cold War. An elaborate 1989 proposal to put Americans on Mars fell through because the 30-year price tag approached half a trillion dollars. Hoping to spread costs, 16 nations are now cooperating to complete the International Space Station by 2006.

But will the first space colonies orbit close to Earth, inhabit the nearby moon, or travel much further to Mars, a planet with its own atmosphere? Bret Drake, head of mission studies at the Johnson Space Center in Houston, believes that by 2025, "we could have human exploration of Mars being conducted routinely." In the twenty-first century, as in the seventeenth, the progression from initial landings to lasting colonization has a logic, a timetable, and a price tag of its own. And no one can predict the outcome in advance. Last time, successful colonies more than paid for themselves by providing crucial resources for their mother country—at least until they sought independence.

Space colonies, like the overseas colonies, may well become self-sufficient. After much costly trial and error, they may even send vital supplies of minerals and food back to Earth. A quarter century ago, planetary scientist

The Puritan Experiment

After more than a generation of costly colonization attempts, England still had little to show for its efforts when Charles I inherited the throne in 1625. Then two forces prompted rapid change: positive publicity about America and negative developments at home. John Smith, long a key promoter of overseas settlement, drew inspiration from the early efforts at Jamestown, Plymouth, and Bermuda. His book *The Generall Historie of Virginia, New-England and the Summer Isles* (1624) predicted future success for these regions. Smith's volume heralding overseas adventures went through six printings in eight years. Ironically, however, its popularity depended in large measure on a combination of worsening conditions in England—religious, political, and economic—that suddenly gave such literature a broad appeal.

Formation of the Massachusetts Bay Company

European Christianity had taken a number of different forms since the religious upheaval sparked by Luther a century earlier. The first Protestants had demanded a reformation of the Roman Catholic church and had questioned papal authority over Christians. Now many non-Catholic English worshippers doubted whether the Church of England (also known as the Anglican Church) had gone far enough toward rejecting the beliefs and practices of Rome. They lamented what they saw as the church's bureaucratic hierarchy, ornate rituals, and fail-

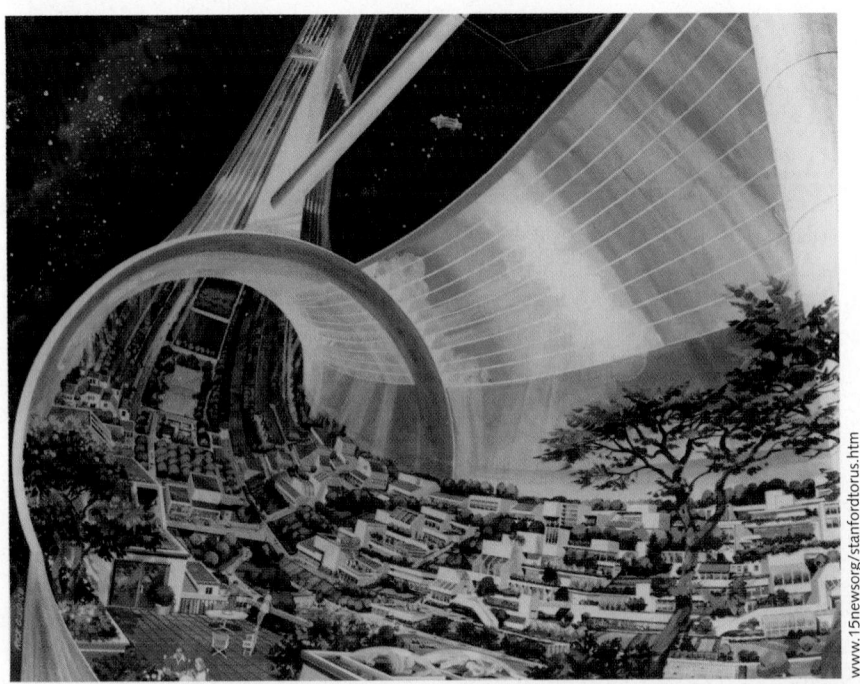

A quarter century ago, this sketch of life inside a vast space colony graced the dust jacket of T. A. Hoppenheimer's book, *Colonies in Space*, with an introduction by science fiction writer Ray Bradbury. Space colonization, like Earth colonization, no doubt will involve imagination as well as money and navigational skills.

T. A. Heppenheimer wrote *Colonies in Space: A Factual and Comprehensive Account of the Prospect for Human Colonization of Space* (1977). He predicted that in the weightless, sun-filled environment of an orbiting colony, "It is entirely reasonable to plan to grow grain in the space farm at a rate of 850 pounds per acre *per day*."

Heppenheimer may well be exaggerating, to make the challenge of launching a colony appear more plausible. In 1600 English propagandist Richard Hakluyt was doing the same thing. To most seventeenth-century Europeans, overseas settlement sounded quite unreasonable—intriguing to fantasize and debate about, but dangerous to undertake. Still, for thousands of people, overseas settlement became their life.

Some argue that colonization may happen again, sooner than we think. If so, who will go into space and under what conditions? Will we depart voluntarily or be forced to move? Will we go with our family and like-minded friends, or will we leave them behind and migrate with strangers? Will some economic or military elite lead the way, or will misfits and dissenters be the first aboard? Will we stay in close touch and plan to return, or will we endure in remote isolation, telling stories of the old country to our children? ■

ure to enforce strict observance of the Christian Sabbath each Sunday. They scoffed at the gaudy vestments of Anglican bishops, elaborate church music, and other trappings of worship unjustified by biblical Scripture. Instead, they praised the stark simplicity that John Calvin had brought to his church in Geneva.

As English Calvinists grew in number, their objections to the Church of England increased. They protested that the Anglican Church, like the Catholic Church, remained inclusive in membership rather than selective. They argued for limiting participation to the devout rather than assuming general access for all. They accused the Church of England of corruption and argued that it should be independent and self-governing rather than tied to the monarchy. This keen desire for further cleansing and purity, so common to reformers, spurred the movement known as Puritanism. Some of the most radical members of this broad religious coalition (including Bradford and the Plymouth pilgrims) became known as Separatists because they were committed to an extreme position: complete separation from what they saw as the corrupt Church of England. But many more Puritans (including most of the reformers who migrated to Massachusetts Bay) resisted separation. They hoped to stay technically within the Anglican fold while taking increased control of their own congregations—a practice known as congregationalism. Unwilling to conform to practices that offended them, these nonseparating Congregationalists remained determined to save the Anglican Church through righteous example, even if it meant migrating abroad for a time to escape persecution and demonstrate the proper ways of a purified Protestant church.

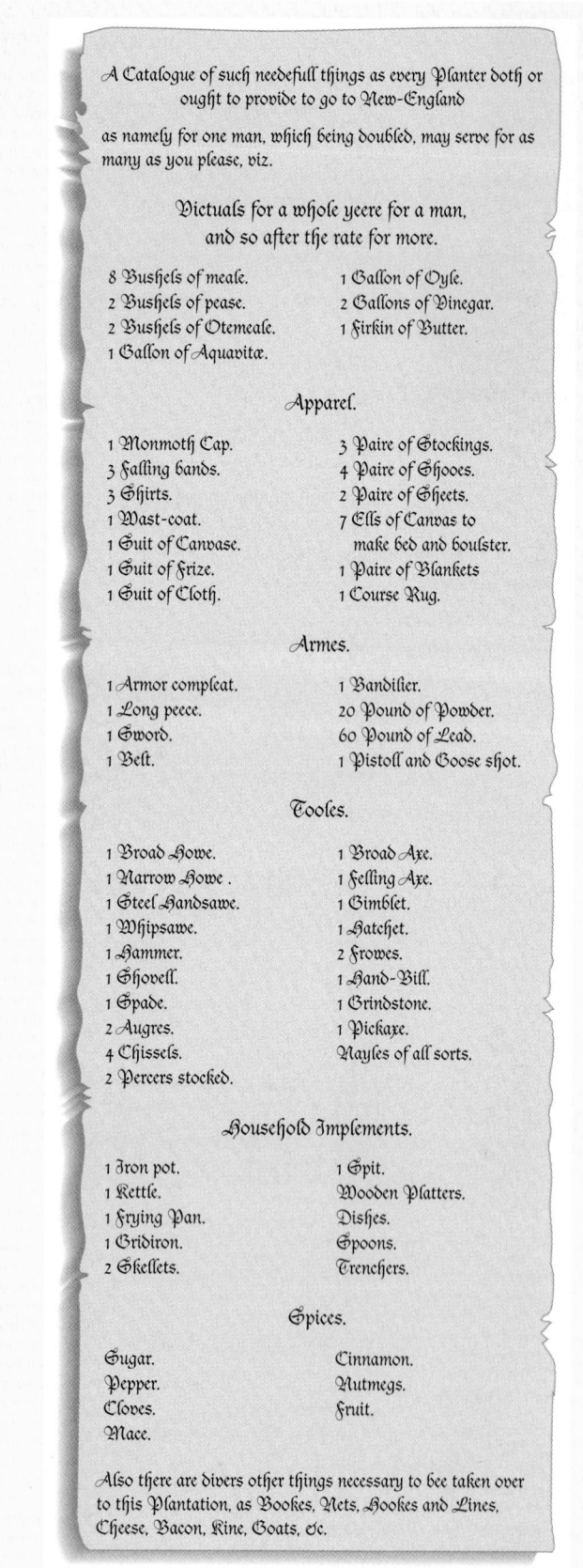

A Catalogue of such needefull things as every Planter doth or
ought to provide to go to New-England

as namely for one man, which being doubled, may serve for as
many as you please, viz.

Victuals for a whole yeere for a man,
and so after the rate for more.

8 Bushels of meale.	1 Gallon of Oyle.
2 Bushels of pease.	2 Gallons of Vinegar.
2 Bushels of Otemeale.	1 Firkin of Butter.
1 Gallon of Aquavitæ.	

Apparel.

1 Monmoth Cap.	3 Paire of Stockings.
3 Falling bands.	4 Paire of Shooes.
3 Shirts.	2 Paire of Sheets.
1 Wast-coat.	7 Ells of Canvas to
1 Suit of Canvase.	make bed and boulster.
1 Suit of Frize.	1 Paire of Blankets
1 Suit of Cloth.	1 Course Rug.

Armes.

1 Armor compleat.	1 Bandilier.
1 Long peece.	20 Pound of Powder.
1 Sword.	60 Pound of Lead.
1 Belt.	1 Pistoll and Goose shot.

Tooles.

1 Broad Howe.	1 Broad Axe.
1 Narrow Howe .	1 Felling Axe.
1 Steel Handsawe.	1 Gimblet.
1 Whipsawe.	1 Hatchet.
1 Hammer.	2 Frowes.
1 Shovell.	1 Hand-Bill.
1 Spade.	1 Grindstone.
2 Augres.	1 Pickaxe.
4 Chissels.	Nayles of all sorts.
2 Percers stocked.	

Household Implements.

1 Iron pot.	1 Spit.
1 Kettle.	Wooden Platters.
1 Frying Pan.	Dishes.
1 Gridiron.	Spoons.
2 Skellets.	Trenchers.

Spices.

Sugar.	Cinnamon.
Pepper.	Nutmegs.
Cloves.	Fruit.
Mace.	

Also there are divers other things necessary to bee taken over
to this Plantation, as Bookes, Nets, Hookes and Lines,
Cheese, Bacon, Kine, Goats, &c.

■ **FIGURE 2.1**
**A 1630 LIST OF ITEMS NEEDED BY EACH ADULT FOR MIGRATION
TO NEW ENGLAND**

An emphasis on instructive preaching by informed leaders lay at the heart of the Puritan movement. Translation of scripture from Latin and its publication into everyday languages the people spoke or read, using the newly invented printing press, had been a central theme of the Reformation. An improved English translation of the Bible in 1611, known as the King James version, provided further access to scripture for all who could read or listen. But James and his bishops, realizing that a "priesthood of all believers" threatened their power, moved to control who could preach and what they could say. A 1626 law prohibited preaching or writing on controversial religious topics such as the conduct of the clergy, the nature of church hierarchy, and the interpretation of Scripture. "There should be more praying and less preaching," wrote one royal supporter, "for much preaching breeds faction, but much praying causes devotion."

Such laws and sentiments only strengthened Puritans' arguments that the religious and political establishment had no interest in allowing people full access to God's word. Why else would the elite encourage sports and recreation on the Sabbath rather than restricting the Lord's Day to religious study and devotion? Puritans believed that the sermon, not the communion sacrament (in which bread and wine signify the presence of the crucified Christ), should form the center of the Christian worship service. Their churches resembled lecture halls, emphasizing the pulpit more than the altar. In preaching, Puritans stressed a "plain style" that all listeners could understand. Moreover, they urged listeners to play an active role in their faith—to master reading and engage in regular study and discussion of scripture. In response to mounting public interest in these practices, Puritan ministers intensified their preaching and published their sermons. In effect, they dared authorities to silence them.

Reprisals came swiftly, led by William Laud, bishop of London, whom Charles I elevated to Archbishop of Canterbury in 1633. Laud instructed all preachers to focus their remarks on biblical passages and avoid writing or speaking about controversial religious matters. The bishop's persecution of Puritan leaders who appeared to disobey these orders only broadened their movement at a time when the king himself was arousing Protestant suspicions. In 1625 Charles I had married Henrietta Maria, Catholic sister of the French king, and had granted freedom of worship to English Catholics, disturbing a wide array of Protestants in the realm. When the House of Commons refused to approve finances for his policies, he arrested its leaders and disbanded Parliament in 1629. He governed on his own for 11 years by levying taxes without parliamentary approval.

As England's church grew more rigid and its monarchy more controlling, the nation's economy also took a turn for the worse. Rents and food costs had risen more rapidly than wages, and workers paid dearly. Jobs grew more scarce after 1625, and several years later, unemployed workers staged local revolts. In 1629 entrepreneurs who viewed New England as a potential opportunity teamed up with disaffected Puritans to obtain a charter for a new entity: the Massachusetts Bay Company. Through a generation of costly trial-and-error experiments, the English had amassed great expertise in colonization. And given the worsening conditions at home, especially among the Puritan faithful, proposals for overseas settlement attracted widespread attention.

"We Shall Be As a City upon a Hill"

During the next dozen years, more than 70,000 people left England for the New World. Two-thirds of them sailed to the West Indies, attracted by the prospect of a warmer climate and a longer growing season. But a large contingent of Puritans (many from the eastern counties of Norfolk, Suffolk, and Essex) embarked from England for the new Massachusetts Bay colony, adjacent to the Plymouth settlement. A loophole in the king's grant permitted them to take the actual charter with them and to hold their company meetings in America. This maneuver took them out from under the usual control of London investors and let them turn the familiar joint stock structure into the framework for a self-governing colony. In 1629 five vessels anchored at Salem. Three years earlier, an advance party had established a post there "for such as upon the account of religion would be willing to begin a foreign plantation."

In England, meanwhile, a Suffolk squire named John Winthrop, whose Puritan commitment had cost him his government post, assumed leadership of the Massachusetts Bay Company. "God will bring some heavy Affliction upon this lande," he predicted to his wife, but the Lord "will provide a shelter & a hidinge place for us and others." In exchange, God would expect great things from these chosen people, as from the Old Testament Israelites. "We are entered into covenant with him for this work," Winthrop told his companions aboard the *Arbella* en route to America in 1630.

Winthrop laid out this higher Calvinist standard in a memorable shipboard sermon titled "A Model of Christian Charity." The values that others merely profess, he explained, "we must bring into familiar and constant practice," sharing burdens, extending aid, and demonstrating patience. "For this end, we must be knit together in this work as one," regardless of social rank. If we fail, he warned, "the Lord will surely break out in wrath against us, and make us know the price of the breach of such a covenant." Far from hiding in obscurity, dedicated Puritans must set a visible example for the rest of the world. Winthrop's listeners understood the biblical reference to Jesus and the Sermon on the Mount (Matthew 5:14) when he concluded, "We shall be as a city upon a hill."

The *Arbella* was one of 17 ships that brought more than 1000 English people to New England in 1630. Choosing Winthrop as governor, the newcomers established Boston and laid out counties with names recalling their homeland: Essex, Norfolk, and Suffolk. By 1634, English arrivals totaled 4000. By the time civil war erupted in England eight years later, nearly 20,000 people had made the journey, eager to escape the religious persecution and denial of parliamentary rights that inflamed partisans against the Royalist forces of Charles I. Whole congregations migrated with their ministers; other people (more than 20 percent) crossed as servants. But most came as independent families with young children. On average, of every 100 newcomers, roughly half

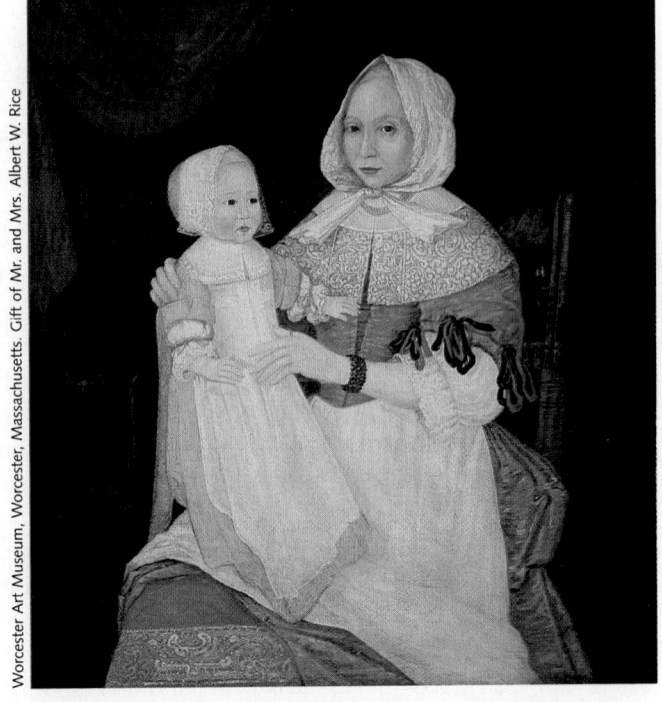

Worcester Art Museum, Worcester, Massachusetts. Gift of Mr. and Mrs. Albert W. Rice

■ Port records for 1635 show that groups leaving London varied markedly, depending on their colonial destination. Young children were common aboard ships heading for New England, as were women and girls. Among passengers for New England, 8 of every 20 were female. In contrast, females made up only 3 in 20 of those going to Virginia and 1 in 20 among people heading for Barbados.

were adults (30 men to 20 women); the other half were all below age 18, divided about evenly between boys and girls.

Earlier settlers traded food, lodging, and building materials to fresh arrivals in exchange for textiles, tools, money, and labor. When new groups of church members wanted to establish a village, they applied for land to the General Court, a legislature made up of representatives elected from existing towns. By 1640, English settlements dotted the coast and had cropped up inland along the Connecticut River, where smallpox had decimated the Indians in 1633. There, English outposts rose at Hartford and Springfield, where English traders hoped to attract furs away from the French and Dutch.

The sheer number of land-hungry settlers drove this rapid expansion. So did friction among newcomers, who competed for scarce resources and complained about price controls and other economic constraints intended to impose civic order. In his initial call to "work as one," Winthrop had worried that migrants would neglect the duties of spiritual regeneration. However, the sharpest dissents came from zealous people who feared that the religious experiment had not gone far enough. Challenging authority lay at the heart of radical Protestantism, for its practitioners stressed inner conviction and personal belief over outward conformity and deference to wealth and status. The more seriously New England's believers took their "errand into the wilderness," the more contentious they became about the proper ways to fulfill God's covenant.

Dissenters: Roger Williams and Anne Hutchinson

Like the biblical Hebrews before them, the Puritans—self-appointed saints—believed that God had chosen them for a special mission in the world. The Almighty, they believed, would watch carefully, punish harshly, and reward mightily. Inevitably, some devout people, raised to question careless ministers or excessive hierarchy, continued to advocate dissenting beliefs in New England. Not everyone accepted the idea that Puritans should dominate Indians or that women should defer to men. Roger Williams, a recent graduate of Cambridge University, and Anne Hutchinson, the talented eldest daughter of an English minister, stand out as two of the earliest and most effective challengers to leadership in the Massachusetts Bay colony.

When Williams arrived in Boston, his Separatist leanings angered Bay Colony authorities, who still hoped to reform the Anglican Church rather than renounce it. But Williams's other contentions proved equally distressing. The young minister argued that civil authorities, inevitably corrupt, had no right to judge religious matters. He even pushed for an unprecedented separation of church and state—to protect the church. He also contended that the colony's land patent from the king had no validity. The settlers, he said, had to purchase occupancy rights from the Native Americans. Unable to silence him, irate magistrates banished Williams from Massachusetts Bay in the winter of 1635. Moving south, he took up residence among the Narragansett Indians and built a refuge for other dissenters, which he named Providence. Still subject to arrest in Boston, he sailed home from New Amsterdam in 1643. Once back in London, he persuaded leaders of England's rising Puritan Revolution to grant a charter (1644) to his independent colony of Rhode Island.

A more explosive popular challenge centered on Anne Hutchinson, who had grown up in England with a strong will, a solid theological education, and a thirst for spiritual perfection. She married a Lincolnshire textile merchant and took an active part in religious discussions while also bearing 15 children. When her Puritan minister, John Cotton, departed for New England, Hutchinson claimed that God, in a private revelation, had instructed her to follow. In 1634 the family migrated to Boston, where Hutchinson attended Cotton's church and hosted religious discussions in her home. The popularity of these weekly meetings troubled authorities, as did her argument that the "Holy Spirit illumines the heart of every true believer." Hutchinson downplayed outward conformity—modest dress or regular church attendance—

Anne Bradstreet: "The Tenth Muse, Lately Sprung Up in America"

The Puritans who migrated to America stressed literacy and education as part of their faith. They wrote down a great deal, and they left extensive records for posterity. But most of their sermons, diaries, and chronicles were drafted by men; few documents about the thoughts and experiences of New England's early migrants come from the pens of women. The poems and reflections of Anne Bradstreet provide a notable exception. "Here you may find," she reminded her children shortly before her death in 1672, "what was your living mother's mind."

The lifelong poet was born Anne Dudley in Lincolnshire, England, in 1612. She already "found much comfort in reading the Scriptures" by age seven. "But as I grew to be about 14 or 15," she recalled, "I found my heart more carnal, and . . . the follies of youth took hold of me. About 16, the Lord . . . smote me with the smallpox . . . and again restored me." That same year, she married Simon Bradstreet, the son of a minister. Two years later, despite a frail constitution, she sailed for Massachusetts Bay with her husband and her father (both future governors of the colony) aboard the Arbella.

Having left England at age 18, Anne Bradstreet was alert to all that seemed strange and different in America. When I "came into this country," she related, "I found a new world and new manners." The young couple set up housekeeping in the town of Cambridge, on the Charles River, but life was difficult at first. Anne suffered from "a lingering sickness like a consumption." Moreover, "It pleased God to keep me a long time without a child, which was a great grief to me and cost me

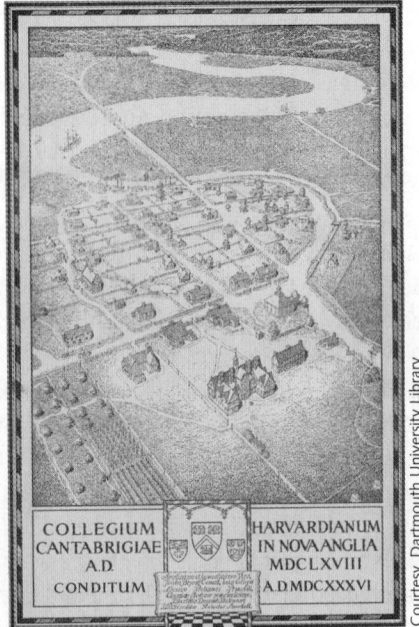

Cambridge looked something like this in the 1660s. The large building in the foreground is Harvard College, founded in 1636, and the smaller brick building beside it is the Indian College, built in 1655. The village was even smaller when Anne Bradstreet resided there briefly after her arrival in Massachusetts Bay.

many prayers and tears." Finally, she bore a son in 1633, and seven more children followed.

As the family grew and moved about, "Mistress Bradstreet" wrote poems and meditations, although detractors hinted that she should put down her quill pen and take up a sewing needle. "If what I do prove well, it won't advance," she lamented in rhyme; "They'l say it's stol'n, or else it was by chance." Nevertheless, a book of her poems was published in England in 1650, hailing her as "The Tenth Muse, Lately Sprung Up in America."

As a writer, Anne Bradstreet was more interested in spiritual improvement than literary grace. "Many speak well," she observed, "but few can do well." Throughout life, she followed a simple creed: "There is no object that we see; no action that we do; no good

that we enjoy; no evil that we feel or fear, but we may make some spiritual advantage" of it. Nothing epitomizes this belief more clearly than "some verses upon the burning of our house, July 10th, 1666." Bradstreet composed the lines on an unburned scrap of paper as she groped to make sense of the calamity. The poem helped her to mourn her loss, take stock of her blessings, and renew her faith. In part, it reads,

In silent night when rest I took,
For sorrow neer I did not look,
I waken'd was with thundring nois
And Piteous shreiks of dreadfull
voice. . . .

I, starting up, the light did spye,
And to my God my heart did
cry. . . .
Then coming out beheld a space
The flame consume my dwelling
place.

And, when I could no longer look,
I blest his Name that gave and took,
That layd my goods now in the
dust:
Yea so it was, and so 'twas just. . . .

When by the Ruines oft I past,
My sorrowing eyes aside did cast,
And here and there the places spye
Where oft I sate, and long did lye.

Here stood that Trunk, and there
that chest;
There lay that store I counted best:
My pleasant things in ashes lye,
And them behold no more
shall I. . . .

Then streight I gin my heart to
chide,
And did thy wealth on earth
abide?
Didst fix thy hope on mouldring
dust,
The arm of flesh didst make thy
trust?. . . .

Thou hast a house on high erect
Fram'd by that mighty Architect. . . .
The world no longer let me Love,
My hope and Treasure lyes Above. ■

as a route to salvation. Instead, she stressed direct communication with God's inner presence as the key to individual forgiveness.

Most Puritans sought a delicate balance in their lives between respected outer works and inner personal grace. Hutchinson tipped that balance dangerously toward the latter. To the colony's magistrates, especially Winthrop, such teaching pointed toward dangerous anarchy—more dangerous when it came from a woman. These officials labeled Hutchinson and her followers as Antinomians (from *anti,* "against," and *nomos,* "law"). But the vehement faction grew, attracting merchants who chafed under economic restrictions, women who questioned men's domination of the church, and young adults who resented the strict authority of their elders. By 1636, this religious and political coalition had gained enough supporters to turn Winthrop out as governor.

Facing complete overthrow, members of the Puritan establishment fought back. They divided the opposition to win reelection for Winthrop, they established Harvard College to educate ministers who would not stray from the fold, they staged a flurry of trials for contempt and sedition (inciting resistance to lawful authority), and they made a special example of Hutchinson herself. After a two-day hearing in which she defended herself admirably, Winthrop sentenced his antagonist to banishment as "a woman not fit for our society." Forced into exile, Hutchinson moved first to Rhode Island and later to the vicinity of Dutch settlements near the Hudson. There she and most of her family were killed by Indians in 1643. A river and a parkway in Bronx, New York, still bear her name.

Expansion and Violence: The Pequot War

Immigration to New England slowed during the 1640s because of religious and political upheaval at home. In England, Puritans and supporters of Parliament formed an army and openly challenged royal authority during the English Civil War. After seizing power, these revolutionaries beheaded Charles I in 1649, abolished monarchy, and proclaimed England a republican Commonwealth. The dramatic struggle preoccupied Puritans in England. Those across the ocean also took heart when they heard news of events at home favorable to their cause.

Nevertheless, word that English Puritans had established a revolutionary commonwealth in their absence shook the settlers' faith that their venture remained at the center of God's plan. They struggled to square such sweeping developments in England with Winthrop's earlier assurance that the eyes of God and humankind would be fixed on New England. Making matters worse, religious and economic controversies intensified as the next generation quickly came of age. Needing new farmland and intellectual breathing room, fresh congregations began to "hive off" from the original settlements like swarms of bees. By 1640, New Hampshire, Rhode Island, and Connecticut each had at least four new towns that would provide the beginnings for independent colonies.

The New York Public Library, Astor, Lenox and Tilden Foundations

■ Captain John Underhill, who directed the dawn raid on a Pequot village in 1637, depicted the massacre in his account the next year. Placing their Indian allies behind them, the English surrounded the palisade and entered the town, firing on unarmed Indians and shooting those who tried to fight their way out.

But the northeastern forest was not an empty wilderness, any more than the Chesapeake tidewater, the Florida interior, or the mesas of New Mexico had been. As the Hutchinsons discovered, newcomers who pushed inland were co-opting the land of longtime residents. Pressure on New England's Native Americans erupted in armed conflict in the Pequot War of 1637, at the height of the Antinomian Crisis. The neighboring Pequot Indians near the mouth of the Connecticut River had been English allies for several years, and a recent smallpox epidemic had weakened them dramatically. But Winthrop, whose son was leading a settlement effort in the area, fanned fears that the Pequots "would cause all the Indians in the country to join to root out all the English."

Recruiting Narragansett and Mohegan Indians to the English side, the colonists unleashed all-out war against the Pequots. The campaign culminated in a dawn raid on a stockaded Pequot town that sheltered noncombatants. The invaders torched the village (at Mystic, Connecticut) and shot or put to the sword almost all who tried to escape. Some 400 Indian men, women, and children died. The Puritans' Indian allies, accustomed to campaigns of capture, adoption, and ritual torture, were shocked by the wholesale carnage. English warfare, they protested, "is too furious, and slaies too many men." Chastened by this intimidating display of terror and weakened by recurrent epidemics, the tribes of southern New England negotiated away much of their land over the next generation, trading furs to the expanding colonists and seeking to understand their perplexing ways.

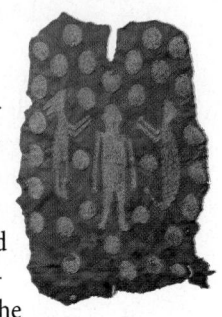

The New York Public Library, Astor, Lenox and Tilden Foundations

MAMUSSE
WUNNEETUPANATAMWE
UP-BIBLUM GOD
NANEESWE
NUKKONE TESTAMENT
KAH WONK
WUSKU TESTAMENT.

Ne quofh'kionumuk nafhpe Wuttinncumoh *CHRIST* noh afcowefit

JOHN ELIOT.

Nahohtôeu ontchetôe Printeuoomuk,

CAMBRIDGE.
Printeuoop nafhpe *Samuel Green.*   MDCLXXXV.

■ **Title page from John Eliot's Indian Bible, 1663**

Having gained the upper hand, the Bible-reading English made gestures to convert their Native American neighbors. Whether the Indians were descended from the Lost Tribe of Israel, as scholars suggested, Puritans believed that "saving the heathen" would almost certainly help them raise funds in London. It would also demonstrate England's zeal to compete with the Catholic Spanish and French in converting souls to Christ. Enthusiastic about these possibilities, the Massachusetts General Court took steps to encourage missionary work. It forbade the worship of Indian gods, mandated the religious and social conversion of local tribes, and set aside land for "praying towns" to encourage "the Indians to live in an orderly way amongst us." On the island of Martha's Vineyard, Reverend Thomas Mayhew, Jr., converted a man named Hiacoomes, who in turn converted several Wampanoag sachems during a 1645 epidemic. In Roxbury, another minister, John Eliot, created a 1200-page Indian Bible. And in Cambridge, officials at Harvard, committed by their charter to the "education of the English and Indian youth of this Country," erected a well-publicized Indian College.

The Chesapeake Bay Colonies

On Chesapeake Bay, settlers' relations with the Indians remained strained at best during the first half of the seventeenth century. In 1608, in an effort to secure the support of Indian leadership, the English performed an elaborate ceremony granting a scarlet cloak and a copper crown to Chief Powhatan. But two years later, suspicious that he was harboring runaway colonists, the English burned the nearest Indian villages and unthinkingly destroyed much-needed corn. One Indian woman leader, taken as a captive, watched English soldiers throwing her children in the river and shooting them in the head before she herself was stabbed to death.

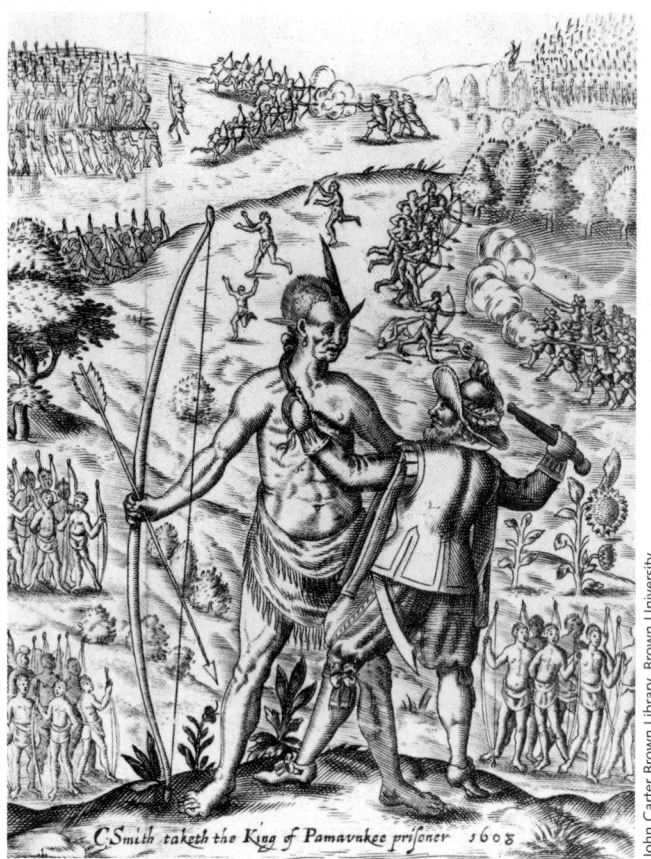

John Carter Brown Library, Brown University

■ Captain John Smith boasted that in 1608 he intimidated Opechancanough with his pistol to disarm the Indians and obtain their corn. Decades later, the Pamunkey leader launched two major attacks on the Jamestown colony. This image of the early incident appeared in Smith's popular *Generall Historie* of 1624.

For both sides, hopes of reconciliation rose briefly in 1614 with the match between Pocahontas, daughter of Powhatan, and John Rolfe, the prominent widower who had introduced tobacco. But the marriage proved brief; Pocahontas died in England three years later, after bearing one child. If leaders intended the wedding alliance as a diplomatic gesture toward peace, it did little to curtail the settlers' bitterness over their lingering dependence on Indian supplies. For their part, the Native Americans resented the encroaching tobacco fields and belligerent tactics of their arrogant neighbors.

The Demise of the Virginia Company

Powhatan's death in 1618 brought to power his more militant younger brother, Opechancanough, the leader of the Pamunkey tribe. His encounters with the English had been frequent and unfriendly. John Smith had even taken him captive at gunpoint to extort food supplies. By 1618, the English tobacco crop was booming, and more newcomers were arriving annually. Over the next three years, 42 ships brought 3500 people to the Chesapeake colony. The influx disheartened the Indians, and Opechancanough and his followers in the Powhatan Confederacy sought ways to end the mounting intrusion.

Briefly, disease seemed to work in the Indians' favor. Immigrants who made the long sea voyage with poor provisions often fell ill in the swampy and unhealthy environment of Jamestown. By 1622, the colony's inhabitants were dying almost as rapidly as newcomers arrived. Sickness had carried off 3000 residents in the course of only three years.

Opechancanough sensed a chance to deliver the finishing blow. He planned a sudden and coordinated offensive against all the settler communities stretched out along the lower James River. On March 22, 1622, his forces attacked the English, surprising the outlying settlements and sparing no one. Of the 1240 colonists, nearly 350 lost their lives. Warned by an Indian, Jamestown survived the uprising, but hope for peaceful relations ended. The attack of 1622 launched a ten-year war in which the Indians showed their versatility by capturing muskets and using them as well as or better than the English.

In London, tales of the disaster fueled opposition to the Virginia Company among disgruntled investors. In 1624 King James annulled the company's charter, making Virginia a royal colony controlled by the crown. In the colony's first 17 years, more than 8500 people, almost all of them young, had embarked for the Chesapeake. By 1624, only 15 of every 100 remained alive.

The colonists placed a bounty on Opechancanough's head, but attempts to ambush or poison him failed. The Indian leader lived on, nursing his distrust of the English. In 1644 he inaugurated a second uprising that killed some 500 colonists. But the English settlement had grown too large to eradicate. By this time old age forced the "Great General" to be carried on a litter. When the English finally captured him and brought him to Jamestown in 1646, Opechancanough was too old to walk unassisted. Still, he remained defiant until shot in the back by one of the Englishmen guarding him.

After two years of brutal warfare, the Pamunkeys and their allies in the Powhatan Confederacy conceded defeat and submitted to English authority. From then on, they would pay a token annual tribute for the privilege to remain on lands that had once belonged to them.

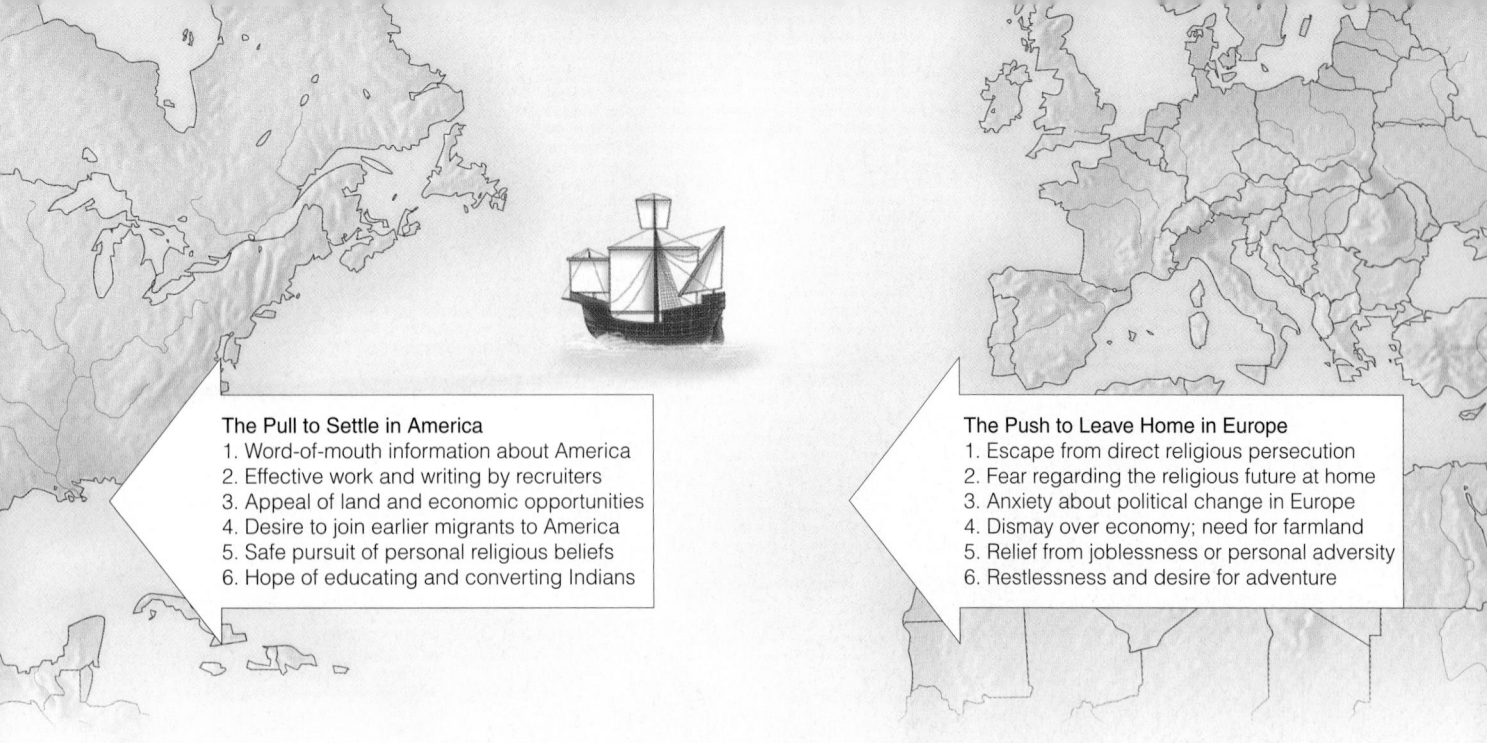

The Pull to Settle in America
1. Word-of-mouth information about America
2. Effective work and writing by recruiters
3. Appeal of land and economic opportunities
4. Desire to join earlier migrants to America
5. Safe pursuit of personal religious beliefs
6. Hope of educating and converting Indians

The Push to Leave Home in Europe
1. Escape from direct religious persecution
2. Fear regarding the religious future at home
3. Anxiety about political change in Europe
4. Dismay over economy; need for farmland
5. Relief from joblessness or personal adversity
6. Restlessness and desire for adventure

■ **FIGURE 2.2**
THE TOUGH CHOICE TO START OVER

With the way cleared for expansion, land-hungry English settlers appeared in ever-increasing numbers in Virginia and neighboring Maryland. By 1660, roughly 25,000 colonists lived near the shores of Chesapeake Bay.

Maryland: The Catholic Refuge

Maryland, the smaller and the younger of the two English colonies on the Chesapeake, owed its beginnings to George Calvert. In a Protestant country, Calvert rose to become a respected Catholic member of England's government. He was named the first Baron of Baltimore, in Ireland, in 1625. Calvert had a keen interest in colonization, and he established a short-lived colony of his own in Newfoundland, welcoming all religious groups. But when attacks by the French defeated that scheme, he sought a safer location.

Calvert (now Lord Baltimore) had followed events in the Chesapeake, and in 1632 he petitioned Charles I for land there. The king granted him 10 million acres adjacent to Virginia, to be named Maryland in honor of the Catholic queen, Henrietta Maria. The Maryland charter, like the one that had governed the Newfoundland colony, gave the proprietor and his heirs unprecedented personal power, especially in the granting of lands to colonists without limitations based on religious belief.

Because Calvert died before the royal charter took effect, his eldest son, the second Lord Baltimore, took charge of the settlement effort. In 1634, the *Ark* and the *Dove* carried more than 200 settlers—both Protestants and Catholics—to the new colony. There, they established a capital at St. Mary's, near the mouth of the Potomac River. With the execution of the king in 1649 and the creation of an anti-Catholic commonwealth in England, the Calvert family provided a haven in Maryland for their coreligionists. However, Catholics never became a majority in the Chesapeake colony.

In 1649, Maryland's assembly passed an Act Concerning Religion, guaranteeing toleration for all settlers who professed a belief in Jesus Christ. This assertion of religious toleration, though limited, proved too broad for many to stomach. In the 1650s supporters of the English Puritan cause seized power in Maryland, repealed the act, and briefly ended the Calverts' proprietorship. But by 1660, with the restoration of the Stuart monarchy in England, proprietary rule returned to the prosperous farming colony.

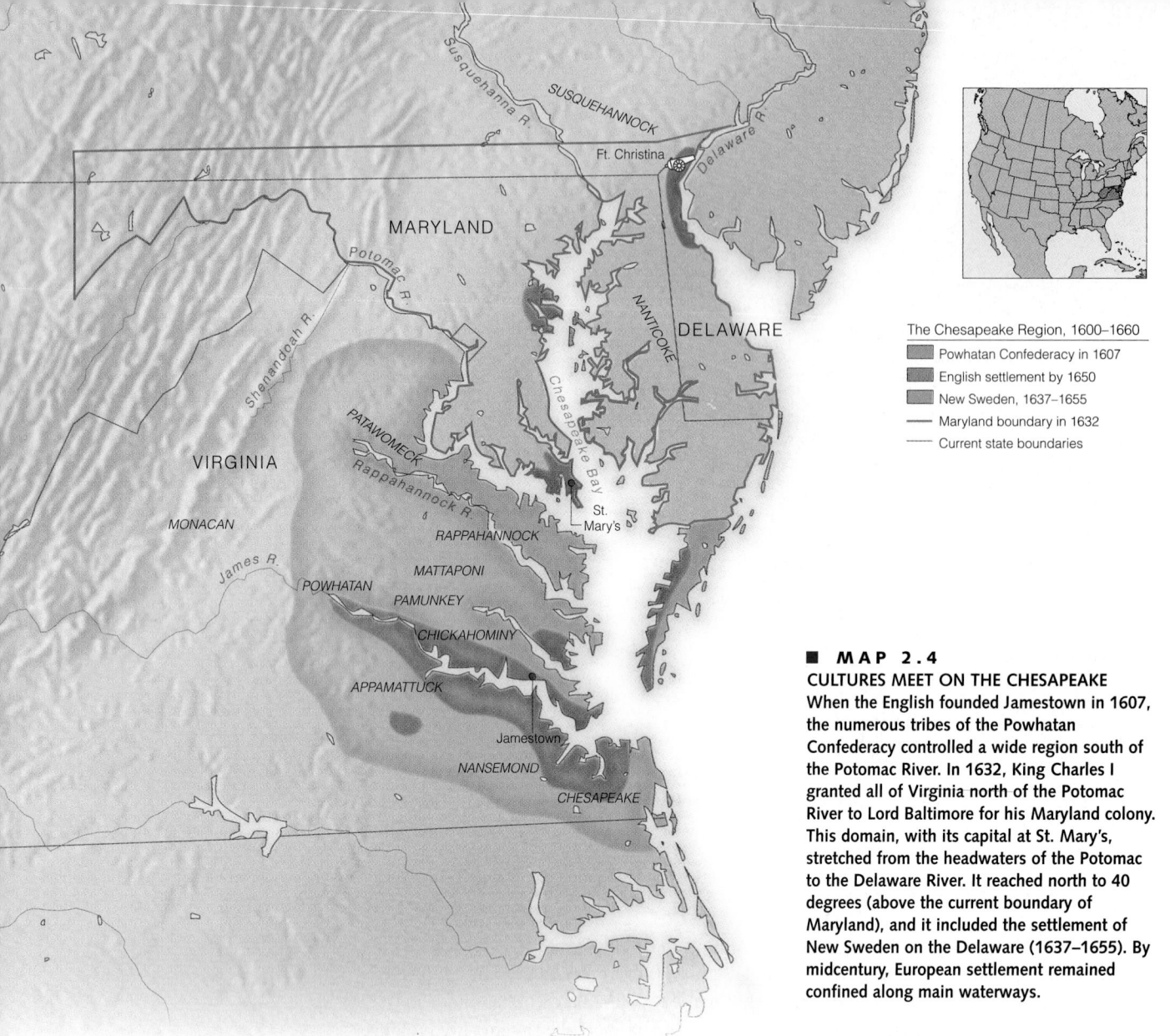

■ **MAP 2.4**
CULTURES MEET ON THE CHESAPEAKE
When the English founded Jamestown in 1607, the numerous tribes of the Powhatan Confederacy controlled a wide region south of the Potomac River. In 1632, King Charles I granted all of Virginia north of the Potomac River to Lord Baltimore for his Maryland colony. This domain, with its capital at St. Mary's, stretched from the headwaters of the Potomac to the Delaware River. It reached north to 40 degrees (above the current boundary of Maryland), and it included the settlement of New Sweden on the Delaware (1637–1655). By midcentury, European settlement remained confined along main waterways.

The Chesapeake Region, 1600–1660
- Powhatan Confederacy in 1607
- English settlement by 1650
- New Sweden, 1637–1655
- Maryland boundary in 1632
- Current state boundaries

Conclusion

D uring half a century, the French, Dutch, and English had all moved to challenge Spanish claims in North America. By 1660, all four of these maritime powers of western Europe had taken aggressive steps to establish permanent footholds on the fringes of the enormous continent. In each instance, the European colonizers benefited first from the presence of knowledgeable Native Americans and then from the sharp decline of those same people through warfare and the onslaught of new diseases.

Granted, warfare with foreign invaders and death from unknown diseases had become a part of Native American history in the preceding century. One need only think of the destruction that followed in the path of Hernando de Soto's expedition through the Southeast. But for the most part, the sixteenth century was an era of intermittent European exploration that was as tentative as it was sweeping. In contrast, the first half of the seventeenth century saw Europeans move from occasional forays to persistent attempts at permanent colonization. As these foreign intruders competed with one another, their tenacious efforts began to yield lasting results.

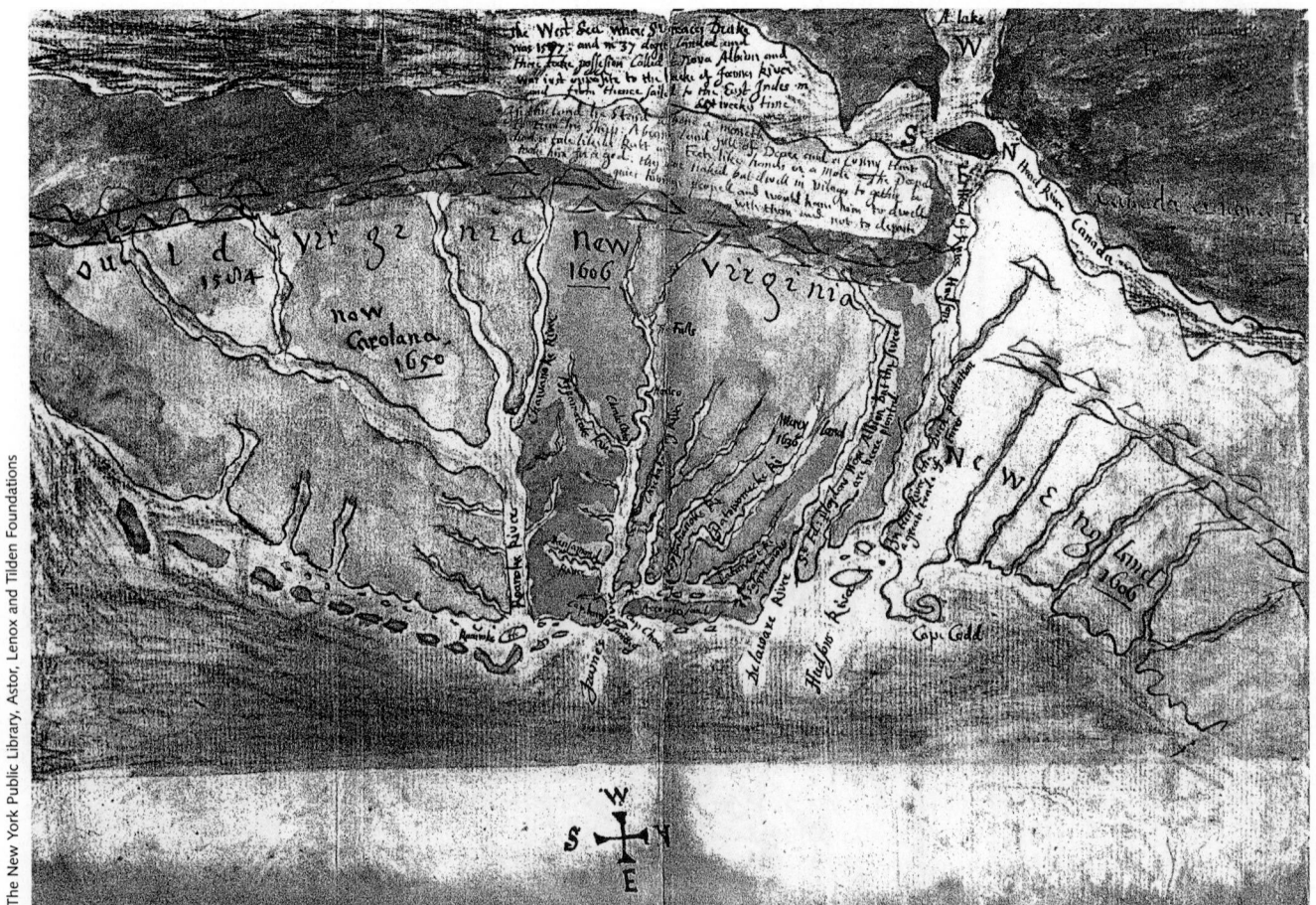

■ By the mid-seventeenth century, most English still had only a vague view of North America. In a 1650 sketch of the Atlantic coast, shown here, John Farrer struggled to piece together the region's geography and recent history. His map, later made into a print, mixed fact and fiction from 70 years of exploring and settlement. Starting in the South (left) Farrer showed the Barrier Islands and the 1584 effort to settle Roanoke Island in "Ould Virginia, now Carolana." In "New Virginia" he drew the James and Potomac Rivers flowing into Chesapeake Bay and noted the founding of Maryland in the 1630s. He correctly placed Swedes along the Delaware River and Dutch on "Hudsons River," doing "a great trade of furs." New England remains vague beyond the hook of "Cape Codd," but "1606" suggests the brief Sagadahoc colony on the coast of Maine.

The most dramatic speculation is in the upper (western) part of the map, beyond the well-defined Appalachian mountains. In 1577, Sir Francis Drake had entered the "West Sea" (Pacific Ocean) and sailed to 37 degrees north latitude, claiming the region around San Francisco Bay as New Albion. Farrer knew that Virginia was in the same latitude and that geographers had speculated about narrow portions of the continent ever since the explorations of Verrazzano. So he repeated the persistent idea that New Albion "was just opposite the backe of James River." Moreover, a Northwest Passage to the Pacific might yet be found if the Hudson and Saint Lawrence Rivers reached the Great Lakes rumored to exist in the interior.

Except for several small pockets on the edges of the continent, Native American societies still held the upper hand. Most had not seen the alien newcomers, learning about them only indirectly, if at all. But on the fringes, stark confrontations had started to occur—small in number but huge in their implications. They involved vastly different languages, lifeways, and beliefs about the world.

Confrontations had also begun among the invaders themselves. After all, they represented rival nations and competing versions of the Christian faith. Although it was clear by 1660 that none would withdraw from North America without a fight, it was also clear that no single nation had decisively obtained the upper hand as yet. Spain, France, Holland, and England each had formidable assets in Europe and on the high seas. All had sponsored colonial settlements that had endured for several generations, and each had begun to taste the seductive fruits of empire in America and elsewhere.

The English, slowest to become involved in overseas colonization, had caught up with their competitors by 1660. Among European countries, England had proven the most aggressive in forming expansive family-based colonies rather than military garrisons or trading outposts. Elizabeth Hopkins and Anne Hutchinson, embarking from England with their husbands and families, exemplified a migration pattern that included thousands of women. Their presence led to the formation of stable households, especially in New England, where the balance of women and men was most even. Women took an immediate role in crucial aspects of domestic manufacture and production, and their numerous children provided additional hands where labor was in short supply. As a result, by 1660 the population of England's fledgling North American colonies had already outstripped that of its rivals, and it was growing at an increasing rate. This emerging superiority in numbers was advantageous in the imperial clashes that lay ahead.

Sites to Visit

Acoma Pueblo

Located near Highway 40 west of Albuquerque, New Mexico, within the Acoma Indian Reservation, the Acoma Pueblo Visitors' Center offers guided tours of "Sky City" that leave in vans from the center. Once on top of the 420-foot mesa, visitors can walk the streets of one of the oldest continuously inhabited sites in North America.

Mission San Luis Park

After the state of Florida acquired 50 acres in northwest Tallahassee in 1983, archaeologists excavated the Apalachee Indian town and Spanish mission that existed there in the seventeenth century. Mission San Luis Park, between Rt. 10 and Rt. 90, contains an outdoor museum with reconstructed buildings, exhibits, and guided tours.

Sainte-Marie Among the Hurons Museum

Overlooking the Wye River near Midland, Ontario, 80 miles north of Toronto on Canada's Georgian Bay, this reconstructed seventeenth-century Jesuit mission site offers canoe trips and candlelight tours in the summer.

The New Netherland Museum and Half Moon Visitor Center

Located in Albany, New York, the museum maintains a full-scale replica of Henry Hudson's ship, the *Half Moon,* which is usually docked at Albany and open for visitors. For information, contact the Main Office at 518-443-1609.

Plimoth Plantation
www.plimoth.org

This living history museum of seventeenth-century Plymouth is located off Route 3 along the coast south of Boston, Massachusetts. It recreates the pilgrim village as it appeared in 1627, with a Wampanoag Indian site nearby. Visit the *Mayflower II* at State Pier on Water Street. Take a virtual tour of the site at www.plimoth.org.

Historic Jamestown
www.history.org/nche/
www.ngdc.noaa.gov/paleo/drought/drght_james.html

At Historic Jamestown you can tour ruins, visit a glass-blowing exhibition, and see excavations of the original fort. Nearby, the Jamestown–Yorktown Foundation runs Jamestown Settlement, with reconstructed ships, fortifications, and Indian dwellings. These sites are seven miles from Williamsburg on Virginia's Colonial Parkway; they can also be approached by ferry across the James River. All are gearing up for the 400th anniversary in 2007. The link to "Virtual Jamestown" is http://www.history.org/nche/. For recent evidence on the severe seven-year Jamestown drought (1606–1612), visit www.ngdc.noaa.gov/paleo/drought/drght_james.html.

Wolstenholme Towne

Archaeologists have excavated this palisaded village, located near Jamestown, which was destroyed in the 1622 Indian attack. The site is located at Carter's Grove Plantation, near Williamsburg. The Winthrop Rockefeller Archaeology Museum next door contains impressive exhibits on English settlement in Virginia.

Historic St. Mary's City

The site of Maryland's first capital lies off Route 5, near the mouth of the Potomac River, in southern Maryland, several hours' drive from Baltimore, Annapolis, and Washington, D.C. Since 1971, an annual summer archaeology field school has worked to excavate additional elements of the town.

For Further Reading

General

Bernard Bailyn, *The Peopling of British North America: An Introduction* (1985).

David Hackett Fischer, *Albion's Seed: Four British Folkways in America* (1989).

Mary Beth Norton, *Founding Mothers and Fathers: Gendered Power and the Forming of American Society* (1996).

Alan Taylor, *American Colonies* (2001).

David J. Weber, *The Spanish Frontier in North America* (1992).

Spain's Ocean-Spanning Reach

Amy Turner Bushnell, *Situado and Sabana: Spain's Support System of the Presidio and Mission Provinces of Florida* (1994).

Ramón A. Gutiérrez, *When Jesus Came, the Corn Mothers Went Away: Marriage, Sexuality, and Power in New Mexico, 1500–1846* (1991).

John H. Hann, *A History of the Timucua Indians and Missions* (1996).

W. Michael Mathes, *Vizcaíno and Spanish Expansion in the Pacific Ocean* (1968).

Jerald T. Milanich, *Laboring in the Fields of the Lord: Spanish Missions and Southeastern Indians* (1999).

France and Holland: Overseas Competition for Spain

Denys Delâge, *Bitter Feast: Amerindians and Europeans in Northeastern North America, 1600–1664* (1993).

W. J. Eccles, *France in America* (1972).

Michael Kammen, *Colonial New York: A History* (1975).

Oliver A. Rink, *Holland on the Hudson: An Economic and Social History of Dutch New York* (1986).

Bruce G. Trigger, *Natives and Newcomers: Canada's "Heroic Age" Reconsidered* (1985).

English Beginnings on the Atlantic Coast

John Demos, *A Little Commonwealth: Family Life in Plymouth Colony* (1970).

Karen Ordahl Kupperman, *Indians and English: Facing Off in Early America* (2000).

Ivor Noël Hume, *The Virginia Adventure: Roanoke to James Towne, An Archaeological and Historical Odyssey* (1994).

Neal Salisbury, *Manitou and Providence: Indians, Europeans, and the Making of New England, 1500–1643* (1982).

Alden T. Vaughan, *American Genesis: Captain John Smith and the Founding of Virginia* (1975).

The Puritan Experiment

David Cressy, *Coming Over: Migration and Communication Between England and New England in the Seventeenth Century* (1987).

William Cronon, *Changes in the Land: Indians, Colonists, and the Ecology of New England* (1983).

Alison Games, *Migration and the Origins of the English Atlantic World* (1999).

Philip F. Gura, *A Glimpse of Sion's Glory: Puritan Radicalism in New England, 1620–1660* (1984).

Alan Heimert and Andrew Delbanco, eds., *The Puritans in America: A Narrative Anthology* (1985).

Edmund S. Morgan, *The Puritan Dilemma: The Story of John Winthrop* (1958).

The Chesapeake Bay Colonies

Wesley Frank Craven, *The Southern Colonies in the Seventeenth Century, 1607–1689* (1949).

James Horn, *Adapting to a New World: English Society in the Seventeenth-Century Chesapeake* (1994).

Edmund S. Morgan, *American Slavery, American Freedom: The Ordeal of Colonial Virginia* (1975).

James R. Perry, *The Formation of a Society on Virginia's Eastern Shore, 1615–1655* (1990).

Helen C. Rountree, *The Powhatan Indians of Virginia* (1989).

Online Practice Test

Test your understanding of this chapter with interactive review quizzes at

www.ablongman.com/jonescreatedequal/chapter2

CHAPTER

3

Controlling the Edges of the Continent, 1660–1715

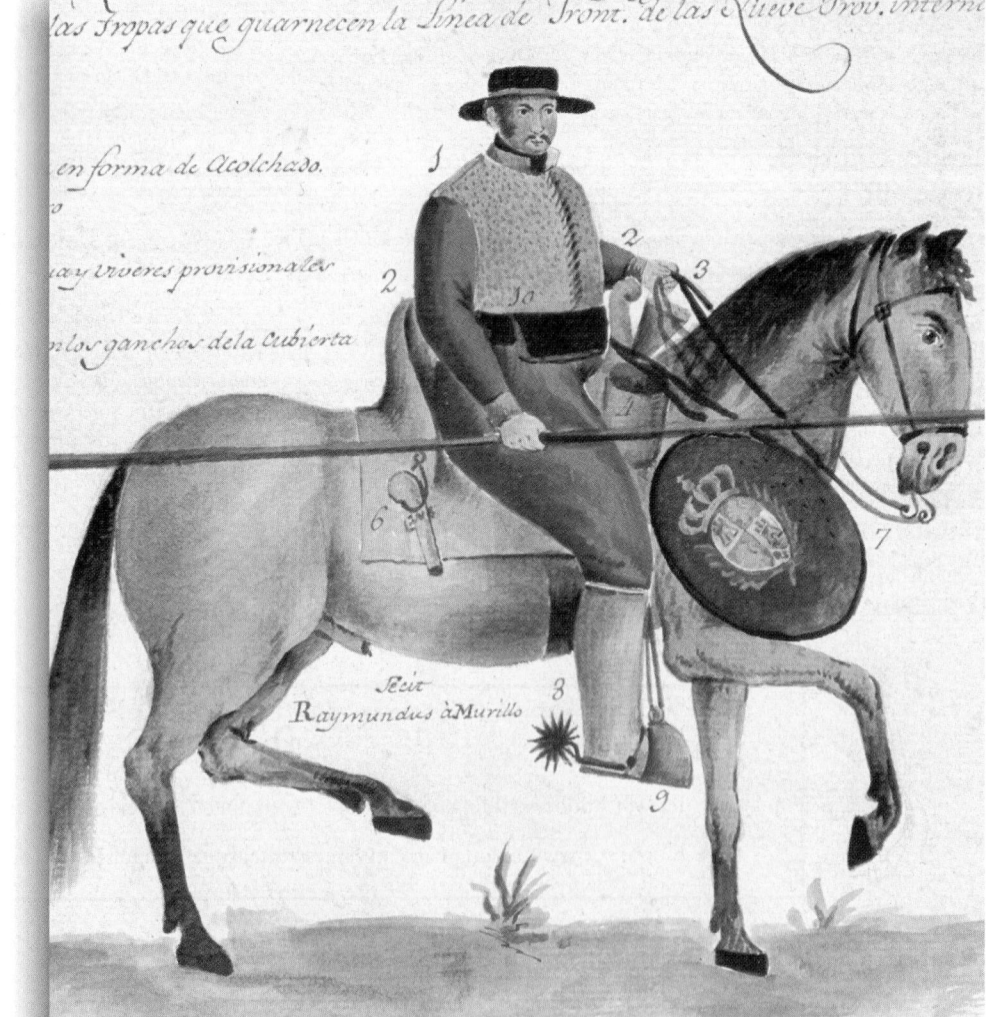

Laurie Platt Winfrey, Inc.

■ Seventeenth-century Spanish frontier guard wearing an arrow-resistant vest.

MARGUERITE MESSIER MADE AN IMPRESSIVE FIGURE ON THE MONTREAL WATERFRONT in April 1704 as she loaded a large canoe. Surrounded by her five children, she worked with her brother, Jean-Michel, to stow food and belongings for their strenuous journey to meet her husband at a new French outpost on the Gulf of Mexico. They were assisted by the guide they had hired to carry them on this daunting wilderness expedition.

At 28, Messier had already been married half her life, having wed explorer–trader Pierre-Charles Le Sueur in 1690 when he was 34 and she was only 14. While her husband traveled often and far, she raised their boy and four girls. She was deeply involved, through family ties, in the dramatic changes taking place throughout the vast North American hinterland claimed by France.

Messier's cousin, an adventurous Canadian named Pierre Le Moyne d'Iberville, had established the French colony of Louisiana near the mouth of the Mississippi River in 1699, and three years later Iberville and his younger brother (Bienville) had started the village of Mobile (near present-day Mobile, Alabama) to serve as the first capital. Messier's husband had long been active in Canada's far-flung western fur trade with the Ojibwe and Sioux Indians living near the Great Lakes. In 1700 he had ascended the Mississippi to the Blue Earth River in what is now Minnesota. Two years later he paddled down the Mississippi with minerals and furs and made his way to the new outpost at Mobile. There he constructed a house for his family; then he accompanied Iberville back to France.

In 1704, confident about the future success of the Louisiana venture, Le Sueur sent word to his wife in Montreal to attempt the inland journey of nearly 2000 miles to Mobile. He himself departed from France aboard the *Pelican* for the same destination, hoping to reunite with his family. With the ice gone from the St. Lawrence, Messier and her party set out from Montreal on April 30, 1704, making their way up river and passing through Lake Ontario and Lake Erie. A year later, they reached the outpost at Kaskaskia in southern Illinois. Heat and sickness took their toll as they descended the Mississippi River. Messier's brother, Jean-Michel, and a daughter, Louise-Marguerite, died in June, two months before the party got to its destination. More bad news awaited them when they finally reached Mobile in August 1705, having covered nearly 2000 miles in 16 months.

The voyage of the *Pelican* had met with disaster. Pierre-Charles Le Sueur had boarded the ship in France, joining missionaries, soldiers, and potential brides recruited to go to Mobile. But at a stopover in Cuba, he had caught yellow fever and died before the ship left Havana. Sixty other passengers also fell ill, and several more died before the immigrants reached Mobile. The town—home to just 160 men and a dozen women— hardly had enough food and shelter for the sickly newcomers, and yellow fever spread quickly. The epidemic swept away 40 residents in two months and decimated nearby Indian villages.

French fort at Mobile, 1705

Still, life at the outpost persisted. Townsmen welcomed the *Pelican*'s eligible young women, ages 14 to 18, and priests celebrated 13 marriages within the first three weeks. By 1705, when Marguerite Messier arrived from Montreal, new children were being born. Moving into the house her late husband had built, Messier determined to stay on and help the colony endure. She sent instructions back to Canada for friends to sell her property and forward the proceeds to her. Meanwhile, she managed a storehouse for her cousins, Iberville and Bienville who had survived the ordeal of the *Pelican,* she made a fresh start in the Louisiana colony.

Many of the changes that took place in North America during Marguerite Messier's lifetime occurred within a broad international context. During the second half of the seventeenth century, the English, Dutch, French, Spanish, and Portuguese were caught up in a race to expand and protect their overseas empires, and they were waging the contest on a global scale. Backed by growing economic and military strength at home, the French planted their flag in the West Indies, West Africa, Madagascar, India, and Ceylon. The Dutch, meanwhile, established a settlement at Cape Town in South Africa in 1652 that helped them challenge Portuguese power in the Indian Ocean and the Spice Islands of the East Indies. But expansion in one region often coincided with contraction somewhere else. By the 1670s, Dutch authorities had been forced to withdraw entirely from North America, leaving that arena of commercial and military competition to their rivals.

With the departure of the Dutch from North America, the three remaining European powers intensified their competition to control the fringes of the continent. In the East, England expanded the number and size of its coastal colonies, and English port towns multiplied along the Atlantic seaboard. On Chesapeake Bay, Anne Arundel (later Annapolis), became Maryland's port of entry in 1668. English newcomers also pressed inland along numerous rivers to found trading towns at the "fall line," the point where falls and rapids provided water power to run grist mills. In the 1670s, a London goldsmith's son named William Byrd established one such town at the falls of the James River on a site that grew to become Richmond, Virginia.

Pushing up from the south, meanwhile, Spain struggled to retain its foothold in Florida and New Mexico and to lay claim to parts of Arizona and Texas as well. New Spanish towns appeared at Albuquerque, El Paso, and Pensacola. Of the three competing powers only France, pressing in from the St. Lawrence Valley, managed to penetrate the interior of the continent extensively. Its government created a string of forts from the Great Lakes to the Gulf of Mexico: Detroit, Peoria, and Mobile all came into being under the French flag.

But the clash between empires would not be the only dynamic at work throughout the continent in these years. The religious strife among Christians that had marked the previous century in Europe continued in North America. Catholic missionaries labored diligently to recruit Native American converts in Canada, Florida, New Mexico, and numerous points in between. Opposed to such activities, Protestants in the English-speaking colonies remained on the alert for any threat—external or internal, real or imagined—that they could decry as a "popish plot". It was a term they used frequently to express their continuing hostility toward the Catholic Church and its leader, the pope in Rome.

Behind all these tensions, one fundamental question recurred in numerous places during the decades after 1660: Who has the right to govern? The structures of control were tenuous almost everywhere, and dissenters and rebels who felt jealous, excluded, or exploited could openly question the legitimacy of those in charge. In congregations, towns, and whole colonies, challenges to authority arose repeatedly, and often they could only be settled by resort to arms. Disruptions, violence, and sudden death were familiar experiences for thousands of people inhabiting North America during these years.

France and the American Interior

For decades before Marguerite Messier traveled from Montreal to Mobile with her family, the potential wealth of the North American interior had intrigued government ministers in France. If French fur traders based in Canada (known as *voyageurs*) could explore and map this vast domain, discovering its resources and befriending its Indian inhabitants, France might control some of the continent's most fertile farmland and keep its extensive natural assets out of the hands of European rivals. If the French could recruit enough Native Americans as loyal allies, they might even threaten the rich mines of the Spanish empire in Mexico and challenge the growing English colonies lying to the east of the Appalachian mountains. But for France to realize such wide ambitions, the French king, Louis XIV, would need to make North American colonization a national priority, and the extent of his commitment remained uncertain.

The Rise of the Sun King

King Louis XIV stood at the center of France's expanding imperial sphere. Indeed, so much seemed to revolve around him that he became known as the "Sun King." He had inherited the French throne in 1643, as a child of five, and in 1661, at age 22, he assumed personal control of a realm of 20 million people. During most of his long rule—from 1661 to his death in 1715 at age 77—Louis dominated European affairs. Always a builder of monuments, he expanded the Louvre in Paris and then dazzled the French nobility and clergy with his opulent new palace at Versailles.

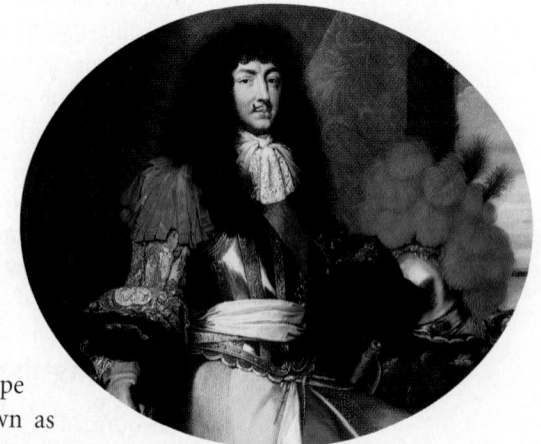

Portrait of Louis XIV

In religion, the Sun King challenged the authority of the Catholic pope on one hand and suppressed the dissent of French Protestants (known as Huguenots) on the other. In politics, he centralized the monarchy's power as never before. His administration consolidated the laws of France, strengthened the armed forces, and expanded commerce. As the government ministries grew in strength, they foreshadowed the modern nation-state, regulating industry, promoting road building, and imposing tariffs and taxes.

Throughout Louis XIV's reign, his officials followed a set of policies known as mercantilism. According to this general system, a government stressed economic self-sufficiency and the importance of a favorable balance of trade. By avoiding foreign debts and drawing in precious metals and other resources from its competitors and its own colonies, a state could pay for wars abroad and costly projects at home. The French mercantilist strategy was to exploit labor efficiently and import raw materials cheaply, while exporting expensive manufactured products, such as glassware, wine, silk, and tapestries, in exchange for foreign gold and silver. France's colonies, like those of Spain and England, were expected to generate much-needed natural resources and to provide eager consumers for the mother country's manufactured goods.

In Paris, finance minister Jean-Baptiste Colbert emerged as the chief architect of this strategy of aggressive mercantilism. At home he taxed foreign imports, removed domestic trade barriers, and improved internal transportation. Moreover, he reduced worker holidays and outlawed strikes. With an eye toward colonial expansion, Colbert improved France's ports and created a code to regulate maritime shipping. He expanded the naval fleet and pressed French sailors into its service. Pushing still harder, he organized overseas trading companies and provided insurance for their expensive ventures. In addition, he sanctioned France's involvement in the African slave trade. Colbert yearned to acquire new territory to increase the empire's self-sufficiency and keep overseas resources out of enemy hands. To that end, he and his successors encouraged French exploration of North America on an unprecedented scale.

The government of Louis XIV assumed direct control over New France (Canada and neighboring Acadia on the Atlantic coast) from a private company in 1663. Colbert hoped to diversify production away from the fur trade and limit settlers from dispersing widely. Therefore, he shipped livestock and tools to help build up the colony's tenuous agricultural base. To establish the power of the king, Colbert dispatched a military governor general to Quebec, along with shiploads of artisans and indentured servants. To promote domestic life and population growth, the government also transported young single women and announced cash incentives for early marriages and large families. Many of the soldiers sent to protect New France from Iroquois and English threats stayed on to establish farms.

On balance, however, Colbert's plans for a prosperous, well-populated colony failed. The small population of New France—ten thousand by 1680—never grew as rapidly as French imperial strategists desired. The harsh winters and short growing seasons hindered the expansion of agriculture. Also, concerns on the part of the king and his ministers played a role in limiting growth. Colbert worried that too much emigration to Canada could depopulate and thereby weaken France at home. In addition, he tried to make sure that the few whom he sent abroad had "suitable" backgrounds as pious and loyal Catholics. "In the establishment of a country," he declared, it was important "to plant good seed."

In contrast to the English, the French did not elect to use their overseas colonies as useful havens for social outcasts, political troublemakers, and religious dissidents. This became clear in 1685, when Louis XIV revoked the Edict of Nantes, which had granted French Protestants their legal rights for nearly a century. The king explicitly forbade these dissenters from traveling to France's colonies. Faced with rising persecution at home, more than 150,000 Huguenots migrated abroad by the early eighteenth century. Several thousand of them found refuge in the new English colonies on America's Atlantic seaboard.

Exploring the Mississippi Valley

Encouraged by the government of Louis XIV, French Canadian explorers probed steadily across the Great Lakes and down the Mississippi River. (They mastered the interior waterways by learning to handle Native American canoes, just as Indian hunters soon learned to ride European horses on the Great Plains.) As early as 1634, some 70 years before Marguerite Messier and her family journeyed through the continental interior, Champlain had sent explorer Jean Nicolet west across Lake Huron to find a route to China. Thinking that Asia might be close at hand, Nicolet even carried a letter of introduction to the Chinese emperor as he paddled through the Straits of Mackinac with his Huron Indian companions. Instead of finding the salt water of the Pacific, they came upon the fresh water of Lake Michigan. They ended up near modern-day Green Bay, Wisconsin. There, Winnebego Indians (today's Ho-Chunk Nation) told of a river called the "Messisipi." When they claimed that the mighty waterway led to a distant sea, Nicolet wondered whether it might flow southwest into the Pacific Ocean.

Rumors of this river circulated among the French on the Great Lakes for a generation. Finally, in 1673, trader Louis Joliet and his associate Jacques Marquette, a Jesuit priest from the St. Ignace mission near Mackinac, entered the upper Mississippi via the Wisconsin River. The two men embarked on what Father Marquette described as a "voyage toward New Mexico." They descended the great stream to the mouth of the Arkansas River, far enough south to suspect that the waterway flowed into the Gulf of Mexico. If it was not an outlet to the Pacific, perhaps the river could still prompt a viable "southern strategy." That is, it might give France a path to the wealth of New Spain and provide French settlers with access to a warm-water port. "The worst thing about Canada," Colbert observed from France, is that the St. Lawrence, "being so far to the north, allows ships to enter only during four, five or six months of the year."

The new governor general in Quebec, Comte de Frontenac, moved to exploit these western prospects, making effective use of an experienced young adventurer: René-Robert Cavelier, Sieur de La Salle. In 1673, to secure control of the growing fur trade on the Great Lakes, La Salle erected Fort Frontenac at the eastern end of Lake Ontario. From there, inspired by word of Joliet's exploits, he and his men pushed west through the Great Lakes to southern Lake

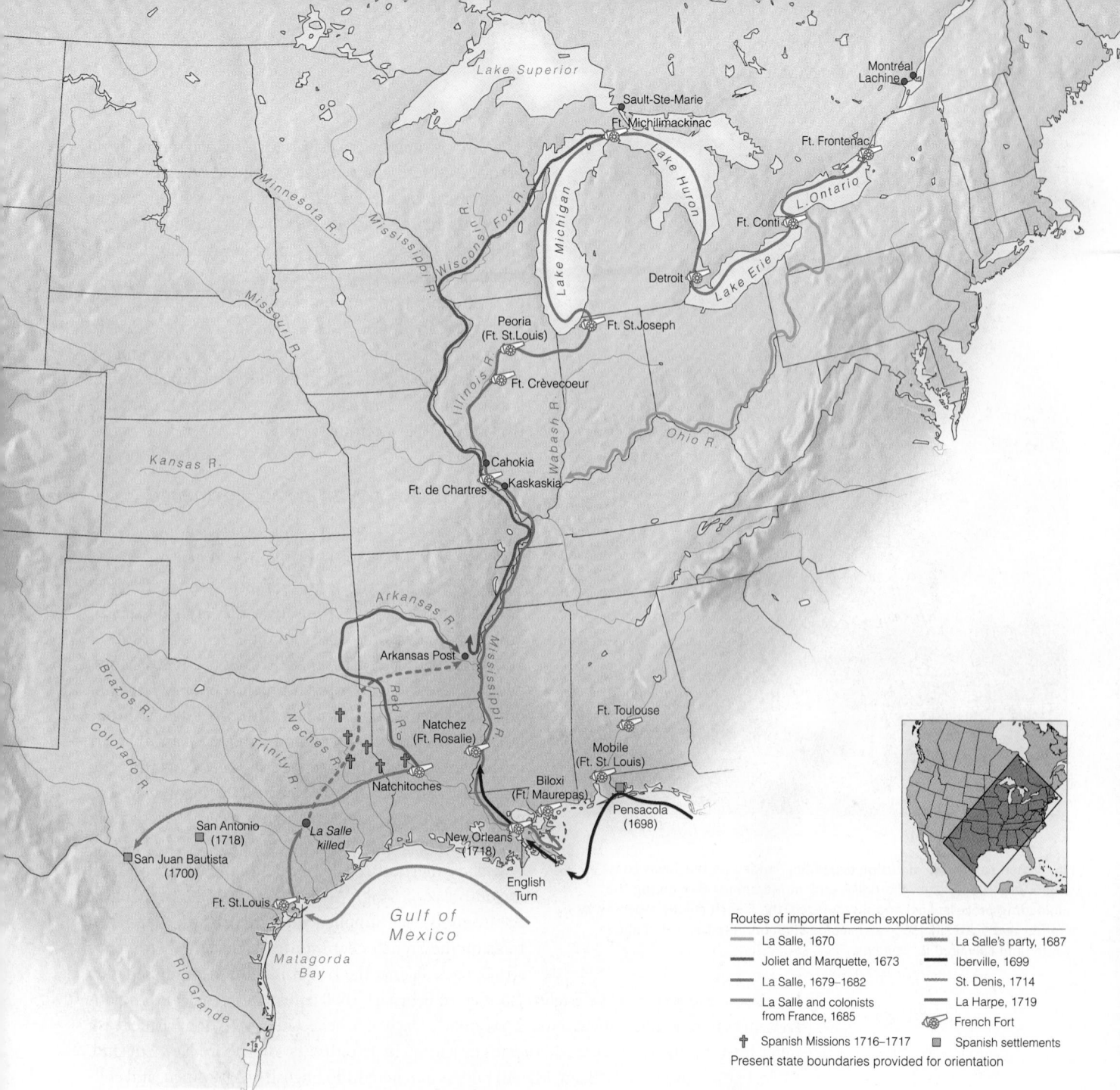

■ **MAP 3.1** FRANCE IN THE AMERICAN INTERIOR, 1670–1720

Routes of important French explorations

—— La Salle, 1670
—— Joliet and Marquette, 1673
—— La Salle, 1679–1682
—— La Salle and colonists from France, 1685
✝ Spanish Missions 1716–1717
—— La Salle's party, 1687
—— Iberville, 1699
—— St. Denis, 1714
—— La Harpe, 1719
⚜ French Fort
◼ Spanish settlements

Present state boundaries provided for orientation

Michigan. After carrying their canoes overland to the Illinois River, they erected several forts on that tributary of the Mississippi. These outposts strengthened French trading ties with local Indians and provided a launching point for more exploration. In 1680 one party dispatched by La Salle traveled down the Illinois River to the Mississippi, which the French called the Colbert. Then turning north, they paddled 500 miles against the Mississippi's strong current all the way to the Falls of St. Anthony: modern-day Minneapolis.

Two years later La Salle himself led a contingent of French and Indians south from the Illinois to explore the lower Mississippi. He returned to confirm that the great river indeed emptied into the Gulf of Mexico. He claimed the rich land drained by all its tributaries for Louis XIV, naming the entire river basin "Louisiana" after his king. Hindered by poor maps and crude navigational instruments, La Salle miscalculated the location of the mouth of the Mississippi.

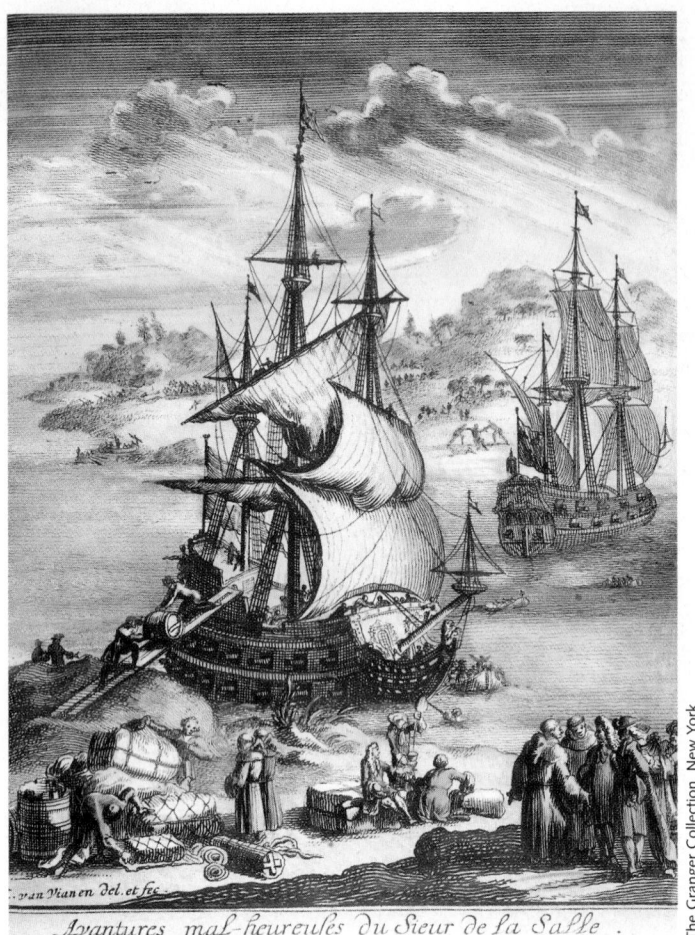

Aventures mal-heureuses du Sieur de la Salle.

The Granger Collection, New York

■ When La Salle's colonizing expedition landed on the Texas coast in 1685, one supply ship, the *Belle*, sank in Matagorda Bay during the unloading process. Lost and discouraged, the French colony faded away within two years. In 1995, archaeologists found the *Belle* in shallow water and salvaged its remains.

Therefore, when he tried to return by sea, sailing from France with four ships and several hundred colonists, he disembarked on the Texas coast early in 1685, mistakenly believing that he was close to the entrance to the river. Slowly, the entire colonization plan unraveled. When one ship sank near shore, the hapless settlers lost valuable supplies and any hope of relocating. Jealous French lieutenants eventually killed La Salle before he could discern the nature of his mistake and locate the whereabouts of the Mississippi River. Most of the colonists he had brought perished in the Texas wilderness, lost like the English settlers at Roanoke a century before.

King William's War in the Northeast

The French colonizers had overreached themselves. They had failed to find a route to the Pacific, to challenge Spanish power in Mexico, or to establish a southern port. Spread thin by the widening fur trade, French Canadians were in a weak position to repel renewed Iroquois attacks along the St. Lawrence River in the 1680s. Moreover, a strengthened Protestant regime emerged in London with the ascent of William III to the English throne in 1689. This transition set in motion more than 100 years of bitter struggle between Protestant England and Catholic France. In North America, the ideological and military contest of these two superpowers stretched out over several generations.

The American conflict began in the Northeast with the outbreak of King William's War in 1689. In that year the Iroquois, well supplied with English arms, launched raids on the French near Montreal. Governor Frontenac struck back against the Iroquois' allies, sending separate forces south to terrorize the English frontier. In February 1690, a force of French and Indians traveling on snowshoes attacked the snowbound village of Schenectady, New York. Farther east, other French joined local Abenaki Indians in setting fire to outposts in northern New England. At Fort Loyal (modern Portland, Maine) raiders butchered 100 English men, women, and children after they surrendered and took others captive. Leaving their dead unburied, the survivors fled south toward Salem and Boston in Massachusetts. Many who experienced the attack viewed it as part of a wider design to undo the Reformation and expand the authority of the Catholic Church, led by the pope in Rome. One wrote fearfully, that there must be "a popish design against the Protestant interest in New England as in other parts of the world."

As the frontier war raged on, bitter New Englanders tried unsuccessfully to seize Quebec. In turn, the French Canadians and their Huron allies conducted punishing raids against Iroquois villages. After eight years of bloodshed, King William's War ended in a stalemate in 1697. The Iroquois realized that staying out of European conflicts would improve their lot. In 1701, therefore, the Iroquois League promised to remain neutral during any future colonial wars between France and England, a pledge they generally honored for more than half a century. The French, having strengthened their position in Canada, could now revive the "southern strategy" of colonization that had so intrigued Colbert and obsessed the adventurer La Salle.

As King William's War closed, a turn in European events opened the door for renewed French efforts in the American heartland. King Carlos II of Spain fell ill without an immediate heir, and the royal courts of Europe competed to determine his successor. Louis XIV, eager to acquire Spain's European realm and American dominions for France, proposed that his grandson, Philip of Anjou, receive the Spanish crown. But England supported an opposing candidate, so the War of Spanish Succession (1701–1714) broke out soon after Carlos died.

Founding the Louisiana Colony

Even before new hostilities erupted in Europe in 1701, Louis XIV and his ministers took steps to secure French claims in the Gulf of Mexico. Given Spain's naval dominance throughout the area, the gulf had long been considered a "Spanish Sea" among the rival colonial powers. By renewing La Salle's plan to create a Louisiana colony, France could strengthen its hand in the impending war over succession to the Spanish throne. A colony on the Gulf of Mexico would provide much more than a southern outlet for the French fur trade; it could serve as a strategic outpost as well. The Spanish had just built a permanent Gulf Coast fortification at Pensacola in western Florida. The French realized that a settlement farther west along the same coast would help them hold onto any new territories in New Spain or the West Indies that might suddenly fall to France through a royal inheritance or a military conquest.

Caught up in the same competition, England also saw advantages to establishing a base on the lower Mississippi. Such a post could challenge Spanish and French claims to the gulf region and increase English trade with the Chickasaws and other southern Indians. In 1698 a London promoter quietly made plans to transport a group of Huguenot refugees to the mouth of the Mississippi. Catching wind of this scheme, the French naval minister, Comte de Pontchartrain, organized his own secret expedition to the Gulf of Mexico under an aspiring Canadian officer, Pierre Le Moyne d'Iberville.

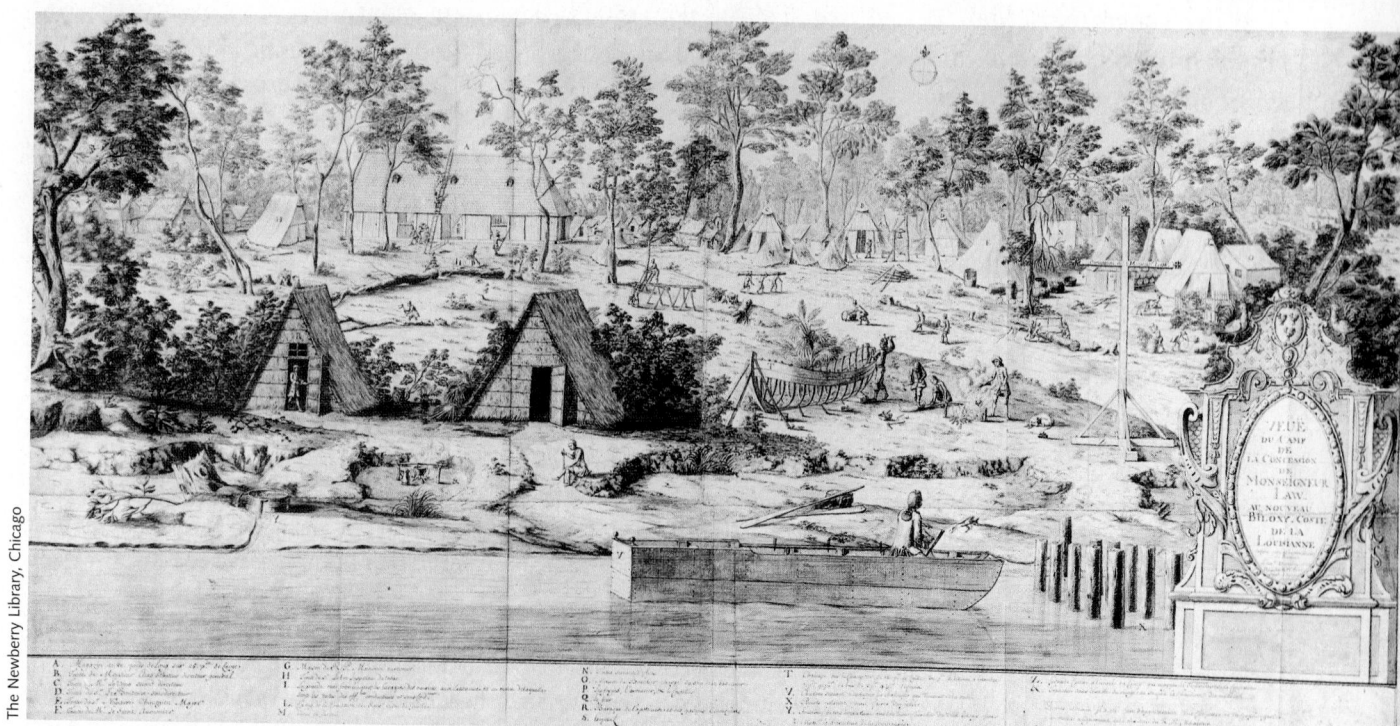

The Newberry Library, Chicago

■ Le Boutaux, *View of the Camp on the Concession of Monseigneur Law at New Biloxi on the Louisiana Coast,* 1720. When the French constructed a new settlement on Biloxi Bay in 1720, colonists still faced crude living conditions along the Gulf Coast. Rats eat our food supplies, one newcomer complained, and "no greens can be raised" in the sandy soil.

During King William's War, Iberville had led the winter raid on Schenectady in 1690 and had later opposed the English at Hudson's Bay and Newfoundland. Coming from a large and well-connected Montreal family, the Le Moynes, Iberville quickly drew several siblings into the gulf colonization plan, including his teenage brother, Bienville. Iberville and his party sailed for the Gulf of Mexico from the French port of Brest in 1699. Their ship entered the mouth of the Mississippi in time to repel the English expedition at a site on the river still known as English Turn. They also managed to build a fort at nearby Biloxi Bay before returning to France.

The two brothers were now well on their way to creating the gulf coast colony that La Salle and his followers had failed to establish. A second voyage let Iberville conduct further reconnaissance of the lower Mississippi. On a third trip, in 1702, he established Fort Louis, near Mobile Bay, giving French traders access to the Choctaw Indians. Young Bienville, placed in charge of Fort Louis, labored to sustain the tiny outpost at Mobile (where the *Pelican* would arrive in 1704). Iberville himself left to pursue other schemes and died an early death in 1706.

Enmeshed at home in the lengthy War of Spanish Succession, France largely ignored its new gulf colony. Epidemics took a heavy toll on the newcomers and an even heavier toll on their Indian neighbors. Sharp divisions separated settlers drawn from Canada and other colonists sent from France. The former had prior wilderness experience, maintained close ties with local Native Americans, and resented the incompetence and haughtiness of newcomers from across the Atlantic. The latter missed the comforts of life in France, complained about the poor living conditions, and looked down on their Canadian counterparts as lacking in education and religious training. However, despite social friction and a chronic lack of supplies from France, the small community at Mobile survived.

North of Mobile, additional French posts began to dot the American interior. They reinforced the territorial claims of France and offered increased trade and protection to neighboring Indians. French traders built the village of Peoria on the Illinois River in 1691. Not far away, Catholic missions sprang up at Cahokia (1697) and Kaskaskia (1703). Between these two missions, the French would later erect Fort de Chartres (1719) overlooking the Mississippi in southern Illinois. Further north, the French established two strategic posts at opposite ends of Lake Huron. In 1689, they laid out a garrison where Lake Huron joins Lake Michigan, expanding their foothold there in 1715 with the construction of Fort Michilimackinac. In 1701, they also created a lasting town on the strait (*le détroit* in French) connecting Lake Erie to Lake Huron. The founder of this outpost—called Detroit—was a Monsieur Cadillac, who foresaw a prosperous future for the village. The powerful Iroquois had pledged their neutrality in 1701, and the new trading post, Cadillac wrote, lay open "to the most distant tribes which surround these vast sweet water seas."

> *Over two generations, the French had established a solid claim on the American interior.*

In 1712 the French crown, its resources depleted by a decade of warfare in Europe granted control over Louisiana to a powerful Paris merchant, Antoine Crozat. Drawing Cadillac from Detroit to the Gulf of Mexico to serve as Louisiana's governor general, Crozat hoped to develop connections to mineral-rich Mexico and to discover precious metals in the Mississippi watershed. But probes on the upper Mississippi, the Missouri, and the Red rivers yielded no easy bonanza. Instead, explorers established three new trading posts among the Indians: Natchitoches on the Red River, Fort Rosalie on the Mississippi (at Natchez), and Fort Toulouse (near modern Montgomery, Alabama) where two streams join to form the Alabama River, flowing southwest to Mobile.

When Louis XIV died in 1715, the colonial population of Louisiana stood at scarcely 300 people. But over two generations, the French had established a solid claim on the American interior. Their position was an ongoing challenge to English and Spanish competitors, for the crescent of wilderness outposts arcing north and then east from the Gulf Coast offered a useful network for additional exploration, Indian trade, and military conquest. French control of the Mississippi Valley remained a real possibility until the era of Thomas Jefferson and Napoleon Bonaparte nearly a century later.

The Spanish Empire on the Defensive

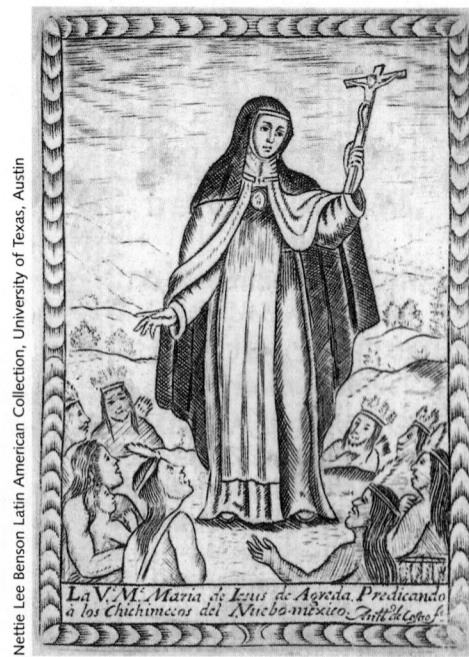

Nettie Lee Benson Latin American Collection, University of Texas, Austin

W hereas France's power expanded during Louis XIV's reign, Spain's overextended empire continued to weaken. This decline opened the door for Louis (leader of the House of Bourbon) to maneuver his own grandson onto the Spanish throne in 1700 as Philip V. Eventually, the resulting new line of Bourbon monarchs brought much-needed changes to the administration of Spain's overseas empire. However, these so-called Bourbon reforms took several generations to devise and implement. Meanwhile, Spanish colonizers struggled to defend vast territorial claims that spread—on paper—from the Gulf of California to the Florida peninsula.

In its remote colonies of New Mexico and Florida, Spain had weak imperial oversight at best. Local administration often proved corrupt, and communication with officials in Spain remained slow and cumbersome. For several generations, the Indian majority had resented the harsh treatment and strange diseases that came with colonial contact. Now, cultural disruptions and pressures from hostile Indian neighbors fanned the flames of discontent. In the late seventeenth century, a wave of Native American rebellions swept the northern frontier of New Spain.

The Pueblo Revolt in New Mexico

The largest and most successful revolt took place along the upper Rio Grande. There, Pueblo Indians from dozens of separate communities (or pueblos) united in a major upheaval in August 1680. They murdered 21 of the 40 friars serving in New Mexico, ransacked their churches, and killed more than 350 settlers. After laying siege to Santa Fe, the rebels drove the remaining Spanish colonists and their Christian Indian allies south out of the province and kept them away for more than a decade. Several thousand refugees ended up at El Paso del Norte, a crossing point on the Rio Grande where the Franciscans had constructed a mission in 1659. These stunned survivors, at what is now El Paso, soon began questioning Indian informants to find an explanation for the fearsome rebellion they had just endured.

■ In the 1630s, missionaries on the Southwest asserted that a nun living in Spain had miraculously appeared to Native American converts. But a generation later, when Indians questioned claims of Christian miracles and European superiority, it resulted in the Pueblo Revolt of 1680.

No single answer existed for the rebellion's source since diverse pressures combined to ignite the Pueblo Revolt of 1680. In retrospect, several factors, stretching back over decades, stand out clearly as providing fuel for the fire. First, a severe drought beginning in 1666 had inflicted a five-year famine with long-lasting effects on the peoples of New Mexico. Second, around the same time, neighboring Apaches and Navajos stepped up their hostilities against the small colonial population and the numerous Pueblo Indians who had been linked with the Spanish over several generations. The attackers were embittered by the continuing Spanish slave raids that took Indian captives to work in the Mexican silver mines. In retaliation these raiding parties, riding stolen Spanish horses, killed livestock and seized scarce food. When Spanish soldiers proved unable to fend off the hit-and-run attacks, their credibility among the Pueblo Indians living alongside the colonists weakened.

Third, a smoldering controversy over religion flared during the 1670s. The mystique surrounding Christianity was damaged when an epidemic struck in 1671 and Spanish missionaries could not stem the sickness through prayer. In response, traditionalist Indian priests regained favor, and they fostered a revival of age-old Pueblo religious customs. Horrified, the Spanish friars and government officials united to punish what they saw as backsliding within a Pueblo population that seemed to have accepted key elements of the Catholic faith. At Santa Fe in 1675, they hanged three Indian leaders for idolatry and whipped and imprisoned 43 others. The Spanish intended to sell the offenders—including a militant leader from San Juan pueblo named Popé—into slavery. However, armed Indians confronted the New Mexico governor and successfully demanded the release of Popé and the other prisoners.

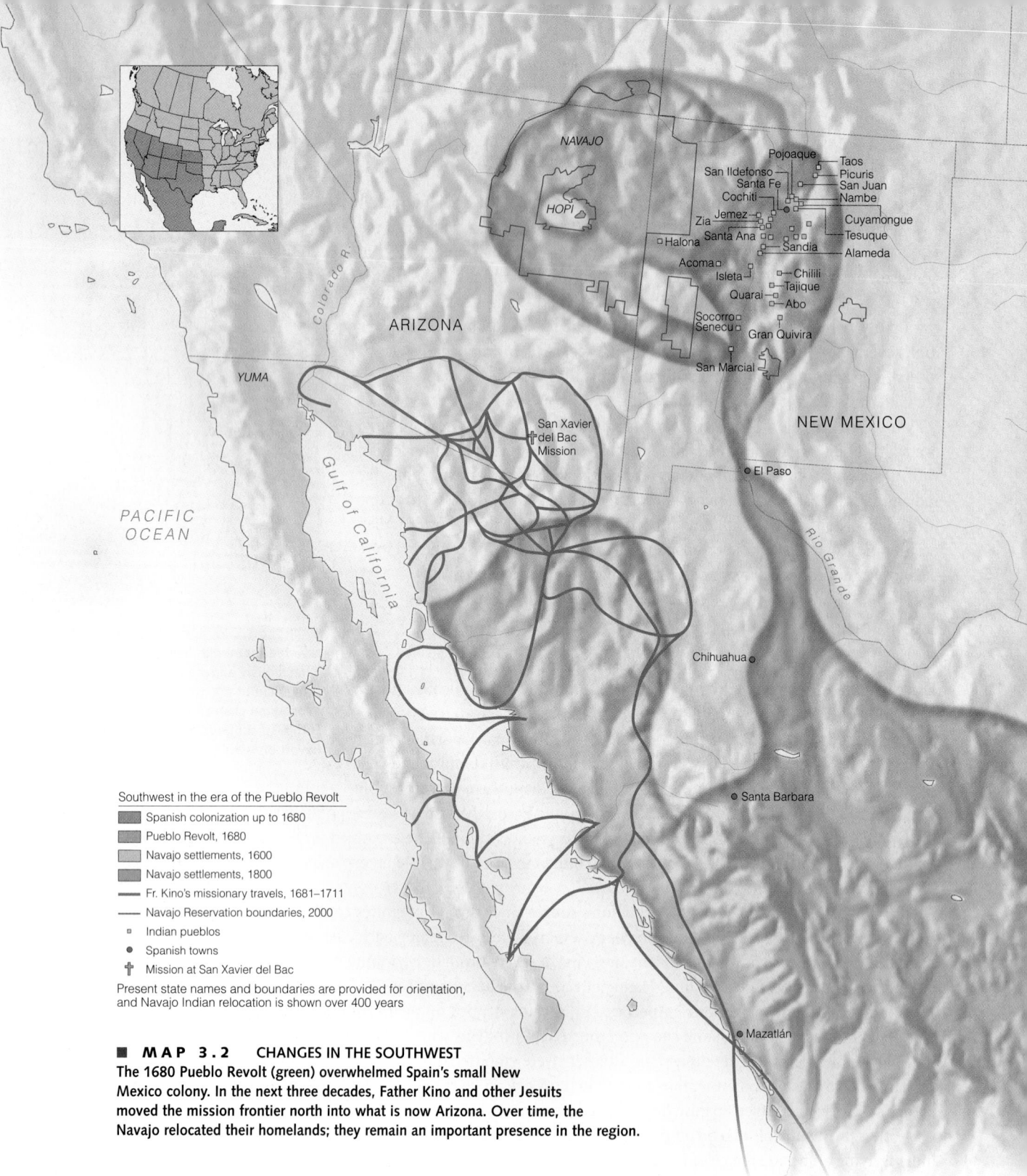

The following are labels on the map:

NAVAJO

HOPI

Pojoaque
San Ildefonso
Santa Fe
Cochiti
Zia
Jemez
Halona
Santa Ana
Acoma
Isleta
Quarai
Socorro
Senecu
San Marcial

Taos
Picuris
San Juan
Nambe
Cuyamongue
Tesuque
Alameda
Sandia
Chilili
Tajique
Abo
Gran Quivira

ARIZONA

YUMA

San Xavier
del Bac
Mission

NEW MEXICO

El Paso

PACIFIC
OCEAN

Gulf of California

Colorado R.

Rio Grande

Chihuahua

Santa Barbara

Mazatlán

Southwest in the era of the Pueblo Revolt

- Spanish colonization up to 1680
- Pueblo Revolt, 1680
- Navajo settlements, 1600
- Navajo settlements, 1800
- —— Fr. Kino's missionary travels, 1681–1711
- —— Navajo Reservation boundaries, 2000
- ▫ Indian pueblos
- ● Spanish towns
- ✝ Mission at San Xavier del Bac

Present state names and boundaries are provided for orientation,
and Navajo Indian relocation is shown over 400 years

■ **MAP 3.2**   **CHANGES IN THE SOUTHWEST**
The 1680 Pueblo Revolt (green) overwhelmed Spain's small New
Mexico colony. In the next three decades, Father Kino and other Jesuits
moved the mission frontier north into what is now Arizona. Over time, the
Navajo relocated their homelands; they remain an important presence in the region.

This confrontation over religion only deepened the divisions within local Indian communities and families. Over several generations, thousands of Pueblo people had converted to
the Christian faith and the Spanish way of life. They had accepted the colonizers' promises of
heavenly rewards, and they feared the reprisals that had followed previous acts of resistance. But
many others felt embittered, especially against the despised encomienda system that granted
control over Native American labor to Spanish newcomers who backed up their claims by force.
These Pueblo malcontents believed that the time for successful opposition was slipping away.

Popé himself, banned from San Juan for disturbing the peace, withdrew to Taos, the north-
ernmost pueblo in New Mexico. From there, he negotiated secretly with like-minded factions

in other pueblos, unifying resistance to Spanish domination. He invoked the spirits of the Pueblo deities, especially the powerful sun spirit known as Po he yemu. He also killed those who threatened to reveal his plot, including his own brother. Popé's militant resolve helped him build an underground movement. In part, he built support around widespread resentment of the encomienda system, used by the Spanish to require Indian communities to supply labor or pay tribute. But two other long-term issues contributed to his success as well. One involved sex and gender; the other combined race and class.

From their earliest encounters, nothing divided the Spanish and Indians more sharply than their contrasting notions of sexuality. For example, Native Americans, like members of most societies around the world, accepted homosexuality. But many Christians considered it an abomination deserving death. More generally, whereas the Pueblos viewed sexuality as a crucial ingredient in social and spiritual life, Christians saw it as a source of sin and embarrassment. Indeed, Franciscans forbade traditional Indian religious ceremonies in part because they included erotic symbols and acts. The ban threatened the very essence of life for the Pueblos, who believed that sexual intercourse yielded not only human children but also bountiful crops, prompting male rains to join with female corn seeds to produce sustenance. Who were these friars who professed celibacy and punished themselves and others with whips for their natural sexual desires? The Pueblos had learned from experience that the same people who prohibited open displays of Indian sexuality occasionally practiced and condoned private acts of rape and molestation. The Indian women whom Spanish priests or soldiers had abused took Popé's side in this cultural clash, covertly supporting his militant design.

The movement also received secret support from numerous *mestizos* and mulattos, mixed-race people whose dark skin and lack of "pure" Spanish blood cost them any chance to rise in the colonial hierarchy. Members of this class included the elderly Pedro Naranjo, son of an Indian woman and a mulatto former slave who had received his freedom in return for joining an early expedition of colonists to New Mexico. At 80 years of age, the bilingual Naranjo could still sign his name in Spanish. He or some other family member may well have worked with Popé behind the scenes to plot the 1680 uprising. Historians have noted a "common report among all the Indians" about an inspirational letter written by a "very tall" and "black" Indian—likely Naranjo. This person was considered a "lieutenant" of the sun spirit, Po he yemu. His letter ordered that "all of them in general should rebel" and threatened destruction on "any pueblo that would not agree to it."

Along with such threats, Popé and his organizers sent runners to each conspiring pueblo in the summer of 1680. The runners delivered knotted ropes so all would know (by untying one knot each day) that the date for the rebellion was August 11. When several messengers were captured on August 9, Popé moved the revolt ahead one day, and his Pueblo warriors swiftly routed their adversaries. Unified in triumph, the zealous victors smeared excrement on Christian altars and bathed themselves to remove the stigma of baptism.

But initial cohesion soon gave way to friction. The successful rebels soon quarreled over who should hold power and how best to return to ancient ways. Kivas would replace churches, and the cross would give way to the kachina. But what other parts of the imported culture should the Indians abandon after eight decades of intermingling with the newcomers? Various Pueblo groups could not agree on which Spanish words, tools, and customs to discard or on which foreign crops and animals they would retain.

In 1681, the Pueblos fended off a Spanish attempt at reconquest. But they remained divided among themselves and more vulnerable than ever to Apache raids. Within a decade, rival factions had deposed Popé, and another Spanish army, under Governor Diego de Vargas, had entered New Mexico. It took the new governor several years to subdue the province, and the Pueblos managed another full-scale rebellion in 1696. But Vargas anticipated the revolt and crushed the opposition with overwhelming force, just as Oñate had done a century earlier. In 1706, several soldiers and their families established the town of Albuquerque on its present site. Learning from previous mistakes, Spanish officials did not reimpose the hated encomienda, with its demand for Native

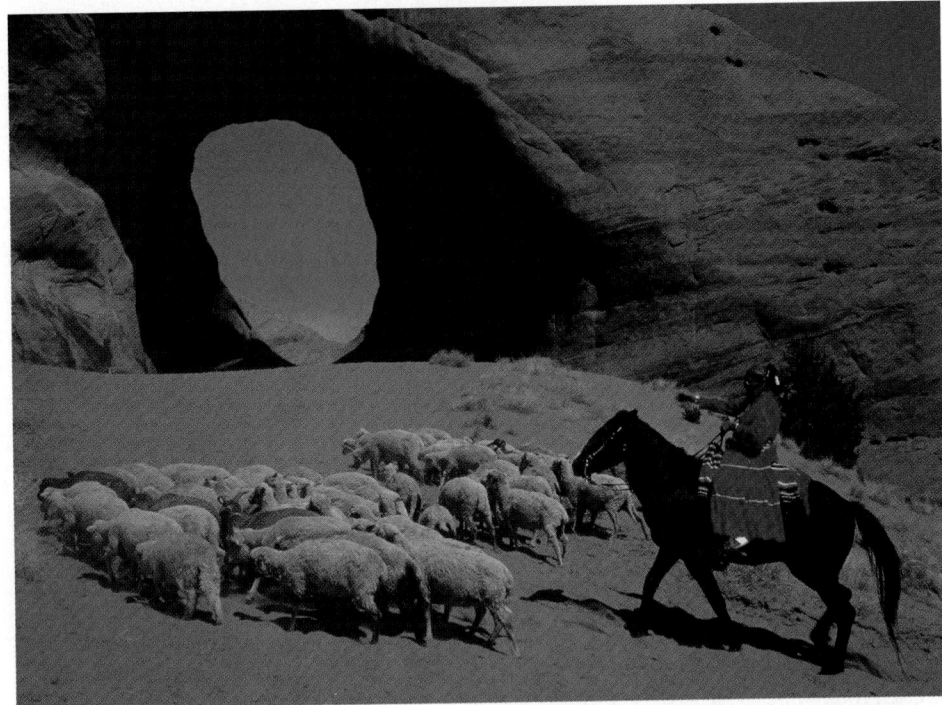

Harald Sund/Getty Images

■ Horses and sheep arrived in the Southwest with the Spanish, and both became central to the Navajo (or Diné) culture in northern Arizona and New Mexico. Navajo women continue to herd sheep and weave their wool into rugs and blankets, as they have done for more than three centuries.

American labor or tribute. A new generation of Franciscan missionaries tolerated indigenous Pueblo traditions as long as the Indians also attended Catholic mass.

Navajos and Spanish on the Southwestern Frontier

The repercussions of rebellion and reconquest along the upper Rio Grande echoed throughout the Southwest. To the north, the Navajos benefited from Pueblo refugees who joined their communities. The Pueblo newcomers had valuable experience as corn farmers. Already known to the Navajos, corn now became an increasingly important food and sacred symbol for them. Moreover, the new arrivals had learned from the Spanish how to plant peach orchards and raise sheep. Pueblo men, long skilled at weaving textiles on stationary looms, showed their Navajo neighbors how to shear sheep, then how to wash the fleece, dye it, card it, and spin it into woolen yarn. Long before the arrival of sheep, Navajo women had always been the weavers in their society. Soon, therefore, women owned the expanding flocks and created wool blankets on their traditional portable looms. The Pueblos also brought more Spanish horses, a key asset that let the Navajos spread their domain west into fine grazing country in what is now northeast Arizona. Farther north, the Utes and Comanches also acquired horses after the Pueblo Revolt. After 1700, the Comanches pressed southeast onto the plains of present-day Texas and honed new skills as mounted buffalo hunters.

The Pueblo Revolt also brought reprcussions for the Spanish, since they had clearly overextended themselves along New Spain's wide northern frontier. Most worried officials agreed that the remote colony of New Mexico needed protection from further upheavals. So, despite their limited resources, authorities in Mexico City sent a few missionary-explorers north near the Gulf of California to spread Christianity and pacify hostile Indians. If possible, they were to extend Spain's geographic knowledge and discover new sources of wealth. In addition, they were to warn of any moves by imperial rivals, for hostile French ships had appeared in the Gulf of California in 1689.

Year by year, these friar-explorers edged north toward what is now southern Arizona until they reached the cactus-studded landscape of the Sonoran Desert in the 1690s. Eusebio Kino, a tireless Jesuit missionary born in Italy and educated in Germany, spearheaded the early exploration of the Arizona region. In 1701, this padre on horseback established a mission at San Xavier del Bac, near the Santa Cruz River below modern Tucson, Arizona. But his incessant travels continued, and the mission fell into disuse after his death in 1711.

During one of his extended explorations, Father Kino visited the Yuma Indians, where the Gila River meets the lower Colorado. He noticed blue seashells that he knew had to have come via overland trade from coastal California. From this he reasoned that California was not an island, as European mapmakers had long supposed. Rather, it was a part of the continent that might be reached by traveling west across the desert above the Gulf of California. Hearing this news, Philip V ordered an outpost to be established on California's upper coast beyond the Baja peninsula. It was the very charge that Sebastián Vizcaíno had failed to complete a century earlier, and once again it went unfulfilled. The Spanish did not take advantage of their improved understanding of the coastal geography until the 1760s.

Meanwhile, Kino's missions languished after his death in 1711. Warfare and sickness eroded the local population of Pima Indians, and attacks by Apache raiders destabilized the entire frontier region. The Spanish finally reinstalled priests at San Xavier del Bac and other missions along the Santa Cruz River in 1732. Four years later, a silver strike at "Arizonac," near present-day Nogales on the U.S.–Mexican border, provided a new name for the region, which would eventually become the state called Arizona.

Borderland Conflict in Texas and Florida

The encounters on Spain's other North American borderland frontiers took different forms, in part because European rivals appeared on the scene. Conflict with the French led the Spanish to found missions in Texas, a land they named after the local Tejas Indians. Still farther east, Indian resentments and war with the English weakened Spanish missions in Florida.

After 1685, Spanish expeditions probed the Gulf Coast region, eager to find and destroy La Salle's French colony. But Indians had already burned the short-lived outpost when the Spanish discovered its whereabouts. (Modern archaeologists have recently rediscovered the site.) In 1693, with any immediate European competition removed, the Spanish postponed attempts to establish a mission in Texas. They renewed their wholehearted commitment to the effort two decades later, when Louisiana's Governor Cadillac (the founder of Detroit) proved eager to open a trade across Texas with the Spanish frontier.

Governor Cadillac sent the Frenchman Louis Saint-Denis from Louisiana to forge ties with Spanish communities south of the Rio Grande. Saint-Denis and two dozen men set out from Natchitoches on the Red River and crossed East Texas, reaching the longtime Spanish outpost at San Juan Bautista, below the modern U.S.-Mexican border, in 1714. Surprised by this intrusion, Spanish authorities swiftly dusted off their plans for colonizing Texas. By 1717 they had established half a dozen small missions on both sides of the Sabine River, the boundary between modern Texas and Louisiana.

The next year, the Spanish took steps to expand their missionary activities and secure the supply route from San Juan Bautista to their distant outposts in east Texas. They built a second cluster of settlements at a midpoint in the trail beside the San Antonio River. Within two decades, a string of missions stretched along the river. Indian converts tended herds of cattle and sheep and constructed aqueducts to irrigate new fields of wheat and corn. The earliest mission, San Antonio de Valero (1718), provided a nucleus for the town of San Antonio. It also strengthened Spanish claims to Texas against the threat of French intrusion. (The same mission, converted into a military post known as the Alamo, became known far and wide for the battle fought there in 1836, when Anglo-Texans pushed for independence from Mexican rule.)

During the second half of the seventeenth century, the Indians of Florida, like the Pueblos in New Mexico, debated whether to reject generations of Spanish rule. The Columbian Exchange had altered their lives in dramatic ways. They ate new foods such as figs, oranges, peas, cabbages, and cucumbers. They used Spanish words such as *azucár* (sugar), *botija* (jar), and *caballo* (horse). The acquisition of metal hoes allowed them to produce more corn than ever before. But expanding contact with missionaries had major drawbacks as well. By 1660 devastating epidemics had whittled away at Native American towns. The Indians still outnumbered the newcomers more than ten to one, but they had to expend enormous energy raising, processing, and hauling food for the Spanish. When colonists at St. Augustine grew fearful of French and English attacks after 1670, they forced hundreds of Indians to perform even more grueling labor: constructing the stone fortress of San Marcos.

Nothing proved more troubling to Florida's Indians than the spread of livestock farming. St. Augustine's elite had established profitable cattle ranches on the depopulated savannas of Timucua, near present-day Gainesville in north central Florida. These entrepreneurs could ship hides to Havana from both Florida coasts. They ignored the colony's requirements to keep cows away from unfenced Indian gardens, and they enforced harsh laws to protect their stock. Any Florida Indian who killed cattle faced four months of servitude; people caught raiding Spanish herds had their ears cut off.

Any Florida Indian who killed cattle faced four months of servitude; people caught raiding Spanish herds had their ears cut off.

Resentment grew among the converts living in Florida's scattered mission villages. Restless Indians wondered whether the English, who had founded their Carolina colony on the Ashley River near modern Charleston in 1670, might make viable allies. The English, less committed to establishing missions than their Spanish rivals, seemed eager to trade for deerskins. In return, they offered the Native Americans a steadier supply of desirable goods than the Spanish could provide. Several Indian communities moved closer to Carolina to test this new alternative for trade. But disillusionment soon set in. When France and Spain joined forces against the English after 1700, Florida's Indians suddenly found themselves caught up in a struggle far larger than they had bargained for.

Ever since the days of Francis Drake, the English had schemed to oust the Spanish from St. Augustine. In 1702 English raiders from Carolina, under Governor James Moore, rampaged through the town. Yet the new stone fortress of San Marcos held firm, protecting the inhabitants. Two years later, Moore devised a more profitable way to disrupt the Spanish colony. With native allies, he invaded Apalachee (near modern Tallahassee). His troops crushed the mission towns, killing hundreds and carrying away more than 4000 Indian captives. Most of them were women and children, whom the English sold as slaves in Carolina and the Caribbean. By 1706 the Spanish settlement at St. Augustine endured, but numerous mission villages in Apalachee and Timucua lay in ruins. "In all these extensive dominions," wrote a troubled Spanish official from St. Augustine, "the law of God and the preaching of the Holy Gospel have now ceased."

England's American Empire Takes Shape

In 1660, as Louis XIV began his long reign in France and Spanish missionaries labored in obscurity in New Mexico and Florida, England experienced a counterrevolutionary upheaval that influenced American colonial affairs dramatically. In the 1640s, amid violent civil war, rebels supporting Puritans and the Parliament had overthrown the ruling Stuart family, beheaded Charles I, and abolished hereditary monarchy altogether.

For a brief period, England became a republican commonwealth without a king. But Oliver Cromwell, the movement's dictatorial leader and self-styled Lord Protector, died in 1658. Pressures quickly mounted to undo the radical Puritan Revolution and return to monarchical government. In May 1660, a strong coalition of conservative interests welcomed the late king's son back from exile and "restored" him to the throne as King Charles II. For this reason, the last three decades of the Stuart dynasty (1660–1688) are remembered in English politics and culture as the Restoration Era.

England's efforts in North America after the restoration of the Stuart monarchy differed sharply from the strivings of France and Spain. Europe's two Catholic powers emphasized geographic exploration and religious conversion. They stretched their claims across vast areas but had less success planting self-sustaining colonial populations. The English, in contrast, focused on precisely this goal along the Atlantic coast.

Monarchy Restored and Navigation Controlled

The shift in London's political winds could hardly have been more sudden, and Charles II moved quickly in 1660 to underscore the end of England's Puritan experiment. He ordered his hangman to burn the revolutionary constitution and parliamentary acts of the preceding government. He also commanded the execution of those responsible for beheading his father in 1649. Several of these individuals (known as regicides) escaped to find sanctuary in Puritan New England, and many who had served the "Good Old Cause" by fighting to end monarchy and strengthen parliament likewise sought refuge across the Atlantic.

The American colonies grew with the arrival of people whose religious and political beliefs had suddenly fallen out of favor at home. But other elements of colonial demographics— early marriage, high birth rates, and a low level of mortality in most places—did even more to prompt expansion up and down the Atlantic coast. Because most colonists still lived within 50 miles of the shoreline, this increase in people steadily broadened the opportunities for seaborne trade. Growing ship traffic, in turn, sparked government desires to regulate colonial navigation to bring mercantilist advantages to the realm.

In 1660 Parliament passed a major Navigation Act designed to promote British shipping and trade. The new law laid out important conditions that shaped England's colonial commerce for generations. First, merchants could not conduct trade to or from the English colonies in foreign-owned ships. Second, key non-English products imported from foreign lands—salt, wine, oil, and naval stores (the tar, pitch, masts, and other materials used to build boats)— had to be carried in English ships or in ships with mostly English crews. Third, the law contained a list of "enumerated articles" produced overseas. The items listed—tobacco, cotton, sugar, ginger, indigo, and dyewoods—could no longer be sent directly from a colony to a foreign European port. Instead, merchants had to ship them to England first and then reexport them, a step that directly boosted England's domestic economy. Another Navigation Act, in 1663, required that goods from the European continent to England's overseas colonies also needed to pass through the island. Moreover, they had to arrive and depart on English ships.

Tabacum latifolium.

Ten years later, yet another navigation measure—the Plantation Duty Act of 1673— tried to close loopholes regarding enumerated articles. The new act required captains to pay a "plantation duty" before they sailed between colonial ports with enumerated goods. Otherwise, colonial vessels carrying such goods had to post bond before leaving harbor to ensure that they would sail directly to England. To enforce these rules, the government sent customs officers to the colonies for the first time. These officials' income depended on the fees they collected and goods they confiscated. Not surprisingly, colonists resented these new intruders as meddling parasites. But almost a century passed before fights over imperial customs collection finally helped spark a revolution.

Backed by the Navigation Acts, English shipbuilding prospered at home and in the tree-rich North American colonies. England's naval and merchant fleets burgeoned. A report to the king claimed that Chesapeake tobacco produced more revenue for the crown "than the East Indies four times over" and boasted that England's growing colonies in America "are his majesty's Indies," for "without charge to him" they had been "raised and supported by the English subjects, who employ above two hundred sail of good ships every year, breed abundance of mariners, and begin to grow into commodities of great value and esteem." Colonial trade, with all its related activities, became a major sector in England's economy.

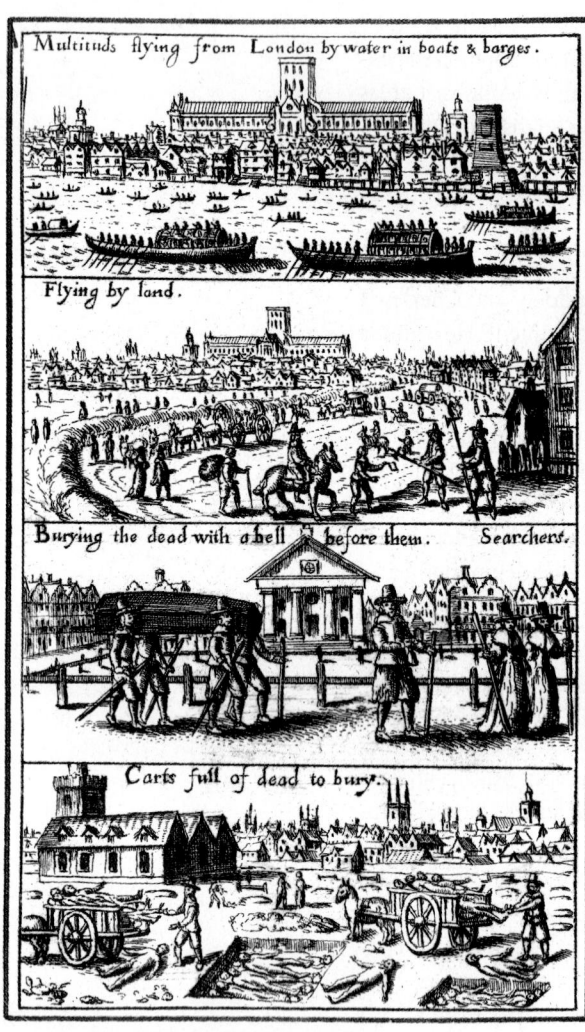

Multituds flying from London by water in boats & barges.

Flying by land.

Burying the dead with a bell before them. Searchers.

Carts full of dead to bury.

■ **Images of the Great Plague in London.**

Even the Great Plague, which swept England in 1665, could not blunt this mercantile growth. And when a catastrophic fire destroyed most of London the next year, the huge loss also provided an opportunity. Planners redesigned the city with the broad streets and impressive buildings that suited the prosperous hub of an expanding empire. The fashionable coffee shops that sprang up as a novelty in late-seventeenth-century London became common meeting places for exchanging news and views about England's increasingly wide and profitable activities overseas. Much of what transpired in English North America was hashed out here, over pipes filled with Virginia tobacco.

Fierce Anglo–Dutch Competition

At the beginning of his reign, Charles II knew he had to build loyalty and strengthen an economy weakened by civil war. The king, with expensive tastes and an impoverished treasury, found that he could reward loyal family members and supporters, at no cost to the crown, by granting them control over pieces of England's North American domain. With this prospect in hand, he and his ministers sought to bolster foreign trade, strengthen the royal navy, and outstrip England's commercial rivals, focusing first on the Dutch.

As London stepped up its search for new profits, English officials moved to strengthen control over existing colonies and establish (or seize) new ones wherever possible. The Navigation Acts cut sharply into the Dutch carrying trade and spurred a decade of renewed warfare between England and Holland. For the most part, these intermittent Anglo–Dutch Wars ended in stalemate. But at the final Peace of Westminster in 1674, the English emerged with two gains in Africa and America that quickly took on huge and lasting significance.

In west Africa, the English captured and held several key coastal outposts: an island at the mouth of the river Gambia (renamed James Fort for the Duke of York) and Cape Coast Castle on the Gold Coast (near Elmina, the African headquarters of the Dutch West India Company). This encroachment challenged Dutch dominance of commerce with Africa for gold and ivory. It also gave England the footholds it needed to force its way into the Atlantic slave trade. Charles II moved quickly to take advantage of the situation. He granted a monopoly to the Royal Adventurers into Africa (1663) and then the Royal Africa Company (1672) to exploit the grim but highly profitable slave traffic. Within several generations, this ruthless initiative reshaped England's American colonies at enormous human cost.

Across the Atlantic, the English had seized the Dutch colony of New Netherland and its poorly defended port of New Amsterdam. Charles II claimed that the land had belonged to England from the time his grandfather endorsed the Virginia Company in 1606. In 1664, the king used his royal prerogative to regain control of this domain. He issued a charter putting the entire region between the Delaware and Connecticut rivers under the personal control of his brother James, Duke of York. That same year, James sent a fleet to claim his prize. When Governor Peter Stuyvesant surrendered the Dutch colony without a fight, both the province and its capital on Manhattan Island each received the name *New York*. Fort Orange on the Hudson became Albany because England's traditional name was *Albion*.

James now controlled an enormous domain that included the Dutch and English settlements on Long Island. He wielded nearly absolute powers over his new dukedom. He never visited New York. But as proprietor, he chose the colony's governor. That official ruled with an appointed council and enforced "the Duke's Laws" without constraint by any assembly. English newcomers to the colony resented the absence of an elected legislature, and the governor finally authorized an elected body in 1683. But the new assemblymen promptly approved a Charter of Liberties, in which they endorsed government by consent of the governed, so the Duke of York disallowed the legislature.

Married women living in the New York colony lost ground in the transition to English rule. Dutch law codes had ensured their full legal status, whereas English common law assigned wives to an inferior status (known as *coverture* or *feme covert*). They could not own property or keep control over money they earned, and they lacked any independent standing before the law.

As the English asserted political control over New York, the Dutch presence remained evident everywhere. Many English married into Dutch families and worshipped in the Dutch Reformed Church. The village of Harlem built a proper road to lower Manhattan in 1669, but an effort to change the town's Dutch name to Lancaster failed. English-speaking New Yorkers borrowed such Dutch words as *waffle, cookie, coleslaw,* and *baas* (boss). Anyone who was bilingual, such as Albany merchant Robert Livingston, had a special advantage. Livingston, an immigrant from Scotland, had learned to speak Dutch in Holland in his youth. His marriage in Albany linked him to powerful Dutch families in the Hudson Valley, and much of his early wealth came from his ability to translate important commercial documents between English and Dutch.

The New Restoration Colonies

Charles II had spurred England's seizure of New Netherland by issuing a charter for control of the contested region to his brother, the Duke of York. To reward supporters, he continued to issue royal charters granting American land. By drawing on England's early claims in North America that dated back to the explorer John Cabot, the king hoped to expand trade and colonization at no cost to the crown. In 1670, for example, he granted a charter to the Hudson's Bay Company. The deal gave the company's proprietors a monopoly on trade, minerals, and land across northern Canada. Farther south, Charles used charters to redistribute control along major portions of the Atlantic coast. His actions prompted an unprecedented scramble for colonial property and profits. Within decades, the English launched important settlement clusters in two regions: the Delaware River valley and the Carolina coast. Each offered lucrative charters to a small network of friends.

Most of these well-placed people belonged to the Councils for Trade and Plantations in London. Created in 1660, these advisory groups linked England's powerful merchants with crown officials. When Charles II issued a charter for Carolina in 1663, five of its eight initial proprietors served on those councils. In 1665, two of these same eight men became the proprietors of New Jersey. In addition, three of the eight played an active role in the Royal African Company, four became founders of the Hudson's Bay Company, and five became initial proprietors of the Bahamas. But Charles reached beyond this small group as well. In 1679 he made New Hampshire a proprietorship (an ill-fated experiment that lasted to 1708). In 1681 he paid off a debt to Quaker aristocrat William Penn by granting him a charter for Pennsylvania. (The generous arrangement included the "Lower Counties" that became Delaware in 1704.)

Charles II had spurred England's seizure of New Netherland by issuing a charter for control of the contested region to his brother, the Duke of York.

Penn's "holy experiment" to create a Quaker refuge benefited from earlier colonization south of New York. Dutch and Swedish settlers had inhabited the lower Delaware Valley for more than a generation. In 1665 the Duke of York carved off a portion of his vast proprietorship, granting the area between the Delaware and the Hudson to two friends: Lord John Berkeley and Sir George Carteret. They named the area New Jersey because Carteret had been born on the Isle of Jersey in the English Channel and had harbored Charles II when he took refuge there in 1649. Berkeley and Carteret promptly announced liberal "Concessions"—a representative assembly and freedom of worship—to attract rent-paying newcomers from England and the existing colonies. But their plans for profit made little headway.

In 1674 the proprietors divided these fertile lands into two separate provinces. East Jersey—where Newark was established in 1666—attracted Puritan families from New England,

Dutch farmers from New York, and failed planters from Barbados. West Jersey was sold to members of the Society of Friends (including William Penn) who inaugurated a Quaker experiment along the Delaware River. Filled with egalitarian beliefs, the Quakers created a unicameral (single body) legislature, used secret ballots, and gave more power to juries than to judges. Their idealistic effort foundered within decades, and by 1702 all New Jersey came under crown control as a royal colony.

But by then, the Quakers had established a foothold in the neighboring colony of Pennsylvania. Its capital, the market town of Philadelphia, laid out by proprietor William Penn in 1682, already had more than 2000 inhabitants. An earnest Quaker, Penn professed pacifism. He made it a point to deal fairly with the Lenni-Lenape (Delaware) Indians. After purchasing their land, he resold it on generous terms to English, Dutch, and Welsh Quakers who agreed to pay him an annual premium, called a quitrent. He also emphasized religious toleration. A growing stream of German Protestants and others facing persecution in Europe began to flow into Pennsylvania after 1700.

Penn drew inspiration from James Harrington, the English political philosopher. Harrington's book *Oceana* (1656) argued that the best way to create an enduring republic was for one person to draft and implement its constitution. After endless tinkering, Penn devised a progressive "Frame of Government" that allowed for trial by jury, limited terms of office, and no use of capital punishment except in cases of treason and murder. But he remained ambivalent about legislative democracy. Settlers resented his scheme for a lower house that could approve acts drafted by the governor but could not initiate laws. In a new Charter of Privileges in 1701, Penn agreed to the creation of a unicameral legislature (that is, having only one chamber, or house) with full lawmaking powers. Disillusioned, Penn then departed for England, writing, "The Lord forgive them their great ingratitude." Penn's expansive proprietorship belonged to his descendants until colonial rule ended in 1776.

Anthony Ashley-Cooper, leader of the Carolina proprietors, also drew inspiration from Harrington, but for a very different undertaking. *Oceana* had stressed that distribution of land determined the nature of any commonwealth, and Ashley-Cooper (later the first earl of Shaftesbury) was eager to establish a stable aristocratic system. With his young secretary, John Locke (later an influential political philosopher), he drew up a set of "Fundamental Constitutions" in 1669. They proposed a stratified society in which hereditary nobles controlled much of the land and wealthy manor lords employed a lowly servant class of "leetmen." Their unrealistic document tried to revive the elaborate feudal hierarchy of medieval times.

The new government framework also endorsed racial slavery, declaring that "Every Freeman of Carolina shall have absolute Power and Authority over his Negro Slaves." This endorsement was not surprising, given the proprietors' involvement with England's new slave-trading monopoly in Africa and their initial recruitment of settlers in 1670 from the sugar island of Barbados. When Carolina colonists founded Charlestown (later Charleston) between the Ashley and Cooper rivers in 1680, the proprietors had already modified aspects of their complicated scheme, setting aside feudalism to encourage greater immigration. Nevertheless, their endorsement of slavery shaped the region's society for hundreds of years.

Bloodshed in the English Colonies: 1670–1690

The appearance of isolated English settlements along the Atlantic coast did little in most places, to alter the traditional rhythms of life. Year after year, the daily challenges of subsistence dominated American life for Indians and colonists alike. The demanding seasonal tasks of clearing fields, planting seeds, and harvesting crops remained interwoven with the incessant chores of providing clothing, securing shelter, and sustaining community.

Over time, however, changing circumstances in America and Europe introduced new pressures up and down the Atlantic seaboard. On occasion after 1670, familiar routines gave way

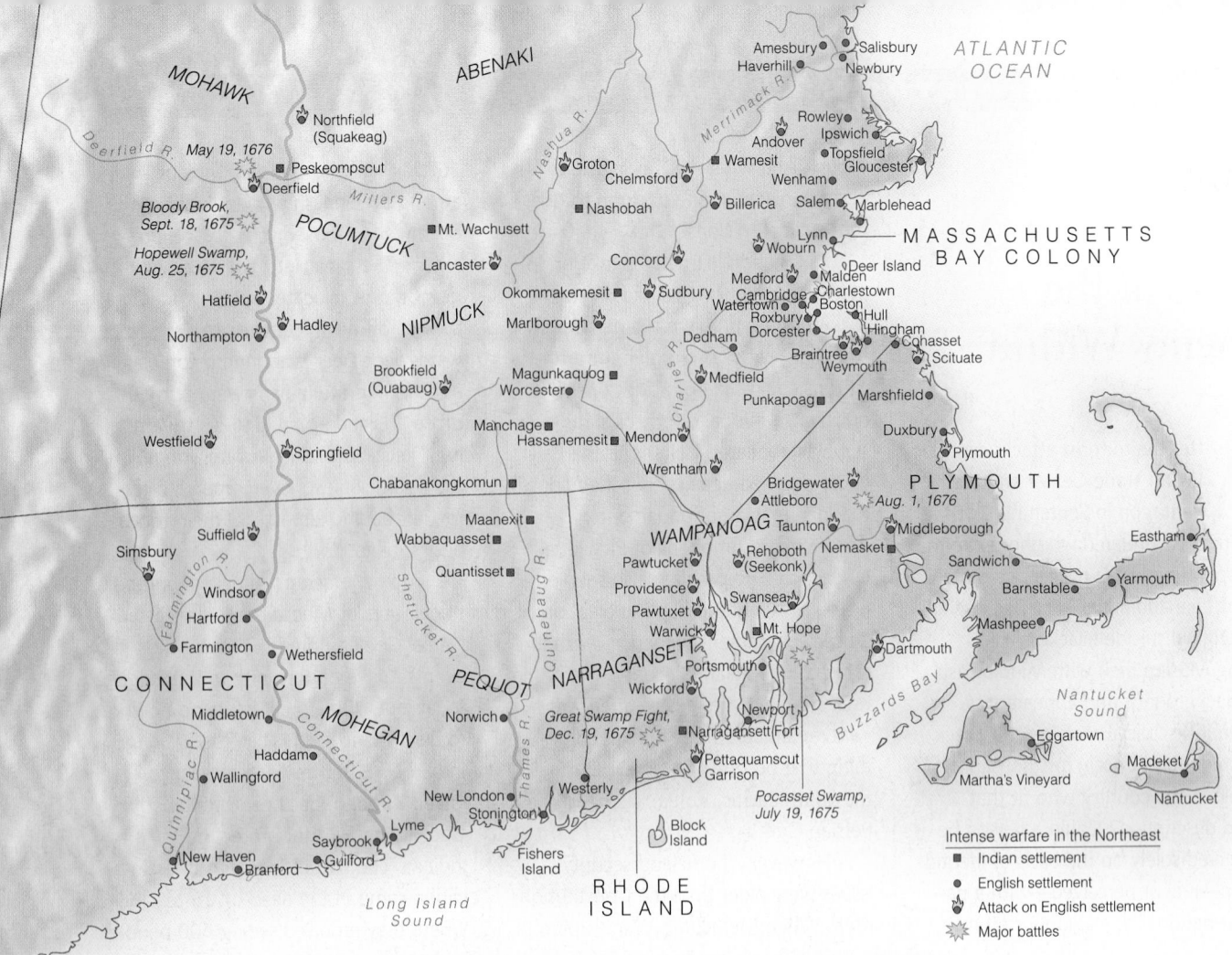

■ MAP 3.3 **METACOM'S WAR IN NEW ENGLAND, 1675–1676** In 14 months of war, New England Indians destroyed more than two dozen colonial towns and suffered their own heavy losses. The brutal conflict ended after the death of Metacom (the Wampanoag leader, also known as King Philip), near Mt. Hope, on August 12, 1676.

to episodes of bloodshed that threatened to tear whole colonies apart. Elsewhere in North America, Pueblo rebels were resisting the Spanish in New Mexico, and Iroquois warriors were challenging the French in Illinois country. The English, with their larger numbers, posed an even greater cultural and economic problem for Indian inhabitants.

In 1675, the Wampanoags and their allies rose up across southern New England in Metacom's War (or King Philip's War). The next year, frontier tensions in Virginia sparked the upheaval known as Bacon's Rebellion. A decade later, events in England prompted further tremors. In London, mounting opposition forced the unpopular James II to surrender the English throne to William of Orange, and Parliament emerged from the "Glorious Revolution" with enhanced powers. In America, the end of rule by the Stuart dynasty was punctuated by controversy and violence in one colony after another. Colonial isolation had already diminished, and European events intruded more forcefully in the decades ahead.

Metacom's War in New England

By 1675 the Native Americans of southern New England, like the Pueblos in New Mexico, had endured several generations of colonization. Yet they disagreed over how much English culture they should adopt. Many Indians used English words for trading, English pots for cooking, and English weapons for hunting. Some had converted to Christianity, living in protected "praying towns." Several young men had enrolled in Harvard's

Homeland Security and Deep Fears of the Enemy Within

After the terrorist attacks on the World Trade Center and the Pentagon in September 2001, Americans wondered whether extremists operating inside the United States might take additional lives. Because all the original suicide hijackers were young Muslim men with Middle Eastern backgrounds and appearances, would it be "racial profiling" to check the credentials closely for thousands of people in the country who fit that broad description? Could a person be suspected solely on the basis of identification—real or perceived—with a particular nationality, religion, or ethnic group? And what kinds of patriotic acts, if any, must one perform to overturn such suspicions?

In a nation learning to take pride in its immigrant origins and diverse make-up, the problem seemed deeply troubling. Feelings ran high, but most citizens could see both sides of the question. National safety, perhaps even survival, appeared to hang in the balance, weighed against cherished constitutional rights and fundamental American presumptions of individual innocence. The problem also seemed novel, as symbolized by the creation of a new government bureaucracy: the Office of Homeland Security. The name itself sounded strange to Americans who remembered war only as something that occurred far away: Europe, the South Pacific, Korea, Vietnam, the Persian Gulf.

However, "homeland security" issues were older than the Constitution itself. When Metacom's War erupted in 1675, it was the Christian Indians living among the English who looked like the enemy and aroused sharp suspicion among Massachusetts colonists. Anxious officials relocated whole "praying towns" of Indian converts to windswept Deer Island in Boston Harbor. "When the Indians were hurried off to an iland at half an hours warning," recalled their advocate, John Eliot, the "pore soules," overcome with terror, left behind almost all "their goods, books, bibles."

After Metacom's attackers burned the villages of Medford and Lancaster, Daniel Gookin noted that the grim events "gave opportunity to the vulgar to cry out, 'Oh, come, let us go down to Deer Island, and kill all the praying Indians.'" Bitter townsfolk never followed through, but they threatened Gookin and Eliot for protecting the Indians. The two men visited the relocation camp in the dead of winter, where they reported seeing 500 people

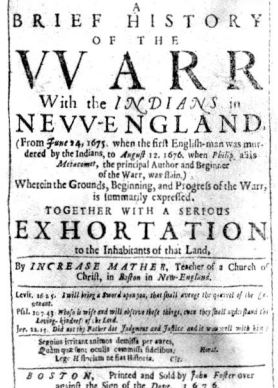

Indian College, where they learned to write English, Latin, and Greek with an eye toward entering the ministry.

Massasoit, the Wampanoag sachem (leader) who had assisted the Pilgrims at Plymouth, made sure that his two sons, Wamsutta and Metacom, learned English ways. The two men raised pigs and fired guns, and the colonists called them Alexander and Philip, after the kings of ancient Macedon. But when Wamsutta died in the 1660s, shortly after succeeding his father, Metacom (now called King Philip) suspected foul play by the English.

Metacom's grievances mounted over the next decade. Colonial traders made the Indians drunk and then cheated them. English livestock trampled Wampanoag corn, and if Indians shot the cattle, colonial courts imposed punishments. Worst of all, colonists now outnumbered the remaining 20,000 Indians in southern New England by more than two to one. When Rhode Island delegates visited Metacom's stronghold near Narragansett Bay, he told them bitterly that "the English should do for us as we did when we were too strong for the English." His own father, Massasoit, had "let them have a hundred times more land" than he now "had for his own people."

The mysterious death of a Christian Indian named John Sassamon sparked open warfare. Sassamon had learned to write English during a brief stint at Harvard. He then crossed back into the Wampanoag world to serve as a secretary for Metacom, who could write his English name only as a labored P, for Philip. Caught between two cultures, Sassamon alerted the English to Metacom's war plans in January 1675. Within days, his corpse was found in a pond near Plymouth. The English accused three Wampanoags of Sassamon's murder, convicted them, and hanged them in early June.

Outraged Indians protested that Sassamon's betrayal of his people and his subsequent death were their own affairs. When a white man shot and wounded a Native American,

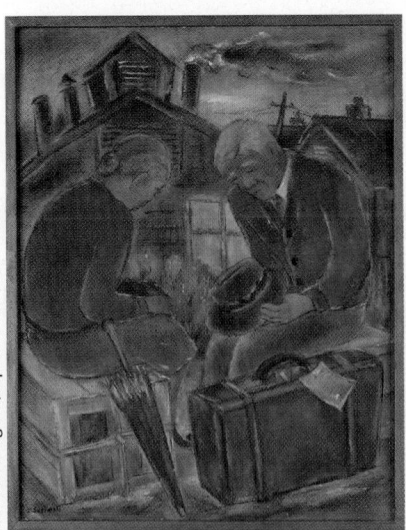

Henry Sugimoto, *Praying for Safety*, c.1942. Gift of Madeleine Sugimoto and Naomi Tagawa, Japanese American National Museum(92.97.44)

Henry Sugimoto was among the artists who documented life in Japanese-American internment camps during World War II.

in need of food and shelter: "The Island was bleak and cold, their wigwams poor and mean, their clothes few and thin." Half the detainees died before spring. With little likelihood that the survivors could "plant or reap any corn" on the barren island, authorities finally freed them. Despite the painful internment, some of the Christian Indians joined the colonial forces in the final months of the war.

For more than two centuries, Native Americans, no matter what their political or religious beliefs, remained subject to recurrent suspicion while Indian Wars raged across the West. In the twentieth century, racial suspicions in wartime shifted to other groups, especially after the Japanese attack on Pearl Harbor during World War II. Fearful of nonwhites in the Pacific War Zone, the U.S. Army removed Aleutian Islanders from their homes in Alaska. And President Franklin Roosevelt signed an executive order that sanctioned the forced relocation of more than 100,000 Americans of Japanese descent living on the West Coast.

Hastily, the U.S. government transported the Japanese Americans to ten barren internment camps in eight western states, trampling the rights of its citizens. Like the Christian Indians in colonial Massachusetts, these victims of wartime hysteria had little time to pack their belongings. Miné Okubo, an art student at Berkeley, remembered being shipped by train to the Central Utah Detainment Center near Topaz Mountain. Finding it "impossible to see anything through the constant dust," Okubo and others sarcastically took to calling the Topaz camp "the jewel of the desert." Reduced to a number by her own government, Okubo made pictures and kept notes of her experience, which she later published as a book: *Citizen 13660*. Some were allowed out to become soldiers, and many lost their lives fighting in Europe. As World War II neared its end, Roosevelt rescinded his order, and the camps emptied. But it took the government a generation to admit that, in this instance, ideas of homeland security had gone badly awry. ■

the long-expected war was under way in earnest. Irate braves raided the town of Swansea, killing nine residents. In the summer and fall, Metacom's warriors ravaged town after town along the Connecticut River valley and closer to the coast. Metacom used the victories to recruit additional Indian allies. The colonists, unprepared after 40 years of peace and unchallenged dominance, were caught off guard. Distrusting even the Christian Indians, Massachusetts officials relocated whole praying towns of Indian converts to windswept islands in Boston Harbor.

By December, the Connecticut and Rhode Island colonies, terrified of being wiped out, united with Plymouth and Massachusetts Bay to create a force of more than a thousand men. An Indian captive led them to a stronghold of the still-neutral Narragansetts in a remote swamp a dozen miles west of Newport, Rhode Island. The colonists surprised and overwhelmed the fortified village, setting it ablaze during the fierce fighting. Indian survivors fled, leaving behind more than 600 dead. Many of the men, women, and children were "terribly Barbikew'd," minister Cotton Mather later recorded.

This "Great Swamp Fight," reminiscent of an earlier battle in the Pequot War, infuriated the Narragansetts, who joined Metacom's growing alliance. During the late winter of 1676, this loose confederacy continued to wreak havoc on New England villages. But as spring arrived, the coalition weakened and the tide turned. Sickness broke out among the fighters, who lacked food and gunpowder. The powerful Mohawks of the Iroquois Confederacy opposed Metacom from the west. In Boston, Christian Indians joined the colonial forces, despite their painful internment. As Metacom's situation worsened, defections and betrayals increased. In August, a former ally shot the resistance leader and delivered the sachem's head to the English.

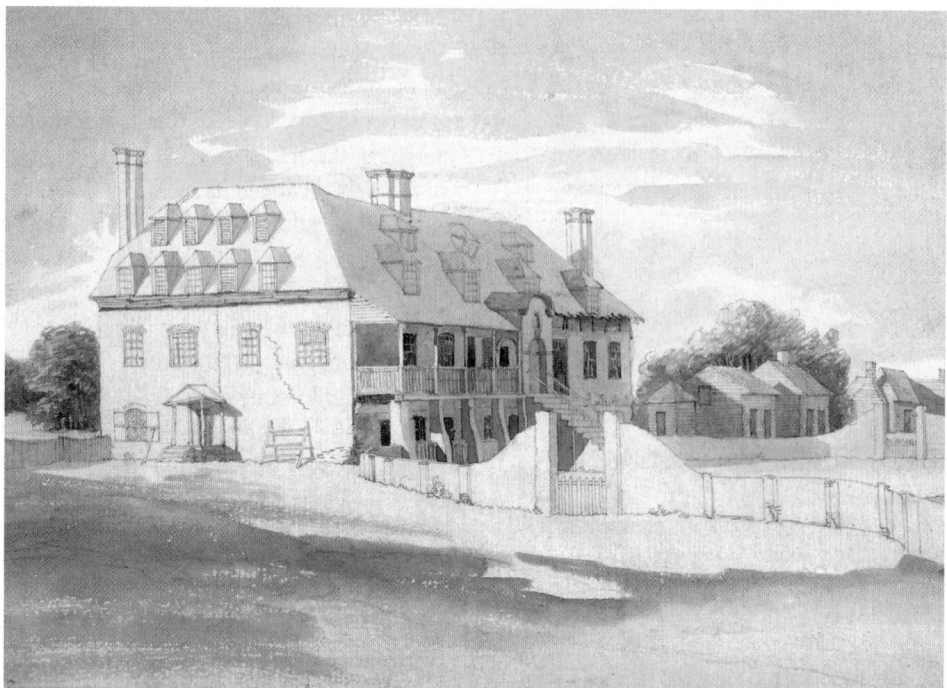

Benjamin Henry Latrobe, *View of Greenspring House*, 1796. The Maryland Historical Society, Baltimore, Maryland (II-33)

■ Green Spring, the largest mansion in Virginia at the time of Bacon's Rebellion, symbolized the autocratic rule of Governor William Berkeley and his "Green Spring Faction." The estate was seized by Bacon's forces in 1676 and later restored by Berkeley's widow.

As the horrific struggle ground to a close, the colonists captured Metacom's wife and child, selling them into slavery in the West Indies along with hundreds of other prisoners of war. New England's remaining Indians became second-class inhabitants, confined to enclaves in the areas they had once dominated. The colonists soon rebuilt and extended their domain. However, the trauma of the war lived on in the minds of the survivors and the sermons of their ministers. For years afterward, Metacom's severed head was displayed on a pole at Plymouth.

Bacon's Rebellion in Virginia

While smoke still billowed over New England, new flames broke out in Virginia. Social unrest had been growing under the stern governorship of Sir William Berkeley. England's wars with the Dutch cut into the tobacco trade and drew enemy ships into Chesapeake Bay. Unfree tobacco workers—more than 6000 indentured Europeans and nearly 2000 enslaved Africans—chafed against their harsh treatment. On the frontier, colonists resented the dependent Indians (Occaneechis, Pamunkeys, and others) who traded furs in exchange for protection from other tribes. Settlers also feared the well-armed Susquehannocks living near the Potomac River. "Consider us," Berkeley wrote to the king in 1667, "as a people press'd at our backes wth Indians, in our Bowills with our Servants . . . and invaded from without by the Dutch."

By 1676 tensions in Virginia reached the breaking point. Officials had increased taxes to pay for fortifications, servant plots and mutinies abounded, and corruption ran rampant among Berkeley's close associates. The aging governor ruled from Green Spring, his huge estate near the capital, Jamestown. Fearing the hostile views of free men who did not own property, Berkeley had revoked their right to vote. He had not dared to call an election in 14 years. He also dreaded outspoken preachers, free schools, and printing presses. "How miserable that man is," he wrote, "that Governes a People where six parts of seaven at least are Poore Endebted Discontented and Armed."

Even wealthy newcomers such as Nathaniel Bacon had trouble gaining access to Berkeley's tight inner circle. When Bacon arrived from England in 1674 at age 27, he received a council seat because of his connections and money. But rivals denied the ambitious gentleman a license to engage in the profitable fur trade. Impatient, Bacon soon condemned Berkeley's ruling Green

Spring faction as sponges who "have sukt up the Publique Treasure." When frontier tensions erupted into racial violence, Bacon threw himself into the conflict, challenging Berkeley's leadership and launching aggressive campaigns. His frontier followers, eager for Indian land, killed friendly Occaneechis as well as hostile Susquehannocks.

The governor, aware of the damage that Metacom's War had inflicted on New England, refused to sanction these raids. He feared "a Generall Combination of all the Indians against us." But Bacon's army continued to grow as backcountry leaders joined landless poor and runaway workers—both black and white—to support his anti-Indian cause. When the desperate governor called for a rare election to assert his strength, Bacon's supporters dominated the new House of Burgesses. Berkeley retreated across Chesapeake Bay and hid on Virginia's eastern shore.

Throughout the summer of 1676, rumors swirled that Bacon might join with malcontents in Maryland and in the newly settled Albemarle region of northeastern North Carolina to carve out an independent enclave and seek aid from the Dutch or the French. The new assembly quickly restored the vote to propertyless men and forbade excessive fees. It limited sheriffs to one year in office and passed other measures to halt corruption and expand participation in government. As an incentive for enlistment in the frontier war, the assembly granted Bacon's recruits the right to sell into slavery any Indians they captured.

For their part, slaves and indentured servants took advantage of the breakdown in public controls to leave their masters and join Bacon. Networks of "news wives" (women who used facts and rumors effectively to fan worker discontent) spread stories of oppressive conditions. In June rebel soldiers talked openly of sharing estates among themselves, and in August they took over Green Spring Plantation, where Berkeley kept 60 horses and 400 head of cattle. A month later, Bacon's army burned Jamestown to the ground.

But by October Bacon was dead, struck down by dysentery, and reinforcements for Berkeley were on the way from England. With armed vessels patrolling the rivers, Berkeley worked up enough nerve to return from the eastern shore. Soon propertied men who had joined with Bacon were changing sides again and receiving amnesty from the governor.

The revolt had been crushed, but the impact of the tumult proved huge. On the frontier, Bacon's violent campaign against the Indians had killed or enslaved hundreds and fostered bitter hatreds. In the Tidewater, the uprising had raised a frightening prospect for wealthy tobacco planters: a unified and defiant underclass of white and black workers. From then on, Virginia's gentry applied themselves to dividing the races and creating a labor force made up of African slaves. In London, the recently formed Royal Africa Company stood ready to further such a design.

The "Glorious Revolution" in England

No sooner had peace returned to New England and Virginia than Stuart policies brought a new round of turmoil on both sides of the Atlantic. In England, debate revived over who would succeed Charles II on the throne. The irreligious Charles, an Anglican in name only, had no legitimate children. Therefore, his brother James, a convert to Catholicism, was first in line to inherit the crown.

In 1678, rumors spread regarding a "Popish Plot" by Catholics to kill the king so that James could take power. The House of Commons, fearful of rule by a Catholic king, urged that James be excluded from the line of succession. Instead of James, House members argued, why not consider James's Protestant daughters by his first marriage: either Mary (recently wedded to her Dutch cousin, William of Orange) or Anne?

Angered by such interference, Charles II dissolved Parliament in 1681 and ruled on his own for the last four years of his life. When he died, the traditional rule of succession prevailed: James II took over the throne in 1685. In France that same year, Louis XIV revoked the Edict of Nantes, which had protected French Protestants. Fear spread among England's Protestant majority that their country's new Catholic ruler, James II, might also sanction persecution of non-Catholics.

These concerns mounted when James disbanded Parliament, raised a standing army, and placed a Catholic in command of the navy. Then in 1688, James's queen gave birth to a male

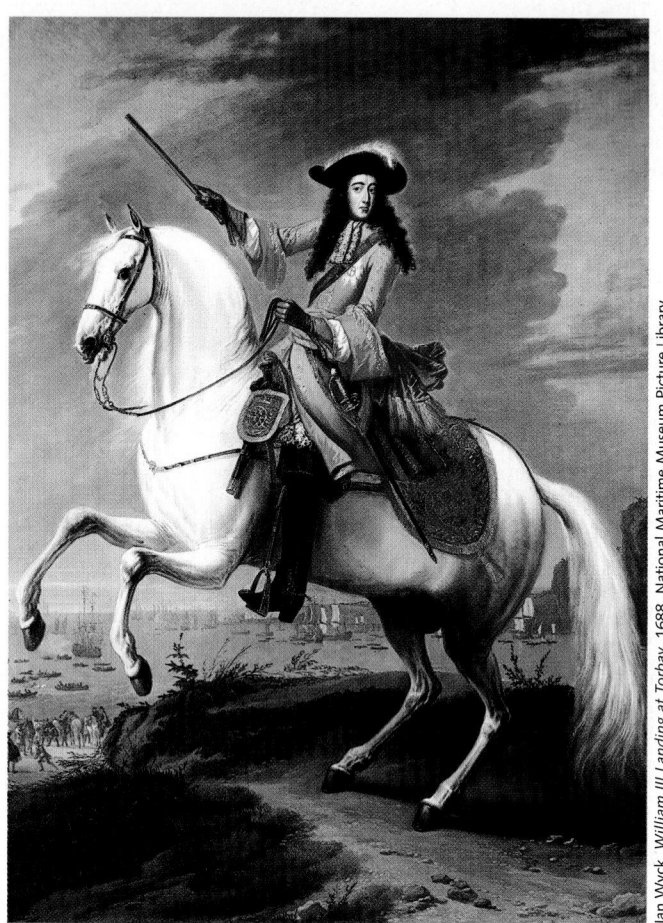

Jan Wyck, *William III Landing at Torbay*, 1688. National Maritime Museum Picture Library

■ Protestants in England and America opposed to King James II welcomed news that William of Orange had arrived from Holland with his army in 1688 to take over the English throne.

heir. Protestant anxieties about a pending Catholic dynasty erupted into open resistance.

United by their fear of Catholicism, rival factions among England's political elite (known for the first time as "Whigs" and "Tories") papered over their differences temporarily. They invited the Protestant William of Orange, James's Dutch son-in-law, to lead an army from Holland and take the English crown. In November 1688, he crossed the English Channel with 15,000 men. Confronting a successful invasion of England (it has never happened since), James abdicated the throne, threw the great seal into the Thames, and escaped into exile. William and Mary were proclaimed joint sovereigns in 1689, accepting a Bill of Rights that limited royal power.

Its position now enhanced, Parliament moved to grant toleration to Protestant dissenters, establish limited freedom of the press, and ensure regular parliamentary sessions. It also imposed limits on any permanent, paid military forces, known as standing armies, because they could accrue their own power and jeopardize civil authority. The English had thus preserved Protestantism and curtailed royal absolutism, all without bloodshed. Parliament hailed King William III as "our great Deliverer from Popery and Slavery." The propertied classes, who benefited most from the peaceful transition, hailed it as "The Glorious Revolution."

The "Glorious Revolution" in America

The succession of James II in 1685 did not bode well for England's American colonies. The new king not only professed the Catholic faith, he also cherished absolute monarchy and distrusted elected assemblies. In colonial affairs, James favored revenue-generating reforms and direct obedience to the crown. He detested the powerful leaders in Massachusetts, for, as Congregationalists, they believed in a decentralized Protestant church. James also resented the fact that they disobeyed the Navigation Acts and asserted their right to self-rule, even after the crown revoked their charter in 1684. Moreover, he rejected the notion that colonists possessed the precious right claimed by the English at home: not to be taxed without giving their consent. The king envisioned an extensive reorganization of the American colonies.

When James assumed the throne, his own colony of New York automatically became a royal province. Convinced of his divine right to set policy, the king nullified the charters of certain colonies in order to bring them under his control. As the cornerstone of his reorganization plan, James linked the New England colonies (plus New York and New Jersey in 1688) into one huge *Dominion of New England*. This consolidation, under an appointed governor general, would make it easier for England to suppress dissent, enforce shipping regulations, and defend the Dominion's frontiers—at least in theory.

In practice, the effort to forge a Dominion of New England proved a disaster. The move met such stiff resistance in America that a similar design for England's southern colonies never materialized. Control of the Dominion went to a military officer, Sir Edmond Andros. The heavy-handed Andros attempted to rule from Boston through a council he appointed, made up of loyal associates, without aid or interference from any elected legislature. He asserted the crown's right to question existing land patents, and he requisitioned a Congregational church for Anglican services. Worse, he offended local leaders by strictly enforcing the Navigation Acts to collect revenue. When participants in democratic town meetings raised objections, he jailed the leaders.

Colonists seethed with resentment toward this revival of Stuart absolutism, which claimed total obedience to the king and his officers as a divine right for the Stuart monarchy. Rumors of French invasions and Catholic plots swirled among staunch Protestants. In April 1689, welcome news that the Protestant William of Orange had invaded England inspired a revolt in Boston. Mobs showed public support for overthrowing the Stuart regime, and local leaders locked Governor Andros in jail.

The success of William and the demise of the Dominion of New England did not end royal efforts to tighten imperial control over New England. The new Massachusetts charter of 1691 consolidated neighboring Plymouth and Maine into the Massachusetts Bay colony. Moreover, it proclaimed that future governors would be appointed by the monarchy, as in other colonies. The men of Massachusetts, who had elected their own governor since the days of John Winthrop, would no longer have that right.

Emboldened by Boston's actions in 1689, New Yorkers ousted their own Dominion officials and set up a temporary government headed by militia captain Jacob Leisler. In Leisler's Rebellion, long-standing ethnic and economic rivalries between English and non-English New Yorkers merged with wider issues of empire. A German Calvinist, Leisler played on Protestant fears of "Popish Doggs & Divells" and on Dutch residents' resentment of English domination to attack the Dominion government.

Leisler's movement also drew on lower-class hostility toward the town's growing elite. His supporters resented their treatment at the hands of the rich. They freed imprisoned debtors and attacked the houses of leading merchants. After a new governor arrived to take charge in 1691, the elite fought back. They lowered artisan wages and executed Leisler as a rebel, although they could find no carpenter willing to provide a ladder for the gallows.

Similar tremors shook the Chesapeake region. In Maryland, where the Catholic proprietor ruled over a large and restive Protestant population, the governing Calvert family waited too long to proclaim its loyalty to King William. Fearing a "Popish" plot, assemblyman John Coode and a force of 250 armed Protestants marched on St. Mary's City and seized the government by force. The "happy Change in England" had replaced divine right rule with a more balanced constitutional monarchy, and Maryland settlers were determined to show their support.

Consequences of War and Growth: 1690–1715

The success of the Glorious Revolution hardly brought peace to England or its empire. On the contrary, warfare marked the reign of William and Mary and also that of Mary's sister, Queen Anne, who ruled from 1702 until her death in 1714. William immediately became involved in bloody campaigns to subdue highland clans in Scotland and overpower Catholic forces in Ireland. Moreover, English involvement against France in two protracted wars on the European continent had implications for colonists and Indians living in eastern North America. The War of the League of Augsburg in Europe became known to English colonists in America as King William's War (1689–1697), and the protracted War of Spanish Succession was experienced in America as Queen Anne's War (1702–1713).

Nowhere was the impact of these imperial wars more evident than in the rapidly growing colonies of the Northeast. Indeed, the earlier bloodshed of Metacom's (King Philip's) War, starting in 1675, had already aroused consternation and soul-searching in Bible-reading New England, and the violent decades that followed were viewed by many as a harsh test or a deserved punishment from the Almighty. They believed that the initial Puritan errand into the wilderness had been closely watched by God. Could it be, ministers now asked from the pulpit, that the Lord had some special controversy with the current generation? As communities grew more prosperous and became caught up in the pursuit of worldly success, were church members forgetting their religious roots and leading less pious lives? Invoking the Old Testament prophet Jeremiah, clerics interpreted personal and collective troubles as God's punishment for the region's spiritual decline.

But such a sweeping explanation of misfortune only raised deeper questions. New Englanders could see clearly that the consequences of rapid change were not spread equally among all towns, congregations, and families. As in most war eras—and moments of economic and demographic growth—some people and localities suffered more than others. Certain individuals and groups seemed to benefit while others fell behind. Some anxious believers saw the hand of Satan in the day-to-day struggles of village life. Others argued that the worldly success and wartime profits of an expanding elite had undermined the community ideals of earlier generations. While flames engulfed isolated Massachusetts communities such as Deerfield and portions of the Maine frontier, fiery passions were also being aroused in older settlements, such as Salem and Boston.

Salem's Wartime Witch Hunt

One of the most memorable disruptions, the Salem witch hunt, occurred in Essex County, Massachusetts, a two-day ride on horseback from the embattled Maine frontier. In 1692 an outburst of witchcraft accusations engulfed Salem Village (now Danvers), a farm community formed as a separate parish in 1672 from the prosperous port of Salem Town, six miles east. The strange episode remains one of the most troubling in American history.

Numerous premodern cultures in Asia, Africa, Europe, and America believed in varieties of witchcraft. Among Christians, the assumption that there are witches who possess supernatural power to inflict harm stretched back for centuries. In the 1600s, witchcraft trials abounded in Europe, and in New England zealous believers had prosecuted scores of supposed witches. They had even executed several dozen people in isolated cases. Three-fourths of those accused (and even more of those executed) were women. Most were beyond childbearing age, often poor or widowed, with limited power to protect themselves in the community. But the hysteria in Salem went far beyond other colonial incidents, with more than 200 people accused and 20 put to death.

Early in 1692, more than half a dozen young women in Salem Village, ranging in age from 9 to 20, began to suffer violent convulsive fits. With reduced appetites and temporary loss of hearing, sight, and memory, they also experienced choking sensations that curtailed their speech. Vivid hallucinations followed. "These calamities first began in my family," wrote Reverend Samuel Parris. A Harvard dropout, Parris had failed as a merchant in Barbados and had later agreed to lead the parish. It was "several weeks before such hellish operations as witchcraft were suspected." The first to appear tormented were Parris's daughter and niece, ages 9 and 11. The children had spent time with Tituba and John, a slave couple of uncertain Indian or African origin whom Parris had brought from Barbados. Tituba often spoke of the supernatural, and soon several of the afflicted girls accused her and two elderly Salem women of witchcraft.

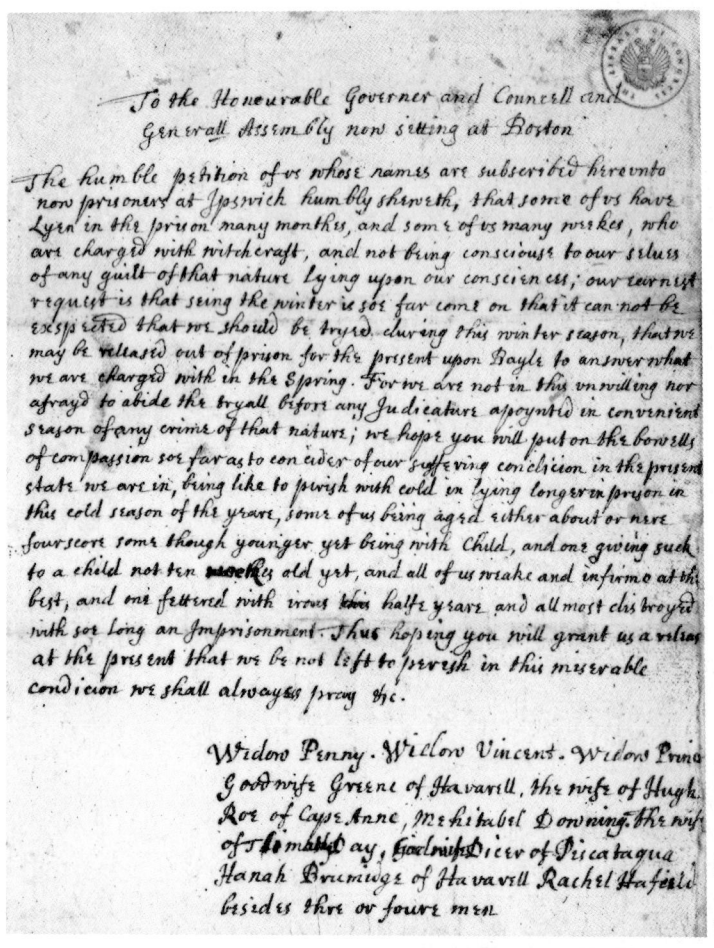

■ A petition from accused women in Salem, addressed to the Governor and General Assembly in Boston.

Library of Congress

By April the girls had accused seven more people. Then some of the seven named others in their elaborate confessions, and the hysteria snowballed. In a world where people considered satanic influence very real, frightened authorities seriously weighed the girls' stories of people appearing to them as devilish specters and apparitions. Overriding tradition, jurists allowed such "spectral evidence" in court. And because all believed that the devil could not inhabit a pious person, protests of innocence from those accused only seemed to confirm the enemy's diabolical ways. The court ordered public hangings of the condemned on Gallows Hill. The hangings continued through September. One poor and elderly farmer, Giles Cory, was pressed to death under heavy stones. Only when accusations reached too high in the social hierarchy and when several accusers recanted their stories did the new governor finally intervene. He emptied the jails, forbade further imprisonments, and pardoned the surviving accused until the tremor could subside.

Why this terrible outburst? Some writers wonder whether the girls' symptoms suggest food poisoning (perhaps from a fungus on rye used in baking bread) or an epidemic of mosquitoborne encephalitis (an inflammation of the brain). Others note political factions within the village. Strained relations between farm families and the more prosperous urban residents of nearby Salem Town may have influenced the craze. Still others emphasize the zeal and gullibility of those first assigned to investigate. Some speculate that the absence of central authority, until Governor Phips arrived in the colony in May, allowed a troubled situation to spin out of control. Finally, commentators stress a perverse psychological dynamic that arises in any witch hunt, ancient or modern. In such cases, accused suspects often can save their own lives by supplying damaging and vivid confessions implicating others rather than by offering heartfelt denials of guilt. One or more of these factors surely came into play.

Yet devastation on the Maine frontier also contributed to what happened in Salem Village. The little Massachusetts town had numerous links to the war zone. George Burroughs, Parris's much-disliked predecessor as minister, had come from Maine. He had returned there when the contentious parish refused to pay him. Traumatized survivors from King William's War—the current conflict with the Abenaki and French—had trickled into the community. Significantly, more than half the young women who had accused others of witchcraft had lost one or both parents in the brutal frontier wars. On February 5, just weeks before the first accusations, attackers had burned the Maine village of York 80 miles north of Salem. The raiders destroyed livestock, killed 48 people, and took 73 captives. Word of the renewed violence no doubt triggered shocking memories among Salem's war refugees, especially the orphans who worked as servants in local households.

Fears deepened in April when one of the accused confessed that the Devil had tempted her while she had been living in Maine. Then the specter of Reverend Burroughs "appeared" to an accuser. Charged with promoting witchcraft and encouraging the hostile Indians (whom the colonists saw as Satan's helpers), Burroughs was arrested in Maine and hanged on Gallows Hill. In Boston, a 17-year-old servant named Mercy Short told of disturbing dreams of the Devil. Short had been captured and orphaned by Indians. She told minister Cotton Mather that in her dreams Satan and his minions had made "hideous assaults" upon her. And, she said, they were "of a tawney, or an Indian colour." Much of what Mather and others recorded as the work of Satan may have spun from posttraumatic stress in a frayed community during wartime.

The Uneven Costs of War

Throughout the 1690s and beyond, England remained entangled in imperial conflict abroad and dynastic struggles at home. The Act of Settlement, passed by Parliament in 1701, ensured that King William, who died the next year, would be succeeded by his wife's sister Anne, who ruled until her death in 1714. King William's War and Queen Anne's War made conflict a constant element in both reigns, and colonists found themselves subject to these winds.

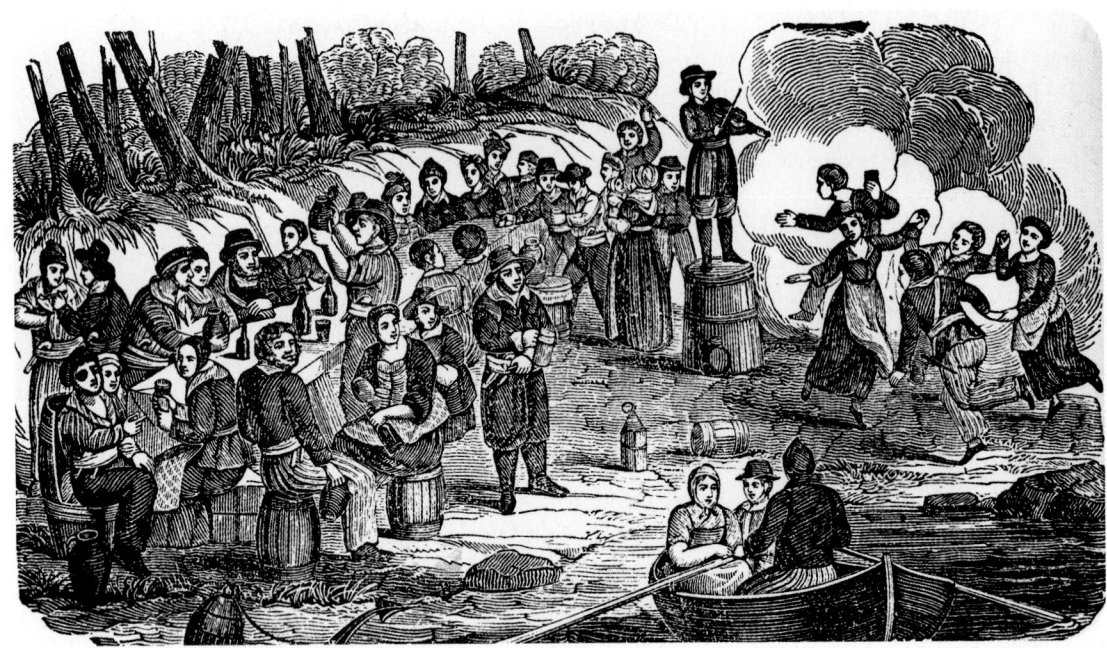

The New York Public Library

■ For protection, the pirate Blackbeard often brought his ship into the shallow waters behind the barrier islands that form North Carolina's Atlantic coast. There, his crew bartered stolen goods at Ocracoke Island and reveled on the beach with local inhabitants.

As in all wars, the burdens fell unevenly. For many colonial families, incessant warfare brought only death and dislocation. But for others, it offered new opportunities. Farmers with access to port towns shifted away from subsistence agriculture and grew crops for commercial sale. In doing so, they exposed themselves to greater financial risks, given transportation costs and market fluctuations. But they hoped to reap large profits.

Overseas trade and wartime smuggling offered investors even higher gains and larger risks. These activities, in turn, boosted demand for sailing vessels. Boston alone supported more than a dozen busy shipyards. They employed hundreds of shipwrights, caulkers, and other skilled workers who crafted hulls, ropes, masts, and sails. Military campaigns, such as the successful ones against the French at Port Royal in Acadia in 1690 and again in 1710, engaged hundreds of colonial soldiers and sailors. When an English fleet of 60 ships carrying 5000 men docked at Boston in 1711, local provisioners (those who sold food and other provisions) reaped the rewards.

The crews of privateers (boats licensed to harass enemy shipping in wartime) made money if they captured a foreign vessel as a prize, and many chose to become buccaneers, pirates who operated for their own gain while avoiding the arm of the law. Englishman Edward Teach (known as Blackbeard) won notoriety as a privateer-turned-pirate, haunting the Carolina coast until his death in 1718. In the brief heyday of buccaneers, numerous colonial sailors also shifted from privateering to pirating.

Everywhere, poorer families were most likely to sink under the burdens of war. Regressive taxes, requiring the same amount from a poor carpenter as from a rich merchant, obviously hurt impoverished people the most. So did high wartime prices for food and other basic necessities. Furthermore, many of the poor men recruited by the military became casualties of combat or disease, increasing the number of widows living in poverty. Such conditions bred discouragement, and struggling communities were struck by the growing distance between rich and poor as towns expanded and interests diverged.

The moral ties and community obligations—known as the social covenant—that Puritan elders had emphasized two generations earlier were loosening. In their place emerged a focus on secular priorities and a new, individualistic spirit. In Boston, troubled ministers decried the hunger and poverty that they saw deepening in their parishes alongside unprecedented displays of wealth. Between 1685 and 1715, the share of all personal wealth in the town controlled by the poorest 60 percent of the population fell from 17 percent to 13 percent. At the same time, the portion belonging to the richest 5 percent climbed from 26 percent to 40 percent. Printers began to publish irate pamphlets protesting these troubling conditions. Angry writers encouraging working people to take political action and charged once-respected elites with studying "how to oppress, cheat, and overreach their neighbours."

No Bostonian wielded more economic power than Andrew Belcher, who first made money supplying provisions to troops during Metacom's War. Each succeeding war brought Belcher larger contracts and greater profits. To the dismay of devout churchgoers and the working poor, he built a mansion on State Street and rode in an imported coach, attended by black slaves dressed in fancy livery. He owned 22 ships and invested in many more. He also repeatedly cornered the wartime grain market, spawning food shortages and raking in inflated profits as prices rose.

In 1710 Belcher asserted his right to ship 6000 bushels of grain on the open market rather than sell flour at home, where people desperately needed bread. Indignant residents rebelled against Belcher's outright defiance of traditional community values. In the dark of night, they disabled his ship by sawing through the rudder. A grand jury declined to indict the protesters. Did ambitious and aggressive merchants such as Belcher cause the city's calamities, or did the townsfolk bring on their own troubles? Using a refrain that recurred in later generations, one godly conservative pointed a finger at the poor and implied they must be sinful if they could not subsist. "There was Corn to be had," he argued; "if they had not impoverished themselves by Rum, they might buy Corn." Only "the Devil's people" lacked food.

Storm Clouds in the South

Peace returned to New England's frontier villages and port towns in 1711, as negotiations began for ending Queen Anne's War in America and the related War of Spanish Succession in Europe. British diplomats managed to gain favorable terms from France and Spain when they signed a treaty at Utrecht two years later. (The formal union of England and Scotland in 1707 under the name *Great Britain* had transformed the *English* empire into the *British* empire.) But London officials could not prevent fresh violence in North America, given the steady expansion of their British colonies. The Wampanoags, Narragansetts, and Abenaki Indians had attempted to roll back the advancement of northeastern settlers into Connecticut, Massachusetts, and Maine. Now Native Americans in the Southeast sought to counter the encroachments of newcomers along the Carolina coast.

By the 1670s, settlers were filtering into what would become the colony of North Carolina. Some were radicals fleeing the Restoration in England. Others, such as John Culpeper, had moved north from the Carolina settlement on the Ashley River, where they disapproved of the hierarchical plans drawn up by Shaftsburg and Locke giving the Carolina proprietors firm control over the new colony. Still others were runaway servants from Virginia and refugees escaping the aftermath of Bacon's uprising. In 1677 these newcomers, led by Culpeper, seized control in the Albemarle region. The proprietors suppressed "Culpeper's Rebellion," but in 1689 they agreed to name a separate governor for the portion of Carolina "That Lies north and east of Cape Feare." Another disturbance, "Cary's Rebellion" in 1710, led to official recognition of "North Carolina, independent of Carolina," the next year. (Surveyors marked off the dividing line with Virginia in 1728.)

In 1680 Native Americans still outnumbered newcomers in eastern North Carolina by two to one, but within 30 years that ratio had been reversed. The Naval Stores Act of 1705, passed by Parliament to promote colonial production of tar and pitch for shipbuilding, drew a stream of settlers to the pine forests of eastern North Carolina. By 1710, English communities existed on Albemarle Sound, at what is now Edenton, and on Pamlico Sound, at Bath (where Blackbeard and other pirates were frequent visitors). Further south, on the site of a

"They Are Really Better to Us Than We Are to Them": Tension on the North Carolina Coast

On one frontier after another from New Mexico to New England, tensions mounted between Indian inhabitants and European intruders. In North Carolina, English settlers William Powell and John Lawson watched as animosities grew from verbal exchanges to open conflict in the Tuscarora War (1711–1713). As colonizers, the two contributed to the escalation and left behind revealing documents about it.

John Lawson provided a published record. In 1700, the young explorer–naturalist made an extensive tour through North and South Carolina, living among the Indians and assessing the land for colonization. His narrative of the journey, A New Voyage to Carolina; Containing the Exact History and Natural History of That Country; Together with the Present State Thereof (London, 1709) became a popular tool for recruiting settlers.

William Powell, Lawson's acquaintance, lacked the skill to be a published writer. But he could look out for his interests. So when angry Indians threatened his household and cursed him for invading their land, he scrawled an account to the governor, with a plea for action. His blunt appeal gives a front-line view of the mounting tensions from one perspective. Some punctuation has been improved, but the

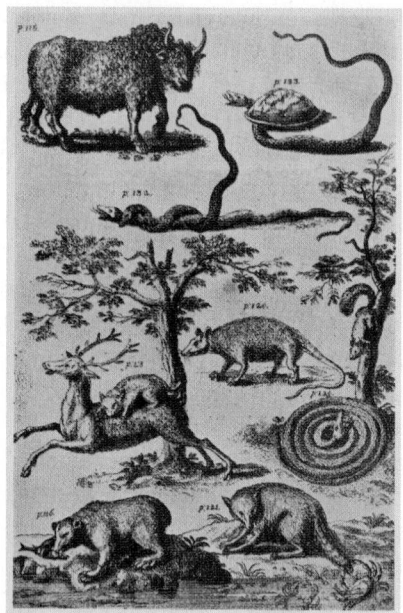

Frontispiece from John Lawson's *New Voyage to Carolina* (London, 1709)

Courtesy, Dartmouth University Library

spelling and language remain as written to the governor.

> October ye 20 1704
> Honorable Sir:
> These Comes to aquaint your honour about the . . . Indians That Came on Thursday Last to my house. There was about sixteen with King Louther all with there guns. I was att worke in the Woods with one Cristopher Gold. I made what hast I could, but they ware to quick for me: for my wife & Children had Left the house. They took away Severall Things that we miss: they have Taken all my Aminition. King Louther strook me with a how. I told him I would Tell yr honour of itt. He said you might kiss his arse. They stod with there guns Cocked So yt I could not gett into my house Tell They had Done what they pleased. I beleve itt is through the Instegation of one John Elderedge for he Told the Indians when I Brought a

Letter to your honour from Mr Lawson that It was to Cutt them of[f] which made them lay [in] wait for me att Seder Island. This they told me & then They Called me sonn of a Bitch & said they would burne my house & when itt was Light Moone the[y] would gather my corne & ye Englishmen's corne. Elderedge Told them further yt the Englishmen would . . . not sell them no Amunition because they would Cutt them of[f]. So we humbly crave that your honour would Take Some Corse or Other with them or Else here will be no Living. . . . Wiliam Powell

Lawson, like Powell, was unsure what the proper "Corse" should be. On one hand, he seems to have been sending messages to the governor urging the English to curtail trade with the Indians. On the other hand, he could write sympathetically about the troubles of Native Americans, whose aggressive new neighbors showed little respect for them:

> They are really better to us than we are to them; they always give us Victuals [food] at their Quarters, and take care we are arm'd against Hunger and Thirst: We do not do so by them (generally speaking) but let them walk by our Doors Hungry, and do not often relieve them.

But eventually, Lawson threw in his lot with Powell and the other settlers. Named surveyor general of North Carolina, he laid out the towns of Bath and New Bern and sketched a precise map of the entire Carolina region to assist further settlement. He soon became a focus of the Indians' resentment. They believed that the naturalist and promoter, "under Colour of being a Surveyor Gen'l, had encroacht too much upon their Territories." When the Tuscarora War erupted in 1711, "they were so enrag'd" that they took Lawson prisoner and put him to death. ∎

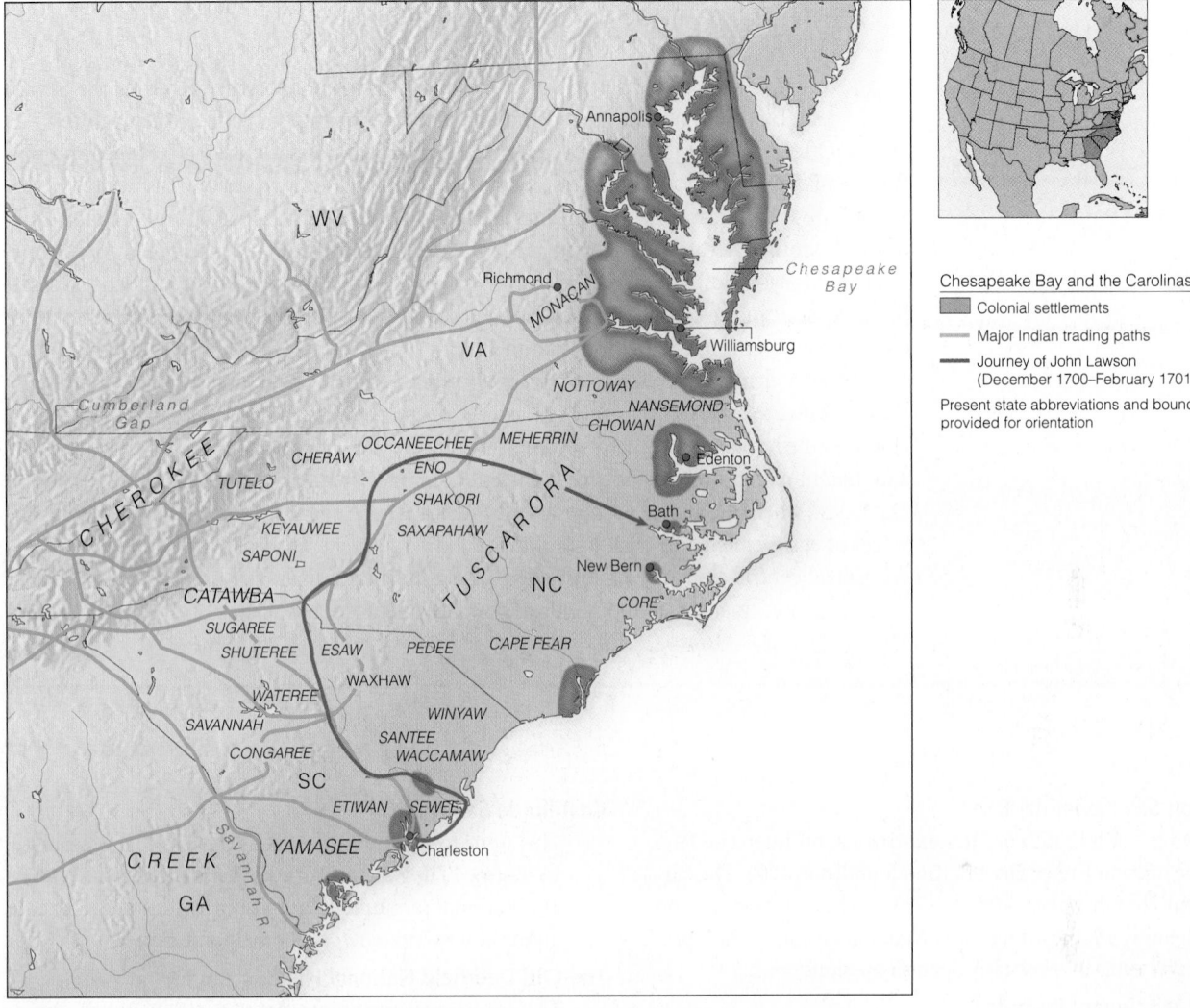

Chesapeake Bay and the Carolinas, c.1710
- Colonial settlements
- Major Indian trading paths
- Journey of John Lawson (December 1700–February 1701)

Present state abbreviations and boundaries provided for orientation

■ **MAP 3.4** **VIRGINIA AND THE CAROLINAS, c. 1710** After John Lawson made a 1,000-mile journey through the Carolina interior (1700–1701), he became an advocate for colonial growth. The expanding settlements of North Carolina and South Carolina pressed the Tuscarora and Yamasee Indians, who staged wars of resistance after 1710.

Native American village at the mouth of the Neuse River, Protestant immigrants from Bern, Switzerland, had staked out the town of New Bern.

All this was too much for the Tuscarora Indians. Frustrated by corrupt traders and land encroachment, they launched a war in 1711 to drive out the intruders. But they had waited too long. Within two years, the settlers—aided by a South Carolina force of several dozen whites and nearly 500 Yamasee Indians—had crushed Tuscarora resistance. Most of the Tuscarora survivors migrated north, where they became the sixth nation within the powerful Iroquois Confederacy.

Yamasee warriors from the Savannah River region helped British colonists quell the Tuscarora uprising. But in 1715 they led their own rebellion against advancing settlers and corrupt traders linked to Charleston. They received support from neighboring Creek Indians, Spanish settlers in Florida, and French traders at the new Alabama outpost of Fort Toulouse. The still-powerful Cherokees in southern Appalachia opted not to join in the Yamasee War. Otherwise, the Indians might have overwhelmed the South Carolina colony.

Conclusion

Along the length of eastern North America, from the Kennebec River to the Savannah, hundreds of settlers and Indians perished during the half-century before 1715. Often the frontier struggles became entwined with wider conflicts between the rival European empires. These wilderness skirmishes seem minute compared with the battles raging in Europe at the same time. (One hundred thousand soldiers clashed when England's Duke of Marlborough defeated the French at Blenheim near the Danube River in 1704. Battle lines stretched for 4 miles, and casualties ran to more than 40,000 killed or wounded.) Despite the small scale of the conflicts in North America, Europe's imperial wars had started to influence developments in the English colonies.

Another element of Europe's expansion overseas—the trans-Atlantic slave trade—had also begun to alter the shape of England's North American colonies. What had seemed only a small cloud on the horizon in the early seventeenth century had grown into an ominous force, with a momentum of its own, by the early eighteenth century. The storm hit hardest along the Southeast Coast, where the arrival of thousands of Africans soon shaped a distinctive and depressing world of enslavement and exploitation that endured for generations. No sooner had the English gained control along the Atlantic edge of North America than they orchestrated a "terrible transformation" that placed thousands in bondage and altered the shape of American history.

Sites to Visit

Mission San Xavier del Bac

Lying 7 miles south of Tucson, Arizona, off Interstate 19 is the mission Father Eusebio Kino founded in 1700. The current church was created in 1783. A short drive south on Highway 19, the Tumacacori National Historical Park preserves ruins of three early Spanish missions.

Jesuit Missionary Records

puffin.creighton.edu/jesuit/relations/

In the late nineteenth century, Reuben Gold Thwaites compiled and edited more than 70 volumes titled *The Jesuit Relations and Allied Documents*. Creighton University has made almost the entire English translation of these valuable documents available on this Web site. The documents are also available on CD-ROM from Quintin Publications.

Fort Toulouse

In 1717, the French built Fort Toulouse where the Coosa and Talapoosa rivers converge, just north of Montgomery, Alabama. On the third weekend each month between April and November, volunteers conduct a French Colonial Living History program in and around the reconstructed French fort, with displays of blacksmithing and musket firing.

The Straits of Mackinac

The Straits of Mackinac joining lakes Huron and Michigan was once a strategic spot. Here, Interstate 75 now links Upper and Lower Michigan. North of the Mackinac Bridge, a memorial at St. Ignace honors Father Marquette. At the south end, Colonial Michilimackinac is a reconstructed village reflecting French and English frontier life.

Castillo de San Marcos

This stone fort guarding St. Augustine, Florida, was built in 1672–1695. The National Park Service maintains this fortress as a national monument and also provides a virtual tour online at www.nps.gov/casa/home/home.htm

The Old Deerfield National Historic Landmark

This site lies just east of Interstate 91 and surrounds a beautiful village in the hills of northwestern Massachusetts. Historic Deerfield, incorporated in 1952, maintains 14 restored houses, open for a self-guided walking tour, and the Flynt Center of Early New England Life displays New England life from 1650 to 1850.

Salem Village Witchcraft

www.nhc.rtp.nc.us:8080/tserve/eighteen/ekeyinfo/salemwc.htm

A good Web introduction to "Witchcraft in Salem Village" appears as part of a project on "Religion and the National Culture" at this Web site of the National Humanities Center. Salem Village (Danvers, Massachusetts) has a memorial to victims of the 1692 witchcraft persecutions.

Eastern North Carolina

www.ah.dcr.state.nc.us/sections/hs/bath/bath.htm

North Carolina's earliest colonial ports at Edenton, Bath, and New Bern (ranging from north to south) still contain rich evidence of eighteenth-century life. This Web site for Historic Bath has links on explorer–naturalist John Lawson, Blackbeard the Pirate, and the Tuscarora War.

For Further Reading

General

Elaine G. Breslaw, *Witches of the Atlantic World: A Historical Reader and Primary Source Book* (2000).

Wesley Frank Craven, *The Colonies in Transition, 1660–1713* (1968).

Elizabeth A. H. John, *Storms Brewed in Other Men's Worlds: The Confrontation of Indians, Spanish, and French in the Southwest, 1540–1795* (1975).

Alvin M. Josephy, Jr., *The Patriot Chiefs: A Chronicle of American Indian Resistance* (1969).

John Lawson, *A New Voyage to Carolina* (1967).

France and the American Interior

Marcel Giraud, *A History of French Louisiana, Volume One: the Reign of Louis XIV, 1698–1715* (1974).

Jay Higginbotham, *Old Mobile, Fort Louis de la Louisiane, 1702–1711* (1977).

Eric Hinderaker, *Elusive Empires: Constructing Colonialism in the Ohio Valley, 1673–1800* (1997).

Robert S. Weddle, *The Wreck of the Belle, the Ruin of La Salle* (2001).

Richard White, *The Middle Ground: Indians, Empires, and Republics in the Great Lakes Region, 1650–1815* (1991).

The Spanish Empire on the Defensive

Ramón A. Gutiérrez, *When Jesus Came, the Corn Mothers Went Away: Marriage, Sexuality, and Power in New Mexico, 1500–1846* (1991).

John H. Hann, *A History of the Timucua Indians and Missions* (1996).

Andrew L. Knaut, *The Pueblo Revolt of 1680: Conquest and Resistance in Seventeenth-Century New Mexico* (1995).

Jerald T. Milanich, *Florida Indians and the Invasion from Europe* (1995).

David J. Weber, editor, *What Caused the Pueblo Revolt?* (1999).

England's American Empire Takes Shape

Joyce D. Goodfriend, *Before the Melting Pot: Society and Culture in Colonial New York City, 1664–1730* (1992).

J. R. Jones, *Country and Court: England, 1658–1714* (1978).

Brendan McConville, *These Daring Disturbers of the Public Peace: The Struggle for Property and Power in Early New Jersey* (1999).

Gary B. Nash, *Quakers and Politics: Pennsylvania, 1681–1726* (1968).

Robert M. Weir, *Colonial South Carolina: A History* (1983).

Bloodshed in the English Colonies: 1670–1690

John Demos, *The Unredeemed Captive: A Family Story from Early America* (1994).

Jill Lepore, *The Name of War: King Philip's War and the Origins of American Identity* (1998).

David S. Lovejoy, *The Glorious Revolution in America* (1972).

Stephen S. Webb, *1676: The End of American Independence* (1984).

Stephen S. Webb, *Lord Churchill's Coup: The Anglo-American Empire and the Glorious Revolution Reconsidered* (1995).

Consequences of War and Growth: 1690–1715

Paul Boyer and Stephen Nissenbaum, *Salem Possessed: The Social Origins of Witchcraft* (1974).

Verner W. Crane, *The Southern Frontier, 1670–1732* (1928).

Carol F. Karlsen, *The Devil in the Name of a Woman: Witchcraft in Colonial New England* (1987).

James H. Merrell, *The Indians' New World: Catawbas and Their Neighbors from European Contact Through the Era of Removal* (1989).

Gary B. Nash, *The Urban Crucible: The Northern Seaports and the Origins of the American Revolution* (1986, abridged edition).

Online Practice Test

Test your understanding of this chapter with interactive review quizzes at

www.ablongman.com/jonescreatedequal/chapter3

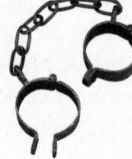
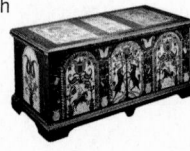
PART TWO

A Century of Colonial Expansion to 1775

O N APRIL 19, 1775, NEW ENGLAND FARMERS BATTLED BRITISH SOLDIERS at Concord Bridge. The confrontation marked the start of the American Revolution. (Each spring in Massachusetts, the date is still set aside as Patriots' Day and celebrated with the running of the Boston Marathon.) But how did colonies that remained weak outposts before 1700 become strong enough to challenge the power of the British empire in the second half of the eighteenth century? The answer is not a simple one. Life changed in dramatic ways during the century before 1775, not only in New England but throughout much of North America.

The rapid spread of Spanish horses across the West allowed Native Americans, such as the Comanche and Sioux, to become mounted buffalo hunters on the Great Plains. The arrival of Russian fur traders disrupted traditional cultures on the Aleutian Islands and the coast of Alaska. At the same time, the gradual success of the new Louisiana colony gave France access to much of the Mississippi River valley. But the potential for a dominant French-speaking empire in America evaporated with the stunning defeat of French forces by the British in the Seven Years' War. As that global conflict ended in 1763, the Spanish also lost ground in North America. After claiming Florida for 200 years, they finally ceded the peninsula to the British, even as they began to extend Spanish missions up the coast of California.

Other changes were even more dramatic. In the eighteenth century race slavery became an established aspect of colonial society in North America. The process began early, well before 1660, and evolved over several generations. In the coastal Southeast, it rapidly took hold as a dominant institution. The English had come late to the trans-Atlantic slave trade, but they became aggressive participants in the lucrative traffic in human beings. English colonizers fashioned harsh slave-based societies in the Caribbean, then in the Chesapeake colonies of Virginia and Maryland, next in North and South Carolina, and finally, after 1750, in the recently established colony of Georgia.

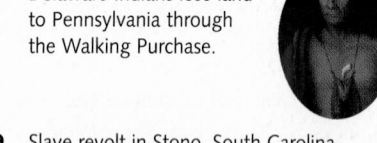

This terrible transformation to mainland colonies based on race slavery had far-reaching results. Thousands of Africans arrived in North American ports in the eighteenth century. Strikingly, they were only a small fraction of the much greater transport of Africans to the Caribbean and Central and South America. Nevertheless, by 1750 there were nearly 250,000 African Americans living in North America. Most lived in the South, and most were enslaved, including several hundred in Spanish East Florida and several thousand in French Louisiana. By 1775 the number exceeded half a million. By then, blacks made up more than 20 percent of the population of the British colonies, and the legal and social constraints that bound them remained tighter than ever.

Newcomers from Europe, as well as from Africa, altered the make-up of Atlantic colonies that had once been almost entirely English. Many of these newly arrived Europeans, unable to afford the cost of passage, had to pledge their labor for a period of years. But in contrast to the Africans, most European migrants came to America voluntarily and were free from obligations within a few years. The Atlantic crossing could be harrowing, of course, but for thousands the long-term advantages outweighed the short-term drawbacks. Artisans of all kinds were in high demand, and land was cheap. Colonial governments ruled with a light hand in comparison to the monarchies of Europe, and they competed with one another to attract newcomers. This competition, in turn, bred relative religious and ethnic tolerance.

Pushed by events in Europe and drawn by opportunities in America, non-English families flocked to Britain's North American colonies. Combined with the African slave trade, this new flow from Europe and the British Isles quickly generated a far more diverse colonial society on the foundations laid by earlier English immigrants. Prior generations of colonists had laid out towns, formed governments, and founded the rudimentary institutions of colonial social life. They had established an ambiguous pattern of interaction with Native Americans that involved warfare and displacement as well as trade and intermarriage. Also, they had located harbors, carved out roads, and started to build an economic infrastructure.

As numbers rose and diversity increased, a series of regional economies emerged along the eastern seaboard. Each sustained the local inhabitants while also serving the wider needs of the British empire. For much of the eighteenth century, the British crown promoted economic growth in the colonies through a workable combination of protectionist controls and benign neglect.

But the British victory over the French brought drastic new problems to eastern North America after 1763. Native Americans lost a valued trading partner and military ally when the French withdrew. Britain faced an enormous war debt and looked to its burgeoning colonies as a source of much-needed revenue. Within little more than a decade, Britain's North American colonists went from resentment and resistance to overt rebellion and an anticolonial war of independence.

1755	Braddock is defeated near Fort Duquesne.
1758	Comanches attack Spanish at San Saba Mission.
1759	Quebec falls to the British.
1760	George III becomes king of England. French surrender Montreal to British.
1763	Treaty of Paris ends the French and Indian War. Proclamation Line limits expansion of British colonies. Pontiac's Rebellion.
1764	Sugar Act; Currency Act.
1765	Quartering Act; Stamp Act. Virginia Resolves; Stamp Act demonstrations. Tenant riots in Hudson Valley.
1766	Stamp Act repealed. Declaratory Act. Bougainville explores the South Pacific.
1767	Townshend Acts.
1768	James Cook makes first of three voyages to explore the Pacific. Massachusetts Circular Letter.
1770	Boston Massacre.
1771	Battle of Alamance ends the Regulator Movement in North Carolina.
1772	Burning of the *Gaspée*.
1773	Boston Tea Party.
1774	Intolerable Acts. First Continental Congress meets. The Suffolk Resolves.
1775	Battles of Lexington and Concord. Spanish enter San Francisco Bay.

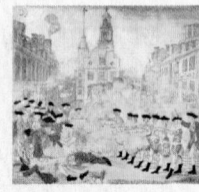

CHAPTER

4

African Enslavement: The Terrible Transformation

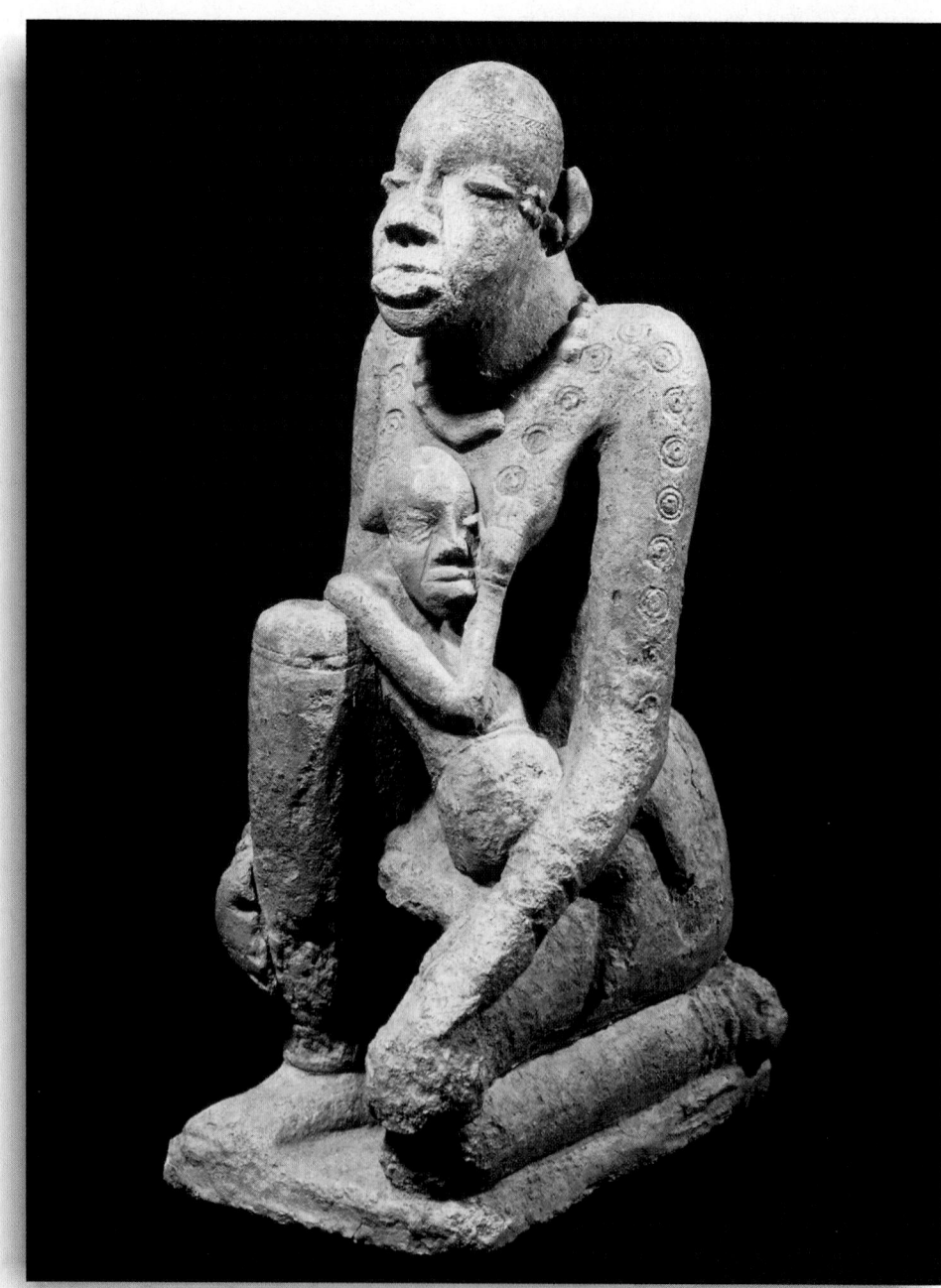

The Menil Collection, Houston

■ Ancient terra-cotta sculpture from Mali depicting an African mother and child.

ON A COOL DAY IN JANUARY 1656, A MULATTO SERVANT NAMED ELIZABETH KEY WENT before the local court in Northumberland County, Virginia. She was 25 years old. The late Colonel John Mottrom, a justice of the peace, had held Elizabeth as a slave, kept in perpetual bondage. She objected strongly, and she wanted to sue the executors of Mottom's estate for her freedom and back pay. Bess, as she was known, presented a threefold argument. First, as the daughter of a free man, she should inherit her father's legal status according to English law. Second, as a baptized Christian, she should not be enslaved. And third, she could produce a document showing that as a small child she had been "put out" to work until she was 14, following local custom. Such contracts for apprenticing a child for a fixed number of years were common in America, where labor was in short supply. But her term of work had expired long ago.

Key was accompanied in court by her white attorney and lover, William Greensted. They had had two children together and would marry six months later, when they finally won a favorable verdict. The executors of Mottrom's estate, eager to show that Bess's father was neither free nor Christian, implied that a Turkish crewman off a visiting ship was the girl's father. But the young couple produced witnesses who testified that Bess was indeed the daughter of Thomas Key, a white man serving in the Virginia General Assembly, and his "Negro woman." One witness, though only 13 at the time of Elizabeth's birth in 1631, told the jury she remembered Bess's mother well. The witness knew that she lived openly with Mr. Key and had heard her say that the girl was Key's daughter.

Other witnesses recalled that Bess Key's mixed parentage "was a common Report amongst the Neighbours." Mrs. Newman, the 80-year-old midwife who had delivered Bess's own children, contributed additional testimony. She recalled that 25 years earlier, Mr. Key was brought to court and "fined for getting his Negro woman with child." Further testimony established that in 1636, not long before he died, Key had bound little Bess to Humphrey Higginson, a member of the Council of State. Higginson "promised to use her as well as if shee were his own Child"; that is, "more Respectfully than a Comon servant or slave." He even stood as her godfather when Bess was christened.

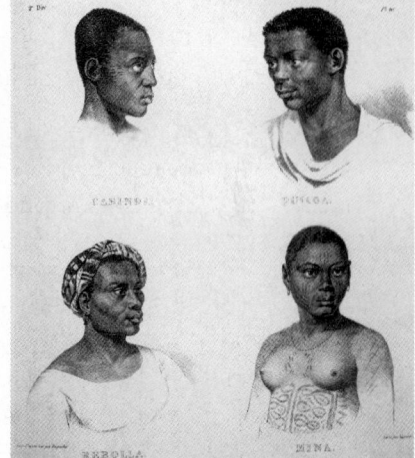

Africans arriving in America often had ornamental scarification (known as "country marks") on their bodies, as well as brands inflicted by slave traders and physical scars from the middle passage.

To be raised in a Christian church was no small matter at a time when Europeans viewed non-Christians captured in wars to be uniquely vulnerable to legal enslavement. For Bess, this circumstance helped her cause greatly, for she proved "able to give a very good account of her fayth." Furthermore, she produced clear evidence that her father had sold her to Higginson for nine years. Mr. Key had demanded that Higginson not dispose of her to any other person, such as to Colonel Mottrom. Rather, he was to give her the usual "freedom portion" of corn and clothes "and lett her shift for her selfe," either in England or Virginia, when her term expired.

The local jury accepted Elizabeth Key's three-part argument and pronounced her free. But the General Court overturned the verdict on appeal, only to be overruled in turn by a committee of the General Assembly. In the end, the committee determined that "Elizabeth ought to bee free." The assemblymen also argued that her last master owed her a "freedom portion," plus back pay "for the time shee hath served longer than Shee ought to have done." Still, the matter generated debate among settlers. Several decades later, Elizabeth's case would have been decided differently. Moreover, the courts of Virginia might well have enslaved her children for life. And their own offspring would have inherited slavery status as well.

A terrible transformation was under way in English colonial culture that would warp American society for centuries to come. It did not become obvious overnight. Instead, it spread gradually, like a cancer, revealing a different pace and pattern in each mainland colony. During the 1620s and 1630s, a few black servants were working alongside white servants in Virginia and New England. All worked for fixed periods of service, with equal expectations of eventually becoming free residents and property holders. But well before the end of the century, a fateful transition had occurred, and the grandchildren of those workers had been separated into two distinct categories based upon skin color and physical appearance, or race. Free blacks persisted in the English colonies, but in most communities they became anomalies, for the tide was flowing against them. From now on, people of African ancestry were to be legally enslaved for life.

The earliest signs of lifetime enslavement definitely predate 1660, and the dark consequences would play out across American history down to the present day. But in scarcely half a century, during the late 1600s and early 1700s, this malignant condition developed from possibility to reality. Elizabeth Key and her children and grandchildren experienced the painful transition first-hand and glimpsed its horrendous consequences.

The Descent into Race Slavery

Some grim transitions in human affairs evolve slowly, even imperceptibly. In the mid-twentieth century, western societies recovering from World War II looked back at the havoc that fascism had spawned in Europe and wondered how Germany had moved from anti-Jewish prejudice, to hatred, to death camps in just two generations. In the mid–twenty-first century, we may look back and wonder how global warming, population expansion, religious fanaticism, weapon proliferation—or some difficulty we cannot now see—went from a negligible problem to a debatable issue to a rampant disaster during our lifetimes. How North American society sank into the pit of race slavery is just such a difficult topic. But the slippery slope sanctioning perpetual servitude based on race demands attention. Nothing shaped colonial cultures more forcefully than the European colonists' gradual commitment to the legalized enslavement of hundreds of thousands of people and their descendants.

The Caribbean Precedent

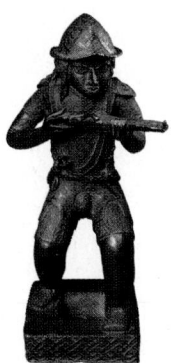

The roots of race slavery in the Americas extend back to the era of Columbus, when warfare, sickness, and exploitation quickly decimated the native populations of the Caribbean after 1492. Hungry for human labor, the Spanish intruders began to import people from Africa to grow crops and dig for gold in the Caribbean islands. As the native population declined sharply through epidemics, the traffic in black newcomers expanded.

Spanish pressure for labor in the New World intensified further with the discovery of additional mines in Mexico and Peru. To meet the growing demand, Spain's king even issued a contract (called the *asiento*) that allowed other European powers—such as Portugal, France, or the Netherlands—to import African slaves to the Spanish colonies. High profits drew eager participation. In the half-century between 1590 and 1640, more than 220,000 people arrived in chains from Africa at the empire's ports in Central and South America.

Meanwhile, the Portuguese purchased enslaved Africans to work their own expanding sugar plantations. They imported more than 75,000 slaves, mostly from the Congo Rver region of West Central Africa, to the Atlantic island of São Tomé in the sixteenth century. And when Portuguese sugar production spread to coastal Brazil, so did the exploitation of African labor. By 1625 Brazil imported the majority of slaves crossing the Atlantic each year and exported most of the sugar consumed in Europe.

Long before the 1660s, therefore, Europeans had set a precedent for exploiting African workers in New World colonies. Over more than a century, Spain and Portugal had learned to purchase, transport, market, and exploit enslaved workers from ports along the West African coast. Moreover, they had found ways to justify in their own minds a deep involvement in this brutal but lucrative system. Religious and secular authorities frowned on actively enslaving people, especially if they were fellow Christians, but purchasing so-called infidels (those who followed other religions or opposed Christianity) could be tolerated, particularly if slavery had already been imposed on them by someone else. These West African victims were non-Christians, and most had already been enslaved by others, captured by fellow Africans in war.

As late as 1660, it was not at all clear that African slavery would gain a prominent place, or even a lasting foothold, in any North American colonies.

Confident in this rationale, the Spanish and Portuguese adapted their laws to accept the enslavement of Africans. Moreover, the condition would be hereditary, passed on from mother to child, and the new labor system had backing from the Catholic Church. Catholic priests occasionally worked to alleviate suffering among Africans in the Americas, and they reached out regularly for the conversion of souls, but the papacy did nothing to condemn the growing traffic. Nor did the Protestant Reformation have a dampening effect. On the contrary, the rising Protestant sea powers of northern Europe proved willing to assist in the slave trade and compete in what historians call the "sugar revolution," growing sugar on a massive scale for expanding Atlantic markets.

Ships of the Dutch West India Company, for example, played an increasing role in the Brazilian trade, transporting both slaves and sugar. Indeed, for a generation in the first half of the seventeenth century, the Dutch ruled the South American colony. When the Portuguese regained control of Brazil at mid-century, they pushed out Dutch settlers who had long experience in managing sugar plantations. These outcasts traveled the islands of the Caribbean, bringing their knowledge with them. Some appeared in the new English possessions of Barbados and Jamaica, and soon they were directing African slaves in cutting, pressing, and boiling sugar cane to make molasses. The thick molasses could then be processed further to make the rum and refined sugar that these English colonies exported. By the 1650s slavery and sugar production were engulfing England's West Indian possessions, just as these twin features had already become central to the New World colonies controlled by Spain and Portugal. But as late as 1660, it was not at all clear that African slavery would gain a prominent place, or even a lasting foothold, in any North American colonies.

Ominous Beginnings

As far back as the sixteenth century, African men had participated in Spanish explorers' forays into the Southeast, and some had remained, fathering children with Indian women. African slaves had helped to establish the small Spanish outpost at St. Augustine in 1565, but a century later no additional coastal colonies had yet appeared on the mainland anywhere south of Chesapeake Bay. Granted, Africans were present farther north in the fledgling settlements of the French, Dutch, and English. But their numbers remained small—several thousand at

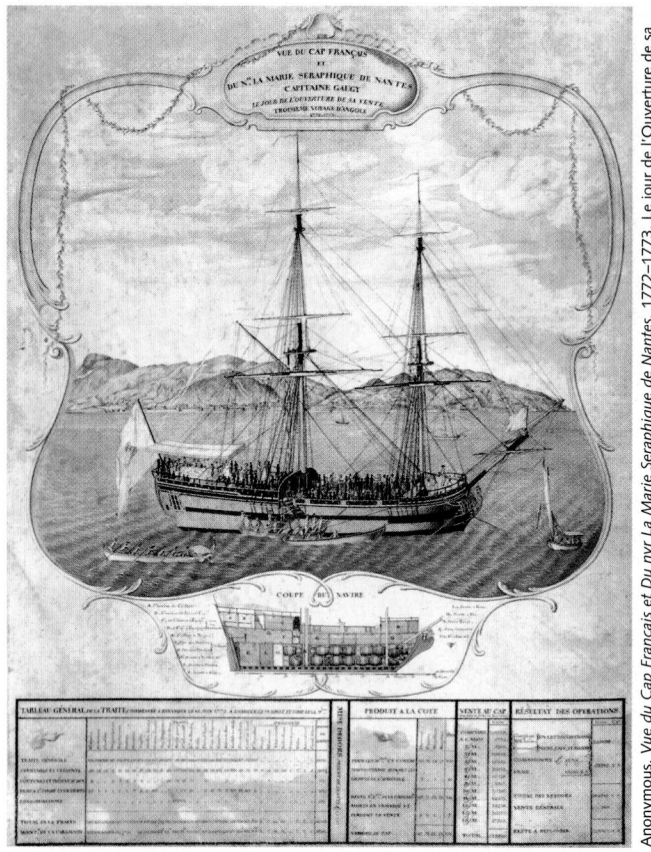

Anonymous, *Vue du Cap Francais et Du nvr La Marie Seraphique de Nantes, 1772–1773. Le jour de l'Ouverture de sa Vente, Troisieme Voyage d'Angole. Musée du Château des Ducs de Bretagne (950.4.3)*

■ **This summary of an African slave-trading voyage shows wealthy planters boarding a French ship upon its arrival in the West Indies in order to buy slaves newly arrived from Angola. The crew has used an iron fence dividing the deck to protect against revolt during the voyage. The captain conducts business under an awning in the stern.**

most—in comparison to the expanding black populations of the older sugar colonies near the equator. In addition, few of these newcomers had come directly from Africa. Most had lived for years in the Caribbean or on the mainland, absorbing the languages, customs, and beliefs of the majority population. So they and their children, like Bess Key, were not viewed as complete outsiders by the European colonists.

The legal and social standing of these few early African Americans remained vague before the 1660s. Local statutes regarding labor were crude and contradictory; their interpretation and enforcement varied widely. Everywhere, workers were in demand, and most black newcomers found themselves indentured for a period of years alongside European servants in a similar unfree condition.

In the Massachusetts Bay colony, early Puritan settlers, casting about for sources of labor and for markets, exchanged goods for slaves in the Caribbean. In 1644, seafaring New Englanders even attempted direct trade with Africa. But the following year, Massachusetts authorities ordered a New Hampshire resident to surrender a black worker he had purchased in Boston. They argued that the man had been stolen from Africa, not captured in war, and should be returned to his home. For the earliest handful of black New Englanders, their standing proved uncertain in a region where religious status mattered far more than language, dress, or outward physical appearance. In 1652 Rhode Island passed a law clearly limiting all involuntary service—whether for Europeans or Africans—to no more than 10 years.

Along the Hudson River, the Dutch colonists had close ties with the sugar islands of the West Indies where race slavery was already an accepted system. In New Netherland, therefore, the laws discriminated against black workers and limited their rights. But the statutes also provided loopholes that permitted social and economic advancement to the community's Africans, most of whom spoke Dutch.

Chesapeake Bay lay even closer to the main routes of the Atlantic slave traffic. In 1619 a Dutch warship that had acquired slaves during a season of raiding in the Caribbean brought more than 20 African men and women to Virginia. They were put up for sale as servants, along with people deported from England to build up the Chesapeake's labor force. Terms of service varied, and some black newcomers earned their freedom quickly and kept it. But others saw their terms extended arbitrarily. In 1640 Virginia's General Court considered punishment for "a negro named John Punch" and two other servants who had escaped to Maryland and had been apprehended together. The Dutchman and the Scotsman each received four additional years of service, but the African was sentenced to unending servitude "for the time of his natural life." That same year, Virginia passed a law that prevented blacks from bearing arms. And a 1643 law taxing productive field hands included African American women but not white women.

These early efforts to separate Africans from Europeans by law set an ominous precedent in the use of skin color as a distinguishing marker. Throughout the 1640s and 1650s, aggressive English tobacco farmers in Virginia and Maryland, in imitation of planters in Barbados, attempted to purchase the labor of Indians and Africans for life. They even claimed rights to the future children of nonwhite women in their possession. Still, rules governing the lives of people of color and their offspring remained ambiguous for several decades, and (as the case of Bess Key makes clear) efforts at exploitation could often be undone in court. But new forces would come into play in the mainland American colonies after 1660, consolidating the transition to hereditary African slavery.

Alternative Sources of Labor

For African newcomers to English North America, their legal status became distinctly clearer and less hopeful in the decades after 1660. This shift was linked to the fact that colonial efforts to exploit two other supplies of affordable workers—captured Native Americans and impoverished Europeans—were running into increasing difficulty. The transatlantic slave trade, already more than a century old, provided certain English colonies with a ready source of African workers at a time when more obvious streams of inexpensive labor were dwindling or drying up.

For labor-hungry colonists, Native Americans had much to recommend them, since they were close at hand and knew the country well. Throughout the century, English newcomers often paid an Indian hunter to keep them supplied with fresh meat. But it was a different matter if European strangers tried to force that neighbor to cut down trees and cultivate unfamiliar crops endlessly, with little or no reward. Native Americans took captives when fighting one another, so colonists could buy Indian prisoners or seize them in frontier warfare. Europeans felt they could enslave such people in good conscience, since they were non-Christians who had been taken captive in war. But Native American numbers were declining steadily, owing to epidemics. And those who did become enslaved knew the countryside well enough to escape. Besides, traffic in Indian slaves worked against other goals of the colonists. It disrupted the profitable deerskin trade, undermined wilderness diplomacy, and sparked conflict on the frontier.

Efforts to maintain a steady flow of cheap labor from Europe ran into different problems. The Great Plague of 1665 devastated the English population, and the London Fire the following year created a new need for workers of all kinds to rebuild the capital. England's labor surplus, which had been a boon to the initial colonies half a century earlier, rapidly disappeared. Those who made their living in English ports by procuring labor for America were forced to nab youngsters off the streets. But even this practice (called by the new word, *kidnapping*) was soon outlawed. The use of indentures persisted, whereby the poor could buy their passage by agreeing to sell their labor for a fixed term. But when these workers reached America, they served for only a few years and then had to be replaced. Moreover, when their terms of indenture expired, they expected "freedom dues" (clothes, tools, and food from their former master) and their own land to farm. Once free, therefore, they competed for acreage that large planters hoped to control.

Equally important, when indentured servants were mistreated, they had little difficulty in relaying their complaints home to other potential workers. The flow of ships back and forth between Europe and North America grew steadily in the century after 1660, so word of places where indentured servants were regularly abused or swindled quickly reached the other side of the Atlantic. As Europeans mulled over private letters, coffeehouse gossip, and sailors' reports, they could adjust their own plans for migration. Depending on what they heard or read, they might postpone a voyage or seek a more promising destination.

In contrast, the African slave trade lacked any similar "feedback loop." People swept up in the growing stream of unfree African labor had no access to information regarding New World conditions. On New World plantations—as in Siberian slave labor camps and German extermination centers in the twentieth century—people and information flowed in only one direction. A mere handful, among hundreds of thousands of enslaved Africans, ever managed to communicate with their homeland. One can only speculate how different the procurement and treatment of colonial labor might have been if generations of Europeans had received no knowledge of conditions in North America, or if Africans had received a great deal. As it was, the brutal treatment of black workers across the Atlantic never had a chance, through accurate feedback, to influence the future flow of deportations from Africa.

Reparations for Slavery?

The small plaque reads, "In memory of the courage, pain and suffering of enslaved African people." But you probably will never see it. In 1993, members of the National Association of Black Scuba Divers lowered it to the bottom of the Atlantic Ocean off Key West, Florida. There it marks the resting place of the *Henrietta Marie,* an English slave ship built in 1699 that sank the next year, during its second voyage. Similarly, civic leaders in South Carolina unveiled a marker at Sullivan's Island in Charleston Harbor. It honors thousands of eighteenth-century Africans who faced enslavement, rather than opportunity, when they arrived at "the Ellis Island of Black America."

Other markers will follow as Americans continue to reexamine the country's long involvement with slavery and the slave trade. But many people now say that memorials, even official apologies, are not enough. Instead, they believe, formal reparations are overdue. The passions stirred by their suggestion show that the matter of slavery in America has not yet been laid to rest.

Payment of reparations—repairing a wrong through some compensation for damages—is an old and honored concept. It can sometimes bring legal satisfaction and moral closure to both the abused and the abuser. And it applies whether individuals, groups, or nations are involved. Germany has paid extensive reparations for Nazi

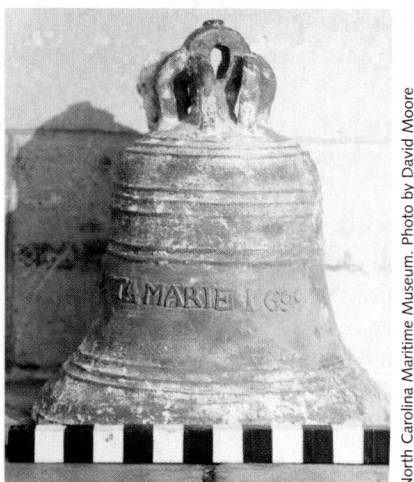

Bell recovered from the *Henrietta Marie,* a slave ship that sank in 1700.

atrocities during World War II, and the German government and private industries are compensating people who were forced to work without pay in slave labor camps.

Inevitably, the issue of reparations sparks controversy whenever it appears. It applies most readily to offenses that are short-lived and recent. For example, after much deliberation, Congress began paying reparations in 1991 to U.S. citizens of Japanese descent who were placed in internment camps during World War II. But reparations have also been argued for human wrongs that lasted much longer and lie buried deeper in the past, such as the enslavement of African Americans over centuries.

Talk of slavery reparations is hardly new. English lawyer James Grahame published a book in 1842 criticizing U.S. hypocrisy and claiming reparations on behalf of African Americans. A generation later it looked as though the country's 4 million slavery survivors

might at least get the simple "freedom dues" that had gone to indentured servants in colonial times for beginning free life after servitude. But promises of "40 acres and a mule" fell through when the federal government refused to redistribute the land of planters who had declared war against the United States. Congressional aid offered through the Freedmen's Bureau proved small and uneven. It was also short-lived. Congress cut off funds for the agency in 1872.

In recent years, opposition to renewed talk of slavery reparations has been swift and varied. How do you calculate such a huge price tag, and who foots the bill? Should compensation go to slavery's descendants (numerous and not always easy to define) or to the African lands that suffered such colossal losses? Would a token payment, spread widely, be useless and insulting all at once? And doesn't the entire notion reopen old wounds and revive talk of victim status long after it is time to move on?

Not so, says John Conyers, a black representative from Michigan who has been prodding Congress for more than a decade to form a commission to study the issue. Frustrated on Capitol Hill, he points to a coalition of lawyers who hope to force the issue in court. They see the primary obstacle not as money but as public ignorance and apathy. Most Americans, they argue, are still in denial about the true nature of slavery and its enormous scope. "We just want the history to be told a little more accurately," Conyers observes. "I think if it's told, we'll have our day in court and we'll win." ■

The Fateful Transition

In general, powerful Chesapeake tobacco planters had opposed challenges to the monarchy from Puritans and Parliament during England's recent civil wars. Many had close ties to the royalists and courtiers (known as "Cavaliers") who had remained faithful to the Stuart cause after King Charles I had been executed and his son had gone into exile. They were encouraged in 1660 by news of the Restoration of Charles II, since he was likely to support their interests and reward their loyalty. These men had noticed the rising profits that sugar growers were making by using slaves in the Caribbean. In Virginia and Maryland, therefore, planters passed a series of laws that sharpened distinctions between servants working for a fixed period and slaves consigned to labor for life. Officials who had objected to the verdict that freed Elizabeth Key in 1656 moved in the following decade to implement their own harsher views as law.

In shaping new legislation, they even challenged long-standing English legal traditions, such as the right of children to inherit their father's status. In 1662 Virginia's General Assembly considered whether any child fathered "by an Englishman upon a negro woman should be slave or Free." In a crucial reversal of precedent, the legislature said that in such cases "all children borne in this country" shall be "held bond or free *only according to the condition of the mother.*" From now on, the infant of any female slave would be enslaved from birth, an obvious boon for masters who wanted additional long-term labor at little cost. Slavery was becoming a hereditary condition.

If enslaved persons accepted Christianity, could they receive their freedom, as sometimes happened in Spanish colonies? A Maryland law of 1664 closed off that prospect. The act made clear that the legal status of non-Christian slaves did not change if they experienced religious conversion. Three years later, Virginia's government agreed that "the conferring of baptisme doth not alter the condition of the person as to his bondage." By taking religion out of the question, legislators shifted the definition of who could be enslaved from someone who was not Christian to someone who did not look European. In 1680, Reverend Morgan Godwyn observed that the "two words, *Negro* and *Slave,*" had already "by custom" grown interchangeable in Virginia. Because nobody could alter their skin color but anyone could change faith, planters moved to categorize colonial workers by their appearance rather than their religion.

In scarcely a generation, black bondage had become a hereditary institution, and the conditions of life had grown markedly worse for African Americans. Europeans receiving wages for work could pay fines for misbehavior; servants indentured for a term could be required to work additional months or years as a punishment. But enslaved Africans, condemned to unpaid labor for life, had no money or time to give up when disciplined for misdeeds, whether real or imagined. Therefore, they found themselves subjected increasingly to corporal punishments: whippings, torture, and even mutilation. In the generation after Elizabeth Key, black slaves—and often free blacks as well—lost their right to accuse, or even testify against, a white person in a court of law. "And further," stated Virginia's formative slave law of 1680, "if any Negro" so much as raises a hand, even in self-defense, "against any Christian, he shall receive thirty lashes, and if he absent himself . . . from his master's service and resist lawful apprehension, he may be killed."

The Growth of Slave Labor Camps

In the second half of the seventeenth century, those who ran the South's emerging staple crop economies undertook a drastic change of course. Step by step, over two generations, tobacco growers in the Chesapeake and rice producers in the new colony of South Carolina embraced the system of hereditary race slavery that had developed in the Caribbean. Within a matter of decades, they made it central to their way of life.

Traditionally, historians had described this change as the rise of plantation agriculture. But for those forced to cut the trees, drain the swamps, and harvest the crops, the shift in production strategy represented—in modern terminology—the emergence of slave labor camps. After all, the plantations of varying sizes that came to dot the southern coastline and the interior river valleys exploited a captive workforce. These people received no wages for their labor, had no legal rights, and could be deported to some other location at any time. This deterioration in

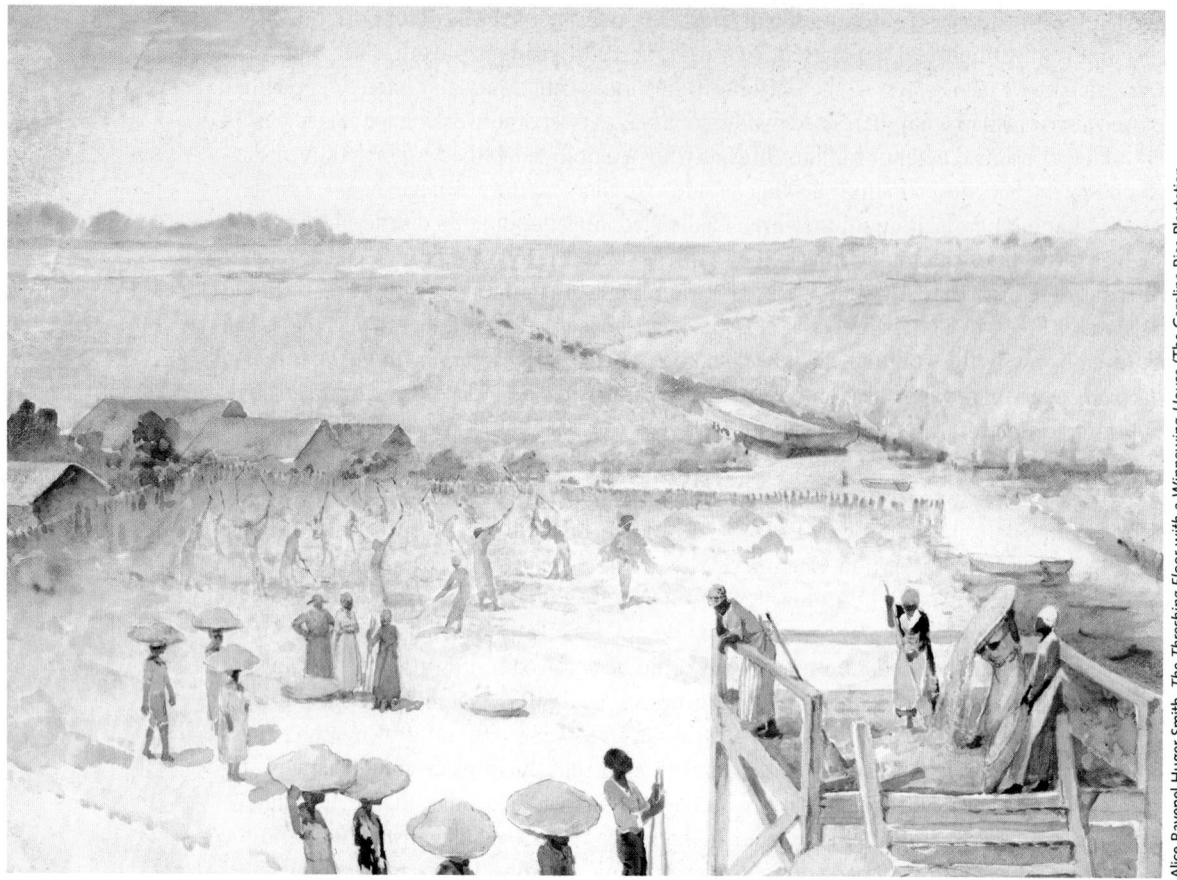

Alice Ravenel Huger Smith, *The Threshing Floor with a Winnowing-House* (The Carolina Rice Plantation Series). Gibbes Museum of Art/CAA, 37.09.22

■ Rice plantations that emerged in coastal South Carolina around 1700 became labor camps where enslaved blacks were confined for generations, without wages or legal rights. In the 1850s, distant descendants of the region's first African workers were still being forced to plant, harvest, and process the huge rice crops that made their masters rich.

conditions occurred first, and most dramatically, in Virginia, where several thousand African Americans lived and labored by the 1670s.

Black Involvement in Bacon's Rebellion

Nothing did more to consolidate Virginia's slide toward race slavery than Bacon's Rebellion, the major uprising that shook the Chesapeake region in 1676 (see chapter 3). The episode pitted aspiring gentry, led by Nathaniel Bacon, against beleaguered Indian groups on the frontier and an entrenched oligarchy in Jamestown. The rebellion underscored the dilemmas inherent in Virginia's reliance on a steady flow of white indentured servants to cultivate tobacco. That labor supply was uneven at best, and employers constantly needed new recruits, since terms of service lasted only several years. Workers who earned their freedom—hundreds every year—were young, armed men who demanded property of their own. Whether they had to take it from rich landholders or neighboring Indians made little difference to them.

These free men, would-be farmers in search of land, made up part of Bacon's following, but a diverse group of unfree workers also proved eager recruits. These ill-treated individuals remained legally bound to large landholders for varying terms, and many of the Africans were undoubtedly bound for life. Together, they raised much of the colony's annual tobacco crop. The backbreaking labor—planting, hoeing, suckering, topping, picking, curing, and packing tobacco—prompted frequent unrest. These ragged workers, however long their term of service might be, had the most to gain and the least to lose from Bacon's revolt. According to the Virginia Assembly, "many evill disposed servants…taking advantage of the loosenes of the tymes…followed the rebells in rebellion." When Bacon fell ill and died in October 1676, many of his wealthier supporters reasserted their loyalty to the colonial government in order to emerge on the winning side. But bound workers who had escaped from their masters continued the fight.

A letter reaching London that fall suggested that at the height of the rebellion Bacon had "proclam'd liberty to all Servants and Negro's." Whether or not Bacon had actually declared freedom to servants and slaves of all sorts, the widespread unrest clearly had given hope to the most downtrodden tobacco pickers, about a quarter of whom were black. As a Royal Commission put it, "sundry servants and other persons of desperate fortunes" had "deserted their masters and run into rebellion on the encouragement of liberty." When military reinforcements arrived in Chesapeake Bay from England in November, their commanding officer, Captain Thomas Grantham, found hundreds of laborers still in active revolt.

Impressed by their strength, Grantham chose to use deceit when he met with eight hundred heavily armed rebels, both white and black, at their headquarters near the York River in Virginia. By distributing brandy and making vague promises regarding pardons and freedom, he persuaded most of the white men to surrender and return home. Only about "Eighty Negroes and Twenty English…would not deliver their Armes." According to Grantham, they threatened to kill him, asserting that they wanted "their hoped for liberty and would not quietly laye downe their armes." But when these last holdouts boarded a sloop to head down river, Grantham managed to lure them within range of his ship's cannons. He disarmed the rebels and chained them below decks for return to their masters.

The Rise of a Slaveholding Tidewater Elite

With Bacon's death and the arrival of British ships, propertied Virginians had narrowly averted a successful multiracial revolution, fueled from below by workers who resented their distressed condition. But it was clear that another revolt might succeed in the future, and the great planters of the Chesapeake region moved to tighten their hold on political and economic power. After Bacon's Rebellion, a strategy of divide and conquer seemed in order. They moved to improve conditions for poor whites in ways that would reduce tension between classes and ensure deference and racial solidarity among Europeans. At the same time, they moved to reduce further the legal status of blacks and solidify their full enslavement. Africans would regularly be forced to serve for life, with increasingly harsh penalties for any show of opposition or dissent.

For precedent, the planters had the model provided by slavery-based colonial societies in the West Indies, including the English sugar island of Barbados. The notion of treating Africans separately, based on their customs, speech, and appearance, became an article of faith among aspiring planters. Their uneasiness continued over importing non-Christian strangers who spoke little, if any, English. But such doubts were more than offset by the prospect of laying claim to the children of slaves and to the lives and labor of all generations to come. In short, enslaved African women gave birth to additional workers, acquired by the master at no extra cost. These same women, moreover, were often more familiar with agricultural tasks than their European counterparts. Besides, planters could exploit black women and men more ruthlessly than they could whites without affecting future labor supplies.

Increasing life expectancy in the Chesapeake region, resulting from sturdier dwellings and more stable living conditions, further motivated planters to move away from a workforce of indentured servants. For a self-interested planter, longer lives meant that a white indentured person, after serving only a few years, would become yet another long-term competitor in the crowded tobacco market. In contrast, Africans enslaved for life would yield profitable service for an increasingly long time. And they would be more likely than ever to produce healthy offspring. Boys and girls who survived childhood could then be forced to clear more land to grow additional crops.

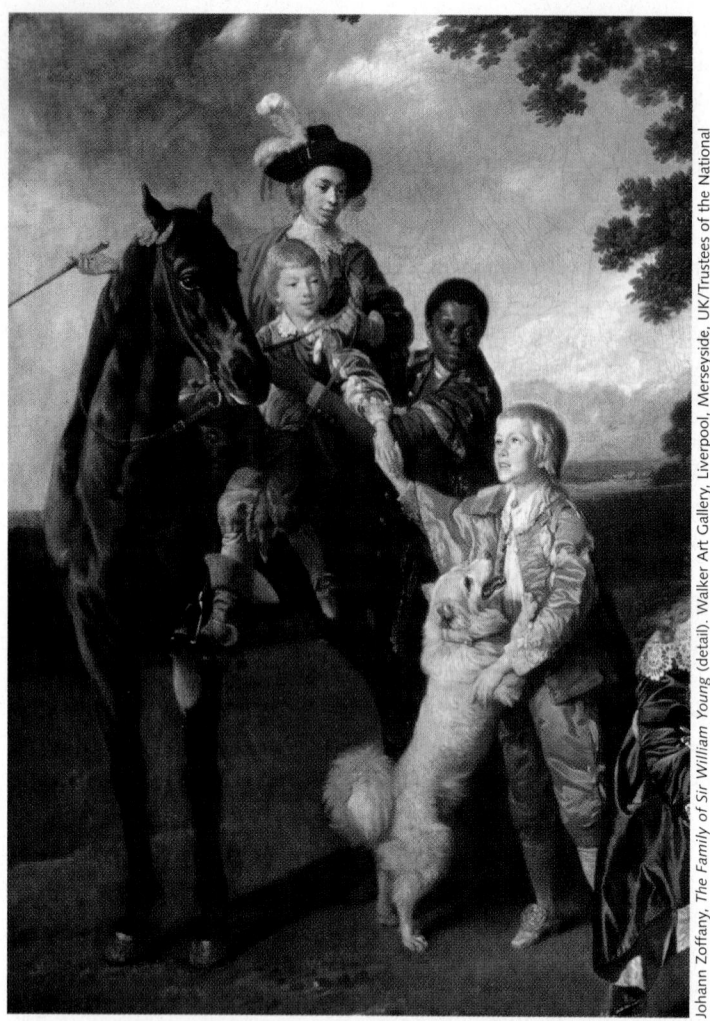

■ A small minority of enslaved Africans became house servants to wealthy families in England and America. Though set apart from the black community and denied entry into white society, many traveled widely and described the outside world to fellow slaves confined to field labor.

Among a circle of wealthy investors, the enticement of such an economic bonanza overcame any cultural anxieties or religious scruples. Seizing the moment, these aggressive entrepreneurs established themselves as the leading families of Virginia. William Byrd was an apt example. The son of an English goldsmith, Byrd took over his uncle's trading post near the falls of the James River at age 18 and soon married into a prominent family. As a frontier resident, he joined briefly in Bacon's uprising. But by the 1680s, he occupied a seat on Virginia's council and held several high financial posts. With his salary, he bought up his neighbors' tobacco and shipped it to England. He then used the proceeds to purchase cloth, kettles, muskets, and beads for the Indian trade. After exchanging these goods for deerskins, he exported the skins at a profit. In return, he imported trade goods from London and slaves and rum from the Caribbean, all of which he sold to small planters for more tobacco so the lucrative cycle could begin again.

In the 1690s, Byrd moved his operations closer to the seat of power, which remained at Jamestown until the capital shifted to nearby Williamsburg in 1699. He established a large estate at Westover, on the north bank of the James River, where he used scores of imported slaves to expand his wealth and launch a family dynasty. By the 1730s, Byrd's son, like other wealthy slave owners, came to fear a "servile war" so violent that it would "tinge our rivers, as wide as they are, with blood."

But for early merchant-planters, the enormous profits offered by slavery outweighed the calculated risks. These ambitious men expected that the English-speaking Africans already present could assist in teaching newcomers to receive orders. They also assumed that slave laborers from diverse African societies could not communicate well enough with one another to cause dangerous disturbances. And of course, having now made skin color a determining feature of social order, they knew that black runaways could be spotted and apprehended readily in the free white community.

Closing the Vicious Circle in the Chesapeake

As the profitability of the slavery option increased, so did its appeal. In 1664 Maryland's governor had been unable to find a hundred planters whose "purses would endure" a scheme in which each bought one slave per year. As yet, there were "nott men of estates good enough to undertake such a buisnesse." But 40 years later, some 4500 people were enslaved in Maryland in a total population of 35,000. And the colony's assembly was taking further measures to encourage the importation of slaves. Growing demand meant that merchants and sea captains who had only occasionally dabbled in the transportation of slaves now devoted more time and larger ships to the enterprise. Expansion of the slave-trading infrastructure made African workers readily available and affordable.

As the supply of enslaved black newcomers grew larger, planters eager to strengthen their position manipulated the established headright system. Traditionally, under this system, the colonial government granted to any arriving head of household 50 acres for every family member or hired hand he brought into the colony. The incentive was intended to spur emigration from Europe, expand the free population, and develop the land through the establishment of family farms. But the wealthy planters who saw African slavery as a profitable labor source also controlled Virginia's legal system. For their own benefit, therefore, they extended the headright system so that a land bonus also went to anyone who purchased an African arrival as a lifelong slave. Thus, before the seventeenth century closed, a Virginia investor buying 20 slaves could also lay claim to headrights worth 1000 acres of land.

To consolidate their new regime, planters worked through the church and the legislature to separate whites from blacks legally and socially. They stigmatized interracial ties and undermined the position of free blacks. A 1691 Virginia statute decried the "abominable mixture and spurious issue" that resulted from "Negroes, mulattoes and Indians intermarrying" with English or other white people, as Bess Key and William Greensted had done. All such couples were "banished from this dominion forever." It also prohibited masters from granting freedom to any black or mulatto unless they provided that person's transportation out of the colony within six months.

Virginia's Negro Act of 1705 further underscored the stark new boundaries. It mandated that white servants who were mistreated had the right to sue their masters in county court. Slaves, in contrast, had no such right. Any enslaved person who tried to escape could be tortured and even dismembered in hopes of "terrifying others from the like practices." When masters or overseers killed a slave while inflicting punishment, they were automatically free of any felony charge, "as if such accident had never happened." And if slaves were killed or put to death by law, the owners would be paid public funds for the loss of their "property." In scarcely 40 years, a dire and long-lasting revolution had transformed the labor system of the Chesapeake with the full backing of the law.

England Enters the Atlantic Slave Trade

By the time planters in North America began to consider aggressively importing African labor in the last decades of the seventeenth century, the trans-Atlantic slave trade had been operating for more than a hundred years. The scope and duration of this forced exodus from Africa remain difficult to conceive. In nearly four centuries, more than 10 million people

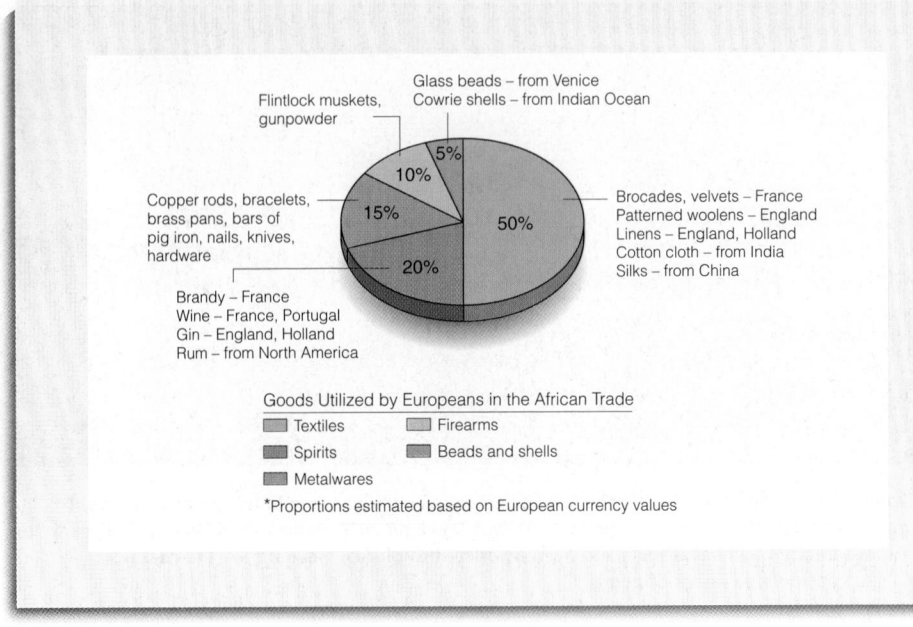

■ **FIGURE 4.1**
GOODS TRADED IN AFRICA As European ship captains expanded trade along the African coast, they tailored their cargoes to suit the demands of local markets.

were torn from their homelands against their will and transported to the Caribbean and to Central, South, and North America. Several million more perished during their abduction. The Atlantic slave trade remains the largest and longest-lasting deportation in human history. By 1700, more Africans than Europeans had already crossed the Atlantic to the Americas. Their numbers grew over the following century as the traffic reached its height and North America became an added destination in the trade.

England took little part in the trade at first. However, the development of Barbados as a lucrative sugar colony and the expansion of English overseas ambitions changed matters quickly after 1640. In 1652 Prince Rupert, a nephew of the late Charles I, visited Gambia in sub-Saharan Africa and saw profits to be made. With the restoration of the English monarchy in 1660, Rupert's cousin Charles II immediately granted a monopoly on African trade to a small group of adventurers, and in 1672 he chartered the powerful new Royal African Company (RAC). The RAC dispatched a steady flow of merchant ships to West Africa. Reaching English outposts along the coast on the first leg of a triangular trade pattern, the ships exchanged textiles, guns, and iron bars for gold, ivory, and enslaved Africans. After a trans-Atlantic "middle passage" of one to three months, the captains sold slaves and took on sugar in the West Indies before returning to England on the final leg of the triangle.

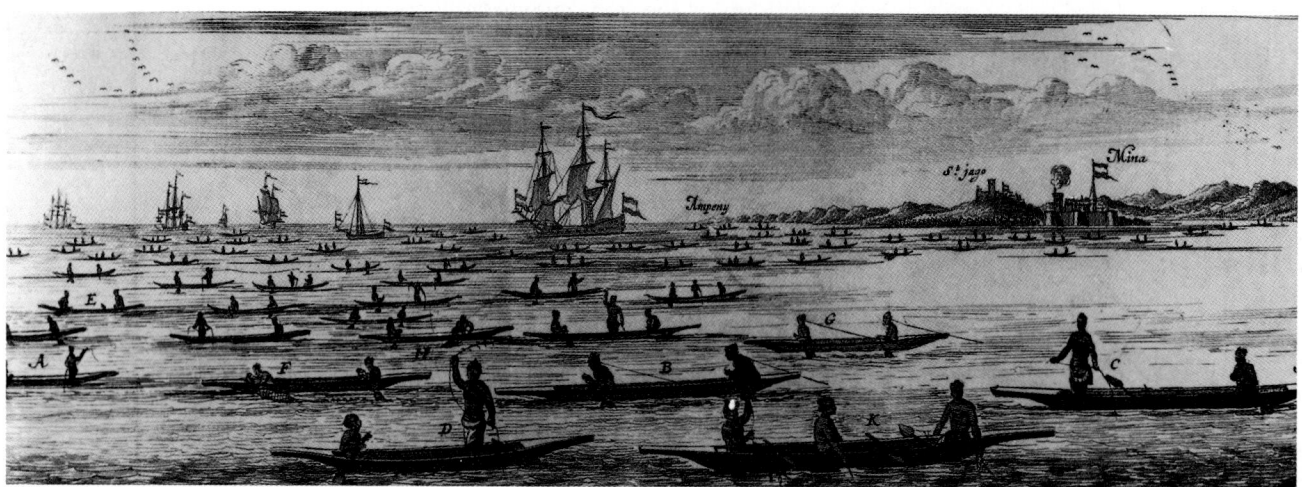

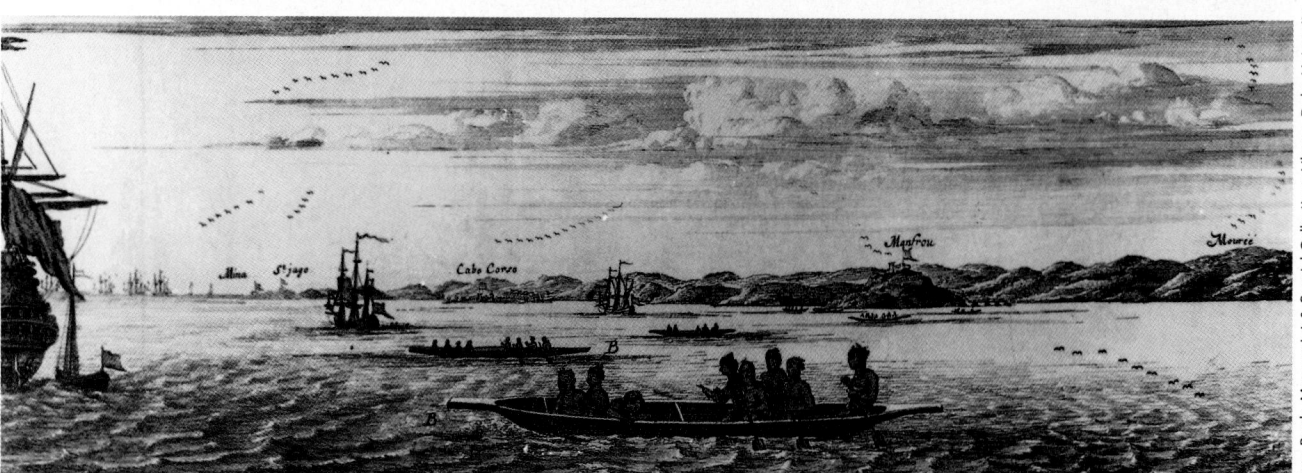

■ Captains anchoring off Elmina on the Gold Coast relied on Africans with fishing canoes (top) to ferry goods and slaves to their ships (bottom). Waves breaking over shallow sand bars made it hard "to carry canoes through without being sunk, overset, or split to pieces," leading to "the death of many...and considerable losses of goods."

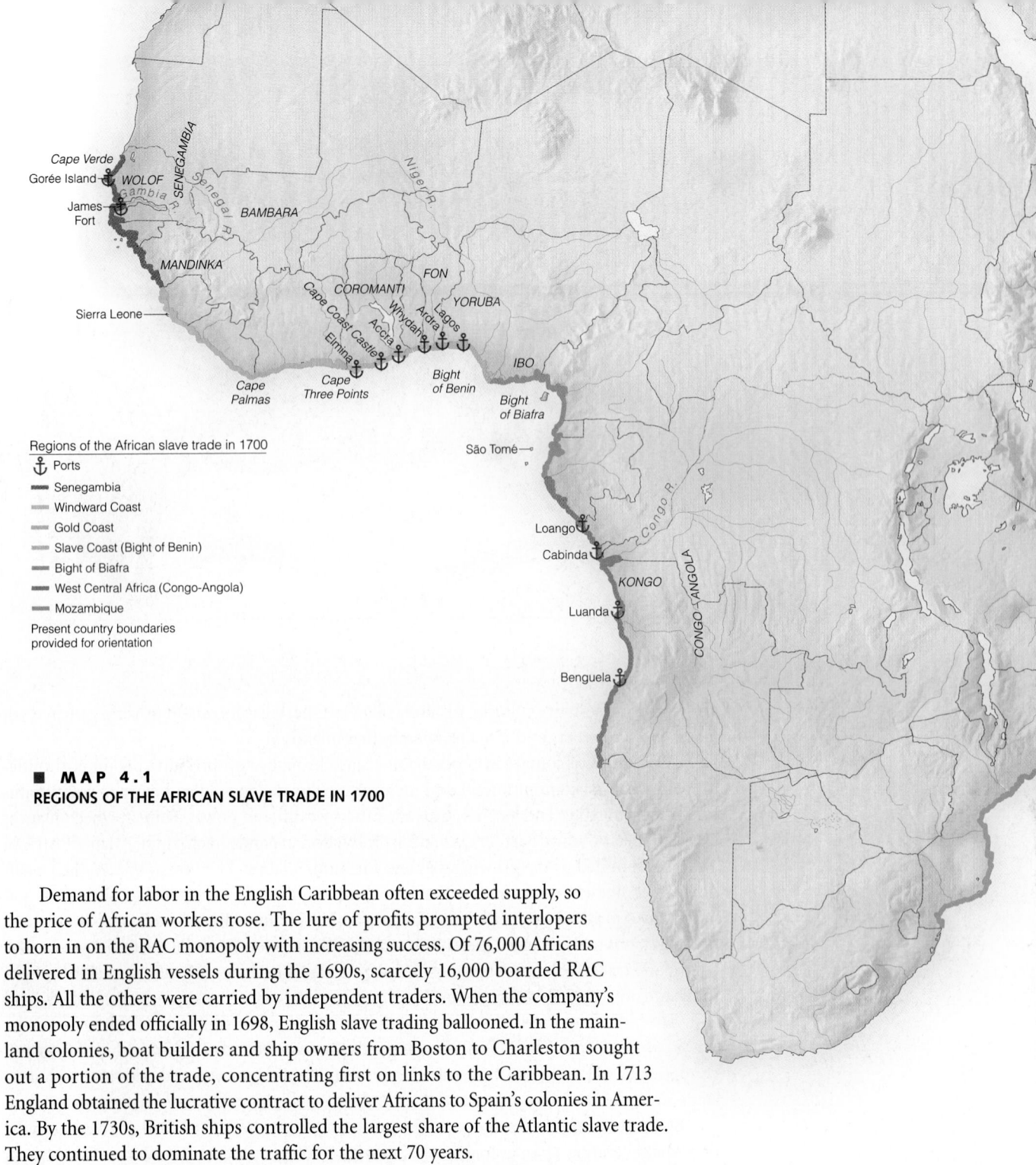

Regions of the African slave trade in 1700

⚓ Ports
▬ Senegambia
▬ Windward Coast
▬ Gold Coast
▬ Slave Coast (Bight of Benin)
▬ Bight of Biafra
▬ West Central Africa (Congo-Angola)
▬ Mozambique

Present country boundaries
provided for orientation

■ **MAP 4.1**
REGIONS OF THE AFRICAN SLAVE TRADE IN 1700

Demand for labor in the English Caribbean often exceeded supply, so the price of African workers rose. The lure of profits prompted interlopers to horn in on the RAC monopoly with increasing success. Of 76,000 Africans delivered in English vessels during the 1690s, scarcely 16,000 boarded RAC ships. All the others were carried by independent traders. When the company's monopoly ended officially in 1698, English slave trading ballooned. In the main-land colonies, boat builders and ship owners from Boston to Charleston sought out a portion of the trade, concentrating first on links to the Caribbean. In 1713 England obtained the lucrative contract to deliver Africans to Spain's colonies in Amer-ica. By the 1730s, British ships controlled the largest share of the Atlantic slave trade. They continued to dominate the traffic for the next 70 years.

The Slave Trade on the African Coast

By the 1680s, it had been two centuries since Portuguese sailors had visited Africa's western shores on both sides of the equator and established a factory at Elmina, in modern-day Ghana. Dozens of depots controlled by rival European powers and their local allies dotted the sub-Saharan coast-line. In the northwest, this string of primary ports and secondary "entrepots" (trading posts) began at the mouth of the Senegal River, just above Cape Verde, the continent's westernmost point. It ended more than 3000 miles to the southeast at outposts below the mouth of the Congo River, in present-day Angola. In between, the coastline curved some 5000 miles from the southwestern edge of the Sahara Desert almost to the Skeleton Coast in present-day Namibia. It embraced diverse geographic environments—from open savannas to thick forests—

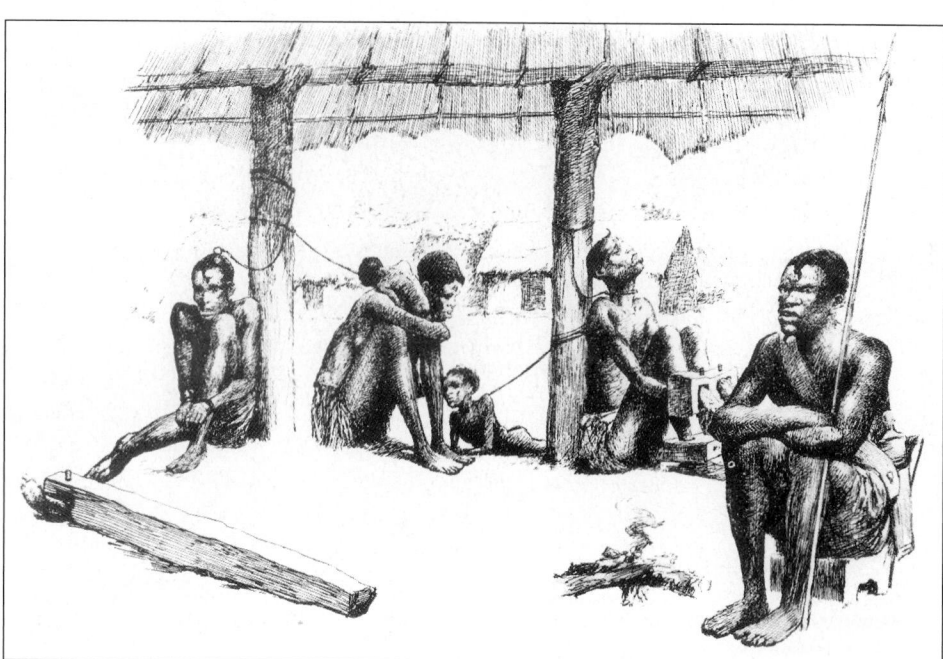

■ Slaves were held as prisoners in the interior before being marched to the African Coast in groups known as coffles.

and scores of distinctive cultures. All along this coastline, villagers caught fish and gathered salt for trade with herders and farmers living farther inland.

Generations of contact with oceangoing ships brought new pressures and opportunities to African coastal communities. Local merchants, who traded gold and ivory to sea captains for imported textiles and alcohol, expanded their wealth and power. Some formed alliances with European trading partners. As sugar production expanded across the Atlantic, African traders responded to the growing demand for human labor. They consolidated their positions near suitable harbors and navigable rivers. From there, they bartered local servants and war captives to white agents (factors). In return, they obtained linen, beads, metalwares, and muskets, items that enhanced their prestige and let them extend their inland trading networks.

Inland traders, alert to the rising demand for slaves in the port towns, annually brought thousands of captives from the backcountry to the coast. The traders traveled by land and water, binding their prisoners together in small groups to form a coffle (from the Arabic word for "caravan"). The overseas goods they received as payment included firearms, gunpowder, and knives, which they used to prosecute additional wars and raids in their homelands and to secure more captives.

By the 1660s and 1670s, the pace of deportation across the Atlantic had doubled from the previous generation to an average rate of nearly 15,000 people each year. It rose steadily to a high of more than 65,000 people per year a century later. As the traffic grew, it became increasingly organized, competitive, and routine. Shrewd African traders played one European vessel against another for the best deals and hid illness among captives. When they saw that a ship was eager to depart, they increased their prices. Hardened European agents stockpiled the wares that African traders most wanted. They also learned to curry favor with local officials and to quell unrest among captives, confined in the holding pens known as barracoons. Experienced captains mastered prevailing winds and currents and modified the holds of their ships to pack in larger cargoes. Increasingly, they timed their ventures to avoid the months when sickness was most rampant in the tropics. Through repeated voyages, improved charts, and accumulated lore, they came to differentiate and exploit half a dozen major slaving regions along Africa's Atlantic coast. On occasion, they even ventured to Mozambique in southeast Africa and the nearby island of Madagascar.

The closest market where Europeans bargained for goods and slaves was Senegambia, or the northern parts of Guinea, between the Senegal River and the Gambia River. Gorée Island, off the coast of Senegal, and James Fort, located in the mouth of the Gambia, served as slave trading centers. The long Windward Coast extending to the southeast beyond Sierra Leone became known for its pepper and grain and for ivory in the south beyond Cape Palmas. Due east on both sides of Cape Three Points stretched the Gold Coast. There, the Portuguese had established Elmina to draw trade from the Asante gold fields in the interior. Farther east, the Slave Coast reached along the Bight of Benin to the huge delta of the Niger River. Trading depots at Whydah, Ardra, and Lagos drew captives from secondary ports in between. Beyond the Niger, where the African coast again turns south near Cameroon, lay the Bight of Biafra. English captains quickly learned the preferences for trade goods in each district, carrying textiles to the Gold Coast, cowrie shells to the Slave Coast, and metals to the Bight of Biafra.

The largest and most southerly region, known as Congo-Angola or West Central Africa, was the only one below the equator. Elsewhere, Europeans did not exert direct control beyond an isolated coastal fortress or trading depot. But here, they held sway over a wider reach. Catholic missionaries had established early footholds. And Portuguese traders had exported slave labor for sugar production, first on the Atlantic island of São Tomé and later in Brazil and the Caribbean. Before 1700, more than half of all Atlantic slaves departed from West Central Africa. In the eighteenth century the proportion remained over one-third.

North of the Congo River, French and English interests came to dominate the slave traffic out of Loango and Cabinda. South of the great waterway, the Portuguese continued to hold the upper hand at Luanda and Benguela. During the entire span of the slave trade, the Congo-Angola hinterland furnished roughly 40 percent of all Atlantic deportees: more than 4.5 million men, women, and children.

The Middle Passage Experience

For every person the exodus was different, a harrowing personal story that depended on the particulars of how old the captives were, where they had lived, and how they were captured. Nevertheless, the long nightmare of deportation contained similar elements for all who fell victim to the trans-Atlantic trade. The entire journey, from normal village life to enslavement beyond the ocean, could last a year or two. It unfolded in at least five stages, beginning with capture and deportation to the African coast. The initial loss of freedom—the first experience of bound hands, harsh treatment, and forced marches—was made worse by the encounters with strange landscapes and unfamiliar languages. Attempts to escape usually proved futile, and initial thoughts of returning home gave way to worries about immediate survival. Hunger, fatigue, and anxiety took a steady toll as coffles of young and old were conveyed slowly toward the coast through a network of traders.

The next phase, sale and imprisonment, began when a contingent reached the sea. During this stage, which could last several months, African traders transferred "ownership" of the captives to Europeans. Many buyers subjected their new property to demeaning inspections and burned brands into their skin. In the confusion, prisoners often lost sight of kinfolk or fellow villagers for a final time. When the buyer was an independent trader, he had the Africans transported through the surf to his waiting vessel. (Their hands were bound, so if a canoe capsized in the waves, it meant certain drowning.) Once aboard, they might languish in the sweltering hold for weeks while the captain cruised the coast in search of additional human cargo.

Often, however, the European purchaser was an agent for a large company. His assignment was to gather up prisoners at small ports and carry them by coastal vessel to a major trade fort. There they were put in irons alongside hundreds of other captives and guarded in a secure spot to prevent escape. For example, the underground dungeon at Cape Coast Castle on the Gold Coast had walls 14 feet thick. A visitor in 1682 observed that the RAC's fortress provided

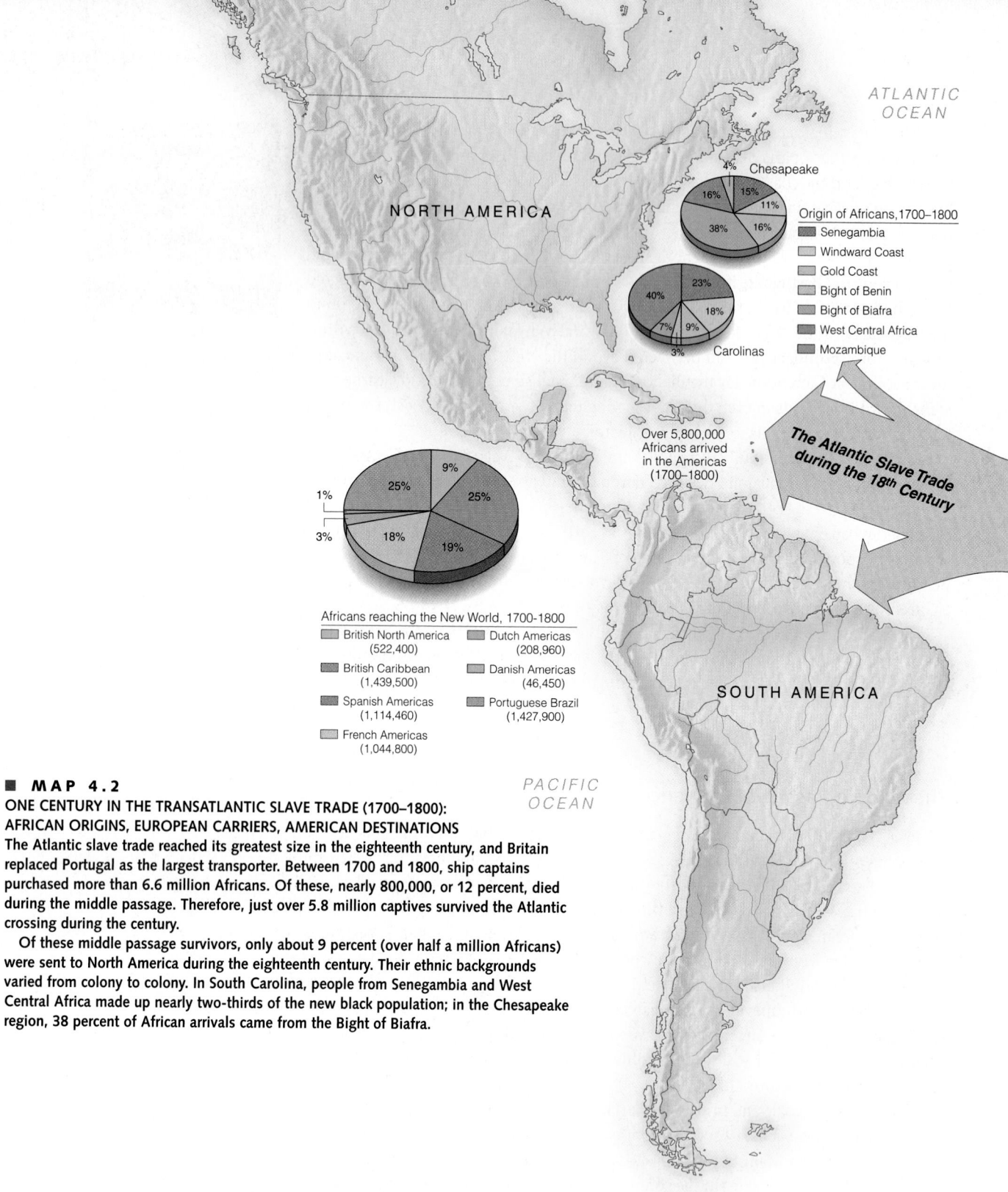

ATLANTIC OCEAN

NORTH AMERICA

Chesapeake

4%
16% 15%
11%
38% 16%

23%
40% 18%
7% 9%
3%
Carolinas

Origin of Africans, 1700–1800
- Senegambia
- Windward Coast
- Gold Coast
- Bight of Benin
- Bight of Biafra
- West Central Africa
- Mozambique

Over 5,800,000
Africans arrived
in the Americas
(1700–1800)

The Atlantic Slave Trade during the 18th Century

9%
25% 25%
1%
3% 18% 19%

Africans reaching the New World, 1700-1800
- British North America (522,400)
- British Caribbean (1,439,500)
- Spanish Americas (1,114,460)
- French Americas (1,044,800)
- Dutch Americas (208,960)
- Danish Americas (46,450)
- Portuguese Brazil (1,427,900)

SOUTH AMERICA

PACIFIC OCEAN

■ **MAP 4.2**
ONE CENTURY IN THE TRANSATLANTIC SLAVE TRADE (1700–1800):
AFRICAN ORIGINS, EUROPEAN CARRIERS, AMERICAN DESTINATIONS
The Atlantic slave trade reached its greatest size in the eighteenth century, and Britain replaced Portugal as the largest transporter. Between 1700 and 1800, ship captains purchased more than 6.6 million Africans. Of these, nearly 800,000, or 12 percent, died during the middle passage. Therefore, just over 5.8 million captives survived the Atlantic crossing during the century.

Of these middle passage survivors, only about 9 percent (over half a million Africans) were sent to North America during the eighteenth century. Their ethnic backgrounds varied from colony to colony. In South Carolina, people from Senegambia and West Central Africa made up nearly two-thirds of the new black population; in the Chesapeake region, 38 percent of African arrivals came from the Bight of Biafra.

"a good security . . . against any insurrection" before a ship arrived and the prisoners could be loaded aboard. According to one English trader, "the negroes were so wilful and loth to leave their own country, that they often leap'd out of the canoes, boat and ship, into the sea, and kept under water till they were drowned." Crew members sometimes raised nets surrounding the deck to prevent such attempts at escape or suicide.

The ship's captain decided when to begin crossing the Atlantic, the harrowing third phase that constituted the middle passage. Drawing on his sponsors' instructions, advice from local agents, and his own experience, he weighed the variables. If he lingered too long to obtain more

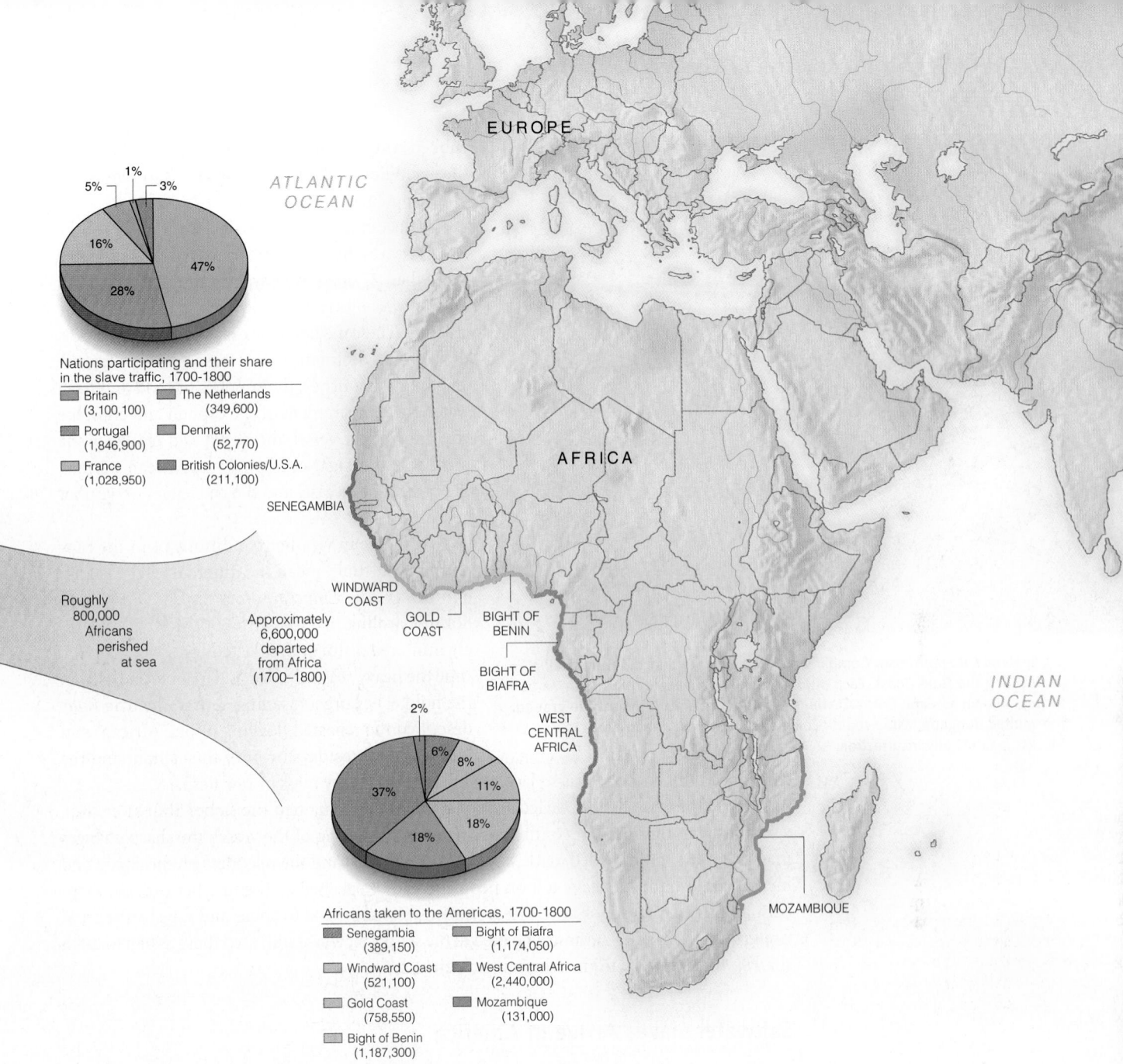

Nations participating and their share
in the slave traffic, 1700-1800

■ Britain (3,100,100)	■ The Netherlands (349,600)	
■ Portugal (1,846,900)	■ Denmark (52,770)	
■ France (1,028,950)	■ British Colonies/U.S.A. (211,100)	

Roughly 800,000 Africans perished at sea

Approximately 6,600,000 departed from Africa (1700–1800)

Africans taken to the Americas, 1700-1800

■ Senegambia (389,150)	■ Bight of Biafra (1,174,050)	
■ Windward Coast (521,100)	■ West Central Africa (2,440,000)	
■ Gold Coast (758,550)	■ Mozambique (131,000)	
■ Bight of Benin (1,187,300)		

slaves at lower prices, he risked depleting his food supplies and raising the death toll among his crew and prisoners. If he departed too soon in an effort to shorten the voyage and preserve lives, including his own, he risked missing a drop in prices or a new contingent of slaves that could absorb his remaining stock of trade goods and bring more profits. He had to balance the danger of late summer hurricanes in the Caribbean against the need to arrive in America when harvests were complete—the time when planters had crops to send to Europe and money or credit to invest in African workers.

The Africans aboard each ship knew nothing of such calculations. Even those who had spent time as slaves among fellow Africans or as fishermen in coastal waters now faced an utterly alien plight, trapped in a strange wooden hull. When the crew finally raised anchor and unfurled the vessel's huge sails, the captives could only anticipate the worst. Already the crowded hold had become foul, and the large wooden buckets used as latrines had taken on a loathsome smell. Now the rolling of the ship on ocean swells brought seasickness and painful chafing from lying on the bare planks. Alexander Falconbridge, who sailed as a surgeon on several slave ships, recorded that "those who are emaciated frequently have their skin and even their flesh entirely

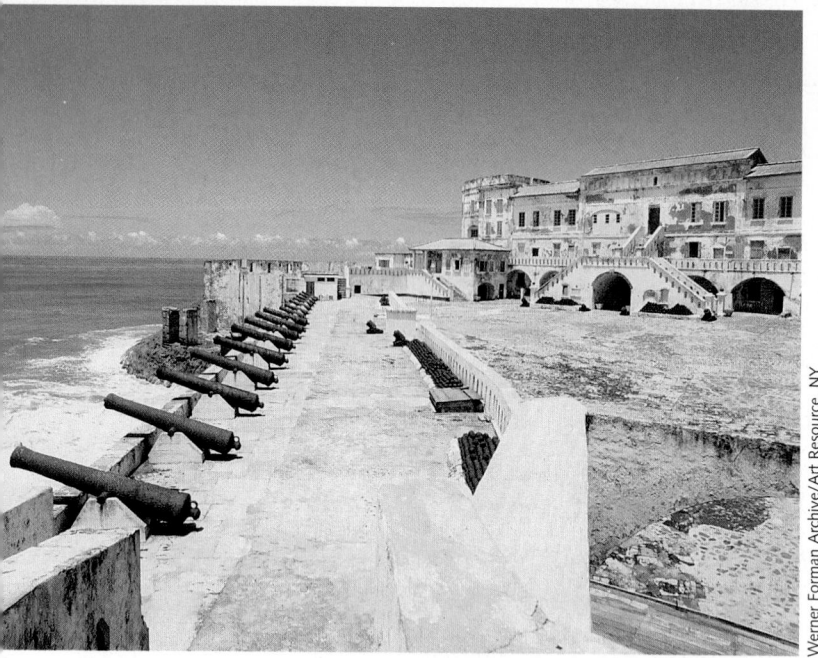

Werner Forman Archive/Art Resource, NY

■ England's Royal African Company maintained more than a dozen small posts along the Gold Coast. Each outpost funneled slaves to this strong 74-gun fortress known as Cape Coast Castle. Cut into rock beneath the parade ground, the vaulted dungeon inside could "conveniently contain a thousand Blacks…against any insurrection."

rubbed off, by the motion of the ship, from the…shoulders, elbows and hips so as to render the bones quite bare."

In its details, every crossing from Africa to the Americas was different. Historians have documented more than 27,000 slave voyages, and in each one an array of variables came into play to shape the Atlantic crossing. These included the exact point of departure, the planned destination, the season of the year, the length of the journey, the supplies of food and fresh water, the temperament of the captain and crew, the condition of the vessel, the health and resolve of the prisoners, the vagaries of piracy and ocean warfare, the ravages of disease, and the challenges of weather and navigation.

A change in weather conditions or in the captain's mood could mean the difference between life and death. The *Emperor,* crossing from Angola to South Carolina in 1755 with 390 Africans aboard, encountered a storm that lasted for a week. By the time the heavy seas subsided, 120 people had died in the hold. The surgeon sailing aboard the brig *Ruby* described the repeated flogging of one African man "for two or three days by both the captain and the chief mate until his body was so lacerated that it was a gory mass of raw flesh."

While the grim details varied, the overall pattern remained the same. Ship after ship, year after year, the attrition continued. The constant rolling of the vessel; the sharp changes in temperature; the crowded, dark, and filthy conditions; and the relentless physical pain and mental anguish took a heavy toll on people already weakened by their earlier ordeals. Pregnant mothers gave birth or miscarried; women were subjected to abuse and rape by the crew. Crews threw the bodies of those who died to the sharks or, worse still, used them as bait to catch sharks, which they fed to the remaining captives.

Saltwater Slaves Arrive in America

For the emaciated survivors of the Atlantic ordeal, two further stages remained in their descent into slavery: the selling process and the so-called time of seasoning. The selling process on American soil varied widely and could drag on for weeks or months. The colonial slave merchant or his agent came aboard soon after the ship dropped anchor, eager to inspect the human cargo. Once he assessed their origins, numbers, and condition, he saw to it that the crew washed and nourished the prisoners, oiled their bodies, and disguised their scars. Then the healthiest were paraded on deck for wealthy buyers or preferred customers. Those not sold immediately were transported to dockside holding pens, where they languished while advertisements circulated announcing their arrival and date of sale. Prospective owners examined and prodded the newcomers. Those purchased were wrenched away from their compatriots and the shipmates with whom they had formed strong links during their shared miseries at sea. Slaves often were auctioned off in groups, or parcels, to ensure sale of the weak along with the strong. Then another journey brought them to the particular slave labor camp where they were fated to work and probably to die.

If slaves arrived in the fall or winter, when spring planting was still a good way off, most newcomers did not begin their forced labor immediately. Instead, they entered a final stage, known as seasoning, which lasted several months or longer. The strangers were distinguished as "saltwater slaves"—in contrast to "country-born slaves" who had grown up in America from birth—and seasoning gave them time to mend physically, regain their strength, and begin absorbing the rudiments of a new language. Inevitably, many suffered from what we would now describe as posttraumatic stress syndrome.

As adults and children recovered from the trauma of the middle passage, they faced a series of additional shocks. Around them they found other Africans who had survived earlier voyages and still spoke their traditional languages. In conversation, they gradually learned where they were and what lay in store for them. They confronted strange foods, unfamiliar tasks, and even new names. They faced alien landscapes and unfamiliar diseases. Worst of all, they encountered a master or his overseer who viewed the seasoning phase as a time to test the spirit of the saltwater newcomers. He made every effort to break the wills of these fresh arrivals and to turn them into compliant bondservants. Repeatedly, the powerful stranger used arbitrary force to demand the slaves' obedience, destroy their hope, and crush any thoughts of resistance.

Survival in a Strange New Land

By 1700 race slavery was accepted throughout the mainland colonies, so Africans found themselves scattered from northern New England to the Carolinas. But their distribution was far from even, for northern locations received only a small portion of the slave traffic to the North American continent. Among roughly 247,000 slaves in the colonies in 1750, only 30,000 (or 12 percent) resided in the North, where they made up just 5 percent of the overall population from Pennsylvania to New Hampshire. More than one-third of these northerners (11,000) lived in the colony of New York, where they made up as much as 14 percent of the inhabitants. All the rest of the people of African descent in North America—some 217,000 men, women, and children by the mid-eighteenth century—lived and worked in the Chesapeake region and the lower South. (Fewer than 5000 of these black southerners resided in French Louisiana.)

African Rice Growers in South Carolina

Throughout the eighteenth century, by far the most North American slaves lived in Virginia or Maryland: 150,000 African Americans by 1750. But the highest *proportion* of enslaved workers lived in South Carolina, where Africans began outnumbering Europeans as early as 1708. By 1750 this black majority (40,000 people) constituted more than 60 percent of the colony's population. Almost all had arrived through the deepwater port of Charleston. Sullivan's Island, near the entrance to the harbor, with its so-called pest house to quarantine incoming slaves and reduce the spread of shipborne disease, has been called the Ellis Island of black America.

What explains the emergence of South Carolina's slave concentration? For one thing, the colony was closer than Virginia to Africa and to the Caribbean. Moreover, it had been founded in 1670, just as the English were embracing plantation slavery and the African trade. Indeed, some of the colony's original proprietors had a stake in the Royal African Company. Also, some of Carolina's influential early settlers came directly from Barbados, bringing enslaved Africans and planter ambitions with them.

In the earliest days of colonization in South Carolina, however, workers of any kind were few in number. The colonists lacked sufficient labor to clear coastal forests and plant crops. Instead, they let their cattle and pigs run wild. With easy foraging and warm winters, the animals reproduced rapidly. The settlers slaughtered them and shipped their meat to the

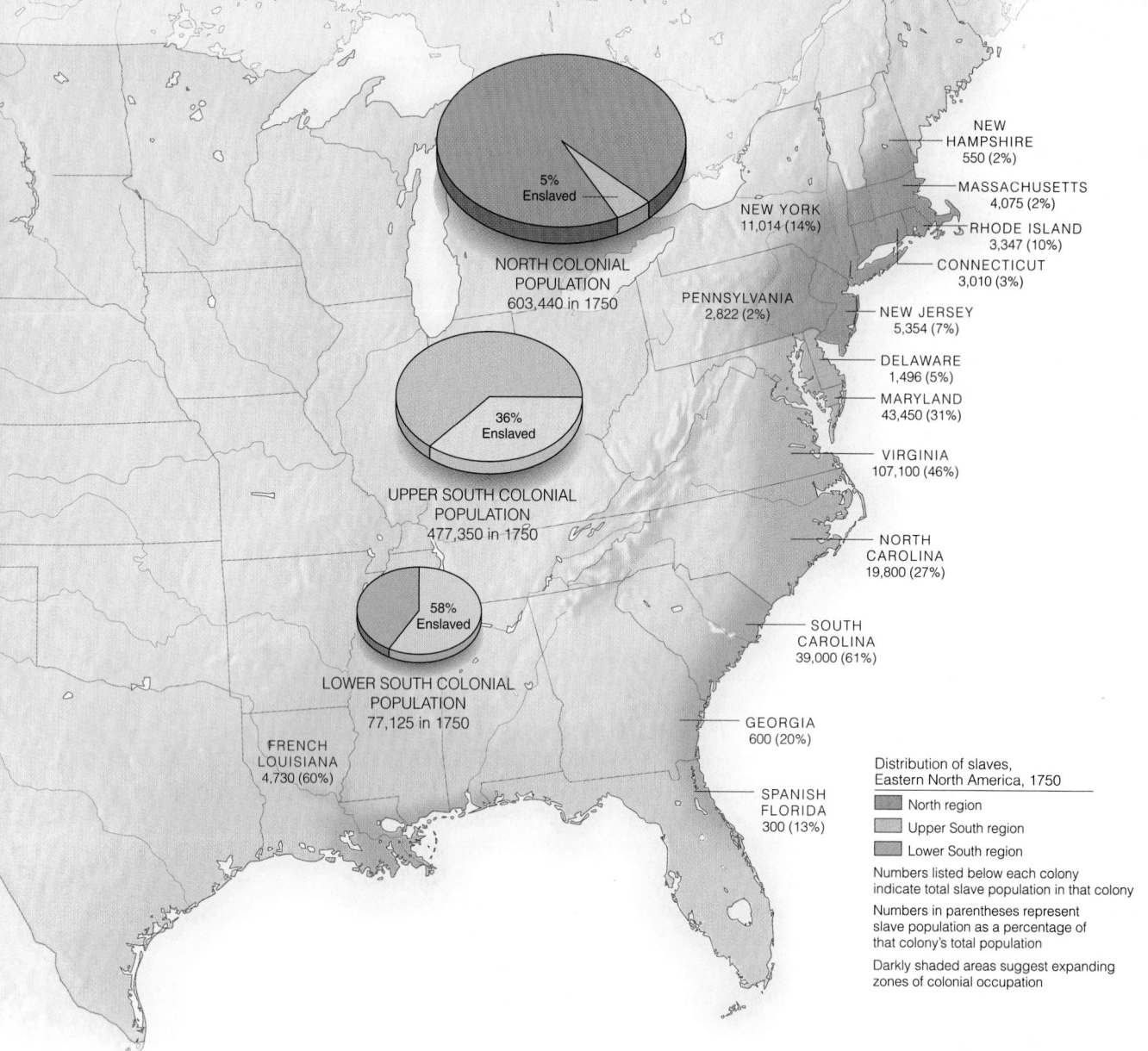

NEW
HAMPSHIRE
550 (2%)

MASSACHUSETTS
4,075 (2%)

NEW YORK
11,014 (14%)

RHODE ISLAND
3,347 (10%)

CONNECTICUT
3,010 (3%)

NORTH COLONIAL
POPULATION
603,440 in 1750

5%
Enslaved

PENNSYLVANIA
2,822 (2%)

NEW JERSEY
5,354 (7%)

DELAWARE
1,496 (5%)

MARYLAND
43,450 (31%)

VIRGINIA
107,100 (46%)

36%
Enslaved

UPPER SOUTH COLONIAL
POPULATION
477,350 in 1750

NORTH
CAROLINA
19,800 (27%)

58%
Enslaved

SOUTH
CAROLINA
39,000 (61%)

LOWER SOUTH COLONIAL
POPULATION
77,125 in 1750

FRENCH
LOUISIANA
4,730 (60%)

GEORGIA
600 (20%)

SPANISH
FLORIDA
300 (13%)

Distribution of slaves,
Eastern North America, 1750

■ North region

■ Upper South region

■ Lower South region

Numbers listed below each colony
indicate total slave population in that colony

Numbers in parentheses represent
slave population as a percentage of
that colony's total population

Darkly shaded areas suggest expanding
zones of colonial occupation

■ **MAP 4.3**

**ENSLAVED PEOPLE LIVING IN NORTH AMERICA IN 1750: DISTRIBUTION BY COLONY, PERCENTAGE
OF TOTAL POPULATION** By 1750 nearly a quarter of a million people lived as slaves in eastern North
America—more than 21 percent of the colonial population. Almost all were Africans or the descendants of
Africans, along with a few thousand Native American and mixed-race slaves. In the North, slaves made up a
small fraction of a large population. By far the greatest number of slaves lived in the Chesapeake area,
where they made up more than a third of the total population. Enslaved people were less numerous but
much more concentrated in the lower South, making up a clear majority of the overall inhabitants. White
settlers had already smuggled several hundred slaves into the fledgling colony of Georgia, even though the
exploitation of slave labor did not become legal there until 1751.

Caribbean, along with firewood for boiling sugar cane and barrels for transporting sugar.
Ship captains also carried enslaved Native Americans to the West Indies and brought back
African slaves.

The new arrivals understood South Carolina's subtropical climate, with its alligators and pal-
metto trees, better than their European owners did. Many of these enslaved newcomers were
already familiar with keeping cattle. Others, obliged to feed themselves, began growing rice in the
fertile swamplands just as they had in West Africa. Slave owners quickly realized that this plant,
unfamiliar to much of northern Europe, held the answer to their search for a profitable staple

crop. Soon, people who had tended their own irrigated rice crops near the Gambia River were obliged to clear cypress swamps along the Ashley and Cooper rivers to grow rice for someone else. Women who had prepared small portions of rice daily for their families in West Africa—pounding the grains with a wooden pestle to remove the husks, then tossing them in a broad, flat basket to winnow away the chaff—now had to process vast quantities of rice for export.

Before long, people in England had developed a taste for rice pudding, and London merchants were shipping tons of Carolina rice to other European countries, where it proved a cheap grain for feeding soldiers, orphans, and peasants. By the middle of the eighteenth centruy, South Carolina's white minority had the most favorable trade balance of any mainland colonists. Their fortunes improved even more when indigo, another African crop, joined rice as a profitable export commodity. Outnumbered by their enslaved workers, South Carolina's landowners passed strict Negro Acts patterned on those of the Caribbean. Legislation prohibited slaves from carrying guns, meeting in groups, raising livestock, or traveling without a pass. Statutes controlled everything from how they dressed to when they shoveled the dung off of Charleston streets. Everywhere, mounted patrols enforced the regulations with brutal severity.

Patterns of Resistance

In South Carolina and elsewhere, enslaved African Americans pushed against the narrow boundaries of their lives. Like any other imprisoned population, they pressed steadily for small indulgences. Then they worked, individually and collectively, to turn occasional concessions into customary rights. And like others held prisoner, they used every possible means to negotiate slivers of freedom, including spreading rumors, refusing to work, breaking tools, feigning illness, and threatening violence. In response, their owners tried to divide them in order to control them. Masters rewarded workers who acted obedient and diligent or who informed on fellow slaves. They imposed harsh punishments—whipping, mutilation, sale, or death—on those suspected of taking food, sowing dissent, or plotting revolt. And they encouraged the formation of black families, not only to gain another generation of laborers at no cost but also to create the emotional ties that they knew would hold individuals in check for fear of reprisals against loved ones.

Owners confined residents in the slave labor camps with curfews and pass systems and kept them from learning to read and from communicating freely with neighbors and relatives. They also refused to allow any impartial system for expressing grievances or appealing arbitrary punishments. Faced with such steep odds, many slaves submitted to the deadening routine of the prison camp to survive. But others resorted to diverse strategies to improve their situation or undermine their masters' dominance. Running away, even for a brief period, provided relief from forced work and deprived owners of the labor they depended on. Frequent newspaper advertisements regarding runaways reveal that thousands risked their lives, alone or in groups, in attempts to escape. Because arson created serious damage and was difficult to detect, some slaves burned down barns at harvest time. Others succeeded in killing their masters or overseers. Such acts of pent-up rage usually proved suicidal, but they also confirmed slave owners' worst fears. Aware that Africans knew how to communicate with one another with drums and could concoct poisons from herbs, white planters became even more fearful of blacks.

Above all, the prospect of open rebellion kept burning in the minds of prisoners and jailers alike. In light of this constant tension, it is hard to untangle episodes of white paranoia from incidents of actual revolt. Many innocent slaves were falsely accused. But countless others did discuss plans for resistance, and a few freedom fighters avoided detection or betrayal long enough to launch serious uprisings. Word of one upheaval, real or imagined, could spark others.

An early wave of slave unrest erupted in the dozen years after 1710, highlighted by violence in New York City in the spring of 1712. The leaders of the conspiracy were "Coromantee," or

June 27, 1734

RUN away on Thursday last from the House of John Richardson, Shoemaker, a new Negroe Girl about 16 or 18 Years of Age, short Stature, branded upon the Breast N R mark'd round the Neck with three Rows like Beads, suppos'd to be a Whedaw Negroe; had on a check'd Cotten Petticoat and a Seersucker Jacket. Her Name is Rose.

Whosoever takes up said Negroe, and brings her to John Richardson aforesaid, or B. Franklin Printer, shall have Twenty Shillings Reward and reasonable Charges paid by   John Richardson.

November 2, 1749

Philadelphia, November 2, 1749.
RUN away three weeks ago, from Marcus Kuhl, of Philadelphia, baker, a Negroe man, named Scipio, wears a blue broad cloth coat, or a black ditto, old shoes, and stockings, of a short stature, plays on the banjou, and sings with it, speaks but indifferent English. Whoever takes up and secures said slave, so that his master may have him again, shall have Fifteen Shillings reward, and reasonable charges, paid by
MARCUS KUHL.

October 26, 1758

Philadelphia, October 24, 1758
RUN away, on the 21st Instant, from Robert Wakely, of this City, a Negro Woman, named Anne, about 18 or 20 Years of Age, is short and well set, and had on a blue Jacket and Petticoat, Ozenbrigs Apron, and an old Cap, but no Shoes or Stockings. Also run away, at the same Time, a Negroe Man, named Frank, belonging to Alexander Collay, of Whitemarsh, about 30 or 35 Years of Age, is a slender middle sized Fellow, and had on a new Wool Hat, Bearskin light coloured Coat, a Snuff coloured Jacket, without Sleeves, a striped Shirt, Leather Breeches, blue Stockings and good Shoes. They are Man and Wife, and supposed to be gone together. Whoever takes up said Negroes, and brings them to either of the Subscribers, shall have fifty Shillings Reward for both, or if put into the next Goal where taken up Forty Shillings, paid by
ROBERT WAKELY, or ALEXANDER COLLAY.

■ **FIGURE 4.2**
RREWARD NOTICES FOR ESCAPED SLAVES, PRINTED IN THE *PENNSYLVANIA GAZETTE* The Philadelphia newspaper published more than 1000 such advertisements between 1728 and 1790. They provide historians with detailed information about the lives of slaves.

Akan people from Africa's Gold Coast region. Several dozen enslaved Africans and Indians, determined to obtain their freedom and kill all the whites in the town, set fire to a building. As citizens rushed to put out the blaze, the rebels attacked them with guns, clubs, pistols, staves, and axes, killing eight and wounding more. When the militia finally captured the insurgents, six of them committed suicide. Authorities condemned 21 others and executed 18. They burned several at the stake, hanged others, and left their bodies on display. Eager to curtail slavery following such unrest, the governor called for "the Importation of White Servants." New York's elected colonial assembly, expressing growing racial hatred, chastised free blacks and prohibited freed slaves from owning property.

A Wave of Rebellion

A second wave of black resistance swept the mainland colonies after 1730, fueled by the largest influx of Africans to date. In Louisiana, the French had moved their capital to the new town of New Orleans on the Mississippi River (1722) and had joined their Choctaw allies in a devastating war to crush the Natchez Indians and seize their lands (1729–1731). As French landowners staked out riverfront plantations, they also imported African slaves. The several thousand black workers soon outnumbered European settlers. Fearful of attack, the whites broke up two presumed slave plots in 1731. One involved a scheme to rebel while Catholic colonists attended a midnight mass on Christmas.

Another apparent plot was revealed by the careless boast of a black servant woman in New Orleans. It included several hundred Bambara newcomers from Senegal who were determined to massacre whites, enslave other Africans, and take control of the region. The leader among eight captured plotters was a man known as Samba Bambara. A former interpreter at Galam on the Senegal River, Bambara had recently lost that post and been deported to Louisiana. There, he became a trusted slave, supervising workers owned by the French Company of the Indies. When torture by fire failed to force confessions from the captives, officials hanged the servant woman and broke Bambara and half a dozen other men on the wheel.

The largest slave uprising in colonial North America broke out in 1739 near the Stono River, 20 miles southwest of Charleston. Several factors fueled the Stono Rebellion. By 1739, blacks exceeded whites nearly two to one among South Carolina's 56,000 people. The proportion of recently imported slaves had reached an all-time high. In addition, working conditions had worsened steadily as rice production expanded. Moreover, for several decades the Spanish in Florida had been luring slaves from South Carolina, knowing that the promise of freedom might destabilize Carolina's profitable slave regime. More than a hundred fugitives had escaped to Florida by 1738, when Florida's governor formed them into a free black militia company at St. Augustine. Hoping to win more defections, he allowed 38 African American households to settle north of the city and build a small fortress—Fort Mose.

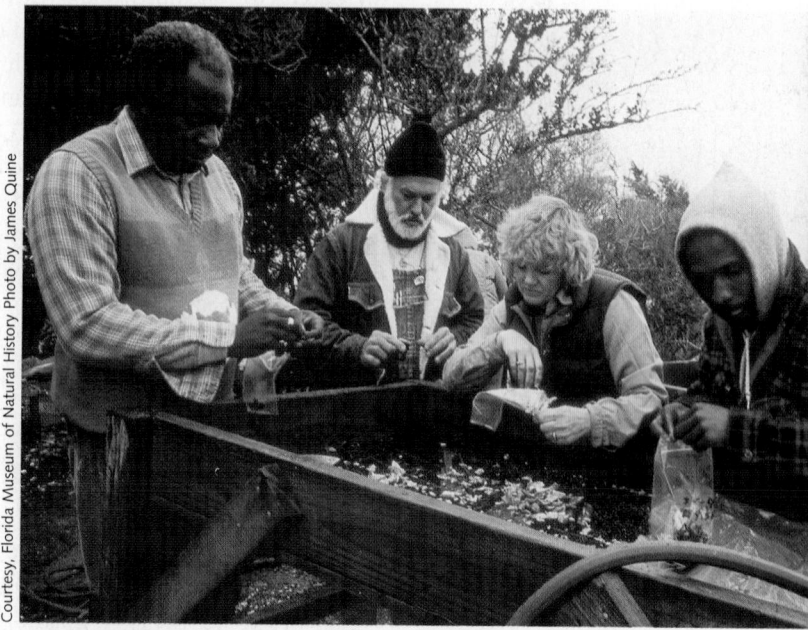

Courtesy, Florida Museum of Natural History Photo by James Quine

■ Archaeologists have recently excavated the site of Fort Mose, near St. Augustine, Florida. Dozens of slaves who escaped from South Carolina received their freedom from the Spanish and established an outpost there in the 1730s.

Meanwhile, the wider commercial rivalries of the British and Spanish continued elsewhere, leading to open warfare between the two Atlantic empires in 1739. The slave uprising at Stono erupted just after word reached Charleston that war had broken out between Spain and Britain. Perhaps this was mere coincidence. Or perhaps the news sparked hopes among slaves that Carolina authorities would be preoccupied and vulnerable, or that Spanish neighbors would assist a revolt in the colony. Other factors may also have influenced the rebels' timing. An epidemic in Charleston had disrupted public activities, and a new Security Act requiring all white men to carry arms to church was to take effect before the end of September.

Early on Sunday, September 9, 1739, 20 slaves from a work crew near the Stono River broke into a local store. There they seized weapons and executed the owners. Led by a man named Jemmy, they raised a banner and marched south, beating drums and shouting "Liberty!" The insurgents burned selected plantations, killed a score of whites, and gathered more than 50 new recruits. But armed colonists overtook them near the Edisto River and blocked their escape to St. Augustine. Dozens of rebels died in the ensuing battle. In the next two days militia and hired Indians killed 20 more and captured an additional 40 people, whom they immediately shot or hanged.

Yet even these reprisals could not quell black hopes. In June 1740 several hundred slaves plotted to storm Charleston and take arms from a warehouse. However, a comrade revealed the plan. According to a report, "The next day fifty of them were seized, and these were hanged, ten a day, to intimidate the other negroes." In November, a great fire of suspicious origin consumed much of Charleston.

Fire also played a role in hysteria that broke out in New York City in 1741. Britain's ongoing conflict with Spain (1739–1743) fanned wild Protestant fears that Jesuit spies and Catholic slaves planned to burn the major towns in English North America. In March, a blaze consumed the residence of New York's governor and a local fort. Other fires soon focused suspicions on a white couple, John and Sarah Hughson, who had often entertained blacks at their alehouse. The Hughsons—thought to fence stolen goods for a black crime ring, the Geneva Boys—were accused of inciting working-class unrest. In exchange for her freedom, Mary Barton, a 16-year-old Irish indentured servant at the Hughsons' tavern, testified that she had overheard the planning of an elaborate "popish plot."

In a gruesome spiral of arrests and executions, New York authorities put to death 34 people, including 4 whites, and banished 72 blacks. On one hand, the debacle recalled the Salem witch trials, as a fearful community engaged in judicial proceedings and killings on the basis of rumors and accusations. On the other hand, the New York Slave Plot recalled Bacon's Rebellion, for evidence emerged of cooperation between impoverished blacks and whites eager to see a redistribution of property. According to his accusers, a slave named Cuffee had often observed that "a great many people had too much, and others too little." He predicted that soon his master "should have less, and that he (Cuffee) should have more." Instead, he was burned at the stake.

The Transformation Completed

Word of the Stono Rebellion and the New York Slave Plot, plus rumors of uprisings in the West Indies, brought renewed hope to enslaved Americans and renewed fear to their captors. The mechanisms for extorting labor from tens of thousands of people were firmly in place. But to maintain this repressive system, local governments and the white population had to keep up constant vigilance and continually threaten blacks. In South Carolina, officials displayed the heads of slain rebels on poles, stepped up night patrols, and passed an even harsher Negro Law.

Some colonists saw slavery as too morally degrading and physically dangerous to maintain, but others found it too rewarding to give up. As in later generations, powerful supporters of the institution suggested modifications in response to calls for outright abolition. For example, white officials in Charleston imposed a heavy duty on new African arrivals for several years, hoping to increase the ratio of white to black slaves in the lowcountry of coastal South Carolina. They also opened a school to provide rudimentary education to a handful of obedient black Christians. At a time of growing humanitarian concerns in Enlightenment Europe, it took great effort to maintain the rationale for enslavement in America. But free people who

"Releese Us out of This Cruell Bondegg"

As researchers pay increasing attention to African bondage in the colonial era, new pieces of evidence continue to appear. This appeal, written in Virginia in 1723 by a mulatto Christian slave, was rediscovered in a London archive in the 1990s and transcribed by historian Thomas Ingersoll. It is addressed to Edward Gibson, the newly appointed bishop of London, whose position gave him religious oversight over all the Anglican parishes in England's American colonies, including Virginia. Gibson, through his pamphlets, had shown an interest in the Christianization of enslaved Africans, but like many contemporary church leaders, he had less interest in the liberation of slaves. This heartfelt document, prepared with great labor and at enormous risk, was simply filed away with the bishop's vast correspondence. It never received a response or prompted any further inquiry into conditions in Virginia.

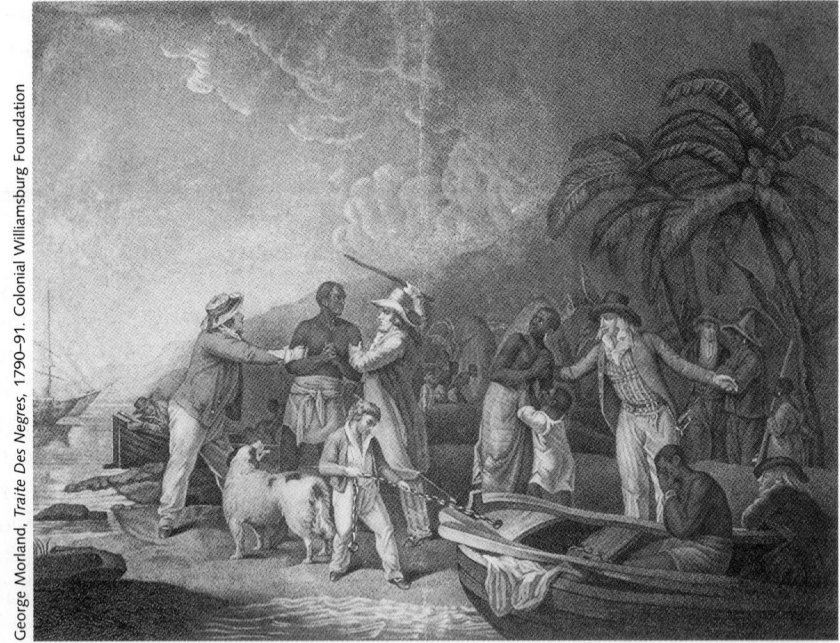

George Morland, *Traite Des Negres*, 1790–91. Colonial Williamsburg Foundation

When abolition of the slave trade finally became a public issue in England in the 1780s, British artists painted scenes criticizing the traffic. But two generations earlier, pleas from New World slaves aroused no response, even from the Bishop of London, who supervised the Church of England in the American colonies.

August the forth 1723

to the Right Raverrand father in god my Lord arch Bishop of Lonnd. . . .

this coms to sattesfie your honour that there is in this Land of verJennia a Sort of people that is Calld molatters which are Baptised and brouaht up in the way of the Christian faith and followes the ways and Rulles of the Chrch of England and sum of them has white fathars and sum white mothers and there is in this Land a Law or act which keeps and makes them and there seed Slaves forever. . . .

wee your humbell and poore partishinners doo begg Sir your aid and assisttancce in this one thing . . . which is that your honour will by the help of our Sufvering [i.e., sovereign] Lord King George and the Rest of the Rullers will Releese us out of this Cruell Bondegg. . . . /and here it is to bee notd that one brother is a Slave to another and one Sister to an othe which is quite out of the way and as for mee my selfe I am my brothers Slave but my name is Secrett/

wee are commandded to keep holey the Sabbath day and wee doo hardly know when it comes for our task mastrs are has hard with us as the Egypttions was with the Chilldann of Issarall. . . . wee are kept out of the Church and matrimony is deenied us and to be plain they doo Look no more upon us then if wee ware dogs which I hope when these Strange lines comes to your Lord Ships hands will be Looket in to. . . .

And Sir wee your humble perticners do humblly beg . . . that our childarn may be broatt up in the way of the Christtian faith and our desire is that they may be Larnd the Lords prayer the creed and the ten commandements and that they may appeare Every Lord's day att Church before the Curatt to bee Exammond for our desire is that godllines Shoulld abbound amongs us and wee desire that our Childarn be putt to Scool and Larnd to Reed through the Bybell

My Riting is vary bad. . . . I am but a poore Slave that writt itt and has no other time butt Sunday and hardly that att Sumtimes. . . . wee dare nott Subscribe any mans name to this for feare of our masters for if they knew that wee have Sent home to your honour wee Should goo neare to Swing upon the gallass tree. ■

Source: Thomas N. Ingersoll, "'Releese Us out of This Cruell Bondegg': An Appeal from Virginia in 1723," *William and Mary Quarterly,* Third Series, 51 (October 1994):776–782.

questioned the institution met stiff resistance from those with vested interests, as the experience of the new colony of Georgia demonstrates.

Voices of Dissent

As race-based slavery expanded numerically and geographically, white colonists treated the continuing presence of free blacks as a contradiction and a threat. As early as 1691, the Virginia assembly passed an act restricting manumissions (grants of individual freedom by masters) because "great inconvenience may happen to this country by setting of negroes and mulattoes free." According to the act, such people fanned hopes of freedom among enslaved blacks by their mere presence. Since most free blacks were quite poor, they were often accused of having links to the slave community and trafficking in stolen goods. Besides, when they grew old and infirm, their care at public expense could constitute "a charge upon the country." By 1723, additional Virginia statutes prevented free people of color from voting, taxed them unfairly, and prevented them from owning or carrying firearms. Lawmakers went on to prohibit manumissions altogether, except when the governor rewarded "meritorious service," such as informing against other enslaved workers.

While the southern slave colonies labored to intimidate, divide, and reduce their free black communities, free blacks in the North faced growing discrimination in their efforts to hold jobs, buy land, obtain credit, move freely, and take part in civic life. Northern slave populations, though small in comparison to those in the South, were growing steadily. As the North's involvement in the Atlantic slave trade expanded, its economic and legal commitment to race slavery increased. Rhode Island's slave ranks jumped from 500 in 1720 to more than 3000 in 1750. Everywhere, new laws made manumission more difficult and African American survival more precarious. In Philadelphia, only 90 slaves gained their freedom between 1698 and 1765. Of the few hundred free blacks living in Boston in 1742, 110 resided in the church-supported almshouse and another 36 in the public workhouse. Only in the century after 1760 did northern free black communities gain the numerical and social strength to offer effective opposition to enslavement.

Whereas free blacks lacked the means to oppose slavery, prominent white Christians lacked the will. Even in Massachusetts, where religion remained a dominant force at the turn of the century and the number of slaves had scarcely reached 1000 people, many leaders already owned black servants. They used them more to flaunt their prosperity than to expand their wealth. When Boston merchants purchased black attendants to serve as coachmen, few citizens objected.

The protests that did appear were ambivalent at best. In 1700 Judge Samuel Sewell questioned African enslavement in a tract titled *The Selling of Joseph*. But he also revealed his sense of superiority and his skepticism that blacks could play a part in "the Peopling of the Land." African Americans, Sewell commented, "can seldom use their freedom well; yet their continual aspiring after their forbidden Liberty, renders them unwilling servants." Reverend Cotton Mather, a slave owner who once berated Sewell as one who "pleaded much for Negroes," was even more ambivalent. In *The Negro Christianized* (1706), the influential Puritan stressed that conversion and Christian instruction, far from earning African slaves their freedom, would make them into "better servants."

The conversion and instruction of slaves, rather than the abolition of slavery, also became a mission for pious English philanthropist Thomas Bray, a well-to-do Anglican committed to religious education and prison reform. In 1699, Bray founded the Society for Promoting Christian Knowledge to organize libraries in the fledgling colonies. The following year, the bishop of London sent Bray to Maryland. He soon returned to England with a desire to train better ministers and to spread the Anglican faith in America among Europeans, Indians, and Africans. In 1701 Bray established the Society for the Propagation of the Gospel in Foreign Parts (SPG).

The SPG strengthened the Church of England abroad in the eighteenth century by providing dozens of ministers to serve in the colonies. But this improved foothold came at a steep price. Southern planters made SPG ministers agree that any promise they offered to slaves regarding heavenly salvation would not include hints of earthly freedom. With few exceptions, the Anglican clergy gave in, strengthening religious support of race slavery. In 1723 a heartfelt petition from a mulatto slave to the bishop of London, in which the author protested "Cruell Bondegg" in Virginia, went unanswered. That same year, Bray set up a trust of "Associates" to carry on his work. With limited success, they focused on converting blacks in the British plantation colonies. By the 1730s, only a few whites in Europe or America dared to press publicly for an end to slavery.

Christian Priber, who arrived in the South in 1735, was one such activist. The idealistic German hoped to start a utopian community in southern Appalachia. But his radical proposal for a multiracial "Paradise" uniting Indians, Africans, and Europeans posed a huge threat to South Carolina authorities. "He enumerates many whimsical Privileges and natural Rights, as he calls them, which his citizens are to be entitled to," wrote a scornful detractor, "particularly dissolving Marriages and allowing Community of Women and all kinds of Licentiousness." Worst of all, according to the coastal elite, this egalitarian haven at the "Foot of the Mountains among the Cherokees" was to be "a City of Refuge for all Criminals, Debtors, and Slaves who would fly thither from [the] Justice of their Masters." Priber's brief career as a social agitator challenging the status quo ended in 1743, when he was arrested and brought to jail in Charleston. He died—or was killed—before his case could be heard in court.

At the same time, a New Jersey tailor and bookkeeper named John Woolman posed a less defiant but more enduring threat to race slavery. In 1743, at age 23, this shy Quaker began to question his role in writing out bills of sale when his fellow Quakers purchased slaves. It struck him forcefully that "to live in ease and plenty by the toil of those whom violence and cruelty have put in our power" was clearly not "consistent with Christianity or common justice." Woolman traveled widely to Quaker meetings, north and south, pressing an issue that most Quakers preferred to ignore. "The Colour of a Man avails nothing," Woolman insisted, "in Matters of Right and Equity." When he drafted *Some Considerations on the Keeping of Negroes* (1754), members of the Quaker Yearly Meeting in Philadelphia published his booklet and circulated it widely in several editions. Four years later, led by Anthony Benezet, this group outlawed slaveholding among its local members. They set a precedent that many Quakers followed in the next generation, and they challenged other denominations to do the same.

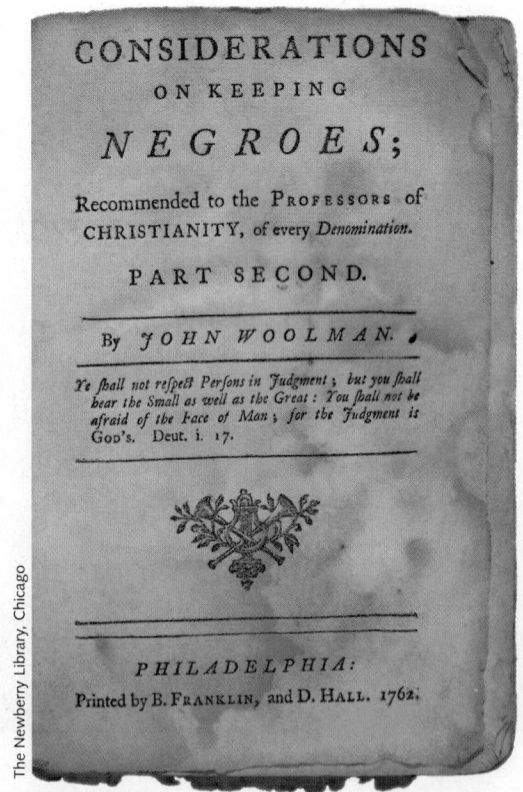

The Newberry Library, Chicago

■ Pennsylvania Quaker John Woolman published a pioneering tract against slavery in 1754. He traveled widely to oppose the institution, and he encouraged people not to use products created by enslaved labor. Benjamin Franklin published the 1762 edition.

Oglethorpe's Antislavery Experiment

The most sustained early challenge to the slavery system in the American South came in the Georgia colony. In 1732 a group of well-connected London proprietors (known as trustees) obtained a 20-year charter for the region between English South Carolina and Spanish Florida. Ten of the 21 initial trustees were members of Parliament. They included James Oglethorpe, who had recently organized and chaired a "committee on jails" to investigate the condition of debtors in English prisons. The trustees foresaw three related purposes—charitable, commercial, and military—for their experimental colony, which they named after King George II. Georgia would provide a haven for England's worthy poor, selected members of the neediest classes who could be transported across the Atlantic and settled on small farms. These grateful newcomers would

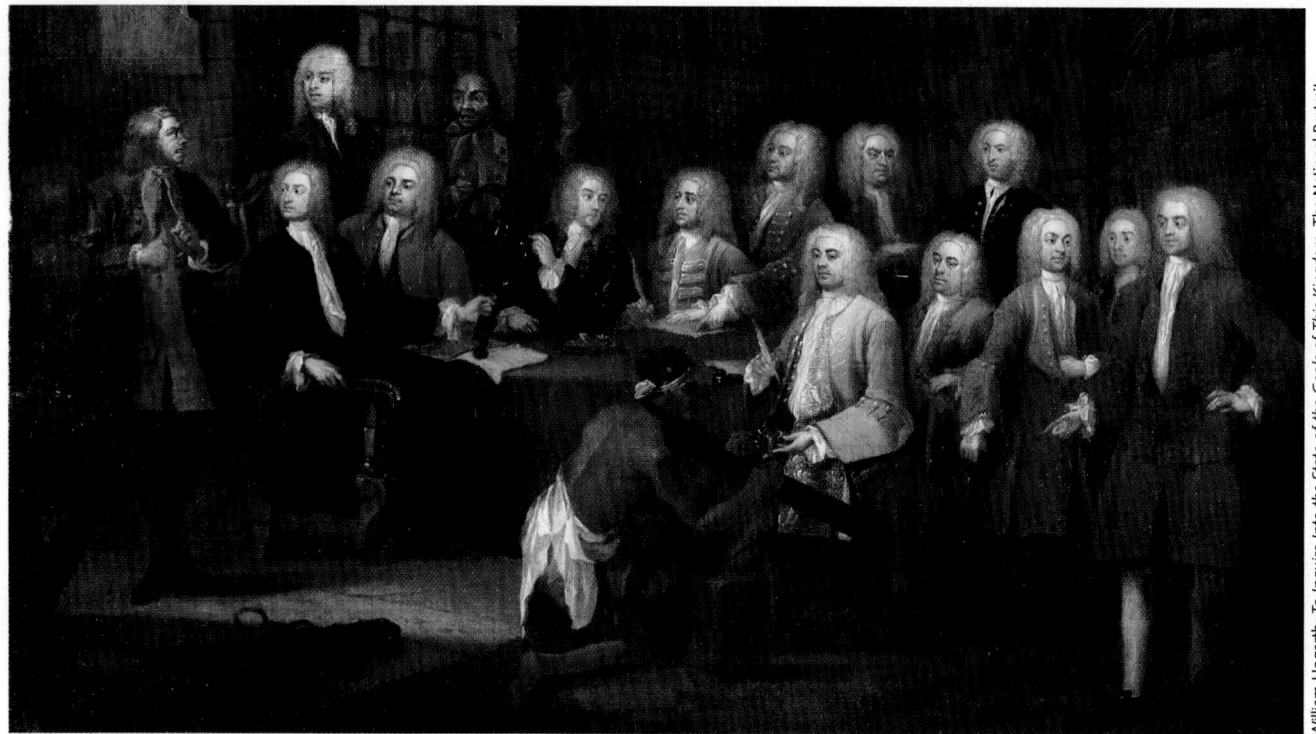

William Hogarth, *To Inquire Into the State of the Gaols of This Kingdom*. The National Portrait Gallery, London

■ In 1729, James Oglethorpe (seated, right front) chaired a Parliamentary committee exposing the harsh conditions in English jails. When William Hogarth portrayed the committee's visit to Fleet Street Prison, the artist showed Oglethorpe's concern for a dark-skinned prisoner, a hint of Oglethorpe's future opposition to slavery in Georgia.

then produce warm weather commodities—olives, grapes, silk—to support the empire. And their prosperity would create a growing market for English goods. Finally, their presence would provide a military buffer to protect South Carolina from further warfare with the Yamasee and Creek Indians and from possible invasion by the Spanish in St. Augustine.

With Oglethorpe as their governor, an initial boatload of 114 settlers arrived in 1733 and began building a capital at Savannah. By 1741 the town, located on a bluff 15 miles up the Savannah River, boasted more than 140 houses. It also had a wharf, a jail, a courthouse (which doubled as a church), and a building for receiving delegations of neighboring Indians. By then, more than a thousand needy English, plus 800 German, Swiss, and Austrian Protestants, had journeyed to Georgia at the trustees' expense. Another thousand immigrants had paid their own way. Like earlier colonizers, Georgia's first arrivals had trouble adjusting to a strange environment. Alligators, rattlesnakes, and hurricanes tested their resolve. Tension over governance only deepened their discouragement.

The idealistic trustees in London declined to accumulate property and profits for themselves in the colony, but they felt justified in controlling every aspect of Georgia's development. For example, they knew that gin was becoming a source of debt and disruption in Europe and that rum and brandy sold by traders was poisoning colonial relations with southeastern Indians. So in 1735 they outlawed the use of every "kind of Spirits or Strong Waters" while still allowing consumption of wine and beer. Georgia's early experiment with prohibition of hard liquor proved difficult to implement, and officials quietly stopped enforcing the law in 1742.

Other efforts at control from above went further. The trustees refused to set up a legislature or to let settlers buy and sell land. Instead, they gave 50 acres to each family they sent over, including a house lot in town to ensure defense for each new village. But they parceled out land with little regard for variations in soil fertility. They also stipulated that owners could pass land on to sons only. Denying daughters the right to inherit, the trustees reasoned, would prevent men from creating large estates simply by marrying women who were likely to inherit big tracts of land. In a further effort to prevent the concentrations of wealth that they saw developing in other colonies, the trustees said that no one could own more than 500 acres. Prohibiting massive estates would allow for thicker settlement and therefore greater manpower to defend the colony militarily.

But the most important prohibition, by far, involved slavery. Oglethorpe began his career as a deputy governor of the Royal African Company, but he died in 1785 opposing the slave trade. His sojourn in Georgia turned him against slavery. In neighboring South Carolina, he saw first-hand how the practice degraded African lives, undermined the morals of Europeans, and laid that colony open to threats of revolt and invasion. More friendly to Indians than to African Americans, Oglethorpe persuaded the trustees to create a free white colony. Specifically, he convinced them to enact a law in 1735 that prohibited slavery and also excluded free blacks. He believed that this mandate would protect Georgia from the corruptions of enslavement while also making it easier to apprehend black runaways heading to Florida from South Carolina.

The Stono Rebellion, and the outbreak of war between England and Spain in 1739, strengthened Oglethorpe's belief that slavery undermined the security of the English colonies by creating internal enemies who would support any foreign attackers. He saw further evidence in 1740, when he failed in a wartime attempt to capture St. Augustine from Spain. Unable to take the Florida stronghold, the governor managed to seize neighboring Fort Mose, which had been erected by anti-English slaves who had escaped from Carolina. But a Spanish force regained the fort, relying heavily on Indian and African American fighters to win a fierce dawn battle. Oglethorpe's army withdrew in disarray, but he had seen the intensity with which ex-slaves would fight the English, their former masters.

The next year, fearing a counterattack, Oglethorpe issued a warning to imperial officials. He predicted that if Spanish soldiers captured Georgia, a colony inhabited by "white

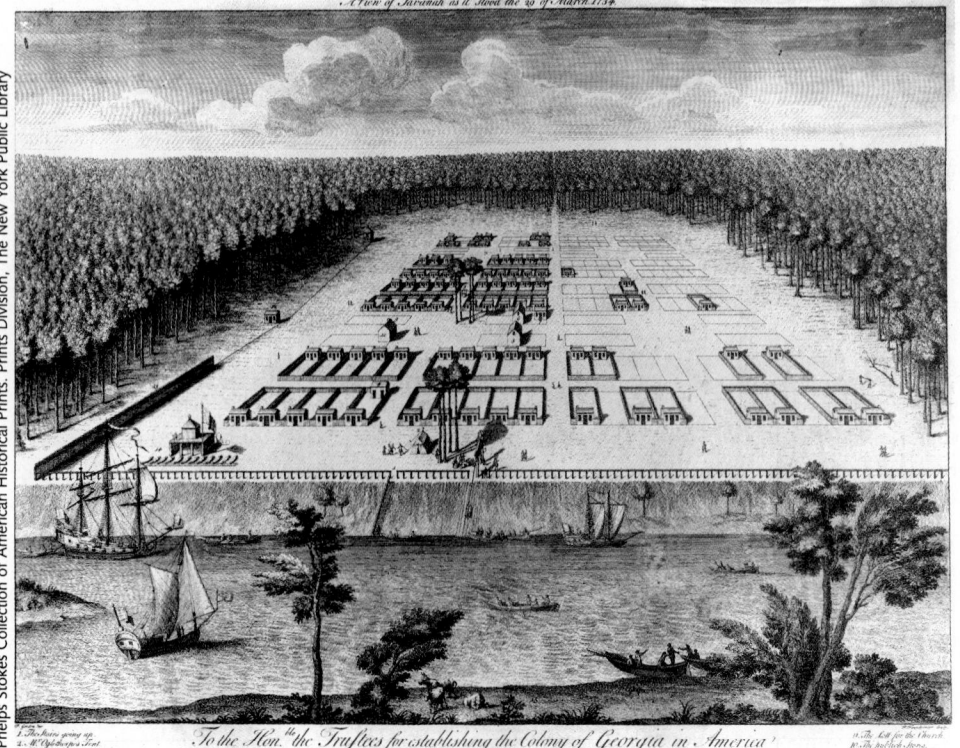

■ Savannah, the capital of Oglethorpe's Georgia, was one year old when this view was sketched in 1734. The following year, Georgia's trustees officially outlawed slavery, creating a sharp contrast with the other British colonies in North America, especially neighboring South Carolina on the opposite bank of the Savannah River.

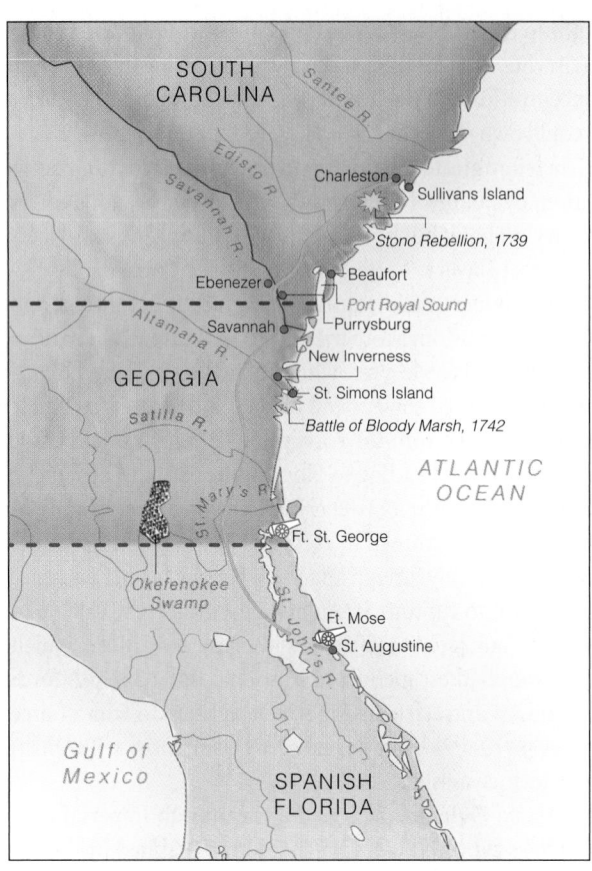

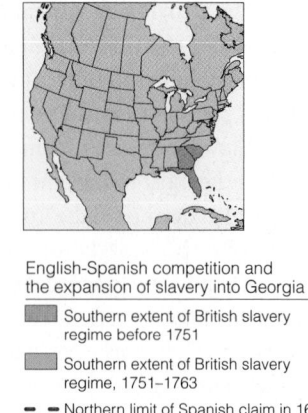

■ **MAP 4.4**
ENGLISH–SPANISH COMPETITION AND THE EXPANSION OF SLAVERY INTO GEORGIA   The Spanish and the British had competing land claims along the southeast coast after 1670. Creation of the Georgia colony in 1732 intensified the rivalry. The Spanish in Florida offered freedom to any slaves who escaped from South Carolina to St. Augustine, sparking the Stono Revolt in 1739. During the war between Britain and Spain (1739–1743) Georgians defeated the Spanish at Bloody Marsh and secured the disputed "Sea Island" region for the British. Within a decade, slavery became legal in Georgia, and scores of new labor camps appeared between the Savannah and the St. Mary's River, producing rice for export.

English-Spanish competition and the expansion of slavery into Georgia
▮ Southern extent of British slavery regime before 1751
▮ Southern extent of British slavery regime, 1751–1763
– – Northern limit of Spanish claim in 1670
– – Southern limit of British claim in 1736
— Path from Charleston to St. Augustine
✸ Major battles
Fort St. George, a British lookout post
Fort Mose, Spanish outpost made up of escaped South Carolina slaves

Protestants and no Negroes," they would then send agents to infiltrate the vulnerable colonies farther north and stir black rebellion. The Spanish, he argued, understood that the thousands of embittered slaves "would be either Recruits to an Enemy or Plunder for them." No sooner had he written his wartime prediction in 1741 than suspicious fires broke out in New York and Charleston.

The End of Equality in Georgia

As Britain's war with Spain continued, few whites could deny the Georgia governor's assertion that slavery elsewhere in British America was a source of internal weakness and strategic danger. In 1742, as the governor had predicted, Spain pushed from Florida into Georgia with an eye toward destabilizing the colonies farther north. Oglethorpe's troops repulsed the invading Spanish force in the crucial Battle at Bloody Marsh on St. Simon's Island. The victory reduced the immediate threat to Britain's North American colonies, especially neighboring South Carolina, where Oglethorpe and his idealistic policies had numerous powerful opponents. These opponents now joined a group of so-called Malcontents in Savannah to question Georgia's continued prohibition against slavery. When this coalition challenged the trustees' antislavery stance, it prompted the first protracted North American debate about enslavement. It dragged on for more than a decade.

In the face of numerous ills—including a sickly climate, poor soil, restrictive land policies, and lack of representative government—a well-organized Georgia faction argued that slavery was the one thing needed for the colony to prosper, since it would provide profits to slaveowners regardless of Georgia's many drawbacks. Not everyone agreed. In 1739 Scottish Highlanders living at Darien on the Altamaha River had contacted Oglethorpe to lay out their practical arguments against importing Africans. Their petition expressed shock "that any Race of Mankind, and their Posterity, Should be sentenced to perpetual slavery." Immigrants from Salzburg, Germany, residing at Ebenezer on the Savannah River drafted a similar statement. But Georgia's Malcontents pushed back. These several dozen English and Lowland Scot adventurers, led by the disgruntled son of a colonial official, wrote letters and circulated petitions demanding the right to import slaves. They drew encouragement and support from powerful merchant-planters in South Carolina. Eager to expand their trade in slaves from Africa and to open up new lands for profitable plantations, these well-to-do Carolinians dreamed of extending their successful rice operations into coastal Georgia.

Oglethorpe warned that the proslavery lobby, hungry to create large estates, seemed bent on "destroying the Agrarian Equality" envisioned in Georgia's initial plan. But the colony's trustees in London grew less unified, committed, and informed over time. Eventually, the persistent efforts of the proslavery pamphleteers bore fruit. In 1750 the trustees gave in on the matter of land titles. They allowed acreage to be bought and sold freely in any amount, which opened the door for the creation of large plantations. From there, it was just one more step to allowing slavery. The trustees finally gave in on the question of bondage, letting Georgians exploit slaves after January 1, 1751. The 1750 law permitting slavery made futile gestures to ensure kind treatment and Christian education for slaves, but the dam had broken. Hundreds of slave-owning South Carolinians streamed across the Savannah River to invest in land. In 1752 the trustees disbanded, their patent expiring, their vision undone. By 1754 Georgia had become a royal colony.

Some argued that Georgia should simply be incorporated into South Carolina. In a sense it was: slave labor camps producing rice and indigo for export soon dotted the lowcountry on both sides of the Savannah River. Georgia's assembly passed a harsh slave code in 1755, based on South Carolina's. Two years later, it legislated a system of patrols to keep the brutal new regime in place. Georgia's effort to counter race slavery in North America had failed, a case of too little too late. After holding out for nearly two decades, the colony fell victim to the same divisive institution that had already taken root more slowly elsewhere along the Atlantic seaboard.

Conclusion

T wo final observations provide a wider Atlantic context regarding the people swept up in the North American portion of the gigantic African traffic. First, their odyssey began comparatively late, for this dimension of the trade did not expand rapidly until after the 1670s. In the broader history of North American immigration, of course, their forced migration from Africa came relatively early. Indeed, the proportion of blacks in the colonial population on the eve of the American Revolution (over 20 percent) was higher than it has ever been in the United States since then. But in terms of the entire African slave diaspora, or dispersion, the influx to English North America occurred long after the traffic to Mexico, Brazil, and the Caribbean was well established.

Second, even at its height, the North American trade remained marginal in relation to the wider Atlantic commerce in African labor. For example, whereas roughly 50,000 enslaved men and women reached all the docks of North America between 1721 and 1740, the small West Indian islands of English Barbados and French Guadeloupe *each* received more than 53,000 Africans during the same period. In the next two decades, while Britain's mainland colonies purchased just over 100,000 Africans, Caribbean Islands such as English Jamaica (120,000) and French Saint Domingue (159,000) absorbed many more slaves.

During this single 40-year span (1721–1760), Brazil bought 667,000 African workers—more than would reach North America during the entire slave trade. All told, scholars currently estimate that some 650,000 Africans were brought to North America over several centuries. They represented roughly 6 percent of the total Atlantic commerce in enslaved people. Still, the number of mainland slaves expanded from scarcely 7000 in 1680 to nearly 29,000 in 1700 and to more than 70,000 in 1720. Half a century later in 1770, because of importation and natural increase, 470,000 individuals were confined to enslavement from New Hampshire to Louisiana.

A century had passed since Elizabeth Key's generation saw the terrible transformation begin. Relative openness had given way to systematic oppression, and slavery's corrosive effects were felt at every level of society. An English visitor to the South in 1759 found provincial planters "vain and imperious," subject "to many errors and prejudices, especially in regard to Indians and Negroes, whom they scarcely consider as of the human species." It took another century before pressures developed that could unseat race slavery, sanctioned by law, as a dominant institution in the land.

Sites to Visit

Colonial Williamsburg

More than half the residents of colonial Williamsburg were black. Increasingly, their lives are being explored and discussed at this reconstructed historic town in tidewater Virginia. The Slave Quarters at nearby Carter's Grove Plantation contain four cabins and provide an interpretation of African American life before the Revolution.

Fort Mose
www.fortmose.org/

Under Spanish protection, slaves who had escaped from colonial South Carolina built Gracia Real de Santa Teresa de Mose, or Fort Mose, on the eastern edge of a marsh, 2 miles north of St. Augustine, Florida. Archaeologists rediscovered the site of this early free black community, and it is being made into an exhibition area.

Africans in America
www.pbs.org/wgbh/aia/home.html

This four-part television series prepared for PBS provides an overview of slavery from its beginnings to the end of the Civil War. Part One deals with "The Terrible Transformation," offering resources and insights on the era from 1450 to 1750.

SeacoastNH.com

Billed as "the biggest website for America's smallest seacoast," this site contains an excellent section on New Hampshire's black history, which stretches back more than 350 years. Links connect to the Portsmouth Black Heritage Trail, which leads to two dozen sites in Portsmouth, describing where black New Englanders lived and worked.

Drayton Hall

This National Trust historic site on the Ashley River outside Charleston, South Carolina, features the oldest plantation house in America open to the public, built by Europeans and African Americans at the time of the 1739 Stono Rebellion. The staff has developed a "Gullah Connection" to explore black culture with local schools.

The Cultural Landscape of the Plantation
www.gwu.edu/~folklife/bighouse/intro.html

American studies professor John Michael Vlach has created this online exhibition using images of plantation buildings from the Library of Congress and linking them with the testimonies of former slaves recorded during the 1930s.

Somerset Place

This is just one of many historic plantations across the South steadily improving the ways in which they present the slave experience. Somerset Place is a huge estate created after the American Revolution beside Lake Phelps, in Creswell, North Carolina. The site has reconstructed slave buildings, and it hosts a biannual black homecoming.

Mel Fisher Maritime Museum

This museum in Key West, Florida, has a Traveling Trunk of artifacts relating to the slave ship *Henrietta Marie*, which sank near Key West in 1700. For rental of these materials, go to www.melfisher.org.

Pictorial Images of the Transatlantic Slave Trade
gropius.lib.virginia.edu/SlaveTrade/index.html

This database from the Virginia Foundation for the Humanities and Public Policy contains numerous images relating to the trans-Atlantic slave trade.

For Further Reading

General

Ira Berlin, *Many Thousands Gone: The First Two Centuries of Slavery in North America* (1998).

David Eltis, *The Rise of African Slavery in the Americas* (2000).

A. Leon Higginbotham, Jr., *In the Matter of Color: Race and the American Legal Process, the Colonial Period* (1978).

Evelyn Brooks Higginbotham, *The Harvard Guide to African-American History* (2001).

John Thornton, *Africa and Africans in the Making of the Atlantic World, 1400–1800* (1992).

Peter H. Wood, *Strange New Land: Africans in Colonial America* (2002).

The Descent into Race Slavery

T. H. Breen and Stephen Innes, *"Myne Owne Ground": Race and Freedom on Virginia's Eastern Shore, 1640–1676* (1980).

Kathleen M. Brown, *Good Wives, Nasty Wenches, and Anxious Patriarchs: Gender, Race, and Power in Colonial Virginia* (1996).

Edward Countryman, ed., *How Did American Slavery Begin?* (1999).

Winthrop D. Jordan, *White over Black: American Attitudes Toward the Negro, 1550–1812* (1968).

Edmund S. Morgan, *American Slavery, American Freedom: The Ordeal of Colonial Virginia* (1975).

The Growth of Slave Labor Camps

Madeleine Burnside, *Spirits of the Passage: The Transatlantic Slave Trade in the Seventeenth Century* (1997).

Clifford Dowdey, *The Virginia Dynasties: The Emergence of "King" Carter and the Golden Age* (1969).

Sylvia R. Frey and Betty Wood, *Come Shouting to Zion: African American Protestantism in the American South and British Caribbean to 1830* (1998).

Allan Kulikoff, *Tobacco and Slaves: The Development of Southern Cultures in the Chesapeake, 1680–1800* (1986).

England Enters the Atlantic Slave Trade

Jay Coughtry, *The Notorious Triangle: Rhode Island and the American Slave Trade, 1700–1807* (1981).

Philip D. Curtin, *The Atlantic Slave Trade: A Census* (1969).

Douglas Grant, *The Fortunate Slave: An Illustration of African Slavery in the Early Eighteenth Century* (1968).

Herbert S. Klein, *The Atlantic Slave Trade (New Approaches to the Americas)* (1999).

James A. Rawley, *The Transatlantic Slave Trade: A History* (1981).

James Walvin, *Black Ivory: A History of British Slavery* (1994).

Survival in a Strange New Land

Kathleen Deagan and Darcie MacMahon, *Fort Mose: Colonial America's Black Fortress of Freedom* (1995).

Michael A. Gomez, *Exchanging Our Country Marks: The Transformation of African Identities in the Colonial and Antebellum South* (1998).

Jane Landers, *Black Society in the Spanish Florida* (1999).

Daniel Littlefield, *Rice and Slaves: Ethnicity and the Slave Trade in Colonial South Carolina* (1981).

Philip Morgan, *Slave Counterpoint: Black Culture in the Eighteenth-Century Chesapeake and Lowcountry* (1998).

Peter H. Wood, *Black Majority: Negroes in Colonial South Carolina from 1670 Through the Stono Rebellion* (1974).

The Transformation Completed

Harold E. Davis, *The Fledgling Province: Social and Cultural Life in Colonial Georgia, 1733–1776* (1976).

Gwendolyn Midlo Hall, *Africans in Colonial Louisiana: The Development of Afro-Creole Culture in the Eighteenth Century* (1992).

Kenneth A. Lockridge, *On the Sources of Patriarchal Rage: The Commonplace Books of William Byrd and Thomas Jefferson and the Gendering of Power in the Eighteenth Century* (1992).

Phillips P. Moulton, ed., *The Journal and Major Essays of John Woolman* (1997).

Betty Wood, *Slavery in Colonial Georgia, 1730–1775* (1984).

Online Practice Test

Test your understanding of this chapter with interactive review quizzes at

www.ablongman.com/jonescreatedequal/chapter4

CHAPTER

5

An American Babel, 1713–1763

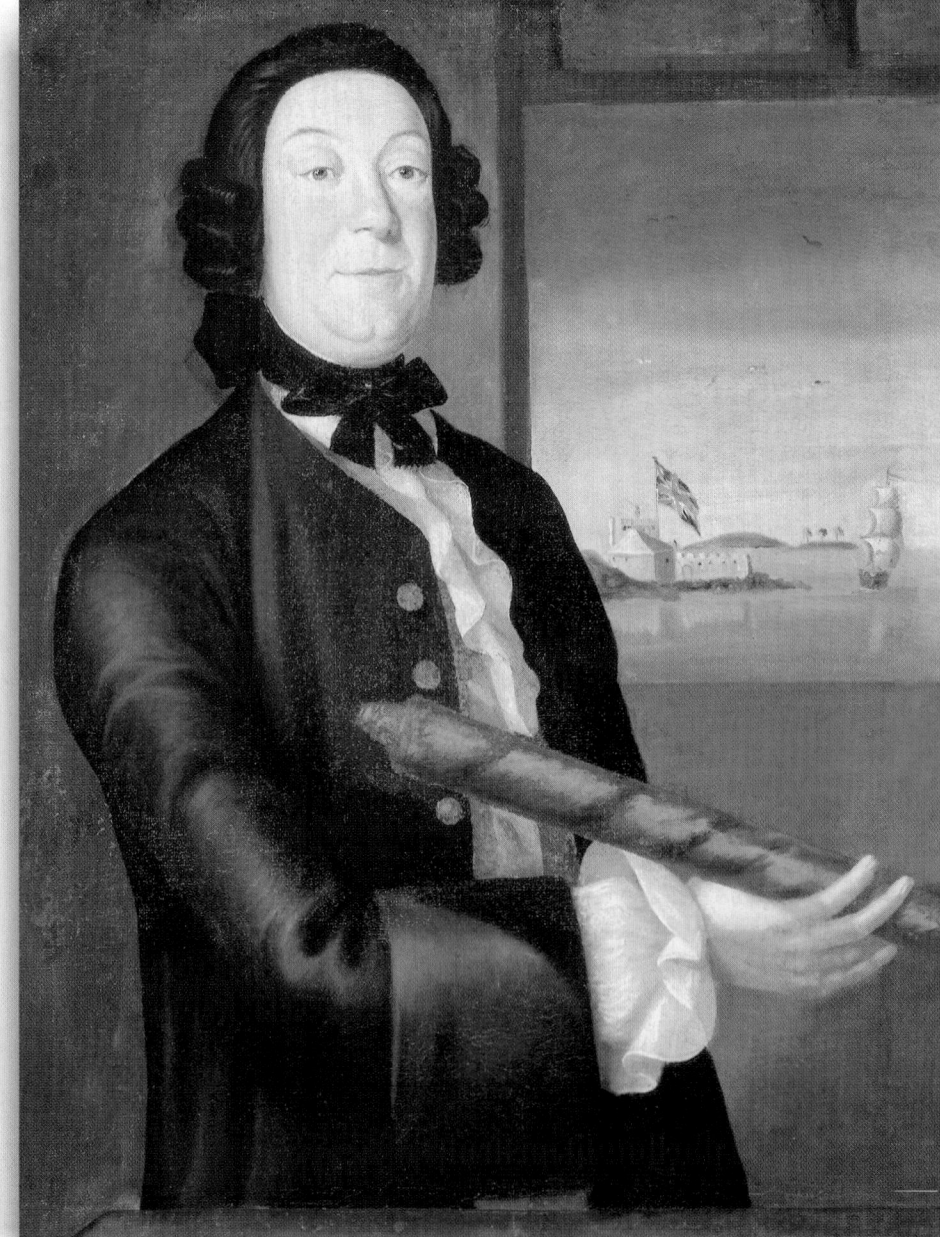

John Greenwood, *Portrait of John Clarke*, 1745–50. Peabody Essex Museum (Acc. #1257 17). Photo by Mark Sexton

■ Captain John Clarke (1701–1764), a Massachusetts merchant, posed for his portrait with Salem's harbor and fort in the background.

IN 1749, PEACE SEEMED A WELCOME PROSPECT IN THE SPANISH SETTLEMENT OF SAN Antonio in south-central Texas. On an August morning, hundreds of people gathered in the plaza in front of the town's presidio, or military post. Captain Turibio de Urrutia, the presidio's commander, was there with a contingent of soldiers. Father Santa Ana, who had presided over the local missions for 16 years, was also present, along with other missionaries and lay residents. Across from them stood four Apache Indian chiefs with several hundred of their people. Between the two groups, in the center of the plaza, Spanish and Indian workers began to dig a deep pit with steep sides. Those attending were about to witness one of the most important events in the town's brief history.

Three decades earlier, in the spring of 1718, a small expedition of Spanish soldiers, missionaries, women, and children had built the presidio and a mission next to the San Antonio River. They constructed rough houses and excavated irrigation ditches to divert river water onto their fields. But they had occupied contested ground, on which the French and Indians also had designs. Undaunted by the failure of LaSalle's Texas colony, the French had established Natchitoches on the Red River in 1716 and New Orleans on the lower Mississippi in 1718. French explorers began probing west along Louisiana's western frontier and trading with Indians in eastern Texas. Then in 1720, Apache bands, moving down from the north under pressure from the Comanches, suddenly made their presence known. When they attacked two San Antonians out looking for missing horses, it marked the start of warfare.

Detail from an eighteenth-century Spanish map showing San Antonio and nearby missions.

Fresh support for the beleaguered settlers arrived at San Antonio in 1731, and additional friars laid out four new missions. But other conflicts arose. Sixteen families who had migrated all the way from the Canary Islands in the Atlantic Ocean received little support from local authorities. Religious leaders jostled with military personnel over how to use scarce resources and deal with raiding parties of neighboring Native Americans. An outbreak of smallpox in 1739 killed scores of mission Indians and forced others to depart in fear, but the cycle of war intensified. When Apache bands stole horses and killed settlers, Spanish officers responded with raids of their own. They captured Apache women and children and sold them into slavery in Mexico.

Captain Urrutia conducted one such campaign northwest from San Antonio in 1745, taking enough captives to earn a profit. Father Santa Ana protested such harsh tactics. When the Apaches retaliated against the presidio, Santa Ana's mission Indians from small local tribes helped fend off the attack. But in the end, the cleric hoped not only to make peace with the Apaches but to draw them into the expanding mission system, where they would accept Christianity, learn Spanish, and take up agriculture under the direction of missionaries. He called on Urrutia to stop selling slaves and provoking reprisals.

At Santa Ana's urging, the captain modified his approach in 1749. During the spring raids and counter-raids, Urrutia used mission Indians as fighters and translators, and he issued orders for humane treatment of the 175 prisoners brought back to San Antonio.

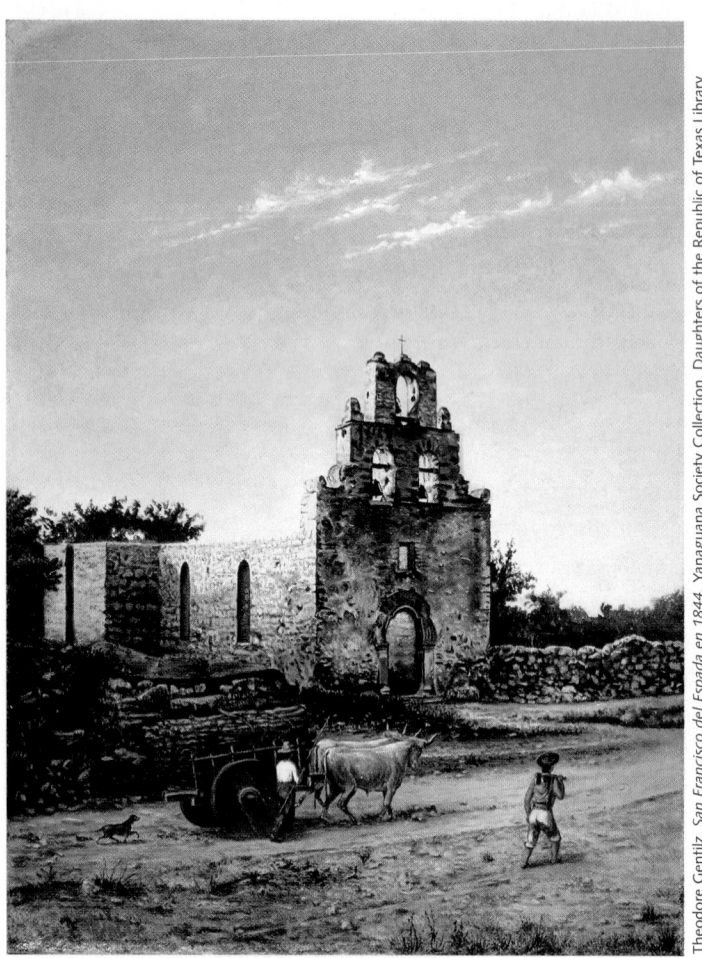

Theodore Gentilz, *San Francisco del Espada en 1844.* Yanaguana Society Collection. Daughters of the Republic of Texas Library at the Alamo

■ Mission San Francisco de la Espada, at San Antonio, had 1100 cattle, 80 horses, and 16 pairs of oxen when this chapel was being constructed in the 1740s. By the time the United States annexed Texas a century later (1845), the church had fallen into disrepair.

Rather than sell them as slaves, the Spanish locked up the men and dispersed the women and children among the missions and local households for "safe-keeping." Then Urrutia and Santa Ana chose two women and a man from among the captives and sent them back to Apache country with a proposal for peace. When the messengers returned with word that four important Apache chiefs were prepared to negotiate, preparations began for a major parley.

On August 16, 1749, Captain Urrutia and Father Santa Ana rode north from San Antonio, accompanied by most of the townsfolk, to welcome the Apache delegation. Both sides were eager for peace, and the negotiations went smoothly. There was ceremonial feasting, important for such occasions, and the four chiefs attended a mass conducted by Father Santa Ana. After two days of discussion through translators, the Spanish released some of their Apache prisoners as a goodwill gesture, and both sides agreed to hold a formal peace ceremony in the presidio plaza the next morning.

The next day all gathered to watch the workers digging the deep pit. Then the longtime adversaries buried their differences in an elaborate symbolic ritual. They lowered a live horse into the hole, along with other emblems of warfare: a lance, a hatchet, and a bundle of arrows. Next, the four chiefs linked hands and walked solemnly around the pit, accompanied first by Captain Urrutia, then by the missionaries, and finally by a resident of the town. Suddenly, at a set moment, all the onlookers grabbed up loose earth and tossed it into the hole. The horse was soon completely buried—a sacrifice for peace in the region—and the ceremony broke up with shouts and celebration.

Though striking, the encounter between the Spanish and Apaches at San Antonio was not unique. During the same era, Europeans and Native Americans met to parley and trade in other colonial towns such as Albany, Philadelphia, Charleston, St. Augustine, Mobile, and New Orleans. Such formal occasions highlight a far wider process of contact and interaction that was going on throughout the North American colonies in the half-century between 1713 and 1763. Everywhere, on a daily basis, the process of colonial expansion brought together Europeans, Africans, and Native Americans in surprising new contacts. Equally important, it forced different peoples *within* each of these three categories, despite contrasting backgrounds and customs, to rub shoulders with one another in unprecedented and unfamiliar ways.

These constant encounters had all been set in motion by the colonization process itself. Spanish missionaries lived among Tejas Indians in eastern Texas; French explorers dominated, and then lost, the Mississippi Valley; escaped African slaves fought militiamen from Georgia on the outskirts of St. Augustine. Some day-to-day meetings proved rewarding—a sound bargain, a helpful remedy, or a happy marriage. But other mixing was strained and uneasy at best—full of verbal misunderstandings, competing claims, and harsh commands.

Everywhere, motives differed, accents jarred, and cultures clashed. In Philadelphia, printer Benjamin Franklin, himself a newcomer from Boston, protested the way in which German-speaking Europeans "swarm into our settlements, and by herding together establish their language and manner to the exclusion of ours."

For many Christians, the new confusions recalled the story of Babel. Despite ambitious plans, the people in that biblical city could not understand one another well enough to work together. Eventually, they scattered abroad across the face of the earth. Bible-reading European-Americans no doubt recalled that tale, especially during the great religious awakening that shook the English colonies in the 1740s, when the prospect of building something new and transcendent seemed close at hand. The German-born utopian Christian Priber even attempted to establish an egalitarian realm in Appalachia where Europeans, Africans, and Native Americans could live peaceably together. Such dreams were not to be, however. Instead, the existing colonies continued to build up regional economies of their own, under British protection, and elements of a dominant Anglo-American culture began to emerge amid the Atlantic Babel's many voices.

New Cultures on the Western Plains

It makes sense that the Apaches chose to bury a horse during their elaborate ceremony at the Spanish presidio in 1749. By this time, the horse, recently introduced to the Indians was transforming life on the Great Plains. It also makes sense that they buried arrows and hatchets rather than guns. Traditionally, the Spanish aspired to make the Indians into loyal subjects and Christian converts. From the time of Spain's arrival in the New World, therefore, official policy had forbidden the sale of firearms to Native Americans.

In contrast, the French, Dutch, and English desired trade at almost any cost. From the beginning, they showed less hesitation about supplying Indians with guns in exchange for furs. Firearms had become familiar to many eastern Indians in the seventeenth century. In the eighteenth century, guns began to spread across the Mississippi River as well. Combined with the

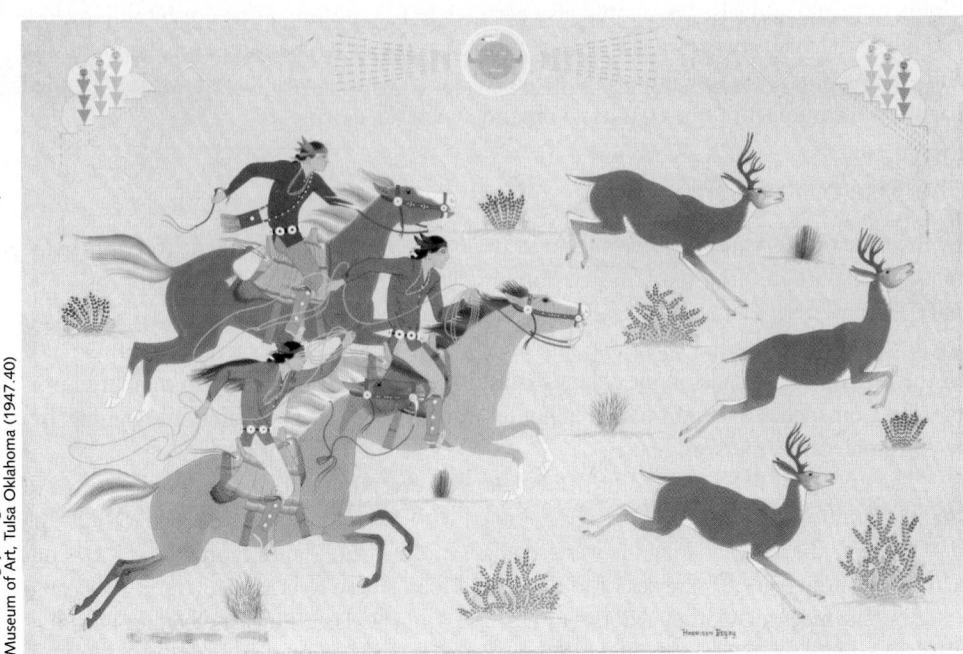

Harrison Begay, "Night Chant Ceremonial Hunt," 1947. Museum purchase, The Philbrook Museum of Art, Tulsa Oklahoma (1947.40)

■ The horse offered new mobility for hunting, as in this modern painting of Navajo riders. Tribes that had once tracked buffalo on foot at the edge of the Great Plains could now pursue herds across miles of open grassland. This was true for the Cheyenne, who were living in fixed villages in what is now South Dakota in the early eighteenth century. "After they got the first horses," recalled John Stands-in-Timber, "they learned there were more of them in the South and they went there after them." Cheyenne life would never be the same again.

movement of horses from the south, this development had enormous consequences. New patterns of warfare altered Indian cultures, and more powerful hunting techniques affected the regional economies and ecologies of the Native American West.

The Spread of the Horse

Although small horses once roamed the ancient West, they migrated into Asia thousands of years ago and became extinct in America. They returned with the early Spanish explorers, but Coronado's soldiers preferred to ride male horses. Only around 1600, when New Mexico's early colonists brought mares north for breeding, did horse herds develop in the Rio Grande valley. After the Pueblo Revolt in 1680, horses taken from the Spanish entered Indian trading networks and rapidly moved north from one culture to another.

By 1690 the Utes had obtained horses and traded them to the Shoshones. Before the mid-eighteenth century, horses had moved west of the Rocky Mountains to the Nez Perce and north to the Blackfeet. The Apaches brought horses east along other routes to the Caddoan cultures near the Red River and then north to the Pawnees, Arikaras, and Hidatsas. Even tribes in the Southeast acquired Spanish horses from the West before they obtained English horses from the Atlantic coast. When La Salle descended the Mississippi in 1682, he met Indians who had heard rumors from the West about a mysterious animal. And when a Chickasaw leader drew a regional map on deerskin in 1723, he showed a Native American leading a horse east of the Mississippi River.

For all Indians, the first horses seemed utterly strange. One elder recalled that "the people did not know what they fed on. They would offer the animals pieces of dried meat." "He put us on mind of a Stag that had lost his horns," another remembered, "and we did not know what name to give him. But as he was a slave to Man, like the dog, which carried our things, he was named the Big Dog." For generations, Native Americans had used dogs to pull provisions and bedding on a travois, an A-frame device made with tent poles. A larger animal could haul bigger loads, including longer tent poles. The long poles, in turn, allowed each family to live in a more spacious tipi.

Whether or not a tribe used tipis as dwellings, it could readily use the horse as a new source of tasty food and as an aid in hunting. The first few horses were far too valuable to risk in warfare. As herds expanded, however, warriors rode into battle, adapting their tactics to take advantage of their new swiftness. On horses, they could conduct lightning raids over long distances to attack rivals. They could also earn respect by stealing horses or by riding close enough to touch an enemy warrior, an act of bravery known as counting coup. Soon, raising and trading horses became important activities, and a family's wealth and status depended partly on the number of horses at its command.

The Rise of the Comanches

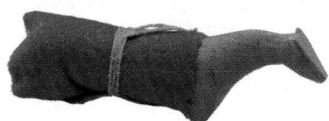

By the time of the American Revolution in the 1770s, mounted Comanche warriors commanded respect and fear across a vast domain. Their territory stretched south nearly 600 miles from western Kansas to central Texas, and it spanned 400 miles from eastern New Mexico to what is now eastern Oklahoma. This area, known as the Comanchería, roughly equaled all the English settlements on the Atlantic coast in size, but its origins were recent and humble. The Comanches' ancestors had been hunter–gatherers on the high plains of Wyoming, living on small game, roots, and berries.

The arrival of the horse around 1690 changed everything. It allowed family bands to migrate southeast from the Rockies. They joined with other Shoshone-speakers to hunt the buffalo herds that grazed along the western edges of the Great Plains. From there, it was not a long ride through the Sangre de Cristo Mountains to northern New Mexico, where they could trade buffalo hides for additional horses at Taos and Santa Fe. The Spanish noted the Shoshone-speaking arrivals in 1706, referring to them as Comanches in their records.

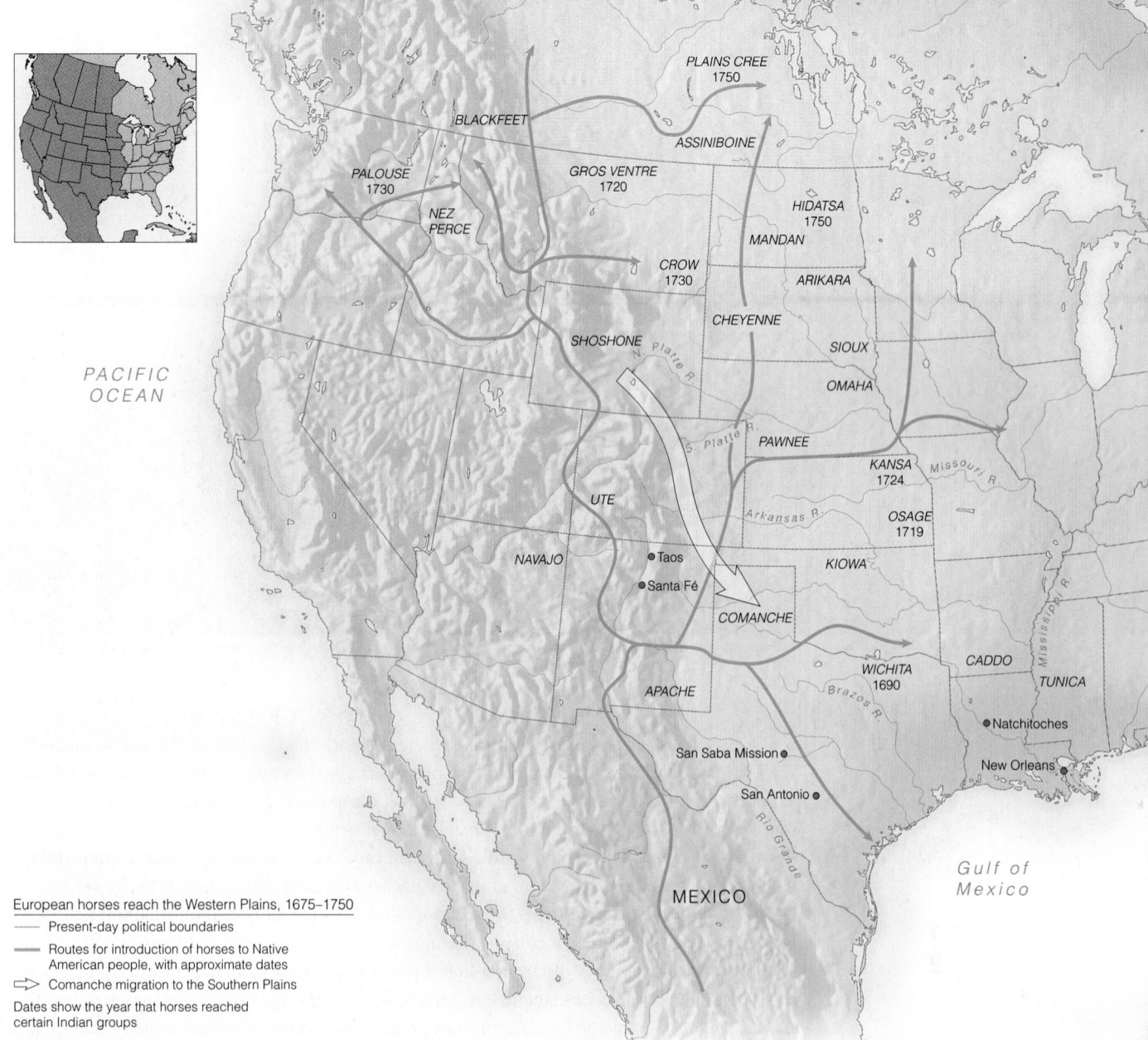

European horses reach the Western Plains, 1675–1750

—— Present-day political boundaries

—— Routes for introduction of horses to Native American people, with approximate dates

⇨ Comanche migration to the Southern Plains

Dates show the year that horses reached certain Indian groups

■ **MAP 5.1**
THE RAPID SPREAD OF SPANISH HORSES ACROSS THE WESTERN PLAINS, 1675–1750

The Comanches were not the first to make their homes in what is now eastern Colorado. For generations, groups of Apaches had settled in the region near the upper reaches of the Platte and Arkansas rivers. Their ancestors had been Athapascan-speakers who had migrated south from Alaska centuries earlier and adjusted well to the warmer climate. Eventually, they had adopted some of the agricultural ways of the Pueblos and learned to ride horses from the Spanish. For Comanche newcomers, the Apache settlements—with their irrigated gardens and herds of horses—provided easy targets. Soon, Comanche raids caused such destruction that the Apaches sought assistance from the Spanish in the New Mexico colony to protect their homeland.

Officials in Santa Fe, fearful about their own defenses, looked for ways to halt Comanche aggression. They also hoped to convert the Apaches to Christianity and stop French traders from moving up the Missouri River onto the Plains. In 1720 the Spanish sent soldiers northeast from Santa Fe to check the latest rumors of French incursions. But they pushed too far. An Indian war party, with French support, routed the force somewhere near present-day North Platte, Nebraska. The Spanish defeat only encouraged the Comanches to launch further attacks on Apache settlements.

Within two decades, the Comanches had hammered their enemies south through one river valley after another: the Arkansas, the Red, the Brazos, the Colorado. Desperate Apache bands

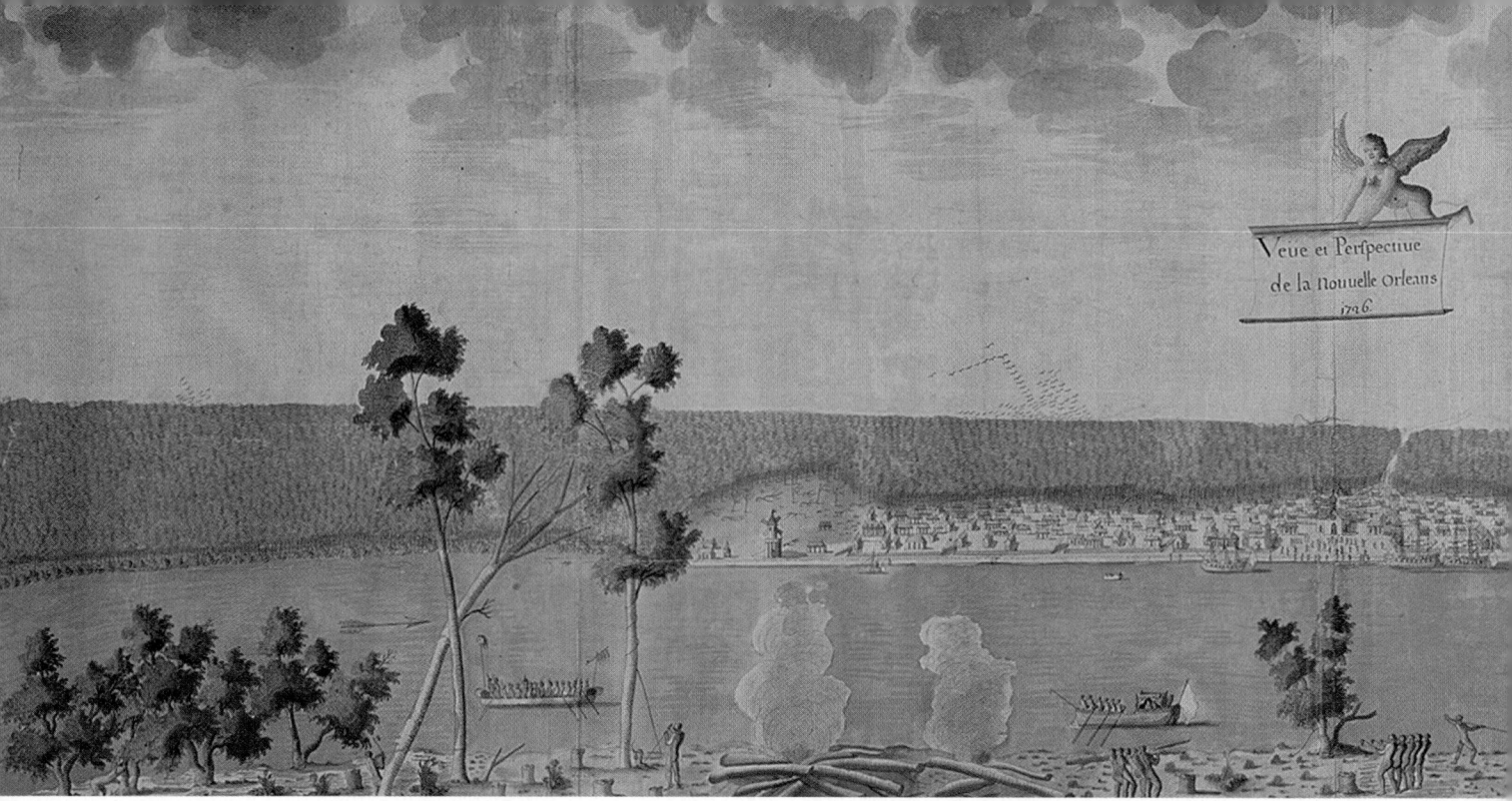

Jean-Pierre Lassus, *Vue et Perspective de la Nouvelle-Orleans*, 1726. C.A.O.M. Aix-en-Provence (France) DFC Louisiane 71 (pf6B)

soon reached the vicinity of San Antonio, where they stole livestock from the new Spanish settlement to survive. Comanche power also pressed the Apaches west, where they raided Spanish outposts in New Mexico. As in Texas, Spanish campaigns against Apache intruders netted captives for the colonial slave trade. When Comanches visited a trade fair at Taos in 1731, they saw first-hand the commerce in Native American captives at the annual *rescate,* or ransoming. Comanche bands then stepped up raids on Apaches and carried the captives to market.

At first, New Mexico resisted the additional trade in slaves. The colony had not been able to protect Apache families or convert them; now it was being asked to buy them. But in the 1740s, officials in Santa Fe discovered that if they turned away Comanche traders, they faced the increasing power of Comanche war parties. So they granted the Comanches access to the *rescate* at Taos in exchange for assurances of peace. With a secure market for their hides, meat, and captives, the Comanches could now focus their raids on central Texas, where their hard-pressed Apache enemies had sealed a pact with the Spanish in 1749.

Not long after they buried the horse in the plaza, the Spanish began plans for a mission and presidio among their new Apache allies. The outpost would lie 150 miles northwest of San Antonio on the San Saba River, near present-day Menard, Texas. But the post had been established for less than a year when the Comanches attacked it in 1758. They returned the next year, capturing 700 horses. "The heathen of the north are innumerable and rich," exclaimed a Spanish officer at San Saba. "They dress well, breed horses, [and] handle firearms with the greatest skill."

Over the next eight years, the Comanche onslaught continued. Their raiders even stole a horse herd from San Antonio itself. Repeated attacks finally forced the Spanish to withdraw from San Saba in 1767. In less than two decades, the Comanches had overrun most of Texas. They continued to absorb smaller Native American groups and swell in numbers. By 1780 they had grown into a proud Indian nation of more than 20,000 people. Their domain, the so-called Comanchería, remained a powerful entity in the Southwest for decades.

The Expansion of the Sioux

Comanche strength depended not only on mounted warfare but also on using the horse as a trade commodity to obtain guns. Because Spanish policy prohibited the sale of firearms to Native Americans, the Comanches looked east for weapons. They quickly discovered that by

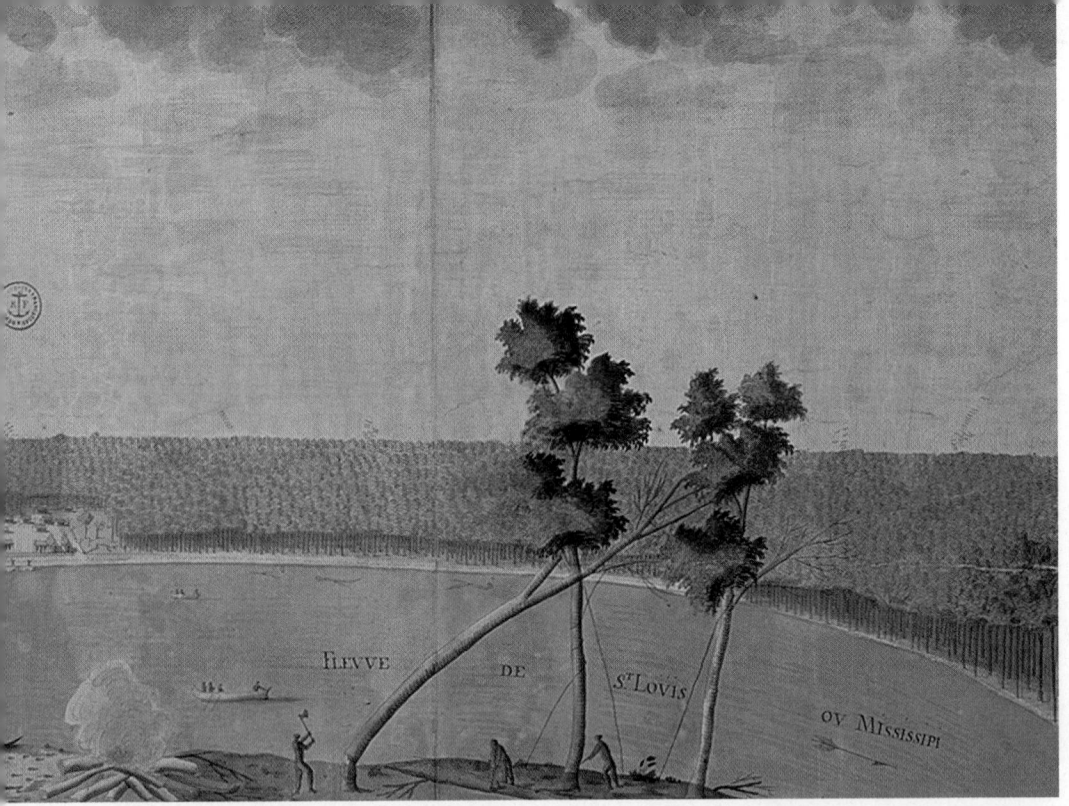

■ By 1726 New Orleans, with 100 cabins and nearly 1000 inhabitants, was receiving shipments of trade goods from France and distributing them up the Mississippi River and its tributaries. Following a Louisiana hurricane in 1722, the levies along the waterfront were expanded, but flooding remains a threat to the low-lying city even today.

selling horses to their eastern allies, such as the Wichita Indians along the Arkansas River, they could receive French muskets from Louisiana in return. But the Comanches were not the only Indian nation to take advantage of the gun frontier as it inched steadily west.

By 1720 the French had established settlements at Peoria, Cahokia, and Kaskaskia in Illinois and at New Orleans, Natchez, and Natchitoches in Louisiana. French traders at these sites provided guns and other metal goods to Indians in exchange for salt, deerskins, beaver pelts, horses, or even war captives to serve as laborers and concubines. Native American groups that took advantage of this trade included the Tunicas beside the lower Mississippi, the Caddos and Wichitas along the Red and Arkansas rivers, and the Osage, Pawnee, and Omaha tribes near the Missouri.

Further north, muskets carried west from French posts on the Great Lakes and south from English bases in subarctic Canada proved more significant than any traffic from Louisiana or Illinois. This northern trade was especially important among the Sioux peoples, who trapped game and gathered wild rice by the lakes of their northern Minnesota homeland. The Comanches had mastered horses and then acquired guns; the Sioux, given their different location, first absorbed firearms and then adopted the horse. But the results proved equally dramatic.

When the Sioux first encountered a gun from French voyageurs in the mid-seventeenth century, they called it *mazawakan*, meaning "mysterious or sacred iron." Initially, they used the few muskets they could obtain to fight their less well-armed Indian neighbors to the north. But in 1682, English agents established an outpost at the mouth of the Nelson River on Hudson Bay, trading muskets to Native Americans for furs. Supplied with shiploads of guns by the Hudson's Bay Company, Cree and Assiniboine Indians pushed southwest, expanding their hunting territory as they depleted the fur supply.

Pressured by these northern rivals, several Sioux bands (the Teton and Yanktonai) migrated to the prairie country of southwest Minnesota, learning to hunt for buffalo on foot. They also sought beaver for an expanding European market. Ready access to firearms facilitated the Sioux migration, giving them a military advantage over tribes to their west. By 1700 French traders, moving from the east, had established direct trade with the Sioux, offering a steady supply of guns and powder in exchange for furs.

For several generations, the Sioux walked between two worlds. In the summers, they followed the buffalo onto the prairies, with dogs pulling travois and women carrying heavy burdens. As cold weather approached, they retreated to the edge of the woodlands to gather

155

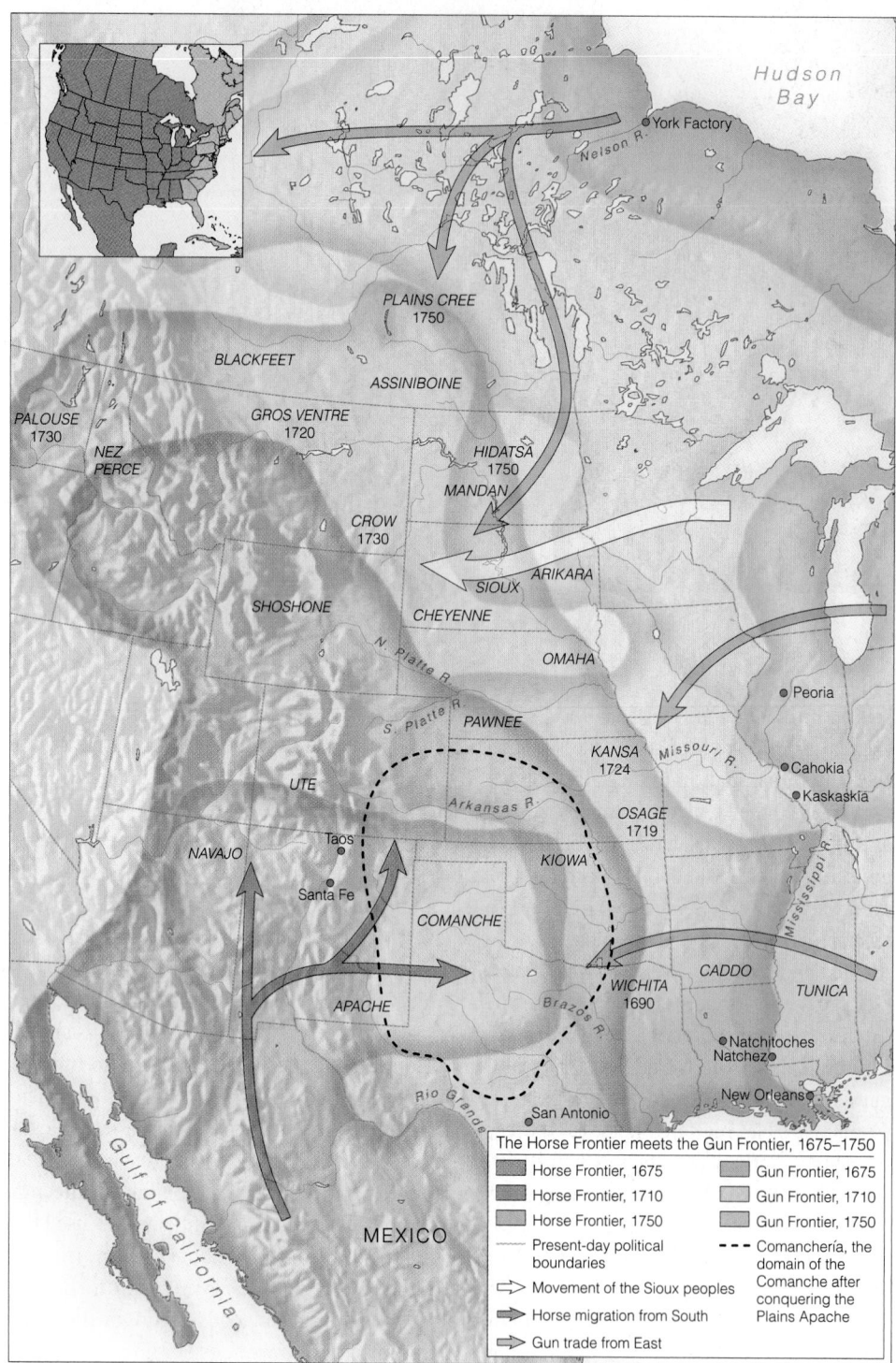

■ MAP 5.2
THE HORSE FRONTIER MEETS THE GUN FRONTIER, 1675–1750

firewood and seek beaver. In the spring, after trading meat and pelts to the French for guns and ammunition, they returned to the edge of the plains. They glimpsed their first horses not long after 1700. But it was several generations before the western Sioux had acquired enough mounts and developed sufficient confidence to drop their old customs and adopt a horse-centered way of life.

By midcentury, the horse frontier on the northern Great Plains had met the gun frontier, just as it had in what is now Texas, Arkansas, and Missouri. Saukamappee, a Cree Indian living with the Blackfeet, remembered vividly the surprise of the initial encounter. When he was a young man, his war party—well armed and on foot—had gone into battle against the Shoshones. "We had more guns and iron headed arrows than [ever] before," he recalled years later. "But our enemies . . . and their allies had Misstutim [Big Dogs, that is Horses] on which they rode, swift as the Deer."

Indian women remembered the arrival of the horse and the gun with ambivalence. These new assets improved food supplies and made travel less burdensome, but the transition brought disadvantages as well. Violent raids became more common, and young men who fought as warriors gained status in the community compared to older men and women. Also, the hard task of processing slain buffalo increased, creating new work for women even as it provided fresh resources for the whole community.

As the overlap of horse and gun proceeded after 1750, Sioux men bearing muskets continued to acquire mounts and fight for control of the buffalo grounds. Their competitors, all of whom had recently acquired horses, now had guns as well. But within several decades, the Sioux had pushed their domain west to the Missouri River. Like the Comanches farther south, they had emerged as the dominant power across a wide portion of the Great Plains—a force to be reckoned with in the century ahead.

Britain's Mainland Colonies: A New Abundance of People

East of the Rockies, horses and guns brought dramatic shifts as the eighteenth century progressed. But east of the Appalachian Mountains, a different force prompted striking change: population growth. Several factors came together to push the demographic curve upward at an unprecedented rate after 1700. From our vantage point in the twenty-first century, the colonial seaports and villages appear tiny, and rural settlement seems sparse. But by the mid-eighteenth century, the coastal colonies represented the largest concentration of people that had ever occupied any portion of the continent.

On both sides of the North Atlantic, steady population growth characterized eighteenth-century life. In Europe, improvements in agriculture led to larger harvests and more fodder for keeping livestock alive through long winters. These changes prompted better diets, and they were accompanied by improvements in food distribution and sanitation that also assisted population growth. But as European numbers rose at a more or less steady pace, the population of Atlantic North America surged. A comparison with England demonstrates how astounding American demographic growth was along the eastern seaboard. England in 1700 had 5.1 million people, and that figure increased a mere 14 percent to 5.8 million by 1750. In the same half century, the colonial population in British North America more than quadrupled, from 260,000 to nearly 1.2 million.

This enormous expansion in numbers contained an additional change. During the first two thirds of the eighteenth century, the Atlantic seaboard colonies made a permanent and dramatic shift away from a population that was almost entirely of English origin. Never before had North America seen such extensive ethnic and racial diversity. As the numerous cultures and languages indigenous to western Europe, western Africa, and eastern North America mixed and mingled, they gave rise to an American Babel.

Population Growth on the Home Front

Natural increase—more births than deaths—played an important role in colonial population growth. Marriages occurred early, and the need for labor created an incentive for couples to have large families. Benjamin Franklin, who rose to become the best-known colonist of his generation, was born in Boston in 1706. He grew up in a household of 17 children. Large

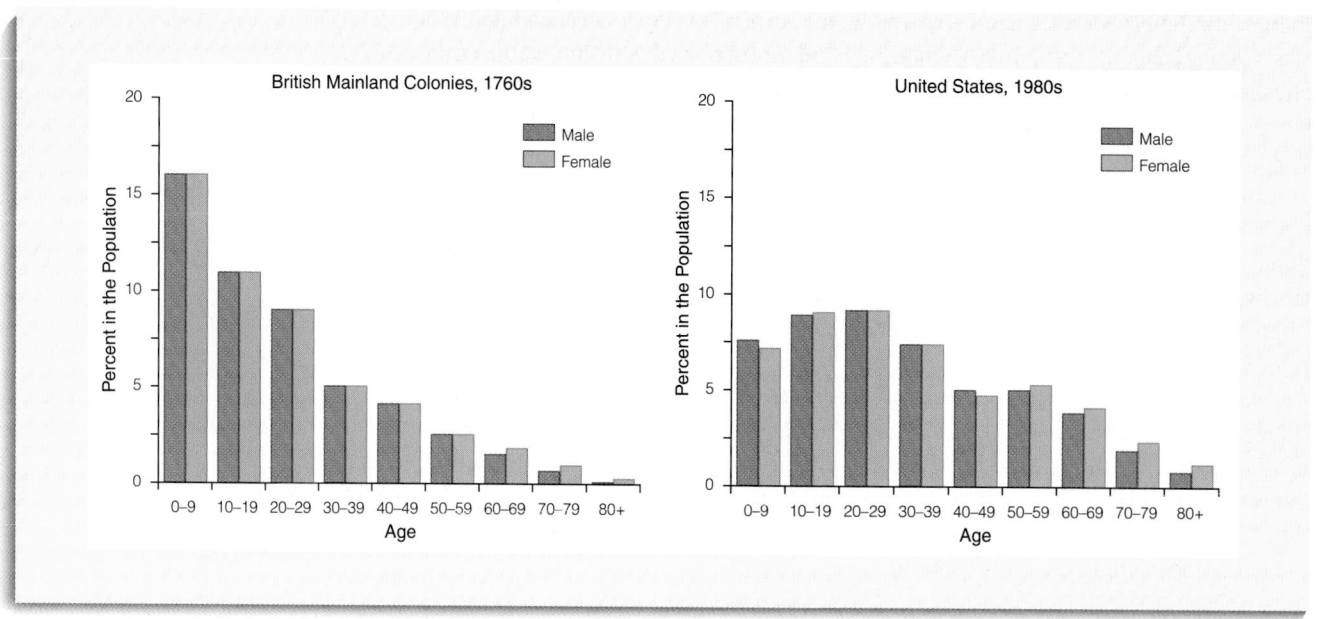

■ **FIGURE 5.1**
COMPARISON OF OVERALL POPULATION STRUCTURE BY GENDER AND AGE: BRITISH MAINLAND COLONIES, 1760s, AND UNITED STATES, 1980s

families had long been commonplace, to compensate for frequent deaths among children. What made the Franklin family unusual was that all the children survived childhood and started families of their own. (Such success would have been highly unlikely in the previous century, when 28 percent of young people in New England died before age 20, and the mortality rate was far higher in Virginia.)

Although a high birth rate typified most preindustrial cultures, it was the low death rate and long average life span that pushed up American population numbers. With no huge urban centers, the colonial populace remained dispersed, so epidemics proved less devastating and of shorter duration than in Europe. Food was plentiful, and housing improved steadily. Newborns who survived infancy could live a long life. Franklin himself lived 84 years, and his publications, the *Pennsylvania Gazette* and *Poor Richard's Almanack,* offered frequent advice and encouragement for readers to become healthy as well as "wealthy and wise."

The 1720s and 1730s proved generally peaceful, in contrast to most earlier decades, so soldiering did not disrupt work and endanger lives among men of military age. For women, death related to pregnancy and childbirth still loomed as a constant threat. (Franklin's own mother was his father's second wife; the first wife died after bearing seven children.) Yet women still outnumbered men among people living into their sixties, seventies, and eighties. Although grandparents often endured far into old age, the average age for the total population stayed remarkably young. In the mid-eighteenth century, fully a third of all people in the British mainland colonies were under age 10, and more than half were under age 20. In the late twentieth century, in contrast, barely one-seventh of all living Americans were below 10 ten years of age, and fewer than one-third were below 20.

The reasons for such a young overall population seem clear. The ratio between men and women was becoming more even over time, the marriage rates for women remained extremely high, and there was no effective means of contraception. Women could resort to sexual abstinence to avoid pregnancy, and mothers could extend the time between births by nursing their infants for a long period (since lactation reduces the chances of conception). Not surprisingly, children abounded.

"Packed Like Herrings": Arrivals from Abroad

Frequent births and improving survival rates were only part of the population story. Immigration—both forced and free—also contributed mightily to the colonies' growth. The unfree arrivals came in two different streams from two separate continents and faced very different prospects. The largest flow of unfree arrivals came from Africa, and these forced migrants faced a bleak new life with few options for improvement. Well before the 1720s, the system of race-based slavery was sanctioned by law. By the 1730s, the expanding trans-Atlantic slave trade brought at least 4000 Africans to the colonies every year, and the rate increased steadily. In 1756, Charleston, South Carolina, received more than 2200 slaves aboard 14 ships (including vessels that bore grimly ironic names such as *Relief, Hope,* and *Success*).

A separate stream of unfree laborers came to the colonies from Europe. It included prisoners forced from crowded jails and also indentured servants unable to pay their own way to America. By comparison to enslaved Africans, the long-term prospects of these European migrants were far more promising. Every year, hundreds of detainees in British jails were offered transportation to the colonies and a term of service laboring in America as an alternative to prison time or execution. In Daniel Defoe's romance *Moll Flanders* (1722), English authorities deport the fictional heroine to Virginia for her crimes as a pickpocket, and she ends up inheriting considerable wealth. Most real-life convicts had no such luck, but most earned their freedom and found ways to blend in to colonial society.

Deported felons joined the larger flow of unfree migrants from Europe: poor people, unable to pay for their own passage, who accepted transportation to America as indentured servants. All were sold to employers to serve as workers, with scant legal rights, until their indenture expired, usually after three to six years. In the 1720s, Philadelphia shippers devised a variation on indentures known as the redemption contract. Under this redemption system, agents in Europe recruited migrants by contracting to loan them money for passage and provisions. On arrival in America, the recruits could then sign a pact with an employer of their own choosing. That person agreed to pay back the shipper, "redeeming" the original loan that had been made to the immigrant. In exchange, the newcomer (called a redemptioner) promised to work for the employer for several years, receiving no more than room and board. After that, the redemptioners were on their own, and their prospects usually improved.

> *Detainees in British jails were offered transportation to the colonies and a term of service as an alternative to prison time or execution.*

Besides Africans who remained unfree for life and Europeans who gained freedom after a period of service, a smaller stream of newcomers involved free families arriving from Europe who could pay their own way. Poor conditions at home pushed these risk-takers to try their luck in the New World, and glowing descriptions of abundant land at bargain rates caught their attention. American land speculators hoped to rent or sell forest tracts to immigrant farmers who would improve the value of the land by clearing acreage, constructing fences, and building homes. For example, Boston merchant Samuel Waldo, infected by this "speculative fever," induced several hundred Germans and Scots to come to America in the 1740s. He transported them to his extensive wilderness lands east of the Damariscotta River, where they became the early inhabitants of what is now Waldoboro, Maine.

Britain's imperial administrators also sought to recruit Europeans to the American colonies. The settlements these immigrants established could bolster colonial defenses against foreign rivals and provide a buffer on the frontier to ward off Indian attacks. In one of many pamphlets for German immigrants, Joshua von Kocherthal explained how South Carolina's proprietors would give a 65-acre plot to each head of household, with the promise of more land if they needed it or if they came with a large group.

Even with such enticements, South Carolina's enslaved African community expanded faster than its free population. By 1760 blacks outnumbered whites 58,000 to 39,000. The next year, fearing the prospect of a slave revolt, the South Carolina government offered a bounty of £4 sterling ($360) to anyone importing a Protestant European, and it provided a smaller amount

"Pastures Can Be Found Almost Everywhere": Joshua von Kocherthal Recruits Germans to Carolina

Joshua von Kocherthal grew up near Heidelberg, capital of the Electoral Palatinate in southern Germany, and trained to be a Lutheran minister. On a visit to London at the start of the eighteenth century, he learned of England's desire to recruit settlers to its American colonies. Because fellow Germans faced hard times at home, he led several groups to New York, where they established Neuberg (Newburgh) on the Hudson River. In 1706, Kocherthal also published a German-language tract promoting migration to South Carolina. The popular booklet went through several editions in his Palatinate homeland east of the Rhine River.

The winter of 1708–1709 was especially harsh in the Palatinate. In the spring of 1709, a stream of desperate refugee families migrated north along the Rhine and then west to England. From there, they hoped to obtain passage across the Atlantic to South Carolina. Many carried Kocherthal's simple pamphlet, and they focused on the numerous advantages outlined in his brochure, especially the abundance of land. According to Kocherthal, the colonial government registered all land grants "to prevent errors or future arguments," and it exempted newcomers from taxes for several years. Best of all, food was plentiful, no feudal obligations or serfdom existed, and members of Protestant denominations had "freedom of religion and conscience."

South Carolina is one of the most fertile landscapes to be found . . . preferable in many respects to the terrain in Germany, as well as in England. . . . Game, fish, and birds, as well as waterfowl such as swans, geese, and ducks, occur there in such plentiful numbers that . . . newcomers can sustain themselves if necessary . . . until they have cleared a piece of land, sown seeds, and gathered in a harvest. . . . Among other things, there can be found in the wild so-called "Indian chickens" [turkeys], some of which weigh about 40 pounds or even more. These exist in incredible numbers. . . .

Hunting game, fishing, and bird-catching are free to anyone, but one shouldn't cross the borders of neighbors or of the Indians [who] live in complete peace and friendship with our families. In addition, their number decreases while the number of our people (namely the Europeans) increases. . . . Lumber can be found there in abundance, especially the most beautiful oaks, but also many of the nicest chestnuts and nut trees which are used by many for building and are considered better than oaks. One can also find beeches, spruces, cypresses, cedars, laurels, myrtle, and many other varieties.

Hogs can be raised very easily in great numbers at little cost, because there are huge forests everywhere and the ground is covered with acorns. . . . Above all, the breeding of horses, cows, sheep, hogs and many other kinds of domestic livestock proceeds excellently, because pastures can

($90) to help the new immigrant get started. These incentives prompted importers to seek out migrants, using kidnapping if necessary, and move them at the least possible expense. Importers' only aim, according to one local observer, was "to deliver as many as possible alive on Shoar upon the cheapest terms, and no matter how they fared upon their Voyage nor in what condition they were landed." More than 3000 newcomers reached South Carolina under this system, but the abuses proved so shocking that it was discontinued after seven years.

Even for those who could pay their own way, the Atlantic passage was a life-threatening ordeal. "The people are packed densely, like herrings," Lutheran minister Gottlieb Mittelberger recorded after a voyage to Pennsylvania. "During the journey the ship is full of pitiful signs of distress—smells, fumes, horrors, vomiting, various kinds of sea sickness, fever, dysentery, headaches, heat, constipation, boils, scurvy, cancer, mouth-rot, and similar afflictions." Despite such hardships, newcomers found economic opportunities awaiting them in America. They often wrote home glowing accounts of colonial life, and their letters helped boost the rising population further. In 1773 English customs officials quizzed 29-year-old Elizabeth McDonald about why she was departing for Wilmington, North Carolina. The unmarried Scottish servant replied that she was setting out "because several of her friends, having gone to Carolina before her, had assured her that she would get much better service and greater encouragement in Carolina than in her own country."

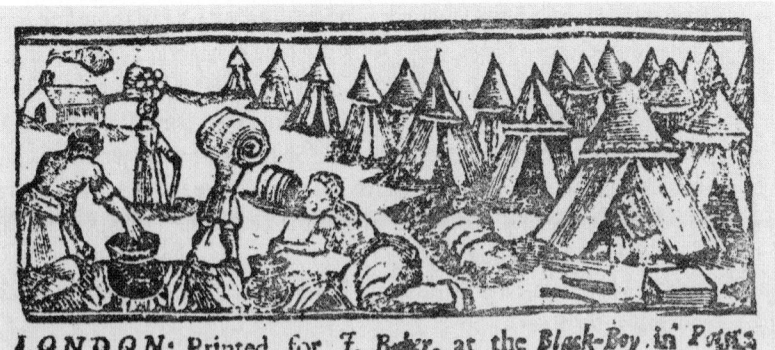

In 1709, roughly 13,000 German immigrants seeking passage to America encamped for months at Blackheath, near London. The British government supplied the Palatines with tents, blankets, bread, and cheese, and churchgoers prayed for their welfare. But other Britons protested that the German strangers took "bread out of the mouths of our native handicraft men and laboring people, and increase the number of our poor which are too many and too great a burden to our nation already." Most of the refugees reached North America, serving as the vanguard for later German migration.

be found almost everywhere, and the livestock can remain in the fields the whole year, as it gets no colder in Carolina in the middle of winter than it does in Germany in April or October. . . . Because of the multiplication of livestock, almost no household in Carolina (after residing there a few years) can justifiably be called poor.

As far as vegetables and fruits are concerned, Indian corn predominates, thriving in such a way that one can harvest it twice a year and grow it wherever one wants to. Our local cereals such as wheat, rye, barley, and oats do well, but above all, rice thrives there as excellently as in any other part of the world, and it grows in such amounts that it can be loaded on ships and transported to other places. And as the inhabitants use rice so much and make much more profit from it than any other cereal, they are most keen on growing rice and there has been very little cultivation of other cereals.

All kinds of our fruits can be planted there, but . . . future arrivals would do well to bring along seedlings of any kind, or at least the seeds. . . . There can already be found different kinds of our local apples. . . . As far as cabbage, beets, beans, peas, and other garden plants are concerned, not only do our local plants grow very well, but there are also many other varieties with excellent taste that are completely unknown to us. . . . Newcomers will do well to acquire all sorts of iron tools and bring these along. . . . If someone has lived in Carolina for a time and he wants to go to another country, he may do so freely at any time. ∎

Source: Translations by Dorothee Lehlbach from Joshua von Kocherthal, *Ausfeuhrlicher und umstaendlicher Bericht von der beruehmten Landschaft Carolina, in dem engellaendischen American gelegen* (Frankfurt: Georg Heinrich Oehrling, 2nd ed., 1709), in the Special Collections Library of Duke University.

Non-English Newcomers in the British Colonies

Colonies that were thoroughly English at their origin became decidedly more varied after 1700. By far the largest and most striking change came from North America's increasing involvement in the Atlantic slave trade. By 1750, some 240,000 African Americans made up 20 percent of the population of the British colonies. Native Americans had been drawn into the mix in small numbers as slaves, servants, spouses, and Christian converts. But roughly four out of five colonists were of European descent. Among them, as among the Africans and Indians, many spoke English with a different accent, or as a second language, or not at all.

No area went untouched by this change. The New England colonies remained the most homogenous, but even there, 30 percent of the residents had non-English roots by 1760. The new diversity, which increasingly characterized American society in future centuries, was most visible in New York because of the colony's non-English origins. A 1703 census of New York City shows that the town had no single ethnic majority. It remained 42 percent Dutch, with English (30 percent) and Africans (18 percent) making up nearly half the population. The rest of the population included a small Jewish community (1 percent) and a growing number of French Protestants (9 percent).

The French New Yorkers had fled to America after Louis XIV ended protection for the Protestant minority of France. When the king revoked the long-standing Edict of Nantes in

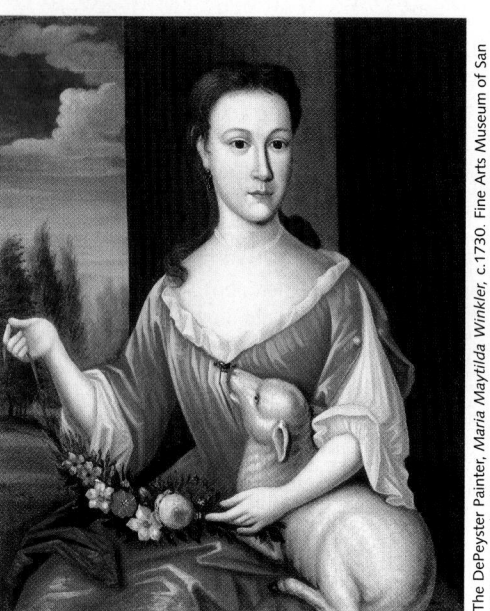

The DePeyster Painter, *Maria Maytilda Winkler*, c.1730. Fine Arts Museum of San Francisco, Gift of Mr. and Mrs. John D. Rockefeller 3rd, 1979.7.34

■ Colonial artists often copied engravings of well-known European pictures and then inserted a likeness of their client's head. That was the case in this New York portrait of Maria Maytilda Winkler, made around 1730 by a Dutch-American "limner," or painter.

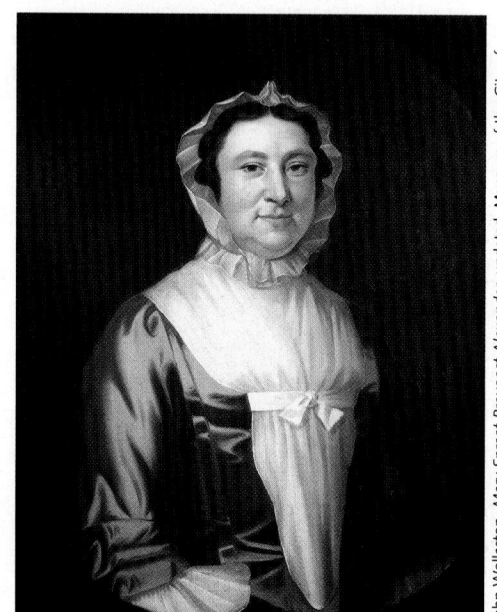

John Wollaston, *Mary Spratt Provoost Alexander*, undated. Museum of the City of New York, Gift of William Hamilton Russell (50.215.4)

■ Like many New Yorkers of her generation, shopkeeper Mary Spratt Provoost Alexander (1693–1760) spoke both Dutch and English. Her Dutch mother had married a Scottish immigrant, and Mary was the wife of a local attorney who also came from Scotland.

1685, he also prohibited Huguenot emigration, but several thousand French Protestants escaped illegally and sought refuge in America. They established small communities such as those at New Rochelle in New York and along South Carolina's Santee River. South Carolina's governor protested against the Huguenots' early political activity: "Shall the Frenchmen, who cannot speak our language, make our laws?" But everywhere, they intermarried with the English and prospered in commerce. By the 1760s, several families with humble Huguenot origins—among them the Faneuils in Boston and the Laurenses, Manigaults, and Ravenels in Charleston—had amassed enormous fortunes.

At a time when France and Great Britain were at war, another infusion of French-speaking refugees, the Acadians, fared less well. In 1755, authorities evicted French colonials from Acadia in British Nova Scotia, fearing they might take up arms for France. Officials burned their homes and deported more than 6000 of them further south, allotting shiploads to the various coastal colonies so that widely dispersed groups could pose no threat. Mistreated for their Catholicism and feared as enemies during wartime, the Acadians struggled to make ends meet. Most had lost all their property. Some, who could not support themselves, were sold into indentured servitude, adults and children alike. Feeling unwelcome in their new homes, many eventually moved on to French Louisiana, where the Acadians, or Cajuns, became a lasting cultural force.

Scotland provided a much larger flow of migrants than France, stemming from two different sources. A growing stream of families, at least 30,000 people by 1770, came from Scotland itself. They were pushed by poverty, land scarcity, famines, and a failed political rebellion in 1745. In addition, a larger group known as the Scots-Irish came from Ulster in Ireland. The British had encouraged these Scottish Presbyterians to settle in Northern Ireland in the seventeenth century, displacing rebellious Irish Catholics. But the Scottish newcomers in Ulster soon faced commercial and political restrictions from Parliament and the Anglican church. By 1770 nearly 60,000 Scots-Irish had opted to leave Ireland for America. Scottish immigrants became farmers and traders throughout the colonies. In Georgia, for example, they established New Inverness (now Darien) on the southern coastal frontier in 1736.

Another stream, German-speaking immigrants from the heart of Europe, nearly equaled the combined flow of Scots and Scots-Irish settlers. They began to arrive shortly after 1700 as religious persecution, chronic land shortages, and generations of warfare pushed whole communities out of the so-called Palatinate in southern Germany and also neighboring Switzerland. Roughly 30,000 migrated in the 1750s alone, and by 1770 the total had reached 85,000. Even more than other European newcomers, these refugees generally came as whole families, and they usually took up farmland on the fringes of the colonies. Germans occupied the Mohawk Valley in New York and the Shenandoah Valley in Virginia, and they fanned out from Germantown across the rich farmland of Pennsylvania. Swiss founded New Bern, North Carolina, in 1710, and migrants from Salzburg established New Ebenezer near Savannah, Georgia, in 1734.

Almost all of the white, non-English newcomers, including several thousand migrants from Wales, were Protestant Christians. Many clung to their language and traditions. (Because the new Pennsylvanians spoke

German, or *Deutsch,* they became known as Pennsylvania Dutch.) But most arrivals learned English, and many of their children intermarried with the English settlers. An eighteenth-century Frenchman wrote of meeting a typical American "whose grandfather was an Englishman, whose wife is Dutch, whose son married a French woman, and whose present four sons have now four wives of different nations."

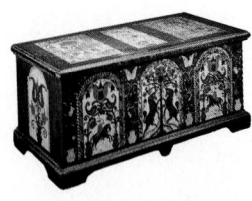

The Varied Economic Landscape

Population growth had consequences, and the changes began at the water's edge. Ships carrying newcomers docked most often at Boston, New York, Philadelphia, or Charleston. Each of these deepwater ports grew from a village to a bustling commercial hub, absorbing manufactured goods from Britain and shipping colonial produce abroad. All four towns spawned secondary ports located on neighboring rivers, where small boats carried on an active coastal trade. Chesapeake Bay, with no single dominant port, was the exception. There, Baltimore, Annapolis, Alexandria, and Newport all expanded. But given the bay's many rivers, Atlantic ships often visited separate riverside plantations and villages to do business.

In Chesapeake Bay and elsewhere, inland commerce was conducted by boat wherever possible. Hartford and Springfield on the Connecticut River, Kingston and Albany on the Hudson, Wilmington and Trenton on the Delaware, and Savannah and Augusta on the Savannah all become active riverside trading centers. Richmond, Virginia, which began as a trading post at the falls of the James River, already had 250 inhabitants when it incorporated as a town in 1742. Trails

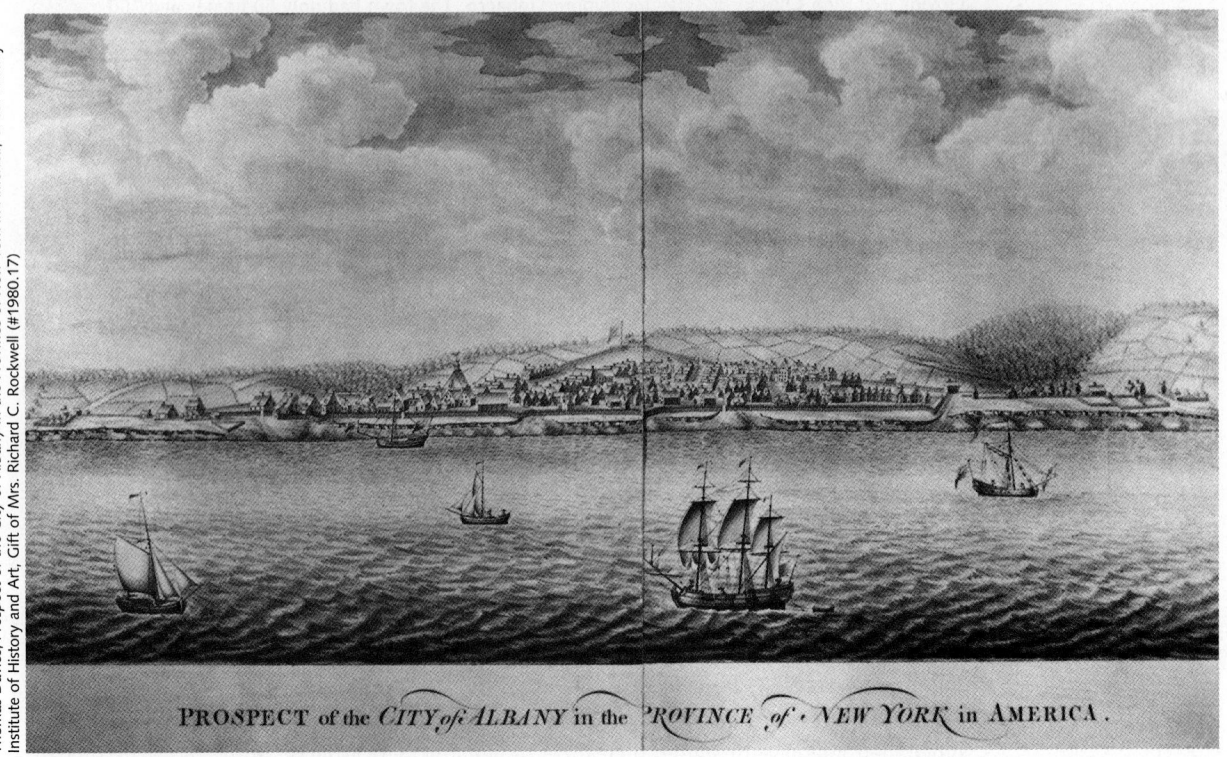

■ Albany, a fur-trading center for generations, prospered in the mid-eighteenth century. The Hudson River town would become the capital of New York in 1797 and the starting point for the Erie Canal, completed in 1825.

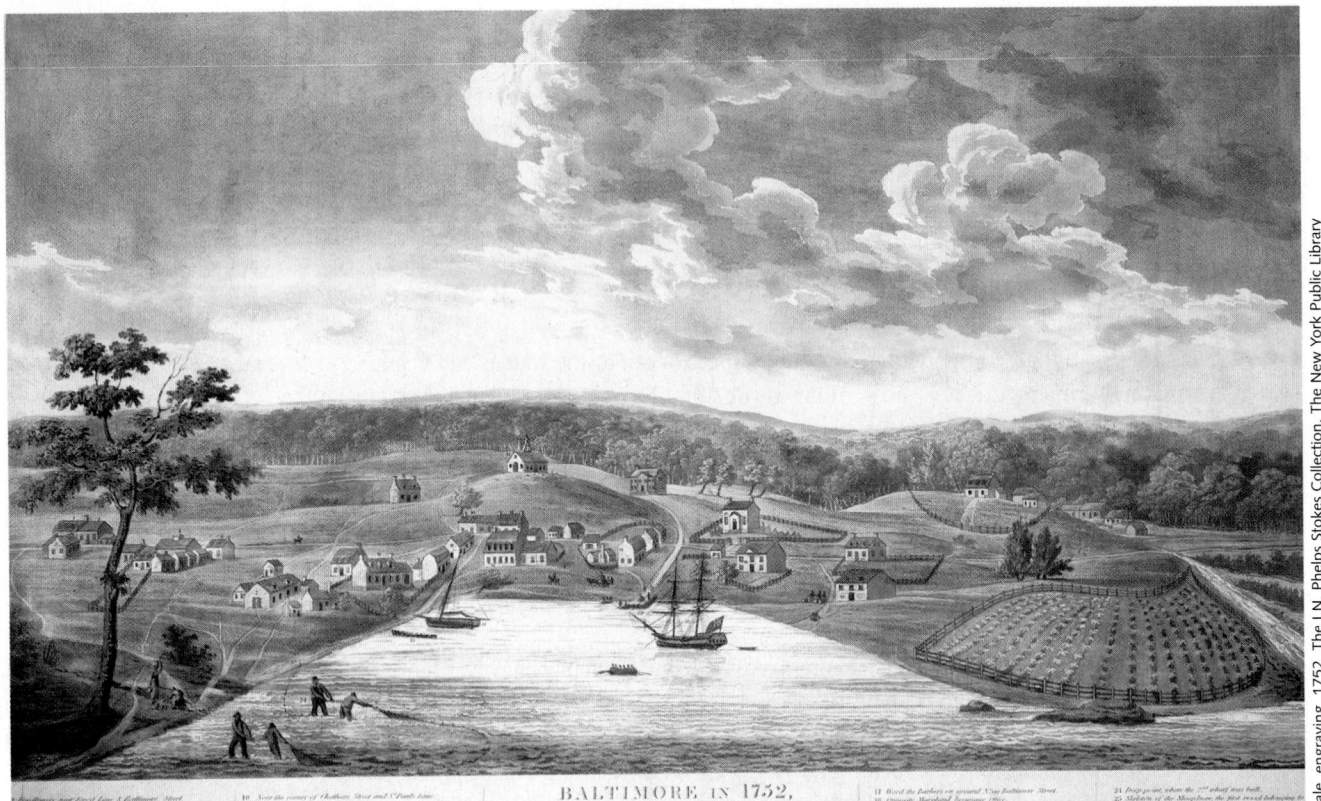

■ **A 1752 sketch of Baltimore by John Moale. In 1729 Maryland planters founded Baltimore to provide a port on Chesapeake Bay for shipping tobacco. The town had only 50 homes and 200 inhabitants when this early sketch was made, but it grew rapidly after that.**

and former Indian paths connected these river-based communities, easing the way for travelers in the hinterland. By the 1740s, a pathway known as the Great Wagon Road headed southwest from Philadelphia to Winchester in Virginia's Shenandoah Valley and then south through gaps in the Blue Ridge Mountains to the Piedmont region of central Carolina.

Widening networks of contact, using boats and wagons, extended inland from the primary ports. And expanding fleets of ships tied each major hub to distant Atlantic ports. As a result, farmsteads and villages that had been largely self-sufficient before 1710 gradually became linked to wider markets. Local production still met most needs. But increasingly, the opportunity existed to obtain a new tool, a piece of cloth, or a printed almanac from far away. These and scores of other items might come from a larger town in the colony or from abroad. The new possibility of obtaining such goods lured farmers to grow crops for market rather than plant only for home consumption.

As local commercial systems gained coherence and strength, a string of regional economies developed along the Atlantic seaboard. Coastal vessels and a few muddy roads linked them tenuously to one another. But geographical and human differences caused each to take on a character of its own, and this distinctiveness increased over the years. Migration patterns reinforced this diversity, since arrivals from Europe often sought out areas where others already spoke their language or shared their form of worship. The growing influx of German farmers through Philadelphia, for example, gave unique traits to life in colonial Pennsylvania. Likewise, the rising importation of Africans helped shape the economy and culture of Chesapeake Bay, and the same held true for coastal South Carolina. Besides the diversity among arriv-

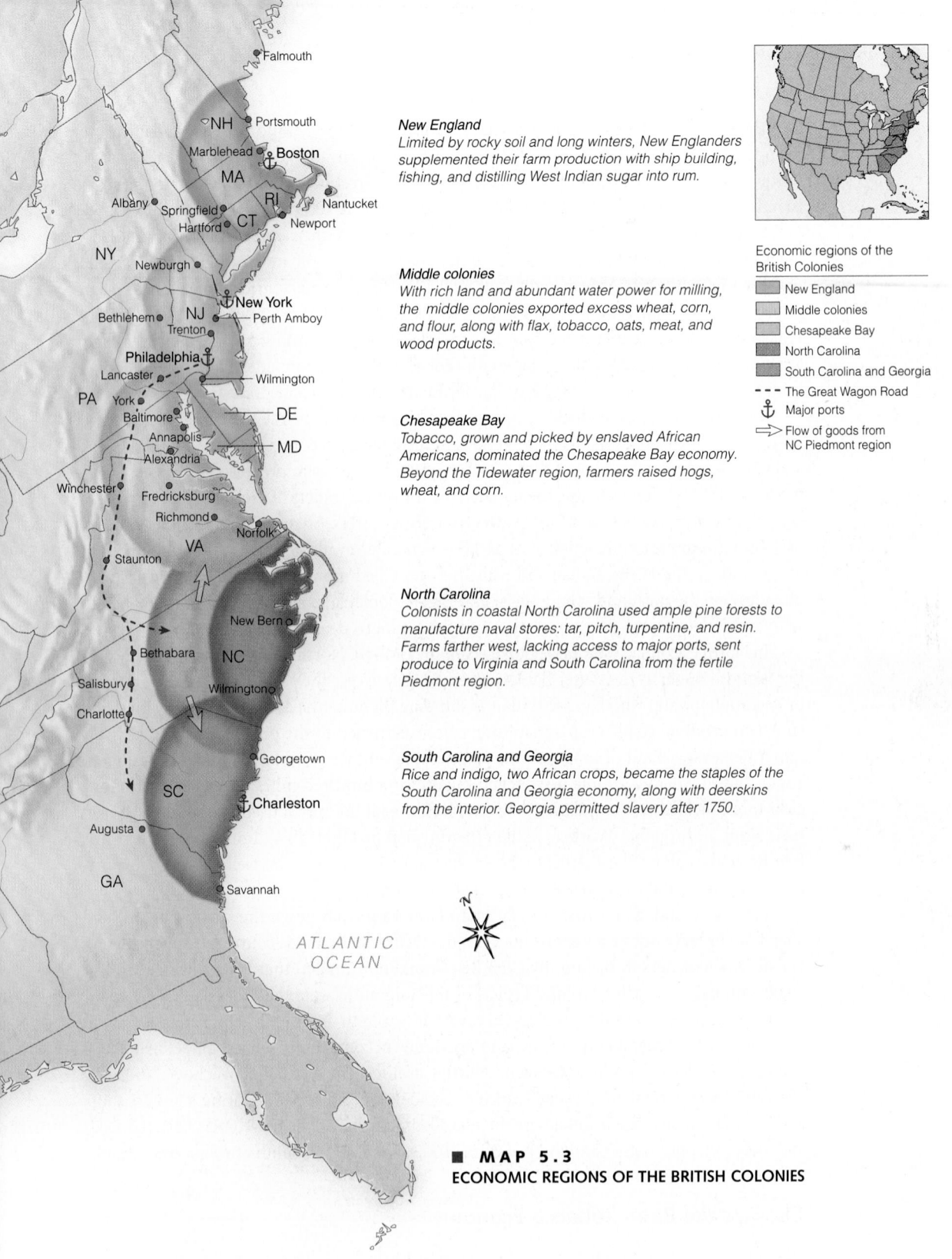

New England
Limited by rocky soil and long winters, New Englanders supplemented their farm production with ship building, fishing, and distilling West Indian sugar into rum.

Middle colonies
With rich land and abundant water power for milling, the middle colonies exported excess wheat, corn, and flour, along with flax, tobacco, oats, meat, and wood products.

Chesapeake Bay
Tobacco, grown and picked by enslaved African Americans, dominated the Chesapeake Bay economy. Beyond the Tidewater region, farmers raised hogs, wheat, and corn.

North Carolina
Colonists in coastal North Carolina used ample pine forests to manufacture naval stores: tar, pitch, turpentine, and resin. Farms farther west, lacking access to major ports, sent produce to Virginia and South Carolina from the fertile Piedmont region.

South Carolina and Georgia
Rice and indigo, two African crops, became the staples of the South Carolina and Georgia economy, along with deerskins from the interior. Georgia permitted slavery after 1750.

Economic regions of the
British Colonies

▢ New England
▢ Middle colonies
▢ Chesapeake Bay
▢ North Carolina
▢ South Carolina and Georgia
- - - The Great Wagon Road
⚓ Major ports
⇨ Flow of goods from
NC Piedmont region

■ **MAP 5.3**
ECONOMIC REGIONS OF THE BRITISH COLONIES

ing peoples, American ecological differences played a role as well. Variations in land and climate contributed to the emergence of five distinctive economic regions along the Atlantic coast.

Sources of Gain in the Southeast

Two related but distinctive regions took shape along the southeastern coast, linked respectively to the two Carolina colonies. The larger of the two centered on the lowcountry of coastal South Carolina. There, the warm current of the Gulf Stream moving north from Florida along the

Sea Islands provided a long growing season. It also assured very mild winters, in contrast to Europe, and this meant that cattle and hogs could forage in the woods unattended for most of the year. As livestock multiplied, settlers sold meat, barrel staves, and firewood to the sugar islands of the West Indies, purchasing African slave labor in return.

Some of the newcomers had grown rice in Africa before their enslavement, and in planting it for their own use they soon demonstrated that the crop, unfamiliar to the English, could thrive in Carolina. Once African know-how made clear the potential for rice cultivation, a system of plantation agriculture, imported from Barbados, took hold quickly after 1700. Rice production spread to Georgia after that colony legalized slavery in 1751. Another African plant, indigo, also took root as a money-making staple crop. For several generations after 1740, cakes of indigo from South Carolina provided the blue dye for England's rising textile industry.

On Charleston's busy docks, casks of deerskins piled up beside the barrels of rice and indigo. The extensive deerskin trade in South Carolina and Georgia depended on the Creek and Cherokee men who hunted the animals and the women who processed the hides. Keeping some skins for domestic use, the Indians sold the rest to traders in exchange for guns, blankets, cloth, knives, kettles, and rum. Native American bearers, often women, carried the heavy packs of skins to the trading posts until packhorses became available in the region. At the height of the trade in the 1730s, Indian and white hunters killed more than a million deer per year, often leaving the meat and selling the skin. When colonial laws against overhunting failed to stem the onslaught, the deer population and the southern deerskin trade declined.

In North Carolina, a second regional economy evolved. North of Cape Fear, the sandy barrier islands known as the Outer Banks prevented easy access for oceangoing vessels and gave protection to pirates who harassed Atlantic shipping. Because the coastal geography hindered efforts to promote staple crop agriculture, colonists turned to the pine forest to make a living. An extensive band of longleaf pine rimmed the southern coastal plain from Virginia to Texas, and in North Carolina it stretched inland for a hundred miles. With labor, this longleaf forest yielded an abundance of naval stores: the tar and pitch used by sailors to protect their ships and rigging. Workers hauled the finished products to Wilmington on the Cape Fear River, the colony's best outlet to the sea. By the 1770s, the port was well known for exporting naval stores, and a dozen sawmills dotted the river.

Further inland, Scots-Irish and German families moved down the Great Wagon Road after 1740 to carve out farms across the Carolina Piedmont on lands controlled largely by several absentee owners in Britain. By 1763 Ben Franklin estimated that Pennsylvania had lost 10,000 families to North Carolina. Typical of this migration were the Moravians, a German-speaking religious group who established towns at Nazareth and Bethlehem, Pennsylvania, in the 1740s. In 1753 members of the expanding Moravian community bought a tract of 100,000 acres near modern-day Winston-Salem, North Carolina. They named it Wachovia, meaning "Peaceful Valley," and within several years they had developed prosperous farms, a pottery shop, and a tannery around their initial settlement, called Bethabara. The newcomers bartered seeds and tools with one another and shipped extra produce overland to South Carolina and Virginia.

Chesapeake Bay's Tobacco Economy

North of the Carolinas, farmers in the colonies bordering Chesapeake Bay committed to tobacco production in the seventeenth century. They clung to that staple crop despite a long decline in its market price. After 1710, demand for tobacco revived and prices rose again, in part because snuff (pulverized tobacco inhaled through the nostrils) became increasingly popular among Europeans. An additional boost came from the French government. It granted a monopoly to a company that bought large amounts of Chesapeake tobacco and distributed it efficiently across Europe. Tobacco prices remained strong, and the leaf continued to dominate the Chesapeake economy. But local conditions in parts of Virginia and Maryland prompted crop diversification as the century progressed.

For one thing, constant tobacco planting depleted the soil and reduced yields. For another, certain soils proved poorly suited for the crop. In addition, most new farmland lay far from any navigable river, and rolling huge casks of tobacco many miles to market became an expensive chore. Wheat and corn thus emerged as important secondary staples. These new crops, along with flax, hemp, and apples for making cider, provided a buffer against poor tobacco harvests. They also spurred related economic activities such as building wagons, making barrels, and constructing mills. These trades, in turn, produced widening networks of local exchange and prosperity for white yeoman families, with or without slaves.

Before 1700, all the mainland colonies could be described as *societies with slaves.* After that, the northern colonies continued to allow enslavement, but they never relied on it. In contrast, the southern colonies, except for certain inland farmlands settled from the north, shifted early in the eighteenth century to become something different: full-fledged *slave societies,* tied economically and culturally to slavery. The system of forced labor created constant tension and violence. But it also created widespread wealth in the white community. In a circular fashion, planters exporting staple crops to Britain reaped sufficient profits to invest in additional African labor to grow more tobacco and rice.

By midcentury, plantation owners remained less wealthy than their counterparts in the West Indies who lived off the profits of slave-grown sugar. But on average, members of the southern elite controlled far more wealth than their counterparts in the North. The profits of the plantation system spread widely through the rest of the European American community. By the 1770s, whites in the South averaged more than twice as much wealth per person as whites in the North. An estimate for 1774 puts the white southerner's average net worth at £93, a sharp contrast to their counterparts in the middle colonies (£46) and New England (£38).

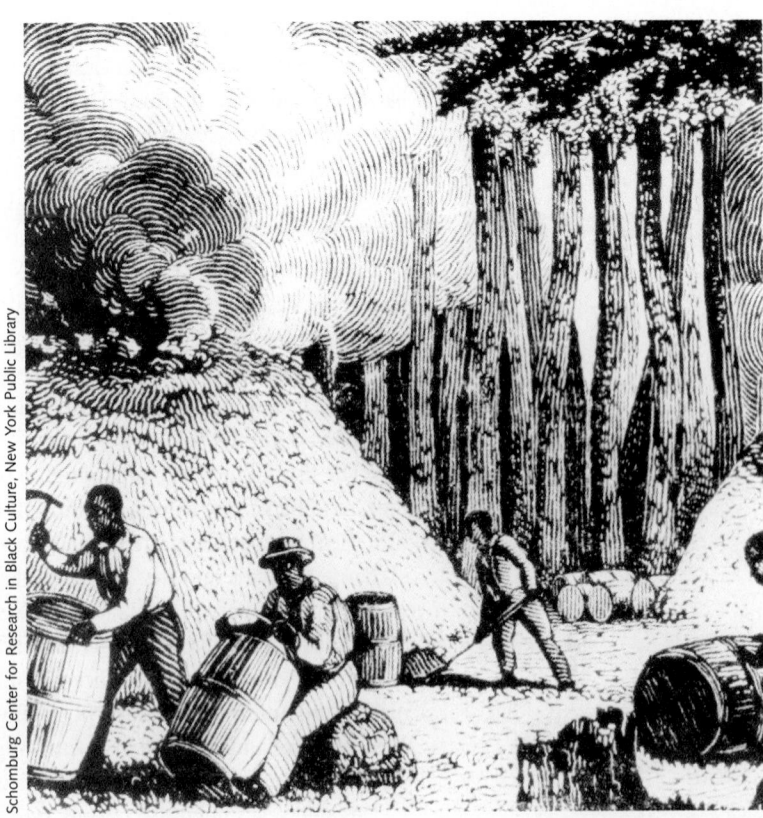

■ **In North Carolina, black workers cut pine trees and then burned the wood in closed ovens to turn pine resin into tar and pitch. These so-called naval stores were sealed into barrels and later used by seamen to protect the ropes on ships.**

New England Takes to the Sea

North of Chesapeake Bay, two overlapping economic regions emerged: the long-established New England colonies and the somewhat newer and more prosperous middle colonies. New England faced peculiar disadvantages, beginning with the rocky soil. Ancient glaciers had strewn stones across the landscape, and it was tedious work to haul them off the fields to build endless stone walls. As imports from London increased, New Englanders found no staple crop that could be sold back directly to Britain to create a balance of trade. All the beaver had been hunted, and much of the best land had been occupied. The region's farm families had adapted well to the challenging environment and short growing seasons. Both men and women worked on handicrafts during the long, hard winters, and networks of community exchange yielded commercial prosperity in many towns. But with a rapidly growing population, each successive generation of parents had less land to pass on to their children. Increasingly, New England's young men with little prospect of inheriting prime farmland turned to the sea for a living.

In timber-rich New England, shipbuilding prospered. Colonists established shipyards at the mouth of nearly every river, drawing skilled carpenters and willing deckhands to the coast. By 1763, Marblehead, Massachusetts, with a fleet of a hundred ships, had grown to 5000 people. That made it the sixth largest town in the 13 colonies, behind only Philadelphia, New York, Boston, Charleston, and Newport, Rhode Island. By 1770, three out of every four ships sailing from New England to a British port was owned by colonial residents. In contrast, in the southern colonies from Maryland to Georgia, the proportion was only one in eight.

On Nantucket Island off Cape Cod, whaling became a new source of income. For generations, the islanders had cooked the blubber of beached whales to extract oil for lamps. In 1715, they outfitted several vessels to harpoon sperm whales at sea and then return with the whale blubber in casks to be rendered into oil. In the 1750s, they installed brick ovens on deck and began cooking the smelly blubber at sea in huge iron vats. This change turned the whaling vessel into a floating factory, and it allowed longer voyages in larger ships. By the 1760s, Nantucket whalers were cruising the Atlantic for four or five months at a time and returning loaded with barrels of oil.

The fishing industry prospered as well. All along the coast, villagers dispatched boats to the Grand Banks, the fishing grounds off Newfoundland. When the vessels returned, laden with fish, the townspeople graded, dried, and salted the catch. They sent the best cod to Europe in exchange for wine and dry goods. Yankee captains carried the lowest grade to the Caribbean sugar islands, where planters bought "refuse fish" as food for their slaves. In return, skippers brought back kegs of molasses to be distilled into rum. By 1770, 140 American distilleries, most of them in New England, produced 5 million gallons of rum annually. Much of it went to colonial taverns and Indian trading posts. But some also went to Africa, aboard ships from Britain and New England. American rum, along with various wines and spirits from Europe, made up one-fifth of the total value of goods utilized to purchase African slaves.

As the New England economy stabilized, it became a mixed blessing for women. On the farm, their domestic labors aided the household economy and helped to offset bad harvests. Mothers taught their daughters to spin yarn, weave cloth, sew clothes, plant gardens, raise chickens, tend livestock, and churn butter. The products from these chores could be used at home or sold in a nearby village to buy consumer goods. While the husband held legal authority over the home, a good wife served as a "deputy husband," managing numerous household affairs, or perhaps earning money as a midwife to help make ends meet. She took charge entirely if her husband passed away or went to sea.

But for all their labors, women seemed to lose economic and legal standing to men as New England towns became larger and more orderly. The creation of public buildings meant that community business was no longer conducted in the home, and so women did not get to participate as frequently as they once had. Networks of local officials, consisting entirely of men, drafted statutes and legal codes that reinforced male privileges. Women found it difficult to obtain credit or receive a business license. In addition, the law barred married women from making contracts, limiting the chance for independent activities outside the home. Increasingly, male apothecaries and physicians with a smattering of formal training shouldered traditional midwives away from the bedside. Even in the port towns, where women outnumbered men, their rights were limited, and poor women faced particular scrutiny. Selectmen and Overseers of the Poor had the power to remove children from a widowed mother and place them in the almshouse.

Economic Expansion in the Middle Colonies

The fifth regional economy, the one that flourished in the middle colonies between New England and Chesapeake Bay, represented the best of two worlds. The Europeans who resettled Indian lands in Delaware, Pennsylvania, New Jersey, and New York found a favorable climate, rich soil, and an abundance of millstreams. Unlike New Englanders, they developed a reliable staple by growing an abundance of grain. They exported excess wheat, flour, and bread as effectively as southerners shipped tobacco and rice. But unlike the planters in Virginia and South Carolina, middle-colony farmers did not become locked in the vicious cycle of making large investments in enslaved workers and exporting a single agricultural staple. Instead, they developed a more balanced economy, using mostly free labor. Besides grain products, they also exported quantities of flaxseed, barrel staves, livestock, and pig iron. Large infusions of money from Britain during its long war against France in the 1750s gave a further lift to this prosperous economy.

Whereas the Chesapeake had no dominant seaport, the middle colonies boasted two major ports of entry. Europeans eager to ply their crafts in America saw little likelihood of competing with unpaid slave artisans in the south. So they flocked to the middle colony seaports instead. Both Philadelphia and New York grew faster than rival ports in the mid-eighteenth century, passing Boston in size in the 1750s. Each city doubled its number of dwellings in the two decades after 1743 as brick structures with slate roofs replaced older wooden homes covered with inflammable cedar shingles. But new houses could not meet the ever-increasing demand. By 1763, Philadelphia had more than 20,000 people, New York had nearly as many, and both cities faced a set of urban problems that had already hit Boston.

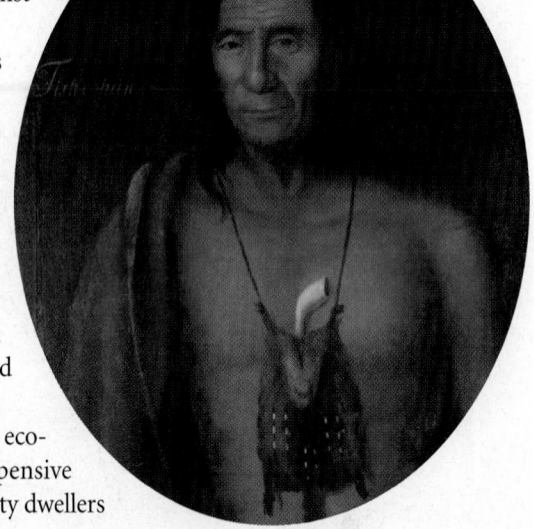

Soon after the Delaware chief, Tishcohan, posed for this 1735 portrait, his people lost valuable land due to Pennsylvania's notorious Walking Purchase.

As the port towns grew, they became more impersonal, with a greater economic and social distance between rich and poor. Large homes and expensive imports characterized life among the urban elite. In contrast, the poorest city dwellers increasingly lacked property and the means to subsist. By the 1760s, Philadelphia's almshouse and the new Pennsylvania Hospital for the Sick Poor were overflowing. In response to the crisis, Philadelphia's Quaker leaders established a voluntary Committee to Alleviate the Miseries of the Poor, handing out firewood and blankets to the needy. They also built a "Bettering House," patterned on Boston's workhouse, that provided poor Philadelphians with food and shelter in exchange for work.

In an effort to limit urban poverty, authorities in New York and Philadelphia continued to move newcomers to the countryside. Dutch and German settlers had already established an efficient farming tradition in the area over several generations. With rising immigration after 1730, the burgeoning region slowly expanded its economic reach far up the Hudson Valley, east into much of Connecticut and Long Island, and south to Baltimore and parts of Maryland.

The farm frontier pushed west as well. The acquisitive Thomas Penn had inherited control of Pennsylvania from his more idealistic father, founder William Penn. In 1737 the young proprietor defrauded the Delaware Indians out of land they occupied west of the Delaware River. In the infamous Walking Purchase, Penn claimed a boundary that could be walked in a day and half. Then Penn's men cleared a path through the woods and sent horsemen along to assist his runners, who covered more than 55 miles in 36 hours. In all, the fast-moving agents took title to 1200 square miles of potential farmland near modern Easton and Allentown, Pennsylvania. Land-hungry settlers pressed the reluctant Delawares west toward the Allegheny Mountains and occupied the rich river valleys of eastern Pennsylvania. Land agents and immigrant farmers called the fertile region "the best poor man's country."

Matters of Faith: The Great Awakening

Philadelphia epitomized the commercial dynamism of the eighteenth-century British colonies. The city was a hub in the fastest-growing economic region on the Atlantic seaboard. Ben Franklin, arriving there in 1723 at age 17, achieved particular success. Within seven years he owned a printing business. Within 25 years he was wealthy enough to retire, devoting himself to science, politics, and social improvement. He created a lending library, developed an efficient stove, promoted schools and hospitals, supported scientific and philosophical organizations, and won fame in Europe for his experiments with electricity. The outburst of scientific inquiry and religious skepticism spreading through European

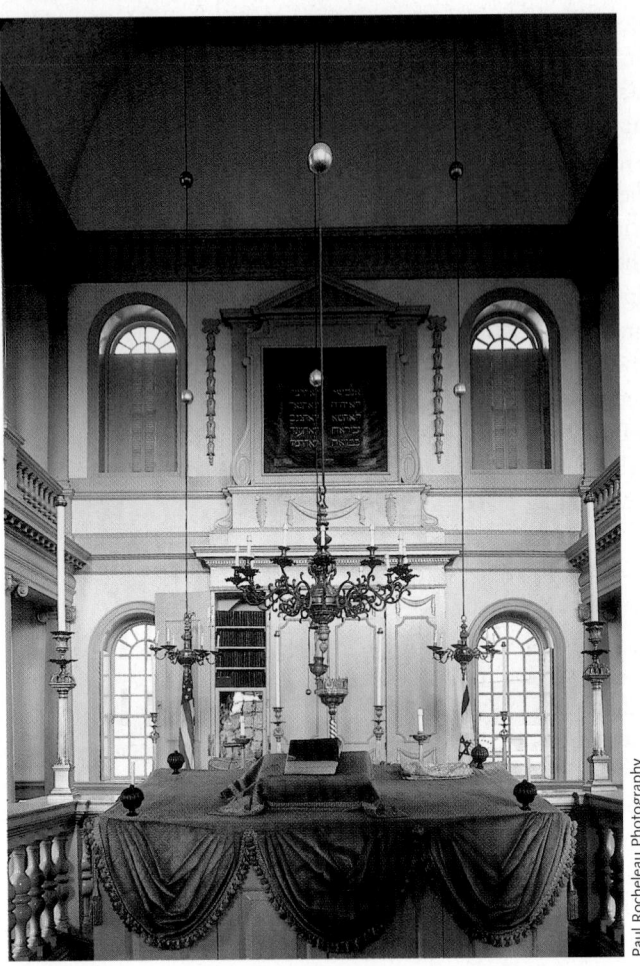

Paul Rocheleau Photography

■ Members of the Jewish community in Newport started Touro Synagogue in 1759, a century after the arrival of their first ancestors in the Rhode Island seaport. Completed in 1763, this gem of colonial architecture is the oldest existing synagogue in the United States.

intellectual circles at the time became known as the Enlightenment. Its spirit of rational questioning and reason was greatly aided by the printing press. In America, Franklin and his fellow printers personified the new Age of Enlightenment.

By 1760 the British mainland colonies had 29 printing establishments, more presses per capita than in any country in Europe. These presses squeezed out 18 weekly newspapers and a variety of public notices, commercial broadsides, fictional pieces, farmers' almanacs, and scientific treatises. They fostered political and business communication throughout the colonies. But they also performed a very different public function, publishing an array of religious material. In Britain's eighteenth-century North American colonies, the spirit of enterprise and worldly achievement existed side by side with a longing for spiritual community and social perfection. The story of another Pennsylvania printer is an apt example.

In 1720, three years before Franklin arrived in Pennsylvania, Conrad Beissel migrated to Philadelphia from the Palatinate in Germany. He lived and preached in nearby Germantown; in 1738 he withdrew farther west to lead a life of unadorned simplicity. Soon other men and women joined him at his retreat near modern-day Lancaster, Pennsylvania. There they created Ephrata Community, the earliest of many wilderness utopias in North America. The communal experiment lasted for more than a generation, supporting itself by operating a printing press. Although Beissel pursued the same trade as Franklin, his experience as a dedicated seeker of spiritual truth represents a very different and important side of colonial life. In the first half of the eighteenth century, colonists witnessed surprising breakthroughs in religious toleration and bitter controversies within the ministry. They also experienced a revivalist outpouring, with roots in Europe and America, that later became known as the Great Awakening. This stirring began in the 1730s, and it gained momentum through the visits from England of a charismatic preacher named George Whitefield (pronounced Whitfield). In most colonies, the aftershocks of the Awakening persisted for a full generation.

Seeds of Religious Toleration

The same population shifts that made Britain's mainland colonies more diverse in the eighteenth century also created a new Babel of religious voices that included many non-Christians. Africans, the largest of all the new contingents, brought their own varied beliefs across the Atlantic. Some slaves from Portuguese Angola had had exposure to Catholicism in their homeland. But most Africans retained as much of their traditional cultures as possible under the circumstances, and they showed skepticism toward initial efforts to plant Christianity among them. An Anglican missionary recalled one black South Carolinian saying that he "preferred to live by what he could remember" from Africa. Christian efforts to convert Native Americans also had mixed results. A minister living near the Iroquois reported that Indians would beat a drum to disrupt his services and then "go away Laughing."

Another non-Christian contingent, Jewish immigrants, remained few in number, with only several hundred families by 1770. Merchants rather than farmers, they established communities in several Atlantic ports, beginning in Dutch New Amsterdam (1654) and Newport

(1658). Most were Sephardic Jews; that is, their ancestral roots were in Spain and Portugal. They came by way of the Caribbean, reaching Charleston in 1697, Philadelphia after 1706, and Savannah in 1733. A few of their children merged into the Protestant culture. In 1743, for example, Phila Franks, daughter of a leading Jewish merchant in New York, wed the son of Stephen DeLancey, a wealthy Huguenot who had married into the city's Dutch aristocracy and then joined the Anglican church. But more than 80 percent of Jewish young people (including a handful of Ashkenazi Jews with ties to central Europe) found partners within their congregations, creating small but lasting communities.

The majority of the colonies' newcomers in the eighteenth century were Christians. A few, such as the Acadians, were Catholics, but the rest had some Protestant affiliation. In the two centuries since the Reformation, numerous competing Protestant denominations had sprung up across Europe. Now this wide array made itself felt in America, as Presbyterians, Quakers, Lutherans, Baptists, Methodists, and smaller sects all increased in numbers. To attract immigrant families, most colonies did away with laws that favored a single established church. Nevertheless, New England remained firmly Congregational, while the merchant elite everywhere, and southern gentry in particular, concentrated increasingly within the Anglican church.

Rhode Island had emphasized the separation of church and state from the start, and Pennsylvania had likewise favored toleration, both as a matter of principle and as a practical recruitment device to attract new settlers. In Europe, Enlightenment thinking gave ideas of religious tolerance greater force as the eighteenth century progressed. So new colonists looked for assurances that they could indeed practice their religion freely and avoid burdensome taxes to support other faiths. In fact, migration from Europe was a demanding ordeal that discouraged the fainthearted. Those willing to take the risk were often people with strong religious hopes and convictions, and various colonies competed to accommodate them. In many places, religious tests still limited who could hold public office, according to the acceptability of their beliefs, but tolerance for competing religious views was definitely expanding.

Ironically, if any institution threatened the growing religious toleration in the colonies, it was the British king's own denomination. The monarch headed the Anglican church, and it had influential American members, including almost every colonial governor. Therefore, repeated talk by the Church of England about installing a resident bishop in America aroused suspicions among loyal colonists who worshipped in other denominations. This was especially true in New England, where Congregationalists had long opposed hierarchies within the Christian faith. Boston, which had 18 churches, rose up against a plan for an Anglican bishop in 1750. In a passionate sermon, Reverend Jonathan Mayhew preached that the town must keep "all imperious bishops, and other clergymen who love to lord it over God's heritage, from getting their feet into the stirrup."

The Onset of the Great Awakening: Pietism and George Whitefield

As relative toleration became a hallmark of the British colonies, no one benefited more than German-speaking Protestant groups. Numerous religious sects, such as the Moravians, Mennonites, Schwenkfelders, and Dunkers, were escaping from persecution as well as poverty at home. Their numbers multiplied after 1730, and hymns in German became a common sound on Sabbath day. In 1743, before any American printer produced an English-language Bible, a press in Pennsylvania put out a complete German edition of Luther's Bible, using type brought from Frankfurt.

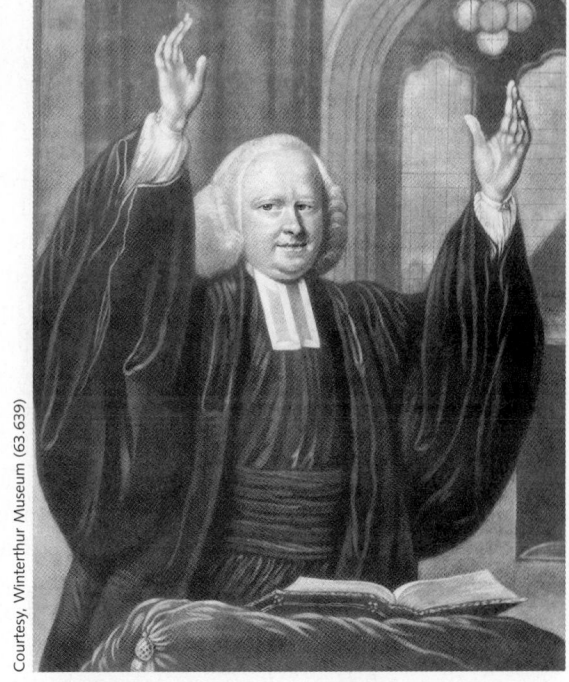

Courtesy, Winterthur Museum (63.639)

■ **When George Whitefield visited America in 1739, his preaching spurred the Great Awakening.**

Sounds Around Us: The Lost World of High Fidelity

George Whitefield was as much a performer as a minister. He preached extemporaneously, mesmerized his listeners, and rarely declined an opportunity to address a crowd. Besides his 7 trips to America, he made 3 tours in Ireland and 15 in Scotland. He preached roughly 18,000 times before his death in New England in 1770, so hundreds of thousands of people heard him on both sides of the Atlantic. Because dozens of his sermons were transcribed and published, we are able to read what he said. But what did he sound like? And for that matter, what did anything sound like in the eighteenth century?

Whitefield had "a clear and musical voice," one listener recalled, "and a wonderful command of it." He squeezed every word for full effect. Some said he could move his listeners to tears with his dramatic enunciation of a single word, such as *Mesopotamia*. England's most famous actor observed, "I would give a hundred guineas if I could only say 'O!' like Mr. Whitefield." Benjamin Franklin, a skeptic and deist in matters of religion, told how he had gone to hear Whitefield preach at Philadelphia's Market Street, determined to hold onto the gold and silver coins he was carrying. "As he proceeded I began to soften," Franklin wrote, "and he finished so admirably that I emptied my pocket wholly into the collector's dish, gold and all."

"The multitudes of all sects and denominations that attended his sermons were enormous," Franklin reported, and their numbers challenged Whitefield's exceptional voice. Ever the rational experimenter, Dr. Franklin set out to measure the preacher's range. He backed down Market Street until he could not hear the sermon distinctly, then calculated the radius of the circle Whitefield could reach, allowed 2 feet for every potential listener, and concluded "that he might well be heard by more than thirty thousand." The estimate may be generous, but it speaks to the strength of Whitefield's operatic voice and the hushed attentiveness of his audience. It also reflects a wider point: the very different quality of hearing three centuries ago.

Of all the five senses, hearing may be the one that historians think and write about least of all. For years they have studied the rich world of musical history, of course, and recently they have awakened to disability history, exploring the complicated saga of social responses across time to hearing loss and other physical impairments. But the broader history of hearing remains so unexamined that few even recognize it as a fit topic of inquiry. Still, if each environment has a distinctive landscape that changes over time, it must have a discernible soundscape as well.

If we could join the residents of Franklin's Philadelphia, or if they could join us, the contrasts in sight, smell, taste, and touch between our two worlds would be fascinating to discuss. When you explore the history of these senses by listing differences, they mount up quickly. The same is true with sound. Rasping handsaws, creaking pump handles, and airy harpsichords would sur-

Collectively, these newcomers were part of a European reform movement to renew piety and spiritual vitality among Protestant churchgoers in an age of increasing rationalism and worldliness. Pietism, as this "Second Reformation" was called, had roots in eastern Germany and stressed the need to restore emotion and intensity to worship that had become too rational, detached, and impersonal. The German pietists reached out after 1700 to inspire Huguenots in France and Presbyterians in Scotland. They influenced reformers in the Church of England such as John Wesley, the founder of Methodism and a teacher at Oxford University. Through Wesley, pietist ideas touched George Whitefield, a lively college student in the class of 1736. Over the next decade, "the boy parson" became the first trans-Atlantic celebrity. Hailed as a preaching prodigy, he sparked a widespread religious awakening in the American colonies.

As a boy growing up in England, George Whitefield left school at 12 to work in the family tavern. But he still managed to attend college, and at Oxford he discovered Wesley and the pietists. He also discovered two other things: the lure of America and his calling to be minister. His mentor, Wesley, had preached briefly in Georgia. So in 1738, at age 23, Whitefield spent several months in the new colony, where he laid plans for an orphanage near Savannah.

Arriving back in England, Whitefield quickly achieved celebrity status. He drew large crowds with fiery sermons that criticized the Anglican church. The evangelist's published *Jour-*

A 10 Cents
LETTER
To the Reverend
Josiah Thomas
Dr. Chauncy,

On Account of some Passages relating to the Rev.
Mr. WHITEFIELD, in his Book intitled *Seasonable*
Thoughts on the State of Religion in New-England.

By *George Whitefield*, A. B.
Late of Pembroke-College OXON.

——*Veniam petimusque damusque vicissim*.] Hor.

B O S T O N: N.E.
Printed and Sold by S. KNEELAND and T. GREEN in *Queenstreet*
1745.

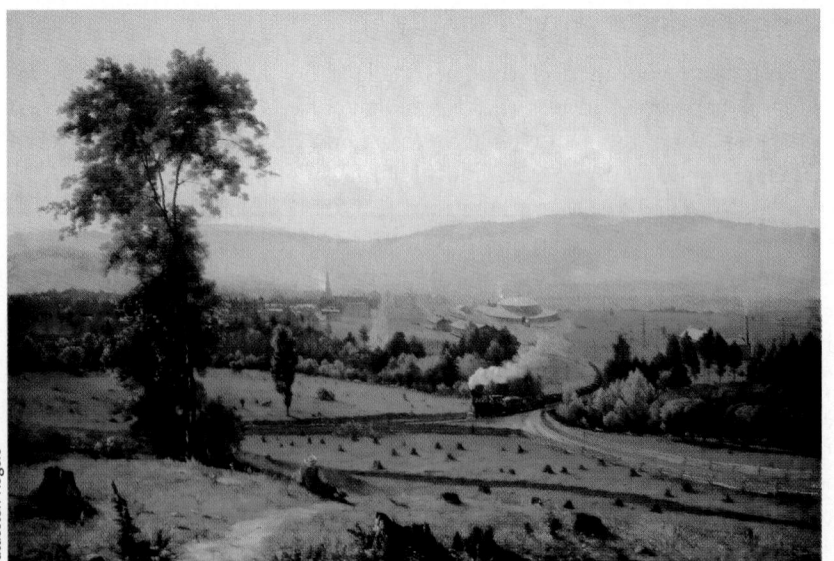

While colonial life featured clear, isolated sounds, modern existence creates constant background noise. This mid-nineteenth-century painting about early industrialization in Pennsylvania suggests the shift. Soon steady noise from the distant factory and the advancing steam engine will blur smaller, sharper sounds.

Tuning of the World (1977). In the preindustrial world (most of history) humans lived in a high-fidelity sound-scape with very little background noise. Distinct sounds traveled clearly and far, whether a tolling bell, a ringing axe, a singing bird, a shouting preacher, or a clap of thunder.

In contrast, we grow up in a low-fidelity world. From birth, our soundscape is filled with a steady array of background noises, large and small, day and night. Even in a rural field or a wilderness campsite, the roar of a snowmobile, the whine of a chainsaw, or the hum of distant tires or a passing jet plane can alter the near silence. The whir and buzz of countless devices is so much a part of our sound envelope that we amplify and blast voices to make them heard. Or we slip on headphones so we can lock out background noise and listen only to what we want to hear. Colonial visitors would marvel at how noisy our world seems but also at how scrambled and indistinct specific sounds become in this modern cacophony. "How do you hear yourselves think?" they might well ask. ■

prise us; droning lawnmowers, honking taxicabs, and pulsating electric guitars would startle them. But with sound, the differences go deeper than simply comparing one set of activities and instruments with another. There is a more fundamental contrast.

Just as the cars, trucks, machines, and factories of our ever-widening industrial world have spawned physical pollution around the globe, they also generate noise as a universal byproduct. These sounds are so numerous and constant that we hardly recognize them as noise pollution because we know no other soundscape. But Murray Schaffer explained the shift in a pioneering work of sound history, *The*

nals, priced at only sixpence, went through six editions in nine months. Moreover, he recruited an experienced publicist, so word of his popularity preceded him in 1739 when he returned to America for an extended tour, the second of seven trans-Atlantic journeys during his career. Building upon religous stirrings already present in the colonies, Whitefield preached to huge and emotional crowds nearly 350 times in 15 months. He made appearances from Savannah to Boston, something no public figure had ever done. "God shews me," he wrote in his journal, "that America must be my place for action."

The timing was perfect. Whitefield, whose brother was a wine merchant, understood the expanding networks of communication and consumption in the British Atlantic world. He saw that in America, as newspapers multiplied and roads increased, he could advertise widely and travel extensively. Other ministers from England had remarked in frustration that most colonists knew "little of the nature of religion, or of the constitution of the church." At times, each person seemed to hold to "some religious whim or scruple peculiar to himself." Whitefield thrived on this vitality and confusion. He had little taste for Protestant debates over church structures and sectarian differences. Instead, he believed that an evangelical minister should simply preach the Bible fervently to a wide array of avid listeners. Everywhere he went, Whitefield served as a catalyst for religious activity.

"The Danger of an Unconverted Ministry"

The heightened commotion in American churches had local origins as well. The same tension felt in European parishes—between worldly, rational pursuits and an emotional quest for grace and salvation—also troubled colonial congregations. Occasional local revivals had taken place in America for decades. The most dramatic "harvest" of committed converts to the church took place in Northampton, Massachusetts, in 1734–1735 under the able guidance of

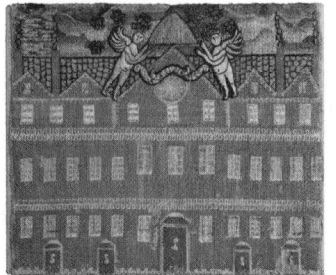

a local minister named Jonathan Edwards. As the colonies' most gifted theologian, Edwards anticipated Whitefield's argument that dry, rote "head-knowledge" made a poor substitute for "a true living faith in Jesus Christ." "Our people do not so much need to have their heads stored," Edwards observed, "as to have their hearts touched."

In a fast-growing society, who would prepare suitable church leaders for the next generation? Candidates for the ministry could train at Harvard College (founded 1636), William and Mary (1693), Yale (1707), or one of several small academies. But these institutions could not instruct a sufficient number and variety of church leaders. The shortage of educated ministers, combined with steady geographic expansion, meant that pulpit vacancies were common. A minister might oversee several parishes, and even if he tended only one parish, it often had broad boundaries. Rural families found it difficult to attend church regularly, and the great distances separating parishioners made it hard for any pastor to travel widely enough to address their needs. Feeling neglected, people voiced their dissatisfaction over the shortage of ministers.

The problem in the pulpit went beyond the matter of quantity. It included the issue of quality as well. Many college graduates had too much "head-knowledge." Their fluency in Latin and Greek often earned them more disdain than respect from down-to-earth congregations. Most foreign-born ministers, such as Anglicans sent from England and Presbyterians from Scotland, had failed to land good positions at home. Some resented their assignments to the colonies, and others felt overwhelmed by the task they confronted. Too often, they showed limited appreciation for the local church members who paid their salaries, and they resented those who criticized their ministries. One such critic was the Scots-Irish immigrant William Tennent, who arrived in Pennsylvania with his family in 1716. Dismayed by the small numbers and cold, unemotional outlook of Presbyterian ministers, Tennent opened a one-room academy in a log house to train his four sons and other young men for the ministry. But local Presbyterian authorities challenged his credentials and disparaged the teachings of his "Log College." Eventually, the school moved and grew, becoming linked to the new College of New Jersey in 1746, which later evolved into Princeton University. But before this happened, Tennent's preacher sons allied themselves with Whitefield and managed to shake the colonial religious establishment to its roots.

One of Tennent's sons, Gilbert, eventually led a Presbyterian church in Philadelphia created by Whitefield's supporters. In 1740, at the time of Whitefield's triumphal tour, young Gilbert Tennent delivered a blistering sermon entitled "The Danger of an Unconverted Ministry" that became a manifesto for the revival. Cutting to the heart of the matter, he condemned the "sad security" offered by incompetent, uncaring, and greedy ministers. "They are as blind as Moles, and as dead as Stones," he charged, "without any spiritual Taste and Relish." He argued that congregations had the right to turn away from these "Orthodox, Letter-learned . . . Old Pharisee-Teachers." It was "an unscriptural Infringment on Christian Liberty," Tennent proclaimed, "to bind men to a particular Minister, against their Judgement and Inclinations."

The Consequences of the Great Awakening

Whitefield hailed Gilbert Tennant and his brothers as "burning and shining lights" of a new kind. All the ministers and worshipers who joined in the movement began to call themselves "New Lights." Opponents, whom they dismissed as "Old Lights," continued to defend a learned clergy, emphasized head-knowledge on the difficult road to salvation, and opposed the disruptions caused by itinerant ministers who moved freely from parish to parish without invitation. The New Lights, in contrast, appealed to people's emotions and stressed the prospect of a more democratic salvation open to all. They defended their itinerant wanderings, which made them more accessible to a broader public and less likely to become set in their ways. "Our Blessed Saviour was an Itinerant Preacher," they reminded their critics; "he Preach'd in no other Way."

Just as New Light preachers moved readily across traditional parish boundaries, they also transcended the lines between different Protestant sects. Their simple evangelical message reached across a wide social spectrum to diverse audiences of every denomination. Moreover, their stress on communal singing, expressive emotion, and the prospects for personal salvation inevitably drew special attention from those on the fringes of the culture, such as young people, women, and the poor. It is important, but not surprising, that New Light ministers and their supporters made headway in spreading Christianity within various African American and Native American communities.

Some of the most zealous New Light men and women tried to transcend the competing denominations altogether and create a broad community of Protestant believers.

Faced with such a broad awakening, members of the religious establishment, once secure as unchallenged leaders within their own church communities, now faced a stark choice. Some reached out to the itinerants who attacked them so vehemently. These powerful churchmen acknowledged their New Light critics and reluctantly welcomed the popular renegades into the local pulpits. Such a strategy might blunt the thrust of the revival, and it would surely raise church attendance. Other Old Lights, however, took the opposite approach; they clung to tradition and stability, challenging their new rivals openly. They condemned itinerancy and disputed the interlopers' right to preach. They mocked the faddish popularity of these overemotional zealots and even banned the New Light itinerants from local districts for the good of the parishioners.

In the end, neither tactic stemmed the upheaval. The arguments of the Great Awakening reverberated through the colonies for a full generation, peaking in the North in the 1740s and in the South during the 1750s and 1760s. But its long-term consequences were mixed. Some of the most zealous New Light men and women tried to transcend the competing denominations altogether and create a broad community of Protestant believers. But for all their open-air preaching, the itinerant reformers could never create such unity, and they left behind no new set of doctrines or institutional structures. Nevertheless, they created an important legacy. First, they infused a new spirit of piety and optimism into American Christianity that countered older and darker Calvinist traditions. Second, they established a manner of fiery and popular evangelical preaching that found a permanent place in American life. Finally, and most importantly, they underscored democratic tendencies in the New Testament gospels that many invoked in later years when faced with other apparent infringements of their liberties.

The French Lose a North American Empire

In 1739 Pierre and Paul Mallet set out up the Mississippi River from New Orleans. The two French Canadians hoped to test rumors that the Missouri River, the Mississippi's mightiest tributary, stretched into New Mexico and to claim the new trading route for France. Far to the east that same year, George Whitefield launched his tour of the English colonies, and the Stono slave rebellion erupted in South Carolina. But in the heart of the French empire thoughts were on expansion. Pausing in the Illinois country to gather seven French Canadian recruits, the Mallet brothers pushed up the Missouri. They finally abandoned the river in northeastern Nebraska, purchased horses at an Omaha Indian village, and set off across the plains. Clanging church bells greeted the French when they reached Santa Fe in July. After a nine-month stay, most of them returned east across the southern plains the next year.

At a stream in central Oklahoma, the explorers exchanged their horses with local Indians for elm bark canoes. (They named the water the Canadian River, a reference to their roots.) Farther east, they stopped at the old Arkansas Post near the mouth of the Arkansas River and then at Fort Rosalie on the lower Mississippi, where Louisiana colonists and their Choctaw allies had put down a revolt by the Natchez Indians a decade earlier. When the Mallet brothers completed their enormous circuit and returned to New Orleans, they brought word from the West of Indian and Spanish eagerness to engage in greater trade. From their perspective, the future of France in America looked bright indeed. But the promise disappeared entirely within their lifetimes.

Prospects and Problems Facing French Colonists

In 1740 French colonists had grounds for cautious optimism. France already claimed a much bigger expanse of North America than Britain or Spain had, and the French wilderness empire ran strategically through the center of the continent. The available resources and potential for agriculture seemed boundless, as a small community of settlers in the Illinois region had already discovered. Moreover, no Europeans had shown greater skill in forging stable and respectful relations with Native American peoples. North of Fort Rosalie and the Arkansas Post, a chain of isolated French forts stretched up the Mississippi River and then east to the lower Great Lakes and the St. Lawrence Valley. These posts facilitated trade with Native Americans and secured ties between Canada and Louisiana. With Indian support, more outposts could be built farther east near the Appalachian mountain chain to contain the English settlers and perhaps one day to conquer them.

At least three problems marred this scenario. First, the French population in America remained small, and the flow of new immigrants paled by comparison to the large number of English settlers. Canada still had fewer than 50,000 colonial inhabitants in 1740, whereas Britain's mainland colonies were rapidly approaching a million. Likewise, the Louisiana colony contained only 3000 French people, living among nearly 4000 enslaved Africans and 6000 Native Americans. Second, colonists lacked sufficient support from France to develop thriving communities and expand the valuable Indian trade. The importation of European goods was still meager and unpredictable, to the dismay of colonists and Native Americans alike. Finally, an ominous trickle of British hunters and settlers was beginning to cross the Appalachian chain. Carolina traders already had strong ties with the Chickasaw Indians living near the Mississippi River, and Virginia land speculators were eyeing lands in the Ohio Valley.

What seemed a promising situation for the French in 1740 was soon put to the test. Britain and France had long been on a collision course in North America. Colonial subjects of the two European superpowers had already clashed in a series of wars, with Indian allies playing crucial roles. After several decades of peace, the conflicts known in English-speaking America as King William's War (1689–1697) and Queen Anne's War (1702–1713) seemed distant memories, but warfare was about to resume. Two more contests, King George's War (1744–1748) and the French and Indian War (1754–1763) preoccupied colonists and Native Americans alike over the next two decades. In 1763 the Treaty of Paris ended the French and Indian War, part of a far wider conflict known in Europe as the Seven Years' War. At that point, less than a quarter century after the Mallet brothers' optimistic journey through the heartlands, the expansive French empire in North America suddenly vanished.

British Settlers Confront the Threat from France

These colonial conflicts of the mid-eighteenth century, generally linked to wider warfare in Europe, had a significant impact on everyone living in the British mainland colonies. A few people took advantage of the disturbances to become rich. They provisioned troops, sold scarce wartime goods, sponsored profitable privateering ventures, or conducted forbidden trade with the enemy in the Caribbean and elsewhere. But many more people paid a heavy price because of war: a farm burned, a job lost, a limb amputated, a husband or father shot in battle or cut down by disease. From London's perspective, the Americans made ill-disciplined and reluctant soldiers. But from the colonists' viewpoint, they received too little respect and inadequate assistance from Britain.

Adding insult to injury, a hard-won victory on North American soil could be canceled out at the peace table in Europe. In 1745, during King William's War, Massachusetts called for an attack on Louisburg, the recently completed French fortress on Cape Breton Island that controlled access to the St. Lawrence River and nearby fishing grounds. Because they had less at stake, other colonies refused to assist the Massachusetts fleet in this endeavor. (George Whitefield, sensing a Protestant crusade against French Catholicism, preached a fiery sermon to the troops before their departure from Boston.) After a lengthy siege, the New England forces prevailed. But the cost was high—dysentery slaughtered the soldiers—and British diplomats soon rescinded the colonial victory. In 1748, at treaty negotiations ending the war, they handed Louisburg back to France in exchange for Madras in India.

Whatever their differences, the American colonists and the government in Britain saw potential in the land west of the Appalachian mountains, and both were eager to challenge French expansion in the region. In 1747, a group of colonial land speculators formed the Ohio Company of Virginia, seeking permission to develop western lands. Two years later the crown granted them rights to 200,000 acres south of the Ohio River if they would construct a fort in the area. Moving west and north, the Virginians hoped to occupy a valuable spot (modern-day Pittsburgh, Pennsylvania) where the Monongahela and Allegheny rivers come together to form the Ohio River. But the French had designs on the same strategic location as they extended their holdings toward the upper Ohio from the Great Lakes region.

> "Everyone cries, a union is necessary, but when they come to the manner and form of the union, their weak noodles are perfectly distracted."

In 1753 the Virginia governor sent a promising young major in the colonial militia named George Washington—at age 21 already regarded as a distinguished soldier—to warn the French to leave the area. The next spring Virginia workers began erecting a fort at the forks of the Ohio, but a larger French force drove them from the site and constructed Fort Duquesne instead. When Major Washington returned to the vicinity with troops in April, he probed for enemy forces. In a skirmish on May 28, 1754, 5 miles east of modern Uniontown, Pennsylvania, his men killed ten French soldiers, the first casualties in what eventually became history's first truly global war. Fearing a counterattack, he fortified his camp, calling it Fort Necessity. With 450 men and meager supplies, he dug in to prepare.

Throughout the British colonies in the early summer of 1754, fears spread about the dangers of French attack and the loyalties of Native American allies. Officials in London requested that all the colonies involved in relations with the Iroquois send delegates to a special congress in Albany, New York, to improve that Indian alliance. Virginia and New Jersey abstained, but seven other colonies sent 23 representatives, who hoped to strengthen friendship with the Iroquois nations and also discuss a design for a union of the colonies.

With these goals in mind, the delegates to the Albany Congress explored and adopted a proposal by Benjamin Franklin. It called for a colonial confederation empowered to build forts and repel a French invasion. The colonies would be unified by an elected Grand Council and a president general appointed by the crown. The delegates hoped the design would be debated by colonial assemblies and implemented by an act of Parliament. But Franklin's far-sighted Albany Plan never received the attention it deserved, and no colonial legislature ever ratified the idea. "Everyone cries, a union is necessary," Franklin wrote, "but when they come to the manner and form of the union, their weak noodles are perfectly distracted."

The main distraction came from Pennsylvania, with word that on July 3 the French had attacked Major Washington at Fort Necessity. After a brief fight, he had no alternative but to surrender to a larger force and then withdraw. But the British colonists were not willing to give up their claims to the Ohio Valley without a fight. Taking the lead, the Virginia government asked for help from Britain in conducting a war against the French and their Native American allies. The crown responded by dispatching General Edward Braddock and two regiments of Irish troops. Early in 1755, his force arrived in Virginia, where preparations were already under way for a campaign to conquer Fort Duquesne. Washington accepted an unpaid position as an aide to Braddock, and in June the combined British and colonial army of 2500 began a laborious march west to face the French.

An American Fight Becomes a Global Conflict

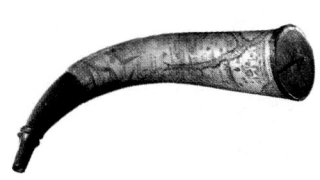

The early stages of the war in America could hardly have been more disastrous for Britain or more encouraging for France. According to his own secretary, the aging Braddock was poorly qualified for command "in almost every respect." A French and Indian force ambushed his column in the forest near Fort Duquesne, cutting it to pieces in the most thorough defeat of the century for a British army. When Braddock died of his wounds during the hasty retreat, Washington oversaw the burial and then wrote in his diary, "We have been most scandalously beaten by a trifling body of men."

Elsewhere, the British fared little better. Indian raids battered the frontiers, spreading panic in the northern colonies. With the local militia away at war, fears of possible slave uprisings swept through the south. The French commander, the Marquis de Montcalm, struck into New York's Mohawk Valley from Lake Ontario in 1756 and then pushed south down Lake Champlain and Lake George in 1757. After a seven-day siege, he took 2000 prisoners at Fort William Henry. In an episode made famous in *The Last of the Mohicans,* his Huron Indian allies killed more than 150 men and women after their release.

The change in British fortunes came with the new ministry of William Pitt, a vain but talented member of the House of Commons. Pitt was an expansionist committed to the growth of the British empire at the expense of France. He brought a daring new strategy to the war effort, and he had the determination and bureaucratic skill to carry it out. In recent contests with France, the military might of the French army in Europe had stymied the British. Now, British forces would instead concentrate on France's vulnerable and sparsely populated overseas colonies. Under Pitt, the British broadened the war into a global conflict, the first in history, taking advantage of their superior naval power to fight on the coasts of Asia and Africa and in North America as well. By 1758, Britain had undertaken a huge military buildup in America (nearly 50,000 troops) and funded it with vast amounts of money.

To win colonial support for his plan, Pitt promised to reimburse the colonies generously for their expenses. In the South, guns, ammunition, and trade goods flowed freely to Britain's Native American allies through Charleston and Savannah, while desperate French officials in Louisiana waited anxiously for supplies that would help them retain the wavering support of their Choctaw and Creek allies. In the North, France lost Louisburg again in July 1758. Fort Frontenac on Lake Ontario fell in August. In November, faced with a powerful force, the French abandoned their valuable position at the Fork of the Ohio, blowing up Fort Duquesne to keep it out of enemy hands. Even without fortifications, the British were glad to possess the strategic site at last. They erected a new post, aptly named Fort Pitt, and laid out the village of Pittsburgh beside it.

In Canada, autumn brought a poor harvest, followed by the worst winter anyone could remember. The Marquis de Montcalm huddled in the provincial capital at Quebec with his ill-equipped army. Ice in the St. Lawrence combined with a British blockade to cut off overseas support from France during the long, cold winter.

In the spring of 1759, the British pressed their advantage, moving against Canada from the West and the South. As Britain's superintendent of Indian affairs in the region, Sir William Johnson had lived among the Iroquois nations for 20 years. His Mohawk Indian wife, Molly Brant,

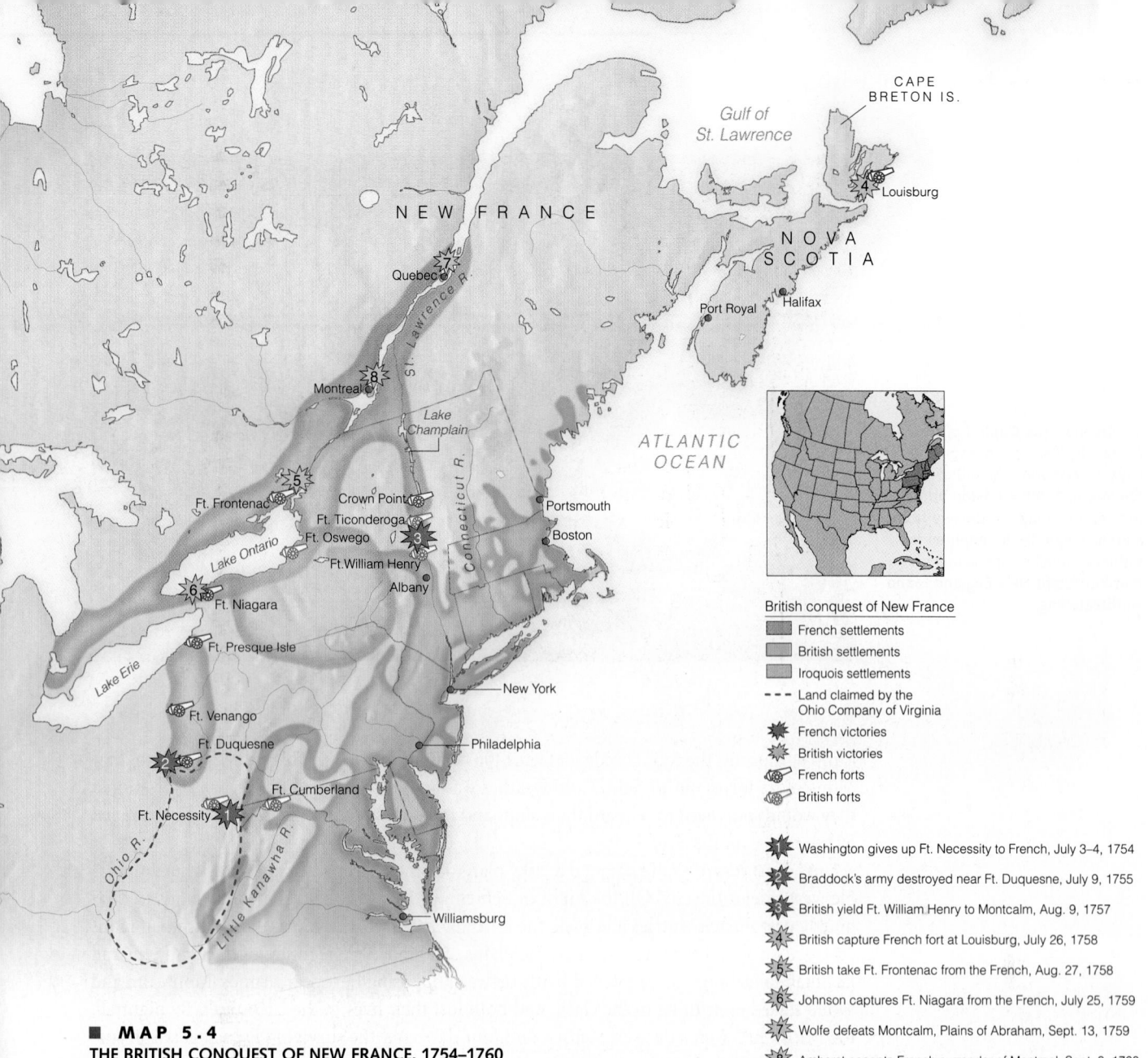

■ **MAP 5.4**
THE BRITISH CONQUEST OF NEW FRANCE, 1754–1760

British conquest of New France
- French settlements
- British settlements
- Iroquois settlements
- - - Land claimed by the Ohio Company of Virginia
- French victories
- British victories
- French forts
- British forts

1 Washington gives up Ft. Necessity to French, July 3–4, 1754
2 Braddock's army destroyed near Ft. Duquesne, July 9, 1755
3 British yield Ft. William Henry to Montcalm, Aug. 9, 1757
4 British capture French fort at Louisburg, July 26, 1758
5 British take Ft. Frontenac from the French, Aug. 27, 1758
6 Johnson captures Ft. Niagara from the French, July 25, 1759
7 Wolfe defeats Montcalm, Plains of Abraham, Sept. 13, 1759
8 Amherst accepts French surrender of Montreal, Sept. 8, 1760

was the sister of Chief Joseph Brant. As British successes mounted, the Mohawks and other Iroquois became increasingly eager to support the winning side in the war. Sensing this, Johnson recruited 1000 formerly neutral Iroquois to join 2000 British regulars on the shores of Lake Ontario. With Johnson in command, they laid siege to Fort Niagara. The fort fell in July, a British victory that effectively isolated enemy posts farther west and obliged the French to abandon them. In August, a British force under Jeffery Amherst captured Ticonderoga and Crown Point on Lake Champlain. The stage was set for an assault on Quebec itself.

Quebec Taken and North America Refashioned

In London, William Pitt knew that capturing Quebec would conquer Canada. Months earlier, he had ordered James Wolfe "to make an attack upon Quebeck, by the River St. Lawrence." Wolfe's flotilla, with 8500 troops, anchored near the walled city in late June. But the French held their citadel despite weeks of heavy shelling. Desperate and sick, Wolfe resorted to a ruthless

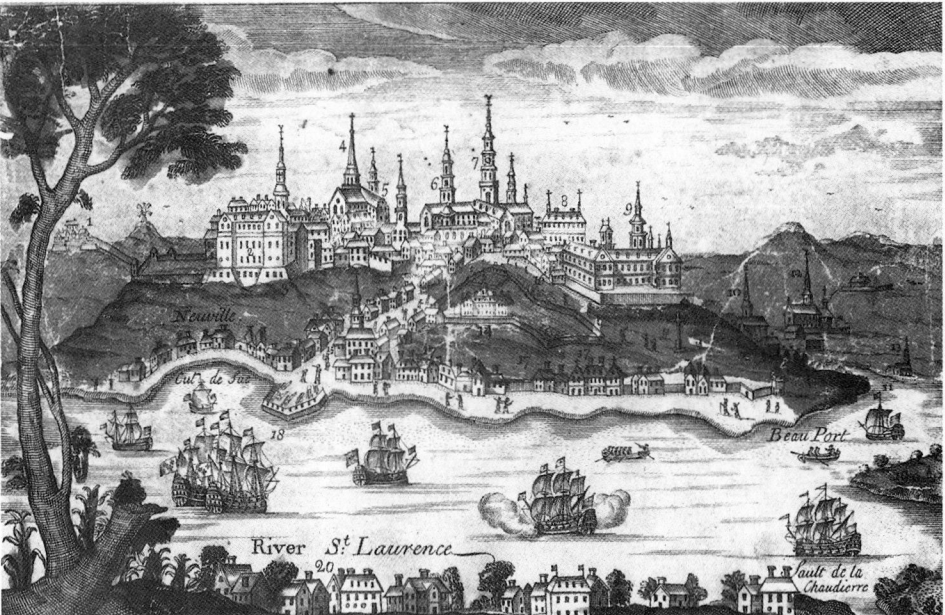

■ *Quebec, the Capital of New France,* by Thomas Johnson. Eager to celebrate the fall of Quebec in 1759, a Boston printer took an old image of the city from a French map. He highlighted the Catholic churches and seminaries that Protestant New England found so threatening.

campaign against the countryside that left 1400 farms in ruins. Even this strategy failed to draw Montcalm's forces out to fight. Cold weather was approaching, and the British realized that they would soon need to reboard their ships and retreat to the Atlantic to avoid being trapped by winter ice on the river.

As a last resort, Wolfe adopted a risky plan to climb a steep bluff and attack the vulnerable west side of the city. On the night of September 12, 1759, he dispatched troops to float quietly past French sentries and scale the formidable cliffs. At daybreak, 12 British battalions emerged on a level expanse known as the Plains of Abraham. The future of the continent and its inhabitants hinged on a pitched battle between opposing European armies. Montcalm and Wolfe staked everything in the clash, and both lost their lives in the encounter. By nightfall, the British had won a decisive victory, and four days later the surviving French garrison surrendered the city of Quebec.

Montreal fell to Britain the following year, and fighting subsided in America. But Pitt continued to pour public money into the global war, and one military triumph followed another. The British conquered French posts in India, took French Senegal on the West African coast, and seized the valuable sugar islands of Martinique and Guadeloupe in the French West Indies. When Spain came to France's aid in 1762, British forces captured the Philippines and the Cuban city of Havana. As Londoner Horace Walpole put it, "Our bells are worn threadbare with ringing of victories." But with 160,000 men under arms, British taxpayers resented the huge costs of the war. Many also worried that the effort to humiliate France and Spain and undo their empires could spark retaliation in the years ahead. Rising criticism pushed Pitt from office, and peace negotiations began.

In a matter of months, the European powers redrew the imperial map of North America. Their complex swaps constituted the largest single rearrangement of real estate in the history of the continent. First, France ceded to Spain the port of New Orleans and all of the Louisiana territory west of the Mississippi River. Then, in the 1763 Treaty of Paris, more transactions followed. Spain turned over East Florida to Britain, receiving back Havana and the Philippines in return. France gave Britain its holdings between the Appalachians and the Mississippi River as well as the parts of Canada not already claimed by the Hudson's Bay Company. In exchange for this vast acquisition, the British returned the sugar islands of Martinique and Guadeloupe to the French. They also allowed France to retain fishing rights off the coast of Newfoundland and two small islands in the vicinity.

Those negotiating the peace agreed that French Canadians could choose between leaving Canada or becoming British subjects. But the Paris treaty made no mention of the thousands of Native Americans whose bountiful homelands were being reassigned. The final results were striking. Britain emerged as the world's leading colonial power, and, after two centuries, the empire of France in North America abruptly disappeared.

Conclusion

For half a century, the complex currents of colonial life had recalled the ancient tale of Babel, as told in the Book of Genesis in the Bible. A confusion of voices, interests, and cultures competed and interacted over a wide expanse in North America. In the process, a string of related economic regions emerged along the eastern seaboard. The colonies that composed these regions varied in ethnic make-up, but they all owed political allegiance to Britain, and they were all expanding rapidly in population. This demographic growth was crucial. Beneath the commercial striving and religious debate, a deeper and less visible change in numbers was underway that would alter the power and place of the Atlantic colonies.

Unprecedented population growth along the Atlantic coast stands out dramatically in hindsight. In 1763 Britain's mainland colonies contained more than 1.6 million people. The figure had quickly come to dwarf all the other population totals on the continent. The Spanish in New Mexico and Texas and the Comanche and Sioux on the Great Plains all controlled wide stretches of territory. But their numbers remained only a minute fraction of the people in the East Coast colonies who had recently managed, despite all their regional differences, to support the British armed forces in ousting the French from North America.

Amazingly, in the 13 years between 1750 and 1763 more than 400,000 people were added to the British mainland colonies. This number of new people—reflecting natural increase and migration combined—exceeded the entire population that had been living in those same British colonies five decades earlier, in 1713. The growth in numbers during the decades to come was equally rapid, and the changes for the continent were even more dramatic and long-lasting.

Sites to Visit

San Saba Mission

The ruins of the mission, abandoned by the Spanish after Comanche attacks in the 1750s, lie 2 miles east of Menard, Texas, off US-190, near the San Saba River. Two miles west of Menard, on Highway 29, the fully restored San Saba Presidio contains a small museum in the rebuilt chapel. Menard is 150 miles northwest of San Antonio.

The Ephrata Cloister

One of America's earliest communal societies was the Ephrata Cloister, founded by Conrad Beissel in 1732. It is located on West Main Street in Ephrata, Pennsylvania, 2 miles west of Highway 222 between Lancaster and Reading. Guided tours include the Meetinghouse, Bake House, and Print Shop.

Winchester, Virginia

Founded in 1744 as a stop on the Great Wagon Road, Winchester is located 70 miles west of Washington, D.C., at Interstate 81, "where the Shenandoah Valley begins and history never ends." Young George Washington worked as a land surveyor in this frontier town, and his office is now a museum.

Old Salem

www.oldsalem.org

This reconstruction of a village founded in 1766 is in Winston-Salem, North Carolina. The site includes the Winkler Bakery, a cemetery, and the Museum of Early Southern Decorative Arts (MESDA). Take a virtual tour of the site at www.oldsalem.org. Nearby is Bethabara, a Moravian community founded in 1753, also open to the public; see www.bethabara.org.

Sermons of the Reverend George Whitefield

www.crta.org/documents/Whitefield.html

The texts of 59 sermons of the Reverend George Whitefield are available online at this Web site. The Bethesda Orphanage, founded by Whitefield in 1740, is located on 650 acres beside the Moon River outside Savannah, Georgia. It is now the Bethesda Home for Boys, America's oldest existing children's home.

The Rice Museum

Located in the Old Market Building in Georgetown, South Carolina, the museum contains dioramas and exhibits describing rice cultivation. The Caw Caw Interpretive Center, west of Charleston on the Savannah Highway (Route 17S) in Ravenel, South Carolina, provides a fascinating view of eighteenth-century rice fields.

Fort William Henry

This fort, at the south end of Lake George, was the location for events in 1757 depicted in *The Last of the Mohicans*. Guided tours relating to the British–French struggle during the Seven Years' War are available at Fort William Henry and at larger Fort Ticonderoga, on Lake Champlain. Both sites are east of Interstate 87, north of Albany, New York. Visit Fort Ticonderoga online at www.fort-ticonderoga.org/.

Seven Years' War Association Journal

www.sywajournal.com/

The online journal of the Seven Years' War Association has links to numerous sites and documents connected to the American portion of the conflict, often known as the French and Indian War. For a Web Index of the French and Indian War, go to www.geocities.com/Athens/Parthenon/1500/fiw.html.

For Further Reading

General

John J. McCusker and Russell R. Menard, *The Economy of British America, 1607–1789* (1991).

Gary B. Nash, *The Urban Crucible: The Northern Seaports and the Origins of the American Revolution* (abridged edition, 1986).

Carla Gardina Pestana, *Liberty of Conscience and the Growth of Religious Diversity in Early America, 1636–1786* (1987).

Marcus Rediker, *Between the Devil and the Deep Blue Sea: Merchant Seamen, Pirates, and the Anglo-American Maritime World, 1700–1750* (1987).

New Cultures on the Western Plains

Gary Clayton Anderson, *Kinsmen of Another Kind: Dakota–White Relations in the Upper Mississippi Valley, 1650–1862* (1984).

Elizabeth A. H. John, *Storms Brewed in Other Men's Worlds: The Confrontation of Indians, Spanish, and French in the Southwest, 1540–1795* (1975).

Frank Raymond Secoy, *Changing Military Patterns of the Great Plains Indians* (1953).

Britain's Mainland Colonies: A New Abundance of People

Kirsten Fischer, *Suspect Relations: Sex, Race, and Resistance in Colonial North Carolina* (2002).

James T. Lemon, *The Best Poor Man's Country: A Geographical Study of Early Southeastern Pennsylvania* (1972).

Harry Roy Merrens, *Colonial North Carolina in the Eighteenth Century: A Study in Historical Geography* (1964).

A. G. Roeber, *Palatines, Liberty, and Property: German Lutherans in Colonial British America* (1993).

Laurel Thatcher Ulrich, *Good Wives: Image and Reality in the Lives of Women in Northern New England, 1650–1750* (1982).

Marianne S. Wokeck, *Trade in Strangers: The Beginnings of Mass Migration to North America* (1999).

The Varied Economic Landscape

Kathryn E. Holland Braund, *Deerskins and Duffels: Creek Indian Trade with Anglo-America, 1685–1815* (1993).

Elaine Forman Crane, *Ebb Tide in New England: Women, Seaports, and Social Change, 1630–1800* (1998).

Margaret Ellen Newell, *From Dependency to Independence: Economic Revolution in Colonial New England* (1998).

Frederick B. Tolles, *Meeting House and Counting House: The Quaker Merchants of Colonial Philadelphia, 1682–1763* (1948).

Daniel Vickers, *Farmers and Fishermen: Two Centuries of Work in Essex County, Massachusetts, 1630–1850* (1994).

Michael Zuckerman, *Peaceable Kingdoms: New England Towns in the Eighteenth Century* (1970).

Matters of Faith: The Great Awakening

Patricia U. Bonomi, *Under the Cope of Heaven: Religion, Society, and Politics in Colonial America* (1986).

Carl Bridenbaugh, *Mitre and Sceptre: Transatlantic Faiths, Ideas, Personalities, and Politics, 1689–1775* (1962).

Philip Greven, *The Protestant Temperament: Patterns of Child-Rearing, Religious Experience, and the Self in Early America* (1977).

Timothy D. Hall, *Contested Boundaries: Itinerancy and the Reshaping of the Colonial American Religious World* (1994).

Jacob R. Marcus, *The Colonial American Jew* (1970).

Mechal Sobel, *The World They Made Together: Black and White Values in Eighteenth-Century Virginia* (1987).

The French Lose a North American Empire

Fred Anderson, *Crucible of War: The Seven Years' War and the Fate of Empire in British North America, 1754–1766* (2000).

Fred Anderson, *A People's Army: Massachusetts Soldiers and Society in the Seven Years' War* (1984).

Francis Jennings, *Empire of Fortune: Crowns, Colonies, and Tribes in the Seven Years' War in America* (1988).

Ian K. Steele, *Betrayals: Fort William Henry and the "Massacre"* (1990).

Daniel H. Usner, Jr., *Indians, Settlers, and Slaves in a Frontier Exchange Economy: The Lower Mississippi Valley Before 1783* (1992).

Online Practice Test

Test your understanding of this chapter with interactive review quizzes at

www.ablongman.com/jonescreatedequal/chapter5

The Limits of Imperial Control, 1763–1775

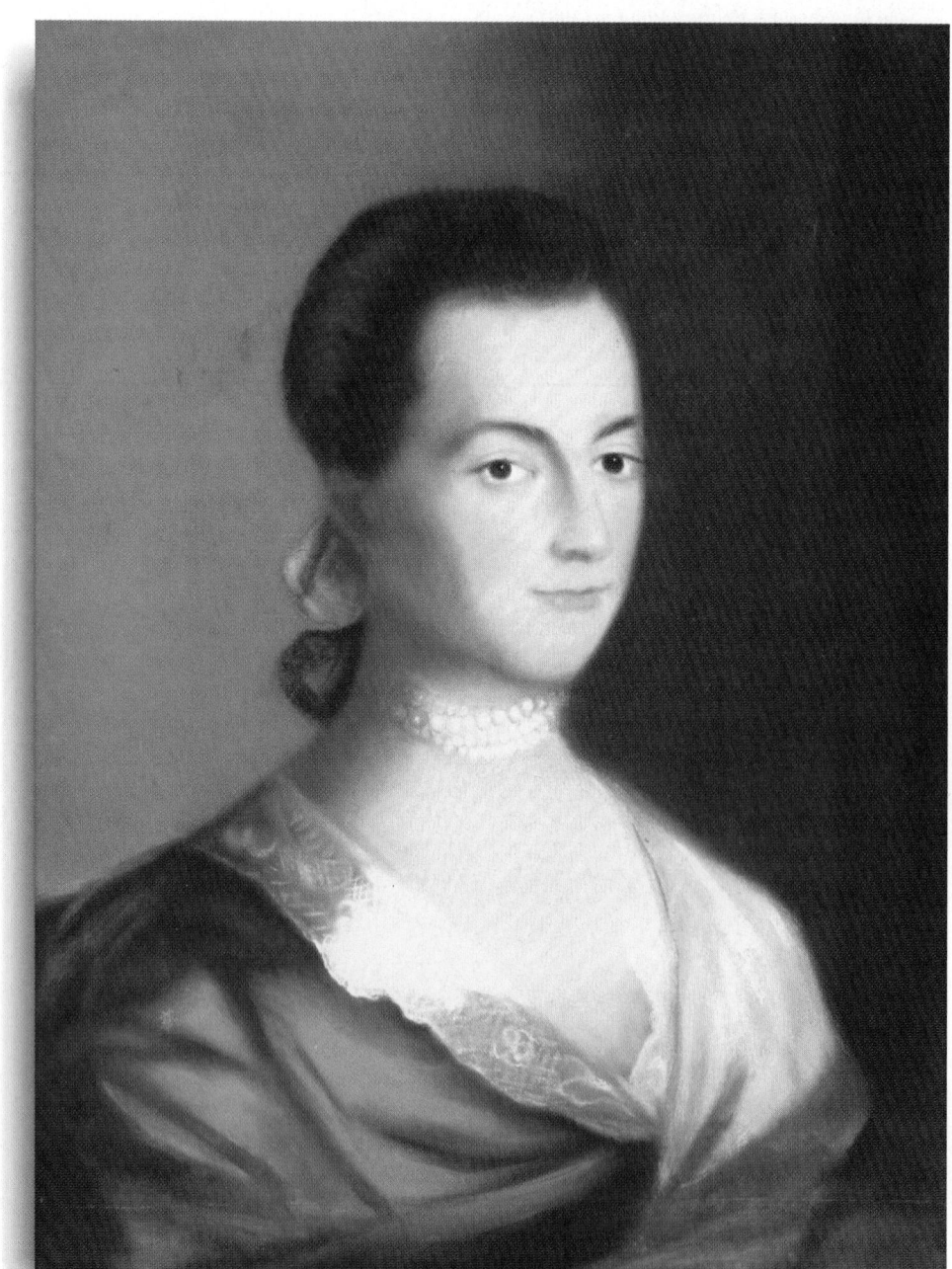

Benjamin Blyth, *Abigail Adams*, c.1766. Courtesy of the Massachusetts Historical Society, MHS #73

■ The astute Abigail Adams (like Barbara Bush in our own time) was the wife of one American president and the mother of another.

B Y THE 1760s, BOSTON HAD GROWN INTO A BUSY SEAPORT OF 16,000 PEOPLE. ALTHOUGH tiny by modern urban standards, the city was much larger and less intimate than it had been a century earlier. The gap between the rich and the poor had expanded steadily, until a mere 5 percent of the city's taxpayers controlled as much wealth as the other 95 percent combined. The Seven Years' War had only worsened the growing inequality. During the war, wealthy Boston families such as the Apthorps and Hancocks multiplied their fortunes, building stately homes and importing elegant fashions. In 1764 young John Hancock, heir to his uncle's vast shipping business, inherited an immense fortune of £80,000.

However, most Bostonians lived in a very different world, made worse by a terrible fire that swept the port in 1760 and the depression that gripped the region after the war ended in 1763. Half the townspeople had lifetime property and savings worth less than £40, and half of those possessed £20 or less. George Hewes, five years younger than Hancock, was born into this other Boston in 1742. Hewes lost his father, a struggling butcher who also sold soap and candles, at age seven. But unlike Hancock, he had no rich uncle. Hewes's mother died in 1755, and when her own father died the next year after a life toiling as a shoemaker, he left behind only £15. George inherited less than £3 from his grandfather, and perhaps his tools and his familiarity with leatherworking as well. The boy became an apprentice shoemaker at age 14.

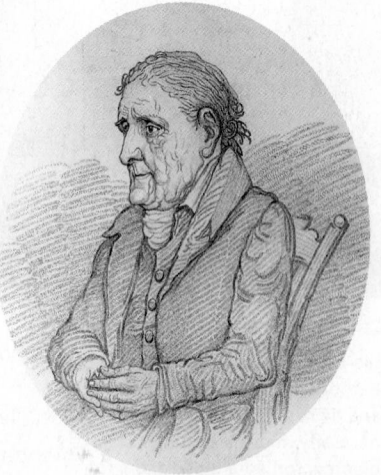

At 93, cobbler George Hewes still recalled his part in the "Boston Tea Party" of 1770.

Despite the town's growth, rich and poor still encountered one another on occasion. If anything those contacts increased during the tumultuous decade that gave rise to the American Revolution. Politics—both imperial and local—heated up in the 1760s, opening up rifts within the ruling elite. Throughout the colonies, British officials and other people who supported the crown's policies became known as Loyalists, or Tories. The wealthy among them saw social and economic dominance as their birthright and scorned their rivals for courting favor with the poor. In contrast, leaders of the emerging opposition (known as Whigs or Patriots) consisted of less conservative—often young and ambitious—members of the educated and professional classes. These people downplayed their rank and privilege to win popular support from those beneath them on the social scale.

In Boston, Hancock was one such person. In 1763, after Hewes repaired an expensive shoe for John Hancock, the merchant invited the young cobbler to a New Year's open house at his impressive mansion. In his old age, Hewes still recalled the occasion vividly. Intimidated by the wealth around him, he remembered being scared "almost to death" when the magnate toasted him and gave him a silver coin.

According to Hewes, the two men met again on very different terms after a decade had passed. In December 1773, the shoemaker painted stripes on his face and then joined other activists, also disguised as Native American warriors, in a risky nighttime action. To protest imperial policies, these patriots in war paint emptied chests of British tea into Boston Harbor. Recalling that night as an elderly man, Hewes was one of the first to refer to the event as a "tea party." And he swore that in the darkness he had rubbed elbows with Hancock himself and had joined him in smashing a crate of tea.

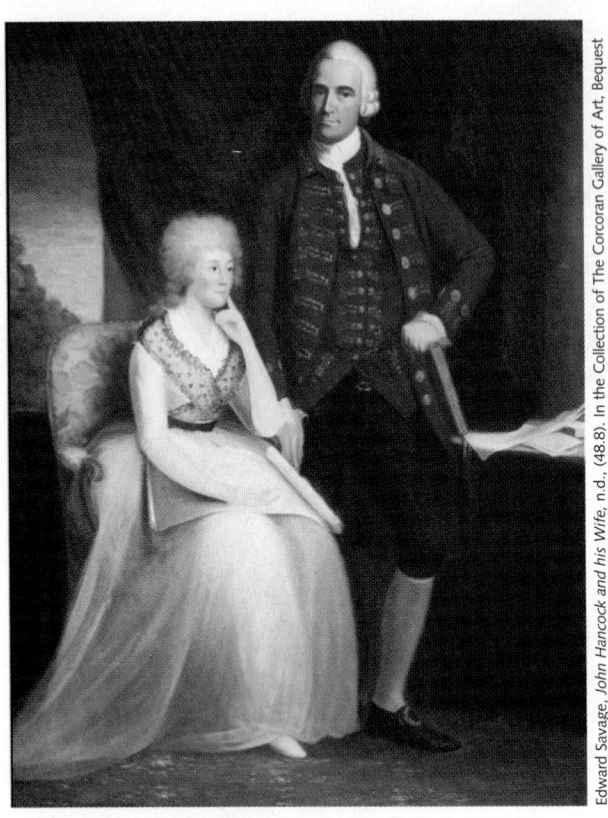

Edward Savage, *John Hancock and his Wife*, n.d., (48.8). In the Collection of The Corcoran Gallery of Art, Bequest of Woodbury Blair

■ Some wealthy colonists, like the Hancocks of Boston, joined the Patriot opposition during the 1760s and 1770s. Gradually, out of necessity, these merchants and planters forged a loose and convenient alliance with colonial artisans and workers who came from a very different world.

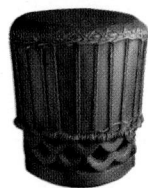

Whether the man beside Hewes—also disguised as an Indian yet wearing a ruffled shirt—was actually Hancock remains doubtful. But symbolically, the two men were now working shoulder to shoulder. They came together across class lines in a coalition that would soon challenge Europe's strongest empire, Britian, and spark the Atlantic world's first successful anticolonial revolution.

Few could have predicted the growth of solidarity between a portion of the colonial elite and a wide spectrum of working people; this implausible alliance developed gradually and imperfectly. During the decade before 1776, there were numerous occasions when class and regional interests still sharply divided the British colonists. Urban artisans, rural farmers, enslaved African Americans, and numerous wives and widows, for example, did not necessarily share common views and concerns. Indeed, they were frequently at odds. Nevertheless, within half a generation enough of these diverse people—many as distant from one another socially as Hancock and Hewes—came together to stage a successful struggle to separate politically from Britain.

What shared experiences and beliefs caused this unstable partnership to emerge against the odds? What events shaped it and prompted it to gather momentum by July 1776, when John Hancock, as president of the Second Continental Congress, applied the first and largest signature to the American colonies' Declaration of Independence? In retrospect, we know that between 1763 and 1775 a significant change in identity took place. Little by little, for the first time, colonists from separate regions and different countries of origin began to speak of themselves as Americans. Gradually, they adopted a term that had previously applied only to Indians. (Indeed, it may be a sign of the increasing identification with North America that they occasionally adopted symbolic Indian garb, as when Hewes and Hancock joined others in dumping tea in Boston Harbor.)

At times, of course, this self-conscious new identification with North America went too far, as in the creation of a *Continental* Congress. In fact, it was not a body of the entire North American continent at all. The tumult and debate that led up to the revolt against Britain touched communities all up and down the Atlantic seaboard, linking them through shared debates and energetic Committees of Correspondence. So it is not surprising that the delegates to Philadelphia boldly called themselves a Continental Congress. Still, the familiar terminology is clearly misleading in any wider, literal sense. Eventually, a new American nation would come to control much of the continent. But that unlikely prospect lay far in the future, and few obvious signs pointed in that direction.

In 1763 thousands of Native Americans in the Midwest, under the leadership of Pontiac, were fighting to assert their own independence from European encroachment. While Indians on the Great Plains, including the Comanche and the Sioux, continued to contend for new territories, other peoples still farther west experienced the initial shocks of colonial contact. Suddenly, inhabitants of the Hawaiian Islands and the Alaskan coast were encountering European intruders for the first time. The rival European empires, meanwhile, competed globally on the high seas, seeking mastery in the Atlantic, the Pacific, and the Indian Oceans. For them, North America, the resources of its rich interior still largely unexplored and unexploited, remained only one piece in a larger puzzle, one prize in a wider imperial game.

Following the departure of the French, the push of rival powers to establish permanent control over the North American continent continued. But the limitations that constrained imperial control were more evident than ever. Geographic ignorance, limited resources, weak bureaucracies, huge distances, strong-willed colonists, and resilient native inhabitants all posed limits for maintaining and expanding far-flung empires. Russia's foothold in Alaska and Spain's presence in California were new and tenuous at best. Spanish dominance at older outposts in Arizona, New Mexico, and Texas remained partial, and Spain's grip on its newly acquired Louisiana territory was even more nominal. East of the Mississippi River, long-term British control finally seemed to be assured. But appearances can be deceiving. Even Britain, secure after its decisive victory over France, would soon be fighting a losing battle to retain much of the American continent that it confidently claimed to control.

New Challenges to Spain's Expanded Empire

With Spain's acquisition of Louisiana from France in 1763, the Spanish held nominal title to the entire West, from the Mississippi to the Pacific. Populated by more than 1 million Native Americans, this expanded empire reached north into the uncharted realms where Russian Siberia faced Alaska. But whether Spain could settle and exploit, or even explore and defend, this vast domain remained an open question. After all, envious rivals were already probing North America's Pacific coast. Exploration voyages by the French and the British challenged Spain's dominance in the Pacific, and Russian colonization in Alaska spurred the Spanish to establish posts along the coast of California. These rivalries, in turn, brought new pressures to bear on the West's diverse Indian peoples, even before the United States emerged as a separate entity with expansionist ambitions of its own.

Pacific Exploration, Hawaiian Contact

Defeat in the Seven Years' War removed the French from North America in 1763. Lamenting the loss and burdened with heavy war debts, France sought fresh prospects in the unexplored

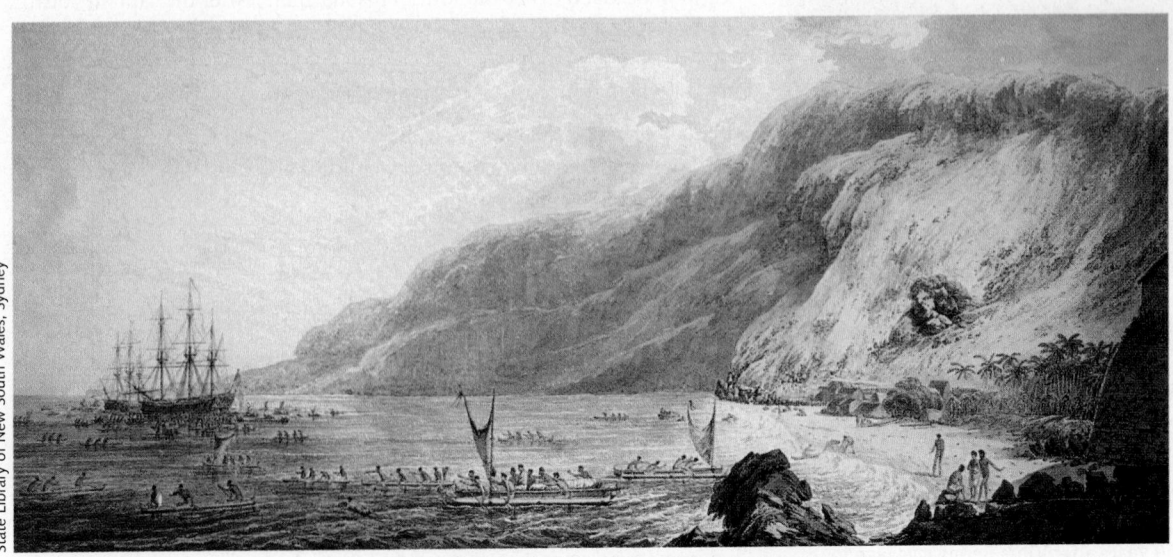

John Webber, *A View of Kealakekua Bay*, c. 1781–1783. Dixson Library, State Library of New South Wales, Sydney

■ When Captain Cook anchored at Hawaii's Kealakekua Bay in 1779, he wrote in his journal that the islanders crowded aboard his two vessels and paddled around them in "a multitude of Canoes." Hundreds of others swam around the ships, along with "a number of men upon pieces of Plank." One such surfboarder is visible in the foreground.

South Pacific. As one Frenchman observed, the discovery of a new continent might furnish "opportunities for profit to equal all that has been produced in America." The task of finding such a bonanza fell to Louis Antoine de Bougainville, a gifted French officer who had served with General Montcalm in Canada during the war. In 1766 Bougainville set out to search for "Terra Australis Incognita," the Pacific's fabled unknown southern land. His voyage marked the first French circumnavigation of the world. Nevertheless, it revealed no continent—only small, lush islands such as Tahiti and Samoa. French hopes for immediate wealth from a new Pacific landmass went unfulfilled.

Not to be outdone, British captains pressed their own Pacific explorations. The most skilled and successful was James Cook, who ranged from the Arctic Circle to Antarctica during three momentous voyages beginning in 1768. In January 1778, during Cook's final voyage, his two vessels happened upon the Hawaiian Islands, eight volcanic isles stretching over 300 miles. More than 13 centuries earlier (A.D. 300–500), seafaring Polynesians had migrated here in remarkable ocean-sailing canoes. They had arrived from the Marquesas Islands far to the south, and their descendants, perhaps as many as 300,000 people, lived in agricultural and fishing communities dominated by powerful chiefs.

The Hawaiians mistook Captain Cook for Lono, a deity they had expected to reappear, and treated him with hospitality and respect. "No people could trade with more honisty," the navigator scrawled in his journal when he departed. During the next 12 months, Cook cruised up the west coast of North America, starting in what is now Oregon. Two centuries had passed since Francis Drake's earlier visit to the California coast. But English mariners still hoped to find a sea passage through North America that might drastically shorten voyages from the Atlantic to Asia. Cook brought an end to the speculation. He encountered a solid coastline that stretched all the way to Alaska. Along the way, he traded with Northwest Coast Indians for sea otter pelts and other furs. In Alaska, he gave his own name to Cook Inlet, near present-day Anchorage. Then he sailed north into arctic waters, pausing at Asia's easternmost tip.

Cook's vessels returned south in 1779, and they were again greeted with fanfare on the big island of Hawaii. But admiration turned to resentment as the English outstayed their welcome at Kealakekua Bay. When an incident of petty pilfering erupted into violence, an angry crowd of Hawaiians killed Cook and four of his mariners. After the captain's death, his two sloops returned to the North Pacific and then stopped at the Chinese port of Macao. There, the crew sold their furs at an enormous profit. They then sailed back to England in 1780 with word of the money to be made selling North American sea otter pelts in China. The voyagers also confirmed a disturbing rumor: Russia already had a foothold in this lucrative Pacific traffic.

The Russians Lay Claim to Alaska

In 1728 Vitus Bering, a Danish captain hired to serve in the Russian naval service, completed a three-year trek east across Siberia. Reaching the Kamchatka peninsula on the Pacific Ocean, he built a boat and sailed north between Asia and America through the strait that bears his name today. The journey ended European speculation that Asia was linked to North America. On a second expedition in 1741, Bering visited the Alaskan mainland and claimed it for Russia. He lost his life on the return voyage after a winter shipwreck on a frozen island.

Bering's crew managed to return to Kamchatka with valuable pelts. Their feat proved that round trips between Russia and America were both possible and profitable. Over the next generation, merchants in Asian Rus-

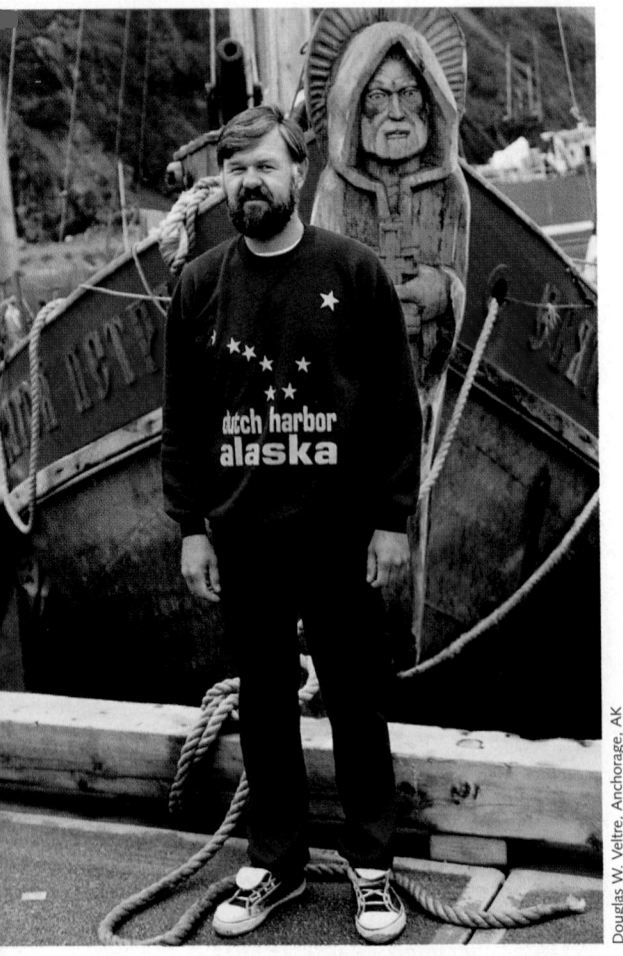

Douglas W. Veltre, Anchorage, AK

■ In 1991, 250 years after Vitus Bering's voyage to Alaska, Russians from Kamchatka sailed replicas of Bering's three small vessels across the North Pacific to Alaska. Aleksandr Maslov-Bering, a descendant of the explorer, poses beside the carved bow of one boat.

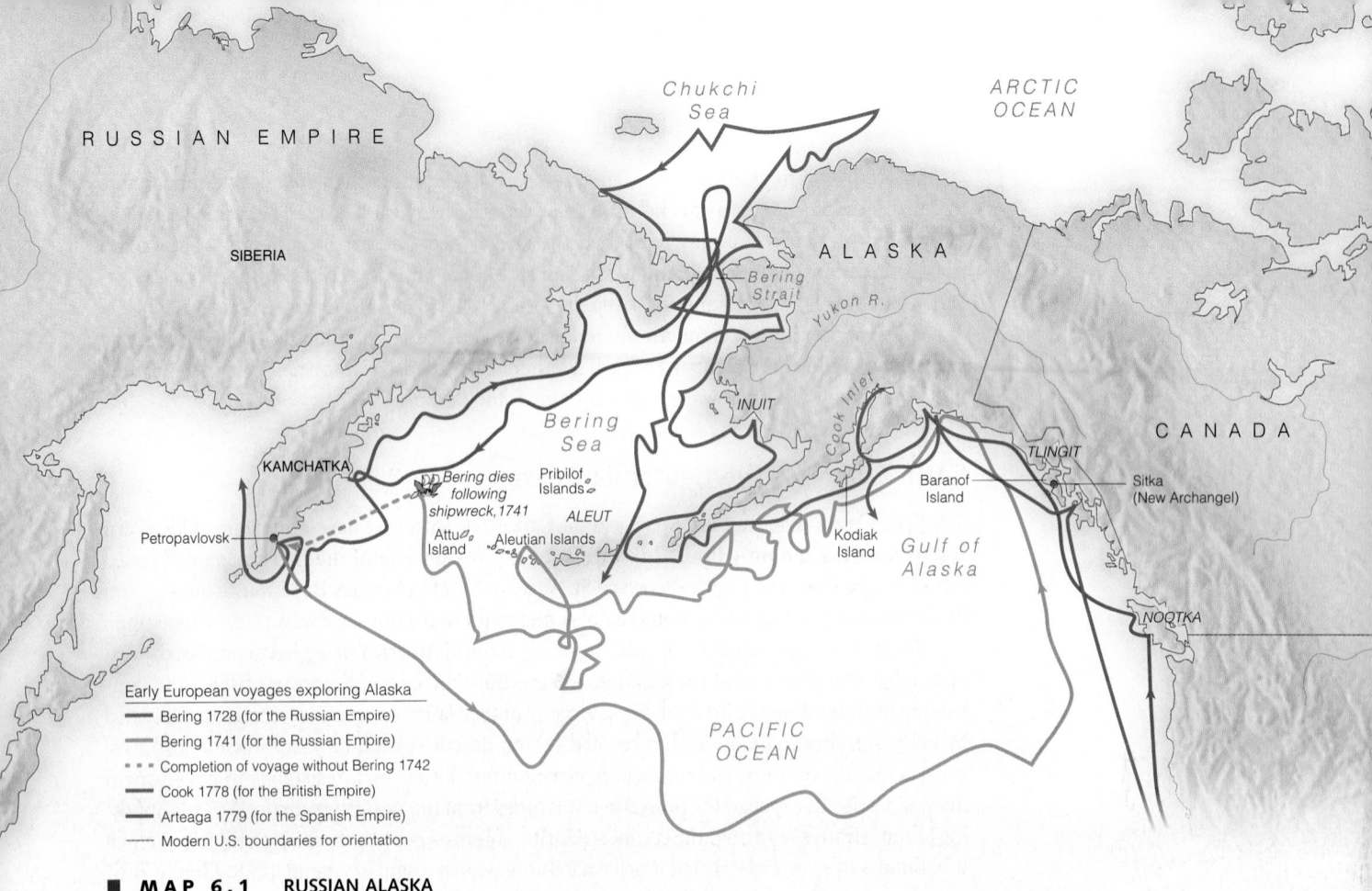

Early European voyages exploring Alaska
— Bering 1728 (for the Russian Empire)
— Bering 1741 (for the Russian Empire)
- - - Completion of voyage without Bering 1742
— Cook 1778 (for the British Empire)
— Arteaga 1779 (for the Spanish Empire)
---- Modern U.S. boundaries for orientation

■ **MAP 6.1** RUSSIAN ALASKA

sia sent several expeditions to Alaska each year, bringing back furs that they traded with the powerful Chinese empire. One typical journey east along Alaska's Aleutian Island chain in 1752 brought back the pelts of 1772 sea otters, 750 blue foxes, and 840 fur seals.

Before reaching Alaska, these rough Russian trappers (known as *promyshlenniki*) had gathered furs in Siberia for generations using a cruel and effective system. They captured native women and children as hostages, then ransomed them back to their men in exchange for a fixed number of furs. In Alaskan waters, the trappers lacked the numbers, the boats, and the skill to collect large supplies of furs on their own. So they put their brutal hostage system into practice there as well. "They beach their vessels and try to take hostages, children and women from the island or nearby islands. If they cannot do this peacefully, they will use force," one Russian captain explained. "No matter where the Natives hunt, on shore or at sea, they must give everything" to the trappers. Native Alaskans resisted these intruders where possible, but many eventually submitted in a desperate effort to survive.

In the quarter century before 1780, 30 different companies sponsored expeditions to Alaskan waters. Harsh conditions and stiff competition between ships made the traffic risky for the Russians and far worse for the Aleutian Islanders. The newcomers, bringing diseases, firearms, and their brutal hostage-taking system, reduced the population of the islands. The remaining Aleuts were forced to overhunt their valuable wildlife, making their own survival even more precarious. As the human and animal population of the Aleutian Islands declined, the Russians pushed farther east in search of new hunters and hunting grounds.

As the voyages from Kamchatka grew longer and more expensive, a Russian organizer named Grigorii Shelikov gave serious thought to establishing an Alaskan base to facilitate operations. Shelikov and a partner formed a new company in 1781, and in 1784, founded a permanent colonial settlement on Kodiak Island east of the Aleutians, despite fierce opposition from the island's native residents. By 1799 the firm would absorb smaller competitors to become the Russian-American Company, with a monopoly from the czar.

In 1790, with the Kodiak base secure, Russians forced more than 7000 island inhabitants to embark on six enormous fur hunts in their versatile two-seat kayaks. That same year, Shelikov hired Alexander Baranov to oversee the Kodiak post and expand operations down the Alaskan coast. In 1799 Baranov established an additional outpost at Sitka in southeast Alaska. When a raid by Tlingit Indians destroyed the fort in 1802, he rebuilt the post. Sitka, called New Archangel at the time, became the capital of Russian America in 1808. From here, Baranov eventually extended the company's reach south toward Spanish California, seeking new hunting grounds and a climate warm enough to grow food crops.

Spain Colonizes the California Coast

The Seven Years' War had left Spain's king, Carlos III, with vast new land claims in western North America and only limited resources to explore or defend them. The Spanish ceded Florida to the British in 1763, evacuating St. Augustine and Pensacola. But Spain acquired from France the port of New Orleans and all of upper and lower Louisiana west of the Mississippi.

The bureaucrats charged with administering Spanish America struggled to oversee the vast and unfamiliar portions of the extended realm. But they faced numerous obstacles in controlling the huge domain. To their dismay, many of the Native Americans were not intimidated by force. Apaches and Comanches resisted several decades of military suppression and slave raids across the Southwest. In addition, clerics offered their own resistance to government designs. Carlos III expelled the powerful Jesuit order from the Spanish realm in 1767 for opposing administrative reform in the colonies. Unruly colonists posed a threat of their own. French inhabitants of New Orleans led a brief rebellion against Spanish rule in 1768. Finally, officials feared challenges in the Pacific from the British and the Russians. It was not until 1812 that Baranov finally established a Russian outpost at Fort Ross on the California coast, just north of San Francisco Bay. But as early as 1759, a Spanish Franciscan had published *Muscovites in California,* warning of Russian settlements.

With the threat of Russians in mind, Spanish leaders in America concentrated on establishing a token presence along the Pacific coast. Responsibility for this difficult task fell to

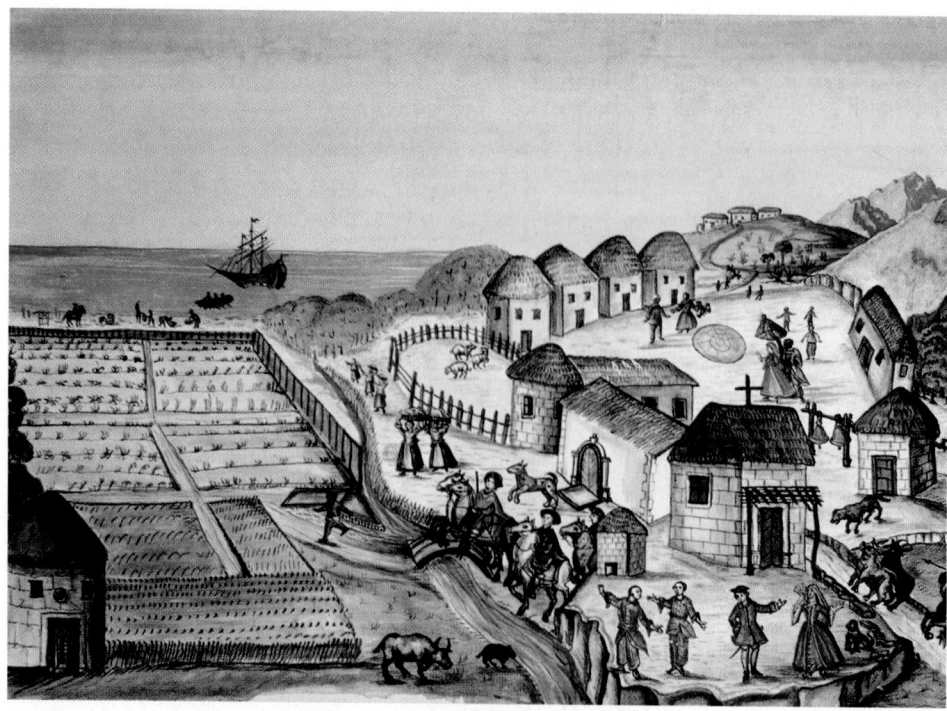

■ Jesuit missionary Ignacio Tirsch drew this view of his mission at the southern tip of Baja California in the 1760s. A Spanish ship that has crossed the Pacific from the Philippines is anchored offshore. When all Jesuits were ejected from Spain's American empire in 1767, Tirsch returned to his home near Prague in eastern Europe.

Czech National Library

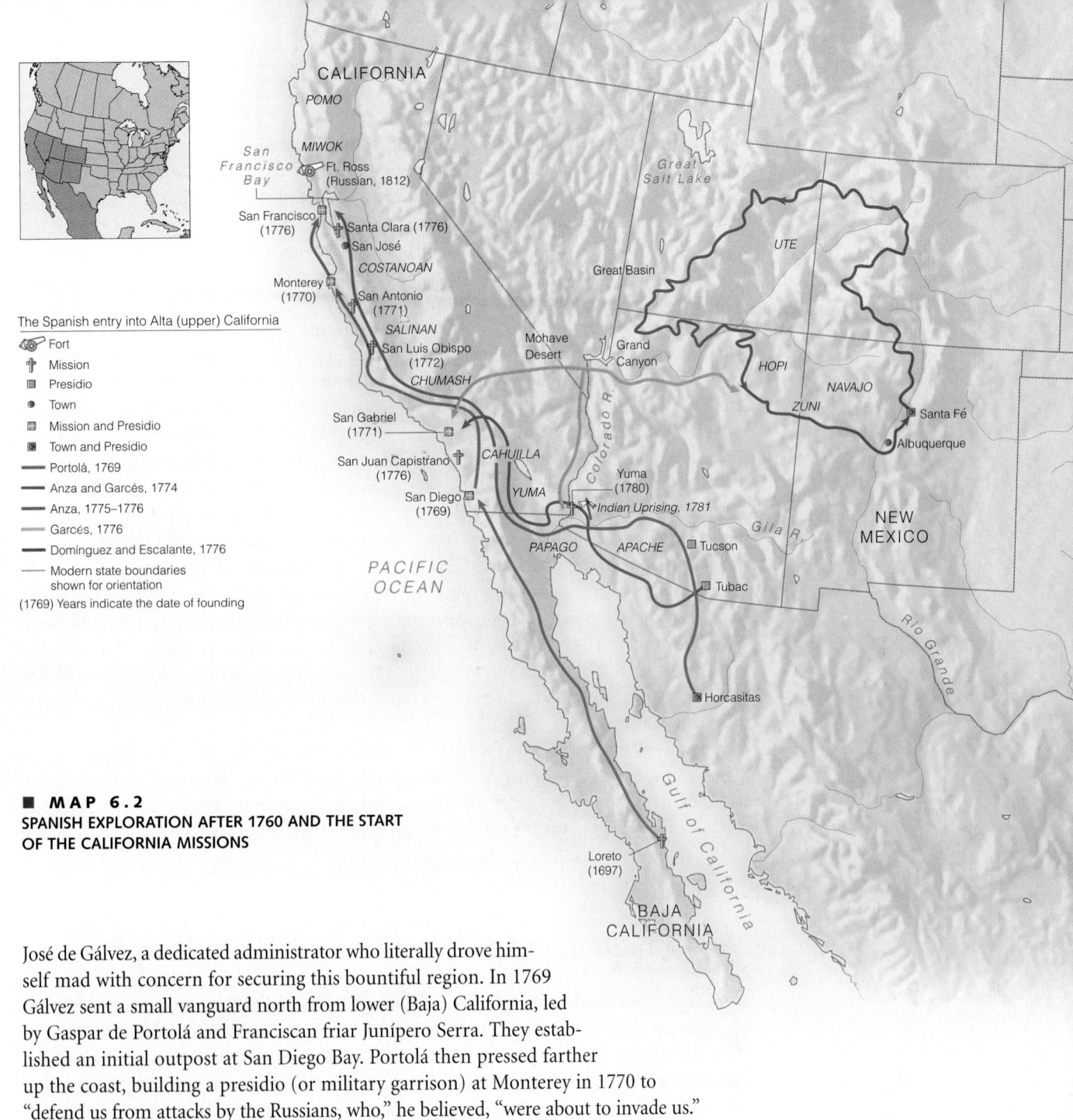

CALIFORNIA

POMO

San
Francisco
Bay

MIWOK Ft. Ross
(Russian, 1812)

San Francisco
(1776)

Santa Clara (1776)

San José

COSTANOAN

Monterey
(1770)

San Antonio
(1771)

SALINAN

San Luis Obispo
(1772)

CHUMASH

San Gabriel
(1771)

San Juan Capistrano
(1776)

CAHUILLA

San Diego
(1769)

YUMA

PACIFIC
OCEAN

Great
Salt Lake

UTE

Great Basin

Mohave
Desert

Grand
Canyon

HOPI

NAVAJO

ZUNI

Santa Fé

Albuquerque

Yuma
(1780)

Indian Uprising, 1781

PAPAGO

APACHE

Tucson

Gila R.

NEW
MEXICO

Tubac

Rio Grande

Horcasitas

Gulf of California

Loreto
(1697)

BAJA
CALIFORNIA

The Spanish entry into Alta (upper) California

🔫 Fort
✝ Mission
▣ Presidio
◉ Town
▣ Mission and Presidio
▣ Town and Presidio
— Portolá, 1769
— Anza and Garcés, 1774
— Anza, 1775–1776
— Garcés, 1776
— Domínguez and Escalante, 1776
---- Modern state boundaries
     shown for orientation
(1769) Years indicate the date of founding

■ **MAP 6.2**
**SPANISH EXPLORATION AFTER 1760 AND THE START
OF THE CALIFORNIA MISSIONS**

José de Gálvez, a dedicated administrator who literally drove himself mad with concern for securing this bountiful region. In 1769 Gálvez sent a small vanguard north from lower (Baja) California, led by Gaspar de Portolá and Franciscan friar Junípero Serra. They established an initial outpost at San Diego Bay. Portolá then pressed farther up the coast, building a presidio (or military garrison) at Monterey in 1770 to "defend us from attacks by the Russians, who," he believed, "were about to invade us."

After the removal of all Jesuits from Spanish America in 1767, numerous Franciscan missionaries, members of a competing Catholic order, expanded their work and took on new responsibilities. Following the lead of Father Serra, other Franciscans soon planted several missions between San Diego and Monterey. These included the San Gabriel mission in 1771, where colonists established the town of Los Angeles ten years later. In 1775 a Spanish captain sailed through the Golden Gate into spacious San Francisco Bay, and the next year a land expedition laid out the presidio and mission of San Francisco. A town sprang up at nearby San José the following year. Isolated Franciscan fathers labored to convert the coast's diverse Indian inhabitants. Meanwhile, Spanish vessels pushed far up the Pacific shoreline. They established contact with the Northwest Coast Indians in 1774, and Captain Ignacio de Arteaga reached the Gulf of Alaska in 1779, 14 months after Captain Cook had been there.

But Spanish ships traveling north from Mexico had difficulty supplying the few dozen settlers in California. Authorities therefore looked to open an overland supply route to the coast from Santa Fe or Sonora. In 1774, Juan Bautista de Anza set out in search of a land route to California from the Sonoran presidio he commanded at Tubac, south of Tucson. Accompanied by a Franciscan named Father Garcés, he forded the Colorado River with the help of Yuma Indians. He then crossed desert and mountains to reach the coast at San Gabriel. The next year, Anza led 240 reinforcements—mostly Spanish women and children—along a similar route, pausing at San Gabriel and heading north to San Francisco Bay.

Further explorations in 1776 proved less successful. Trying to find a usable route between California and New Mexico, Father Garcés meandered through the southwestern deserts. He traveled north along the Colorado River from Yuma country and then probed west across the Mohave Desert and east near the Grand Canyon without success. Two other Franciscans, Fathers Domínguez and Escalante, left Santa Fe on horseback in July 1776. They headed northwest across Colorado and Utah in search of a more northern route to avoid hostile Indians and lead to Monterey on the Pacific coast. But no such trail existed, and eventually they turned back. Instead of a west-flowing river, their five-month, 1800-mile trek revealed the huge expanse of the Great Basin. A passable route linking Santa Fe to the West Coast would have to wait for another half century.

Moreover, the Sonoran path to California that Anza had established proved short-lived. The same Yuma Indians who had helped his party cross the Colorado River in 1774 quickly grew to resent the Spanish trespassers. The last straw came in the summer of 1781, when a party of Spanish soldiers and settlers arrived at the river, heading for California with nearly a thousand head of livestock. When a sergeant demanded food from the Yumas, he reported that "the Indians screamed out to me that the cows and horses destroyed their mesquite [trees] and corn fields." The irate inhabitants asked him why the animals "were not fenced in," and within weeks they retaliated. Father Garcés and more than 100 Spanish men, women, and children died in the bloody Yuma Revolt, and hopes for a rapid expansion of the Spanish colony in California died with them.

Despite all these problems, the tiny California settlements endured. With difficulty, Spain managed to retain some control over its recently expanded North American empire. The same could not be said for the British in their own newly enlarged empire farther east. They had taken Canada from the French, and their military might dominated the Atlantic world. But their fortunes in North America were about to change.

New Challenges to Britain's Expanded Empire

In September 1760, French forces at Montreal submitted to British commander Jeffery Amherst in the final surrender of the Seven Years' War. For Native Americans living east of the Mississippi, the French defeat had an immediate impact. General Amherst, who despised Indians as "treacherous" and "contemptible," intended to alter Native American relations in the interior to reflect the new balance of power.

Immediately, Amherst dispatched James Grant to South Carolina with instructions "to chastise the Cherokees," who had taken up arms against the growing number of English traders and settlers in western Carolina. With 2800 soldiers—and more than 80 blacks to tend 700 packhorses and 400 beef cattle—Grant invaded Cherokee country in 1761. His men burned 15 villages and destroyed 1500 acres of beans and corn. The attackers had orders "to put every Soul to Death" without sparing women or children. The Indians who escaped Grant's force retreated in defeat.

With the Cherokees chastened in the South, Amherst turned his attention to the Indians living north of the Ohio River. Here his harsh policies brought a sudden retaliation from the Native Americans that took many lives and cost Amherst his command. And if Indians in the Midwest posed fresh challenges to Britain's expanded American empire, so did the colonists themselves.

Midwestern Lands and Pontiac's War for Indian Independence

As soon as the British unseated their French competitors in the Ohio River Valley, they prohibited traffic with Indians in such goods as knives, tomahawks, muskets, lead, and powder.

They also cut back on the use of ceremonial gifts. When the French were still powerful, the British had been generous, but now, one Native American complained, "you Look on us as Nobody." As French traders withdrew, the British took over their strategic posts at Detroit and at Michilimackinac. English settlers built new forts in the Ohio Valley and erected massive Fort Pitt over the ruins of Fort Duquesne. Indians at Niagara Falls commented in dismay at "so many Men and so much artillery passing by."

In 1761 wary Senecas proposed a preemptive strike against the British intruders. They failed to recruit their former enemies—the Ottawas, Potawatomies, and Hurons—so the plan died. But the next year brought poor harvests, a harsh winter, and a deadly epidemic. Hard conditions, plus the lack of French trade, weakened these "three fires" of the Great Lakes region and made them more willing to take up arms. Then, early in 1763, rumors spread through the Indian communities regarding peace negotiations in Europe. Reportedly, France would cede Louisiana to Spain and give up Canada and the entire Midwest to Great Britain. Among Native Americans, this shocking news undercut moderate leaders who were willing to accommodate the English and strengthened the hand of war factions.

Word that a remote treaty in Paris might disrupt the entire region also drew attention to Neolin, a Delaware Indian prophet who urged a return to ancient ways and a separation from the corrupting Europeans. Neolin's vision of gaining independence from white control by driving out the British held wide appeal for Native Americans in the Midwest. Among those influenced by it was Pontiac, a militant Ottawa warrior. In April, Pontiac addressed a great council of more than 400 Ottawas, Potawatomies, and Hurons, meeting secretly within 10 miles of Fort Detroit. Invoking the Delaware Prophet's vision, he told the gathering that the Master of Life resented the British and wanted them removed: "Send them back to the lands which I have created for them and let them stay there." By May, he had mobilized a coalition and laid siege to Detroit.

Pontiac's uprising ignited other attacks, as Indians from 18 nations joined in a widespread war of liberation. By mid-June 1763, both Detroit and Fort Pitt were under siege. Moreover, the British had lost every other Ohio Valley and Great Lakes outpost. As Indian raiding parties ravaged white communities in western Virginia and Pennsylvania, embittered settlers responded with indiscriminate racial killing. In December, white men from Paxton Creek descended on families of peaceful Conestoga Indians near Lancaster, Pennsylvania, executing more than 30 Christian converts in cold blood. When eastern Pennsylvanians protested this outrage, the "Paxton Boys" marched on Philadelphia to demand increased protection on the

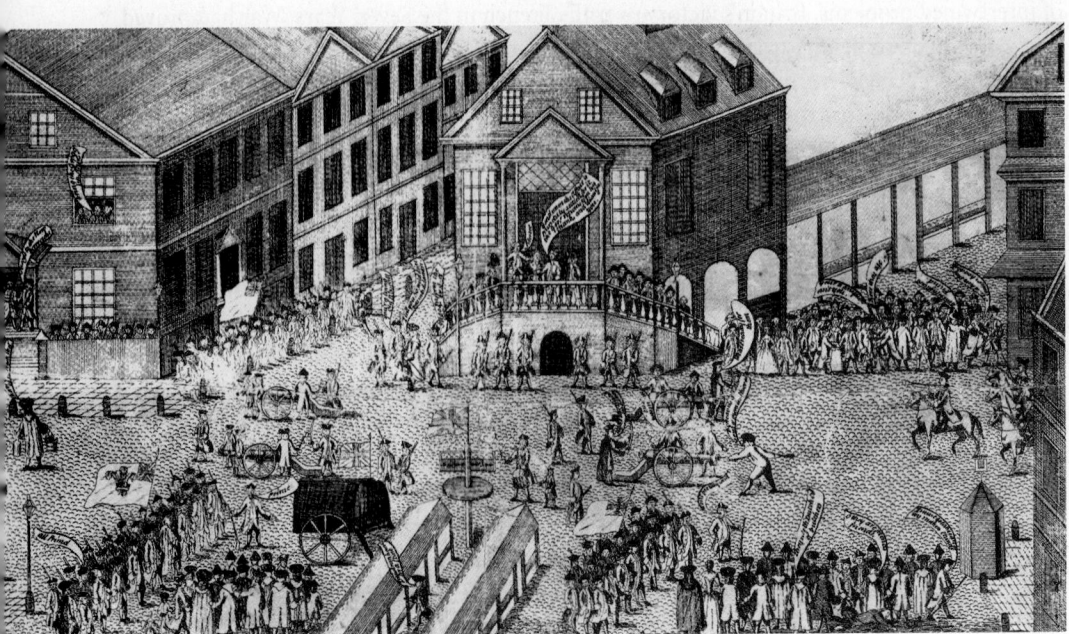

■ Violence on Pennsylvania's frontier prompted turmoil in Philadelphia, where Quakers had pressed for peaceful relations with Native Americans. In 1764 the Paxton Boys marched to the city to demand support for frontier settlers from the government. Ironically, as this cartoon shows, local pacifists prepared to resist them with force.

frontier. General Amherst ordered his officers to take no Indian prisoners, spread smallpox if possible, and treat the Native Americans as "the vilest race of beings that ever infested the earth." They deserved extermination, he ranted, "for the good of mankind."

The violence ended in a stalemate. Without French support, Native American munitions ran short, and Detroit and Fort Pitt endured. Indian militancy waned, and fighters deserted the coalition. Then in 1765, Pontiac was assassinated by a Peoria Indian in Illinois. Although the Native Americans had not won, they also had not lost, for the costly uprising prompted a shift in British policy. To avoid further expensive warfare, officials moved to restore the Indian trade, keep squatters and debt evaders out of Indian country, and prevent colonial speculation in western lands. In October 1763, Major General Thomas Gage replaced Amherst in command of British forces.

In England, the crown went further. Late in 1763, it issued a proclamation forbidding colonial settlers from moving west across the Appalachian Divide. They were not to go past the headwaters of the familiar rivers that ran east into the Atlantic Ocean. Beyond that line, where the streams flowed west into the Mississippi River or south into the Gulf of Mexico, all the land east of Spanish Louisiana would be reserved for Native Americans and a few authorized British soldiers, Indian agents, and traders.

In practice, the Proclamation Line of 1763, drawn in London, had only limited success. But it managed to frustrate aspiring members of Virginia's gentry, such as George Washington and Thomas Jefferson. These prominent men were investors in land companies that speculated in large western tracts, hoping to obtain property cheaply from Native Americans and sell small parcels to eager settlers at a steady profit. One place they did this was Kentucky, a region that had been disputed among Indians for generations.

Conflicting treaties in 1768 only sharpened the disagreement. At the Treaty of Hard Labor in South Carolina, the Cherokees retained control of the Kentucky region for hunting. Yet at the Treaty of Fort Stanwix in New York, the Iroquois ceded the same area to the British in exchange for a large payment. They did so even though the Kentucky lands were not theirs to sell. Virginia investors, hoping that this latter deal would open the region for purchase, pressed their case. But the British government, fearful of sparking unified Indian opposition and additional warfare, denied the Virginians' wishes and aroused their resentment.

Grenville's Effort at Reform

In 1763, the same year as the Proclamation Line, King George III also appointed Robert Grenville to head a new government in London. Grenville's ministry immediately faced a series of intertwined problems. Britain's victory over the French in the Seven Years' War had proved costly, nearly doubling the national debt to a staggering £146 million. As England's postwar depression deepened, returning soldiers swelled the ranks of the unemployed. Aggressive imperialists objected to what they saw as a timid peace settlement with France. In addition, rural mobs protested a new tax on domestic cider, imposed to help whittle away at the war debt.

No one promoted opposition to the government more than John Wilkes, a flamboyant member of Parliament (MP) who published an outspoken periodical. In issue number 45 of the *North Briton*, Wilkes attacked the king's peace settlement and the king himself. Grenville reacted quickly, issuing a general warrant to search the homes of all those connected to the paper. He also arrested the publisher, despite his status as an MP. Angered by the government's sweeping suppression of dissent, protesters made "Wilkes and Liberty!" and "45" into popular rallying cries.

Pressured at home, Grenville set out to impose order on Britain's growing American colonies through a series of reforms. The first step was to maintain a considerable military presence. Even with the Proclamation Line in place, Grenville's ministry kept nearly 7000 troops in North America. Leaving them there could help enforce peace with the Indians, protect the newly acquired territories of Canada and Florida, and keep young British men employed overseas rather than jobless at home. Grenville also saw another positive aspect to this move that helped to justify it. Strapped for funds, he considered paying for the trans-Atlantic forces with money drawn from the very colonies these troops were defending?

Raising money in this way would also remind the British colonies of their subordination to the sovereign power of Parliament. Colonists had grown wealthy by sidestepping the elaborate Navigation Acts and trading illegally with foreign powers, even during wartime. Sympathetic colonial juries had looked the other way. Worse, American legislatures had used their power of the purse to withhold money from any British governor who ignored local interests. Finally, lax customs officers assigned to colonial ports often collected their salaries while remaining in England, without even occupying their posts.

As a preliminary step, Grenville ordered absentee customs officials to their colonial stations and dispatched 44 navy ships to assist them. Next, he moved his first reform through Parliament: the American Duties Act of 1764, also known as the Revenue Act or the Sugar Act. The new law increased the duty on sugar and other products, such as wine, spirits, cloth, coffee, and indigo, entering the empire from non-British ports. But most important, it cut in half the long-standing import duty of sixpence per gallon on foreign molasses. Officials hoped that New England rum distillers, who had been secretly importing cheap molasses from the French West Indies without paying customs, would be willing to pay threepence per gallon to import the ingredient legally. If fully enforced, the act would reduce smuggling and boost revenues while saving merchants from the heavy costs of bribing port officials and courtroom participants.

> *"What has America done," protested critics, "to be stripped of so invaluable a privilege as the trial by jury?"*

To ensure compliance, the Sugar Act strengthened the customs officers' authority to seize goods off arriving ships, and it established the first of several vice-admiralty courts. The court sat at Halifax, Nova Scotia, so defendants had large travel expenses and no hope of a favorable local jury. Instead, they faced a single appointed judge and no jury. Shockingly, a captain or shipowner accused of smuggling was presumed guilty until he could prove his innocence. If he failed to do so, he lost his seized property. "What has America done," protested critics, "to be stripped of so invaluable a privilege as the trial by jury?"

Additional statutes followed quickly. The Currency Act of 1764 prohibited colonial assemblies from issuing paper money or bills of credit to be used as legal tender to pay off debts. The move only worsened the money shortage in British America, where trade languished in a postwar depression. A lopsided trade balance was already draining gold and silver from the colonies to England annually, and colonial merchants had to pay Grenville's new duties using the same scarce hard money.

The next year, after resentful New Yorkers refused to provide firewood for General Gage's troops, Parliament passed a Quartering Act that obliged colonists to assist the army. Soldiers could not be quartered in private homes, as Gage had requested, but officers could requisition vacant barns and other buildings as temporary quarters when regular barracks and alehouses could not accommodate all their men. The local governor was to supply the soldiers, at colonial expense, with certain basic necessities they would expect at any inn: firewood, candles, bedding, salt, vinegar, utensils, and rations of beer and cider. Colonial assemblies had willingly voted such support during the Seven Years' War. However, these peacetime requisitions, ordered by a distant Parliament, seemed to challenge their authority and smacked of indirect taxation.

The Stamp Act Imposed

There was nothing indirect about Grenville's most important reform: the Stamp Act. Early in 1765, Parliament approved the new statute "for raising a further revenue" to pay for "defending, protecting, and securing" the British colonies in America. Grenville patterned his legislation on a similar law already in place in England. The new act was a complex measure that required stamps (rather like those on modern packs of cigarettes) to appear on a wide variety of articles in America after November 1, 1765. The list included all legal contracts and commissions, plus countless other paper documents from land deeds and liquor licenses to servant indentures and academic degrees. Newspapers, pamphlets, almanacs, playing cards, and dice also had to bear a stamp.

Colonial lawyers and printers were supposed to purchase these stamps from designated agents and pass the additional cost on to their clients and customers. The official stamp distributor in each colony would receive a handsome fee equaling 7.5 percent of all stamp sales. The British Exchequer (Treasury) anticipated taking in at least £100,000 per year, to be held in a separate account and spent only for government operations in America.

The proposed stamp bill generated little debate in Parliament. William Pitt, the leader of the opposition party and a friend of the colonists, did not even attend the session. Only Isaac Barré, a veteran of the Quebec campaign, protested. Claiming to "know more of America than most of you," Barré challenged the assertion of Stamp Act supporters that England had nurtured and protected the colonies from earliest times. He defended the Americans as true "Sons of Liberty": loyal British subjects protective of their rights and quick to "vindicate them, if ever they should be violated."

But Grenville countered Barré's claims. Americans, the minister argued, had nothing to fear from England. Granted, colonists had no actual representation in the Parliament that had enacted this tax. But in this they were like the majority of subjects in England. Most of them did not have the right to cast a ballot, yet all of them were said to be "virtually" represented by MPs, who supposedly had the interests of the entire country at heart. If members of Parliament could look out for nonvoting subjects at home, surely they could provide the same sort of "virtual representation" for all British subjects throughout the realm.

Whether or not they spoke for colonists in America, most MPs viewed Grenville's stamp measure as appropriate, moderate, and well conceived. They saw no legal distinction between external duties used to regulate trade and enforce the nation's navigation acts and internal taxes imposed by Parliament within the colonies themselves to raise revenue. Besides, because the stamp tax applied to numerous daily articles used throughout the colonies, it would be widely and evenly distributed. Even better, revenues would grow steadily and automatically as colonial economic activity continued to expand.

So as not to cause alarm in the colonies, Parliament set initial stamp prices in America lower than those charged in England, although it could always raise the rates as colonists grew accustomed to the tax. Moreover, the tax was to be gathered quietly by Americans themselves in the course of doing business rather than extracted from individual citizens by tax collectors. In drafting the act, the ministry had consulted agents serving as lobbyists for the American colonies in London, including Benjamin Franklin. According to these public figures, prominent colonists were eager to accept the lucrative stamp distributorships. No one predicted the upheaval that the Stamp Act would instigate. But it soon unleashed a storm of organized, militant resistance in the colonial ports where the stamps were to be sold.

The Stamp Act Resisted

At first, most colonial assemblies had mixed responses to the burdensome new tax. But in late May, the youngest member of the Virginia House of Burgesses—a rising country attorney named Patrick Henry—galvanized American resistance to the Stamp Act. Henry introduced a series of fiery resolves regarding the mandate. The House session was winding down, and many conservative members who endorsed Parliament's right to impose taxes had already departed from Williamsburg. With impressive oratory, the 28-year-old Henry managed to gain narrow passage of five separate resolutions. Young Thomas Jefferson recalled listening to the heated debate from a hallway, with other students from the College of William and Mary.

Henry's fifth and most provocative resolve asserted that Virginia's assembly had the "sole exclusive right and power to lay taxes" on the colony's inhabitants. The resolution passed by just one vote. In fact, opponents reintroduced it the next day, after Henry himself left town, and voted it down. But the spark had been struck. Within a month, distant newspapers were reprinting Henry's "Virginia Resolves." The papers included not only the resolution that had been voted down but also two ominous-sounding ones that had been drawn up but never introduced for a vote, since approval seemed unlikely. According to these two added resolutions, Virginians were "not bound to yield obedience" to any such tax, and anyone arguing otherwise must "be deemed an enemy" to the colony.

In Massachusetts, the assembly took a different approach. It issued a call for each colony to send delegates to a Stamp Act Congress in New York in October 1765 to "implore relief" from Parliament. Local citizens, inflamed by Virginia's resolutions and squeezed by an economic depression, prepared to take more direct action. In Boston, a small group of artisans and merchants known as the Loyal Nine mobilized to halt the new tax before it could even be implemented. They hatched a plan to force the designated stamp distributor, Andrew Oliver, to resign before the stamps arrived from England.

The Loyal Nine persuaded Ebenezer McIntosh, leader of the well-organized Pope's Day demonstrations in that city's South End, to join forces with North End rivals in a demonstration against Oliver. On August 16, a crowd of several thousand hanged an effigy of Oliver and tore down his newly erected Stamp Office. That night, the protesters ransacked Oliver's elegant house, drinking his wine and smashing his furniture. The next day, Oliver resigned his appointment.

As word of the protest spread, crowds took to the streets in scores of towns. Often the mobs were encouraged by local leaders who opposed the Stamp Act. These prominent citizens had started to organize themselves in secret groups, which they called the Sons of Liberty, borrowing the phrase first used by Isaac Barré in Parliament. With speeches and additional prompting, they aroused angry demonstrators. The crowds, in turn, forced the resignation of potential stamp distributors in ports from New Hampshire all the way down to the Carolinas. When a shipment of stamps finally arrived in New York City, a crowd of nearly five thousand risked open warfare to confiscate the hated cargo on Guy Fawkes Day, November 5.

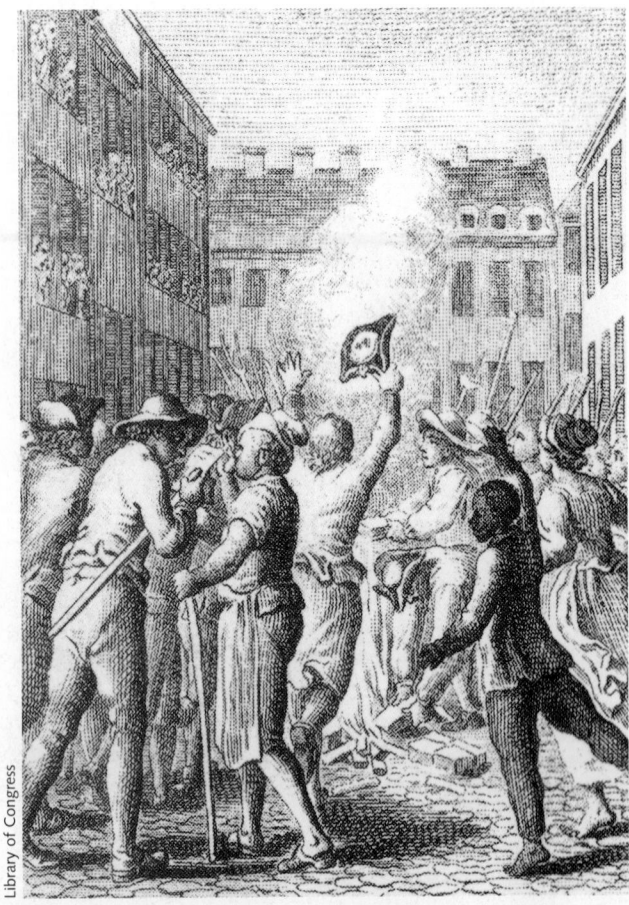

Library of Congress

■ Lawyers and artisans in the Sons of Liberty encouraged demonstrations against the Stamp Act. But they ran the risk, suggested here, that poor workers, black slaves, and women in the crowds might give their own meanings to the shouts of "Liberty!"

Throughout the second half of 1765, the Sons of Liberty promoted street violence against specific targets. But they quickly learned that they could not always contain and control the demonstrations, since the debtors, sailors, blacks, and women drawn to such crowds all had separate grievances of their own. For example, on August 26 in Boston, just 10 days after the raid on Oliver's house, a second mob launched a broader assault. Without sanction from the Loyal Nine or the Sons of Liberty, the crowd went after the homes of several wealthy office holders, including the house of Lieutenant Governor Thomas Hutchinson. Because he also served as chief justice of the Superior Court, Hutchinson had offended townspeople by issuing numerous warrants for debtors and collecting large fees for administering bankruptcies. He recounted how he fled when "the hellish crew fell upon my house with the Rage of devils and…with axes split down the doors." By the time the assault ended, the attackers had pillaged Hutchinson's entire estate.

In South Carolina several months later, the spirit of insurrection also went well beyond the careful boundaries intended by the Sons of Liberty. They were pleased when Charleston artisans hanged a stamp distributor in effigy, with a sign reading, "Liberty and no Stamp Act." And they gave tacit approval when white workers harassed the wealthy slave trader and potential stamp distributor Henry Laurens with chants of "Liberty, Liberty!" Soon, however, enslaved African Americans also took to the streets, raising their own defiant cry of "Liberty, Liberty!" Fearing an insurrection by South Carolina's black majority, the same people who had sanctioned earlier street demonstrations quickly shifted their focus, believing that ideas of freedom had spread

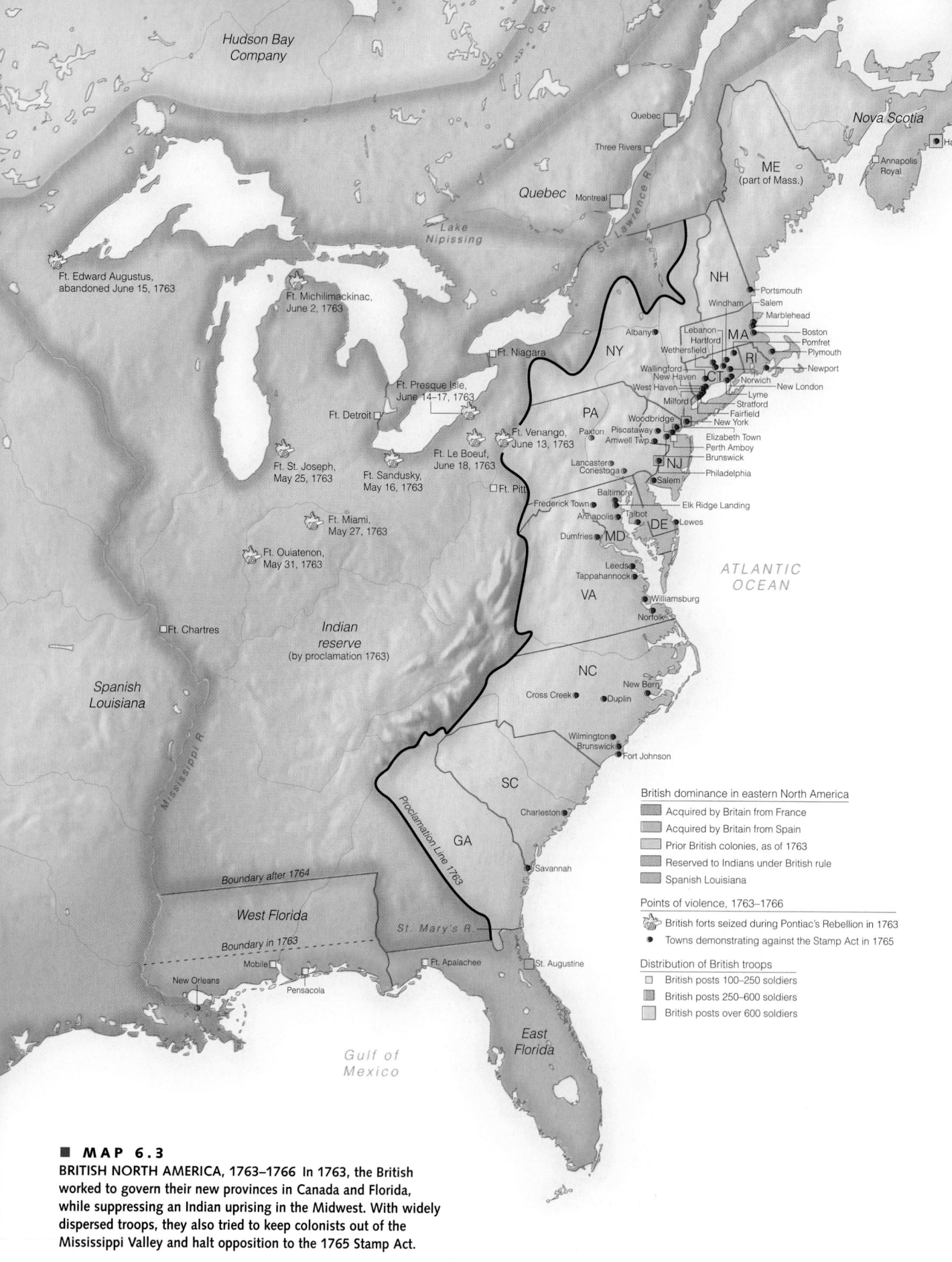

Hudson Bay
Company

Nova Scotia

Quebec

Three Rivers

■ Halifax

Annapolis
Royal

Quebec

Montreal

ME
(part of Mass.)

Lake
Nipissing

St. Lawrence R.

NH

Ft. Edward Augustus,
abandoned June 15, 1763

Ft. Michilimackinac,
June 2, 1763

Albany

Portsmouth
Windham
Salem
Marblehead

Ft. Niagara

NY

Lebanon
Hartford
Wethersfield

Boston
Pomfret
Plymouth

MA

RI

Ft. Presque Isle,
June 14–17, 1763

Wallingford
New Haven
West Haven
Milford

CT

Norwich

New London

Newport

Ft. Detroit

PA

Lyme
Stratford
Fairfield

Ft. Venango,
June 13, 1763

Woodbridge

New York

Ft. Le Boeuf,
June 18, 1763

Paxton

Piscataway
Amwell Twp.

Elizabeth Town
Perth Amboy

Ft. St. Joseph,
May 25, 1763

Ft. Sandusky,
May 16, 1763

Lancaster
Conestoga

Brunswick

NJ

Salem

Philadelphia

Ft. Pitt

Frederick Town

Baltimore

Elk Ridge Landing

Ft. Miami,
May 27, 1763

Annapolis
Dumfries

Talbot

DE

Lewes

MD

Ft. Ouiatenon,
May 31, 1763

Leeds
Tappahannock

ATLANTIC
OCEAN

Williamsburg

Ft. Chartres

Indian
reserve
(by proclamation 1763)

VA

Norfolk

Spanish
Louisiana

NC

New Bern

Cross Creek

Duplin

MISSISSIPPI R.

Wilmington
Brunswick

Fort Johnson

SC

Charleston

Proclamation Line 1763

GA

Boundary after 1764

Savannah

West Florida

Boundary in 1763

St. Mary's R.

Mobile

Ft. Apalachee

St. Augustine

New Orleans

Pensacola

East
Florida

Gulf of
Mexico

British dominance in eastern North America

- Acquired by Britain from France
- Acquired by Britain from Spain
- Prior British colonies, as of 1763
- Reserved to Indians under British rule
- Spanish Louisiana

Points of violence, 1763–1766

- British forts seized during Pontiac's Rebellion in 1763
- Towns demonstrating against the Stamp Act in 1765

Distribution of British troops

- British posts 100–250 soldiers
- British posts 250–600 soldiers
- British posts over 600 soldiers

■ **MAP 6.3**
BRITISH NORTH AMERICA, 1763–1766 In 1763, the British
worked to govern their new provinces in Canada and Florida,
while suppressing an Indian uprising in the Midwest. With widely
dispersed troops, they also tried to keep colonists out of the
Mississippi Valley and halt opposition to the 1765 Stamp Act.

too far. The colonial assembly banned further importation of Africans temporarily, while local leaders expanded slave patrols and placed Charleston briefly under martial law.

Elsewhere, too, the colonial elites took steps to contain the turbulence. Many moved—often reluctantly—toward more radical positions, joining the Sons of Liberty and ridiculing the British concept of virtual representation. Colonial assemblies condemned Grenville's intrusive reforms, and the Stamp Act Congress passed resolutions vehemently protesting both the Sugar and Stamp acts. But even as they challenged Parliament, these same local leaders counseled caution and restraint. They stressed their continuing loyalty to the crown and moved to control the violence, some of which was directed at them. Such moderation appealed to cautious merchants in Boston, New York, and Philadelphia. Reluctantly, they agreed to stop ordering goods from Britain. As they saw it, British exporters, feeling the boycott's economic pinch, might use their political strength to force a repeal of the Stamp Act and defuse the tense situation.

When politics in London prompted Grenville's sudden removal from office, hopes rose in America for a possible compromise resolving the Stamp Act crisis. In March 1766, these hopes were nearly fulfilled. The new ministry of Lord Rockingham, responding to merchant pressure as predicted, and also to the compelling rhetoric of William Pitt, persuaded Parliament to repeal the Stamp Act. But colonial victory had a hollow ring to it, for the repeal bill was accompanied by a blunt Declaratory Act. In it, the members of Parliament declared clearly that they reaffirmed their power "to make Laws…to bind the Colonists and People of America…in all Cases whatsoever."

"The Unconquerable Rage of the People"

As news of Stamp Act repeal spread, the Sons of Liberty organized elaborate celebrations in British America. In Charleston and Philadelphia, citizens staged public "illuminations," placing lighted candles in the windows of their homes. In Boston, they lit so many fireworks that the town shone like day, and John Hancock treated the public to casks of Madeira wine. But word of the Declaratory Act had a sobering effect. Clearly, the problems surrounding colonial taxation and representation remained unresolved. The atmosphere of mutual suspicion and righteous indignation that had erupted during the Stamp Act crisis divided colonists further in the years ahead.

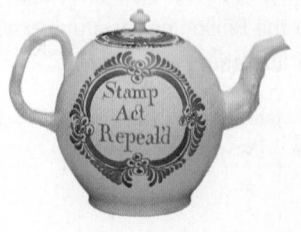

A flurry of pamphlets from colonial presses broadened awareness of the issues, sharpened arguments, and inspired new coalitions. For the first time, colonists from separate regions and different countries of origin began to identify themselves as Americans, gradually adopting a term that had previously applied only to Indians. Most importantly, as colonial leaders collaborated with one another, they discovered a shared viewpoint that gave heightened meaning and importance to each new event. This emerging ideology had a logic of its own, with common assumptions and unifying principles. It also had deep roots stretching back into earlier periods in English history.

Expanding the Framework for Revolution

The radical ideas that had emerged during England's Civil War in the 1640s, when English subjects briefly overthrew their monarchy and proclaimed a Puritan Commonwealth, lived on long after the Restoration in 1660. Decades later, the English Whigs who led the Glorious Revolution invoked some of these same principles when they limited the monarchy's power and strengthened Parliament's authority in 1688. Succeeding generations of mainstream publicists hailed the rights of all freeborn English subjects and congratulated themselves that Great Britain (as England and Scotland became known in 1707) had achieved a truly balanced government. They drew on the ancient Greek philosopher Aristotle to explain their accomplishment.

Aristotle, his modern readers noted, had observed a cycle in politics. He believed that too much power vested in a king could eventually corrupt the monarchical form of government.

Movement Building Against the Odds

Few popular protests, no matter how novel, start from scratch. Social movements regularly build on their predecessors. Even when protesters address new issues, they borrow many of their strategies from the past. Consciously or unconsciously, they adopt tactics that have proven effective at other times in undermining powerful opponents and rallying public support. Old songs are rewritten for fresh causes or adopted by new generations. The Civil Rights anthem "We Shall Overcome" began as a slave protest song and spread into the modern labor movement before returning to the black freedom struggle in the 1950s. In the late twentieth century, it circled the globe from Poland to South Africa to the Philippines as a universal hymn of liberation.

But each era of conflict contributes its own fresh additions to the arsenal of protest. Nineteenth-century slavery opponents and advocates for women's rights raised the ancient art of petition writing to a form of public demonstration. Withholding local tax payments also became a viable protest action. Author Henry David Thoreau went to jail for this act in 1846, as a gesture to oppose the Mexican–American War. In a famous essay, Thoreau popularized the general idea of civil disobedience and influenced the nonviolent protest tactics of Mahatma Gandhi in India a century later. In the twentieth century, American autoworkers and civil rights activists perfected the sit-in, drawing inspiration from Gandhi.

The Atlantic world of the late eighteenth century made key contributions to the list of effective protest tactics. Strikes, the organized work stoppages that became a central weapon for organized labor in the industrial era, draw their name from earlier acts by British deck hands. As far back as the 1760s, militant sailors in London would "strike" (take down) the sails and the horizontal yardarms of their square-rigged ships. By keeping vessels in the world's busiest port, they could halt English trade until their demands were met.

In North America, meanwhile, colonists experimented with the same boycott tactics used more recently by farm workers, environmentalists, and opponents of movie violence and record industry obscenity. Groups of irate colonists combined in formal associations, using their collective buying power to withhold purchases of certain imported goods. These nonimportation agreements were intended to cripple commerce with Britain until the government altered its policies. Such associations, though supposedly voluntary, put heavy social pressure on nonmembers who refused to join, ignoring them at church and in the streets. (Such boycotts, both commercial and social, did not earn their current name until a century later, when Irish protesters used them effectively against a landlord named Captain Boycott in 1880.)

Unbounded royal power sooner or later led to a tyranny, misrule by a despot wielding absolute control. When nobles then asserted themselves against the tyrant (as English barons had done when they forced King John to sign the Magna Carta in 1215), the resulting aristocracy could easily turn corrupt as well. Abuse of power by such an oligarchy of self-serving nobles could then prompt the common people, known as the commons, to rise up. If the commons gained sway, they might build a democracy, but it too could degenerate, leaving only anarchy. Such a "mobocracy" only paved the way for an opportunistic leader to once more seize the scepter of royal power and start the cycle over again.

Confident Whigs claimed that England had halted this vicious cycle by balancing the power of the nation's three estates: the king epitomized the legitimate interests of monarchy, the House of Lords represented the aristocracy, and the House of Commons represented the rest of the population. A few of the more radical Whig theorists continued to oppose this consensus view long after 1700, however. Calling themselves the Real Whigs, these skeptics argued that the existing mixed government—which claimed an ideal and lasting balance between monarchy, aristocracy, and commons—was actually much less perfect and more vulnerable than most people suspected.

A truly balanced government, they argued, is hard to achieve and difficult to maintain, for if power inevitably corrupts, then schemers who obtain undue control can readily disrupt such a fragile system. So its protection, these critics argued, demanded constant vigilance. They urged

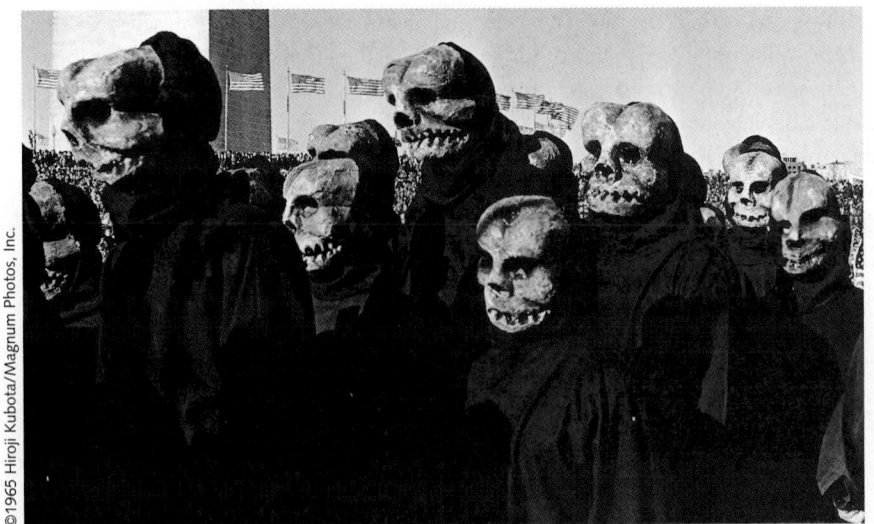

Ever since the era of the Boston Tea Party, Americans have organized symbolic demonstrations to challenge official policies and attract public attention. In November 1965, protestors in Washington, DC, donned death masks to draw media coverage to a rally opposing the Vietnam War.

attacking an abortion clinic can be viewed as a wake-up call by those committing the act. But they can also provoke a strong backlash in public opinion. For movements building a broad base of support, therefore, it often seems best if violence and deadly force come first from the powers that be. That was true when British soldiers fired into a Boston crowd on March 5, 1770, and equally true two centuries later when troopers on horseback attacked peaceful civil rights marchers at Selma, Alabama, on March 9, 1965.

So colonial protesters, like modern antiglobalization activists, preferred mock hangings to real ones. And like their descendants with cell phones, they stressed coordination, knowing that communication was essential to the movement's success. It is no surprise that printer Ben Franklin and messenger Paul Revere played central roles. The Committees of Correspondence that linked Whig leaders in separate colonies have present-day counterparts in the campus networks that spur anti-sweatshop activism. ■

Colonists also went beyond nonimportation agreements to engage in concerted attacks on property. But these volatile actions rarely spun far out of control. If there was one thing that the protesters knew from experience and passed on to their successors, it was the need for patience in building a movement. Premature or excessive action by a few enthusiasts could draw down reprisals, turn away potential supporters, and discredit the cause. So organizers who worked to stir up cautious or complacent citizens also worked to rein in overzealous dissidents.

In any era, deadly acts of violence such as seizing a federal arsenal, bombing a public building, or

citizens to watch for the two surest signs of decay: the concentration of wealth in few hands and the political and social corruption that inevitably follows. Where others saw grandeur and stability in England's exuberant growth, these Real Whigs perceived sure signs of danger in the powerful new Bank of England, the expanding stock market, and the rise in public debt.

No Real Whigs proved more vigilant than John Trenchard and Thomas Gordon. The two men sensed around them the same luxury and greed that had undermined the Roman Republic. They pored over the works of ancient historians and social critics, including the Roman statesman Cato, whose correspondence described and challenged corrupt behavior. In 1721 they published *Cato's Letters: Essays on Liberty,* in which they cautioned against "the Natural Encroachments of Power" and warned that "public corruptions and abuses have grown upon us."

One abuse that offended Trenchard and Gordon was Britain's expanding patronage system. New public positions seemed designed to reward loyal support, and too many people appeared to gain office through political ties rather than through skill or training. The two writers warned that this system of patronage, when carried to an extreme, put private advancement ahead of the public good. Far from being independent civil servants, the patronage appointees supported and protected some important figure high up in the government. They dutifully filled a post (often in the colonies) and took direction from their patron in exchange for the chance to line their pockets with public money.

The authors of *Cato's Letters* saw each individual act of corruption as representing a dangerous precedent, if unopposed. They reminded their readers that tyranny is often imposed through small, subtle steps, for "if it is suffered once, it is apt to be repeated often; a few repetitions create a habit." Soon, before the citizens realize that they are losing their liberties, the permanent "Yoke of Servitude" is in place, supported by military force, and all hope of successful protest has disappeared. Equally insidious, would-be tyrants may actually "provoke the People to Disaffection; and then make that Disaffection an Argument for new Oppression…and for keeping up Troops." The encroachment of power over liberty, Trenchard and Gordon concluded, is "much easier to prevent than to cure."

Though these writers attracted only limited attention in England, they earned a wide American following. The popularity of *Cato's Letters* and related tracts continued to spread in the colonies during the 1760s, for colonists saw disturbing parallels between the warnings of Real Whig authors and current events in America. Throughout history, the essayists warned, corrupt ministers have encouraged expensive wars, negotiated damaging treaties, and promoted "worthless and wicked" officials whose only qualification is to "show stupid alacrity to do what they are bid." When tainted by corruption, a government might deny adequate representation, initiate unjust taxes, or replace jury trials with arbitrary proceedings such as the vice-admiralty courts. If public officials curtailed freedoms of press or religion, that only confirmed their schemes to consolidate power. Moreover, weak and unprincipled ministers might advise the monarch poorly or keep citizens' pleas from reaching their king's ears. If the populace relaxed its guard, these ministers might even sanction a standing army in peacetime to impose arbitrary rule over their own population.

> *During the 1760s, colonists saw disturbing parallels between the warnings of Real Whig authors and current events in America.*

According to Real Whig doctrine, ordinary people must be alert but circumspect; a measured response to these threats was all-important. After all, one stubborn or mistaken act by officials did not necessarily indicate a pattern of conspiracy. Also, it could be counterproductive to raise alarms too often. So prudent citizens should turn first to accepted, legal methods of appeal and redress. If the system was functioning properly, claims of real abuses would bring forth proper corrections. Even if forced to take to the streets as a last resort, crowds should be organized and purposeful, not riotous and uncontrolled. They should threaten property before people and hang effigies, not actual office holders.

For the most part, the Stamp Act demonstrations had followed this logic of restraint and had gained the desired effect. "In every Colony," wrote John Adams, "the Stamp Distributors and Inspectors have been compelled, by the unconquerable Rage of the People, to renounce their offices." But did individual demands for liberty have limits? If so, what were they? Could slaves seek liberty from their masters? What about wives from their husbands? Could tenants press for redress from rich landlords, or debtors from powerful creditors? Such questions generated widespread, heated debate in the turbulent quarter-century ahead.

Rural Unrest: Tenant Farmers and Regulators

For a growing number of colonists, international events in the years after 1765 seemed to confirm the views that the Real Whigs had passed down. When John Wilkes was repeatedly elected to Parliament but expelled from the Commons for his radical views, his English supporters cried foul and demanded political reform. Americans saw Wilkes as their champion. In 1768, when troops in London fired on a huge mob protesting Wilkes's imprisonment—killing half a dozen people and wounding innocent bystanders—colonists joined in condemning "the massacre of St. George's Field." South Carolina's Assembly even tried to contribute public money to support Wilkes. Similarly, Americans embraced the short-lived cause of Pasquale Paoli, who fought to free the Mediterranean island of Corsica from domination by Genoa.

Many colonists christened their sons after Wilkes or Paoli, and Pennsylvanians named new towns after these overseas heroes. The two men seemed to embody a broader struggle of liberty against tyranny. But often that contest flared up closer to home as well. Local occurrences, large and small, seemed to fit a pattern described by the Real Whigs. On the religious front, for example, New England colonists bemoaned rumors that the Church of England—which had persecuted their Puritan ancestors—hoped to install an American bishop in Boston. Similar talk of a resident bishop in Virginia, where the Church of England had long dominated, also provoked debate. Controversy intensified with the work of Virginia's Separate Baptist ministers, who won over thousands of recruits with their staunch opposition to the colony's established church.

After 1765, as local controversies simmered, the "Rage of the People" often seemed to boil up from below, especially in rural areas, where most colonists lived. "The People, even to the lowest Ranks, have become more attentive to their Liberties," John Adams observed with some worry, "and more determined to defend them" than ever before. For example, while stamp protesters demonstrated in New York City, aggrieved tenant farmers staged a violent revolt against powerful landholders in the Hudson River Valley. They chose an Irish immigrant named William Prendergast as their leader, established a council, and organized militia companies with elected captains. Calling themselves Levellers, they broke open local jails to free debtors, and they set up their own people's courts to try captured gentry.

British troops finally suppressed the Hudson Valley revolt, but not before the land rioters proclaimed themselves Sons of Liberty and sought aid from Stamp Act rebels in New York City. A participant named Moss Kent recalled that "when they went to New York they expected to be assisted by the poor people there." However, leaders in New York City's antistamp protests rebuffed the request for assistance from upriver. These prominent figures were also Hudson River land moguls who had evicted scores of tenants from their manors. Such men proved "great opposers of the Rioters," according to one observer, "as they are of opinion no one is entitled to Riot but themselves." (For example, one New York judge condemned land rioters who were brought before him, even while he was taking an active role in the Stamp Act Congress.) A special court convicted Prendergast of high treason and sentenced him to be disemboweled and then beheaded. Luckily for him, the king spared his life.

While tenant farmers protested in the Hudson Valley, unrest also shook the Carolinas in the interior region known to colonists as the backcountry, or the Piedmont. In South Carolina, the absence of civil government beyond the coastal parishes fostered lawlessness and disunity among white settlers until the governor extended circuit courts into the interior in 1769. In North Carolina, migrants seeking land were moving south from Virginia and Pennsylvania into the fertile backcountry in a steady stream. When they arrived in the Piedmont, they found a local elite already in place. Appointed to county offices by the governor, these officials possessed strong family and financial ties to powerful planters and merchants farther east. (Their high-handed and self-serving ways epitomized, at the local level, the sorts of corruption that had long troubled Real Whig pamphleteers.)

The newcomers disliked the grasping officeholders and corrupt courts. As their numbers rose, they protested against inadequate representation for backcountry counties in the colonial assembly. They began organizing into local groups to better "regulate" their own affairs, and they soon became known as Regulators. These small farmers, many of them in debt after moving to a new region, protested loudly against regressive taxes that imposed the same burden on all colonists, regardless of their wealth or poverty. The Regulators' discontent turned into outrage when they heard that coastal planters who dominated the assembly had voted public funds to build a stately mansion in New Bern for William Tryon, the colonial governor. By this act, the slaveholding elite in eastern North Carolina would establish the colony's permanent capitol building on the coast, rather than in the expanding interior town of Hillsborough. What's more, farmers who would never see the stately mansion would bear most of the cost of constructing it.

The decision to erect "Tryon's Palace" at public expense confirmed the worst suspicions of backcountry settlers. The governor and his associates, they decided, were concerned primarily with their own wealth, at the expense of the public interest. Hundreds, then thousands, of aroused Piedmont farm families joined local alliances that swelled into the well-organized Regulator Movement. They filed petitions, withheld their tax money, closed courts, and

"Exert Your Selves This Once in Our Favour": Petition Signed by 30 North Carolina Regulators, October 4, 1768

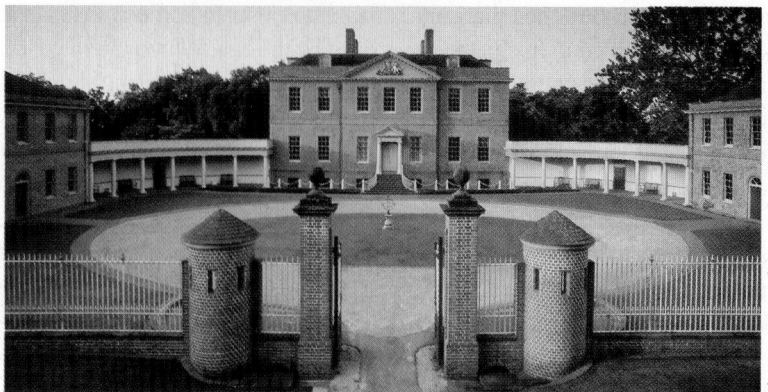

Tryon Palace, the governor's mansion in New Bern, North Carolina, erected in 1768.

Photo courtesy of Tryon Palace Historic Sites & Gardens

In the 1760s, corruption prevailed among appointed officials in central North Carolina. Often holding numerous offices at once, these men managed elections, controlled courts, and gathered taxes. Apparently not all the tax money they collected made it to the public treasury. Nevertheless, any farmer who resisted payment might lose the plow horse or the milk cow that sustained the family. It could be "seized and sold" to cover a small tax payment or minor debt, with "no Part being ever Return'd" from the proceeds.

Banding together to better regulate their own affairs, these farmers sought relief through every possible legal means. But by 1768, when this document was created, these organized Regulators had exhausted most avenues of peaceful protest. The western counties where they resided were badly underrepresented in the colonial assembly. As a new session prepared to convene in November, they fired off a final round of petitions. They assured the legislators that they were law-abiding citizens willing to pay their legal share of taxes. And they begged for the appointment of honest public officials who would protect their interests. (For greater readability, editorial corrections have been made in this emotional petition.)

To the Worshipful House of Representatives of North Carolina

Your Poor Petitioners [have] been Continually Squez'd and oppressed by our Publick Officers both with Regard to their fees as also in the Laying on of Taxes as well as in Collecting. . . . Being Grieved thus to have our substance torn from us [by] . . . such Illegal practices, we applied to our public officers to give us some satisfaction . . . which they Repeatedly denied us.

With Regard to the Taxes,. . . we labour under Extreem hardships. . . . Money is very scarce . . . & we exceeding Poor & lie at a great distance from Trade which renders it almost Impossible to gain sustenance by our utmost Endeavours. . . .

To Gentlemen Rowling in affluence, a few shillings per man may seem triffling. Yet to Poor People who must have their Bed and Bedclothes, yea their Wives Petticoats, taken and sold to Defray, how Tremenious [tremendous] . . . must be the Consequences. . . . Therefore, dear Gentlemen, to your selves, to your Country, and in Pity to your Poor Petitioners, do not let it stand any longer to Drink up the Blood and vitals of the Poor Distressed.

After seeking relief from existing taxes, the petitioners went on to question new burdens, such as the law imposing an additional tax "to Erect a Publick Edifice" for Governor Tryon in New Bern.

Good God, Gentlemen, what will become of us when these Demands come against us? Paper Money we have none & gold or silver we can Purchase none of. The Contingencies of Government Must be Paid, and . . . we are Willing to Pay, [even] if we [must] sell our Beds from under us. And [yet] in this Time of Distress, it is as much as we can support. . . . If, therefore, the Law for that Purpose can be happily Repealed, . . . May the God of Heaven Inspire you with sentiments to that Purpose.

We humble Begg you would . . . Use your Influence with our Worthy, Virtuous Governor to discontinue . . . such Officers as would be found to be ye Bane of Society, and [instead to] Put in the Common Wealth [officials willing] to Encourage the Poor and . . . to stand [up] for them. This would Cause Joy and Gladness to Spring from every Heart. This would cause Labour and Industry to prevail over Murmuring Discontent. This would Raise your poor Petitioners . . . to a flourishing Opulent and Hoping People. Otherwise . . . disatisfaction and Melancholy must Prevail over such as Remain, and Numbers must Defect the Province and seek elsewhere an Asylum from Tyranny and Oppression. . . .

We leave it to you . . . in your great Wisdom . . . to pass such Act or Acts, as shall be Conducive to the welbeing of a whole People over Whose welfare ye are plac'd as Guardians. . . . For the Lords Sake, Gentlemen, Exert your selves this once in our favour. ■

Source: William S. Powell, James K. Huhta, and Thomas J. Farnham, eds., *The Regulators of North Carolina: A Documentary History, 1759–1776* (Raleigh: State Dept. of Archives and History, 1971), 187–189.

harassed corrupt office holders, protesting the "unequal chances the poor and weak have in contentions with the rich and powerful."

Both sides dug in their heels. In 1771 Governor Tryon finally called out the militia, marching a thousand men into the Piedmont. After defeating several thousand irate farmers at the battle of Alamance in May 1771, Tryon imposed his will on the dissenters. Half a dozen captured leaders were hanged publicly in Hillsborough, and Tryon forced residents to swear an oath of loyalty. Many refused, migrating farther south to backcountry Georgia or west to the Appalachian Mountains. Their leader, a Quaker named Herman Husband, barely escaped with his life, as Prendergast had done in New York. In North Carolina, just as in the Hudson Valley, well-to-do members of the Sons of Liberty dismissed the organized and militant farmers as misguided rabble.

A Conspiracy of Corrupt Ministers?

Numerous sharp divisions—some leading to armed conflict—continued to separate colonists of different classes and regions. But ill-timed steps by successive administrations in London attracted widening attention throughout British America, prompting uneasy new alliances. Colonists familiar with the dire warnings of Real Whig pamphleteers asked themselves a question: in the weak and short-lived ministries that succeeded Grenville's, were the leaders simply ill-informed, or were they actively corrupt? A widening array of colonists wondered whether some official conspiracy existed to chip away at American liberties. Even loyal defenders of the crown expressed frustration with new policies, fearing that they were too harsh to calm irate colonists, yet too weak to force them into line. "It's astonishing to me," wrote a beleaguered supporter from Boston, "after the Warning and Experience of the Stamp Act Times; that any new Impositions should be laid on the Colonies," especially "without even so much as a single Ship of Warr" to back up new measures.

Parliament's first new imposition after repeal of the Stamp Act was the Revenue Act of 1766. The act offered an additional reduction in the duty on molasses, from threepence per gallon to a single penny, in hopes of further discouraging smuggling and raising revenue. Colonial merchants reconciled themselves to this measure as an external tax designed to regulate imperial trade. They paid the new duty, and customs revenues rose. But Real Whigs reminded them that compliance with even the most innocuous measure could set a dangerous precedent.

The skeptics had a point, for Parliament soon imposed new hard-line measures. These distasteful statutes, put in motion by Chancellor of the Exchequer Charles Townshend before his sudden death in 1767, sparked angry responses from colonists. The most telling came from John Dickinson, a moderate Philadelphia lawyer who drafted a series of widely circulated "Letters from a Farmer in Pennsylvania." Urging colonists to respond "peaceably—prudently—firmly—jointly," he dismissed any distinction between external and internal taxation. He also rejected the idea that Americans had virtual representation in Parliament. "We are taxed without our own consent," Dickinson proclaimed to his readers. "We are therefore—SLAVES."

The Townshend Duties

In search of additional funds for the Exchequer, Townshend persuaded Parliament to pass the Revenue Act of 1767, which created new duties on colonial imports of glass, paint, lead, paper, and tea. Proceeds were to be spent in the colonies for "the administration of justice, and the support of civil government," a seemingly benevolent gesture. But Dickinson and other colonists pointed out what these two phrases actually meant. "The administration of justice" cloaked expanded searches of American homes and shops in which customs officers used hated "writs of assistance" to ferret out smuggled goods. "The support of civil government" ensured that governors and appointed office holders could draw their pay directly from the new duties instead of depending on an annual salary grant from the local assembly. In short, the new act removed

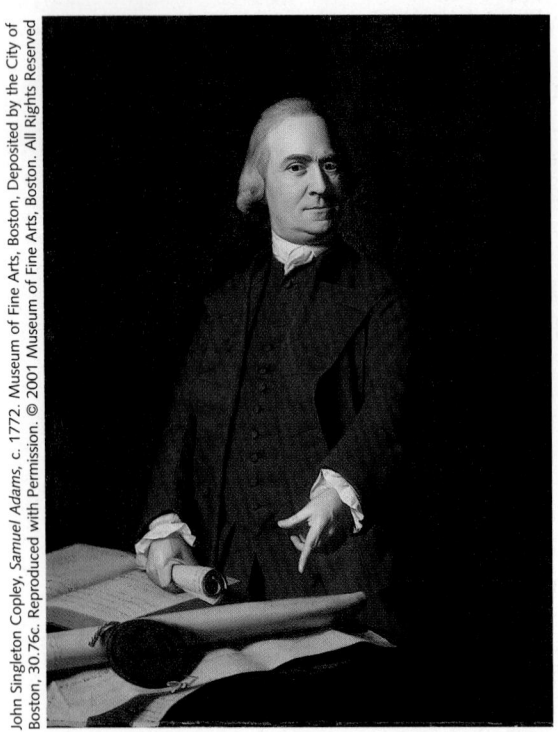

■ **Portrait of Samuel Adams by John Singleton Copley.**

from colonial legislatures one of their strongest bargaining tools in dealing with the crown: the power to pay or withhold yearly salaries for key officials sent from Britain.

Similar acts and instructions followed. Asserting its sovereignty, Parliament disciplined the New York Assembly for its "direct disobedience" in refusing to comply with the Quartering Act of 1765. The crown instructed governors in America, now less dependent for their salaries on colonial lower houses, to disapprove any further measures from legislatures asserting their traditional control over how members were chosen, what their numbers should be, and when they would meet. Equally galling, the Customs Act of 1767 established a separate Board of Customs for British North America. Ominously, the commissioners would live in Boston rather than London. To strengthen the board's hand in customs enforcement, Britain moved in 1768 to expand the number of vice-admiralty courts in North America from one to four. It supplemented the court in Halifax (established by the Sugar Act of 1764) with new courts in Boston, Philadelphia, and Charleston. Furthermore, to look after its troublesome mainland colonies, the British government created a new American Department, overseen by Lord Hillsborough. It also began to move British troops in America from remote frontier outposts to major Atlantic ports, both as a cost-cutting measure and as a show of force.

Whereas most people in England viewed these measures as legal, timely, and efficient, many Americans found them threatening, especially when considered as a whole. In February 1768, the Massachusetts legislature, led by 46-year-old Samuel Adams, petitioned the king for redress. The legislators also circulated a call to other lower houses to voice similar protests. Condemning the Townshend Revenue Act as unconstitutional, they argued that it imposed taxation without representation. By removing control of the governors' salaries from colonial legislatures, they said, Parliament set the dangerous precedent of making royal officials "independent of the people." Lord Hillsborough demanded an immediate retraction of this provocative "Circular Letter" and ordered the dissolution of any other assembly that took up the matter.

In June, just as word arrived of the Wilkes Riot in London, events in Boston took a more radical turn. Defying Hillsborough, the Massachusetts assembly voted 92 to 17 against rescinding its circular letter. "The 92" became instant celebrities, and their opponents were vilified by the Sons of Liberty. On June 5, a dockside crowd faced down a "press-gang" from a British warship and protected local sailors from being forced (or "pressed") into naval service. Five days later, customs officials seized John Hancock's sloop, *Liberty,* and demanded that he pay import duties for a cargo of Madeira wine. This move sparked a huge demonstration as citizens dragged a small customs boat through the streets and then burned it on Boston Common. "Hancock and Liberty" became a rallying cry—"as 'Wilkes and Liberty' is in London!" "Let us take up arms immediately and be free," Sam Adams was heard to say; "We shall have thirty thousand men to join us from the Country."

Emotions ran high. But most leaders sensed that any escalation of the violence would be premature and perhaps suicidal. They managed to rein in demonstrations and initiate efforts to expand their base of support. Organizers turned their attention to implementing a boycott of British goods proposed the previous fall. Spurred by an energetic press, nonimportation plans took hold rapidly. These plans called upon colonists to refrain from imported luxuries and opt instead for virtuous self-sufficiency. The idea held broad appeal, as did the prospect that nonviolent resistance might reverse British policies.

As the nonimportation movement expanded, it drew in men from small towns previously untouched by the imperial controversy. It also engaged women of all ranks in sacrificing for the cause. Self-proclaimed Daughters of Liberty took to making, wearing, and selling homespun garments. Local associations sprang up, pledging to forgo imported tea and London fashions. A dozen colonial assemblies voted to halt importation of selected goods. In New York, the value of imports from Britain shrank from £491,000 to just £76,000 in a single year.

Elsewhere, the novel boycott exerted less impact, but the damage to English shipping proved substantial. Britain was losing far more revenue in colonial trade than it was gaining through the expanded customs duties. Soon influential exporters in England were pressing the government for relief. When Lord North established a new ministry in January 1770, he received the king's consent to work toward a better arrangement with the colonies. On March 5, 1770, North persuaded Parliament to repeal all the Townshend Duties except the one on tea. The move defused the colonial boycott, but it offered too little too late. Like the earlier Declaratory Act, this measure reaffirmed Parliament's disputed right to tax the colonists at will. Moreover, it came at the exact moment when violence and bloodshed were escalating in America.

The Boston Massacre

After the *Liberty* riot in June 1768, tensions had mounted in Boston, especially with the arrival in October of two regiments of British soldiers, well armed and dressed in their traditional red coats. Paul Revere, a local silversmith and member of the Sons of Liberty, crafted an ominous engraving entitled "British Ships of War Landing Their Troops." According to Real Whig beliefs, any appearance by a standing army in peacetime constituted danger, and the issue of how to house and feed unwanted troops quickly became a political hot button. The soldiers pitched their tents on Boston Common, a central gathering place for boisterous crowds. Artisans in a sluggish economy welcomed the increased business that the men in uniform generated, but numerous unemployed workers resented the soldiers' "moonlighting," trying to earn extra pay by applying for local jobs.

In Paul Revere's image of the 1770 Boston Massacre, soldiers defend the hated customs house by moonlight, while a sniper fires from a window clearly labeled "Butcher's Hall." The partisan engraving spread an anti-British view of the bloody event.

With 4000 armed men encamped in a seaport of scarcely 16,000, confrontation seemed inevitable. When rowdy American youths harassed the intruders as "redcoats" and "lobsterbacks," British officers ordered their men not to retaliate. Their refusal to fight only prompted more taunts. Affairs "cannot long remain in the state they are now in," wrote one observer late in 1769; "they are hastening to a crisis. What will be the event, God knows."

In February 1770, the answer came. When a hostile crowd threatened a customs informer, he fired back, killing 11-year-old Christopher Seider. The boy's elaborate funeral brought crowds of demonstrators into the streets. On Friday, March 2, protesters reappeared after a run-in between local workers and job-seeking soldiers. Rumors spread during the weekend that a larger confrontation between the two sides was looming. On Monday morning, a scrawled notice of unknown origin appeared on a wall. It read, "to Inform ye Rebellious people in Boston that ye Soldjers . . . are Determend to Joine to Gether and Defend them Selves against all who Shall Oppose them."

Regardless of who actually posted the notice, both sides were ready for a fight. Around 9 P.M. on March 5, a crowd gathered outside the customs house, where a harassed sentry struck a boy with his rifle butt. As witnesses pelted the guard with snowballs, he called for help. As seven fellow soldiers pushed through the mob to assist him, firebells summoned more townspeople to the scene. The British loaded their rifles and aimed at the crowd, their bayonets fixed.

Into this tense standoff marched a brash contingent of several dozen sailors from Dock Square. Led by Crispus Attucks, an ex-slave, they arrived waving banners and brandishing clubs. Attucks was an imposing figure, standing 6 feet 2 inches. The son of a black man and an Indian woman, he had run away from his master two decades earlier and then taken up a life at sea. John Adams assumed the unpopular task of defending the British soldiers at the trial resulting from this incident. He told the court that "Attucks appears to have undertaken to be the hero of this night." Damning the soldiers and daring them to fire, Attucks pressed his band of sailors to the front, waving a long stick in the moonlight.

A slave witness named Andrew, who had climbed a post to get a better view, testified that Attucks "threw himself in, and made a blow at the officer," shouting, "kill the dogs, knock them over." Adams later showed the court how with one hand the sailor "took hold of a bayonet, and with the other knocked the man down." In the mayhem, a British gun went off, prompting a volley of fire from the other soldiers. The crowd recoiled in disbelief at the sight of their dead and wounded neighbors lying in the street, but they stayed past midnight to demand that the soldiers be jailed for murder. According to a printed report, Attucks and four others had been "killed on the Spot." The anti-British cause had its first martyrs, joining young Christopher Seider.

By grim coincidence, the bloody episode on King Street occurred only hours after Lord North addressed the House of Commons to urge removal of most Townshend Duties. His effort at reconciliation immediately became lost in a wave of hostile publicity. In Boston, Paul Revere captured the incident in an inflammatory engraving that circulated widely. The Sons of Liberty quickly named the event of March 5 the Boston Massacre and compared its martyred victims to the Wilkes demonstrators who had perished in London during the Massacre at St. George's Field. "On that night," John Adams remarked, "the foundation of American independence was laid."

The *Gaspee* Affair

As the 1770s unfolded, citizens in Boston commemorated "Massacre Day" each year with orations. According to speakers, the bloodshed on March 5 had revealed a dark scheme among British cabinet ministers. They seemed intent, the orators proclaimed, to drive America into a state of rebellion, "whereby they might hope to gratify both their malice and avarice."

Besides the aggression of a standing army, the overzealous conduct of customs officers gave colonists further cause for distrust. As traffic with Britain revived, after the repeal of most Townshend Duties and the end of the colonial boycott of English goods, so did the likelihood of conflict between merchants and customs inspectors. In the Delaware River region, local residents thrashed and jailed a customs collector in 1770. The next year, protesters stormed a customs schooner at night, beat up the crew, and stole their sails. Tensions ran especially high in Rhode Island. In 1769 Newport citizens seized the sloop *Liberty*—which crown agents had confiscated from John Hancock the year before and converted into a customs vessel—and scuttled it. In June 1772, the *Gaspee,* another customs boat said to harass local shipping, ran aground near Pawtuxet. In a midnight attack, more than a hundred raiders descended on the stranded schooner in half a dozen boats, driving off its crew and setting fire to the vessel.

The destruction of the *Gaspee* renewed sharp antagonisms between the two sides. Alarmed, the Earl of Hillsborough, secretary of state for the American colonies, sent a royal commission from London to investigate and to transport suspects to England for trial. But many of the attackers, such as John Brown of Providence, came from important Rhode Island families. Even a £500 reward could not induce local inhabitants to name participants. Besides, colonists viewed the order to deport accused citizens to England as a denial of their fundamental right to trial by a jury of their peers. They took action.

Again, Virginia's House of Burgesses led the way, as it had in the Stamp Act crisis. In March 1773, Patrick Henry, Thomas Jefferson, and Richard Henry Lee pushed a resolution through that body establishing a standing committee to look into the *Gaspee* affair and to keep up "Correspondence and Communication with our sister colonies" regarding the protection of rights. Following Virginia's example, ten other colonial legislatures promptly established their own Committees of Correspondence. In Massachusetts, similar committees sprang up linking individual towns. Within months a new act of Parliament, designed to rescue the powerful East India Company from bankruptcy, gave these emerging communication networks their first test.

Launching a Revolution

In 1767, before Parliament imposed the Townshend Duties, Americans had imported nearly 870,000 pounds of tea from England. But the boycott movement cut that amount to less than 110,000 pounds by 1770 as colonists turned to smuggling Dutch blends and brewing homemade root teas. When nonimportation schemes lapsed in the early 1770s, purchase of English tea resumed, even though a duty remained in effect.

Encouraged by this apparent acceptance of parliamentary taxation, Lord North addressed the problem facing the East India Company. The ancient trading monopoly owed a huge debt to the Bank of England and had 18 million pounds of unsold tea rotting in London warehouses. Moreover, many MPs held stock in the company. In May, Parliament passed a new law designed to right the situation and bail out the ailing company.

The Tempest over Tea

The Tea Act of 1773 let the struggling East India Company bypass the expensive requirement that merchants ship Asian tea through England on its way to colonial ports. Now they could send the product directly to the colonies or to foreign ports, without paying to unload, store, auction, and reload the heavy chests. Any warehouse tea destined for the colonies would have its English duty refunded. These steps would reduce retail prices and expand the tea market. They would also quietly confirm the right of Parliament to collect a tea tax of threepence per pound.

The company promptly chose prominent colonial merchants as consignees to receive and distribute more than 600,000 pounds of tea, for which they would earn a hefty 6 percent commission. But wary colonists in port towns, sensing a repetition of 1765, renewed the tactics that had succeeded against the Stamp Act. Sons of Liberty vowed to prevent tea-laden ships from docking, and crowds pressured local distributors to renounce participation in the scheme. "If they succeed in the sale of that tea," proclaimed New York's Sons of Liberty, "then we may bid adieu to American liberty."

In Boston, where tea worth nearly £10,000 arrived aboard three ships in late November, tension ran especially high. The credibility of Governor Thomas Hutchinson, who had taken a hard line toward imperial dissent, had suffered in June when Benjamin Franklin published private correspondence suggesting the governor's willingness to trim colonial rights. When two of Hutchinson's sons were named tea consignees, the appointments reinforced townspeople's suspicions of an elaborate plot. The governor could have signed papers letting the three vessels depart, but that would give victory to the local opposition. Instead, he determined to unload and distribute the tea, by force if necessary. One could scarcely buy a pair of pistols in Boston, a resident observed on December 1, "as they are all bought up, with a full determination to repel force by force."

On December 16, the largest mass meeting of the decade took place at Boston's Old South Church. A crowd of 5000, including many from other towns, waited in a cold rain to hear whether Hutchinson would relent. When word came in late afternoon that the governor had refused, the cry went up, "Boston Harbor a teapot tonight!" Following a prearranged plan, 150 men, disguised as Mohawk Indians and carrying hatchets, marched to the docks and boarded the ships.

As several thousand supporters looked on, this disciplined crew spent three hours methodically breaking open hundreds of chests of tea and dumping their contents overboard. The

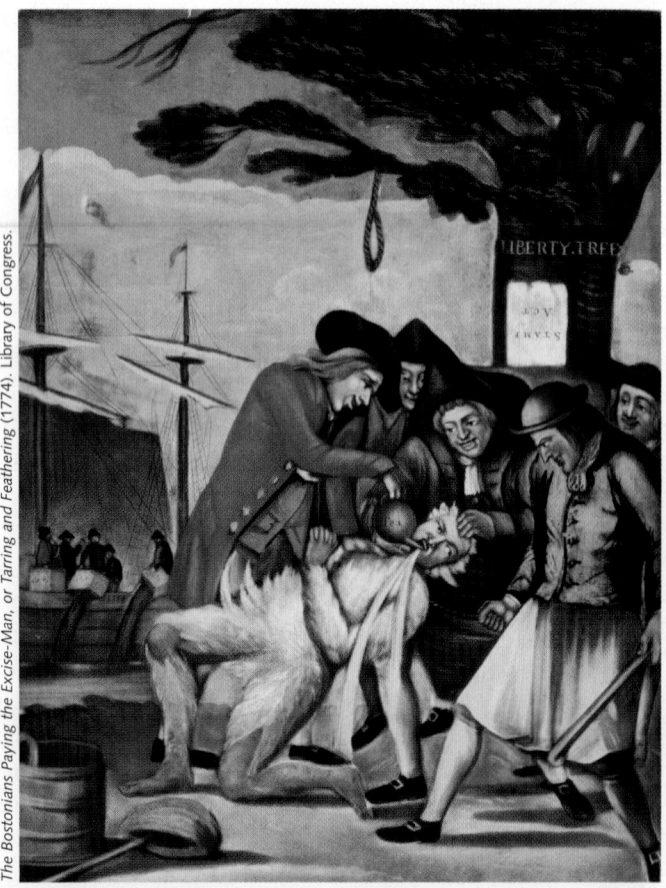

The Bostonians Paying the Excise-Man, or Tarring and Feathering (1774). Library of Congress.

■ A 1774 London cartoon expressed anger that Boston's Sons of Liberty, defying British authority, could overturn the Stamp Act, abuse revenue agents, dump East India Company tea, and use their "Liberty Tree" to hang officials in effigy.

quasimilitary operation proved swift, efficient, and well organized. It united participants reflecting all levels of society—from merchants such as Hancock to artisans such as Hewes—and news of it spurred similar acts of defiance in other ports. "This destruction of the Tea is so bold, so daring, so firm," John Adams wrote in his diary the next day, "it must have so important Consequences, and so lasting, that I can't but consider it as an Epocha in History." Sixty years later, as one of the oldest veterans of the Revolution, George Hewes still recalled with special pride his role in "the destruction of the tea."

The Intolerable Acts

"The crisis is come," wrote British general Thomas Gage, responding to the costly Tea Party in Boston Harbor; "the provinces must be either British colonies, or independent and separate states." Underestimating the strength of American resolve, Parliament agreed with King George III that only stern measures would reestablish "the obedience which a colony owes to its mother country." Between March and June 1774, it passed four so-called Coercive Acts to isolate and punish Massachusetts.

The first of the Coercive Acts, the Boston Port Act, used British naval strength to cut off the offending town's sea commerce—except for shipments of food and firewood—until the colonists paid for the ruined tea. By the Administration of Justice Act, revenue officials or soldiers charged with murder in Massachusetts (as in the Boston Massacre) could have their trials moved to another colony or to Great Britain. The Quartering Act gave officers more power to requisition living quarters and supplies for their troops throughout the colonies. Most important, the Massachusetts Government Act removed democratic elements from the long-standing Massachusetts Charter of 1691. From now on, the assembly could no longer elect the colony's Upper House, or Council; the governor would appoint that important body instead. In addition, colonists would have to get written permission from him to hold town meetings.

Lord North's government went even further. It replaced Hutchinson with Gage, installing the commander of British forces in America as the governor of Massachusetts and granting him special powers and three additional regiments. It also secured passage of the Quebec Act. The new legislation addressed nagging problems of governance in Canada after a decade of English rule. It accommodated the Catholic faith and French legal traditions of Quebec's inhabitants. Moreover, it multiplied the size of the colony several times over to draw scattered French settlers and traders under colonial government. Suddenly, Quebec took in the entire Great Lakes region and all the lands north of the Ohio River to the east bank of the upper Mississippi River.

Expanding the province of Quebec to the Ohio River might extend British government to French wilderness outposts and help to regulate the Indian trade there. But as American land speculators in Virginia and elsewhere quickly realized, the move also challenged the western claims of other colonies. The Quebec Act appeared to favor French Catholics and Ohio Valley Indians—both recent enemies of the crown—over loyal English colonists. Resentment ran especially high in New England, where Protestants had long associated Catholicism with despotism. The Quebec Act, which denied that province a representative assembly and jury trials in civil cases, set an ominous precedent for neighboring colonies.

The Coercive Acts and the Quebec Act—lumped together by colonial propagandists as the Intolerable Acts—brought on open rebellion against crown rule. Competing pamphlets debated the proper limits of dissent. In *A Summary View of the Rights of British America*, Jefferson went beyond criticisms of Parliament to question the king's right to dispense land, control trade, and impose troops in America. Sympathy for the economic and political distress of Massachusetts mounted in other colonies. Sam Adams and his Boston colleagues had proven their ability to mobilize large and determined crowds; now they needed to foster wider cooperation among distant colonies that were less directly threatened. At the same time, they had to build resolve among wealthy merchants and cautious gentry. Within months, Massachusetts had called for a congress of all the colonies. It also established its own Provincial Congress at Concord, a small vil-

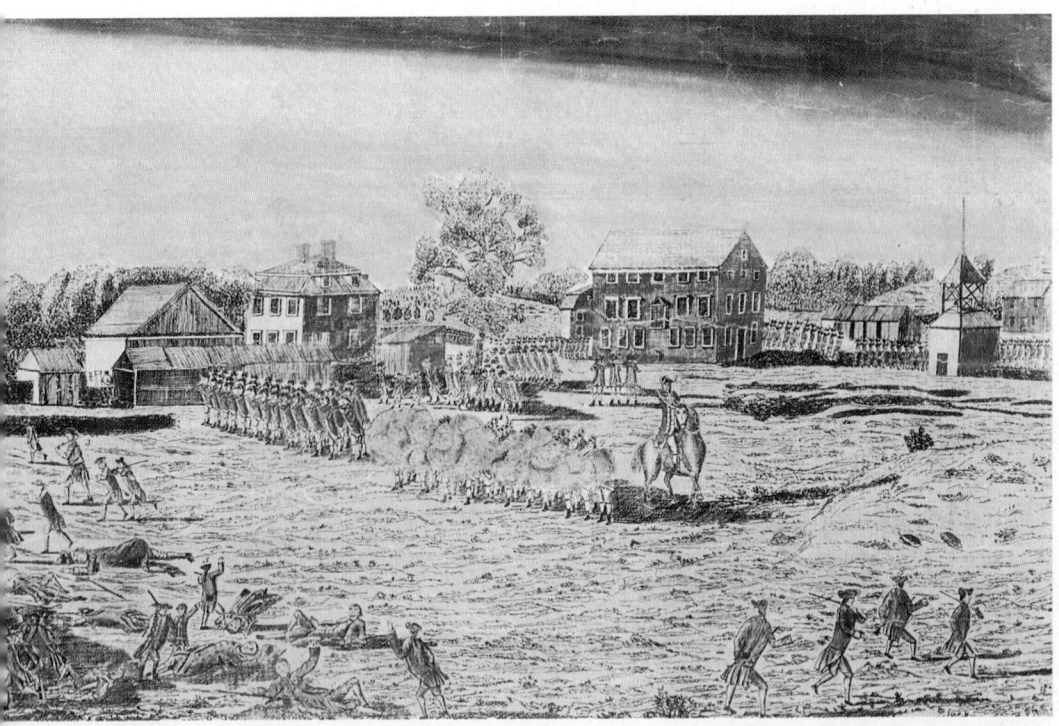

lage that lay 17 miles west of Boston and British naval power. Operating as a de facto government, the Massachusetts Provincial Congress reorganized the colonial militia into units loyal to its own Committee of Public Safety. These farmer-soldiers became known as Minutemen for their quick response to Gage's repeated efforts to capture patriot gunpowder supplies.

From Words to Action

While Massachusetts chafed under these new restrictions, shifting coalitions in each colony, ranging from conservative to radical, vied for local political control. Extralegal committees, existing outside the authorized structure of colonial government, took power in hundreds of hamlets. In Edenton, North Carolina, 51 women signed a pact to abstain from using imported products for the "publick good." London cartoonists mocked the action as the "Edenton Ladies' Tea Party," but women in other colonies made similar agreements to boycott British textiles and tea. Towns instructed their representatives to provincial assemblies to support Massachusetts' call for an intercolonial congress. During the summer, all colonies except Georgia selected representatives to the First Continental Congress. In September 1774, 56 delegates convened at Carpenters Hall in Philadelphia. Most had never met before, and they differed as much in their politics as in their regional manners.

At first the delegates disagreed sharply over how best to respond to the Intolerable Acts. Joseph Galloway, a wealthy lawyer and commercial land speculator from Pennsylvania, urged a compromise with Britain modeled on the Albany Congress of 1754. His plan called for the creation of a separate American parliament, a grand council with delegates elected by the colonial legislatures. The less conservative delegates voiced opposition to this idea for a federation of the colonies, under a president-general appointed by the king. Led by Patrick Henry of Virginia, they managed to table the Galloway Plan by a narrow vote.

When Paul Revere arrived from Boston on October 6, bearing a set of militant resolves passed in his own Suffolk County, further rifts appeared. Southern moderates, while expressing sympathy for Massachusetts, still resisted calls for a nonexportation scheme that would withhold

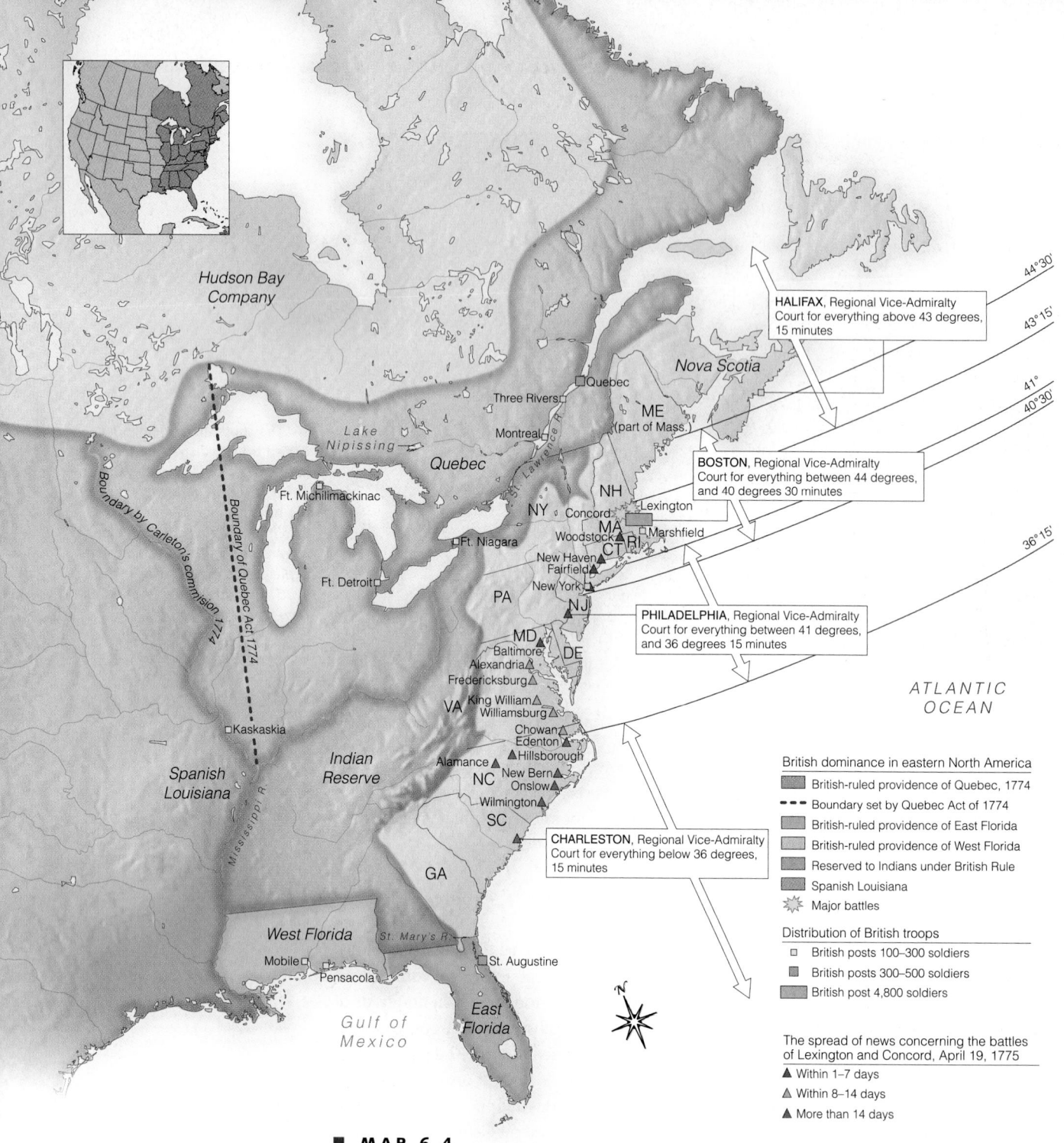

Hudson Bay
Company

Boundary by Carleton's commission

Boundary of Quebec Act 1774

Ft. Michilimackinac

Lake
Nipissing

Quebec

Three Rivers

Quebec

Montreal

St. Lawrence R.

Ft. Niagara

Ft. Detroit

Kaskaskia

Spanish
Louisiana

Indian
Reserve

Mississippi R.

Woodstock

New Haven
Fairfield

New York

PA

NJ

MD

Baltimore
Alexandria
Fredericksburg

VA

King William
Williamsburg

Chowan
Edenton

Alamance

Hillsborough

NC

New Bern
Onslow

Wilmington

SC

GA

West Florida

Mobile

Pensacola

St. Mary's R.

Gulf of
Mexico

East
Florida

St. Augustine

Nova Scotia

ME
(part of Mass.)

NH

NY

Concord

Lexington

MA

Marshfield

CT   RI

44°30'

43°15'

41°
40°30'

36°15'

ATLANTIC
OCEAN

HALIFAX, Regional Vice-Admiralty
Court for everything above 43 degrees,
15 minutes

BOSTON, Regional Vice-Admiralty
Court for everything between 44 degrees,
and 40 degrees 30 minutes

PHILADELPHIA, Regional Vice-Admiralty
Court for everything between 41 degrees,
and 36 degrees 15 minutes

CHARLESTON, Regional Vice-Admiralty
Court for everything below 36 degrees,
15 minutes

N

British dominance in eastern North America

- British-ruled providence of Quebec, 1774
- - - Boundary set by Quebec Act of 1774
- British-ruled providence of East Florida
- British-ruled providence of West Florida
- Reserved to Indians under British Rule
- Spanish Louisiana
- Major battles

Distribution of British troops

- British posts 100–300 soldiers
- British posts 300–500 soldiers
- British post 4,800 soldiers

The spread of news concerning the battles
of Lexington and Concord, April 19, 1775

- Within 1–7 days
- Within 8–14 days
- More than 14 days

■ **MAP 6.4**
BRITISH NORTH AMERICA, APRIL 1775   Rising colonial unrest brought strong countermeasures. The
British government organized regional vice-admiralty courts to punish smugglers; it greatly expanded
Quebec in 1774; and it reallocated troops to the Boston area. When warfare erupted there in April 1775,
the news spread throughout the colonies within weeks.

American tobacco, rice, and indigo from Great Britain. But by the time the Congress adjourned
in late October, it had issued a Declaration of Rights and passed a range of measures that seemed
to balance competing views. On one hand, the Congress endorsed the fiery Suffolk Resolves, which
condemned the Coercive Acts as unconstitutional and spoke of preparation for war. On the other,
it humbly petitioned the king for relief from the crisis and professed continued loyalty. But in
practical terms, Galloway and the more conservative members had suffered defeat. Most importantly, the delegates signed an agreement to prohibit British imports and halt all exports to Britain

except rice. They called for local committees to enforce this so-called Association, and they set a date—May 10, 1775—for a Second Congress.

Before delegates could meet again in Philadelphia, the controversy that had smoldered for more than a decade on both sides of the Atlantic erupted into open combat. Predictably, the explosion took place in Massachusetts. The spark came in the form of secret orders to General Gage, which he received April 14, 1775. The confidential letter from his superiors in London urged him to arrest the leaders of the Massachusetts Provincial Congress and regain the upper hand before the strained situation grew worse. He was to use force, even if it meant the outbreak of warfare.

On April 18, Gage ordered 700 elite troops from Boston to row across the Charles River at night, march 10 miles to Lexington, and seize John Hancock and Sam Adams, who had taken refuge with Hancock's relatives. Next, the soldiers were to proceed 7 more miles to Concord to capture a stockpile of military supplies. Alerted by signal lanterns, express riders Paul Revere and William Dawes eluded British patrols and spurred their horses toward Lexington along separate routes to warn Hancock and Adams. Bells and alarm guns spread the word that the British were coming. By the time the British soldiers reached Lexington, shortly before sunrise, some 70 militiamen had assembled on the town green. When the villagers refused to lay down their arms, the redcoats dispersed them in a brief skirmish that left eight militiamen dead.

The British column trudged west to Concord and searched the town for munitions. Four hundred Minutemen who had streamed in from neighboring communities watched from the outskirts of town. By 11 A.M., a fire had broken out in the village. The Minutemen advanced in double file, with orders not to fire until the British fired first. At the small bridge over the Concord River, British regulars opened fire. "The shot heard 'round the world" killed two men. The Americans loosed a volley in return, killing three. By noon, British forces were retreating in disarray. Exhausted, hungry, and short of ammunition, the redcoats made easy targets for the more than 1000 Americans who shot at them from behind stone walls. A relief party prevented annihilation, but the British suffered severe losses: 73 killed and 200 wounded or missing. They encamped briefly at Bunker Hill, but lacking the foresight and strength to retain that strategic height, they soon returned to Boston. The Americans, with only 49 dead, had turned the tables on General Gage, transforming a punitive raid into a punishing defeat.

Conclusion

For the British, festering administrative problems in America had suddenly become a military emergency. A decade of assertive but inconsistent British policies had transformed the colonists' sense of good will toward London into angry feelings of persecution and betrayal. The years of incessant argument and misunderstanding reminded many, on both sides of the Atlantic, of watching a stable, prosperous household unravel into mutual recrimination. A once-healthy family was becoming increasingly dysfunctional and troubled. The assertive children grew steadily in strength and competence; the aging parents chafed at their diminished authority and respect.

Predictably, authorities in London found the once-dependent colonists to be ungrateful, intemperate, and occasionally even paranoid. With equal assurance, the American subjects saw Parliament, government ministers, and eventually the king himself as uninformed, selfish, and even deceitful. For the aggrieved colonists, the moment had come to declare loyalties and muster sustained resistance. They would receive suitable recognition within the family, or they would leave home for good. Britain's overseas empire, which had expanded steadily for two centuries, now seemed on the verge of splitting apart.

From the perspective of Britain's mainland colonies, rapid economic and demographic growth had been a fact of eighteenth-century life. It had created serious growing pains, generating strong tensions across boundaries of region, race, and class. In 1676, near the beginning of this growth process, the colonial tensions that generated Bacon's Rebellion in Virginia had been focused into war against the Indians and conflict against the ruling colonial elite, with independence little more than a remote ideal for a few. A century later, the equation had changed, and the limits of imperial control in North America had become increasingly evident. Colonists could overcome their regional and ethnic differences, and political independence no longer seemed implausible. With effort, class hostilities and urban-rural divisions could also be overcome. Redirecting these long-standing local resentments against the distant and powerful British crown could increase the sense of unity among people with very different personal backgrounds and resources.

Nor would British colonists be alone if they mounted a rebellion. On one hand, they could make the unlikely choice of liberating half a million slaves, empowering colonial women, and embracing the anti-British cause of Pontiac and numerous Native Americans. Such revolutionary moves would increase their strength dramatically in one direction. On the other hand, they could also take a more cautious and less democratic route. If men of substance could gain control of the forces that were being unleashed, they might curb potential idealism among slaves, women, tenant farmers, and the urban poor, giving precedence instead to policies and practices that would win powerful European allies.

Bacon's rebels, after all, had never managed to muster French or Dutch support as hoped. But the new Sons of Liberty might well succeed in enlisting vital support from the continent of Europe in an American fight for independence from Britain. France, recently evicted from North America, and Spain, anxious about British designs in the Pacific, might both be willing allies, despite their commitment to monarchy. Such an alliance, if it ever came about, could push the limits of British imperial control to the breaking point.

Sites to Visit

Anza-Borrego Desert State Park
anza.uoregon.edu

This isolated and beautiful state park covers 600,000 acres 80 miles east of San Diego, California. The Web site, which focuses on the exploration of Alta, California, 1774–1776, contains maps, resources, and documents in both English and Spanish concerning Juan Bautista de Anza's two overland expeditions.

Baranov Museum

Located near the ferry landing in Kodiak, Alaska, the Baranov Museum is housed in one of the few remaining structures from the Russian colonial era. In Fairbanks, the modern University of Alaska Museum, located on Yukon Street overlooking the campus, provides a rich introduction to the region's history and cultures.

Fort Ross State Historic Park

This reconstruction of the outpost built by the Russians on the northern California coast in the early nineteenth century is located on a scenic bluff 11 miles northwest of the town of Jenner on Highway 1, about a two-hour drive from San Francisco.

Pontiac Marker

In 1977, Michigan placed a marker concerning Pontiac on a building at 3321 East Jefferson Avenue, near the Renaissance Center in downtown Detroit. It commemorates the Battle of Bloody Run, in July 1763, which marked the height of Pontiac's siege of Detroit. The city of Pontiac, named for the Ottawa leader, lies 25 miles northwest.

Boston's Freedom Trail

This 2.5-mile self-guided walking tour begins at Boston Common. Stops include the Boston Massacre site, the Old South Meeting House where the Boston Tea Party began, Paul Revere's house, and the Granary Burial Ground, where Revere, John Hancock, Samuel Adams, and Crispus Attucks are all buried.

Colonial Williamsburg
www.history.org

This tourist site in Virginia, suitable for all ages, features shops, homes, and public buildings as they existed in the 1770s. In the Capitol Building on Duke of Gloucester Street, Patrick Henry stirred the House of Burgesses to oppose the Stamp Act in 1765. There are regular tours and candlelight evening programs.

Tryon's Palace

Governor William Tryon erected this building in New Bern, North Carolina, in 1768 over the protests of Regulators. The Georgian mansion, with a handsome garden overlooking the Trent River, served as the colony's first capitol. Now restored, Tryon Palace Historic Sites and Gardens is 112 miles east of Raleigh, the current capital.

Alamance Battleground

At this site, located on Route 62 near Burlington, North Carolina, Governor Tryon's forces defeated the Regulators in 1771. In historic Hillsborough, 30 miles east, a plaque on a hillside at the end of King Street on the east side of the town marks the site where Regulator leaders were hanged.

For Further Reading

General

Jack P. Greene, ed., *Colonies to Nation: A Documentary History of the American Revolution* (1975).

Merrill Jensen, *The Founding of a Nation: A History of the American Revolution, 1763–1776* (1968).

Pauline Maier, *From Resistance to Revolution: Colonial Radicals and the Development of American Opposition to Britain, 1765–1776* (1972).

Robert Middlekauff, *The Glorious Cause: The American Revolution, 1763–1789* (1982).

Alfred F. Young, ed., *The American Revolution: Explorations in the History of American Radicalism* (1976).

New Challenges to Spain's Expanded Empire

John Francis Bannon, *The Spanish Borderlands Frontier, 1513–1821* (1970).

Richard Hough, *Captain James Cook* (1994).

John L. Kessell, *Spain in the Southwest: A Narrative History of Colonial New Mexico, Arizona, Texas, and California* (2002).

Mark Santiago, *Massacre at the Yuma Crossing: Spanish Relations with the Quechans, 1779–1782* (1998).

Barbara Sweetland Smith and Redmond J. Barnett, eds., *Russian America: The Forgotten Frontier* (1990).

New Challenges to Britain's Expanded Empire

John K. Alexander, *Samuel Adams: America's Revolutionary Politician* (2002).

John L. Bullion, *A Great and Necessary Measure: George Grenville and the Genesis of the Stamp Act, 1763–1765* (1982).

Gregory E. Dowd, *A Spirited Resistance: The North American Indian Struggle for Unity, 1745–1815* (1992).

Edmund S. Morgan and Helen M. Morgan, *The Stamp Act Crisis: Prologue to Revolution*, 3rd ed. (1995).

Peter D. G. Thomas, *British Politics and the Stamp Act Crisis: The First Phase of the American Revolution, 1763–1767* (1975).

Peter D. G. Thomas, *John Wilkes: A Friend to Liberty* (1996).

"The Unconquerable Rage of the People"

Bernard Bailyn, *The Ideological Origins of the American Revolution* (1967).

Edward Countryman, *A People in Revolution: The American Revolution and Political Society in New York, 1760–1790* (1981).

Ronald Hoffman, *A Spirit of Dissention: Economics, Politics, and the Revolution in Maryland* (1973).

Marjoleine Kars, *Breaking Loose Together: The Regulator Rebellion in Pre-Revolutionary North Carolina* (2002).

Rachel N. Klein, *Unification of a Slave State: The Rise of the Planter Class in the South Carolina Backcountry, 1760–1808* (1990).

A Conspiracy of Corrupt Ministers?

Bernard Bailyn, *The Ordeal of Thomas Hutchinson* (1974).

Woody Holton, *Forced Founders: Indians, Debtors, Slaves, and the Making of the American Revolution in Virginia* (1999).

John Shy, *Toward Lexington: The Role of the British Army in the Coming of the Revolution* (1965).

Peter D. G. Thomas, *The Townshend Duties Crisis: The Second Phase of the American Revolution, 1767–1773* (1987).

John W. Tyler, *Smugglers and Patriots: Boston Merchants and the Advent of the American Revolution* (1986).

Launching a Revolution

David Hackett Fischer, *Paul Revere's Ride* (1994).

Benjamin Woods Labaree, *The Boston Tea Party* (1964).

Philip Lawson, *The Imperial Challenge: Quebec and Britain in the Age of the American Revolution* (1989).

Peter D. G. Thomas, *Tea Party to Independence: The Third Phase of the American Revolution, 1773–1776* (1991).

Alfred F. Young, *The Shoemaker and the Tea Party: Memory and the American Revolution* (1999).

Online Practice Test

Test your understanding of this chapter with interactive review quizzes at

www.ablongman.com/jonescreatedequal/chapter6

Additional Photo Credits

Page 185: Courtesy, American Antiquarian Society

Page 186: Hunterian Museum and Art Gallery, University of Glasgow

Page 193: The I.N. Phelps Stokes Collection of American Historical Prints. Prints Division, The New York Public Library

Page 199: Peabody Essex Museum. Photograph by Mark Sexton

Page 211: Amos Doolittle, *The Battle of Lexington, Plate I,* 1775. The Connecticut Historical Society, Hartford, CT (Acc. #1844.10.1)

1776 Thomas Paine, *Common Sense.*
Declaration of Independence.
Washington crosses the Delaware.
New Jersey gives women the right to vote.

1777 Burgoyne surrenders
at Saratoga.

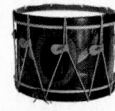

1778 U.S. forges an alliance with France.

1779 Sullivan's campaign against the Iroquois.

1780 Charleston falls to the British.

1781 Cornwallis surrenders
at Yorktown.
Articles of
Confederation
are ratified.

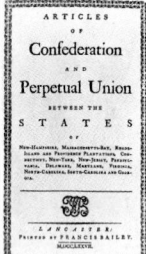

1783 Treaty of Paris.
Newburgh Conspiracy
is thwarted.

1785 Land Ordinance of 1785.

1786 Shays's Rebellion.

1787 Constitutional Convention meets in
Philadelphia.
Constitution of the United States is signed.
Northwest Ordinance creates Northwest
Territory.

1789 George Washington is elected the first
president of the U.S.
U.S. Constitution
goes into effect
after ratification
by nine states.

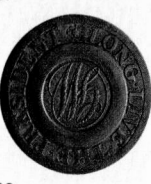

1789 Judiciary Act of 1789.

1790 First U.S. Census enumerates population
of 4 million.
Congress restricts citizenship to "free
white persons."
Northern states take steps
to abolish slavery.
Miami Chief Little Turtle scores victory
over U.S. troops.

PART THREE

The Unfinished Revolution, 1775–1803

I N 1775, GREAT BRITAIN STILL POSSESSED ALL OF NORTH AMERICA EAST of the Mississippi River, from Hudson Bay to the Gulf of Mexico. If the British could suppress the troublesome rebellion along the Atlantic seaboard, their prospects for expansion in America looked promising. Farther west, Spain had recently acquired the vast Louisiana Territory from France. The Spanish retained their dominance in the Southwest, and they were finally beginning to expand their claim to California by building a series of new missions and presidios.

By 1803, however, the broad picture had changed markedly. In the Pacific Ocean, Europeans had encountered the Hawaiian Islands for the first time, Russian fur traders had consolidated their hold in Alaska, and Spanish vessels along the Pacific coast faced increasing competition from the ships of rival nations. The British still held Canada and Florida, but the 13 rebellious colonies had become an independent republic and had started to acquire new territories. The most spectacular acquisition was the Louisiana Territory, which the United States purchased in 1803, after Spain returned the region to the control of France.

Few could have foreseen such an unlikely series of events in such a brief span of time. Thomas Jefferson drafted the Declaration of Independence in 1776 at age 33. His generation had reluctantly become the effective leaders of a revolutionary movement by the mid-1770s. They contended ably with those who pushed for greater democratization, those who desired the stability of military rule, and even those who longed for the protection of the British monarchy.

These unlikely revolutionary leaders were by no means united in all their views and actions. They argued fervently over constitutional issues, domestic policies, and foreign alignments. Most managed to reap personal rewards from the new society's collective success. And they saw to it that these rewards reached far beyond their own households. Urban artisans, frontier farmers, and immigrant newcomers benefited from the removal of monarchy.

Such positive developments inspired optimism for many, both at home and abroad. Yet although the revolutionary era fulfilled the expectations of numerous citizens, it failed to meet the hopes and aspirations of many Americans. Many American merchants and planters, indebted to British interests before 1776, gained by the separation from Great Britain as creditors and investors in the new society. Many frontier farmers and army veterans, on the other hand, faced burdensome debts after the Revolutionary War.

Women worried that the numerous written constitutions of the period were unresponsive to their interests. In 1776 only New Jersey gave the vote among property holders to "all free inhabitants," including women. But this provision was undone a generation later, in 1807, when New Jersey men objected to the idea of women having the right to vote. From New Hampshire to Georgia, committed "Daughters of Liberty" had made possible colonial boycotts through their industry and had managed families, farms, and businesses during the dislocations of war. Female access to education and the courts improved somewhat in the last quarter of the eighteenth century, but for most American women the advances were more symbolic than real.

For African Americans the disappointments were greater still. British offers of freedom prompted thousands of southern slaves to take up the Loyalist cause at great personal risk. Other free blacks and slaves, primarily in the North, shouldered arms for the Patriots, drawn by the rhetoric of liberty and the prospect of advancement. Even though they had chosen the winning side, they reaped few benefits. Although the number of free blacks expanded after the Revolutionary War, the African slave trade to the United States resumed and gained official protection. Slavery itself gained renewed significance with the transition to cotton production in the South and a federal constitution that sanctioned the power of slaveholders. Even in the North, where gradual emancipation became the norm by the end of the century, free blacks found their welcome into white churches and schools to be so half-hearted that many set about organizing their own separate institutions.

Eastern Indians, like African Americans, had good reason to distrust the Revolution and its leaders. The majority, including most Iroquois and Cherokee warriors, sided with the British and paid a steep price in defeat. Throughout the Mississippi Valley, Native Americans who still remembered the benefits of French trade and British military support faced relentless pressure as American speculators, soldiers, and settlers dissected their homelands. Some government officials promised that the newly acquired lands beyond the Mississippi would become an Indian Territory, providing lasting refuge for displaced eastern tribes. If so, what was to become of the Native American nations that already inhabited the western plains?

Like most political upheavals, the American Revolution left many questions unanswered and much business unfinished. Even the new federal government itself, in operation for little more than a decade by 1803, remained a work in progress. The specific roles and relative power of the government's three separate branches spurred endless debate, as did the proper place of the military and the most suitable direction for foreign policy. The Constitution ratified in 1789 seemed promising, but it remained an uncertain and largely untested framework.

1791	Bill of Rights is ratified. Saint Domingue slave revolt. Alexander Hamilton, "Report on the Subject of Manufactures." Samuel Slater constructs first spinning machine on U.S. soil. Bank of the United States is chartered.
1792	Washington is reelected president. Mary Wollstonecraft, *Vindication of the Rights of Woman*.

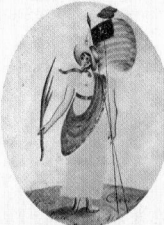

1793	Washington issues Neutrality Proclamation. Eli Whitney invents the cotton gin.

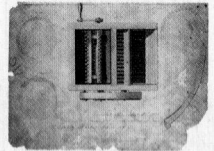

1794	U.S. troops defeat forces of Ohio Confederacy. Whiskey Rebellion.
1795	Jay's Treaty. Treaty of San Lorenzo.
1796	Washington's farewell address. John Adams is elected president.
1797	XYZ Affair.
1798	Quasi War with France (to 1800). Alien and Sedition Acts. Kentucky and Virginia Resolutions (1798–1799).
1799	Seneca Leader Handsome Lake proclaims gai'wiio, or "Good Message."
1800	Thomas Jefferson is elected president. Gabriel plot is exposed in Richmond, Virginia.
1801	Judiciary Act of 1801. War against Barbary pirates. Spain secretly cedes Louisiana Territory to France.
1803	Louisiana Purchase. *Marbury v. Madison*.

Revolutionaries at War, 1775–1783

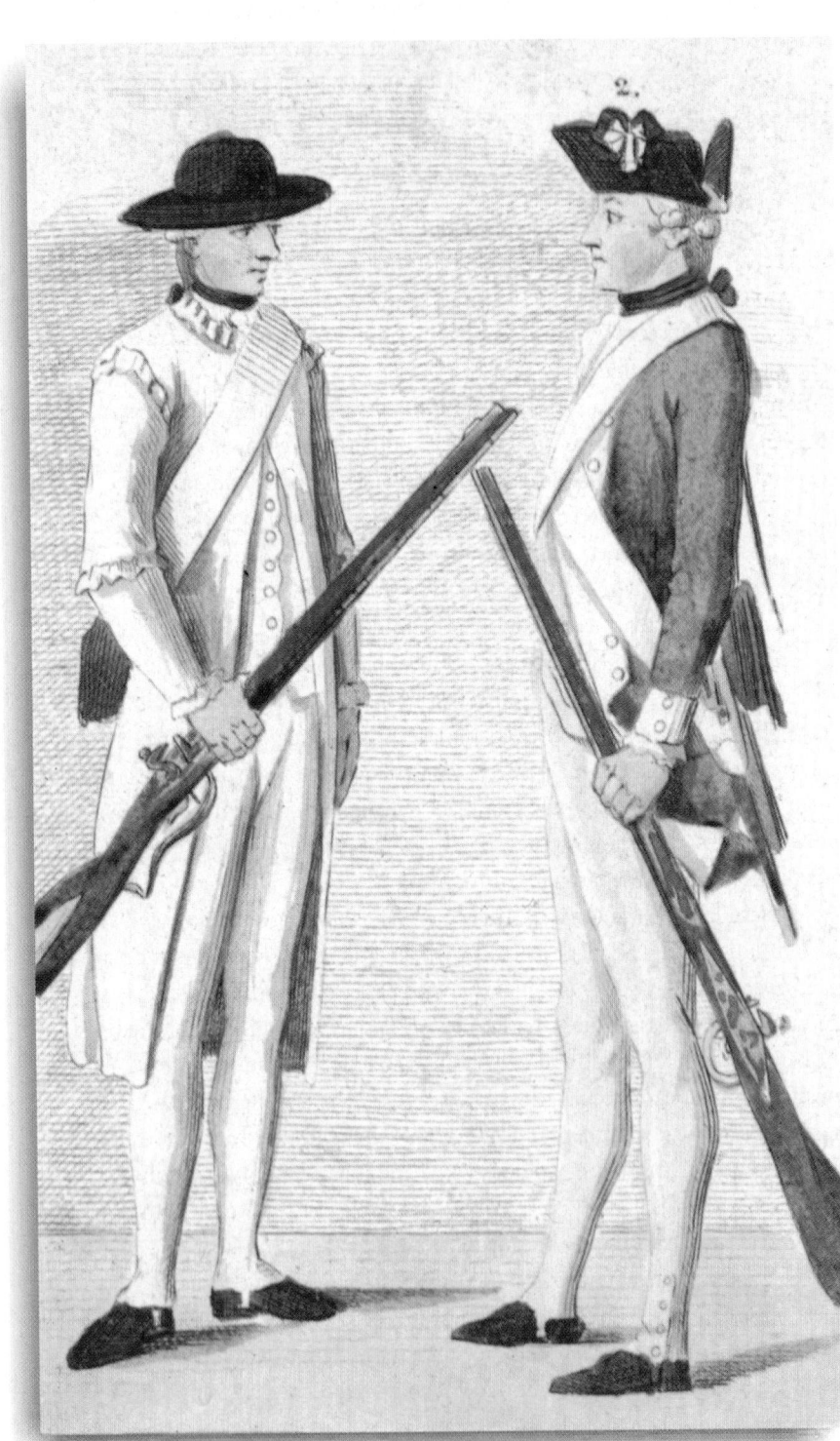

American sharpshooter and Pennsylvania regular infantryman, 1784

I N 1775, AFRICAN-BORN THOMAS PETERS WAS A 37-YEAR-OLD SLAVE IN WILMINGTON, North Carolina. As a young man, this Yoruba speaker had been taken from what is now Nigeria and shipped to Louisiana aboard the slave ship *Henri Quatre*. Forced to cut sugar cane in the French colony, Peters rebelled repeatedly. For this, he endured whipping, shackles, branding, and exile. His owner sold him to a merchant on North Carolina's Cape Fear River, where he received his English name, learned to operate a grist mill, and started a family. Still enslaved, Peters was working as a millwright and living with his wife, Sally, age 22, and their 4-year-old daughter, Clairy, by the eve of the Revolutionary War.

During the 15 years between Peters's abduction from Africa in 1760 and the outbreak of hostilities between America and Britain in 1775, nearly 225,000 people had streamed into the British mainland colonies. More than half came from the British Isles (125,000), and another 15,000 arrived from Europe, mostly German-speaking settlers landing in Philadelphia. But the remaining 85,000 newcomers—or 4 in every 10—had all been purchased in Africa and enslaved in the coastal South. Thomas Peters, entering from Louisiana, was among the recent arrivals in British America.

In the summer of 1775, Peters must have heard talk about possible slave revolts in Virginia and the Carolinas. Before the end of the year, he certainly knew that Virginia's governor, Lord Dunmore, had offered freedom to slaves who would take up arms for the British. The following March, ships of the Royal Navy arrived at the Cape Fear River. The fleet carried a strike force under the command of Sir Henry Clinton, and it offered to provide safe haven for any slaves escaping from Patriot masters. For two months, the ships cruised the Lower Cape Fear, and Thomas and Sally Peters realized that the opportunity would not last. Joining numerous other black families, they risked arrest to gain their personal liberty by bolting to the British vessels.

Peters was with General Clinton when the British fleet tried to take Charleston, South Carolina, in June 1776. Throughout the war, he served in a unit called the Black Pioneers. He was wounded twice and rose to the rank of sergeant. In October 1783, as defeated Loyalists left New York at the end of the Revolutionary War, the British officer in command of Peters's company swore out a certificate attesting to his service and affirming that he had "gained the good wishes of his officers and comrades." By serving, Peters had earned the promise of a farm in British Canada. He joined other members of the Black Pioneers aboard the *Joseph James* in New York harbor, bound for Nova Scotia. With him were Sally, Clairy, and 18-month-old John. Departing in November 1783, the ship was blown off course by foul weather. The ex-slaves spent the winter sheltered at Bermuda before finally joining 3500 other black Loyalists in Nova Scotia the following May.

But reaching Nova Scotia did not mark the end of Thomas Peters's odyssey. In 1790, after he and others had been denied the promised farmland, he ventured to London as an

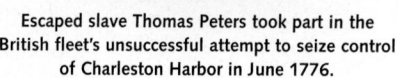

Escaped slave Thomas Peters took part in the British fleet's unsuccessful attempt to seize control of Charleston Harbor in June 1776.

advocate for these former slaves. He protested their treatment, petitioned for relief, and met with British abolitionists who were planning a colony of former slaves in West Africa. Eager to take part in the effort, he returned to Canada and led 1200 African Americans to Sierra Leone, where he died at Freetown in 1792. In 32 years, Peters had seen New Orleans, Wilmington, Charleston, New York, Halifax, and London. He had escaped after 16 years of enslavement and then gone to war, fighting for his belief in freedom and for the safety of family and friends.

Though Thomas Peters's saga is unusual, it helps to illustrate an overriding point about the Revolutionary War. Although it has often been represented as such a simple "family affair," the American War of Independence was not, in fact, a clear, two-sided struggle in which unified English colonists joined together to oppose the English monarchy and Parliament. Instead, like most revolutions, it was a conflict fought by loose and shifting coalitions.

After decades of intensive migration, the mainland colonies had become increasingly complex (and in many ways non-English) societies. At a personal level, innumerable options existed to create fresh personal alliances, marrying someone who differed in language, ethnicity, religion, or class. Similarly, in a time of strife, there were countless possibilities for forging political "marriages of convenience" between different regions, groups, and interests. Where would merchants and sailors, wives and widows, servants and slaves, farmers and shopkeepers wind up in the emerging alignment between the Patriots (or rebels) on one hand and the Loyalists (or Tories) on the other? And what about dozens of other possible groupings, such as debtors, Catholics, young people, or frontier dwellers? Given the diversity of people with a stake in the outcome of the war, almost any combination seemed plausible.

Within each small community, and within the Atlantic theater as a whole, alliances often proved the old adage that "My enemy's enemy is my friend." No doubt Thomas Peters escaped servitude to join the British in part because the man who had been holding him in slavery was a leading member of the local Sons of Liberty. Likewise, powerful colonial merchants like John Hancock and Henry Laurens threw in their lot with the crowds in the streets in part because they had grown disillusioned with the political and commercial controls exerted by Parliament. On the international scale, the monarchies of France and Spain eventually swallowed their dislike for American rhetoric to join in a war that allowed them an opportunity to attack their longstanding rival, Britain. On the other hand, many Cherokee and Iroquois Indians, disillusioned by contact with land-hungry settlers, cast their lot with the British forces from overseas.

Precisely because the alliances were so numerous and complex, they often remained problematic and incomplete. Not all Iroquois warriors or African slaves sided with the British, and by no means all New England merchants or Virginia planters embraced the Patriot cause. In a landscape marked by uncertainty, large numbers of people at all levels of society opted for cautious neutrality as long as they could, while others shifted their allegiance as the winds changed. It was even possible, as the dramatic case of Benedict Arnold made clear, to betray a post of trusted leadership on one side and assume a position of authority on the other.

Not surprisingly, given so many complexities and uncertainties, the final outcome of the conflict remained a source of constant doubt. Looking back, Americans often view the results of the Revolutionary War as inevitable, perhaps even foreordained. In fact, the end result—and thus independence itself—hung in the balance for years.

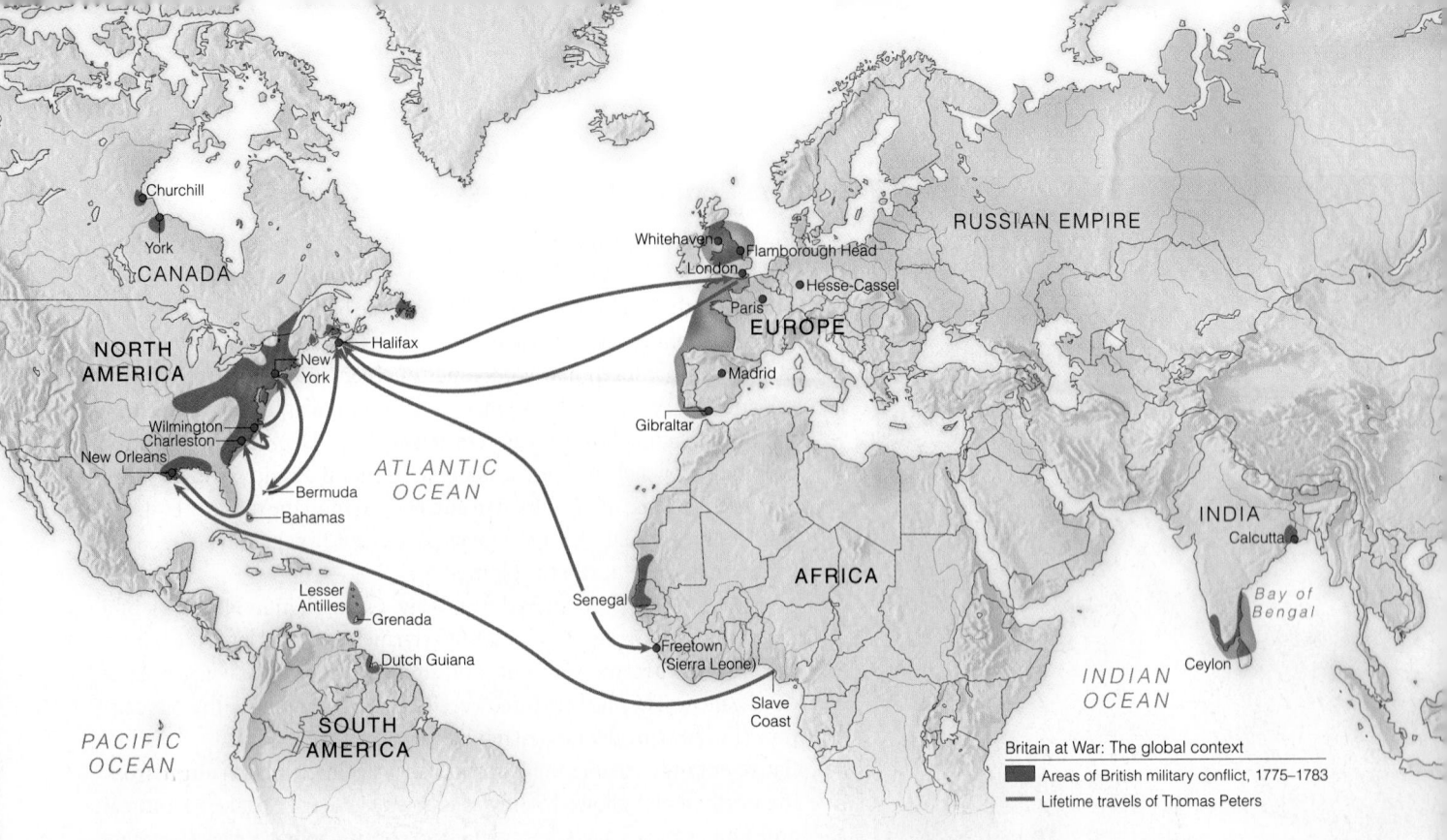

■ **MAP 7.1**

BRITAIN AT WAR: THE GLOBAL CONTEXT, 1778–1783 For Britain, the war that began in 1775 expanded into a worldwide conflict against rival European powers within three years. By 1783, the British lost American colonies while expanding their hold in India. The lifetime journey of African-born Thomas Peters, shown here, is clearly exceptional, but extensive movements figured in many lives during these years of warfare. General Cornwallis, for example, went on to serve the British in India after his defeat at Yorktown in 1781.

Declaring Independence

New England's Minutemen had rallied swiftly at Lexington and Concord to harry the British. They moved equally quickly to spread news of their success in all directions. A ship carrying the Patriot version of events arrived in England two weeks before the dispatches of General Gage. Word reached Charleston, South Carolina, by early May and soon spread west beyond the Appalachian Mountains. When hunters exploring the bluegrass region heard the news, they named their campsite Lexington, now a city in modern-day Kentucky.

In the ensuing months, Congress took the initial steps to form a Continental Army. It also launched efforts to force the British out of Boston and to pull Canada into the rebellion. If these predominantly Protestant rebels hoped to draw the French Catholics of Quebec into their revolt, would free whites also be eager to include the blacks of Boston, Williamsburg, and Charleston in the struggle for liberty? Or would it be British officials who recruited more African Americans and furnished them with arms? After all, determined ex-slaves like Thomas Peters represented a serious threat to their former masters and a stark reminder to other slave owners who contemplated joining the colonists' rebellion. The answers to such questions became clear in the 15 months between the skirmish at Lexington and the decision of Congress to declare political independence from Britain in July 1776.

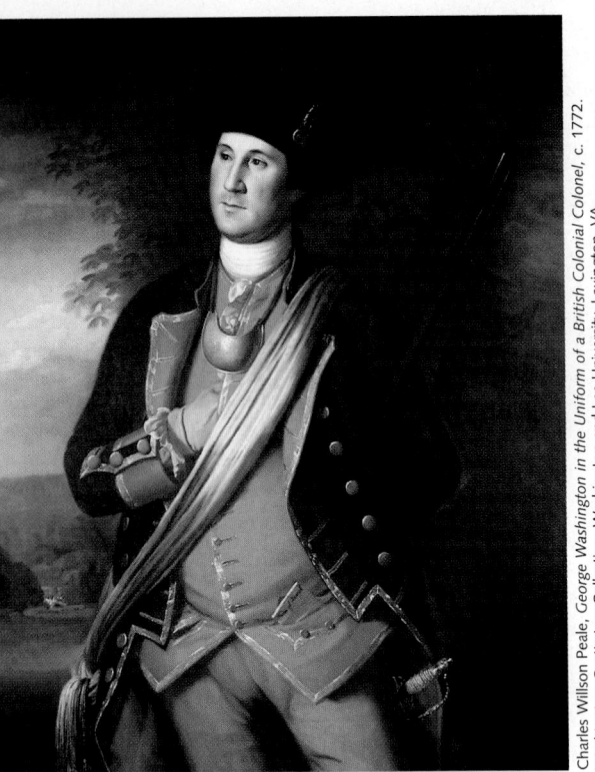

Charles Willson Peale, *George Washington in the Uniform of a British Colonial Colonel*, c. 1772. Washington-Custis-Lee Collection, Washington and Lee University, Lexington, VA

■ In June 1775, Congress selected a wealthy Virginia planter to command its army. The choice of George Washington reassured southern slave owners and disappointed blacks and whites in the North who saw slavery as a contradiction in the struggle for freedom.

The Continental Congress Takes Control

Enthusiasm ran high in Philadelphia in May 1775 as the second Continental Congress assembled amid cheers and parades. Delegates moved quickly in the weeks that followed to put the beleaguered colonies on a wartime footing. They instructed New York to build fortifications. They also paid for a dozen new companies of riflemen—recruited in Pennsylvania, Maryland, and Virginia—to be sent north to aid the Minutemen surrounding Boston. They created an Army Department under the command of a New York aristocrat, General Philip Schuyler, and approved an issue of $2 million in currency to fund the military buildup. The Congress also took important steps to ensure a coalition between the southern and the northern colonies.

In late May, word arrived from Lake Champlain in New York of a victory for the Green Mountain Boys (farmers led by Ethan Allen, from the area that became Vermont) and soldiers under Benedict Arnold of Connecticut. They had captured Fort Ticonderoga, along with all its cannon (heavy arms the new Army Department needed badly). This initiative not only secured the Hudson Valley against a British attack from the north; it also allowed Schuyler to propose a strike against Montreal and Quebec via Lake Champlain and the Richelieu River. Congress approved the assault, to be led by General Richard Montgomery. It also approved a daring scheme submitted by Arnold. He planned to lead separate forces up the Kennebec River. They would assist Montgomery in seizing Quebec and winning Canada before the region could become a staging ground for British armies.

But no single action by Congress had greater implications for coalition building among the colonies than the one taken on June 15, 1775. That day, members voted unanimously to appoint George Washington, a 43-year-old delegate from Virginia, "to command all the continental forces." Colonel Washington already headed a committee that was drawing up regulations to run the new army, and he had notable military experience. But his strongest asset may have been his southern roots. Northern delegates—especially John Adams, who had nominated Washington—sensed the need to foster colonial unity by placing a non–New Englander in charge of the army outside Boston. For their part, Southerners sensed keen regional differences, particularly over slavery. They appeared jealous, as one delegate noted, "lest an enterprising New England general, proving successful, might with his victorious army" enforce control over "the southern gentry."

In military and political terms, the selection of Washington proved auspicious. The tall, imposing planter from Mount Vernon emerged as a durable and respected leader in both war and peace. At another level, however, putting a slaveholder in command signaled the beginning of an important alliance between the well-to-do regional leaders of the North and South. Although no one could foresee it at the time, this alliance would contribute to the particular shape of the Federal Constitution a dozen years later, and the bond endured sufficiently to shape the governing of the country until the middle of the next century.

"Liberty to Slaves"

The selection of Washington strengthened the hand of plantation owners in the emerging coalition across regions. But in so doing, it signaled a limit to the prospects for any major or lasting American coalition across racial lines. The move sent a stronger message than Congress realized to some half a million African Americans, increasing their skepticism about the Patriot cause and spurring many of them—including Tom Peters, no doubt—to risk siding with the British.

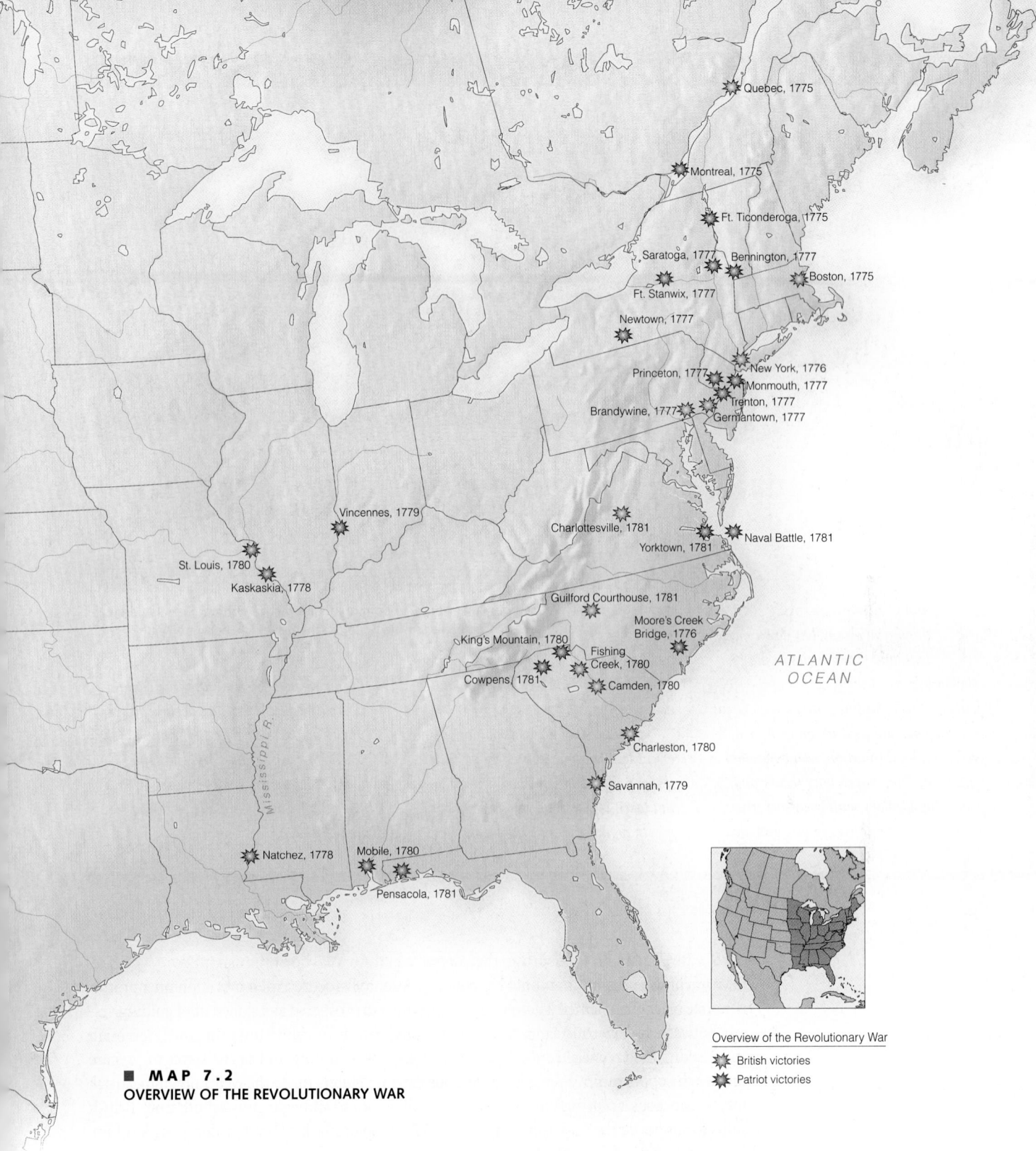

■ MAP 7.2
OVERVIEW OF THE REVOLUTIONARY WAR

Overview of the Revolutionary War

* British victories
* Patriot victories

For their part, the British gave increasing thought to the idea of befriending enslaved Africans in order to undermine rebellious planters. In June 1775, the British commander in America, Thomas Gage, wrote to London: "Things are now come to that crisis, that we must avail ourselves of every resource, even to raise the Negros, in our cause." One Lutheran minister who spoke to black house servants near Philadelphia the next year noted that they "secretly wished that the British Army might win, for then all Negro slaves will gain their freedom. It is said that this sentiment is almost universal among the Negroes in America."

In the South, rumors of liberation swept through the large African American community during 1775. Slaveholding rebel authorities countered with harsh measures to quell black

"Revoking Those Sacred Trusts Which Are Violated": A Declaration Signed by 15 Grand Jury Members in South Carolina, May 1776

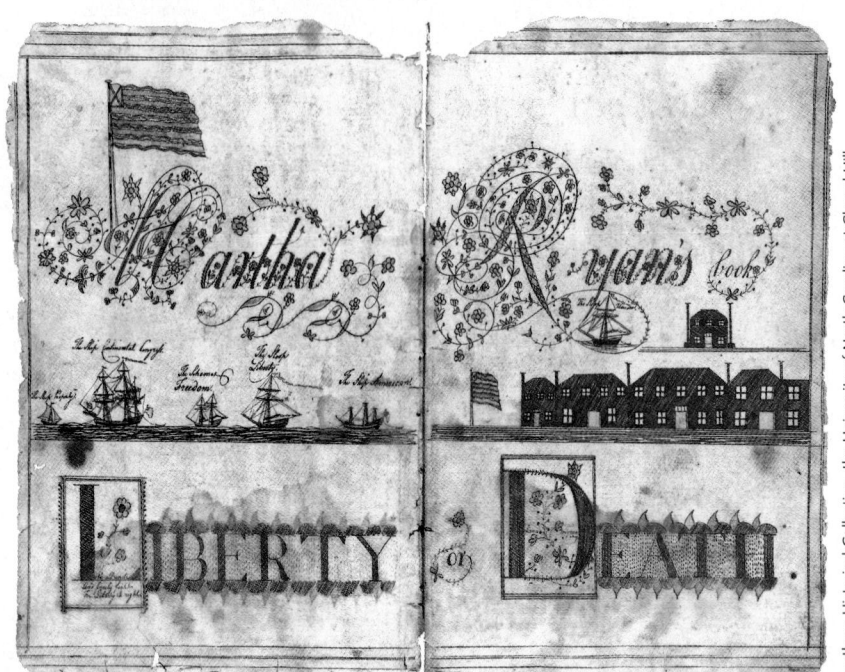

Young Martha Ryan used her cipher-book to do more than practice writing. She also drew American ships and flags and embellished the popular rallying cry, "Liberty or Death."

Throughout the late spring of 1776, provincial assemblies, town meetings, and grand juries in the 13 colonies began issuing their own pronouncements regarding a break with Great Britain. The authors drew on historical precedent, legal tradition, and emotional sentiment. They mixed lofty theory and Real Whig ideology with local concerns. They also incorporated rhetoric and ideas from current pamphlets, speeches, and newspaper essays.

At least 90 of these proclamations survive. Most are more impressive for their strong feelings than for their literary merit. But taken together, they suggest the sentiments, arguments, and words that were in the air when Jefferson drafted the Declaration of Independence. This document was drawn up and signed by 15 members of the Cheraw District grand jury who came together for their regular court session in Long Bluff, South Carolina, on Monday, May 20, 1776.

unrest. In Charleston that spring, they deported an African-born minister, David Margate, for preaching a sermon that hinted at equality. Also, they focused their attention on a prominent free black man named Thomas Jeremiah, who had prospered as a skilled pilot guiding vessels between treacherous sand bars into the busy South Carolina port. In April, Jeremiah supposedly told an enslaved dockworker of a great war coming and urged slaves to prepare to seize the opportunity. Weeks later, nervous Patriot planters made the well-known free black into a scapegoat, accusing him of involvement in a plot to smuggle guns ashore from British ships to support a slave uprising. In August 1775, despite a lack of hard evidence against him, Jeremiah was publicly hanged and then burned.

That September, a Georgia delegate to Congress made a startling comment. If British troops were to land on the southern coast with a supply of food and guns, he said, and offer freedom to slaves who would join them, 20,000 blacks from Georgia and South Carolina would materialize in no time. In November, the beleaguered royal governor of Virginia, Lord Dunmore, attempted just such a scheme. Dunmore issued a proclamation granting freedom to the slaves of rebel masters who agreed to take up arms on behalf of the king. Hundreds responded to Dunmore's proclamation. They formed the Ethiopian Regiment and wore sashes proclaiming "Liberty to Slaves."

The Presentments of the Grand Jury of and for the Said District

I. When a people, born and bred in a land of freedom and virtue . . . are convinced of the wicked schemes of their treacherous rulers to fetter them with the chains of servitude, and rob them of every noble and desirable privilege which distinguishes them as freemen,—justice, humanity, and the immutable laws of *God,* justify and support them in revoking those sacred trusts which are so impiously violated, and placing them in such hands as are most likely to execute them in the manner and for the important ends for which they were first given.

II. The good people of this Colony, with the rest of her sister Colonies, confiding in the justice and merited protection of the King and Parliament of *Great Britain,* ever . . . esteemed such a bond of union and harmony as the greatest happiness. But when that protection was wantonly withdrawn, and every mark of cruelty and oppression substituted; . . . self-preservation, and a regard to our own welfare and security, became a consideration both important and necessary. The Parliament and

Ministry of *Great Britain,* by their wanton and undeserved persecutions, have reduced this Colony to a state of separation from her . . . as the only lasting means of future happiness and safety. . . . Cast off, persecuted, defamed, given up as a prey to every violence and injury, a righteous and much injured people have at length appealed to *God!* and, trusting to his divine justice and their own virtuous perseverance, taken the only and last means of securing their own honour, safety, and happiness.

III. We now feel every joyful and comfortable hope that a people could desire in the present Constitution and form of Government established in this Colony; a Constitution founded on the strictest principles of justice and humanity, where the rights and happiness of the whole, the poor and the rich, are equally secured; and to secure and defend which, it is the particular interest of every individual who regards his own safety and advantage.

IV. When we consider the publick officers of our present form of Government now appointed, as well as the method and duration of their appointment, we cannot but declare our entire satisfaction and

comfort; as well in the characters of such men, who are justly esteemed for every virtue, as their well-known abilities to execute the important trusts which they now hold.

V. Under these convictions, . . . we . . . recommend it to every man . . . to secure and defend with his life and fortune a form of Government so just, so equitable, and promising; . . . that the latest posterity may enjoy the virtuous fruits of that work, which the integrity and fortitude of the present age had, at the expense of their blood and treasure, at length happily effected.

VI. We cannot but declare how great the pleasure, the harmony, and political union which now exists in this District affords; and having no grievances to complain of, only beg leave to recommend that a new Jury list be made for this District, the present being insufficient.

And lastly, we beg leave . . . that these our presentments be printed in the publick papers.— PHILIP PLEDGER, Foreman [and 14 other signatures] ■

Source: Pauline Maier, *American Scripture: Making the Declaration of Independence* (New York: Knopf, 1997), 229–231.

The Struggle to Control Boston and Quebec

In the North, British forces had been confined in Boston ever since the Battle of Lexington. They would remain isolated on the town's main peninsula, supported by the Royal Navy, for nearly a year. In early July 1775, Washington arrived at nearby Cambridge to take up his command and oversee the siege of Boston. He quickly set out to improve order among his men. He tightened discipline, enforced punishments, and calmed regional jealousies. He removed nearly a dozen incompetent officers. In addition, he wrote scores of letters to civilian political leaders and the president of Congress to muster support for his meager army.

The Massachusetts legislature alone received 34 messages from the new commander. Washington made clear that nearly everything was in short supply, from tents and uniforms to muskets and cannon. He dispatched 25-year-old Henry Knox, a former bookseller and future general, to retrieve the ordnance captured at Ticonderoga. The Patriots' siege of Boston, he informed Congress, could not succeed without heavy fieldpieces to bombard the city from the heights at Dorchester and Charlestown that lay across the water.

Even before Washington's arrival, the British and the Americans had vied for control of these strategic heights. Indeed, the British General Gage drew up plans to secure Charlestown peninsula by seizing its highest point, Bunker Hill. But the Patriots learned of the scheme. On the night of June 16, 1775, they moved to fortify Breed's Hill, a smaller knoll 600 yards in front of Bunker Hill. The next afternoon, 1500 well-entrenched but inexperienced Patriot volunteers confronted the full force of the British army as thousands watched from the rooftops of Boston.

Although Gage might easily have sealed off Charlestown peninsula with his naval power, he instead used 2500 British infantry, weighed down by heavy packs, to launch three frontal attacks up Breed's Hill from the shoreline. The first two charges fell back before withering volleys at close range. Finally, with adjoining Charlestown ablaze and rebel powder supplies exhausted, a third assault overran the hill and dislodged the Americans. Mistakenly, the engagement became known as the Battle of Bunker Hill. Although it was technically a British victory, success came at a terrible price. Forty-two percent of British troops (1054 men) were wounded or dead—the worst casualty figures of the entire war. Gage lost his command, replaced in October by General William Howe. The Royal Army itself lost its aura of invincibility.

As Washington used the last half of 1775 to organize his rudimentary army in Cambridge, Henry Knox pursued his mission to retrieve the captured British ordnance from Ticonderoga. Using oxen, sledges, and local volunteers, he managed to haul 43 heavy cannon east, across trails covered with snow and ice, from the Hudson Valley to the coast. His men delivered the guns in late winter, and in March 1776 the Americans moved to secure Dorchester Heights. As at Breed's Hill, they made their surprise move at night. But this time, they had cannon that could reach far enough to bombard their enemies huddled in Boston. The British General Howe, who had commanded the charges at Breed's Hill and seen the devastation, drew back from a similar assault on Dorchester Heights. Instead, he evacuated his army, retreating by ship to Halifax, Nova Scotia. There, he made plans to attack the rebels again at New York, where Loyalist support was stronger.

As Washington's forces laid siege to Boston, other Americans converged on British troops in Canada. General Montgomery's troops seized Montreal in November 1775. They then descended the St. Lawrence River to join Benedict Arnold's men, who had struggled north toward Quebec under brutal winter conditions. As one combined force, under Montgomery, they attacked the walled city during a fierce snowstorm on the night of December 30. But their assault failed, and Montgomery perished in the fighting. Smallpox had already broken out in the American ranks, and it spread to new arrivals during the next five months. When British reinforcements showed up at Quebec in May, the Americans beat a hasty retreat toward Lake Champlain. They left behind most of their baggage and hundreds of sick companions.

Hundreds more died of smallpox during the withdrawal of the shattered army, and others spread the deadly pox further as they returned to their New England homes. "I got an account of my johns Death of the Small Pox at Canada," one New Hampshire father scrawled in his diary after learning that his 24-year-old son had died while fighting against the King's forces. "He was shot through his left arm at Bunker Hill." Now, "in defending the just Rights of America," John had been taken "in the prime of life by means of that wicked Tyranical Brute (Nea worse than Brute) of Great Britan." In thousands of American households, strained loyalty was turning to explosive anger.

"Time to Part"

In January 1776, a brilliant pamphlet, *Common Sense,* captured the shifting mood and helped propel Americans toward independence. British corsetmaker Thomas Paine, age 39, had endured a long series of personal and economic failures in England before sailing to Philadelphia. To this passionate man, with his gift for powerful and accessible prose, America represented a fresh start. Arriving late in 1774, Paine poured his energy into bold newspaper essays. In one, he argued that African American slaves deserved freedom and ample land to become productive citizen–farmers.

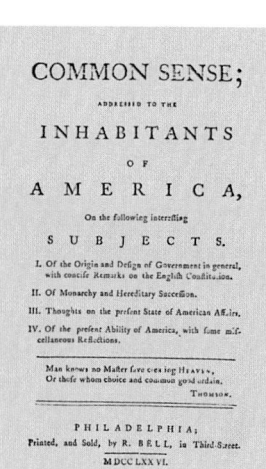

COMMON SENSE;

ADDRESSED TO THE

INHABITANTS

OF

AMERICA,

On the following interesting

SUBJECTS.

I. Of the Origin and Design of Government in general, with concise Remarks on the English Constitution.

II. Of Monarchy and Hereditary Succession.

III. Thoughts on the present State of American Affairs.

IV. Of the present Ability of America, with some miscellaneous Reflections.

Man knows no Master save creating HEAVEN, Or those whom choice and common good ordain.
THOMSON.

PHILADELPHIA;

Printed, and Sold, by R. BELL, in Third-Street.

MDCCLXXVI.

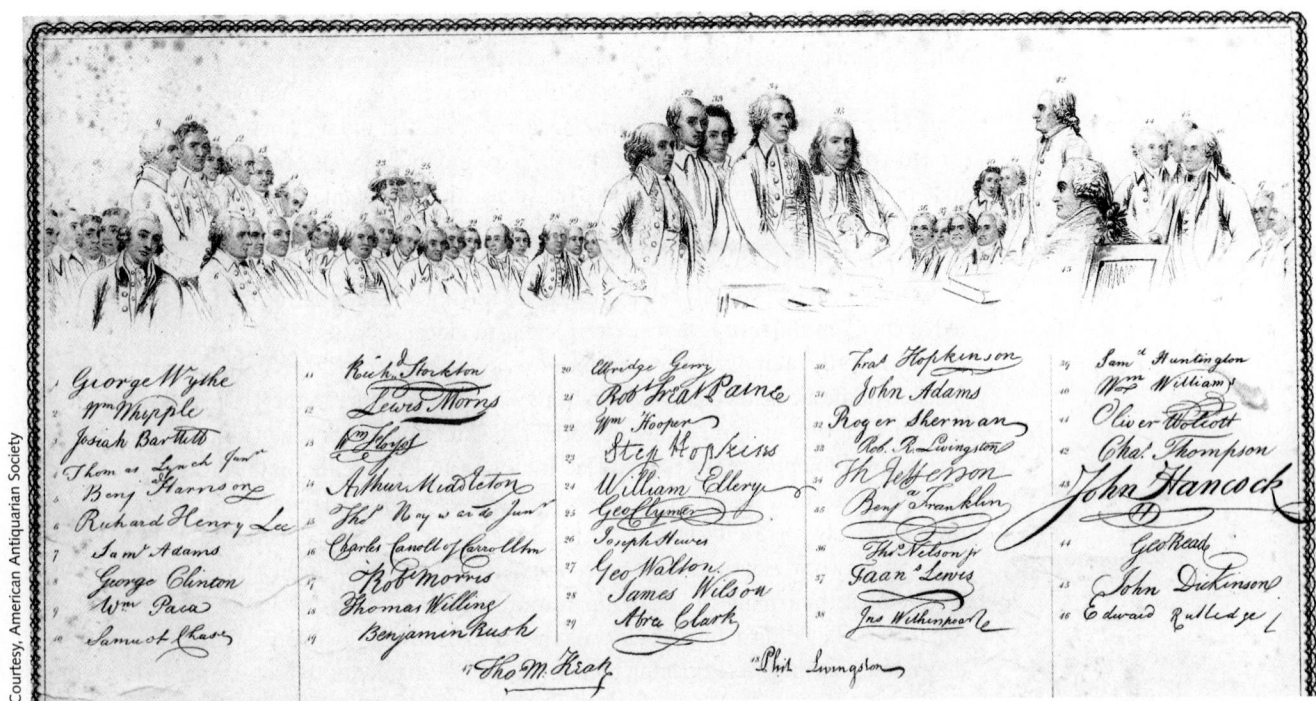

Courtesy, American Antiquarian Society

■ John Trumbull spent years gathering portraits for his famous painting, *The Declaration of Independence.* This engraving identifies individuals in the painting with their signatures. The artist placed the Drafting Committee in the center (31–35). He omitted signers for whom he had no likeness, and he included several non-signers, such as John Dickinson.

Paine's *Common Sense* was a wildly popular tract, selling 120,000 copies in three months and reaching all sorts of readers. In it, the author promised to lay out "simple facts, plain arguments, and common sense" on the precarious American situation. He then proceeded to lambaste "the so much boasted constitution of England." Not stopping there, he went on to attack hereditary monarchy and the divine right of kings. "One honest man," Paine proclaimed, is worth more to society "than all the crowned ruffians that ever lived." He urged the creation of an independent constitutional republic that could become "an asylum for all mankind." "Reconciliation is now a fallacious dream," he argued: "'TIS TIME TO PART."

Thousands of Paine's avid readers agreed. In the spring of 1776, one colony after another instructed its representatives to vote for independence. But many among the well-to-do still held strong social and economic ties to London; they feared the loss of British imperial protection and the startling upsurge of democratic political activity among the lower orders. At first, Congress vacillated. But with no sign of accommodation from England, most members agreed with Robert Livingston of New York that "they should yield to the torrent if they hoped to direct its course." In early June, young Livingston, age 30, joined the committee assigned to prepare a formal statement declaring independence from Great Britain. The Committee of Five also included Benjamin Franklin, John Adams, Roger Sherman, and the second youngest member of the Continental Congress, Thomas Jefferson.

The 33-year-old Jefferson had recently returned to Philadelphia from Virginia, where his mother had died suddenly in March. Personally independent for the first time, he willingly took responsibility for crafting the document. He framed a stirring preamble, drawing on British philosopher John Locke's contract theory of government. Locke (1632–1702) believed that the sovereign power ultimately resided not in government but in the people themselves, who chose to submit voluntarily to civil law to protect property and preserve basic rights.

According to Locke, rulers held conditional, not absolute, authority over the people. Citizens therefore held the right to end their support and overthrow any government that did not fulfill its side of the contract. For any people facing "a long train of abuses," Jefferson wrote, "it is their right, it is their duty, to throw off such government and to provide new guards for their future security." He went on to catalogue the "repeated injuries and usurpations" committed by King George III. Meanwhile, on July 2, Congress voted on the statement affirming that "these United Colonies are, and of right, ought to be, Free and Independent States." Twelve colonies voted to approve a resolution, with the New York delegation abstaining until it could receive further instructions from home. Having made the fundamental decision, the delegates then considered how to "declare the causes" behind their momentous choice to separate from Great Britain.

Over the next two days, all the Congress members edited the draft declaration submitted by the Committee of Five. They kept Jefferson's idealistic assertion that "all men are created equal." But they removed any reference to slavery, except for the charge that the king had "excited domestic insurrections amongst us," a veiled reference to the Thomas Jeremiah debacle in Charleston and to Lord Dunmore's proclamation. With other changes in place, they finally voted to approve the revised Declaration of Independence on July 4, 1776.

John Hancock, the president of the Congress, signed the document with a flourish, and printers hastily turned it into a published broadside. The other signatures (contrary to folklore) came two weeks later, after New York had offered its approval. Then 56 delegates gathered to sign their names to "The unanimous declaration of the thirteen United States of America." They did so at great risk. As they endorsed the document with their signatures, they knew that they were opening themselves to face charges of treason, punishable by death.

The British Attack New York

While the Continental Congress debated whether to declare independence, the British sharpened their strategies for suppressing the rebellion. Strangling the revolt with a naval blockade appeared impossible, given the length of the American coastline. But two other alternatives emerged in the first year of open warfare. These options shaped British intentions throughout the rest of the conflict. One design involved a southern strategy. It rested on the assumption that loyalty to the crown remained strongest in the South. If the British could land forces below Chesapeake Bay, Loyalist support might enable them to gain the upper hand and push north to reimpose colonial rule elsewhere.

In June 1776 troops under General Henry Clinton arrived off the Carolina coast with such a mission in mind. But Loyalists had already lost a battle to the Patriots at Moore's Creek Bridge near Wilmington, North Carolina, in February, and the British ships sailed to South Carolina instead. On June 28, they bombarded Sullivan's Island, at the mouth of Charleston harbor. But the Americans' cypress log fortress withstood the cannon fire, and the attackers withdrew. The British did not renew their southern design for several years, concentrating instead on a separate northern strategy.

According to Britain's alternative northern plan, troops would seize New York City and then divide the rebellious colonies in two at the Hudson River. By advancing upriver while other forces pushed south from Canada, they would take control of the entire Hudson Valley. Then, having sealed off New England, they could finally crush the radicals in Massachusetts who had spearheaded the revolt while restoring the loyalties of inhabitants farther south. Lord George Germain, the aggressive new British cabinet minister in charge of American affairs, favored this plan. An overwhelming strike, he asserted, could "finish the rebellion in one campaign."

Early in 1776, Germain set out to generate a land and sea offensive of unprecedented scale. He prodded the sluggish Admiralty for ships, and when he could not raise troops swiftly at home, he rented them from abroad. Empress Catherine of Russia declined a request for 20,000 soldiers, but the German states produced 18,000 mercenaries. Eventually, 30,000 German troops traveled to America, so many of them from the state of Hesse-Cassel that onlookers called all of them Hessians. Canada, having already repulsed Montgomery's American invasion, could provide a loyal staging ground in the north. "I have always thought Hudson's River the most proper part of the

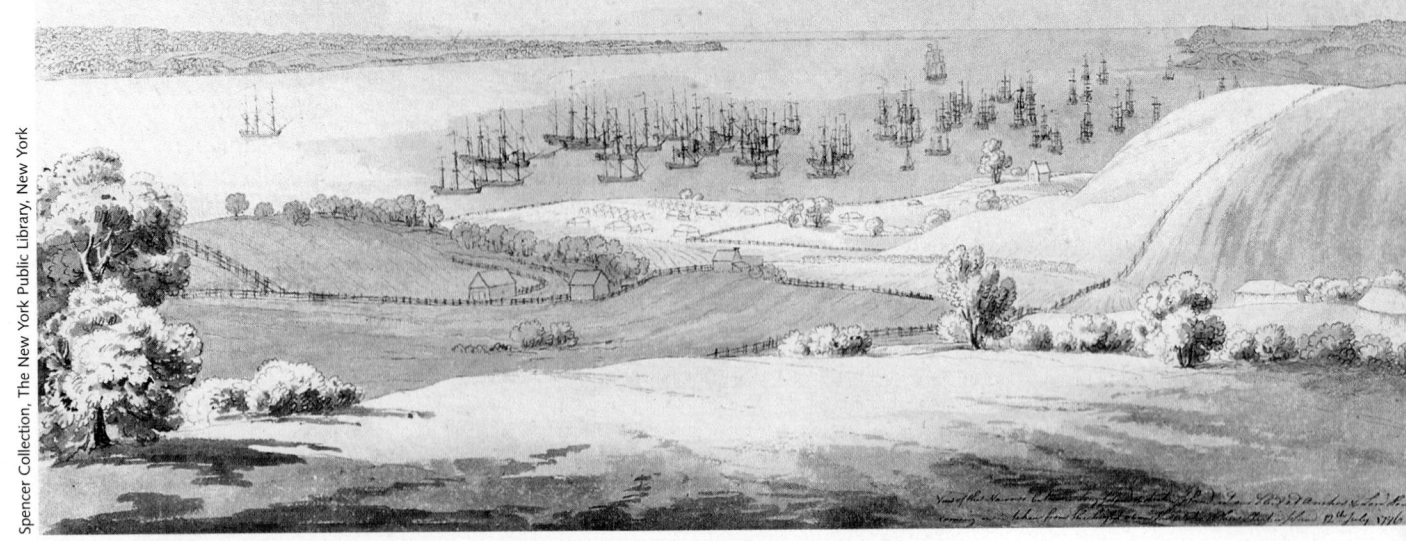

■ In July 1776 the largest expeditionary force that the British had ever assembled arrived by sea at New York Harbor. British officer Archibald Robinson sketched part of the fleet and the initial camp at Staten Island. By September, the troops had seized Long Island and occupied New York City.

whole continent for opening vigorous operations," observed "Gentleman Johnny" Burgoyne, the dapper and worldly British general who arrived at Quebec with reinforcements in May 1776.

But plans for a strike south from Canada had to wait. Britain made its first thrust toward the mouth of the Hudson River by sea, using nearly 400 ships. In June, a convoy under General William Howe sailed from Halifax to Staten Island, New York, with 9000 soldiers. By mid-August, the general had received 20,000 reinforcements from across the Atlantic. His brother, Admiral Richard Howe, hovered nearby with 13,000 sailors aboard 70 naval vessels.

On orders from Congress, General Washington moved south to defend New York City, a difficult task made harder by ardent Loyalist sentiment. Rumors swirled of a Loyalist plot to kidnap the general or even take his life. A bodyguard named Thomas Hickey, implicated in the Tory scheme, was hanged before a huge crowd of anxious onlookers in late June. Intrigue aside, Washington's army lacked the numbers, equipment, and naval support to defend New York properly. The general weakened it further by dividing his troops between Manhattan and Brooklyn Heights on nearby Long Island.

A month after Congress members signed the Declaration of Independence, the commander nearly lost his entire force—and the cause itself. General Howe moved his troops by water from Staten Island to the Brooklyn area and then outflanked and scattered the poorly trained Americans in the Battle of Long Island on August 27. Remarkably, the British leader called off a direct attack that almost certainly would have overrun the American batteries on Brooklyn Heights. Perhaps Howe remembered yet again the heavy toll that a similar assault had taken on his forces at Bunker Hill. When his equally cautious brother failed to seal off the East River with ships, rebel troops escaped disaster by slipping back to New York City in small boats under cover of night and fog.

"Victory or Death": Fighting for Survival

Washington's narrow escape to Lower Manhattan from Long Island in August 1776 was only the first of numerous retreats. His army left New York City on September 15. (Congress counseled the American forces against destroying the town as they departed, but a suspicious fire devastated much of the city a week later.) The rebels withdrew from upper Manhattan and Westchester in October and from Fort Washington and Fort Lee on the Hudson—with heavy losses—in November. The Americans "fled like scared rabbits," one Englishman wrote. "They have left some poor pork, a few greasy proclamations, and some of that scoundrel Common Sense man's letters, which we can read at our leisure."

With winter at hand, the ragged Continental forces retreated southeast toward Philadelphia, plagued by deserting troops and low morale. But thanks to the unlikely success of one desperate maneuver—recrossing the Delaware River by night—they survived to renew their efforts in 1777. By the end of the next campaign season, two and a half years after the skirmish at Lexington, their powerful adversaries stumbled badly. Still, it was a long 14 months between the painful withdrawal from New York City and a stunning victory that finally came at Saratoga, 185 miles up the Hudson.

A Desperate Gamble Pays Off

As the American army retreated from New York late in 1776, General Howe repeatedly failed to press his advantage. The British commander and his brother had received a commission from Lord North, who headed the government in London, permitting them to negotiate a peace settlement with the Americans whenever possible. They hoped that a strong show of force, without a vicious offensive that might alienate civilians, could bring the enemy to terms. Howe's troops captured General Charles Lee, second in the American command, as they chased Wash-

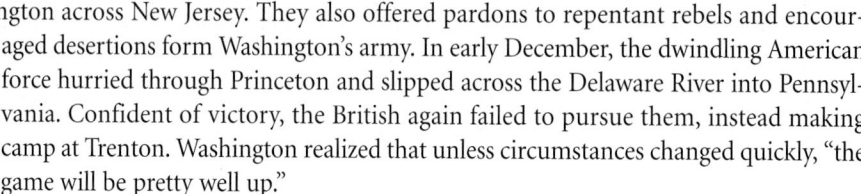

ington across New Jersey. They also offered pardons to repentant rebels and encouraged desertions form Washington's army. In early December, the dwindling American force hurried through Princeton and slipped across the Delaware River into Pennsylvania. Confident of victory, the British again failed to pursue them, instead making camp at Trenton. Washington realized that unless circumstances changed quickly, "the game will be pretty well up."

Distressed by civilian talk of surrender, Tom Paine again took up his pen. In the *Pennsylvania Journal* for December 19, he launched a new series of essays called "The American Crisis." The series began with the ringing words, "These are the times that try men's souls." Paine mocked "the summer soldier and the sunshine patriot" who shrank from extreme trials, and he chided Lord North's administration for so underestimating "our abilities and disposition." Just when Britain "supposed us conquered," Paine predicted hopefully, "we rose the conquerer."

Action soon followed words. On Christmas Day 1776, Washington issued a new code phrase for sentinels: "Victory or Death." He ordered Paine's words read aloud to the troops. Then, after dark, his men recrossed the windswept Delaware River in a driving snowstorm and advanced on Trenton. Overconfidence, holiday festivities, and the foul weather had left the enemy unprepared. The Americans inflicted a startling defeat, killing several dozen and capturing more than 900 Hessian soldiers.

Few Patriot soldiers could converse with their German-speaking captives, but they could see first-hand that their opponents had superior resources. Both the British and their Hessian mercenaries possessed standardized equipment and ample supplies. The Americans, in contrast, were expected to provide their own firearms, and soldiers who brought a blanket from home earned a bonus. On enlisting, they were generally offered 40 shillings a month and a new issue of clothes, but the cost of their outfit came out of their pay at 10 shillings per month. Food was poor, rifle balls were makeshift, and gunpowder was so scarce that earlier in the year Benjamin Franklin had seriously proposed the use of bows and arrows. Most soldiers had signed up to serve for a brief term and return home, and many had joined the previous January for a one-year stint.

Washington knew that numerous enlistments expired on December 31 and that men would leave if the brief offensive halted. So he advanced again on December 30. Howe sent fresh troops forward under Charles Cornwallis to confront the rebels, pinning them down at Trenton. But when the British paused before attacking, the Americans left their campfires burn-

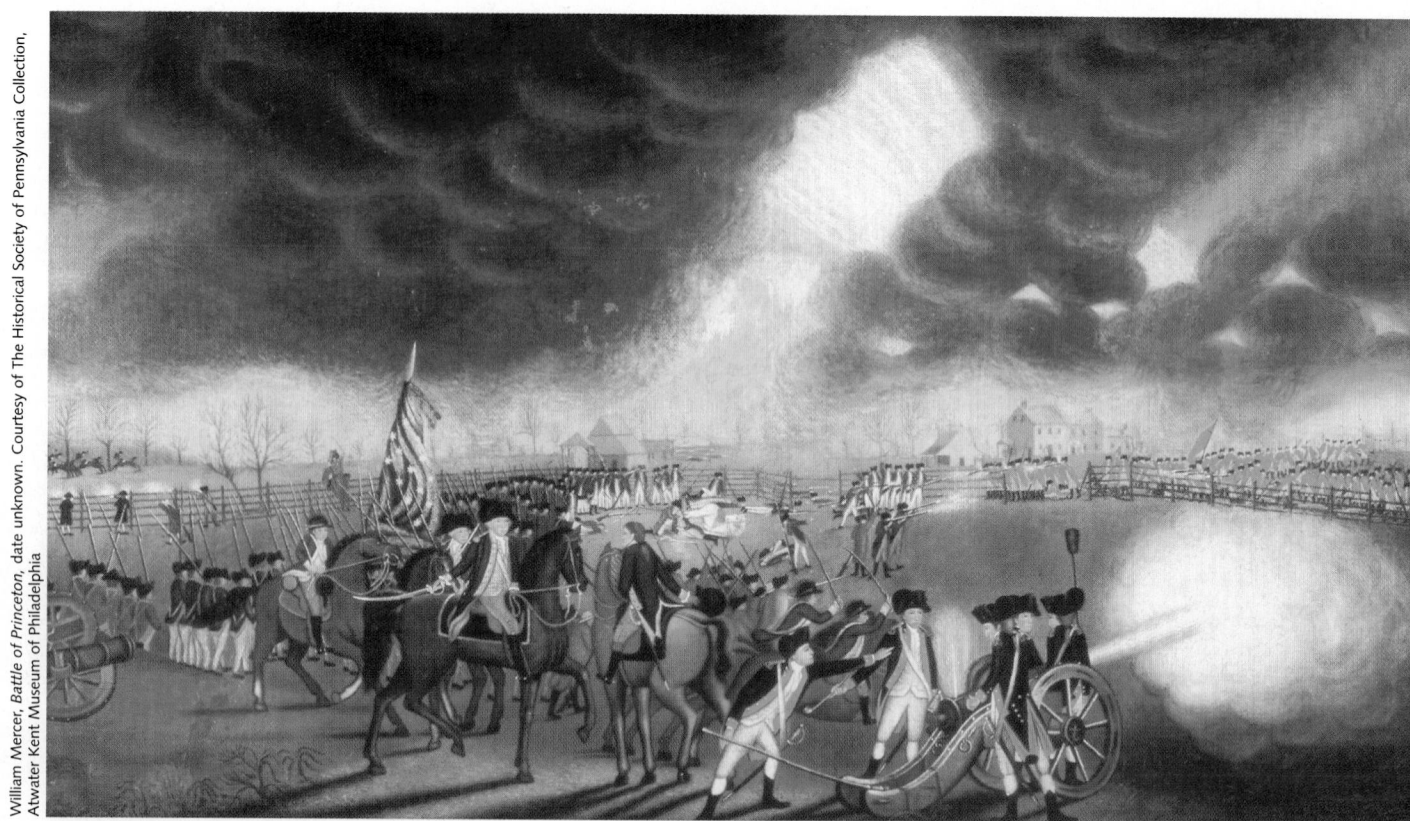

William Mercer, *Battle of Princeton*, date unknown. Courtesy of The Historical Society of Pennsylvania Collection, Atwater Kent Museum of Philadelphia

■ **This picture showing the noise and movement of the American victory at the Battle of Princeton was created by deaf painter William Mercer, whose father, Brigadier General Hugh Mercer, died in the battle.**

ing and slipped out of reach. They then circled behind Cornwallis to surprise and defeat his reinforcements at Princeton on January 3. It was not the last time that Washington bested Cornwallis. But for now, the victories at Trenton and Princeton restored a glimmer of hope for the tattered Continental Army as it took up winter quarters at Morristown, New Jersey.

When Howe withdrew his forces from much of New Jersey, anxious civilians who had sworn their loyalty to the crown felt deserted. Public sentiment again swung toward the rebels. More importantly, news of the victories spurred support for the American cause overseas in France. Eager to see their powerful rival bogged down in a colonial war, the French dispatched secret shipments of munitions to aid the revolutionaries. One young aristocrat, the idealistic Marquis de Lafayette, was already on his way from France to volunteer his services to General Washington. But it took a larger show of success to draw forth an official French commitment to the American cause.

Breakdown in British Planning

Among the Americans, two years of grim conflict had dampened the initial zeal for rebellion that had prompted citizen soldiers to enlist. Washington believed that the armed resistance could scarcely continue unless many more men made longer commitments to fight. They needed better pay, he insisted, and tighter discipline. Congress members reluctantly agreed. Though opposed in principle to a professional standing army, Congress expanded the commander's disciplinary powers and approved a bonus for men who enlisted for three-year terms.

Faced with a slumping economy, numerous recruits answered the call, including recent immigrants and unemployed artisans. All lacked training, supplies, and experience; many also lacked immunity to smallpox. Most of the enemy soldiers had acquired immunity from the devastating disease in Europe by surviving frequent epidemics. In contrast, Washington's rural recruits came from isolated townships and had never been exposed to the disease. When smallpox broke out among the American soldiers at Morristown, the commander promptly ordered inoculation. Because the process brings on a mild case of the disease, he anxiously counted the days until his rebuilding army could be ready to fight. "If Howe does not take advantage of our weak state," Washington commented in April 1777, "he is very unfit for his trust."

Despite the Americans' vulnerability, the British were slow to move. By seeking both a decisive blow and a negotiated settlement in 1776, they had achieved neither objective. George Germain and his colleagues in Lord North's ministry had fallen victim to contradictions in their own cumbersome planning process. They had also underestimated the persistence of Washington's army. During the campaigns of 1777, the British learned further hard lessons about the difficulty of the task facing them and the need for tight coordination of plans.

General Burgoyne, returning to London for the winter, won government support for a major new offensive. He planned to lead a large force south from Canada via Lake Champlain, using the Hudson Valley to drive a wedge through the rebellious colonies. In support, a combined British and Indian force would strike east from Lake Ontario, capturing Fort Stanwix (east of modern-day Syracuse, New York) and descending the Mohawk River to meet Burgoyne at Albany. Howe would push north from New York City to complete the design.

But General Howe had formed a different plan. Assuming Burgoyne would not need his help in the Hudson Valley, he intended to move south against Philadelphia. The two generals never integrated their separate operations, and the results were disastrous. In one six-month span, the British bungled their best chance for victory and handed their enemies an opening that permanently shifted the course of the war.

Saratoga Tips the Balance

The isolated operations of Burgoyne and Howe got off to slow starts in late June 1777. Howe used up two months in moving his troops by sea from New York harbor to the headwaters of Chesapeake Bay. This delay gave the Americans time to march south to check the British advance on Philadelphia. But at the Battle of Brandywine Creek (September 11, 1777), Howe bested Washington once again, using the same flanking maneuver that had worked so well on Long Island the year before. The British general finally marched into Philadelphia in late September, only to find that the rebel Congress had retreated to York, Pennsylvania.

With pacifist Quakers and active Tories in the area, Washington could count on little support from local militia. Nevertheless, he launched a surprise attack against the large Hessian garrison at Germantown just north of Philadelphia on the morning of October 4. He hoped to repeat his previous success at Trenton. However, dawn fog created so much confusion that the inexperienced Patriot troops "ran from victory," according to American general Anthony Wayne. Yet as Washington led his battered army to winter quarters at nearby Valley Forge, the defeats at Brandywine and Germantown seemed worth the price. The Americans had gained needed combat experience and had made Howe pay heavily in men and in time for his hollow capture of Philadelphia. "Now," Washington wrote expectantly, "let all New England turn out and crush Burgoyne."

Moving south from Canada in late June, "Gentleman Johnny" saw little likelihood of being crushed. His huge army consisted of 7200 soldiers, with 1500 horses to haul baggage and heavy equipment. The British officers believed their force to be irresistible and foresaw little danger. General Burgoyne even brought his mistress along on the campaign. Weakened by tensions in their own command and knowing the British were on the march, the Americans fell back from Crown Point and Ticonderoga on Lake Champlain.

But as British supply lines lengthened, the crown's army grew less invincible. Burgoyne's soldiers were forced to expend valuable time cutting a roadway through the wilderness. Also,

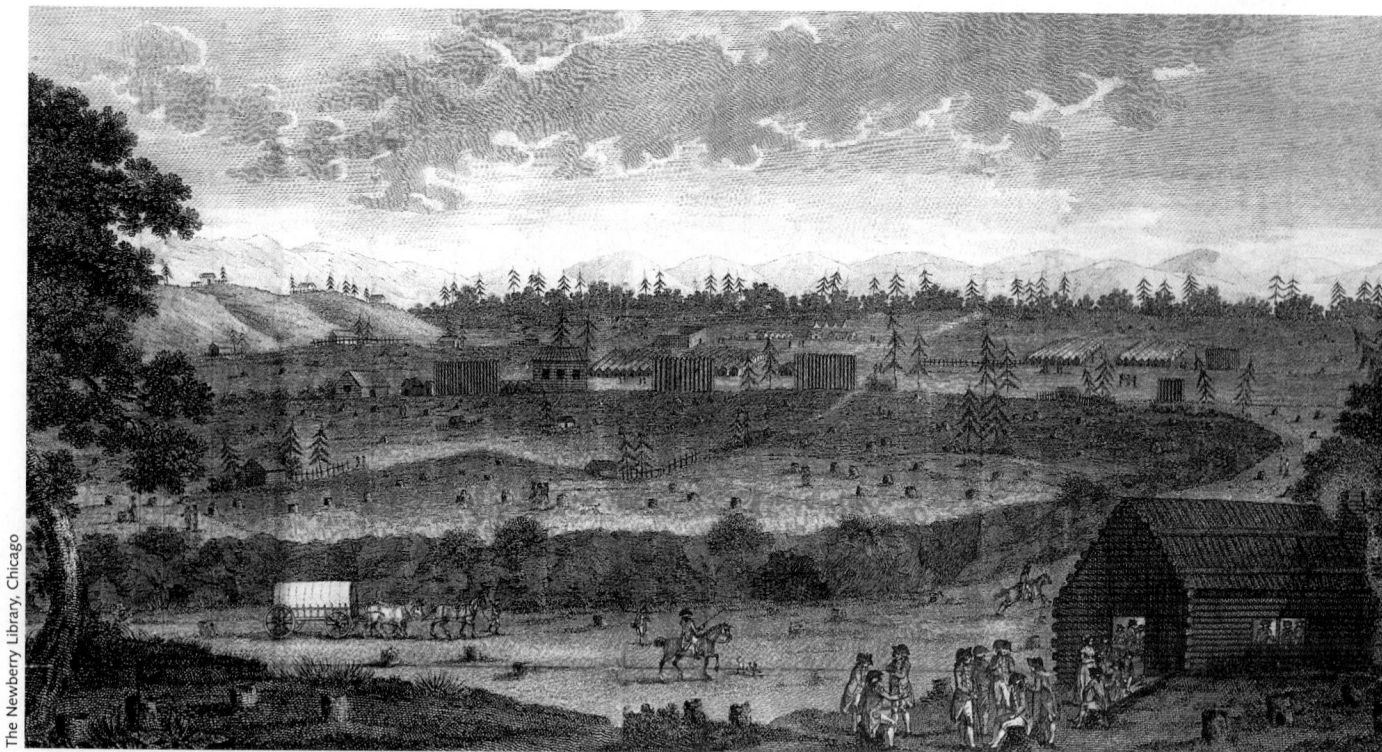

The Newberry Library, Chicago

■ The surrender of Burgoyne's army at Saratoga, New York, in October 1777 put more than 5000 British soldiers in American hands. Fearing that they would fight again if allowed to return to England, Congress ordered them held at this camp in Virginia until the end of the war. Many escaped and chose to settle in America.

the reinforcements anticipated from the west never arrived; Benedict Arnold turned them back at Fort Stanwix. Even worse, a British unit of 600 sent east to forage for corn and cattle was badly mauled by militia near Bennington. With cold weather approaching and his supplies dwindling, Burgoyne pushed toward Albany, unaware that Howe would not be sending help up the Hudson to meet him.

As Burgoyne's situation worsened, the American position improved. An arrogant British proclamation demanding submission from local residents only stiffened their resolve and drew out more rebel recruits. The Americans' strength grew to nearly 7000 in September after Congress gave command in the Hudson Valley region to Horatio Gates. The new general was an ambitious English-born officer who harbored resentments toward his American superior, Washington, and toward the much-admired Benedict Arnold. While Burgoyne's army crossed to the Hudson River's west bank at Saratoga, Gates's American forces dug in on Bemis Heights, 10 miles downstream.

On September 19, 1777, Patriot units under two aggressive officers, Benedict Arnold and Daniel Morgan, confronted the enemy at Freeman's Farm, not far from Saratoga. In the grueling battle, British forces suffered 556 dead or wounded, nearly twice the American losses. Gates's refusal to commit reinforcements prevented the Patriots from achieving total victory. Nevertheless, he claimed success and saw to it that his nemesis, Arnold, later lost his command.

In the weeks that followed, the American ranks swelled with new recruits who sensed a chance to inflict losses on Burgoyne's forces. On October 7, the beleaguered British tried once more to smash southward, only to suffer defeat in a second battle at Freeman's Farm. Morgan and Arnold once again played key roles, though Arnold suffered a crippling leg wound. When Burgoyne's entire army of 5800 surrendered at nearby Saratoga ten days later, Gates took full credit for the stunning triumph.

Uncanny Similarities: Britain's Vietnam?

Does history repeat itself? Never exactly, of course, yet sometimes the general similarities can be striking. This applies not only to small incidents but also to larger historical events such as the American Revolution. Consider the following six paragraphs:

The **British** had emerged victorious from a major world war just decades earlier. They took pride in their commercial dynamism, military strength, and cultural power. Also, they felt justifiably confident that their political institutions tended more toward liberty than those of their competitors. Still, step by step, they let themselves be drawn into a difficult conflict on a distant continent. At the time, the political and economic reasoning for entering combat made sense to most **British** leaders, especially because they were engaged in an ongoing struggle for global power with their major rival, **France.**

But **British** forces soon discovered that they were unable to exert their full military superiority. Instead, they needed to work incessantly to win the "hearts and minds" of the people (a phrase coined by John Adams). They found the population in the theater of war to be deeply divided politically, although it was often difficult to determine just who supported the **British** presence and who opposed it.

Commandeering local resources might alienate the very people they hoped to support. But supplying a large modern army with food and equipment across a wide ocean posed unprecedented logistical problems. Moreover, **British** recruits who had little personal stake in the conflict had to fight on unfamiliar terrain alongside soldiers of several nationalities. Career army officers found it difficult to maintain high morale among the **British** troops when facing a highly motivated citizen army opposed to colonialism of any kind.

France, the rival superpower, provided extensive support to the enemy's war effort to increase the capacity and willpower of a determined people's army. Officers, diplomats, and politicians in **France** hoped to keep large portions of the **British** army and navy tied up in a long and expensive war. That way, troops and resources were unavailable for engagements in other parts of the world.

At home, despite well-intentioned efforts, charges of corruption and inefficiency within the **British** bureaucracy and military establishment weakened the war effort. Opposition to the war slowly expanded within vocal portions of the **British** public. As casualties rose and the nation's deficit spending increased, the war became a divisive domestic issue. After years of fighting, successful enemy offensives underscored the army's weak position. The **British** concentrated their final efforts in the southern part of the country, where support remained strongest.

Finally, successive defeats (and a desire to protect **British** interests elsewhere in the world) prompted

Forging an Alliance with France

Ever since declaring independence, Congress had maneuvered to win international recognition for the new nation and aid for its military cause. While claiming neutrality, the Dutch supplied gunpowder for the rebellion through their West Indian island of St. Eustatius. In November 1776 they fired cannon there to salute an American ship—the first foreign acknowledgment of American sovereignty. Weeks later, Benjamin Franklin arrived in France as part of a commission sent to seek wider European support.

It was one thing for the Dutch Republic to recognize fellow republicans; it was quite another for the French king, Louis XVI, to endorse a revolution that opposed monarchy. Some in France, like the young marquis de Lafayette, felt enthusiasm for the American cause as an expression of rational enlightenment beliefs. But others, such as France's foreign minister, Comte de Vergennes, saw the colonists' revolt as an opportunity to avenge old grievances against Britain and undermine British power. Uncertain about the rebellion's chances for success, especially after the fall of Philadelphia, the government in Paris moved cautiously. It confined itself to substantial but covert assistance in the form of money and arms.

Word of the American victory at Saratoga suddenly gave Franklin more room to maneuver. When he hinted to the French that he might bargain directly with London for peace, Vergennes moved immediately to recognize American independence. France agreed to renounce

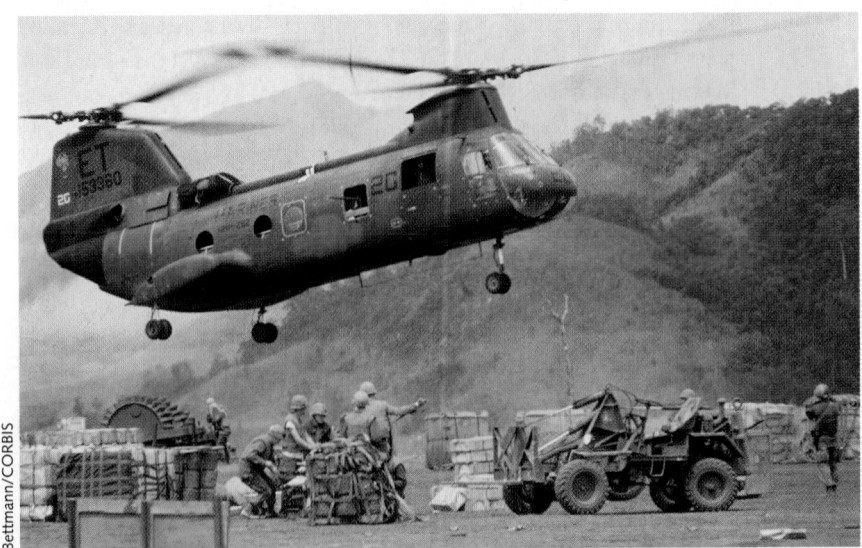

Bettmann/CORBIS

American soldiers in Vietnam, like the British in America two centuries earlier, had superior arms but faced huge logistical problems moving heavy supplies to a distant war zone.

the full-scale evacuation of the army. As the troops departed, they were accompanied by thousands of civilians who had remained loyal supporters. After nearly a decade, the **British** and their enemies negotiated a peace treaty in Paris, and the long war came to a conclusion. But ill will lingered between the

two countries for another generation before they finally resumed peaceful commerce.

This seems a brief and plausible overview of events, at least from a British perspective. But now try going over these six paragraphs again. This

time, for each use of the word *British* read *American,* and for *France* read *the Soviet Union.* Surprisingly, two centuries after the War of Independence, the United States found itself in a situation that bore remarkable similarities to the British position during the American Revolution. Again, a powerful English-speaking empire (this time an informal one) seemed to have overextended its reach across a western ocean.

Americans now have three decades of perspective on the Vietnam War. In a new generation that did not experience the conflict first-hand, many feel a keen interest in understanding its lessons. For historians, comparison is a traditional tool for such inquiry. They often seek out similarities between two historical people or episodes and then test the comparison, seeing where it works best, where it breaks down, and where it leads to new comparisons or deeper insights. Could learning more about Vietnam possibly help to put the American Revolution in a new light—and vice versa? ■

forever any claim to English land in North America, and Franklin promised that the Americans would help defend French holdings in the Caribbean. Both parties pledged to defend the liberty of the new republic, and each agreed not to conclude a separate peace with Great Britain or to cease fighting until U.S. independence had been ensured by formal treaty. In May 1778 the Continental Congress approved this alliance. The next month, France entered the war, adding its enormous wealth and power to the American cause. A year later, Spain—unwilling to ally itself directly with the upstart republic but eager to protect its vast American assets from Great Britain—entered the war on the side of France.

For the British, what had been a colonial brushfire swiftly flared into a global conflict reminiscent of the Seven Years' War. These new hostilities with France meant possible invasions at home. Equally worrisome, they meant inevitable attacks on outposts of Britain's empire around the world, from the Mediterranean Straits of Gibraltar to India's Bay of Bengal. Over several years, French ships seized Senegal in West Africa, took Grenada in the West Indies, and burned trading factories at Churchill and York on Hudson Bay. London's annual war expenditures climbed from £4 million in 1775 to £20 million in 1782.

As these costs mounted, British domestic opposition to the war in America intensified. Some members of Parliament pushed for a swift settlement. In 1778 a peace commission led by Lord Carlisle offered concessions to the Continental Congress, hoping to tear the French alliance apart. But the Carlisle Commission failed to win a reconciliation. Other Britons went

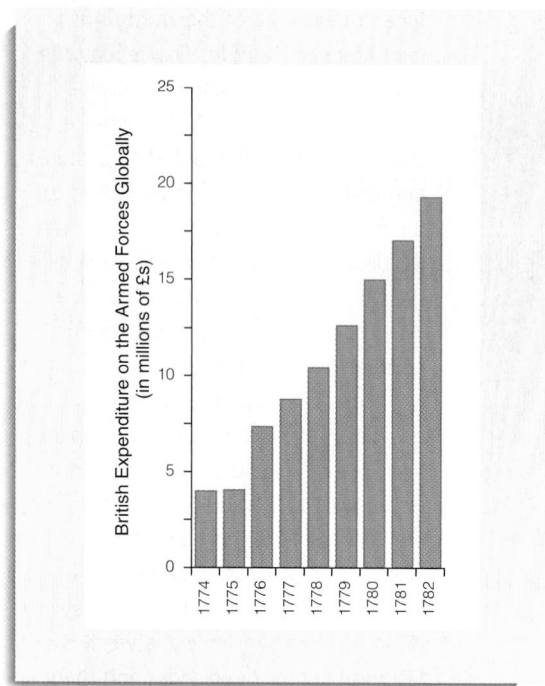

■ FIGURE 7.1
BRITISH GOVERNMENT EXPENSES ON ARMED FORCES
THROUGHOUT THE WORLD (IN MILLIONS OF POUNDS),
1775–1782   Britain's war budget soared after France
entered the conflict in 1778, but major resources flowed
toward India and the Caribbean, limiting the share available
for North America.

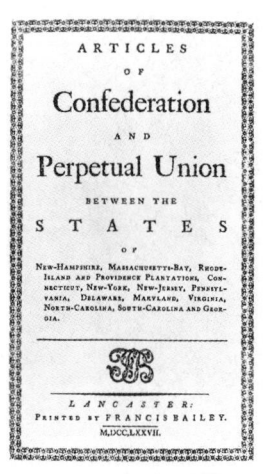

further in opposing the American war. Their diverse reasons included fear of French power, desire for American trade, disgust over war profiteering, hatred of government corruption, ties to friends in America, and idealistic belief in the revolution's ideals. They drank toasts to General Washington and openly supported the American cause.

Faced with growing economic and political pressure, the king and his ministers briefly considered withdrawing all troops from the rebellious colonies and focusing on the French threat. But instead, when General Howe resigned as commander-in-chief in America, they instructed his successor, Sir Henry Clinton, to retreat from Philadelphia to New York and devote his main resources to attacking the French in the Caribbean. Over the next four years, discontent within Britain continued to escalate, and no strategy proved sufficient to pacify the Americans or to crush their rebellion.

Legitimate States, a Respectable Military

E ven with a new French alliance in hand, the rebellious American states faced serious challenges on both the civilian and military fronts in the struggle to secure lasting independence. They had thrown out their colonial governors and embarked on a dangerous war, but two fundamental questions still confronted them: How would the once-dependent colonies govern themselves? And even if they devised new forms of self-governance, how could they shape a military force strong enough to defend themselves but not so unchecked as to overthrow their new civil governments? Their colonial experience had taught them to trust representative legislatures over strong executive authority. They had also learned another lesson: Any standing army, even one's own, could pose a danger if not under civilian control. For people who often cited ancient history, one well-known story drove this point home. Colonists knew how Rome's military commander, Julius Caesar, and his legion crossed the Rubicon in 49 B.C. and helped destroy the Roman Republic they had sworn to defend.

The Articles of Confederation

The Continental Congress that the rebelling states created had taken prompt initiative. Without clear authority, it had declared independence, raised an army, issued currency, borrowed money from abroad, and negotiated an alliance with France. Then it moved to bring greater stability and legitimacy to its work. In November 1777, one month after the victory at Saratoga, it approved Articles of Confederation and presented this formal plan for a lasting and unifying government to the states for ratification. In every region, citizens were already debating how much authority each new state government would have in relation to the larger federation. Who would have the power to levy taxes, for example, and who would control the distribution of land?

The Articles declared "The United States of America" to be a "firm league of friendship" between the 13 former colonies that had each become a new state. The final document proposed a weaker confederation than the one outlined in an earlier draft by John Dickinson. According to the finished charter, each state would retain its sovereignty and independence, plus all rights and powers not "expressly delegated" to the Confederation Congress. Indeed, it implied such a loose arrangement of states that the French considered sending 13 separate ambassadors to America. And several European proposals to end the war suggested negotiating separately with each state.

According to the Articles, Congress could not collect taxes or regulate trade; it could only requisition funds from the states. Their proportions would vary depending on relative population. Moreover, the Confederation had no separate executive branch; executive functions fell to various committees of the Confederation Congress. In addition, to the dismay of land speculators, the Congress would not control the western domains that several large states had claimed. Maryland, a small state without western claims, protested this arrangement and refused to ratify. To win approval, drafters changed the plan and granted the Confederation control of western lands. After four years, the Articles finally won ratification in 1781.

Given the importance of the states, the task of designing new state governments seemed a higher priority to many than inventing a confederation structure. Some leaders in the Continental Congress returned home to help implement this reconstruction process. In May 1776, for example, two of Jefferson's friends in the Virginia delegation in Philadelphia departed for Williamsburg. They left their younger colleague behind, but they carried his written draft for a possible state constitution. Those already at work in Virginia accepted Jefferson's proposed preamble, and on June 29, 1776, Virginia led the way, adopting the first republican state constitution.

Virginia had already pioneered in another respect. Two weeks earlier, Virginia representatives approved a Declaration of Rights drawn up by George Mason. In language anticipating Jefferson, Mason affirmed that "all men are by nature equally free and independent," possessing inherent rights "to the enjoyment of life and liberty, with the means of acquiring and possessing property, and pursuing and obtaining happiness and safety." He affirmed the revolutionary concepts that all power derives from the people and that magistrates are their servants. He went on to endorse trial by jury, praise religious freedom, and condemn hereditary privilege. Over the next eight years, each state adopted a similar bill of rights to enumerate the fundamental limits of government power.

Creating State Constitutions

Though diverse, the 13 states shared practical needs. Each had removed a functioning colonial government and needed to reestablish the rule of law under a new system. To do so, they drew on principles they had learned in the previous decade and on English common-law traditions. Britain possessed no written constitution, but the colonists had been ruled under published charters, and they shared a belief in the value of such clear and open arrangements. Thus they readily envisioned an explicit controlling document, or constitution, for each new state. Besides, the novel idea that government flowed from the people—as an agreement based on the consent of the governed—called for some all-encompassing, written legal contract.

A new written constitution, whether for a state or a union of states, represented something more fundamental and enduring than a regular law. It needed to be above day-to-day legal statutes and political whims. Somehow, the people, through chosen representatives, had to prepare a special document that citizens would affirm, or ratify, only one time. After the new government structure was in place, the constitution itself would be difficult, though not impossible, to change.

In 1779, Massachusetts legislators, under pressure from the public, fixed upon a method for providing the elevated status and popular endorsement for such a new document. Local voters in town meetings chose representatives for a specific constitution-drafting convention. These delegates, building on a model suggested by John Adams, crafted a suitable document, and their proposed constitution was then submitted to all the state's free men (regardless of race or property) for ratification. This widened constituency was intended to give special weight to the endorsement process.

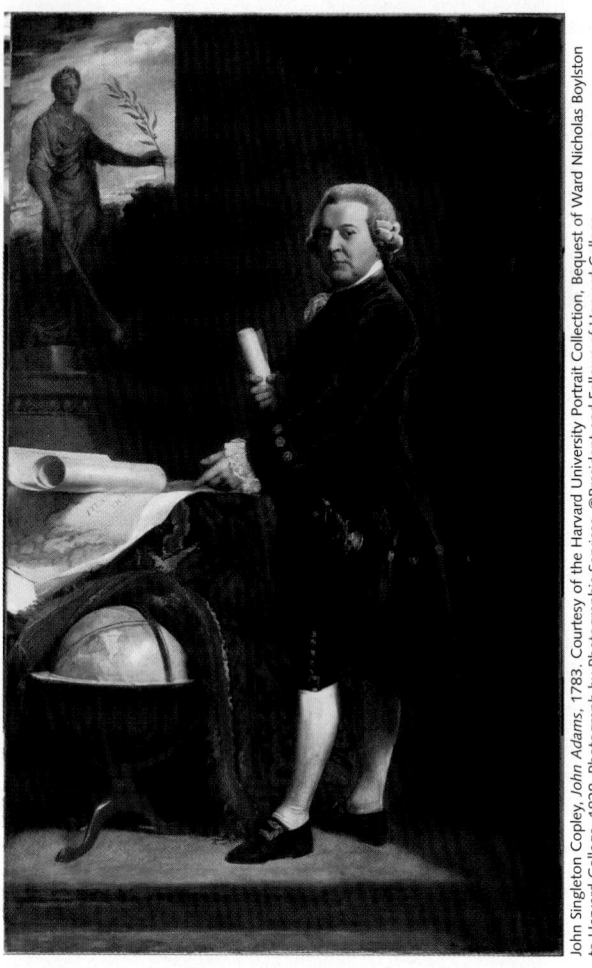

After independence, Americans had to create their own governments, and states experimented with new forms. John Adams of Massachusetts was part of a unique generation of lawyers who became skilled in the art of constitution-making.

John Singleton Copley, *John Adams*, 1783. Courtesy of the Harvard University Portrait Collection, Bequest of Ward Nicholas Boylston to Harvard College, 1828. Photograph by Photographic Services. ©President and Fellows of Harvard College

Approval of the Massachusetts document was hotly debated. Many objected to the limits on popular power that were part of Adams's novel design. A reluctant revolutionary, Adams had dismissed Tom Paine as "ignorant, malicious, short-sighted." He had even composed a tract titled *Thoughts on Government* to counter the democratic enthusiasm of Paine's *Common Sense*. In his pamphlet, Adams argued that "interests" (like-minded groups), rather than people, should receive equal representation. In addition, he proposed sharing legislative responsibilities between a house, a senate, and a chief executive. Property requirements for these offices were steep, so wealthy interests would have power far beyond their numbers. The Massachusetts state constitution, ratified by a narrow margin, implemented these ideas. They signaled a turn away from the strongest popular radicalism of 1776 and foreshadowed the more conservative balance of interests that Madison championed in the federal Constitution drafted in 1787.

This extended experiment in constitution writing was exhilarating and unprecedented. Never before in history, John Adams observed, had several million people had numerous opportunities "to form and establish the wisest and happiest government that human wisdom could contrive." Initial state efforts yielded varied results as citizens debated novel approaches to self-government. By 1780, the desire of prominent and well-established elites to rein in democratic power was evident. Yet in comparison to the overseas monarchy they had rejected, even the most conservative new state constitutions seemed risky and bold.

At least three common threads ran through all the documents. First, fearing executive might, drafters sharply curtailed the strength of state governors. These men no longer had the power to dismiss assemblies, raise armies, declare war, fill offices, or grant privileges. Colonial governors had been appointed from above, by proprietors or the crown, and they could serve terms of any length. In contrast, state governors would now be elected annually, usually by the assembly. Moreover, their service was subject to impeachment and controlled by term limits. In Pennsylvania, the most radical of the new constitutions did away with a single governor altogether, placing executive power in the hands of a 12-member council elected by the people.

Second, whether out of political belief or an effort to mobilize broad support for the revolutionary cause, drafters expanded the strength of the legislature and increased its responsiveness to the popular will. They enlarged the size of assemblies and increased the frequency of elections to allow greater local involvement. They also reduced property requirements for holding office and changed limits on the right to vote to allow wider participation.

Third, the constitution-makers feared the possible corruptions that came when people held more than one office at the same time. Having experienced these glaring conflicts of interest first-hand, they stressed the separation of executive, legislative, and judicial posts. The decision to prevent members of the executive branch from also holding a legislative seat removed any prospect for a cabinet-style government along the lines of the British model.

Tensions in the Military Ranks

A new republican order, whatever its nature, could not defend itself without a suitable fighting force. Just as defunct colonial administrations gave way to new state governments after serious debate, colonial militia companies transformed into state militia amid intensive arguments. In the state militias, and in Washington's army, controlled and paid by the Continental Congress, inevitable tensions emerged from the start. Heated discussions erupted as to what constituted equitable pay, appropriate discipline, suitable tactics, and a proper distribution of limited supplies. Others argued over whether wealth, popularity, vision, military experience, political savvy, European training, or influential ties should play a role in determining who received, or retained, the cherished right to command.

Two basic tensions underlay all of these debates. One involved the stresses arising between educated gentry and citizen soldiers when different, even opposing, social ranks joined in a coalition across class lines to confront a common enemy. The other concerned strains within the upper levels of society, as status-conscious members of the upper classes wrestled with what constituted appropriate service and recognition for men of their standing. Should they serve in the military at all, and if so, how much should they defer to older soldiers, seasoned frontiersmen, foreign-born officers, or civilian authorities without taking offense.

One heated topic involved the election of officers. Wealthy gentry assumed that they would command their state militia, while citizen soldiers demanded the right to choose their own leaders. Another source of tension concerned an old European tradition—the right of any prosperous individual to buy exemption from military service or to send a paid substitute. Back in December 1776, as Washington's army had retreated into Pennsylvania, militia in Philadelphia had chastised "Gentlemen who formerly Paraded in our Company and now in the time of greatest danger have turn'd their backs." They asked whether state authorities meant "to force the poorer kind into the field and suffer the Rich & the Great to remain at home?"

Three years later, some of these same Philadelphia militia, bitter that the burdens of the war always fell disproportionately on the poor, took part in what became known as the Fort Wilson Riot. Staging a demonstration in October 1779 spurred by soaring food prices, they intentionally marched passed the stately home of James Wilson, where wealthy Patriots had gathered. "The time is now arrived," the demonstrators' handbill proclaimed, "to prove whether the suffering friends of this country, are to be enslaved, ruined and starved, by a few overbearing Merchants,. . . Monopolizers and Speculators." Shots were exchanged, and six died in the melee at "Fort Wilson." (Wilson himself went on to become a leader of the 1787 Constitutional Convention.)

Subtle class divisions had also beset the Continental Army, where jealousies over rank plagued the status-conscious officer corps. Congressional power to grant military commissions, often on regional and political grounds, only intensified disputes. Also, Americans representing Congress abroad were empowered to promise high military posts to attract European officers. Some of these recruits served the American cause well, such as Johann de Kalb and Friedrich von Steuben (both born in Germany) and Thaddeus Kosciusko and Casimir Pulaski from Poland. In France, at age 19, the Marquis de Lafayette secured a commission to be a major general in America, and he assisted Washington impressively throughout the war.

However, other foreign officers displayed arrogance and spread dissension. Irish-born Thomas Conway, for example, courted congressional opponents of Washington and encouraged the desires of General Horatio Gates to assume top command. Whether or not a concerted "Conway Cabal" ever existed, Washington managed to defuse tensions from Valley Forge during the hard winter of 1777–1778. His numerous letters helped to patch frayed relations with Gates and consolidate his position with Congress.

Another rival for command of the army, English-born Charles Lee, met disfavor several months later, when Washington ordered him to attack the rear guard of Clinton's army as it withdrew from Philadelphia to New York. Lee mismanaged the encounter at Monmouth, New Jersey, on June 28, 1778, and only Washington's swift action stopped a premature retreat. The Battle of Monmouth ended in a draw, but American troops claimed victory and took pride in their swift recovery and hard fighting.

Shaping a Diverse Army

The army's improved effectiveness came in large part from the efforts of Friedrich von Steuben, a European officer recruited by Benjamin Franklin after charges of homosexuality disrupted his German military career. He had arrived at Valley Forge in February 1778, offering to serve without pay. There he found soldiers with poor food, scant clothing, and limited training. Many Americans still wanted to see a more democratic citizen army, with elected officers and limited hierarchy. But Washington hoped to mold long-term soldiers into a more "Europeanized" force, using stern discipline to train the Continental Line. Steuben provided the chance to do so. Shouting in several languages—he spoke no English—the newcomer worked energetically to drill soldiers who, in turn, trained others. A written drill manual was drawn up, and the strict training paid off. Alexander Hamilton, who observed the routine and later fought beside Steuben at Yorktown, wrote that "unquestionably to his efforts we are indebted for the introduction of discipline in the Army."

New discipline helped boost morale. Still, terms of service and wage levels remained sources of contention for American soldiers. So did the disparities in treatment and pay between officers and enlisted men. There were other grievances as well. Congressional committees overseeing the war effort appeared inept. Officers with political appointments frequently proved incompetent, and civilians often expressed indifference or hostility toward militia. A steady shortage of new recruits added to the frustrations of enlisted men.

Arguments also persisted over who could serve in the army. Women organized in diverse ways to assist the war effort, making uniforms and running farms and businesses for absent husbands. A few American women, such as Deborah Sampson of Massachusetts, disguised themselves as men and fought. Far more accompanied the troops to cook and wash in the camps. Earning scant pay, they carried water to the weary and wounded on the battlefield. Serving in these capacities, they formed a significant presence in both armies. For example, when Burgoyne launched his campaign from Canada, 2000 women accompanied his 7200 troops.

As many as 20,000 women, many of them wives, may have accompanied the American army during the war. Washington reluctantly accepted the presence of women in camp, reasoning that they freed men for "the proper line of their duty." Mary Hays, wife of a Pennsyl-

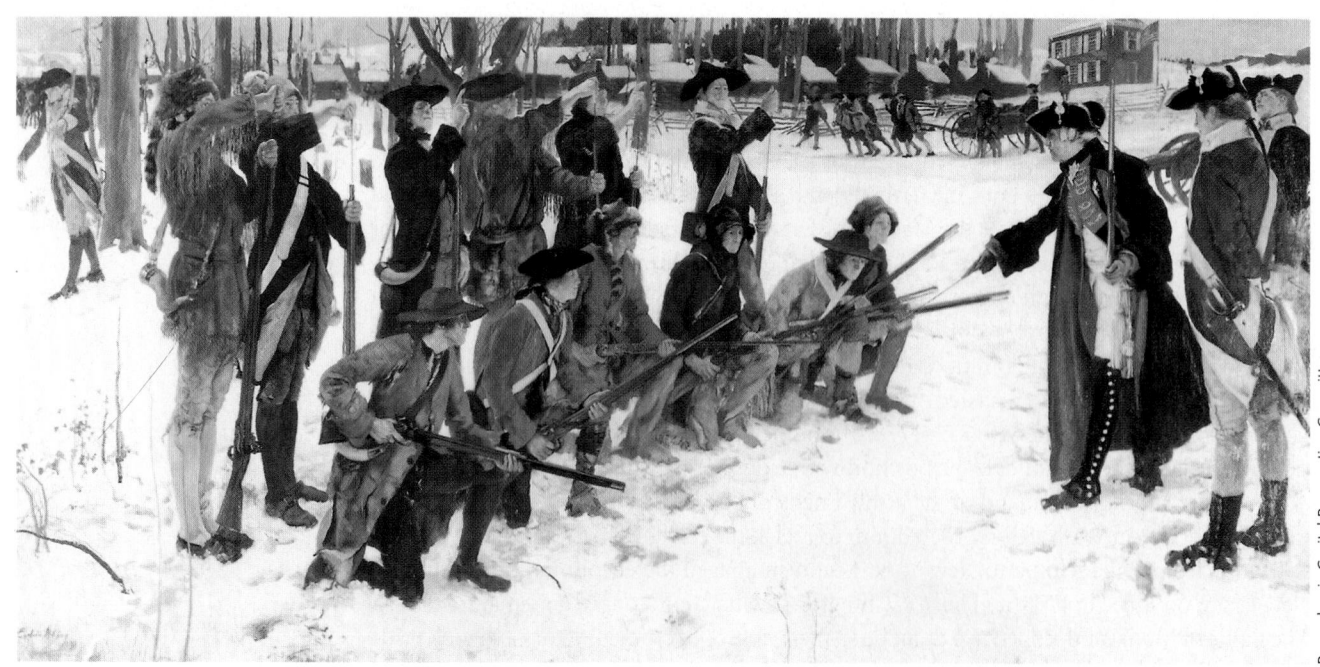

Pennsylvania Capitol Preservation Committee

■ More than a century after the grim winter at Valley forge, artist Edwin Abbey composed this mural of Steuben drilling Washington's soldiers in February 1778.

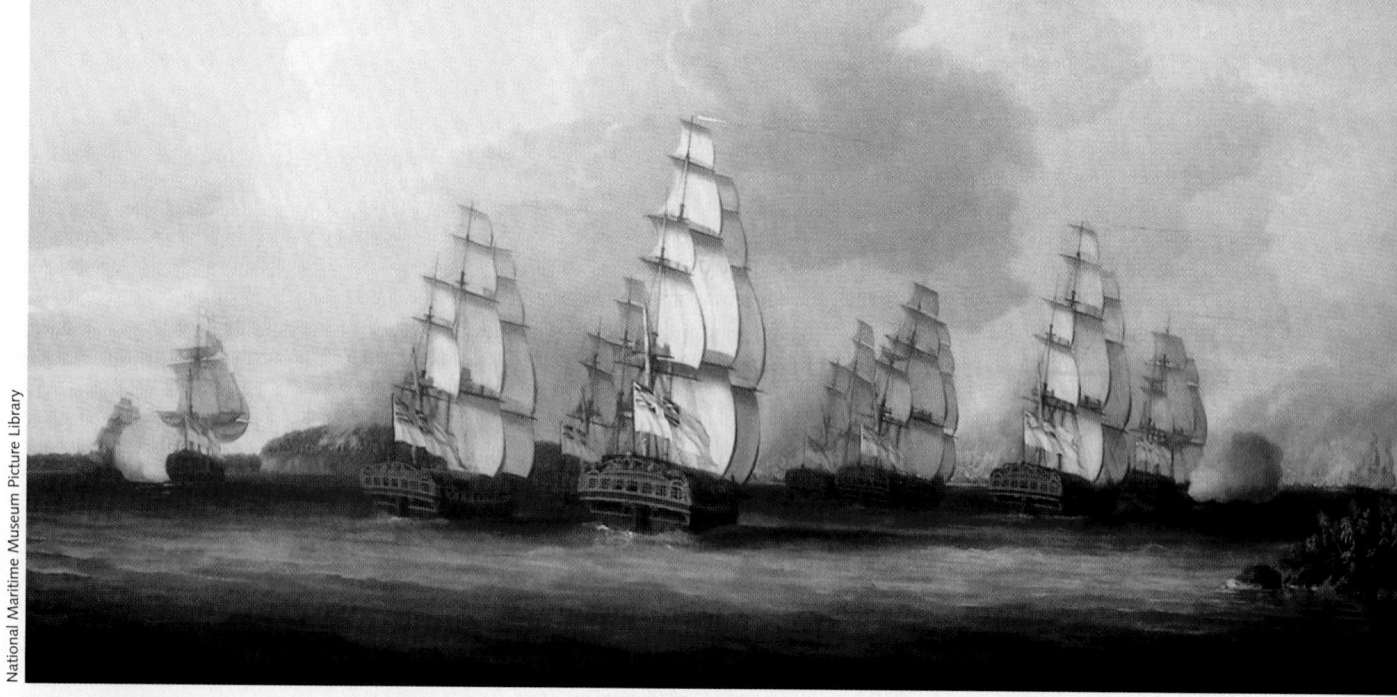

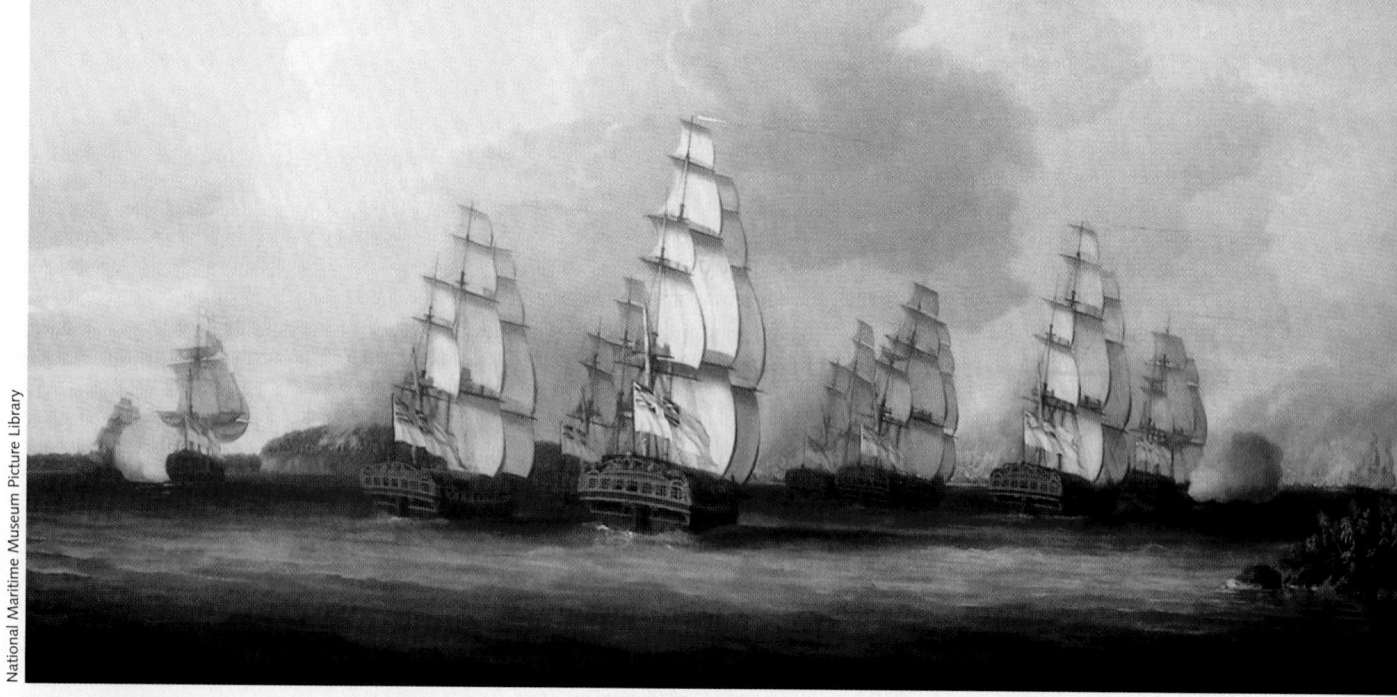

■ When British ships trapped an expedition from Massachusetts along the Maine coast in August 1779, the 40 American vessels retreated up the Penobscot River. Before fleeing into the woods, the crews set fire to their boats, creating a spectacular blaze. "When they Blew up," one sailor wrote, "Shott and Timber flew verey thick up and Down the River."

vania soldier, embodied the women's effort and commitment. She endured the winter at Valley Forge and later hauled pitchers of water on the battlefield at Monmouth. When her husband was wounded, she is said to have set down her jug and joined his gun crew, earning folk legend status as the cannon-firing "Molly Pitcher."

After petitioning to fight, free blacks were allowed to join the revolutionary army. Rhode Island even formed an African American regiment. But repeated proposals to arm southern slaves met with defeat. South Carolina and Virginia went so far as to move in the opposite direction, offering to give away slaves captured from Tory planters as a bonus to white recruits. Thus it is no surprise that thousands of enslaved people, especially in the South, risked their lives to escape to British lines.

The War at Sea

Even as the Americans' army grew into a respectable force, their lack of naval strength proved a constant disadvantage. As early as October 13, 1775, the Continental Congress had agreed to arm two vessels to prey on British supply ships on the Atlantic. In retrospect, the vote marked the birth of the American navy. At the time, however, many delegates still held out hope for reconciliation with Britain. Samuel Chase, a cautious lawyer from Maryland, thought a new navy would be large enough to provoke British resentment and retaliation but far too small to be effective. He objected that it was "the maddest Idea in the World to think of building an American Fleet."

Despite such objections, Congress promptly appointed a committee to acquire sailing craft for "protection and defense." Most of the 13 states built up their own small navies for local purposes, only adding to the confusion. The lack of central coordination proved deadly. When Massachusetts sent its ships "down east" along the Maine coast to challenge a Loyalist buildup at Castine in 1779, British vessels cornered the fleet at Penobscot Bay and crushed the enterprise.

Despite its strength, the British navy was stretched thinner as more European powers joined the fray: France in 1778, Spain in 1779, and Holland in 1780. The English feared possible invasion, and French corsairs harassed Britain's coastline, joined by American captains. One of these captains, a Scottish immigrant named John Paul Jones, arrived in European waters from America in early 1778, just as Franklin signed the pact with France. In April, Jones led a night raid on the port of Whitehaven in his native Scotland. He inflicted slight damage on the Irish Sea town, but the propaganda triumph of an American success in British waters proved huge. The brazen young captain won an even greater victory the next year off Flamborough Head on England's east coast. Jones and his crew—including men of 11 nationalities—were sailing an aged French ship named the *Bonhomme Richard* in tribute to Benjamin Franklin's "Poor Richard." In a fierce battle, they managed to board Britain's sleek new H.M.S. *Serapis* and capture the larger, heavily armed British frigate before their own vessel sank.

In all, the Continental Navy equipped more than 50 vessels and captured nearly 200 British craft as prizes. But these numbers pale in comparison to the activities of American privateers. More than a thousand private ship owners obtained licenses from Congress to seize enemy ships and divide the proceeds among themselves and their crew. With international commerce curtailed, shipowners and sailors were eager to try their luck at this tempting opportunity. Average pay aboard privateers was higher than on a government vessel, and discipline was less strict. In 1778 nearly 10,000 men were engaged in privateering aboard several hundred vessels. Their small, quick boats swarmed the Atlantic like troublesome gnats, frustrating England's mighty navy. According to one estimate, by war's end the British had surrendered 2000 ships, 12,000 men, and goods valued at £18 million. Moreover, because privateering drew merchant investors directly into the Patriot war effort, it helped bind the coastal elite more firmly to the American cause.

The Long Road to Yorktown

By July 1778, Clinton's British forces had returned to New York City, and their situation had not improved. Frustrated in New England and the middle tier of states, Clinton revived the southern strategy discussed at the beginning of the war. A southern plan offered numerous potential benefits. Because the region produced staple crops, it held more economic value for Britain than the North did. Less thickly settled than the North, the South was more vulnerable. In addition, it supposedly contained a wide array of Loyalists who would offer their support. The recently acquired colonies of East and West Florida had never rebelled, and the British army might win back Georgia and the Carolinas with a sufficient show of force. Success there would open up Virginia for reconquest.

Furthermore, the South's warm weather allowed longer campaigns and easier provisioning of troops. A lengthy growing season meant more fodder for the wagon horses and cavalry mounts so essential to any large military operation. The region's long Atlantic coastline, far from New England privateers, lay open to the British. Clinton knew that Washington's distant, land-based army would have trouble defending it. Moreover, nearly 500,000 enslaved African Americans posed a constant threat to Patriot planters and represented potential support for British invaders. Finally, the same whites who dreaded slave rebellion also feared war with Native Americans, as Jefferson had explained in the Declaration of Independence. So the possible use of Indian allies also entered Britain's strategic calculation.

Indian Warfare and Frontier Outposts

Most Native Americans in eastern North America remained loyal to the British during the Revolutionary War. Exceptions existed, such as the Oneida, Tuscarora, and Catawba, but Indians in many regions had long-standing grievances about the encroachments of colonial whites. In southern Appalachia, colonial land investors and settlers had defied the king's Proclamation

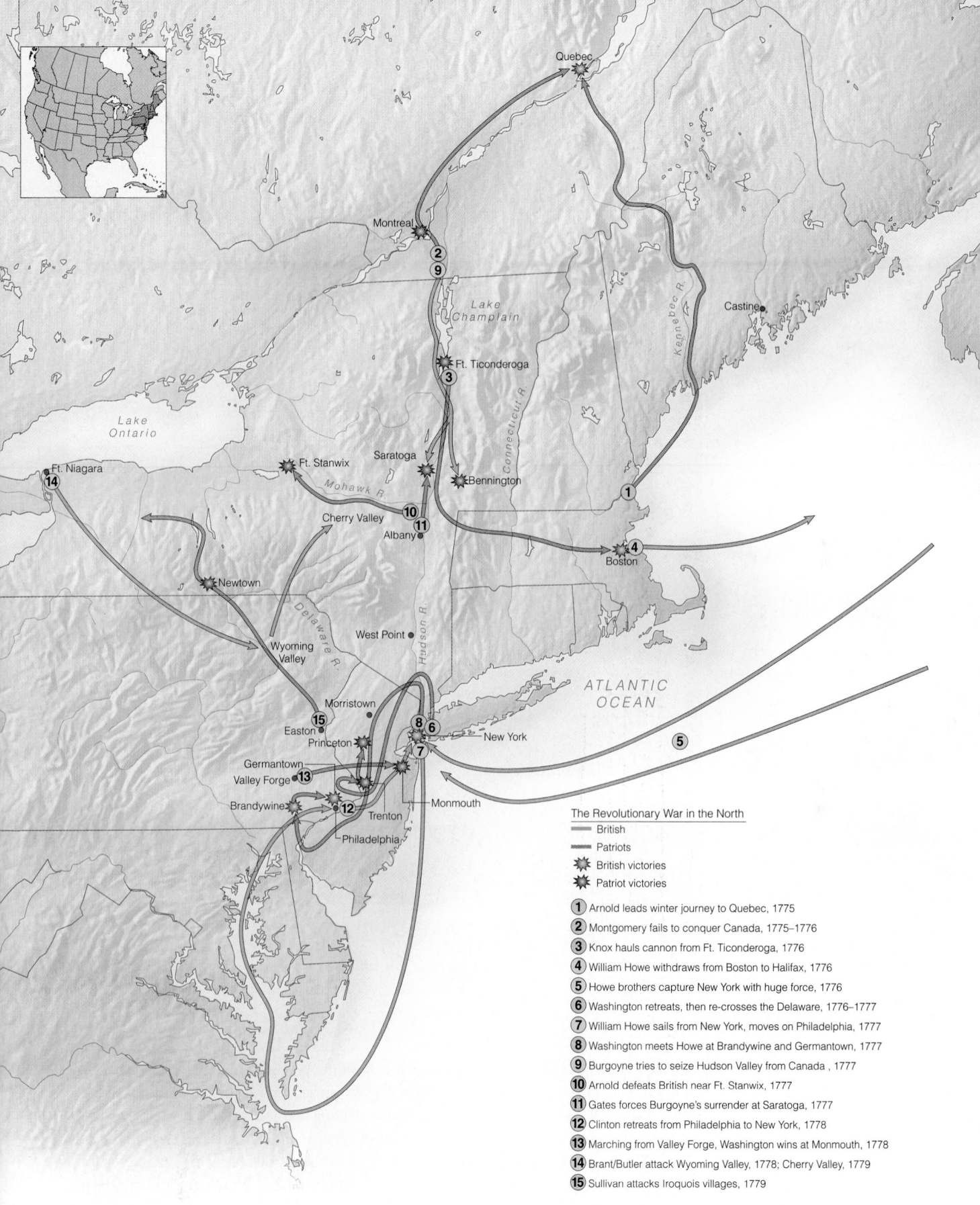

Quebec

Montreal

2
9

Lake
Champlain

Kennebec R.

Castine

Ft. Ticonderoga
3

Lake
Ontario

Connecticut R.

Ft. Niagara
14

Ft. Stanwix

Saratoga

Bennington

Mohawk R.

Cherry Valley

10
11

Albany

1

Boston
4

Newtown

Delaware R.

West Point

ATLANTIC
OCEAN

Wyoming
Valley

Morristown

Easton
15

Princeton

8 **6**

7

New York

5

Germantown

Valley Forge **13**

Monmouth

Brandywine

12

Trenton

Philadelphia

The Revolutionary War in the North

— British
--- Patriots
✹ British victories
✸ Patriot victories

1 Arnold leads winter journey to Quebec, 1775

2 Montgomery fails to conquer Canada, 1775–1776

3 Knox hauls cannon from Ft. Ticonderoga, 1776

4 William Howe withdraws from Boston to Halifax, 1776

5 Howe brothers capture New York with huge force, 1776

6 Washington retreats, then re-crosses the Delaware, 1776–1777

7 William Howe sails from New York, moves on Philadelphia, 1777

8 Washington meets Howe at Brandywine and Germantown, 1777

9 Burgoyne tries to seize Hudson Valley from Canada , 1777

10 Arnold defeats British near Ft. Stanwix, 1777

11 Gates forces Burgoyne's surrender at Saratoga, 1777

12 Clinton retreats from Philadelphia to New York, 1778

13 Marching from Valley Forge, Washington wins at Monmouth, 1778

14 Brant/Butler attack Wyoming Valley, 1778; Cherry Valley, 1779

15 Sullivan attacks Iroquois villages, 1779

■ **MAP 7.3**
THE REVOLUTIONARY WAR IN THE NORTH

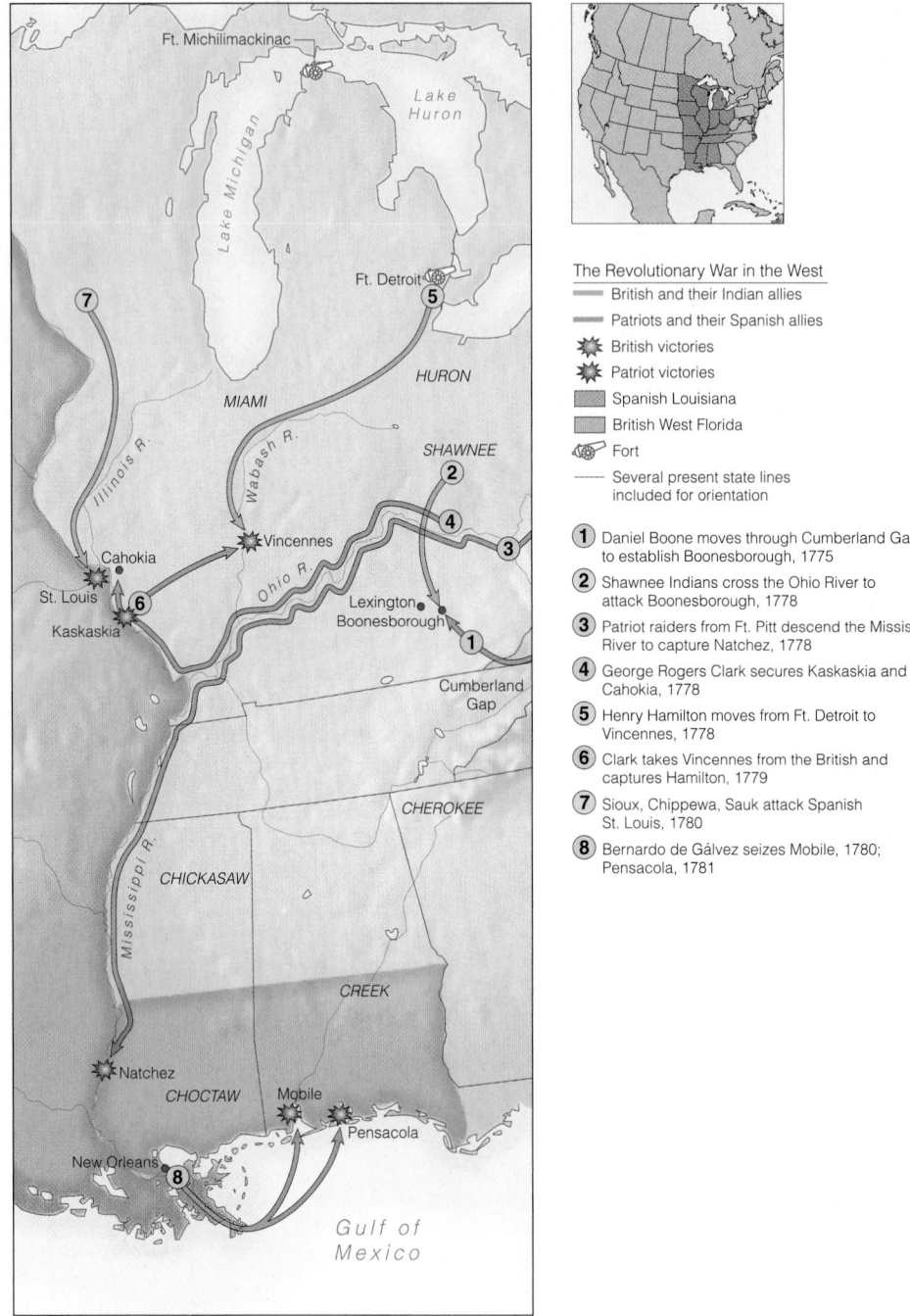

The Revolutionary War in the West
— British and their Indian allies
— Patriots and their Spanish allies
✦ British victories
✦ Patriot victories
▨ Spanish Louisiana
▨ British West Florida
⚙ Fort
---- Several present state lines
    included for orientation

① Daniel Boone moves through Cumberland Gap to establish Boonesborough, 1775

② Shawnee Indians cross the Ohio River to attack Boonesborough, 1778

③ Patriot raiders from Ft. Pitt descend the Mississippi River to capture Natchez, 1778

④ George Rogers Clark secures Kaskaskia and Cahokia, 1778

⑤ Henry Hamilton moves from Ft. Detroit to Vincennes, 1778

⑥ Clark takes Vincennes from the British and captures Hamilton, 1779

⑦ Sioux, Chippewa, Sauk attack Spanish St. Louis, 1780

⑧ Bernardo de Gálvez seizes Mobile, 1780; Pensacola, 1781

■ **MAP 7.4**
THE REVOLUTIONARY WAR
IN THE WEST

Line for more than a decade. At Sycamore Shoals on the Watauga River in 1775, North Carolina speculators led by Richard Henderson illegally purchased much of the Cherokees' territory. A young war chief named Dragging Canoe, defying his more conservative elders, vowed to turn the region into a "dark and bloody ground." True to his word, he laid siege to the new "Over-Mountain" Watauga settlement in July 1776. Whites struck back, organizing separate expeditions from four southern states. In all, 6000 troops pushed into the mountains, laying waste to Cherokee villages.

Meanwhile, Daniel Boone (an agent for Henderson) led settlers through Cumberland Gap in western Virginia to establish a fort on the Kentucky River at Boonesborough in 1775. By 1777, these pioneer families faced constant warfare against Indian adversaries who were fighting for their homelands. The Native Americans were also being urged on by Henry Harri-

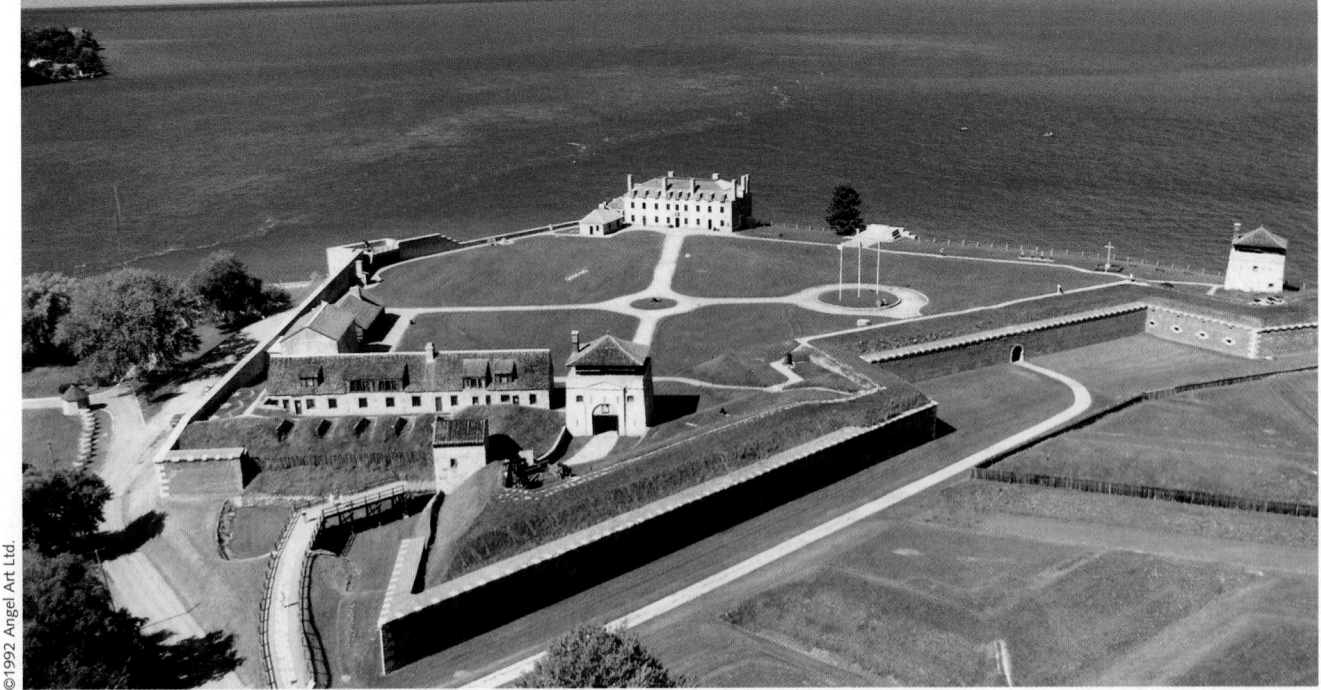

■ The British used Fort Niagara (on the southwest edge of Lake Ontario, at the mouth of the Niagara River) to launch attacks on American settlements and to shelter Indian allies. During the harsh winter of 1779–1780, 5000 Iroquois refugees, made homeless by the scorched-earth campaign of General John Sullivan, camped near the fort in five feet of snow.

son, the British commandant at far-off Detroit. In one six-month span, Harrison, who became known as the Scalp Buyer, received 77 prisoners and 129 scalps from this frontier warfare.

Along the upper Ohio, the violence escalated, despite efforts by Indian elders to maintain neutrality. Not all deaths occurred in battle. Americans killed Shawnee leader Cornstalk and his son during a truce in 1777. The next year, they murdered the neutral Delaware leader, White Eyes, although they had recently hinted to him and other Native Americans in Ohio Country that the Indians might one day "form a state" and have "representation in Congress." Four years later, at the village of Gnadenhutten (south of modern-day Canton, Ohio), militia from Pennsylvania massacred 100 peaceful Delaware men, women, and children who had been converted to Christianity by missionaries of the Moravian church.

By then, conflict had also flared farther north, much of it involving Native Americans. Joseph Brant, a mixed-race Mohawk leader educated in New England and loyal to the British, pushed south from Fort Niagara on Lake Ontario. Joined by a Loyalist band under John Butler, Brant and his men attacked poorly guarded frontier settlements. First in the Wyoming Valley of northeastern Pennsylvania and later in New York's Cherry Valley, the raiders killed hundreds of settlers.

In the summer of 1779, American General John Sullivan, fresh from fighting the British in Rhode Island, received a new assignment: lead a punitive campaign to annihilate Indian towns as a reprisal for the Cherry Valley slayings. His revenge-minded army of more than 4000 marched into Iroquois Country, pushing aside resistance from Brant and Butler at Newtown (Elmira, New York). Sullivan's troops destroyed 40 villages of the four tribes in the Iroquois Confederacy most linked to the British cause: the Mohawk, Onondaga, Cayuga, and Seneca. They avoided towns of the two Iroquois groups sypathetic to the Americans—the Oneida and Tuscarora—but elsewhere they chopped down orchards, torched crops, burned 160,000 bushels of corn, and sent several thousand Indian refugees streaming toward Fort Niagara. Hunger and retaliatory raids haunted the region until the end of the war.

While the British were passing arms and supplies to the divided Iroquois Confederacy through Fort Niagara, they were also using several western posts to arm other Indian allies and seek an advantage in the interior. Soldiers at Fort Michilimackinac recruited Sioux, Chippewa, and Sauk warriors for an unsuccessful attack on Spanish-held St. Louis in 1780. At Fort Detroit, Harrison continued to equip war parties of Ottawa, Fox, and Miami Indians to attack American settlers migrating into the Ohio Valley.

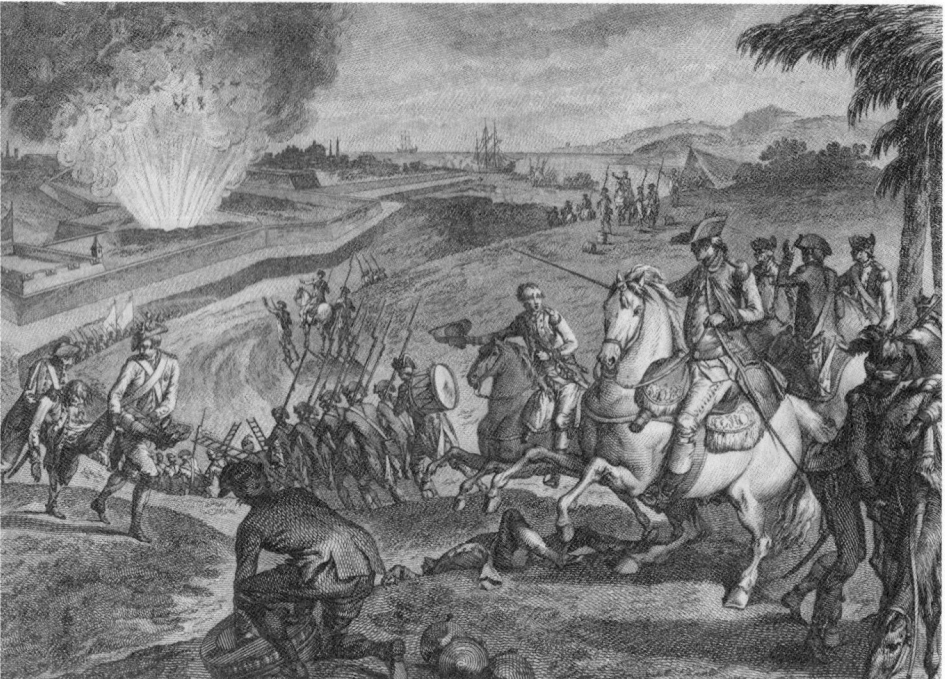

■ In 1781, 7600 Spanish and French troops under Bernardo de Gálvez laid siege to Pensacola. The turning point came on May 8, when a Spanish shell struck the British powder magazine. The explosion left 100 dead or wounded (many of them Pennsylvania Loyalists), and the British promptly surrendered the port and all of West Florida.

In 1778, with support from his home state of Virginia, a young Patriot surveyor named George Rogers Clark organized a foray west to counter these raids and lend support to Spanish and French allies in the upper Mississippi Valley. He secured the settlements at Kaskaskia and Cahokia on the Mississippi River, and in February 1779 he led a grueling winter march to the fort at Vincennes in southern Indiana. In surprising that outpost on the Wabash River, Clark managed to capture Henry Harrison, but he failed to seize Detroit.

The Unpredictable War in the South

The rebel war effort beyond the Appalachian Mountains also expanded south. In 1778 a Patriot party setting out from Fort Pitt managed to descend the Ohio and Mississippi rivers unnoticed. The raiders captured Natchez on the Lower Mississippi and seized property in British West Florida. But it was the energetic governor of Spanish Louisiana, Bernardo de Gálvez, whose moves proved decisive. Living in New Orleans, Gálvez maintained a careful neutrality between the Americans and their British rivals through 1778. But when Spain allied with France and declared war on Britain the next year, the governor acted quickly to keep the British from gaining ground on the Gulf Coast.

Moving from west to east, Governor Gálvez drove the British from the Mississippi River in 1779, seized their fort at Mobile in 1780, and conquered Pensacola, the capital of British West Florida, in 1781. His plan to retake St. Augustine with American help came to nothing. Still, his troops had reasserted Spain's control over the entire Gulf Coast and protected Spanish interests in the Gulf of Mexico. The fall of Mobile and Pensacola also cut British supply lines to the southeastern interior. The move hurt Creeks and Cherokees, who depended on their ally's assistance. Without additional guns, knives, and powder, the Indians could offer little assistance in Britain's ambitious plan to win back the South and regain the upper hand in the war for eastern America. It was support the British could ill afford to lose.

Still, the crown's forces regained control of most of Georgia from the rebels in 1778. The next year, they blocked American and French efforts to retake Savannah. Early in 1780, British generals Clinton and Cornwallis ferried troops by sea from New York to South Carolina aboard more than a hundred ships. By May, this army had isolated Charleston and forced the capitulation of 5500 American troops. The surrender was the largest loss of American men and

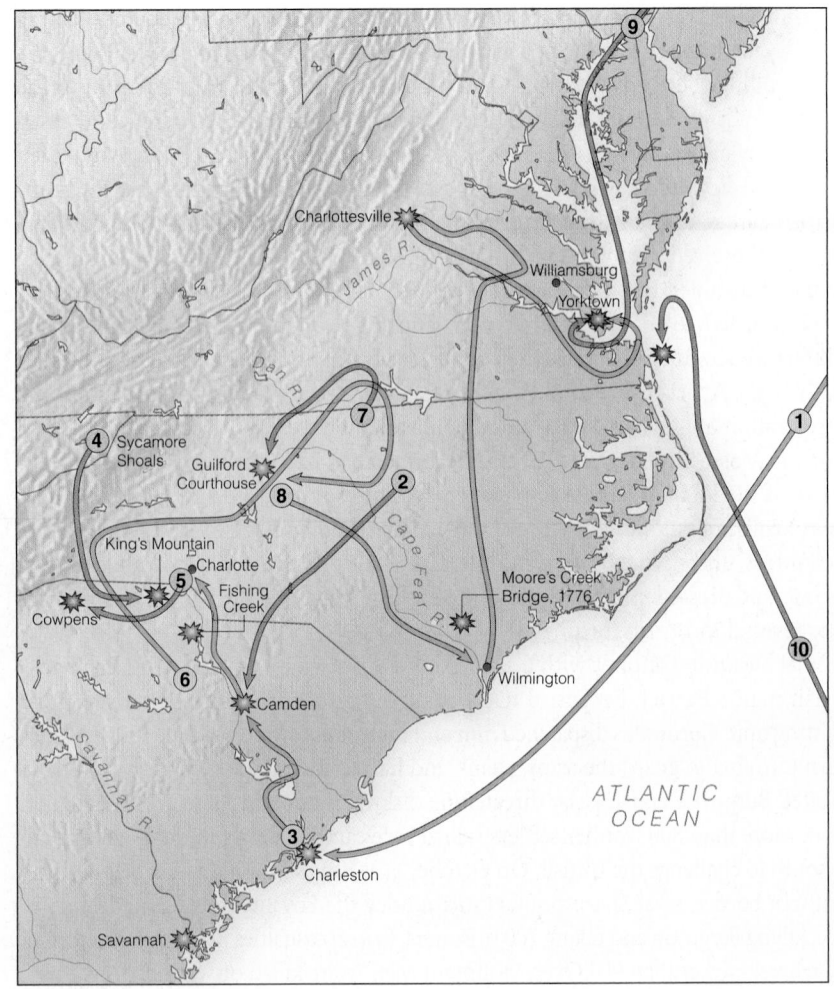

The Revolutionary War in the South

- British and their Loyalist allies
- Patriots and their French allies
- 💥 British victories
- 💥 Patriot victories

1 Clinton and Cornwallis force surrender of Charleston, May 1780

2 Gates moves the American army to Camden, August 1780

3 Cornwallis bests Gates at Camden and moves North, August 1780

4 Americans defeat Ferguson at Kings Mountain, October 1780

5 Morgan meets British at Cowpens, defeats Tarleton, January 1781

6 Cornwallis pursues Greene's army across the Dan River, February 1781

7 Greene confronts Cornwallis at Guilford Courthouse, March 1781

8 After a retreat to Wilmington, Cornwallis moves to Virginia, April 1781

9 Washington moves south, pins Cornwallis at Yorktown, August 1781

10 De Grasse from West Indies, defeats the British fleet, September 1781

■ **MAP 7.5**
THE REVOLUTIONARY WAR IN THE SOUTH

weapons during the entire conflict. (Not until the Civil War—at Harpers Ferry, Virginia, in 1862—and World War II—at Bataan in the Philippines in 1942—were comparable numbers of U.S. Army soldiers obliged to lay down their arms.) For disappointed Patriots, the fall of Charleston nearly offset the triumph at Saratoga. One soldier wrote that the defeat delivered "a rude shock to the Independence of America."

A confident Clinton returned to New York, leaving Cornwallis in command in South Carolina. Throughout that summer, fierce fighting erupted across the state. Banastre Tarleton's green-coated British dragoons (mounted troops), along with their Loyalist supporters, went head to head against the guerrilla bands led by Thomas Sumter, Andrew Pickens, and Francis Marion. In June, Congress appointed Horatio Gates to take command of southern operations, and he hurried to the Carolinas with fresh troops.

On August 16, 1780, in a poorly calculated move, Gates's army confronted Cornwallis at the South Carolina garrison town of Camden, 120 miles north of Charleston. The Americans, short on rest, food, and leadership, suffered another huge defeat. The British killed or wounded eight hundred and took a thousand prisoners. Two days after the Camden disaster, as Gates fled north ahead of his troops, Tarleton's cavalry landed another blow. They surprised Sumter's band of 800 partisans at Fishing Creek near the Catawba River and took 300 prisoners. The dragoons inflicted 150 casualties and freed several hundred Loyalists and British regulars while suffering almost no losses themselves.

That September, as Washington absorbed word of the defeats at Camden and Fishing Creek, he received yet another "rude shock." Benedict Arnold—in command of West Point, the key outpost controlling the Hudson River—had plotted to defect and yield the post to the British. A gifted and admired leader in battle, Arnold was also brash, self-centered, and easily affronted. Troubled by his war wounds and passed over by Congress for promotion, Arnold felt increasingly alienated from the Patriot cause. His scheme was revealed by the American capture of his British contact, Major John André. The major was hanged as an enemy spy, but Arnold escaped and received command of British troops.

These setbacks troubled not only General Washington but also Congress. Its members stood firmly committed to maintaining civilian control over the American army. They appointed military leaders and supervised their funds, reviewing countless problems of the war effort on a daily basis. Apart from Arnold's treason, Congress rarely faced disloyalty among officers, but frustration and disobedience among enlisted men were more common. Early in 1780, soldiers from Massachusetts, New York, and Connecticut had mutinied in separate incidents. Members of the Pennsylvania and New Jersey Lines soon staged similar strikes over disputed terms of enlistment. After five years of war, a harried Congress also faced soaring inflation, scarce resources, and sinking citizen morale. Cornwallis had reason for optimism as he divided his troops and pressed into North Carolina in the fall of 1780. But the next 12 months saw a dramatic reversal in British fortunes.

That reversal began in October with a surprising Patriot victory in the southern backcountry. British major Patrick Ferguson had organized South Carolina Loyalists into a successful fighting unit. Cornwallis dispatched him and his troops toward the Blue Ridge Mountains in western Carolina to guard the army's flank and harry rebel supporters. Overconfident, Ferguson repeated Burgoyne's mistake by threatening disloyal mountain settlers with hangings and retribution. More than 800 frontier settlers rallied at Sycamore Shoals in the Watauga Valley and raced south to challenge the British. On October 6, at King's Mountain just below North Carolina's southern border, these sharpshooters surrounded the Loyalist troops and decimated the entire force, killing Ferguson and taking 700 prisoners. British casualties in the one-sided affair exceeded 300, whereas fewer than 90 "Over-Mountain Men" were killed or wounded.

The Final Campaign

A shrewd change in leadership followed the American victory at King's Mountain. Congress realized its mistake in appointing Gates to the southern command, and it turned to Washington to suggest a replacement. He selected Nathanael Greene, an experienced Rhode Islander who soon proved more than a match for Cornwallis. General Greene arrived in Charlotte, North Carolina, in December 1780, taking charge of a tattered army of 1600. The British, stung by their losses at King's Mountain, postponed designs on North Carolina. This gave the new commander precious weeks to reorganize his American force.

Greene used his time wisely. Earlier, he had served as the army's quartermaster general, overseeing supplies, and he quickly realized that his soldiers had pressing needs. He swiftly ordered one town to make shoes for his men, another to sew uniforms. He also dispatched scouts to explore possible river crossings and paths of retreat, necessary for the elusive "fugitive war" he planned to conduct. Shocked by the violence of partisan warfare and conscious of the need to win public support, he urged restraint on such experienced guerrilla fighters as Sumter and Marion while weaving them into his overall plans.

Going against traditional practice, Greene decided to divide his small army and send half his men into South Carolina under the seasoned Daniel Morgan to harass the British flank. "It makes the most of my inferior force," he explained, "for it compels my adversary to divide his, and holds him in doubt as to his own line of conduct." Cornwallis took the bait and dispatched Tarleton in pursuit. He caught up with Morgan at Hannah's Cowpens, west of King's Mountain, on January 17, 1781.

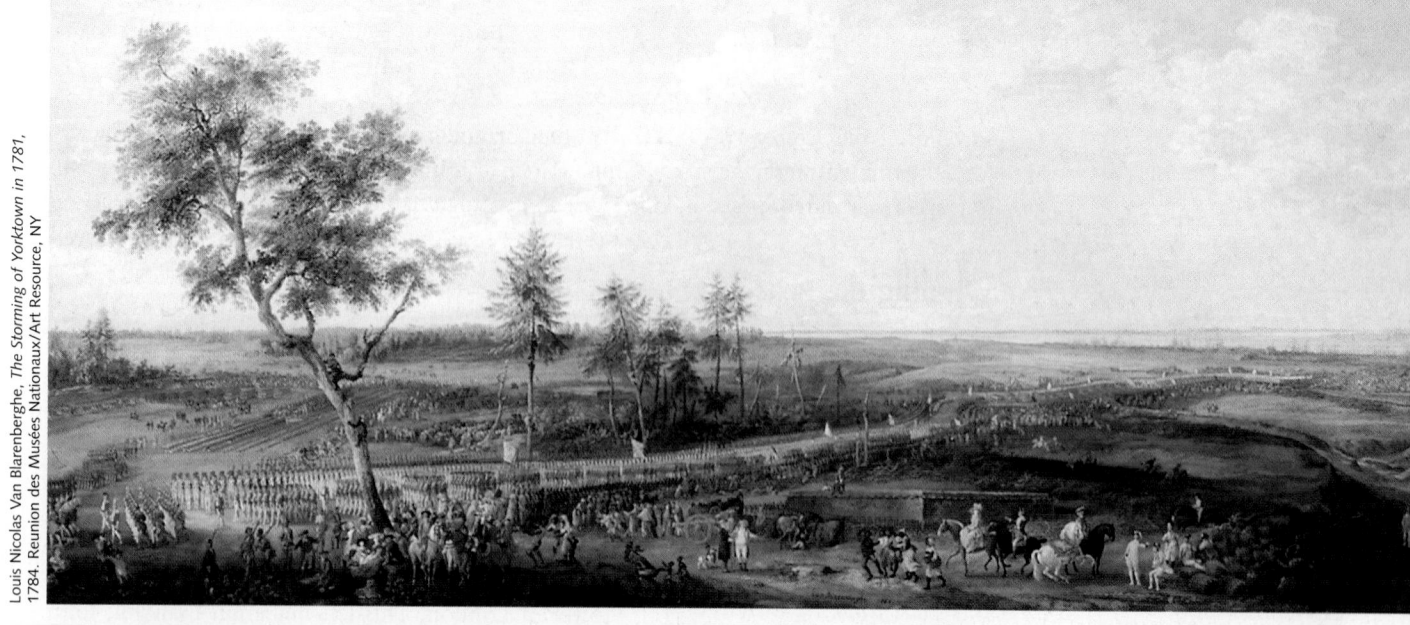

Louis Nicolas Van Blarenberghe, *The Storming of Yorktown in 1781*, 1784. Reunion des Musées Nationaux/Art Resource, NY

■ The joint American-French victory at the siege of Yorktown, Virginia, in October 1781 ended British hopes for preventing American independence. As Cornwallis's troops marched out to lay down their arms, a band played "The World Turned Upside Down." "Finally," Lafayette wrote proudly, "everything came together at once, and we had a sensational turn of events. . . .The play is over."

The outnumbered rebel militia lacked experience and discipline, but Morgan shrewdly turned this weakness to an advantage at the Battle of Cowpens. He stationed the militia units in front of his Continental forces with orders to fire two rounds and fall back. Sensing an enemy retreat, the British force of 1100 advanced too far too fast. Morgan's men promptly overwhelmed them. Tarleton managed to escape, but he left behind 100 dead, 800 prisoners, and most of his horses and ammunition. Morgan's force suffered only 148 casualties, mostly wounded militia. He rightly called the battle of Cowpens "a devil of a whipping."

Though frustrated, Cornwallis clung to the belief that "a successful battle may give us America." He discarded all excess baggage and pursued the rebel army 200 miles across North Carolina. Greene directed a speedy retreat over swollen rivers to the Virginia border, then doubled back to confront the weary British in the Battle of Guilford Courthouse on March 15. Although the American forces eventually withdrew from the field, Cornwallis sustained such heavy losses that he was forced to alter his plans.

The British retreated to the coast at Wilmington, North Carolina, and then marched north in early summer 1781 to Yorktown, Virginia. There, Cornwallis hoped to obtain reinforcements by sea, rally Loyalists in the Chesapeake region, and divide the rebelling colonies once and for all. The design's success hinged on continued naval superiority and timely support from General Clinton in New York. But Cornwallis could be assured of neither.

In mid-August, the French fleet in the Caribbean set out for Chesapeake Bay. It planned to spend eight weeks in American waters, assisting the combined French–American army, located near New York. "Employ me promptly and usefully," French admiral De Grasse urged, so that "time may be turned to profit." Suddenly Washington had access to impressive naval power. He seized his chance. He sent word south to Lafayette in Virginia to keep Cornwallis contained at Yorktown. Then, to hold Clinton's forces in New York, he ordered his men to make a show of building roads and baking ovens, as if preparing for a lengthy siege of the city. Behind this disguise, French and American soldiers slipped away, secretly marching south to lay a trap for the British army.

De Grasse reached Chesapeake Bay with two dozen ships at the end of August. On September 5, he repulsed a British fleet off the mouth of the bay, dashing Cornwallis's hopes for relief by sea. When 9000 Americans and 7800 French converged on Yorktown in late September, they outnumbered their 8000 opponents by more than two to one. The trap had been sprung, and the siege proved brief. Plagued by sickness and shortages of food and munitions, the British army surrendered on October 19, 1781. For Washington and his army, Yorktown was a stunning victory. Intermittent warfare continued for another year. But the Americans finally had powerful leverage to bargain for peace and force Britain to recognize their independence.

Winning the Peace

After Yorktown, the fighting in America gave way to diplomacy in Europe. Indeed, the final phase of the war played out in European courts. There, the maneuvering was almost as complicated and risky as it had been on the battlefield. As one representative, the American Congress dispatched Henry Laurens, its former president, to the Dutch Republic. The South Carolinian was to negotiate a loan and a commercial treaty with the United Province of the Netherlands, but the British captured Laurens at sea. They salvaged the incriminating documents Laurens tried to throw overboard and then locked him in the Tower of London. This left Benjamin Franklin, John Adams, and John Jay as the key American players. Often at odds, the three men nevertheless managed to achieve a final triumph that proved as unlikely and momentous as Washington's victory in Virginia. They did it, wrote the immodest Adams, "in spite of the malice of enemies, the finesse of Allies, and the mistakes of Congress."

For the British, the road to the peace table had been long and unpleasant. Early feelers about a negotiated settlement—from the Howes in 1776 and the Carlisle Commission in 1778—had not mentioned independence. But conditions changed drastically after Yorktown. Domestic unrest in Britain had already boiled into riots, and the expanded war was going poorly in India and the West Indies. "O God, it is all over!" Lord North muttered when he received the news of Cornwallis's defeat in Virginia. Within months, Sir Guy Carleton replaced Clinton in command of the remaining British forces in America, the hawkish Lord Germain stepped down from the Cabinet, and North resigned after 12 years as prime minister. Even the king spoke briefly of abdicating. But instead, he approved a new ministry more suited to the rising antiwar sentiment in Parliament. The Earl of Shelburne became prime minister in July 1782. Even before he assumed office, he had authorized peace discussions with his old acquaintance, Benjamin Franklin.

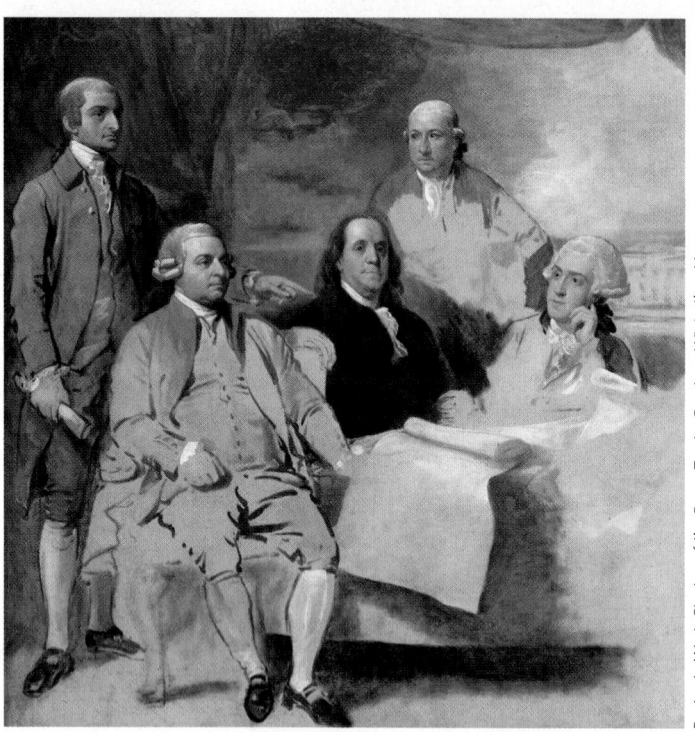

■ The final American victory in the War of Independence came at the peace table, when negotiators John Jay, John Adams, and Benjamin Franklin won favorable terms in the 1783 Treaty of Paris. Benjamin West's unfinished painting also includes the absent Henry Laurens (rear) and Franklin's grandson (right), the delegation's secretary.

Benjamin West, Signing of the Peace Treaty. Courtesy, Winterthur Museum

Franklin was in a difficult position. The crucial alliance he had negotiated with France stated that the Americans would not sign a separate peace with Britain. Moreover, Congress, grateful for vital French military and financial support, had instructed the American negotiators to defer to the wishes of Vergennes, the French foreign minister. The Americans did not realize that the minister's own agenda differed sharply from their own. Balancing the desire to reduce British power against the crippling costs of the war, Vergennes had already entertained thoughts of a truce that would leave London in control of all the territory it currently held in America. This consisted of Penobscot Bay in Maine (with its valuable supplies of naval timber), New York City, and parts of the lower South. Vergennes opposed the Americans' republican principles, and he resented their desire to expand their boundaries and gain the right to fish the Grand Banks off Newfoundland. He refused to treat the American diplomats as equal partners. To strengthen the French position, he also hoped to keep the weak new governments dependent on France whether the American states remained united or broke apart, as most European observers thought likely.

The American peace commission, though cautioned from home and belittled abroad, ultimately elected to chart its own course. The three commissioners fared surprisingly well in the treacherous waters of European diplomacy, starting with Franklin's first informal talks with the British. He laid out four "necessary" points, leading with the recognition of American independence. To this he added the removal of British troops, the right to fish in Newfoundland waters, and the revision of the Canadian border, which the Quebec Act of 1774 had pushed south to the Ohio River.

Franklin then noted some "desirable" items, no doubt intended to position the Americans for later bargaining. The British, he suggested, should consider paying an indemnity for war damages. In doing so, they would officially acknowledge their own blame for the war. Perhaps they should cede Canada to the United States as well. For their part, the British sought compensation for the American Loyalists who had been driven from their homes and the right to collect old debts that colonists had owed to British merchants before 1776.

After helping Washington at Yorktown, French admiral De Grasse had sailed back to the Caribbean to seize Great Britain's wealthiest colony, Jamaica. But British admiral George Rodney had intercepted his ships and taken De Grasse prisoner. Word of the naval victory strengthened Britain's negotiating hand and weakened France's position. Hoping to disrupt the American–French alliance and to reestablish profitable trade with their former colonies, the British negotiated preliminary peace terms with the Americans in November 1782. In return for independence, troop withdrawal, and fishing rights, the Americans agreed vaguely that their Congress would "recommend" that individual states approve compensation for confiscated Loyalist property.

On the Canadian boundary question, the Americans scored another success, but one that came at the expense of Indian nations. By giving up their bid for all of Canada, the negotiators persuaded Britain to relinquish the Ohio Valley and accept a northern boundary for the United States defined by the Great Lakes and the St. Lawrence River. In the west, the United States would reach to the Mississippi River, and Americans would gain free navigation on the waterway, despite Spanish opposition. In the south, the 31st parallel, above East and West Florida, would provide the American boundary.

The diplomats endorsed the final peace terms at Versailles, France, in September 1783. Amid all the other treaty terms, the British yielded East and West Florida to Spain. In the process, however, they made no mention of the Indians who had served as allies in the American conflict. Abandoned, the Native Americans had to confront their new situation alone. To end up "betrayed to our Enemies & divided between the Spaniards and the Americans is Cruel & Ungenerous," protested the Creek leader, Alexander McGillivray. His people had been "most Shamefully deserted."

Conclusion

The War for Independence that began at Lexington had lasted eight years. Like any lengthy armed struggle, it took a heavy toll on combatants and non-combatants alike. Personal survival itself was far from certain, as encounters with sickness and the enemy carried off enlisted men. American forces lost an estimated 25,000 soldiers over eight years. The number seems small in modern terms, but comparable losses in the present military service, as a proportion of the current United States population, would total more than 2 million people.

For those who avoided death, lesser dangers abounded. Separations were frequent, and uprooting from home became commonplace. Losses of property proved extensive, and indebtedness appeared to be widespread. Some, of course, managed to benefit from the precarious circumstances. During the war years, whether by determination, foresight, or simple good fortune, they expanded their wealth, gained their freedom, or enhanced their reputation. But other individuals and families, through lost opportunities, poor choices, or bad luck, suffered from the winds of war. Despite constant uncertainties at the individual level, a makeshift revolutionary army, learning as it marched, had forced the British to concede American independence.

As in all wars, some of the most decisive action occurred far from the battlefield. In London, weakness and inconsistency in the chain of command, combined with a lumbering bureaucracy and divided public sentiment, undermined the British war effort. In Europe, skillful American diplomats built the international alliances needed to secure victory and won peace terms that promised survival to the new confederation of states. Meanwhile, a flurry of constitution-writing unprecedented in history had launched more than a dozen newly independent states, and the Articles of Confederation, approved after long delay, had knit them together into a formal league with a common Congress. The new and difficult art of republican self-government remained a work in progress, with some of the most difficult and contentious choices still to come.

As the former slave Thomas Peters climbed aboard the *Joseph James* with his family and other Loyalists to leave New York in 1783, pressing problems still confronted all those who had had a stake in the conflict. Some of the white settlers, Indian allies, and African Americans who had taken the British side chose to withdraw altogether. They joined the massive evacuation engineered by royal ships from St. Augustine, Savannah, Charleston, and New York. But all who stayed did not celebrate for long. The fragile unity built on fighting a common enemy was soon be strained to the limit, as new debates erupted over the meaning and direction of the unfinished revolution.

Loyalties fluctuated with the fortunes of war, and even those far from the fighting became entangled in the web of confrontations, debts, and reprisals that played out year after year. The story of Thomas Peters and his family serves to underscore the point that no one could predict clearly the ultimate outcome of protracted warfare in America.

Sites to Visit

The Saratoga National Historical Park

The National Park Service maintains a visitor center and has arranged a self-guided battlefield tour that includes the locations for the British and American camps during the crucial engagement of October 1777 at this park, which is located 10 miles south of Saratoga Springs, New York, on Route 50.

Brandywine Battlefield State Park

This park is located on Highway 202 west of Philadelphia, Pennsylvania, not far from the borders of Delaware and Maryland. (At nearby Chadds Ford, the Wyeth Museum celebrates three generations of one of America's great artistic families.)

The Continental Congress
memory.loc.gov/ammem/bdsds/bdsdhome.html

This Web site on the Continental Congress in the American Memory series of the Library of Congress contains materials dating from 1774.

Virginia Runaways Project
www.uvawise.edu/history/runaways/index.html

This digital database of runaway slave and servant advertisements from eighteenth-century Virginia newspapers contains full transcripts and images of all runaway ads placed in Virginia newspapers from 1736 to 1790, including those for slaves who responded to Lord Dunmore's proclamation.

The Cowpens National Battlefield
www.nps.gov/cowp/index.htm

The actual site of the battle where Daniel Morgan's troops defeated Banastre Tarleton's British forces (January 17, 1781) is located 10 miles west of Gafney, South Carolina, off Highway I-85. The battle was dramatized in Hollywood's film *The Patriot* (see www.patriotresource.com).

Spy Letters of the American Revolution
www.si.umich.edu/spies/index-timeline.html

This Web site, maintained by the Clements Library at the University of Michigan, contains 12 facsimiles and transcriptions of spy letters contained in the Sir Henry Clinton collection and provides some context for each letter.

Old Fort Niagara
www.oldfortniagara.org/

This New York State Historic Site overlooks Lake Ontario at the mouth of the Niagara River. Built by the French in 1727, the fort is located just off the Robert Moses Parkway, not far from Niagara Falls, at Youngstown, New York.

The Birth of the Navy of the United States
www.history.navy.mil/faqs/faq31-1.htm

Visit the Naval Historical Center Web site to learn about the history of the U.S. Navy.

For Further Reading

General

Colin G. Calloway, *The American Revolution in Indian Country: Crisis and Diversity in Native American Communities* (1995).

Edward Countryman, *The American Revolution* (1985).

Don Higginbotham, *The War of American Independence* (1971).

Sidney Kaplan and Emma Nogrady Kaplan, *The Black Presence in the Era of the American Revolution* (revised edition, 1989).

Piers Mackesy, *The War for America, 1775–1783* (1965).

Robert Middlekauff, *The Glorious Cause* (1982).

Mary Beth Norton, *Liberty's Daughters: The Revolutionary Experience of American Women, 1750–1800* (1980).

Ray Raphael, *A People's History of the American Revolution: How Common People Shaped the Fight for Independence* (2001).

Gordon S. Wood, *The Creation of the American Republic, 1776–1787* (1969).

Alfred F. Young, ed., *Beyond the American Revolution: Explorations in the History of American Radicalism* (1993).

Declaring Independence

Eric Foner, *Tom Paine and Revolutionary America* (1976).

Ira D. Gruber, *The Howe Brothers and the American Revolution* (1972).

Pauline Maier, *American Scripture: Making the Declaration of Independence* (1997).

Charles Patrick Neimeyer, *America Goes to War: A Social History of the Continental Army* (1996).

Richard A. Ryerson, *The Revolution Is Now Begun: The Radical Committees of Philadelphia, 1765–1776* (1978).

Hal T. Shelton, *General Richard Montgomery and the American Revolution* (1994).

"Victory or Death": Fighting for Survival

Wayne Bodle, *The Valley Forge Winter: Civilians and Soldiers at War* (2002).

R. Arthur Bowler, *Logistics and the Failure of the British Army in America, 1775–1783* (1975).

Stephen Conway, *The British Isles and the War of American Independence* (2000).

Sylvia R. Frey, *The British Soldier in America: A Social History of Military Life in the Revolutionary Period* (1981).

Richard M. Ketchum, *The Winter Soldiers* (1973).

Max M. Mintz, *The Generals of Saratoga: John Burgoyne and Horatio Gates* (1990).

Legitimate States, a Respectable Military

Paul Adams, The *First American Constitutions: Republican Ideology and the Making of the State Constitutions in the Revolutionary Era* (1980).

Elisha P. Douglass, *Rebels and Democrats: The Struggle for Equal Political Rights and Majority Rule During the American Revolution* (1955).

Jonathan R. Dull, *A Diplomatic History of the American Revolution* (1985).

James S. Leamon, *Revolution Down East: The War for American Independence in Maine* (1993).

Samuel Eliot Morison, *John Paul Jones: A Sailor's Biography* (1959).

The Long Road to Yorktown

Robert M. Calhoon, *The Loyalists in Revolutionary America, 1760–1781* (1973).

Barbara Graymont, The *Iroquois in the American Revolution* (1972).

Max M. Mintz, *Seeds of Empire: The American Revolutionary Conquest of the Iroquois* (1999).

Richard B. Morris, *The Peacemakers: The Great Powers and American Independence* (1965).

Steven Rosswurm, *Arms, Country, and Class: The Philadelphia Militia and the Lower Sort During the American Revolution* (1987).

J. Barton Starr, *Tories, Dons, and Rebels: The American Revolution in British West Florida* (1976).

Carl Van Doren, *Mutiny in January: The Story of a Crisis in the Continental Army* (1943).

Online Practice Test

Test your understanding of this chapter with interactive review quizzes at

www.ablongman.com/jonescreatedequal/chapter7

Additional Photo Credits

Page 219: Henry Gray, *The Morning After the Attack on Sullivan's Island, June 1776.* Gibbes Museum of Art/Carolina Art Association, 1907.002.0001

Page 221: Courtesy, The West Point Museum

Page 226: Library of Congress

Page 230: Collection of the Museum of Early Southern Decorative Arts; Winston-Salem, North Carolina

Page 232: The Bostonian Society

CHAPTER

8

New Beginnings:
The 1780s

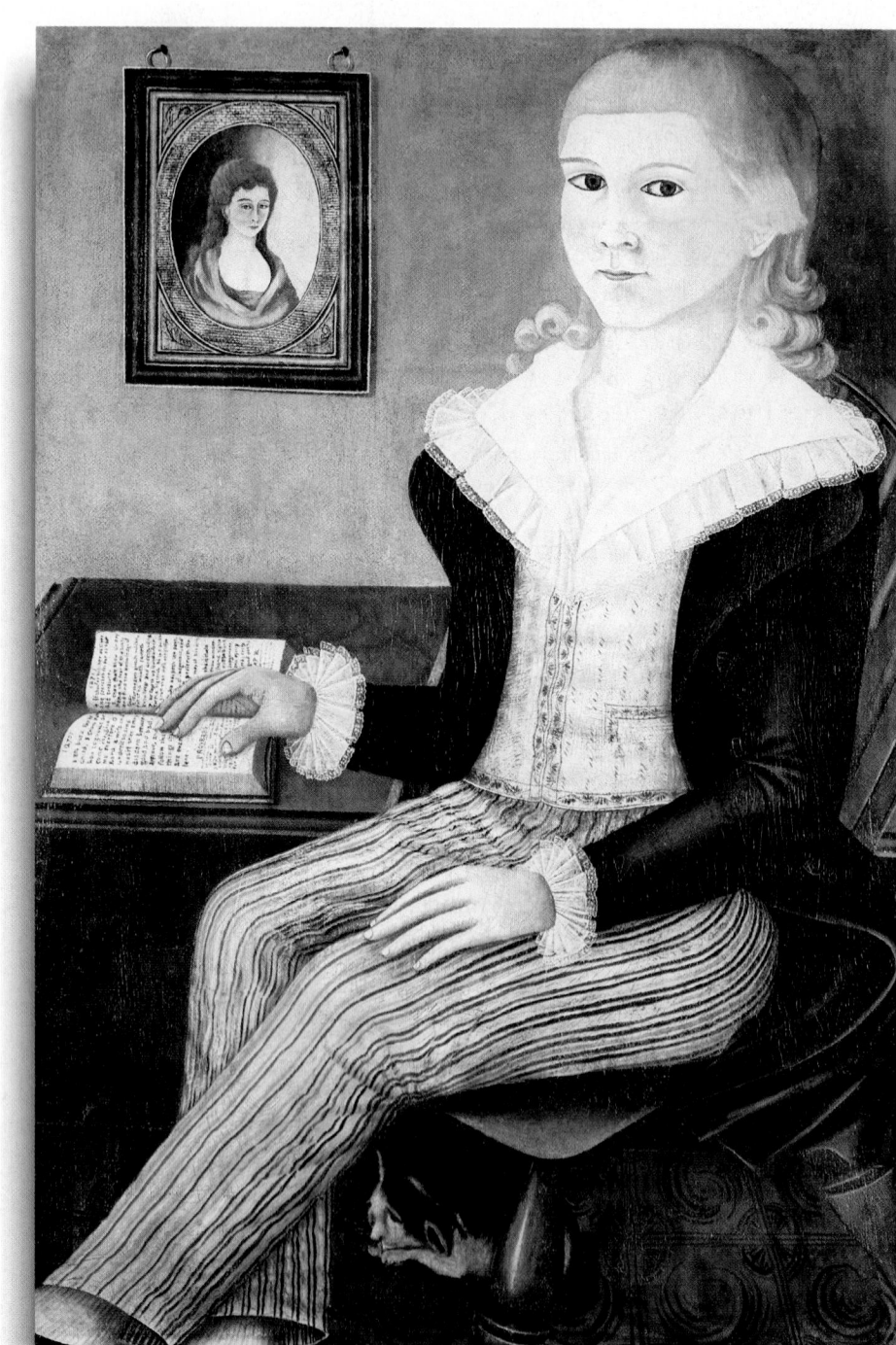

Unidentified Artist, *Jonathan Knight*, c.1797. Collection of American Folk Art Museum, New York, New York, Promised gift of Ralph Esmerian (P1.2001.3). Photo courtesy Sotheby's, New York

■ Jonathan Knight, c. 1797.

LUIS SALES SERVED AS A CATHOLIC MISSIONARY TO THE INDIANS ON THE PENINSULA OF Baja California from 1772 to 1790. His darkest times occurred in 1781. One fateful day, he recalled, "there entered the port of Loreto" a small vessel bringing families across the narrow Gulf of California "from Sonora, infected with the small-pox." Immediately, the sickness "spread like lightning through all the missions," causing "havoc which only those who have seen it can believe. The towns and missions were . . . deserted, and bodies were seen in the road." Some who had watched loved ones break out in sores and die painful deaths insisted on "throwing themselves into the sea at the onset of the disease." Others, in desperation and fear, "cast themselves into mudholes, others into fire, and still others set about burning the pustules with live coals." Many Indians crowded into caves, Sales remembered, and "when they noticed any infected with the disease," they "fled to another cave," deserting the sick and spreading the illness. Time and again, "the poor little children, abandoned beside the dead, died without help."

While Father Sales ministered to survivors, the dozen families who had unwittingly brought the disease moved north along the peninsula to Alta (or Upper) California. Their destination was the San Gabriel Mission, built ten years earlier. They finally reached the outpost in late summer, "arriving with some little children recently coming out with smallpox." Mission leaders immediately quarantined them in a separate camp. Still, during that autumn, the Spanish-speaking newcomers managed to establish a village named Our Lady of the Angels, the start of modern-day Los Angeles. A census that year showed that this frontier band of "recruits, colonists, and families" contained a variety of Indian, black, and Spanish adults with several dozen mixed-race children. On their journey from Sonora, they had unintentionally spread destruction in their wake.

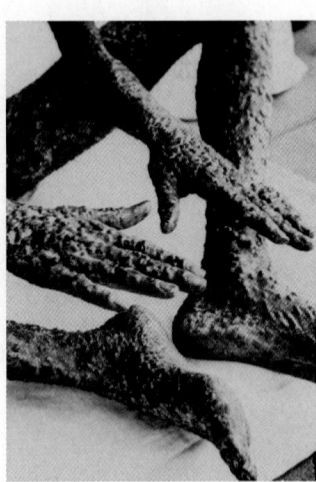

Smallpox was among the deadliest of all epidemic diseases until its eradication in 1979.

The torment Sales described was only a tiny part of a far wider swath of destruction created by this deadly disease. Between 1775 and 1782—the exact years of the Revolutionary War—a huge smallpox epidemic ricocheted relentlessly across broad sections of North America. At times the epidemic entwined itself with the war, traveling on supply ships and moving with marching troops. In the Northeast, it struck during the siege of Boston and the attack on Quebec. In the South, it cut down hundreds of Virginia slaves who had escaped at the start of the war to join Governor Dunmore, when he promised emancipation to slaves who would desert their rebel masters and fight for Britain. The disease found additional victims during the British siege of Charleston, South Carolina, in 1780.

Like the wartime violence, smallpox erupted first in Massachusetts. But the devastating contagion spread far more widely than the destruction caused by the war. Whereas the American army remained "continental" in name only, the great smallpox epidemic proved

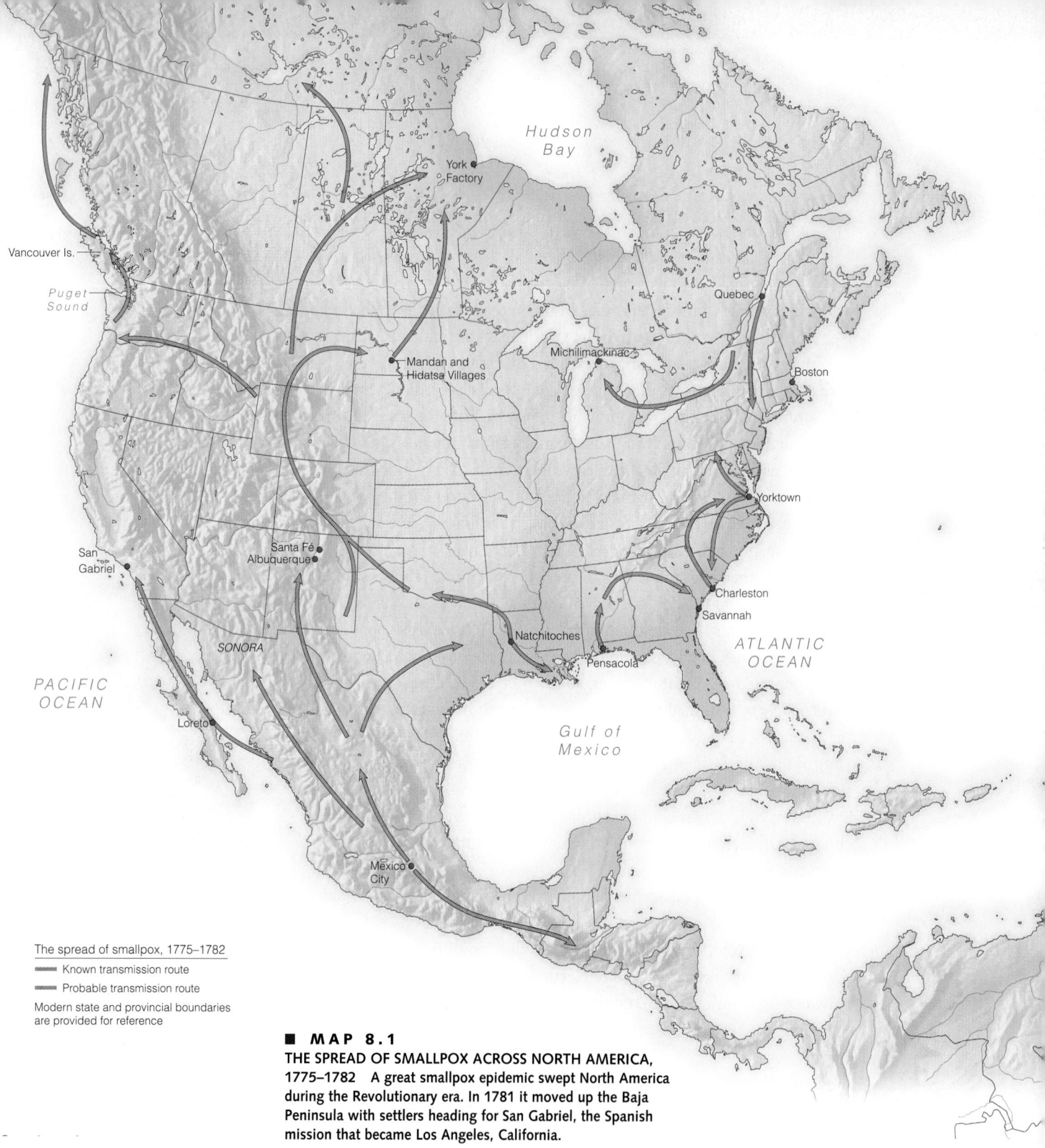

The spread of smallpox, 1775–1782
━━━ Known transmission route
━━━ Probable transmission route
Modern state and provincial boundaries
are provided for reference

■ **MAP 8.1**
THE SPREAD OF SMALLPOX ACROSS NORTH AMERICA,
1775–1782 A great smallpox epidemic swept North America
during the Revolutionary era. In 1781 it moved up the Baja
Peninsula with settlers heading for San Gabriel, the Spanish
mission that became Los Angeles, California.

truly continental in scope. It soon gained a foothold in New Orleans, Mexico City, and even
the far-flung trading posts that dotted the Canadian interior. In 1781 the disease menaced
Virginia as French and American troops completed their successful campaign against the
British at Yorktown. At the same time, it ravaged Indian villages as far away as the Northwest Coast. Within another year, as the War of Independence ended in the East, the
transcontinental epidemic also drew to a close.

The contagion left a patchwork of destruction from the Atlantic to the Pacific. The smallpox losses were greatest among Native Americans, and few groups or regions remained untouched. British sea captain George Vancouver, probing the Northwest Coast near the head of Puget Sound in 1792, observed numerous skulls, ribs, and "other vestiges of the human body in many places promiscuously scattered about the beach." Vancouver's pilot, Peter Puget, pressed farther into the sound that is now named for him. There he found deserted villages that only a dozen years earlier had bustled with people. In its eight-year course, the fearsome virus took more than 130,000 North American lives, many times the total lost on battlefields during the Revolution. In different ways, these two events exerted a drastic and lasting impact on the continent and its people.

As the dual scourges of epidemic and war subsided, fresh problems confronted North America's inhabitants. Despite the successful bid for independence by England's mainland colonies, the question of which European powers would exert the most influence on various parts of the huge continent remained unresolved. British power ruled Canada; Spanish authority claimed much of the West; and in Paris, despite the approach of the French Revolution, some still dreamed of restoring the Mississippi Valley to the control of France. In the North Pacific, Russians sent by Empress Catherine the Great intruded on the Alaskan coast. And lucrative new trade with China was soon luring sea captains from several nations, including the United States, to the Northwest coast. Ships from Atlantic ports could barter for sea otter pelts near Puget Sound and then cross the Pacific to deliver this "soft gold" to the Chinese in exchange for tea and porcelain. In the fertile woodlands between the Appalachian Mountains and the Mississippi River, Indians whom Pontiac had sought to unify a generation earlier once again endured sudden transfers of their ancestral land between distant powers. But now the rapid incursion of American settlers added new urgency and desperation to their situation.

Farther east, inhabitants of the Atlantic seaboard faced an array of thorny problems after warfare and smallpox loosened their grip. Many black Americans had escaped from servitude, won their freedom through military service, or been freed by masters who saw a conflict between slavery and the Revolution's rhetoric of equality. But half a million people remained legally enslaved. During the Revolutionary War, they had seen that armed rebellion in the name of liberty could succeed, and they were potential allies for any European power seeking to disrupt the fragile new society.

In addition, members of the Confederation's Continental (or national) Congress in Philadelphia had a restless army to pay, a weak government to reform, and enormous war debts to confront. When they imposed unprecedented taxes to pay off war bonds accumulated by wealthy speculators, irate farmers and veterans protested that Congress was gouging "the Many" to enrich "the Few." As these dissenters—increasingly numerous and desperate—showed signs of success in pressuring state governments to provide debt relief and issue paper money, wealthy creditors reacted forcefully. Like-minded men maneuvered to create a new and stronger central government that could support their interests and override state-level economic measures that favored the common people. Sidestepping the existing government, they drafted a new constitution at a closed convention in Philadelphia in 1787, and they campaigned successfully for its ratification by 1789. The reins of power, which nearly slipped from the hands of established American leaders during the tumultuous 1770s, had been securely restored by the end of the 1780s, in the face of bitter and varied opposition.

Beating Swords into Plowshares

At first, in the wake of military victory over Britain, the short-term survival of the new United States of America seemed assured, thanks to years of intense fighting and skillful diplomacy. The former colonies had banded together under the Articles of Confederation, duly ratified in 1781, which placed specific governmental powers in the hands of an elected national legislature, or Continental Congress. But deeper questions persisted. Who would benefit most from independence, and who would chart the direction of the new republican experiment? Should power rest primarily with the victorious army, the wealthy merchants, or the artisans and farmers who had provided the backbone of the revolutionary movement? And should authority be consolidated in the hands of a well-educated, new national elite, or should it be widely dispersed, with local communities and regions empowered to manage their own affairs?

Equally important, what did the newly emerging cultural patterns mean for the fledgling society? In these postwar years, scientific, educational, and humanitarian undertakings flourished. Literary endeavors also prospered, and lending libraries sprang up. "At no time did Literature make so rapid a progress in America, as since the peace," boasted a Massachusetts periodical in 1785. "It must afford real pleasure to every son of science, that our swords are beaten into ploughshares, and that the torch of Learning now shines with such lustre in this western hemisphere." This Biblical reference of turning from war and swords to peacetime activities like plowing was particularly compelling to a nation that had endured nearly a decade of war.

Will the Army Seize Control?

After their triumph at Yorktown, Washington's men had moved north to press British forces to evacuate New York City. More than 10,000 American troops and 500 officers encamped at Newburgh, on the Hudson River. With victory at hand, the soldiers looked forward to returning to civilian life. But they were also eager to receive their pay, long overdue because the protracted war had exhausted public finances. Clearly, they could negotiate best for the promised wages while they were still together and still on a wartime footing. Their bargaining position would weaken sharply once peace arrived and they laid down their weapons. Officers were especially reluctant to disband without clear assurances of money and status. In 1780 they extracted from the Congress a promise of half pay for life, in imitation of the European model. In December 1782, with no sign of the money in sight, the disgruntled officers sent a delegation to Philadelphia to press their claims.

Within Congress, the men around financier Robert Morris, including James Wilson and Alexander Hamilton, wanted to bolster and centralize the Confederation's finances. To that end, they sought a new "continental impost"—a duty of 5 percent on imported goods—to raise money from the states. In the short run, revenue from the impost would help make the Confederation government solvent. But the measure would also strengthen that government in the long run, for the new income would allow it to assume responsibility for paying off state war debts. In turn, this economic commitment would tie the interests of wealthy citizens to the Confederation government's survival and success. Morris even threatened to resign his position as secretary of commerce if the "nationalists" did not get their way. Rumblings from the officer corps would help these politicians push through the impost measure, crucial to their long-term goals. So they quietly encouraged the military dissidents in Newburgh.

In late February 1783, anonymous petitions—penned by the staff of Washington's old rival, Horatio Gates—circulated among officers encamped at Newburgh. These inflammatory "addresses" suggested that officers should sit tight, neither fighting nor laying down their arms, until Congress guaranteed their future payments. If the government met their demands, they would be like "lambs," General Henry Knox wrote privately to a fellow general. But if not, they would become "tigers and wolves." Such phrases suggest the veiled

Demobilization: "Turned Adrift Like Old Worn-Out Horses"

Joseph Plumb Martin was born in western Massachusetts in 1760, and he took up arms in the Revolution before his sixteenth birthday. He served faithfully in the Continental Army and was encamped at West Point, New York, when peace finally arrived. Later, in a compelling narrative of his wartime experiences, he recalled the demobilization process from the perspective of a common soldier.

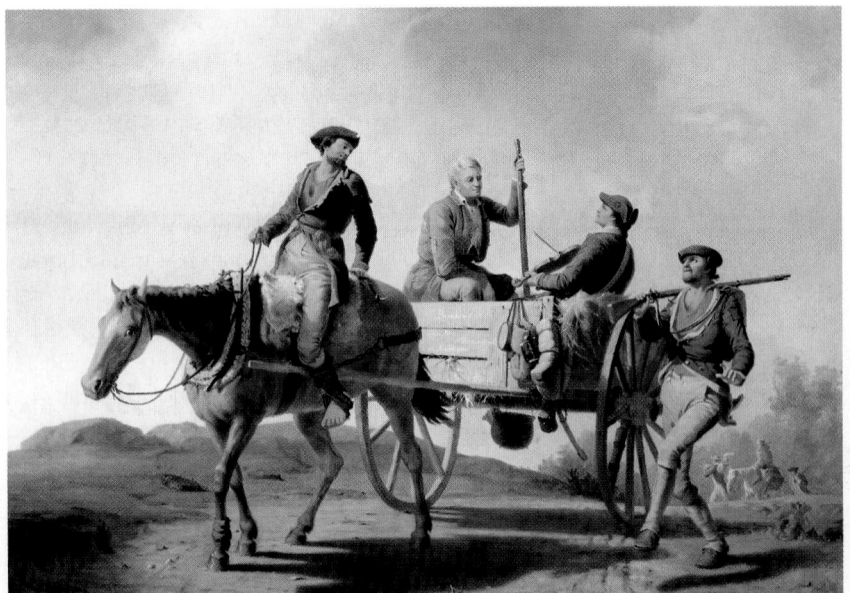

William Ranney painted *Revolutionary War Veterans Returning Home* in 1848, when the United States was at war with Mexico. The image offered a positive reminder of earlier American military success. But in reality, soldiers leaving the Continental Army in 1783 had little reason to laugh and sing.

William Ranney, Veterans of 1776 Returning from the War, c. 1848. Dallas Museum of Art, The Museum League Fund, Special Contributors and General Acquisitions Fund

[On April 19, 1783,] we had general orders read which satisfied the most skeptical, that the war was over and the prize won [after] eight tedious years. But the soldiers said but little about it; their chief thoughts were closely fixed upon their situation. . . . Starved, ragged and meager, not a cent to help themselves with, and no means or method in view to remedy or alleviate their condition. This was appalling in the extreme. . . .

At length, the eleventh day of June 1783, arrived. "The old man," our captain, came into the room, with his hands full of papers. . . . He then handed us our discharges, or rather furloughs, . . . permission to return home, but to return to the army again if required. This was policy in government; to discharge us absolutely in our present pitiful, forlorn condition, it was feared, might cause some difficulties. . . .

Some of the soldiers went off for home the same day that their fetters were knocked off; others stayed and got their final settlement certificates, which they sold to procure decent clothing and money. . . . I was among those. . . . I now bid a final farewell to the service. I had obtained my settlement certificates and sold some of them and purchased some decent clothing, and then set off from West Point. . . .

When those who engaged to serve during the war enlisted, they were promised a hundred acres of land, each. . . . When the country had drained the last drop of service it could screw out of the poor soldiers, they were turned adrift like old worn-out horses, and nothing said about land to pasture them upon. . . . Congress did, indeed, appropriate lands, . . . but no care was taken that the soldiers should get them. [Instead,] a pack of speculators . . . were driving about the country like so many evil spirits, endeavoring to pluck the last feather from the soldiers. The soldiers were ignorant of the ways and means to obtain their bounty lands. . . . It was, soldiers, look to yourselves; we want no more of you.

We were, also, promised six dollars and two thirds a month. . . . And what was six dollars and sixty-seven cents of this "Continental currency," as it was called, worth? It was scarcely enough to procure a man a dinner. . . . I received one month's pay in specie while on the march to Virginia, in the year 1781, and except that, I never received any pay worth the name while I belonged to the army. . . . It is provoking to think of it. The country was rigorous in exacting my compliance to *my* engagements . . . but equally careless in performing her contracts with me, and why so? One reason was that she had all the power in her own hands and I had none. Such things ought not to be.

After the war, Martin settled on the Maine frontier, and a speculator bought his right to 100 acres of bounty land in Ohio. In 1818, as a disabled laborer with a large family, he successfully petitioned Congress for a small pension to support the household. He died poor in 1850. ■

Source: James Kirby Martin, ed., *Ordinary Courage: The Revolutionary War Adventures of Joseph Plumb Martin,* 2nd ed. (New York: Brandywine Press, 1999), pp. 159–164.

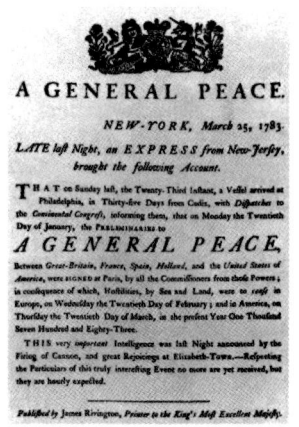

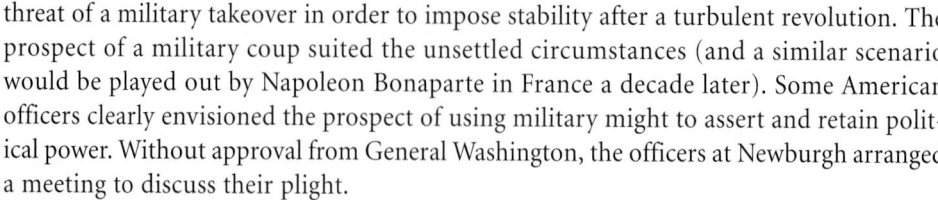

threat of a military takeover in order to impose stability after a turbulent revolution. The prospect of a military coup suited the unsettled circumstances (and a similar scenario would be played out by Napoleon Bonaparte in France a decade later). Some American officers clearly envisioned the prospect of using military might to assert and retain political power. Without approval from General Washington, the officers at Newburgh arranged a meeting to discuss their plight.

If the plotters hoped to draw Washington into the scheme, they were sorely disappointed. He did attend the officers' meeting on March 15, but he used his commanding presence to discredit the ill-advised plan. His eyes weakened by endless wartime correspondence, he drew a pair of spectacles from his pocket. Few had seen him wear glasses, and the gesture underscored the commander's years of dedication and sacrifice. He read a letter from Congress containing assurances of support, and he urged his officers not to take any actions that would undermine the honor they had earned. Finally, he agreed to draft a reasoned request to Congress, stressing the army's needs. His leadership prevailed, and the officers disavowed the "infamous propositions."

Within weeks, Congress offered assurances of back wages for the officers. However, promise of half pay for life met stiff opposition from congressmen who worried about its costliness. The plan was exchanged for a guarantee of full pay to officers for the next five years, and all parties accepted the compromise. In April 1783, word spread that preliminary articles of peace had been signed in Paris. By June most soldiers were headed home.

The Society of the Cincinnati

By quieting his officers, Washington had averted the threat of a military coup. The commander's strong stance against the suspected Newburgh conspiracy reminded his admirers of the story of Roman general Cincinnatus, well known to people at that time. In the early Roman Republic, the Senate called Cincinnatus from his farm to command an army against the Aequians. After defeating the invaders, he put down his sword and took up his plow again rather than seize power as a military ruler. His selfless action earned him the lasting respect of the Roman people. The familiar story of Cincinnatus appealed to Washington. At a crucial moment in the republic's earliest days, the American general had bravely urged fellow officers to respect the fragile principle of civilian control over the military.

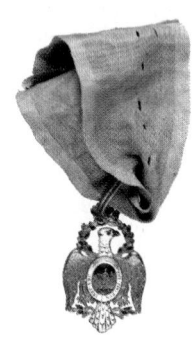

Thomas Jefferson praised Washington's action. He wrote to him admiringly that "the moderation and virtue of a single character has probably prevented this revolution from being closed as most others have been by a subversion of that liberty it was intended to establish." Still, Jefferson and others worried that some military officers might yet meddle in politics while hiding behind the noble name of Cincinnatus. Their fears soon seemed confirmed. In May 1783, as demobilization got under way, General Knox announced formation of the Society of the Cincinnati. The new organization invoked the name of the famous Roman, in a plural form, to put its members in the best light. It was open only to officers in the Continental army at the war's end, plus former officers and invited honorary members.

Some onlookers believed that the "Cincinnati Club" was no more than a social fraternity for men united by their war experience. Benjamin Franklin assumed those joining the society had been drawn together simply by the lure of ceremony and recognition. Perhaps, he mused, these officers had "been too much struck with the Ribbands and Crosses they have seen . . . hanging to the buttonholes of Foreign Officers." But others sensed a more sinister purpose. After all, members contributed an entire month's salary to a charitable fund that resembled a political war chest. Also, the society's state chapters maintained contact with each other through newsletters concerning "the general union of the states." Most ominously, participants endorsed hereditary membership so that the eldest sons of Continental officers would join the society down through the generations.

For skeptics, the society appeared to plant the seeds of a self-perpetuating ruling class. In a scathing pamphlet titled *Considerations on the Society or Order of Cincinnati . . . with*

Remarks on Its Consequences to the Freedom and Happiness of the Republic, Judge Aedanus Burke of South Carolina protested that the organization revealed a "thirst for power" and created a "race of hereditary patricians, or nobility." Critics such as Burke argued that the society would spawn a separate aristocracy of the very kind Americans had fought to erase.

Jefferson and other friends of Washington, who was automatically a member, urged the general not to accept a leadership position in the new organization. Struck by this "violent and formidable" opposition, Washington suggested changes in the society, including doing away with the hereditary and honorary memberships. However, he never played a central role in the organization, and his well-publicized alterations were never implemented. The Cincinnati exerted influence as a pressure group before receding from politics in future generations.

Renaming the Landscape

The controversy over the Society of the Cincinnati represented part of a larger debate about the direction of postwar life. The victors in any revolutionary struggle must move quickly to solidify their success, heal internal differences, and fulfill bold promises. In the wake of the revolutionary war, many Americans—despite continuing disagreements—set out to build a national culture and a shared identity. Those who had fought or had endured hardship because of the war wanted to create a country that would justify their sacrifices and uphold the ideals of the revolution. Citizens of the new Confederation would strive to match all that they still admired about European culture and, at the same time, separate themselves from all that they distrusted or rejected. Like the Puritans before them, they aspired to provide new models for the Atlantic world.

> *One zealous professor went so far as to rewrite nursery rhymes to eliminate offending words.*

They began with names. Everywhere, people christened new towns, counties, streets, and schools and renamed old ones. Just as citizens had stripped away royal statues and coats of arms at the beginning of the war, they replaced numerous British names, such as those of hated prewar governors. Dunmore County in Virginia, named after Lord Dunmore, received the Indian name *Shanando* (later spelled *Shenandoah*). Tryon County, New York, which had celebrated Governor William Tryon, became Montgomery County, after the American general who died at Quebec. A frontier town in what would become Vermont, named after Governor Thomas Hutchinson of Massachusetts, took its new name, Barre, from Isaac Barré, a parliamentary supporter of the American cause.

Political leaders rediscovered and popularized Christopher Columbus as well. Their reasoning was simple: For generations, the English had downplayed the explorer's importance as they contested Spanish claims in the Western Hemisphere. Now, American writers coined the ringing term *Columbia* for their land to stress its separation from Britain. In South Carolina, citizens named their new capital Columbia in 1786. That same year, in Philadelphia, an Irish immigrant named Mathew Carey launched an ambitious new periodical called *The Columbian Magazine.* Five years later, supporters of the proposed national capital christened it the District of Columbia. In New York City, King's College had been founded with a royal charter in 1754 and had served as an army hospital during the Revolutionary War. But when the school reopened in 1784 under local governance, it was called Columbia College (later Columbia University).

Most people in the new republic found any references to royalty distasteful. One zealous professor at Columbia College went so far as to rewrite nursery rhymes to eliminate offending words. Children should no longer hear that a pie filled with singing blackbirds appeared "before the king." The "dainty dish" would be "set before the Congress" instead. King Street in Boston quickly became State Street. Still, royal figures who had aided the revolution received their due. At the Falls of the Ohio River, settlers named their new town Louisville, honoring America's wartime alliance with King Louis XVI of France.

Farther up the Ohio River, in 1790, General Arthur St. Clair renamed a village near Licking Creek, calling it Cincinnati. He hoped to honor all his fellow officers in the controversial society and to invoke Cincinnatus, the Roman general. Such classical references cropped up everywhere. In 1789, for instance, citizens of Vanderheyden's Ferry on the Hudson River voted to rename their town Troy, New York, after the citadel that the Greeks captured in Homer's *Iliad.* "I find not the least resemblance," complained one newspaper editor, "between the old city of that name and this small village." (The trend of putting ancient names on small towns continued well into the nineteenth century. Settlers along the Mississippi River, known as "the Nile of America," invoked famous Egyptian cities when they laid out Cairo, Illinois; Memphis, Tennessee; and Alexandria, Louisiana.)

Of all the new names, those honoring individual war heroes became the most popular. Citizens hailed foreign supporters of the revolution—such as Lafayette, Pulaski, and Steuben—by using their names on streets and towns. They saluted American officers the same way. Washington's name was used most often, but those of Montgomery, Wayne, Greene, Lincoln, Mercer, Marion, and others popped up as well. North Carolina named one of its trans-Appalachian forts on the Cumberland River Nashborough, after General Francis Nash, who had died at the battle of Germantown. Citizens changed the fort's name to *Nashville* in 1784. Two years later, inhabitants of a site on the Tennessee River named their new town Knoxville in honor of General Henry Knox, who had become the Confederation's secretary of war the previous year.

An Independent Culture

New names were just part of the story. Many Americans felt that their whole language needed to be made more independent and accessible. Noah Webster, a schoolteacher who had fought against General Burgoyne, believed that "as an independent nation, our honor requires us to have a system of our own, in language as well as government." In his *American Spelling Book* (1783), Webster championed a simple, uniform written language that rejected English conventions. Words such as *colour* and *labour* lost their silent *u, theatre* became *theater,* and *plough* was shortened to *plow.* The New Englander followed this success with an influential grammar book and a popular reader. Webster went on to produce *An American Dictionary of the English Language* (1828) that incorporated 5000 new words, many of them reflecting Indian origins (*tomahawk*) and American nature (*rattlesnake*).

Webster also joined other reformers in lobbying state legislatures for copyright laws that would protect the literary works that poured from the pens of ambitious writers. Philip Freneau, a classmate of James Madison at Princeton, drafted a poem titled "The British Prison Ship" (1781), about his war experiences. Authors living near Hartford, known as the Connecticut Wits, made similar nationalistic contributions. Timothy Dwight, future president of Yale College, created a poetic allegory, "The Conquest of Canaan" (1785), and Joel Barlow composed an epic poem titled "The Vision of Columbus" (1787), heralding a bright future for citizens of the new nation.

> Each rustic here, that turns the furrow'd soil,
> The maid, the youth, that ply mechanic toil,
> In freedom nurst, in useful arts inured,
> Know their just claims, and see their rights secured.

Increasingly, the land itself captured the imagination of Americans. In 1784 a Connecticut silversmith engraved the first map of the new United States and a a recent Yale graduate, Jedidiah Morse, published *Geography Made Easy,* which went through 25 editions. (Five years later, Morse created *The American Geography* and earned his reputation as the "Father of American Geography.") In Pennsylvania, naturalist William Bartram distributed seeds

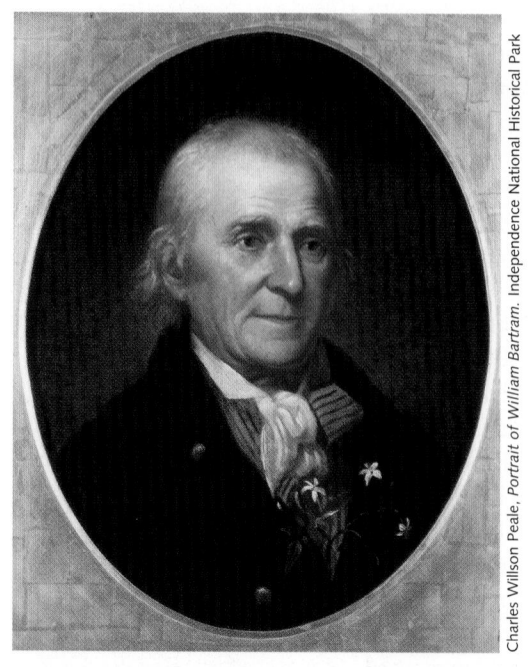

Charles Willson Peale, *Portrait of William Bartram.* Independence National Historical Park

■ When Pennsylvania botanist William Bartram explored the Southeast, Indians called him Pucpuggy—"the flower gatherer." Years later, Charles Willson Peale painted the naturalist holding a flower.

from an experimental garden that his father, Quaker botanist John Bartram, had developed beside the Schuylkill River. The younger Bartram also drafted a pioneering nature book about his travels throughout the Southeast. In nearby Philadelphia, versatile painter and patriot Charles Willson Peale launched a museum to promote interest in art and the natural world. He gathered specimens, mastered taxidermy, and originated the practice of displaying stuffed animals in a model of their natural habitat. "Sir," George Washington wrote to Peale from Mount Vernon, "you will receive by stage the body of my gold pheasant packed in wool." At Monticello, Thomas Jefferson also corresponded with Peale and continued to pursue his own fascination with the American landscape. He promoted exploration, tested new crops, and tried his hand at archaeology by excavating ancient Indian mounds.

In *Notes on the State of Virginia* (1785), Jefferson detailed his region's geography, society, and natural history. He also challenged the theories of famous French naturalist Comte de Buffon regarding the vitality of New World species. Buffon had declared, without first-hand knowledge, that America's weak soil and dubious climate prompted the inevitable degeneration of plants and animals, including people. Jefferson and others disagreed. Hector St. John de Crèvecoeur, a Frenchman who made his home in America, had already argued the opposite case. In 1782 he published *Letters from an American Farmer*. In the book's most famous essay, "What Is an American?" Crèvecoeur proclaimed that poor European immigrants became revitalized "in this great American asylum." "Every thing has tended to regenerate them," he wrote. "In Europe they . . . withered; and were mowed down by want, hunger, and war; but now, by the power of transplantation, like all other plants, they have taken root and flourished!"

According to Crèvecoeur, free people flourished in America not only because of "new laws" but also because of "a new mode of living, a new social system" that nurtured community growth. Crèvecoeur's argument had merit: Voluntary associations bent on improving local conditions sprang up everywhere. Of course, societies for bettering jails, assisting debtors, and building libraries had existed in port cities before independence. But a new generation revived many of these charities after the war and created new ones at an unprecedented rate. Earnest reformers launched more than 30 new benevolent organizations between 1783 and 1789. Some provided relief for the physically and mentally ill. Others offered aid to strangers and immigrants. Still others granted charity to the poor and disabled or lobbied to reform harsh penal codes.

In 1785 prominent New Yorkers John Jay and Alexander Hamilton joined like-minded citizens to form a Society for the Promotion of the Manumission of Slaves. Society members decried slavery as "disgraceful" and "shocking to humanity." And in Connecticut, citizens banded together to stop the abuse of liquor. Members of this early temperance organization protested that the state's residents consumed 400,000 gallons of rum annually and that communities paid dearly in both financial and moral terms. Meanwhile, the new Massachusetts Humane Society dedicated itself to assisting people in "suspended animation" between life and death, whether from drowning, drinking, heatstroke, or other causes. The society provided crude lifesaving equipment along waterfronts. It also constructed huts, stocked with food and firewood, to aid shipwreck survivors on isolated coastlines. Similar efforts to reform and improve the new nation sprang up everywhere. Amid such optimism, no sooner had the former British colonists disentangled themselves from the British Empire than they began to speak of shaping an expansive empire of their own.

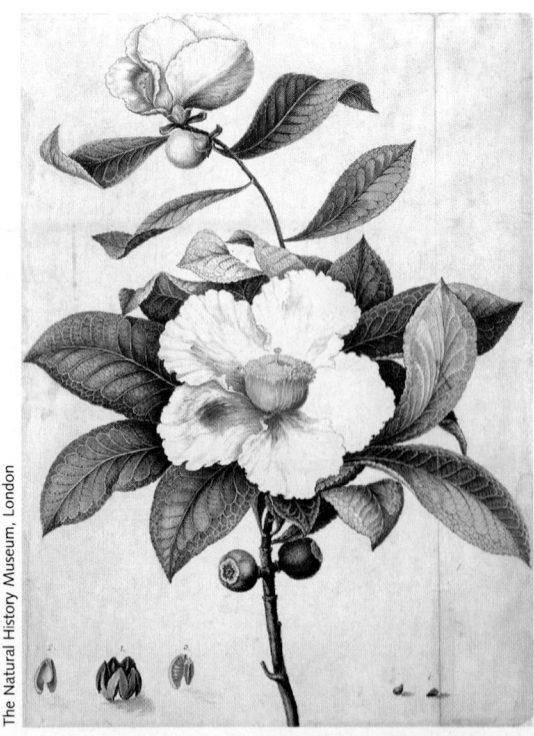

The Natural History Museum, London

■ Exploring near the Altamaha River in Georgia, William Bartram and his father found "several curious shrubs, one bearing beautiful good fruit." They named it the Franklin tree after their scientist friend in Philadelphia, Benjamin Franklin. William drew a watercolor of the rare plant and saved seeds to protect the species.

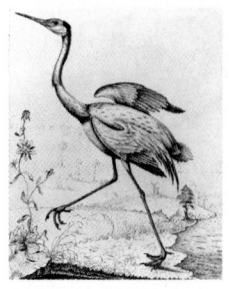

Competing for Control of the Mississippi Valley

"It has ever been my hobby-horse," John Adams wrote in 1786, "to see rising in America an empire of liberty, and a prospect of two or three hundred millions of freemen, without one noble or one king among them. You say it is impossible. . . . I would still say, let us try the experiment." Westward expansion became a persistent American theme. But during the postwar decade, interest and activity centered mostly on the land just beyond the eastern mountains, territory reserved for Indians by the British until they ceded the lands to the United States at the end of the Revolution. There, countless tributaries of the Mississippi River flowed west from the Appalachian ridges toward the interior of the continent.

In the South in the 1780s, pioneer families searching for land pushed west along an old buffalo trail and Indian trading path. Passing through Cumberland Gap, where southwest Virginia now touches Kentucky, they spread out across parts of the lower Mississippi Valley, a region that eventually became known as the Old Southwest. These aspiring homesteaders promptly faced resistance from Native American inhabitants and their Spanish supporters. At the same time, north of the Ohio River, other American settlers were flocking to newly claimed lands that lay between the Allegheny Mountains and the Upper Mississippi, a vast, wooded expanse later remembered as the Old Northwest. They, too, met stiff opposition from Native Americans defending their homelands and from the Indians' British allies in neighboring Canada. By the time the Constitutional Convention met in Philadelphia in the summer of 1787, the Continental Congress of the existing Confederation government was busy revising an elaborate plan to draw this territory into the union.

Disputed Territory: The Old Southwest

For a generation, as part of wider reforms within its American empire, Spain had been rebuilding its position north of the Gulf of Mexico and east of Texas in the Old Southwest. The Spanish had acquired Louisiana from France in 1763 and had conquered West Florida. In a 1783 treaty, Britain gave back East Florida to the Spanish and agreed that Spain would retain West Florida as well. The Spanish occupied St. Augustine, Pensacola, New Orleans, and Natchez, not to mention St. Louis farther north. Because they controlled both banks of the lower Mississippi and dominated the gulf with their navy, the Spanish controlled who could use the huge river as an access route to the Atlantic. Mississippi Valley settlers knew that if they carried their produce downstream to New Orleans, they could then ship it to the West Indies and Atlantic ports more cheaply than they could haul bulky commodities east across the Appalachian Mountains. Besides, merchants in Louisiana paid for goods in Spanish silver, and settlers upriver needed the hard currency.

Since 1763, the Spanish had let British subjects navigate freely on the Mississippi, so trans-Appalachian fur traders had become accustomed to using this thoroughfare. And during the Revolutionary War, Spain's American allies had retained access to the river. But Spain was shocked when Britain, through its separate treaty with the United States in 1783, granted the Americans a generous southern boundary: the 31st parallel. The treaty terms also included the right of Americans to navigate the Mississippi.

Spain had good reason to claim that its West Florida province stretched north *above* 31 degrees at least to the mouth of the Yazoo River and perhaps as far as the Tennessee River. Moreover, the Spanish felt that they should be the only ones to decide whose boats had access to the Mississippi. To be sure, the Spanish in New Orleans had grown dependent on foreign produce arriving by river from the north. But they also feared American expansion into the Mississippi Valley. Spanish authorities debated whether to co-opt the newcomers and profit from their trade or resist settlers pushing from the east.

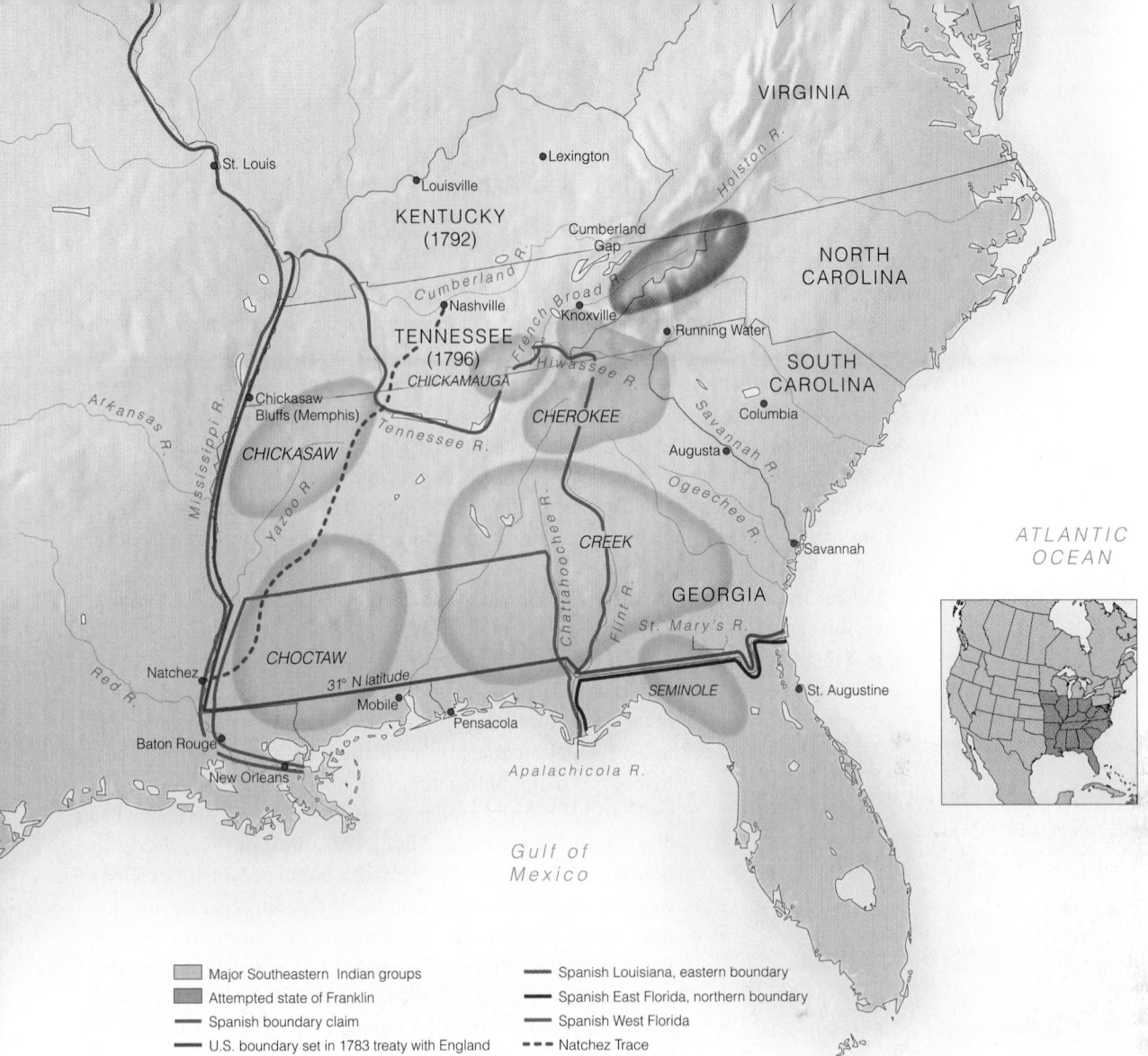

■ **MAP 8.2**

SOUTHERN LAND DEBATES AFTER 1783 Following the Revolution, competing forces collided in the trans-Appalachian South. The United States claimed land reaching the Mississippi River down to 31 degrees latitude, and the Spanish claimed territory north to the Tennessee River. Although major Indian tribes continued to possess much of the region, coastal states also claimed sweeping jurisdiction. In Georgia, for instance, settlement remained confined near the Savannah River, but the state sold speculators large tracts as far west as the Yazoo River.

For its part, the new Confederation had the force of numbers working to its advantage. The Proclamation Line of 1763 had dammed up colonial expansion for two decades. After the war, Americans migrated by the thousands to three existing centers of Anglo settlement in the Old Southwest. By 1785, 10,000 settlers clustered along the Holston, Watauga, and French Broad rivers above Knoxville. Nearly three times that many newcomers had already staked claims to the rich land south of the Ohio River between Lexington and Louisville. In addition, another 4000 were clearing farms along the Cumberland River around Nashville. These Americans took advantage of the fact that Spain had not negotiated an explicit boundary treaty of its own with the United States in 1783. As the flow of settlers increased, some talked aggressively about pushing even farther. They imagined establishing a foothold on the Mississippi at Chickasaw Bluffs (modern Memphis) or perhaps seizing Natchez or New Orleans.

American Claims and Indian Resistance

The weak Confederation government lacked power to constrain the westward push. And state governments, with little money to pay war veterans, had instead given them paper vouchers with which to claim frontier farmland. In the southern states, powerful land speculators pressed their legislatures to support expansion. Georgia, unlike many other states, had not relinquished its western lands to the Confederation. The state's so-called Yazoo claim embraced a region of 35 million acres. This vast expanse stretched west from the Chattahoochee River (Georgia's present boundary with Alabama) to the Mississippi River and from the lower border of modern-day Tennessee to the 31st parallel. "I look forward to a time, not very far distant," wrote Judge George Walton, when Georgia "will be settled and connected . . . from the shores of the Atlantic to the banks of the Mississippi." By 1789, Walton had been elected governor of the state, and the land business boomed. During his tenure, Walton signed warrants for huge tracts up to 50,000 acres, sometimes selling unusable or even nonexistent acreage.

Unlike Georgians, pioneers from Virginia and the Carolinas faced a rugged mountain barrier. But they still trekked west through Cumberland Gap, seeking land of their own or land that they could improve and then sell to later arrivals. In the decade after the war, backwoodsman Daniel Boone worked as a surveyor for these migrants in the trans-Appalachian region of Virginia that became Kentucky in 1792. He accumulated more than 20,000 acres of his own, only to lose much of it in litigation with other claimants. During that same decade, North Carolina issued more land patents than it had created during the entire colonial era, most of them deeds for homesteads west of the mountains. Some of North Carolina's western landholders tried to create their own separate jurisdiction, calling themselves residents of the mountain state of Franklin. Without recognition from the Confederation government, their venture soon failed. Instead, all of North Carolina's western territory—from the Appalachians to the Mississippi—became the state of Tennessee in 1796.

Native American southerners, living in all these lands, suddenly found themselves caught between the competing claims of Spain and the United States. Ravaged by the recent smallpox epidemic and the bitter war and utterly ignored during peace negotiations, they endured the increasingly aggressive acts of state legislatures and frontier settlers from the east. The Cherokees, Creeks, Choctaws, and Chickasaws—numbering roughly 40,000 people—all debated over which leaders and strategies to follow. Some responded to their new situation by selecting leaders with European-American ties. Among the Creeks, for example, Alexander McGillivray rose to prominence. The son of a wealthy Scottish trader and a Creek woman, he had been raised on his father's Georgia plantation before becoming the Creeks' spokesperson in 1782. The fact that he owned 50 slaves and kept a wine cellar may have boosted his bargaining power with Spanish and American officials. However, it also separated him from the needs and lives of those he represented.

The renegade Cherokee warrior Dragging Canoe, who had split with tribal elders before the Revolution broke out, offered a different approach. Hundreds of militant Indians, discouraged by the compromises of their leaders, had joined his band of guerrilla fighters known as the Chicamaugas. After Americans burned the Chicamauga encampments at Lookout Mountain in the closing days of the Revolutionary War, the

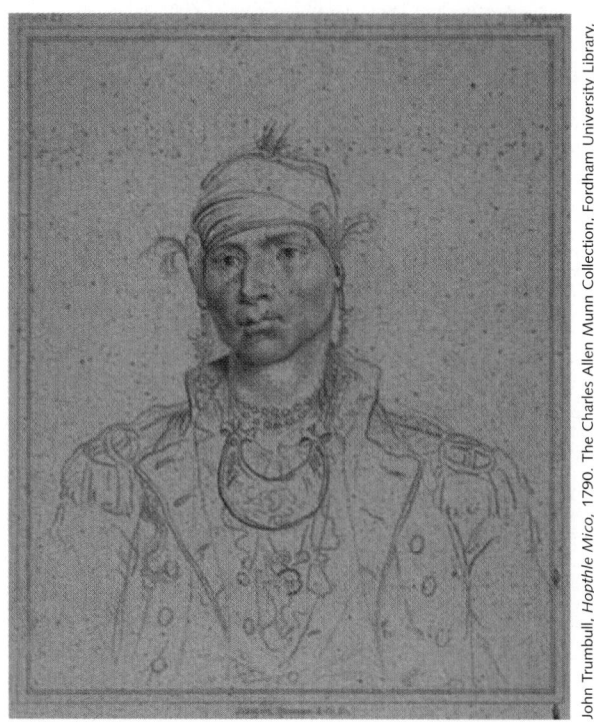

John Trumbull, *Hopthle Mico*, 1790. The Charles Allen Munn Collection, Fordham University Library, Bronx, New York (Catalog #3)

■ In 1790 American artist John Trumbull paused from painting scenes commemorating the Revolution in order to sketch members of a Creek Indian delegation visiting New York City from Georgia. In this picture of an important Native American orator, a medal presented by the American government is visible amid the ruffles of his shirt.

Indians erected five new villages nearby on the Tennessee River, including Dragging Canoe's headquarters at Running Water Town.

From this well-protected location—near where Alabama, Georgia, and Tennessee now meet—the Chicamaugas recruited allies and led forays to stop American encroachment. They drew aid from the Spanish when possible, sending delegations as far as St. Augustine. When Anglo frontiersmen murdered Old Tassel, a moderate Cherokee leader, during a truce in 1788, Indian support for the militant Chicamaugas increased. But Dragging Canoe died in 1792 before he could build a strong alliance with Indians north of the Ohio River. They, too, struggled with the steady incursions of newcomers and the disintegration of their way of life.

"We Are Now Masters": The Old Northwest

Like their neighbors in the South, most Native Americans in the North had sided with the British during the Revolutionary War. So Americans lost no time in claiming northern Indian domains ceded by Britain in the 1783 Treaty of Paris. "We are now Masters of this Island," General Philip Schuyler boasted to the Iroquois, "and can dispose of the Lands as we think proper." Britain refused to vacate western forts at Oswego, Niagara, Detroit, and Michilimackinac on the pretext that Americans still owed prewar debts to London merchants. Even so, the British could provide little material support to the Indians of the region, who felt betrayed by the terms of the Paris treaty.

American delegations moved quickly to draft treaties with the Iroquois and the Ohio Valley tribes. Delegates bluntly asserted the right of the new United States government to Indian lands. The Congress of this recently established Confederation government instructed these negotiators to deal with the Native Americans as dependents rather than equals, calling them children rather than brothers. The treaty makers even took hostages to force the Indians to accept their terms. Ordinary Americans sealed these claims with a surge of migration into western Pennsylvania and beyond. "The Americans . . . put us out of our lands," Indian leaders complained to the Spanish governor at St. Louis in 1784, "extending themselves like a plague of locusts in the territories of the Ohio River which we inhabit."

Clearly, the British and the Indians had lost the upper hand. However, Americans initially remained divided among themselves over who would control the region. One by one, the states of Massachusetts, New York, Connecticut, and Virginia ceded separate territorial claims—dating from their early colonial charters—to the Confederation government. However, Connecticut retained economic control over a "western reserve" of 4 million acres south of Lake Erie that it used to satisfy claims from the state's war veterans. Similarly, Virginia held onto land rights for an even larger "military district" to repay soldiers and war victims.

These western land acquisitions transformed the Confederation. For the first time, it became more than a league of states. With lands of its own to organize and oversee, the Confederation government took on attributes of a sovereign ruling body. As the number of cessions increased, Congress put Thomas Jefferson in charge of a committee to draft a plan to administer this national domain. Before he departed for Europe to replace Benjamin Franklin as the American minister to France, Jefferson drew up an orderly design for western land distribution.

This document became the basis for the Land Ordinance of 1785. Jefferson knew that in the South, where hired surveyors often staked out piecemeal claims on a first-come, first-served basis, the best property had gone to wealthy investors. Moreover, boundary litigation over odd-shaped and overlapping lots had proved endless. To avoid these complications, the 1785 ordinance called for surveyors to lay out a grid of adjoining townships, beginning at the point where the Ohio River flowed out of Pennsylvania. A township would contain 36 numbered sections, each 1 mile square (640 acres). This grid plan shaped all future American land policy and left a permanent mark on the country's landscape. As its most far-reaching innovation, the ordinance reserved the income from one valuable section near the heart of every township—square number 16—to support public education.

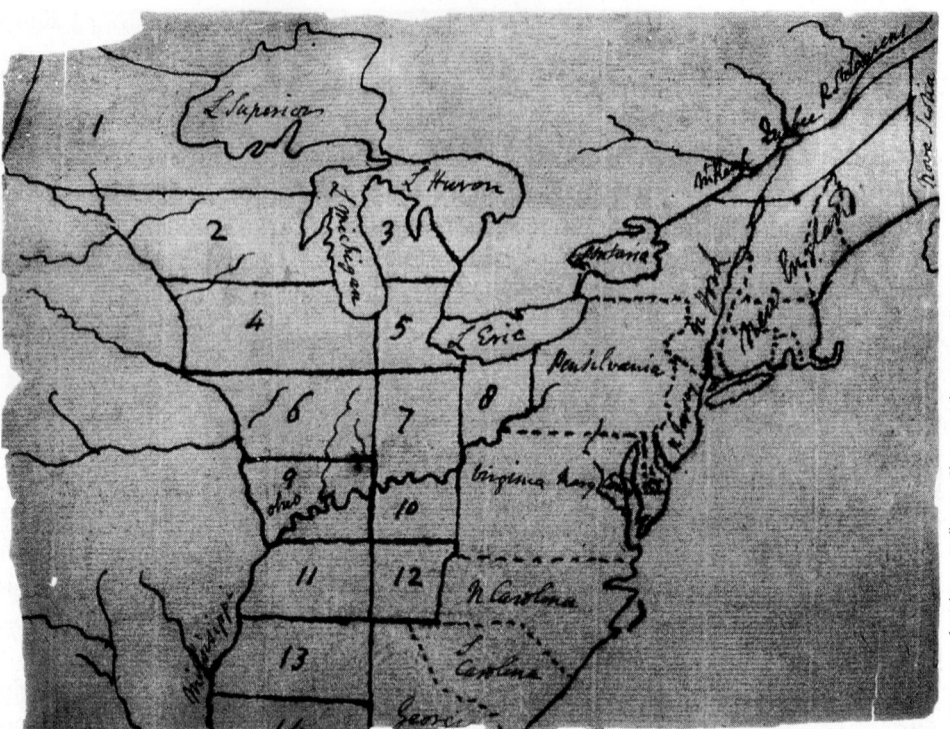

■ A sketch by Congressman Thomas Jefferson shows his proposal to divide the new interior territories into 14 states (with Number 7 to be named Saratoga after the crucial Revolutionary War victory). By suggesting numerous compact states, Jefferson hoped to maximize the Congressional voting power of western farmers. Others, eager to limit western power in Congress, pushed successfully for fewer, larger states.

But orderly surveying and public education were just parts of Jefferson's plan. Hoping to populate the region with self-sufficient yeomen farmers, he proposed that the government give away land in small parcels rather than sell it in large blocks that only wealthy speculators could afford. He envisioned self-government for these enterprising settlers, not colonial rule. For Jefferson, the more weight these independent farmers obtained in the American government the better, so he urged the rapid entry of numerous new territories into the union on an equal footing with the 13 original states. He suggested creating up to 14 small, rectangular districts in the west, with elaborate names such as Metropotamia. At least nine would be north of the Ohio River, and each could become a separate state with voting rights in Congress.

According to Jefferson's report "Government for the Western Territory," the first settlers to arrive in each district were to form their own temporary governments. And when the local population reached 20,000, residents could call a convention, frame a constitution, and send a delegate to Congress. When the district's population equaled the number of free inhabitants living in the smallest of the 13 original states, that district could enter the union if certain conditions were met. Each new state must agree to support a republican form of government, remain part of the Confederation, and accept a share of the federal debt. It must also agree to exclude slavery after 1800. Once Jefferson left for France, Congress accepted his report. However, it then modified the plan greatly. In the Land Ordinance of 1785, Congress removed his call for numerous districts, ignored his suggestion of ornate names, dismissed the notion of free land, and dropped the idea of ending slavery.

The Northwest Ordinance of 1787

Surveying the vast wilderness north of the Ohio River into neat geometric squares raised untold practical and diplomatic problems. The task would take years to complete. Almost immediately—and long before the initial ordinance could take hold—political shifts produced an entirely new law from Congress: the Northwest Ordinance of 1787. This law determining how territories north of the Ohio River would be governed contained a number of additional changes to Jefferson's original plan. For example, it reversed direction on the slave question once again, introducing an immediate prohibition of slavery north of the Ohio River. However, it made arrangements to deport fugitive slaves back to their owners in slaveholding states.

In various ways, the new ordinance proved less democratic than earlier versions. Congress cut the possible number of new states from the Northwest, specifying there could be only three to five new states. This move limited the potential political weight of the vast territory. In addition, the ordinance increased property requirements for citizens who wanted to vote or hold office. It also slowed the process by which new states could gain admission to the union. Eventually, Congress granted statehood to five new entities—Ohio (1803), Indiana (1816), Illinois (1818), Michigan (1837), and Wisconsin (1848)—but the process took more than half a century. Minnesota, part of which was also in the original cession from Britain, did not become a state until 1858.

Most members of Congress feared the prospect of democratic governance and local control in the Old Northwest, giving a strong voice to people with different regional interests. And they worried that aggression by settlers could spark expensive Indian wars. To retain control over the region, they provided for the appointment of territorial officials—a governor, a secretary, and three judges—instead of allowing elected governments. Even when territorial legislatures formed, the governor would have veto power over their actions. James Monroe, head of the committee that moved the bill through Congress, wrote candidly to Jefferson, "It is in effect to be a colonial gover[nme]nt similar to wh[at] prevailed in these States previous to the revolution."

These changes benefited eastern land speculators most, some of whom were members of Congress. They hoped to control these lands for profit. What they did not want was to see numerous western states emerge quickly to play a powerful role in the national government. In 1786, former army officers in New England, joined by five surveyors who had seen the promising region first-hand, organized the Ohio Company to buy up western land. They dispatched a clever Massachusetts minister named Manasseh Cutler to lobby Congress to sell a huge tract to the company at bargain rates. Cutler joined forces with congressional insiders associated with another venture, the Scioto Company. Together, they engineered a deal providing 1.5 million acres to the Ohio Company and another 5 million acres for the Scioto investors.

Whatever suspicious bargains surrounded congressional passage of the Northwest Ordinance of 1787, the new law still granted basic rights to western residents. These guarantees—following state bills of rights—included religious freedom, trial by jury, and access to common-law judicial proceedings. Most important, the western territories were assured of full entry into the union as equal states rather than receiving dependent status as permanent colonies. This system established an orderly method for bringing new regions of settlement into the union. The same process, first used when Vermont became the fourteenth state in 1791, remained in use as late as 1959, when the Pacific territories of Alaska and Hawaii received statehood.

Courtesy, Monroe County Historical Commission, Monroe, MI

■ Marie-Thérèse Lasselle (1735–1819) witnessed a generation of transitions in the Great Lakes region. She and her husband ran a trading post at Kekionga on the Maumee River (now Fort Wayne, Indiana). Long after the Revolutionary War drove them to Detroit, she created this self-portrait, using watercolor on embroidered silk.

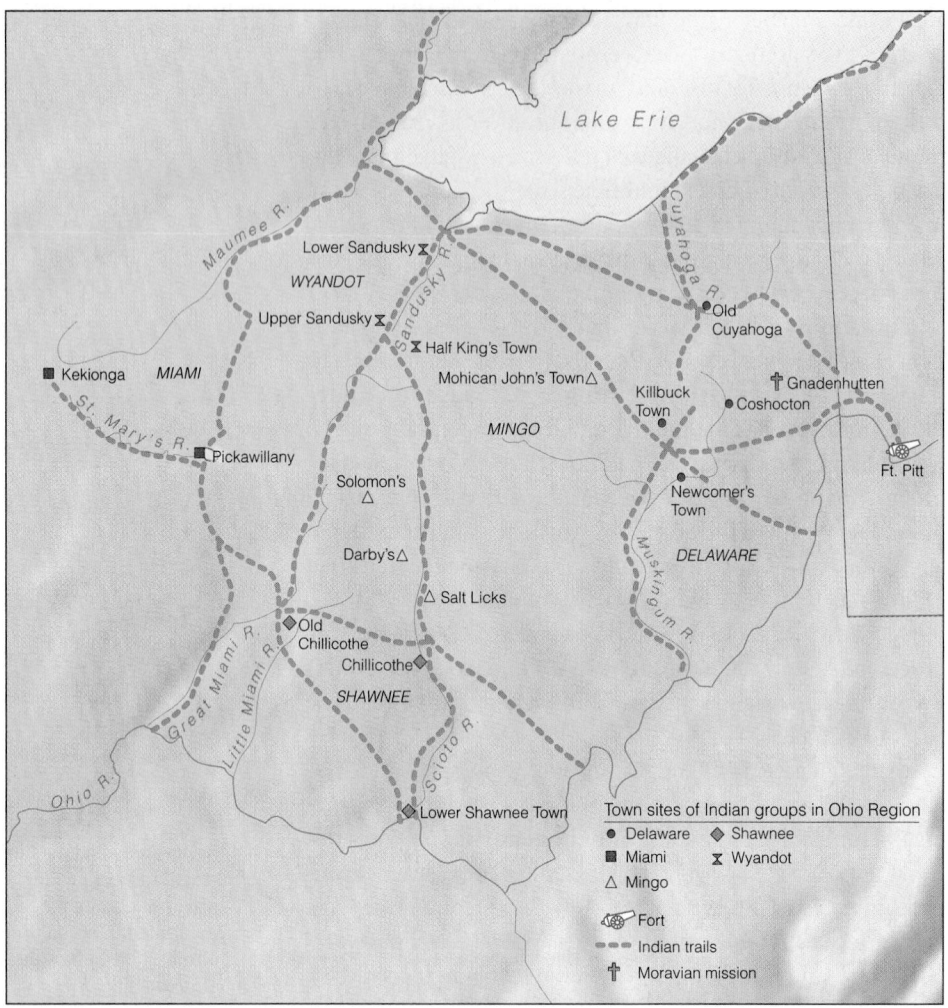

■ MAP 8.3
NATIVE AMERICAN OHIO BEFORE 1785 For centuries, what is now Ohio was a land of Native American villages, set by rivers. Key eighteenth-century Indian towns and trails are shown here. (In 1781 whites massacred Christian Indians at the Moravian mission of Gnadenhutten.)

Creditors and Debtors

The end of the Revolutionary War brought widespread economic depression. The money spent by foreign armies for goods and services dried up, and the split with Britain disrupted established patterns of commerce. When peace returned, merchants and artisans scrambled to find new markets and to locate new routes of profitable trade. At the same time, those who had preserved their holdings or made money during the war snapped up foreign goods that had been scarce during the fighting. These purchases—whether for luxury goods or more necessary items—drained hard currency away from the states and increased the Confederation's debt.

Citizens everywhere felt the brunt of the postwar slump as prices dropped and the money supply shrank. As credit tightened, merchants called in their loans and unpaid bills. But the people who had taken on debts earlier, when higher prices prevailed, had more difficulty in paying them off. Families, especially poor artisans and subsistence farmers, suddenly faced the threat of foreclosure and loss of their property. They fought back in local elections, state legislatures, and even the streets. Violence broke out in state after state, from New Hamp-

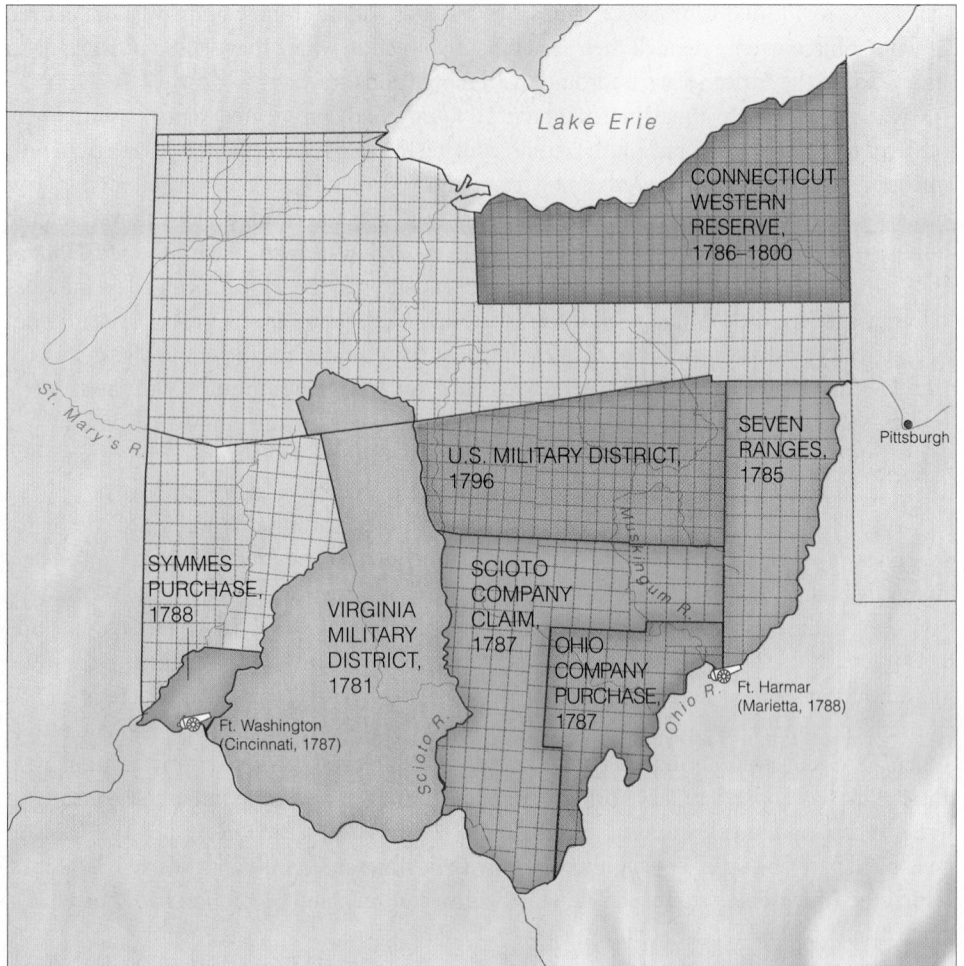
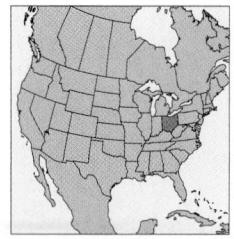

■ **MAP 8.4**
SETTLERS' OHIO, AFTER 1785   Starting in 1785, the American government imposed a novel grid system on the territory northwest of the Ohio River. Rectangular property lines and geometric state boundaries laid out by surveyors later overlay the natural landscape of the American West.

shire to Georgia, as hard-pressed people, many of them veterans, decried fiscal policies that seemed to favor the moneyed classes. When armed conflict erupted in Massachusetts, wealthy merchants raised an army to suppress the revolt. They succeeded, but they feared similar conflicts in the future. After all, democratic forces had shown that they had the strength to win control in a number of the state legislatures. The Massachusetts rebellion therefore helped prompt a drastic effort to restructure and strengthen the national government through a special, closed-door convention in Philadelphia.

New Sources of Wealth

As diplomats finalized the Peace Treaty of 1783, the British government managed to fire one parting shot at the former colonies. To nurture Britain's maritime trade and punish New England shippers, it imposed restrictions on the Americans' trade with the British West Indies. The move barred American ships from a key portion of Britain's imperial commerce, forcing merchants to seek out new avenues of trade. In 1784 an American vessel entered the Baltic Sea and established trade relations with Russia. Meanwhile, the New England whaling towns of Nantucket and New Bedford rebuilt their war-ravaged fleets and stepped up their search for whales to provide oil for American lamps. Sea captains had no trouble finding sailors in need of work. Ship owners extended their reach in any direction where they sensed possible profits, even into the African slave trade and the remote China trade.

Early in 1783, a Savannah merchant named Joseph Clay commented that a "vast number" of slaves had fled Georgia and South Carolina during the war. As rice plantations renewed production, African workers were "exceeding scarce and in demand." Sensing a profit, foreign slave traders shipped 15,000 Africans to the two states by 1785. American captains moved to grab a share of the trade. The seaports of Bristol, Newport, and Providence in Rhode Island, as well as Boston and Salem in Massachusetts, all sent ships to the west African coast in hopes of renewing a trade that had been interrupted during the war. True, antislavery sentiment had increased with the idealism of the Revolution. And several states, including Massachusetts, Rhode Island, and even Virginia, had passed laws outlawing slave imports. But these developments did not prevent American sea captains from transporting Africans to the Spanish West Indies and to Georgia and South Carolina. "The Negro business is a great object with us," Clay reported in 1784. "It is to the Trade of this Country, as the Soul to the body."

Although American merchants had taken part in the African trade and other commerce for generations, their ships had rarely, if ever, ventured outside the Atlantic. That changed dramatically in the decade after Yorktown. John Ledyard, an American who had sailed with Captain Cook in the Pacific, convinced financier Robert Morris of the profits to be made by opening new trade routes to the Orient. The project would take an enormous investment—ten times the amount needed to send a ship to Europe—but the potential rewards were irresistible. "I am sending some Ships to China," Morris announced to John Jay, "in order to encourage others in the adventurous pursuits of Commerce." His first vessel, a former privateer renamed the *Empress of China,* left New York harbor for Canton by way of the Indian Ocean early in 1784. It carried almost 30 tons of ginseng root—242 casks procured from the mountains in the "back part of Virginia"—highly prized by the Chinese. The ship also carried 2600 furs, which the Chinese used to line fashionable winter clothing, and $20,000 in hard currency, a huge drain on New York's economy.

In six months, the American vessel reached Canton, China's outlet for foreign commerce. "The Chinese had never heard of us," one sailor noted, "but we introduced ourselves as a new Nation, gave them our history, with a description of our Country," and stressed the mutual advantages of trade, "which they appear perfectly to understand and wish." The Chinese called the strangers "the new people." They called their country "the flowery flag kingdom" because to them the stars on the American flag resembled blossoms. Business proved brisk, and in May 1785 the *Empress of China* returned to New York loaded with tea, chinaware, and silk. Morris and his partners raked in a hefty 20 percent return on their investment.

Other traders took notice. In 1787 the Browns, wealthy merchants in Providence, diverted their slave ship, the *General Washington,* from the African trade to the China tea trade. That same year, six Boston investors sent two vessels—the *Columbia* and the *Lady Washington*—around Cape Horn at the tip of South America to trade for furs on the American Northwest Coast. Within five years, their captains, Robert Gray and William Kendrick, had pioneered new Pacific routes for American ships.

Captain Gray traded cloth and iron goods for sea otter pelts with the Nootka Indians. Then he took the *Columbia* across the Pacific, pausing at the Hawaiian Islands for supplies. Reaching Canton in 1789, Gray found 70 foreign ships in the harbor, 14 of them American. He traded profitably and proceeded home through the Indian Ocean, making the *Columbia* the first American ship to circumnavigate the globe. Because Gray's voyage affirmed the rewards of trade along the Northwest Coast, a diplomatic controversy flared the following year at Nootka Sound, on the west side of Vancouver Island. Although Spain protested British and American trading activities in the area, Gray was back on the Northwest Coast by 1792. He entered a powerful stream—where the states of Washington and Oregon now meet—and named it the Columbia River, after his ship. When he planted the American flag at the mouth of this major

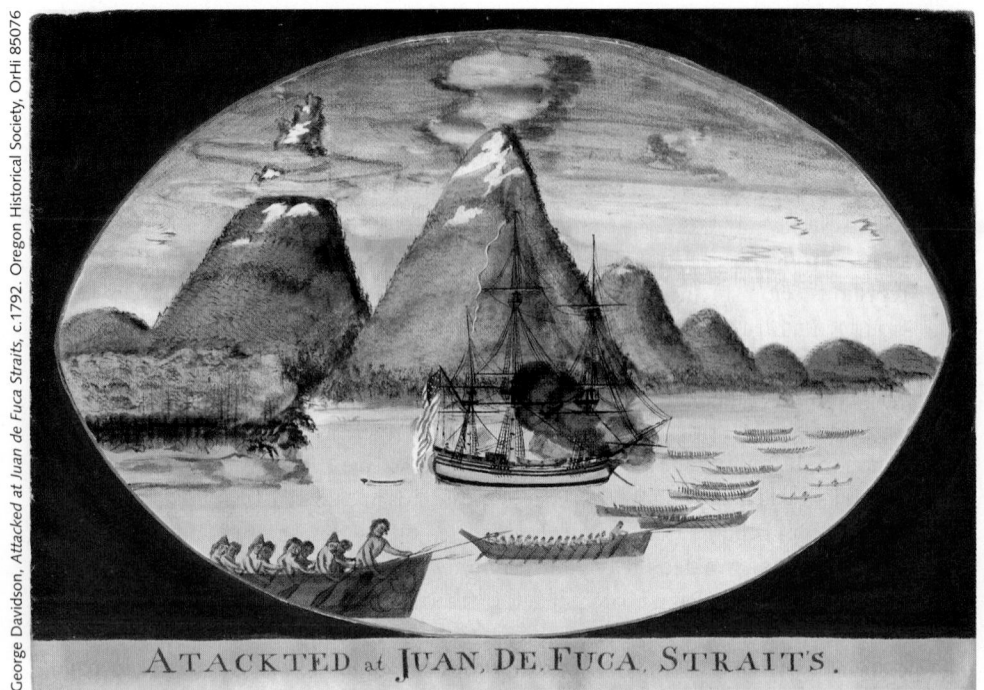

George Davidson, *Attacked at Juan de Fuca Straits*, c.1792. Oregon Historical Society, OrHi 85076

ATACKTED at JUAN. DE. FUCA. STRAITS.

■ This painting on glass shows Northwest Coast Indians menacing the American ship *Columbia* from their large war canoes. Captain Robert Gray was conducting trade for sea otter pelts to transport across the Pacific Ocean to China, where the soft fur was highly valued.

waterway, his action foreshadowed later territorial claims by the United States in the Oregon region. At the same time, Captain Kendrick, sailing in the *Lady Washington,* anchored off the Japanese island of Honshu, hoping to gain access for American trade. But Japan remained closed, and Kendrick's objective was not realized for another 62 years.

While American merchants probed for new markets from the Baltic to the Pacific, they also moved to strengthen their economic and political position at home. Peacetime brought forth a variety of ingenious schemes, many of which foundered in the troubled economy. But one practice attracted wide interest among the wealthiest people in town after town. Paying only a small fraction of the original value, they bought up a variety of loan certificates, paper notes, and wartime securities issued by state governments and the Continental Congress. Certificates issued to soldiers and officers at the end of the war rapidly became part of this speculative market as the original recipients sold their notes to prosperous speculators in return for ready cash. As a result, such holdings accumulated increasingly in the hands of the well-to-do. In Maryland, for example, the claims on $900,000 owed by the state became concentrated in the possession of only 318 people by 1790. Moreover, 16 of these people controlled more than half of the total value, and the 8 largest holders possessed 38 percent. As their speculative holdings increased, these few wealthy investors maneuvered to influence political events. They realized that the people who controlled the reins of power at the state and national levels would determine whether and how the various notes of credit might be redeemed. With this in mind, they purchased large quantities of these notes for a fraction of their face value. These men stood to reap enormous profits from any government that would pay interest on, and then buy back, all these paper arrangements at their original high value.

"Tumults in New England"

The few people who had acquired most of the paper securities wanted their holdings redeemed for hard money. But the majority of citizens, faced with rising debts amid an economic downturn, resented the heavy taxes needed to pay interest on the debt to these wealthy speculators. Favoring much easier credit, they urged their states to issue new paper money. This conflict was familiar from colonial times, when many merchants and planters, in debt to British firms, had chafed under Britain's tight fiscal policies. But the views of local elites had shifted when they gained control over their own state governments. They now wanted to limit paper money in ways that favored their new position as powerful creditors and holders of wartime certificates. Their opponents argued that issuing paper money could take the pressure off cash-strapped farmers and help retire enormous war debts. In seven states, these advocates of economic relief carried the day. State government presses put additional notes in circulation.

Local battles over debt, credit, and currency issues hit hardest in the Northeast for several reasons. During the war, Americans had foiled British plans to isolate and crush New England's rebellious colonists. Indeed, the region had prospered. Yankee farmers sold provisions to the Continental Army at hefty prices. French forces stationed at Newport in 1780 paid for food and firewood in gold coins. And throughout the war, numerous New England ships, known as privateers, fought with an eye on profit, hauling captured enemy vessels into local ports as prizes. In 1783, however, Britain's move to ban American ships from the British West Indies cut off the lucrative trade that New Englanders had created. For generations, these American captains had sold fish, grain, and lumber to the islands in exchange for hard currency. Sudden exclusion from Britain's Caribbean colonies dried up the flow of much-needed cash into New England and undermined the region's economy.

These changes had an immediate impact. In New Hampshire courts, debt cases rose six-fold from 1782 to 1785. Even if the debts themselves were not large, the heavy costs of traveling to court and paying high legal fees pushed thousands of families into insolvency. As long as the courts remained open, judges routinely ordered the seizure and sale of property. Embittered farmers watched as their horses, cows, wagons, and household goods disappeared in auction at low prices. Hard times often spark drastic responses, and New England's pot soon boiled over. Early in 1787, from his desk at Mount Vernon, Washington's secretary noted that the "tumults, insurrections, and *Rebellion* in New England have of late much engrossed the minds of the people here."

Newspaper accounts told of disturbing events in Rhode Island. There, rural politicians seeking relief for indebted farmers swept into power during the elections of April 1786. Their triumph freed the assembly from its longtime domination by rich Providence merchants. The newcomers, elected on their paper money platform, wasted no time in implementing their ballot box revolution. Their region had a withered economy, and the state government carried a burdensome war debt. To address these matters, assemblymen approved a huge outlay of paper money: £100,000. The assembly planned to distribute the legal tender among the towns and lend it to citizens on equitable terms. The revenue received back in taxes as the economy rebounded would then be used to pay off the state's debts and retire the paper currency. To ensure the plan's success, legislators declared the money as legal tender that all creditors had to accept as payment. And if any creditors refused to accept the paper money, debtors could deposit the funds with the county court. The judge would then advertise that the debt had been paid.

Many merchants closed their stores rather than accept payments in the new medium of exchange.

Not surprisingly, creditors and speculators resented Rhode Island's currency law. Moreover, they fumed at the new legislature's unwillingness to assume a share of the national debt and pay off wealthy bond holders, as other states had done. Without control over the legislature, these speculators feared they would be left holding all the continental securities they had acquired. They took swift action. Though heavily outnumbered, members of the moneyed class in Providence used their economic strength to fight back. Many merchants closed their stores rather than accept payments in the new medium of exchange. Some even left the state to avoid being forced to accept debt payments in paper money. When judges who favored the merchants' cause finally declared the new statute unconstitutional, creditors everywhere sighed with relief. Their newspapers condemned the "Rogue Island" currency law as a dire example of the dangers of democracy.

The Massachusetts Regulation

In Massachusetts and New Hampshire, unlike Rhode Island, wealthy merchants in coastal centers retained control over the new state assemblies. They therefore had the power to resist public pressure to generate more paper money. Such a policy might provide relief for an expanding backcountry population hit hard by the economic downturn and the scarcity of circulating currency, but it did not suit the interests of these creditors. Instead, it was the enforcement of debt collection by the courts that would best expand merchants' holdings and improve their standing in international trade. As in other states, a small contingent of wealthy speculators had bought up, at bargain rates, most of the public securities and certificates issued during the war. They anticipated enormous windfall profits if a government they controlled could redeem these notes, in gold and silver, at their full face value.

In New Hampshire, by 1785, securities valued at nearly £100,000 belonged to just 4.5 percent of the state's adult male population: 1120 men among approximately 25,000. A mere 3 percent of this group—34 men—controlled more than a third of this vast speculative investment. Most of these men had close ties to the prevailing government, situated in Exeter, near the coast. When farmers organized conventions to voice their economic grievances, merchants infiltrated and disrupted their meetings. In September 1786, 200 citizens, many of them armed war veterans, marched on Exeter to demand money reforms before conditions "drive us to a state of desperation." Officials organized cavalry units to confront the desperate citizens, arresting their leaders from the crowd "as a butcher would seize sheep in a flock." As soon as the state's governor, General John Sullivan, had suppressed the dissenters, he issued a proclamation forbidding further conventions. He then wrote to Massachusetts governor James Bowdoin, offering to help crush similar unrest in the neighboring state.

Early in 1786, the Commonwealth of Massachusetts had imposed a heavy direct tax

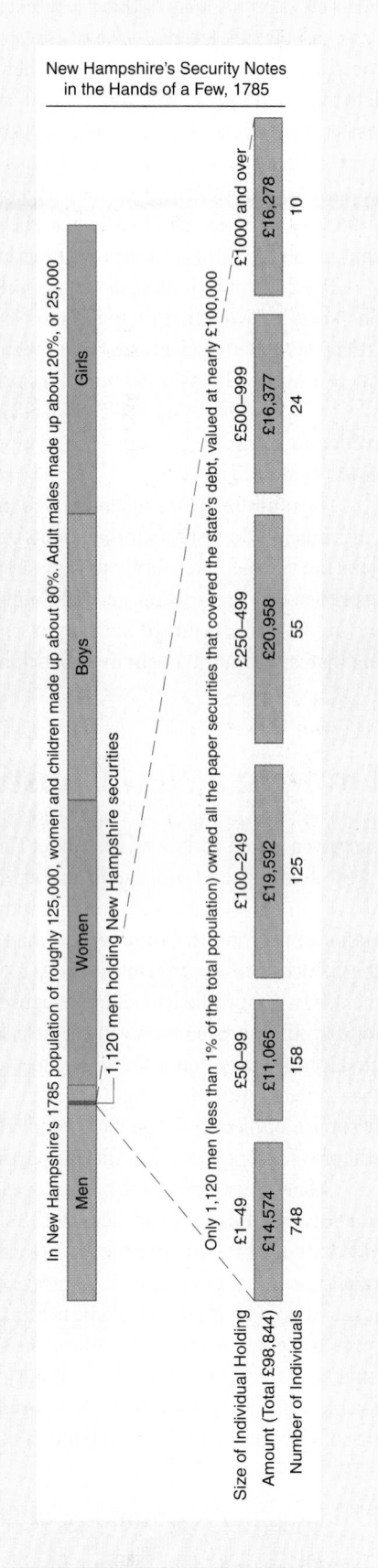

New Hampshire's Security Notes in the Hands of a Few, 1785

In New Hampshire's 1785 population of roughly 125,000, women and children made up about 80%. Adult males made up about 20%, or 25,000.

Only 1,120 men (less than 1% of the total population) owned all the paper securities that covered the state's debt, valued at nearly £100,000

1,120 men holding New Hampshire securities

Size of Individual Holding	£1–49	£50–99	£100–249	£250–499	£500–999	£1000 and over
Amount (Total £98,844)	£14,574	£11,065	£19,592	£20,958	£16,377	£16,278
Number of Individuals	748	158	125	55	24	10

■ **FIGURE 8.1**
CONCENTRATION OF SECURITY NOTES IN THE HANDS OF A FEW: THE EXAMPLE OF NEW HAMPSHIRE IN 1785

on its citizenry, stipulating that people pay it in hard currency. Western farmers lacked sufficient cash and already faced a wave of foreclosures for debt. They protested the tax law at town meetings and county conventions. When their complaints fell on deaf ears, they took actions into their own hands, "regulating" events as the North Carolina Regulators had done two decades earlier. The Massachusetts Regulation became known as Shays's Rebellion when Daniel Shays, a revolutionary officer who had served with distinction under Lafayette, emerged as one of its popular leaders. At first, these New England Regulators focused on closing the courts. In August 1786, 1500 farmers marched against the Court of Common Pleas in Hampshire County and shut it down. The next month, another band closed the court in Worcester.

The confrontation escalated as winter set in. By January the next year, more than 1000 Shaysites, knowing that their allies in New Hampshire had been defeated, moved to seize the federal arsenal in Springfield. But Governor Bowdoin had mobilized an army, financed largely by wealthy merchants in Boston. This private militia overpowered the westerners and forced all who did not flee to sign an oath of allegiance. Disarmed but not silenced, the dissidents succeeded in defeating Bowdoin in the next election and extracting some relief from the new governor, John Hancock.

The unrest in New England played into the hands of those advocating a stronger national government. (Some of their opponents even suspected that ardent nationalists had helped provoke the violence specifically to rally support for their cause.) In a typical letter, Henry Knox expressed fear to his fellow general, John Sullivan, that "we are verging fast to anarchy." Writing in May 1787, he urged Sullivan to send delegates from New Hampshire to a crucial meeting that was about to begin in Philadelphia.

Drafting a New Constitution

Even before Yorktown, Alexander Hamilton, Washington's youthful Caribbean-born aide-de-camp, had proposed a convention to restructure the national government. Now he worked with another young nationalist, James Madison, and their energetic supporters to bring it about. Congress had made earnest efforts toward reform, but any changes to the Confederation's governing articles required approval from all 13 states. Thus, vital amendments—which would let Congress regulate commerce, raise revenue, and establish a judiciary, for example—proved nearly impossible. For some powerful leaders, especially merchants and creditors, a major political revision seemed in order. They were willing to alter the Articles of the Confederation, which governed the United States, or perhaps even scrap them, in favor of some modified structure that would reflect their worldview and serve their own interests yet still prove acceptable to a sufficient portion of the people.

"Many Gentlemen both within & without Congress," wrote Madison, desire a "Convention for amending the Confederation." Still, it would take impressive leadership—Madison provided much of it—to seize the initiative and then generate enough momentum to change the rules of national government. Extensive compromise, both between elite factions and toward resistant popular forces, would be necessary at every stage. After all, it would take an enormous push to engineer such a convention, to guide it to restructure the government along nationalist lines, and finally to persuade voting Americans to ratify the proposed changes and accept their legitimacy. To begin such a task, would-be reformers needed to recruit the enormous prestige of George Washington and obtain the acquiescence of a stymied Congress.

Philadelphia: A Gathering of Like-Minded Men

The path began at Mount Vernon in 1785 when Washington hosted commissioners appointed by Maryland and Virginia to resolve state boundary disputes regarding the Potomac River.

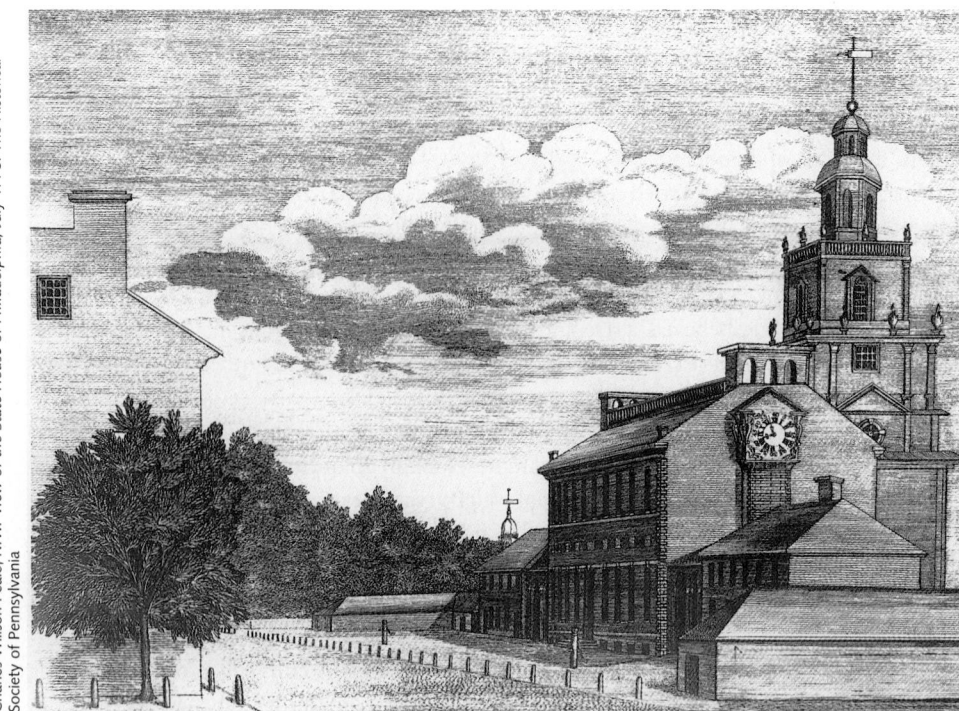

Charles Willson Peale, *N.W. View of the State House of Philadelphia*, July 1778. The Historical Society of Pennsylvania

■ In July 1787 *Columbian Magazine* published "A N.W. View of the State House in Philadelphia," drawn by Charles Willson Peale during the Revolutionary War. Once again, the country was in turmoil, and readers were eager for a glimpse of the place where delegates were meeting in secret session to alter the government.

During the gathering, these men (including James Madison) scheduled a broader meeting on Chesapeake trade for the next year at Annapolis, Maryland. They invited all the states to send representatives. Only 12 delegates from five states showed up at Annapolis in September 1786, but news of the serious unrest in New England prompted talk of a more extended meeting. Alexander Hamilton, as a representative from New York, persuaded the other delegates to call for a convention in Philadelphia the following May to discuss commerce and other matters. Madison won endorsement for the proposal from the Virginia legislature and then from Congress. Reform-minded congressmen, such as James Monroe, saw an opportunity to amend and improve the existing Confederation structure. But when the states sent delegates to Philadelphia the following spring, many of the appointees felt that amendments might not go far enough. They were open to the more sweeping changes that Madison and other nationalists had in mind. So the gathering called to consider commercial matters and propose improvements to the Articles of Confederation soon became a full-fledged Constitutional Convention, a private meeting to design and propose an entirely new structure for governing the United States.

Madison reached Philadelphia in early May 1787. He immediately began drafting plans for drastic change and lobbying delegates, some of whom came early to attend a secret gathering of the Society of the Cincinnati. On May 25, when representatives from seven states had arrived, they launched the convention and unanimously chose Washington as the presiding officer. Participants agreed that they would operate behind closed doors and each state delegation would have one vote. There would be no public discussion or official record of their proceedings. Soon, delegates from 12 states had joined the gathering. Only Rhode Island opted not to send representatives.

The 55 delegates had much in common. All were white, male, and well educated, and many already knew one another. These members of the national elite included 34 lawyers, 30 public creditors, and 27 members of the Society of the Cincinnati. More than a quarter of the participants owned slaves, and nearly a dozen had done personal business with financier Robert Morris of the Pennsylvania delegation. Not surprisingly, all seemed to agree that the contagion of liberty had spread too far. Indeed, Elbridge Gerry of Massachusetts called the current situation "an excess of democracy."

Specifically, these men feared recent legislation that state assemblies had adopted to assist hard-pressed citizens: laws that delayed tax collection, postponed debt payments, and issued paper money. Most delegates hoped to replace the existing Confederation structure with a national government capable of controlling finances and creating creditor-friendly fiscal policy. To be effective, they believed, a strengthened central government must have greater control over the states. Only Robert Yates and John Lansing of New York and Luther Martin of Maryland staunchly resisted expanding central power.

Many of the delegates, especially those from the large states, thought that the national legislature should be based on proportional representation according to the number of inhabitants rather than each state receiving equal weight regardless of its population. Also, most wanted to see the single-house (unicameral) Congress of the Confederation replaced by an upper and lower house that would reflect the views and values of different social classes. John Adams had helped create such a two-house (bicameral) system in the Massachusetts constitution, thereby limiting pure democracy and giving more political power to propertied interests. Besides calling for checks within the legislative branch itself, Adams had also laid out strong arguments for separating, and checking, the powers of each competing branch of government. For a sound and lasting government, Adams had argued in earlier essays, the legislative branch should be balanced by separate executive and judicial branches that are equally independent. Most delegates agreed with this novel system of checks and balances, intended to add stability and remove corruption.

Compromise and Consensus

The Philadelphia gathering, which lasted through the entire summer, would later be known as the Constitutional Convention of 1787. Even as a general consensus emerged within the small meeting, countless personal, practical, and philosophical differences persisted. Hamilton delivered a six-hour speech in which he staked out an extremely conservative position, no doubt intended to make other proposals look more moderate and therefore acceptable. He underscored "the imprudence of democracy" and stressed a natural separation between "the few and the many"—the "wealthy well born" and the "turbulent and changing" people. Hamilton's conservative oration called for the chief executive and the senators to be chosen indirectly, by elected representatives rather than by the people themselves, and he recommended that these high officials should serve for life. Such ideas undoubtedly appealed to many of his listeners, but all of the delegates knew that a majority of citizens would never accept such proposals. Pierce Butler of South Carolina, invoking ancient Greece, urged members to "follow the example of Solon, who gave the Athenians not the best government he could devise but the best they would receive."

This attentiveness of convention members to what the public would accept is illustrated by their approach to voting rights. Even delegates who wanted to limit the vote to property holders realized that various state constitutions, responding to popular pressure, had already distributed suffrage more broadly. Property ownership was no longer a universal voting requirement, and states varied on whether religion, race, or gender could determine eligibility. James Wilson of Pennsylvania, second only to Madison in working to build a practical nationalist majority in the convention, pointed out that "it would be very hard and disagreeable" for any person, once franchised, to give up the right to vote. Accordingly, the delegates proposed that in each state all those allowed to vote for the "most numerous branch of the state legislature" would also be permitted to cast ballots for members of the House of Representatives. But they shied away from accepting direct election for the Senate or the president, and they deferred suffrage matters to the states.

Time and again during the 16-week convention, these like-minded men showed their willingness to bargain and compromise. Lofty principles and rigid schemes often gave way to balancing and improvisation. The unlikely creation of the electoral college for selecting a president is one example. Delegates who differed over the length for the chief executive's term of office and right to run for reelection also disagreed on the best method of presidential selection. Some of them suggested that ordinary voters should elect him; others proposed that the state governors, or the national legislature, or even electors chosen by state legislators should choose the chief executive.

Finally, the aptly named Committee on Postponed Matters cobbled together an acceptable system: a gathering (or "college") of chosen electors from each state would cast votes for the presidency. This electoral college plan had little precedent, but it managed to balance competing interests. Under the scheme, state legislatures would set the manner for selecting electors. The least populous states would get a minimum of three electoral votes, and states with more people would choose more electors in proportion to their numbers, giving them added weight in the decision. The people could also participate in the voting process, though only if their state legislatures called for it. And if no candidate won a majority in the electoral college, the House of Representatives had the right to determine the president, with each state having one vote. The system was far from elegant or democratic, but it placated varied interests, and it won prompt approval.

Questions of Representation

As deliberations stretched across the long, hot summer of 1787, two central issues threatened to unravel the convention: political representation and slavery. Questions of representation pervaded almost every discussion, pitting large states such as Virginia, Pennsylvania, and Massachusetts against the less populated states. Madison's well-organized Virginians offered a comprehensive blueprint outlining a new national government that would have three separate branches. This design, called the "Virginia Plan," recommended a bicameral national legislature with proportional representation in each body. The House of Representatives would be chosen by popular election, the Senate by state legislators.

Madison's system clearly favored populous states. Not surprisingly, a coalition of small-state delegates led by William Paterson of New Jersey submitted an alternative "New Jersey Plan." This less sweeping revision built on the current Articles of Confederation. It called for a continuation of the existing unicameral legislature, in which each state received an equal vote. A committee chaired by Benjamin Franklin managed to break the impasse. The idea of an upper house, or Senate, would be retained, and each state, whatever its size, would hold two senate seats. Seats in the House of Representatives would be determined proportionally, according to the relative population of each state. Moreover, this lower house would have the power to initiate all bills dealing with finance and money matters.

As deliberations stretched across the long, hot summer of 1787, two central issues threatened to unravel the convention: political representation and slavery.

To implement proportional representation in a fast-growing society, the delegates provided for a national census every 10 years. No European country had attempted a regular periodic headcount, so the census represented a radical innovation at the time. This in turn raised a thorny question. Should slaves—people enumerated in the census yet denied the rights of citizens—be counted in determining a state's proportional representation in the national government? Slaveholding states wanted their human property to count because that would give those states more representation. The convention resolved this dilemma in mid-July with

Equal Representation?

The ratified Constitution was an approved blueprint, not a finished house. In the name of "We, the people of the United States," the new plan affirmed citizen representation in government. The tradition had grown during generations of local self-rule in the colonies, and debate over the issue had sparked rebellion from British rule. Regular elections allowing the choice of "representative" public officials would be central to the new framework. But each state government held the right to decide how "the people" would be defined in election matters. And no one knew how the proposed federal court system might rule on these issues. Everywhere, concerned onlookers wondered how representation would work in the new republic.

After all, the majority of inhabitants found themselves excluded from the franchise on the basis of age, gender, or race. Status as a slave or servant, lack of sufficient property, military status, tax classification, criminal record, or length of residency could also be factors in denying the vote. But to many in the ruling elite, broadening the franchise appeared a dangerous proposition. "Democracy," Elbridge Gerry had told the Constitutional Convention, is "the worst . . . of all political evils." (Later, when he served as governor of Massachusetts, Gerry's name became associated with the art of drawing voting districts in strange shapes to assure political advantage, a practice known ever after as *gerrymandering*.)

Struggles over the right to vote have expanded the franchise and the

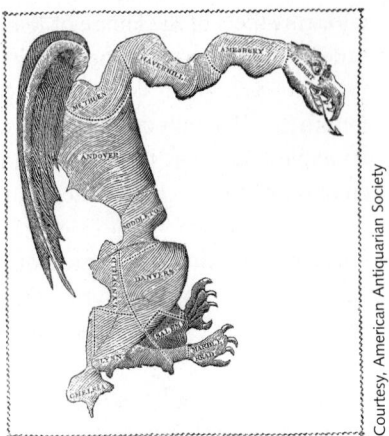

Courtesy, American Antiquarian Society

Voting districts linked together in strange ways for political advantage have been known as a "gerrymander" ever since 1812, when a cartoonist suggested that the arrangement designed by Elbridge Gerry to connect counties in Massachusetts resembled "a new species of Monster."

federal government's role in guaranteeing that right through amendments to the Constitution itself. After the bloody Civil War, the Fifteenth Amendment (1870) granted that a citizen's voting rights could not be "denied or abridged . . . on account of race, color, or previous condition of servitude" (gender was not mentioned), and it empowered Congress to enforce the article. But Congress shirked this assignment and tolerated new devices for black disfranchisement. Similarly, Congress failed to protect Native American voting rights, even after a 1924 act granted Indians the rights of citizenship. Meanwhile, women mounted a suffrage campaign of their own, leading to passage of the Nineteenth Amendment (1920), removing voting restrictions "on account of sex."

As enfranchisement expanded, so did the proliferation of devices to inhibit voting and limit its value. In the segregated South, poll taxes, literacy tests, and outright intimidation all

became tactics for preventing black voter registration and participation. So did racial gerrymandering. When Charles Gomillion, a sociologist at Tuskegee Institute, registered hundreds of black voters in Macon County, Alabama, during the 1950s, the white legislature fought back. It redrew the boundaries of the city of Tuskegee to exclude most black voters, "gerrymandering" them into adjacent precincts where their votes would count for little. In a landmark case (*Gomillion v. Lightfoot,* 1960), the Supreme Court ruled such redistricting unconstitutional. When Congress, pressured by the Civil Rights Movement, passed the Voting Rights Act of 1965, the idea of "one person, one vote" gained a legal foothold in the land. Each person should be able to register freely, cast a secret ballot, and have that vote tallied fairly. But in addition, one citizen's vote should *count* as much as another.

In one way, the framers of the Constitution anticipated the problem of uneven representation, for they mandated a new census every ten years. This headcount would allow state and federal legislators to reapportion representation every decade in a rapidly growing society, with courts overseeing the disputes. But in another way, the framers, through their electoral college system, created a time bomb of sorts. What would happen if a presidential candidate received the majority of the popular vote but only a minority of votes in the electoral college? Such an unlikely event occurred once in 1876, with chaotic results, and again in 2000. Both times, millions of voters suddenly realized that in selecting a president each ballot does not have equal weight. This ensures that the debate over how American leaders are selected will continue for years to come. ■

a "three-fifths" formula that Madison had proposed in earlier legislation. The odd recipe made every five enslaved people equivalent to three free people in apportionment matters.

In an ironic twist, the same week the Constitutional Convention delegates approved the notorious three-fifths clause, the existing government of the United States leaned in the opposite direction. Meeting in New York, members of th Confederation's Congress passed the Northwest Ordinance, which outlawed slavery in the new territory above the Ohio River. Because there was much contact between the two meetings, some scholars speculate that powerful Southerners agreed to give away the prospect of slavery north of the Ohio River in exchange for more support of slavery within the new plan taking shape in Philadelphia.

Slavery: The Deepest Dilemma

During the debate over the three-fifths clause, Madison commented that the greatest division in the United States "did not lie between the large & small States: it lay between the Northern & Southern," owing to "the effects of their having or not having slaves." This highly charged issue continued to simmer beneath the surface for most of the summer.

In late August, with most other matters resolved, delegates could no longer postpone questions surrounding slavery. Yet again, a committee deliberated, and a bargain was struck. But this time, hundreds of thousands of human lives were at stake. Planter delegates from Georgia and South Carolina refused to support any document that regulated the slave trade or curtailed slavery itself. And, they asserted, such a charter could never win acceptance at home. In part they were bluffing. In fact, constraints against slavery had wide popular appeal in the expanding backcountry of the Deep South, where independent farmers outnumbered planters, ministers questioned slavery, and pioneers wanted national support in confronting powerful Indians.

Yet few delegates challenged the proslavery posture, possibly because strong antislavery opinions could have prolonged or even deadlocked the convention. The weary delegates were eager to complete their work and fearful of unraveling their hard-won consensus. Rather than force the matter, even those who disapproved of slavery rushed to compromise. In doing so, they heaped a huge burden on generations of Americans to come. Southern delegates dropped their protests against giving Congress the power to regulate international shipping. In exchange, the framers approved a clause protecting the importation of slaves for at least 20 years. They also added a provision governing fugitive slaves that required the return of "any person held to service or labor." Through a calculated bargain, delegates had endorsed slavery and drawn the South into the union on terms that suited that region's leaders. The word *slave* never appeared in the finished document.

In early September, the convention members put the finishing touches on their proposal and prepared to present it to the public. Most still had qualms about the document they had created and wondered whether Americans would accept it. Winning state-by-state approval would involve an uphill battle, especially given the delegates' resistance to the idea of a bill of rights. George Mason, who had drawn up Virginia's Declaration of Rights 11 years earlier, reminded members that such a set of guarantees "would give great quiet to the people." But in the convention's closing days, fellow delegates voted down his suggestion overwhelmingly.

Without a bill of rights, Mason and Gerry refused to endorse the final document, along with Edmund Randolph of Virginia. Other delegates who

In a crucial decision, members of the Constitutional Convention elected to protect the slave trade and preserve slavery. One African American who had already taken matters in her own hands was Mumbet, a slave in Massachusetts and widow of a Revolutionary War soldier. In 1781 she sued for her freedom on the grounds that "all were born free and equal." Her court victory proved a landmark in New England. Proudly, she took the name Elizabeth Freeman.

dissented had already departed. Of the 74 delegates chosen at the convention's outset, 55 actually attended the proceedings, and only 39 agreed to sign the finished plan. These small numbers made it more important than ever to end on a note of unanimity. By polling the state delegations instead of individual delegates, the document's authors shrewdly hid the three dissenting votes. This allowed them to assert, in article VII, that their task—framing a new constitution for the United States—had been approved "by the unanimous consent of the States present" on September 17, 1787.

Ratification and the Bill of Rights

Having negotiated an alternative structure for a strengthened central government, committed nationalists now faced their most difficult task: winning public acceptance for a document that defied existing law. After all, the proposed constitution ignored the fact that the Articles of Confederation—the document governing the United States at the time—could be amended only with the approval of all 13 states. Instead, the text drafted in Philadelphia stated that ratification (acceptance through voting) by conventions in any nine states would make the new document take effect in those places. Moreover, the proposed ratification process left no room for partial approval or suggested revisions. Each state, if it wanted to enter the debate at all, had to accept or reject the proposed frame of government as offered.

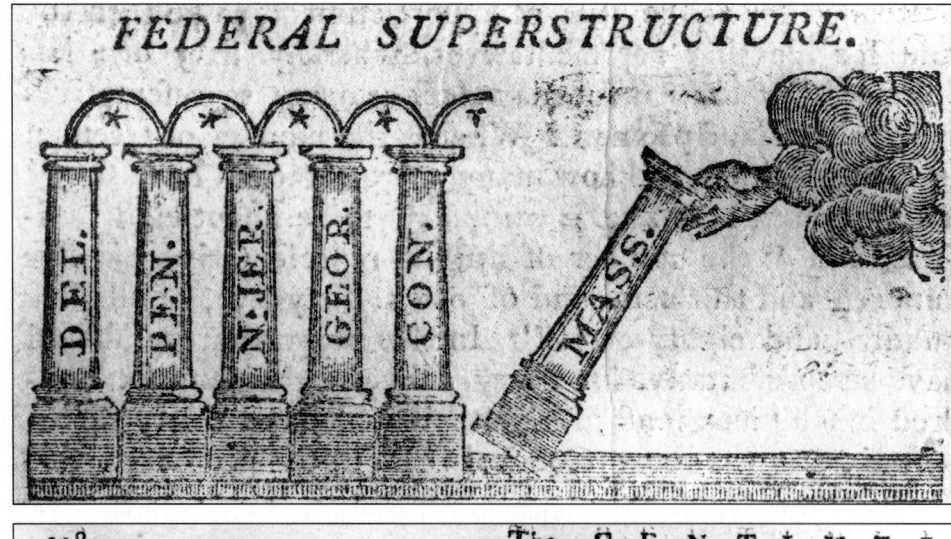

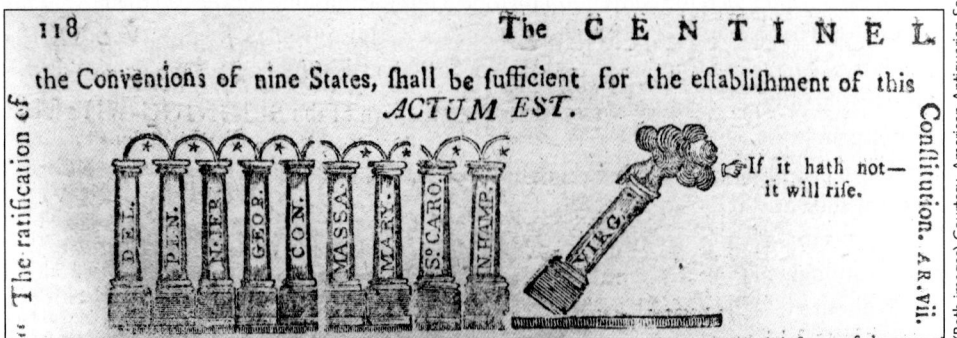

(Both images) Courtesy, American Antiquarian Society

■ In 1788 newspapers tracked ratification of the new "federal superstructure" state by state. Massachusetts ratified the proposed Constitution in March—apparently aided by the Hand of God! New Hampshire provided the "ninth and sufficient pillar" in June, followed by Virginia four days later.

The Campaign for Ratification

The Confederation Congress had acquiesced in allowing the convention to occur in the first place. Most congressional representatives had expected the meeting to produce proposals for amending the current government, not discarding it. But now that the Philadelphia conclave had ended, the Congress sitting in New York City balked at endorsing the revolutionary document. To avoid a lengthy and troublesome debate, proponents of the new constitution urged Congress simply to receive the frame of government as a possible proposal and then transmit it to the states without an endorsement. Congress did so on September 28, 1787, and the document's advocates portrayed the unanimous vote as an expression of approval.

Supporters had no time to lose because Pennsylvania's assembly was set to adjourn on the next day. An early victory in that large and central state would be crucial in building momentum before an organized opposition developed. So they hired a courier to rush the congressional letter of transmittal from New York to Philadelphia. There, the assembly faction dominated by Robert Morris quickly moved to schedule a state ratifying convention. When opposition members saw that they could not defeat the motion on short notice, 19 of them walked out of the chamber, hoping to prevent a vote that would begin the ratification the process. But proponents dragged back two of them to have enough members for a legal vote. Over the next three months, towns and counties elected delegates, a convention met, and Pennsylvania voted to approve the new plan. Delaware had already approved unanimously on December 7, and New Jersey and Georgia promptly followed suit. By the end of January, Connecticut had also ratified. Other states had called elections and scheduled conventions. Only Rhode Island, which had not sent delegates to the drafting convention, refused to convene a meeting to debate ratification.

By seizing the initiative early, the proponents of the new framework shaped the terms of debate. The drafters, anything but a cross-section of society, worked to portray themselves as such. They noted that their document began with the ringing phrase, "We the people of the United States," a last-minute addition by Gouverneur Morris of New York. And Madison told the public that the text sprang from "*your* convention."

Most important, in a reversal of logic and contemporary usage, the nationalists who supported the new constitution took for themselves the respected name of *Federalists*. They gave their opponents, a diverse assortment of doubters and critics, the negative-sounding term *Anti-Federalists*. The Federalists then used their ties to elite leaders and influential editors to wage a media war for public support. They dashed off letters, prepared pamphlets, and published essays praising the proposed constitution.

The strongest advocacy came from the pens of Alexander Hamilton and James Madison. The two men composed 80 essays for the New York press under the pen name *Publius*. John Jay added five more, and in the spring of 1788 the collection appeared as a book titled *The Federalist*. In the most famous piece, "Number 10," Madison challenged the widely accepted idea that a republic must be small and compact to survive. Turning the proposition around, he argued that minority opinions would fare better in a large nation, where diverse competing interests would prevent a unified majority from exerting control.

Dividing and Conquering the Anti-Federalists

Opponents of the new plan found themselves on the defensive from the start. Many of them had supported some government change, and most conceded the presence of economic difficulties. But the Federalists' dire predictions of impending chaos struck them as exaggerated. "I deny that we are in immediate danger of anarchy," one Anti-Federalist writer protested.

Richard Henry Lee, president of the Confederation Congress, condemned the Federalists as a noisy "coalition of monarchy men, military men, aristocrats and drones." Other prominent figures joined him in opposition: George Clinton in New York; Luther Martin, Samuel

Chase, and William Paca in Maryland; and Patrick Henry, George Mason, and Benjamin Harrison in Virginia. Though not always sufficiently forceful or committed, such notables became the spokespeople for a far wider array of skeptics.

Many critics of the proposed constitution protested the plan's perceived threat to local political power. Despite Madison's reassurances in Federalist Number 10, they believed that local and state governments represented voters more fairly and responded to their needs and concerns more quickly than a distant national authority could. For some critics this belief expressed a radical democratic principle; for others it represented their firm provincial bias. In short, Anti-Federalists were too diverse to speak with a single voice. Their ranks included many subsistence farmers living at a distance from any navigable river or urban market. These self-sufficient yeomen were joined by numerous war veterans who saw their rights to direct influence in republican government diminished by the proposed system. A wide variety of indebted people also opposed ratification, on the grounds that a strong national government would favor the interests of bond holders and foreign creditors ahead of the economic well-being of ordinary people.

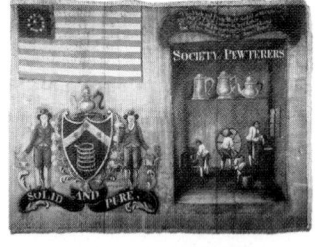

But if Anti-Federalists were numerous in the remote countryside, Federalists predominated in the coastal commercial centers. Using a variety of tactics, they pressed their advantages in the fight to control state ratifying conventions. They lured prominent Anti-Federalist delegates with hints of high office in the proposed national government. They also intimidated less prominent figures by ridiculing them as Shaysite extremists. Meanwhile, in state after state, they forged coalitions linking large commercial farmers living near towns and rivers with aspiring artisans and city-based entrepreneurs. Through intensive politicking, they garnered approval in Massachusetts in February 1788, but only by a thin margin (187 votes to 168 in the ratifying convention). This commitment from "the Bay State" helped to sway Maryland in April, South Carolina in May, and New Hampshire in June.

In July 1788 celebrations hailed the new Constitution. "Columbus" on horseback led New York City's parade, followed by artisan groups. The silk banner of the pewterers proclaimed that under the Federal Plan, "All Arts Shall Flourish in Columbia's Land, And All Her Sons Join as One Social Band."

The Federalists could now claim the nine states they said they needed to implement their plan, and the approved Constitution became the law of the land. But in Massachusetts, they had triumphed only by promising to add a bill of rights, giving explicit written protection for valued civil liberties. They had to make similar assurances during the summer to secure slim majorities in Virginia (89 to 79) and New York (30 to 27). North Carolinians had voted down the proposed frame of government at their first ratifying convention because it lacked a bill of rights. A second North Carolina convention, called in 1789, withheld approval until a bill of rights had actually been introduced into the first Federal Congress as proposed amendments to the Constitution. In 1790, Rhode Island narrowly voted approval for the new framework (34 to 32) rather than risk being left in economic and political isolation.

Adding a Bill of Rights

In a society consisting of almost 3 million people, the franchise remained a limited privilege, open primarily to white men with property. All told, only about 160,000 voters throughout the country took part in choosing representatives to the state ratifying conventions. And only about 100,000 of these people—less than 7 percent of the entire adult population—cast votes for delegates who supported the Constitution. Fully aware of these slim numbers, the Federalists knew they would have to fulfill their promise to incorporate a bill of rights. Madison, goaded by Jefferson from his post in Paris, promised Virginians that he would push for the inclusion of specific rights as amendments to the Constitution. In making this promise, he had several motives. First, he hoped to ensure his own election to the nation's new House of Representatives. Second, he wanted to stave off the prospect that discontented states would call a second national convention "for a reconsideration of the whole structure of government."

In compiling a list of protections, or bill of rights, Madison drew from scores of proposals for explicit amendments put forward by the state ratifying conventions. He selected those, mostly dealing with individual rights, that could pass a Federalist-dominated Congress and would not dilute any of the proposed new government's powers. He set aside suggestions for limiting the government's right to impose taxes, raise a standing army, or control the time and place of elections. True to his word, he pushed 12 less controversial statements through the Congress as constitutional amendments, despite congressional apathy and opposition. Within two years, three-fourths of the states ratified ten of these short but weighty pronouncements. Hence, the first ten amendments—the Bill of Rights—quickly became a permanent part of the U.S. Constitution.

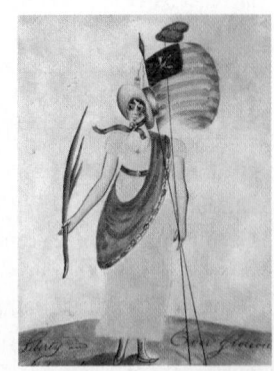

Many of the protections provided by the Bill of Rights harked back to lessons learned in the colonists' earlier struggle with Parliament. The ten amendments guarded the right of the people to bear arms, limited government power to quarter troops in private homes, and banned unreasonable searches or seizures. They also guaranteed crucial legal safeguards by ensuring the right to trial by jury, outlawing excessive bail and fines, and prohibiting "cruel and unusual punishments." The First Amendment secured freedom of speech and of the press, protected people's right to assemble and petition, and prohibited Congress from meddling in the exercise of religion. By securing these freedoms, Madison engineered a final set of compromises that ensured the acceptance and longevity of the Constitution he had done so much to frame.

Conclusion

The War for Independence exhausted the new nation. Defeating the British and managing the difficult task of demobilization and reconstruction consumed American energy and resources in the 1780s. So did the new western domain, where Americans had to balance prospects for national expansion against the military threats posed by European empires and Native American groups that asserted old and competing claims in the region. Also, economic differences set aside during the war reemerged in the years after Yorktown, so questions of wealth and property loomed large. How should the public debt be handled? Should slavery and the African slave trade be allowed to continue?

Over all these matters hovered the basic issue of governance. Independence from Britain meant an end to monarchy for Americans. They were keenly aware that they were sailing in uncharted waters as they experimented with constitution-making at every level. Acceptance of the Articles of Confederation in 1781 was a major accomplishment, and all assumed that the structure would demand further revision and adjustment. However, few could foresee that it would be set aside for a more centralized federal design within eight years.

The fierce debate over ratification of the new constitution raised fresh uncertainties about the long-term survival of the union. Much hinged on selection of the first president for the newly constituted nation. Only a few years earlier, Madison—then a young representative serving in Philadelphia—had met George Washington as the general journeyed south toward Yorktown in 1781. Now the fellow Virginian, 19 years Madison's senior, was the overwhelming favorite to become the first chief executive of the new republic.

Sites to Visit

Washington's Newburgh Headquarters

For 16 months in 1782–1783, the farmhouse of Jonathan Hasbrouck served as Washington's headquarters in Newburgh, New York, 12 miles north of West Point. The state of New York purchased the stone building on Lafayette Street in 1850 and opened it as the first publicly operated historic site in the United States.

Fraunces Tavern

Here, at 54 Pearl Street near the tip of Manhattan, Washington bid farewell to his officers in 1783. From 1785 to 1787, while New York served as the capitol city, the building held the departments of foreign affairs, the treasury, and war. Now it houses a museum with exhibits relating to the eighteenth century.

Mount Vernon

www.mountvernon.org/

During the nineteenth century, concerned women rallied to preserve Mount Vernon, George Washington's estate on the Potomac River. It is still maintained by the Mount Vernon Ladies' Association. If you cannot visit the plantation itself, eight miles south of Alexandria, Virginia, you can visit the Web site.

Independence National Historical Park in Philadelphia

Covering 45 acres and containing 20 buildings, this site includes Independence Hall, where the Constitutional Convention met in the summer of 1787. The Visitor Center is at Third and Walnut Streets. On the Market–Frankfurt Subway, use the 5th St. and Market station.

The Natchez Trace Parkway

Running 444 miles from Natchez, Mississippi, to the outskirts of Nashville, Tennessee, this one-time Chickasaw Indian trail became a pathway for boatmen returning north after floating their goods down the Mississippi. It is now a scenic road maintained by the National Park Service.

Congress and the Constitution

memory.loc.gov/ammem/bdsds/bdsdhome.html

The Continental Congress and the Constitutional Convention are the subjects of a rich Web site created by the Library of Congress in its American Memory series.

James Madison: His Legacy

www.jmu.edu/madison/madison.htm

The James Madison Center at James Madison University in Virginia maintains this Web site, which provides ready access to materials on Madison's life and interests, along with links to numerous documents and Web sites.

Historic Bartram's Garden

www.ushistory.org/tour/index.html

This Web site is part of LibertyNet's Virtual Tour of Historic Philadelphia. The garden itself, located at 54th Street and Lindbergh Boulevard, is run by the John Bartram Association, named for William's botanist father. Visit http://www.bartramtrail.org/ to learn more about backpacking Bartram's Trail through the South.

For Further Reading

General

Merrill Jensen, *The New Nation: A History of the United States During the Confederation, 1781–1789* (1948).

Richard B. Morris, *The Forging of the Union, 1781–1789* (1987).

Kenneth Silverman, *A Cultural History of the American Revolution* (1976).

Larry E. Tise, *The American Counterrevolution: A Retreat from Liberty, 1783–1800* (1998).

Gordon S. Wood, *The Creation of the American Republic, 1776–1787* (1969).

Beating Swords into Plowshares

Elizabeth A. Fenn, *Pox Americana: The Great Smallpox Epidemic of 1775–82* (2001).

Richard H. Kohn, *Eagle and Sword: The Federalists and the Creation of the Military Establishment in America, 1783–1802* (1975).

Henry F. May, *The Enlightenment in America* (1976).

George R. Stewart, *Names on the Land*, 4th ed. (1982).

Competing for Control of the Mississippi Valley

Gregory Evans Dowd, *A Spirited Resistance: The North American Indian Struggle for Unity, 1745–1815* (1992).

R. Douglas Hurt, *The Ohio Frontier: Crucible of the Old Northwest, 1720–1830* (1996).

Peter S. Onuf, *Statehood and Union: A History of the Northwest Ordinance* (1987).

John Sugden, *Blue Jacket: Warrior of the Shawnees* (2000).

Arthur Preston Whitaker, *The Spanish American Frontier, 1783–1795* (1927, reprinted 1969).

Creditors and Debtors

E. James Ferguson, *The Power of the Purse: A History of American Public Finance, 1776–1790* (1961).

Jackson Turner Main, *The Anti-Federalists: Critics of the Constitution, 1781–1788* (1961).

Edmund S. Morgan, *Inventing the People: The Rise of Popular Sovereignty in England and America* (1988).

David P. Szatmary, *Shays' Rebellion: The Making of an Agrarian Insurrection* (1980).

Drafting a New Constitution

Charles A. Beard, *An Economic Interpretation of the Constitution of the United States* (1913).

Donald A. Grinde, Jr., and Bruce E. Johansen, *Exemplar of Liberty: Native America and the Evolution of Democracy* (1991).

Leonard W. Levy and Dennis J. Mahoney, eds., *The Framing and Ratification of the Constitution* (1987).

John P. Kaminski, ed., *A Necessary Evil? Slavery and the Debate Over the Constitution* (1995).

Jack N. Rakove, *Original Meanings: Politics and Ideas in the Making of the Constitution* (1996).

Ratification and the Bill of Rights

Akhil Reed Amar, *The Bill of Rights: Creation and Reconstruction* (1998).

Saul Cornell, *The Other Founders: Anti-Federalism and the Dissenting Tradition in America, 1788–1828* (1999).

Michael Kammen, *A Machine That Would Go by Itself: The Constitution in American Culture* (1986).

Robert A. Rutland, *The Ordeal of the Constitution: The Antifederalists and the Ratification Struggle of 1787–1788* (1966).

Garry Wills, *Explaining America: The Federalist* (1981).

Online Practice Test

Test your understanding of this chapter with interactive review quizzes at

www.ablongman.com/jonescreatedequal/chapter8

Additional Photo Credits

CHAPTER

9

Revolutionary Legacies, 1789–1803

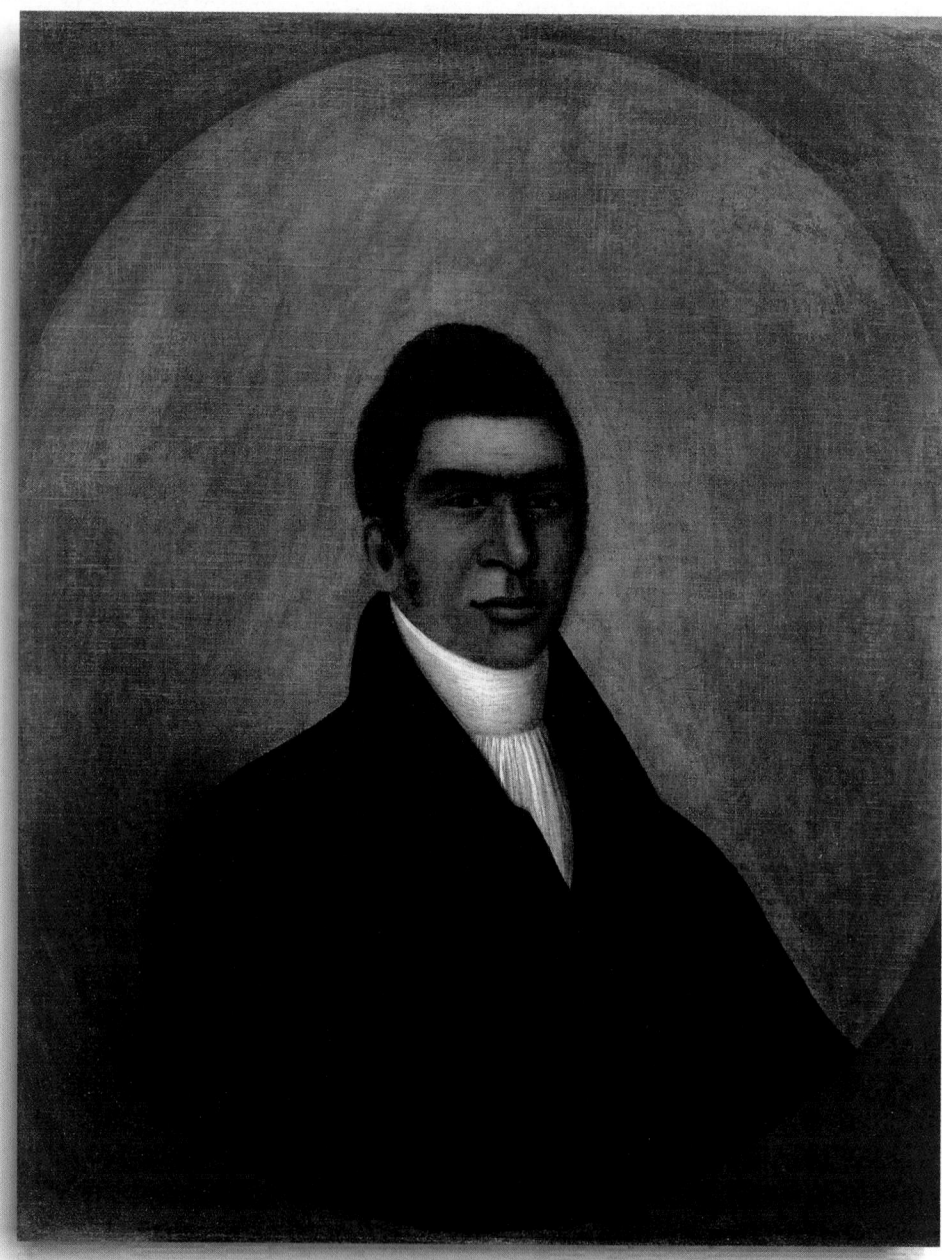

Joshua Johnson, *Portrait of a Cleric*, c. 1805–1810. Bowdoin College Museum of Art, Brunswick, Maine (Acc. #1963.490). Museum Purchase, George Otis Hamlin Fund

■ *Portrait of a Cleric*, c. 1805–1810 by Joshua Johnson

THE AMERICAN REVOLUTION DESTROYED ONE INDIAN CONFEDERATION AND LED TO THE creation of another. The Six Nations of the Iroquois Confederacy—which consisted of the Seneca, Cayuga, Oneida, and Mohawk nations of present-day New York state had suffered greatly during the war. Then, in the late 1780s, some tribal members migrated westward and northward, away from their ruined fields and still smoldering villages. Regrouping in Detroit, they sought to forge a new political alliance, this time with other Indians living along the Ohio River and in the Great Lakes region. Mohawk leader Joseph Brant (born Thayendanegea) urged the Algonquians, Shawnees, Delawares, Miamis, and Weas, among others, to join in common purpose, to resist U.S. territorial aggression, even as each group retained its separate identity. Together, he claimed, western Indians could "eat out of one bowl with one spoon." Unity would bring strength, he explained: "Whilst we remain disunited, every inconvenience attends us. The Interest of any one Nation should be the Interests of us all, the welfare of the one should be the welfare of all the others."

The European Americans were determined to rid themselves of the persistent military threat posed by Indian and British forces in the Northwest Territory and so launched a concerted campaign against Indians in the area that is present-day Ohio, Indiana, and Michigan. Under the leadership of Miami chief Little Turtle (Michikinikwa), and with support from the British, this Ohio Confederacy held off the advances of the American army. In August of 1794 the forces of General "Mad" Anthony Wayne overwhelmed those of Little Turtle. The Ohio confederation of Indians lay in ruins until a new generation of leaders arose.

The Ohio Confederacy offers some intriguing parallels to the coalition of colonies during the Revolution and to the union of the states afterward. Before the Revolution, Benjamin Franklin had marveled at the cohesion of the Six Nations (the precursor of the Confederacy), drawing inspiration from the Indians' example. He noted, "If Six Nations of Ignorant savages" could create a union, then 13 colonies led by white men should be able to do so also. Patterns of leadership in the Confederacy were in some ways similar to those of the Patriots. Joseph Brant, in his call for unity, was the Thomas Jefferson—the political theorist—of the Confederacy. Little Turtle was its George Washington, a leader skilled in both political negotiation and military warfare.

Soon after the war, Brant pointed to lessons that the Indians learned from the United States in creating the Ohio Confederacy: with political unity came military strength. Indians, like the colonists, sought to overcome regional and cultural differences among themselves. In both cases, disparate groups found common ground in their fight against a common enemy—Great Britain in the case of the thirteen colonies, the United States in the case of the Ohio Confederacy.

Artist Gilbert Stuart painted this portrait of Mohawk leader Joseph Brant, born Thayendanegea, in 1786.

Indians and European Americans soon discovered that neither the Ohio Confederation nor the new United States could function as completely independent political entities. In the early 1790s the Indians relied heavily on the British for guns and artillery. And until 1815, the United States found itself mired in European conflicts, its trade and domestic politics shaped by ongoing wars between France and Britain.

From 1775 to 1800, the Great Lakes region, or Northwest Territory west of the Appalachian Mountains and east of the Mississippi River, was a vast middle ground, where Indian villagers coexisted with British traders and French trappers. The cultures of these groups intermingled. For example, Brant had visited England in the mid-1770s, and he had been educated at a Christian school in Connecticut, so he was comfortable with certain European and American customs related to dress and diet. After the Revolution, the incursion of European American settlers into this "middle ground" disrupted Native hunting practices. Squatters from the East did not want only to cultivate the land; they wanted to own it. Violence escalated in an endless cycle of raids and retaliation. The U.S. citizens who settled in the area that is today Michigan, Indiana, Ohio, and Kentucky—the trans-Appalachian West—were the vanguard of the new, expanding republic. At the same time, they drew the army of the infant nation into a costly, bloody war.

One U.S. official labeled these European American migrants "white savages," suggesting that they would make more trouble for the country than the "tawny ones" would. Indeed, the Revolution had spawned a number of new groups who would challenge colonial ideas about race, gender, wealth, and standing in the community. White settlers were being compared to Indians in the Northwest Territory. In New England and the Upper South, another new class— free people of color—struggled to assert their rights. Throughout the colonies, some women maintained a high degree of political engagement; New Jersey even granted well-to-do women the right to vote, if only for a brief period. Artisans also sought to wield new political clout. "White savages," free blacks, women voters, artisan–politicians—they all revealed both the social tensions mounting in the new republic and the promise it offered to these same groups.

> *The Revolution had spawned a number of new groups who would challenge colonial ideas about race, gender, wealth, and standing in the community.*

The country's natural landscape and resources, as well as its sheer size, shaped both economic and political development. Leaders continued to disagree over whether such a huge country could remain a unified republic of well-informed voters. James Madison argued that a large population dispersed over a wide area would prevent any single group from tyrannizing smaller and diverse groups. Regional economic activity—cotton cultivation in the South and commercial development in the North—demonstrated the young nation's potential as a producer of goods. Also, the country's physical expanse allowed people to leave their homes in the East, migrate, regroup, and begin life anew in the West. Geographic mobility remained a hallmark of the American experience.

The first census of the United States, conducted in 1790, tallied 4 million people. Of this number, 750,000 were black. People of various ethnicities clustered together in pockets throughout the states. German-born people accounted for one-third of all Pennsylvanians, and almost one-fifth of New York residents were Dutch. Numbers of Northerners and Southerners were about equal. However, ethnic and regional differences proved less significant in shaping the emerging two-party system than the persistent split between urban-based merchants and rural interests such as southern planters. Moreover, policy differences between these wealthy propertied white men—proponents of a strong federal government versus supporters of states' rights and local authority—could not account for all the domestic turmoil that rocked the young republic in its early years. The Revolution unleashed enormous creative energy as some people, unfettered by restrictions imposed by the Crown, pursued new economic opportunities. In contrast, many artisans and small farmers continued to stagger under a burden of debt and new federal taxes. For them, the Revolution was a betrayal of their vision for America.

The impulse for association so evident in the U.S. union of states and in the Indians' Ohio Confederacy permeated everyday American life. In effect, ordinary people put into practice the grand theories of the Revolution. Exhorting their brothers and sisters to join in religious fellowship, revivalists formed new spiritual communities. Reform groups wrote constitutions for themselves in an effort to commit their principles to paper. Temperance advocates joined together and called on men and women to cast off the tyranny of drink; the reformed drunkard was considered as noble as the patriot.

Most dramatically, opponents of slavery kept alive the rhetoric and the ideals of the Revolution. In 1800 Gabriel, an enslaved blacksmith in Richmond, Virginia, plotted a rebellion to seize the city. His actions gave voice to the egalitarian principles articulated in Philadelphia in 1776 and then in Saint-Domingue in 1791, when slaves had staged a bloody revolt against their French masters. (In 1804 they renamed the country Haiti.) Gabriel's rebels used the words of the Founding Fathers to justify their actions, rallying around the cry, "Death or Liberty." One even compared himself to George Washington in his struggle to "obtain the liberty of [his] countrymen." Gabriel's plans to kill all whites except abolitionists failed when informants betrayed him to Richmond authorities. Yet Gabriel's rebellion, even though unsuccessful, is indicative of the struggle of almost all Americans, regardless of creed or color, wrestled with the legacy of the Revolution.

Competing Political Visions in the New Nation

In the first two decades of the life of the new nation, domestic politics remained entwined in relations with the great European powers. For all their bold talk of freedom and liberty, the heirs of the Revolution continued to formulate public policies based upon the models offered by Great Britain and France specifically. Some Americans found much to admire in British traditions of social order and stability, traditions shaped by a strong central authority in the form of a monarchy. Other Americans derived inspiration from the French Revolution, which began in 1789; they believed that, for all its bloody excesses, the revolution represented an ideal of true democracy, an ideal at odds with entrenched privilege in the form of monarchies and aristocracies. The British model appealed to Federalists, supporters of a strong central government. In contrast, the French model appealed to Anti-Federalists, soon to be called Democratic-Republicans, supporters of the rights of the states and of the active participation of ordinary citizens in politics. These divergent views shaped both foreign and domestic policy in the 1790s.

Within this contentious atmosphere, George Washington assumed the presidency in 1789, backed by the unanimous endorsement of the Electoral College. Even today, he has the distinction of being the only president in U.S. history to be elected unanimously. The early days of his administration provided some evidence that even his political foes shared his core beliefs. Support for Washington appeared to be widespread: When the new president traveled from his home in Virginia to the capitol in New York, cheering throngs of citizens lined the route, and parades of artisans marked celebrations in the largest towns.

Neither the ratification of the Constitution nor Washington's election silenced the continuing debate over civil liberties and the nature of the national government. Responding to the concerns of the Anti-Federalists, Congress quickly passed ten amendments, collectively called the Bill of Rights, to the Constitution. Ratified by the necessary number of states in 1791, the

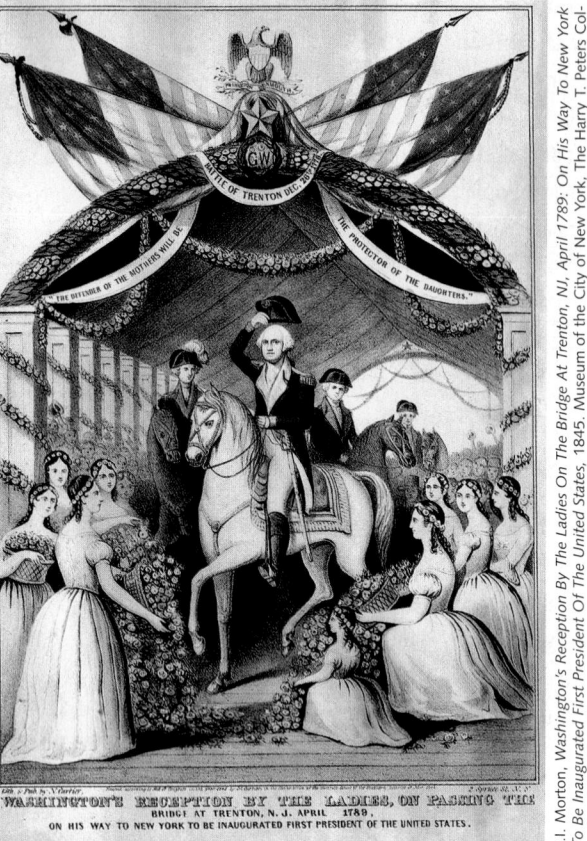

J.I. Morton, Washington's Reception By The Ladies On The Bridge At Trenton, NJ, April 1789: On His Way To New York To Be Inaugurated First President Of The United States, 1845. Museum of the City of New York, The Harry T. Peters Collection (56.300.847)

WASHINGTON'S RECEPTION BY THE LADIES, ON PASSING THE BRIDGE AT TRENTON, N. J. APRIL 1789.
ON HIS WAY TO NEW YORK TO BE INAUGURATED FIRST PRESIDENT OF THE UNITED STATES.

■ Founders of the new nation identified citizenship with economic independence. By this definition, women, children, slaves, and others dependent on property owners could not become citizens. However, drawing on their privileged status, white women sought to carve out a place for themselves in the young republic. This scene shows the women and girls of Trenton, New Jersey, greeting the newly elected president George Washington en route to his inauguration in New York City, the temporary capital. The girls sang as he passed by, "Virgins fair and Matrons grave,/Those thy conquering Arms did save."

amendments were intended to protect white men from the power of government, whether local, state, or national. The Judiciary Act of 1789 established a national, federal court system that included a five-member Supreme Court and the office of attorney general, charged with enforcing the nation's laws. The new republic was taking shape as the founders had hoped. It would be a nation of laws, with the executive, legislative, and judicial branches of government checking one another's power.

Like other political leaders of the time, Washington believed that ideological differences between political leaders should never become institutionalized in the form of separate political parties. These leaders believed politicians should debate issues freely among themselves, without being bound by partisan loyalty to one view or political candidate over another. However, by the late 1790s, the intense rivalry between Alexander Hamilton, Washington's secretary of the treasury, and Thomas Jefferson, his secretary of state, had produced a two-party system that proved remarkably durable. Representing two competing political visions, Hamilton and his supporters (known as Federalists) and Jefferson and his supporters (called Democratic-Republicans) disagreed on foreign diplomacy and domestic economic policies. Hamilton advocated a strong central government that would promote commerce and manufacturing. In contrast, Jefferson favored states' rights bolstered by small, independent farmers who would serve as the nation's moral and political center. These opposing viewpoints represented a continuation of the debate over the proper role of government, a debate that had shaped the Constitution. The Democratic-Republicans were the political heirs of the Anti-Federalists, and the Federalists continued to support the power of the federal government.

In 1792 Washington ran for and won a second term, although his rivals for office (his own vice president, John Adams, and New York governor George Clinton) all lacked party designations in the contest. Four years later, Washington declined to run for a third term. His successor was John Adams, an unabashed Federalist who rankled Jefferson and other more egalitarian-minded citizens. Between 1789 and 1800, the clash between the Federalists and the Democratic-Republicans reverberated on the high seas, in Indian country, and in the halls of Congress.

Federalism and Democratic-Republicanism in Action

In 1793, France and England went to war over territorial claims in Europe and the West Indies. At the outbreak of the war, President Washington issued a Neutrality Proclamation. The United States, he declared, would remain on the sidelines of the conflict. Nevertheless, the two combatants drew the new country into the struggle, and few Americans could resisit taking sides.

In the 1790s many Americans followed closely the dramatic events unfolding in France. At first, U.S. support for that country's revolution was widespread; by imposing constitutional constraints on their king, Louis XVI, the French seemed to be engaged in a heroic struggle, much like that of the Patriots of 1776 who had challenged the absolute power of the English crown. However, in 1792, French revolutionaries beheaded the king and launched what came to be known as the Reign of Terror, executing aristocrats and presumed opponents of the revolution—wealthy people tied to the monarchy through kin ties and economic interests.

In the United States, public opinion toward the revolution shifted in response to the Reign of Terror. Many Americans abhorred the carnage. In their eyes, the blood-soaked Place de la Concorde in Paris, where heads rolled off the guillotine platform and into baskets with the rhythmic precision of drumbeats, represented the end of order and humanity. Federalist politicians hoped to take advantage of these views, claiming that the bloody excesses of the French Revolution represented an argument in favor of a moderate and stable central government for the United States, one like that of Great Britain.

Tensions between France and the United States took a turn for the worse when France's first envoy to the United States, Citizen Edmund Genet, ignored the Neutrality Proclamation and tried to enlist American support for French designs on Spanish Florida and British Canada. Genet was eager to raise an army among Americans who lived on the borders of these territories. The French thought they would find support among men who hoped to free the Mississippi River from Spanish control and open it to U.S. commercial interests.

Nor did Britain endear itself to its former American subjects during these years. Pursuing French military forces in 1793, the British navy seized 300 American merchant ships plying the West Indian seas, forcing American sailors into service. In a practice known as impressment, British sea captains boarded American ships and captured sailors at gunpoint. England claimed that it was simply reclaiming its own sailors, who had deserted from the Royal Navy in response to U.S. captains who offered them higher wages. Meanwhile, along the United States' northern border, British officials were supplying the Indians of the Ohio Confederacy with guns, alcohol, and encouragement in their fight against the Americans. Nevertheless, Alexander Hamilton and the Federalists continued to proclaim their support of Britain against France. These proponents of strong central government feared that the French would aid and encourage violent anti-Federalist tendencies, such as those that had motivated Shays's Rebellion in 1786. Thomas Jefferson and other Democratic-Republicans condemned the French Reign of Terror but admired the French spirit embodied in their motto: *egalité* and *fraternité* (equality and brotherhood).

> *As secretary of the treasury, Hamilton took bold steps to advance the commercial interests of the new nation.*

As secretary of the treasury, Hamilton took bold steps to advance the commercial interests of the new nation. Hamilton wanted the wealthy to invest in American rather than European manufacturing enterprises. He believed that if government promoted a robust economy that benefited successful businesspeople and investors, then, eventually, the poorest people would prosper as well. For example, tariffs protecting domestic manufacturers would provide employment to artisans. In 1789, Hamilton persuaded Congress to enact the first U.S. tariff on imported goods to encourage home manufactures and to raise money for the treasury. (Between 1790 and 1860, the tariff yielded two-thirds of the national government's income.)

Hamilton also sought to strengthen the federal government through monetary policy. At his prodding, in 1790 Congress agreed to fund the national debt—that is, to assume responsibility for repaying the government's creditors and for paying the interest on it (a total of $54 million). It also assumed responsibility for debts that the individual states had incurred during the Revolution. To pay for all this, federal officials stepped up debt collection and imposed new taxes on individuals. In 1791 Congress also issued a 20-year charter to the first Bank of the United States. Hamilton had argued that this institution, modeled after the Bank of England, would help stimulate the economy by circulating surplus funds held by the government. He intended that the bank would serve the interests of urban-oriented manufacturers.

In his "Report on the Subject of Manufactures" (1791), Hamilton argued that factories stimulated economic growth. They used labor-saving machinery, promoted foreign emigration, and freed the United States from dependence on European-made goods in times of war, he pointed out. They also spurred a demand for consumer products and furnished "greater scope for the diversity of talents and dispositions which discriminate men from each other." Hamilton also advocated the employment of poor women and children in factories. He especially admired the way British employers hired women and children in their own textile mills.

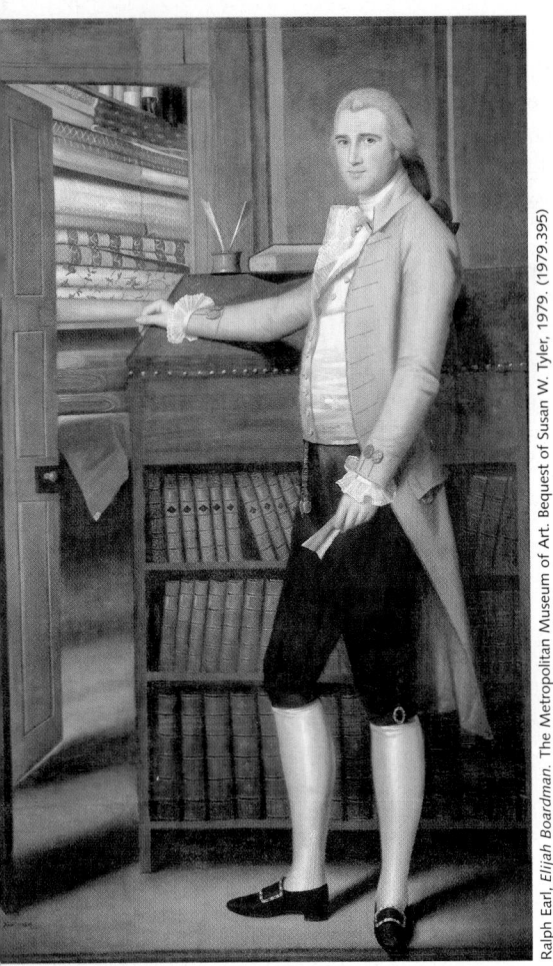

Ralph Earl, *Elijah Boardman.* The Metropolitan Museum of Art. Bequest of Susan W. Tyler, 1979. (1979.395)

■ Elijah Boardman of New Milford, Connecticut, poses at his desk in 1789. The portrait highlights Boardman's success as a merchant. His business prospered because wealthy Americans wanted to dress fashionably, as he did, with his ruffled sleeves, silk stockings, and fancy shoe buckles. In the background are some of the colorful, luxurious fabrics he sold. By the late eighteenth century, New England merchants were at the center of a thriving worldwide exchange of goods between Europe, the United States, and China. Their profits helped to finance the country's industrial revolution.

An advocate of agricultural interests and the power of individual states, Jefferson disagreed with Hamilton on all these issues. Jefferson bitterly opposed the Bank of the United States, arguing that only the states could issue charters for financial institutions. He favored a lower tariff, arguing that high-priced imports hurt farmers and other small consumers. More generally, Jefferson objected to the idea that fiscal policy should serve as a tool for nation building. The leader of the Democratic-Republicans believed that the government should not interfere in the lives of its citizens by imposing higher taxes on individual households or on imported goods. He was not interested in extending government aid to manufacturers or other businesses. According to Jefferson, governments, like individuals, should exercise restraint in their spending and should avoid accumulating debt. Hamilton and Jefferson's opposing views of government shaped the American political party system for generations to come.

Planting the Seeds of Industry

When the "Report on the Subject of Manufactures" came out, in 1791, New England was already moving in the direction that Hamilton advocated. That same year, Samuel Slater, a 21-year-old English inventor, arrived in the United States. With financial support from Moses Brown, a wealthy merchant of Providence, Rhode Island, Slater constructed the first cotton thread spinning machine on American soil. To launch his Steam Cotton Manufacturing Company, Slater hired seven boys and two girls (between ages 7 and 12) to operate the machinery.

Nevertheless, during the late eighteenth century, most manufacturing took place in individual households. For example, working in sheds called ten footers (so called because of their length), master shoemakers employed journeymen (skilled workers) and apprentices (young boys learning the trade) as well as their own wives and children. Throughout New England and the Mid-Atlantic, families processed wheat, pork, hides, and cheese and made soap, candles, and leather. From 1800 to 1810, Philadelphia textile factories turned out 65,000 yards of cloth annually, but households in the region produced nearly four times that much. These small home-based producers shared similar values with yeoman (small property-owning) farmers; both groups prized property ownership and the independence of their households.

In 1793 Massachusetts-born Eli Whitney invented the cotton gin. This machine gave a tremendous boost to both the southern plantation system and the fledgling northern industrial system. By quickly removing the seeds from cotton balls and cleaning other impurities from raw cotton, the cotton gin fostered the emergence of a new cotton economy. Planters rushed to meet the nearly insatiable demand for cotton from mill owners in both England and New England. Southern slaveholders expanded their holdings into Alabama and Mississippi, where fresh, fertile lands beckoned. Between 1793 and 1815, annual cotton production soared from 3 million to 93 million pounds.

In the 1790s undeniable signs of an emerging manufacturing economy appeared, especially along the "fall line," the region where the Piedmont's hills meet the broad coastal plain. Stretching from New England to New York, New Jersey, and Pennsylvania, this area had all the ingredients for an American Industrial Revolution: water power from rushing rivers, a faltering agricultural economy that western producers would soon eclipse, capital from successful merchants, and a dense population to serve as both workers and consumers.

Many people marveled at U.S. energy, productivity, and diversity. Especially in the North, the sounds of industry attested to American ingenuity and ambition. On a visit to the United States in 1794, an Englishman named Henry Wansey found Boston "a very flourishing place, full of business and activity." Its docks groaned under "casks of sugar and rice, bags of cotton and wool, pipe staves, lumber, iron bars, bags of nails, and, in short, every article of commerce." The Boston Duck and Sail Cloth Manufactory, an imposing structure 180 feet long and two stories high, employed as many as 400 people. Boston and its environs also boasted distilleries and factories that turned out wallpaper, nails, woolen goods, carpets, and paper. Sawmills and flour mills dotted the countryside. Throughout the North, silversmiths, booksellers, hairdressers, and makers of toys, fine carriages, and furniture, among others, produced luxury goods and provided a variety of services.

Yet Wansey also saw evidence of labor problems to come. The expanding American economy yielded many jobs preferable to those of factory and domestic work, prompting high rates of labor turnover. In New York City, textile artisans brought over from Lancashire, England, proved unreliable. They left the factories at the first opportunity, eager to buy land of their own and thus "arrive at independence." And in Newark, New Jersey, wealthy women had trouble retaining domestic servants. Poorer women were eager to take advantage of economic opportunities that did not require them to wait on their social betters hand and foot. They resented the deference demanded of them in the domestic-employer relationship. When their employees "stipulated that they shall sit at table [and dine] with their masters and mistresses," the mistresses were horrified at this breach of social etiquette.

By the mid-1790s Hamilton and his supporters were praising the regional economic growth and specialization that protective tariffs nourished. In the South, the growing reliance

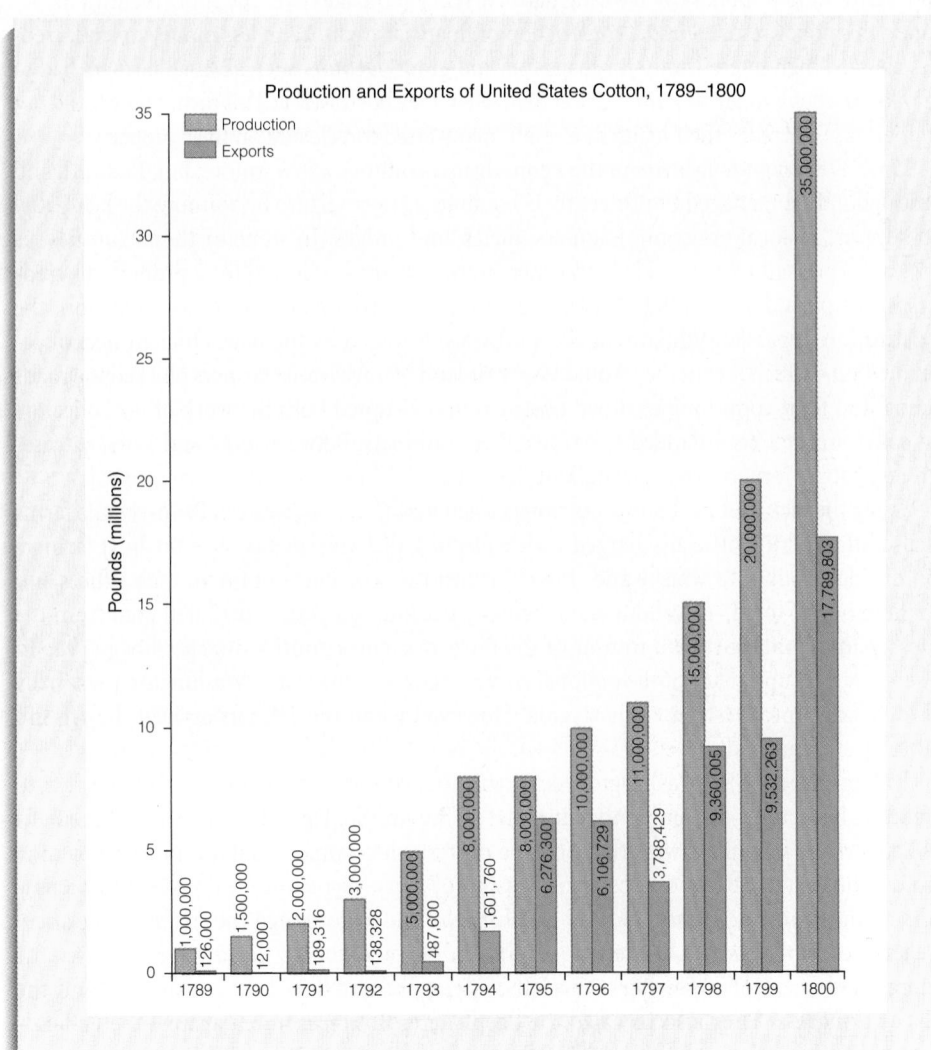

Production and Exports of United States Cotton, 1789–1800

■ **FIGURE 9.1**
EXPORTS OF UNITED STATES COTTON, 1784–1800

Sources: Stuart Brucey, *Cotton and the Growth of the American Economy, 1790–1860* (1967), pp. 14–15; Timothy Pitkin, *A Statistical View of the Commerce of the United States of America* (1835), p. 111.

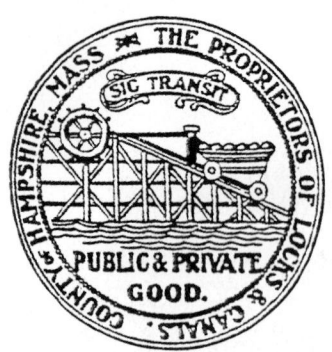

■ This logo advertises the Hampshire machine. A precursor of the canal lock, the machine consisted of a pulley that carried a canal barge in a cart up an inclined plane. Invented in 1795, it was used on the Connecticut River in western Massachusetts. However, it proved too cumbersome in the long run. Most canals used locks, sections closed off with gates so that the water level could be raised or lowered.

on slaves for cotton, the newly crowned king of crops, further accelerated that growth. Tar, pitch, and turpentine produced in North Carolina, tobacco from Virginia and the Carolinas, and wheat grown in the Mid-Atlantic states, revealed the richness of the new nation's natural resources. Freed from colonial restrictions, the New England shipbuilding industry thrived, constructing masts, boards, planks, and barrels from the forests of Maine and New Hampshire. Miners extracted iron from the land; mariners pulled fish from the sea. Innovations in transportation facilitated growth. Since the Revolution, construction had begun on 11 canals. In addition, the Lancaster Turnpike, a 62-mile road, connected Philadelphia to its outlying areas. Privately financed by stockholders, the venture yielded a profit of 15 percent annually (because of tolls) for its investors and furthered settlement of the western part of the Mid-Atlantic region.

Echoes of the American Revolution in the Countryside

Despite Hamilton's optimism about the economy, Washington's administration faced violent resistance to its policies from certain quarters. In the West, American soldiers suffered a series of humiliating defeats in battles with Indians until they finally subdued Little Turtle and his warriors at the Battle of Fallen Timbers in 1794. That same year, farmers and grain distillers in southwestern Pennsylvania refused to pay their federal taxes, prompting Washington to send militiamen to quell the protest. Known as the Whiskey Rebellion, this uprising was sparked by the new 7-cents-a-gallon tax on whiskey. It was the culmination of a lengthy rural protest against Hamilton's "hard money" policy. By favoring hard currency (coinage) over the more plentiful paper money, this policy resulted in the constriction of financial credit. With less money to lend, creditors charged high interest rates for loans they did grant. Debtors such as small farmers had to repay loans when money was even scarcer than when they borrowed it. This meant they could not pay their taxes or repay their loans; as a result, many faced foreclosure on their property.

Until 1787, debtor-farmers in the Pennsylvania counties of Westmoreland, Bedford, and Huntingdon had managed to protect their holdings against seizure by winning the sympathy and support of local tax commissioners, juries, and judges. In some of these counties, as many as 43 percent of all taxable landowners were in danger of losing their property to creditors in the period 1782–1792. But by providing for a federal system of tax collection, the Constitution bypassed sympathetic local officials. Enraged by the new, efficient tax collection methods, which meant they would lose their land, Pennsylvania farmers blocked the roads leading into their communities. Road obstructions disrupted both the work of tax collectors and court proceedings intended to enforce their authority. Between 1787 and 1795, 62 cases of road obstruction occurred throughout the state.

Using the tactics of the Stamp Tax rioters a generation earlier, western Pennsylvania farmers also attacked the officials charged with collecting the whiskey tax. The tax hurt farmers who distilled grain into whisky and shipped it east for sale. They set fire to their offices and ran them out of town. To subdue the rebellion, Washington gathered 13,000 men from the states' militias and sent them to four of the most resistant counties in September 1794. To underscore the supremacy of the national government over the states, Washington personally led the troops into western Pennsylvania. However, when the soldiers arrived they found that the protesters had dispersed.

In November 1794 Washington devoted most of his annual address to Congress to defending his actions as commander-in-chief of the militia. He indirectly charged the defiant Pennsylvania distillers with treason. The protests, he claimed, had been incited by men who demonstrated "an ignorance or perversion of facts, suspicions, jealousies and accusations of the whole government." Yet Washington failed to gauge the extent of country dwellers' economic distress. By defying federal authority so openly, the farmers expressed the general grievances of westerners who felt underrepresented in state legislatures and the halls of Congress. They also revealed the deep current of resentment against the Federalists running through rural America. Another uprising in rural Pennsylvania—this one cen-

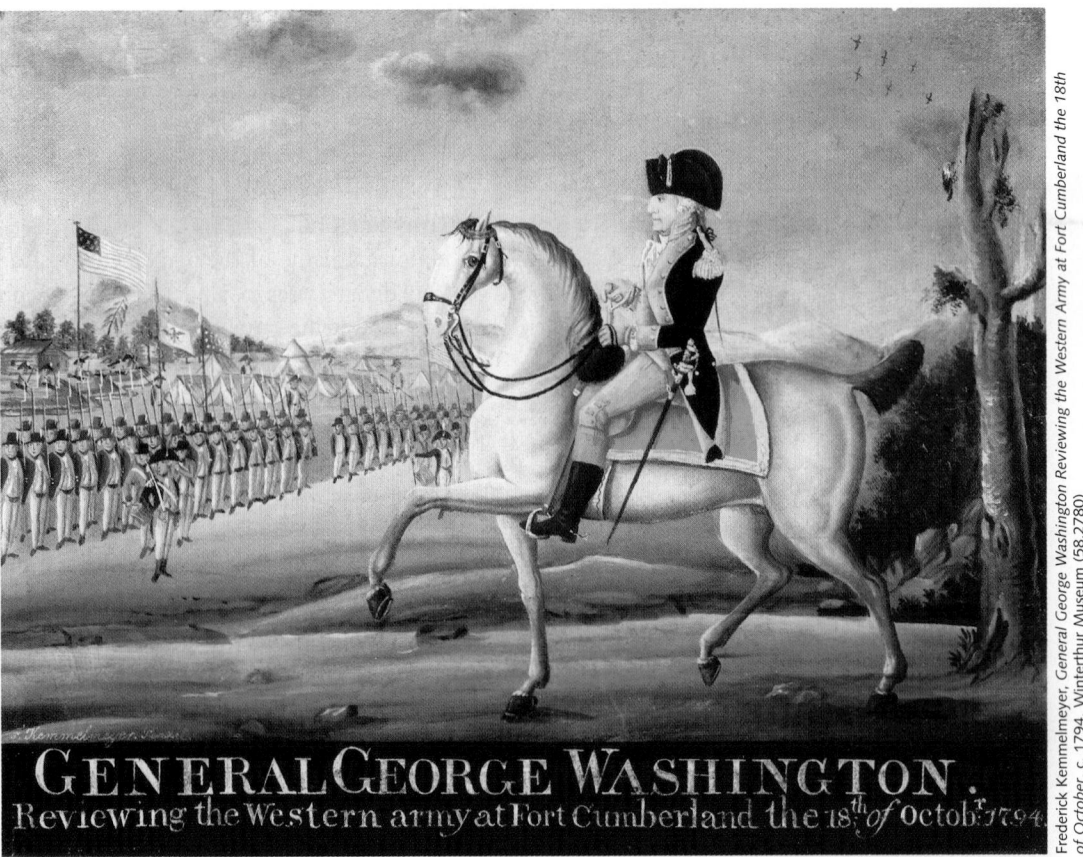

Frederick Kemmelmeyer, General George Washington Reviewing the Western Army at Fort Cumberland the 18th of October, c. 1794. Winterthur Museum (58.2780)

■ This 1794 painting seemingly evokes the American Revolution, when General Washington reviewed American troops. However, in this scene, President Washington is surveying some of the 13,000 state militiamen he commanded in an effort to suppress the Whiskey Rebellion in western Pennsylvania. Farmers objected to the new government tax on whiskey. With cries of "Liberty and No Excise," the protesters harassed federal tax collectors, reminiscent of anti–Stamp Act demonstrations three decades before. The Whiskey Rebellion melted away quickly. Critics objected to Washington's willingness to use such a huge force against the protesters.

tered in the southeastern part of the state in 1799—violently affirmed popular opposition to federal taxes. Protesters charged that "Congress and the government" intended to "rob the people" and reduce them to the status of European peasants, "poor as snakes." Yet, like the Whiskey Rebellion, these civil disturbances sputtered and then failed, leaving the authority of the federal government intact.

Securing Peace Abroad, Suppressing Dissent at Home

In 1795 the president sent Chief Justice John Jay to England to negotiate a key treaty. The negotiations were intended to address the problems of British forts in the Northwest, American debts owed to British creditors, British seizure of American ships and sailors in the West Indies, and the right of individual Americans to trade freely with European belligerents in wartime. Jay obtained a treaty but failed to extract meaningful compromises from England. Pro-British in his political leanings, he found it difficult to press that country for concessions. He was also hampered by the fact that Hamilton—in an effort to thwart the treaty—had supplied the British with secrets related to Jay's bargaining strategy.

In the treaty that bore his name and that the Senate eventually ratified, England grudgingly agreed to evacuate its northern forts and to stop seizing American ships. More ominously, Jay acquiesced to English demands that individual Americans pay the debts they had owed to English creditors since before the Revolution. The Americans believed that their victory in the war exempted them from longstanding financial obligation to their English creditors. The Democratic-Republicans took alarm at these developments. In their view, the new agreement humiliated all Americans and threatened southern planters in particular.

TABLE 9-1		
The Election of 1796		
Candidate	Political Party	Electoral Vote
John Adams	Federalist	71
Thomas Jefferson	Democrat-Republican	68
Thomas Pinckney	Federalist	59
Aaron Burr	Democrat-Republican	30

Western agricultural interests gained as a result of the Pinckney Treaty of 1795, negotiated by American diplomat Thomas Pinckney. The formal name of the agreement was the Treaty of San Lorenzo. Under this agreement, Spain allowed the United States to navigate the Mississippi River freely and to land goods at New Orleans free of taxes for three years. Yet this measure hardly placated the Democratic-Republicans, still smarting over what they considered Jay's humiliating treaty with the British.

With their eye on the next presidential election, the Democratic-Republicans began a vigorous campaign in favor of their own candidate, Thomas Jefferson. They contrasted Jefferson, the friend of the small farmer, with the Federalists' choice, Massachusetts's John Adams, advocate of a strong central government run by the well-educated and the well-born. Jefferson's party expressed particular dismay over Washington's haste to crush the rebellious Pennsylvania farmers in 1794 and over Jay's Treaty. Yet, backed by the New England states, Adams won the election, though narrowly. Because he received the second largest number of electoral votes—68 to Adams's 71—Jefferson became the new vice president according to the terms of the Constitution then in effect (Article II, Section I).

In his farewell address, printed in newspapers but not delivered in person, Washington reviewed his years in office. Most memorably, he warned against the "insidious wiles of foreign influence" and against alliances with foreign powers that could compromise America's independence and economic well-being. "Europe has a set of primary interests which to us have none or a very remote relation," he wrote. "Why, by interweaving our destiny with that of any part of Europe, entangle our peace and prosperity in the toils of European ambition, rivalship, interest, humor, caprice?"

Nevertheless, upon assuming the presidency in 1797, Adams found that European powers still had a hold on American domestic and foreign relations. France began to seize American merchant vessels (300 of them by mid–1797) in retaliation for what it saw as favoritism toward England in Jay's Treaty. In October of that year, the new president sent John Marshall and Elbridge Gerry to join the U.S. ambassador to France, Charles Pinckney, to negotiate a new treaty with France. However, French intermediaries (referred to only as X, Y, and Z in the Americans' dispatches) demanded that the three U.S. commissioners arrange for a loan of $12 million to France and pay a $250,000 bribe. Only then would the envoys be allowed to speak to the foreign minister, Charles Talleyrand. The sentiments of the American public, outraged at the idea of paying a bribe and willing to defend their new nation against all aggressors, were captured in the cry, "Millions for defense, but not one cent for tribute." Adams called the commissioners home.

In the next two years, tensions escalated on both the domestic and international stage. Federalists throughout the country called for war against France, and the Adams administration sought to shore up the country's military forces by creating a navy and the Marine Corps. Hoping to rid U.S. coastal waters of French "pirates," ships that were seizing American vessels, in May 1798 Congress authorized American ships to seize "armed vessels under authority or pretense of authority from the Republic of France." Over the next two years, the undeclared so-called Quasi War pitted the American navy against its French counterpart.

The major players in this drama—Adams, Talleyrand, and his successor, Napoleon—were all determined to avoid outright war. They succeeded. The two nations signed a treaty, called the Convention of 1800, in Paris. This agreement dissolved the Franco-American Alliance

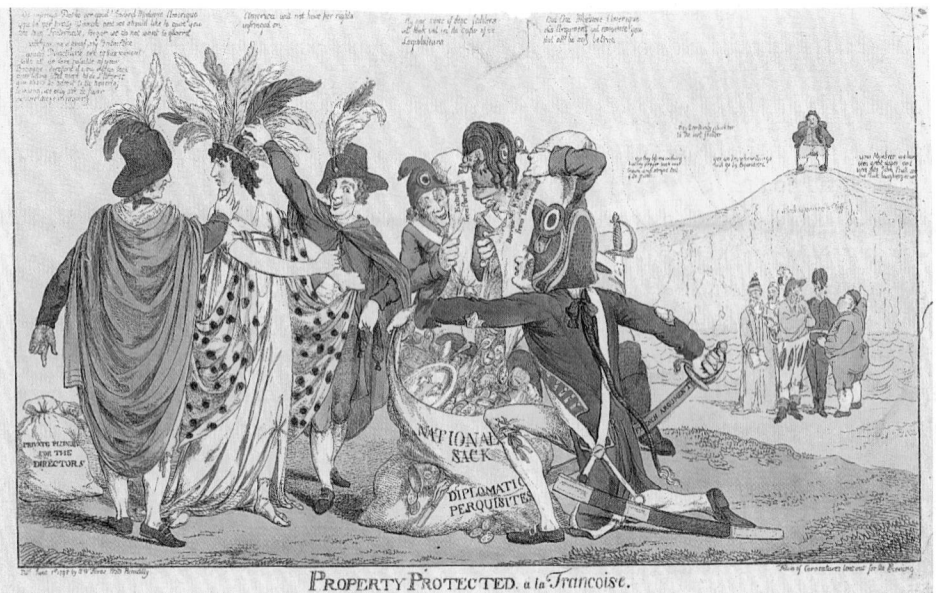

PROPERTY PROTECTED. a la *Francoise.*

◼ In 1798 Americans reacted indignantly to news that France had demanded a bribe and a large loan before its ambassadors would agree to meet with American envoys. In this political cartoon, America is portrayed as an innocent young woman assaulted by French diplomats. The incident precipitated an undeclared war on the high seas, called the Quasi War, between the two countries.

that the two nations had created during the Revolution, provided restitution for American shippers damaged by French aggressors, and secured a permanent peace between the United States and France. French privateers and naval vessels were removed from the U.S. coastline.

Conflicts continued to simmer on the domestic front. Soon after Adams's inauguration, the Federalist-dominated Congress moved to suppress the rising chorus of dissent among rural people, Democratic-Republican leaders, and newspaper editors. Such dissent, they charged, amounted to sedition—an act of insurrection against the government. Foreign influences were whipping up disloyalty among the populace and endangering the security of the new nation, the Federalists claimed. To eradicate this perceived threat, Congress passed the Alien and Sedition Acts in 1798. These new laws made it more difficult for immigrants to become resident aliens, gave the president the power to deport or imprison aliens, and branded as traitors any people (U.S. citizens included) who "unlawfully combine or conspire together, with intent to oppose any measure or measures of the government of the United States."

Even though the Alien and Sedition Acts were unconstitutional—they violated the First Amendment's guarantee of freedom of speech—the Federalist-dominated Supreme Court upheld them. Consequently, Democratic-Republicans were by definition guilty of treason, for they advocated policies and supported candidates opposed by the Federalists, the party in power.

Ten newspaper editors were convicted, and many others charged and jailed, under the Sedition Act. Their convictions suggested the increasing influence of newspapers as conduits of information and as shapers of strong political opinion. Between 1790 and 1810, the number of newspapers in the country ballooned from 90 to 370. But editors were not the only targets of the new laws against sedition. Some Democratic-Republican lawmakers also spent time in jail because their speech offended their partisan rivals. Matthew Lyon, a congressman, went to prison for suggesting that President Adams showed "unbounded thirst for ridiculous pomp, foolish adulation, and selfish avarice."

In 1798 and 1799 the state legislatures of Kentucky and Virginia issued a series of resolutions condemning the Alien and Sedition Acts. Outraged at what they saw as the Federalists' blatant power grab, the two legislatures proposed that individual states had the right to declare such measures "void and of no force." Thomas Jefferson (for Kentucky) and James Madison (for Virginia) wrote the actual resolutions. In declaring that states could essentially nullify federal laws, the two Founding Fathers unwittingly laid the theoretical framework for Southerners to ignore congressional authority in the future.

Civil Liberties Under Siege During Wartime and Other National Crises

Passed by Congress in 1798, the Alien and Sedition Acts severely curtailed freedom of speech among immigrants and native-born Americans alike. Supporters of these measures feared that the nation would soon be embroiled in a war with France and that all critics of the Federalist government, including Democratic-Republicans, must be silenced. During several other periods in American history, government officials have advocated the suspension of civil liberties on the grounds of national security. Immigrants and political radicals have proved especially vulnerable to these measures in times of crisis.

Soon after the outbreak of Civil War, in April 1861, President Abraham Lincoln suspended the writ of habeas corpus (that is, he denied arrested persons the right to petition for their freedom in federal court) in the states of Pennsylvania, Delaware, and Maryland and in the District of Columbia. Military authorities had the power to arrest people suspected of aiding the Confederacy and to detain suspects indefinitely without formally charging them with a crime. Two years later Lincoln extended the suspension to all other states under Union control.

During World War I, Congress passed the Entry and Departure Controls Act. The law made it easier for government officials to target noncitizens "whose presence was deemed contrary to public safety." During the Red Scare of 1919–1920, some Americans feared that the recent Russian Revolution would inspire the spread of communism in the United States. Officials cited the act in their attempts to deport thousands of immigrants, many of whom were labor and political radicals.

The outbreak of war with Japan in 1941 led President Franklin D. Roosevelt to sign Executive Order 9066. This measure resulted in the relocation of more than 110,000 West Coast Japanese immigrants and Japanese American citizens to internment camps. In two different cases, *Hirabayashi v. United States* and *Korematsu v. United States,* the Supreme Court upheld the government's position. However, in 1988 Congress awarded restitution payments of $20,000 to each of 60,000 surviving internees.

After World War II, tensions surrounding the Cold War led to suppression of the rights of U.S. communists and other people suspected of disloyalty toward the United States. Under the Internal Security Act of 1950, communists had to register with the government. Many other Americans lost their jobs because they expressed, or were charged with expressing, views critical of U.S. policies on any number of subjects, including civil rights and foreign affairs.

During the Vietnam War in the late 1960s and early 1970s, President Richard Nixon's administration sought to suppress antiwar sentiment in the United States. High-ranking officials, including Attorney General John Mitchell and Federal Bureau of Investigation head J. Edgar Hoover, monitored

People of Color: New Freedoms, New Struggles

In the late eighteenth century, North American elites demonstrated an emerging preoccupation with matters of race as a means of categorizing people and distinguishing groups from each other. Spanish officials in colonial New Mexico conducted a 1790 census that divided the population into a variety of groups based on ethnicity: Spanish, Indian, Mestizo (Spanish and Mexican Indian), *coyote* (Spanish and New Mexican Indian), mulatto (a person of African plus Spanish or Indian heritage), *genizaro* (children of acculturated Indians), and *color quebrado* and *lobo* (both designating some form of mixed-race parentage). In the United States, a 1790 naturalization law limited naturalized U.S. citizenship to "free white persons," thereby belying the oft-heard claim that all men were equal under the law.

The crosscurrents of the revolutionary legacy showed themselves most obviously in the status of African Americans after the war. To some extent, people's fate depended on where they lived and labored. Soon after the United States won its independence from England, all the northern states lay the groundwork for the abolition of slavery. In the Upper South, citing the egalitarian principles of the Revolution, some planters also freed their enslaved workers. But overall, economics rather than principles influenced these decisions. The North and Upper South had

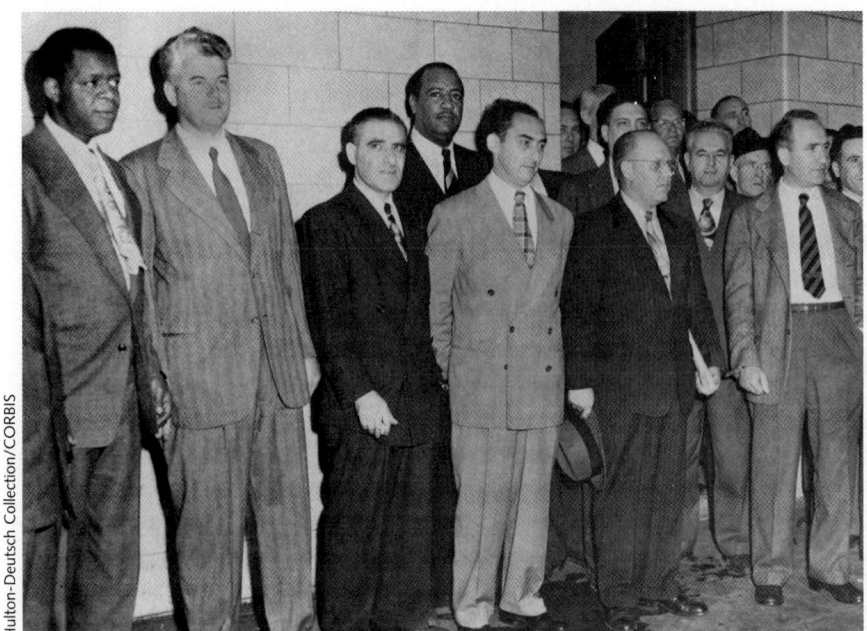

Convicted leaders of the American Communist Party.

the activities of, and kept secret files on, antiwar activists.

In the late twentieth century, the rise of terrorist activity around the world resulted in several laws designed to detect and apprehend people suspected of such activity. The 1978 Foreign Intelligence Act, and its expansion in 1994, authorized electronic wiretapping and eavesdropping and covert physical searches in the effort to collect information related to terrorism. In 1996 Congress passed the Antiterrorism and Effective Death Penalty Act, which targeted immigration offenses, including possession of a false driver's license or passport.

In response to the terrorist acts of September 11, 2001, President George W. Bush proposed that foreign nationals accused of terrorism be tried by military tribunals. Constitutional rules of evidence would not apply in these special courts. Meanwhile, the Justice Department enacted new guidelines allowing officials to eavesdrop on people in federal custody and to listen in on conversations between these prisoners and their lawyers. In October 2001 Congress passed the U.S.A. Patriot Act of 2001. This act expanded the government's authority to monitor and destroy terrorists' sources of funding, to wiretap and engage in other forms of surveillance activity, and to detain immigrants suspected of terrorism.

Americans who applaud these measures argue that "the Constitution is not a suicide pact" and that stringent measures are needed to protect the security of the United States and its citizens. Critics counter that the suspension of legal rights in the name of national security might eventually erode civil liberties for all Americans. ∎

---

been accustomed to using bound workers of all kinds, including white indentured servants, youthful apprentices, and slaves. With changes in the economy, owners of grist mills and other enterprises now wanted paid labor. Paid laborers offered a flexible workforce; they could be hired and fired at a moment's notice.

Even free African Americans faced an uphill struggle in their efforts to achieve political rights and economic well-being. Free people of color found their employment options limited as white men competed with them for jobs and political representation. When they emerged from bondage, freed people created educational and religious institutions that affirmed their sense of community and shared heritage. However, chronic underemployment and persistent white prejudice, sanctioned by law, condemned many black men and women to poverty. Lacking full citizenship rights, they saw the Revolution as an unfulfilled promise rather than a glorious achievement.

Blacks in the North

For many northern blacks, the Revolution continued to resonate in their memories and their hopes. Gad Asher, seized from his home on the western coast of Africa around 1750, had been forced to work as a slave for a ship carpenter in East Guilford, New Jersey. During the Revolution, Asher had served as a soldier in his master's place. His owner promised him the money he would earn as a Continental soldier. Yet when Asher came home after the war, his master reneged on the promise. Eventually, Asher managed to earn enough money on his own to buy his freedom. In 1785 he and his wife had a son, Jeremiah. The youngster loved to hear his father and two other African American veterans talk of the "motives which had prompted them to 'endure hardness'" while fighting the British. Recalled Jeremiah many years later,

> I was so accustomed to hear these men talk, until I almost fancied to myself that I had more rights than any white man in the town. Such were the lessons taught me by the old black soldiers of the Revolution. Thus, my first ideas of the right of the colored man to life, liberty, and the pursuit of happiness, were received from these old veterans and champions for liberty.

Between 1790 and 1804, all the northern states abolished slavery. Some, such as New York and New Jersey, did so gradually, stipulating that the children of slaves must serve a period of time (as long as 28 years in certain states) before they could gain their freedom. In 1800, over 36,500 blacks in the North were still enslaved, and some 47,000 were free. Pennsylvania did not liberate its last slave until 1847. Yet throughout the North, blacks—whether enslaved or free— were only a small percentage of the total population, ranging from less than 1 percent in Vermont to almost 8 percent in New Jersey. Most black men worked as farm hands or manual laborers, most black women as domestic servants or laundresses. Nevertheless, some whites saw black men as rivals for their jobs and as a threat to the well-being of the white population.

At both the state and national levels, most free blacks lacked basic citizenship rights. In 1792, two years after Congress limited naturalization to white aliens, it restricted the militia to white men. State legislatures in New England and the Mid-Atlantic region imposed various other restrictions on free people of color. These measures limited blacks' right to vote, serve on juries, and move from place to place. Rectifying an "oversight" in their state constitutions, New Jersey and Connecticut later took special pains to disfranchise African American men. Massachusetts offered free blacks the most rights, including the right to vote (for men) and the right of blacks and whites to intermarry.

As slaves, blacks had served in a variety of skilled capacities in the North. Yet as free people, they faced mounting pressures in trying to live independently. Certain jobs, such as those with the federal postal service, remained closed to them by law. And municipal authorities refused to grant them licenses to ply their trades, such as wagon driving. Lacking the means to buy tools and equipment and the ability to attract white customers, many black artisans had to take menial jobs.

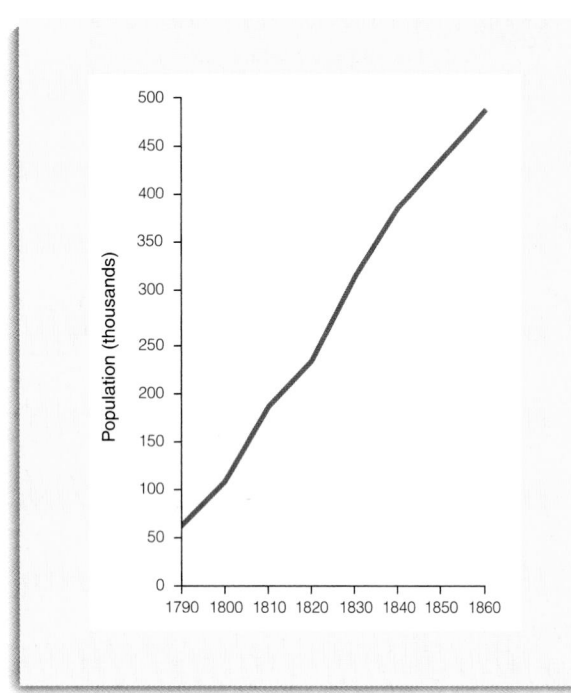

■ **FIGURE 9.2**
FREE BLACKS AS A PERCENTAGE OF TOTAL POPULATION IN SELECTED SOCIETIES

Source: The New York Public Library African American Desk Reference, p. 38.

Blacks' experiences in New York City are an apt example. In 1790 the free black population in that city amounted to about 1000 people; ten years later that number had more than tripled. In 1800 about 38 percent of male free heads of household in New York made their living as artisans. By 1810 that number had fallen to 29 percent, and it continued to drop in the years that followed. Increasingly, free black men took jobs as laborers, sailors, and domestic servants, and black women worked mostly as domestic servants and laundresses.

Still, free blacks in the North set about creating their own households and institutions. They moved out of the garrets and back rooms in houses owned by whites and set up housekeeping on their own. In Boston in 1790, one in three blacks lived outside white households;

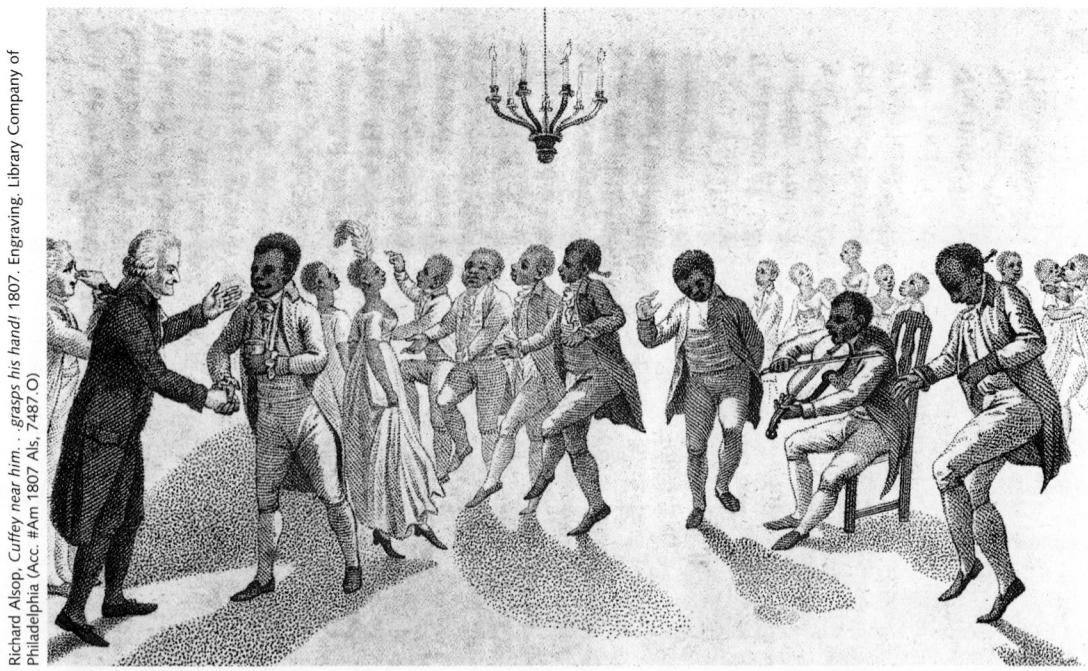

Richard Alsop. *Cuffey near him. . grasps his hand!* 1807. Engraving. Library Company of Philadelphia (Acc. #Am 1807 Als, 7487 O)

■ Massachusetts Governor John Hancock sponsored a celebration for Boston blacks in 1793. This picture appeared in a local periodical, *American Mercury,* accompanied by a satirical poem. The poet ridiculed blacks and the "motley scenes" they produced: "loud to anarchy their voices raise." New England blacks felt the tension between their newly won freedom and old forms of prejudice and subordination that endured after emancipation. Often isolated from each other in the workplace, they appreciated the opportunity to come together, enjoy each others' company, and, in this case, to dance, in the poet's words, "to the sweet Tune of Freedom born anew."

30 years later, eight in ten did so. In response to efforts of white Methodists to segregate church seating, Philadelphia black leaders formed the Free African Society in 1787. The first independent black church in the North, St. Thomas Protestant Episcopal Church, was founded in Philadelphia in the early 1790s. Absalom Jones, an African American preacher, headed the new church. In 1794 the Bethel African Methodist Episcopal Church, a branch of the Methodist denomination, was dedicated.

Black people also continued to celebrate their own festivals, some of which originated in the colonial period: Pinkster (based on the Jewish and Christian celebration of Pentecost) in New York and Training Day, Negro Election Day, and Coronation Day in New England. Usually conducted in late spring or early summer, these events featured parades in which black people came together to strut their finery, play drums and other African musical instruments, and proclaim their identity as a free people. In Massachusetts, blacks celebrated "Negro Election Day" by choosing their own "governors" and "judges," unofficial but influential community leaders (often African-born). In Providence, slaves and free people of color joined with small numbers of Narraganset Indians in Negro Election Day celebrations. The festivals gave men and women alike an opportunity to escape the confines of the workplace, even if only for a short time, and eat, drink, and dance with other people of color.

Manumissions in the South

In 1782 the Virginia state legislature lifted a 59-year-old ban on manumission, a process by which owners released selected people from bondage. Over the next ten years, approximately 10,000 Virginia slaves gained their freedom through manumission. Some planters believed

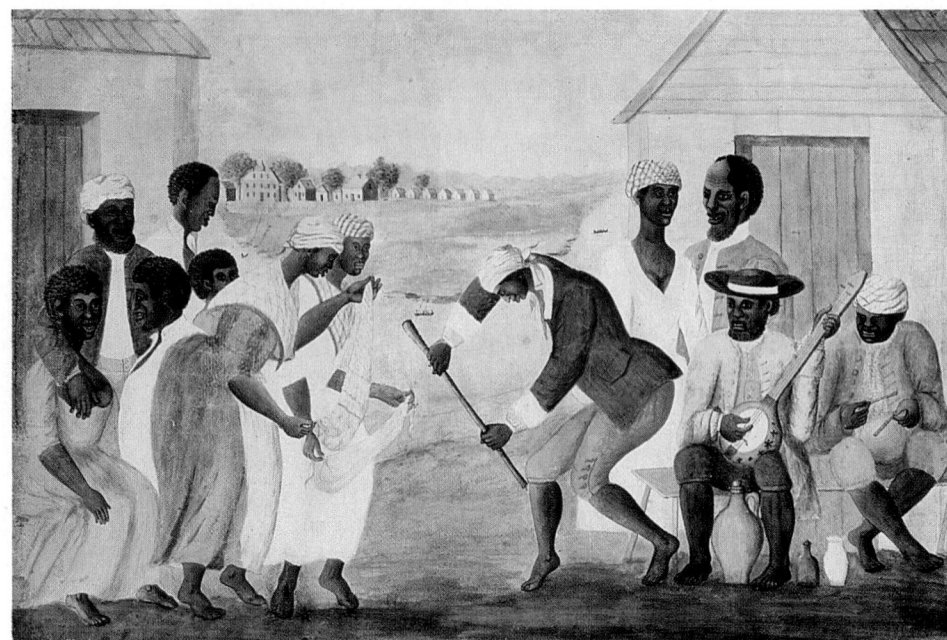

■ An anonymous artist captured this scene, probably in the slave quarters of a South Carolina plantation, in 1800. It is unknown what kind of entertainment or celebration the musicians and dancers are engaged in. The two men on the right are playing musical instruments of west African origin: a banjo and a *quaqua,* or skin-covered gourd used as a drum. On large lowcountry plantations especially, Africans and their descendants preserved traditional musical forms and social rituals.

The Old Plantation, c. 1790–1800. Abby Aldrich Rockefeller Folk Art Museum. Colonial Williamsburg Foundation, Williamsburg, VA

that the Revolution was the will of God, and they came to believe that slavery violated their religious principles. Some, taking to heart the rhetoric of the Revolution, objected to the glaring contradiction between the ideal of liberty and the reality of bondage. In 1802 a Maryland woman freed her slaves because, she said, the institution went against "the inalienable Rights of Mankind."

In the Upper South, especially, private manumissions dramatically increased the free black population. There, the emergence of a more diversified economy, including craft shops and grist mills, had lowered slave prices and encouraged abolitionist sentiment among some lawmakers, clergy, and slave owners. Between 1790 and 1810, the free black population in Baltimore increased from around 325 to over 5600.

Virginia planters George Washington and Robert Carter were unusual in terms of the numbers of slaves they manumitted (several hundred) and their efforts to ease the transition to freedom for people who possessed neither land nor financial resources. Providing for manumission in his will, Washington arranged apprenticeships for younger freed blacks and pensions for aged ones. In 1792 Carter granted his older slaves small plots of land. In general, however, newly emancipated men and women had difficulty finding employment as free workers. Nor was their freedom guaranteed: the 1782 Virginia manumission law provided that black debtors could be returned to slavery. The next year, Maryland went out of its way to stipulate that manumitted blacks were not "entitled to the rights of free men" except in their ability to own property. In southern cities, free people of color had to compete with both whites and enslaved laborers for work. The latter group, especially, formed a pool of cheap labor that limited the economic opportunities of all free workers, white and black alike.

Not all southern blacks achieved freedom through manumission. Some slaves, inspired by the growing community of free people of color in their midst and by the example of the black revolutionaries in the Caribbean island of Saint-Domingue in 1791, freed themselves. They ran away, heading for the anonymity of a nearby town or a haven such as Philadelphia or New York. Despite the growth in the free black population, the number of slaves actually increased in the Upper South, from over 520,000 in 1790 to almost 650,000 in 1810. In the South, slavery proved to be an extraordinarily durable institution.

Continuity and Change in the West

Later generations of Americans claimed that the western fringe of European American settlement—the ever-receding frontier—was the most American of all places. There, it was said, with a great deal of hard work, the rugged sons and daughters of the Revolution and their descendants could carve a living out of the land and prosper independently of landlords and creditors. Yet this image was more fantasy than reality. In certain key respects, western communities tended to duplicate their eastern counterparts. The opening of federal lands proved a boon for speculators, who extended credit to homesteaders and profited from the sale of small land parcels. Charged high prices for their purchases and forced to buy expensive supplies transported across the Appalachians, some settlers rapidly sank into debt. Westerners, like their eastern counterparts, needed money and business savvy—and in some cases political connections—to succeed.

Many native-born men and women and German and Scots-Irish immigrants who followed the Shenandoah Valley south brought with them, or bought, enslaved workers to toil on river docks and in cotton fields. The late-eighteenth-century trans-Appalachian West (modern-day Ohio, Indiana, Kentucky, and Tennessee) thus offered few African Americans a fresh start. Even in the Northwest Territory, where slavery was prohibited by law, African Americans faced the same kind of prejudice that shaped social relations in the East. Rather, than extend the bounds of liberty, western settlement solidified ideas about white supremacy.

From the Canadian border to Georgia, the trans-Appalachian West had become a cultural battlefield. European Americans warred against Indians, but Indian leaders also disagreed bitterly with one another about how to respond. Should they defend their hunting grounds to the last man, woman, and child? Seek refuge elsewhere? Capitulate completely to an alien culture? Or embrace some combination of these alternatives? The true history of the West during this period reveals the dangers of generalizing about "Americans," "Indians," and "foreigners." Yet one generalization does hold true: the abundance of natural resources and the vastness of the land, combined with the clash of cultures and the prevalence of armed men of all backgrounds, made life particularly dangerous in the borderlands.

Indians Wars in the Great Lakes Region

Many Indians residing in the Northwest Territory in the 1790s were refugees from the East, victims of the Revolutionary War. As they resettled in villages, they managed to retain some elements of their cultural identity. These groups included the Ottawas, Ojibways, Wyandots, Algonquians, Delawares, and what remained of the Iroquois Confederacy. They also included peoples who had long occupied the area that today is called the Great Lakes region and the Upper Midwest (Map 9.1): the Miamis, Weas, Piankashaws, Potawatomis, Menominees, Kickapoos, Illinois, Peorias, Kaskaskias, Fox, Winnebagos, Sauks, and Shawnees.

In the seven years immediately after the Revolution, thousands died in Indian–white clashes in this region. What caused this violence? By encouraging European Americans to stake their claim to the area, the Northwest Ordinance inflamed passions on both sides: whites' determination to occupy and own the land and Indians' equal determination to resist this incursion. In 1790, under orders from President Washington, Brigadier General Josiah Hamar led a force of about 1500 men into the Maumee River Valley in the northwest corner of modern-day Ohio. Orchestrating two ambushes in September, Miami chief Little Turtle and his men killed 183 of Hamar's troops, driving the general back in disgrace. The next year, Washington chose another officer, General Arthur St. Clair, to resume the fight. St. Clair's men met Little Turtle's warriors in November near the upper Wabash River and slightly south of the site of Hamar's defeat. During this engagement, 600 whites died.

Washington tried once more to find a commander equal to Little Turtle. This time he chose General Anthony Wayne, a Revolutionary War hero dubbed "Mad Anthony" for his

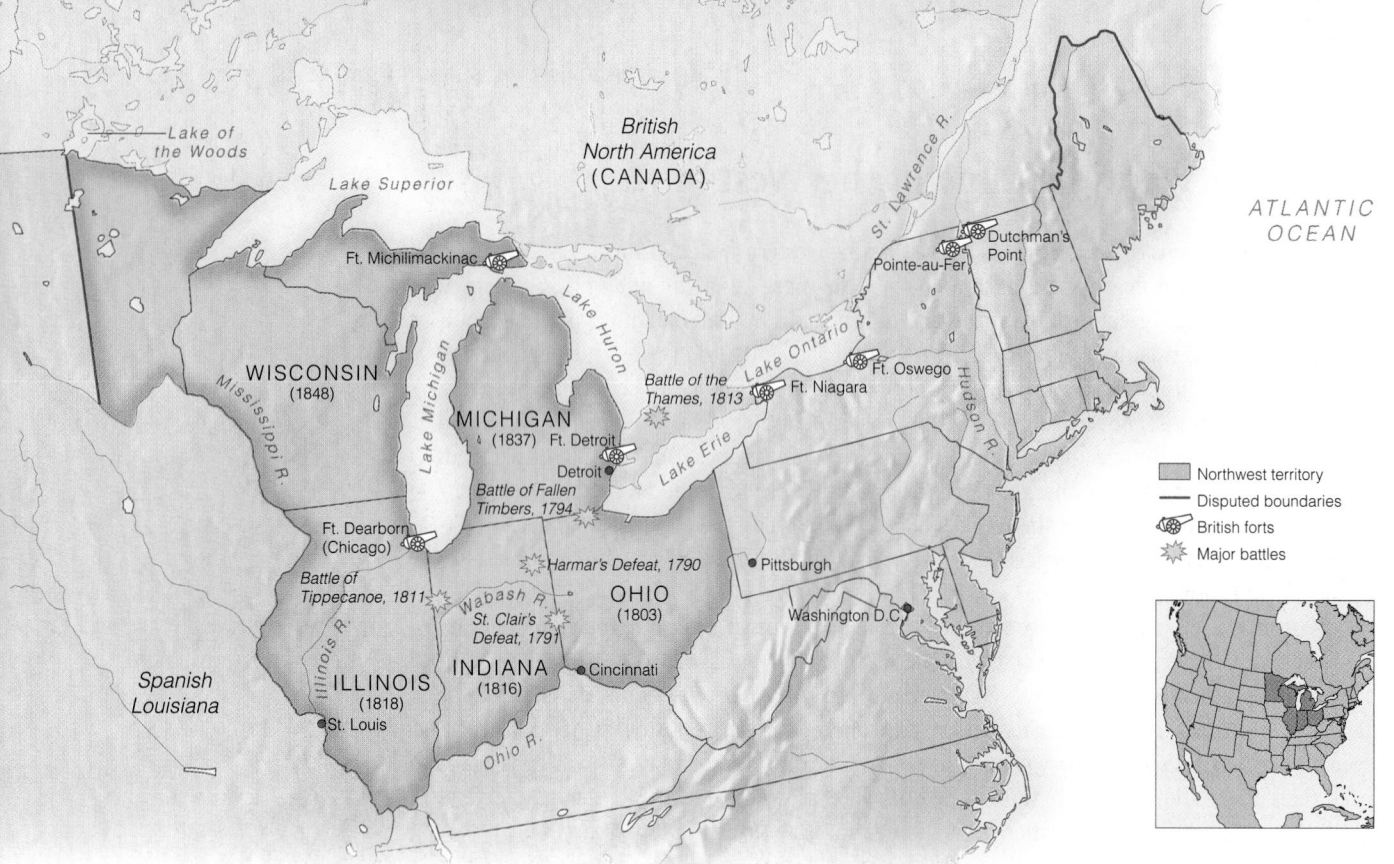

■ **MAP 9.1**

THE NORTHWEST TERRITORY After the Revolution, the Northwest Territory became a battleground. Indians—both long-term residents and newcomers—as well as European American squatters and speculators vied for control of the land. The Northwest Ordinance of 1787 provided for territorial governments before an area could apply for statehood. The present-day states of Ohio, Indiana, Michigan, Illinois, and Wisconsin were carved out of the Northwest Territory. All had gained statehood by 1848, but only after almost sixty years of bloodshed between Indians and U.S. troops in the region.

bold recklessness. Wayne mobilized a force of 3000 men and constructed a string of new forts as well. Alarmed by this new offensive, Little Turtle urged his warriors and the Ohio Confederacy to make peace. Instead, they chose a new leader, a warrior named Turkey Foot. When the anticipated encounter came in August 1794, at the British Fort Miami on the Maumee River (near the western shore of Lake Erie), the Indians found themselves surrounded. They sought refuge in the fort, but the British would not let them enter, refusing to become involved in a wider war with the Americans. Hundreds of Indians perished as Wayne's forces closed in.

The withdrawal of British support helped to doom the Ohio Confederacy, which was less a union of Indians than a lopsided alliance between Indians and their British benefactors. On August 3, 1795, 1100 Indian leaders met at Fort Greenville (in western Ohio) and ceded to the United States a vast tract of Indian land: all of present day Ohio and most of Indiana. Little Turtle helped negotiate the agreement.

Indian Acculturation in the West

Various Indian groups differed in their responses to the European Americans who settled among them or attempted to persuade—or force—them to "acculturate" by adopting the customs and habits of whites. According to European Americans, men farm and herd sheep and cattle; women milk cows, keep chickens, tend the garden, spin thread, and weave cloth. However, in the "middle ground" throughout the West, newly arrived settlers and indigenous peoples traded foodways, folk remedies, and styles of dress. Even Joseph Brant and Little Turtle picked and chose among European American (and, in Brant's case, English) cultural

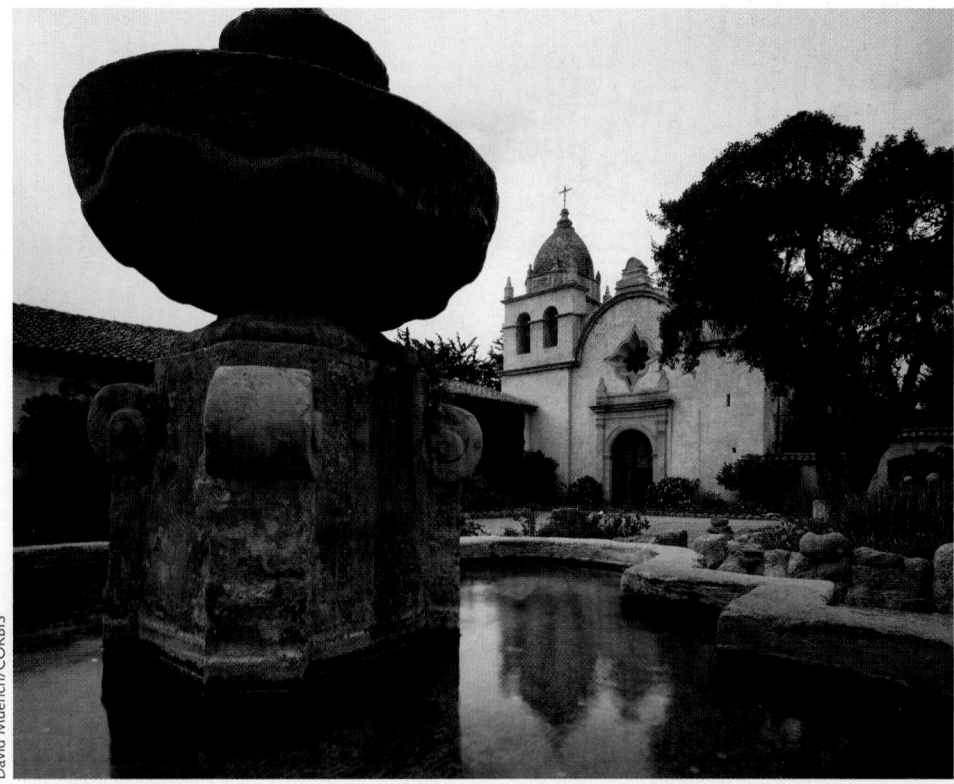

David Muench/CORBIS

■ Mission San Carlos Borromeo in Carmel, California. In the foreground is the mission's central courtyard. In the background is the *ranchería,* where Indians lived. In this and other missions along the California coast, Indians maintained separate residences in traditional-style dwellings. Even Indians who worked and prayed at the missions attempted to preserve their own customs related to clothing, food, and kinship and family relations.

traits. Little Turtle drank tea and coffee, kept cows, and shunned leather breeches in favor of white men's clothing. The fact that his wife made butter suggested that she was skilled in the ways of European American homemakers. Little Turtle himself appealed to Quaker missionaries to help the Miamis adapt to stock raising and the plow. The white population was advancing "like oil on a blanket," he pointed out, and the Indians were disappearing "like snow before the sun."

Adopting some habits of European Americans—for example, liquor consumption—amounted to self-destruction. On the "middle ground," alcohol was a prized trade item. Moreover, European Americans and Indians often used it to lubricate political negotiations and cultural rituals. Yet conflicts over liquor, and tensions vented under the influence of liquor, became increasingly common—and deadly. Some Indian leaders, such as Joseph Brant and Little Turtle, who came to view the drinking of alcohol as a full-blown crisis among their people, believed that Indians must reject the white man's bottle if they were to survive. Others placed their priorities elsewhere and continued to indulge in alcohol. In 1799 Seneca leader Handsome Lake (Skanyadariyoh) emerged from an alcohol-induced coma to proclaim *Gai'wiio,* or Good Message. This message urged Indians to accept certain elements of whites' culture (stock tending and individual homes) while retaining traditional rituals and languages.

But liquor was not the only crisis facing the Indians, as the experience of the Five Civilized Tribes in the southeastern United States revealed. This group included the Cherokee, Chickasaws, Chocktaws, Creeks, and Seminoles. The migration of whites into their hunting grounds had depleted their game supply and devastated their crop fields. After the Revolution, the Cherokees appealed to the federal government for aid. Some of the other groups, unable to hunt for food, took up agriculture. Men, using plows, replaced women, who had relied on hoes. Protestant missionaries encouraged Indian women to learn to spin thread and weave cloth.

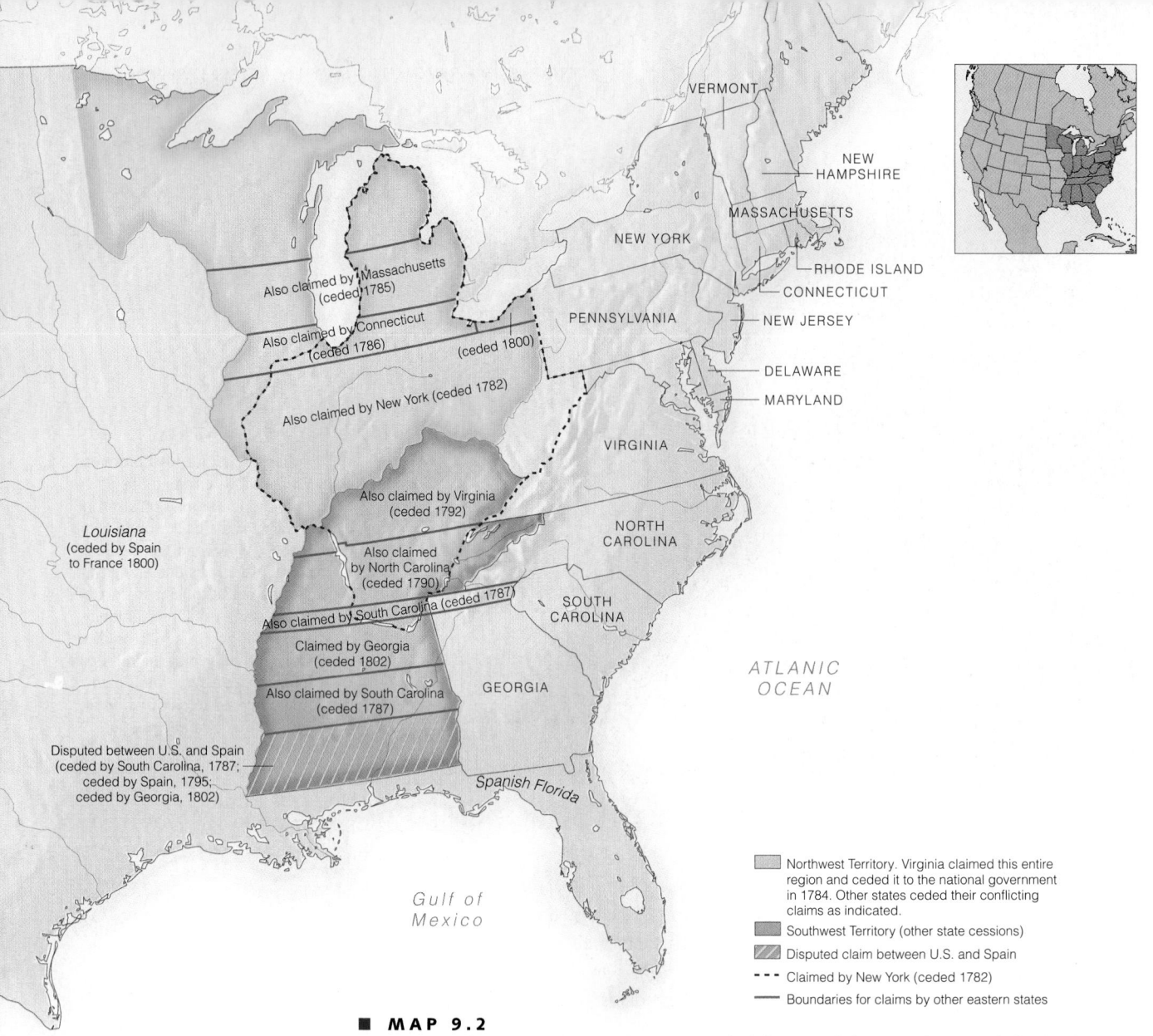

■ MAP 9.2

WESTERN LAND CLAIMS OF THE STATES Several of the original thirteen colonies, including Massachusetts, Connecticut, New York, Virginia, South Carolina, North Carolina, and Georgia claimed land west of the Appalachian mountains. By 1802, these states had ceded their western lands to the federal government. The Land Ordinance of 1785 provided that this expanse be auctioned off in parcels no less than 640 acres each, with a minimum price of one dollar per acre—too expensive for many family homesteaders, thus opening the way for investors to purchase and profit. Hoping to raise money through land sales, the federal government did not object to speculation.

The southeastern groups only gradually accepted the idea of keeping livestock, for they retained cultural scruples against eating certain kinds of animals. The Cherokees, for example, believed that people would assume the characteristics of the animals they ate, so they discouraged the consumption of pork and other pig products. Yet in 1796, when a federal Indian agent toured Creek country, he noted signs of "civilization": black slaves (most of them runaways from southern plantations) hard at work in the fields and fences that protected crops from cattle and other beasts. The willingness of members of the Five Civilized tribes to accommodate themselves to European American law and divisions of labor allowed them to stay in their homeland and retain key elements of their cultural identity. Later generations of southwestern Indian leaders challenged this strategy of accommodation.

In southwest and far west borderland areas, Spanish officials met with mixed success in their attempts to convert Indians to Christianity and encourage them to engage in sedentary farming. For example, between 1772 and 1804, Spanish priests established five missions among the Chumash, hunter-gatherers living in permanent villages along the California coast. When large numbers of the Indians moved to these settlements, they forfeited their traditional kin and trade networks, and their distinctive culture began to fade. Birth rates plummeted due to disruptions in family life (more women than men lived in the missions), and mortality rates increased dramatically as the Spanish introduced new diseases.

In contrast, along the Texas Gulf Coast, the Spanish made little headway in their efforts to bring the Karankawas Indians into the missions. Members of this nomadic tribe arrived at the mission gates only when their own food reserves were low; in essence, the Karankawas simply included the missions in their seasonal migrations between the Gulf Coast and the coastal prairie.

Land Speculation and Slavery

The West was not necessarily a place of boundless economic opportunity for all people who settled there. When Americans poured into the trans-Appalachian West after the Revolution, they often carried alcohol and guns, staples of trade among all groups. These items proved a lethal mix, injecting violence into commercial and diplomatic relations among a variety of cultural groups. Moreover, land speculators sought to make large profits from family homesteaders forced to buy property at inflated prices. And too, many European American migrants brought their slaves west in a bid for economic self-sufficiency or profit-making, or both. For all these reasons, in several respects the West soon came to resemble society on the eastern seaboard, with its hierarchies based on class, ethnicity, and race.

Eager investors and creditors thwarted many homesteaders' quest for cheap land. Post-Revolutionary-era schemes such as the Ohio Company of Associates foreshadowed the significance of land speculation in shaping patterns of settlement and property ownership in the West. With backing from wealthy investors, the Ohio Company quickly bought up tracts of land and then sold parcels to family farmers at inflated rates. A similar venture was initiated in Georgia in 1795, when speculators bribed state legislators for the right to resell huge tracts to the west of the state, land that the state did not even own. The state legislature passed the so-called Yazoo Act (named for a Georgia river) because of these bribes. The act resulted in the defrauding of thousands of buyers, whose land titles were worthless.

By protecting slavery and opening territory new territory to European America settlement, the new nation condemned southern blacks to a kind of legal bondage that stood in stark contrast to revolutionary principles. Many settlers relied on slave labor. By the late eighteenth century, Kentucky slaves numbered 40,000—more than 18 percent of the state's total population. In isolated settlements, where farmers owned just one or two slaves, African Americans faced a kind of loneliness unknown on large plantations in the East. In 1793, near Newport, Kentucky, slaves Moses and Humphrey informed their master, James Taylor, that "there are no colored people here, we have no women to wash for us, on Sundays we stalk about without being able to talk to anyone." Where white planters embraced new kinds of opportunity in the new territories, their slaves experienced backbreaking toil unrelieved by companionship or family ties.

Patterns of land use directly affected the spread of slavery into the West. Despite eastern planters' use of European soil conservation techniques (crop rotation, use of manure as fertilizer), many of them had to contend with depleted soil in the Upper South. Generations of tobacco growers had worn out the land, depriving it of nutrients. As a result, many growers

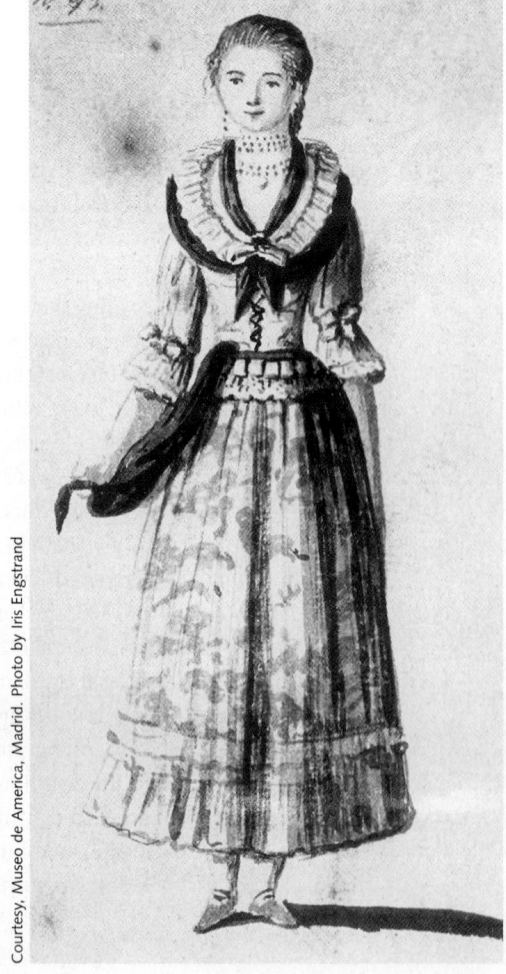

Courtesy, Museo de America, Madrid. Photo by Iris Engstrand

■ In 1791, an artist made this sketch of the wife of a Spanish soldier stationed at the presidio, or military garrison, in Monterey, California. Many elite Spaniards in the Americas went to great lengths to dress like their European counterparts. This woman is wearing the elegant dress, elaborate jewelry, and dainty shoes that befit her status. One eighteenth-century resident of New Mexico wrote that, despite the hot climate, European Americans "will go up to their ears in debt simply to satisfy their pride in putting on a grand appearance." However, most *nuevomexicanos* adopted some elements of Indian-style clothing, such as practical leather moccasins and garments made of buckskin and coarse woolens.

were forced to abandon tobacco. Some of them moved west into Indian lands (Mississippi Territory) to cultivate cotton. The scarcity of labor motivated slave owners to push workers to the limits of their endurance. Slaves prepared the ground for cultivation, rooted out tree stumps, and cleared brush. Then slaves followed the rhythms of the cotton-growing season: planting in the spring, hoeing in the summer, and harvesting in the fall. Slaves on cotton plantations worked in gangs under the sharp eye of a white overseer or black driver. Men, women, and children labored as human hoeing machines, growing as much cotton as quickly as possible. In contrast, slaves who worked in rice fields were organized under the task system: each day, once they completed a certain amount of field work, they were allowed to devote time to cultivating their own gardens and tending their own chickens. Whether working on a gang or task system, blacks and Indian captives of war remained vulnerable to certain Indian tribes such as the Cherokee, which actively practiced slavery.

Even many free people of color found a less than hospitable welcome in the West. In 1802 delegates to the first Ohio territorial convention moved to restrict blacks' economic and political opportunities, even though fewer than 400 were living in Ohio at the time. One proposal read that "no negro or mulatto shall ever be eligible to hold any office, civil or military, or give oath in any court of justice against a white person." Although slavery was outlawed in Ohio and other territories, blacks still lacked the right to vote. Soon after Ohio became a state in 1803, the legislature took steps to prevent the in-migration of free blacks altogether.

Several other Midwestern territories and states followed Ohio's example. In 1803 the territorial legislature of Indiana passed a "black law" prohibiting blacks or Indians from testifying in court against white people. Black families in the Northwest were also vulnerable to kidnapping: some white men seized free blacks and sold them as slaves to plantation owners in the South. Moreover, whites took advantage of poor blacks by "indenturing" their children. Under this arrangement, a white man or woman controlled the labor of a black youth for a stipulated number of years. In Indiana, terms of indenture for any black person could last as long as 90 years.

Shifting Social Identities in the Post-Revolutionary Era

The nation's founders had argued for an egalitarian society, one in which people prospered according to their talents and ambition. Of course, their definition of egalitarianism encompassed only white men. Still, it was a revolutionary idea and led to challenges of social hierarchies after the Revolution. These hierarchies included institutions such as the patriarchal (male-headed) family, established Protestant denominations, power systems based on social standing, and ideas about race and gender. Several writers applauded these leveling tendencies. They argued that authority of all kinds—fathers over families, clergy over congregations, political leaders over citizens—was suspect and counter to revolutionary ideas. Ordinary men and women penned letters to local newspapers, glorifying common laborers and questioning the claim to power of "the marchent, phesition [physician] the lawyer and divine [minister] and all the literary walkes of life, the Jutical & Executive oficeers & all the rich who live without bodily labour." This letter writer's creative spelling suggests that even people lacking in formal education felt free to voice their opinions on political issues of the day.

In the early nineteenth century, voluntary reform organizations multiplied across the nation, transforming the professions, the religious landscape, slavery, the rights of women, and a host of other American institutions. In the years immediately after the Revolution, both the possibilities and limitations of reform became clear. Some groups—for example, white working men—sought to advance their own self-interest without showing much concern for the plight of African American laborers. In other cases, people banded together to target the behavior of a specific group: drunkards, slave owners, the irreligious, or prostitutes. These moral reform groups welcomed diversity among members, as long as new converts supported the cause.

The Search for Common Ground

As people embraced a common cause with like-minded others, a variety of groups emerged. Manumission and temperance societies had appeared during the Revolution. Other kinds of associations sprang up and multiplied after the war. For example, in southwestern Pennsylvania, tax resisters formed the Mingo Creek Society. The organization offered mediation services for citizens who felt "harassed with suits from justices and courts, and wished a less expensive tribunal." In New York, 15 women formed the Society for the Relief of Poor Widows and Small Children. Often, free people of color in the North and South created new churches designated as "African," a testament to a shared heritage that predated their transportation to America and enslavement.

Americans redefined the family to accommodate new circumstances and ideas. Some whites who chose to live in Indian villages (known as white Indians) felt they had found new families. Wrote Mary Jemison, a captive and then willing member of the Senecas, "It was my happy lot to be accepted for adoption." She described her initiation ceremony in these terms: "I was received by the two squaws to supply the place of their brother in the family; and I was ever considered and treated by them as a real sister, the same as though I had been born of their mother."

In some instances the family metaphor extended to religious ties. Members of Baptist and Methodist congregations referred to themselves as brothers and sisters. They called their preachers "elder brother" or, in some places in the South, "Daddy." The Shakers, a sect founded by Englishwoman Ann Lee in the 1770s, forbade sexual intercourse between male and female members. In this group, the church itself replaced traditional family relationships.

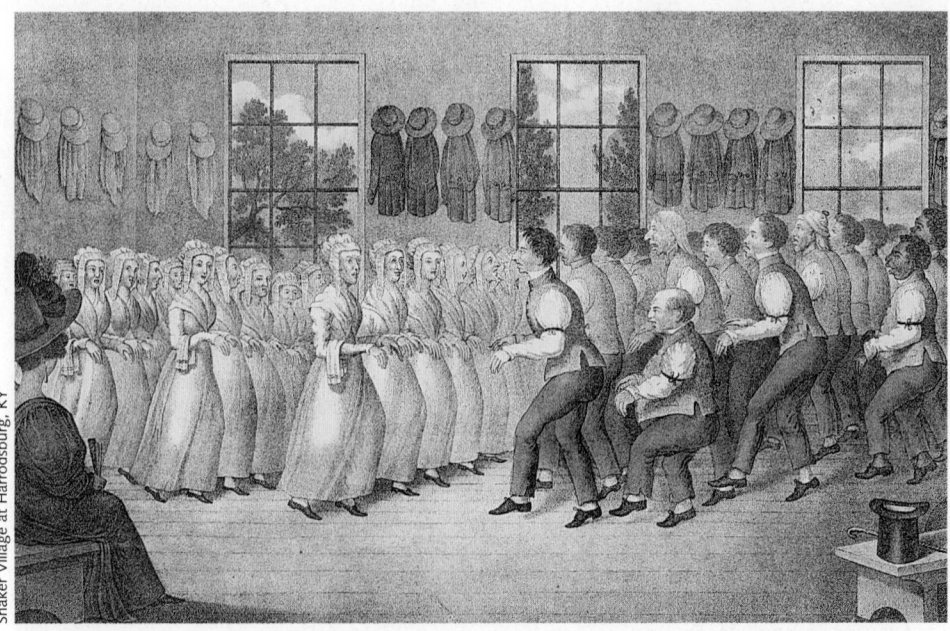

Shaker Village at Harrodsburg, KY

■ Men and women participate in a Shaker worship service in New Lebanon, New York. The formal name of the church was the United Society of Believers in Christ's Second Appearance. The group's more familiar name derived from their peculiar worship style, which involved trembling and shaking. Founded in 1787, the New Lebanon community was the church's largest. Members of the group reconfigured traditional family relations. They forbade marriage but, like several other Protestant denominations, encouraged congregants to call each other brothers and sisters.

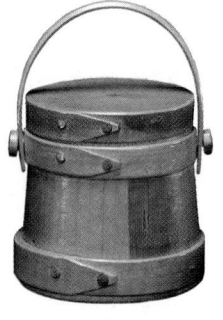

Artisan–Politicians and the Plight of Post-Revolutionary Workers

In the decades after the Revolution, residents of port cities along the eastern seaboard grew accustomed to public parades marking special occasions: a visit from George Washington, the ratification of the Constitution, the Fourth of July. Most of these parades consisted of groups of artisans marching together, carrying the banners of their respective occupations. As one example, the bricklayers' flag declared, "Both Buildings and Rulers Are the Works of Our Hands."

Proud of their role in the Sons of Liberty and other revolutionary organizations, bricklayers—along with tanners, carpenters, glassblowers, weavers, and other groups of artisans—proclaimed themselves the proud citizens of the new nation. In some respects, these groups resembled the guilds of Europe: members of one craft united and caring for one another in mutual obligation. In other respects, American worker organizations were unique, for they built on a distinct revolutionary heritage that stressed the equality of all (white) freeborn men. Master artisans in several cities—including Boston, Albany, Providence, Portsmouth, Charleston, Savannah, and New York—created organizations called the General Society of Mechanics and Tradesmen that brought together skilled workers from a variety of fields. The proliferation of newspapers let these artisans participate in a new, more open public forum. Such participation in turn helped gain them influence within local politics. In some towns, as many as 85 percent of adult men owned property of some kind and thus were eligible to vote. Indeed, artisans' organizations soon became quasi-political groups, extending their reach in ways that pre-Revolutionary trades-based associations had not.

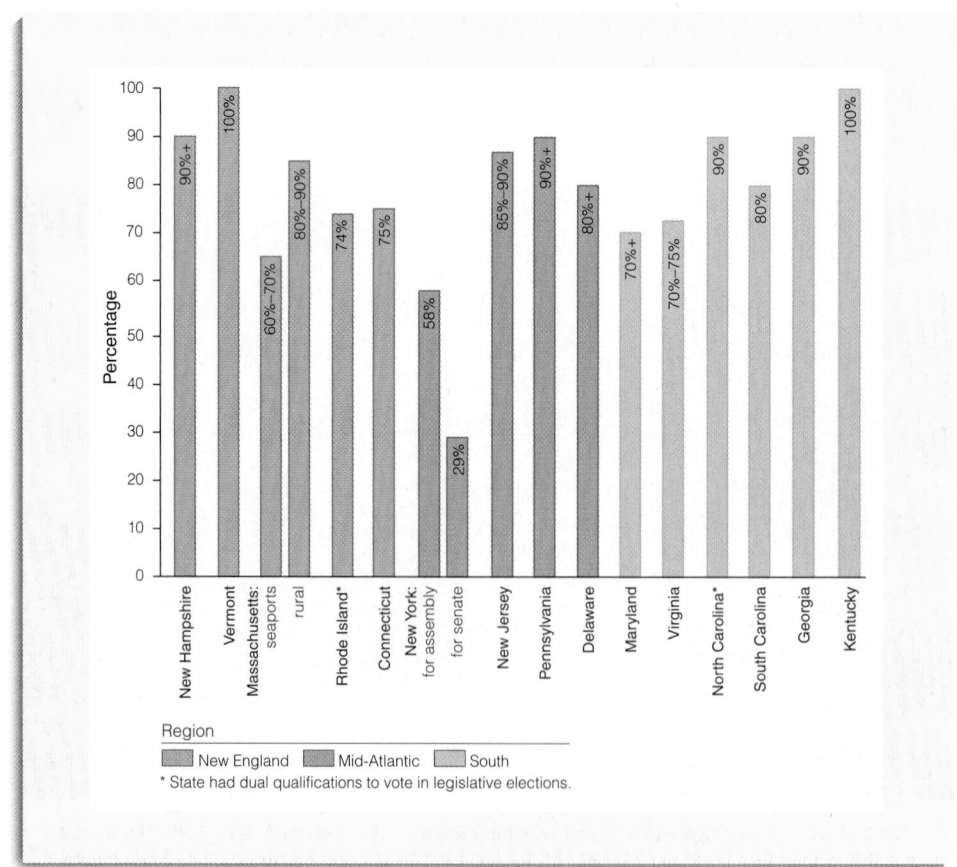

■ **FIGURE 9.3**
PERCENTAGE OF WHITE MEN ELIGIBLE TO VOTE IN THE UNITED STATES, 1792

Source: Robert J. Dinkin, Voting in Revolutionary America: A Study of Elections in the Original Thirteen States, 1776–1789 (1982), pp. 36–39.

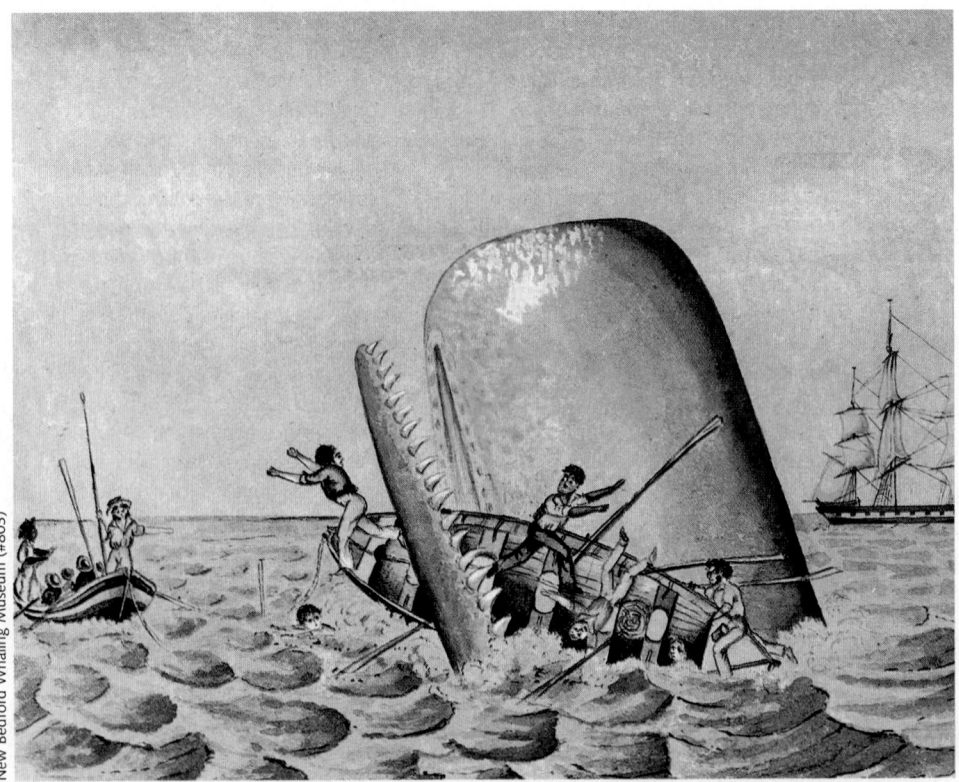

New Bedford Whaling Museum (#803)

■ After the Revolution and well into the early nineteenth century, African Americans, both enslaved and free, served as sailors in disproportionate numbers. This picture suggests the dangers faced by all men who labored on whaling ships. By the 1790s, American whalers were searching for sperm whales as far away as the South Pacific. These whales were the source of several prized substances, including sperm oil (a fuel), spermaceti (used to make candles), and ambergris (an ingredient in expensive perfumes). During the heyday of the sperm whale industry, American fleets were killing 10,000 whales annually.

Still, these organizations exhibited their own brand of elitism. Although commerce flourished in the 1790s, not all members of the laboring classes prospered. Journeymen in particular faced an uncertain future. In Philadelphia in the 1790s, half of the journeymen shoemakers eventually established their own shops, but only 10 percent of their tailor counterparts managed to do so. Dockworkers and other kinds of laborers struggled to find year-round employment. Meanwhile, more and more free men of color were drawn to sailing. Although they had little chance to rise within the ranks of a ship's command, they accepted the seafaring life because it was the steadiest work they could find.

As the country expanded and developed methods and systems of transport, the canal worker replaced the skilled artisan as the typical laborer. The diggers who constructed the canals of the early 1790s included men from all walks of life: part-time farmers, indentured servants, slaves, and white transients. Moving around in search of work, they led an unsettled existence that contrasted greatly with the more predictable life of urban artisans.

The plight of menial laborers (in the countryside and the cities) suggests the ironies that accompanied the decline of indentured servitude and the rise of the "free laborer." To be sure, master artisans attained a degree of economic independence that many other workers did not. But for men and women who lacked skills, money, and wealthy patrons,

A Sailmaker Discusses "Means for the Preservation of Public Liberty" on the Fourth of July, 1797

Urban skilled artisans (also called mechanics) played a significant role in the American fight for independence. In the years after the conflict, many artisans remained active in politics. They believed that the success of the new nation depended on the ability of its citizens to remain informed about and engaged in the political process.

In a speech delivered on July 4, 1797, a New York sailmaker, George James Warner, warned that citizens must strive to preserve the hard-won gains of the Revolution.

We must guard as a most valuable privilege, the freedom and rights of election. WHEREVER the wealthy by the influence of riches, are enabled to direct the choice of public officers, *there* the downfall of liberty cannot be very remote. It is our own fault if an influence so dangerous, has become in any measure prevalent among us. It would not be the case if the people did not consent to become the dupes of design. It is because tradesmen, mechanics, and the industrious classes of society consider themselves of TOO LITTLE CONSEQUENCE to the body politic that *any thing* belonging to the system of oppression at all obtains. We ought to spurn from us with disdain, the individual who would not solicit our vote, from motives of personal consideration. He ought not to be listened to, who would *demand* it as the price of friendship, or who would *expect* it from regard to his superior riches. It too often happens that men only capable of attracting public notice by an ostentatious display of their wealth, are deemed best qualified to protect the rights of the people, and consequently receive their suffrages; while our choice ought only to be directed to men of TALENTS and VIRTUE whatever their situation in life might be. The *possession* of riches is not necessarily accompanied by superior understanding or goodness of heart. On the contrary, the experience of ages confirms this opinion, that a state of mediocrity is more favorable to them both.

If, instead of improving on it original plan, our government, at any future period, should be irresistibly impelled in an unalterable course toward despotism, the dividing line between the *rich* and the *poor* will be distinctly marked, and the *latter* will be found in a state of vassallage [slavery] and dependence on the former.

Be it your care then, my fellow-citizens, to guard with unceasing vigilance against the growth of this evil; assume the native dignity of your character and maintain with a modest but determined spirit, the liberty of opinion. Suffer no one to DICTATE imperiously what line of conduct you are to pursue; but at the same time let no one be sacrificed at the alter of public vengeance, for a candid and liberal expression of his sentiments. . . .

We must endeavor to acquaint ourselves with the political situation and relative interests of our country. Without this information, we shall either be unable to form an accurate opinion on our own, or often become the dupes of the designing. The PUBLIC PRINTS naturally present themselves as the vehicles of this necessary knowledge. Those conducted in a spirit of liberality, yet alto-

freedom often meant financial insecurity and, in some cases, reliance on public or private charity. Those who did find work usually had the kinds of jobs that came with the booming economy of the late eighteenth century: moving goods from one place to another, building new structures, and providing personal services for the merchants who profited from all this commercial activity. In the coming years, trade associations for skilled white artisans would take pains to distance themselves from workers whom post-Revolutionary prosperity had left behind.

"Republican Mothers" and Other Well-Off Women

Some well-educated women in the United States read English writer Mary Wollstonecraft's *Vindication of the Rights of Women* published in England and in the United States in 1792. In that manifesto, Wollstonecraft argued that young men and women should receive the same

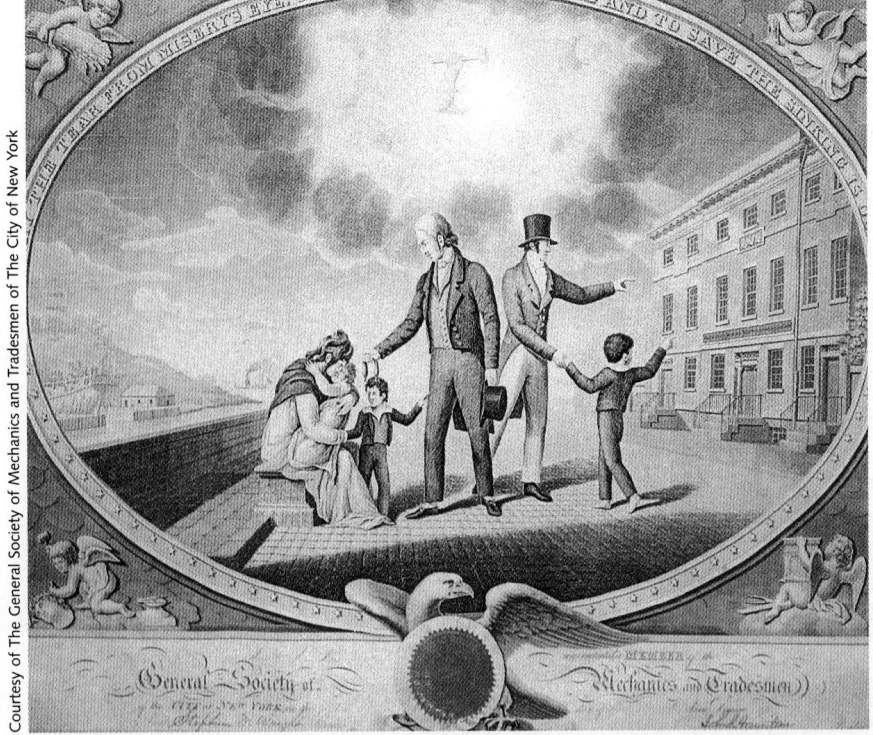

Courtesy of The General Society of Mechanics and Tradesmen of The City of New York

The New York City Mechanics' Society was founded in 1785 and incorporated in 1792. The society included many different kinds of artisans. In addition to representing the interests of skilled artisans, it served as a mutual aid association, lending money to members and distributing charity to the poor. This certificate of membership combines the traditional symbol of arts and crafts, the arm and hammer, with images of American patriotism (the eagle in the center foreground) and prosperity (waterways and fields on the left, urban townhouses on the left). Children are prominently featured here. In 1820 the General Society opened a school for the children of its members, and began offering classes to women in 1821.

gether consonant to the principles on which our revolution was achieved, should employ the public attention and meet its decided support. It will be found, that a JUST and EQUAL GOVERNMENT will ever derive additional stability, as the PEOPLE obtain a more general knowledge of its principles and operations. The result is, that every

sincere friend to our NATIONAL CONSTITUTION, ought sedulously to promote the dissemination of this knowledge, as a barrier to the risings of sedition, as well as to the encroachments of arbitrary power.

In his speech, Warner also called for "the practice of all the moral virtues" and the education of children "as to the

RIGHTS which they possess, and the DUTIES which they owe society." Warner himself became active in New York's Democratic-Republican party. ■

Source: George James Warner, *Means for the Preservation of Public Liberty* (New York, 1797); reprinted in Howard B. Rock, *The New York City Artisan, 1789–1825* (Albany: State University of New York Press, 1989), pp. 6–11.

kind of education. She objected to a special female curriculum that exclusively emphasized skills such as needlepoint and musical accomplishments; this "false system of education," she charged, left women "in a state of perpetual childhood."

In 1801 an anonymous "American Lady" published an essay titled "A Second Vindication of the Rights of Women." In it, she claimed that "a good kitchen woman [that is, a household drudge], very seldom makes a desirable wife, to a man of any refinement." The anonymous "American Lady" and others who shared her opinion celebrated a new kind of woman—the "Republican mother"—who provided cultured companionship for her husband and reared her children to be virtuous, responsible members of society. This image of womanhood led to a new notion: that well-off women should dedicate themselves to tending the home fires rather than aspiring to a more public role in business or politics.

Prior to the Revolution, women tended to bear many children, since additional hands were needed to labor in the fields. The decline in white women's fertility rates after the Revolution suggested that the economy had shifted. Factory managers and bookkeepers did not need to rely on the paid labor of their offspring. And some women could now buy products their grandmothers had made at home. In particular, a small but influential group of well-to-do women in the cities were shedding their roles as producers of candles, soap, and textiles. Instead, they became consumers of these staples and of luxury goods, and they managed household servants. As "Republican mothers," these women participated in the public life of the new nation as the guardians of the home and the socializers of children.

But the idea of the "Republican mother" also suggested a more radical notion. If such a woman wanted to earn the respect accorded all intelligent human beings, she must strive for an education equal to that of men's. In the 1790s a number of academies for "young ladies" opened in New England, including Sarah Peirce's in Litchfield, Connecticut, and Susanna Rowson's in Medford, Massachusetts. Many female academies catered to boarders, students living away from home. These schools offered courses in such "womanly pursuits" as needlework, etiquette, and music. But many also offered a classical curriculum consisting of mathematics, foreign languages, and geography. This system of study encouraged young women to think for themselves. In this respect, female academies challenged the view that women were intellectually inferior to and necessarily dependent on men.

Some elite women—like the anonymous "American Lady" and Alice Izard of Charleston, South Carolina—did not share this more radical viewpoint. For example, in opposition to Woll-

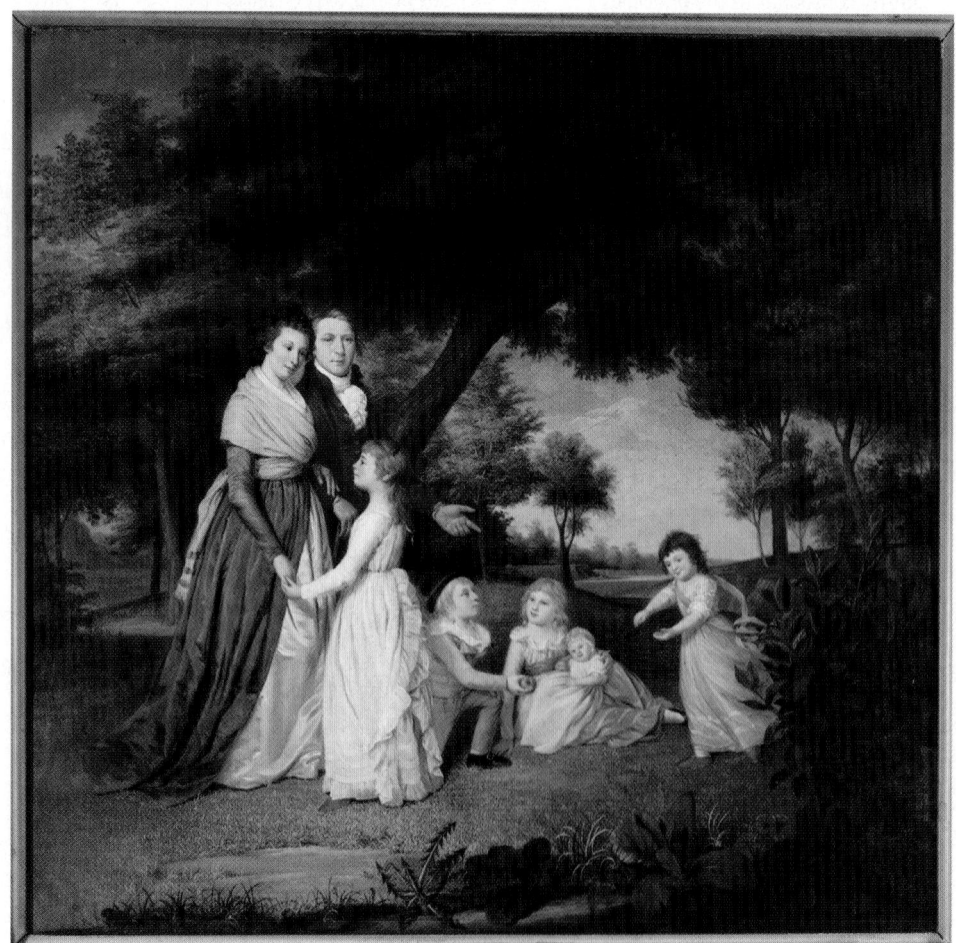

■ James Peale completed this painting of his family in 1795. Peale came from a distinguished family of artists. The picture represents the ideal of post-Revolutionary citizenship and family life. Husband and wife are both featured prominently, although their roles differ. The husband represents the household in the public, political sphere. The wife, a devoted mother, is responsible for preparing the children to be virtuous citizens of the new republic. Growing up in a well-to-do home, these playful children are exempt from the hard labor associated with childhood in the colonial period and, in the 1790s, still characteristic of childhood among enslaved, rural, and poor families.

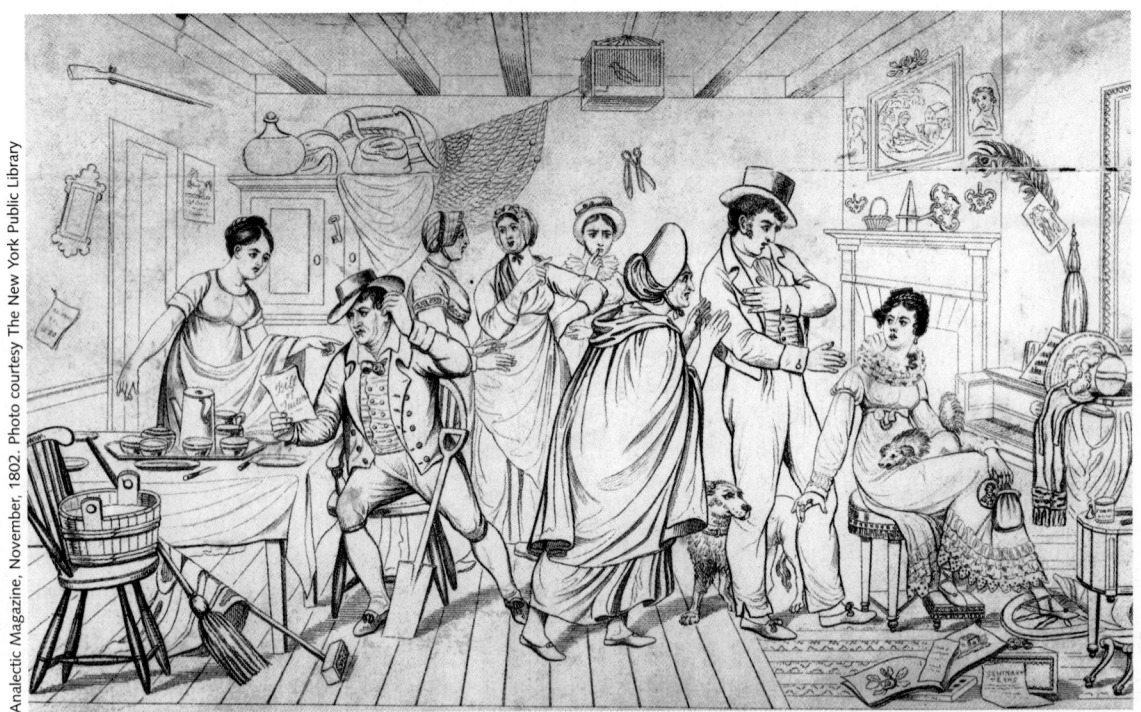

Analectic Magazine, November, 1802. Photo courtesy The New York Public Library

■ With the Revolution came a heightened awareness of the significance of women's education. Private academies offered instruction to elite young women. This engraving, titled *Return from a Boarding School*, appeared in the November 1802 issue of *Analectic Magazine*. The fashionably dressed student, on the right, sits at the piano and greets visitors while her father, on the left with her mother, agonizes over the tuition bill. The shovel, washtub, and broom indicate that the parents are hard-working, simple people. Yet the parlor, with its birdcage, furniture, and carpets, suggests that the household values both prosperity and sociability.

stonecraft's argument in favor of equal education for young men and women, Izard expressed disgust with notions of female equality. "It is not by being educated with Boys, or imitating the manners of Men that we shall become more worthy beings," she proclaimed. Women need not attain public glory, she wrote, to gain "domestic honor and true praise."

Alice Izard was not alone in her beliefs. After the Revolution, many American women, even those of modest means, eagerly read advice manuals written by both native and foreign-born authors. These manuals stressed the importance of good manners over formal education. And even graduates of the new female academies often renounced aspirations to public life once they married and assumed household responsibilities. Wrote Eliza Southgate Bowne, a defender of women's education, "I believe I must give up all pretension to *profundity*, for I am much more at home in my female character."

Other women were more sympathetic to Wollstonecraft's arguments regarding women's equality with men. As the author of a series of essays on women's rights such as "On the Equality of the Sexes," published in *Massachusetts Magazine* in 1790, Judith Sargent Murray was the intellectual heir of Abigail Adams. With a notable lack of success, Adams had urged her husband, John, to secure married women's property rights in the Constitution. By arguing for the inherent equality of men and women, Murray echoed Wollstonecraft and laid the groundwork for the women's rights movement to come. The white women of means who came of age after the Revolution keenly felt the ties that bound them together, even as those ties limited their participation in the public sphere, especially after the wartime emergency had passed.

A Loss of Political Influence: The Fate of Nonelite Women

The Revolution gave elite white women a rationale for speaking out in the realm of politics. Yet the war had a very different impact on other groups of women. For example, among the Cherokees, the introduction of a European American division of labor lessened women's customary political influence as leaders and diplomats. European Americans believed that only men should serve in positions of authority, and so Cherokee women felt pressured to refrain from taking part in political negotiations and to subordinate themselves to men. In 1787 one Cherokee leader (called a War Woman, or Beloved Woman) wrote to Benjamin Franklin. She was confident in her own ability to participate in postwar Indian–white negotiations. Out of respect for Franklin, and in the diplomatic tradition of her people, she enclosed in the letter some of the same tobacco used in the peace pipes of Cherokee warriors. She lectured Franklin, "I am in hopes that if you Rightly consider that woman is the mother of All—and the woman does not pull Children out of Trees or Stumps nor out of old Logs, but out of their [women's] Bodies, so that they [men] ought to mind what a woman says."

By the end of the century, only men had the power to negotiate treaties and land transactions. Still, some women managed to resist this new arrangement. Nancy Ward, the "Beloved Woman of Chota," participated in a treaty conference in Hopewell, South Carolina, in 1785. Speaking as the "mother of Cherokee warriors," she became a powerful person in her own right, not just because of her ties to male leaders. In the early nineteenth century she mobilized other Cherokee women, and together they spoke out forcefully against the practice of selling Cherokee lands to whites.

In the West, Indian women registered the brunt of ongoing conflicts between their own people and European American settlers. In New Mexico, female Indian captives from Plains tribes (such as the Apache, Comanche, and Kiowa) became *indios servientes* in Hispanic households. In some cases their masters set them to work tending sheep, an occupation that had been reserved for men in traditional native cultures. In the East, Native American women dispossessed of their land pieced together a meager existence. For example, in Natick, Massachusetts, women turned to weaving and peddling baskets and brooms, while their men scrounged for wage labor. Many Indian women, such as Hannah Freeman, a Lenape woman in rural Pennsylvania, depended on white farmers for seasonal work. Born in southeastern Pennsylvania 1731, Freeman spent her lifetime moving or being moved from Pennsylvania to New Jersey to Delaware and back again as her family sought refuge from whites and struggled to make a living. By the 1790s, she was an itinerant laborer; her biographer noted that "she has been moving from place to place making baskets &c and staying longest where best used but never was hired or recd wages except for baskets." In 1800 she entered the Chester County Poorhouse, where she died two years later.

> *Commercial development, combined with race and gender discrimination, offered only modest possibilities for many impoverished women and women of color.*

For some Americans, the postwar years brought unprecedented opportunities to buy, sell, and trade. However, commercial development, combined with race and gender discrimination, offered only modest possibilities for many impoverished women and women of color. Like other free blacks, Chloe Spear of Boston "worked early and late" at a number of jobs, such as laundering and ironing clothes. Eventually, she managed to purchase her own home. In Rhode Island, Elleanor Eldrige started her work career at age ten in 1795. Thereafter, she worked as a domestic servant, spinner, weaver, dairymaid, and nurse. She finally went into business, first as a soapboiler and then as a wallpaperer and house painter. However, like many free blacks, Eldrige remained vulnerable to the machinations of white men who tried to defraud her of her hard-won earnings.

Some white women also felt the effects of fluctuations in the market economy. In Philadelphia in the mid-1790s, two former servants—Polly Nugent (married to a blacksmith who had just lost his job) and Grace Biddle (newly widowed)—had to plead for assistance from their former mistress, Elizabeth Drinker. The city's "Bettering House" for indigent people housed men and women, blacks and whites. Many women had neither the resources nor the opportunities to improve their lot after the Revolution.

The Election of 1800: Revolution or Reversal?

The campaign of 1800 pitted Thomas Jefferson and his vice-presidential running mate, Aaron Burr, against the incumbent, John Adams, and his vice-presidential nominee, Charles Pinckney. Certain elements of the campaign were predictable. The Democratic-Republicans blasted Alexander Hamilton's economic policies and the Adams administration's military buildup. Jefferson's party also condemned the Alien and Sedition Acts' effect of silencing Adams's political opponents. For their part, the Federalists portrayed Jefferson as a godless supporter of the French Revolution. They also charged that he had fathered children by one of his slaves, Sally Hemings. (Two centuries later, DNA evidence suggested that this charge might be true.)

Jefferson prevailed in the 1800 election, but his victory did not come easily. The electoral college allowed delegates to vote separately for president and vice president, and as a result Jefferson tied with Burr. Each man received 73 votes. Then the decision went to the House of Representatives, which was dominated by Federalists. After a series of tied votes, Jefferson finally gained a majority. His selection in February 1801 marked the orderly transfer of power from the Federalists to the Democratic-Republicans, a peaceful revolution in American politics.

As chief executive, Jefferson did little to change the direction of the country. Aware of his razor-thin victory, he retained many Federalist appointees. And his eagerness to expand the boundaries of the United States—which culminated in the Louisiana Purchase of 1803—solidified the Hamiltonian principles that favored commerce and trade over agrarian values.

TABLE 9-2

The Election of 1800

Candidate	Political Party	Electoral Vote
Thomas Jefferson	Democrat-Republican	73
Aaron Burr	Democrat-Republican	73
John Adams	Federalist	65
Charles C. Pinckney	Federalist	64

The Enigmatic Thomas Jefferson

Who was Thomas Jefferson? In 1800 Jefferson, the presidential candidate, wrote, "I have sworn upon the altar of God eternal hostility against every form of tyranny over the mind of man." Yet Jefferson's own views on ordinary people were less heroic. Specifically, his support for slavery and the assimilation of Indians provided justification for whites' violent assault on both groups in the early nineteenth century.

Many Americans know Jefferson as the author of the Declaration of Independence. But he also sought to justify slavery as a central institution in the new republic. In his *Notes on the State of Virginia* (1785), Jefferson searched for a rationale to exclude nonwhite men from the new body politic. His stereotypical views of all blacks (for example, he believed they lacked imagination and intelligence) suggested what we today would call scientific racism.

Jefferson wrote much about the noble calling of the yeoman farmer. Yet he assigned the task of tilling the soil on his own estate (Monticello, near Charlottesville, Virginia) to his enslaved workers. When he did acknowledge the abolitionist sentiment, he warned of a possible race war between aggrieved blacks and their white masters. Such a war, he said, would "produce convulsions, [and] probably never end but in the extermination of one or the other race."

The president's views on Indians also did nothing to reverse the course of aggression in the West. He believed that land ownership created the stable institutions necessary for civilized behavior. He told the Delawares,

> When once you have property, you will want laws and magistrates to protect your property and persons, and to punish those among you who commit crimes. You will find that our laws are good for this purpose. You will wish to live under them; you will unite yourselves with us, join in our great councils, and form one people with us, and we shall all be Americans. You will mix with us by marriage. Your blood will run in our veins and will spread with us over this great island.

Yet the system of private property, and the violent methods that whites used to enforce it, spelled the destruction of traditional Indian ways of life. Jefferson's views on assimilation sounded idealistic. But in practical terms, they paved the way for seizures of Indian lands and the forced migrations that removed the Five Civilized Tribes from their homelands in the nineteenth century. Though committed to a political union of disparate states, Jefferson despised what he considered to be racial differences between groups of people.

It is tempting to excuse Jefferson's racist beliefs by saying he merely reflected his time. But in fact, a significant number of Jefferson's contemporaries were voicing their misgivings about slavery. While Jefferson acknowledged their arguments, he did not share their beliefs. A citizen of a trans-Atlantic "republic of ideas," he corresponded with political thinkers—from John Adams to the Marquis de Lafayette—who understood the inherent tension between freedom for whites and slavery for blacks. Obviously, Jefferson knew that some of the northern states (Massachusetts and Vermont among them) had written constitutions that incorporated the sentiments of the Declaration of Independence. These states had interpreted the document in ways that justified the abolition of slavery. Moreover, a notable number of Jefferson's wealthy Virginia compatriots (including George Washington) had chosen to free their slaves, either by their own hand or through provisions of their wills, to practice in their own households what they preached to British tyrants.

Jefferson lived in an age when revolutionary enthusiasm was sweeping the western world. Challenges to slavery had rocked Europe; France outlawed the practice in 1794, although Napoleon later reinstated it. Abolition had also transformed the Western Hemisphere with the successful rebellion of the Saint-Domingue slaves in 1791. The United States provided the political theory and rhetoric to inspire abolitionists around the globe, but within the new nation, the debate over the institution of slavery continued to rage. The southern states, in particular, took decisive steps to solidify the institution within their own boundaries.

Protecting and Expanding the National Interest: Jefferson's Administration to 1803

As president, Jefferson reconsidered his original vision of the United States: a compact country in which citizens freely pursued modest agrarian interests without interference from the national government or distractions from overseas conflicts. Indeed, during his years in office, the federal government moved toward increasing its own power.

In early 1801, just before Jefferson assumed the presidency, the Federalist-dominated Congress had strengthened the national court system by passing the Judiciary Act of 1801. The act created 16 circuit (regional) courts, with a judge for each, and bolstered support staff for the judicial branch in general. President Adams appointed these judges (so-called midnight judges because they were appointed right before Jefferson took office). Before stepping down,

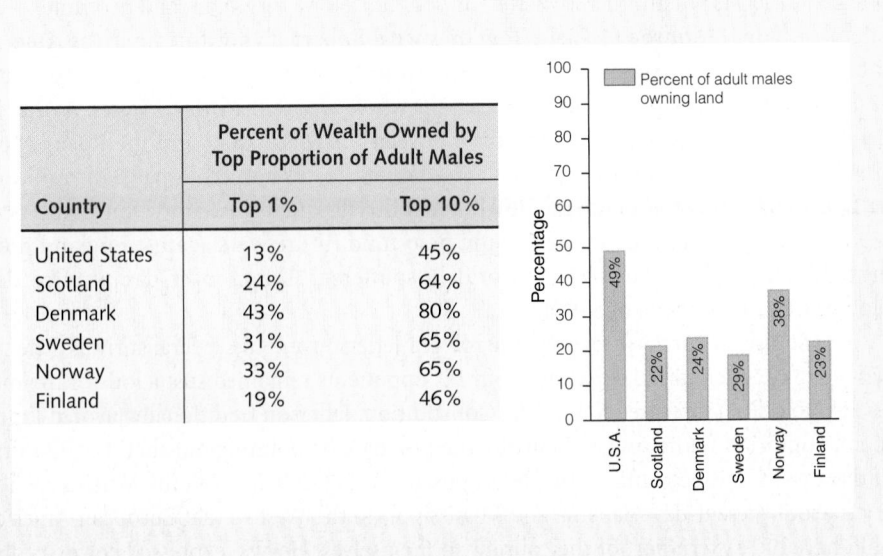

Country	Percent of Wealth Owned by Top Proportion of Adult Males	
	Top 1%	Top 10%
United States	13%	45%
Scotland	24%	64%
Denmark	43%	80%
Sweden	31%	65%
Norway	33%	65%
Finland	19%	46%

■ **FIGURE 9.4**
DISTRIBUTION OF WEALTH IN THE UNITED STATES AND EUROPE, 1798

Source: Lee Soltow, *Distribution of Wealth and Income in the United States in 1798* (1989), p. 238.

Adams had also appointed Secretary of State John Marshall as chief justice of the Supreme Court. Adams's last-minute acts had long-term consequences.

Marshall remained on the bench for 34 years. He presided over the court when it rendered its landmark *Marbury v. Madison* decision in 1803, which established the judiciary's right to declare acts of both the executive and legislative branches unconstitutional. When Jefferson assumed the presidency, the actual document listing Adams's choices for "midnight judges" had not yet been finalized. Jefferson ordered the new secretary of state, James Madison, to withhold the appointments. One of the nominated judges, William Marbury, petitioned the Supreme Court to force Madison to approve Adams's appointments to the bench. The Court refused to do so, arguing that the basis of Marbury's suit, Section 13 of the Judiciary Act of 1789, was unconstitutional. With this decision, the Court thereby established the principle of judicial review—the notion that the justices could invalidate any state or congressional statute they deemed unconstitutional. Chief Justice Marshall declared, "It is emphatically the province and duty of the judicial department to say what the law is."

In the realm of international affairs, Jefferson asserted his own authority. Challenges from foreign powers prompted the Democratic-Republican president to take bold steps to protect U.S. economic and political interests abroad and along its own borders. In 1801 Jefferson's administration launched a war against pirates in North Africa when Tripoli (modern-day Libya) demanded ransom money for kidnapped American sailors. (Together, the North African kingdoms of Tunis, Tripoli, Algeria, and Morocco were known as the "Barbary States." The war against Tripoli, which spanned four years, revealed the extent of U.S. trade interests even at this early point in the nation's history. The United States signed a peace treaty with Tripoli in 1805 and paid $60,000 for the release of the American captives. The plight of these captives, many of whom had been enslaved, transfixed whites at home. For the first time, whites contemplated a form of slavery that confounded traditional notions of skin color and legal status.

At the beginning of the nineteenth century, the European powers continued their operations in the territory west of the United States. In 1801 Napoleon persuaded the King of Spain to secretly cede the trans-Mississippi region called Louisiana to France. Retaining control of New Orleans, Spain denied Americans the right to use that city as a depository for goods awaiting shipment. In 1803 Jefferson sent his fellow Virginian, and prominent Anti-Federalist, James Monroe to Paris. Together with Robert Livingston (there as American ambassador), Monroe set out to secure American trading rights to New Orleans. To the president's surprise, Napoleon agreed to sell the whole area to the United States. At the time, Louisiana included most of the territory between the Mississippi and the Rocky Mountains—a total of 828,000 square miles. The United States agreed to pay $15 million for the Louisiana Purchase. Frustrated by his inability to quell the Saint-Domingue revolt, Napoleon believed that the money would help fund future wars against England. Referring to his failed ventures in the New World, he sputtered, "Damn sugar, damn coffee, damn colonies. . . . I renounce Louisiana."

The Louisiana Purchase reversed the roles of Jefferson and his Federalist rivals. The president advocated territorial expansion, but his opponents remained suspicious of the move. Devoted to a strict interpretation of the Constitution, Jefferson traditionally favored limiting federal authority. Yet he sought to justify the purchase by pointing out that it would finally rid the area of European influence. He proposed shifting Indians from the Mississippi Territory (part of present-day Alabama and Mississippi) to the West so that European Americans could have the eastern part of the country to themselves. He also expressed curiosity about the geography and natural resources of the new acquisition. For their part, the Federalists feared

■ **MAP 9.3**
THE BARBARY STATES   The Barbary states included the small kingdoms of Morocco, Algeria, Tunis, and Tripoli in northern Africa. Before the Revolution, Great Britain paid the states protection money each year; in return, Barbary pirates agreed not to loot British ships or capture their sailors for ransom. This arrangement covered the ships of the American colonies as well. After the Revolution, the Barbary states dealt directly with the United States. Tripoli insisted that the United States pay more money. President Jefferson refused. The ensuing U.S.–Tripoli war ended in 1805; the treaty signed that year freed the U.S. of protection payments.

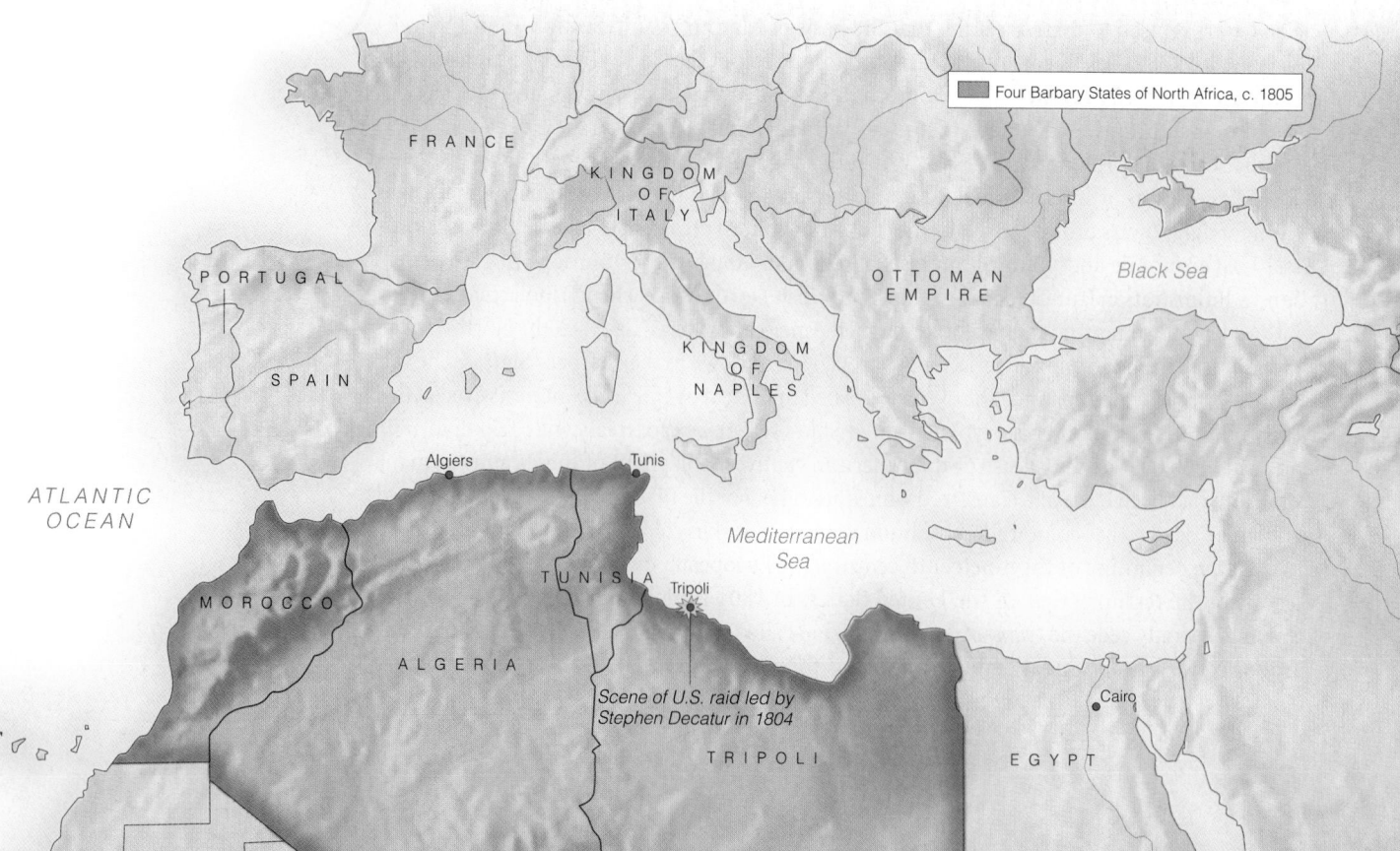

that Louisiana would benefit mainly agrarian interests and eventually dilute New England's long-standing political influence and power. They suspected Jefferson of attempting to expand the influence of his own political party.

Neither the Democratic-Republicans nor the Federalists expressed much concern about the fate of the many Indian and Spanish-speaking inhabitants of Louisiana. All these peoples became residents, if not citizens, of the United States when the Senate approved the purchase in October 1803.

Conclusion

In his first inaugural address, Jefferson spoke about partisan politics. He cautioned, "Every difference of opinion is not a difference of principle." Indeed, Jefferson felt that partisan conflicts obscured a broad, common ground uniting all leaders of the new republic: "We have called by different names brethren of the same principle. We are all Republicans, we are all Federalists." Jefferson was suggesting that all political leaders shared essentially the same views about the role of government and the importance of economic opportunity for ordinary people. Most office holders, regardless of party affiliation, remained committed to the "pursuit of happiness," which they defined as the right to own private property. These leaders also expressed suspicion of groups that professed religious beliefs that lay outside the mainstream of Protestantism or liberal Deism (a general belief in God without ties to a particular religious denomination). They considered slavery not a moral issue, but a political issue that individual states must address. They united behind the idea that women, as well as black and Indian men, should have no formal voice in governing the nation.

Despite these common principles shared by many political leaders in the post-Revolutionary period, this era saw the rise of two opposing camps—those favoring local control and those supporting federal authority. Many people defined political interests in "either-or" terms: either the French system of political equality *or* the British monarchy; either the individual states *or* the federal government; either the farm *or* the factory. Such thinking promoted a narrow view of the United States, a society of great economic and ethnic diversity. For example, certainly the country was large and prosperous enough to accommodate the views of people who believed that both manufacturing and farming were crucial for national growth and development, or who believed that the states and the federal government could share power in a way that enhanced the rights and well-being of all citizens. Yet the machinery of government ran most efficiently on a two-party system. A candidate's political victory depended on his winning more votes than his opponent, and the electoral system provided no avenues for different groups to share power. This system made it extremely difficult for people who had no place in it to find their own political voice and claim the Revolutionary legacy as their own.

At the same time, the new nation gave white men opportunities practically unknown in the rest of the world. Regardless of their background, many white men could aspire to own property and to participate in the political process. The federal government supported economic growth by facilitating territorial expansion, technological innovation, and the protection of private property. As much for the prosperity it promoted as for the noble ideas it nourished, the Revolution continued to inspire liberation movements within the United States and throughout the world.

Sites to Visit

Thomas Jefferson
www.pbs.org/jefferson/

This site is the companion to the Public Broadcasting System series on Jefferson. The site includes material on how people understand Jefferson today.

Archiving Early America
earlyamerica.com

Old newspapers provide a window into issues of the past. This site includes the Keigwin and Matthews collection of early newspapers.

Alexander Hamilton
odur.let.rug.nl/~usa/B/hamilton/hamilxx.htm

This site, from a Hypertext of American History, examines Hamilton's life and influence in the United States during the early national period.

The XYZ Affair
gi.grolier.com/presidents/aae/side/xyzaffr.html

This site examines the XYZ affair.

The Whiskey Rebellion
www.whiskeyrebellion.org

This site devoted to the 1794 Whiskey Rebellion includes a narrative of events and a timeline.

Native Languages of the Americas
www.geocities.com/bigorrin/miam.htm

This site provides information on the language of the Miami and Illinois Indians, a dialect of the same Algonquian language spoken in Indiana and later in Oklahoma.

The Avalon Project at the Yale Law School
www.yale.edu/lawweb/avalon/quasi.htm

This site explores the Quasi War between the United States and France.

The Marshall Cases
odur.let.rug.nl~usa/D/1801-1825/marshallcases/marxx.htm

John Marshall, and the cases he heard, shaped the form and function of the judicial system in the United States.

National Museum of the American Indian
www.si.edu/nmai

The Smithsonian Institution maintains this site, which provides information about the museum that is dedicated to the history and culture of Native Americans.

For Further Reading

General Works

Joyce Appleby, *Inheriting the Revolution: The First Generation of Americans* (2000).

Joseph J. Ellis, *Founding Brothers: The Revolutionary Generation* (2000).

Lester D. Langley, *The Americas in the Age of Revolution: 1750–1850* (1996).

Philip Morgan, *Slave Counterpoint: Black Culture in the Eighteenth-Century Chesapeake and Lowcountry* (1998).

Richard White, *The Middle Ground: Indians, Empires, and Republics in the Great Lakes Region, 1650–1815* (1991).

Competing Political Visions in the New Nation

Joyce Appleby, *Capitalism and the New Social Order: The Republican Vision of the 1790s* (1984).

Terry Bouton, "A Road Closed: Rural Insurgency in Post-Independence Pennsylvania," *Journal of American History* 87 (Dec. 2000):855–887.

Albert Bowman, *The Struggle for Neutrality: Franco-American Diplomacy During the Federalist Era* (1974).

John Hoadley, *Origins of American Political Parties, 1789–1803* (1986).

James Roger Sharp, *American Politics in the Early Republic: The New Nation in Crisis* (1995).

James Morton Smith, *Freedom's Fetters: The Alien and Sedition Laws and American Civil Liberties* (1956).

People of Color: New Freedoms, New Struggles

Ira Berlin, *Slaves Without Masters: The Free Negro in the Antebellum South* (1981).

Graham R. Hodges, *Root and Branch: African-Americans in New York and East Jersey, 1613–1863* (1999).

James O. Horton and Lois Horton, *In Hope of Liberty: Culture, Community, and Protest Among Northern Free Blacks, 1700–1860* (1997).

Leon Litwack, *North of Slavery: The Negro in the Free States, 1790–1860* (1961).

Shane White and Graham White, *Stylin': African-American Expressive Culture from Its Beginnings to the Zoot Suit* (1998).

Continuity and Change in the West

Henry W. Bowden, *American Indians and Christian Missions: Studies in Cultural Change* (1981).

Gregory Evans Dowd, *A Spirited Resistance: The North American Indian Struggle for Unity, 1745–1815* (1992).

R. David Edmunds, *Tecumseh and the Quest for Indian Leadership* (1984).

Robert V. Hine and John Mack Faragher, *The American West: A New Interpretive History* (2000).

Reginald Horsman, *Expansion and American Indian Policy, 1783–1812* (1992).

Dorothy V. Jones, *License for Empire: Colonialism by Treaty in Early America* (1982).

James P. Ronda, *Lewis and Clark Among the Indians* (1984).

Shifting Social Identities in the Post-Revolutionary Era

Nathan O. Hatch, *The Democratization of American Christianity* (1989).

Jacqueline Jones, *American Work: Four Centuries of Black and White Labor* (1998).

Linda Kerber, *Women of the Republic: Intellect and Ideology in Revolutionary America* (1980).

William G. McLaughlin, *Cherokee Renascence in the New Republic* (1986).

Billy G. Smith, *The "Lower Sort": Philadelphia's Laboring People, 1750–1800* (1990).

The Election of 1800: Revolution or Reversal?

Doron Ben-Atar and Barbara B. Oberg, eds., *Federalists Reconsidered* (1998).

David B. Davis, *The Problem of Slavery in the Age of Revolution, 1770–1823* (1975).

Joseph J. Ellis, *American Sphinx: The Character of Thomas Jefferson* (1996).

Peter S. Onuf, *Jefferson's Empire: The Language of American Nationhood* (2000).

Anthony F. C. Wallace, *Jefferson and the Indians: The Tragic Fate of the First Americans* (1999).

Online Practice Test

Test your understanding of this chapter with interactive review quizzes at

www.ablongman.com/jonescreatedequal/chapter9

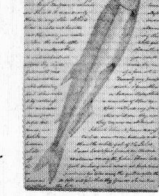

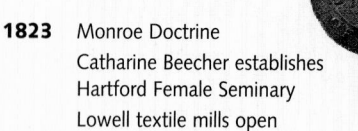

PART FOUR

Expanding the Boundaries of Freedom and Slavery, 1803–1848

IN THE FIRST HALF OF THE NINETEENTH CENTURY, FEW IF ANY NATIONS ON earth could rival the United States' remarkable record of growth. At its founding, the country consisted of 4 million people living in 13 states that hugged the eastern seaboard of North America. By the mid-nineteenth century, the nation's population had grown to 22.5 million people as a result of reproduction, foreign immigration, and the conquest of indigenous and Spanish-speaking peoples. Because of a mix of diplomatic pressure and military aggression, dramatic geographic expansion accompanied the burgeoning population growth. By 1850 the country sprawled the breadth of the continent to the Pacific Ocean.

Territorial expansion, economic growth, and increasing ethnic diversity profoundly shaped American politics in the first half of the nineteenth century. Innovations in transportation (the steamboat), communication (the telegraph), and the production of crops and textiles (reapers and mechanical looms) allowed Americans to move materials, people, and information more quickly and to produce food and goods more efficiently. Meanwhile, the immigration of large numbers of western Europeans, the rapid expansion of the free black population, and the conquest of Spanish-speaking peoples in the Southwest in 1848 challenged the United States' view of itself as an exclusively Anglo-Protestant nation.

Some citizens declared that the United States had a God-given duty and God-given right to expand its borders in opposition to the British and Russians in the Northwest and in opposition to Spain and later Mexico in the South and Southwest. Thus, territorial expansion brought the United States into conflict with other countries and groups that claimed the land. America's victory in the War of 1812 secured the nation's Great Lakes border and at the same time proved that American soldiers and sailors were the equal of England's seasoned fighting forces. In 1823, fearful that European powers would take advantage of independence movements in Latin America, the United States issued the Monroe Doctrine, stating that the era of colonization of the Americas was over.

Nevertheless, Indian tribes continued to resist the incursion of European Americans who believed that land was a commodity to be wrested from native peoples and then bought and sold. In the southern part of the country, the Five Civilized Tribes and other Native American groups occupied territory coveted by both gold seekers and cotton growers. Many American voters demanded that their political leaders work to expand the nation's boundaries through a variety of means: treaty, negotiation, or military force.

Andrew Jackson, who assumed the presidency in 1828, seemed a fitting symbol and a representative politician of the age. Determined to expand the power of the executive branch of government, Jackson claimed to represent the interests of ordinary people in his political battles against the Second Bank of the United States and the Supreme Court and in his forceful removal of Indian tribes from the Southeast to Indian Territory (present-day Oklahoma). Like other politicians of the time, Jackson conceived of citizenship as a system of rights and privileges for white men only.

Still, European Americans trumpeted the arrival of a new era of egalitarianism. Western settlers laid claim to political power, and suffrage restrictions based on property ownership crumbled in the wake of egalitarian legislation and rhetoric. Americans were restless, moving out west and back east again, around the countryside, and in and out of cities. Believing that people could and should work together to reform society, many created reform associations, embraced new religious beliefs, and joined political parties. New forms of association yielded new kinds of communities in an era characterized by great geographic mobility.

At the same time, two distinct power systems coalesced to ensure that certain groups would monopolize the political and economic life of the country. In the South, cotton planters launched an aggressive defense of the institution of slavery. In the North, an emerging class system extended the differences between the political influence and material well-being of factory owners and machine operatives.

For the country, therefore, growth brought great promise and great peril. Abolitionists, associations of working people, nativists (people hostile to immigrants), women's rights advocates, and a variety of other groups proclaimed their agendas for social change. Most significantly, by 1848 it was becoming more difficult for national legislators to resolve the question of whether to allow slavery in the territories. As passions rose, few could imagine a political compromise that would satisfy abolitionists and proslavery advocates alike. As mid-century approached, more and more Americans seemed prepared to express their convictions—or their prejudices and resentment—through violent means.

1826	American Society for the Promotion of Temperance founded
1827	Workingmen's Party founded in Philadelphia
1828	*Cherokee Phoenix* begins publication
1829	Gold discovered on Cherokee lands in Georgia
1831	Nat Turner leads slave rebellion in Virginia William Lloyd Garrison publishes *The Liberator*
1832	Nullification crisis *Worcester v. Georgia* Jackson vetoes Second Bank of the United States Black Hawk War 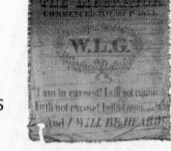
1833	Great Britain abolishes slavery National Road completed
1834	Cyrus McCormick patents reaper First strike at Lowell mills Whig Party organized
1835	Alexis de Tocqueville, *Democracy in America* Texas revolts against Mexico
1836	Congress passes gag rule on antislavery petitions Republic of Texas founded
1837	Panic of 1837 John Deere invents steel plow
1838	Pennsylvania revokes black male suffrage Cherokee removal begins; Trail of Tears
1840	Liberty Party founded
1841	John Tyler assumes presidency after death of William Henry Harrison Supreme Court rules in favor of *Amistad* Africans
1844	Mormon leader Joseph Smith killed by mob in Nauvoo, Illinois
1845	Irish potato famine Frederick Douglass, *Narrative of the Life of Frederick Douglass* Texas becomes twenty-eighth state 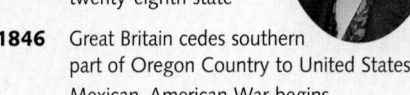
1846	Great Britain cedes southern part of Oregon Country to United States Mexican–American War begins
1847	United States wins battles of Buena Vista, Vera Cruz, Mexico City Capture of San Patricio soldiers, Battle of Churubusco
1848	Treaty of Guadalupe Hidalgo ends Mexican–American War Women's Rights convention in Seneca Falls, New York Popular revolutions sweep Europe

CHAPTER

10

Defending and Expanding the New Nation, 1803–1818

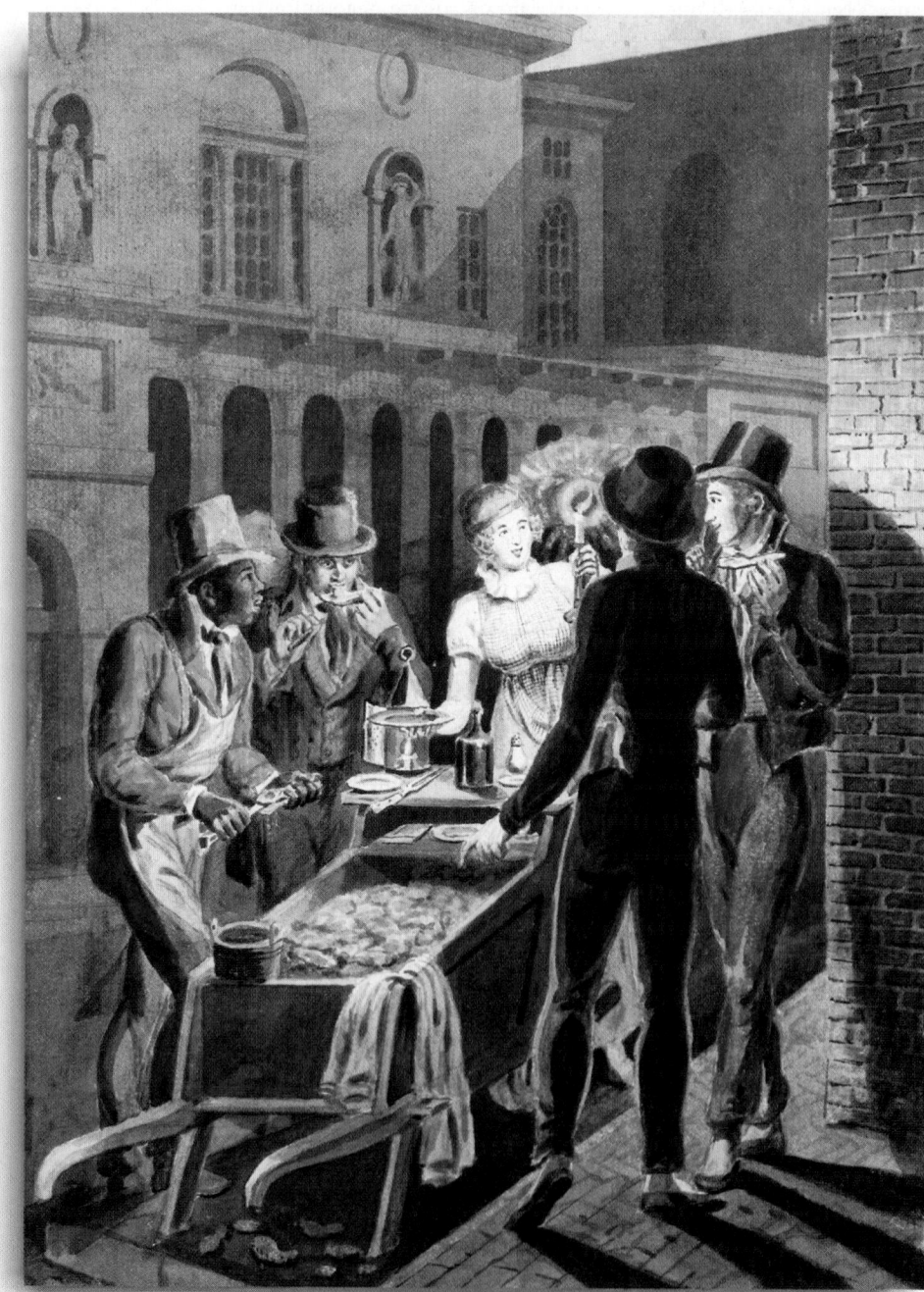

John Lewis Krimmel, *Night Life in Philadelphia—an Oyster Barrow in front of the Chestnut Street Theater*, c.1811–1813. The Metropolitan Museum of Art, Rogers Fund, 1942 (42.95.18). Photograph ©1982 The Metropolitan Museum of Art

■ *Night Life in Philadelphia: An Oyster Barrow in Front of the Chestnut Street Theater, 1811–12.*

IN EARLY NOVEMBER 1804 A GROUP OF SOLDIERS WORKED FEVERISHLY TO CONSTRUCT A rough military garrison on the north bank of the Missouri River, near several Mandan Indian villages and what is today Washburn, North Dakota. The soldiers knew they had to work quickly. Within a month, winter would descend on the Northern Great Plains, and the temperature would plummet. In fact, not long after Fort Mandan was completed, the temperature registered at 45 degrees Fahrenheit below zero.

The garrison provided shelter for an expedition party led by Meriwether Lewis and William Clark. Both captains in the U.S. Army, Lewis and Clark had been commissioned by President Thomas Jefferson to explore the upper reaches of the newly acquired Louisiana Territory, which had doubled the size of the country. With the ultimate goal of reaching what is today Oregon, their party spent the winter at Fort Mandan and joined the buffalo hunts and nightly dances sponsored by their hosts, the Mandan Indians. Between November 1804 and March 1805, Lewis and Clark also found time to record their observations on all manner of things natural and cultural. In their journals and their letters to President Jefferson, they described the language of the Hidatsa Indians and the beadwork of the Arikaras, the medicinal properties of native plants, and the contours of the Missouri River. In a shipment prepared for the president, they included deer horns, pumice stones, the pelt of a white weasel, and an assortment of live animals. (Sadly, only a magpie and a prairie dog survived the journey to Washington, D.C.)

Lewis and Clark's trek took 28 months to complete and covered 8000 miles. Along the way, the two men assured the Indians they met that their expedition's purpose was purely scientific. However, Jefferson had also commissioned them to chart a waterway passage to the Northwest. The president hoped to divert the profitable fur trade away from Canada and into the hands of Americans by locating a river connecting the Northwest directly to eastern U.S. markets. Jefferson also instructed Lewis and Clark to initiate negotiations with various Indian groups, to pave the way for miners and ranchers to move into the area.

Throughout their journey, Lewis and Clark expressed awe of the magnificence of the land—its physical beauty and its commercial potential. While camped at Fort Mandan, Lewis described the Missouri: "This immence river so far as we have yet ascended waters one of the fairest portions of the globe, nor do I believe that there is in the universe a similar extent of country, equally fertile, well watered, and intersected by such a number of navigable streams." When the expedition's official report was published in 1814, it caused a sensation. Americans swelled with pride at the bounteous expanse called the Upper Louisiana.

Lewis and Clark's party consisted of a diverse group of people, including British and Irish enlisted men, and Lewis's African American slave, York. At Fort Mandan, the group picked up Toussaint Charbonneau, a French Canadian, and his 15-year-old wife, Sacajawea,

Captain Meriwether Lewis posed in Indian dress for this watercolor completed in 1807 by French artist C. B. J. Févret de Saint-Mémin.

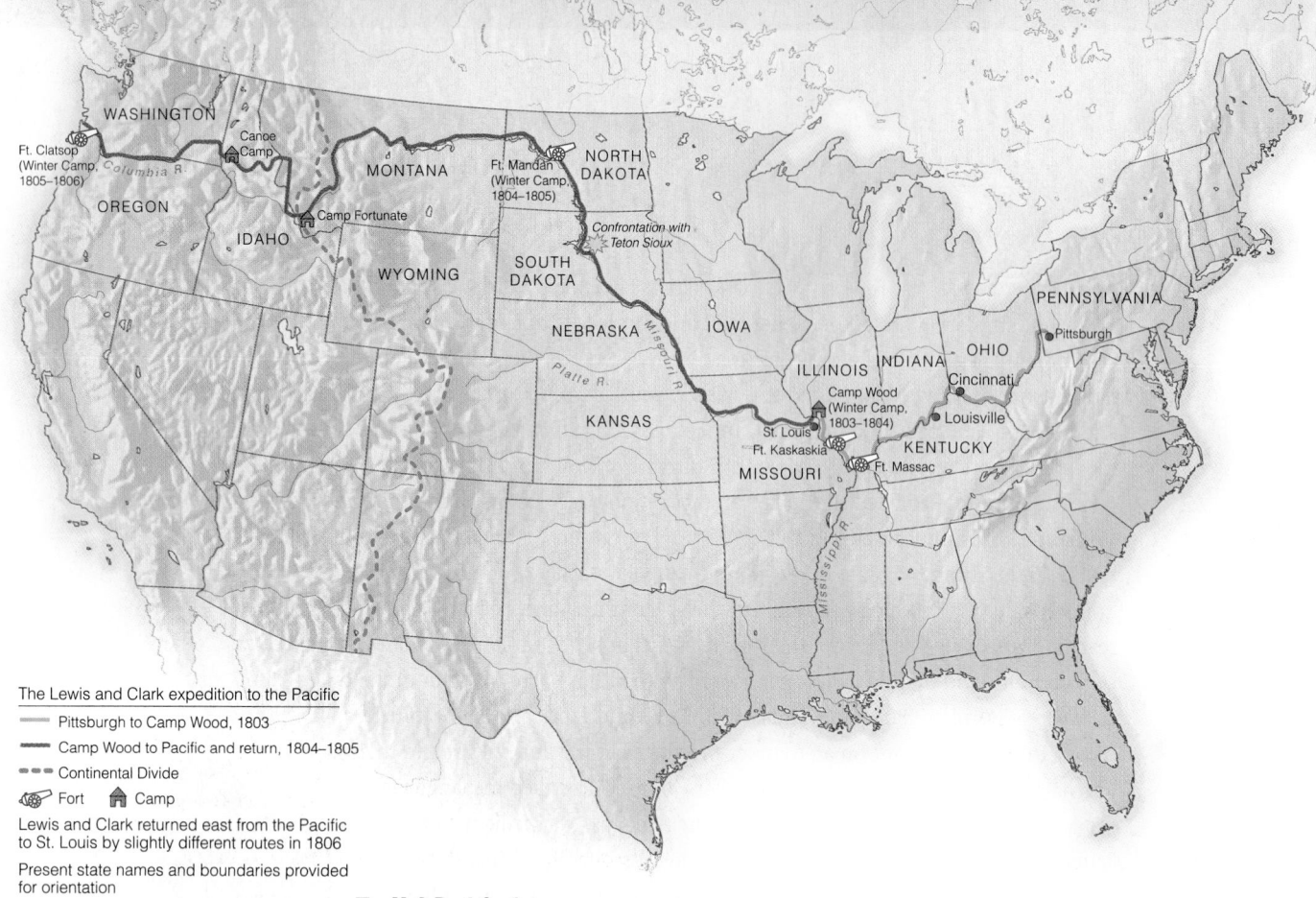

The Lewis and Clark expedition to the Pacific

— Pittsburgh to Camp Wood, 1803

▬▬ Camp Wood to Pacific and return, 1804–1805

■ ■ ■ Continental Divide

🔫 Fort   🏠 Camp

Lewis and Clark returned east from the Pacific to St. Louis by slightly different routes in 1806

Present state names and boundaries provided for orientation

■ **MAP 10.1**

LEWIS AND CLARK This map, showing the route of the Lewis and Clark expedition, suggests the importance of interior waterways in facilitating travel and exploration in the West. Spain feared, rightly, that the Americans would use western rivers to establish trade links with the Indians and thereby challenge Spain's northern border with the United States.

Source: From Stephen Ambrose, *Undaunted Courage.*

a Shoshone Indian. The explorers came to rely on Sacajawea's skills as an interpreter. And because women never traveled with Indian war parties, Sacajawea's presence reassured suspicious Native Americans that the goal of the expedition was peaceful. White men were fond of boasting that "they were great warriors, and a powerful people, who, if exasperated, could crush all the nations of the earth." Indians heard these threats frequently and so were not inclined to look kindly upon an expedition of white men.

Lewis and Clark failed in their mission to locate a commercial route across the Rocky Mountains; the terrain proved too rugged. However, by sponsoring this and other major exploration parties, the federal government signaled its intention to help European Americans settle the West. The expedition also revealed that control of western waterways would be crucial to America's attempt to explore the interior of the continent and to establish trading relations with the Indians. The exploitation of waterways and water power proved a key component in the new nation's economic growth and development. In sum, the Lewis and Clark expedition yielded information that furthered westward migration, commercial development, and scientific knowledge about the western landscape.

During the first two decades of the nineteenth century, the United States faced a number of challenges from within and outside its borders, challenges that had long-lasting political and economic effects. Indians in general were a persistent threat to the new nation. Indeed, in the Great Lakes region, various tribes maintained political and military alliances with Great Britain. Nevertheless, in this period the United States successfully met its most severe test to date: a war with England that raged from 1812 to 1815. The effects of this so-called Second

American Revolution were far-reaching. The conflict eliminated the British from the Northwest once and for all. Its military heroes, including Andrew Jackson and William Henry Harrison, went on to illustrious political careers. The war also spurred industrialization and stimulated commerce. In the South, the cotton plantation system began to shape the political and economic life of the entire region.

Some Europeans who visited the United States during these years criticized Americans for their crudeness and their lack of accomplishment in literature, architecture, road building, and manners. Yet after the War of 1812, American patriotism soared. The country now stretched from New Orleans to the Canadian border—an enormous expanse blessed with rich natural resources. Its military leaders were the equal of, if not superior to, the finest European officers. However, some Americans began to see a threat to their sense of themselves as a unique people. That threat—the expansion of human bondage—would come not from the outside but from within their own borders.

The British Menace

In the election of 1804, Democratic-Republican Thomas Jefferson and his vice-presidential running mate, George Clinton, a former governor of New York, easily bested their Federalist opponents, Charles C. Pinckney and Rufus King. Jefferson had gained widespread favor among the voters through the Louisiana Purchase. And his decision to repeal the federal excise tax on whiskey that had so angered farmers in the West secured his popularity. On the eve of his second term, he no doubt imagined himself examining the specimens and reading the reports that Lewis and Clark sent back from the West. Yet the ongoing squabbling between France and England and the increasing aggression of the British navy toward American sailors demanded his attention.

Developments overseas preoccupied Jefferson during his second term in office. England and France continued to challenge each other as the reigning powers of Europe. In 1805 the British navy, under the command of Lord Nelson, defeated the French and Spanish fleets in the Battle of Trafalgar off the coast of Spain. That same year, France reveled in its own triumph on land when Napoleon conquered the Austrian and Russian armies at the Battle of Austerlitz. Supreme on the seas, England in 1806 passed the Orders in Council, which specified that any country that wanted to ship goods to France must first send them to a British port and pay taxes on them. Many Americans believed that England's policies amounted to acts of military and economic aggression against the United States.

■ Lewis and Clark were not only explorers; they were also pioneering naturalists committed to gathering, recording, and studying plants and animal life in the West. William Clark drew this sketch of a eulachon, also called a candlefish, as part of his journal entry for February 25, 1806. Pacific Indians dried the oily fish and used it as a torch.

William Clark, Eulachon (T. Pacificus), 1806, Voorhis Journal #2. William Clark Papers, Missouri Historical Society Archives

TABLE 10-1		
The Election of 1804		
Candidate	Political Party	Electoral Vote
Thomas Jefferson	Democratic-Republican	162
Charles C. Pinckney	Federalist	14

The Embargo of 1807

Not content to control trade across the Atlantic as decreed by the 1806 Orders in Council, the British also seized sailors from American ships, claiming that these men were British seamen who had been lured away from their own vessels by American captains promising them higher wages. In some cases these claims were probably true. However, U.S. political leaders charged that an estimated 6000 U.S. citizens had been seized by the British navy between 1808 and 1811, including an unknown number of African Americans, many of whom were working as mariners. Seafaring appealed to free men of color because it paid good wages. In the early

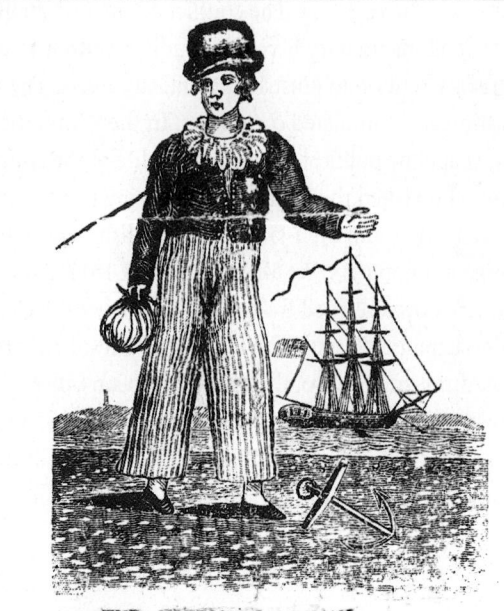

THE MPRESSMENT OF AN

American Sailor Boy,

SUNG ON BOARD THE BRITISH PRISON SHIP CROWN PRINCE, THE FOURTH OF JULY, 1814
BY A NUMBER OF THE AMERICAN PRISONERS.

THE youthful sailor mounts the bark,
  And bids each weeping friend adieu ;
Fair blows the gale, the canvass swells :
  Slow sinks the uplands from his view.

Three mornings, from his ocean bed,
  Resplendent beams the God of day :
The fourth, high looming in the mist,
  A war-ship's floating banners play.

Her yawl is launch'd ; light o'er the deep,
  Too kind, she wafts a ruffian band :
Her blue track lengthens to the bark,
  * ʼʼae soon on deck the miscreants stand.

Around they throw the baleful glance :
  Suspense holds mute the anxious crew—
Who is their prey ? poor sailor boy !
  The baleful glance is fix'd on you.

Nay, why that useless scrip unfold ?
  They damn'd the " lying yankee scrawl,"
Torn from thine hand, it strews the wave—
  They force thee trembling to the yawl.

Sick was thine heart as from the deck,
  The hand of friendship wav'd farewell ;
Mad was thy brain, as far behind,
  In the grey mist thy vessel fell.

One hope, yet, to thy bosom clung,
  The captain mercy might impart ;

Vain was that hope, which bade thee look,
  For mercy in a Pirate's heart.

What woes can man on man inflict,
  When malice joins with uncheck'd power ;
Such woes, unpitied and unknown,
  For many a month the sailor bore !

Oft gem'd his eye the bursting tear,
  As mem'ry linger'd on past joy ;
As oft they flung the cruel jeer,
  And damn'd the " chicken liver'd boy."

When sick at heart, with " hope defer'd,"
  Kind sleep his wasting form embrac'd,
Some ready minion ply'd the lash,
  And the lov'd dream of freedom chas'd.

Fast to an end his miseries drew :
  The deadly hectic flush'd his cheek :
On his pale brow the cold dew hung,
  He sigh'd, and sunk upon the deck !

The sailor's woes drew forth no sigh ;
  No hand would close the sailor's eye :
Remorseless, his pale corse they gave,
  Unshrouded to the friendly wave.

And as he sunk beneath the tide,
  A hellish shout arose ;
Exultingly the demons cried,
  " So fare all Albion's Rebel Foes !"

■ This poem was published in the United States during the War of 1812 to highlight the plight of American sailors pressed into service by British sea captains. The poem tells the story of a young lad ripped from his shipmates and subjected to scorn and abuse by British sailors. After he dies, his corpse is thrown into the ocean. His tormentors exclaim, "So fare all Albion's [England's] Rebel Foes!"

nineteenth century, black mariners' pay equaled that of their white counterparts. And in this line of work, a man's skill, not the color of his skin, determined the nature of his job. With limited economic opportunities on shore, black sailors accepted the danger and long absences from home. However, neither black nor white sailors had bargained for enforced service in His Majesty's Royal Navy.

Seizure, or impressment, reminded Americans of their pre–Revolutionary War days, when British "press gangs" prowled the docks of American port cities and seized colonial merchant sailors. In 1807 the tensions over this practice erupted into violence. Just ten miles off the shore of Virginia, the American ship *Chesapeake* came under attack from a British vessel. British naval officers claimed that the Americans were harboring four British deserters. In the ensuing exchange of cannon fire, 3 Americans were killed and 18 wounded. Jefferson demanded that England leave American sailors and ships alone, but he was rebuffed.

In 1807 President Jefferson decided to place an embargo on all exports to the European powers in an effort to force those nations to respect the rights of Americans on the high seas. The move aroused intense opposition in Federalist-dominated New England, where the regional economy depended heavily on foreign trade. The Embargo Act passed by Congress halted the shipment of goods from the United States to Europe. Because Europe—including England—relied heavily on American grain and timber, Jefferson hoped that the move would force England to respect American independence. The president saw this measure as preferable to either war or capitulation to England, but the New England states, which were particularly hard hit by the embargo, saw the matter quite differently. As the effects of the embargo took hold, the New England grain growers saw the markets for their products dry up, and the shipbuilding industry, which made heavy use of timber, ground to a standstill. Southern tobacco and cotton planters faced similar hardship because of the embargo. By 1808 some of them had joined with Northerners to circumvent the embargo by moving their goods through Canada and then to Europe.

The embargo seemed only to intensify, not lessen, tensions between England and the United States.

Yet Jefferson held his course. He prodded Congress to enforce the unpopular act, but his efforts provoked a backlash. Ordinary citizens compared him to George III, and New England politicians threatened to take their states out of the union. Despite all the uproar, the embargo did benefit Americans in some ways. Specifically, it encouraged New Englanders to rely more on goods produced locally and less on foreign imports. Jefferson had advocated a policy that had an unanticipated effect: it promoted industrialization at home. At the same time, the embargo seemed only to intensify, not lessen, tensions between England and the United States.

On the Brink of War

Both the Federalists and the Democratic-Republicans suffered a blow to their leadership in 1804. That year, the Federalist party lost one of its original leaders with the death of Alexander Hamilton at the hand of his rival, Aaron Burr. Both successful New York attorneys, the two men had risen together through the political ranks in the 1780s and 1790s. Burr served as Jefferson's running mate in the election of 1800; four years later he ran for governor of New York. Incensed by a report that Hamilton had claimed he was "a dangerous man, and one who ought not to be trusted with the reins of government," as well as "still more despicable rumors," Burr challenged his antagonist to a pistol duel in Weehawken, New Jersey, in July 1804. (Many European American men, especially in the South, considered dueling a means to preserve their honor in response to a perceived insult leveled at them or at a family member.) As the combatants faced off, Burr fired at Hamilton. Mortally wounded, Hamilton died the next day. As a result, Burr's political career lay in ruins. In 1807 he stood trial for treason, charged with conspiring to create an empire for himself out of the territory Spain held west of the Mississippi. Acquitted of the charges, he nevertheless fled the United States for Europe.

Jefferson declined to run for a third presidential term in 1808, and he left office in March 1809 upon the inauguration of the new president, James Madison. Soon after Madison took office, Congress repealed the embargo and replaced it with the Non-Intercourse Act, which eased the complete ban on exports to Europe. This measure permitted American exporters to ship their goods to all European countries except for France and England, still at war with one another. New Englanders opposed even this limited embargo.

Meanwhile, the Federalists' influence in Congress was waning. The partisan division within Congress—the Federalists, with their emphasis on a strong national government, against the localist Democratic-Republicans—gradually eased. That division had emerged in response to the ratification of the Constitution and debates over the direction of the new nation. By 1810 a new split had emerged—between young, hotheaded representatives from the West and their more conservative seniors from the eastern seaboard. The western group, or "war hawks," called on the nation to revive its former glory. Americans must uphold U.S. honor, they declared, by opposing European, especially British, claims to military dominance. The war hawks also yearned to vanquish the Indians who impeded settlement of the area west of the Mississippi.

In 1810 Congress passed legislation called Macon's Bill No. 2. Under its provisions, if either France or England agreed to resume trade with the United States, then the Americans would resume trade with that country and refuse to trade with the other. France's emperor Napoleon seized this offer to reestablish economic ties with the United States. Outraged, England began to contemplate war not only with its arch enemy, France, but also with the upstart United States. The new nation had positioned itself directly in the middle of a conflict between the two major European powers.

Looking eastward, the war hawks saw an England determined to defile the honor of their young nation. Looking westward, these same men saw an equally threatening menace: the rise of an ominous Indian resistance movement that blended military strength with native spirituality. The movement was led by Shawnee brothers Tecumseh and Tenskwatawa. Tenskwatawa (also known as the Prophet) claimed that he had a vision in which he received a message from the world's creator. In the Prophet's words, the creator stated that European Americans "grew from the scum of the great water, when it was troubled by an evil spirit and the froth was driven into the woods by a strong east wind." The Prophet declared to other Indians, "They are numerous, but I hate them. They are unjust; they have taken away your lands, which were not made for them."

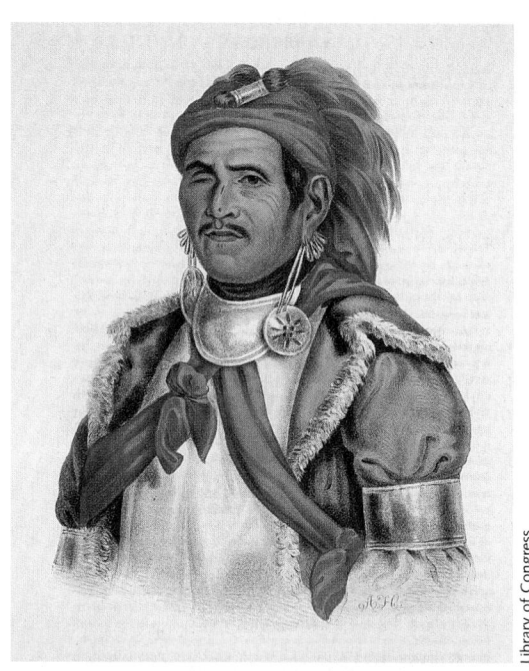

Library of Congress

■ This lithograph of the Prophet (Tenskwatawa) was based on an 1824 painting of the Shawnee mystic and holy man. Early in life, he suffered an accident with bows and arrows, losing his right eye. He and his older brother Tecumseh called on all Indians to resist the encroachment of their lands by whites and to renounce the way of life followed by whites, including the use of liquor. After the Indians' defeat at the Battle of Tippecanoe in 1811, the Prophet retreated to Canada. He returned to the United States in 1826. By that time he no longer wielded influence as a leader of the Shawnees.

In 1808 the two brothers founded Prophet's Town in Indiana. They envisioned a sovereign Indian state and the preservation of Native American culture. Tenskwatawa spoke of a time and place where Indians would reject alcohol and scorn "the food of whites" as well as the "wealth and ornaments" of commercial trade. Tecumseh set out to deliver the message to as many Indian groups as possible, traveling the broad swath of territory from Florida to Canada.

In his journey south, Tecumseh found the Creek nation in Muskogee Territory particularly receptive to his message of Indian solidarity. By that time the Creeks had lost millions of acres of land to the Americans. Tecumseh deputized a relative, Seekaboo, to remain with the Creeks and instruct them in the religion of Tenskwatawa. He could not know that, within a few years, Tenskwatawa's message would spark armed conflict between the Creeks and American troops.

Meanwhile, in 1809, the territorial governor of Indiana, William Henry Harrison, plied a group of Indian leaders with liquor, then got them to agree to sell 3 million acres to the U.S. government for just $7600. Upon hearing of the deal, Tecumseh decried a new form of American aggression: "treaties" between U.S. officials and Indians who lacked the authority to sell their people's homeland. "All red men," Tecumseh proclaimed, "[must] unite in claiming a common and equal right in the land, as it was at first, and should be yet; for it never was divided, but belongs to all, for the use of each."

In November 1811 Harrison led 1000 U.S. soldiers in an advance on Prophet's Town. But before they could reach the settlement, several hundred Shawnees under the command

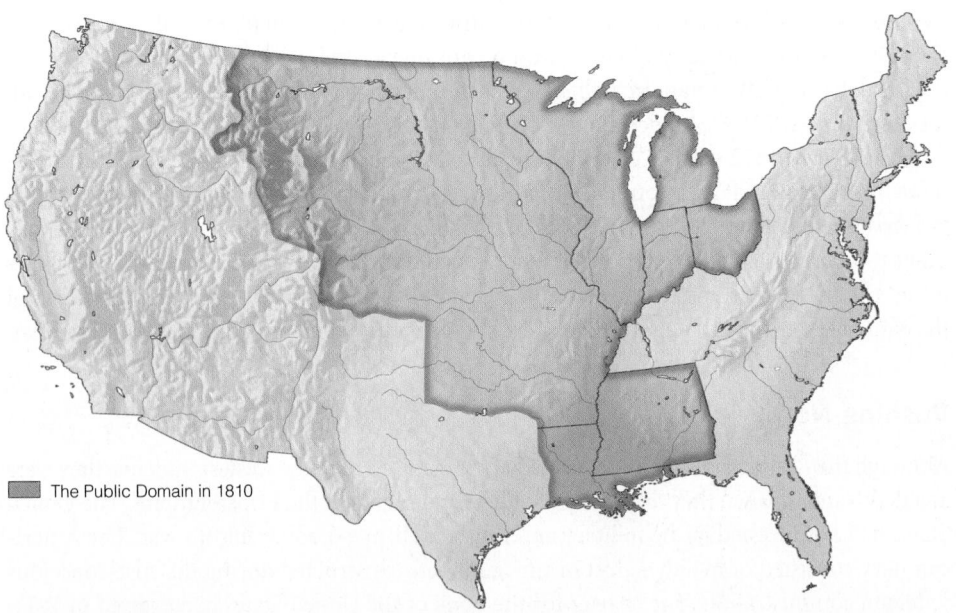

■ MAP 10.2

THE PUBLIC DOMAIN IN 1810   This map indicates the expanse of western lands owned by the U.S. government in 1810, after the Louisiana Purchase. American war veterans received land warrants in return for military service in the Revolutionary War and the War of 1812. A warrant entitled the bearer to settle a specific number of acres of unoccupied lands. Warrants could be transferred, sold, and traded like stocks and bonds. After the War of 1812, the government issued 29,186 land warrants for a total of 4.8 million acres.

Source: After Charles O. Paulin, *Atlas of Historical Geography* (Washington, DC), Plate 57.

of Tenskwatawa attacked their camp on the Tippecanoe River. The Indians suffered a sound defeat, and Harrison burned Prophet's Town to the ground. A Potawatomi chief, Shabonee, who fought at the Battle of Tippecanoe, later recalled the false sense of superiority that had inspired the Indians' doomed attack on Harrison and his men. According to Shabonee, the Indians believed, "the white soldiers are not warriors. Their hands are soft. Their faces are white. One half of them are calico [fabric] peddlers. The other half can only shoot squirrels." Warriors or not, the Americans had a distinct advantage over the Indians: better guns. Clearly, military technology, not just determination, would shape the western conflict.

The War of 1812

The defeat of the Shawnees at Tippecanoe only inflamed western war hawks' passions and stiffened their resolve to break the back of Indian resistance altogether. But to achieve this goal, the United States would have to invade Canada and eliminate the British arms suppliers who had been trading with the Indians. Claiming the mantle of patriotism, western and southern members of the House of Representatives agitated for a war that would eliminate both the British threat on the high seas and the Canada-based Indian–British alliance. These Americans wanted a war that would win for them a true independence once and for all. "On to Canada! On to Canada!" became the rallying cry of the war hawks.

In a secret message sent to Congress on June 1, 1812, President Madison listed Americans' many grievances against England: the British Navy's seizure of American citizens, the blockades of American goods, and continued conflict "on one of our extensive frontiers," the result of "savages" who had the backing of British traders and military officials. Madison left it up to Congress whether the nation would continue to endure these indignities or would act "in defense of their natural rights." Seventeen days later, the House voted 79 to 49 and the Senate voted 19 to 13 to declare war on England and, by extension, the western Indians.

The War of 1812 united Americans behind a banner of national expansion. But, at the same time, it exposed dangerous divisions between regions of the country and between political viewpoints. Many New Englanders saw the conflict as a plot by Virginia Democratic-Republicans primarily to aid France in opposition to England and to add agrarian (that is, slave) states to the Union. In an ironic twist, the New England Federalists—usually staunch defenders of the national government—argued that states should control their own commerce and militias.

Pushing North

Although the Americans were better armed and organized than the western Indians, they were at a disadvantage when they took on the soldiers and sailors of the British Empire. The United States had not invested in the military and thus was ill-prepared for all-out war. The American navy consisted of merely a fleet of tiny gunboats constructed during the cost-conscious Jefferson administration. The charter for the Bank of the United States had expired in 1811, depriving the country of a vital source of financial credit. Suffering from a drop in tax revenues as a result of the embargo on foreign trade, the nation lacked the funds to train and equip the regular army and the state militias. Nevertheless, in the fall of 1812, the Americans launched an ambitious three-pronged attack against Canada, striking from Niagara, Detroit, and Lake Champlain. All three attempts failed miserably.

Lacking united, enthusiastic support on the home front, the Americans' offensive got off to a bad start. Yet some people, even in Federalist New England, believed that all Americans should support the war, regardless of the potential outcome. Writing from a Federalist stronghold in December 1812, Abigail Adams (the wife of former president John Adams) acknowledged to a correspondent that her home state of Massachusetts "had much to complain of" because the war had severely disrupted trade. However, she added, "that cannot justify [Massachusetts] in paralyzing the arm of Government [that is, opposing federal trade policies], when raised for her defense and that of the nation." She warned against "a house divided against itself," which she believed could be the nation's undoing.

In the West, the British moved to take advantage of divisions on American soil. They cemented their long-standing alliance with the Indians, who possessed both military prowess and an abiding hatred of the land-hungry Americans. In late 1812, Tecumseh (who had accepted a commission as a brigadier general in the British army) and British General Isaac Brock captured Detroit. Indians also participated in England's successful raid on Fort Dearborn (Chicago). In at least two cases, when U.S. soldiers marched into Canada, they lost their advantage when state militia members refused to cross the border. Leaders of these militias claimed that their sole purpose was to defend their states from attack, not invade foreign territory.

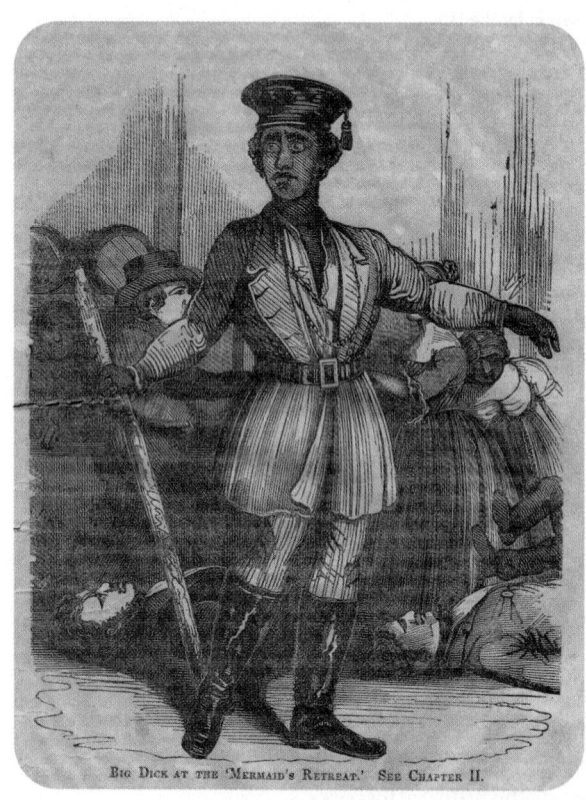

BIG DICK AT THE 'MERMAID'S RETREAT.'   SEE CHAPTER II.

■ In 1815 approximately 6000 American prisoners of war were confined to Britain's dank Dartmoor Prison in Devonshire, England. Many of them were African Americans, who represented one-fifth of all sailors who fought in the war. Among that group was Richard Crafus. An imposing man, Crafus earned the title "King Dick" by serving as the leader of the central barracks at Dartmoor, where blacks were held. He strolled through the cell block, carrying a large club and settling disputes between the prisoners.

Courtesy, Dartmouth University Library

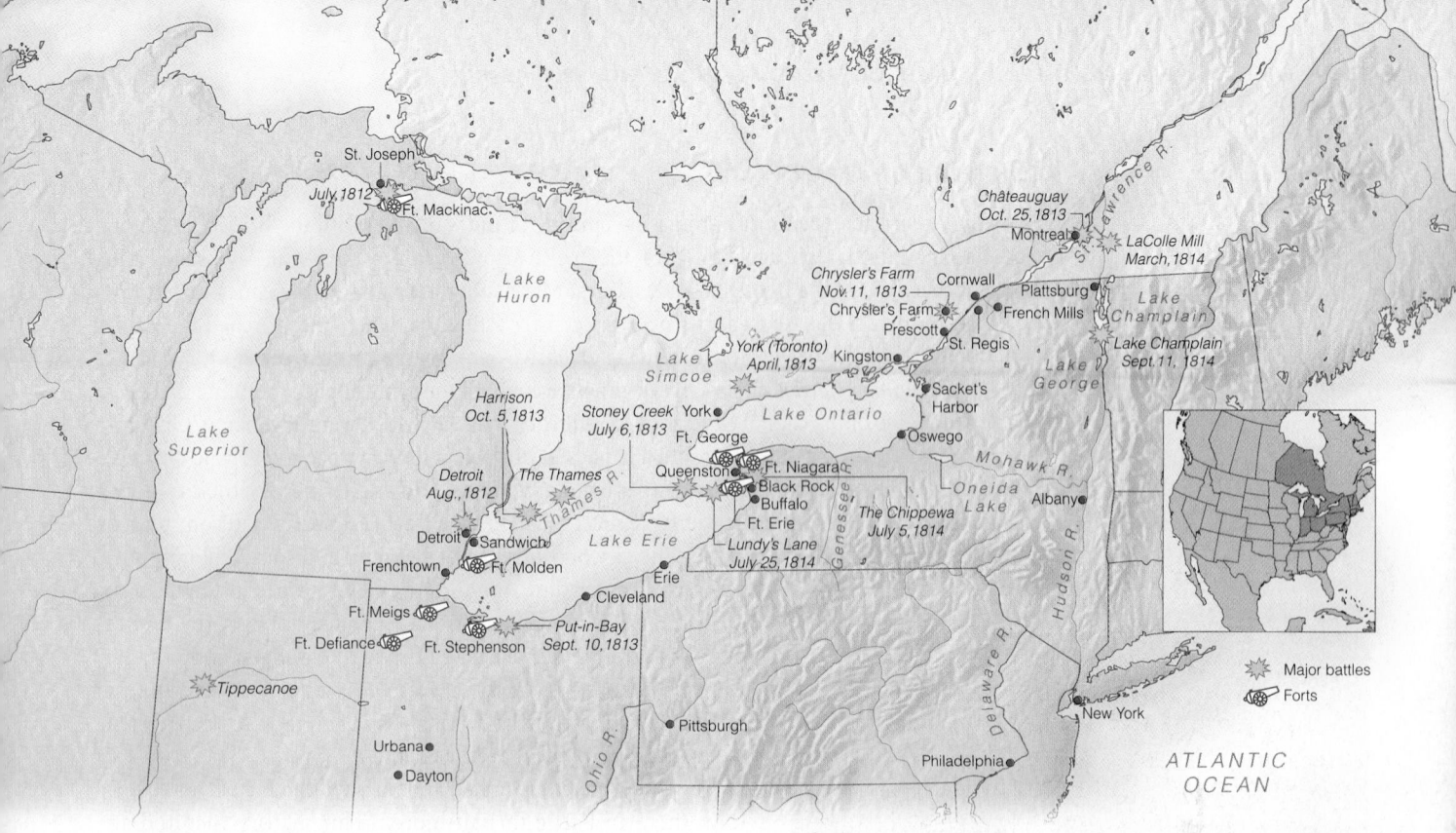

■ **MAP 10.3**

THE NORTHERN FRONT, WAR OF 1812 Much of the fighting of the War of 1812 centered in the Great Lakes region. It was there, the war hawks charged, that the British were inciting Indians to attack American settlements. Conducted in 1812 and 1813, the campaign against Canada was supposed to eliminate the British threat and, some Americans hoped, win Canadian territory for the United States.

Yet the Americans scored some notable successes in 1813. That September, Commodore Oliver H. Perry defeated a British fleet on Lake Erie. Exhilarated, he declared, "We have met the enemy and they are ours." But Perry's victory came at a steep price. Shortly before the engagement, about a third of all the officers and men in the American fleet had fallen victim to a typhus epidemic. Then the battle started. By the end of the day, of the 100 men who had reported for duty that morning, 21 were dead and more than 60 wounded.

Perry's hard-won victory forced the British back into Canada, over Tecumseh's objections. General William Henry Harrison followed in hot pursuit. British Colonel Henry Proctor marched his troops to eastern Ontario, leaving Tecumseh to try holding the Americans at bay. At the Battle of the Thames (that October), Harrison defeated the Indians. Many perished, Tecumseh among them. A group of Kentucky soldiers skinned what they mistakenly believed to be his corpse. His body was never found.

Later that autumn, an American campaign against Montreal failed. The Americans trudged back into New York state, the British close behind them. Flush with their victory in Montreal, the British captured Fort Niagara and set Buffalo and other nearby towns aflame.

By mid–1814, the English had also crushed Napoleon. This success freed up 15,000 British troops, who promptly sailed for North America. Still, in July 1814 the Americans, under the leadership of Major General Jacob Brown and Brigadier General Winfield Scott, managed to defeat the British at the Battle of Chippewa, across the Niagara River from Buffalo. But by the end that year, the Americans had withdrawn to their own territory and relinquished their goal of invading and conquering Canada. The arrival of fresh British troops forced the Americans to defend their own soil.

Fighting on Many Fronts

For the Americans, the most humiliating episode of the war came with the British attack on the nation's capital. On August 24, 1814, the British army, backed by the Royal Navy, sailed into Chesapeake Bay. At the Battle of Bladensburg, Maryland, they scattered the American troops they encountered. The Redcoats then advanced to Washington, where they torched the Capitol building and the White House, causing extensive damage to both structures.

The *Baltimore Patriot* carried an eyewitness account of the confusion surrounding the spectacle. Residents of the capital city had received word that the British were advancing. On Sunday, August 21, public officials frantically packed up their books and papers. Private citizens, also gathered up their furniture and other belongings and left town. By Tuesday, the city stood nearly empty. As a ragtag American force succumbed to the British, President Madison "retired from the mortifying scene, and left the city on horseback." His aides and some military officers accompanied him. As it turned out, he escaped just in the nick of time: by Wednesday flames had engulfed not only the capitol but also Monroe's residence. Disorganized, hungry, and hot, the American troops had put up scant resistance. The eyewitness reported, "Our army may with truth be said to have been beaten by fatigue, before they saw the enemy."

Yet the Americans rallied and pursued the British and overtook them in battle in Baltimore. (This victory inspired an observer, Francis Scott Key, to write "The Star Spangled Banner" as he watched "the bombs bursting in air" over Baltimore's Fort McHenry.) The Americans scored another crucial victory in September, when U.S. naval commander Thomas McDonough crushed the British fleet on Lake Champlain near Plattsburgh, New York.

In the Southeast, Tecumseh's message of Indian unity had resonated with particular force among Native Americans once the war broke out. Some Cherokees and Choctaws cast their lot with the United States. However, a minority of Creeks were emboldened by Tenskwatawa's message, "War now. War forever. War upon the living. War upon the dead; dig up their corpses from the grave; our country must give no rest to a white man's bones." By 1813, a group of warriors called Red Sticks (for their scarlet-painted weapons) stood ready to do battle with the Americans. Yet they faced opposition from some of their own people, the White Sticks, who counseled peace. The Red Sticks finally decided to attack Fort Mims (in what is now Alabama). In response, Andrew Jackson, leader of the Tennessee militia, received a commission as major general. His mission was to retaliate against the Indians.

Jackson had a history as a speculator in Indian lands in Mississippi Territory. Even in a country where anti-Indian sentiment ran high, his views were extreme. He called Native Americans "savage bloodhounds" and "blood thirsty barbarians." After the attack on Fort Mims, he vowed, "I must destroy those deluded victims doomed to distruction by their own restless and savage conduct." He boasted about collecting the scalps of all his Indian victims.

Jackson's 3500 troops laid waste to Creek territory. Regiments of Cherokee, Choctaw, and Chickasaw Indians, as well as White Sticks, helped them. During a monumental battle in March 1814,

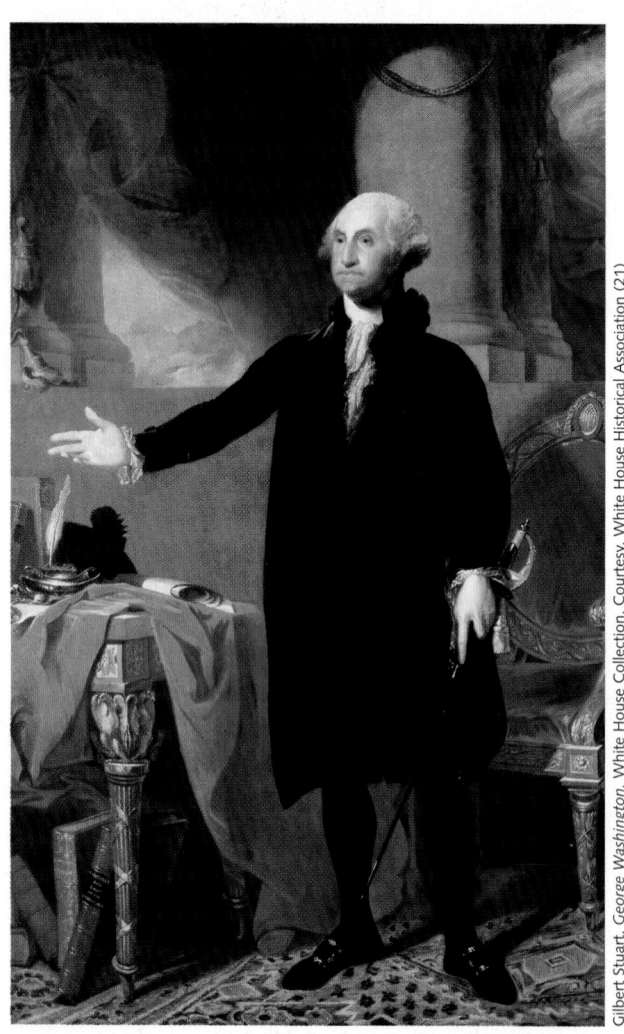

Gilbert Stuart, *George Washington*. White House Collection, Courtesy, White House Historical Association (21)

■ Dolly Madison, wife of the president, helped to rescue this famous painting of George Washington by artist Gilbert Stuart when the British invaded Washington in August 1814. The full-length portrait hung in what was then called the President's House. She later wrote a friend that the British attack had rendered her "so unfeminine as to be free from fear." She had hoped to remain in the mansion "if I could have had a cannon through every window, but alas! Those who should have placed them there, fled."

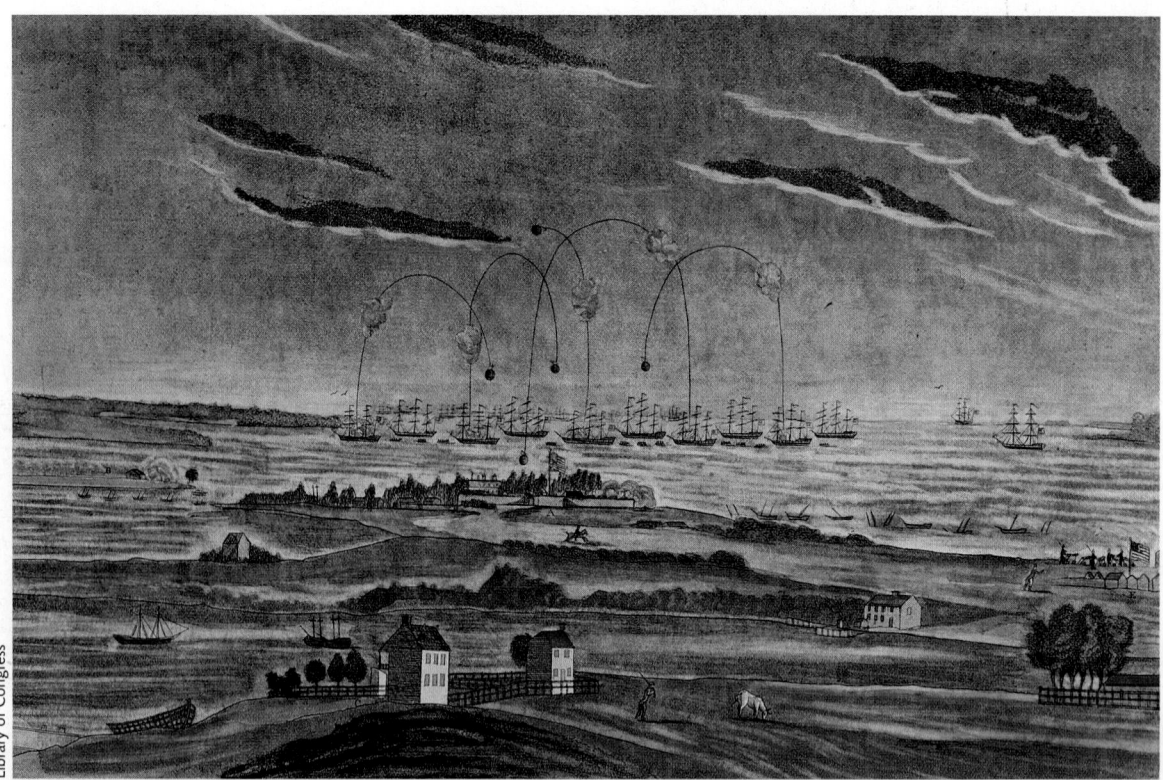

Library of Congress

■ This engraving, published in 1814, depicts the bombardment of Fort McHenry by British warships in September of that year. When he witnessed the battle, Francis Scott Key, a Washington lawyer, was aboard a prisoner exchange boat in Baltimore Harbor. He was seeking release of a friend captured by the British. After penning the poem "The Star Spangled Banner," Key set the words to music, using the tune of a popular English drinking song. Congress declared the song the national anthem in 1931.

more than three-quarters of the 1000 defending Red Sticks and a number of Indian women and children died at Horseshoe Band (in modern-day Alabama). Jackson survived the battle thanks to the intervention of a Cherokee soldier. Some American soldiers took their victory to a brutal extreme; they flayed the corpses of their victims and made horse bridles out of their skin.

Yet Jackson insisted on praising his soldiers as a civilizing force. They were only reclaiming the land from a band of savages, he explained. In a postbattle speech to the men under his command, he declared,

> In their places a new generation [of Indians] will arise who know their duties better. The weapons of warfare will be exchanged for the utensils of husbandry; and the wilderness which now withers in sterility and seems to mourn the desolation which overspreads it, will blossom as the rose, and become the nursery of the arts.

In the Treaty of Horseshoe Bend that followed the massacre, the Americans forced the Creek Nation to give up 23 million acres. The remnants of the Red Sticks fled to the swamps of Florida. There they eventually regrouped in the company of fugitive slaves, as Seminoles (from the Spanish *cimarrones,* or runaway slaves).

Jackson next marched to New Orleans to confront the British. Knowing he would be facing some of Europe's finest soldiers, he assembled 7000 men, U.S. soldiers and militiamen from the states of Louisiana, Kentucky, and Tennessee. Two Kentucky regiments consisted of free Negro volunteers, about 400 men in total. The Battle of New Orleans, fought on January 8,

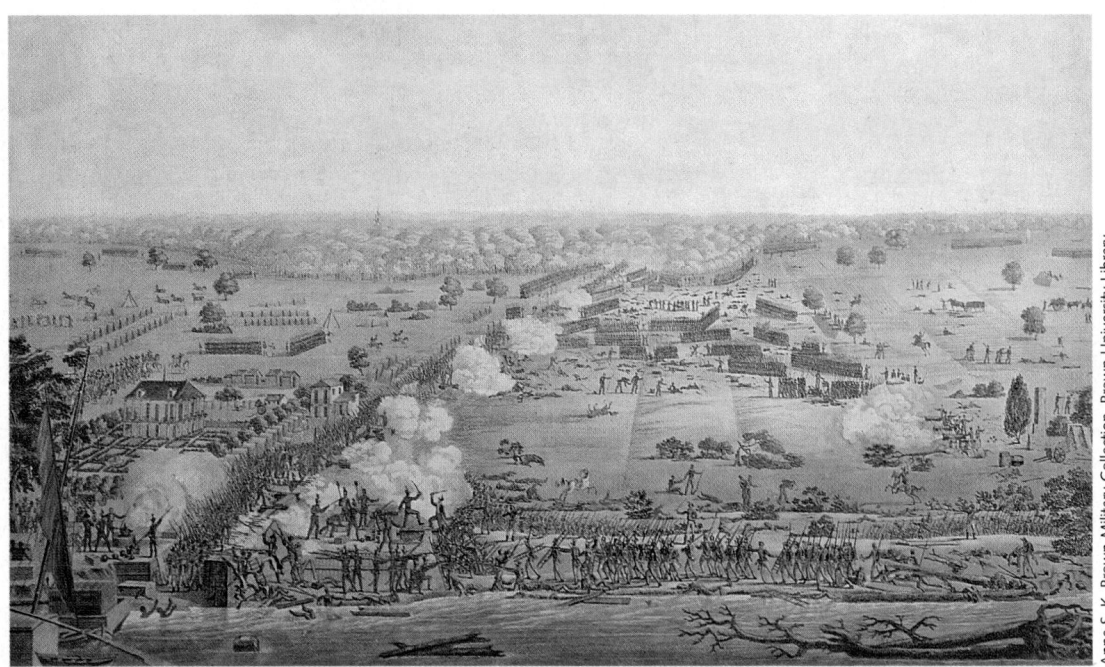

Anne S. K. Brown Military Collection, Brown University Library

■ **A scene from the Battle of New Orleans.**

1815, began with a ferocious assault by British soldiers. But within just half an hour, 2000 of them lay dead or wounded. The Americans lost only 70. They had vanquished the army of Europe's greatest military power.

An Uncertain Victory

American and British negotiators had signed a peace agreement that ended the war two weeks before "Old Hickory" defeated the British in New Orleans. (Jackson received his nickname when one of his soldiers called him "tough as hickory.") Later, many Americans associated Andrew Jackson with the war's decisive battle and most glorious victory. The Battle of New Orleans might have been a glorious victory for the Americans, but it was hardly the decisive battle of the war.

In the fall of 1814 Madison had decided to end the war. He dispatched John Quincy Adams, son of former president John Adams, to the Belgian city of Ghent to start negotiations. Representative Henry Clay and three other American envoys accompanied Adams. At first, English representatives to the meeting made two demands. The Americans, they said, must agree to the creation of an Indian territory in the upper Great Lakes region. They must also cede much of the state of Maine to England. The Americans refused, and the negotiations dragged on.

In the meantime, the New England states had grown increasingly impatient with what they called "Mr. Madison's war." As with the embargo, they saw the effort as a mistake and a threat to their regional commercial interests. In December 1814, Massachusetts, Connecticut, Rhode Island, New Hampshire, and Vermont sent delegates to a gathering in Hartford, Connecticut, to consider a course of action. The delegates demanded that the federal government give their states financial aid to compensate for the revenue they had lost as a result of disrupted trade. Some delegates even hinted that their states wanted to secede from the union. Although most delegates shied away from the idea, the majority of them apparently wanted to leave that possibility open.

Back in Ghent, the British had reversed their initial position by late December. They had lost recent battles in upper New York and in Baltimore and, as always, were still worried about new threats from France. They dropped their demands for territory and for an Indian buffer state in the upper Midwest. They also agreed to an armistice that, in essence, represented a draw: both combatants would retain the same territory they had possessed when the war began. The British made no concessions to the Americans' demands that they stop impressing American sailors and supplying the western Indians with arms or that they revoke the Orders in Council. Still, most U.S. citizens considered the war a great victory for the United States. After 1815, the Americans and the British never again met each other across a battlefield as enemies.

Some of the American soldiers and sailors who had survived the conflict paid a high price. For example, Benjamin F. Palmer was an American sailor imprisoned in an English jail from 1813 to 1815. There he subsisted on meager rations and witnessed unspeakable cruelties, including the murder of inmates by guards. In all probability, the Treaty of Ghent did not change Palmer's views of the British soldiers' "Brutal & Savage Barbarity." In total, 6000 American combatants had died or suffered wounds in the war. Yet survivors felt that they and their dead fellows had preserved the nation's honor.

Many Indians saw matters quite differently. For them, the War of 1812 had only stiffened white settlers' determination to take native peoples' land. Andrew Jackson, the Indian-hater and Indian-killer, would aggressively pursue a national political career. And so, the Battle of Horseshoe Bend signaled not only a continuation of bloodshed but also a terrifying sign of things to come. American nationalism came at the expense of vast Indian homelands and thousands of lives on both sides.

The "Era of Good Feelings"?

In 1816 the Democratic-Republicans nominated James Monroe for president, to run against Federalist candidate Rufus King. Although Monroe only narrowly won his party's endorsement, he soundly defeated King in the general election. Monroe benefited from several developments that had mortally wounded the Federalist party: the War of 1812 victory, presided over by a Democratic-Republican chief executive; the New England Federalists' flirtation with secession (and treason) during the war years; and the strong nationalist tendencies of both the Jefferson and Madison administrations, which had stolen the Federalists' thunder.

Addressing Congress in December 1817, Monroe expressed optimism about the state of the nation. The country's boundaries were secure, and the Indians had little choice but to retreat farther and farther west. The president predicted that, shortly, "Indian hostilities, if they do not altogether cease, will henceforth lose their terror." Equally inspiring, the Americans had once again defied the British Empire and won. Two treaties with Britain—the Rush–Bagot of 1817 and the Convention of 1818—set the U.S.–Canadian border at the 49th parallel and provided that the two countries would jointly occupy Oregon Territory for ten years.

Monroe called on Congress to acknowledge "the vast extent of territory within the United States [and] the great amount and value of its productions" and to facilitate the construction of roads and canals. It was this "happy situation of the United States," in Monroe's words, that ushered in what some historians called "The Era of Good Feelings." Although voters continued to disagree over some issues of the day—such as the national bank, sectionalism, and internal improvements—they did not necessarily express those disagreements in the form of bitter partisan wrangling. In any case, the term "good feelings" can be applied only to a

TABLE 10-2

The Election of 1816

Candidate	Political Party	Electoral Vote
James Monroe	Democratic-Republican	183
Rufus King	Federalist	34

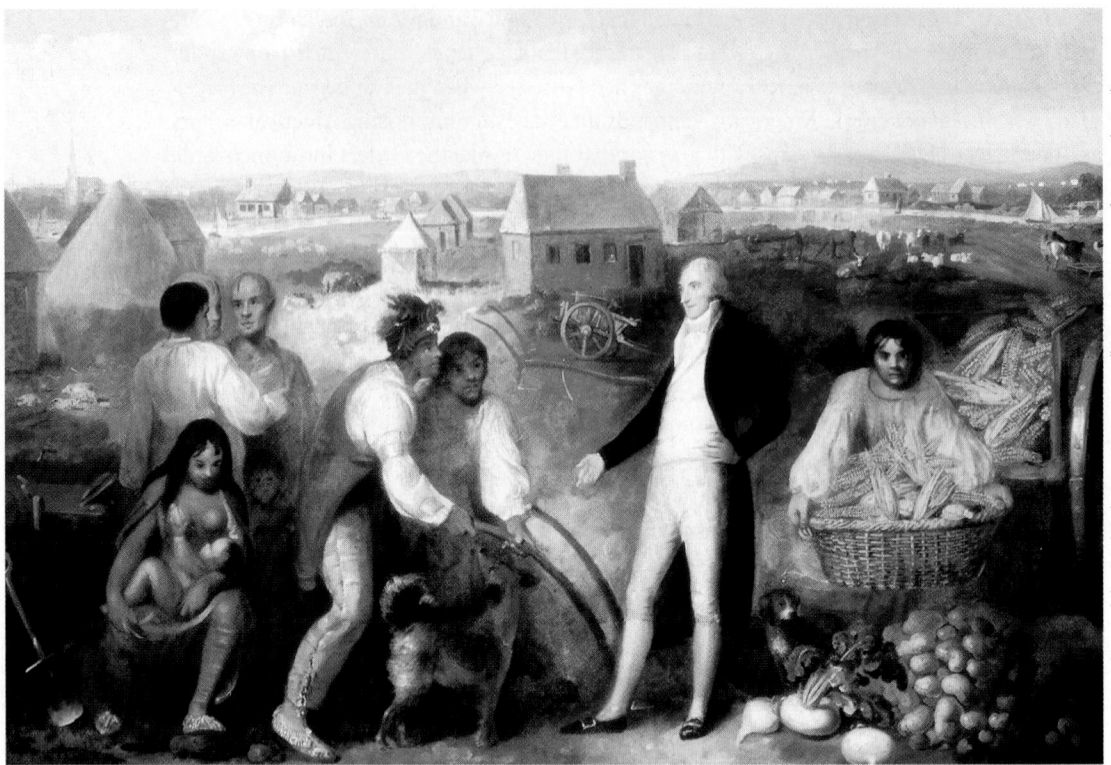

Benjamin Hawkins and the Creek Indians, c. 1805. Greenville County Museum of Art, South Carolina

■ Southeastern Indians varied widely in their willingness to adopt European American ways. Some argued that the best way to preserve their community and remain on the land of their forebears was to accommodate themselves to white practices of trade, textile production, and farming. This 1805 painting shows Benjamin Hawkins, a government Indian agent, at a Creek settlement near Macon, Georgia. Hawkins expresses evident satisfaction with the Indians' neat cabins, well-tended fields, flocks of sheep, and bountiful harvest of vegetables.

narrow group of enfranchised citizens, men who shared common beliefs about territorial expansion and economic development.

The War of 1812 yielded little in the way of material gains for the United States or concessions from England. Yet it permanently reshaped American social, political, and economic life. The nation exploited the vulnerable southeastern Indians and hastened their removal from their homeland. Many veterans of the war gained land grants, military glory, and political influence in return for their sacrifices. Although the war had disrupted foreign trade, it also gave home manufacturers a tremendous boost. The textile industry spearheaded a revolution in industry. And a new class of workers—factory operatives (machine tenders)—emerged to symbolize both the promise and the hazards of machines.

Praise and Respect for Veterans After the War

American veterans of the War of 1812 won the praise of a grateful nation. Even the British expressed a grudging respect for Americans' fighting abilities. One British naval officer admitted, "I don't like Americans; I never did, and never shall like them." He further declared that he had "no wish to eat with them, drink with them, deal with them, or consort with them in any way." But, he said, he would rather not fight with them either, for they were "an enemy so brave, determined, and alert, and in every way so worthy of one's steel, as they have always proved." To reward veterans for their service, Congress offered them 160-acre plots of land in the territory between the Illinois and Mississippi rivers. These grants did much to encourage families to emigrate west and establish homesteads.

Cherokee Women Petition Against Further Land Sales to Whites in 1817

In traditional Cherokee society, men took responsibility for foreign affairs while women focused on domestic matters, leading to a roughly equal division of labor. However, European American diplomats, military officials, and traders dealt primarily with Indian men. As a result, beginning in the eighteenth century, Cherokee women's traditional influence was eroding within their own communities. In this new world, Indian warriors wielded significant power.

Nevertheless, Cherokee women insisted on presenting their views during the crisis of 1817–1819, when men of the group were deciding whether to cede land to U.S. authorities and move west. The following petition was supported by Nancy Ward, a Cherokee War Woman. This honorific title was bestowed on women who accompanied and attended to the needs of war parties. Ward had supported the colonists' cause during the American Revolution.

Amovey [Tennessee] in Council 2nd May 1817

The Cherokee Ladys now being present at the meeting of the Chiefs and warriors in council have thought it their duties as mothers to address their beloved Chiefs and warriors now assembled.

Our beloved children and head men of the Cherokee nation we address you warriors in council we have raised all of you on the land which we now have, which God gave to us to inhabit and raise provisions we know that our country has once been extensive but by repeated sales has become circumscribed to a small tract, and [we] never have thought it our duty to interfere in the disposition of it till now, if a father or mother was to sell all their lands which they had to depend on which their children had to raise their living on which would indeed be bad and to be removed to another country we do not wish to go to an unknown country [to] which we have understood some of our children wish to go over the Mississippi but this act of our children would be like destroying your mothers. Your mothers your sisters ask and beg of you not to part with any more of our lands, we say ours[. Y]ou are our descendants and take pity on our request, but keep it for our growing children for it was the good will of our creator to place us here and you know our father the great president [James Monroe], will not allow his white children to take our country away for if it was not they would not ask you to put your hands to paper for it would be impossible to remove us all for as soon as one child is raised, we have others in our arms for such is our situation and will consider our circumstance.

Therefore children don't part with any more of our lands but continue on it and enlarge your farms and cultivate and raise corn and cotton and we your mothers and sisters will make clothing for you which our father the president has recommended to us all we don't charge anybody for selling any lands, but we have heard such intentions of our children but your talks become true at last and it was our desire to forewarn you all not to part with our lands.

Nancy Ward to her children[:] warriors to take pity and listen to the talks of your sisters, although I am very old yet cannot but pity the situation in which you will hear of their minds. I have great many grand children which I wish they do well on our land.

In addition to Nancy Ward, 12 Cherokee women signed the petition. Their names suggest the varying degrees of assimilation to white ways on the part of Cherokees in general. Petitioners included Cun, o, ah and Widow Woman Holder, as well as Jenny McIntosh and Mrs. Nancy Fields.

It is unclear what effect, if any, this petition had on Cherokee male leaders. The Cherokee nation did halt land cessions to whites between 1819 and 1835. ■

Source: Cherokee Women to Cherokee Council, May 2, 1817, series 1, Andrew Jackson Presidential Papers, Library of Congress Manuscripts Division, Washington, D.C. Reprinted in Nancy F. Cott, Jeanne Boydston, Ann Braude, Lori Ginzberg, and Molly Ladd-Taylor, eds., *Root of Bitterness: Documents of the Social History of American Women* (Boston: Northeastern University Press, 1996), pp. 177–178.

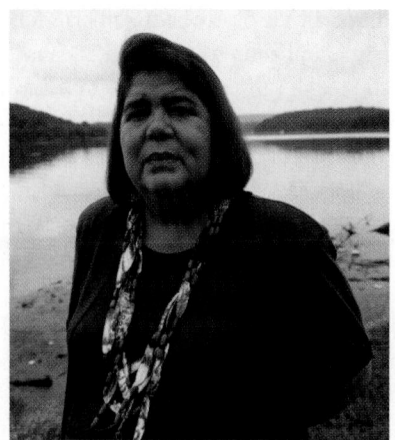

Wilma Mankiller, Cherokee Chief

Peter Turnley/CORBIS

Some military heroes of the war parlayed their success into impressive political careers. Andrew Jackson won election to the presidency in 1824, William Henry Harrison, in 1840. Winfield Scott served in a war against Mexico in 1848 and ran for president in 1852.

But European American veterans were not the only ones to gain status and influence within their own communities as a result of the conflict. A Cherokee leader named the Ridge also earned the gratitude of American officials for his contributions to the war effort. (His original Indian name, Kah-nung-da-tla-geh, means "the Man Who Walks on the Mountaintop.") The Ridge accepted the government's attempts to press the Cherokees to adopt European American ways. When the Ridge married a Cherokee woman named Susanna Wickett in the early 1790s, the couple settled in a log cabin (in northwest Georgia) rather than in a traditional Cherokee dwelling made of hardened clay daubed onto a wooden frame. During the war against the Red Sticks, the Ridge served under Andrew Jackson and earned the title of major. For the rest of his life, the Cherokee leader was known as Major Ridge. His wife devoted herself to tending an orchard, keeping a garden, and sewing clothes, tasks traditionally performed by European American but not Native American women. Eventually, the family prospered and bought African American slaves. They eventually became Christians as well.

The Ridge's battlefield experiences earned him the respect of other Cherokees who embraced the "civilization" program that missionaries and government officials promoted. At the same time, the Ridge vehemently resisted U.S. officials' attempts to persuade the Cherokee to give up their lands to whites and move west. Emerging as a leader of the Cherokee nation after the War of 1812, he criticized members of his group who had abandoned their lands in favor of a new life in the West. He declared, "I scorn this movement of a few men to unsettle the nation, and trifle with our attachment to the land of our forefathers." The Ridge believed that his people should adopt some elements of white culture but should also hold fast to their native lands in opposition to white settlers and politicians.

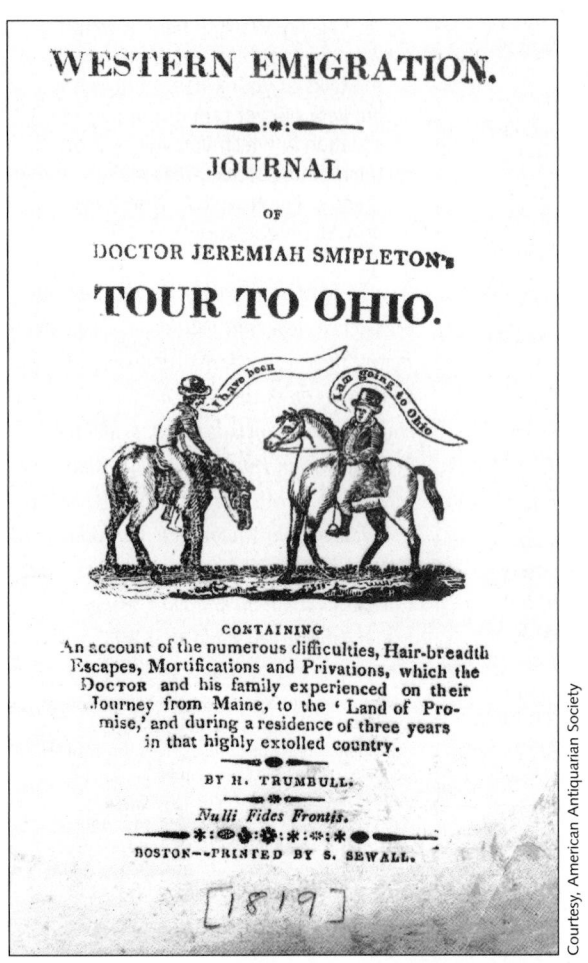

Courtesy, American Antiquarian Society

■ This cartoon, c. 1810, reveals two sides to the western emigration question. On the right, a well-dressed Easterner sets out for Ohio. He encounters a dejected, ragged migrant returning home. The men's horses tell a larger story about the failed dreams and hardship endured by many western emigrants. In the caption the artist cautions travelers on "the impropriety and folly of emigrating" from New England to the "Western Wilderness."

A Thriving Economy

The Embargo of 1807 and the War of 1812 stimulated home manufactures—especially the production of cloth and other goods in private households and factories. Home manufacturing resulted in a significant shift in the national economy—from reliance on imported goods to the production of those goods at home. The experiences of one rural Massachusetts family demonstrate the impact this shift had on individuals. Before the war, Lucy Kellogg and her sister worked at home, braiding straw hats to be sold at market. The war ruined their straw business, since economic hardship among New Englanders meant fewer people could afford to buy hats. In response, the sisters invested in cotton looms, which they used to make cloth. They secured cotton thread from the Massachusetts factories that had sprung up during the war to compensate for the lack of English textile imports. The Kellogg sisters found a ready market for their shirts, gingham dresses, and bed tickings. Still, their family was restless, moving briefly to New Hampshire but then returning to Worcester, where they resumed farming.

The end of the war saw up an upsurge in this kind of internal migration. New Englanders, especially, pushed west in search of new opportunities. Between 1800 and 1820, the population of Ohio grew from 45,000 to 581,000. Nevertheless, some emigrants expressed disillusion with the hardships and rigors of western life. Clearing the land of trees and then living in an isolated cabin did not appeal to everyone. John Stillman Wright initially sold his New York State farm in 1818 and settled in Ohio with high hopes. Later, he published *Letters from the West*, which recounted "the cruel disappointment and vain regret, which so many thousands are now enduring."

New means of transportation—and new means to fund them—facilitated the movement of goods, people, and ideas from the East to the West (and, in some cases, back again). Indeed, riding in stagecoaches, wagons, and boats and on horseback, Americans seemed to be on the move constantly. In 1807 an entrepreneur named Robert Fulton piloted the *Clermont,* a new kind of boat powered by steam, up the Hudson River from New York City. Within a few years, such vessels were plying the western waterways: the Columbia, Sacramento, Colorado, and Mississippi rivers and their tributaries. Steamboats traveled up river, against the current, ten times faster than keelboats, which had to be pushed, pulled, or hauled by men or mules.

New improvements in land transportation also stimulated economic growth. The profits that the Philadelphia and Lancaster Turnpike raked in by charging travelers tolls inspired other local private corporations to invest in roads. By 1810 several thousand such corporations were building roads up and down the East Coast. Funding came from a variety of sources, both public and private. Philadelphia textile mill owners financed transportation links with the city's hinterland (rural areas to the west) to bring their goods to the largest number of customers. Individual cities also invested in routes westward. The state of Virginia authorized a board of public works to expend funds for roads and other internal improvements. Western politicians flexed their political muscle in 1806 by securing congressional authorization for the building of the Cumberland (later National) Road, which snaked through the Allegheny Mountains and ended at the Ohio River.

> *New improvements in land transportation also stimulated economic growth.*

The acceleration of commerce in the West, combined with the disruption in trade from Europe that had come with the embargo and war, stimulated manufacturing throughout the United States. Philadelphia's growth proved particularly dazzling. During the War of 1812, the city's craft producers did not have to worry about foreign competition. Local merchant-financiers, who otherwise might have been pouring their money into trade ventures, began to invest in manufacturing. As early as 1808, the city's new factories had compensated for the glass, chemicals, shot, soap, lead, and earthenware that no longer flooded in from England. Philadelphia soon took the lead in production of all kinds, whether carried out in factories, artisans' shops, or private homes. Metalworking, ale brewing, and leather production counted among the array of thriving industries that made Philadelphia the nation's top industrial city in 1815.

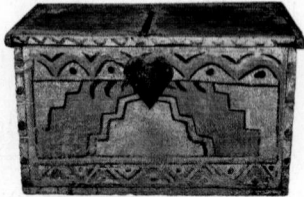

Still, in 1820, about two-thirds of all Philadelphia workers labored in small shops employing fewer than six people. Only 10 percent were employed in establishments larger than nine people. Moreover, because of an influx of English and Irish immigrants in the late eighteenth century, the city never developed a mechanized textile industry along the lines of New England's. Many of these newcomers were skilled textile workers; they continued to work in small shops rather than tend machines in large factories like New England textile workers.

Transformations in the Workplace

Even the earliest stages of the industrial revolution transformed the way people lived and worked. Some crafts—for example, the production of leather, barrels, soap, candles, and newspapers—expanded from small shops with skilled artisans into larger establishments with unskilled wage earners. In these cases, production was reorganized; now wage earners under the supervision of a boss replaced apprentices and journeymen who had formerly worked alongside a master artisan. These workers performed a single task many times a day instead of using their specialized skills to see a production process through to completion.

While skilled artisans were alarmed at the prospect of being reduced to mere "hands" tending machines, the sons and daughters of many New England farmers eagerly took new jobs in the mills. They appreciated the opportunity to escape close family supervision, to live on their own, and to earn cash wages. Some farm hands and manual laborers considered factory work, no matter how grueling and ill-paid, preferable to plowing fields, digging ditches, and

Revolutions in Transportation

The introduction of commercial steamboat service in 1807 marked a new era in seafaring transportation. Until that time, improving the speed of ships involved adding more sails while still relying on windpower. With the invention of the steam-powered boat, shippers were no longer at the mercy of the wind and the currents.

Over the generations, American prosperity has depended on moving things—whether barrels of flour, new computers, or people—over long and short distances. New forms of power such as steam, electricity, and gasoline, combined with innovations in technology and engineering, produced revolutions in transportation.

The first railroads also relied on steam engines; they challenged wagons and horses as the most efficient means of moving across land. During the Civil War, northern and southern armies used railroads to move men, weapons, and supplies to battlefields. This task was complicated by the South's lack of a standard railroad gauge, (that is, a uniform track size) necessitating unloading goods from one train and loading them onto another.

By the end of the nineteenth century, five transcontinental railroad lines spanned the entire breadth of the United States. During this time, two specific innovations transformed rail travel and transport. The Pullman sleeping car allowed passengers to travel long distances in comfort. Refrigerated cars allowed farmers to ship fresh vegetables, fruits, and meat to distant markets and consumers.

In the 1880s the first streetcars ran on electric power. Gasoline-powered engines propelled automobiles (developed in the 1890s) and airplanes, inaugurated by the first successful flight of brothers Orville and Wilbur Wright in 1903. By the 1920s, automobiles were the chief means of passenger transportation, and trucks rivaled trains as means of shipping foodstuffs and manufactured goods. Commercial airline service began in the 1950s. In the late twentieth century, shippers introduced a system called containerization, a form of transportation linking land, sea, and water. Containers of uniform size could be loaded onto ships, trucks, or trains, facilitating the international trade necessary to a global economy.

Various means of conveyance relied on new developments in engineering. Locks adjusted the water level of canals that were integral to freight transportation in the eastern United States in the first half of the nineteenth century. Crucial to the westward migration of thousands of Americans during that period were interstate roads. Costing $6.82 million, the gravel-paved Great National Pike stretched from Cumberland, Maryland, to Vandalia, Illinois. Begun in 1806, it took 34 years to complete. The first transcontinental railroad, finished in 1869, was an engineering marvel, with trestles spanning deep chasms, tracks running alongside rivers, and tunnels burrowing through mountains.

hauling lumber. Chauncey Jerome, a young Connecticut man, lamented that few opportunities were open to him in rural areas: "There being no manufacturing of any account in the country, the poor boys were obliged to let themselves to the farmers, and it was extremely difficult to find a place where they would treat a poor boy like a human being."

New England rapidly became the center of mechanized textile production in the United States. By the late eighteenth century, Boston shippers were making handsome profits by supplying Alta Californio (the area north of San Diego, encompassing present-day California, Nevada, and parts of Arizona and Utah) with cloth, shoes, and tools, selling Western otter pelts in China, and returning home laden with Chinese porcelains and silks. These profits financed New England's mechanized textile industry. By 1813, 76 cotton mills housing a total of over 51,000 spindles had cropped up within the vicinity of Providence, Rhode Island.

Faced with a shortage of adult men (many were moving west), New England mill owners sought other local sources of labor. The Rhode Island system of production had relied on child spinners working in small mills. This system gave way to the Lowell model, based in Waltham and Lowell, Massachusetts, which brought young women from the surrounding countryside to work in gigantic mills. Many of the women were eager to earn cash wages and to escape the routine of farm life. Still, New England mill owners realized that they had to reas-

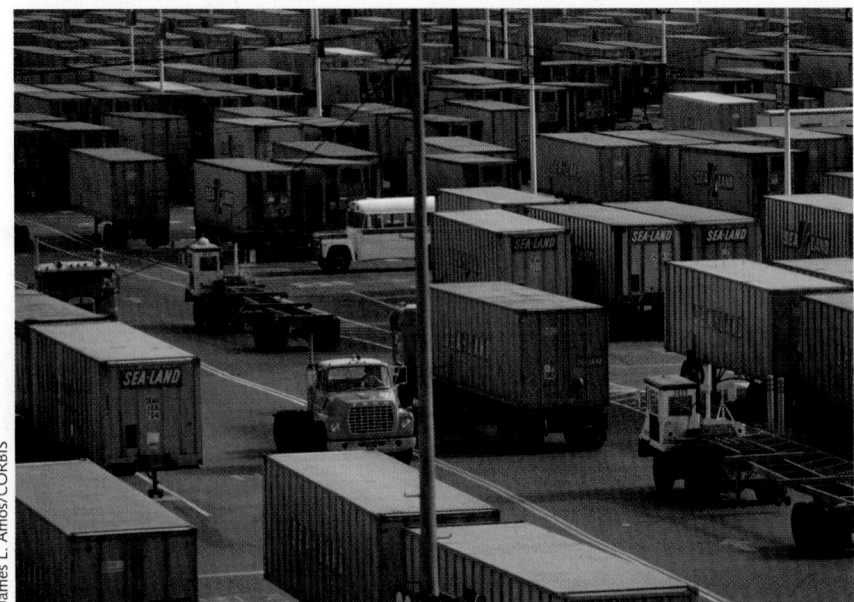
Modern transportation containers

Beginning in 1900, the largest cities constructed systems of underground tunnels for streetcars. Between 1900 and 1930, states and counties paved 700,000 miles of roads and highways. The Federal Aid Highway Act of 1956 established the interstate highway system. By the end of the twentieth century, the total highway mileage in the United States was 4 million miles, with about 46,000 of that number part of the interstate system. By this time almost 200,000 miles of pipeline carried various fuels and gases from Alaska to the continental United States and within and between states.

In 2000, approximately 125 million cars, 70 million trucks, 700,000 buses, and 200,000 aircraft were in use in the United States. The proliferation of vehicles put tremendous strains of the environment. Environmental regulations increased fuel efficiency, especially for newer vehicles; between 1970 and 2000, average miles per gallon on cars increased from 13.5 miles to 21.3 miles. In the early twenty-first century, the United States accounts for one-fourth of all fossil fuel emissions in the world. These emissions increase pollution in American cities and greenhouse gases worldwide.

In early 2002, President George W. Bush's administration announced a shift in federal policy, from a quest for ever-more fossil-fuel–efficient cars to the development of vehicles powered by hydrogen-based fuel cells. However, scientists predicted that this particular revolution in transportation was still decades in the future. ■

sure Yankee parents that their daughters would find the factories to be safe, attractive places to work. Mill owners offered the young women housing in dormitory-like boardinghouses staffed by older women, called matrons, who looked after them.

Some New Englanders were unsettled by the social changes that accompanied these new ways of working. Factories encouraged parents to put their children to work rather than sending them to school. The new production system also widened the economic inequality between owners and wage hands. Colonial communities, where men and women, rich and poor, had worked together in the fields, gave way to mill towns. There, the wives of owners lived lives of privilege and leisure compared with the women who toiled at looms or spindles all day.

Nevertheless, New England had not yet developed what might be called a factory working class. Many people went back and forth between farm and factory, depending on their own fortunes and inclinations. Some workers were neither suited for nor inclined to work in or around the mills; they quit or were fired. One account in the contract books of the Pomfret Manufacturing Company in Massachusetts revealed that a 14-year-old girl named Sukey Blois was hired on May 7, 1807. The details of her hiring are followed by the words, "Quit May 10."

These transformations in the workplace and in social relations disturbed some white laborers in particular. They feared for their own status as freeborn, proud sons (and grandsons) of

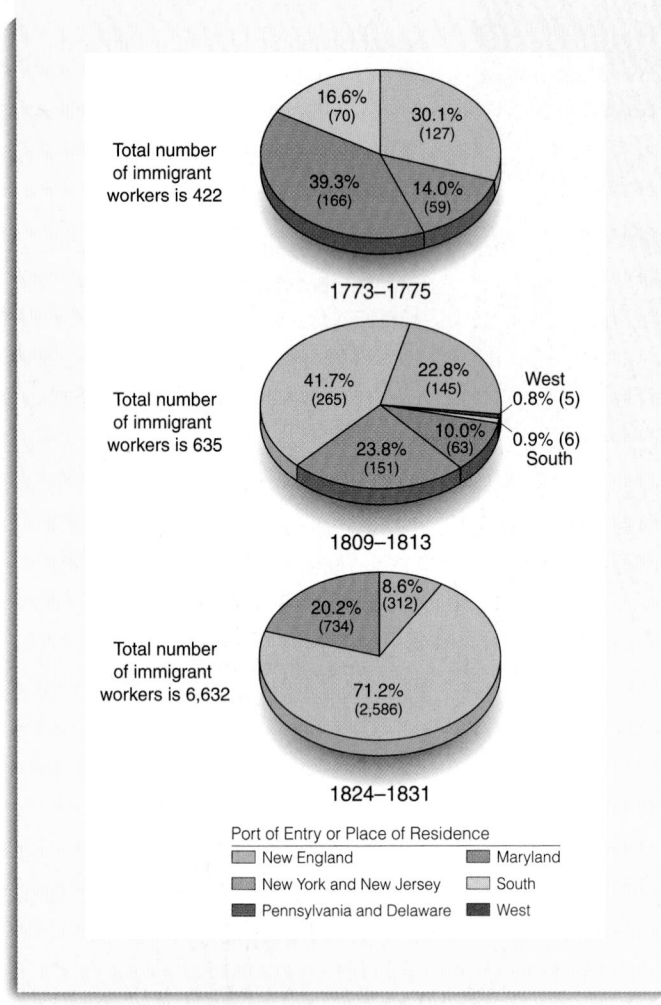

■ FIGURE 10.1
GEOGRAPHIC LOCATIONS OF BRITISH IMMIGRANT TEXTILE WORKERS, 1770s–1831

Source: David J. Jeremy, *Transatlantic Industrial Revolution: Diffusion of Cotton Power-Loom Weaving Technology* (Cambridge, MA: MIT Press, 1981), p. 156.

the Revolution. To them, the factory represented a loss of independence; they were becoming mere "hands" to tend machines. In 1806 striking Philadelphia shoemakers charged, "The name of freedom is but a shadow." The court ruled that by joining together to withhold their labor from their employer, these workers were guilty of conspiring to raise their own wages.

Some whites went so far as to claim that they were "wage slaves." No longer in charge of their own work lives, they felt condemned to long hours and low pay. The contrast between the ideal of household independence—a father and husband who owned property and could provide comfortably for his family—and the reality of men, women, and children working for pitiful wages in a noisy, dirty factory was profoundly demeaning to these men. They claimed that toiling for puny wages was not all that different from laboring as slaves.

Black men and women continued to suffer the stigma of slavery. Regardless of legal status, all blacks were descendants of slaves. This stigma determined the jobs for which blacks were hired and the pay they received. The 7500 free blacks who lived in New York City in 1810 were about only 8 percent of the city's total population. But they made up fully 84 percent of all black people in the city (the rest were enslaved children who would not gain their freedom until they became adults). They struggled to earn a living, and they had limited employment options. One job that was open to them was the dangerous, dirty work of cleaning chimneys. Black men served as master chimney sweeps and employed youths of their own race as assistants and apprentices. In an attempt to control the sweeps, the New York City Council tried to insist that they purchase expensive licenses to ply their trade. In response, a group of master chimney sweeps decried a double standard; resenting what they considered unreasonably high licensing fees, they declared that they wanted to be treated "in the same manner as you have thought proper

to do in respect to Cartmen, porter, measurer &c." Realizing that they had to protect themselves, they established their own mutual aid society, the United Society of Chimney Sweeps. Some members asserted their equality with white men of the city by noting that they too had "served in the revolutionary war & some of them received wounds." Their efforts proved short-lived, however. Eventually, the use of machinery eroded black men's monopoly on this kind of work. Most black men could not afford to purchase the machines, which eliminated the need for skilled labor.

Chimney sweeps plied their trade by walking the streets and calling out loudly, "Sweep O! Sweep O!" to potential customers. In 1816 the New York City Common Council moved again to restrict the sweeps' work. The council outlawed "crying aloud or singing in the public streets." Those who persisted, council members warned, would be deprived of their licenses. In other cities as well, municipal officials, backed by white laborers, sought to regulate the behavior of black men who worked outdoors, whether it was pulling carts, cleaning streets, peddling goods, or emptying chamberpots. Whites claimed that black outside workers were noisy and disorderly. These complaints revealed the hypocrisy of white people, who relegated blacks to the most disagreeable jobs and then criticized these workers for not pursuing other (better) kinds of work.

In the coming years, some white workers embraced the cause of temperance as a means of distancing themselves from poor people in general and poor blacks in particular. White men's own sober behavior, they claimed, was far superior to that of the rowdy poor, especially black men and women who had to make their living by working outdoors, singing and "crying" for customers—practices that whites linked to drunken, disorderly behavior. White men in cities increasingly associated productive labor with inside work performed by people who practiced punctuality, thrift, and sobriety. Poor people of both races remained vulnerable to the charge of vagrancy. According to an observer in the New York *Independent Mechanic* in 1811, vagrants "infest our streets, by day, shocking the delicacy of our females, and disgusting the feelings of everyone, who is not as debased as the wretches themselves."

Industrialization was not confined to New England; the southern states encouraged the development of textile mills as well. Yet in the South, industrialization had different social consequences. By 1816, England had begun to dump its accumulated stores of textiles in the United States, selling them at bargain rates and putting hundreds of American mills out of business. Some New England factory owners moved their operations to the South, hoping to find cheaper land and labor. The southern mills used white wage hands, enslaved workers, or a combination of the two.

Many owners of southern industrial establishments sought to piece together their labor forces on the basis of the availability of different kinds of labor: enslaved and free, black and white, male and female, young and old. Thus, ironworks, gold and coal mines, brickworks, hemp factories, salt-processing plants, and lumber, railroad, and canal camps often employed men of both races, enslaved and free. In southern cities, white artisans concerned about losing their livelihood protested the use of skilled slave labor. But their complaints fell on deaf ears. Most members of city councils and regulatory boards owned slaves themselves, and they had no intention of giving up their enslaved workers so that white artisans could find jobs.

Southern industry always reflected developments in the plantation economy. For example, when cotton prices rose, slave owners kept their slaves working in the fields. Thus, planters discouraged any kind of large-scale manufacturing that might disrupt the agrarian society they had built so carefully over so many years.

However, in 1816 neither southern nor northern congressmen foresaw that the differences between their two regions would intensify over the coming years. That year Congress debated whether to impose a tariff on foreign goods. The proposed tax would require importers of such goods to pay duties of 20 to 25 percent of the value of the total. A young representative from South Carolina, John C. Calhoun, spoke in favor of the tariff bill. The South, he explained, might someday have to rely heavily on manufacturing. Calhoun, therefore, was open to a tariff that would raise the price of goods manufactured in the United States. In contrast, Representative Daniel Webster of New Hampshire opposed the measure. The tariff, he said, would further harm the New England shipping industry by dampening foreign trade altogether. The Tariff of 1816 passed and became law. Within a few years these two men reversed their positions on the tariff as the North became more rigidly associated with manufacturing and the South with staple crop agriculture.

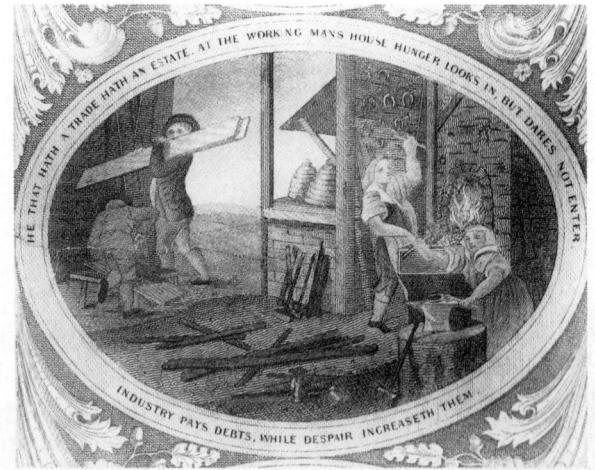

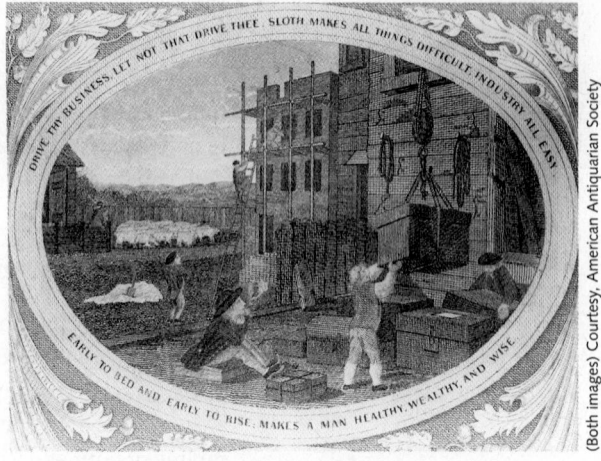

(Both images) Courtesy, American Antiquarian Society

■ In the early nineteenth century, many skilled artisans worried that economic growth and development would erode their independence. They sought to portray themselves as upright and virtuous citizens and, by extension, superior to poor people who lacked either self-discipline or steady employment. These engravings feature sayings from Benjamin Franklin published in *Poor Richard Illustrated: Lessons for the Young and Old on Industry, Temperance, Frugality &c.*

The Rise of the Cotton Plantation Economy

The growth and spread of the cotton economy redefined the institution of slavery, the southern political system, and, ultimately, all of American history. With the invention of the cotton gin and the acquisition of the Louisiana Territory, cotton production boomed, and with it the enslaved population. About 700,000 slaves resided in the United States in 1790; just two decades later, that figure had jumped to 1.1 million. In 1790 plantations produced 3000 bales (about 300 pounds each) of cotton; 20 years later, that number hit 178,000. On the eve of the Civil War, in 1860, the southern states were growing 4 million bales of cotton. Behind these figures lay a human drama of immense proportions.

Beginning in 1808, the United States outlawed the importation of new slaves. However, the astounding profitability of cotton heightened the demand for slave labor. Although South Carolina had banned its own trans-Atlantic slave trade in 1787 (that is, outlawed the importation of slaves into the state), the state reopened the trade in 1803. Between those years, annual exports of cotton had risen from less than 10,000 pounds to more than 6 million. Between 1803 and the imposition of the national ban five years later, South Carolina imported 35,000 Africans. (This number far exceeded the number of slave importations in any other five-year period in the state's history.) However, other states began to rely on the domestic slave trade—the forced migration of slaves from the upper South to the lower South.

The institution of slavery was marked by sharp regional variations. Between 1800 and 1820, those variations reflected the impact of cotton cultivation on local economies. At the same time, the contours of an African American culture emerged. This culture had certain characteristics regardless of place, such as strong ties that bound nuclear and extended family members, rich oral and musical traditions heavily influenced by West African customs, and individual and collective resistance to slavery. White people as a group understood little of this culture; they viewed black people primarily as workers who would never become citizens. As U.S. military strength and nationalistic pride grew, southern planters imposed a harsher, more regimented system of slavery on the black population. The tension between the rhetoric of freedom and the reality of slavery shaped southern—and American—life for the next four decades.

Regional Economies of the South

Throughout the South, shifts in production methods transformed the demographic and economic make-up of specific regions. For example, by the early nineteenth century, the Chesapeake tobacco economy had declined as a result of worn-out lands and falling prices. In its place arose a more diversified economy based on crafts, the cultivation of corn and wheat, and the milling of flour and wheat. Owners put enslaved men to work making barrels and horseshoes while their wives, sisters, and daughters labored as spinners, weavers, dairymaids, personal servants, and livestock tenders.

The lower South states of Georgia and South Carolina also saw their economies change during this period. The indigo export business never recovered from the Revolution, when it was outlawed by the Continental Congress to deprive foreign countries of the prized dye. European customers now had to turn to Louisiana and Central America for indigo. In contrast, the lowcountry (coastal) South Carolina rice economy recovered and flourished after the war. Technical advances in tidal rice production boosted the size of rice holdings, and ambitious planters bought up the land of neighboring small farmers. In a particularly rich rice district, All Saints Parish, one out of two slaves lived on a plantation with more than a hundred slaves in 1790; 30 years later, four out of five lived on such large establishments. In these areas, the plantation owners themselves often lived elsewhere, and black people constituted almost the entire population.

Adding to the wealth of South Carolina was the rapid development of cotton cultivation, especially in the state's interior, away from the coast. In 1810 fully half of the state's population lived away from the coast. There, prosperous cotton planters began to rival their

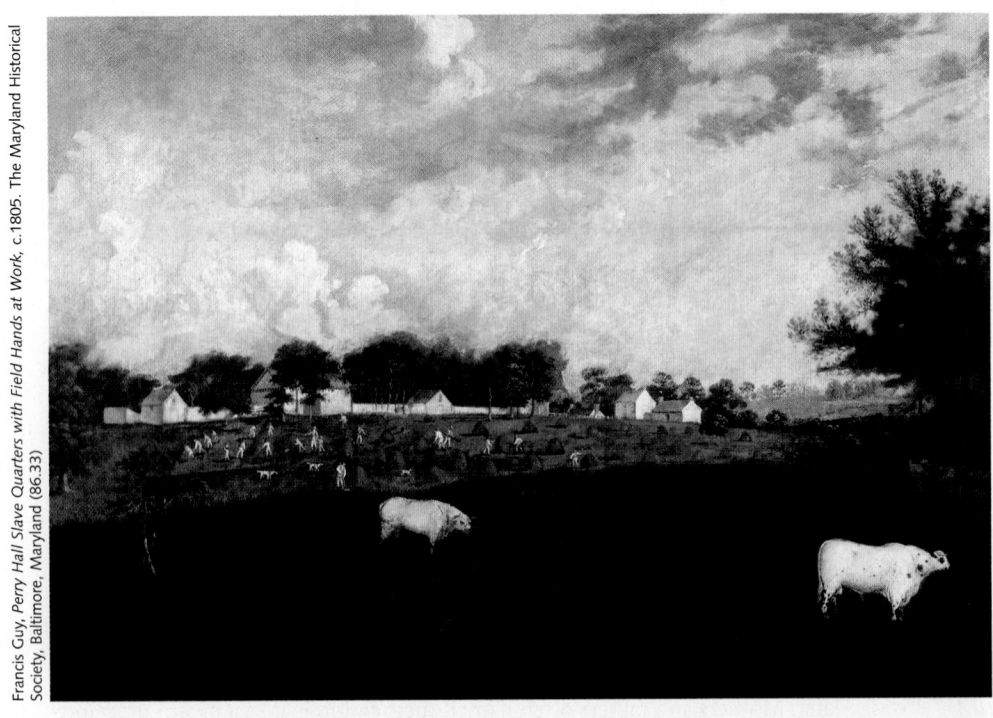

Francis Guy, *Perry Hall Slave Quarters with Field Hands at Work*, c.1805. The Maryland Historical Society, Baltimore, Maryland (86.33)

■ This painting (c. 1805) by Francis Guy is titled *Perry Hall Slave Quarters with Field Hands at Work*. Enslaved workers, organized in a gang, cultivate tobacco on a Chesapeake plantation. After the turn of the century, the center of the plantation staple crop economy moved south and west. The Chesapeake region of Maryland and Virginia developed a more diversified economy than that of the rich cotton lands of Alabama and Louisiana.

lowcountry rice-growing counterparts in social status and political influence. Meanwhile, Charleston's population grew more diverse, as refugees from Saint-Domingue (current-day Haiti) arrived in the 1790s and as the free black population grew.

Southern slaveholders supported territorial expansion because they understood that a thriving staple-crop economy relied on the cultivation of fresh lands. Cotton planters rushed into the Louisiana Territory after 1803. They accelerated an economic process that had begun in the late eighteenth century: the replacement of a frontier exchange economy with plantation agriculture. (Sugar dominated the New Orleans region; cotton, the rest of the Lower Mississippi valley.) No longer able to serve as traders in this frontier territory, slaves remained confined to their masters' estates. Their owners forbade them to sell or buy goods and to own firearms. By 1800, slaves in lower Louisiana were producing 4.5 million pounds of sugar annually and more than 18,000 bales of cotton.

The reaches of the Lower Mississippi took on an increasingly multicultural flavor. A strong Spanish influence persisted as a vestige of colonial days. French-speaking planter–refugees and their slaves from revolutionary Saint-Domingue came to New Orleans while the city was still in French hands (1800 to 1803). Between 1787 and 1803, nearly 3000 slaves arrived to be sold in New Orleans—some imported clandestinely from Africa, others bought from the Spanish in West Florida, still others transported from the Chesapeake region. In 1803 and afterward, American planters began to import even larger numbers of slaves from the North. Slave owners who settled in Natchez, on the banks of the Mississippi River, grew cotton—and grew rich.

Black Family Life and Labor

Between 1790 and 1861, approximately 400,000 Africans were imported into the territory that became the United States. Yet by 1860, the black population had grown to more than 4 million— a tenfold increase in 160 years. These numbers suggest a tremendous rate of natural increase. Some planters continued to buy slaves brought into the country illegally after 1808. But most of the increase stemmed from births. The preferences of both slaveowners and slaves account for this development. Unlike their Latin American and West Indian counterparts who preferred to work large numbers of male slaves to death, southern planters encouraged black women to bear many children. At the same time, enslaved African Americans valued the family as a social unit; family ties provided support and solace for a people deprived of fundamental human rights. Even under harsh conditions, black people fell in love, married (albeit informally, without the sanction of law), had children, and reared families. Despite the lack of protection from local, state, and national authorities, the slave family proved to be a remarkably resilient institution.

The stability of individual slave families depended on several factors, including the size and age of the plantation and the fortunes and life cycle of the slaveowner's family. Very large or long-established plantations had more two-parent slave families compared to small or newer holdings, which tended to have more unrelated people. Slave families were broken up when whites died and their "property" bequeathed to heirs. Slaves might also be sold or presented to other family members as gifts. For example, a slaveowner might present a slave to a son or daughter getting married and setting up a new household. In these instances, whites' family ties came at the expense of blacks' family ties. Ultimately, slaveowners prized the natural increase of their workers but had little respect for the family feeling that black people nourished within their own communities.

> *Enslaved African Americans valued the family as a social unit [providing] support and solace for a people deprived of fundamental human rights.*

Still, enslaved men and women struggled to retain some control over their own lives. Slaves tended to be exogamous—that is, they married outside their circle of cousins and other close relatives. To keep from being sold, slave girls at times felt compelled to demonstrate their fertility to their owners. Many of them had their first child with an enslaved man in their late teens, then entered stable marriages later. Mothers and fathers often named their children after a parent or grandparent. On the Good Hope Plantation in Orangeburg, South Carolina, five slave children were born between 1804 and 1819. Flora and Clarinda were each named for their mother's mother, Sambo for his mother's father, and Primus and July for their fathers.

Many slave families suffered disruption in response to the growing demand for slaves in the fresh cotton lands of Alabama and Mississippi. The forced migration from upper South to lower South necessarily severed kin ties, but slaves often reconstituted those ties in the form of symbolic kin relationships. For example, families adopted new, single members of the slave community, and the children called these newcomers "Aunt" or "Uncle." Slaves throughout the South tended to have large families, and they preferred to live in units consisting of two parents with children. However, they adapted their household structures to the available housing. On the Oakland Plantation in West Feliciana Parish, Louisiana, the slave quarters consisted of 15 cabins that housed various forms of families. In 1811, four married couples and their children lived alone, but other cabins consisted of single people, a married couple only, or households of extended family and adopted kin. Established in 1809, this plantation had fewer nuclear families than long-established rice plantations in South Carolina did, for example.

After the Civil War, southern blacks combined their work and family lives by laboring within their families in the fields. Under slavery, however, owners showed little or no inclination to take family relationships into account when they parceled out work assignments to men, women, and children. Rather, those assignments, and the conditions under which slaves performed them, reflected the size and crops of a particular plantation. An estimated 75 percent of antebellum slaves worked primarily as field hands. On large plantations the division of labor could be quite specialized. Men served as skilled carpenters, blacksmiths, and barrelmakers, and women worked as cooks, laundresses, nursemaids, and personal maids.

Rice slaves continued to work under the task system. Each day, after they completed a specific assigned task, they spent their time as they chose, within limits. The women washed clothes and cleaned the living quarters. The men hunted and fished. Both men and women visited friends and worked in their own gardens. Slaves jealously guarded their limited forms of freedom. One white man in Georgia described a slave who had completed his appointed task for the day: "His master feels no right to call on him," leaving him "the remainder of the day to work in his own corn field."

Even in the cotton-growing regions, where blacks labored under the regimented gang system, slaves tried to work for themselves in the little free time they had on Saturday afternoons and Sunday. In Louisiana, one white observer noted that the slave man returning to his living quarters after a long, hot day in the fields "does not lose his time. He goes to work at a bit of the land which he has planted with provisions for his own use, while his companion, if he has one, busies herself in preparing some for him, herself, and their children." Family members who grew or accumulated a modest surplus—of corn, eggs, vegetables— in some cases could sell their wares in a nearby market or to slaves on another plantation.

Some slaves appropriated goods from their master's storeroom and barn and sold or traded them to other slaves or to poor whites. This kind of labor benefited individual slaves and their families. These transactions often took place under the cover of darkness. Planters complained of slaves who stole their cattle, hogs, chickens, sacks full of cotton, farm equipment, and stores of ham and flour. In 1806 planters in lowcountry South Carolina, along the Combahee River, railed against a problem that would grow worse in the coming years: "pedling boats which frequent the river . . . for the purpose of trading with The Negroe Slaves, to the very great loss of the Owners, and Corruption of such slaves." Thus slaves' various forms of labor fell into at least three categories: work performed at the behest of and directly under the supervision of whites, labor performed by and for family members within the slaves' living quarters, and the sale (or sometimes clandestine exchange) of goods with masters, other slaves, and poor whites.

Resistance to Slavery

In 1817 the New Orleans City Council decreed that slaves could sing and dance at a stipulated place—Congo Square—every Sunday afternoon. Thereafter, a variety of groups came together to make music. These groups included recent émigrés from Saint-Domingue and slaves

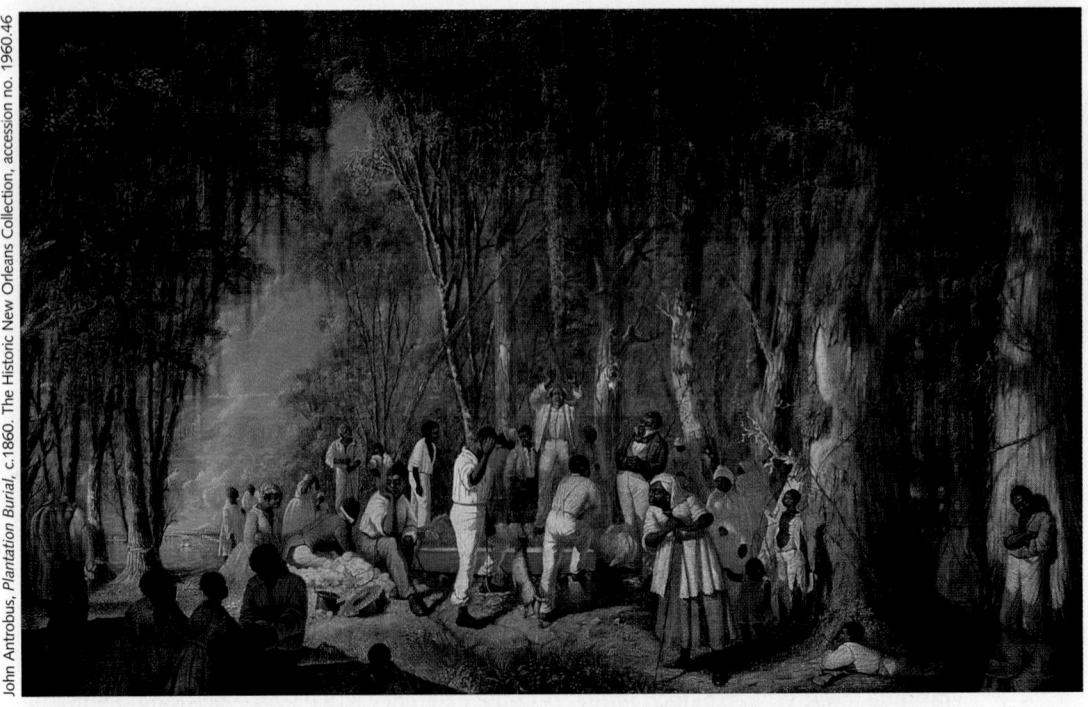

John Antrobus, *Plantation Burial*, c.1860. The Historic New Orleans Collection, accession no. 1960.46

■ British artist John Antrobus titled his 1860 painting *Plantation Burial*. Held at night, after the workday, slave funerals provided an opportunity for the community—including slaves from nearby plantations—to come together in mourning. Planters remained suspicious of such gatherings, which were marked by African musical forms and religious rituals. Whites feared that slaves would conspire under the cover of darkness.

newly imported from Africa; slaves from neighboring plantations, in town for the day; and free people of color (Creoles), who often blended Spanish and French classical music traditions. One eyewitness declared that the Congo Square musicians "have their own national music, consisting for the most part of a long kind of narrow drum of various size." In towns and on plantations throughout the South, black people drew from West African musical styles, using drums as well as banjolike instruments, gourd rattles, and mandolins. From Congo Square and other southern places flowed the roots of several uniquely American musical styles: the blues, gospel, ragtime, jazz, swing, and rock 'n' roll.

In their artistic expression, dress, hairstyles, and language, slaves sought to preserve their cultural uniqueness and create an existence that slaveholders could not touch. In the South Carolina lowcountry, slaves spoke Gullah. Originally a pidgin—a blend of words and grammatical structures from West African languages and English—Gullah later developed into a more formal Creole language. Slaves throughout the United States also mixed West African religious beliefs with Christianity. Nevertheless, they showed little interest in some of the essential features of European American Protestantism, including the concept of original sin and the possibility of eternal damnation in the afterlife. Many West African groups believed in a close relationship between the natural and supernatural worlds. In slave quarters, spiritual leaders not only preached a Christianity of equality but also told fortunes and warned away "haunts" (spirits of the dead).

In gatherings of many kinds, enslaved Americans affirmed their bonds with one another and their resistance to bondage. For example, funerals provided opportunities for music and expressions of group solidarity. The rich oral tradition that characterized slave life preserved collective memories of Africa and the lore of individual families and kin networks.

Black resistance to slavery took many forms. Slaves might work carelessly in an effort to resist a master's or mistress's demands. During the course of their workday, some slaves broke hoes and other farm implements. A cook might burn the biscuits, thus spoiling a special dinner party for her mistress. Striking out more directly, the African-influenced "conjurer"—often a woman who had a knowledge of plants and herbs—could wreak havoc on a white family by concocting poisons or encouraging disruptive behavior among slaves.

Slaves also stole goods from their masters and at times stole themselves by running away. (This practice was more common among young, unmarried men than among those who had family obligations.) Some slaves revolted. In St. Charles and St. John the Baptist parishes in Louisiana, an 1811 revolt of 400 slaves cost two whites their lives and left several plantations in flames. Under the leadership of a free man of color, Charles Deslondes, the original group acquired new members as they marched toward New Orleans. U.S. troops cut their advance short, killing 66 of them. In the Southeast in 1817 and 1818, 400 to 600 runaway slaves converged on the swamps of central Florida, uniting with Indian refugees from the Red Stick War. Together, they raided Georgia plantations until Andrew Jackson and his soldiers halted them in April 1818.

To justify their own behavior, masters and mistresses created a number of myths about the black people they exploited. Whites had a vested interest in believing that their slaves felt gratitude toward them. Skilled in the so-called deference ritual, some slaves hid their true feelings and acted submissively in the presence of white people. Owners and overseers alike interpreted this behavior as a sign of black contentment.

Yet most whites understood that danger could lurk beneath the surface of the most accommodating slave. Therefore, the prevailing stereotypes of black men and women encom-

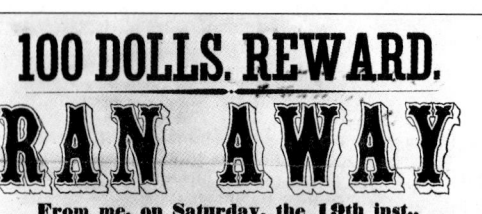

100 DOLLS. REWARD.

RAN AWAY

From me, on Saturday, the 19th inst.,

Negro Boy Robert Porter,

aged 19; heavy, stoutly made; dark chesnut complexion; rather sullen countenance, with a down look; face large; head low on the shoulders. I believe he entered the City of Washington on Sunday evening, 20th inst. He has changed his dress probably, except his boots, which were new and heavy.

I will give **$50** if taken and secured in the District of Columbia, or **$100** if taken north of the District, and secured in each case and delivered before the reward shall be good.

Dr. J. W. THOMAS.

Pomunky P. O., Charles Co., Md.

Chicago Historical Society, ICHi-22005

■ From colonial times through the abolition of slavery in 1865, runaways were a persistent problem for slaveholders. This advertisement was published in the Centerville, Maryland, *Times and Eastern-Shore Public Advertiser.* Typically, the owner describes the runaways in terms of their height, skin color, and other distinguishing characteristics. For example, Sam supposedly rolls his eyes "when spoken to." Runaways tended to be young men. This group of four, three men and a woman, probably had to go their separate ways, eventually, to avoid detection.

passed two caricatures: "Sambo" and "Mammy" were childlike and grateful, and "Nat" and "Jezebel" were surly, cunning, dangerous, and unpredictable. One Kentucky slave, Susan, was described by a planter in 1822 as "the biggest devil that ever lived." Susan reportedly poisoned a stud horse and set a stable on fire, causing $1500 worth of damage, after managing to escape from handcuffs.

Although some planters boasted of their fatherly solicitude for their slaves, in fact, slaveowners harbored deep fears about the men and women they held in bondage. These fears explain the barbaric punishments that some owners inflicted on men, women, and children. Whip-wielding overseers made pregnant women lie down in a trench in the fields, presumably so that the lash would not harm the fetus. Even in "respectable" southern families, slave owners branded, mutilated, and beat enslaved workers for resisting discipline or to deliver a warning to other potentially defiant slaves. In the slave South, American cries of freedom, equality, opportunity, and the blessings of citizenship rang hollow.

Conclusion

In the first two decades of the nineteenth century, striking historical developments stirred the spirit of American nationalism. The Louisiana Purchase magnified the natural wealth of the young nation, and the federal government encouraged citizens to exploit that wealth through trade and settlement. Both the Embargo of 1807 and the War of 1812 freed the country from the British menace in the West and on the high seas. The war also bolstered the American economy by stimulating technological innovation and the growth of manufacturing. Territorial expansion combined with economic development created new jobs for a burgeoning population. Unlike the rigidly class-conscious nations of Europe, America seemed to offer limitless possibilities—at least for propertied white men, the only people entitled to the full rights of citizenship.

Southern cotton planters and northern factory owners derived their newfound prosperity from very different sources: staple crop agriculture on one hand and the emerging industrial system on the other. At the same time, these two groups had much in common. As they expanded their operations, whether sprawling plantations or gigantic mill complexes,

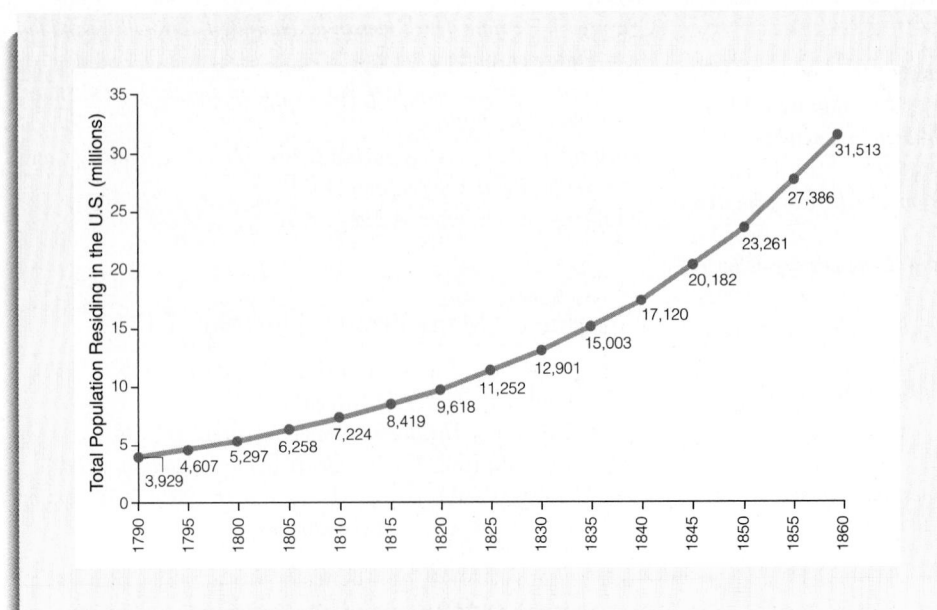

■ **FIGURE 10.2**
ESTIMATED POPULATION OF THE UNITED STATES, 1790–1860

Source: Historical Statistics of the United States, p. 7.

they displaced smaller landowners and raised land prices. Members of both elite groups proved restless entrepreneurs, eager to move around to find the freshest lands and the cheapest labor. Their personal wealth and their political power set them apart from the people under them— the slaves and wage earners—who produced that wealth. And both the southern "lords of the lash" and the northern "lords of the loom" depended on large numbers of slaves to grow cotton. Thus, the fluffy white fiber of the cotton boll is perhaps a most fitting symbol of the emerging American economy. Producing and processing it yielded tangible benefits for a few and created a new, harsher world of work for many.

Sites to Visit

The Lewis and Clark Expedition

www.cp.duluth.mn.us/~tmcs/lewsclrk1.htm

This site offers assorted materials treating the expedition that explored the Louisiana Territory.

The Barbary Treaties

www.yale.edu/lawweb/avalon/diplomacy/barbary

This site includes the texts of treaties between the United States and the Barbary states, 1786–1816.

Documents from the War of 1812

www.yale.edu/lawweb/avalon/diplomacy/britian/br1814m.htm

This site includes important documents from the War of 1812.

Whole Cloth: Discovering Science and Technology Through American Textile History

www.si.edu/lemelson/centerpieces/whole_cloth/

The Jerome and Dorothy Lemelson Center for the Study of Invention and Innovation and Society for the History of Technology assembled this site. It includes excellent activities and sources related to early American manufacturing and industry.

Indian Affairs: Laws and Treaties

www.library.okstate.edu/kappler/

This digitized text at Oklahoma State University includes preremoval treaties with the Five Civilized Tribes and other groups.

For Further Reading

General

Stephen E. Ambrose, *Undaunted Courage: Meriwether Lewis, Thomas Jefferson, and the Opening of the American West* (1996).

Joanne P. Melish, *Disowning Slavery: Gradual Emancipation and "Race" in New England, 1780–1860* (1998).

Theda Perdue, *Slavery and the Evolution of Cherokee Society, 1540–1866* (1979).

Carroll Pursell, *The Machine in America: A Social History of Technology* (1995).

Howard B. Rock, *Artisans of the New Republic: The Tradesmen of New York City in the Age of Jefferson* (1979).

Donald J. Weber, *The Spanish Frontier in North America* (1992).

The British Menace

W. Jeffrey Bolster, *Black Jacks: African-American Seamen in the Age of Sail* (1997).

Thomas J. Fleming, *Duel: Alexander Hamilton, Aaron Burr and the Future of America* (1999).

Bradford Perkins, *Prologue to War: England and the United States, 1805–1812* (1961).

Burton Spivak, *Jefferson's English Crisis: Commerce, Embargo, and the Republican Revolution* (1974).

John Sugden, *Tecumseh: A Life* (1998).

Fighting on Many Fronts: The War of 1812

Donald R. Hickey, *The War of 1812: A Forgotten Conflict* (1989).

Walter Lord, *The Dawn's Early Light* (1972).

Robert V. Remini, *The Battle of New Orleans* (1999).

Robert Allen Rutland, *The Presidency of James Madison* (1990).

David C. Skaggs and Larry L. Nelson, eds., *The Sixty Years' War for the Great Lakes, 1754–1814* (2001).

The "Era of Good Feelings"?

James H. Broussard, *The Southern Federalists, 1800–1816* (1979).

Theda Perdue, *Cherokee Women: Gender and Culture Change, 1700–1835* (1998).

Kirkpatrick Sale, *The Fire of His Genius: Robert Fulton and the American Dream* (2001).

Ronald Schultz, *The Republic of Labor: Philadelphia Artisans and the Politics of Class, 1720–1830* (1993).

Cynthia Shelton, *The Mills of Manayunk: Industrialization and Social Conflict in the Philadelphia Region, 1787–1837* (1986).

George Rogers Taylor, *The Transportation Revolution, 1815–1860* (1951).

The Rise of the Cotton Plantation Economy

Eugene D. Genovese, *Roll, Jordan, Roll: The World the Slaves Made* (1976).

Charles W. Joyner, *Down by the Riverside: A South Carolina Slave Community* (1984).

Ann Patton Malone, *Sweet Chariot: Slave Family and Household Structure in Nineteenth-Century Louisiana* (1992).

Michael Mullin, *Africa in America: Slave Acculturation and Resistance in the American South and British Caribbean* (1992).

Jeffrey Robert Young, *Domesticating Slavery: The Master Class in Georgia and South Carolina, 1670–1837* (1999).

Online Practice Test

Test your understanding of this chapter with interactive review quizzes at

www.ablongman.com/jonescreatedequal/chapter10

Expanding Westward: Society and Politics in the "Age of the Common Man," 1819–1832

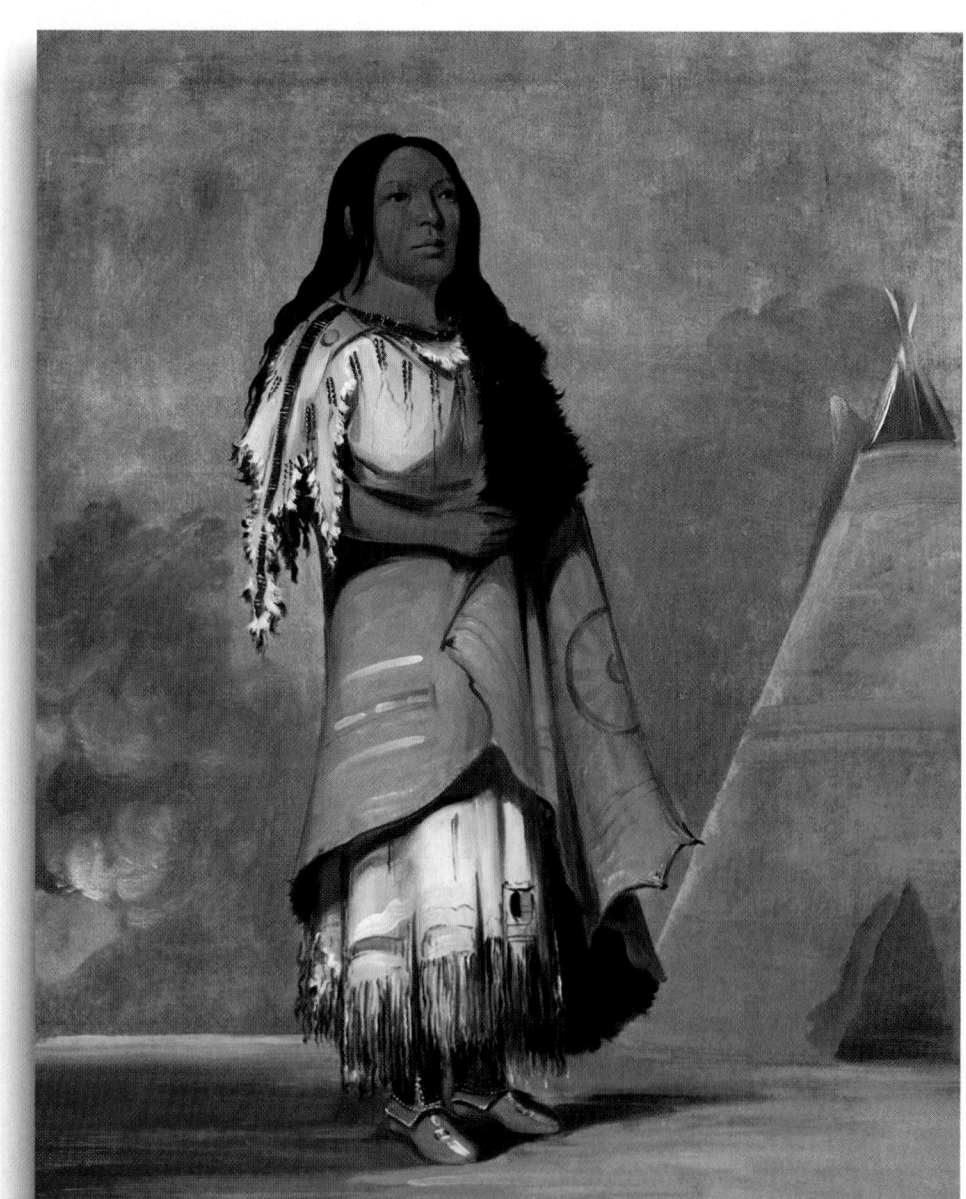

Smithsonian Institution, American Art Museum/Art Resource, NY

■ "Woman Who Strikes Many," Blackfeet, 1832.

CAMPAIGNING FOR POLITICAL OFFICE IN TENNESSEE IN THE 1820s WAS NOT AN ACTIVITY for the faint of heart. Candidates competed against each other in squirrel hunts, the loser footing the bill for the barbecue that followed. A round of speechmaking often was capped by several rounds of whiskey drinking enjoyed by candidates and supporters alike. Into this boisterous arena stepped a man unrivaled as a campaigner. David Crockett ran successfully for several offices, including local justice of the peace in 1818, state legislator in 1821 and 1823, and U.S. congressman in 1827, 1829, and 1833. The plainspoken Crockett knew how to play to a crowd and rattle a rival. He bragged about his skill as a bear hunter and ridiculed the fancy dress of his opponents. He condemned closed-door political caucuses (small groups of party insiders who hand-picked candidates) and praised grassroots democracy. Crockett claimed he could out-shoot, out-drink, and out-debate anyone who opposed him. If his opponent lied about him, why, then, he would lie about himself: "Yes fellow citizens, I can run faster, walk longer, leap higher, speak better, and tell more and bigger lies than my competitor, and all his friends, any day of his life." Crockett's blend of political theater and folksy backwoods banter earned him the allegiance of voters like him—men who, though having little formal education, understood the challenges of carving a homestead out of the dense thickets of western Tennessee.

Crockett's raucous brand of campaigning appealed to Westerners, that is, at this point in history, European Americans living just west of the Appalachian Mountains. His social betters might sniff that he was a rough, ignorant man—in the words of one Tennessee political insider, "more in his proper place, when hunting a Bear in the cane Brake, than he will be in the Capital." But newspaper reporters and defeated opponents alike grew to respect his ability to champion ordinary farmers. As a politician, Crockett spoke for debtors, squatters, and militia veterans of the Revolutionary War. He scorned the well-born in favor of men who could shoot down and skin a wolf.

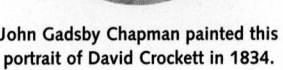

John Gadsby Chapman painted this portrait of David Crockett in 1834.

During the 1820s, European American settlers in the trans-Appalachian West transformed the style and substance of American politics. Beginning with Kentucky in 1792, western states began to relax or abolish property requirements for adult male voters. Even the English that Americans spoke changed. New words introduced into the political vocabulary reflected the rough-hewn, woodsman quality of western electioneering: candidates hit the campaign trail, giving stump speeches along the way. They supported their party's platform with its planks (positions on the issues). As legislators, they voted for pork-barrel projects that would benefit their constituents at home. Emphasizing his modest origins, David Crockett became widely known as Davy Crockett. (It is hard to imagine anyone calling the Sage of Monticello Tommy Jefferson.)

These developments reflected the movement of European Americans westward. In 1790, 100,000 Americans (not including Indians) lived west of the Appalachian

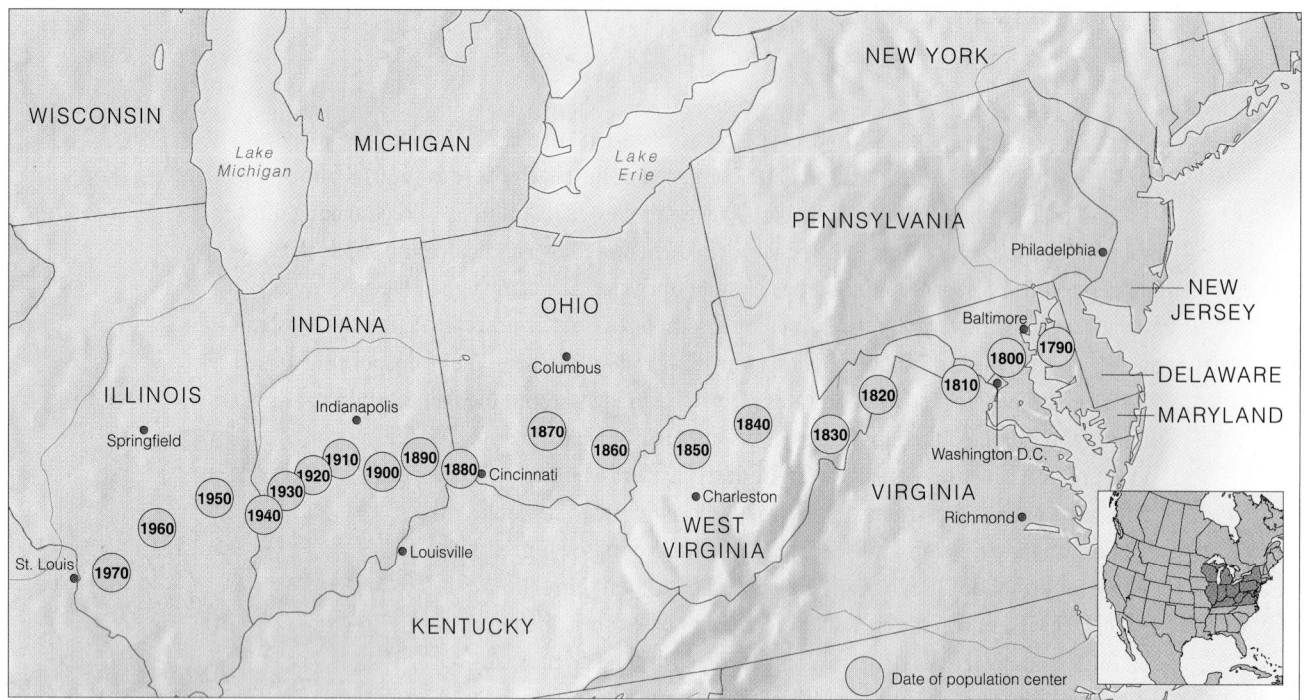

■ **MAP 11.1**
THE CENTER OF POPULATION MOVES WEST, 1790–1970   In 1830 most European Americans still lived
along the eastern seaboard. Yet the statistical center of the country had shifted dramatically westward as
settlers moved across the trans-Appalachian West. Migrants from the South sought out the fresh cotton
lands of Alabama and Mississippi, while New Englanders created new communities in the Upper Midwest.
Migration to areas such as Wisconsin and Georgia was contingent on the removal of Indians from those
areas, either by treaty or by military force.

Mountains; half a century later that number had increased to 7 million, or about 4 out of
10 Americans.

Western settlers attacked what they considered to be centralized, eastern-based institutions
of wealth and privilege. They scorned a six-person Supreme Court that could overturn the laws
of Congress and the individual states; the privately held Second Bank of the United States, which,
its critics charged, enriched its own board of directors at the expense of indebted farmers; and
federally sponsored internal improvements, such as turnpikes and canals, which, many western
homesteaders believed, served the interests of well-connected merchants and financiers.

Western voters rejoiced with the 1828 election of Andrew Jackson to the presidency;
here, they claimed, was a man who would battle eastern financiers and at the same time
support white settlers' claims to Indian lands in the West. Jackson held out the promise that
ordinary men would have a political voice and access to expanding economic opportunities.
Indeed, during these years, voter participation in presidential elections soared, from 25 percent of eligible voters in 1824 to 50 percent in 1828.

During his two terms in office (1828–1836), Andrew Jackson so dominated the American political landscape that historians have called him the symbol of an age and the representative man of his time. Born in humble circumstances, orphaned at age 14, Jackson
achieved public acclaim as a lawyer, a military officer, and, finally, president. In promoting a
strong central government, and the authority of the chief executive in particular, he fought
against foreign military forces (the British in the War of 1812) and Native Americans, and
he clashed with southern states' rights advocates. Jackson backed up his vision with the use

of violence and, at times, contempt for the law. Nevertheless, Jackson's view appealed strongly to workers and small farmers, men who resented what they called entrenched eastern privilege in politics and the economy.

Yet democracy had its limits during this period, for most people could not vote. Native Americans remained barred from even the rudiments of formal citizenship. White married women, who could neither own property nor vote, found themselves second-class citizens. Almost all free people of color, whether in the North, South, or Midwest, likewise lacked basic rights—to vote, serve on juries, or send their children to public school.

Further complicating this age was the rise of social classes. Acquiring great economic and political significance, the class system seemed to mock the idea of equality. The outlines of this system appeared in the 1820s in the Northeast, where business and factory managers received salaries, not hourly wages, and their wives were full-time homemakers and mothers. New forms of popular literature, such as the *Ladies Magazine,* published in Boston, glorified the middle-class family, especially the pious wife and mother who held moral sway over it.

The "age of the common man" was thus rife with irony. Jackson himself embodied many apparent contradictions. An Indian-fighter, he adopted a young Indian boy as his ward. A foe of privilege, he was a slave owner. A self-professed champion of farmers and artisans, he expressed contempt for their representatives in Congress. He also took steps to expand the power of the executive branch. The 1820s in general revealed these larger contradictions as national leaders pursued a more democratic form of politics on one hand and supported a system based on class and racial differences on the other. The resulting tensions shaped American society and politics in the third decade of the nineteenth century.

The Politics Behind Western Expansion

As the United States gained new territory through negotiation and conquest and people moved west, the nation felt the impact. Western debtors' economic distress echoed in eastern centers of finance. Congressional debates over whether Missouri should be admitted to the Union as a slave or free state sent shock waves throughout the country. Of the political conflict over the fate of slavery in the territories, the elderly Thomas Jefferson wrote, "This momentous question, like a firebell in the night, awakened and filled me with terror. I considered it at once as the death knell of the Union."

As new states were carved out of the west, gaining national influence in Congress, traditional methods of choosing candidates and the old political parties of Democratic-Republicans and Federalists came under fire. Parties began to choose their presidential nominees in conventions, not in caucuses of legislators. Rejecting practices that favored the wealthy, more and more states abolished the requirement that would-be voters and office holders had to own property. "The people must be heard!" became a rallying cry.

However, the opening of the West to European American settlement, which invigorated white men's democracy, also sowed seeds of economic and political conflict. Settlers made their way not through empty territory but through Native American homelands. Once in the West, most of these settlers faced the same kinds of conflicts that increasingly preoccupied Easterners, especially those between masters and slaves and debtors and creditors.

The Missouri Compromise

In 1819 the United States consisted of 22 states. Slavery was legal in half of them. Late that year, the territory of Missouri applied for statehood. This move set off panic in both the North and South because a twenty-third state was bound to upset the delicate balance of senators

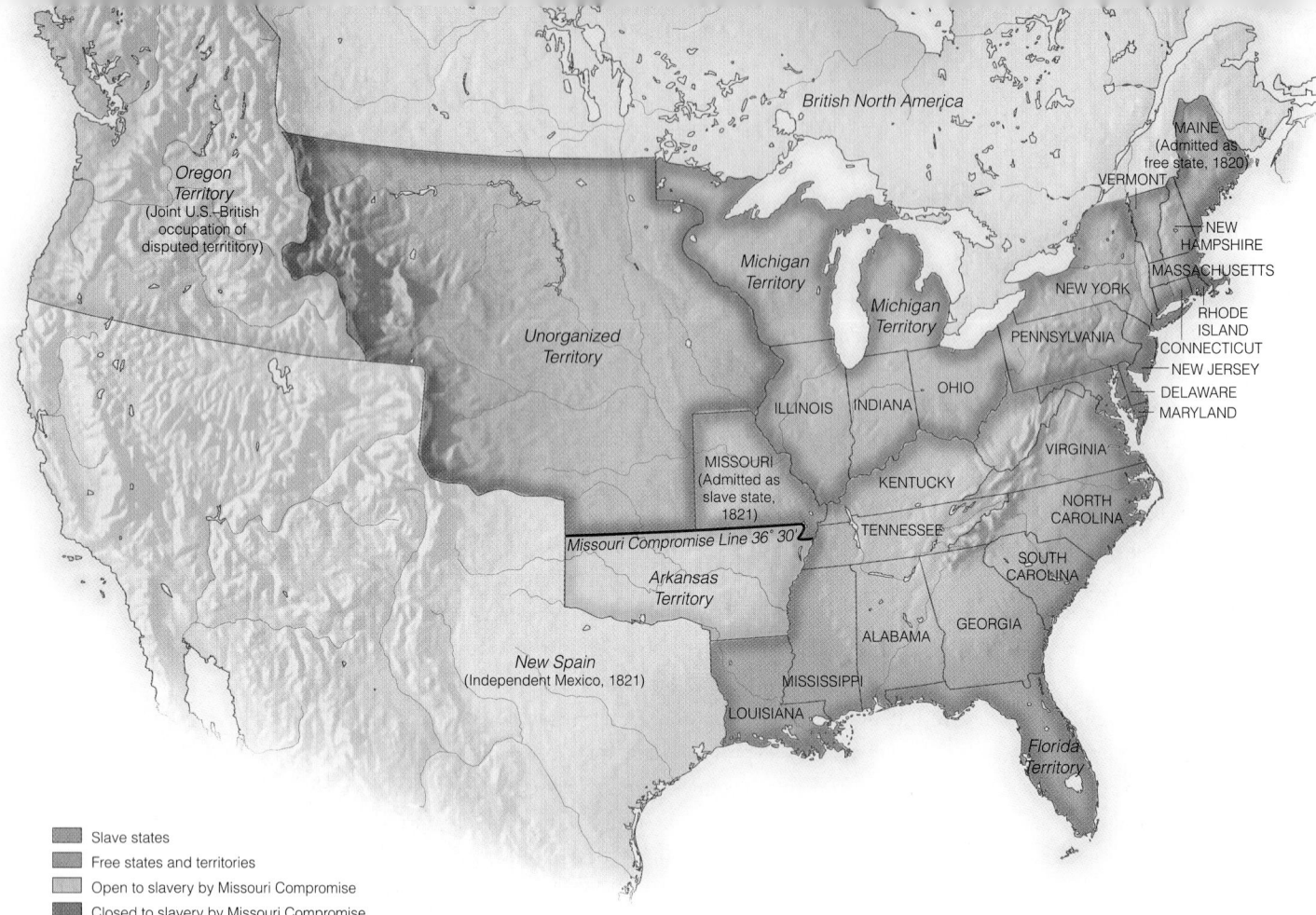

■ **MAP 11.2**

THE MISSOURI COMPROMISE Missouri applied for statehood in 1819, threatening the balance between 11 free and 11 slave states. According to a compromise hammered out in Congress, Missouri was admitted as a slave state, and Maine, formerly part of Massachusetts, was admitted as a free state. Slavery was banned above the 36°30′ parallel.

Legend:
- Slave states
- Free states and territories
- Open to slavery by Missouri Compromise
- Closed to slavery by Missouri Compromise

between slave and free states. Representative James Tallmadge of New York proposed a compromise: no slaves would be imported into Missouri in the future, and the new state would gradually emancipate the enslaved men and women living within its borders. The Tallmadge Amendment was defeated in the House as Southerners resisted this blatant attempt to limit the spread of slavery. The debate over the future of Missouri occupied Congress from December 1819 to March 1820.

In the Senate, Rufus King of New York claimed that Congress had the ultimate authority to set laws governing slavery. However, his colleague William Pinckney of Maryland retorted that new states possessed the same rights as the original 13; that is, they could choose whether to allow slavery. Maine's application for admission to the Union suggested a way out of the impasse. Speaker of the House of Representatives Henry Clay of Kentucky proposed a plan calling for Missouri to join the Union as a slave state. At the same time, Maine, originally part of Massachusetts, would become the twenty-fourth state and be designated a free one. In the future, slavery would be prohibited from all Louisiana Purchase lands north of latitude 36°30′, an area that included all territory north of present-day Missouri and Kansas. The House and the Senate finally approved the compromise, which maintained the balance between the number of slave and free states.

The day Congress sealed the compromise, Secretary of State John Quincy Adams walked home from the Capitol with Senator John C. Calhoun of South Carolina. The two men engaged in a muted but intense debate over slavery. Calhoun claimed that the institution "was the best guarantee to equality among the whites." Slavery, he asserted, demonstrated that all white men were equal to one another and superior to all blacks. Unnerved by Calhoun's comments,

Adams concluded that the debate over Missouri had "betrayed the secret of [Southerners'] souls." By reserving backbreaking toil for blacks, wealthy planters fancied themselves aristocratic lords of the manor. Adams confided in his diary that night, "They look down upon the simplicity of a Yankee's manners, because he has no habits of overbearing like theirs and cannot treat negroes like dogs."

Adams acknowledged that the compromise had kept the number of slave and free states in balance. Still, he reflected, slavery "taints the very sources of moral principle." Would it not have been better to confront the issue squarely and amend the Constitution in favor of free labor in all new states admitted to the Union? Adams feared that the North-South conflicts over the issues might someday imperil the nation itself. He concluded ominously, "If the Union must be dissolved, slavery is precisely the question upon which it ought to break." Five years later, Adams won the presidency of the United States. Elected separately by the voters, his vice president was none other than John C. Calhoun. Over the next four years, the two men managed to maintain an uneasy political alliance.

Ways West

Through land grants and government financing of new methods of transportation, Congress encouraged European American migrants to push their way west and south. The Land Act of 1820 enabled westerners to buy a minimum 80 acres at a price of $1.25 an acre in cash—even in those days, a bargain homestead. Built with the help of government legal and financial aid, new roads and canals, steamboats, and, after the early 1830s, railroads facilitated migration. Between 1820 and 1860, the number of steamboats plying the Mississippi River jumped from 60 to more than 1000. Canals linked western producers to eastern consumers of grains and cattle and connected western consumers to eastern producers of manufactured goods. Shipping costs and times between Buffalo and New York shrank. Cities such as Rochester and Syracuse, New York, and Cincinnati, Ohio, flourished because of their geographic position along waterways.

Americans took a variety of routes West. One route was taken in the 1820s by desperate planters moving out of the exhausted lands of the Upper South (the states of Virginia and Maryland), the Carolinas, and Georgia, westward into Alabama, Arkansas, Louisiana, and Mississippi. This migration across the Appalachian Mountains furthered the nationalist idea of the "expansion of liberty and freedom," a view held by many white men regardless of political affiliation. Yet it also spread slavery. The sight of slave "coffles"—groups of men, women, and children bound together in chains, hobbling down a city street or a country road—became increasingly common in this western region. In 1821 Virginia, North Carolina, South Carolina, and Georgia had produced two-thirds of the nation's cotton crop; the rest came from recently settled areas. Just a dozen years later the proportions shifted: Tennessee, Louisiana, Alabama, Mississippi, and Florida together produced two-thirds of all cotton, and the remaining one third came from older areas. The race to riches in the western portions of the South went to planters who had the most slaves and the most money to drain swamps and build the levees needed to hold back springtime river flooding. Soon a new planter elite—men and women who presided over vast slave holdings and lorded over their poor-white neighbors—dominated the lower Mississippi Valley.

European Americans also migrated across the border into Mexican territory. In 1821 Spain approved the application of a U.S. citizen, Moses Austin, to settle 300 American families on 200,000 fertile acres along the Colorado and Brazos river bottoms in southeastern Texas. Austin died soon after, but his son Stephen carried on his legacy. Within two years, the younger Austin had received permission (now from the government of newly independent Mexico) to bring in another 100 families. These settlers, together with squatters, numbered about 1500 people. Although the Mexican constitution prohibited slavery, some of the newcomers brought their slaves with them, and some free people of color came on their own. All these migrants from the United States called themselves Texians to distinguish themselves from the *Tejanos*, or Spanish-speaking

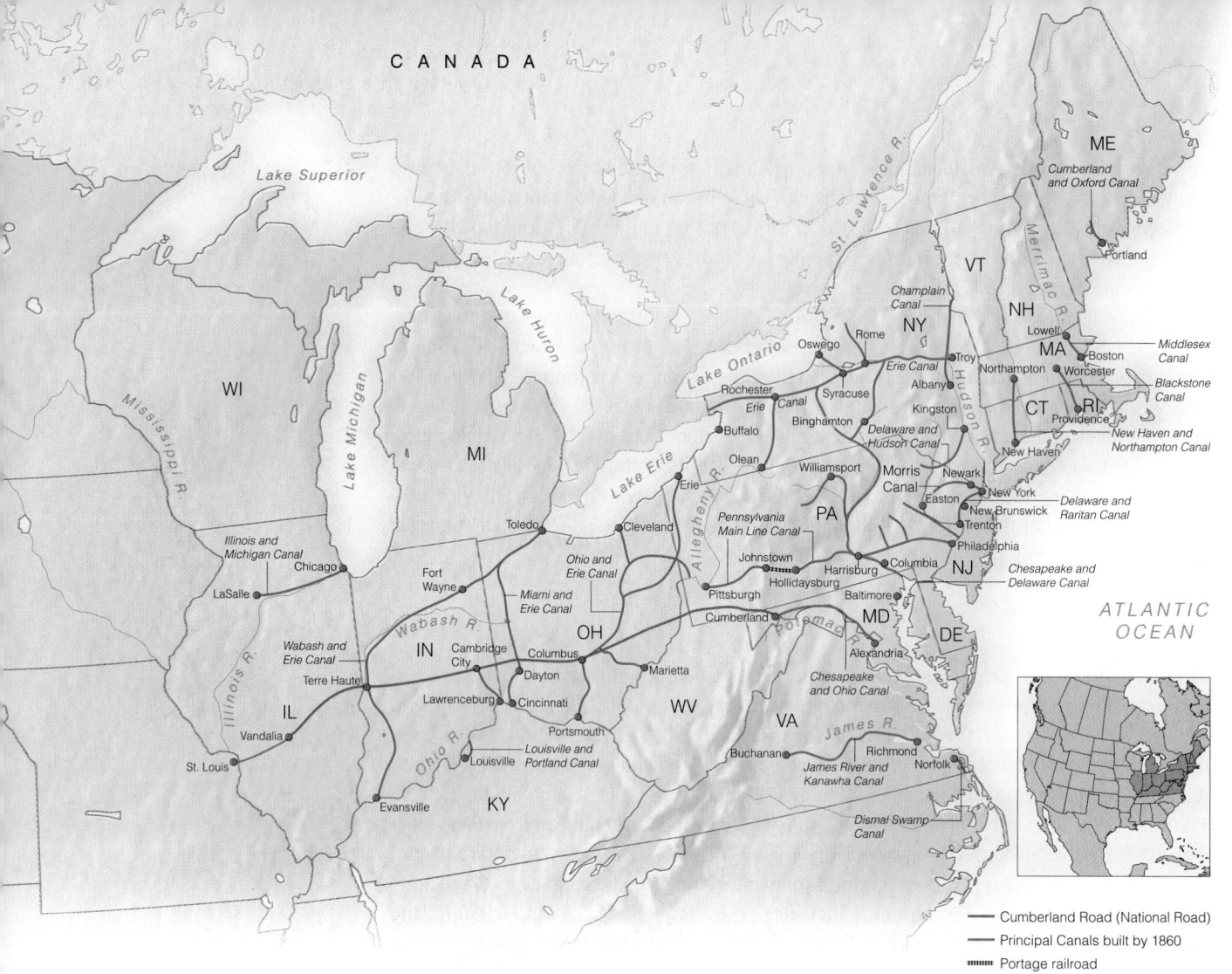

■ **MAP 11.3**

PRINCIPAL CANALS BUILT BY 1860 Many canals were expensive ventures and, in some cases, engineering nightmares. The Erie Canal had a competitive advantage because it snaked through the Mohawk Valley, the only major level pass through the mountain chain that stretched from Canada to Georgia. In contrast, the Pennsylvania Main Line Canal, which ran from Harrisburg to Pittsburgh, used a combination of inclined planes and steam engines in ten separate locations to haul boats up and down the Allegheny Mountains.

residents of the region. These newly arrived Texians agreed to adopt the Catholic faith and become citizens of Mexico. Eager for settlers to improve the land, Mexican authorities made it clear they would welcome new settlers "from hell itself," in the words of one official.

By late 1821 Mexico's independence had nullified the trade embargo that Spain had imposed on Mexico and on cities to the north, including Santa Fe and Albuquerque in New Mexico Territory. Ambitious people of all stripes rushed into New Mexico, including European American merchants who brought ready-made cloth (in the process displacing Hispanic and Native American textile producers), U.S. soldiers who claimed "God-given rights of conquest," and mountain men intent on harvesting animal pelts from the New Mexico Rocky Mountains.

In the 1820s, 900 additional families sponsored by Austin arrived in Texas. They were followed by 3000 squatters. This mass migration raised well-founded fears among Mexican officials that they would lose authority over the American newcomers within their borders.

The Panic of 1819 and the Plight of Western Debtors

In 1819 a financial panic swept across the nation, followed by an economic depression. The Second Bank of the United States played a major role in triggering this economic downturn, which came to be called the Panic of 1819. Granted a twenty-year charter by Congress

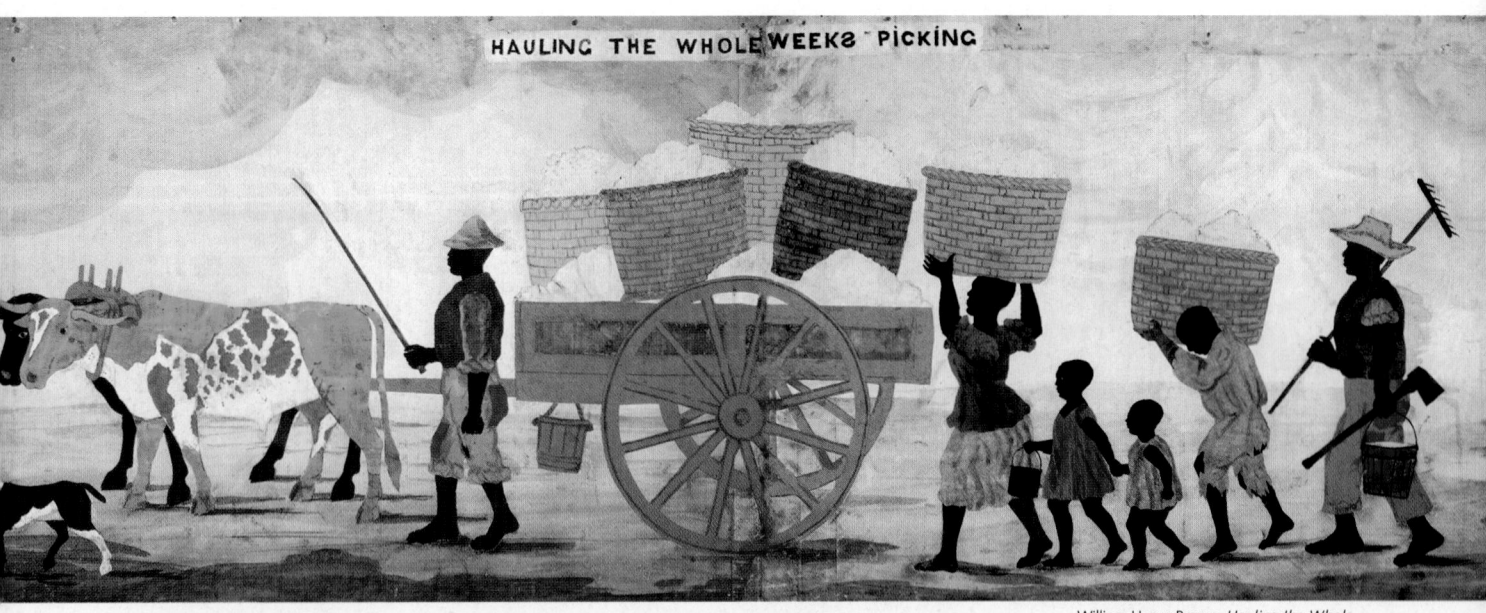

HAULING THE WHOLE WEEKS PICKING

■ The rich bottomlands of the Mississippi Delta proved ideal for growing cotton. After the forced removal of the Five Civilized Tribes from the Old Southwest, slave owners established expansive plantations in the delta. This scene, painted in 1842 by artist William Henry Brown, shows a group of slaves bringing in "the whole weeks picking" of cotton on the Vick plantation near Vicksburg, Mississippi.

William Henry Brown, *Hauling the Whole Weeks Picking*, 1842. The Historic New Orleans Collection, (1975.93.1 & 1975.93.2)

in 1816, the Bank resembled its predecessor, seeking to regulate the national economy through loans to state and local banks. In 1819 the Bank clamped down on small, local "wildcat" banks, which had extended credit to many people who could not repay their loans. Many homesteaders were not self-sufficient farmers but producers of staple crops or proprietors of small enterprises. They relied on credit from banks and local private lenders. As a result, the Bank's crackdown on wildcat banks had a devastating impact on western households. Debtors unable to meet their obligations had their mortgages foreclosed, their homes seized, and their crops and equipment confiscated. Ruined by the Panic of 1819, many western farmers developed an abiding hatred of the Bank of the United States and a deep resentment of eastern financiers.

Davy Crockett's own family history suggests the plight of families dependent on bank credit to create homesteads out of western territory. The son of a propertyless squatter, Crockett had an intense fear of debt. Although he campaigned as a hunter and a farmer, he had built several enterprises on land he leased or owned on Shoal Creek in south central Tennessee: a water-powered grist mill, a gunpowder factory (worked by slaves), an iron ore mine, and a liquor distillery. For each venture, he had to borrow money from local creditors. Spending much of his time away from home, Crockett relied on his wife, Elizabeth, and his children to manage these businesses. (He had nine children by Elizabeth and three by his first wife, Polly, who died in 1815.)

The depression of 1819 cut off Crockett's sources of credit, and in 1822 a flash flood swept away his grist mill and powder factory. Without milled grain, the distillery could no longer operate. Creditors immediately set upon the family, demanding payment of their debts. The Crocketts were fortunate enough to own land they could sell, using the proceeds to repay their debts. Nevertheless, they decided to move further west, to a remote area on the banks of the Obion River in northwest Tennessee. There they started over. Crockett described the area as a "complete wilderness" (although he noted that it was also "full of Indians who were hunting"). The region still showed the effects of an earthquake that had occurred in 1811. With its downed trees and thick brambles, the fissure-riddled landscape presented challenges to

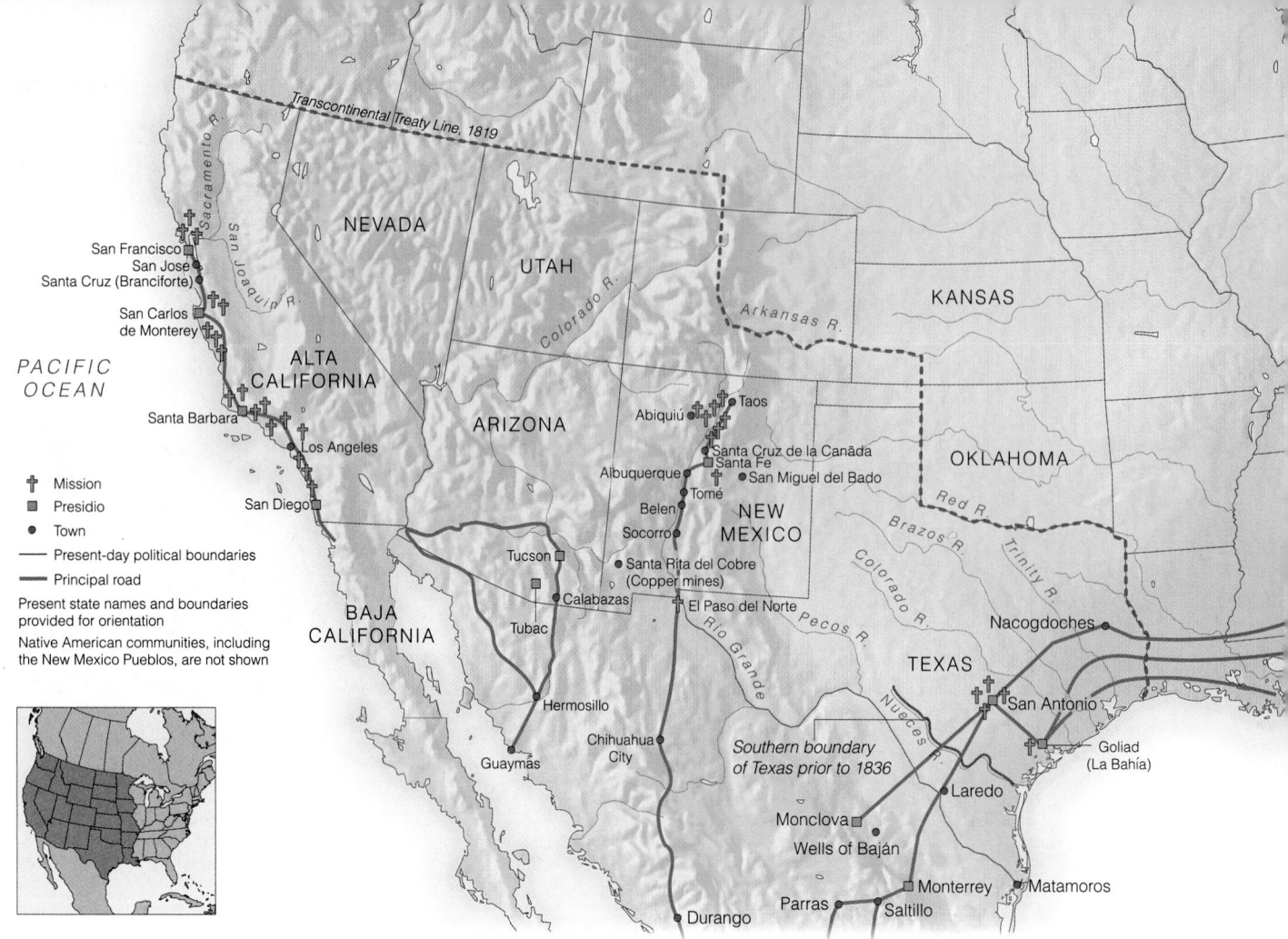

■ MAP 11.4

MEXICO'S FAR NORTHERN FRONTIER IN 1822 This map shows Mexico's far northern frontier in 1822. When Moses Austin died suddenly in 1821, the task of supervising the settlement of in-migrants from the United States fell to his son Stephen. The Mexican government authorized the younger Austin to act as empresario of the settlement. He was responsible for the legal and economic regulations governing the settlements clustered at the lower reaches of the Colorado and Brazos rivers.

the farmers who ventured there. Once again, Crockett needed bank loans, this time to buy flour and seed for cotton.

Many western settlers engaged in the same sort of cycle: borrowing to improve their land, then selling out and moving on. Unable to pay their debts, the least fortunate among them were thrown in jail. In several states, politicians urged the abolition of debtors' prison. They pointed out that jailing people who owed money did little to ensure that the debt would be repaid. New York state legislators passed such a law in 1831 in response to a group of well-to-do petitioners who argued that debtors' prison was "useless to the creditor—oppressive to the debtor—injurious to both."

Crockett advocated a system that would allow local sheriffs to buy debtors' property at bankruptcy auctions and then sell it back to the former owners. He denounced the bankers and other creditors, men who "had gone up one side of a creek and down another, *like a coon,* and pretended to grant the poor people great favors" in making them loans that the moneylenders knew they could not afford to repay. Then these creditors demanded their money and wiped out families, taking their land and livestock. Too often, according to Crockett, the backwoods farmer was burdened by debt and vulnerable to depressions and scheming creditors alike.

The Panic of 1819 caused widespread economic distress. Small farmers who lost their land through foreclosure could not produce crops for the eastern market, contributing to the rise in the price of food. Deprived of credit, small shopkeepers also felt the effects of the depression.

With rising unemployment, consumers could not afford to buy cloth, and as the demand for cotton fell, southern plantation owners, too, felt the contraction. Within a few years Andrew Jackson would capitalize on the fears and resentments of working men, farmers, planters, and tradesmen, as he championed the "common man" in opposition to what debtors called the "eastern monied interests." In doing so he would transform the two-party system.

The Monroe Doctrine

James Monroe won reelection easily in 1820. The depression did not affect his popularity. He also benefited from the disorganization of his opponents and from the demise of the Federalist party. Congressman John Randolph of Virginia suggested that the voters were unanimous on only one issue: their indifference to Monroe. As it turned out, the president's 231–1 victory in the Electoral College was the last chapter in the so-called Era of Good Feelings.

On the international front, Monroe's second term opened on a tense note. Foreign nations had started claiming land or promoting their own interests near U.S. borders. The United States remained especially wary of the Spanish presence on its southern and western borders. In 1818, President Monroe authorized General Andrew Jackson to broaden his assault on the Seminole Indians—a group composed of Native Americans and runaway slaves—in Florida. For the past two years, U.S. troops had pursued fugitive slaves into Spanish-held Florida. Now Jackson and his men seized the Spanish fort at Pensacola and claimed all of western Florida for the United States. The United States demanded that Spain either suppress the Seminole population or sell all of east Florida to the United States. With the Transcontinental Treaty of 1819, Spain gave up its right to both Florida and Oregon (although Britain and Russia still claimed land in Oregon). In 1822 General Jackson became the first governor of Florida Territory.

In 1821 the czar of Russia forbade non-Russians from entering the territory north of the fifty-first parallel and the open sea 100 miles off the coast of what is now Canada and Alaska. The Russians had established trading posts up

TABLE 11-1		
The Election of 1820		
Candidate	**Political Party**	**Electoral Vote**
James Monroe	Democratic-Republican	231
John Quincy Adams	Democratic-Republican	1

and down that coast, some almost as far south as San Francisco Bay. Meanwhile, the crowned heads of Europe were cracking down on popular rebellions (in Italy in 1821 and Spain in 1823). Rumors circulated that these monarchs were planning new invasions of Latin America.

Fearful of an alliance between Russia, Prussia, Austria, Spain, and France, President Monroe and Secretary of State John Quincy Adams formulated a policy that became a landmark in American diplomatic history. Adams rejected a British proposal that Great Britain and the United States join forces to oppose a further Spanish encroachment in Latin America. He convinced Monroe that the United States must stand alone against the European powers—Spain in the South and Russia in the Northwest—if it hoped to protect its own interests in the Western Hemisphere. In his annual message to Congress in December 1823, the president declared that the era of Europe's colonization of the Americas had ceased. Henceforth, he said, foreign nations would not be allowed to intervene in the Western Hemisphere.

The United States conceived the so-called Monroe Doctrine as a self-defense measure aimed specifically at Russia, Spain, and Britain. With the Russo-American Treaty of 1824, Russia agreed to pull back its claims to the area north of 54°40′, the southern tip of the present-day Alaska panhandle. However, the United States did not have the naval power to back up the Monroe Doctrine with force.

In its earliest form, the doctrine was more a statement of principle than a blueprint for action. The United States sought to discourage European powers from political or military meddling in the Western Hemisphere. The doctrine would have greater international significance in the late nineteenth century, when the United States developed the military might to enforce it.

The Strange Career of the Monroe Doctrine

What U.S. president was responsible for relocating several hundred suspected Taliban and Al Qaeda terrorists from Afghanistan to Cuba in early 2002? President George W. Bush had ultimate authority for the decision, of course; he claimed that intelligence officers needed to interrogate the men in a secure U.S. military installation, away from war-torn Afghanistan. Yet indirectly, at least, the detainees found themselves in steel cages on the shores of Guantanamo Bay because President James Monroe had announced his famous doctrine to the world almost 180 years before.

At the time, Monroe and his secretary of state, John Quincy Adams, saw threats to U.S. economic interests and national security. Both Russia and Great Britain were making territorial claims in the Northwest, in what was called Oregon Country. To the south of the

United States, a number of Spanish colonies had won, or were about to win, their independence: Chile in 1818, Mexico in 1821, Brazil in 1822, and Venezuela in 1824. The Monroe administration hoped to convince Spain, France, and Portugal not to take advantage of this unstable situation.

However, over the years, the purpose of the doctrine shifted from trying to keep the European powers from recolonizing any part of the Americas to justifying U.S. territorial acquisition and attempts to police and intervene in the domestic affairs of Latin American countries. For example, Presidents Tyler and Polk cited the doctrine to further the nation's continental expansion, including the conquest of Texas and California. In the mid–1890s, Secretary of State Richard Olney justified the U.S. decision to intervene in a border dispute between Britain and Venezuela by proclaiming, "Today the United States is practically sovereign on this continent and its fiat is law . . . its infinite resources combined with its isolated position render it master of the situation and practically invulnerable as against any or all other powers."

The American victory over Spain in the War of 1898 gave policymakers an opportunity to gain influence over Cuban domestic matters. The Platt Amendment to the Cuban–American Treaty of 1903 restricted the freedom of the newly independent Cuban government. Under pressure from the United States, Cuba incorporated into its constitution provisions that barred a foreign power (other than the United States) from intervening in Cuban political and economic affairs and gave the United States the right to buy or lease sites for naval installations (including the site at Guantanamo Bay). In 1934 President Franklin D. Roosevelt nullified most provisions of the Platt Amendment, but the United States retained its right to the base at Guantanamo. This decision was part of U.S. actions to claim small but geographically critical land holdings around the globe to use for military purposes: imperial claims to Guam, Hawaii, and the Philippines in addition to the base in Cuba, for example.

Theodore Roosevelt devised his famous policy called the Roosevelt Corollary to justify military intervention into Central American countries that

Andrew Jackson's Rise to Power

The election of 1824 provided a striking contrast to the bland affair four years earlier. In 1824 the field of presidential nominees was crowded, suggesting a party system in disarray. In the spirit of openness, secretive congressional caucuses no longer nominated presidential candidates. Instead, a number of states backed their "favorite sons" in the presidential race. Although all the candidates called themselves "Democratic-Republicans," the label meant little more than the fact that most politicians sought to distance themselves from the outmoded "Federalist" label, which hearkened back to the post-Revolutionary period, rather than pointing forward to the nation's new challenges. Secretary of State John Quincy Adams threw his hat in the ring. Other nominees included Representative Henry Clay of Kentucky and Andrew Jackson, now a senator from Tennessee. Jackson received the highest number of electoral votes (99), but no candidate achieved a majority. As a result, the election went to the House of Representatives. The Twelfth Amendment to the Constitution, adopted in 1804, provided for separate electoral balloting for the office of vice president, and John C. Calhoun won that vote.

Clay withdrew from the race. He had promised Jackson his support but then endorsed Adams, whom the House subsequently elected. When Adams named Clay secretary of state,

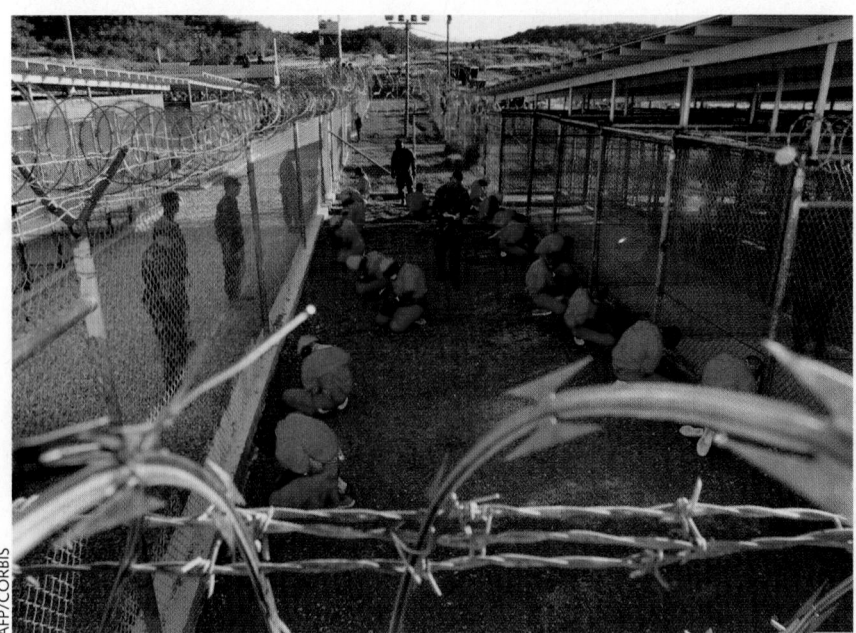

Guantanamo Bay with Al-Qaeda prisoners

communist nation. Presidents John F. Kennedy and Ronald Reagan cited the Monroe Doctrine in pushing Congress to authorize the use of force against the spread of communism in Latin America. Yet by 1989 President George Bush felt no need to justify his administration's action in Panama, when U.S. troops forcibly seized dictator Manuel Noriega and returned him to the United States to stand trial on charges of drug smuggling.

Over the generations, the Monroe Doctrine has proved a flexible policy, providing justification for almost any action the United States deemed necessary to its self-interest, broadly defined. Detaining Al Qaeda members at the Guantanamo naval station, for example, allows U.S. authorities to hold them securely, without the dangers of keeping them on American soil, where democratic traditions and constitutional rules might complicate the situation. This state of affairs exemplifies both the strength and the weakness of the Monroe Doctrine; the United States controls a small piece of Cuba, but the communist regime there stubbornly endures. ■

were indebted to American banks or businesses. Under Roosevelt's Big Stick policy, U.S. marines landed in Nicaragua in 1912 and remained in the country until 1933. The stated purpose of the occupation was to make certain that Nicaragua paid off its debts to U.S. banks. A guerrilla group led by General Augusto Cesar Sandino led an armed resistance against the American troops. In the mid–1970s, members of a resistance movement fighting the repressive Somoza regime in Nicaragua called themselves Sandinistas in honor of the general, who was killed by Nicaraguan government troops in 1934.

As a result of the revolution led by Fidel Castro in 1959, Cuba became a

Jackson's supporters cried foul. The election, they charged, amounted to nothing more than a corrupt deal between two political insiders.

Haunted by these charges, Adams served his four-year term under a cloud of public distrust. A member of a respected New England family and the son of former president John Adams, the new chief executive had served with distinction in Monroe's cabinet. Still, Adams proved ill suited to the rough-and-tumble world of what came to be called the New Democracy. Adams held strong political views; he advocated a greater federal role in internal improvements and public education, a variation on Henry Clay's "American System," a set of policies which promoted a national bank, public funding of canals and turnpikes, and a high tariff to protect domestic manufactures.

Adams's party, which called itself the National Republicans, faced a formidable challenge in the election of 1828. Having seethed for four long years, Andrew Jackson's

TABLE 11-2

The Election of 1824

Candidate	Political Party	Popular Vote	Electoral Vote
John Quincy Adams	Democratic-Republican	108,740	84
Andrew Jackson	Democratic-Republican	153,544	99
William H. Crawford	Democratic-Republican	46,618	41
Henry Clay	Democratic-Republican	47,136	37

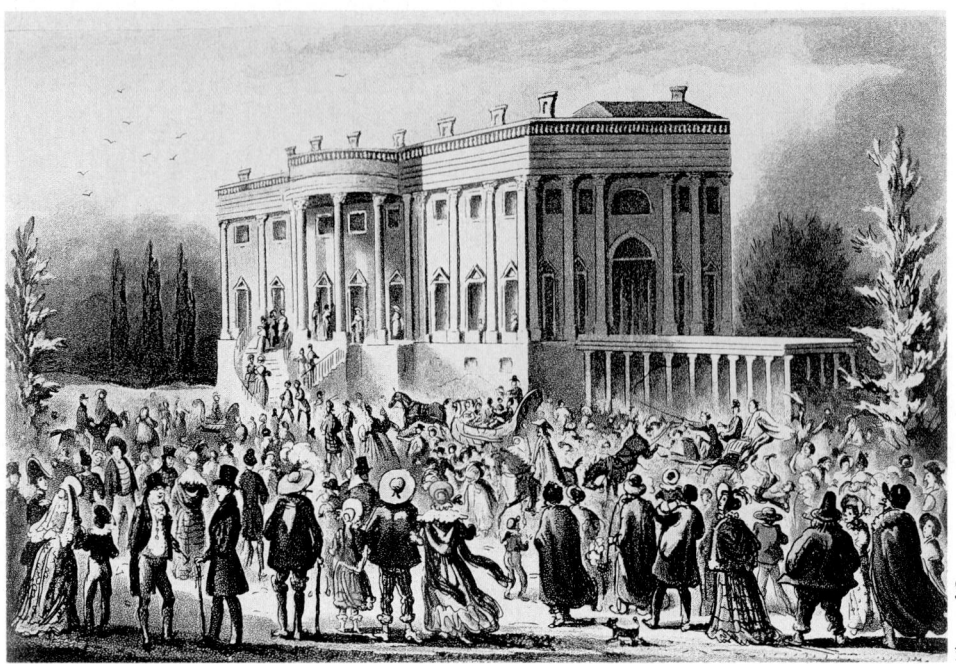

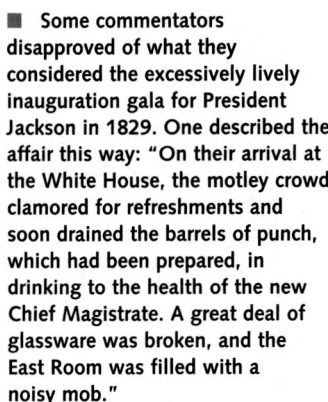

■ Some commentators disapproved of what they considered the excessively lively inauguration gala for President Jackson in 1829. One described the affair this way: "On their arrival at the White House, the motley crowd clamored for refreshments and soon drained the barrels of punch, which had been prepared, in drinking to the health of the new Chief Magistrate. A great deal of glassware was broken, and the East Room was filled with a noisy mob."

Library of Congress

supporters (the Democratic-Republicans) now urged "the people" to reclaim the White House. The campaign was a nasty one. Jackson's opponents attacked his personal morality and that of his wife and his mother. Jackson's supporters countered with the charge that Adams himself was corrupt and that he and his cronies must be swept from office. At campaign rallies, Jacksonians waved about brooms to signal their disgust with the current administration.

By the time of the 1828 election, the Democratic-Republicans and their rivals had developed sophisticated national organizations. They sponsored local entertainments such as parades and barbecues. These gatherings brought out the vote and cultivated party loyalty. With the decline of state laws regulating voter qualifications, ordinary people in the South and the West cast ballots for the first time. The "Hero of the Battle of New Orleans" won a stunning victory, accumulating a record 647,292 popular votes. His supporters hailed the well-to-do slaveholder as the president of the "common" (meaning white) man.

In office, Jackson tightened his party's grip on power by introducing a national political spoils system. Through this process, successful candidates rewarded their supporters with jobs and tossed their rivals out of appointed offices. The spoils system let the Democratic-Republicans—now called the Democrats—build a nationwide political machine. Not surprisingly, it also provided fertile ground for corruption.

TABLE 11-3			
The Election of 1828			
Candidate	Political Party	Popular Vote	Electoral Vote
Andrew Jackson	Democratic	647,292	178
John Quincy Adams	National Republican	508,064	83

Federal Authority and Its Opponents

When Americans defeated the British in the War of 1812, they ensured the physical security of the new nation. However, the war's end left a crucial question unanswered: what role would federal authority play in a republic of states? During Andrew Jackson's tenure, Congress, the chief executive, and the Supreme Court all jockeyed for influence over one another and over the states. To be sure, some groups, such as the Cherokee nation, challenged federal power. But these efforts failed against the sheer determination of Andrew Jackson. During his term in office, Jackson claimed a broad popular mandate, the authority the people gave him to act, in his effort to increase the power of the presidency.

At the same time, militant southern sectionalists regarded the growth of federal executive and judicial power with alarm. If the president could impose a high tariff on the states and if the Supreme Court could deny the states the authority to govern Indians within their own borders, might not high-handed federal officials someday also threaten the South's system of slavery?

Judicial Federalism and the Limits of Law

In a series of notable cases, the Supreme Court, under the leadership of Chief Justice John Marshall, sought to limit states' power to control people and resources within their own boundaries. In *McCulloch v. Maryland* (1819), the Court supported Congress's decision to grant the Second Bank of the United States a 20-year charter. The state of Maryland had imposed a high tax on notes issued by the bank. Declaring that "the power to tax involves the power to destroy," the Supreme Court ruled the state's action unconstitutional. The court justices held that, although the original Constitution did not mention a national bank, Congress retained the authority to create such an institution. This fact implied that Congress also had the power to preserve it. This decision relied on what came to be called a "loose construction" of the Constitution to justify "implied powers" of the government. Under a "loose" construction, or interpretation, of the Constitution, the federal government reserved for itself forms of authority not explicitly stated in the Constitution. Similarly, in deciding *Cohens v. Virginia* (1821), the Court limited the power of individual states. The Cohens had been convicted of illegally selling lottery tickets. The Supreme Court upheld their conviction but also asserted its own authority to review state legislation that affected the federal government's powers.

In 1832 a case involving the rights of the Cherokee nation brought the Court head to head with President Jackson's own brand of federal muscle-flexing. With the expansion of cotton cultivation into upland Georgia in the early nineteenth century, white residents of that state increasingly resented the presence of their Cherokee neighbors.

At the same time, some Cherokees worked and worshipped in ways similar to European Americans: they cultivated farmland, converted to Christianity, and established a formal legal code. A census authorized by the Cherokee Nation in 1828 enumerated the population and provided evidence of the group's conformity to whites' ways. For example, the 2600 residents of Georgia's Coosewaytee District owned a total of 295 slaves, 2944 black cattle, 1207 horses, 4965 swine, 113 looms, 397 spinning wheels, 461 plows, and several sawmills, grist mills, and blacksmith shops. Two missionary schools had a total of 21 Cherokee pupils. On July 4, 1827, Cherokee leaders met in convention to devise a republican constitution. In the grand tradition of the Patriots of 1776, the group proclaimed itself a sovereign nation, responsible for its own affairs and free of the dictates of individual states.

By the late 1820s certain white people, including the president, were calling for the removal of the Cherokee from the Southeast. The 1829 discovery of gold in the Georgia hills brought 10,000 white miners to Cherokee territory in a gold rush that the Indians called the "Great Intrusion." Whites, it seemed, were less interested in Indian assimilation and religious conversion than they were in the riches to be extracted from Indian land. President Jackson saw the very existence of the Cherokee nation as an affront to his authority and a hindrance to Georgia's economic well-being. He resented the fact that the Cherokee considered themselves a sovereign nation, independent of the U.S. president. Jackson also feared that the Cherokee would prevent whites from mining or farming land within Indian borders. Jackson, in fact, favored removing all Indians from the Southeast to make way for whites. He declared that Georgia should be rid of "a few thousand savages" so that "towns and prosperous

	Census of 1809	Census of 1824	Percent of Change 1809–1824
Cherokee Population	12,395	16,060	30%
Negro slaves	583	1,277	119
Whites	314	215	-29
Schools	5	18	260
Students	94	314	234
Gristmills	13	36	177%
Sawmills	3	13	333
Blacksmith shops	—	62	—
Stores	—	9	—
Tanyards	—	2	—
Powder mills	1	1	—
Looms	429	762	78%
Spinning wheels	1,572	2,486	58
Wagons	30	172	473
Plows	567	2,923	416
Threshing machines	—	1	—
Horses	6,519	7,683	18%
Cattle	19,165	22,531	18
Swine	19,778	46,732	136
Sheep	1,037	2,566	147
Goats	—	430	—

■ **FIGURE 11.1**
CHEROKEE NATION INTERCENSUS CHANGES, 1809–1824

Source: Douglas C. Wilms, "Cherokee Land Use in Georgia Before Removal," in William L. Anderson, ed., *Cherokee Removal: Before and After* (Athens: University of Georgia Press).

farms" could develop there. In 1830, with the president's backing, Congress passed the Indian Removal Act. The Act provided for "an exchange of lands with the Indians residing in any of the states or territories, and for their removal west of the river Mississippi."

Outraged by this naked land grab, the Cherokee Nation refused to sign the removal treaties specified by Congress as part of the Indian Removal Act. In a petition to Congress in 1830, members of the group declared, "We wish to remain on the land of our fathers. We have a perfect and original right to claim this, without interruption or molestation." In a message to his own people in 1831, Cherokee leader John Ross invoked the promise of President Jackson himself. Ross noted that the president had claimed two years earlier that *"so far as we had rights we should be protected in them."*

Citing both the treaties that guaranteed them a right to the land and the "laws of the United States made in pursuance of treaties," the Cherokee Nation appealed to the Supreme Court. In an effort to protect their land titles, the Indian nation had first tried to take its case to Georgia courts, but Georgia refused to allow it to press its claim. The Georgia legislature maintained that it had authority over all the Indians living within the state's borders, and that the Cherokee nation lacked jurisdiction over its own people.

The Cherokee hoped that the Supreme Court would support their position that they were an independent entity, not bound by the laws of Georgia. In a set of cases—*Cherokee Nation v. Georgia* (1831) and *Worcester v. Georgia* (1832)—the Court agreed that Georgia's

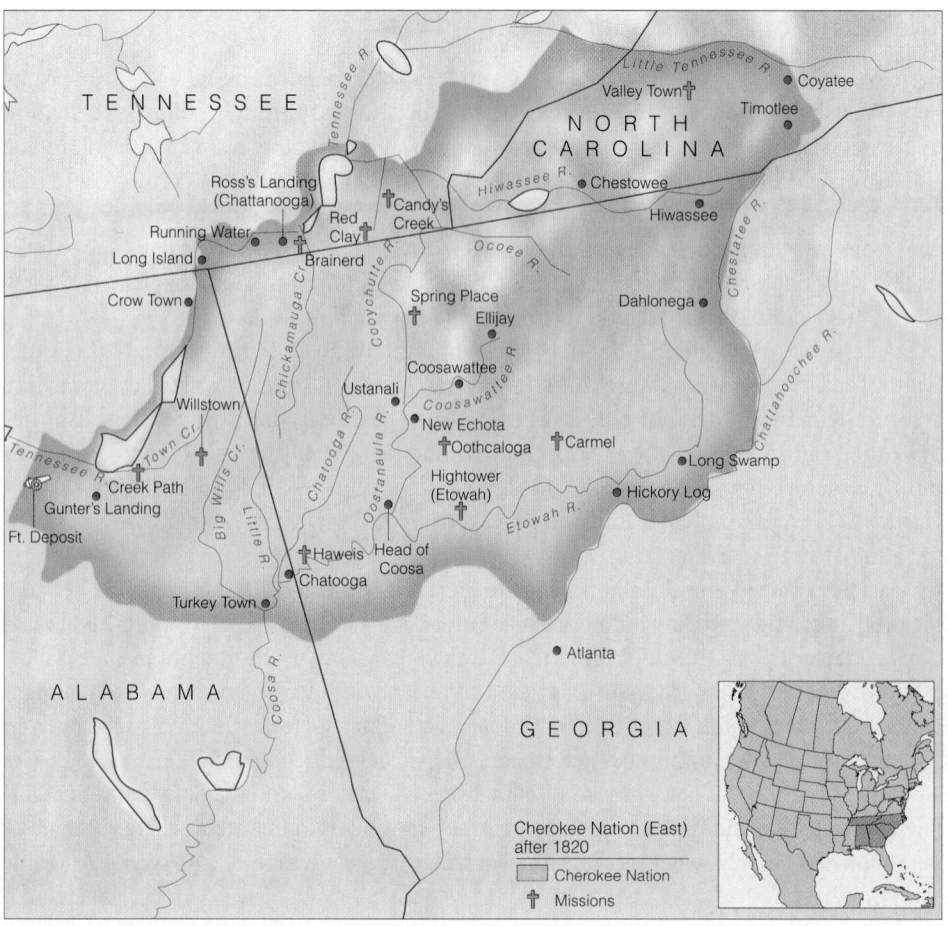

■ MAP 11.5

THE CHEROKEE NATION AFTER 1820   This map shows the Cherokee nation on the eve of removal to Indian Territory (present-day Oklahoma). The discovery of gold in the region sparked a constitutional battle over control of Cherokee land. In 1832 the Supreme Court ruled that the federal government had ultimate authority over Indian nations. The state of Georgia ignored the ruling and sought to enforce its own laws in Cherokee territory.

authority did not extend to the Cherokee Nation. The Court proclaimed that Indian self-governing bodies were "domestic dependent nations" under the authority of the U.S. government, not the individual states. Under this ruling, Georgia lacked the authority to force Indians from their land. More generally, the states must defer to the federal government in issues related to the welfare and governance of the Indians. Governor Wilson Lumpkin of Georgia rejected these Supreme Court rulings. In 1832 he declared, "It is due to the sovereign character of every State of the Union to maintain its territorial rights and policy over its own population." Jackson, too, ignored the Court's display of judicial authority. Of the *Worcester* decision, Jackson declared, "John Marshall has made his decision. Now let him enforce it."

Some of the president's own supporters protested his determination to deprive landowners—even Indian landowners—of their personal property. Davy Crockett announced that he was voting his conscience and opposing Jackson's Indian removal policy. Declared Crockett, "I believed it was a wicked, unjust measure, and that I should go against it, let the cost to myself be what it might." Nevertheless, in 1832 the president sent troops to Georgia to begin forcing the Indians out of their homeland.

The "Tariff of Abominations"

Besides engineering the removal of the Cherokees, Jacksonian Democrats continued the post–War of 1812 policy of high tariffs. In 1828 they pushed through Congress legislation that raised fees on imported manufactured products and raw materials such as wool. Facing a disastrous decline in cotton prices after the Panic of 1819, Southerners protested: to survive, they had to both sell their cotton on the open world market and buy high-priced supplies from New England or Europe. In their view, the higher the tariff on English goods, the less likely the English were to continue to purchase their cotton from southern planters. Southerners dubbed the 1828 legislation the "Tariff of Abominations."

A renewal of the tariff four years later moderated the 1828 rates. But by this time, South Carolina politicians were in no mood to sit back and accept what they saw as the arrogant wielding of federal power. They drew on past precedents in developing a theory called nullification—the idea that individual states had the authority to reject, or nullify, federal laws. The Virginia and Kentucky Resolutions of 1798 and 1799 and the Hartford Convention of New England states during the War of 1812 had previously raised the issue of state sovereignty.

Led by Senator John C. Calhoun, the nullifiers met in a convention in 1832 and declared the tariff "null and void" in South Carolina. But Jackson struck back swiftly. In his Nullification Proclamation of December 10, 1832, he argued that states' rights did not include nullification of federal laws or secession from the Union. The president then sent a token military and naval force to South Carolina to intimidate the nullifiers. Henry Clay, now senator from Kentucky, brokered a compromise agreement: a 10 percent reduction in the Tariff of 1832 over a period of eight years. This compromise finally eased tensions, and the South Carolina nullifiers retreated for the time being. However, they continued to maintain "that each state of the Union has the right, whenever it may deem such a course necessary . . . to secede peaceably from the Union."

The "Monster Bank"

The repository of federal funds ($10 million), the Bank of the United States in the 1830s had 30 branches and controlled the money supply by dictating how state banks should repay their loans: in paper notes or in currency. After the expiration of the charter of the first Bank of the United States in 1818, Americans relied on a combination of state bank notes and on coins minted by the individual states as well as by foreign countries. Congress attempted to relieve the chaotic money and state-banking system by chartering a Second Bank of the United States in 1816. As a central (though privately held) institution, the bank also aided economic growth and development by extending loans to commercial enterprises.

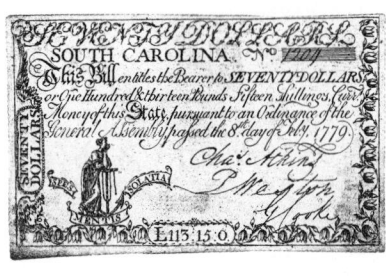

In 1832, Jackson vetoed a bill that would have renewed the charter of the Second Bank of the United States, which was due to expire in 1836. Somewhat contradictorily, Jackson claimed to represent the interests of small lenders such as farmers, but he also advocated hard money (currency in the form of gold or silver, not paper or credit extended by banks). Traditionally, small lenders objected to hard money policies, which kept the supply of currency low and interest rates for borrowers high. Jackson also objected to the bank's work as a large commercial institution. For example, he blamed the bank for precipitating the Panic and Depression of 1819 by withholding credit from small banks, causing them to recall their loans and, in some cases, fail.

José Agustin de Escudero Describes New Mexico as a Land of Opportunity, 1827

In the early nineteenth century, many people believed that the West afforded abundant economic opportunities for those willing to work hard. However, in most areas of the trans-Appalachian West, farming was a risky venture. Farmers needed cash or credit to hire hands—or to buy slaves—to clear dense underbrush and make other improvements on the land. Floods and droughts could wipe out a year's hard work and ruin even the most industrious family.

Nevertheless, certain frontier livelihoods did not take large investments in labor or equipment. In 1827, José Agustin de Escudero, a lawyer from the Mexico state of Chihuahua, visited the northern reaches of his country and reported on the partido system of sheep raising in the colony of New Mexico. He reported that the quality and expanse of the land meant that young men of modest means could prosper after a few years without securing large loans.

It can be asserted that there were no paupers in New Mexico at that time, nor could there be any. At the same time, there were no large-scale stockmen who could pay wages or make any expenditure whatever in order to preserve and increase their wealth in this branch of agriculture. A poor man, upon reaching the age when one generally starts a family, would go to a rich stockman and offer to help him take care of one or more herds of sheep. These flocks were composed of *a thousand* ewes and *ten* breeding rams, which were never separated from the herd as is the practice of stock raisers in other countries. Consequently, in each flock, not a single day would go by without the birth of two or three lambs, which the shepherd would put with the ewe and force the female to suckle without the difficulties which he would have had with a larger number of offspring. The shepherd would give the owner ten or twenty per cent of these sheep and an equal amount of wool, as a sort of interest, thus preserving the capital intact.

From the moment he received the flock, the shepherd entered into a contract in regard to the future increase, even with his own overseer. As a matter of fact, he usually contracted it at the current market price, two reales per head [an advance from the stockman], the future increase to be delivered in small numbers over a period of time. With this sum, which the shepherd had in advance, he could construct a house, and take in other persons to help him care for and shear the sheep, which was done with a knife instead of shears. The milk and sometimes the meat from the said sheep provided him sustenance; the wool was spun by his own family into blankets, stockings, etc., which could also be marketed, providing an income. Thus the wealth of the shepherd would increase until the day he became, like his overseer, the owner of a herd. He, in turn, would let out his herds to others after the manner in which he obtained his first sheep and made his fortune. Consequently, even in the homes of the poorest New Mexicans, there is never a dearth of sufficient means to satisfy the necessities of life and even to afford the comfort and luxuries of the wealthiest class in the country.

José de Escudero was a visitor to, not a resident of, New Mexico. It is possible that he oversimplified the partido shepherds' self-sufficiency in this region. Soon after winning its independence from Spain, Mexico opened New Mexico to U.S. traders. By the mid–1820s, traders were leading mule trains along the Santa Fe Trail, which ran from Franklin, Missouri, to Santa Fe, New Mexico. In his account here, de Escudero indirectly highlights the roles of wives and mothers (as spinners and weavers of cloth) in preserving the economic independence of the shepherds' households.

Nevertheless, de Escudero's observations suggest that a combination of factors, including the nature of the landscape itself (in this case suitable for sheep grazing) and the amount of initial capital necessary to the enterprise (in this case a minimal amount of cash), were crucial elements in providing young men and their families with economic opportunities on the frontier. ■

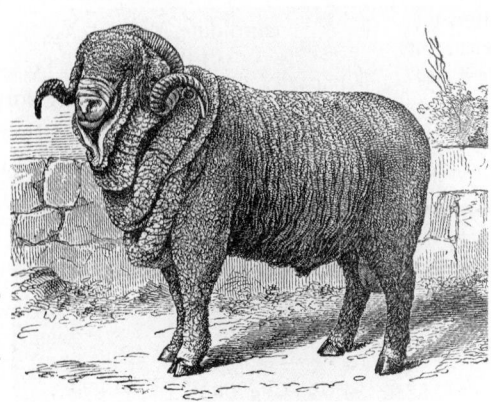

Library of Congress

Merino sheep.

Source: H. Bailey Carroll and J. Villasana Haggard, trans. and ed., *Three New Mexico Chronicles* (Albuquerque, 1942): 41–42.

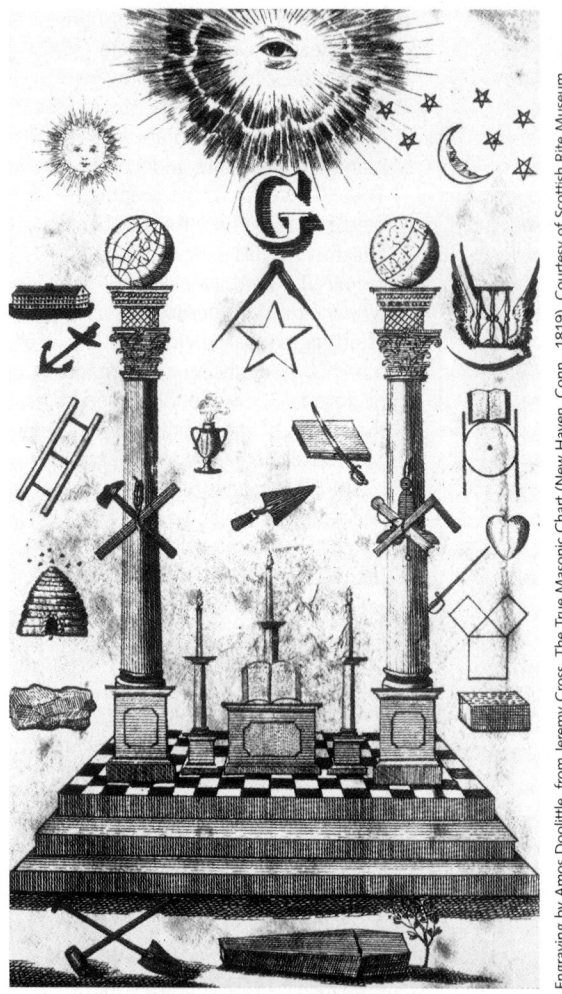

Engraving by Amos Doolittle, from Jeremy Cross, The True Masonic Chart (New Haven, Conn., 1819). Courtesy of Scottish Rite Museum of Our National Heritage, Library, 14.I, C951,1820a. Photography: John Miller Documents, Van Gorden-Williams Library

■ Many political leaders in the New Republic, including George Washington, were members of the Masons, a fraternal order. The Masons drew their members from a cross-section of the male, primarily urban population, including merchants, artisans, and sailors. The order relied on secret rituals and on symbols such as those in this engraving, which appeared mysterious and threatening to outsiders. In 1831 the Anti-Masonic party became the first party to select its presidential candidate at a convention, where it also adopted a party platform.

Jackson condemned the bank as a "monster" intent on devouring hardworking people and enriching a few eastern financiers. In his veto message to Congress, he denounced the bank as an instrument of privilege, one that granted favors to the well-born and well-connected. He fumed, "The humble members of society—the farmers, mechanics, and laborers—who have neither the time nor the means of securing like favors to themselves, have a right to complain of the injustice of their Government."

By vetoing the bank bill, Jackson angered members of Congress and his own cabinet. They had urged him to recharter the bank because they believed the credit system was necessary for economic progress and expansion. Convinced that Jackson had overextended his reach, his opponents seized on the issue as a sign of the chief executive's political vulnerability. Harboring presidential ambitions himself, Henry Clay was certain that the bank controversy would prove Jackson's downfall.

However, Clay, the "Great Compromiser," badly miscalculated. Congress upheld Jackson's veto of the Bank (the Bank closed when its chapter expired in 1836). Nominated for president by the National Republicans in 1832, Clay drew support from merchants who had benefited from Bank of the United States loans and from the sizable contingent of Jackson-haters. Yet a new player, the Anti-Masonic party, entered the fray and complicated matters for Clay, as it drew some of the anti-Jackson sentiment away from him. This group accused the Masons, a secret fraternal order, of subverting American democratic values. Jackson himself was a member of the Masons, prompting the new party to call into question the president's devotion to the "common man."

The Anti-Masonic party gained some favor in New England and the Mid-Atlantic states, where rumors flew about the Masons' secret rituals and alleged clandestine political influence. Still, Jackson won in a landslide against Clay. The president carried not only his stronghold, the West, but also the South and substantial parts of New York, Pennsylvania, and New England. The Anti-Masonic candidate, William Wirt, won only Vermont.

While in office, Jackson used his veto power a total of 12 times. All his predecessors *combined* had used it just 10 times. When his opponents finally formed a political party in 1834, they called themselves Whigs, after the English antimonarchist party. In choosing this name, their intention was to ridicule "King Andrew." In the words of the states' rights advocates, Jackson's high-handed manner was "rather an appeal to the loyalty of subjects, than to the patriotism of citizens." The Whigs opposed the man who had built up the power of the presidency in defiance of Congress and the Supreme Court.

TABLE 11-4

The Election of 1832

Candidate	Political Party	Popular Vote	Electoral Vote
Andrew Jackson	Democratic	687,502	219
Henry Clay	National Republican	530,189	49
John Floyd	Independent		11
William Wirt	Anti-Masonic	33,108	7

Real People in the "Age of the Common Man"

Universal white manhood suffrage set a new standard for political involvement in the United States. Now, white men could vote and run for office regardless of their class or religion. However, as the voting public expanded, those excluded from it charged that white men's rights came at their expense. White men had the freedom to move west and settle the land because Indians lost their own claim to the land. White men could buy and sell slaves because African American men and women lacked the power to control their own work and keep their families together. White men pursued their careers and stations in the public sphere because women were restricted to the domestic sphere. Together, Indians, blacks, and white women constituted about 70 percent of the American population in the 1820s. Thus, in the "age of the common man," less than one-third of the adult population had the right to vote.

In the early 1830s, a wealthy Frenchman named Alexis de Tocqueville visited the United States and wrote about the contradictions he saw. In his book *Democracy in America* (published in 1835), de Tocqueville noted that the United States lacked the rigid hierarchy of class privilege that characterized European nations. However, he also noted some sore spots in American democratic values and practices. He commented on the plight of groups deprived of the right to vote, whose lack of freedom stood out starkly in the otherwise egalitarian society of the United States. He sympathized with the southeastern Indians uprooted from their homelands. He raised the possibility that conflicts between blacks and whites might eventually lead to bloodshed. He even contrasted the situation of young unmarried white women, who seemed so free-spirited, with that of wives, who appeared cautious and dull. He concluded, "In America a woman loses her independence forever in the bonds of matrimony." In other words, de Tocqueville saw America for what it was: a blend of freedom and slavery, of independence and dependence.

Wards, Workers, and Warriors: Native Americans

Population growth in the United States—and on the borderlands between the United States and Mexican territory—put pressure on Indian societies. Yet different cultural groups responded in different ways to this pressure. Some, like the Cherokees, conformed to European American ways and became sedentary farmers. Others were forced to work for whites. Still others either waged war on white settlements and military forces or retreated further and further from European American settlements in the hope of avoiding clashes with the intruders.

Nevertheless, prominent whites continued to denigrate the humanity of all Indians. In the 1820s Henry Clay claimed that Indians were "essentially

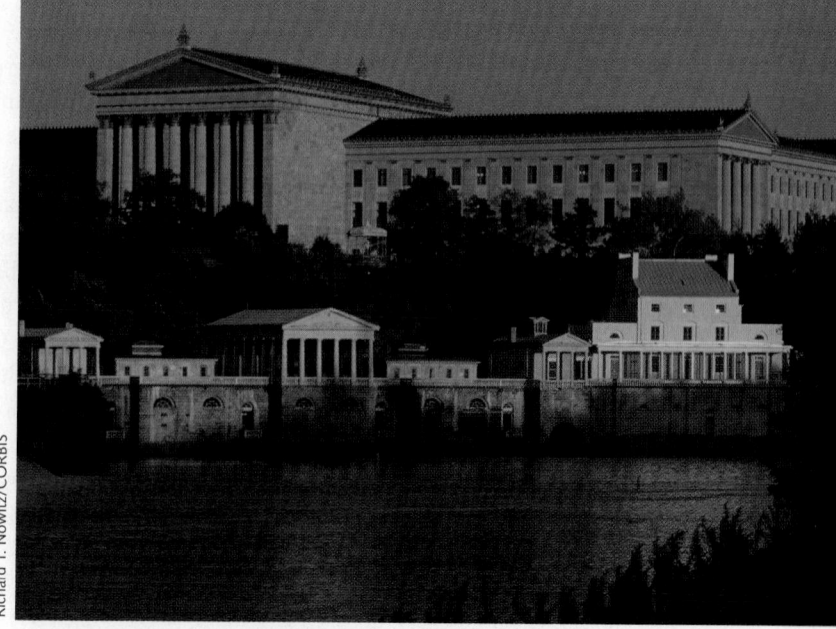

Richard T. Nowitz/CORBIS

■ This photo of the Fairmont Waterworks in Philadelphia shows the effects of Greek architecture on American public buildings in the early nineteenth century. Designed by Frederick C. Graff, the waterworks were completed in 1822. Numerous banks, colleges, commercial buildings, and large private homes built during this period were designed in the Greek Revival style. The United States saw itself as the embodiment of democracy, a form of government characteristic of some early Greek city-states.

inferior to the Anglo-Saxon race . . . and their disappearance from the human family will be no great loss to the world." In 1828 the House of Representatives Committee on Indian Affairs surveyed the Indians of the South and concluded that "an Indian cannot work" and that all Indians were lazy and notable for their "thirst for spirituous liquours." According to the committee, when European settlers depleted reserves of wildlife, Indians as a group would cease to exist.

Members of the Cherokee Nation bitterly denounced these assertions. "The Cherokees do not live upon the chase [for game]," they pointed out. Neither did the Creeks, Choctaws, Chickasaws, and Seminoles—the other members of the Five Civilized Tribes, so called for their varying degrees of conformity to white people's ways.

Charting a middle course between the Indian and European American worlds was Sequoyah, the son of a white Virginia trader–soldier and a Cherokee woman. A veteran of Andrew Jackson's campaign against the Creeks in 1813–1814, Sequoyah moved to Arkansas in 1818, part of an early Cherokee migration west. In 1821 he finished a Cherokee syllabary (a written language consisting of syllables and letters, in contrast to pictures, or pictographs). The product of a dozen years' work, the syllabary consisted of 86 characters. In 1828 the *Cherokee Phoenix*, a newspaper based on the new writing system, began publication in New Echota, Georgia.

Sequoyah's written language enabled the increasingly dispersed Cherokee Indians to remain in touch with each other on their own terms. At the same time, numerous Indian cultural groups lost their struggle to retain even modest control over their destinies. In some areas of the continent, smallpox continued to ravage native populations. In other regions, Indians became wards of, or dependent on, whites, living with and working for white families. Other groups, living close to whites, adopted their trading practices. In Spanish California, the Muquelmne Miwoks in the San Joaquin delta made a living by stealing and then selling the horses of Mexican settlers.

In other parts of California, Spanish missionaries conquered Indian groups, converted them to Christianity, and then forced them to work in the missions. In missions up and down the California coast, Indians worked as weavers, tanners, shoemakers, bricklayers, carpenters, blacksmiths, and other artisans. Some herded cattle and raised horses. Indian women cooked for the mission, cleaned, and spun wool. They wove cloth and sewed garments.

Nevertheless, even Indians living in or near missions resisted the cultural change imposed by the intruders. Catholic missionaries complained that Indian women such as those of the Chumash refused to learn Spanish. But by abandoning their native tongue, these women would have lost much—positions of influence within their own religious community—and gained little because positions of authority were dominated by Spanish-speaking men. The refusal among some Indians to assimilate completely signaled persistent, deep-seated conflicts between native groups and incoming settlers. In 1824 a revolt among hundreds of newly converted Indians at the mission *La Purisima Concepción* north of Santa Barbara revealed a rising militancy among native peoples.

After the War of 1812, the U.S. government had rewarded some military veterans with land grants in the Old Northwest. Federal agents tried to clear the way for these new settlers—farmers as well as miners with their eye on the rich lead deposits in northern Illinois and southern Wisconsin—by ousting Indians from the area. Overwhelmed by the number of whites, some Indian groups such as the Peorias and Kaskaskias gave up their lands to the interlopers. However, the Kickapoos along the Wabash and Illinois rivers, together with the Winnebagos, Sauks, and Fox, took a stand against the white intrusion. In 1826 and 1827 the Winnebagos attacked white families and boat pilots living near Prairie du Chien, Wisconsin. Two years later, the Sauk chief Black Hawk (known to Indians as Ma-ka-tai-me-she-kia-kiak) assembled a coalition of Fox, Winnebagos, Kickapoos, and

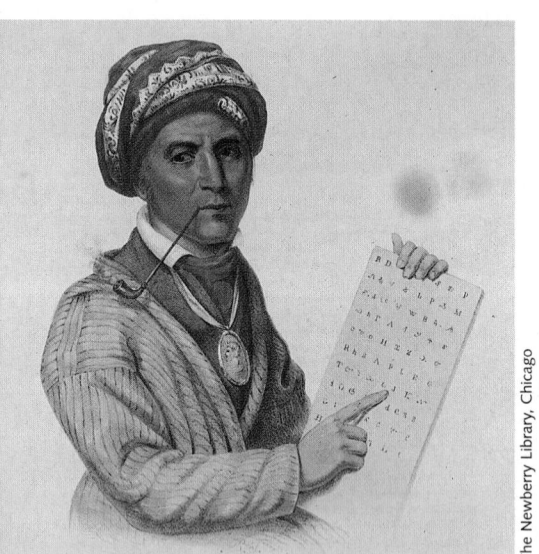

The Newberry Library, Chicago

■ Artist Charles Bird King painted this portrait of Sequoyah while the Indian leader was in Washington, D.C., in 1828. Government officials honored him for developing a written form of the Cherokee language. He is wearing a medal presented to him by the Cherokee nation in 1825. He later settled permanently in Sallisaw, in what is today Sequoyah County, Oklahoma.

Potawatomis. Emboldened by the prospect of aid from British Canada, they clashed with federal troops and raided farmers' homesteads and miners' camps.

In August 1832 a force of 1300 U.S. soldiers and volunteers struck back, attacking an encampment of Indians on the Bad Axe River in western Wisconsin. The soldiers killed 300 Indian men, women, and children. The massacre, the decisive point of what came to be called the Black Hawk War, marked the end of armed Indian resistance north of the Ohio River and east of the Mississippi. If the United States did not have justice on its side, it at least had superior military might. In the courts and on the battlefield, Indian cultures were under siege.

Slaves and Free People of Color

In 1820 the U.S. population included 1.5 million slaves. A decade later that figure had grown to 2 million, almost entirely from natural increase. In the same ten-year period, the number of free blacks increased from 99,281 to 137,529 in the North as a result of emancipation. The figure rose from 134,223 to 182,070 in the South. The large free black population in the Upper South was scattered in rural areas, whereas the small numbers of their Lower South counterparts were concentrated in the cities.

Overall, however, the proportion of free blacks within the southern population declined. True, some masters freed their slaves, and some slaves managed to run away or buy their freedom. The free population also grew by natural means. But within the South, whites perceived free blacks as an unwelcome and dangerous presence, especially given the possibility that they would conspire with slaves to spark a rebellion. For these reasons some states began to outlaw private manumissions (the practice of individual owners freeing their slaves) and to force free blacks to leave the state altogether.

One free black who inspired such fears was Denmark Vesey. Born on the Danish-controlled Island of Saint Thomas in 1767, Vesey was a literate carpenter as well as a religious leader. In 1799 he won $1500 in a Charleston lottery and used some of the money to buy his freedom. In the summer of 1822, a Charleston, South Carolina, court claimed to have unearthed evidence of a "diabolical plot" hatched by Vesey together with plantation slaves from the surrounding area. The judges charged that Vesey and his coconspirators aimed "to trample on all laws, human and divine; to riot in blood, outrage, and rapine . . . and conflagration, and to introduce anarchy and confusion in their most horrid form."

The judges' claims provide a laundry list of whites' fears about free men of color. In their account of the testimony, they suggested that Vesey drew inspiration from the Saint Domingue slave revolt that freeman Toussaint L'Ouverture had led in 1791. They claimed Vesey closely followed congressional debates during the Missouri Compromise crisis of 1819 and 1820. They implicated members of Charleston's African Methodist Episcopal Church, an independent body founded in 1818, which whites believed provided fertile ground for black insurrectionists. Finally, the judges took note of one witness who claimed that, "even whilst walking through the streets in the company with another, he [Vesey] was not idle; for if his companion bowed to a white person he would rebuke him, and observe that all men were born equal." Notions of freedom and equality had explosive potential in the slave South.

Yet the historical record strongly suggests that no plot ever existed. Black "witnesses" who feared for their own lives provided inconsistent and contradictory testimony to a panel of judges. Authorities never located any material evidence of a plan, such as stockpiles of weapons. Under fire from other Charleston elites for rushing to judgment, the judges redoubled their efforts to embellish vague rumors of black discontent into a tale of a well-orchestrated uprising and to implicate growing numbers of black people. As a result of the testimony of several slaves, 35 black men were hanged and another 18 exiled outside the United States. Of those executed, Vesey and 23 other men said nothing to support even the vaguest charges of the court.

The uncovering of the Vesey "plot" prompted whites throughout the South to crack down on meetings, religious or otherwise, among slaves and free people of color. In Charleston, a new white group calling itself the South Carolina Association sought to restrict the movements of free blacks and return fugitive slaves to their owners. The city's African Methodist Episcopal Church was shut down and its preacher, Moses Brown, hounded out of South Carolina.

In the North, some blacks were granted the right to vote after emancipation in the late eighteenth century; however, many of those voting rights were lost in the early nineteenth century. New Jersey (in 1807), Connecticut (1818), New York (1821), and Pennsylvania (1838) all revoked the legislation that had let black men cast ballots. In several instances, the political party in power feared that black voters would swing the election to their opponents. Free northern blacks continued to suffer under a number of legal restrictions. Most were not citizens and therefore perceived themselves as oppressed like the slaves in the South.

A new group of black leaders in the urban North began to link their fate to that of their enslaved brothers and sisters in the South. In Boston, North Carolina–born David Walker published his fiery *Walker's Appeal to the Coloured Citizens of the World* in 1829. Walker called for all blacks to integrate fully into American society, shunning racial segregation whether initiated by whites or by blacks themselves. Reminding his listeners of the horrors of the slave trade, he declared that black people were ready to die for freedom: "I give it as a fact, let twelve black men get well armed for battle, and they will kill and put to flight fifty whites." Walker ended by quoting the Declaration of Independence. Whites, he argued, had demonstrated more cruelty and tyranny toward blacks than Great Britain had ever shown toward the colonies.

Also in Boston, Maria Stewart, a charismatic black preacher, became the first American-born woman (of any background) to lecture in public. In 1832 and 1833 she delivered a series of stirring addresses. She argued that free blacks in the North were not much better off than enslaved blacks in the South. "Knowledge is power," she exhorted her audience, urging them to pursue education on their own.

Northern black leaders disagreed among themselves on the issues of integration and black separatism—for example, whether blacks should create their own schools or press for inclusion in the public educational system. A few leaders favored leaving the country altogether, believing that black people would never find peace and freedom in the United States. Founded by whites in New Jersey in 1817, the American Colonization Society (ACS) paid for black Americans to settle Monrovia (later Liberia) on the west coast of Africa. The group claimed that foreign colonization would bring American blacks "unspeakable blessings." The ACS drew support from a variety of groups: whites in the Upper South who wanted to free their slaves but believed that black and white people could not live in the same country and some slaves and free people of

> *Northern black leaders disagreed among themselves on the issues of integration and black separatism.*

color convinced that colonization would give them a fresh start. A small number of American-born blacks settled in Liberia. However, most black activists rejected colonization. They had been born on American soil, and their forebears had been buried there. Maria Stewart declared, "But before I go [to Africa] the bayonet shall pierce me through."

Northern whites sought to control black people and their movements. Outspoken black men and women such as Walker and Stewart alarmed northern whites who feared that if blacks could claim decent jobs, white people would lose their own jobs. African Americans who worked outdoors as wagon drivers, peddlers, and street sweepers were taunted and in some cases attacked by whites who demanded deference from blacks in public. In October 1824 a mob of white men invaded a black neighborhood in Providence, Rhode Island. They terrorized its residents, destroyed buildings, and left the place "almost entirely in ruins." The catalyst for the riot had come the previous day, when a group of blacks had refused to yield the inside of the sidewalk— a cleaner place to walk—to white passersby. These blacks were arrested, but a jury found the defendants not guilty. Noting the unabashed racism of white Northerners and the unwillingness of white Southerners to acknowledge the terrible consequences of slavery,

Alexis de Tocqueville wrote, "There is something more frightening about the silence of the South than about the North's noisy fears."

The South's silence was broken in 1831 when white Southerners took steps to reinforce the institution of slavery, using both violent and legal means. That year Nat Turner, an enslaved preacher and mystic, led a slave revolt in Southampton, Virginia. In the 1820s the young Turner had looked skyward and had seen visions of "white spirits and black spirits engaged in battle . . . and blood flowed in streams." Turner believed that he had received divine instructions to lead other slaves to freedom, to "arise and prepare myself, and slay my enemies with their own weapons." In August he and a group of followers that eventually numbered 80 moved through the countryside, killing whites wherever they could find them. Ultimately, nearly 60 whites died at the hands of Turner's rebels. Turner himself managed to evade capture for more than two months. After he was captured, he was tried, convicted, and sentenced to death. A white man named Thomas Gray interviewed Turner in his jail cell and recorded his "confessions" before he was hanged.

> *In the early nineteenth century, work was becoming increasingly identified as labor that earned cash wages.*

Published in 1832 by Gray, *The Confessions of Nat Turner* reached a large, horrified audience in the white South. According to Gray, Turner said that he had exhibited "uncommon intelligence" when he was a child. As a young man, he had received inspiration from the Bible, especially the passage "Seek ye the kingdom of Heaven and all things shall be added unto you." Perhaps most disturbing of all, Turner reported that, since 1830, he had been a slave of "Mr. Joseph Travis, who was to me a kind master, and placed the greatest confidence in me; in fact, I had no cause to complain of his treatment to me." Turner's "confessions" suggested the subversive potential of slaves who were literate and Christian and those who were treated kindly by their masters and mistresses.

After the Turner revolt, a wave of white hysteria swept the South. In Virginia near where the killings had occurred, whites assaulted blacks with unbridled fury. The Virginia legislature seized the occasion to defeat various antislavery proposals. Thereafter, all the slave states moved to strengthen the institution of slavery. For all practical purposes, public debate over slavery ceased.

Legal and Economic Dependence: The Plight of Women

In the political and economic realms, the egalitarian impulse rarely affected the status of women in a legal or practical sense. Regardless of where they lived, enslaved women and Indian women had almost no rights under either U.S. or Spanish law. Still, legal systems in the United States and the Spanish borderlands differed in their treatment of women. In the United States, most of the constraints that white married women had experienced in the colonial period still applied in the 1820s. A husband controlled the property that his wife brought to the marriage, and he had legal authority over their children. Indeed, the wife was considered her husband's possession. She had no right to make a contract, keep money she earned, or vote, run for office, or serve on a jury. In contrast, in the Spanish Southwest, married women could own land and conduct business on their own. At the same time, however, husbands, fathers, and local priests continued to exert much influence over the lives of these women.

European American women's economic subordination served as a rationale for their political inferiority. The "common man" concept rested on the assumption that only men could ensure American economic growth and well-being. According to this view, men had the largest stake in society because only they owned property. That stake made them responsible citizens.

Yet women contributed to the economy in myriad ways. Although few women earned cash wages in the 1820s, almost all adult women worked. In the colonial period, society had highly valued women's labor in the fields, the garden, and the kitchen. However, in the early nineteenth century, work was becoming increasingly identified as labor that earned cash wages. This attitude proved particularly common in the Northeast, where increasing numbers of workers labored under the supervision of a boss. As this belief took root, men began valuing women's contributions to the household economy less and less. If women did not earn money, many men asked, did they really work at all?

In these years, well-off women in the northeastern and mid-Atlantic states began to think of themselves as consumers and not producers of goods. They relied more and more on store-bought cloth and household supplies. Some could also afford to hire servants to perform housework for them. Privileged women gradually stopped thinking of their responsibilities as making goods or processing and preparing food. Rather, their main tasks were to manage servants and create a comfortable home for their husbands and children. They saw their labor as necessary to the well-being of their families, even if their compensation came in the form of emotional satisfaction rather than cash.

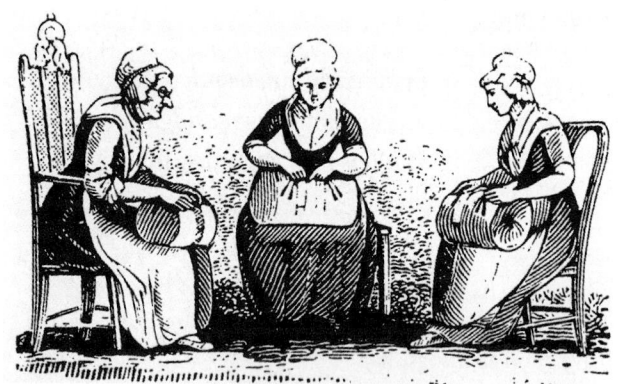

In contrast, women in other parts of the country continued to engage in the same forms of household industry that had characterized the colonial period. In Spanish settlements, women played a central role in household production. They made all of their family's clothes by carding, spinning, and weaving the wool from sheep. They tanned cowhides and ground blue corn to make tortillas, or *atole*. They produced their own candles and soap, and they plastered the walls of the home.

In the Spanish mission of San Gabriel, California, the widow Eulalia Pérez cooked, sewed, ministered to the ill, and instructed children in reading and writing. As housekeeper, Pérez kept the keys to the mission storehouse. She also distributed supplies to the Indians and the *vaqueros* (cowboys) who lived in the mission. She supervised Indian servants as well as soap makers, wine pressers, and olive oil producers.

At Mission San Diego, Apolonaria Lorenzana worked as a healer and cared for the church sacristy and priestly vestments. Lorenzana devoted her life to such labors, from the time she arrived in Monterey as a child of seven (in 1800) until her death in the late nineteenth century. Although the priests tried to restrict her to administering the mission hospital, she took pride in her nursing abilities, "even though Father Sánchez had told me not to do it myself, but to have it done, and only to be present so that the servant girls would do it well."

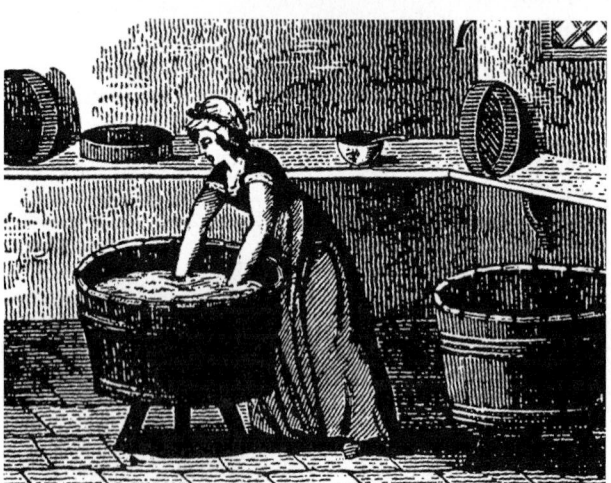

■ The plight of needlewomen became representative of the hazards faced by female workers in the new urban commercial economy of the late eighteenth and early nineteenth centuries. Many women worked at home, sewing garments that they returned to a "jobber" for payment. The labor, often performed by candlelight in ill-lighted tenements, was tedious and ill-paid. Laundry work also took up much of women's time.

Indian women also engaged in a variety of essential tasks. Sioux and Mandan women, though of a social rank inferior to men, performed a great deal of manual labor in their own villages. They dressed buffalo skins that the men later sold to traders. They collected water and wood, cooked, dried meat and fruit, and cultivated maize (corn), pumpkins, and squash with hoes made from the shoulderblades of elk. These women worked collectively within a network of households rather than individually within nuclear families.

In many communities, women, regardless of ethnicity, were paid in kind for their work—that is, they received food and shelter but not money. Nevertheless, some women did work for cash wages during this era. New England women and children, for example, were the vanguard of factory wage-earners in the early manufacturing system. In Massachusetts in 1820 women and children constituted almost a third of all manufacturing workers. In the largest textile factories, they made up fully 80 percent of the workforce.

The business of textile manufacturing took the tasks of spinning thread and weaving cloth out of the home, where such tasks often were performed by unpaid, unmarried daughters, and relocated those tasks in factories, where the same workers received wages. The famous "Lowell mill girls" are an apt example. Young, unmarried white women from New Hampshire, Vermont, and Massachusetts, these workers moved to the new company town of Lowell, Massachusetts, to take jobs as textile machine operatives. In New England, thousands of young men had migrated west, tipping the sex ratio in favor of women and creating a reserve of female laborers. But to attract young women to factory work, mill owners had to reassure them (and their parents) that they would be safe and well cared for away from home. To that end, they established boarding houses where employees could live together under the supervision of a matron—an older woman who served as their mother-away-from-home.

Company towns set rules shaping employees' living conditions as well as their working conditions. In the early 1830s, a posted list of "Rules and Regulations" covered many aspects of the lives of the young women living at the Poignaud and Plant boardinghouse at Lancaster, Massachusetts. The list told the women how to enter the building (quietly, and then hang up "their bonnet, shawl, coat, etc. etc. in the entry") and where to sit at the dinner table (the two workers with greatest seniority were to take their places at the head of the table). Despite these rules, many young women valued the friendships they made with their coworkers and the money they made in the mills. Some of these women sent their wages back home so that their fathers could pay off the mortgage or their brothers could attend school.

> *The new delineation between men's and women's work and workplaces intensified the drive for women's education begun after the Revolution.*

But not all women wage-earners labored in large mills. In New York City, single women, wives, and widows toiled as needleworkers in their homes. Impoverished, sewing in tiny attics by the dim light of candles, these women were at the mercy of jobbers—merchants who parceled out cuffs, collars, and shirt fronts that the women finished. Other urban women worked as street vendors, selling produce, or as cooks, nursemaids, or laundresses.

The new delineation between men's and women's work and workplaces intensified the drive for women's education begun after the Revolution. If well-to-do women were to assume domestic responsibilities while their husbands worked outside the home, then women must receive their own unique form of schooling, or so the reasoning went. Most ordinary women received little in the way of formal education. Yet elite young women had expanded educational opportunities, beginning in the early nineteenth century. Emma Willard founded a female academy in Troy, New York, in 1821, and Catharine Beecher established the Hartford (Connecticut) Female Seminary two years later. For the most part, these schools catered to the daughters of wealthy families, young women who would never have to work in a factory to survive. Hailed as a means to prepare young women to serve as wives and mothers, the schools taught geography, foreign languages, mathematics, science, and philosophy, as well as the "female" pursuits of embroidery and music.

Out of this curriculum designed especially for women emerged women's rights activists, women who keenly felt both the potential of their own intelligence and the degrading nature of their social situation. Elizabeth Cady, an 1832 graduate of the Troy Female Seminary, later went on to marry Henry B. Stanton and bear seven children. But by the 1840s she strode onto the national stage as a tireless advocate of women's political and economic rights.

Ties That Bound a Growing Population

The Founding Fathers had disagreed among themselves about whether democracy could still thrive in a large nation, where news necessarily traveled slowly and people remained isolated from their neighbors. However, by the 1820s few Americans doubted that the nation could grow and still preserve its democratic character. In fact, westward expansion seemed to promote democracy. Now, more ordinary white men than ever participated in the political process.

At the same time, population growth and migration patterns disrupted old bonds of community. When people left their place of birth, they often severed ties with their family and

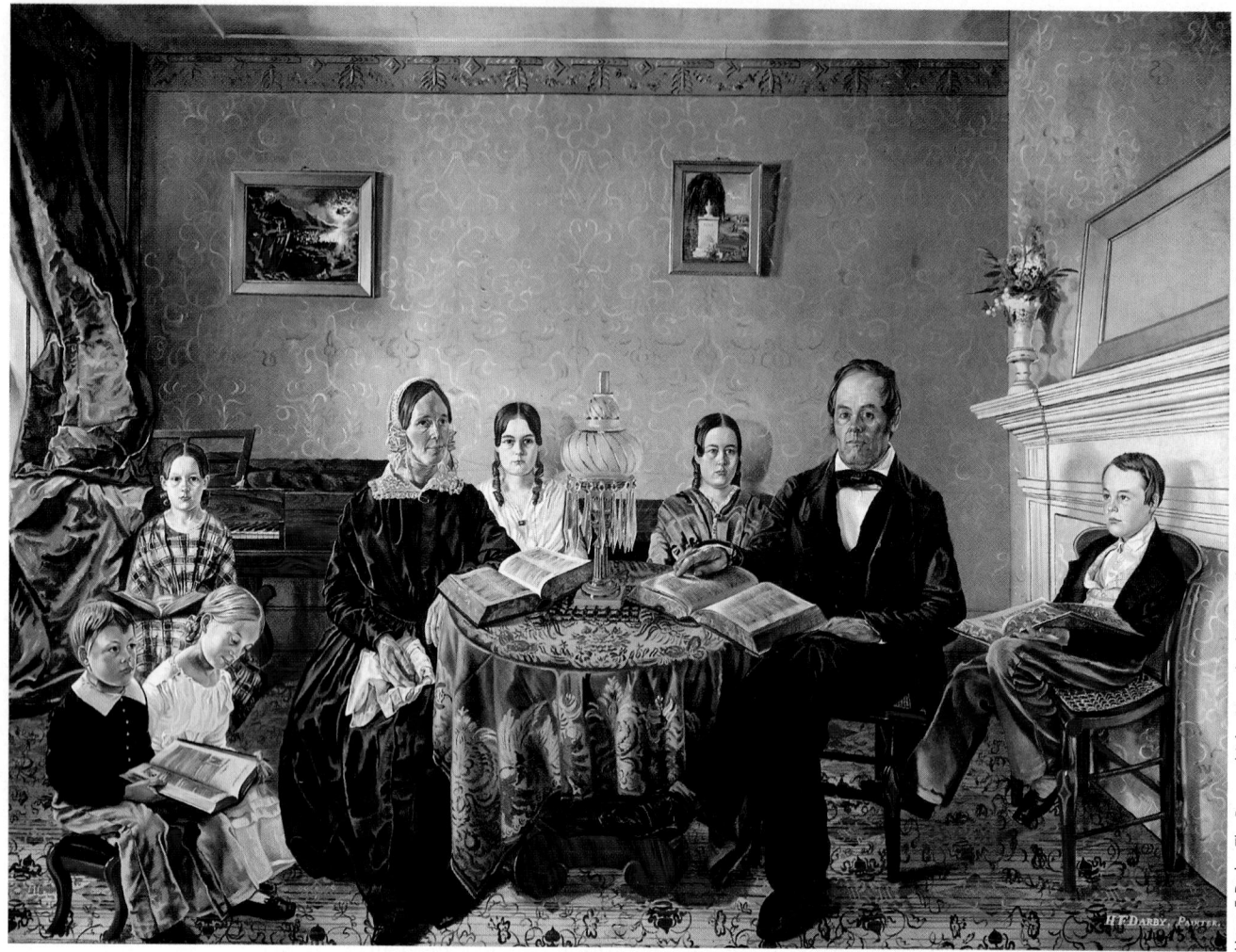

■ The Rev. John Atwood and family reading the Bible, 1845.

original community. New forms of social cohesion arose to replace these traditional ties. By the 1830s, for example, the national party system of Democrats and Whigs claimed the allegiances of white men from all sections of the country. Indeed, when one English visitor to New York state observed the "furious acrimony of party spirit," he suggested that Americans cared more for the trappings of partisan loyalty—"the spirit of electioneering"—than for ideas themselves.

In addition, new religions sought to make sense of changing political and economic landscape. High literacy rates among the population created a new community of readers, a far-flung audience for periodicals as well as for a new, uniquely American literature. Finally, opinionmakers used the printed word to spread new ideas and values across regional boundaries. These ideas, such as glorification of male ambition, helped knit together far-flung segments of the population, men and women who began to speak of an "American character."

New Visions of Religious Faith

New forms of religious faith arose in response to turbulent times. During the Indian Wars in the Old Northwest, a Winnebago prophet named White Cloud helped Black Hawk create a coalition of Winnebagos, Potawatomies, Kickapoos, Sauks, and Fox Indians. A mystic and medicine man, White Cloud preached against the white man and exhorted his followers to defend their way of life, an Indian way that knew no tribal boundaries. White Cloud, the religious leader, and Black Hawk, the military leader, surrendered together to federal troops on August 27, 1832, signifying the spiritual component in the Indians' militant resistance to whites. Through the rest of the nineteenth century, a number of Indian groups found inspiration, and in some cases common ground, in the teachings of Indian religious leaders.

New religious enthusiasms took hold in other parts of the country as well. In the late 1820s and early 1830s, the Second Great Awakening swept western New York. The fervor of religious revivals so heated the region that people began to call it "the Burned-Over District." Hordes of people of various Protestant denominations attended week-long prayer meetings, sat together on the "anxious bench" for sinners, and listened, transfixed, as new converts told of their path to righteousness.

What explains this wave of religious enthusiasm? A major factor was a clergyman named Charles Grandison Finney who managed to tap into the wellspring of hope and anxiety of the time. A former lawyer, Finney preached that people were moral free agents, fully capable of deciding between right and wrong and doing good in the world. Finney's message had great appeal during this period of rapid social, economic, and technological change. In New England and New York, for example, canals were bringing new kinds of goods to rural areas and longtime residents were departing for the Midwest. Traditional social relationships seemed threatened.

Finney believed that people could control their own destinies and that they should work through earthly institutions to do it. In one sermon, he declared, "The church must take the right ground in regard to politics. . . . The time has come that Christians must vote for honest men." Of course, not all Christians agreed on what constituted the "right ground" in politics. But Finney sought to link the life of the spirit with political and reform efforts, and many men and women responded enthusiastically.

Throughout the country, religious institutions also grappled with questions about slavery. As the fear of possible black uprisings spread, white clergy in the South began to turn away from their former willingness to convert anyone. Instead, they began seeking respectability in

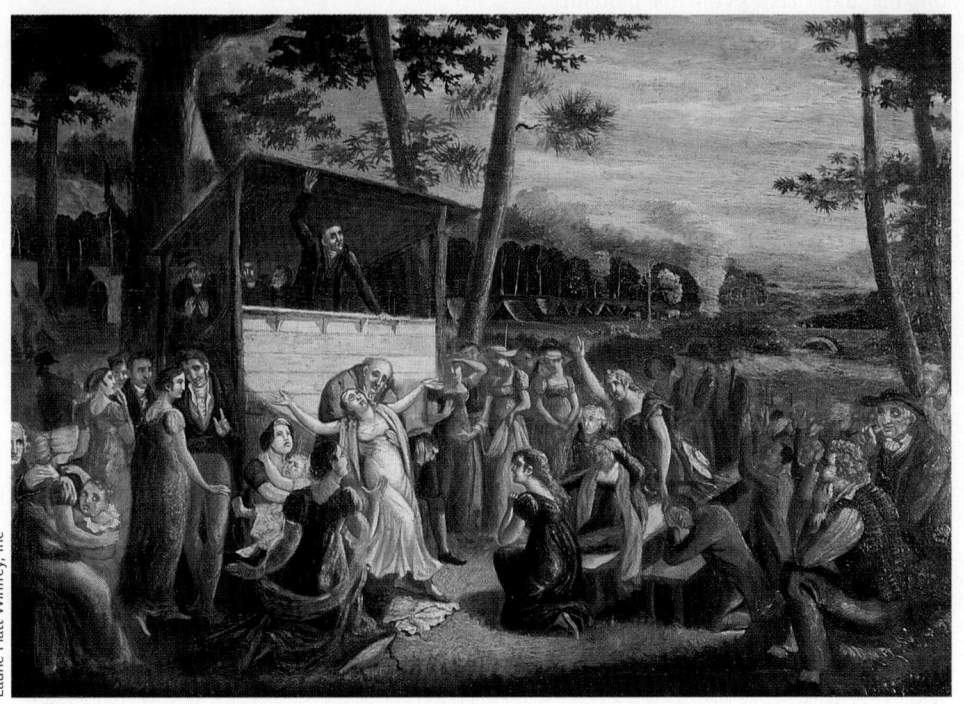

Laurie Platt Winfrey, Inc

■ The long-lived religious revival called the Second Great Awakening swept through the United States in the 1820s and 1830s. Charles Grandison Finney, an itinerant preacher, helped lead the movement. He urged listeners to consider themselves "moral free agents" with control over their own destinies. Services conducted outdoors, called "camp meetings," provided settings for mass audiences to engage in emotional release and personal testimonials of newly found faith.

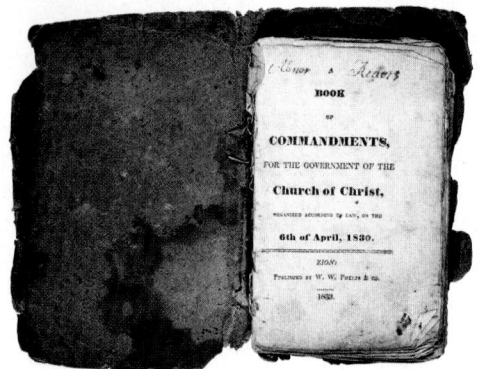

the eyes of the well-to-do, slave-owning class. Incorporating masculine imagery into their sermons, they used the language of militant patriotism to distance themselves from the white women, slaves, and free people of color in their congregations. At a western revival in 1824, one itinerant Methodist minister described his military service in the War of 1812; he had helped to vanquish not only the British but also "the merciless savages of the forest, and to secure and perpetuate the liberties secured to us by our forefathers." These preachers strove to reinforce the power of husband over wife, parent over child, and master over slave, relations that defined the typical plantation household.

Elsewhere, some church leaders sought to purge Christianity of what they saw as its too-worldly nature and to revive the primitive church that Jesus and his disciples had established. On April 6, 1830, a young farmer named Joseph Smith, Jr., founded the Church of Jesus Christ of Latter-Day Saints (also called the Mormons) in Fayette, New York. Smith said that, in a vision, he had received the text of a holy book originally written by a Native American historian more than 1400 years earlier. Transcribed from tablets presented to him by an angel named Moroni, the text was called the *Book of Mormon.* Together with the Old and New Testaments, it formed the basis of a new faith. Over the next few years, the Mormon Church grew rapidly, claiming 8000 members by the mid-1830s. However, the young church also aroused intense hostility among mainstream Protestant denominations that regarded the new group's theology and textual inspiration with suspicion. It was almost impossible for religious institutions to escape the worldly realm of politics and social fragmentation.

Literate and Literary America

In 1828 a young widow named Sarah Hale broke new ground for women. She became the first woman to edit an American periodical when she accepted responsibility for editing the *Ladies Magazine,* published in Boston. Once a hatmaker but now a published poet and novelist, Hale aimed "to make females better acquainted with their duties and privileges" through the articles in her magazine. Between 1825 and 1850, thousands of other magazines cropped up and then disappeared, the product of a growing audience of literate (and literary) city-dwellers. But the *Ladies Magazine,* later renamed *Godey's Lady's Book,* lived an uncommonly long life under Hale's editorial guidance.

The *Ladies Magazine* appealed primarily to well-off white wives and mothers in the Northeast, the South, and the West. They identified with its message promoting motherhood and the virtues of piety and self-sacrifice. The *Ladies Magazine* and other publications portrayed women as especially devout and thus powerful: men might claim as their domain "the government and the glory of the world," wrote Hale in 1832, "but nevertheless, what man shall become depends upon the secret, silent influence of women." That influence, Hale and other men and women like her believed, derived from women's roles as nurturers and caretakers.

Indeed, many of the poems and short stories published in the *Ladies Magazine* and other women's periodicals came under the category of sentimental literature. Such writing was calculated to appeal to readers' emotions, rather than their intellect, as their titles reveal: "Burial of a Motherless Infant," "The Blind Mother and Her Children," and "The Harp of the Maniac Maiden" (about a young girl's descent into insanity).

Just as sentimental fiction and poetry attracted a large readership among women, a number of male writers staked their claim to emerging American literature. Washington Irving, James Fenimore Cooper, and William Cullen Bryant all explored regional histories and landscapes in their works. In *Rip Van Winkle* (1819) and the *Legend of Sleepy Hollow* (1820), Irving wrote about the legends of upstate New York. Cooper explored the western New York middle ground contested by the British, Americans, French, and Indians in the late eighteenth century in such works as *The Spy* (1821) and *Last of the Mohicans* (1826). Bryant, inspired by the sight of the Illinois plains in 1832, penned "The Prairies." This praise-song to the vast plains described them as beautiful and "quick with life" ("The graceful deer/Bounds to the woods at my approach"). As the vanguard of a new generation of male American authors, these writers began a literary "American Renaissance."

Along with this new American literary tradition, small towns across the nation began publishing newspapers to educate, inform, and entertain readers. News stories about national elections and legislation, about foreign monarchs and conflicts, reached log cabins in the West as well as elegant townhouses in Boston and Philadelphia. Wrote Washington Irving in 1820, "Over no nation does the press hold a more absolute control than over the people of America, for the universal education of the poorest classes makes every individual a reader."

Newspapers, books, and magazines promoted a set of values that writers claimed described an enduring American character. The ideal American supposedly was ambitious—ready to seize opportunity wherever it could be found—and at the same time devoted to home and family. In fact, these values strongly resembled those adopted by the British middle classes at the same time. Indeed, the United States spawned its own brand of middle-class sensibility called Victorianism, after the English queen who reigned from 1837 to 1901.

Four core values defined early American Victorianism. First, the Victorians believed in the significance of the individual. People should be judged on the basis of their character, not on the circumstances of their birth. This belief, however, generally applied only to white men. Second, individuals should have the freedom to advance as far as their talents and ambition took them; no person should claim advantages over others by virtue of a noble title or aristocratic lineage. Third, work was intrinsically noble, whether performed by a canal digger wielding a pick-axe or a merchant using a quill pen. All people, regardless of their trade, deserved to reap the fruits of their labor. Finally, men and women occupied separate but complementary spheres. American society could be orderly and stable only if men could find a haven from the heartless world of work in their own homes. There, wives tended the hearth and infused the household with their love, self-sacrifice, and religious devotion.

Victorians often saw work as an individualistic endeavor, with men, women, and children earning wages for the number of hours they worked or for each task they performed. However, not all groups embraced Victorian attitudes. The Sioux and Mandan, among other Indian tribes, favored a communal way of life that valued community over the individual. Likewise, Spanish-speaking settlers of tight-knit adobe pueblos prized the close cooperation of men and women: *compadres* (godfathers) with *comadres* (godmothers). These settlers lived their lives according to the seasonal rhythms of agriculture and stock-raising.

In the South, slaveholders straddled both positions. They idealized both profit-seeking individualism and a traditional way of life based on community ties. These white men and women eagerly raked in the financial gains that flowed from their control over staple crop agriculture. Yet in their public pronouncements, they scorned the exclusive pursuit of profit. They held their loyalties to family, kin, and community above the crass emphasis on cash that Yankees espoused. As conflicts between Indians and whites revealed, differences in values were far more than theoretical abstractions. Ultimately, they could wreak death and destruction, as northerners and southerners soon discovered.

Freed from the arduous household labor required of the colonial housewife, the idealized mother of the nineteenth-century emerging middle classes devoted herself to providing religious instruction to her children. This mother, portrayed in *Godey's Lady's Book,* teaches her daughter to pray. The well-appointed bedroom suggests a life of physical comfort and ease.

Conclusion

Western settlement infused American politics with raw energy in the 1820s. Andrew Jackson was the first in a long line of presidents who boasted of their humble origins and furthered their careers by denouncing what they called the privileges enjoyed by wealthy Easterners. The western impulse for grassroots politicking shaped in political reforms, such as those that gave voters more power in nominating candidates for office and electing members of the Electoral College. The challenges faced by western settlers in establishing homesteads and paying their debts emerged as national, not purely local issues. Through the sheer force of his personality, Andrew Jackson exemplified these dramatic changes in the political landscape. Almost single-handedly, he extended the limits of executive power and remade the American party system in the process.

However, the contradictions in Jacksonian politics became glaring in the coming years. As the nation expanded its borders and diversified its economy, distinctions between social classes sharpened. The country also staked its claim to foreign territory, using violence to advance democratic values. Meanwhile, the North and South eyed each other with increasing distrust. And the contrast between those who moved from place to place voluntarily and those who were forced to move became even more dramatic.

Sites to Visit

The Second Bank of the United States, 1816–1936
odur.let.rug.nl/~usa/E/usbank/bank04.htm
> The political conflict surrounding the Second Bank of the United States contributed to the rise of the Whig party.

The Erie Canal
www.syracuse.com/features/eriecanal
> This site presents the Erie Canal as "the super highway of pre–Civil War America."

The Cherokee Nation
www.cherokee.org/culture/history.asp
> This is the official Web site of the Cherokee Nation based in Talequah, Oklahoma.

Commerce on the Prairie
www.ukans.edu/carrie/kancoll/books/gregg/contents.htm
> This University of Kansas site includes information on life and commerce on the frontier between the United States and Mexico.

Pioneering the Upper Midwest: Books from Michigan, Minnesota, and Wisconsin, ca. 1820–1910
memory.loc.gov/ammem/umhtml/umhome.html
> This Library of Congress site looks at first-person accounts, biographies, promotional literature, ethnographic and antiquarian texts, colonial archival documents, and other works from the seventeenth to early twentieth century. It covers many topics and issues related to Americans and the settlement of the Upper Midwest.

The Settlement of African Americans in Liberia
www.loc.gov./exhibits/african/perstor.html
> This site contains images and text relating to the colonization movement sponsored by the American Colonization Society.

African American Women Writers from the Nineteenth Century
digital.nypl.org.schomburg/writers_aa19/toc.html
> The New York Public Library–Schomburg Center for Research in Black Culture site contains texts of nineteenth-century African American literature by women.

For Further Reading

General

Stuart R. Blumin, *The Emergence of the Middle Class: Social Experience in the American City, 1760–1900* (1989).

Daniel Feller, *The Jacksonian Promise: America, 1815–1840* (1995).

D. W. Meinig, *The Shaping of America: A Geographical Perspective on 500 Years of History. Vol. 2: Continental America, 1800–1867* (1993).

Melvyn Stokes and Stephen Conway, eds., *The Market Revolution in America: Social, Political, and Religious Expressions, 1800–1880* (1996).

Anthony F. C. Wallace, *The Long, Bitter Trail: Andrew Jackson and the Indians* (1993).

David J. Weber, *The Spanish Frontier in North America* (1992).

The Politics Behind Western Expansion

William J. Cooper, *The South and the Politics of Slavery, 1828–1856* (1978).

James W. Covington, *The Seminoles of Florida* (1993).

Mark Derr, *The Frontiersman: The Real Life and Many Legends of Davy Crockett* (1993).

Ernest R. May, *The Making of the Monroe Doctrine* (1976).

Timothy Matovina, *Tejano Religion and Ethnicity: San Antonio, 1821–1860* (1995).

Ronald E. Shaw, *Canals for a Nation: The Canal Era in the United States, 1790–1860* (1990).

Federal Authority and Its Opponents

William W. Freehling, *Prelude to Civil War: The Nullification Controversy in South Carolina, 1816–1836* (1966).

Michael D. Green, *The Politics of Indian Removal: Creek Government and Society in Crisis* (1982).

Michael F. Holt, *Political Parties and American Political Development from the Age of Jackson to the Age of Lincoln* (1992).

Lawrence Frederick Kohl, *The Politics of Individualism: Parties and the American Character in the Jacksonian Era* (1989).

Marvin Meyers, *The Jacksonian Persuasion: Politics and Belief* (1968).

Robert V. Remini, *Andrew Jackson and His Indian Wars* (2001).

Real People in the "Age of the Common Man"

Virginia Marie Bouvier, *Women and the Conquest of California, 1542–1840: Codes of Silence* (2001).

Thomas Dublin, *Transforming Women's Work: New England Lives in the Industrial Revolution* (1994).

Albert L. Hurtado, *Intimate Frontiers: Sex, Culture and Gender in California* (1999).

Jack Larkin, *The Reshaping of Everyday Life, 1790–1840* (1988).

Walter Licht, *Industrial America: The Nineteenth Century* (1995).

David Walker, *David Walker's Appeal, in Four Articles* (1965 ed.).

Julie Winch, *Philadelphia's Black Elite: Activism, Accommodation, and the Struggle for Autonomy, 1787–1848* (1988).

Ties That Bound a Growing Population

Jeanne Boydston, *Home and Work: Housework, Wages, and the Ideology of Labor in the Early Republic* (1990).

Richard L. Bushman, *Joseph Smith and the Beginnings of Mormonism* (1984).

Charles Hambrick-Stowe, *Charles Grandison Finney and the Spirit of American Evangelism* (1996).

Nathan O. Hatch, *The Democratization of American Christianity* (1989).

Christine L. Heyrman, *Southern Cross: The Beginnings of the Bible Belt* (1997).

Paul E. Johnson, *A Shopkeeper's Millennium: Society and Revivals in Rochester, New York, 1815–1837* (1978).

Walter Benn Michaels and Donald E. Pease, eds., *The American Renaissance Reconsidered* (1985).

Online Practice Test

Test your understanding of this chapter with interactive review quizzes at

www.ablongman.com/jonescreatedequal/chapter11

Additional Photo Credits

Page 359: John Gadsby Chapman, *Davy Crockett*, date unknown. Art Collection, Harry Ransom Humanities Research Center, The University of Texas at Austin (neg. #65.349)

Page 363: Courtesy, Janice L. and David Frent

Page 374: Eric P. Newman Numismatic Education Society

Page 379: The American Numismatic Society, New York

Page 386: Reproduced by permission of The Huntington Library, San Marino, California

Page 387: Courtesy, Dartmouth University Library

Peoples in Motion, 1832–1848

■ Richard Caton Woodville's *War News from Mexico*, 1848.

I
N THE SPRING OF 1847 JANNICKE SAEHLE LEFT HER HOME IN BERGEN, A CITY ON THE
western coast of Norway, and boarded a ship bound for New York City. From New
York, the young woman traveled by steamship up the Hudson River to Albany. There
she boarded a train to Milwaukee, Wisconsin. Although arduous, the journey had its pleasures. Piloted by a charming captain, the steamship resembled, in Saehle's words, "a complete house four stories high, and very elegantly furnished, with beautiful rugs everywhere."
On the train, the passengers enjoyed each other's company as well as "the noteworthy
sights that we rushed past." By the summer Saehle was living with and working as a domestic servant for a Norwegian family, the Torjersens, in Koshkonong in southeastern Wisconsin. Founded in 1840, Koshkonong was a rapidly growing settlement of Norwegian
immigrants farming the fertile prairie.

Jannicke Saehle was eager to make a new life for herself in the United
States. For just a few months of service in the Torjersen household,
she received the harvest of 3 acres of wheat for three years. In
the fall she found a job washing and ironing at a tavern in
Madison. For the first five weeks she earned a dollar a
week. Then she received a raise of $.25 a week, with the
promise of another raise, and relief from washing, at the
end of the winter. Although she could not speak English, she was pleased to "enjoy the best treatment" from
the tavern owners and patrons. However, hoped to leave
the tavern and work as a domestic servant for a local family, the Morisons. Saehle believed this new position would
be comfortable; with the Morisons she could "live more
peacefully and have a room by myself."

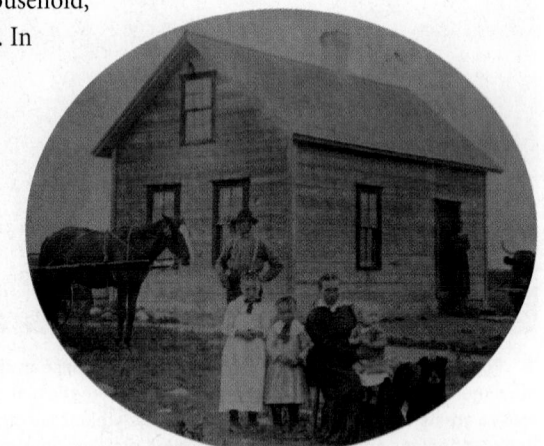

Norwegian immigrants to the United States, 1880s.

In September 1847, Jannicke Saehle wrote of her good
fortune in America in a letter to her family back in Nor-
way. She described "the superabundance of food" in the Torjersen home. On his 40-acre
farm Torjersen kept swine and produced "tremendous amounts" of wheat, potatoes, beans,
cabbage, cucumbers, onions, and many other kinds of vegetables. At the Madison tavern
she had "food and drink in abundance" and dined on the same fare served to the guests:
for breakfast, "chicken, mutton [lamb], beef or pork, warm or cold wheat bread, butter,
white cheese, eggs, or small pancakes, the best coffee, tea, cream and sugar." For supper she
feasted on "warm biscuits, and several kinds of cold wheat bread, cold meats, bacon, cakes,
preserved apples, plums, and berries, which are eaten with cream, and tea and coffee."
Saehle felt heartbroken to see excess food thrown to the chickens and pigs, for, she wrote,
"I think of my dear ones in Bergen, who like so many others must at this time lack the nec-
essaries of life."

During the 1840s, more than 13,000 immigrants from Norway, Sweden, and Denmark
arrived in the United States, a sixfold increase over the number of Scandinavians who had

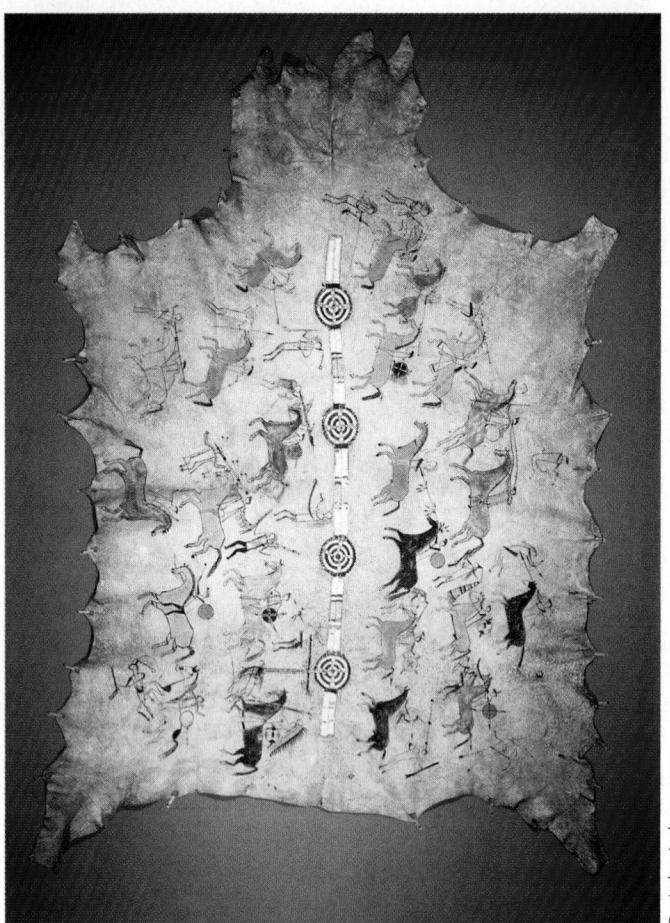

Deutsches Ledermuseum

■ **Plains Indians developed new art forms in response to the westward movement of European American trappers, missionaries, and settlers. Native artists used picture writing to describe violent encounters between Indians and intruders. They etched pictures on sandstone or painted them on cliffs or clothing. These battle pictographs, painted on a Cheyenne buffalo robe c. 1845, bear similarities to other images produced by Flathead artists. Scholars believe that these drawings formed a language understood by a variety of Indian groups from Canada to the American Southwest.**

arrived the decade before. This migration continued to increase over the course of the nineteenth century. In the 1880s, more than 655,000 Scandinavians, fleeing poverty and military conflict, came to America. Many traveled to Wisconsin and Minnesota, where they farmed small homesteads and found the cold winter climate similar to that of their homeland.

In the rural upper Midwest, clashes between Indians and white settlers shaped the experiences of many immigrants. Newcomers to Minnesota, especially, did not fare well; there the great Sioux uprising of 1862 resulted in the deaths of hundreds of Indians and immigrant settlers, Swedes and Norwegians prominent among them. However, by the late 1840s, settlers in Wisconsin such as Jannicke Saehle had little reason to fear the Indians whose ancestral lands they occupied; the U.S. army's destruction of a band of Sauk Indians under the leadership of Black Hawk in 1832 had opened up much of the area to whites.

In the 1830s and 1840s, patterns of settlement and employment among immigrant groups varied widely in the United States. For example, most Irish immigrants lacked the resources to move much farther west than the eastern seaboard ports where they landed. In contrast, many Germans arrived with enough money to buy farmland in the Midwest or take up a trade in eastern cities. Nevertheless, Norwegian immigrants had much in common with other groups that came to the United States in these years. Many relied for jobs and housing on compatriots who had already arrived. The newcomers found employment in expanding regional economies. Communities of immigrants built their own religious institutions and mutual aid societies.

In the 1830s and 1840s, the United States was home to many peoples in motion. Groups of Indians in the Southeast and Midwest and slaves in the upper South were forced at gunpoint to move from one region of the country to another. From western Europe came poor and persecuted groups drawn to the United States by the demand for labor and the promise of religious and political freedom. Some Americans eagerly pulled up stakes and moved to nearby cities or towns in search of better jobs. Migrants with enough resources made the long journey across the Sonoran Desert in the Southwest or to the Oregon Territory in the Northwest.

Population movements and economic change generated new forms of community and group identity. Some immigrants and migrants left behind old identities and created new ones for themselves in their new homes. In their native lands, many newcomers to the United States had lived and labored as peasants under the control of aristocratic landlords. Now in America these immigrants worked as wage earners or as small farmers. Urban workers founded the National Trades Union, an organization that tried to help laboring people wield political influence. Women and men who believed in their power to change society banded together for any number of causes—including those that challenged basic institu-

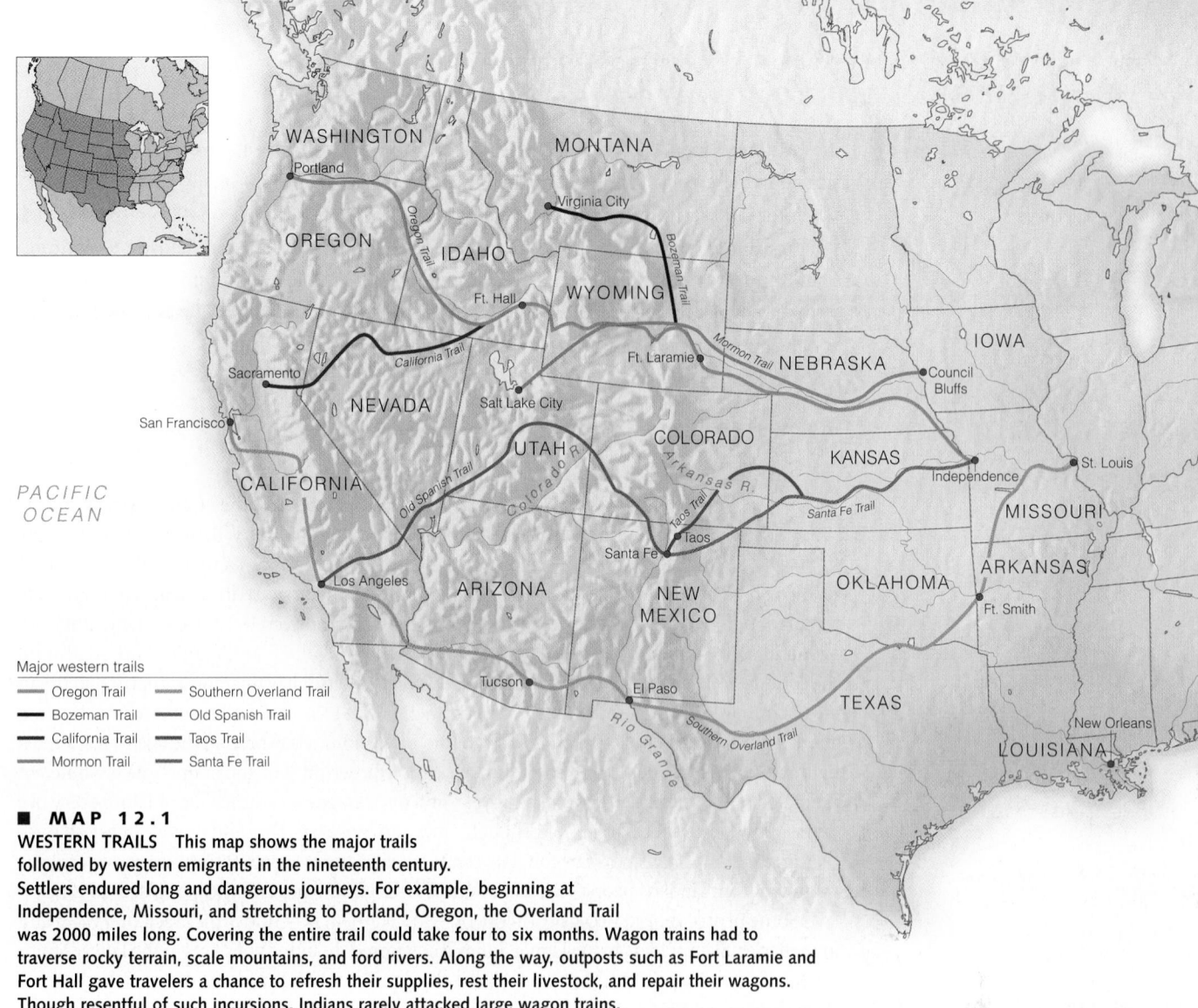

■ MAP 12.1
WESTERN TRAILS   This map shows the major trails
followed by western emigrants in the nineteenth century.
Settlers endured long and dangerous journeys. For example, beginning at
Independence, Missouri, and stretching to Portland, Oregon, the Overland Trail
was 2000 miles long. Covering the entire trail could take four to six months. Wagon trains had to
traverse rocky terrain, scale mountains, and ford rivers. Along the way, outposts such as Fort Laramie and
Fort Hall gave travelers a chance to refresh their supplies, rest their livestock, and repair their wagons.
Though resentful of such incursions, Indians rarely attacked large wagon trains.

tions such as the nuclear family, slavery, and white supremacy. Some reformers established
new communities based on alternative notions of marriage and child-rearing.

Partisan politics also entered a new era. By 1836, the so-called Second Party system had
emerged, as Jacksonian Democrats squared off against the Whigs on familiar issues including
tariffs and new systems of transportation. A coalition of anti-Jackson forces, the Whigs, sought
to craft an economic program that would appeal to the largest number of voters. Less concerned with the purity of their ideas than with success at the ballot box, the Whigs saw their
policies as a means to winning elections and not necessarily as ends in themselves.

The choices offered by the Whigs and Democrats failed to represent what many groups
saw as their pressing political and economic interests. Many Americans turned to violence to
advance or defend their causes. The deep-seated resentments or lofty aspirations among various ethnic and religious groups and social classes provoked bloodshed. Urban mobs vented
their wrath against African Americans, abolitionists, and Irish immigrants and other
Catholics. The government itself sponsored violence, which peaked in the late 1830s with the
forced removal of southeastern Indians to the West, and again in the late 1840s, when the
United States wrested a vast expanse of land from Mexico. Indeed, within the larger society,
physical force seemed to be an acceptable means of resolving disputes; tellingly, politicians of
all persuasions followed Andrew Jackson's lead and staked their claim to national leadership
on the basis of their records as soldiers, military officers, and Indian-killers.

Although industrial machines such as locomotives and textile looms grew more sophisticated in these years, farming remained the primary occupation for many people. However, when the land refused to yield crops, millions of people had to move on—from the blighted potato fields of Ireland, the rocky soil of New England, or the worn-out fields of the cotton South. In search of new economic opportunities, some people moved into lands belonging to other people. In the territory occupied by native Spanish speakers in Texas or by Indians in the Southeast, people stood ready to fight—and die—for the land.

Mass Migrations

When foreign visitors called Americans a "restless" people, they were referring to patterns of both immigration and migration within the country. Between 1830 and 1850, 2.3 million immigrants entered the United States, up from a total of 152,000 during the two previous decades. In the 1840s, 1.7 million immigrants arrived (in 1850 the country's total population stood at 27 million people). Most newcomers came from Ireland, Germany, England, Scotland, and Scandinavia. In the United States itself, individuals and families moved around the country with almost dizzying speed in search of better jobs. They migrated from rural to urban areas, from one city to another, out west and then back to the east. In Boston, in any one year, about a third of the population left the city to find a new home elsewhere. In the late 1840s, almost half of all urban residents moved within a 12-month period. For the country as a whole, an estimated one family in five moved every year, and on average every family moved once every five years. Many westward migrants had enough money to move overland and buy a homestead once they arrived in Wisconsin or Oregon. However, much of the population turnover in urban areas stemmed from landless people's relentless quest for higher wages and cheaper places to rent.

Some people moved because other people forced them to—under the crack of a whip and in manacles. Slave traders in the Upper South transported thousands of slaves to the Lower South for sale "on the block." Indians underwent the equivalent of a middle passage (the horrific slave ship voyages between Africa and the Americas) when U.S. soldiers forced them to walk from their homelands in the southeast to Indian Territory (now the state of Oklahoma).

Europeans marveled at Americans' apparent willingness to search out new opportunities. But to some Americans, moving meant the death of dreams and the loss of hope for a better life.

Newcomers from Western Europe

By the early nineteenth century, life had become more precarious than ever for the long-suffering people of Ireland. Over the generations, small farm plots had been subdivided among heirs to the point that most holdings consisted of less than 15 acres each. At the same time, the population of Ireland had grown exponentially—to more than 4 million people in 1800. England treated Ireland like a colony that existed purely for the economic gain of the mother country (or, in the eyes of the Irish, an occupying power). A series of English laws and policies mandated that farmers export most of the island's grain and cattle, leaving the impoverished people to subsist mainly on a diet of potatoes. Then, beginning in 1845, a blight devastated the potato crop. In the next five years, 1 million people died and another million fled to the United States. The great Irish migration had begun.

Increasing numbers of poor Irish had settled in the United States before the potato famine of the mid–1840s. In the 1820s, about 50,000 such immigrants arrived; the following decade saw a spike in numbers to more than 200,000. Yet a more dramatic increase was yet to come. As the 1840s and 1850s unfolded, 1.7 million Irish men, women, and children emigrated to the United States. This exodus continued over the next century as more than 4.5 million Irish arrived. Many immigrants were single women who found work as servants and sent money back to Ireland. As Margaret McCarthy wrote in a letter to her parents back home in County

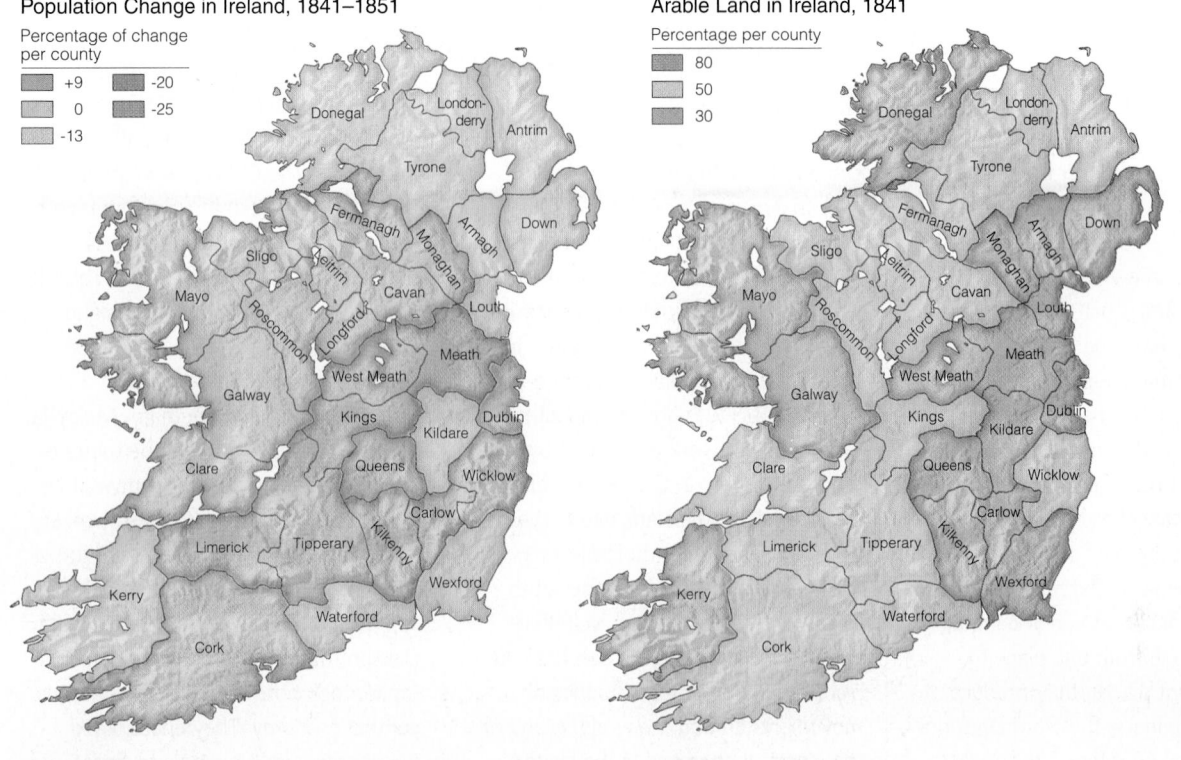

Population Change in Ireland, 1841–1851

Percentage of change per county

+9
0
-13
-20
-25

Arable Land in Ireland, 1841

Percentage per county

80
50
30

■ **MAP 12.2**
POPULATION CHANGE IN IRELAND, 1841–1851   During the famine of the late 1840s, some counties in Ireland lost more than one-quarter of their population to out-migration. However, emigration rates in some of the very poorest counties were not always high. People there were too poor to pay for passage to the United States. The county of Kerry, in the country's southwestern corner, is an example.

Pauperism in Ireland, 1847–1851

More than 50% of population pauper for over 1 year by Poor Law Union

Cork, in 1850, the newcomers embraced "this plentyful Country where no man or woman ever Hungerd or ever will and where you will not be Seen Naked."

By the 1870s, the Irish constituted fully 20 percent of the population of New York City, 14 percent of Philadelphia, and 22 percent of Boston (the "hub of Gaelic America"). The newcomers quickly formed mutual aid associations and other community organizations. In cities across America, the Sisters of Mercy, a Roman Catholic order founded in Dublin, established homes to provide lodging for single women and day nurseries for the children of working mothers.

Most Irish immigrants lacked the resources to move much farther west than the eastern seaport cities where they landed, and they soon realized that their struggle against poverty, discrimination, and religious persecution would not end in the United States. The arrival of large numbers of Irish immigrants in the 1830s threatened the jobs of native-born Protestants, who reacted with resentment and violence. Employers posted signs outside their doors reading "No Irish Need Apply." Despised for their Roman Catholicism and their supposed "clannishness," the Irish competed with African Americans for the low-paying jobs at the bottom of the economic ladder. At times, anti-Irish sentiment reached violent extremes. In 1834 a mob destroyed the Ursuline convent

Diasporas

Almost all of the Irish men, women, and children who emigrated from their homeland in the nineteenth century came to the United States. In this respect, the Irish exodus was somewhat unusual. Over the last four and a half centuries, many peoples have participated in transoceanic mass migrations. Yet most of those migrations have been characterized by a scattering of peoples to different countries. Since its beginnings, the United States has been a major host, but not the only one, to immigrants as well as forced migrants.

When specific ethnic or cultural groups disperse from one place to many different places, they produce a diaspora. Originally, the word *Diaspora* (with a capital *D*) referred to the dispersal of Jewish communities out of Palestine and into Europe and Africa 2000 years ago. Now scholars use the term more generally to refer to many kinds of population dispersals in the past and today. These migrations are the result of two historical phenomena. The first is an emerging world economy with its intense demand for labor, especially in the mining, agricultural, and industrial sectors. The second phenomenon is the desire among specific peoples to flee poverty and persecution and to seek out land, jobs, and religious and political freedom elsewhere.

The African diaspora reveals the effects of a forced migration. Between 1500 and 1850 slave traders transported 12 million Africans to the Western Hemisphere. An estimated

one-tenth of that number died during the Middle Passage. Of the survivors, 10 million were taken to the Caribbean or Latin America and fewer than 450,000 to the area that is now the United States. Yet by 1865, the U.S. African American population accounted for 30 percent of all people of African descent in the Western Hemisphere. Why? American slaveholders encouraged their slaves to have families. In addition, cotton cultivation in the United States was not as unhealthful as other kinds of work performed by slaves elsewhere in the hemisphere. Thus, African Americans had higher fertility rates and lower mortality rates than their counterparts to the south.

Over the generations, voluntary migration to the United States has taken place among other mass population movements around the world. Many of the groups that arrived in the United States between 1880 and 1920, such as Italians, Russian Jews, and Germans, also sent immigrants to other parts of the world. In the twentieth century, political and religious conflict in their homeland propelled Greek emigrants to many different countries. They settled in New York, Philadelphia, Chicago, Los Angeles, and San Francisco, but others migrated to such diverse places as Dakar, Senegal; Kinshasa, Zaire; Addis Ababa, Ethiopia; and Sydney and Melbourne, Australia. Their modern dispersal was similar to that of Lebanese emigrants, who went not only to the United States but also to Latin America, Africa, and Australia.

In some cases, governments have encouraged their citizens to search widely for work to increase the flow of cash into their own countries. When

China began to trade with the rest of the world in 1845, that country sponsored a mass out-migration among men. Those men were supposed to work abroad temporarily and send their earnings home. The Chinese who arrived in the United States in the mid-nineteenth century were part of a larger mass migration that sent 400,000 men also to Canada, Australia, and New Zealand. Between 1845 and 1900, 1.5 million Chinese went to Southeast Asia (Indonesia, Thailand, Vietnam, Malaysia, and Singapore) to work in the mines or the fields. Another half million went to Peru, Cuba, and Chile. Chinese workers in all these countries tried to save to send money back home to their families.

In the early twentieth century, officials on the island of Okinawa, part of Japan, took note of their faltering agricultural economy. They encouraged able-bodied young people to find employment elsewhere and send their wages to families back home. Beginning in 1900, Okinawa immigrants arrived in Hawaii to work on sugar plantations. Over the next decades other Okinawans moved to California to labor in the fruit and vegetable fields and to the Philippines to grow Manila hemp. Others went to Canada, Brazil, Argentina, Bolivia, Mexico, Cuba, Paraguay, and the islands of Micronesia.

In the 1980s, the Ferdinand Marcos government in the Philippines made a series of agreements with other countries to accept Filipino workers. Marcos saw the wages the migrants sent home as a means to boost the national economy. However, by that time, the worldwide demand for male workers in the

in Charlestown, near Boston, after terrifying the women and children residents and ransacking the building. In 1837 a group of Boston City Guards (a fraternal order) assaulted the Montgomery Guards, the first Irish military company in the city. (Local military companies often functioned as social groups for men of all ages.) The attackers accused the immigrants of lacking patriotism because they had created a group based on ethnic loyalties.

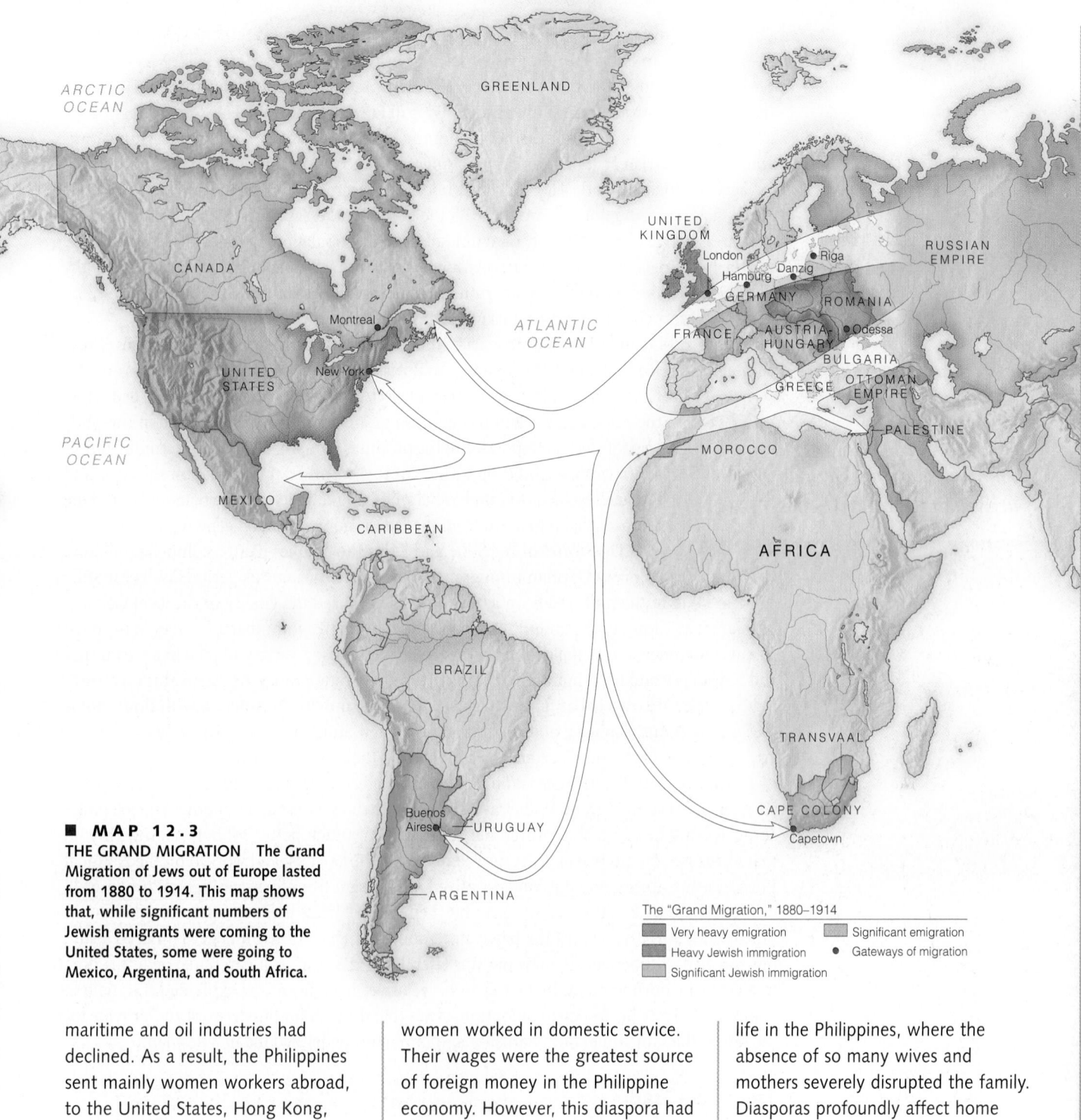

■ **MAP 12.3**
THE GRAND MIGRATION The Grand Migration of Jews out of Europe lasted from 1880 to 1914. This map shows that, while significant numbers of Jewish emigrants were coming to the United States, some were going to Mexico, Argentina, and South Africa.

The "Grand Migration," 1880–1914

■ Very heavy emigration ■ Significant emigration
■ Heavy Jewish immigration ● Gateways of migration
■ Significant Jewish immigration

maritime and oil industries had declined. As a result, the Philippines sent mainly women workers abroad, to the United States, Hong Kong, and Europe. Most of these immigrant women worked in domestic service. Their wages were the greatest source of foreign money in the Philippine economy. However, this diaspora had severe consequences for domestic life in the Philippines, where the absence of so many wives and mothers severely disrupted the family. Diasporas profoundly affect home countries as well as host countries. ■

Nevertheless, by the 1850s, the Irish had gained a measure of influence. They filled many high positions in the U.S. Catholic church and became active in the Democratic party. They claimed that their white skin entitled them to distance themselves from blacks and lay claim to full American citizenship. More than one hundred years later, the election of the first Catholic president of the United States—John Fitzgerald Kennedy of Boston, a descendant of famine-era immigrants on both his mother's and father's side of the family—became a milestone in the Irish rise to political power.

The hardship endured by the Irish in the early nineteenth century mirrored the political and economic distress of many other people living in Europe at the time. The Revolutions of 1848 stemmed from a rising nationalist fervor among Germans, Italians, Czechs, and Hungarians against the Austrian Empire. Popular uprisings in France, Germany, and parts of Italy struck out against monarchy and called for constitutional government. In England and Germany, new textile factories could not accommodate all the urban workers who sought jobs. Europeans in rural areas also fell on particularly hard times. Dramatic population increases made food scarce, and the Industrial Revolution put artisans out of work. In an effort to bolster their power, wealthy landholders consolidated their estates from the holdings of peasant farmers. In the process, the demand for farm labor decreased, pushing many people off the countryside.

Between 1831 and 1850, more than half a million Germans arrived in the United States. Those numbers exploded in the next few decades. An uprising against the authoritarian Prussian state had failed in 1848, and German intellectuals, farmers, and workers alike fled across the ocean. Like Scandinavian immigrants, many Germans settled in the Midwest. Some had responded to the promises of railroad land and recruiting offices scattered through Europe. These offices promised transportation subsidies and low-interest loans to immigrants who bought land from the railroads—land the railroads had purchased from the federal government on generous terms.

> *Between 1831 and 1850, more than half a million Germans arrived in the United States.*

The stories of the Stille and Krumme families paint a compelling picture of many German immigrants' experience during this period. Wilhelm Stille came to Ohio in the mid–1830s. In letters home, he praised the vitality of the local German immigrant community, the bountiful soil, and the "feel for freedom" that infused even the most recent newcomers. Over the next few years Stille worked at a variety of jobs in a steam mill and a distillery and for a merchant. Scraping together some money, he started his own trading business. He traveled as far away as New Orleans and South America with flour, potatoes, string beans, cabbage, onions, and apples. Then Stille married a young woman newly arrived from Switzerland. Together the couple tried their hand at farming.

Meanwhile, Wilhelm's sister Wilhelmina, who had accompanied him to America, married another German immigrant, Wilhelm Krumme. Wilhelmina missed her mother and felt guilty about leaving her. But, she assured her mother, "I'm much better off here than with you, that's because you can live in peace over here." Wilhelmina's husband worked on the National Road, crushing rocks, and the couple received money sent from their families in Europe. Still, in the early 1840s a national depression hit them hard: "These are bad times now, there's not much work and if you work the pay is not good." In 1841 Wilhelmina gave birth to a son, but she died of tuberculosis a few months later. Within a year, Wilhelm remarried, this time to a German-born woman. In a letter to his relatives back home, he explained that he had almost had to give his son up for adoption; it was that difficult for him to work and provide for the boy at the same time. Both hardship and opportunity defined life in a new land.

The Slave Trade

Between 1800 and 1860, the average price of slaves quadrupled, revealing a growing demand for bound labor. The slave market responded accordingly. In the last three decades before the Civil War, approximately 670,000 people were bought and sold. As many as one out of every ten slave children in the Upper South was sold to the Lower South (many to cotton planters) between 1820 and 1860. Slave households in Virginia bore the brunt of these forced separations. There, an estimated three quarters of the people sold never saw their spouse, parents, or children again.

Owners sold slaves for a variety of reasons. Some they considered poor workers or too "uppity." Occasionally, a mistress decided to rid herself of the sight of a slave woman whom her husband had sexually abused. Selling slaves also generated ready cash for masters who wanted to build a new house, divide an estate, or settle a debt. Moses Grandy, for example,

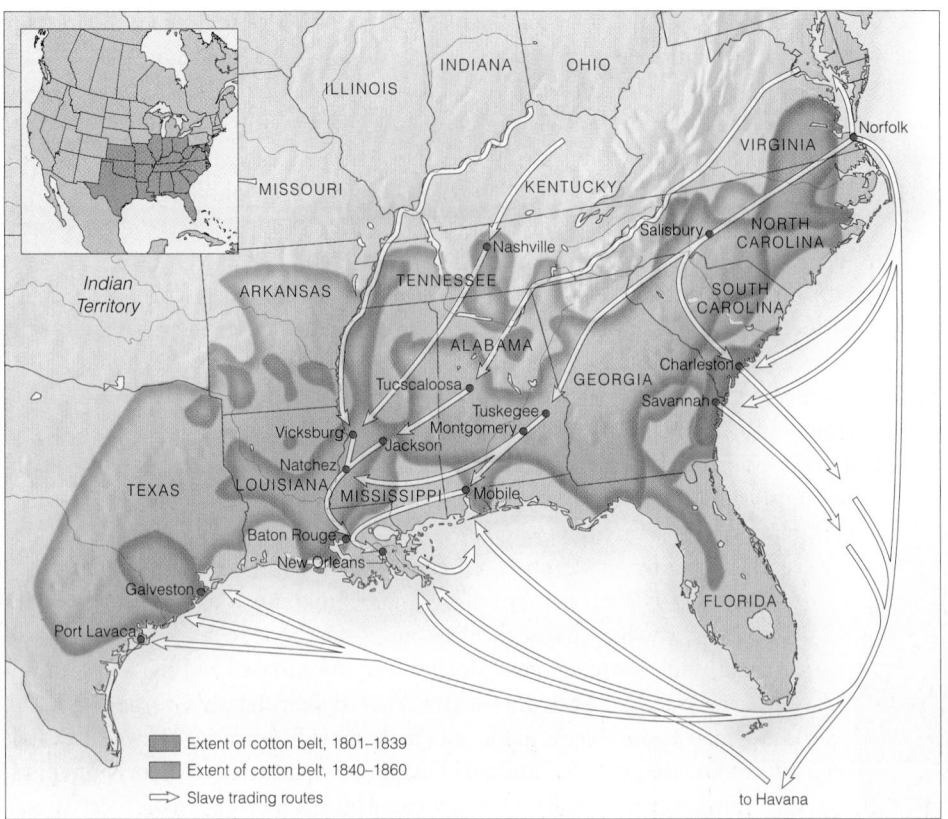

■ **MAP 12.4**

EXPANSION OF THE COTTON BELT AND SLAVE TRADING ROUTES, 1801–1860   This map shows the spread of cotton cultivation and routes followed by traders in transporting slaves from the upper South to the new plantations of the Southwest. After Texas won its independence from Mexico in 1836, the new republic legalized slavery. Many white landowners believed that they could not grow cotton without the use of slave labor.

was sold because his master, who had failed to pay his mortgage, needed the cash. A later sale separated Grandy from his wife: standing on a sidewalk one day, he saw his wife in chains, in a coffle passing by. He recalled the scene in his autobiography, *Narrative of the Life of Moses Grandy, Late a Slave in the United States of America* (1844):

> Mr. Rogerson was with them on his horse, armed with pistols. I said to him. "For God's sake, have you bought my wife?" He said he had; when I asked him what she had done, he said she had done nothing, but that her master wanted money. He drew out a pistol and said that if I went near the wagon where she was, he would shoot me. I asked for leave to shake hands with her which he refused, but said I might stand at a distance and talk with her. My heart was so full that I could say very little. . . . I have never seen or heard from her from that day to this. I loved her as I love my life.

The slave trade became big business. Many wealthy traders made regular trips between the Upper and Lower South. Owners of slaves who worked in the sawmills and grist mills of Virginia and Maryland realized they could profit handsomely by selling blacks to cotton planters in Mississippi and Alabama. A large slave trade establishment such as Franklin and Armfield, for example, had operations in Alexandria, Virginia (where slaves languished in pens until traders could ship them south), in Natchez, Mississippi, and in New Orleans, Louisiana. The pace of buying and selling picked up in late fall, after slaves had harvested grains and tobacco in the upper South and cotton in the lower South. Traders transported men, women, and children by boat down the eastern seaboard or down the Mississippi River or chained and forced them to walk as much as 20 miles a day for seven or eight weeks at a time in the chill autumn air. Eventually, slaves stood on the block in the markets of New Orleans, Natchez, Charleston, and Savannah, where white men inspected them for health, strength, and compliance.

The European American slave owners who had moved to Texas in the 1820s took their slaves with them. When Mexico abolished slavery in 1829, some European American masters freed their slaves but then forced them to sign lifelong contracts that kept them in a state akin to bondage. Nevertheless, some free people of color—men such as John Bird—saw Texas as a place of opportunity. He had brought his family to Texas from Virginia because he hoped that they "would be received as citizens and entitled as such to land."

Indeed, during this period, voluntary migrations of African Americans formed the counterpoint of the slave trade as runaways and free people of color made their way out of the old slave states. An estimated 50,000 enslaved workers tried to escape each year, but few made it to the North and freedom.

Some southern free people of color headed to northern cities. By 1850, more than half of all Boston blacks had been born outside Massachusetts. Of those migrants, about one-third had been born in the South, most in Virginia, Maryland, and the District of Columbia. Slave runaways who lived in fear of their safety and their lives eluded census takers, but by midcentury as many as 600 fugitives lived in Boston.

Regardless of their place of origin, many migrants took up residence with other blacks, who helped ease the newcomers' transition to city life. These boarding arrangements strengthened ties between the enslaved and the free communities. For example, when authorities arrested the runaway George Latimer in Boston in 1842, free blacks in that city took immediate action. They posted signs condemning the police as "human kidnappers." Some tried to wrench him physically from his captors. Still others sponsored protest meetings in the local African Baptist Church and made common cause with white lawyers sympathetic to abolitionism. Finally a group of blacks and whites raised enough money to buy Latimer from his owner and free him. Out of this campaign came a 150-pound antislavery petition containing the names of thousands of Massachusetts citizens. The petition, ignored by Congress, called for legislation forbidding the complicity of state officials in apprehending fugitive slaves.

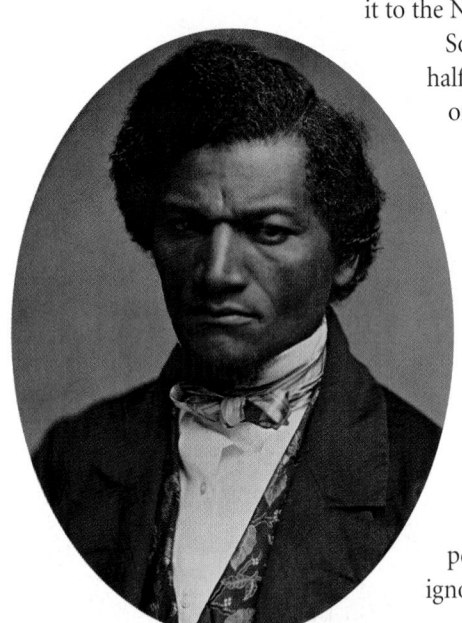

Born a slave in Maryland in 1818, Frederick Douglass became a leading abolitionist speaker, editor, and activist. Not content to condemn southern slaveholders exclusively, he also criticized northern employers for not hiring blacks. Trained as a ship caulker, Douglass faced job discrimination in the shipyards of New Bedford, Massachusetts, where he and his wife, Anna, settled soon after he escaped slavery and they moved north (in 1838).

Meanwhile, throughout the urban North, whites began eyeing blacks' jobs. Irish immigrants in particular desperately sought work. Skilled black workers found it increasingly difficult to ply their trades as cooks, hotel and boat stewards, porters, brickmakers, and barbers. In 1838, 656 black artisans in Philadelphia reported that they had to abandon their work because white customers would no longer patronize them. White factory owners in Philadelphia preferred white laborers. In that same city, a bustling site of machine shops and textile factories, almost no blacks did industrial labor of any kind. Shut out of ship-caulking work in New Bedford, Massachusetts, fugitive slave Frederick Douglass warned of the consequences of an economic system that condemned all blacks to lowly, ill-paid labor, "Men are not valued in this country, or in any country, for what they *are*; they are valued for what they can do." Douglass understood that whites would judge blacks on the basis of their jobs as menial laborers and not on the basis of their rights as American citizens. These judgments, he predicted, would lead to further discrimination and hardship among blacks.

Trails of Tears

In 1835 President Andrew Jackson made a puzzling declaration. The removal of eastern Indian groups to Indian Territory, he said, would ensure their "physical comfort," "political advancement," and "moral improvement." Rarely have a chief executive's words contrasted so starkly with reality.

Throughout the 1830s, the U.S. government pursued the policy of removing Indians from the Southeast by treaty or by force. The 1832 Treaty of Payne's Landing, negotiated by the

Seminole Indians and James Gadsden, a representative of Secretary of War Lewis Cass, aimed to force the Seminoles out of Florida and into Indian Territory (present-day Oklahoma). The federal government promised to give individual Indians cash, plus blankets for the men and dresses for the women, in exchange for their lands. Government authorities also hoped to recapture the large number of runaway slaves who had sought refuge in Seminole villages, deep in the swamps of central Florida.

Three years later, many of the Indians had departed for the West. But a small number withdrew deeper into the Everglades and held their ground. They were led by a young man named Osceola, who with his followers waged a guerrilla war (based on ambush tactics rather than traditional conventions of European American warfare) against U.S. troops. Accustomed to meeting the enemy on a battleground, U.S. army troops failed to dislodge significant numbers of Indians who had hidden themselves in the swamps. Referring to the twin military goals of removing the Indians and capturing runaway slaves, General Thomas S. Jesup expressed his frustration with the military operation: "We have committed the error of attempting to remove them when their lands were not required for agricultural purposes, when the greater portion of their country was an unexplored wilderness, the interior of which we were as ignorant of as the interior of China." Osceola's resistance, called the Second Seminole War, dragged on for seven years. Eventually, the government forced 3000 Seminoles to move west, but not until it had spent $20 million, and 1500 U.S. soldiers had lost their lives.

The Choctaws of the southern Alabama–Mississippi region, the Chickasaws directly to the north of them, and the Creeks in central Georgia and Alabama suffered the same fate in the 1830s. The Creeks remained bitterly divided among themselves on the issue of removal. Creek leader Eneah Emothla organized a violent resistance movement against government soldiers. Emothla's actions gave the government a pretext for forcibly relocating 15,000 of his people, more than a fifth of whom died as a result of the operation.

The threat of removal also provoked intense conflict within the Cherokee Nation. Cherokee Indians, Major Ridge, his son John Ridge, and Elias Boudinot, leaders of the so-called Treaty Party, urged their people to give up their homeland and rebuild their nation in the West. John Ross and others like him opposed the Ridges and Boudinot. The Cherokees must remain in Georgia at all costs, Ross insisted. He claimed that he spoke for a majority of Cherokees. To silence him, the U.S. government threw him in prison. Then it concluded negotiations with the Treaty Party, which agreed to sell Cherokee land to the federal government for $5 million. Elias Boudinot said, "We can die, but the great Cherokee Nation will be saved." Within a few years, the Ridges and Boudinot died at the hands of anti–Treaty Party Cherokee assassins.

In 1838 General Winfield Scott, with 7000 troops under his command, began rounding up the citizens of the Cherokee Nation. U.S. troops held men, women, and children in concentration camps before forcing them to march west. During the period from 1838 to 1839, nearly 16,000 Indians began a journey that they called the Trail on Which We Cried. Four thousand of them died of malnutrition and disease in the course of the 116-day forced march. U.S. troops confiscated or destroyed the material basis of Cherokee culture: sawmills, cotton gins, barns, homes, spinning wheels, meetinghouses, flocks, herds, and the printing press used to publish the *Cherokee Phoenix*.

Rebecca Neugin later recalled the arrival of army troops at her house. "My father wanted to fight," she said, "but my mother told him that the soldiers would kill him if we did and we surrendered without a fight. They drove us out of our house to join other prisoners in a stockade." The soldiers let Rebecca's mother take a few cooking utensils with her; the family lost everything else. Still, Neugin's family remained

The Cherokee Elias Boudinot was educated at missionary schools in North Carolina and Connecticut. As editor of the *Cherokee Phoenix*, Boudinot clashed with Principal Chief John Ross on the issue of forced removal to the West. Ross believed that the paper's editorial policy should reflect the official Cherokee position on the matter. Boudinot resigned in protest. In 1835, Boudinot, with his cousin John Ridge, and Major Ridge, defied Ross and other leaders and signed the Treaty of New Echota. Although the treaty did not have the approval of the Cherokee Nation, it paved the way for the Trail of Tears, 1838–1839.

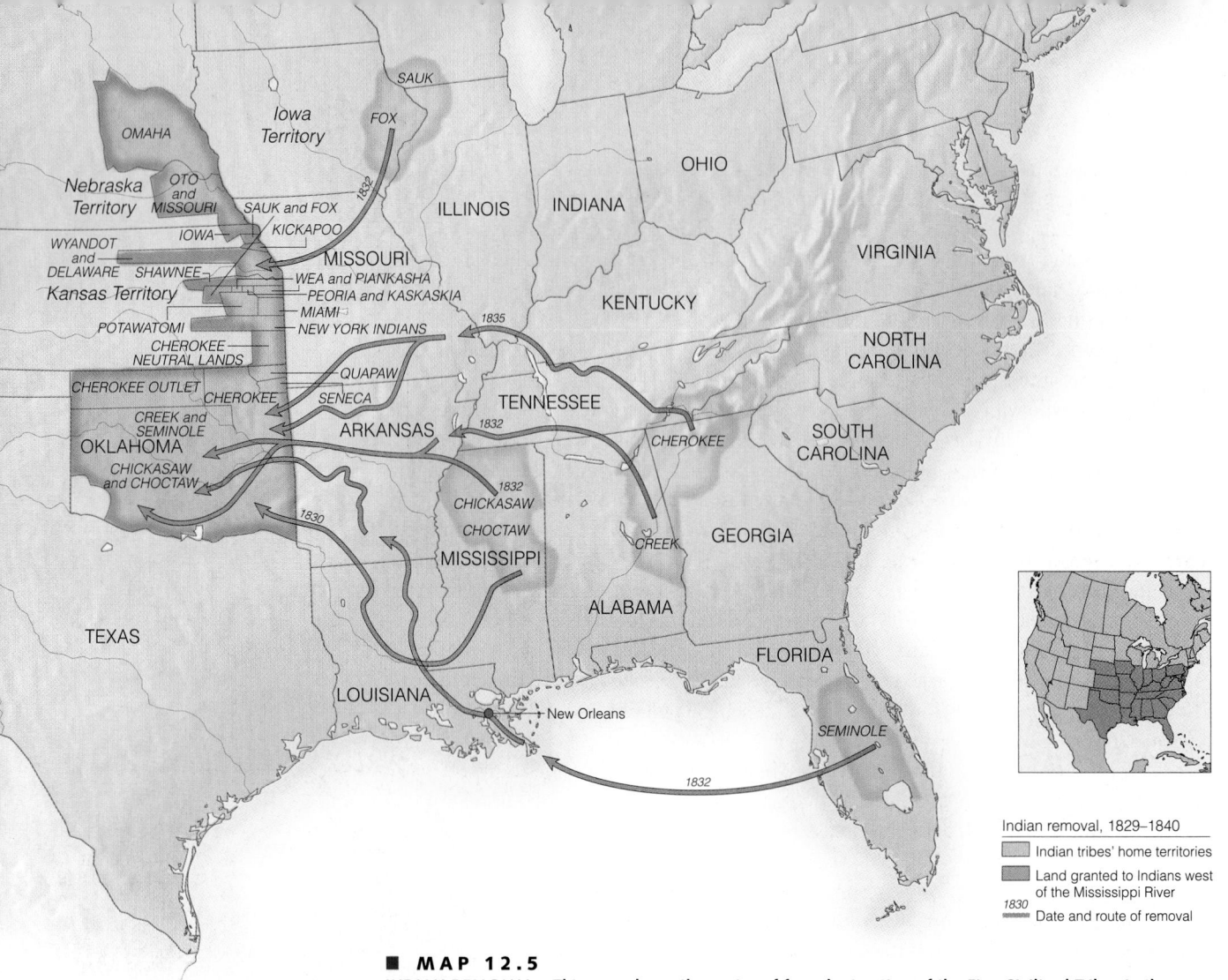

■ MAP 12.5

INDIAN REMOVAL This map shows the routes of forced migration of the Five Civilized Tribes in the 1830s. By the 1870s, several groups of Plains Indians, including the Cheyenne, Arapaho, Comanche, and Kiowa, had joined them in Indian Territory (present-day Oklahoma).

intact. Many others did not. A soldier who participated in the operation saw children "separated from their parents and driven into the stockade with the sky for a blanket and the earth for a pillow."

U.S. officials claimed that troops had carried out the removal with "great judgment and humanity." However, an internal government report completed in 1841 revealed that the United States had reneged on even its most basic treaty promises. "Bribery, perjury, and forgery, short weights, issues of spoiled meat and grain, and every conceivable subterfuge was employed by designing white men." Many government agents seized goods such as blankets and food intended for Indians and sold these goods for profit. Military authorities suppressed the report, and the public never saw it.

Migrants in the West

For many native-born migrants seeking a new life west of the Mississippi, the road proved neither smooth nor easy. For example, the Mormon community moved west, seeking refuge from religious persecution. The founder of the church, Joseph Smith, had aroused the anger of his neighbors in Nauvoo, Illinois. They took alarm at the Nauvoo Legion, a military company formed to defend the Mormon community. They also heard rumors (for the most part true) that Smith and other Mormon leaders engaged in plural marriage. Through this practice the Mormon Church granted men permission to marry more than one wife.

TABLE 12-1

Outfitting a Party of Four for the Overland Trail

Area	Item	Amount	Unit Cost ($)	Cost ($)	Weight (lb.)
Transport	Wagon	1	90.00	90.00	
	Oxen	4 yoke	50.00/yoke	200.00	
	Gear		100.00	100.00	
Food	Flour	600 lb.	2.00/100 lb.	12.00	600
	Biscuit	120 lb.	3.00/100 lb.	3.60	120
	Bacon	400 lb.	5.00/100 lb.	20.00	400
	Coffee	60 lb.	7.00/100 lb.	4.20	60
	Tea	4 lb.	50.00/100 lb.	2.00	4
	Sugar	100 lb.	10.00/100 lb.	10.00	100
	Lard	200 lb.	6.00/100 lb.	12.00	200
	Beans	200 lb.	8.00/100 lb.	16.00	200
	Dried fruit	120 lb.	24.00/100 lb.	28.80	120
	Salt	40 lb.	4.00/100 lb.	1.60	40
	Pepper	8 lb.	4.00/100 lb.	.32	8
	Saleratus	8 lb.	4.00/100 lb.	.32	8
	Whiskey	1 keg	5.00/keg	5.00	25
Goods	Rifle	1	30.00	30.00	10
	Pistols	2	15.00	30.00	10
	Powder	5 lb.	.25/lb.	1.25	5
	Lead	15 lb.	.04/lb.	.60	15
	Shot	10 lb.	.10/lb.	1.00	10
	Matches			1.00	1
	Cooking utensils			20.00	25
	Candles and soap	65 lb.	From home	from home	65
	Bedding	60 lb.	From home	from home	60
	Sewing kit	10 lb.	From home	from home	10
	Essential tools			from home	20
	Clothing			from home	100
			Totals	$589.69	2216

In 1844 the Nauvoo Legion destroyed the printing press owned by a group of rebellious church members who objected to what they considered Smith's authoritarian tactics. Civil authorities charged Smith and his brother Hyrum with the destruction of private property and arrested and jailed the two men in the nearby town of Carthage. In June 1844 an angry mob of non-Mormons broke into the jail and lynched the brothers.

By 1847, Brigham Young, who had inherited the mantle of leadership from Smith, determined that the Mormons could not remain in Illinois. Migrants, some of them pushing handcarts loaded with personal belongings, set out for the West. Several thousand settled at the base of the Wasatch Mountains on the edge of the Great Salt Basin, in what is present-day Utah. By 1852, 10,000 Mormons lived in Salt Lake City. With their large numbers and church-inspired discipline, the community prospered. They created an effective irrigation system and turned the desert into a thriving agricultural community.

The Mormons had not settled an uninhabited wilderness. Around Salt Lake, Canadian trappers, Paiute Indians, and Spanish speakers from New Mexico crossed paths, some to hunt, others to gather roots and berries, herd sheep, or trade captives. A variety of cultural groups mingled with and reacted to one another in diverse ways, from intermarriage to savage brutality. Here, one might hear the sounds of a Mexican's guitar, the song of a man half-Mohawk and "half American Scotch," or the lament of an Indian woman taken captive and forcibly separated from her children.

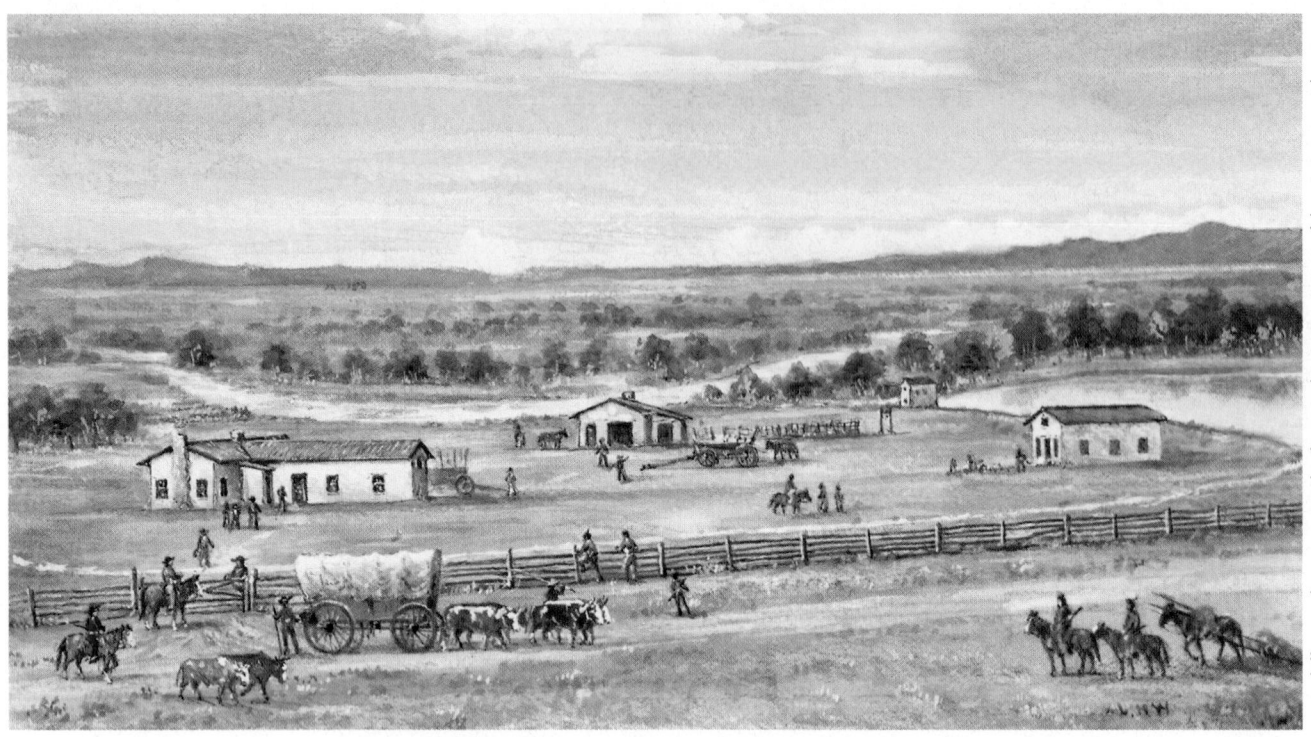

Scotts Bluff National Monument, Nebraska. United States Department of the Interior, National Park Service

■ This picture of the Whitman mission at Waiilatpu, Oregon, in 1845, shows the missionaries' house on the left, a mill in the background, a blacksmith shop in the right center, and a gathering place for worshippers on the far right. By this time the Whitmans had turned their attention from converting Indians to preaching to European American emigrants recently arrived from the East.

A Christmas dinner celebrated near Great Salt Lake around this time revealed the multicultural mix of western life. The guests included Osborne Russell (a European American trader), a Frenchman married to a Flathead woman, and various other intermarried Cree, Snake, and Nez Percé Indians. The group feasted on the meat of elk and deer, a flour pudding, cakes, and strong coffee. After the meal, the women cleared the table. The men smoked pipes and then went outside and conducted target practice with their guns.

Other European Americans also migrated to the Northwest during this period. Protestant missionaries initially settled Oregon beginning in 1834. But in contrast to the Mormons, these northwestern colonists found themselves in the midst of hostile Native Americans. One young doctor and his wife from western New York, Marcus and Narcissa Whitman, established a mission near present-day Walla Walla, Washington. There they encountered the Cayuse Indians and what Narcissa Whitman called "the thick darkness of heathenism." Deciding that white settlers offered a more fertile field for converts, the Whitmans encouraged emigrants from the East to move to Oregon. More than a thousand did so during the "Great Migration" of 1843.

The U.S. government aided this westward movement when it commissioned its Topographical Corps of Engineers to survey the Oregon Trail. That task fell to an expedition headed by John Charles Frémont, educated in mathematics and engineering. From 1843 to 1844, members of Frémont's expedition, including several Indian scouts and fur trappers, took precise measurements of the terrain using barometers and field telescopes.

Their final report had immense practical value for the emigrants, for it mapped the way west and provided crucial information about pasture, sources of water, and climate. In addition to detailing plant and animal life, the *Report of the Exploring Expeditions to the Rocky Mountains* described a middle ground where "well-dressed" Indians spoke fluent Spanish, where whites employed Indian labor to grow their wheat and irrigate their fields, and where German immigrants were following a variety of "agricultural pursuits."

The Oregon settlements founded by missionaries were fragile affairs. Discouraged and overwhelmed by homesickness, Narcissa Whitman eagerly awaited copies of the latest *Mothers' Magazine* sent to her by female relatives in the East. After 1843, the influx of newcomers brought her some consolation but also brought outbreaks of measles, to which the Native Americans had no immunity. An ensuing epidemic among the Cayuse claimed many lives. In 1847, blaming the missionaries for the deaths of their people, several Indians attacked the Whitman mission, killing 12 whites, including Narcissa and Marcus Whitman.

New Places, New Identities

The Midwest and the borderlands between U.S. and Spanish territories were meeting places for many different cultures. Leaving established communities behind, some migrants challenged rigid definitions of who was black, Indian, Hispanic, or European American. Moving from one place to another enabled—or forced—people to adopt new individual and group identities.

People who fell into one racial category in the east sometimes acquired new identities in the west. Some people classified as "black" in the south became "white" outside the region. In 1831, George and Eliza Gilliam decided to leave their home in Virginia and make a new life for themselves in western Pennsylvania. Eliza died in 1838, and George remarried nine years later. He prospered over the course of his lifetime. He worked as a doctor and druggist and invested in and sold real estate. George and his second wife, Frances, eventually moved to Illinois, and the couple finally settled in Missouri. Several of the Gilliam children attended college in Ohio. In 1870, the census listed the value of his estate at $95,000 (the equivalent of $2 million dollars today).

For George Gilliam and his family, the move west produced an American success story. Yet this migration story was unusual in at least two respects. First, the Gilliams left behind a large amount of property, including slaves, when they moved from Virginia in 1831. Second, in leaving Virginia, they became white.

George Gilliam was the son of a white father and a black mother. Although he and his first wife Eliza were very light-skinned, the commonwealth of Virginia classified them both legally as black. Beginning their married life near Petersburg, they were well aware of Virginia's tightening restrictions on free people of color; black men could not vote or enter certain professions such as the law or the ministry. Convicted of a crime, even free blacks could be sold into slavery and sent south. The year the Gilliams left Virginia, the state legislature enacted an additional law making it illegal to teach black children, whether slave or free, to read and write. Though connected by blood to several elite white families, the Gilliams faced at best an uncertain future in Virginia, where local officials knew who they were and who their parents were. In contrast, the public records in their new home states of Pennsylvania, Illinois, and Missouri listed family members as white. Outside the slave South, the Gilliams managed to reinvent themselves and embrace opportunities sought by many other Americans in this era of migration.

Throughout the West, migrants forged new identities as a matter of course. For example, many people straddled more than one culture in the western borderlands. In 1828 Mexican military officer Jose Maria Sanchez described the *Tejano* settlers (Spanish-speaking natives of Mexico) he met in the province of Tejas (Texas): "Accustomed to the continued trade with the North Americans, they have adopted their customs and habits, and one may say truly that they are not Mexican except by birth, for they even speak Spanish with a marked incorrectness."

In other provinces of northern Mexico, European American Protestant traders and travelers mingled with native Spanish speakers. For example, in Santa Fe, New Mexico, Gertrudis Barceló owned a saloon that served as a meeting site for people of many cultures. There European American men could attend a nighttime fandango (dance), play monte (a card game), listen to Spanish music, and socialize with native Spanish speakers. A center of politics, business, and social life, the saloon broke down barriers based on religion, language, and even preconceived notions of personal morality as men and women came to gamble, drink, and carouse.

Leaving established communities behind, some migrants challenged rigid definitions of who was black, Indian, Hispanic, or European American.

In some cases new relationships led to marriage and, ultimately, the creation of households that blended Catholic and Protestant, Spanish and European American cultures.

In parts of the West, traditional social identities yielded to new ones, based less on a single language or ethnicity than on a blend of cultures and new ways of making a living from the land. The 1830s and 1840s marked the height of the Rocky Mountain fur trade. The trade could generate huge profits for the eastern merchants who controlled it; for example, the Rocky Mountain Fur Company sold 168 packs of beaver pelts for $85,000 in 1832—more than $1 million today. However, individual trappers fared more modestly. They ranged freely across national boundaries and cultures, going wherever the bison, bear, and beaver took them. These men demonstrated a legendary ability to navigate among Spanish, French, European American, and Native American communities. Westerners coined new terms to describe the people representative of new kinds of cultural identity within trading communities. Some white men became "white Indians," and the children they had with Indian women were called "métis" (mixed bloods). William Sherley "Old Bill" Williams, a convert to the religion of the Osage Indians of the southeastern Plains, was not unusual in the ways he crossed cultural boundaries. He married an Osage woman, and when she died, he wed a New Mexican widow. His third wife was a Ute woman. Williams's life story suggests the ways that Indian and Hispanic women could serve as cultural mediators between native peoples and European American traders.

A Multitude of Voices in the National Political Arena

The increasing diversity of the American population, combined with specialized regional economies, heightened tensions within and between different groups and sections of the country. The Second Party system, which replaced the Federalist–Anti-Federalist rivalry of the early nineteenth century, was characterized by intense competition between the Jacksonian Democrats and anti-Jackson Whigs. But this new system could not accommodate the old or new conflicts based on race, religion, ethnicity, regional loyalties, and political beliefs. Social and cultural disputes spilled out of the courthouse and the legislative hall and into the streets. Public demonstrations ran the gamut from noisy parades to bloody clashes. During these displays, resentments between ethnic and religious groups, arguments over political issues, and opposition to reformers often blended together.

Specific interests—the white laboring classes, abolitionists, southern slave owners, and nativists (people hostile to immigrants)—sought to find their own political voices. Yet as national parties, the Democrats and Whigs refrained from facing, head-on, controversial issues such as slavery. Deprived of what they considered effective representation on the national level, some Americans grew increasingly frustrated by their own lack of political clout. Their grievances set off a full-blown political crisis and led to party realignment once again in the 1850s.

Whigs, Workers, and the Panic of 1837

Ill with tuberculosis, Andrew Jackson did not run for a third term in 1836. The Democrats nominated Jackson's vice president and friend Martin Van Buren for president. As his running mate, they chose Col. Richard M. Johnson, the self-proclaimed killer of Tecumseh. The Jackson-haters, led by Senator Henry Clay and other Congressmen formed a political party called the Whigs. They drew their support from several groups: advocates of Clay's American System, states' rights southerners opposed to Jackson's heavy-handed use of national power, and merchants and factory owners in favor of the Second Bank of the United States. Evangelical Protestants from the middle classes also joined the anti-Jackson forces; they objected to his rhetoric stressing class differences because they believed that individual religious conviction, not a group's material status, should shape politics and society. Still somewhat disorganized, these allied groups fielded three candidates: Hugh White of Tennessee, Senator Daniel Webster of Massachusetts, and General William Henry Harrison of Indiana. Benefiting from the Whigs' disarray, Van Buren narrowly won the popular vote but swept the Electoral College.

TABLE 12-2

The Election of 1836

Candidate	Political Party	Popular Vote	Electoral Vote
Martin Van Buren	Democratic	765,483	170
William Henry Harrison	Whig		73
Hugh L. White	Whig	739,795	26
Daniel Webster	Whig		14
W.P. Magnum	Independent		11

In northeastern cities, political candidates of all persuasions began to court the allegiance of workers aligned with a new trade union movement. Urban traders and laborers had become a political force in their own right. The spread of the factory system threatened the livelihoods of artisans in a number of trades. Immigration increased workers' anxieties. People worried about making a living tended to favor the Democratic Party, which spoke against class privilege and the wealthy. In the late 1820s and early 1830s, a variety of trade organizations had formed to advance the interests of skilled workers (the "producing classes," they called themselves). These unions pressed for a ten-hour workday, the abolition of paper money (so that workers would receive their wages in hard currency rather than bank notes) and debtors' prisons, and higher wages. In some cities, though representing only a minority of workers, these unions fielded their own candidates through Workingmen's Parties. In other places, workers counted on the Democrats to advance their interests at the polls. However, once in office, politicians often were indifferent to the demands of urban laboring people.

In some cases, journeymen protesting long hours and low wages took their grievances to the streets. In New York City in 1834, groups of sailors, bakers, shoemakers, carpet weavers, locksmiths, stonecutters, and hatters staged boisterous work stoppages. In October of that same year, the stonecutters turned their fury on a building under construction. They smashed windows and caused much damage until "a strong posse of watchmen" made them disperse.

The founding of the National Trades Union (NTU) in 1834 made workers more politically visible. The union represented workers as diverse as jewelers, butchers, bookbinders, and factory workers. In Philadelphia in the early 1830s, for example, the local NTU organization, called the General Trades Union, consisted of 50 trade societies and supported a number of successful strikes. Both Whigs and Democrats professed allegiance to the union, but neither party went out of its way to represent the interests of workers over other groups, such as farmers and bookkeepers.

But even larger troubles loomed for the trade union movement. In the course of his term, Van Buren had to grapple with the effects of a major depression, the Panic of 1837. Brought on by overspeculation—in canals, turnpikes, railroads, and slaves—the panic deepened when large grain crops failed in the West. British creditors worsened matters when they recalled loans they had made to American customers.

The depression, which lasted until the early 1840s, devastated the NTU and its constituent organizations. Up to one-third of all Americans lost their jobs when businesses failed. Those fortunate enough to keep their jobs were in no position to press for higher wages. Not until the Civil War era did members of the laboring classes recapture political momentum at the national level.

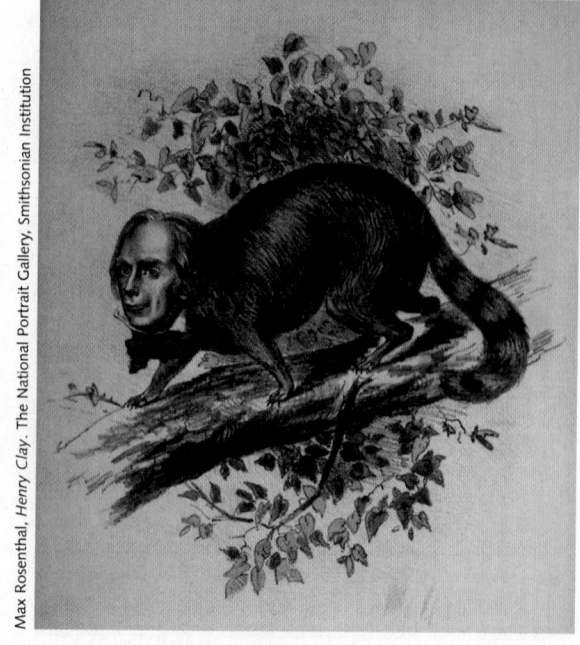

Max Rosenthal, *Henry Clay*. The National Portrait Gallery, Smithsonian Institution

■ Henry Clay had a distinguished career as statesman and politician for more than four decades. He was President John Quincy Adams's secretary of state. He served as speaker of the House of Representatives for a longer term than anyone else in the nineteenth century. He represented Kentucky in the Senate. A prominent Whig leader, he promoted "the American System" of tariffs and federal subsidies for transportation projects. By 1840, members of both parties were boasting of their (supposed) humble origins. Here Clay is portrayed as the "Old Coon" because the Whigs had adopted the raccoon as their symbol for the election of 1840.

Suppression of Antislavery Sentiment

In 1831 a Boston journalist named William Lloyd Garrison launched *The Liberator,* a newspaper dedicated to "immediate emancipation" of all slaves. Two years later, a group of 60 blacks and whites formed the American Anti-Slavery Society (AA-SS). That same year, Great

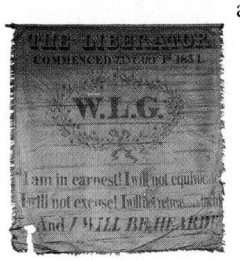

Britain had abolished slavery in the West Indies. This move encouraged like-minded Americans eager to cooperate with their British counterparts to abolish slavery everywhere. In the United States, the abolitionist movement enlisted the energies of a dedicated group of people who believed not only that slavery was immoral but also that the federal government must take immediate steps to destroy this "peculiar institution."

The position of the AA-SS was clear: "the slaves ought instantly to be set free, and brought under protection of law." The *Declaration of Sentiments of the American Anti-Slavery Society* strongly condemned southern slaveholders and supporters of African American colonization. Indeed, it criticized the latter group for encouraging American blacks to move to Africa—in the words of the AA-SS, a "delusive, cruel and dangerous" scheme. A well-organized movement, the society sponsored an aggressive campaign against slavery, gathering hundreds of names on antislavery petitions to present to Congress. The group also distributed antislavery literature throughout the North.

The society drew moral and financial support from northern communities of free people of color as well as from white women and men. All the supporters showed a great deal of courage

> *The American Anti-Slavery Society sponsored an aggressive campaign against slavery, gathering hundreds of names on antislavery petitions, to present to Congress.*

within a larger American society indifferent to the issue of slavery. Activists such as Maria Stewart and David Walker had laid the foundation for the abolitionist movement. Well-to-do black leaders, including Henry Highland Garnet, Charles Lenox Remond, and his sister Sarah Parker Remond, spoke out on behalf of southern blacks in chains. Fugitive slaves, including Frederick Douglass, Solomon Northup, and William and Ellen Craft, electrified northern abolitionist audiences with their first-hand accounts of the brutality of slavery and of their own daring escapes from bondage.

Douglass's autobiography, *Narrative of the Life of Frederick Douglass* (1845), immediately gained an enthusiastic audience among abolitionists on both sides of the Atlantic. Within five years of its publication the book had sold 30,000 copies. An American tale of determination and self-education, the *Narrative* is also a literary classic. In one passage Douglass describes standing on the banks of the Chesapeake Bay, watching sailboats "robed in purest white" skimming along the water:

> I have often, in the deep stillness of a summer's Sabbath, stood all alone along the lofty banks of that noble bay, and traced, with saddened heart and tearful eye, the countless number of sails moving off to the mighty ocean. The sight of these always affected me powerfully. My thoughts would compel utterance; and there with no audience but the Almighty, I would pour out my soul's complaint.

Large and charismatic, Douglass had a compelling speaking style. He soon became a much-sought-after abolitionist speaker in the Northeast, the Midwest, and England.

A few white women also became active in the abolitionist cause. Sarah and Angelina Grimké, for example, left the household of their slave-owning father in Charleston, South Carolina, and moved to Philadelphia. The Grimké sisters spoke before groups composed of men and women, blacks and whites in the North, an act offensive to many other whites. They were struck by what they considered the similar legal constraints of slaves and white women. White men considered both groups to be unworthy of citizenship rights, childlike in their demeanor, well-suited for domestic service, and inherently unintelligent. Also in the North, local associations, such as the Female Antislavery Society of Andover, Massachusetts, mobilized women who then fired off letters to the *Liberator* and other publications. In these letters, they urged other women to respond to "the sighs, the groans, the deathlike struggles of scourged sisters in the South. . . . We feel that woman has a place in this God-like work."

Such activities provoked outrage not only from southern slave owners but also from anti-abolitionists and their allies in Congress—in other words, most northern whites. In Washington, D.C., the House of Representatives imposed a gag rule on antislavery petitions, forbidding them to be read aloud or entered into the public record. Supporters of slavery also resorted to violence. In 1834 a mob of whites attacked a school for young women of color operated by a white teacher, Prudence Crandall, near New Haven, Connecticut. A local paper charged that the school was fostering "levelling [egalitarian] principles, and intermarriage between whites and blacks." The next year in Boston a different mob attacked the *Liberator* founder, William Lloyd Garrison himself, tying a rope around him and parading him through the streets of that city while onlookers jeered. In 1837 in Alton, Illinois, a group of whites murdered outspoken abolitionist Rev. Elijah P. Lovejoy. Hounded out of Missouri because of his antislavery pronouncements, Lovejoy had moved directly across the river to Alton, in free-state Illinois, where he published the *Alton Observer* and organized the Illinois Anti-Slavery Society. The mob had destroyed his printing press before turning on Lovejoy. After the killing, Garrison and others hailed Lovejoy as a martyr.

Throughout the North, anti-abolitionist mobs voiced the fears of whites who believed that every black man who had a job took one from a white man. Antiblack riots broke out in New York City, Philadelphia, and Cincinnati in 1834, and again in Philadelphia in 1842. White workers attacked blacks so often in the 1830s and 1840s that bricks became known as "Irish confetti" because of the way immigrants used them as weapons.

Still, these dramatic episodes had little noticeable impact on the two major political parties. In 1840 the Democrats renominated Van Buren, although many people blamed him

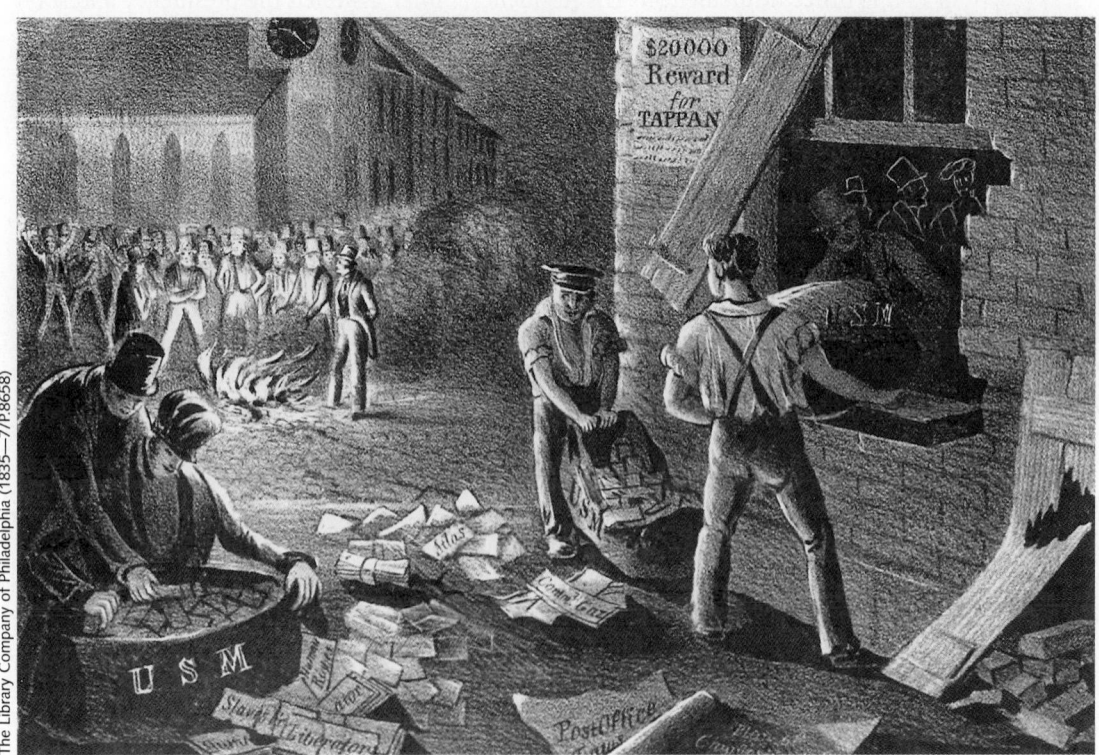

The Library Company of Philadelphia (1835–7/P.8658)

■ The artist titled this print *"New Method of Assorting the Mail, as Practised by Southern Slave-Holders."* In July 1835, a proslavery mob broke into the U.S. post office in Charleston, South Carolina, and burned abolitionist literature. The sign on the side of the building offers a "Reward for Tappan." The brothers Arthur and Lewis Tappan were wealthy New York City merchants who funded abolitionist activities. Southern slaveholders hoped to stem the north–south flow of abolitionist literature, which took the form of sermons, pamphlets, periodicals, and resolutions.

for the depression. Eager to find a candidate as popular as Andrew Jackson, the Whigs selected William Henry Harrison; his supporters called him "Old Tippecanoe" in recognition of his defeat of Indians at the battle of the same name in 1811. As Harrison's running mate the Whigs chose John Tyler, who had been both governor of and a senator from Virginia. To counter their reputation as well-heeled aristocrats, which in fact they were, the Whigs promoted Harrison as a simple, humble man living in a log cabin and drinking hard cider. They rallied around the slogan "Tippecanoe and Tyler Too."

The election of 1840 represented the triumph of style over substance in political electioneering as the two major parties ignored the growing controversy over slavery. That year abolitionists meeting in Albany, New York, founded a new party, the Liberty Party, dedicated to eradicating slavery. Although it garnered only 7000 votes for its candidate, James G. Birney, in the general election, the party soon gained the ability to swing local elections in favor of antislavery candidates. Still, Whigs and Democrats dominated the campaign of 1840. The two major parties were well organized and evenly matched. They used symbols, songs, and imagery in innovative ways to build party loyalty. Sloganeering substituted for meaningful discussion of the issues of the day.

TABLE 12-3			
The Election of 1840			
Candidate	Political Party	Popular Vote	Electoral Vote
William Henry Harrison	Whig	1,274,624	234
Martin Van Buren	Democratic	1,127,781	60
James G. Birney	Liberty	7,069	

By this time, the Whigs had gained strong support among wealthy southern planters, who worried that Van Buren would not protect their interests in slavery. Harrison won the election, but he contracted pneumonia at his inauguration and died within one month of taking office. Ridiculed as "His Accidency," Tyler assumed the presidency and soon lost his core constituency, Whigs who favored a strong central government, by vetoing bills for both a national bank and higher tariffs. The new president represented members of the Whig party who were ardent supporters of states' rights. As a result, he proved a poor standard-bearer for the numerous nationalist-minded Whigs. Tyler learned a hard lesson: that members of his own party were a loose coalition of groups with varying views on a range of issues rather than a unified party bound to a single idea or principle.

Abolitionists could claim few victories, either real or symbolic, during these years. However, they did take heart from the *Amistad* case. In 1839 Spanish slave traders attempted to transport 53 illegally purchased Africans to Havana, Cuba, on a ship named *Amistad*. En route to Havana, the Africans, under the leadership of a young man named Cinqué, rebelled, killed the captain, and took over the ship. Soon after, U.S. authorities captured the ship off the coast of Long Island. President Van Buren wanted to send the blacks to Cuba. However, a federal district court judge in Hartford, Connecticut, ruled that because the African slave trade had been illegal since 1808, the Africans had been wrongfully enslaved. The U.S. government appealed the case to the Supreme Court.

To publicize the *Amistad* case, abolitionists produced a play, "The Black Schooner or the Private Slaver '*Amistad*.'" To raise funds, Philadelphia black leader Robert Purvis paid to have Cinqué's portrait painted; then antislavery activists sold copies for $1 each. In 1841 former president John Quincy Adams argued the Africans' case before the high court. The court ruled in their favor. Of the original 53 men, women, and children, 35 had survived the ordeal (the rest died), and they returned to Africa. Slavery advocates and abolitionists alike pondered the question: Could the law be used to dismantle slavery?

Nativists as a Political Force

Among the active players on the political scene were the nativists, who opposed immigration and immigrants. The immigrants who came to the United States were a varied group in terms

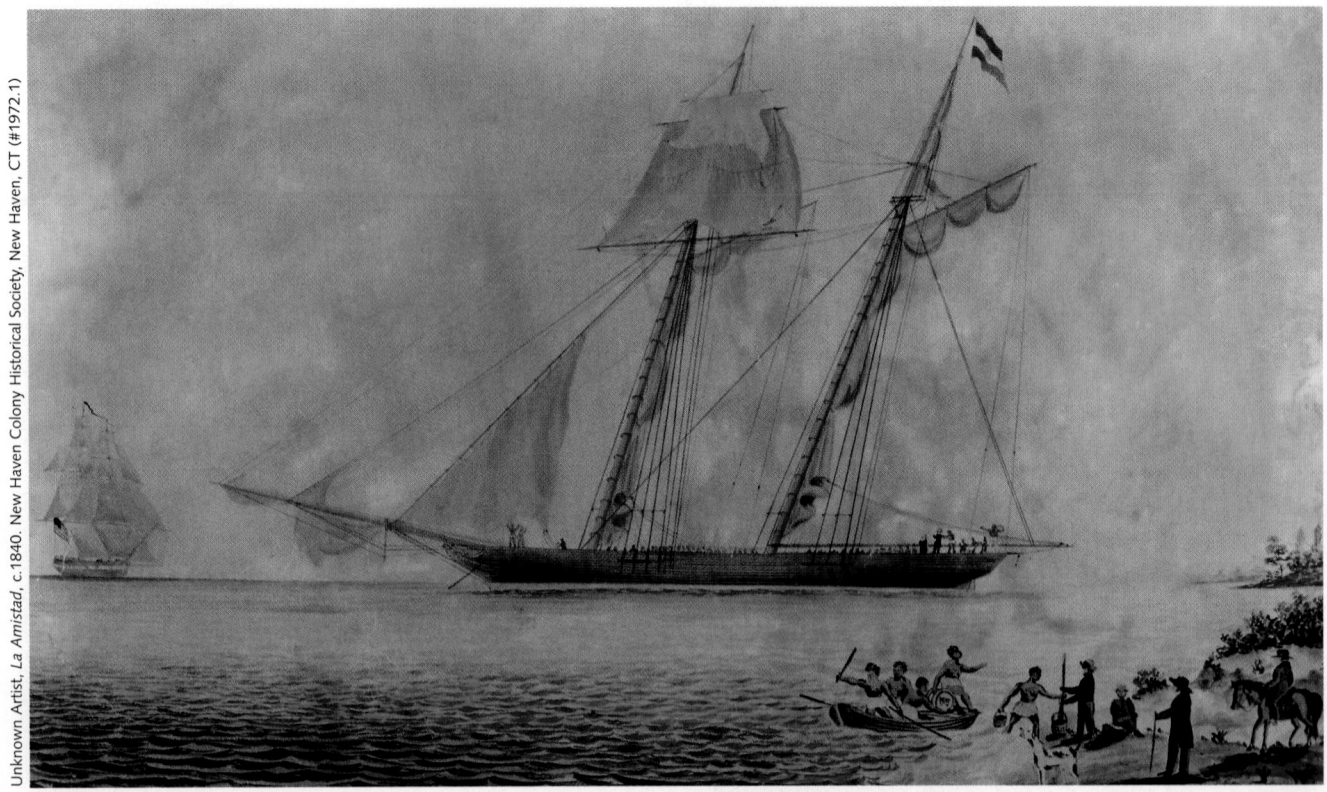

Unknown Artist, *La Amistad*, c.1840. New Haven Colony Historical Society, New Haven, CT (#1972.1)

■ Abolitionists hailed the eventual freeing of the *Amistad* captives as one of their few successes in the fight against slavery before the Civil War. This picture shows the Spanish slave ship, commandeered by the captives under the leadership of Cinqué, anchored off Culloden Point, Long Island, in 1839. Initially charged with the murder of the ship's captain, the Africans were held in New Haven, Connecticut, until a U.S. Supreme Court ruling led to their release and return to Africa in 1842.

of their jobs, religion, and culture. Some farmed homesteads in Michigan, and others worked in northeastern factories. But to nativists, these distinctions made little difference: all immigrants were foreigners and thus unwelcome. Some nativists were also temperance advocates calling for the prohibition of alcohol; they objected to the Irish drinking in taverns and the Germans drinking in their *Biergarten*. Protestants worried that large numbers of Catholic immigrants would be loyal to the pope in Rome, the head of the Catholic Church, and thus undermine American democracy. Members of the working classes, black and white, feared the loss of their jobs to desperate newcomers who would accept low, "starvation" wages. But nativists objected just as much when immigrants kept to themselves—in their Catholic schools or in their German *Turnverein* (gymnastics clubs). They also complained when immigrants participated in U.S. politics as individual voters and members of influential voting blocs.

Samuel F. B. Morse, the artist and inventor, was among the most vocal nativists. In the early 1840s he ceased painting portraits and turned his creative energies to developing a form of long-distance electric communication. Congress financed construction of the first telegraph line, which ran from Washington to Baltimore. In May 1844, Morse sent a message in code, "What hath God wrought!" and the modern telegraph was born. The precursor of all later communication innovations, the telegraph revolutionized the spread of information and tied the country together.

Morse was convinced that Catholic immigrants in particular (mostly the Irish) were a grave threat to American democracy. In his book *Imminent Dangers to the Free Institutions of the*

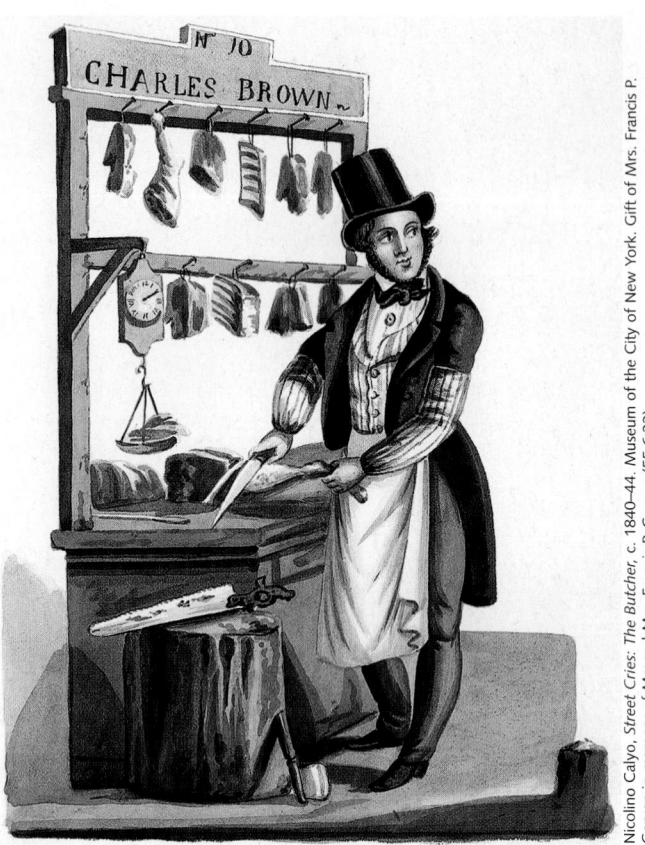

Nicolino Calyo, Street Cries: The Butcher, c. 1840–44. Museum of the City of New York. Gift of Mrs. Francis P. Garvan in memory of Mr. and Mrs. Francis P. Garvan (55.6.22)

■ Nicolino Calyo's **Street Cries: The Butcher, c. 1840–1844.**

United States (1835), Morse charged that Catholics favored "monarchical power" over republican governments. Catholicism was like a cancer, he wrote, "We find it spreading itself into every nook and corner of the land; churches, chapels, colleges, nunneries and convents are springing up as if by magic every where." In his fears, Morse expressed nostalgia for a simpler past, even as his technical ingenuity paved the way for the modern world.

In 1844, an openly nativist political organization, the American Republican Party, made substantial gains in New York, Philadelphia, and Boston. The party elected six of its candidates to Congress and dozens of others to local political offices. In 1849, nativists founded the Order of the Star-Spangled Banner. Also called the Know-Nothing Party, the group got its name by cautioning its members to profess ignorance when asked about its existence. The Know-Nothings drew their support from a broad spectrum of the native-born population, including Whigs who saw immigrants as the backbone of the Democratic party. Native-born Democrats who shared that view also supported the Know-Nothings.

Anti-Catholic prejudices in particular helped to justify territorial expansion. Many U.S. Protestants believed the government was justified in seizing the land of Spanish-speaking Catholics in the West. They claimed religious and cultural superiority over Hispanics. As Protestant explorers, traders, and travelers reported on their experiences in the Southwest, they condemned what they called the region's "ignorant, priest ridden peasantry," in the words of one writer for *Harper's Magazine.* They also disdained Hispanic material culture: adobe houses revealed "the power of mud," suggested one European American. Albert Pike, a native New Englander, called the Santa Fe region "bleak, black, and barren." Other Protestants disdained what they considered "a people infatuated with the passion" for gambling. Protestant stereotypes of Mexican Roman Catholics set the stage for the U.S. conquest of northern Mexico in the late 1840s. However, not just in the West, but all over the continent, nativists' ideas had violent consequences.

In the 1830s and 1840s, violence in the form of military action or urban riots pitting anti-abolitionists against abolitionists, workers against employers, or nativists against immigrants constituted a widespread form of political expression. However, the opposing sides in some riots were not nearly so clear-cut. For example, with the demise of the Philadelphia General Trades Union, the laboring classes fell to fighting among themselves, venting their ethnic and religious differences. In May 1844, in the Philadelphia suburb of Kensington, Irish Catholic immigrant cloth weavers and native-born Protestant artisans brawled in the streets for four days. Protestant artisans came together to urge temperance, protest the increasing prominence of Irish politicians in the Democratic Party, and advocate the use of the King James Version of the Bible in the public schools. Catholic clergy disapproved of that translation, which, they claimed, public school teachers imposed on Catholic school children with the aid of taxpayers' dollars. The May riot, fueled by the emergence of the nativist American Republican Party, left several native-born workers dead and the Irish workers' churches and homes in shambles. Thus, ethnic animosity, anti-Catholicism, and nativism, as well as the temperance cause (widely associated with pre–Civil War reform) blended to produce often violent conflict.

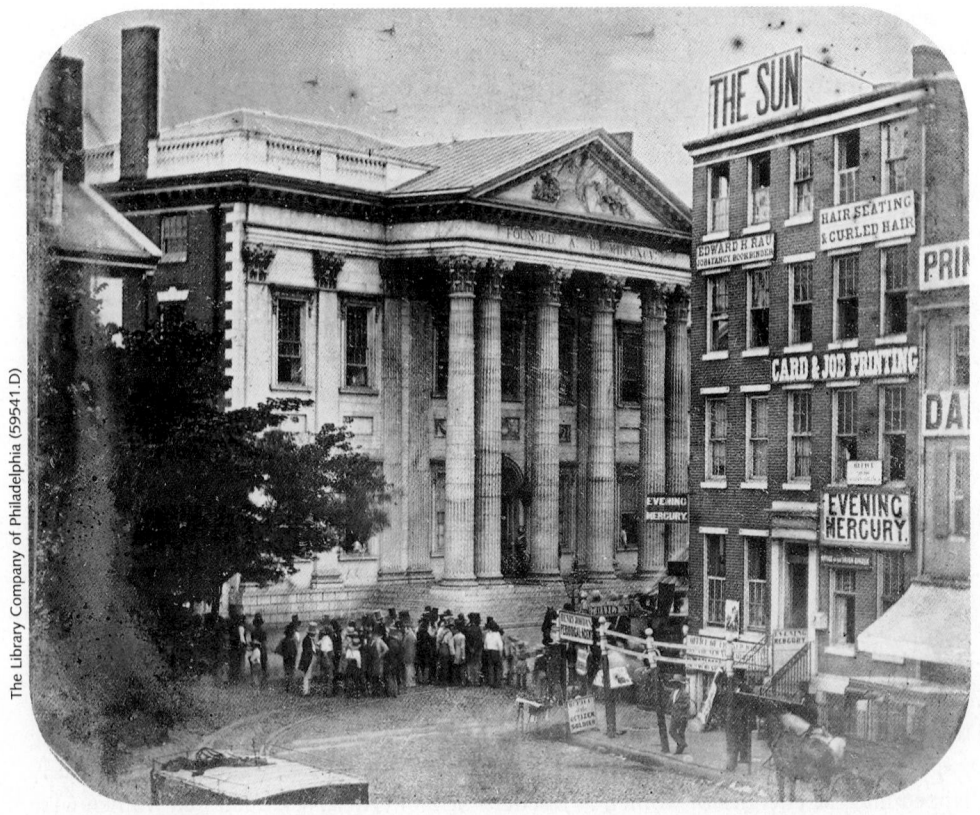

■ Taken on May 9, 1844, this daguerreotype is one of the first American photographs to record an urban civil disturbance. A crowd gathers outside Philadelphia's Girard Bank, at the corner of Third and Dock streets. At the time, soldiers called in to quell the riot were occupying the bank. Called the Bible Riots, the clash between Protestant and Catholic workers revealed tensions arising from nativism, temperance activism, and the use of the Protestant version of the Bible in the public schools.

Reform Impulses

In August 1841 writer Lydia Maria Child recorded a striking scene in New York City: a march sponsored by the Washington Society, a temperance group, was snaking its way through the streets. The procession stretched for 2 miles and consisted of representatives from "all classes and trades." The marchers carried banners depicting streams and rivers (the pure water favored over liquor) and poignant scenes of the grateful wives and children of reformed drunkards. Stirred by the martial sounds of trumpets and drums, Child wrote that the music was "the voice of resistance to evil." She added, "Glory to resistance! for through its agency men become angels."

Inspired by Charles Grandison Finney's faith in the "perfectibility" of human beings and heartened by the rapid pace of technological progress, many Americans set about trying to "make angels out of men," in Child's words. In the process, various reform associations targeted personal habits such as dress and diet, conventional beliefs about sexuality and the status of women, and institutions such as schools, churches, and slavery. Their efforts often brought women out of the home and into public life. Marches and meetings also led to encounters between different cultural groups: Christian missionaries and non-Christians, rich and poor, native-born and immigrants. Yet not all Americans shared the reformers' zeal. Even those who did rarely agreed about the appropriate means to transform society.

Public Education

In the eyes of some Americans, a growing nation needed new forms of tax-supported schooling. As families moved from one area of the country to another, public education advocates pointed out, children should be able to pick up in one school where they had left off in another. Members of a growing middle class wanted to provide their children with schooling beyond basic literacy instruction (reading and writing skills) and had the resources to do so. Factory owners, for their part, supported education that would produce a self-motivated, disciplined labor force.

Horace Mann, a Massachusetts state legislator and lawyer, was one of the most prominent educational reformers. In 1837 Mann became secretary of the first state board of education. He stressed the notion of a common school system available to all boys and girls regardless of class or ethnicity. In his annual report of 1848, he noted, "Education, then, beyond all other devices of human origin, is the great equalizer of the conditions of men—the balance-wheel of the social machinery." In an increasingly diverse nation, schooling promoted the acquisition of basic knowledge and skills. But it also provided instruction in what Mann and others called American values: hard work, punctuality, and sobriety.

How exactly would educators teach reading and writing skills and moral values? The dictionary of Connecticut's Noah Webster (published in 1828) and the McGuffey's *Reader* series, first published in 1836, provided a way. In his books, William H. McGuffey, a college professor and Presbyterian minister, combined lessons in reading with lessons in moral behavior: "Beautiful feet are they that go/Swiftly to lighten another's woe." Over the next 20 years, the McGuffey series sold more than 7 million copies.

By the 1840s, public school systems attended by white children had cropped up across the North and the Midwest. Urban districts, using tax revenues to support schools, sought to educate as many pupils as possible. These districts pioneered in grading classrooms, imposing uniform standards for curricula and teachers' qualifications, and regimenting pupils to make schooling more "efficient." Toward that end, local school boards eagerly tapped into the energies of women as teachers. School officials claimed that women were naturally nurturing and could serve as "mothers away from home" for small children.

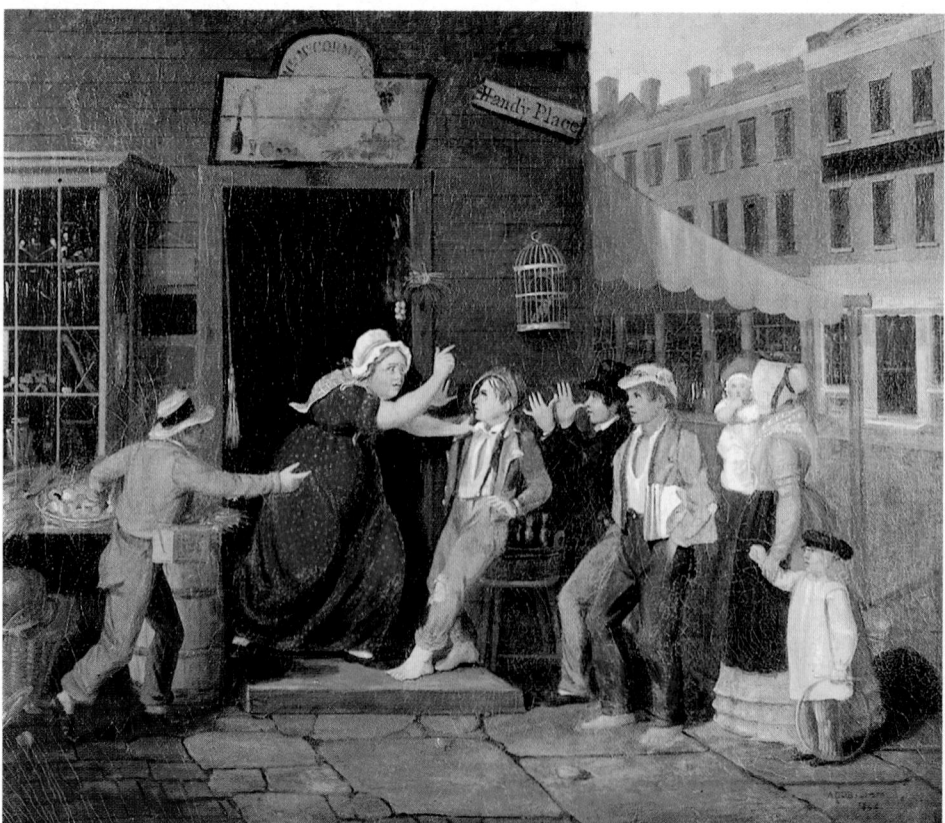

■ Artist Albertis Browere titled this 1844 painting *Mrs. McCormick's General Store*. These barefoot boys are getting into trouble. Reformers advocated universal, compulsory schooling as one way to rid street corners of young mischief makers. Had these youngsters lived in the country, they probably would have been working in the fields.

Albertus del Orient Browere, *Mrs. McCormick's General Store*, 1844. Fenimore Art Museum, Cooperstown, New York (N-0387.55)

Furthermore, schools could pay women only a fraction of what men earned. Between the 1830s and 1840s, the number of female schoolteachers in Massachusetts jumped more than 150 percent.

In 1846 writer and educator Catharine Beecher urged unmarried women to devote themselves to teaching. That year, she created a Board of National Popular Education, which sent New England teachers to the Midwest. By 1847 she had enlisted the services of 70 young Protestant women to serve as teacher–missionaries in Illinois, Indiana, Iowa, Wisconsin, Michigan, Tennessee, and Kentucky. Beecher expected these young women to endure hardship cheerfully. Many tried to do so. Dutifully reporting from her new home in what she described as "a newly organized county," one teacher wrote, "I came expecting to make sacrifices, and suffer privations." She found her pupils to be "ragged and dirty in the extreme" and unschooled in proper classroom decorum.

Other forms of education also multiplied. Lyceums—informal lectures offered by speakers who traveled from place to place—attracted hordes of adults regardless of their formal education. By the mid–1830s, approximately 3000 local lecture associations, mostly in New England and the Midwest, were sponsoring such series. In addition, local agricultural fairs offered informal practical instruction to rural people.

> *Despite the lofty goals of Mann and other reformers, public schooling did not offer a "common" experience for all American children.*

The number of colleges more than doubled (46 to 119) between 1830 and 1850. Founded in 1837, Mount Holyoke, a college for women in Massachusetts, and Oberlin in Ohio, which accepted black men as well as women of both races, were unusual for their liberal admission policies. Most colleges were supported by a specific religious denomination or cultural group. In Indian Territory, for example, the Cherokee National Council founded the Cherokee Female Seminary in 1851. With a classical curriculum similar to that of Mount Holyoke, the school was intended for the daughters of wealthy, assimilated Cherokees.

In an ironic twist, innovations in education heightened differences in status. Despite the lofty goals of Mann and other reformers, public schooling did not offer a "common" experience for all American children. Almost exclusively, northern white children benefited from public school systems. Slightly more than one-third of all white children attended school in 1830; twenty years later, the ratio had increased to more than one half. In northern cities, these proportions were considerably higher; there reformers were able to provide elementary-school instruction for relatively large numbers of white children, both immigrant and native-born.

By contrast, few black children had the opportunity to attend public schools. In the South, slave children were forbidden by law to learn to read and write. Recalled one former slave many years later, "dey [owners] didn't teach 'em nothin' but wuk [work]." By the 1830s, schools for even the children of free people of color had to meet in secret. In the North, many black households needed the labor of children to survive, resulting in black school-attendance rates well below those of whites. Throughout the Northeast and Midwest, black children remained at the mercy of local officials, who decided whether they could attend the schools their parents' tax dollars helped to support.

In the late 1840s, Benjamin Roberts, a black man, launched a series of lawsuits against the Boston School Committee on behalf of his five-year-old daughter Sarah. Roberts demanded that the city's schools be integrated. The abolitionist-politician Charles Sumner argued the Roberts case before the state's highest court, but lost. However, in 1855, the Massachusetts legislature would outlaw segregated schools.

All over the country, education remained an intensely grassroots affair, belying the reformers' call for uniform systems. Local communities raised money for the teacher's salary, built the schoolhouse, and provided wood to heat the building. Southern states did not develop uniform public education systems until the late nineteenth century. Lacking local, popular support for tax-supported schooling, poor white children remained illiterate, while wealthy parents hired tutors for their own children or sent them to private academies.

Formal training for professionals also changed during this period. New state licensing and certification standards meant that people preparing to become physicians and lawyers must receive specialized training. As these professions came to insist on formal educational standards for practitioners, some women lost some of their traditional roles such as midwifery and healing. By the 1830s, almost all states required that doctors be licensed. The only way to attain such a license was to attend medical school, and these schools still excluded women. In regions of the country where medical schools appeared, the self-taught midwife gradually yielded to the formally educated male physician. In contrast, in rural communities of black and white Southerners, Native Americans, and Hispanics, women continued to practice time-honored ways of midwifery and healing.

Alternative Visions of Social Life

The crosscurrents of reform showed up most clearly in debates about sexuality, the family, and the proper role of women. For example, reformer Sylvester Graham argued that even husbands and wives must monitor their sexual activity. Sexual excess between husband and wife, he claimed, caused ills ranging from headaches, chills, and impaired vision, to loss of memory, epilepsy, insanity, and "disorders of the liver and kidneys." Graham also promoted a diet of special crackers made of wheat flour (now called Graham crackers) and fruit (in place of alcohol and meat) in addition to a regimen of plain living reinforced with cold showers.

Other reformers disagreed with Graham's notion that people must repress their sexuality to lead a good and healthy life. Defying conventional standards of morality, sponsors of a number of experimental communities discouraged marriage-based monogamy (a legal commitment between a man and a woman to engage in sexual relations only with each other) and made child-rearing the responsibility of the entire community rather than just the child's parents. These communities were communitarian—seeking to break down exclusive relations between husband and wife, parent and child, employer and employee—in an effort to advance the well-being of the whole group, and not just individuals within it. These communities were also utopian, seeking to forge new kinds of social relationships that would, in the eyes of the reformers, serve as a model for the larger society.

The crosscurrents of reform showed up most clearly in debates about sexuality, the family, and the proper role of women.

Many of these communities explicitly challenged mainstream views related to property ownership and the system of wage labor as well as rules governing relations between the sexes. The Scottish industrialist and socialist Robert Owen founded New Harmony in Indiana in 1825 basing his experiment on principles of "cooperative labor." In 1826 Owen released his "Declaration of Mental Independence, " which condemned private property, organized religion, and marriage. By this time, 900 persons had joined the New Harmony order.

The community at Nashoba, Tennessee, was more radical still, at least in theory. In 1825 a Scottish immigrant and heiress named Frances Wright established the settlement a few miles from Memphis, on land that the U.S. government had seized from the Chickasaws. A liberal thinker on many issues such as slavery and the roles of women, Wright wanted to prepare slaves for a life of freedom. Inspired by Owen, she embraced his program. Yet Nashoba, isolated in the Tennessee swamps, was an unhealthy site for everyone, white and black, young and old. The slaves resented the labor the community required of them before they could gain their freedom. Outsiders recoiled at what they considered the loose morality of the experiment, especially Wright's apparent approval of interracial sexual relations. Newspapers denounced her as a "voluptuous preacher of licentiousness," intent on converting the whole world "into a universal brothel." When Nashoba collapsed in the late 1820s, Wright joined the Owenites in New Harmony. She later moved to New York City, where she became a public lecturer, speaking out on behalf of workers and against the legal subordination of women.

Several other prominent communitarian experiments that challenged conventional marital relations were vehemently criticized, and participants were sometimes physically attacked by their neighbors. Salt Lake City Mormons, who practiced plural marriage, continued to meet intense hostility from outsiders.

Another group, the Oneida Community, founded in upstate New York near Utica in 1848 by John Humphrey Noyes, went even further than the Mormons in advocating an alternative to monogamy. At its peak, Oneida consisted of 300 members who endorsed the founder's notion of "complex marriage," meaning communal sexual unions and community-regulated parent–child relations. Charges of adultery eventually forced Noyes to flee the country and seek refuge in Canada.

Numerous moral reforms overlapped with and reinforced each other. For example, women's rights advocates often supported temperance. Husbands who drank, they pointed out, were more likely to abuse their wives and children. Sarah and Angelina Grimké gained prominence as both abolitionists and advocates for women's rights. They also followed Sylvester Graham's program, and for a short time they sported "bloomers" (loose fitting pants, popularized by dress reformer Amelia Bloomer) in place of cumbersome dresses.

Abolitionism and women's rights reinforced each other and spawned overlapping political movements in Europe as well as in the United States. Beginning in the 1820s, European women reformers began challenging a host of institutions, including slavery, capitalism, and the nuclear family. By the late 1840s, abolitionism, socialism, and utopianism helped inspire the European revolutions of 1848.

In the United States, women's rights advocates made some progress independent of the abolitionist movement. For instance, in 1839, Mississippi passed the nation's first Married Women's Property Law. The ruling was intended to protect the fortunes of the married daughters of wealthy planters. In 1848 both New York and Pennsylvania passed legislation giving married women control over any real property (land) or personal property they brought to marriage. But the organized women's rights movement drew its greatest inspiration from the abolitionist cause.

Elizabeth Cady Stanton, who played an active role in a local Female Anti-Slavery Society, is an apt example. Together with other American women, Cady Stanton attended the 1840 World Anti-Slavery Convention in London. Male leaders of the British and Foreign Anti-Slavery Society relegated the women delegates to a balcony and excluded them from the formal deliberations. Eight years later, Cady Stanton worked with Lucretia Mott, a Quaker minister; Susan B. Anthony, a young women's rights activist; and other similarly inclined men and women to organize a women's rights convention at Seneca Falls, New York.

Massachusetts resident Margaret Fuller explored many reform impulses of the day during her brief life (1810–1850). Educated in the classics by her father at home (in Cambridge), in the 1830s she embraced a new intellectual sensibility called Transcendentalism. Fuller cultivated friendships with two other famous Transcendentalists living in the Boston area: Ralph Waldo Emerson and Henry David Thoreau. Transcendentalists

Margaret Fuller was one of the foremost American intellectuals of the antebellum period. Throughout her life she remained conscious of an inner struggle between her passionate self, desiring an active life, and her intellectual self, wanting to engage in study and debate with other scholars. She explored Transcendentalism, feminism, social reform, and finally the revolutionary fervor of Italian nationalism.

believed in the primacy of the spirit and the essential harmony between people and the natural world. They took their inspiration from European Romantics, who celebrated the beauty of nature in art, music, and literature. Transcendentalists also encouraged engagement with the world: in Emerson's words, "I will not shut myself out of this globe of action, and transplant an oak into a flower-pot." In 1840, Fuller began editing *The Dial,* the transcendentalist movement's magazine.

In the early 1840s, Fuller sponsored study groups among her female neighbors in Boston. By pondering questions such as "What is beauty?" and "What is truth?" the groups sought to discover the "connection between nature and the affections of the soul." Fuller also lent her moral support to a Transcendentalist community named Brook Farm, in West Roxbury, Massachusetts. There, men and women shared equally in the home chores and fieldwork. However, most members preferred thinking to laboring, and the venture failed in 1846.

Around this time, Fuller published *Woman in the Nineteenth Century,* one of the first feminist essays written by an American. "I would have Woman lay aside all thought, such as she habitually cherishes, of being led and taught by men," wrote Fuller. She then embraced the role of investigative journalist, writing about the plight of slaves, Indians, and imprisoned women for the New York *Tribune.* In 1847, the newspaper sent her to Italy to report on the Italian unification movement. Returning home in 1850, Fuller; her new husband, Italian revolutionary Giavanni Angelo, Marchese d'Ossoli; and their son drowned off the shore of Fire Island, New York, when their ship sank. In just two decades of her adult life, Margaret Fuller had embraced a spectrum of social ideas, from reformist to revolutionary.

The United States Extends Its Reach

In the mid–1840s, the editor of the *New York Morning News* declared that the United States had a "manifest destiny" to "overspread the continent" and claim the "desert wastes." Those inhabiting the "desert wastes"—Mexican settlers and a variety of Indian groups—apparently would have little say in the matter. The term *manifest destiny* soon became a catchall phrase, justifying American efforts not only to conquer new territory but also to seek out new markets for its goods across the oceans. With its growing population and increasingly specialized regional economies, the country strove to expand both geographically and economically.

International political developments and technological innovations led to expanded opportunites for trading. In 1846 Britain repealed its exclusionary Corn Laws, which had protected its own agricultural markets from foreign competition. As a result, farmers in the U.S. Midwest had fresh incentive to produce wheat for export. The invention of the clipper ship, which ushered in "the golden age of American shipping," also helped in the expansion of global trade. Narrow-bodied vessels, topped with large sails on towering masts, the new ships "clipped off" the miles. American merchants used them to import tea from China and wool from Australia. Investors from the eastern United States financed trading companies that marketed antelope skins, beaver pelts, and cured beef to places as far away as Cuba. They eyed Asian ports hungrily, an impulse that would result in U.S. seizure of Pacific island naval waystations in the late nineteenth century.

Within the United States, many groups advocated the expansion of the country's borders. Among all American exports to foreign countries, cotton was king, accounting for half of the total goods shipped after 1840. Southern planters and northern merchants alike made huge profits from the cotton trade. In 1840 English textile manufacturers depended on the fiber, and the American South produced about three-quarters of their supply. No wonder then that southern slave owners were eager to extend their land holdings into Texas. They were joined in that hope by residents of the western states, men such as Davy Crockett, hoping to press into the fresh lands of the far West and Southwest. Little did they know that their interest would evetually lead to all-out war.

The Lone Star Republic

In the early 1830s, the Mexican government grew alarmed by the growing number of American emigrants to Texas. Worried that the settlers would refuse to pledge allegiance to Mexico, that country closed the Texas border to further in-migration. By 1835 only one out of every eight residents of Texas was a *Tejano* (that is, a native Spanish speaker); the rest, numbering 30,000, hailed from the United States. The U.S.-born Texians, together with some prominent *Tejanos,* had become increasingly well armed and militant. They organized volunteer patrols to attack Indian settlements. These forces became the precursor of the Texas Rangers, a statewide organization of law enforcement officers.

In 1836 the Texians decided to press for independence from Mexico. Only by becoming a separate nation, they believed, could they trade freely with the United States, establish their own schools, and collect and spend their own taxes. The pro-independence Texians included Davy Crockett. He had lost his congressional race in 1835, partly because of his opposition to Jackson's Indian removal policies. Crockett moved to Texas in late 1835; he hoped to revitalize his political career there and also find work as a land agent.

In early February 1836, Crockett and the other armed Texians retreated to a Spanish mission in San Antonio called the Alamo. The next month, a military force led by Antonio López de Santa Anna, president of the Republic of Mexico and a general in the army, battled them for 13 days. All 187 Texians died at the hands of Santa Anna and his men (the Mexican leader lost 600 of his own troops). Historians disagree on whether the Alamo defenders died fighting or were executed by Mexican soldiers.

In April a force of Texians and their *Tejano* allies, including military leader Juan Seguin, surprised Santa Anna and his men at the San Jacinto River and killed another 600 of them. The victors captured Santa Anna and declared themselves a new nation.

Sam Houston, former U.S. congressman from Tennessee and commander-in-chief of the Texian army, became president of the Republic of Texas (also called the Lone Star Republic) in 1837. Some *Tejanos* who objected to Mexican high-handedness joined in supporting the new republic. They resented restrictions imposed by Mexico limiting trade between the Mexican states and the United States. For these reasons a number of prominent *Tejano* leaders, including Jose Antonio Navarro, Francisco Ruiz, and Lorenzo de Zavala, signed their names to the Texas Declaration of Independence. De Zavala became vice president of the new republic.

In New Mexico and other northern territories of Mexico, many Spanish speakers had long felt abandoned by the Mexican government, which had made no provisions for their self-government and, as in the case of Texas, inhibited trade relations with the United States. In 1835 one New Mexico newspaper editorialized, "The rain of brute force has been replaced by reason. We can be sure that Americans will not take the land by bullets. Their weapons are their industry, their liberty, and their independence. Mexico has left us in a deplorable state, a deplorable darkness." Although other Mexican provinces protested the way they were treated by the government, Texas was the only Mexican state to launch a successful rebellion against Mexico.

Texas's independence raised the fears of U.S. abolitionists and blacks living in the new republic. In contrast to Mexico, which had abolished slavery in 1829, Texas approved a constitution that not only legalized slavery but also prohibited free blacks from living in the country. Greenbury Logan, a black man who owned a farm near Austin, petitioned to stay. He wrote, "Every privilege dear to a free man is taken away." But vigilantes forced him to leave. They also forced out many *Tejanos.* Among them was Juan Seguin, who had helped defeat Santa Anna at the Battle of San Jacinto and was now the mayor of San Antonio. Not until 1981 did another *Tejano,* Henry Cisneros, hold the office of mayor of the city of San Antonio.

The Election of 1844

As an independent republic, Texas became a hotly contested political issue in the United States. During the election of 1844, politicians began to debate whether the United States should annex Texas. Van Buren was outspoken in his opposition to the idea. As a result,

TABLE 12-4			
The Election of 1844			
Candidate	Political Party	Popular Vote	Electoral Vote
James K. Polk	Democratic	1,338,464	170
Henry Clay	Whig	1,300,097	105
James G. Birney	Liberty	62,300	

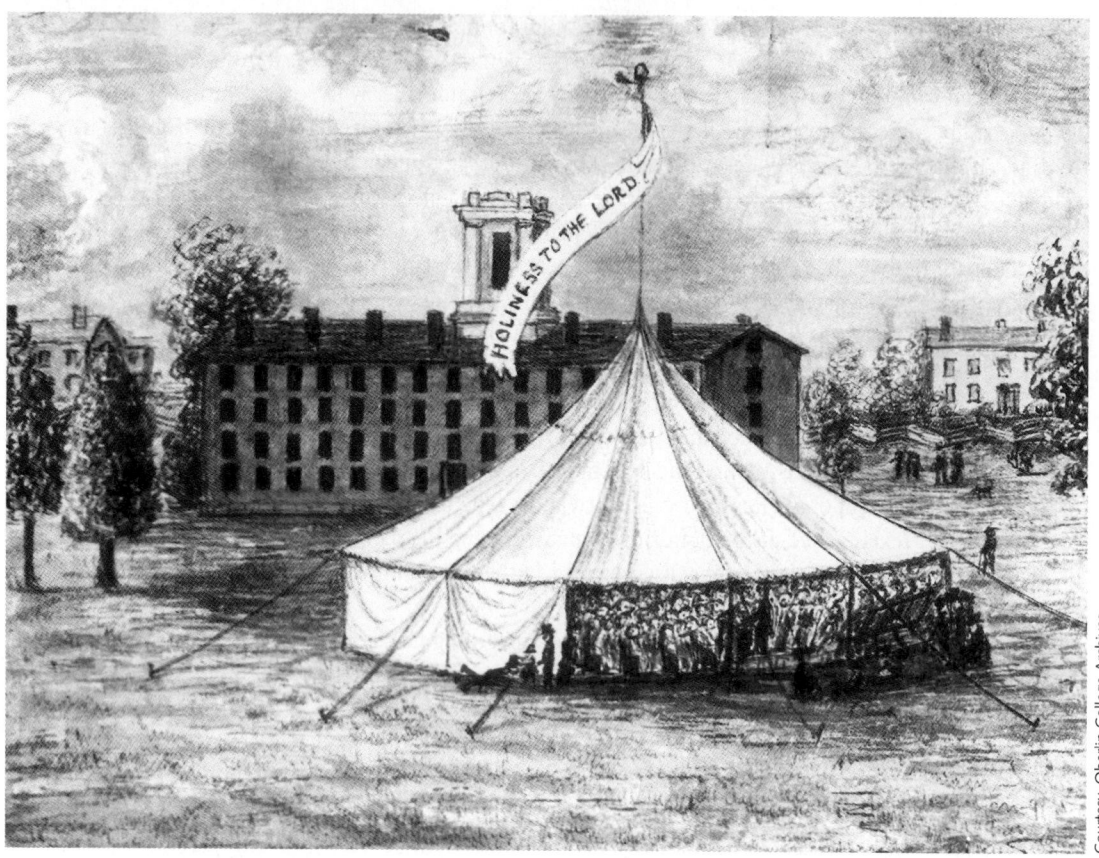

■ In the mid–1840s, the Liberty Party moved this big tent around the country, holding their meetings and conventions in it. Charles G. Finney had used the tent for his religious revivals the decade before. Above the tent flew a banner that read "Holiness to the Lord." Some critics objected to the party's "mixing up" of religion and politics. Responded one party member, "Mix them, and mix them, and keep mixing, until they ceased to be mixed, and politics became religion and religion, politics."

the frankly expansionist Democrats spurned the former president as a candidate and nominated James K. Polk of Tennessee. They called for "the reannexation of Texas" and the "reoccupation of Oregon." Their rallying cry became "54°40′ or Fight," a reference to their desire to own the area (expressed in terms of its longitude and latitude coordinates) claimed by the British in present-day Canada south of Alaska and west of the Continental Divide. Kentucky congressman Henry Clay received the Whig nomination after he announced he was against the annexation of Texas. But under pressure from southerners, he later changed his mind, to the disgust of party leaders.

Neither the Democrats nor the Whigs had shown an interest in addressing the issue of slavery directly in the last presidential election. Yet in 1844 the controversy over the annexation of Texas made it impossible for the two parties to ignore the growing controversy over bound labor. Under the banner of the young Liberty Party, some abolitionists charged that territorial expansion would mean the continued growth and prosperity of the slave system; they pointed to the public pronouncements of southern planters, who were outspoken in their desire to expand their slaveholdings into the fertile lands of Texas. In 1844 the Liberty Party once again nominated James G. Birney as its presidential candidate.

The Liberty Party revealed a major split within the abolitionist movement in general. One faction within that movement was represented by the prominent abolitionist William Lloyd Garrison, editor of the *Liberator* and a founder of the American Anti-Slavery Society. Garrison had alienated his conservative supporters with several controversial principles. Specifically, he believed that women had a right to participate equally in the abolitionist movement with men. He also saw all political institutions and parties as inherently corrupt, since they upheld the U.S. Constitution, a document Garrison believed legitimized slavery. Another abolitionist faction was represented by members of the Liberty Party, men who believed that political action, far more than moral suasion (appealing to people's sense of justice and humanity) would halt the spread of slavery. By upholding abolitionism but rejecting Garrison's views, Liberty men claimed that slavery was ultimately a political issue, one that should rightfully claim the attention of all political parties.

For their part, Democrats and Whigs believed, correctly, that most voters would ignore slavery when they cast their ballots. Thus members of both parties tried to silence both sides of the slavery debate. They turned a deaf ear to the proslavery advocates on one hand and squelched northern abolitionist opinion by ignoring petitions to Congress on the other. In the end, Polk won the election. The expansionists had elected one of their most ardent champions to the highest office in the land.

Still, Polk was not interested in going to war with Great Britain over the vast territory of Oregon. In 1846 the two countries reached a compromise. Britain would accept the 49th parallel as the border between Canada and the United States and retain the disputed islands off the coast of Vancouver. The United States settled for one-half of its original claim to Oregon. Therefore, it was free to turn its full attention to extending its southern and western borders.

War with Mexico

Texas leaders wanted to become part of the United States. In 1845, as one of his last acts as president, Tyler invited Texas to become the twenty-eighth state. He also understood

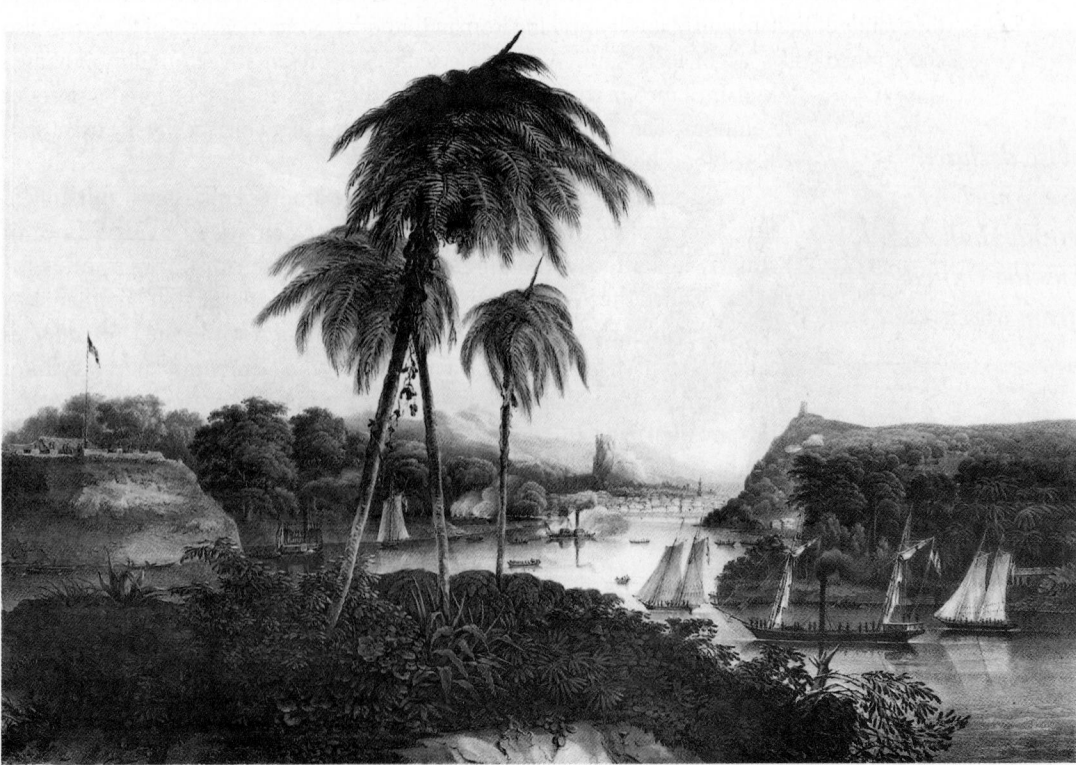

Joseph Vollmering, *The U.S. Naval Expedition Under Comore. M.C. Perry, Ascending the Tuspan River,* 1848. Amon Carter Museum, Forth Worth, Texas (1976.33.2)

■ This painting shows the U.S. Navy going up the Tuxpan River in Mexico during the U.S.–Mexican War. Located on the Gulf coast halfway between Vera Cruz and Tampico, Tuxpan was the last significant Mexican port to be seized by U.S. forces by the spring of 1847. Commodore M. C. Perry assembled a formidable force of Marines and infantry to take over the town on April 19, 1847.

that annexing Texas was a way to goad Mexico into open hostilities; Mexico had warned the United States that such a move would mean war. A joint resolution of both houses of Congress confirmed Texas statehood in December of 1845.

The boundaries between Mexico and the new state of Texas Mexico remained in dispute. Mexico recognized the Nueces River as the boundary for Texas. In contrast, Texians and U.S. politicians envisioned the boundary hundreds of miles to the west at the Rio Grande. Complicating matters further, the new president, James K. Polk, had sent an envoy, John Slidell, to purchase California and a disputed section of Texas from Mexico. Mexico refused the deal. Nevertheless, around this time, Polk wrote in his diary that if he could not acquire all of New Mexico and California through diplomatic negotiation, he was determined to obtain them by force. The stage was set for war.

Armed conflict broke out in January 1846. U.S. troops, under the command of General Zachary Taylor (a veteran of wars against Tecumseh, the Seminoles, and Black Hawk), clashed with a Mexican force near the mouth of the Rio Grande near Matamoros. Taylor had deliberately moved his troops across the Nueces River into disputed territory; his intention was to provoke an armed response from Mexico. A skirmish ensued, 11 Americans were killed, and Taylor pulled back. Polk used this military action as justification for a declaration of war against Mexico. The president declared, "American blood has been shed on American soil."

Not all Americans supported the war. Transcendentalists and others objected to what they saw as a naked land grab. Refusing to pay taxes for what he considered a war to expand slavery, Henry David Thoreau went to jail. He explained his actions in an essay, "Civil Disobedience," published in 1848. He wrote, "It is not desirable to cultivate a respect for the law, so much as for the right. The only obligation which I have a right to assume is to do at any time what I think right."

Nativists also objected to the war, fearing that the United States would have to assimilate thousands of Indians and Spanish-speaking Roman Catholics. Some members of Congress also condemned Polk's "act of aggression." A newly elected U.S. Representative from Illinois named Abraham Lincoln, together with a few other legislators, sponsored a series of resolutions. The "Spot Resolutions" demanded that Polk specify the exact spot where bloodshed had occurred.

The Wilmot Proviso declared that "neither slavery nor involuntary servitude shall ever exist" in territories the United States acquired from Mexico.

Predictably, opponents of slavery were among Polk's most outspoken critics. Soon after the outbreak of war, Representative David Wilmot of Pennsylvania attached an amendment to a bill appropriating money for the war. Called the Wilmot Proviso, the measure declared that "neither slavery nor involuntary servitude shall ever exist" in territories the United States acquired from Mexico. Though a member of the Democratic party, Wilmot spoke primarily as a white Northerner; he wanted to preserve the West for "the sons of toil of my own race and color." Wilmot's views show how racial prejudice and antislavery sentiment coexisted in the minds of many white Northerners. The House approved the Proviso, but the Senate did not. Abandoning party loyalty, southern Democrats claimed that Congress had no right to deprive slaveholders of their private property anywhere in the nation.

Meanwhile, Polk launched a three-pronged campaign against Mexico. He sent Taylor into northern Mexico and ordered General Stephen Watts Kearny into New Mexico and then into California. Following the third directive of the campaign, General-in-Chief of the U.S. Army Winfield Scott coordinated an amphibious landing of 10,000 soldiers at Vera Cruz, on the Gulf of Mexico coast. Marching west, Scott's men followed in the footsteps of the Spanish conquistadors of the sixteenth century. Mexican forces tried to defend their homeland using guerrilla tactics. But U.S. soldiers overcame them by terrorizing civilians. Scott acknowledged that the men under his command had "committed atrocities to make Heaven weep and

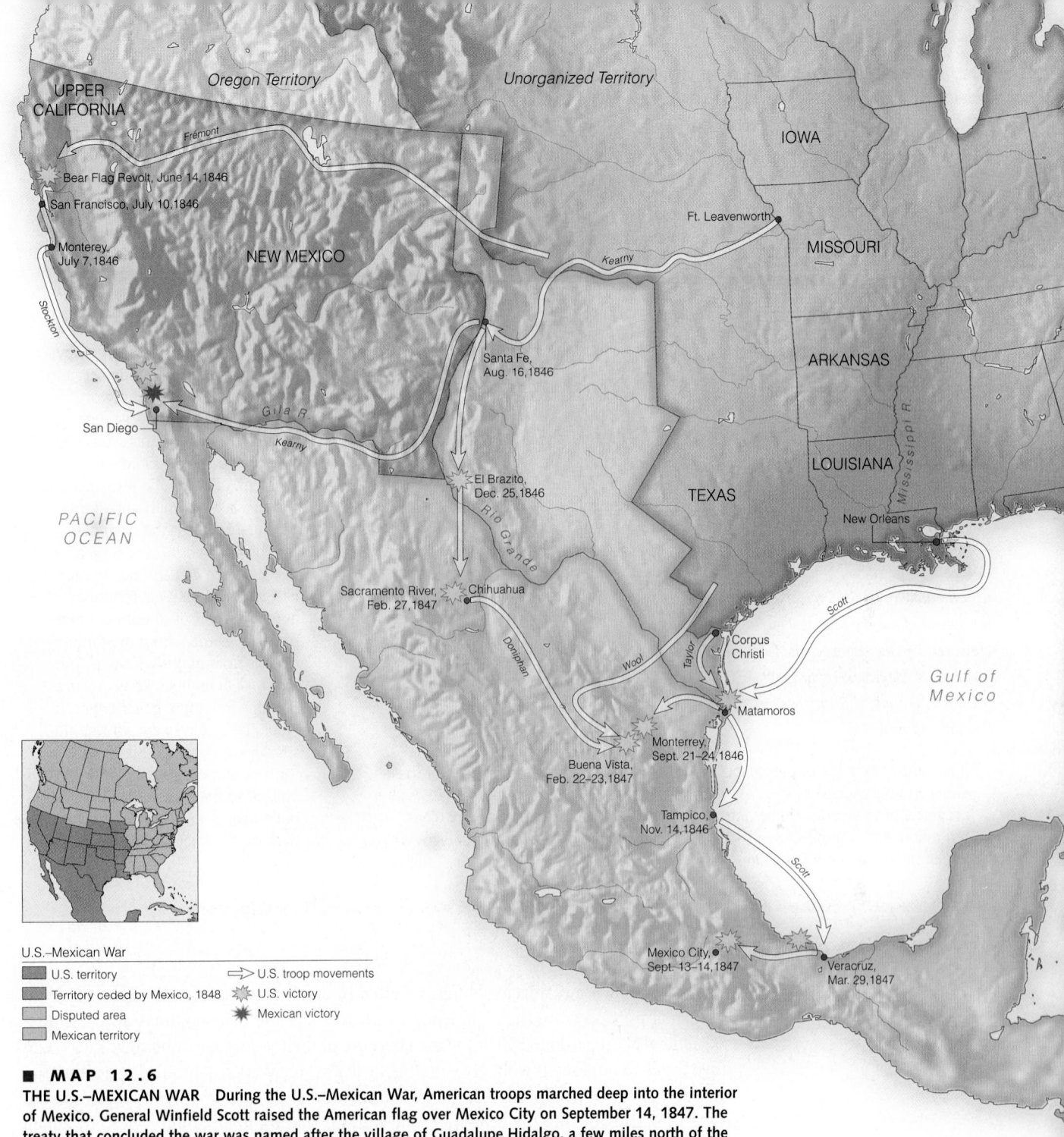

■ **MAP 12.6**

THE U.S.–MEXICAN WAR During the U.S.–Mexican War, American troops marched deep into the interior of Mexico. General Winfield Scott raised the American flag over Mexico City on September 14, 1847. The treaty that concluded the war was named after the village of Guadalupe Hidalgo, a few miles north of the Mexican capital. The U.S. army withdrew the last of its troops from foreign soil in July 1848.

every American of Christian morals blush for his country. . . . Murder, robbery and rape of mothers and daughters in the presence of tied-up males of the families."

Along the way, at the Battle of Churubusco in August 1847, U.S. forces encountered a battalion of Irish immigrants who had originally served with the United States but were now fighting for Mexico. The San Patricio Battalion (St. Patrick's Company) consisted primarily of Irish-born men who had deserted from the U.S. army and defected to Mexico. Some had recoiled at the atrocities committed by U.S. troops on Mexicans; others wanted to ally with Catholic Mexico in opposition to Protestant America. Court martial

Senator John C. Calhoun Warns Against Incorporating Mexico into the United States

In January 1848, Senator John C. Calhoun delivered a speech, addressing his remarks to President Polk and to his fellow lawmakers. He urged them to resist calls to incorporate all of a conquered Mexico into the United States. Calhoun favored the spread of slavery into new territories. However, here he expresses the fear that residents of Mexico were incapable of becoming suitable U.S. citizens for "racial" reasons.

It is without example or precedent, either to hold Mexico as a province, or to incorporate her into our union. No example of such a line of policy can be found. We have conquered many of the neighboring tribes of Indians, but we never thought of holding them in subjection—never of incorporating them into our Union. They have either been left as an independent people amongst us, or been driven into the forests.

I know further, sir, that we have never dreamt of incorporating into our Union any but the Caucasian race—the free white race. To incorporate Mexico, would be the first instance of the kind of incorporating an Indian race; for more than half of the Mexicans are Indians, and the other half is composed chiefly of mixed tribes. I protest such a union as that! . . .

Sir, it is a remarkable fact, that in the whole history of man, as far as my knowledge extends, there is no instance whatever of any civilized colored races being found equal to the establishment of free popular government, although by far the largest portion of the human family is composed of these races. . . . Are we to associate with ourselves as equals, companions, and fellow-citizens, the Indians and mixed race of Mexico? Sir, I should consider such a thing as fatal to our institutions.

Calhoun then moves on to another theme. He disputes the notion that Mexico can begin as a territory and then work its way up to statehood, following the standards Congress set for other western territories.

You can establish a Territorial Government for every State in Mexico, and there are some twenty of them. You can appoint governors, judges, and magistrates. You can give the people a subordinate government, allowing them to legislate for themselves, whilst you defray the cost. So far as the law goes, the thing is done. There is no analogy between this and our Territorial Governments. Our Territories are only an offset of our own people, or foreigners from the same regions from which we came. They are small in number. They are incapable of forming a government. It would be inconvenient for them to sustain a government, if it were formed; and they are very much obliged to the United States for undertaking the trouble, knowing that, on the attainment of their majority—when they come to

trials of captured San Patricio soldiers resulted in death sentences for 70 of them. Heeding formal protests from the archbishop of Mexico and the British ambassador of Mexico, General Scott pardoned 50 of the men because of their young age or because they could prove they had not fought willingly with the Mexicans. Yet Mexico continued recruiting San Patricio soldiers for the duration of the war. In all, more than 4800 Irish-born soldiers served in the U.S. army during the U.S.–Mexican War. Of that number, about 4 percent ended up fighting for the Mexicans.

In September 1847 Mexico City surrendered, and the war ended. Mexico had been in no shape to resist superior U.S. firepower. The United States paid for Scott's victory with 13,000 lives and $100 million. The Mexicans lost 20,000 lives.

In the Treaty of Guadalupe Hidalgo (approved by the Senate in 1848) Mexico agreed to give up its claims to Texas. The United States gained all of Texas and half of the territory of Mexico: the area west of Texas, comprising present-day New Mexico, Arizona, and California. Male residents of areas formerly held by Mexico were given one year to decide whether to stay in the United States and become citizens or return to Mexico. They were also entitled to retain their titles to the land, a provision that proved difficult to enforce in the face of European American land hunger.

The U.S. government paid Mexico $18,250,000. Of that amount, $15 million was designated as payment for land lost; the rest was restitution to U.S. citizens who might bring claims against

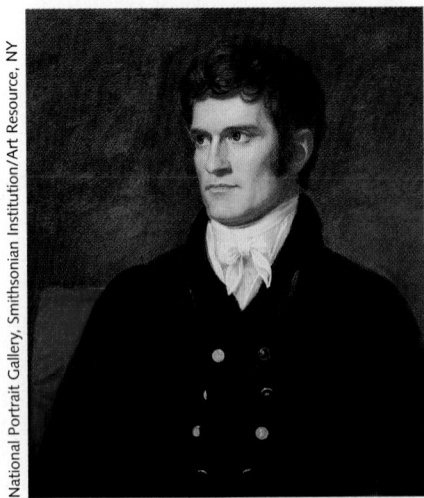

Portrait of John C. Calhoun by Charles Bird King, c. 1818–1825.

manhood—at twenty-one—they will be introduced to an equality with all other members of the Union. It is entirely different with Mexico. You have no need of armies to keep your Territories in subjection. But when you incorporate Mexico, you must have powerful armies to keep them in subjection. You may call it annexation, but it is a forced annexation, which is a contradiction in terms, according to my conception. You will be involved, in one word, in all the evils which I attribute to holding Mexico as a province. In fact, it will be but a Provincial Government, under the name of a Territorial Government. How long will that last? How long will it be before Mexico will be capable of incorporation into our Union? Why, if we judge from the examples before us, it will be a very long time. Ireland has been held in subjection by England for seven or eight hundred years, and yet still remains hostile, although her people are of kindred race with the conquerors. A few French Canadians on this continent yet maintain the attitude of hostile people; and never will the time come, in my opinion, Mr. President, that these Mexicans will be reconciled to your authority. . . . Of all nations of the earth they are the most pertinacious—have the highest sense of nationality—hold out the longest, and often even with the least prospect of effecting their object. On this subject also I have conversed with officers of the army, and they all entertain the same opinion, that these people are now hostile, and will continue so. . . .

We make a great mistake, sir, when we suppose that all people are capable of self-government. We are anxious to force free government on all; and I see that it has been urged in a very respectable quarter, that it is the mission of this country to spread civil and religious liberty over all the world, and especially this continent. It is a great mistake. None but people advanced to a very high state of moral and intellectual improvement are capable, in a civilized state, of maintaining free government; and amongst those who are so purified, very few, indeed, have had the good fortune of forming a constitution capable of endurance.

Calhoun also warns that "these twenty-odd Mexican States" would eventually have power in Congress. He asks his listeners whether they would want their own states "governed by" these peoples. ■

Source: Clyde A. Milner, ed., *Major Problems in the History of the American West: Documents and Essays* (1989), pp. 219–221.

Mexico for damaged or destroyed property during the war. Americans had conflicting views of the treaty. Abolitionists saw it as a blood-drenched gift from American taxpayers to slaveholders. Others argued that Polk had squandered a rare opportunity to seize all of Mexico.

Conclusion

In the 1830s and 1840s, mass population movements affected almost every aspect of American life. Immigrants from western Europe helped to swell the nation's labor force in midwestern farming communities and eastern cities. The arrival of the Roman Catholic Irish provoked a backlash among native-born Protestants and spawned a nativist political movement. Reformers in the United States and Europe went back and forth across the Atlantic, exchanging ideas related to women's rights, abolitionism, and utopian communities. As European Americans pushed the boundaries of the country west and south, they clashed with Indians and with foreign powers that claimed those lands as their own. Thus migration and immigration had profound consequences for American politics, economy, ideas, and society.

Most striking was the restlessness among land-hungry slave owners and antislavery forces alike. The war with Mexico in general and the clash over the Wilmot Proviso in particular opened a new chapter in the debate over slavery. In considering the Proviso, Congressmen gave up their party loyalties as Democrats or Whigs and began to think of themselves as Southerners and Northerners. When Wilmot proclaimed that he wanted to preserve the West for his "own color," he revealed that even antislavery Northerners did not necessarily embrace black people as equals. When Southerners indicated that even the vast expanse of Texas would not satisfy their desire for land, they revealed that the conflict over slavery was far from over. In fact, that conflict was about to enter a new and ominous stage.

Sites to Visit

The American Whig Party, 1834–1856
odur.let.rug.nl/~usa/E/uswhig/whigsxx.htm

This site explores the rise and fall of the anti-Jackson Whig Party.

The Alexis de Tocqueville Tour: Exploring Democracy in America
wwww.tocqueville.org/

Text and images are part of this companion site to C-SPAN's recent programming on de Tocqueville.

America's First Look into the Camera: Daguerreotype Portraits and Views, 1839–1862
memory.loc.gov/ammem/daghtml/daghome.html

The Library of Congress's daguerreotype collection consists of more than 650 photographs from the 1839–1864 period. The collection includes portraits, architectural views, and some street scenes.

Important Black Abolitionists
www.loc.gov/exhibits/african/influ.html

This Library of Congress exhibit includes pictures and text related to African American abolitionists.

On the Trail in Kansas
www.ukans.edu/carrie/kancoll/galtrl.htm

This Kansas collection site provides primary sources and images related to the Oregon Trail and European Americans' early movement westward.

The Era of the Mountain Men
www.xmission.com/~drudy/amm.html

This site includes private correspondence from early settlers in the area west of the Mississippi River.

Exploring *Amistad*
amistad.mysticseaport.org/main/welcome.html

The Mystic Seaport Museum in Mystic, Connecticut, maintains this site, which includes collections of historical documents related to the slave revolt aboard the *Amistad* and the trial that followed.

The Trail of Tears
www.americanwest.com/pages/indians.htm

A site on the forced migration of Cherokees from their home in the Southeast to Indian Territory.

The American Presidency: A Glorious Burden
americanhistory.si.edu/presidency/index.html

The Smithsonian Institution maintains this site on American presidents.

"Been Here So Long": Selections from the WPA American Slave Narratives
newdeal.feri.org/asn/index.htm

A site devoted to the interviews of former slaves conducted in the late 1930s.

The Roberts Case and the Efforts to Desegregate Boston Schools
www.sjchs-history.org

This site explores the legal challenge to racial segregation in Boston's schools during the late 1840s.

The Mexican–American War Memorial
sunsite.dcaa.unam.mx/revistas/1847

Images and text explore the causes, course, and outcome of the Mexican–American War.

For Further Reading

General

Michael Holt, *The Rise and Fall of the American Whig Party: Jacksonian Politics and the Onset of the Civil War* (1999).

Michael Morrison, *Slavery and the American West: The Eclipse of Manifest Destiny and the Coming of the Civil War* (1997).

Mary P. Ryan, *The Cradle of the Middle Class: The Family in Oneida County, New York, 1790–1865* (1983).

Charles G. Sellers, *The Market Revolution: Jacksonian America, 1815–1846* (1991).

Edward H. Spicer, *Cycles of Conquest: The Impact of Spain, Mexico, and the United States on the Indians of the Southwest, 1533–1960* (1962).

Harry L. Watson, *Liberty and Power: The Politics of Jacksonian America* (1990).

David J. Weber, *The Spanish Frontier in North America* (1992).

Mass Migrations

Jennifer S. H. Brown, *Strangers in Blood: Fur Trade Company Families in Indian Country* (1980).

Kathleen Neils Conzen, *Immigrant Milwaukee, 1836–1860: Accommodation and Community in a Frontier City* (1976).

Frederick Douglass, *The Narrative of the Life of Frederick Douglass, An American Slave* (1845).

John Ehle, *Trail of Tears: The Rise and Fall of the Cherokee Nation* (1988).

John Mack Faragher, *Women and Men on the Overland Trail* (1979).

Walter Johnson, *Soul by Soul: the Inside of the Antebellum Slave Market* (1999).

Philip J. Schwarz, *Migrants Against Slavery: Virginians and the Nation* (2001).

A Multitude of Voices in the National Political Arena

Donald B. Cole, *Martin Van Buren and the American Political System* (1984).

Paul A. Gilje, *The Road to Mobocracy: Popular Disorder in New York City, 1763–1834* (1987).

Daniel Walker Howe, *The Political Culture of the American Whigs* (1979).

Lawrence F. Kohl, *The Politics of Individualism: Parties and the American Character in the Jacksonian Era* (1989).

Richard P. McCormick, *The Second American Party System: Party Formation in the Jacksonian Era* (1966).

David R. Roediger, *The Wages of Whiteness: Race and the Making of the American Working Class* (rev. ed., 1999).

Reform Impulses

Charles Capper, *Margaret Fuller: An American Romantic Life* (1992).

Jed Dannenbaum, *Drink and Disorder: Temperance Reform in Cincinnati from the Washington Revival to the Women's Christian Temperance Union* (1984).

Michael D. Fellman, *The Unbounded Frame: Freedom and Community in Nineteenth-Century America Utopianism* (1969).

Howard Jones, *Mutiny on the Amistad: The Saga of a Slave Revolt and Its Impact on American Abolition, Law, and Diplomacy* (1987).

Carl Kaestle, *Pillars of the Republic: Common Schools and American Society, 1780–1860* (1983).

Henry Mayer, *All on Fire: William Lloyd Garrison and the Abolition of Slavery* (1998).

Shirley J. Yee, *Black Women Abolitionists: A Study in Activism, 1828–1860* (1992).

The United States Extends Its Reach

Arnoldo De Leén, *The Tejano Community, 1836–1900* (1982).

Richard Griswold Del Castillo, *The Treaty of Guadalupe Hidalgo: A Legacy of Conflict* (1990).

Robert W. Johannsen, *To the Halls of the Montezumas: The Mexican War in the American Imagination* (1985).

David Alan Johnson, *Founding the Far West: California, Oregon, and Nevada, 1840–1890* (1992).

Paul D. Lack, *The Texas Revolutionary Experience: A Political and Social History, 1835–1836* (1992).

Ramón Ruiz, ed., *The Mexican War: Was It Manifest Destiny?* (1963).

Online Practice Test

Test your understanding of this chapter with interactive review quizzes at

www.ablongman.com/jonescreatedequal/chapter12

Additional Photo Credits

Page 391: Museum Collections, Minnesota Historical Society (Neg. #6640)
Page 400: Samuel J. Miller, *Frederick Douglass*, 1847–52. Major Acquisitions Centennial Endowment, 1996.433.
    Photograph ©The Art Institute of Chicago
Page 401: Archives and Manuscripts Division of the Oklahoma Historical Society, 19615.43
Page 408: Massachusetts Historical Society, MHS (neg. #0031)
Page 411: Courtesy, Milwaukee County Historical Society
Page 414: The Newberry Library, Chicago
Page 417: Bettmann/CORBIS
Page 420: Benjamin W. Thayer Lithography Company, *Henry Clay's Grand March*, 1844. National Portrait
    Gallery, Smithsonian Institution, Washington, DC/Art Resource, NY

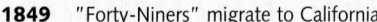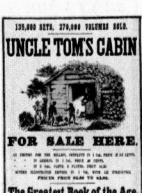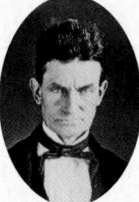
PART FIVE

Disunion and Reunion

THE CIVIL WAR WAS THE COUNTRY'S GREATEST POLITICAL AND MORAL crisis. By 1860 the two-party system could no longer contain the dispute between proslavery and antislavery forces. That dispute centered on the fate of slavery in new territories to the west. Several dramatic developments—the secession of southern states from the union, the formation of the Confederate States of America, and a Confederate attack on a federal fort in Charleston Harbor—precipitated all-out war. In the spring of 1861 few people could have anticipated that the conflict would drag on for four long years and claim more than 600,000 lives.

The Second Party System, based on divisions between Whigs and Democrats, unraveled in the 1850s. Both parties represented coalitions of groups that expressed cultural, not sectional, sensibilities. Yet a series of events led to a realignment of parties into northern and southern camps. Many Northerners chafed under the Fugitive Slave Act of 1850, which required that all citizens assist law enforcement agents in retrieving runaway slaves for their owners. The founding of the Republican party in 1854 gave a political voice to Northerners hoping to preserve the western territories for family farmers who would not have to compete for land and labor with large slaveholders. In 1857 the Supreme Court ruled that black people had no rights that any court was bound to respect. Violent conflicts between proslavery and antislavery forces in Kansas and a failed raid by abolitionists on Harpers Ferry, Virginia (in 1859), revealed that legislators' resolutions and maneuverings were insufficient to stave off bloodshed.

In pursuing a militant nationalism, Confederates hoped to compensate for their relative weakness in terms of population and industrial capacity compared with the North. They believed that they could use a large, docile black labor force to grow food and serve as a support system for the army. They anticipated that European nations, dependent on southern cotton, would extend them diplomatic recognition and that white civilians would rally to the defense of their homeland no matter what the price in money or blood. Confederates also believed that western Indians would gladly assist them in their cause against a hated U.S. army and that brilliant southern generals could outstrategize a huge, lumbering invading army indefinitely. On all these counts they miscalculated, but their miscalculations were revealed gradually.

During the war, white Southerners had to contend with two major unanticipated consequences of the conflict. First, war mobilization efforts across the South necessitated the centralization of government and economic policymaking. Principled states' rights supporters opposed these efforts. Second, slaves and free blacks alike proved traitorous to the Confederate cause. In myriad ways—running away from their owners and spying for the enemy, slowing their work pace in the fields, and fighting for the Union army—black people served as combatants in the war. They fought for their families and their freedom and for a country that would grant them full citizenship rights. In the North, only in late 1862 did President Abraham Lincoln announce that the United States aimed to destroy slavery, but violent antidraft, antiblack riots in several cities showed that the northern population was deeply divided over emancipation.

Soon after the end of the war, in April 1865, congressional Republicans began to challenge President Andrew Johnson's plan for reconstructing the South; they considered it too lenient toward the former Confederate states. In 1867 these political leaders had enough votes to enact their own plan, calling for the enfranchisement of black men in the South, the reorganization of southern state governments under leadership loyal to the Union, and the enactment of a labor contract system between southern landowners and black laborers.

Members of the Republican party backed a strong Union, a federal system in which the central government would ensure that individual men could pursue their own self-interest in the marketplace of goods and ideas. Yet the Civil War era exposed the limits of the Republican vision. The Plains Indians sought not citizenship but freedom from federal interference altogether. Women and working people challenged various components of the Republican ideal, with its emphasis on unbridled individualism and federal subsidies of business. African Americans aspired to own property, vote, and send their children to school, just as other nineteenth-century Americans did. They wanted to farm their own land and care for their own families free from white intrusion. Yet congressional Republicans did not enact large-scale land redistribution programs; most felt that once the rebels were subdued and slavery abolished, their duty was done.

Civil strife persisted into the postwar period. Union generals turned from quelling the southern rebellion to putting down armed resistance among the Plains Indians. Former rebels formed vigilante groups to attack black voters and their allies in the South. By the early 1870s most Northerners had lost interest in the welfare of the former slaves and acquiesced as former Confederates reclaimed state governments. The last occupying forces withdrew from the South in 1877. In welding the country together as a single economic and political unit, the Republicans had triumphed. However, white Southerners retained control over their local social and political affairs. The revolution to secure African American civil rights was stalled for nearly 100 years.

1864	Fort Pillow massacre of African American (Union) soldiers. Sand Creek (Colorado) massacre. Sherman's March to the Sea.
1865	Freedmen's Bureau is formed. Confederacy is defeated. Lincoln is assassinated; Andrew Johnson becomes president. Thirteenth Amendment is ratified.
1866	Civil Rights Act of 1866. National Labor Union is founded. Equal Rights Association is founded. Ku Klux Klan is organized. Congress approves Fourteenth Amendment.
1867	National Grange is founded. U.S. purchases Alaska from Russia. Reconstruction Act of 1867.
1868	Johnson is impeached and acquitted. U.S.–China Burlingame Treaty. Colored Labor Union is founded. Fourteenth Amendment is ratified
1869	Congress approves Fifteenth Amendment. Transcontinental Railroad is completed. National Woman Suffrage Association and American Woman Suffrage Association are formed. Knights of Labor is founded.
1870	Fifteenth Amendment is ratified.
1871	Ku Klux Klan Act.
1872	Apex Mining Act of 1872. Congress creates Yellowstone National Park. Susan B. Anthony attempts to vote. Crédit Mobilier scandal.
1873	Timber Culture Act. Onset of depression.
1874	Freedman's Savings Bank fails.
1875	Civil Rights Act. Resumption Act. Whiskey Ring is exposed.
1876	Battle of Little Big Horn. Contested presidential election between Rutherford B. Hayes and Samuel J. Tilden.
1877	Compromise of 1877. California Workingmen's Party is formed. Great Railroad Strike.

The Crisis over Slavery, 1848–1860

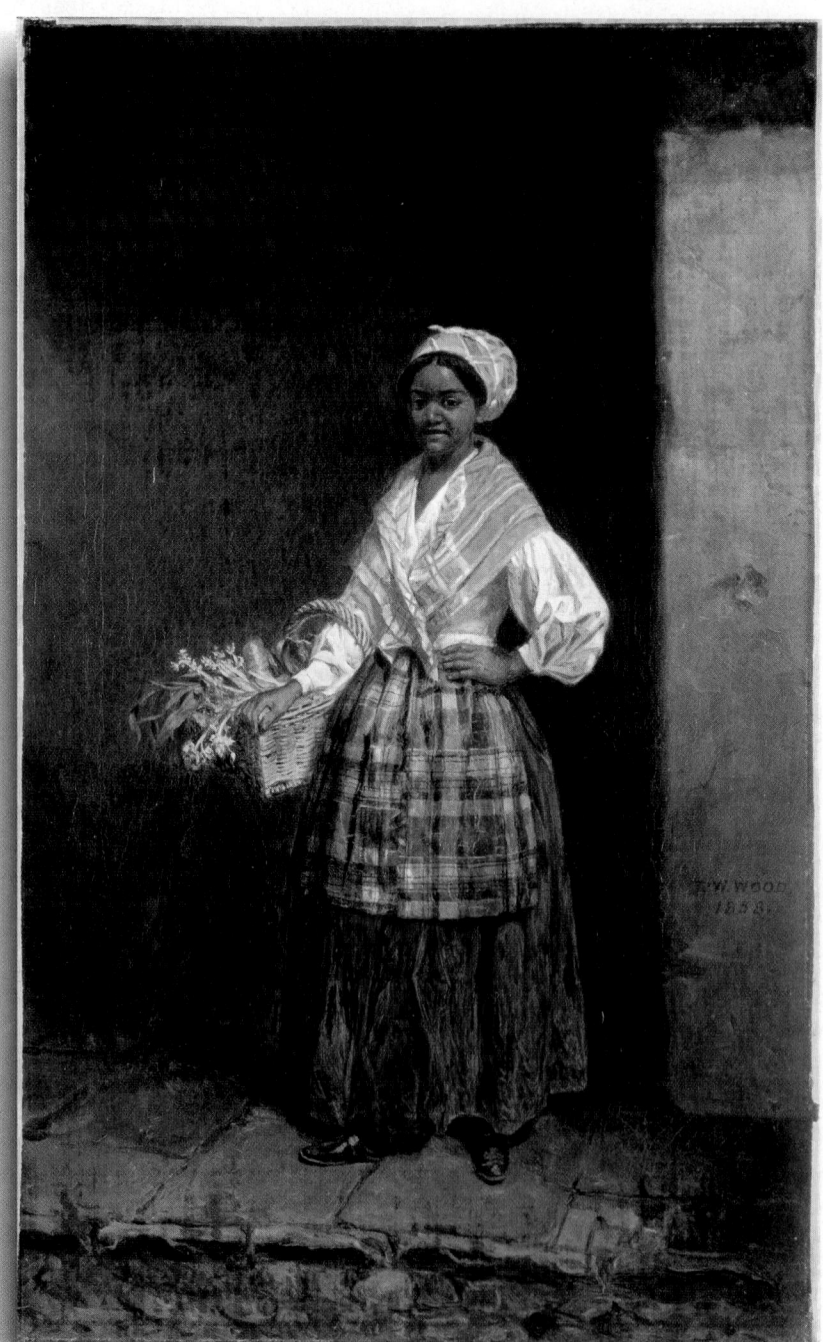

Thomas Waterman Wood, American 1823–1903. *Market Woman,* 1858. Oil on canvas, 23-3/8 × 14-1/2 in. Fine Arts Museums of San Francisco, Mildred Anna Williams Collection, #1944.8

■ T.W. Wood, *Market Woman,* 1858. Wood's portrait depicts an African American woman going about one of her daily chores—going to market.

ON JANUARY 24, 1848, HENRY WILLIAM BIGLER TOOK A BREAK FROM BUILDING A sawmill for John Sutter in California's Sacramento Valley and penned in his pocket diary, "This day some kind of mettle was found . . . that looks like goald." GOLD! News of the discovery at Sutter's mill spread like wildfire. By 1848 immigrants from all over the world and migrants from all over the United States had begun to pour into the foothills of the Sierra Nevada Mountains. Dubbed "the Forty-Niners," they had journeyed westward across the mountains, from the tenements of New York City and the great plantations of Mississippi; north from Mexico; and over the oceans, from western Europe, China, and South America. Equipping themselves with simple mining tools, the Forty-Niners began to dig for buried treasure, determined to stake a claim and make a fortune. And so they sang:

> I'll scrape the mountains clean, my boys,
> I'll drain the rivers dry,
> A pocket full of rocks bring home,
> So brothers, don't you cry!

During the Gold Rush years of 1848 to 1859, various cultural groups were thrown in close proximity to each other. Men from Belgium, France, Germany, Scotland, Chile, and Long Island learned to appreciate flour and corn tortillas (*tortillas de harina* and *tortillas de maiz*) and beef cooked in chile, staples of the Mexican diet. The disproportionate number of men permitted small numbers of women to challenge European American gender conventions. A gold miner might take a break from washing his clothes, straighten his aching back, and watch a Mexican woman and her daughter, well mounted on their horses, rounding up a herd of near-wild cattle. An-Choi, a Chinese immigrant woman, earned a tidy sum by opening a brothel

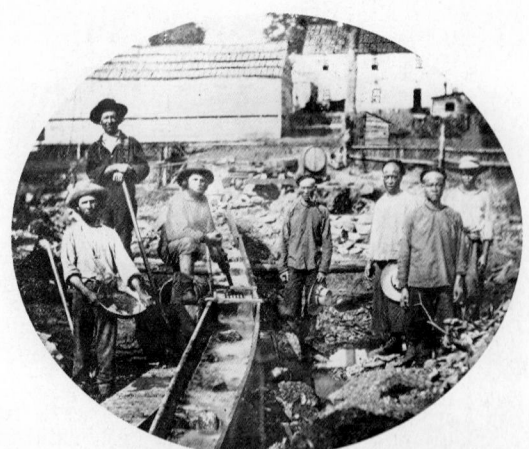

Chinese and European American miners pan for gold in the Auburn Ravine in California in 1852.

that catered to gold miners. Biddy Mason, an enslaved woman, successfully sued for her freedom and became the first African American homesteader in Los Angeles.

California came to be part of the United States as a result of the U.S.-Mexican War. In the 1848 Treaty of Guadalupe Hidalgo, Mexico agreed to hand over territory stretching from Texas northwest to California. As a result, the United States obtained a vast expanse of land—almost 530,000 square miles—called the Mexican Cession.

In addition to the land, the nation added to its population large numbers of men, women, and children already living in the area—13,000 Spanish speakers and 100,000 Indians (all former Mexican citizens) in California alone. After 1848 many new settlers streamed into California, and the migrants pressed for statehood, granted in 1850. By that year 90,000 new European American settlers lived in the state. Prominent among the Forty-Niners were Chinese immigrants—20,026 had arrived in California by 1852. Within two decades their numbers would swell to 50,000. From the American South came both free and enslaved African Americans; between 1850 and 1852, the California black population more than tripled from almost 700 people to over 2200. Rapid growth meant that, soon after the beginning of the Gold Rush, California had surpassed the minimum population necessary for statehood—60,000 people.

California became a state in 1850, but only after a bitter Congressional debate over the extension of slavery. The resulting Compromise of 1850 included several provisions bearing on the issue of slavery: California would be admitted as a free state; slave-trading would be outlawed in the District of Columbia; carved out of the Mexican Cession, the Utah and New Mexico territories could decide for themselves whether or not to legalize slavery. Finally, a new, harsh, fugitive slave law provided for the capture and return of slaves who found their way to free states in the north or west, including California. Though called a compromise, in fact these provisions inflamed the passions on both sides of the slavery debate—abolitionists in the North and slaveowners in the South.

Despite California's status as a free state, the principle of free labor was often violated. For example, in 1850 the state enacted a law with the misleading title, "An Act for the Government and Protection of the Indians," which provided for the indenture or apprenticeship of Indian children to white men for indeterminate periods of time. The law also allowed for the hiring out, to the highest bidder, of adult Indians deemed guilty of vagrancy. Indians in the region belonged to the Uto-Aztecan, Hokan, Penutian, Yukian, and Athabascan language families. Nevertheless, European Americans ignored these distinctions and called all Indians by the contemptuous term "Diggers," denounced them as lazy and uncivilized, and denied them the rights accorded American citizens.

Though a free state, California also enacted discriminatory legislation against African Americans. The state's Fugitive Slave Law of 1852 decreed that, regardless of his or her current status, a black person who entered the state as a slave and thereafter attempted to remain on free soil was a fugitive slave. That year, three African American gold miners, Robert Perkins, Carter Perkins, and Sandy Perkins, all former slaves who had been freed by their owner, were arrested under the law and ordered re-enslaved in their native Mississippi.

Moreover, some European Americans continued to hold people against their will illegally. Thomas Shearon, a quartz-mining entrepreneur from Nashville, Tennessee, defied the state constitution by using slave labor in the vicinity of San Francisco.

Other California labor systems revealed that the principle of free labor was not carried out in practice. Chinese immigrants to California entered the country organized in companies, or district associations, indebted to merchants for their transportation and bound to work for an employer until the debt was repaid. Fearing competition from cheap labor, alarmed European Americans labeled these Asian workers "coolies" (i.e., enslaved laborers). By 1852 the Chinese in California (almost all of them men) had been pushed out of mining as a result of the discriminatory Foreign Miners Tax, a measure leveled with special force against both Chinese and Mexican miners.

Although the Treaty of Guadalupe Hidalgo guaranteed U.S. citizenship rights to Mexicans, those rights were not enforced under the law. Many Mexicans found them-

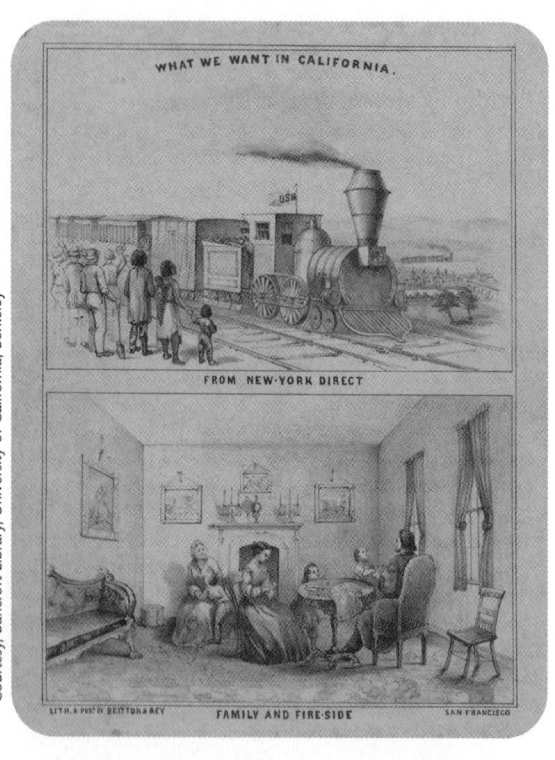

■ This pair of cartoons, titled "What We Want in California," suggests that migrants from the East hoped to reestablish a middle-class ideal in their new home. Above, an Indian family watches the arrival of a train from New York. Below, a European American family relaxes in a well-appointed parlor.

selves vulnerable to violence and land dispossession perpetrated by the growing European American majority. Delegates to California's constitutional convention in 1849 stipulated that only white *Californios* (descendants of the original Spanish colonists) were entitled to vote, over the objections of the 8 *Californios* among the 48 delegates in attendance. The majority of delegates also approved a measure prohibiting Indians and blacks from testifying against white people in court.

At mid-century the legal, economic, and cultural tensions among different groups in California mirrored tensions within the country as a whole. Rapid population growth, the coming together of many different cultures, and dramatic economic changes all fueled the conflict over slavery. The controversy surrounding California statehood revealed that awkward and unjust Congressional "compromises" would satisfy neither side in a debate that was becoming increasingly strident and even violent. All over the nation, in the pages of the popular press, on the streets of Boston, in the cotton fields of Alabama, no less than in the courts of California, Americans gradually united around a radical proposition: that the question of whether or not human beings could be held as private property was an issue on which there could be no compromise.

Regional Economies and Conflicts

It is tempting to view the decade of the 1850s with an eye toward the impending firestorm of 1861. However, in the early 1850s, few Americans could have anticipated the Civil War. At mid-century the United States was going through a period of rapid transition. New developments such as railroads, the factory system, and more efficient farm equipment led to significant changes in regional economies and began to give shape to an emerging national economy. Annexation of land in the Southwest and West and the conquest of Indians on the Plains produced wrenching social upheavals for Native Americans in those regions. Meanwhile, Americans continued to wrestle with the role of slavery in this rapidly changing society.

Native American Economies Transformed

On the Plains, Indians confronted wrenching transformations in their way of life. Forced to relocate from the Southeast to Indian Territory (present-day Oklahoma), the Five Southern ("Civilized") Tribes, the Cherokee, Choctaw, Creek, Chickasaw, and Seminole, grappled with the task of rebuilding their political institutions. By the 1850s the Cherokees had established a new capital at Talequah, along with public schools. They published a Cherokee newspaper (the *Advocate*) and created a flourishing print culture in their own language.

To the north and west of Indian Territory, Plains Indian tribes such as the Sioux, Kiowahs, and Arapahos exploited the horse, which had been introduced by Europeans in the Southwest in the seventeenth century. By raiding, trading, and breeding, these groups increased their stock of horses, which they used to hunt bison and transport their lodges and food from site to site. With abundant food and the means to trade with whites, these groups prospered for a brief period in the mid-nineteenth century. Their beadwork and animal skin painting exemplified the artistic vitality of their cultures.

In the 1850s U.S. officials negotiated treaties with various Plains Indian groups to enable European Americans to move west without fear of attack. Most settlers were bent on heading straight for California or the Northwest, traversing the Plains, which they called the Great American Desert in the mistaken belief that the absence of trees there demonstrated the infertility of the soil. The Fort Laramie Treaty of 1851 and the Treaty of Fort Atkinson three years later provided that the government could build roads and establish forts along western trails and that, in return, Indians would be compensated with supplies and food for their loss of hunting

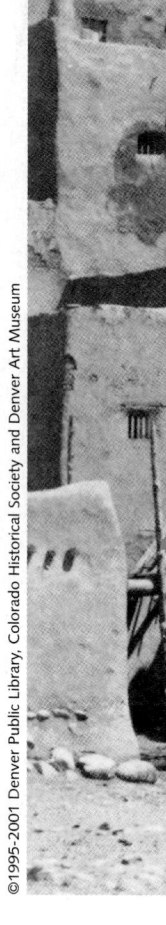

rights in the region. A young Cheyenne woman, Iron Teeth, recalled "the government presents" to her people in these terms: "We were given beef, but we did not care for this kind of meat. Great piles of bacon were stacked upon the prairies and distributed to us, but we used it only to make fires or to grease robes for tanning." She and her family sought out other items from government trading posts: "brass kettles, coffee-pots, curve-bladed butcher knives, boxes of black and white thread."

Thus as whites moved west in large numbers to "scrape the mountains clean and drain the rivers dry," they overran the fragile settlements of Indians and disregarded U.S. treaties and tribal boundaries. Taking leave of the Fort Laramie conclave of 1851, Cut Nose of the Arapahos had declared, "I will go home satisfied. I will sleep sound, and not have to watch my horses in the night, or be afraid for my women and children. We have to live on these streams and in the hills, and I would be glad if the whites would pick out a place for themselves and not come into our grounds." But within a generation, the Plains Indians were beseiged by the technology, weaponry, and sheer numbers of newcomers heading west.

Land Conflicts in the Southwest

In the mid-nineteenth century the United States gained control over a vast expanse of land, provoking legal and political conflicts over the rights and labor of the people who lived there, both natives and newcomers. Under the terms of the Treaty of Guadalupe Hidalgo, Mexico ceded not only California but also the province of New Mexico, territory that included the present-day states of New Mexico, Arizona, Utah, Nevada, and southern Colorado. In 1853 the United States bought an additional tract of land from Mexico, 55,000 acres located in the area south of the Gila River (in present-day New Mexico and Arizona). Overseen by the U.S. secretary of war, a Mississippi planter named Jefferson Davis, the agreement was called the Gadsden Purchase (after James Gadsden, a railroad promoter and one of the American negotiators).

The presence of so many Mexicans in this region prompted fears that any new state carved from the territory would remain under political control of Spanish speakers. European Americans charged that Mexicans were "not Americans, but 'Greaser' persons ignorant of our laws, manners, customs, language, and institutions," and consequently "unfit for statehood." New Mexico did not become a state until 1912.

The outcome of the U.S.-Mexican War—the U.S. seizure of present-day Texas and the area west of it—intensified rather than lessened conflicts over the land. Newly arrived European Americans battled native *Tejanos* (people of Mexican origin or descent) for political and economic supremacy. White migrants from the southern United States brought their slaves with them to the region, claiming that the institution of slavery was crucial for commercial development. With their irrigated fields, Mexican and Indian farmers had already demonstrated that crops could grow in the Southwest, suggesting that the slave system could also flourish there. German immigrants came to central and east Texas, founding towns with German names such as Fredericksburg, Weimar, and Schulenburg. During the 1850s, commercial farming continued to replace subsistence homesteading as the cattle industry spread and the railroads penetrated the region. Although European Americans monopolized the courts and regional political institutions, *Tejanos* retained cultural influence throughout Texas, dominating the cuisine and styles of music and architecture.

U.S. courts tended to disregard the land titles held by *Californios* and *Tejanos*. In the early 1850s California authorities battled Mexican social bandits such as Joaquin Murrieta, who, with his men, raided European American settlements. Murrieta and others argued that they were justified in stealing from privileged European Americans who, they claimed, disregarded the lives and property of Mexicans. In 1859 in the Rio Grande Valley of Texas, tensions between the *Tejano* majority and groups of European American law enforcement officers called the Texas Rangers

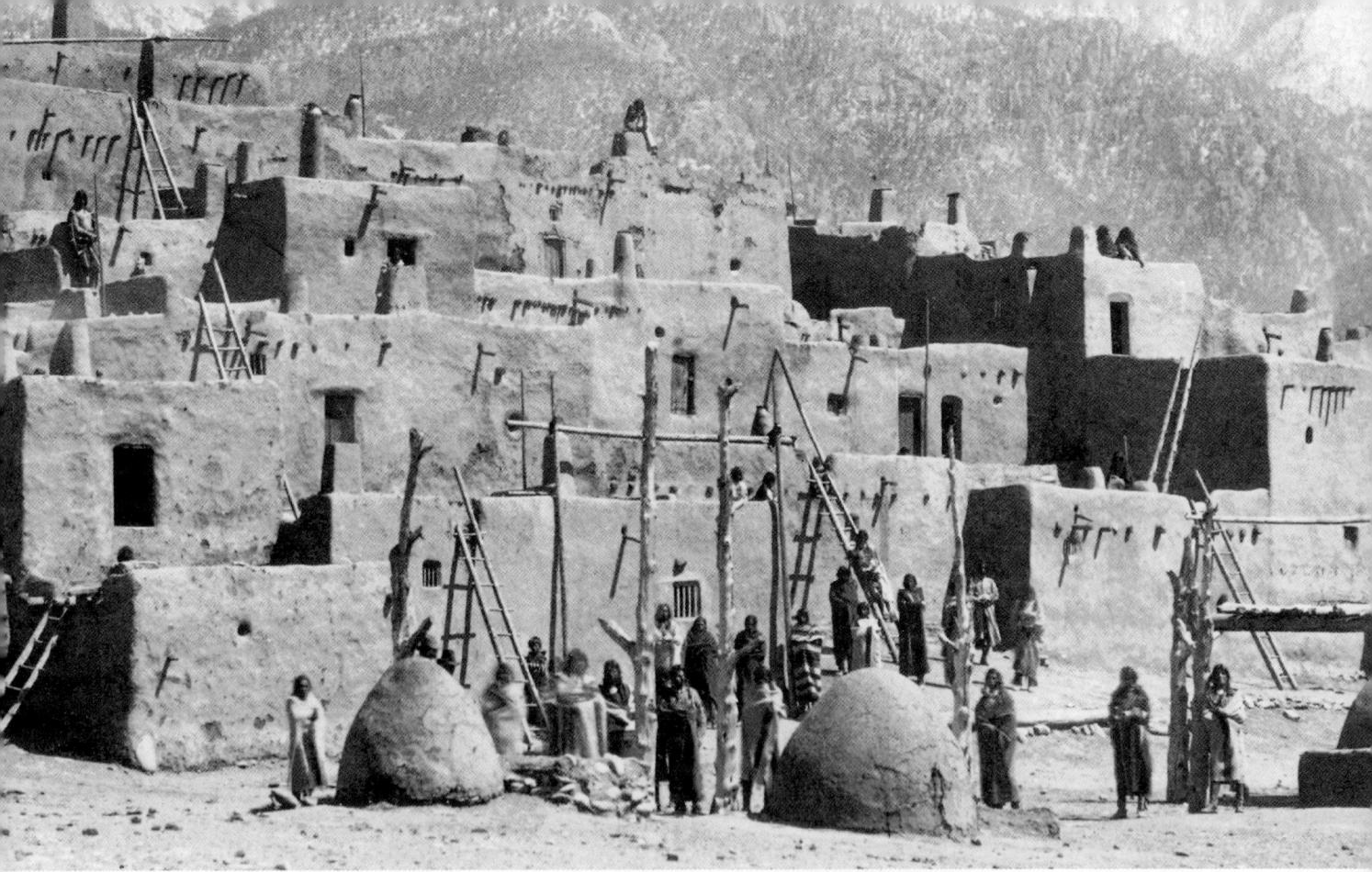

■ Dwellings of U.S. residents varied greatly depending on regional cultures. The Pueblo Indians of the Southwest took their name from the multilevel, rectangular, flat-roof clay houses where they lived. (*Pueblo* is the Spanish word for "village.") These structures have receding terraces connected by wooden ladders. In the forefront of this pueblo in Taos (present-day New Mexico) are clay beehive ovens. Farmers, hunters, and gatherers, the Pueblo Indians became residents of the United States as a result of the Treaty of Guadalupe Hidalgo in 1848.

erupted into full-scale warfare. Juan Cortina, who had fought on the side of Mexico during the Mexican War, orchestrated attacks on European Americans and their property in the vicinity of Brownsville. U.S. retaliation led to Cortina's War, pitting the Mexican leader against a young U.S. colonel, Robert E. Lee. Cortina himself became a hero to *Tejanos.* "You have been robbed of your property, incarcerated, chased, murdered, and hunted like wild beasts," he declared, "to me is entrusted the work of breaking the chains of your slavery."

Ethnic and Economic Diversity in the Midwest

The Yankee Strip (named for the northeasterners who migrated there) ran through northern Ohio, Indiana, and Illinois and encompassed the entire states of Michigan, Wisconsin, and Minnesota. Here migrants from New England settled and established public schools and Congregational churches. Immigrants from western Europe also made a home in this region—the Germans, Belgians, and Swiss in Wisconsin, the Scandinavians in Minnesota. At times cultural conflict wracked even the smallest rural settlements. In some Wisconsin villages, equally matched numbers of Yankees and Germans contended for control over the local public schools, with the group in power posting notices for school board elections in its own language, hoping that its rivals would not show up at the polls. Yankees complained that the Scandinavian farmers put their wives to work in the fields and that Germans took their children with them to *Biergarten* (places where beer was served).

The lower Midwest, including the southern portions of Ohio, Indiana, and Illinois, retained strong cultural ties to the southern states. In this region, many settlers had migrated from the South. Though residing in free states, they maintained broad support for the institution of slavery. In some cases they outnumbered their Yankee counterparts and managed to shape the legal system in a way that reflected a distinct antiblack bias. For example, Indiana's state constitution, approved in 1851, prohibited black migrants from making contracts with whites, testifying in trials that involved whites, voting, and entering the state.

Most rural midwestern households followed the seasonal rhythms characteristic of traditional systems of agriculture. However, by the mid-nineteenth century family farming had become dependent on expensive machinery and hostage to the national and international grain markets. John Deere's steel plow (invented in 1837) and Cyrus McCormick's horse-drawn mechanical reaper (patented in 1854) boosted levels of grain production. Yet these devices also required farmers to invest an ever-greater proportion of their profits in technology and in labor provided by hired hands. In Titibawassee, Michigan, an immigrant recently arrived from Germany bought land and eastern-made farm machinery, noting proudly that his new steam engine (purchased at a cost of $2135) "has 10 horse power and is arranged so that the power can be used in two ways so that if grinding grain does not pay, I will saw wood." Improved agricultural efficiency meant that the Midwest, both upper and lower, was fast becoming the breadbasket of the nation.

Regional Economies of the South

At mid-century the South Atlantic states encompassed a number of regional economies. Bolstered by the high price of cotton on the world market, slave plantations prospered in the Black Belt, a wide swath of fertile soil stretching west from Georgia. In many areas of the South, planters concentrated their money and energy on cotton, diverting slaves from nonagricultural labor to toil in the fields. During the 1850s, enslaved Virginia sawmill laborers, South Carolina skilled artisans, and Georgia textile mill operatives all found themselves reduced to the status of cotton hands. In some cases, white laborers took their places in mills and workshops. In other parts of the South, slaves combined field work with nonagricultural work. For example, on expansive low-country South Carolina rice plantations, slaves worked in the fields, but they also processed the raw material, preparing it for market.

Even modest farmers shared with the great planters a southern way of life that prized the supremacy of whites over blacks.

Increasingly, northern critics described the South as a land of economic extremes, with wealthy planters enjoying their white-columned mansions while degraded blacks slaved obediently in the fields. The reality was more complicated. Even among whites, there were huge variations in material conditions and daily experiences. A large amount of wealth in land and slaves was concentrated among a small percentage of the white population, and many non-slaveholding whites were tenant farmers, leasing their land, mules, and implements from wealthy planters. In some areas as many as one of five farms was operated by tenant farmers.

At the same time, about half the total southern white population consisted of yeoman farmers, families that owned an average of 50 acres and produced most of what they consumed themselves, with the occasional help of a hired hand (a leased slave or a wage-earning white person). In upcountry Georgia and South Carolina, yeoman farmers maintained local economies that were little affected by the cotton culture of the great planters in the Black Belt. These families grew what they needed: corn for themselves and their livestock and small amounts of cotton that the women spun, wove, and then sewed into clothing. Men and women alike labored in neighborhood networks of exchange, trading farm produce such as milk and eggs for services such as shoemaking and blacksmithing. Nevertheless, even modest farmers shared with the great planters a southern way of life that prized the independence of white households and the supremacy of whites over blacks.

The institution of slavery discouraged immigrants from moving to the rural South in large numbers. German artisans realized that slave labor would undercut their own wages, and Scandinavian farmers understood that they could not compete with large planters in terms of landowning or slave owning. However, the ethnic diversity of southern port cities offered a

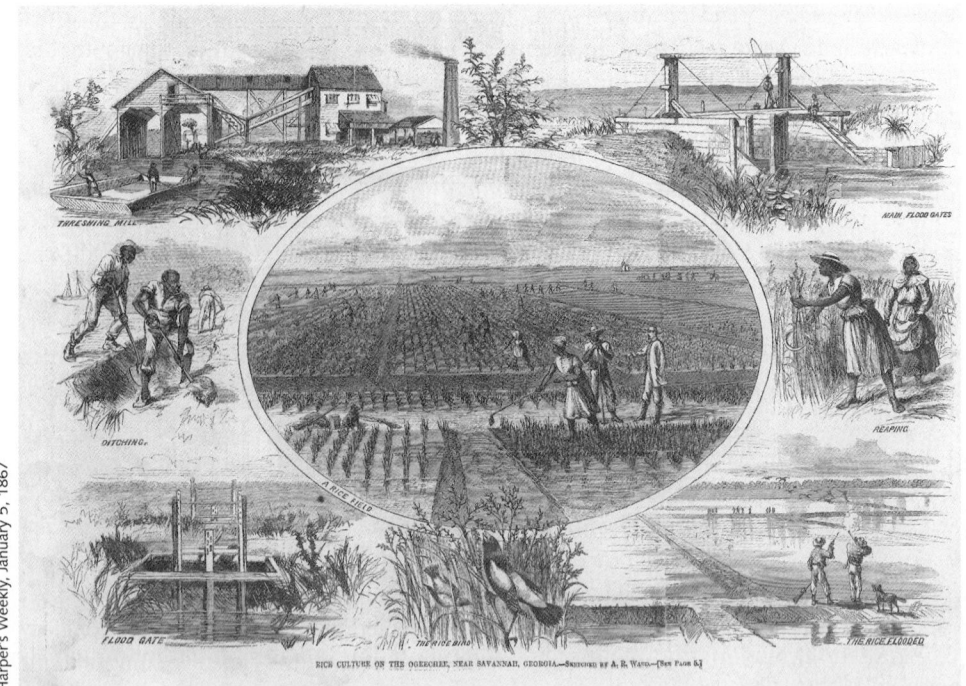

Harper's Weekly, January 5, 1867

■ This wood engraving from *Harper's Weekly* suggests the specialized nature of rice cultivation in the low country of South Carolina and Georgia. Rice growers used complex systems of dikes, ditches, and floodgates to grow the grain and threshing mills to process it. Masters assigned their enslaved workers daily tasks; after completing those tasks, men and women could spend time raising crops or tending livestock for their own use.

striking contrast to the countryside, where native-born Protestants predominated. In 1860, 54 percent of all skilled workers and 69 percent of unskilled workers in Mobile, Alabama, were immigrants. On assignment from the *New York Times* in the 1850s, journalist Frederick Law Olmsted noted that in New Orleans, German and Irish workers labored shoulder-to-shoulder with slave artisans, and although white immigrants "were rapidly displacing the slaves in all sorts of work," it was still possible to glimpse an "Irishman waiting on negro masons."

Throughout the slave states, black people continued to challenge the underpinnings of white supremacy. On the backroads of the plantation counties, late at night, poor workers of both races colluded to deprive the planter elite of their ill-gotten gain. Slaves swapped hams pilfered from smokehouses and bags of cotton lifted from storehouses for cash and goods offered by landless whites. In the vicinity of Augusta, Georgia, planters formed the Savannah River Anti-Slave Traffick Association in response to "the extensive and growing traffick unlawfully carried on with slaves by white persons and chiefly by Retailers of Spiritous Liquors."

Southern blacks were a diverse group. In the cities, planters allowed highly skilled slaves to hire themselves out and keep part of the money they earned for themselves. In their pride of craft and in their relative freedom to come and go as they pleased, these people inhabited a world that was neither completely slave nor completely free. Located primarily in the upper South and in the largest towns, communities composed of free people of color supported churches and clandestine schools, mocking the white notion that all black people possessed a childlike temperament and were incapable of caring for themselves. During the 1850s, the population of Virginia's free people of color increased from 54,333 to 58,042; in North Carolina the number increased from 27,463 to 30,463. The reality of southern society was not captured by the simple picture of white prosperity and black enslavement. Not all black people were enslaved field hands, and not all whites were privileged landowners. The widespread mythology masked a more complicated social reality.

A Free Labor Ideology in the North

In reaction to the southern slave system, the rural areas of the Northeast and Mid-Atlantic spawned a potent free labor ideology, which held that workers should reap what they sow, unfettered by legal systems of slavery and indentured servitude. Free labor advocates glorified the family farmer, the sturdy landowner of modest means, the husband and father who labored according to the dictates of the season and owed his soul—and his vote and the land he tilled—to no master. Nevertheless, the reality that sustained this ideal was eroding in the North during the 1850s.

More and more northerners were earning wages by working for bosses, rather than tilling their own land. Faced with competition from Midwestern farmers and burdened by unfavorable growing conditions imposed by rocky soil and a long winter, New Englanders were migrating to nearby towns and mill villages and to the West. By 1860 the region's textile and shoemaking industries were largely mechanized. From New Hampshire to Rhode Island, growing numbers of water-powered factories perched along the fall line, where rivers spilled swiftly out of the foothills and into the coastal plain. The all-white factory workforce included men and women, adults and children, Irish Catholics and native-born Protestants, failed farmers and young men and women eager to leave the uncertain, hardscrabble life of the countryside for the promise of the mill towns.

And yet the process of industrialization was an uneven one. For example, rural shoemaking workers labored at home, producing shoes for merchant capitalists who provided the raw materials and paid them by the piece. In contrast, in the huge new shoe factories of Lynn, Massachusetts, one worker at a Singer sewing machine (adopted by the John Woolredge Company for shoemaking) achieved the same output as 11 people doing the same task by hand in their homes. In the seaport cities, wage earning had become the norm, although many men and women continued to toil in the hope that they might eventually work for themselves. Thus the seamstress aspired to own a dress shop, the hotel waiter a tavern, the journeyman carpenter a small business.

In New York, Boston, Cincinnati, and elsewhere, large numbers of Irish newcomers successfully challenged small numbers of black workers for jobs at the lowest echelons of the labor force. In 1853 fugitive slave Frederick Douglass noted with dismay, "White men are becoming house-servants, cooks and stewards on vessels—at hotels. They are becoming porters, stevedores, hod-carriers, brickmakers, whitewashers and barbers, so that blacks can scarcely find the means of subsistence." Stung by the contempt of Yankee Protestants, impoverished Irish Catholics sought to assert their equality through race. They distanced themselves from African Americans by claiming a white skin as a badge of privilege over the former slaves, a badge of equality with the native born.

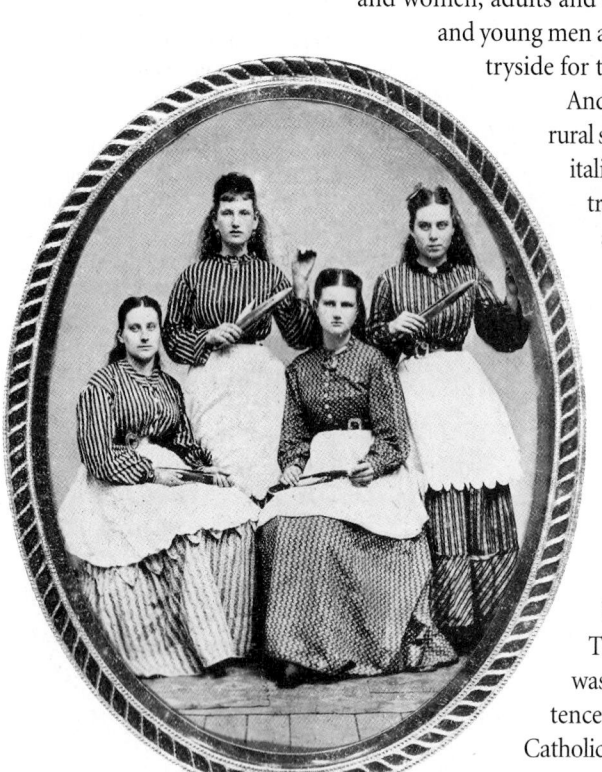

■ Maine textile workers, with their shuttles, pose for a formal portrait around 1860. Although women factory workers developed a collective identity distinct from that of middle-class wives, most young, native-born women eventually married and withdrew from the paid labor force. Many male factory workers were skeptical that women could or should play an effective role in labor organizations such as unions. Nevertheless, women workers in a number of industries, including textiles and shoes, formed labor organizations in the antebellum period.

Although Northerners in general contrasted themselves to the "backward slave South," their region of the country retained elements of unfree labor systems. New Jersey did not emancipate the last of its slaves officially until 1846, and throughout the North, vestiges of slavery lingered through the mid-nineteenth century. As a group of disproportionately poor people, blacks in New England, the Mid-Atlantic, and the Midwest were vulnerable to labor exploitation, including indentured servitude and a system of "apprenticeship" whereby black children were taken from their parents and forced to work for whites. In Delaware, an African American charged with a petty crime could be "disposed as a servant" by court authorities to the highest bidder for a term of seven years.

Many nonslave workers did not receive pay for their labors. As is the case today, wives and mothers throughout the country performed almost all of their work in the home without monetary compensation, although the measure of a white man was rendered more and more in cash terms. On farms and in textile mills such as those of Pawtucket, Rhode Island, children played a key role in the livelihood of individual households but received little or nothing in cash wages. Some members of the white working classes began to condemn "wage slavery," a system that deprived them of what they considered a fair reward for their labors and left them at the mercy of merchant capitalists and factory bosses. These workers charged that they were paid so little by employers, their plight was similar to that of black slaves in the South.

Different regions developed specialized economies. In turn, these regions relied on each other for the production of staple crops and manufactured goods. The result was a national economy. Southern slaves produced the cotton processed in New England textile mills. Midwestern farmers grew the grain that fed eastern consumers. California Forty-Niners discovered the gold that expanded the national currency supply. Yet these patterns of economic interdependence were insufficient to resolve the persistent political question: Which groups of people are entitled to American citizenship, with all the rights and privileges that the term implies?

Individualism Vs. Group Identity

Throughout the country, racist ideas and practices began to exert greater force. People were defined ever more strongly on the basis of their nationality, language, religion, and skin color. They were more and more limited in their legal status and the jobs they could obtain. Degrading images of legally vulnerable groups—blacks, Chinese, Hispanos—became a part of popular culture, in the songs people sang and the pictures they saw in books and magazines. Through these means, native-born Americans of British stock sought to distance themselves from people of color and from immigrants.

Paradoxically, some writers also began to highlight the idea of American individualism during this time. Such authors extolled what they considered to be the universal qualities embedded in American nationhood. They believed that the United States consisted not of distinctive and competing groups, but of a collection of individuals, all bent on pursuing their own self-interest, variously defined. They believed that the "representative" American was ambitious and acquisitive, eager to make more money and buy new things.

Yet not everyone could afford to embrace this optimistic form of individualism. Many who were marginalized found emotional support, and in some cases even political power, in a strong group identity. For example, on the Plains, the Sioux Indians resisted the idea that United States officials could carve up territory and sell land to individual farmers at the expense of a people that pursued the buffalo across artificial political boundaries. During negotiations at Fort Laramie in 1851, Black Hawk, a leader of the Oglala

TABLE 13-1

Nativity of Residents of the Boston Area, 1860

Country of Birth	Middlesex County	Norfolk County	Suffolk County
United States	166,126	83,693	125,439
England	4,273	2,494	4,472
Ireland	38,098	19,138	48,095
Scotland	1,272	607	1,440
Wales	28	34	61
Germany	629	1,159	1,290
France	187	133	397
Spain	39	9	59
Portugal	19	62	38
Belgium	5	6	19
Holland	67	17	177
Turkey	4	1	6
Italy	29	26	258
Austria	24	21	44
Switzerland	28	55	125
Russia	4	4	38
Norway	28	11	68
Denmark	26	18	97
Sweden	98	41	259
Prussia	150	103	744
Sardinia	1	1	64
Greece	3	3	10
China	9	5	4
Asia	19	13	29
Africa	----	2	20
British America	4,784	1,563	7,503
Mexico	6	1	2
South America	24	18	44
West Indies	59	27	149
Sandwich Islands	15	9	10
Atlantic Islands	39	5	260
Bavaria	33	246	250
Baden	73	331	663
Europe[a]	133	6	165
Hesse	14	32	107
Nassau	----	4	18
Poland	----	2	78
Wurttemberg	16	38	142
Australia	1	----	10
Pacific Islands	1	7	8
Other countries	----	5	38
Total foreign	50,238	26,257	67,261
Total population	216,354	109,950	192,700

[a] Not specified.

Source: Oscar Handlin, *Boston's Immigrants* (New York: Atheneum, 1972), p. 245.

Sioux, condemned the whites with his understatement, "You have split my land and I don't like it." In contrast to the Plains Indians, who wanted no role in American politics, African Americans and white women strove for full citizenship rights. These groups looked forward to the day when each person was accorded the same rights and was free to pursue his or her own talents and ambitions.

Putting into Practice Ideas of Social Inferiority

Everywhere, European American men sought to achieve or preserve the most stable, well-paying, and appealing jobs for themselves. By promoting ideas related to the inferiority of African Americans, Hispanos, and immigrants, white men could justify barring these groups from the rights of citizenship and landownership as well as from nonmenial kinds of employment. In Texas, Mexican leader Juan Cortina condemned Anglo interlopers whose "brimful of laws" facilitated the seizure of *Tejanos'* land by U.S. law enforcement agents and the courts. In California, U.S. officials justified the exclusion of blacks, Indians, Chinese, and the poorest Mexicans from citizenship rights by claiming that members of these groups were nonwhite or, in the words of one state judge writing in 1854, "not of white blood." (Of course, the concept of "white blood" has no scientific basis because the different blood types—A, B, AB, and O—are found among all peoples.)

> *The precarious social status of various groups was revealed in patterns of their work.*

The precarious social status of various groups was revealed in patterns of their work. In California, white men pursued opportunities on farms and in factories while increasing numbers of Chinese men labored as laundrymen and domestic servants. Indians toiled as field hands under white supervision. In rural Texas, Anglos established plantations and ranches while more and more Mexicans worked as *vaqueros* (cowboys), shepherds, sidewalk vendors, and freighters. In Massachusetts mill towns, white men and women served as the forefront of an industrial labor force while many African Americans of both sexes and all ages were confined to work in kitchens and outdoors as sweepers, cart drivers, and hawkers of goods.

Despite the divergent regional economies that shaped them, emerging ideologies of racial inferiority were strikingly similar. European Americans persisted in focusing on physical appearances, and they stereotyped all Chinese, Mexicans, and African Americans as promiscuous, crafty, "degraded," and intellectually inferior to whites. They characterized these groups as "cheap labor" who got by with little money: the Chinese supposedly could subsist on rice, Mexicans on beans and *tortillas,* blacks on the "fatback" of the pig. Such prejudices, in places as diverse as Boston, San Antonio, and San Francisco, prevented many people of color from reaching the limits of their own talents in mid–nineteenth-century America.

"A Teeming Nation"—America in Literature

Ideas about ethnic and racial difference coexisted with notions of American individualism, which stressed forms of universal equality. The variety of voices that gave expression to the national ideals of personal striving and ambition suggested the growth, energy, and vitality of the United States in the 1850s. In the Northeast, writers such as Ralph Waldo Emerson, Henry David Thoreau, Herman Melville, and Walt Whitman each crafted a unique writing style. At the same time, these men promoted a robust sensibility attuned to the challenges posed by the rigors of both the external world of natural beauty and the inner world of the spirit.

Some forms of literature offered an explicit critique of American materialism, with its love of things. According to Emerson, people were too concerned about material possessions; as he put it, things were "in the saddle," riding everyone. During the 1850s, Thoreau's work became more explicitly focused on nature. In his book *Walden* (1854), he described swimming in the Massachusetts pond of the same name: "In such transparent and seemingly bottomless water, reflecting the clouds, I seemed to be floating through the air as in a balloon." An apprecia-

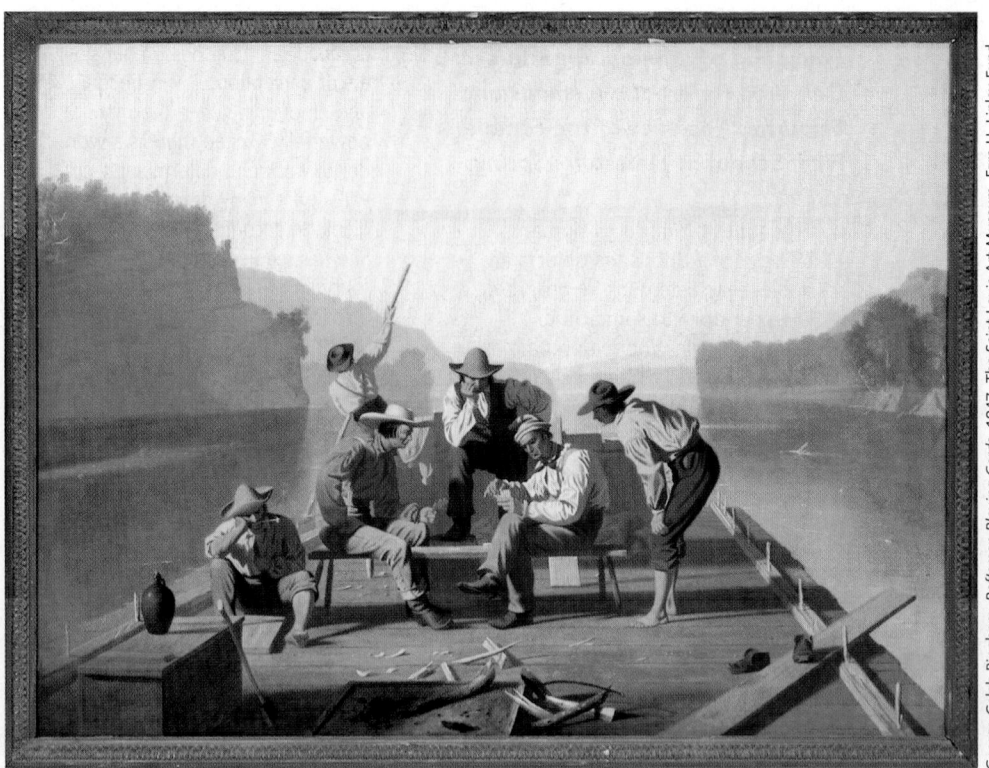

George Caleb Bingham, *Raftsmen Playing Cards*, 1847. The Saint Louis Art Museum, Ezra H. Linley Fund

■ **Just as American writers explored questions of national identity, American artists portrayed everyday scenes related to the vitality of American enterprise and democracy. This painting, *Raftsmen Playing Cards* (1847), was one from George Caleb Bingham's series of pictures of Missouri rivermen. A contemporary observer speculated that the youth on the right is "a mean and cunning scamp, probably the black sheep of a good family, and a sort of vagabond idler." Large rivers such as the Missouri and Mississippi remained powerful symbols of freedom in the American imagination.**

tion of the wonders of nature—wonders that could be felt and tasted, as well as seen—amounted to a powerful force of democratization; anyone and everyone could participate. In turn, Thoreau actively supported the abolition of slavery; his love of nature formed the foundation of his belief in the universal dignity of all people in general and the cause of freedom for black people in particular.

In contrast, other writers celebrated busy-ness, whether in the field or workshop. In the introduction to his book of poetry titled *Leaves of Grass* (1855), Walt Whitman captured the restlessness of a people on the move: "Here is not merely a nation but a teeming nation of nations. Here is action untied from strings necessarily blind to particulars and details magnificently moving in vast masses." To Whitman, the expansiveness of the American landscape mirrored the American soul, "the largeness and generosity of the spirit of the citizen." His sensuous "Song of Myself" constituted an anthem for all Americans poised, gloriously diverse in their individuality (and their sexuality), to exploit the infinite possibilities of both body and spirit: "I dote on myself, there is a lot of me and all so luscious."

Challenges to Individualism

Many men and women remained skeptical of—and, in some cases, totally estranged from—the wondrous possibilities inherent in Whitman's phrase, "Me, Me going in for my chances." In northern cities, individualism spawned the kind of creative genius necessary for technological innovation and dynamic economic change, but it had little meaning for Native Americans

Professor Howe on the Subordination of Women

Antebellum southern elites prized what they called "natural" hierarchical social relations: the authority of fathers and husbands over daughters and wives, parents over children, rich over poor, and whites over blacks. According to slaveholders, clergy, and scholars, these relationships provided social stability and ensured that the weak and dependent would receive care from the rich and powerful. In July 1850, George Howe, professor of biblical literature at the Theological Seminary at Columbia, South Carolina, addressed the graduating class of a private women's academy. Howe suggested that the roles of women (elite white women) were enduring and never-changing.

The Endowments, Position and Education of Woman. An Address Delivered Before the Hemans and Sigourney Societies of the Female High School at Limestone Springs

The duties of life to all human beings are arduous, its objects are noble—each stage of its progress is preparatory to some other stage, and the whole a preparation to an interminable existence, upon which, in one sense, we are hereafter to enter, and in another, have already entered. Others may slightly regard the employments, trials and joys of the school girl. I am disposed to put on them a higher value. Our wives, sisters, and our mothers were in the same position yesterday. You will occupy a like [position] with them tomorrow. Whatever of virtue, of patient endurance, of poignant suffering, of useful labor, of noble impulse, of generous endeavor, of influence exerted on society for its good, has been exhibited in their example, in a few short years we shall see exhibited also in yours.

To woman, . . . there must be ascribed . . . acuteness in her powers of perception, . . . instincts . . . and emotions. When these are powerfully excited there is a wonderful vigor and determination of will, and a ready discovery of expedients to accomplish her wishes. She has readier sympathies, her fountain of tears is nearer the surface, but her emotions may not be so constant and permanent as those of man. She has greater readiness and tact, purer and more noble and unselfish desires and impulses, and a higher degree of veneration for the virtuous and exalted, and when she has found the way of truth, a heart more constant and more susceptible to all those influences which come from above. To the gentleness and quiet of her nature, to its affection and sympathy, that religion which pronounces its benediction on the peace-makers and the merciful, which recommends to them the ornament of a meek and quiet spirit, which, in the sight of the Lord, is of a great price, addresses itself with more force and greater attraction than it addresses man. Born to lean upon others,

in the West, most of whom were desperately seeking a collective response to new threats in the form of cattle ranchers and the U.S. Cavalry. On the Great Plains, groups such as the Mandan and Pawnee performed ceremonies and rituals that celebrated kinship and village life above the individual.

African Americans in the North forged a strong sense of group identity. Though they rejected notions of white people's "racial" superiority, blacks had little choice but to think of themselves as a group separate and distinct from whites. Their sense of group solidarity was manifested in everyday life and in political rhetoric and action. In northern cities, blacks took in boarders and joined mutual-aid societies in order to affirm the collective interests of the larger black community. In contrast, well-to-do whites were increasingly emphasizing the sanctity of the nuclear family, composed solely of parents and children. Black leaders criticized the racist laws and ideas that affected the lives of black men, women, and children. For example, the charismatic Boston preacher Maria Stewart denounced the twin evils of racial and gender prejudice for condemning all black women to a life of menial labor: "How long shall the fair daughters of Africa be compelled to bury their minds and talents beneath a load of iron pots and kettles? The [white] Americans have practised nothing but head-work these 200 years, and we have done their drudgery."

Some groups of women embraced a collective identity of womanhood, although the definition of that identity took several forms. For example, in the North, writers such as Catherine Beecher articulated a vision of female self-sacrifice fueled by family obligations and emotional relationships. Beecher declared that self-sacrifice formed the "grand law of the sys-

rather than to stand independently by herself, and to confide in an arm stronger than hers, her mind turns more readily to the higher power which brought her into being . . . .

Providence, then, and her own endowments mark out the proper province of woman. In some cases she may strive for the mastery, but to rule with the hand of power was never designed for her. When she thus unsexes herself she is despised and detested by man and woman alike. England's Queen Victoria at the present moment, if not more feared, is far more beloved in the quiet of her domestic life, than Elizabeth was, the most feared of her female Sovereigns.

Howe ends his address by drawing an implicit comparison between the South and the North. Like many Southerners, he associated the North with labor radicalism, abolitionism, and challenges to the "natural" position of women.

When women go about haranguing promiscuous assemblies of men, lecturing in public, either on infidelity or religion, on

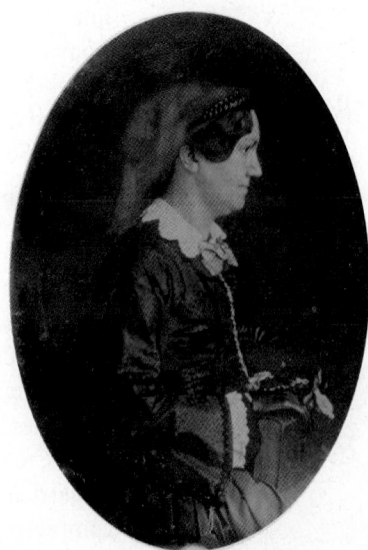

Louisa McCord was the member of an elite slaveholding family in South Carolina. She was an ardent supporter of slavery. Though an accomplished essayist herself, she believed that white women should remain subordinate to their fathers and husbands. In 1856 she wrote, "The positions of women and children are in truth as essentially states of bondage as any other, the differences being in degree, not kind." She added that the "true definition of slavery" thus "applies equally to the position of women in the most civilized and enlightened countries."

slavery, on war or peace—when they meet together in conventions and pass resolutions on grave questions of State—when they set themselves up to manufacture a public opinion for their own advantage and exaltation—when they meet together in organized bodies and pass resolutions about the "rights of woman," and claim for her a voice and a vote in the appoint-

ment of civil rulers, and in the government, whether of Church or State, she is stepping forth from her rightful sphere and becomes disgusting and unlovely, just in proportion as she assumes to be a man. ■

Source: George Howe, *The Endowments, Position and Education of Woman. An Address Delivered Before the Hemans and Sigourney Societies of the Female High School at Limestone Springs,* July 23, 1850 (Columbia, SC: I.C. Morgan, 1850), pp. 5, 9, 10–11.

tem" by which women should live their lives. Through poetry, short stories, and novels for popular audiences, other women writers posited an alternative to the world of masculine daring and individualism.

Informed by religious devotion and sustained by labors of love in the home, this female world offered an alternative to the individualism necessary to profit-seeking, whether on the family farm or in the bank or textile mill. As consumers of store-bought food and goods, antebellum housewives believed they were deprived of the satisfactions supposedly enjoyed by their grandmothers and associated with maintaining a colonial household—churning butter, spinning flax, making candles, and weaving cloth. Yet middle-class women believed they could take pride in rearing virtuous citizens and caring for overworked husbands. Sarah Willis Parton (Fanny Fern) cautioned her readers in a series of sketches published in 1853 (*Fern Leaves from Fanny's Portfolio*) that marriage is "the hardest way on earth of getting a living. You never know when your work is done."

Well-to-do white women in the Northeast yearned to be productive and useful although they stood outside the cash-based market economy. Nevertheless, other groups of women cherished different kinds of aspirations. Organizers of the country's first conference devoted to the status of women, the Seneca Falls Convention held in upstate New York in 1848, derived inspiration from the abolitionist movement and protested the efforts of white men to exclude women from formal participation in it. Elizabeth Cady Stanton and Lucretia Mott recalled the humiliation they felt when they found themselves relegated to a women's gallery at the World Anti-Slavery Convention in London in 1840. In their demands for women's rights they

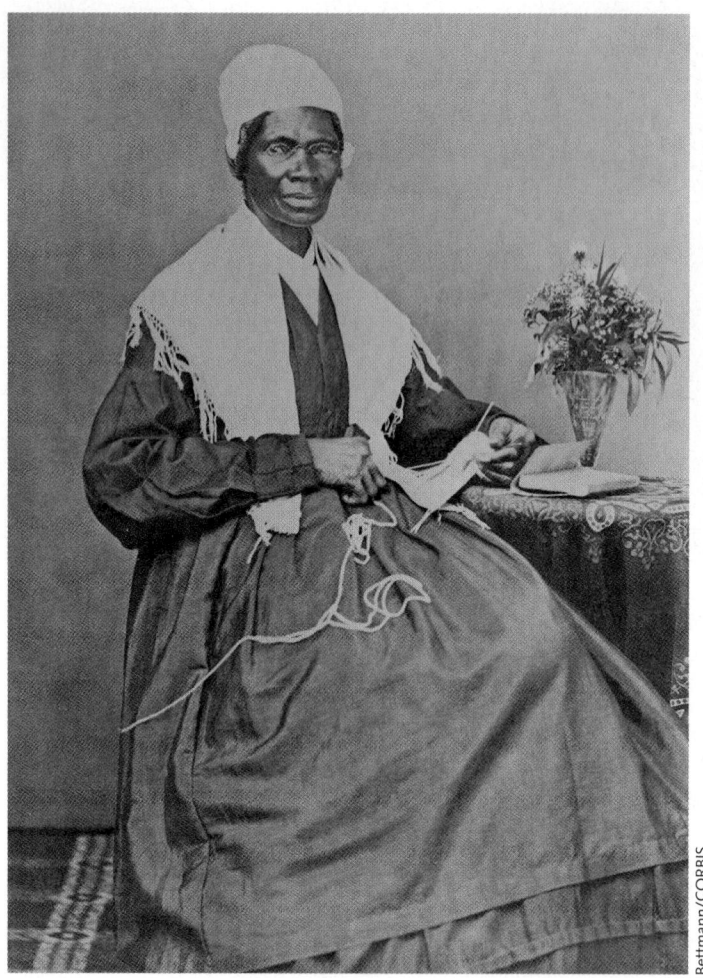

Bettmann/CORBIS

■ Isabella Baumfree was born into slavery in New York State in 1797. Thirty years later she escaped from bondage and became a preacher. In 1843 she changed her name to Sojourner Truth. A powerful orator, she spoke on behalf of abolitionism and urged white women's-rights activists to embrace the cause of enslaved women. Truth sold small cards, called *cartes de visite,* to support herself. On this card, a portrait taken in 1864, she notes that she must sell her image ("the Shadow") to make a living.

linked the plight of the slave with the plight of free women, arguing that white men exploited and denigrated members of both groups. Stanton, Mott, and others received crucial support from African American leaders such as Sojourner Truth and Frederick Douglass.

Delegates to Seneca Falls (including Douglass) approved a document called the "Declaration of Sentiments," modeled after the Declaration of Independence: "When in the course of human events . . . . We hold these truths to be self-evident: that all men and women are created equal." This group of women thus claimed for themselves a revolutionary heritage and all the rights and privileges of citizenship: to own property in their own names, to vote, to attend schools of higher learning, and to participate "in the various trades, professions, and commerce." In the process they expressed at least an implied kinship with the freedom fighters of France, Italy, and Germany who also launched struggles for self-determination during the fateful year of 1848.

Many women, including enslaved workers throughout the South and hard-pressed needleworkers toiling in cramped New York City tenements, could not devote themselves full time to the care of hearth and home, nor could they aspire to a career of public agitation. In her autobiographical novel, *Our Nig; or, Sketches from the Life of a Free Black, in a Two-Story White House, North* (1859), Harriet Wilson wrote bitterly of the fate of women such as her mother, a woman "early deprived of parental guardianship, far removed from relatives . . . left to guide her tiny boat over life's surges alone and inexperienced." Like the book's main character, Alfrado, Wilson herself had suffered at the hands of tyrannical white women employers, but at the end of the story Alfrado achieves a measure of dignity and independence for herself by setting up a small business. She thus offered an explicit challenge to both the arrogance of propertied white men and the homebound sentimentality of wealthy white women.

In sum, there was no single, transcendent American identity in the mid-nineteenth century. And yet, critiques of the dominant culture could at times uphold its lofty ideals while condemning everyday reality. In his 1852 speech "The Meaning of July Fourth for the Negro," delivered in Rochester, New York, Frederick Douglass took the country to task for failing to live up to the principles embodied in the Declaration of Independence: "Stand by those principles," he exhorted his listeners, "at whatever cost." His words foreshadowed a great war.

The Paradox of Southern Political Power

Slavery needed to expand to survive. Decades of intensive cultivation were exhausting the cotton fields in the South. The planter elite was counting on the admission of new territories as slave states to preserve their threatened power in Congress. To slave owners, northern-sponsored efforts to block their expansion amounted to a death sentence for all that the white South held dear. In defense of the slave system, the white South had to mount a strong offense or die.

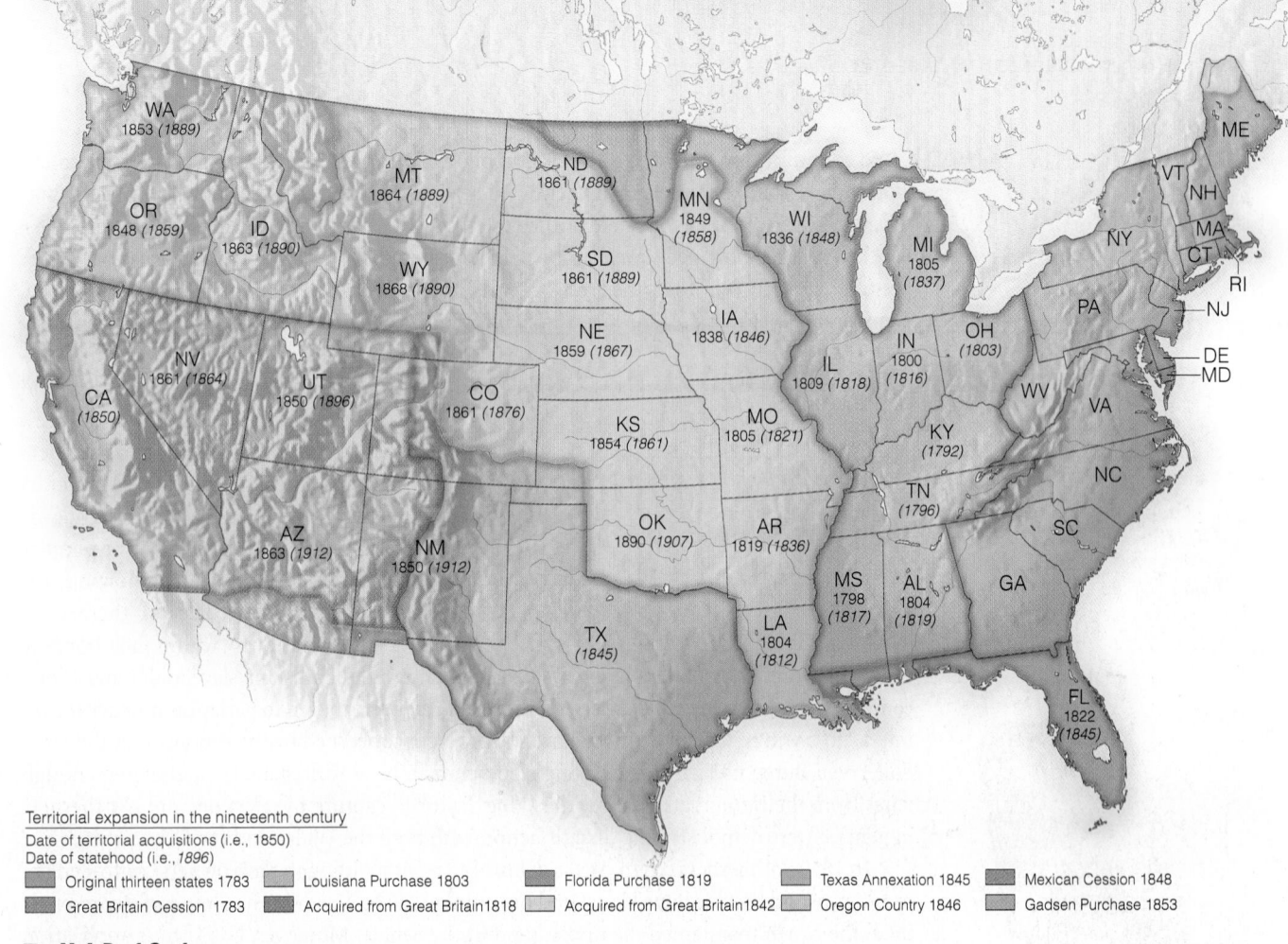

Territorial expansion in the nineteenth century

Date of territorial acquisitions (i.e., 1850)
Date of statehood (i.e., 1896)

Original thirteen states 1783 · Louisiana Purchase 1803 · Florida Purchase 1819 · Texas Annexation 1845 · Mexican Cession 1848

Great Britain Cession 1783 · Acquired from Great Britain 1818 · Acquired from Great Britain 1842 · Oregon Country 1846 · Gadsen Purchase 1853

■ MAP 13.1

TERRITORIAL EXPANSION IN THE NINETEENTH CENTURY   As a result of the Mexican War (1846–1848), the United States won the territory west of Texas by conquest. In 1853, James Gadsden, U.S. ambassador to Mexico, received congressional approval to pay Mexico $15 million for 55,000 square miles in present-day southern Arizona and New Mexico. That year marked the end of U.S. continental expansion.

In the early 1850s, proslavery forces maintained firm control over all branches of the federal government. Nevertheless, southern planters felt increasingly defensive as the country expanded westward. In 1850 a writer for *DeBow's Review,* a mouthpiece for the planter class, offered a peculiar combination of bravado and anxiety. Boasting of the South's agricultural capacity and resources so integral to "the welfare of humanity at large," the writer nonetheless claimed that the region's "undisturbed progress" depended on "a firm adherence to the compromises of the constitution" and warned against "the abolition excitement," which would necessarily upset the delicate balance between slave and free states.

Gradually, this tension between southern strength and southern fears led to the fraying and then unraveling of the Jacksonian American party system, which had relied on a truce maintained between Whigs and Democrats on the issue of slavery. A new party, the Republicans, fused the democratic idealism and economic self-interest of native-born Northerners in such a powerful way that white Southerners believed that the institution of slavery was in danger of succumbing to the Yankee onslaught. And so a clash of ideas gradually slipped out of the confines of the polling place and into the realm of armed conflict.

The Party System in Disarray

In 1848, eight years after the appearance of the antislavery Liberty party, cracks in the second two-party system (which pitted the Whigs against the Democrats) intensified with the founding of the Free-Soil party. Free-Soilers challenged the prevailing notion that the Whigs and Democrats could continue to smooth over the question of slavery in the territories with a variety of patch-work policies and piecemeal compromises. The Free-Soil platform promoted a forthright no-slavery-in-the-territories policy and favored the Wilmot Proviso (introduced in Congress in 1846), which would have banned slavery from all land acquired as a result of the Mexican War. In the presidential election of 1848, the Free-Soil party nominated former President Martin Van Buren, Democrat of New York. At the same time, Free-Soilers extended their appeal to the Whig party by supporting federal aid for internal improvements, free western homesteads for settlers, and protective tariffs for northern manufacturers.

Nevertheless, the two major parties persisted in avoidance politics. The Democrats chose General Lewis Cass as their standard-bearer, a man known as the "father of popular sovereignty" because he favored allowing citizens of new states to decide for themselves whether to permit slavery within their borders.

TABLE 13-2

The Election of 1848

Candidate	Political Party	Popular Vote	Electoral Vote
Zachary Taylor	Whig	1,360,967	163
Lewis Cass	Democratic	1,222,342	127
Martin Van Buren	Free-Soil	291,263	----

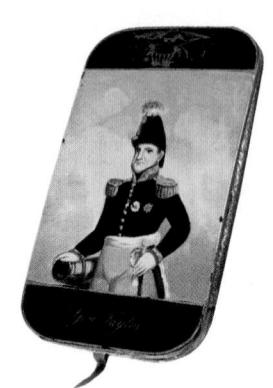

The Whigs put forth General Zachary Taylor, although the Louisiana slaveholder and Mexican War veteran had never held elected office. Still, Taylor managed to parlay his military record into a close win in the fall of 1848. Slaveholders were concerned by the support that the Free-Soiler Van Buren had garnered among Democrats in New York State. He had drawn enough votes from the Democrats to allow the Whig Taylor to capture the election, and Northerners in general were demonstrating dissatisfaction with both the Whigs and the Democrats.

In 1849 Southerners confronted a disturbing reality. Although slave owners controlled the presidency and the Supreme Court and outnumbered the North in the House of Representatives, the North maintained the upper hand in the Senate. Moreover, California's application for statehood in 1849 raised the specter of an unbalanced federal system consisting of 16 free states and 15 slave states. And the abolitionist threat appeared in other guises as well: the territories of Utah and New Mexico apparently preparing to ban slavery once they became states, abolitionists clamoring for the immediate emancipation of all slaves, and black men and women, including former slave Harriet Tubman, working with abolitionists in the upper South and the North to facilitate the escape of slaves through a network of safe stops called the Underground Railroad. The "railroad" consisted of northerners, white and black, who sheltered fugitives from southern slavery in their flight to the North or, in some instances, to Canada.

The Compromise of 1850

Against this backdrop of sectional controversy, Congress debated the terms under which California would enter the Union in 1850. In their physical demeanor, the three principals in the Senate debate revealed that the effort to placate those on both sides of the slavery question was on the verge of exhaustion. John C. Calhoun, dying of tuberculosis, argued that the North must concede that the South had the right to its own property, regardless of whether that property took the form of land or human beings. Together, the frail Henry Clay, age 73, and Daniel Webster, 68 years old and racked with disease, sought to wring concessions from both sides.

A young Democratic senator from Illinois, Stephen Douglas, helped to cobble together a complicated agreement that proved workable enough in the short run but only prolonged the showdown over slavery. Under the Compromise of 1850, California would enter the Union as a free state that year. New Mexico and Utah would eventually submit the slavery question to voters and thus put the idea of popular sovereignty to a practical test. The federal government would abolish the slave trade in Washington, D.C. (a move that did not affect the status of slaves already living there), and shore up the Fugitive Slave law of 1793 with a new, harsher measure.

The Fugitive Slave Law of 1850 essentially did away with the notion of the North as free territory, for it required local and federal law enforcement agents to retrieve runaways no matter where they sought refuge in the United States. Blacks were denied a trial or the right to testify on their own behalf. Fugitive slave commissioners earned $10 for each runaway they returned to a claimant. By compelling ordinary citizens to aid in the capture of alleged fugitives, the law brought the issue of slavery to the doorstep of northern whites. In the fall of 1850, Millard Fillmore, who had assumed the presidency in July of that year after Taylor died in office, signed the bill.

TABLE 13-3			
The Election of 1852			
Candidate	Political Party	Popular Vote	Electoral Vote
Franklin Pierce	Democratic	1,607,510	254
Winfield Scott	Whig	1,386,942	42
John P. Hale	Free-Soil	155,210	----

Despite these dramatic events, the presidential campaign of 1852 was a lackluster affair. The Democrats nominated an unknown lawyer, Franklin Pierce. Although he hailed from New Hampshire, Pierce supported slavery. The Whigs turned their back on President Fillmore and chose as their nominee General Winfield Scott, who had gained fame during the Mexican War of 1848. Yet the Whigs split into regional factions during the election; Northerners resented Scott's support of the Fugitive Slave Law, and Southerners doubted Scott's devotion to slavery. This split foreshadowed the end of national political parties and the emergence of regional parties, an ominous development indeed.

Expansionism and Political Upheaval

The interests of southern planters affected not only domestic politics, but debates and policies related to foreign affairs as well. Even as Congress was heatedly discussing the Compromise of 1850, Southerners were contemplating ways to extend their reach across and even beyond the continental United States. They wanted to find new fresh, fertile lands for cotton cultivation, and, they hoped, to incorporate those lands into the United States. Such expansion would also help to bolster the political power of slaveowners in Congress by someday adding new slave states to the Union.

In 1850 the United States and Great Britain signed the Clayton–Bulwer Treaty, agreeing that neither country would seek to control the rights to any canal spanning the Panama–Nicaragua isthmus. In 1848 President Polk had made a gesture to buy Cuba from Spain, an offer that was rebuffed but one that did not discourage two privately financed expeditions of proslavery Americans from making forays into Cuba in an effort to seize the island by force on behalf of the United States. In 1854 the American ambassadors to Great Britain, France, and Spain met in Ostend, Belgium, and issued a statement declaring that, if Spain would not sell Cuba, the United States would be justified in taking control of the island. According to the Americans, the Monroe Doctrine gave license to the United States to rid the western Hemisphere of European colonial powers. Noting that two of the three ambassadors hailed from slave states, abolitionists charged that the Ostend Manifesto was just one more ploy to extend the power of slaveholders throughout the northern hemisphere.

In 1855 a young proslavery American adventurer, Tennessee-born William Walker, gathered a band of 58 mercenaries and managed to capture Granada, Nicaragua. Declaring himself president of Nicaragua, Walker encouraged the institution of slavery and won U.S. recognition for his regime in 1856. Walker was driven out of the country a year later, but his arrogance and bold move helped to set the stage for the Nicaraguan anti-American movement that would resurface in the twentieth century.

Political maneuvering and military might combined to advance the march of European Americans across the American continent, fueling popular notions of "manifest destiny," as if expansion were preordained by God and not furthered by rifles and bayonets. In 1853, Congress authorized the Gadsden Purchase, 30 million acres of land within the present-day states of New Mexico and Arizona. But, at least in a commercial sense, expansion failed to stop at the edge of the continental United States. Americans saw the Pacific Ocean as a trade route and East Asia as a trading partner. Commodore Matthew Perry commanded a fleet of U.S. Navy ships that steamed into Tokyo Harbor. The treaty Perry helped arrange with Japan in 1854 protected American whaling ships, sailors, and merchants in that part of the world and opened the door to an increase in trade later in the century.

By the mid-1850s the uniting of the continent into what would eventually become the 48 contiguous states was a source of sectional tension as well as national pride. Fewer and fewer Northerners supported what they considered proslavery charades, so-called legislative compromises. And the territory of Nebraska, poised on the brink of statehood, forced national lawmakers to confront again the political problem of the expansion of slavery. Once more Senator Douglas from Illinois stepped in to fill the breach left by the dying generation of great compromisers. Committed to the idea of a transcontinental railroad traversing the Nebraska Territory, Douglas adhered to the traditional (if increasingly unlikely) goal of mutual accommodation between North and South, free and slave states, but he believed that such accommodation demanded a constant process of negotiation and flexibility on both sides. Thus he argued that the gigantic territory be split into two new states, Kansas and Nebraska, whose respective voters would decide the issue of slavery for themselves. His proposal necessitated that part of the Missouri Compromise of 1820, the part that forbade slavery above the 36–30 line, would have to be repealed.

The Kansas–Nebraska Act became law in 1854. The Act enraged northern Free-Soilers, forced to watch the dismantling of the 1820 agreement. They became convinced that what they called the Slave Power Conspiracy would stop at nothing until slavery overran the entire nation. The measure also had a profound effect on the Plains Indians, for it deprived them of fully one-half the land they had been granted by treaty. Specifically, the act wrought havoc on the lives of Ponca, Pawnee, Arapahoe, and Cheyenne on the southern and central plains. European American settlers poured into the region, provoking Indian attacks. In September 1855, 600 American troops staged a retaliatory raid against an Indian village, Blue Water, in Nebraska, killing 85 Sioux and leading to an escalation in violence between Indians and settlers in the area. Among the young warriors involved in these battles was Crazy Horse, who became a famous leader of the Sioux in the coming years.

In their impatience with the two major parties, Free-Soilers were not alone in the early 1850s. The American party, founded in 1852, departed from the bland consensus embodied by the Whigs and Democrats and built its movement on nativism—the belief that Americans must rule America—in the North and South. The party explicitly condemned the growing political influence of immigrants, especially Roman Catholics. It derived its nickname, the Know-Nothings, from members' habit of claiming "I know nothing" when asked about their organization. With its ranks filled with former Whigs, the party tapped into a deep wellspring of resentment against immigrants on the part of urban, native-born workers as well as Protestant farmers anxious about retaining their influence in public affairs. Candidates for office who appealed to Irish voters ran the risk of incurring the Know-Nothing charge that Catholic priests were in league with "the worst class of American politicians, designing demagogues, selfish office-seekers, and bad men, calling themselves Democrats and 'Old Line Whigs'!" During the early 1850s, the Know-Nothings revealed that anxiety over immigration was not limited to northeastern cities; the loosely organized party was responsible for bloody clashes—native born against newcomer—in Baltimore, Louisville, St. Louis, and New Orleans.

The Republican Alliance

The rapid rise of the Know-Nothings further indicated that voters had grown disillusioned with the two-party system. Confirmation of that fact appeared on March 20, 1854, in the small town of Ripon, Wisconsin, when a group of disaffected Whigs created a new party called the Republicans. One core idea informed the party: that slavery must not be allowed to spread into the western territories. From this base the Republicans built an organization so powerful that it would capture the presidency within six years.

The genius of the Republican party resided in its ability to create and maintain an alliance between groups with vastly different goals. Now forced by the Fugitive Slave Act of 1850 to serve

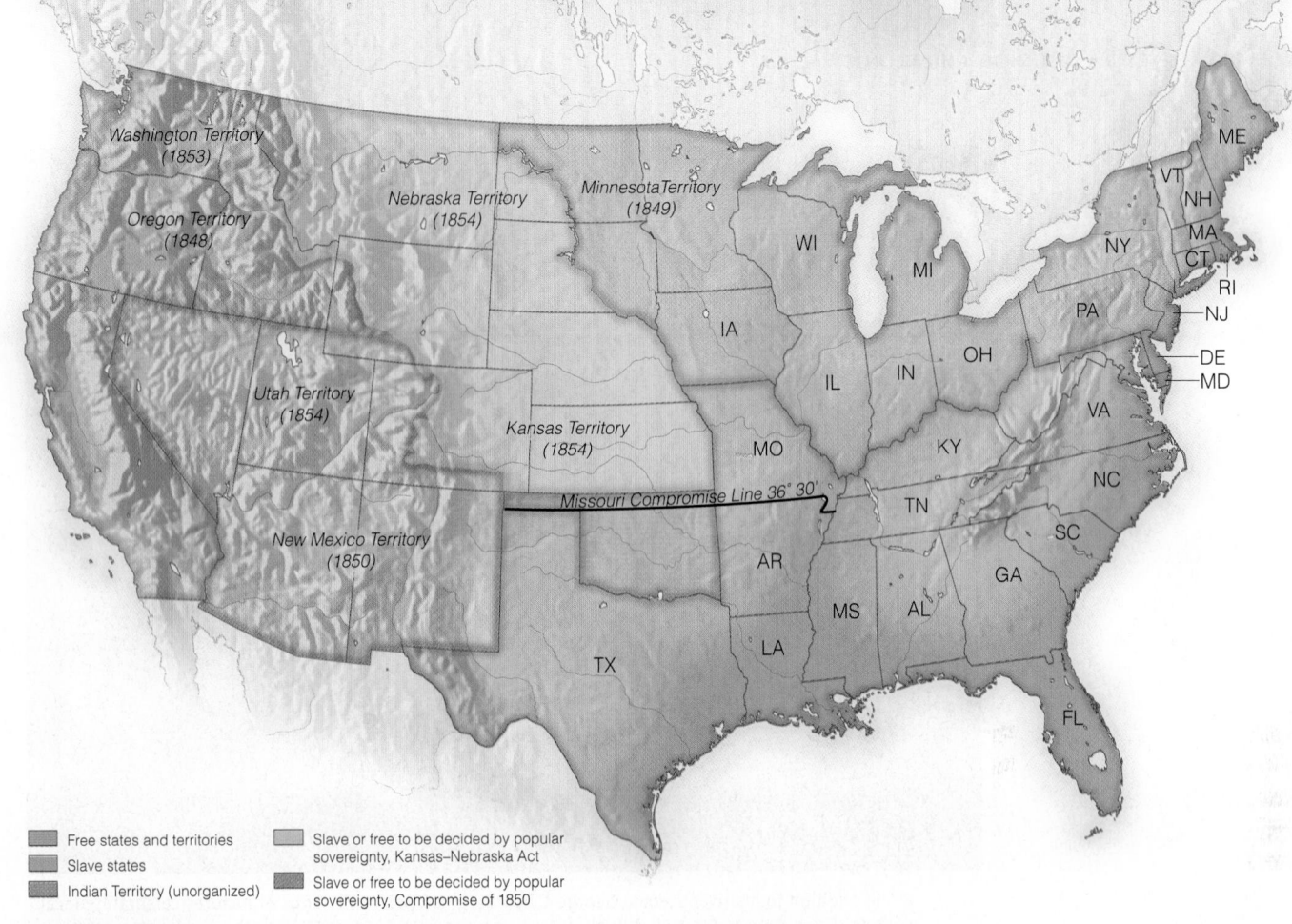

▮ Free states and territories	▮ Slave or free to be decided by popular sovereignty, Kansas–Nebraska Act
▮ Slave states	
▮ Indian Territory (unorganized)	▮ Slave or free to be decided by popular sovereignty, Compromise of 1850

■ MAP 13.2

THE KANSAS–NEBRASKA ACT, 1854 Stephen A. Douglas, senator from Illinois, proposed the Kansas–Nebraska Act of 1854. Douglas hoped to ensure that any transcontinental railroad route would run through Illinois and benefit his constituents. To secure southern support for the measure, proponents of the bill repealed the Missouri Compromise of 1850. As a result of the act, settlers displaced many Plains Indians from their lands. In the mid–1850s, the territory of Kansas became engulfed in an internal civil war that pitted supporters of slavery against abolitionists.

slaveholders (by returning runaway slaves to them) and fearful of the potential of slaveholding Southerners to capture their party, some northern Democrats cast their lot with the Republicans. From the ranks of antislavery men—the long-suffering adherents of the Liberty and Free-Soil parties—came another wing of the Republicans. These party members openly proclaimed their belief in the power of the federal government to halt the relentless march of slavery and ensure that, throughout the land, free soil would be tilled by free labor, free men and women.

Yet antislavery Republicans were by no means unified on major issues apart from the extension of slavery. Many Northerners were willing to tolerate slavery as long as it could be confined to the southern states; they cared little or nothing for the rights of black people, slave or free. And in fact, in the Midwest, Republicans saw no contradiction in calling for the end of slavery in one breath and for the end of black migration to the area in the next. Likewise, members of various northern white working classes feared the encroachment of slavery into the free states. These white men believed that, given the chance, black people would gladly abandon the South in favor of economic opportunities in the North. As job competitors, blacks would force whites to work for less money than they were accustomed to, or would push whites out of jobs altogether—at least those were the fears of white men who sought to block all blacks from moving north. For these reasons white Republicans could dislike slavery as an institution and at the same time approve of the discriminatory legislation that limited the economic and geographical mobility of black people.

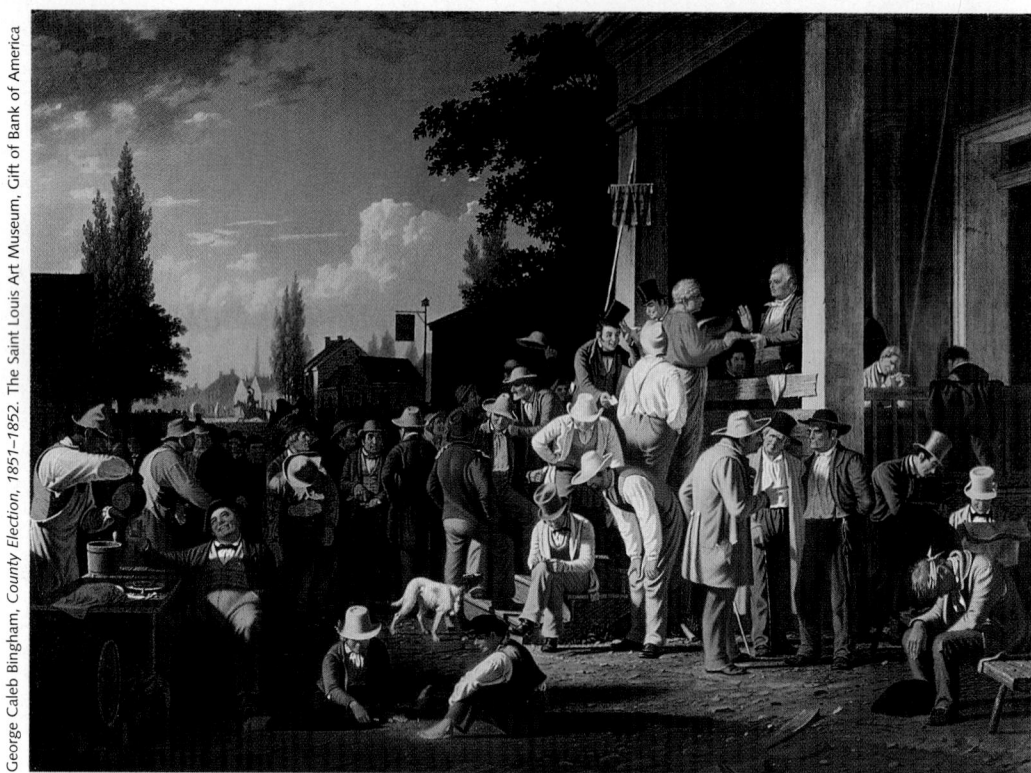

George Caleb Bingham, *County Election*, 1851–1852. The Saint Louis Art Museum, Gift of Bank of America

■ In addition to his river scenes, George Caleb Bingham painted a series of pictures celebrating local politics. Titled *County Election,* this piece was completed in 1851–1852. Bingham had lost a campaign to become a congressional representative from Missouri in 1846. This scene suggests that election day is an opportunity for the men of the county to come together and eat and drink, swap information, and close deals.

Many northern merchants supported the Republicans' claims for the power of the federal government above that of the states. Still, some of the wealthiest and most influential in the cities of Philadelphia and New York maintained overtly racist views and retained cultural ties with southern slaveholders. Juxtaposed to these groups of whites were northern blacks, like those in Boston who in 1856 offered only limited support for the new party: "We do not pledge ourselves to go further with the Republicans than the Republicans will go with us," they vowed.

From the ranks of the newly formed Illinois state Republican party emerged a formidable leader capable of bringing all of these factions together. Born in 1809 in Kentucky, Abraham Lincoln came from a modest background and followed a checkered path into Illinois Whig politics: from youthful plowhand and log-splitter, to local postmaster and county surveyor, and finally self-taught lawyer and member of the state legislature (1834–1842). Although his 6-foot 4-inch frame and humble background drew ridicule from wealthy people—a Philadelphia lawyer described him as "a tall rawly boned, ungainly back woodsman, with coarse, ill-fitting clothing"—Lincoln made good use of his oratorical gifts and political ambition in promoting the principles of free soil.

The presidential election of 1856 revealed the full dimension of the national political crisis. The Democrats nominated James Buchanan, a "dough-face" (i.e., proslavery Northerner) from Pennsylvania, with John Breckinridge of Tennessee as his running mate. In their platform they took pains to extol the virtue of sectional compromise on the slavery issue, by this time a very unpopular position. Meanwhile, the enfeebled Whigs could do little but stand by helplessly and declare as their "fundamental article of political faith, an absolute necessity for avoiding geographical parties," another plank decidedly out of favor with a growing number of voters. The Know-Nothings cast their lot with former President Millard Fillmore. They offered voters little more than the ringing declaration that only "*native*-born citizens should be selected for all state, federal, and municipal offices of government employment, in preference to all others."

Drawing on former members of the Free-Soil and Whig parties, respectively, the Republicans nominated John C. Frémont of California for president and William Dayton of New Jer-

TABLE 13-4

The Election of 1856

Candidate	Political Party	Popular Vote	Electoral Vote
James Buchanan	Democratic	1,832,955	174
John C. Frémont	Republican	1,339,932	114
Millard Fillmore	American	871,731	8

sey for vice president. Their platform stated in no uncertain terms the party's opposition to the extension of slavery, as well as Republican support for a transcontinental railroad and other federally sponsored internal improvements such as rivers and harbors. The document also included the bold, noble rhetoric—in favor of "the blessings of liberty" and against "tyrannical and unconstitutional laws"—that would be the hallmark of the Republican party in the decade to come.

Despite his nickname "Old Fogy," Democratic candidate James Buchanan won the election. Nevertheless, the fact that the Republican Frémont carried 11 of the 16 northern states boded well for the Republican party and ill for the slaveholders' union. In Illinois, Frémont had benefited from the tireless campaigning of Abraham Lincoln, who electrified ever-growing crowds of people with the declaration that "the Union must be preserved in the purity of its principles as well as in the integrity of its territorial parts."

The Deepening Conflict over Slavery

Only a small subset of Americans—adult white men—participated directly in the formation of new political parties that set the terms for congressional debates over territorial expansion and slavery. Nevertheless, during the 1850s, increasing numbers of ordinary people were drawn into the escalating conflict over the South's "peculiar institution" as some Northerners mounted concerted challenges, violent as well as peaceful, to the Fugitive Slave Law. The western territory of Kansas became a bloody battleground as abolitionists and proslavery forces fought for control of the new state government.

Sites of struggle over the slavery issue included the streets of Boston, the Supreme Court of the United States, political rallies in Illinois, and a federal arsenal in Harpers Ferry, Virginia. No longer would the opposing sides confine their disagreements to congressional debates over the admission of new states. Nor would words be the only weapons. The country was rushing headlong into nationwide armed conflict.

The Rising Tide of Violence

The Fugitive Slave Law of 1850 caused fear and alarm among many Northerners. In response to the measure, some African Americans, hiding in northern cities, fled to Canada, often with the aid of conductors on the Underground Railroad. In the summer of 1854 the National Emigration Convention of Colored Peoples drew more than 100 black leaders to Cleveland, where they debated the merits of migration to Canada, the West Indies, Central and South America, or Liberia in Africa.

Abolitionists, white and black, made dramatic rescue attempts on behalf of men and women sought by their self-proclaimed southern owners. In Boston in 1851, a waiter named Shadrach Minkins (he called himself Frederick Jenkins) was seized at work and charged with running away from a Virginia slaveholder. During a court hearing to determine the merits of the case, a group of blacks stormed in, disarmed the startled authorities, and, in the words of a sympathetic observer, "with a dexterity worthy of the Roman gladiators, snatched the trembling prey of the slavehunters, and conveyed him in triumph to the streets of Boston." Shadrach Minkins found safety in Montreal, Canada, and a Boston jury refused to convict his lawyers, who had been accused of masterminding his escape. The spectacular public rescue of Minkins, and other such attempts, both successful and unsuccessful, throughout the North, brought the issue of slavery into the realm of public performance in northern towns and cities.

In Cincinnati, Ohio, a group of African American men met to press demands for equal rights and to declare that "we sympathize deeply with the man *Shadrach* of Boston, who fled from the American Fiery Furnace, to its contrast—the snows of Canada." Throughout the North, African American conventions responded to the slavecatchers' provocation, providing a forum not only for leaders such as Frederick Douglass of New York and John M. Langston of Ohio but also for barbers, farmers, and other workers.

Black women remained conspicuous for their absence from these formal conventions. Delegates to the meeting in Troy, New York, in 1855 cast out the lone woman in attendance, Barbery Anna Stewart; several men objected to her presence "on the ground that this is not a Woman's Rights Convention." Nevertheless, black and white women working together became prominent supporters of the abolitionist cause. Though unable to vote, they made public speeches and petitioned politicians, and they coordinated local boycotts of products made by slave labor.

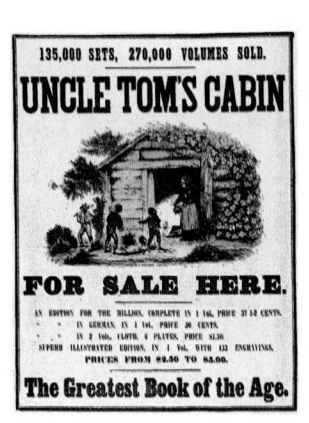

Gradually, the war of words over slavery cascaded out of small-circulation abolitionist periodicals and into the consciousness of a nation. In particular, author Harriet Beecher Stowe managed to wed politics and sentiment in a most compelling way. Her novel *Uncle Tom's Cabin* (1852) sold more than 300,000 copies within 10 months and a million copies over the next seven years. The book, originally serialized in a magazine, *The National Era*, introduced large numbers of Northerners to the sufferings of an enslaved couple, Eliza and George. Slavery's greatest crime, in Stowe's eyes, was the forced severance of family ties between husbands and wives, parents and children.

Southern slaveholders were outraged at Stowe's attempt to portray their way of life as an unmitigated evil; a South Carolina slave-holding woman, Louisa McCord, wrote "We proclaim it [slavery], on the contrary, a Godlike dispensation, a providential caring for the weak, and a refuge for the portionless." Another Southerner, George Fitzhugh, took this argument to its logical conclusion. In his book *Cannibals All! Or, Slaves Without Masters* (1857), Fitzhugh claimed that civil society demanded the enslavement of the masses, whether white or black: "Some were born with saddles on their backs, and others booted and spurred to ride them—and the riding does them good." Fitzhugh also argued that slaves, whom he claimed were cared for by benevolent planters, were better off than northern factory workers, whom he asserted were exploited and neglected by indifferent employers.

A roving reporter for the *New York Times*, Frederick Law Olmsted, expressed in journalistic terms what Stowe had described in her novel: cruel aristocrats lording over plantations operated by degraded slaves and non-slaveholding whites mired in sloth, ignorance, and poverty. Olmsted seemed most concerned about effects of slavery on whites; in one of his dispatches he quoted a Louisiana planter, who believed that the institution's "influence on the character of the whites was what was most deplorable." Thus in the 1850s the issue of slavery became a staple of both mainstream periodicals and the best-seller list. Few people could ignore the controversy.

As increasing numbers of Americans read the starkly drawn images of the South produced by northern printing presses, the territory of Kansas was becoming engulfed in a regional civil war. Proslavery settlers, aided and abetted by their compatriots (called Border Ruffians) from Missouri, installed their own territorial government at Shawnee Mission in 1855. Opposing these proslavery settlers were the Free-Soilers, some of whom had organized into abolitionist groups, such as the New England Emigrant Aid Company, and armed themselves with rifles. Antislavery groups called the guns Beecher's Bibles, after Brooklyn's Reverend Henry Ward Beecher, Harriet Beecher Stowe's brother and a fundraiser for abolitionist forces in Kansas.

Systems of Unfree Labor

The controversy over slavery ultimately precipitated the Civil War, the bloodiest conflict in the nation's history. Yet the abolition of slavery (with the ratification of the Thirteenth Amendment in 1865) did not eradicate forms of coerced labor. Indeed, systems of unfree labor—in which individuals are forced to work without compensation and for the benefit of someone else—have characterized the whole sweep of American history.

In the seventeenth century, most tobacco field workers in the Chesapeake region were indentured servants. These young men and women received passage from Europe to the colonies. In return, they bound themselves to a master for a stipulated amount of time (usually seven years). Apprentices, children and young people, labored for a master artisan until they reached age 21.

Beginning in the late seventeenth century, the institution of slavery spread throughout the colonies. This system, which depended on the labor of Africans and their descendants, differed in crucial ways from indentured servitude and apprenticeship. Slaves remained slaves for life, and they had no rights under law. Children took the status of their enslaved mother.

States outside the South had emancipated their slaves by the mid-nineteenth century. However, forms of bound labor persisted. In some Mid-Atlantic and New England small towns, local officials sold the labor of impoverished men, women, and children to the highest bidder, thereby relieving taxpayers of the expense of supporting them. Poor people confined to workhouses were forced to toil at many different kinds of jobs,

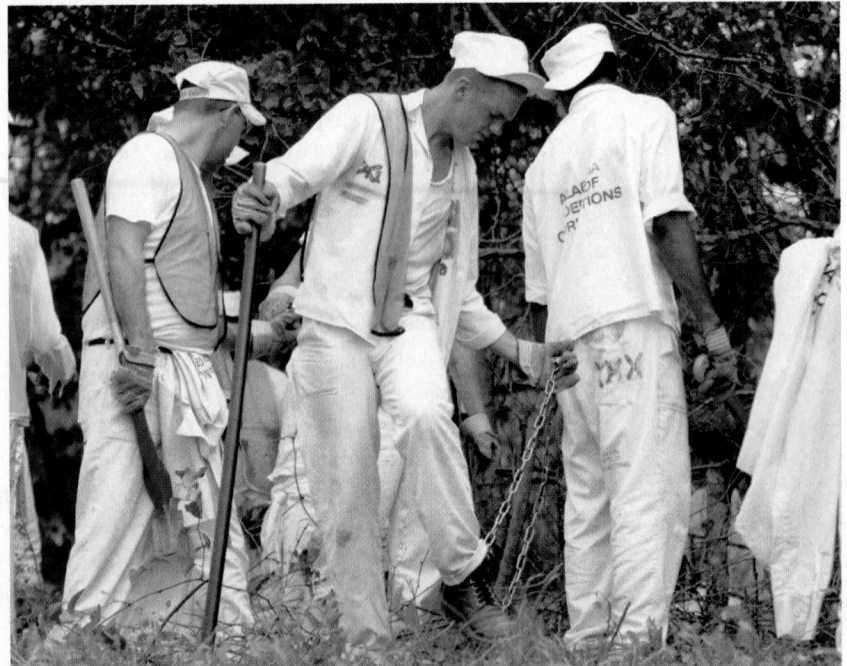

Shackled inmates work to clear brush along a highway near Prattville, Alabama. A 1996 settlement prevented the state from shackling inmates together on a "chain gang," but shackling of individual convict laborers was still permissible.

such as growing crops, spinning thread, weaving cloth, and producing handicrafts. In some cases, ship captains kidnapped sailors and forced them to work for no pay on long voyages. Indian and African American children remained at risk as labor-hungry whites forcibly "apprenticed" them with the aid of the courts.

By the late nineteenth century, peonage characterized the southern staple crop economy as well as the rural extractive sector (logging, sawmills, turpentine production, and mining). Held against their will, sharecroppers and railroad workers alike labored in isolated rural areas where law enforcement agents were few and far between. The outlawing of peonage in 1911 failed to end this practice.

The southern states also pioneered in the use of convict labor, a means of channeling petty criminals (and random, innocent young African American

men) into the rough and dangerous work of building roads through swamps and digging coal out of the earth. Convict labor officials often demonstrated a reckless disregard for human life. Unlike slave owners, prison officials and the private individuals who leased convicts had few incentives to treat these workers in a humane way.

In the early twenty-first century, coerced labor persists. Some illegal immigrants continue to indenture themselves to smugglers and remain indebted to these smugglers for many years. Prisoners perform a variety of tasks for private companies, including entering data into computers and taking hotel reservations by phone. American labor unions publicize the fact that some products consumed in this country have been manufactured by unfree workers abroad, such as prisoners in China and child laborers in Pakistan and Vietnam. ■

AP/Wide World Photos

This dangerous situation soon gave way to terrorism and insurrection on both sides. In 1855, in retaliation for a proslavery raid on the "Free-Soil" town of Lawrence, Kansas, an Ohio abolitionist named John Brown, together with his four sons and two other men, hacked to death five proslavery men at Pottowatamie Creek. The massacre only strengthened the resolve of proslavery advocates, who in the next year drew up a constitution for Kansas, which effectively nullified the principle of popular sovereignty over the issue of slavery. Called the Lecompton Constitution, the document decreed that voters might approve or reject slavery, but even if they chose to reject it, any slaves already in the state would remain slaves under the force of law. By throwing his support behind the Lecompton Constitution, President Buchanan alienated northern members of his own party, and the Democrats descended into north–south factionalism.

The spilling of blood over slavery was not confined to the Kansas frontier. In 1856 Senator Charles Sumner of Massachusetts, an outspoken abolitionist, delivered a speech on the floor of the United States Senate condemning "The Crime Against Kansas" (the Lecompton Constitution) and the men who perpetrated it, men he characterized as "hirelings picked from the drunken spew and vomit of an uneasy civilization," men who (like his own colleague Senator Butler of South Carolina) loved slavery the way that degenerates loved their prostitutes. Shortly after this speech, Congressman Preston S. Brooks of South Carolina, a relative of Senator Butler, leapt to the defense of the white South and attacked Sumner on the floor of the Senate, beating him into unconsciousness with a cane. This was "southern chivalry" and "southern honor," fumed an outraged northern press: a defenseless man beaten almost to death by a bully armed with a club. Soon, "Bleeding Kansas" became a rallying cry for abolitionists everywhere. They contemplated the necessity of defending themselves and their interests in the courtrooms of New England and the small towns of the West no less than in Congress.

The *Dred Scott* Decision

Across the street from the Capitol, proceedings in the Supreme Court were more civil but no less explosive. In 1857 a former slave named Dred Scott sued in federal court, claiming that he was a citizen of Missouri and a free man. Scott maintained that he had become free once his master had taken him onto free soil (the state of Illinois and the territory of Wisconsin). In the case of *Dred Scott v. Sanford* (1857), the court ruled that even residence on free soil did not render a slave a free person, for, regardless of their status, black people had "no rights which the white man was bound to respect." With this single decision, then, Chief Justice Roger B. Taney and the Court threw off the hard-won balance between slave and free states. In effect, the Court declared unconstitutional the Compromise of 1820, which had banned slavery in the region north of Missouri's southern boundary, because, the justices held, slave owners could not be deprived of their property without due process. This decision threatened the precarious freedom of the South's quarter million free people of color and extended the reach of slavery into the northern states.

Most white people residing outside the South never read the Court's ruling, but if they had, they probably would have agreed with the justices' claim that, since the earliest days of the Republic, blacks "had been regarded as beings of an inferior order, and altogether unfit to associate with the white race, either in social or political relations." At the same time, northern opinion makers warned that the decision made Northerners complicit in the slave system. Of the "slave power," the *Cincinnati Daily Commercial* thundered, "It has marched over and annihilated the boundaries of the states. We are now one great homogeneous slaveholding community." Convening in Philadelphia, black leaders expressed the hope that white Northerners would condemn the Scott decision and "make common cause with us . . . and striking for impartial liberty, they will join with us in our efforts to recover the long lost boon of freedom."

Even nonabolitionists had good reason to fear the long-term implications of the ruling, for it suggested that the institution of slavery was about to spill out of the confines of the southern states and into the rest of the country. Free white men and women feared competing with slaves in the workplace, whether in the West or East. In 1857 a depression hit the northeastern and midwestern states, as the discovery of California gold produced inflation in the East.

Businesses failed and debtors had a difficult time repaying their creditors. In New England, shoemakers responded to these economic pressures, and to the labor-saving machinery installed by their employers, by banding together and forming a union. Members of the new organization, called the Knights of St. Crispin, believed their future looked bleak. They reasoned that they would not be able to seek new economic opportunities out West if that part of the country were dominated by southern planters and cheap slave labor. Like other members of the northern laboring classes, the shoemakers also feared a mass migration of blacks out of the South and into the North. As a result, national unions such as the ones formed by bookbinders and printers in 1850 began to take precautionary measures by barring free people of color from apprenticeship positions and from certain workplaces altogether.

The Lincoln–Douglas Debates

Against this backdrop of economic turmoil and political conflict, the congressional elections of 1858 assumed great significance. In particular, the Senate contest in Illinois pitted

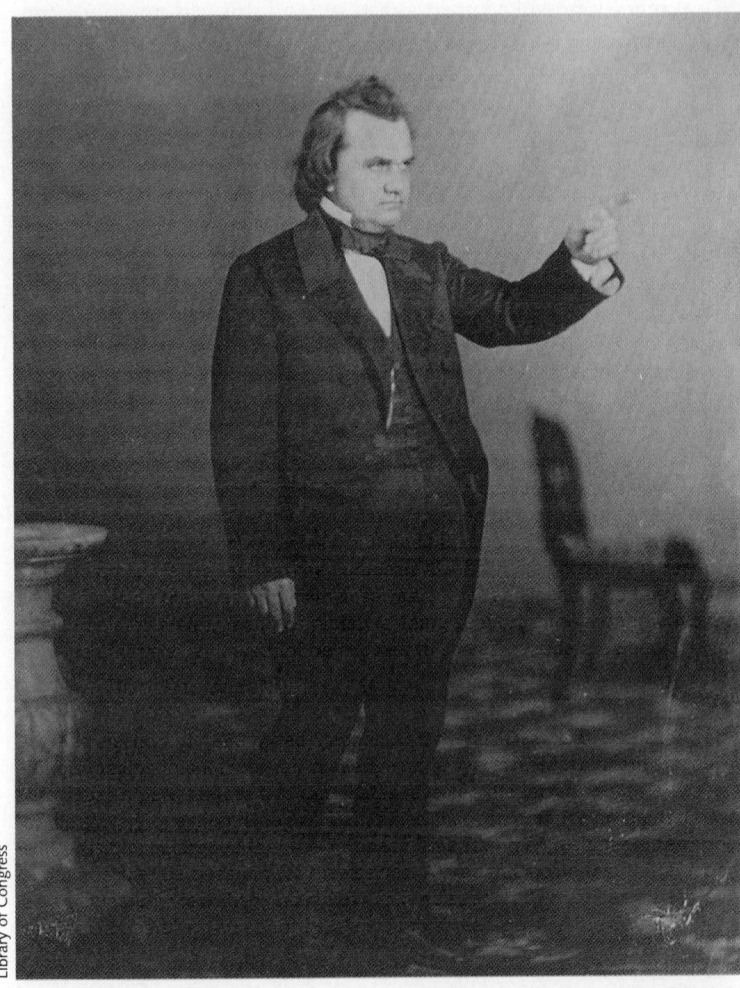
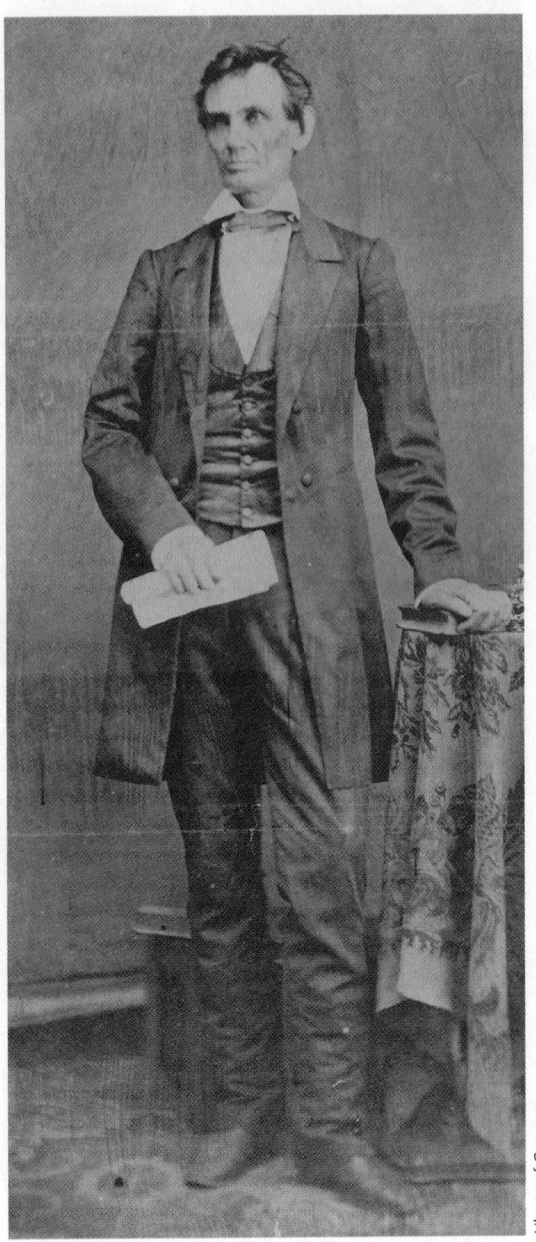

■ The election of 1858 pitted Stephen A. Douglas, Democratic senator from Illinois, against his Republican challenger, a lawyer named Abraham Lincoln. The debates between the two candidates revealed the increasing divisiveness of the slavery question. Douglas maintained that compromise on the issue was still possible; he argued that the European American men residing in territories should decide the question for themselves. Although Lincoln lost this election, he articulated a view that was rapidly gaining support throughout the North: the idea that slavery must not be allowed to spread outside the South.

incumbent Stephen A. Douglas against challenger Abraham Lincoln. In a series of seven public debates, the two men debated the political conflict over slavery as it had been shaped during the tumultuous decade after the Mexican War. Though no friend of the abolitionists, Douglas was quickly falling from favor within the Democratic party; the Supreme Court had nullified his proposal for popular sovereignty in the territories, and he had parted ways from his southern brethren when he denounced Kansas's Lecompton Constitution. Yet in the last debate between Lincoln and Douglas, held in Alton on October 15, 1858, Douglas declared, "I care more for the great principle of self-government, the right of the people to rule, than I do for all the negroes in Christendom."

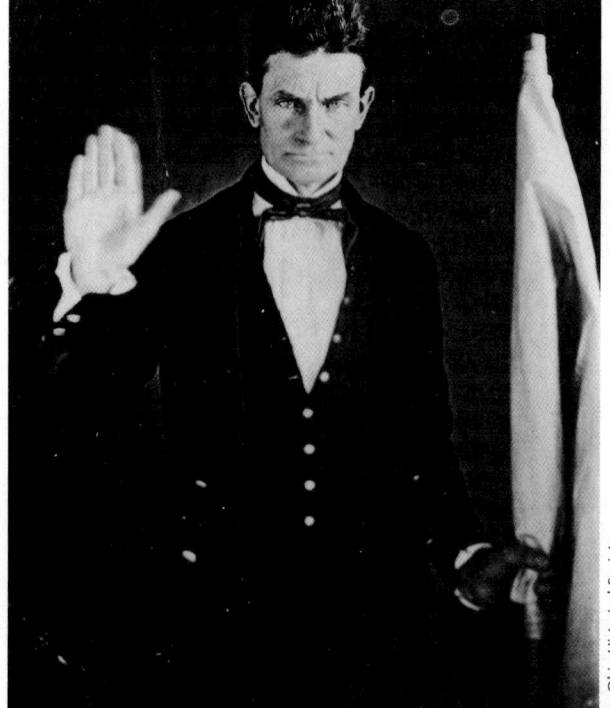

■ Augustus Washington, son of a former slave, took this picture of John Brown in 1846, 13 years before the raid on Harpers Ferry, Virginia. A pioneer daguerreotypist, Washington operated a successful studio in Hartford, Connecticut. After the passage of the Fugitive Slave Law in 1850, Washington emigrated with his family to Liberia, an African settlement for American freeborn blacks and former slaves, founded as a republic in 1847.

The Ohio Historical Society

Lincoln ridiculed the doctrine of popular sovereignty, which he maintained was as thin as the "soup that was made by boiling the shadow of a pigeon that had starved to death." He had no desire to root out slavery in the South, but, "I have said, and I repeat, my wish is that the further spread of [slavery] may be arrested, and that it may be placed where the public mind shall rest in the belief that it is in the course of ultimate extinction." According to a reporter present, this last remark provoked great applause. And this was no minor confrontation between two candidates; it is estimated that in six of the seven debates the two men spoke before crowds exceeding 10,000 people each. Lincoln lost the election (in which blacks were not allowed to vote as a matter of Illinois law), but, more significantly, he won the loyalty of Republicans all over the North and put the white South on notice that the days of compromise were over. Meanwhile, with the admission as free states of Minnesota in 1858 and Oregon in 1859, Congress began to reflect a distinct antislavery bias.

Harpers Ferry and the Presidential Election of 1860

On a Sunday night in October 1859, John Brown and 19 other men (including at least five African Americans) launched a daring attack on the federal arsenal in Harpers Ferry, Virginia. They had received guns and moral support from some of the North's leading abolitionists, and their plan was to raid the arsenal and distribute firearms to slaves in the surrounding area, thereby inciting a general rebellion that, they hoped, would engulf the rest of the South. The Virginia militia cornered Brown and his men, but not before the insurrectionist had killed seven people (including a free man of color) and injured ten others. Within two days a U.S. Marine force, commanded by Lieutenant Colonel Robert E. Lee, had captured Brown and his surviving followers.

Two weeks later Brown stood in a Virginia courtroom and declared that his intention indeed had been "to free the slaves." Brown was convicted of several charges: treason against the United States for his raid on the federal arsenal, murder, and inciting an insurrection. On December 2, 1859, before being led to the gallows, Brown handed a scrap of paper to one of his guards: "I John Brown am now quite *certain* that the crimes of this *guilty land: will* never be purged *away:* but with Blood." Brown failed as the instigator of a slave rebellion, but he succeeded as a prophet.

The raid on Harpers Ferry cast a shadow over the party conventions held in the summer of 1860. By then it was apparent that the national party system had all but disintegrated. Southerners in effect seceded from the Democratic party by walking out of their Charleston convention rather than supporting Stephen Douglas as candidate for president. Within a few weeks, representatives of both the northern and the southern wings of the party reconvened in separate conventions in Baltimore; Northerners gave the nod to Douglas and Southerners chose as their standard-bearer John C. Breckinridge, a proponent of extending slavery into the territories and annexing Cuba. Representing the thoroughly discredited strategy of compromise was the candidate of the Constitutional Union party, John Bell of Tennessee.

TABLE 13-5

The Election of 1860

Candidate	Political Party	Popular Vote	Electoral Vote
Abraham Lincoln	Republican	1,865,593	180
Stephen A. Douglas	Democratic	1,382,713	12
John C. Breckinridge	Democratic	848,356	72
John Bell	Constitutional Union	592,906	39

In Chicago, the Republicans lined up behind the moderate Abraham Lincoln and agreed on a platform that had something for everybody, including measures to boost economic growth (as promoted by Henry Clay's American System earlier in the century): a proposed protective tariff, a transcontinental railroad, internal improvements, and free homesteads for western farmers. The Republicans renounced the Know-Nothings. Lincoln himself had taken the lead in admonishing Republicans who sought to curtail the voting rights of European immigrants, such as the Germans and Scandinavians. Lecturing members of his own

TABLE 13-6

U.S. Population, by Nativity and Race, for Regions, 1830–1860

Year	Total	White Total	White Native	White Foreign Born	Negro Total	Negro Slave	Other Races
Northeast							
1860	10,594,268	10,438,028	8,419,243	2,018,785	156,001	18	239
1850	8,626,851	8,477,089	7,153,512	1,323,577	149,762	236	----
1840	6,761,082	6,618,758	----	----	142,324	765	----
1830	5,542,381	5,417,167	----	----	125,214	2,780	----
Midwest							
1860	9,096,716	8,899,969	7,357,376	1,542,593	184,239	114,948	12,508
1850	5,403,595	5,267,988	4,617,913	650,075	135,607	87,422	----
1840	3,351,542	3,262,195	----	----	89,347	58,604	----
1830	1,610,473	1,568,930	----	----	41,543	25,879	----
South							
1860	11,133,861	7,033,973	6,642,201	391,772	4,097,111	3,838,765	2,277
1850	8,982,612	5,630,414	5,390,314	240,100	3,352,198	3,116,629	----
1840	6,950,729	4,308,752	----	----	2,641,977	2,427,986	----
1830	5,707,848	3,545,963	----	----	2,161,885	1,980,384	----
West							
1860	618,976	550,567	406,964	143,603	4,479	29	63,930
1850	178,818	177,577	150,794	26,783	1,241	26	----
1840	----	----	----	----	----	----	----
1830	----	----	----	----	----	----	----

Source: Historical Statistics of the United States from Colonial Times to 1957 (Washington, D.C.: U.S. Department of Commerce, 1960) pp. 11–12.

party in Massachusetts, he declared, "I have some little notoriety for commiserating the oppressed condition of the negro, and I should be strangely inconsistent if I could favor any project for curtailing the existing rights of white men, even though born in different lands, and speaking different languages from myself."

Yet Republicans held out little hope for other groups demanding the rights and protection that flowed from American citizenship. Spanish-speaking residents of California, Chinese immigrants, free people of color throughout the North, Indian tribes from North Carolina to the northwestern states, the wives and daughters of men all over the country—these groups were not included in the Republicans' grand design for a country based on the principles of free labor.

Abraham Lincoln was elected president in 1860, although he received support from only 40 percent of the men who cast ballots. Lincoln won the Electoral College, and he also received a majority of votes. However, ten southern states had refused to list him on the ballot; in that region of the country he received almost no votes. Stephen Douglas won almost 30 percent of the popular vote; together, Douglas and Breckenridge outpolled Lincoln (2.2 million votes to 1.85 million). Nevertheless, the new president had swept New England, New York, Pennsylvania, and the upper Midwest. Regional (northern and southern) interests took precedence over national political parties.

Lincoln and his party represented the antislavery sentiments of northern family farmers. The South took heed of this dramatic shift in the national political landscape. By the end of 1860 South Carolina had seceded from the Union, and the nation headed toward war.

Conclusion

During the 1850s, Americans on both sides of the slavery issue began to voice their opinions, and their frustrations, in ever more dramatic ways. Ultimately, these deep feelings led to war. People all over the country came to feel that the debate over slavery had relevance to their lives. In the slave states, black workers remained yoked to a system that denied their humanity and mocked the integrity of their families. In the nonslave states, free people of color understood that northern racial prejudice was but a variation of the slaveholders' theme of domination. New England farm families looking to move west were convinced that western homesteads would not improve their economic security if these homesteads were surrounded by plantations cultivated by large numbers of enslaved workers. Although they expressed little regard for the rights of blacks, enslaved or free, the northern laboring classes feared that the expansion of slavery into the western territories would limit their own economic opportunities; whether shoemakers, wagon drivers, or seamstresses, they could not possibly compete with bound workers in the labor market. The Republicans drew inspiration from the anxieties of all these groups, and the party's platform beckoned toward a future full of hope, a future that would fulfill the long-thwarted promise of the young country as a "republic of equal rights, where the title of manhood is the title to citizenship."

In contrast, southern whites of various classes agreed on a rallying cry that stressed independence from Yankee interlopers and freedom from federal interference. Yet this uni-

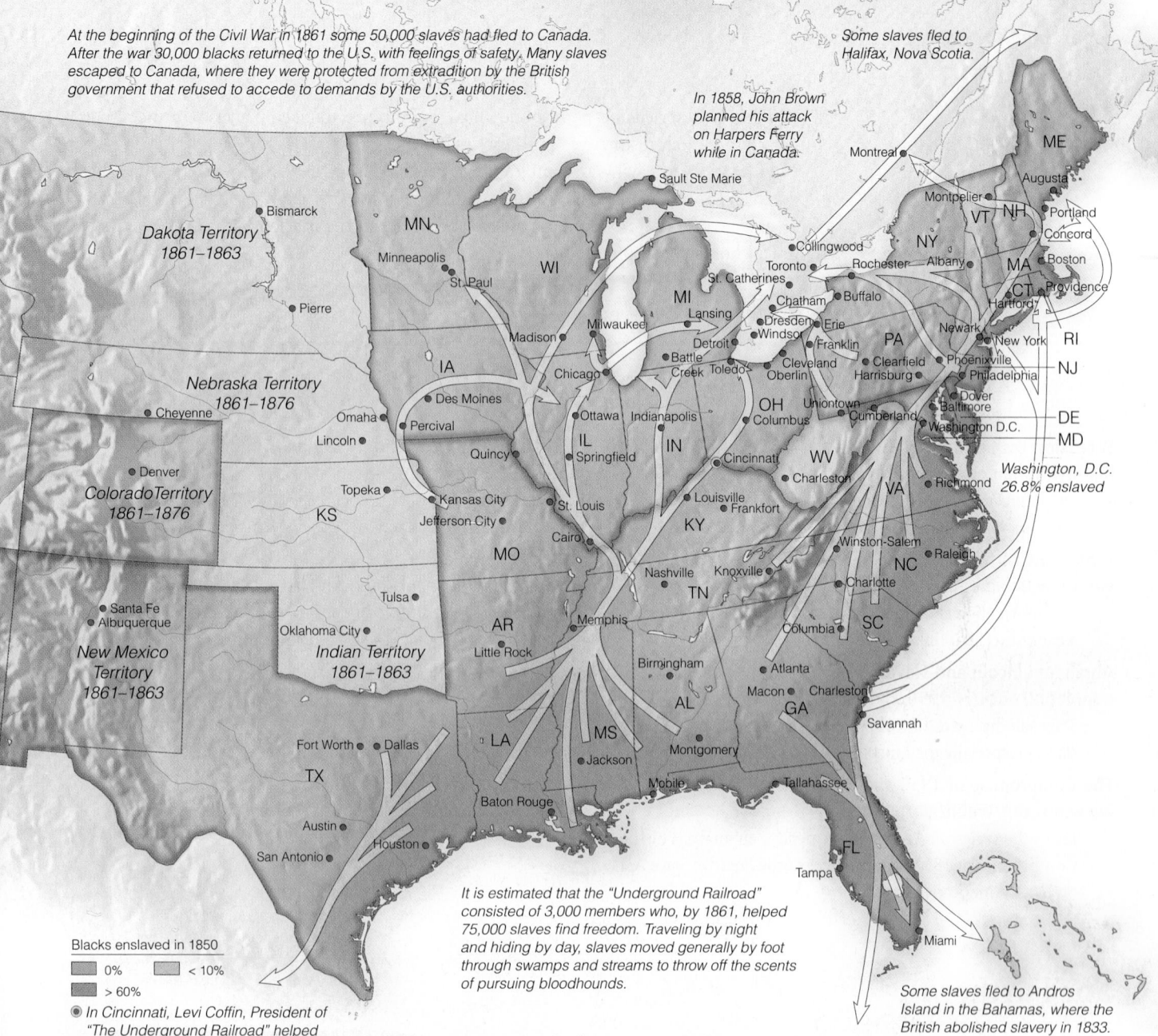

At the beginning of the Civil War in 1861 some 50,000 slaves had fled to Canada. After the war 30,000 blacks returned to the U.S. with feelings of safety. Many slaves escaped to Canada, where they were protected from extradition by the British government that refused to accede to demands by the U.S. authorities.

Some slaves fled to Halifax, Nova Scotia.

In 1858, John Brown planned his attack on Harpers Ferry while in Canada.

Washington, D.C. 26.8% enslaved

It is estimated that the "Underground Railroad" consisted of 3,000 members who, by 1861, helped 75,000 slaves find freedom. Traveling by night and hiding by day, slaves moved generally by foot through swamps and streams to throw off the scents of pursuing bloodhounds.

Some slaves fled to Andros Island in the Bahamas, where the British abolished slavery in 1833.

Blacks enslaved in 1850
- 0%
- < 10%
- > 60%

In Cincinnati, Levi Coffin, President of "The Underground Railroad" helped more than 300 slaves escape.

■ **MAP 13.3**

THE UNDERGROUND RAILROAD   The Underground Railroad consisted of a network of people who helped fugitives in their escape from slavery en route to the North or Canada. An escaped slave named Harriet Tubman made an estimated 19 separate trips south to help an estimated 300 slaves escape to freedom. Like Tubman, most "conductors" on the Underground Railroad were blacks, many of them free men and women living in the North.

fying rhetoric carried different meanings for different groups of southerners. The owners of large plantations were desperate to preserve their enslaved labor forces, and also hungry for fresh lands and renewed political power; these men scrambled to maintain their own privileges in the face of growing northern influence in Congress. Nonslaveholding farmers sought to produce all household necessities themselves and remain independent of the worldwide cotton market economy so crucial to the wealth of slave masters and mistresses. Yet almost all southern whites, rich and poor, stood allied, determined to take up arms to protect their households and their distinctive "southern way of life."

On the eve of the Civil War, complex forces roiled an ethnically diverse society. Ultimately the North and South marched into combat, each side united enough to mobilize huge armies. However, wartime strains would expose the fault lines in the free labor coalition as well as in the slaveholders' republic.

Sites to Visit

Secession Era Editorial Project

history.furman.edu/~benson/docs/

Furman University is digitizing editorials about the secession crisis and already includes scores of them on this site.

John Brown trial links

www.law.umkc/edu/faculty/projecs/ftrials/Brown.html

For information about the John Brown trial, this site provides a list of excellent links.

Abraham Lincoln and Slavery

odur.let.nl/~usa/H/1990/ch5_p6.html

This site discusses Lincoln's views and actions concerning slavery, especially the Lincoln–Douglas debate.

The Compromise of 1850 and the Fugitive Slave Act

www.pbs.org/wgbh/aia/part4

From the series on Africans in America, an analysis of the Compromise of 1850 and the effect of the Fugitive Slave Act on black Americans.

The 1850s: An Increasingly Divided Union

nac.gmu/mmts/50proto.html

A tutorial skill development site of the Multi-Media Thinking Skills project that focuses on events in the 1850s leading to the Civil War.

Words and Deeds in American History

leweb2.loc.gov/ammem/mcchtml/corhome.html

A Library of Congress site containing links to Frederick Douglass; the Compromise of 1850; speeches by John C. Calhoun, Daniel Webster, and Henry Clay; and other topics from the Civil War era.

Harriet Beecher Stowe and Uncle Tom's Cabin

xroads.virginia.edu/~HYPER/STOWE/stowe.html

This site provides both text and descriptions of Stowe's important books and information about the author's life.

For Further Reading

General Works

Eric Foner, *Free Labor, Free Soil, Free Men: The Ideology of the Republican Party Before the Civil War* (1970).

William W. Freehling, *The Road to Disunion* (1990).

Robert V. Hine and John Mack Faragher, *The American West: A New Interpretive History* (2000).

James Oliver Horton and Lois E. Horton, *In Hope of Liberty: Culture, Community and Protest Among Northern Free Blacks, 1700–1860* (1997).

Nancy Isenberg, *Sex and Citizenship in Antebellum America* (1998).

Regional Economies and Conflicts

Joan Cashin, *A Family Venture: Men and Women on the Southern Frontier* (1991).

Christopher Clark, *The Roots of Rural Capitalism: Western Massachusetts, 1780–1860* (1990).

Steven Hahn, *The Roots of Southern Populism: Yeoman Farmers and the Transformation of the Georgia Upcountry, 1850–1890* (1983).

Albert Hurtado, *Indian Survival on the California Frontier* (1988).

Susan Lee Johnson, *Roaring Camp: The Social World of the California Gold Rush* (2000).

John D. Majewski, *A House Dividing: Economic Development in Pennsylvania and Virginia Before the Civil War* (2000).

David Montejano, *Anglos and Mexicans in the Making of Texas, 1836–1986* (1987).

Shifting Collective Identities

Tomás Almaguer, *Racial Faultlines: The Historical Origins of White Supremacy in California* (1994).

Bonnie S. Anderson, *Joyous Greetings: The First International Women's Movement, 1830–1860* (2000).

Mary H. Blewett, *Men, Women, and Work: Class, Gender, and Protest in the New England Shoe Industry, 1780–1910* (1988).

Yong Chen, *Chinese San Francisco, 1850–1943: A Trans-Pacific Community* (2000).

Frances Levine, *Our Prayers Are in This Place: Pecos Pueblo Identity over the Centuries* (1999).

David Roediger, *The Wages of Whiteness: Race and the Making of the American Working Class* (1991).

The Paradox of Southern Political Power

Avery O. Craven, *The Growth of Southern Nationalism, 1848–1861* (1953).

Lacy K. Ford, *Origins of Southern Radicalism: The South Carolina Upcountry, 1800–1860* (1988).

Robert E. May, *The Southern Dream of a Caribbean Empire, 1854–1861* (1973).

Stephanie McCurry, *Masters of Small Worlds: Yeoman Households, Gender Relations, and the Political Culture of the Antebellum South Carolina Low Country* (1995).

Leonard Richards, *The Slave Power: The Free North and Southern Domination, 1780–1860* (2000).

The Deepening Conflict over Slavery

David Herbert Donald, *Lincoln* (1995).

William E. Gienapp, *The Origins of the Republican Party, 1852–1856* (1987).

Michael F. Holt, *The Rise and Fall of the American Whig Party: Jacksonian Politics and the Onset of the Civil War* (1999).

Stephen Oates, *To Purge This Land with Blood: A Biography of John Brown* (1984).

Manisha Sinha, *The Counterrevolution of Slavery: Politics and Ideology in Antebellum South Carolina* (2000).

Albert J. Von Frank, *The Trials of Anthony Burns: Freedom and Slavery in Emerson's Boston* (1998).

Online Practice Test

Test your understanding of this chapter with interactive review quizzes at

www.ablongman.com/jonescreatedequal/chapter13

"To Fight to Gain a Country": The Civil War

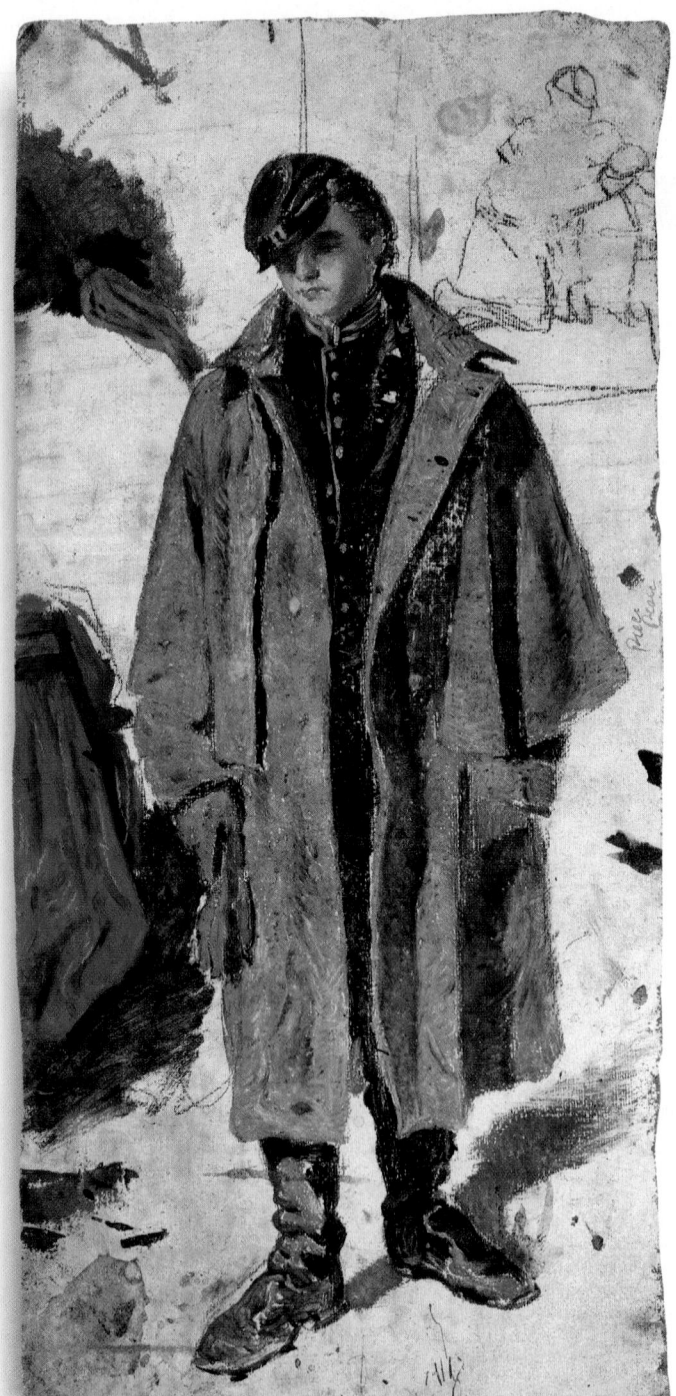

Winslow Homer, *Young Union Soldier: Separate Study of a Soldier Giving Water to a Wounded Companion*, 1861. Cooper-Hewitt, National Design Museum, Smithsonian Institution. Gift of Charles Savage Homer, Jr. (1912-12-110). Photo by Ken Pelka

■ Winslow Homer's painting *Young Union Soldier: Separate Study of a Soldier Giving Water to a Wounded Companion*, 1861.

PENSACOLA, FLORIDA, WAS THE SITE OF A DRAMATIC COURT MARTIAL TRIAL IN April 1862, when five men were charged with treasonous acts against the Confederate States of America. "Possessed of information well calculated to aid the enemy," and thus capable of "giving intelligence" to the enemy, the defendants had endangered the security of Confederate troops stationed in the area, according to the chief prosecutor. At the conclusion of the three-day hearing, the court convicted the men and ordered that two of them, alleged ringleaders, be hanged. Later, the presiding officer claimed that "high Military Necessity" had mandated the swift trial and stern verdict: coastal communities were engulfed in a "general stampede" as planters tried to move slaves and livestock out of the way of the encroaching Union army. According to the officer, at stake in this trial was the very fate of the would-be new nation.

By 1862, Confederate leaders knew full well that the war for southern independence would be a hard and long one. Indeed, the Pensacola court martial provided striking evidence of the political and military challenges faced by southern nationalists, for all of the defendants—George, Robert, Stephen, Peter, and William—were runaway slaves. The specific charges lodged against them read, "That the said slaves are intelligent beings possessing the faculties of Conveying information which would prove useful to the enemy and detrimental to the Confederate States." Clearly, these five men were combatants in the war, as threatening to the well-being of the Confederacy as any Yankee sharpshooter in a blue uniform. The charges also suggest that the Confederates were forced to repudiate elements of their own proslavery beliefs, which held that black people were childlike and servile, incapable of acting on their own, and grateful for the guidance and protection of southern whites.

Sgt. F. L. Baldwin, a Union soldier, poses with an American flag as a backdrop.

The Pensacola slaves were assigned a defense lawyer, who attempted to show that they had not actually encountered any Union soldiers and so had had no opportunity to divulge information related to Confederate troop movement. Technically, then, they were not guilty of spying. In court, however, the accused men did admit that, ever since President Abraham Lincoln had taken office in early 1861, three white men in the vicinity (a whiskey seller, an employee of the slaves' master, and a shingle maker) had been encouraging them to seek their freedom behind Union lines.

Prosecuting officers believed that "strong measures" were needed to prevent the nefarious activities of "spies whether white or black." These officials therefore were unprepared for the firestorm of criticism that followed the announcement of the verdict. The owner of the slaves, General Jackson Morton, expressed outrage that two of his men were marked for summary execution. In a formal complaint to Confederate authorities, Morton denounced the hearing as "vulgar and improper." By the time the controversy faded, an impressive array of Confederate military officers (from sentinels to a lieutenant, a captain, a colonel, a major

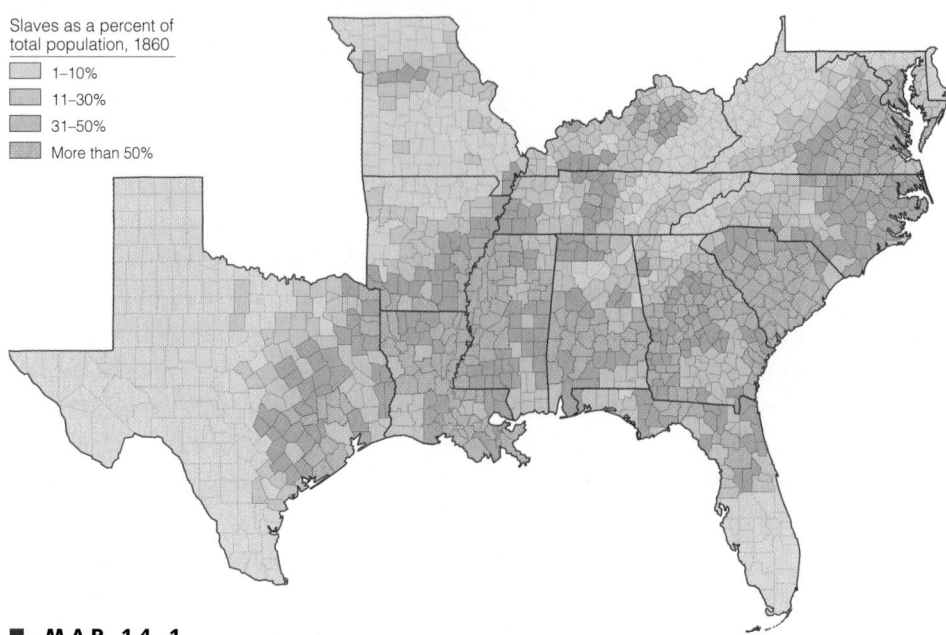

Slaves as a percent of
total population, 1860

▢ 1–10%
▢ 11–30%
▢ 31–50%
▢ More than 50%

■ **MAP 14.1**

SLAVERY IN THE UNITED STATES, 1860   In the South, the areas of the greatest concentration of slaves were also the areas of greatest support for the Confederacy. During the war, the Appalachian mountain region and the Upper Piedmont—the area between the mountains and the broad coastal plain—were home to people loyal to the Union and to people who became increasingly disaffected with Confederate policies as the war dragged on.

general, and a general) had had to justify their actions in convening the trial. The Confederate adjutant and inspector general took time out from more pressing matters to review the case for the secretary of war. In the words of one Confederate official, "The sacrosanctity of slave property in this war has operated most injuriously to the Confederacy."

Though at a distinct disadvantage compared to the North in terms of troops and materiel, the white South managed to fight on for four long bloody years. Early on, politicians hailed slaves as a tremendous asset, an immense, easily managed labor force that would grow food and dig trenches. Instead, African American men and women became freedom fighters, a source of subversion in the heart of the Confederacy. In October 1862, in response to the crisis of wartime slave management, the Confederate Congress passed a measure that exempted from military service one white man for every 20 slaves on a plantation. Many slave owners used this law to shield themselves or their sons from combat duty. In turn, the Twenty-Negro Law inflamed resentment among non–slave-owning, small farmers who charged that this rich man's war was actually a poor man's fight. Even within the ranks of the elite, conflicts over military strategy and national mobilization policies hobbled the Confederate effort. Many slaveholding women gradually came to see the sacrifice of their husbands, brothers, and sons as too high a price to pay for southern independence.

As defenders of slavery, the Confederates cast themselves as rebels in an age when the principle of individual rights was gaining ground. The citizens of France, Germany, and Italy were agitating on behalf of modern, democratic nation-states, and systems of serfdom and slavery throughout Europe and the Western Hemisphere were under siege. By early 1865, leading southern politicians and strategists had initiated a public debate over the possibility of offering slaves their liberty in return for military service. In acknowledging that African American men might serve as effective soldiers (as 179,000 of them had demonstrated in the Union army), the Confederates tolled their own death knell. White Southerners were fighting for their own nation, but African Americans were fighting to gain their own country as well.

The Republican conduct of the war revealed the party's long-range, guiding principles. Yet not all non-Southerners embraced the party's brand of nationalism. Several groups objected to a strong federal government, one that would weld the country together geographically as well as economically. The Lincoln administration met bitter resistance from Indian tribes as diverse as the Santee Sioux of Minnesota, the Cheyenne of Colorado, and the Navajo and Apaches of the Southwest. In northeastern cities, Irish immigrants battled federal draft agents and attacked black women, men, and children, their supposed competitors in the workplace. The Civil War, then, was less a "brothers' war" between the white farmers of the North and South exclusively and more a conflict that pitted diverse groups against each other over the issues of slavery, territorial expansion, federal power, and local control. Yet by the end of the war in April 1865, for the time being at least, the Republican vision of a union forged in blood had prevailed, at the cost of more than 600,000 lives.

Mobilization for War, 1861–1862

On December 20, 1860, less than eight weeks after Abraham Lincoln was elected president of the United States, South Carolina seceded from the Union, determined, in the words of its own Declaration of Independence, to "resume her separate and equal place among nations." By February 1, 1861, Mississippi, Florida, Alabama, Georgia, Louisiana, and Texas (all states dependent on slave-based staple crop agriculture) had also withdrawn from the United States of America. Three days later, representatives of the seven states met in Montgomery, Alabama, and formed the Confederate States of America. They also adopted a new constitution for their new nation. Though modeled after that of the United States, this document invoked the power of "sovereign and independent states" instead of "we, the people."

Delegates to the Montgomery convention elected as their president Jefferson Davis, a wealthy Mississippi planter with an impressive record of public service. Davis was a graduate of West Point, a veteran of the Mexican War, and a former United States congressman and senator. He had also held the position of secretary of war in the Franklin Pierce administration. Chosen vice president was a former Whig from Georgia, Alexander H. Stephens. In devising a cabinet, Davis bypassed some well-known radical secessionists—"fire eaters" such as William Lowndes Yancey (of Alabama) and Robert Barnwell Rhett, Jr. (of South Carolina)—on the assumption that the builders of a new nation would need skills different from the destroyers of an old one.

The Secession Impulse

In some respects, the Civil War seems difficult to explain, for the two sides shared a great deal. Most of the people North and South were English-speaking Protestants with deep roots in the culture of the British Isles. Together they celebrated a revolutionary heritage, paying homage to George Washington and the other Founding Fathers.

Why then was the white South, especially the slave South, so fearful of Abraham Lincoln? Although Lincoln enjoyed a broad Electoral College victory—180 votes to 123 for his opponents combined—the popular vote margin was slim. Six out of ten Americans cast their ballots for a candidate other than Lincoln in the 1860 presidential election. Together, Stephen A. Douglas and John C. Breckinridge polled 366,484 more votes than did the lanky lawyer from Illinois. Lincoln received no votes from the Deep South (he was not on the ballot in those states),

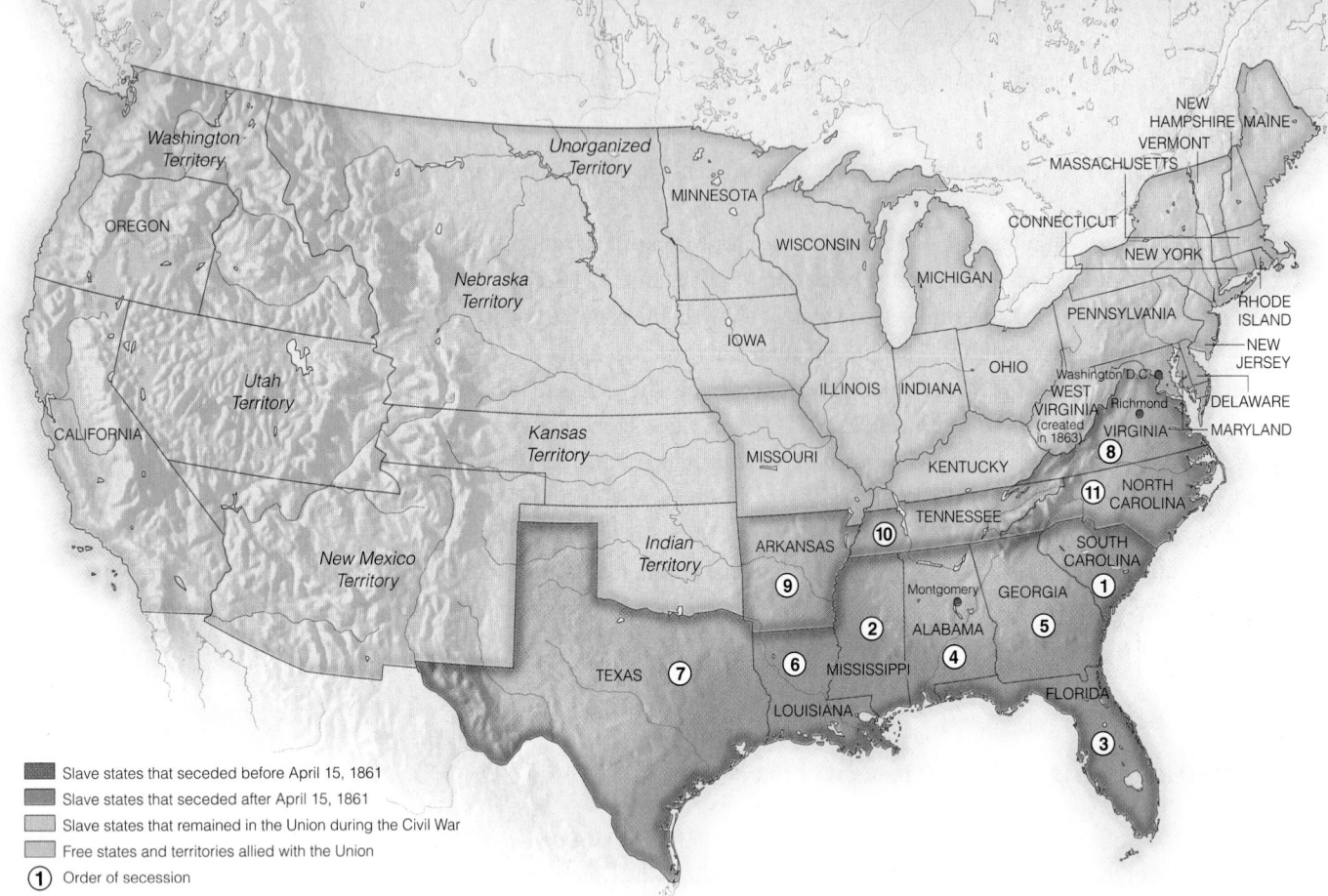

Slave states that seceded before April 15, 1861
Slave states that seceded after April 15, 1861
Slave states that remained in the Union during the Civil War
Free states and territories allied with the Union
① Order of secession

■ **MAP 14.2**
THE SECESSION OF SOUTHERN STATES, 1860–1861   The southern states seceded from the Union in stages, beginning with South Carolina in December 1860. Founded on February 4, 1861, the Confederate States of America initially consisted of only that state and six Deep South states. The four upper South states of Virginia, Arkansas, Tennessee, and North Carolina did not leave the Union until mid-April, when Lincoln called for 75,000 troops to put down the civil rebellion. The slave states of Delaware, Maryland, Kentucky, and Missouri remained in the Union, but each of those states was bitterly divided between Unionists and Confederate sympathizers.

and five upper South states gave him only 4 percent of his popular vote total (and those came mostly from German immigrants in or near St. Louis). The Republicans failed to capture either the House of Representatives or the Senate, and the Supreme Court remained within the southern camp, with five of its nine justices determined to protect the institution of slavery.

Political support for Lincoln thus appeared slim, and he did not seem likely to invoke his authority to move against slavery. He had made it clear that, as president, he would possess neither the authority nor the desire to disturb slavery as it existed in the South. However, he summed up his philosophy before the secession crisis this way: "As I would not be a *slave,* so I would not be a *master.* This expresses my idea of democracy. Whatever differs from this . . . is not democracy."

Not surprisingly, then, southern elites felt threatened by Lincoln in particular and the Republicans in general, pointing to the new president's oft-repeated promise to halt the march of slavery into the western territories. Although he was in no position to achieve this goal by executive order, Lincoln did have the power to expand the Republican base in the South by dispensing patronage jobs to a small group of homegrown abolitionists. He could also make appointments to the Supreme Court as openings became available. The Republican party was not a majority party; it was a sectional party in that its power was all in the North and the Upper Midwest. Ominously for the South, this sectional party had managed to seize control of the executive branch of government. The antebellum balance of power between slave and free states had tipped decisively in favor of the North.

Slaveowners reasoned that it was only a matter of time before the North—what some southern whites called the Anti–Slave Power Conspiracy—spread its tentacles all over the South. According to this view, John Brown's 1859 raid on the federal arsenal at Harpers Ferry, Virginia, was just the first in a series of planned attacks on the slave South. Moreover, some Southerners feared that the swearing in of (what they saw as) the ugly, uncouth new president would encourage the growth of any number of northern evils, from labor unionism and women's rights to free love and dress reform (promoted by the infamous "Bloomer women," who wore pants instead of skirts). Submission to "Black Republicans" would bring the South only humiliation and degradation.

Two last-ditch efforts at compromise failed to avert a constitutional crisis. In December 1860, as South Carolina was seceding and other states were preparing to join it, neither northern Republicans nor lower South Democrats showed any interest in a series of proposed constitutional amendments that would have severely curtailed the federal government's ability to restrict the interstate slave trade or the spread of slavery. Called the Crittenden Compromise (after its sponsor, Senator John J. Crittenden, a Whig from Kentucky), this package of proposed amendments was defeated in the Senate on January 16, 1861. A peace conference, organized by the Virginia legislature and assembled in February, revised the Crittenden Compromise, but key players were missing: the seven Confederate states and five northern states. Congress rejected the conference's recommendations at the end of February. By this time many Americans, radicals and moderates, Northerners and Southerners, were in no mood to compromise on the issue of slavery, especially its extension into the Western territories.

Lincoln was faced with the task of cobbling together a cabinet composed of representatives of his Republican coalition. Shrewdly, he named four party leaders who had challenged him for the presidential nomination the previous year (William H. Seward as secretary of state, Edward Bates as attorney general, Simon Cameron as secretary of war, and Salmon P. Chase as secretary of the treasury). He appointed Montgomery Blair (from strategically located Maryland) as postmaster general. In his inaugural address of March 4, Lincoln appealed to the South to refrain from any drastic action, invoking the historic bonds of nationhood, the "mystic chords of memory, stretching from every battle-field, and patriot grave, to every living heart and hearthstone."

In his inaugural address of March 4, Lincoln appealed to the South to refrain from any drastic action.

For the most part Lincoln's plea for unity fell on deaf ears. However, among the Southerners who initially resisted the secessionists' call to arms was the West Point graduate and Mexican War veteran Robert E. Lee of Virginia. As late as January 1861, Lee maintained that the framers of our Constitution would never have "exhausted so much labor, wisdom, and forbearance in its formation" if they had intended the Union to be so easily dismantled. Later, after Virginia seceded, Lee cast his lot with the Confederacy: "I cannot raise my hand against my birthplace, my home, my children," he declared. By his home Lee meant the Commonwealth of Virginia, not the collection of disaffected states.

Indeed, in early April, the Confederacy was a rhetorical powerhouse, full of blustering firebrands. But it was also a poor excuse for an independent nation, with only one-third of the U.S. population and almost no industrial capacity. Over the next few weeks, as the seven Confederate states attempted to coax the upper South to join their revolution, Lincoln emerged as an unwitting ally in their effort.

Located in Charleston Harbor, Fort Sumter was one of two Union forts in southern territory, and in the spring of 1861 it was badly in need of supplies. On April 12, Lincoln took the high moral ground by sending provisions but not troops to the fort. The Confederates found the move provocative nonetheless and began firing on the fort. After a 33-hour Confederate bombardment, the heavily damaged fort surrendered without a fight. In response, many white Southerners, such as Mary Boykin Chesnut, the wife of a high Confederate official, cheered and embraced the "pomp and circumstance of glorious war."

Alabama Secession Convention Occupations

Occupation of Delegate	Cooperationists	Secessionists	Total
Farmer or Planter	20	118	38
Lawyer	10	22	32
Physician	2	3	5
Merchant	2	2	4
Farmer-Lawyer	3	1	4
Clergyman	3	1	4
Teacher	2	—	2
Judge	—	2	2
Sheriff	—	1	1
Manufacturer	1	—	1
Cotton factor	—	1	1
Factor-Merchant	1	—	1
Farmer-Manufacturer	1	—	1
Farmer-Merchant	—	1	1
Unknown	1	2	3
Total	46	54	100

Alabama Secession Convention Property Holding*

Value of Property Held by Delegate	Cooperationists	Secessionists	Total
Real Property			
Less than $10,000	31	20	51
$10,000–$24,999	8	17	25
$25,000–$49,999	4	9	13
$50,000–$99,999	1	4	5
$100,000 and above	1	2	3
Total	45	52	97
Personal Property			
Less than $10,000	19	6	25
$10,000–$24,999	12	10	22
$25,000–$49,999	8	14	22
$50,000–$99,999	5	13	18
$100,000–$199,999	—	7	7
$200,000 and above	1	2	3
Total	45	52	97

*Three delegates not found in manuscript census; hence, 97 rather than 100 is the total here.

■ FIGURE 14.1
DELEGATES TO THE ALABAMA
SECESSION CONVENTION

Three days after the capture of Fort Sumter, Lincoln (anticipating a conflict no longer than 90 days) called for 75,000 northern volunteers to quell a civil uprising "too powerful to be suppressed by the ordinary course of judicial proceedings." By the end of the month he had ordered a blockade of southern seaports. Condemning these moves as acts of "northern aggression," the upper South, including Virginia (deprived of its western part, which now formed a new state called West Virginia), Tennessee, Arkansas, and North Carolina all seceded from the Union by May 20. Grateful for the newfound loyalty of Virginia and eager to appropriate the Tredegar Iron Works (in Richmond), the Confederacy moved its capital from the down-at-the-heels Montgomery to the elegant Richmond on May 11.

The process by which the southern states left the Union foreshadowed the political rifts the new nation faced in the horrific years to come. With the exception of Tennessee, which placed the secession question before its state legislators, all of the states elected delegates to special secession conventions; acting separately, each of these bodies ultimately ratified an ordinance of secession. Some white Southerners (especially Union sympathizers called Unionists) refused to vote for convention delegates at all, considering the whole enterprise illegal. Other voters supported delegates who initially favored cooperating with other southern states in the hope that the South could broker some compromise on slavery with the North, but then later, in the heat of the moment, changed their minds and voted to secede. Most of the delegates to the North Carolina secession convention were slave owners, hardly a representative group from that state of yeomen. During the war, poor Southerners would charge that wealthy slave owners protected their own economic interests while ignoring those of ordinary people. Moreover, a core of Unionists would prove active traitors to the Confederate cause.

Only Texas, Virginia, and Tennessee submitted their ordinances directly to the voters for approval, and although secession gained overwhelming approval in all three cases, it was not clear that those victories represented the will of the people. Moreover, certain segments of the southern population early demonstrated that they would withhold their support from the Confederacy; yeoman farmers in the upcountry, Louisiana sugar planters dependent on world markets for their product, and people in the hill country of east Tennessee all voted for Unionist delegates to their respective state conventions. The Border States of Missouri, Kentucky, Maryland, and Delaware remained within the Union, but among their residents were many outspoken people who openly sympathized with the South.

Commissioners from individual states helped to coordinate the secession process and justify the collective decision to leave the United States. As a group, the commissioners maintained that northern Republicans intended to dishonor and degrade southern white men. The commissioners highlighted slavery as the cause of secession, maintaining that Lincoln's election threatened to provoke a rebellion among the slaves and thus destroy a way of life for all southern white men and women. Stephen Hale, Alabama's commissioner to Kentucky, declared that the Republicans' "new theory of government" was a direct attack on southern property rights. A Republican administration, he declared, would lead to "all the horrors of a San Domingo servile insurrection." Southern whites, Hale maintained, were in danger of losing not only their slaves but also their lives. This overheated rhetoric paved the way to war.

Preparing to Fight

Poised to battle each other, the South and the North faced similar challenges. Both sides had to inspire—or force—large numbers of men to fight. Both had to produce massive amounts of cannon, ammunition, and food. And both had to devise military strategies that would, they hoped, ensure victory. In early 1861 white Southerners were boasting of the stockpiles of cotton that, if needed, would serve as leverage for military support, diplomatic recognition, and financial assistance from the great European powers. Plantations brimming with hogs and corn, it was hoped, would sustain both masters and slaves, in contrast to the North, where cotton mills would lie idle and workers would soon descend to poverty and starvation.

In defense of secession, white Southerners emulated the rhetoric of 1776—high tariffs on imported manufactured goods were latter-day taxes imposed without representation—and thus drew inspiration from the

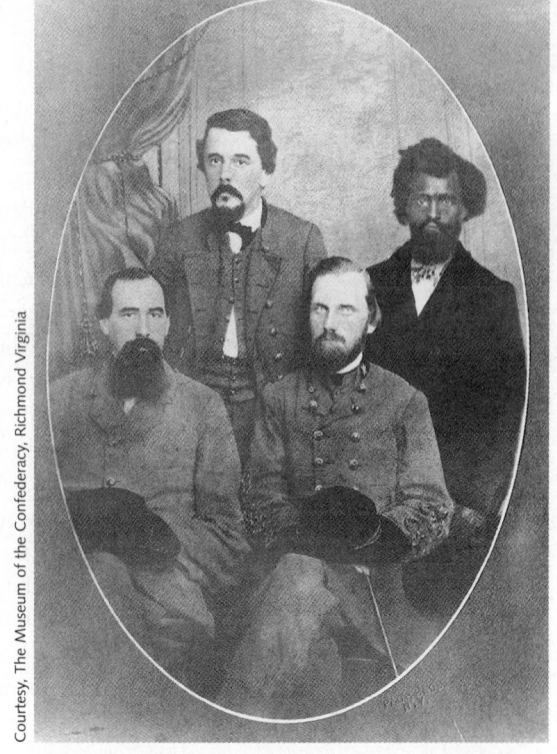

Courtesy, The Museum of the Confederacy, Richmond Virginia

This picture shows three Confederate surgeons, along with their African American servant, at the hospital in Lynchburg, Virginia. Confederate officials used enslaved men and women in a variety of capacities—as menial laborers, cooks, and laundresses in army camps, aides in hospitals, railroad hands, and industrial laborers.

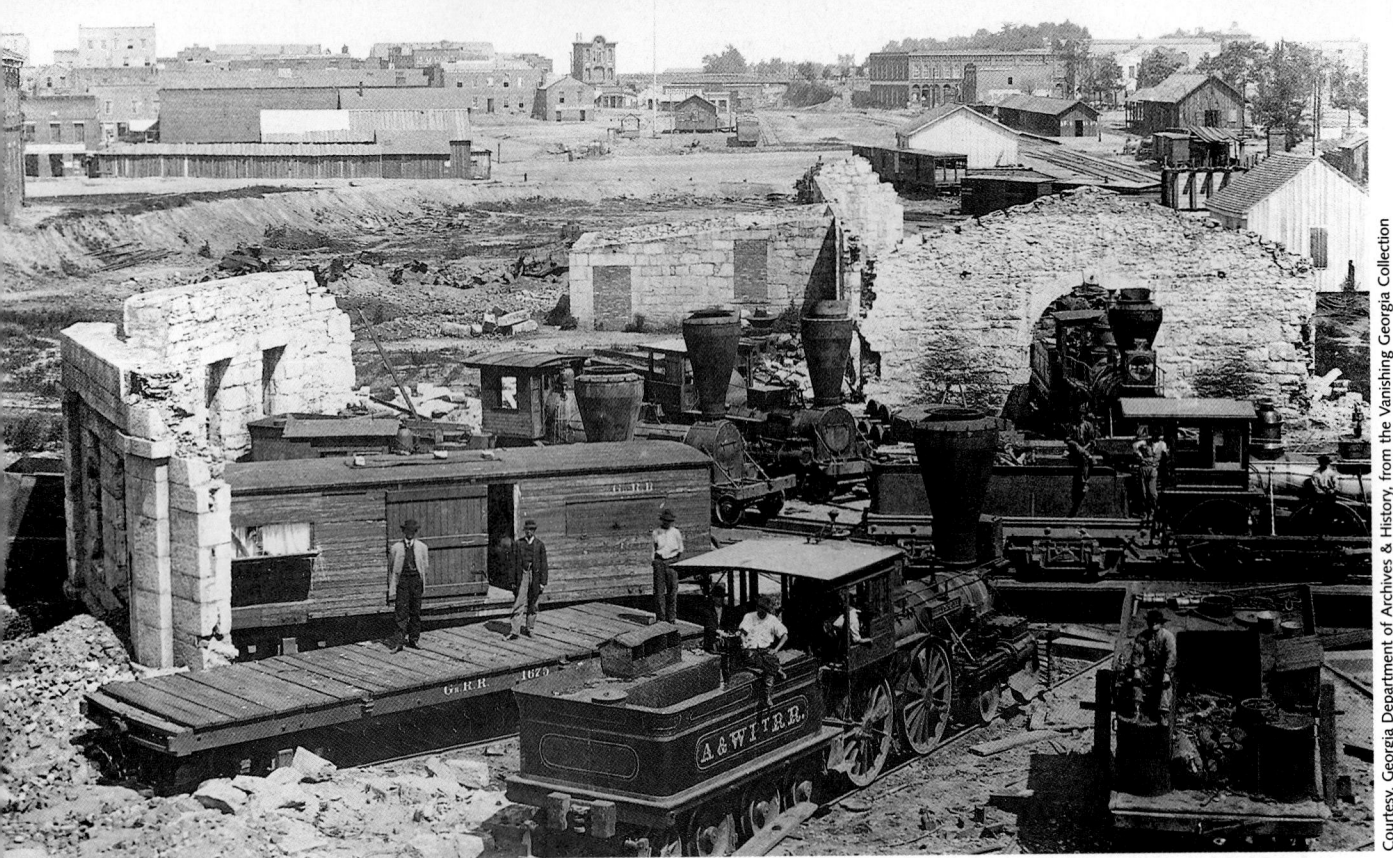

■ The Confederacy impressed large numbers of enslaved men and women into service. Black men worked on trains and on railroad maintenance crews. This photo shows a Georgia train roundhouse destroyed by General William T. Sherman's men on their march to the sea in late 1864. By forcing slaves to work far from home and in nonagricultural jobs, Confederate officials unwittingly contributed to the dismantling of slavery, a system that depended on controlling large numbers of blacks on plantations.

creation of the nation they now sought to dismantle. At the same time, however, Vice President Stephens acknowledged the revolutionary nature of the Confederacy. Repudiating the words of a famous Virginian, Thomas Jefferson, who had declared equality among men to be a "self-evident truth," Stephens boldly asserted, "Our new government is founded upon exactly the opposite idea; its foundations are laid, its cornerstone rests, upon the great truth that the negro is not equal to the white man; that slavery . . . is his natural and normal condition."

From the beginning of the war, Confederates aimed for a strategy calculated to draw on their strengths. They would fight a purely defensive war, a war of "annihilation," by overwhelming Union armies that ventured into Confederate territory. Small units of troops would be deployed around the South's 6000-mile border (a "dispersed defensive" tactic). Seasoned officers such as Robert E. Lee and Thomas J. Jackson would lead the charge to crush the Yankees. Finally, the South could command 3 million black people (a third of its total population of 9 million), all of whom, it was assumed, would do the bidding of planters and military men. Whereas the North would have to conquer the South to preserve the Union, the Confederacy would only have to survive to win its independence. White Southerners likened themselves to the Patriots of the American Revolution, boldly waging a defensive war against an arrogant, powerful enemy.

At first, the North was inclined to think little past the numbers: in 1860, it possessed 90 percent of the manufacturing capacity and three-quarters of the 30,000 railroad miles in the United States. Its population, 22 million, dwarfed that of the South. More than 1 million Northerners were employed in factories and workshops, compared to 110,000 Southerners. The North retained control of the (admittedly less than formidable) U.S. Navy and all other resources of the federal government, including a bureaucratic infrastructure to facilitate troop deployment and communication. Its diversified economy yielded grain as well as textiles; it could not only mobilize a large army but count on feeding it as well.

Early on, the North had a plan, but one that could hardly be dignified by the term *strategy*. It would defend its own territory from Southern attack and target Confederate leaders, under the assumption that latent Union sentiment in the South would arise to smash the rebellion before it went too far. Union gunboats positioned along the East Coast and up and down the Mississippi River would seal off the Confederacy from foreign supply lines (the so-called Anaconda Plan proposed by General-in-Chief Winfield Scott in the summer of 1861). The North would also launch a political offensive calculated to undermine Confederate sympathizers by bolstering Unionist sentiment everywhere. For example, from the beginning of the war, Lincoln made clear that he would continue to appeal to slaveholders loyal to the Union, whether those slaveholders lived in the Border States or deep in the heart of the Confederacy.

Northerners also invoked a Revolutionary heritage to justify their cause. However, they downplayed the issue of unjust taxation and instead stressed the glories of the Union—in Lincoln's words, "the last, best hope of mankind" in an age of kings and emperors. In an address to the nation on July 4, 1861, the president declared that the nation preceded—and thus created—the Union. He maintained that no person should be enslaved to another person and that all people must have equal opportunities to succeed in life, regardless of their background or skin color. The war, he argued, was "essentially a people's contest": its purpose was "to lift artificial weights from all shoulders . . . to afford all an unfettered start, and a fair chance in the race for life." Northerners as a whole found these words uplifting. In contrast, Confederates urged white Southerners to die so that other people would remain enslaved. This message, however, lost its appeal among nonelite Southerners over the coming months and years.

Barriers to Southern Mobilization

On July 21, 1861, at Manassas Junction (Bull Run), about 30 miles southwest of Washington, D.C., Union and Confederate forces encountered each other on the field of battle for the first time. This was the fight that earned Thomas "Stonewall" Jackson his nickname and burnished his reputation, for Union troops skirmished briefly with the enemy and then turned and fled back to the capital, disgraced. In the coming weeks, Northerners gave up the idea that the effort to suppress the rebels would be an easy one, and Lincoln began to reorganize the country's officer corps and fortify its armies. Contrary to the expectations of the women who had accompanied the Union forces out of the nation's capital, planning to lunch while they observed the first battle of the war, this fight was no picnic, military or otherwise.

To win this initial victory, the Confederates had relied on the massing of several huge forces: those of Generals Joseph Johnston and P. G. T. Beauregard, as well as Stonewall Jackson. Consequently, southern military strategists decided they must continue to defend southern territory while going on the offensive against the Yankees (the "offensive-defensive" strategy was used for the duration of the conflict). In other matters, however, the South learned life-and-death lessons more slowly. Only gradually did the central paradox of the Confederate nation become abundantly clear: that a country

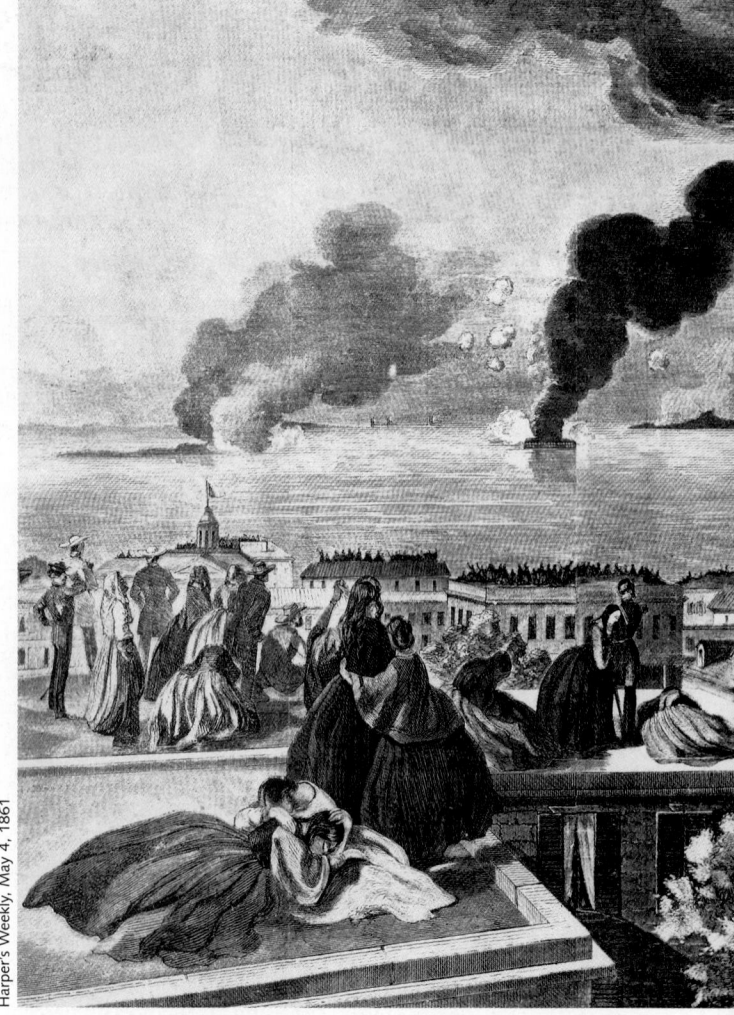

Harper's Weekly, May 4, 1861

■ This drawing, titled "The House-Tops of Charleston during the Bombardment of Sumter," appeared in the May 4, 1861, issue of *Harper's Weekly*, about three weeks after the event. Many Confederate women sent their husbands and sons into battle with great displays of patriotism. However, those parades and parties often masked deep fears. Noted one woman of her husband's departure, "It has always been my lot to be obliged to shut up my griefs in my own breast."

A Virginia Slaveholder Objects to the Impressment of Slaves

During the Civil War, some southern slave owners bitterly resisted Confederate slave impressment policies. On December 4, 1861, John B. Spiece, an Albemarle County, Virginia, slaveholder and lawyer, wrote to the Confederate attorney general and protested government policy.

Dr Sir, Although a stranger to you, yet in consequence of the excitement and distress in this section of the country, in reference to a certain matter; I am constrained to address you, not merely on my own account; but on behalf of a large number of most respectable citizens.. . .

A practice has prevailed for some considerable time in *this* section of the country of impressing into service of the confederate army, the horses wagons and *slaves* belonging to the people.

The "Press masters" will go to their houses, and drag of their property to Just Such an extent as they choose; until it has not only created great excitement and distress; but bids fair to produce wide spread ruin. And I am told that these "Press masters" are paid by the Government the enormous price of *two dollars and fifty cents for each team with they impress;*—hence their anxiety and untiring exertions to increase the number;—thus making thirty or forty dollars pr day—

While I do not controvert the right of the Government to impress into its service *wagons and teams;* yet I do controvert the right to impress *Slaves*—It does seem to me that no one can be impress'd into military service of any kind, unless he is subject to military duty: because this whole business is relating to the Army, and is purely a military matter.—

The people in this section of the country are much attached to their slaves, and treat them in a humane manner—consequently they are exceedingly pained at having them dragged off at this inclement season of the year, and exposed to the severe weather in the mountains of north western Virginia.. . . Some have already died, and others have returned home afflicted with Typhoid fever, which has spread through the family to a most fatal and alarming extent.—

I am a practicing lawyer myself, but these "Press masters" will hear nothing from any one residing amongst the people.—

Therefore Sir, in consequence of the distress produced by the causes before mentioned, I am constrained to write to you; requesting you if you please, to give your opinion upon the questions involved.

To wit—If a man's wagon and team should be impress'd into Service, can his slave be impress'd to drive the said team—

Secondly—If a man has neither wagon or team can his slave be impress'd to drive some other team (*some* of the "Press masters" yield this *last* point, whilst others do not, and contend that they can impress just as many slaves as they choose from any plantation, taking all the negro men if they think proper.)—

---

founded on an agrarian ideal of "states' rights" needed to industrialize its economy and centralize its government operations to defeat the Union.

The first weeks of the war revealed that the South would pursue its antebellum aims of conquering western territory for slavery. An early victory of Texas forces over Union troops in New Mexico led to the formation of what slaveholders in that region called the Confederate Territory of Arizona. Over the next year the Confederates launched successful assaults on the cities of Albuquerque and Santa Fe, in present-day New Mexico. However, southern troops amounted to little more than a band of plunderers; in Rio Abajo, for example, farmers and ranchers switched their allegiance to the Union after the rebels raided their homesteads.

Deprived of money raised from customs duties (the blockade brought a halt to established patterns of overseas trade), the Confederacy relied on floating bonds ($400 million worth), raising taxes, and a 10 percent tax on farm produce. The Confederate Treasury printed money at a furious rate ($1 billion over the course of the conflict), but its value declined precipitously; near the end of the war one Confederate dollar was worth only 1.6 cents.

Raising a volunteer army and impressing slave labor (forcing slaves to labor for the military) met with stiff resistance from various quarters of southern society. For yeoman farm families, long defensive of the independence of their own households, Confederate mobilization efforts came as a rude shock. Antebellum Southerners believed that white fathers should pro-

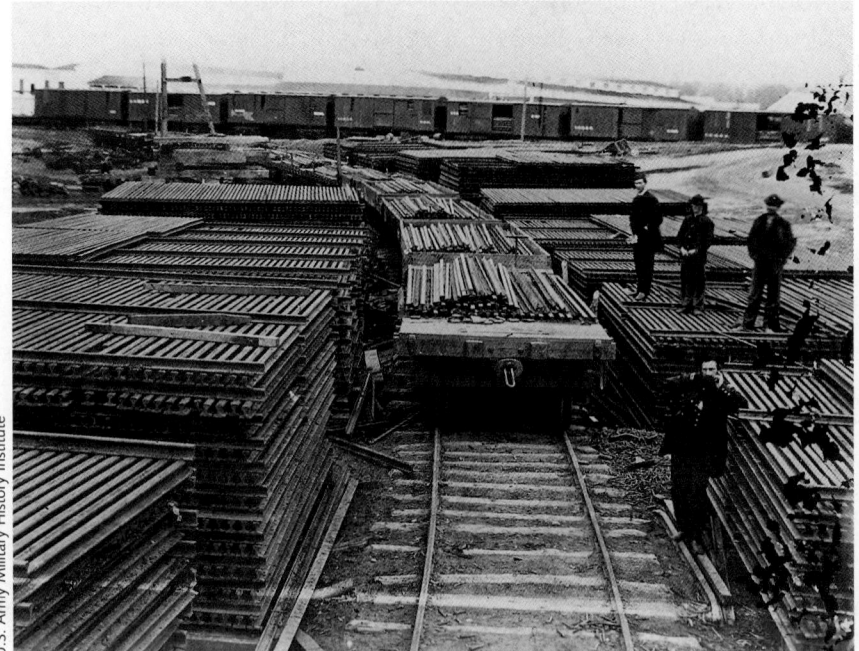

Stockpile of rails at Alexandria, Virginia

Some few of the people have not been able to sow their grain this fall:—and there is deep dissatisfaction amongst the people—therefore I deem it proper and expedient that the authorities should know it—

Spiece goes on to cite the laws of the Commonwealth of Virginia, as amended in 1860, "by which it seems there is no power to impress Slaves." In the absence of Confederate congressional legislation to that effect, he argues, government authorities

lack the legal right to take slaves from their owners. Spiece concludes his letter by suggesting that in taking slaves far from their homes, Confederate authorities were endangering the security of the would-be-new nation.

There is also a serious evil in impressing slaves for the service in North western Virginia:—whilst there they get to talking with *Union men* in disguise, and by that means learn the original cause of the difficulty between North & South: then return home and inform other negroes:—not long since one of my neighbors negro men went to his master, and desired to let him go again to the north western army—adding "I wish you to let me go further than I went before["]—I have the honor to be most respectfully your Obt Servt.

It is unknown whether Confederate officials responded to Spiece's letter. ■

Source: Ira Berlin, Barbara J. Fields, Thavolia Glymph, Joseph P. Reidy, and Leslie S. Rowland, eds., *Freedom: A Documentary History of Emancipation, 1861–1867*, Series 1, Vol. 1, *The Destruction of Slavery* (1985), pp. 782–783.

tect and retain control over their dependents at all times. In August 1861, the attorney general of Virginia reluctantly informed the Confederate secretary of war that the residents of Shenandoah County, with a white population of 12,800, were balking at the call for 10 percent of its population in volunteers. Likewise, resentful of the impressment of the few slaves from their area, farmers in Randolph County, Alabama, pointed to the sacrifices of their own women and children, "industriously engaged on their farms," their necks reddened by the sun, while in the city wealthy whites (and their slaves) went about business as usual.

Some masters stood on principle in their efforts to keep their enslaved men and women out of the clutches of Confederate "press agents." Planters also expressed a well-founded fear that slaves impressed for a wide range of tasks, whether saltmaking or chopping trees or tending brick kilns, were difficult to control now that plantation discipline had been loosened. All over the South, white men resisted the idea that they must relinquish their slaves to the Confederacy to preserve the institution of slavery.

The Confederate call for volunteers failed to produce the number of soldiers (and menial laborers) needed to fight the Union, and so in March 1862 Davis received congressional authorization to implement a military conscription law (all men between ages 18 and 35 were called up for three years of service), the first draft on the North American continent. (By September the upper age had been raised to 45.) The law also exempted certain kinds of workers, such as railroad employees, schoolteachers, miners, and druggists, and allowed the buying of

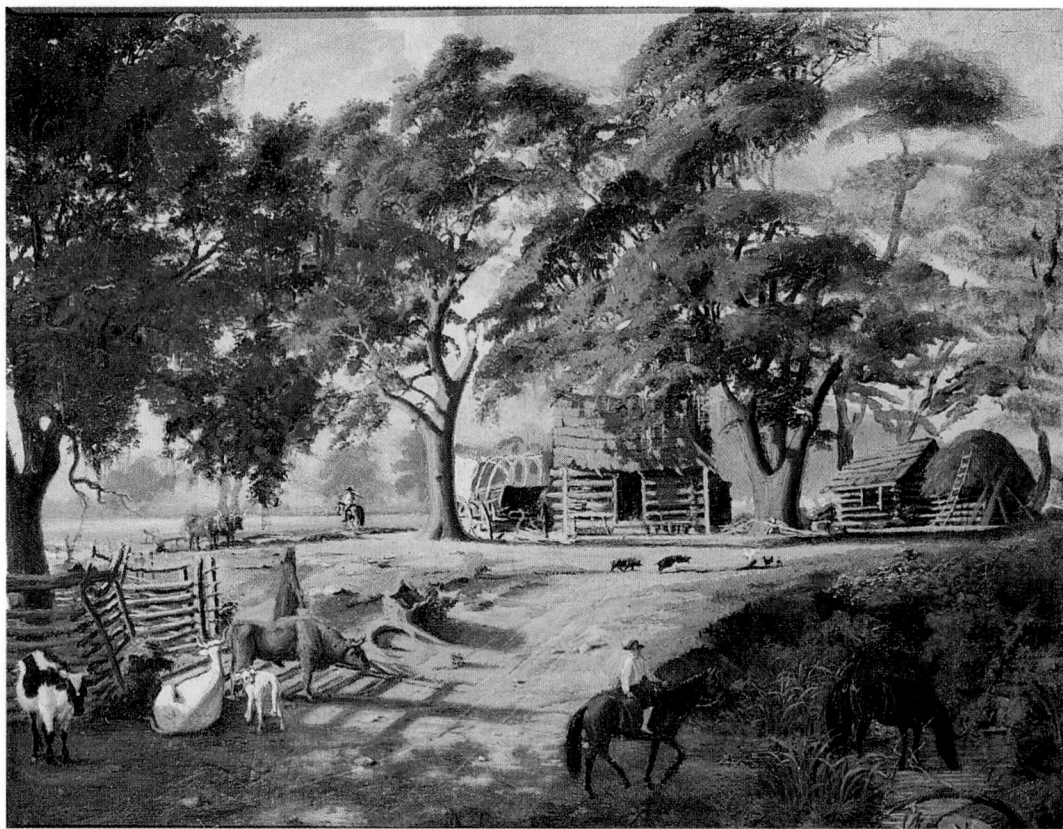

Carl G. von Iwonski, *Block House, New Braunfels*. Yanaguana Society Collection. Daughters of the Republic of Texas Library

■ Farmer's cabin, Block House, New Braunfels.

"substitutes" by draftees who could afford the $300 price for them. This last type of exemption allowed wealthy men to pay someone to fight in their place.

These provisions provoked anger not only among ordinary citizens but also among principled states' rights advocates such as governors Joseph Brown of Georgia and Zebulon Vance of North Carolina. Brown exempted large numbers of men from the draft, claiming that the Confederacy posed a greater threat to states' rights than did the Union. On January 1, 1862, 209,852 southern men were present for duty. Yet the northern force was more than twice as large, with 527,204.

In Confederate encampments, antebellum identities gave way to wartime necessity. Reduced to the status of menial laborers, washing their own clothes and cooking their own meals, digging trenches and hauling wood, some sons from elite families felt demeaned by their new responsibilities. Soon after the war began, Colonel Jonathan A. Winston complained to the commander of the Confederate post at Yorktown, Virginia, that his men were "laboring in the unloading of Ships"—a poor use of their time, he thought, and a job better suited to slaves. However, there were too few blacks in the immediate area to meet all the needs of the army and the needs of the white soldiers themselves. For the purposes of war, white men must serve other white men.

Indians and Immigrants in the Service of the Confederacy

Just as the Confederates failed in their attempt to use fully the labor of enslaved workers, so they failed to reap much gain from the vaunted military prowess of Indians, especially those in Indian Territory (present-day Oklahoma). In 1861, southern military officials appealed to the Cherokees and the other Five Tribes for support, promising them arms and protection from

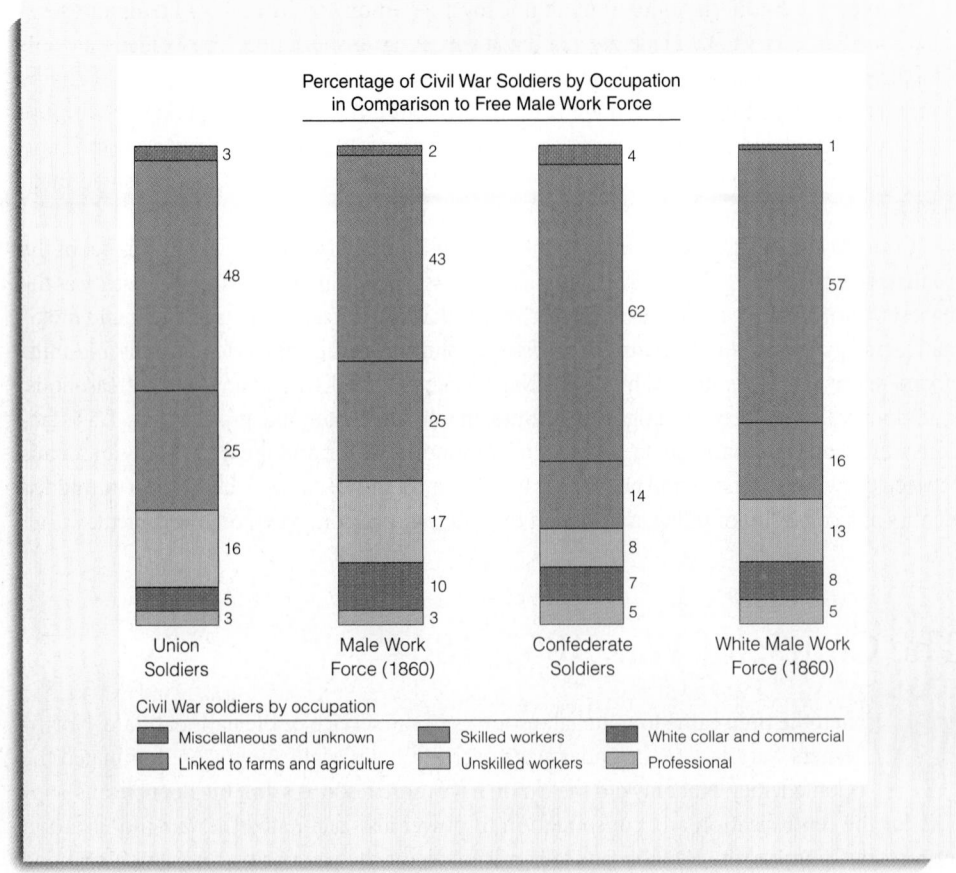

Percentage of Civil War Soldiers by Occupation in Comparison to Free Male Work Force

Civil War soldiers by occupation

- Miscellaneous and unknown
- Linked to farms and agriculture
- Skilled workers
- Unskilled workers
- White collar and commercial
- Professional

■ **FIGURE 14.2**
OCCUPATIONAL CATEGORIES OF UNION AND CONFEDERATE SOLDIERS

Union forces in return. Only gradually and reluctantly did Cherokee leader John Ross commit his men to the Confederacy: "We are in the situation of a man standing alone upon a low naked spot of ground, with the water rising all around him."

More devoted to the Confederate cause was Stand Watie, the brother of Elias Boudinot (one of the Cherokee leaders to have signed the original removal treaty). Backed by many Cherokee slaveholders, Stand Watie proceeded to mobilize what he called the "United Nations of Indians" as a fighting force on behalf of the Confederacy. Among those responding to the call to arms were Chocktaw and Chickasaw men, who formed Company E of the 21st Mississippi Regiment, "the Indian Brigade."

Although Indian Territory was considered of great strategic value to the Confederacy, southern military officials at times expressed frustration with the traditional battle tactics of Indian warriors. They were unused to military encounters that pitted long, straight rows of men on foot against each other. At the Battle of Elkhorn Tavern (Pea Ridge) in March 1862, Indian troops abandoned the battlefield in the face of cannon fire, leading their commander, Albert Pike, to demand that in the future they be "allowed to fight in their own fashion" rather than "face artillery and steady infantry on open ground." Yet most Confederate generals, like George Washington during the Seven Years' War, measured Indians by European American standards of what made a "proper" soldier on the battlefield. In the summer of 1862 the Confederacy lost its advantage in Confederate territory; the Cherokee and Creek were divided in their loyalties, with some joining Union forces and all "undisciplined . . . [and] not very reliable." By this time, the Comanche and Kiowa, resentful of the Confederacy's broken promises (guns and money diverted from them), had joined Union troops and were threatening to invade Texas.

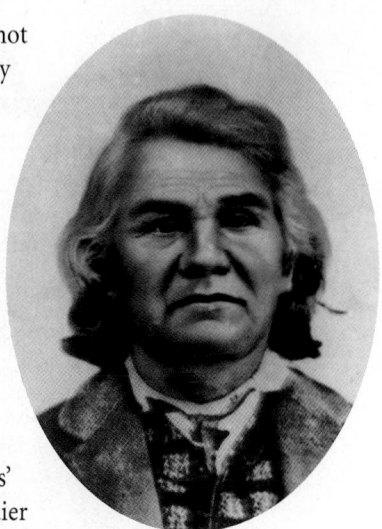

Stand Watie

Even on the southern home front, ethnic loyalties among white men could disrupt services deemed necessary to Confederate manufacturing and transportation. The Confederate railroad director in Selma, Alabama, contended with a labor force of immigrants (most probably from Germany and Ireland), men who "do not feel identified in any great degree with the South" and who demanded high wages. They were constantly threatening to run away to Union lines, where they believed they could make more money and enjoy the luxuries denied them in war-torn Alabama.

Complicating the Davis administration's attempts to mobilize for war was the refusal of the Confederates to form a political party system, on the assumption that unity among whites was the highest priority. However, the lack of parties meant that real differences over military and diplomatic strategy were reduced to infighting between shifting groups of elected officials and military men. Davis and members of his cabinet were quick to label dissent of any kind as treasonous, squelching legitimate debate on significant issues. In wartime Richmond, pro- and anti-Davis factions were made and unmade on the basis of rumor, innuendo, and the friendships and feuds between the wives of officers and politicians. In this respect the white South clung to an outmoded identity as a collection of individuals bound to yield to no person, party, or government.

The Course of War, 1862–1864

When the time came to marshal resources in the service of the national state, Northerners were at a distinct advantage over the states' rights men who dominated the Confederacy. Not only did the Union have more resources, but the Republicans' support for the centralization and consolidation of power also facilitated the war-mobilization process. In Congress, the Republicans took advantage of their majority status and expanded federal programs in the realm of the economy, education, and land use. However, like Davis, Lincoln encountered vehement opposition to his wartime policies. Meanwhile, on the battlefield, Union losses were mounting. The United States confronted an uncertain fate.

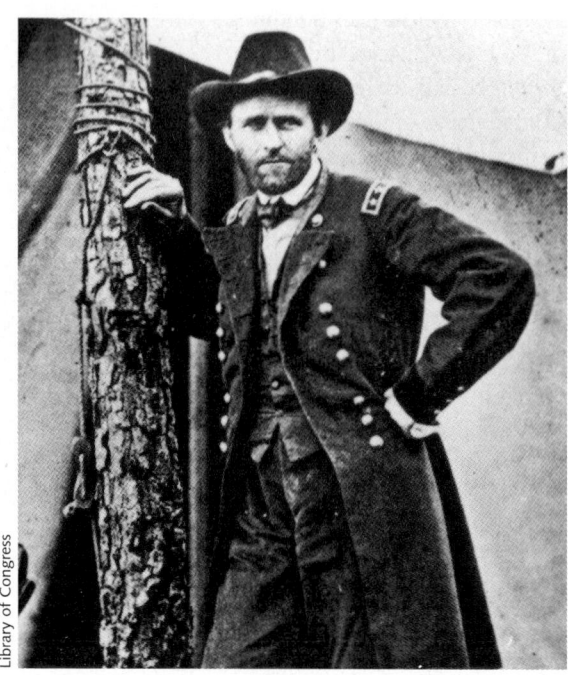

■ **Ulysses Grant**

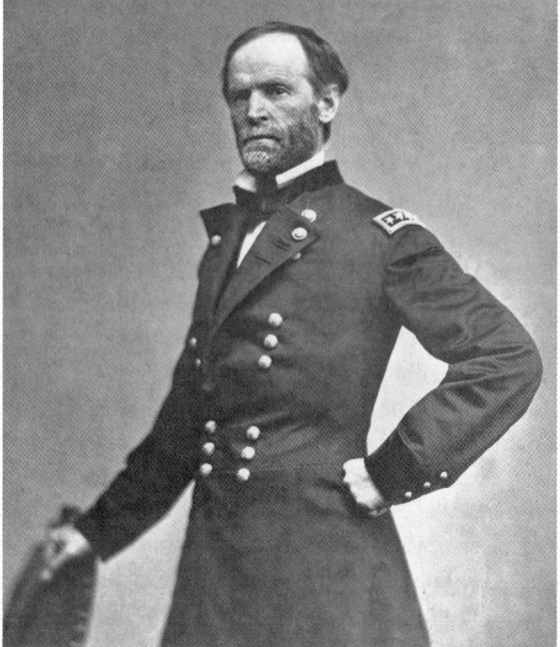

■ **William Sherman**

Library of Congress

Library of Congress

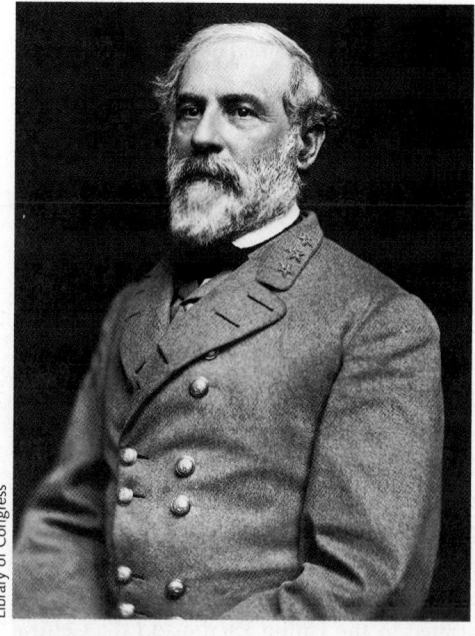

Library of Congress

■ Robert E. Lee

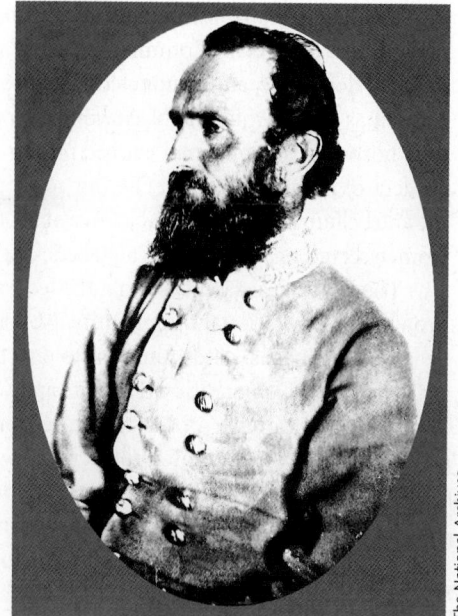

The National Archives

■ Stonewall Jackson

The Republicans' War

Worried about disloyalty in the vicinity of the nation's capital, on April 27, 1861, Lincoln gave General Winfield Scott the power to suspend the writ of habeas corpus (a legal doctrine designed to protect the rights of people arrested) in Baltimore. By the end of the year, this policy, which allowed the incarceration of people not yet charged with a crime, was being applied in almost all of the loyal United States. Chief among those targeted were people suspected of interfering with war mobilization of men and supplies. Democrats stepped up their opposition to the president, denouncing him as a tyrant and a dictator. Meanwhile, from the other side of the political spectrum, abolitionists expressed their frustration with the administration's conciliatory policy toward the South in general and toward Unionist slaveholders in particular. Claimed Frederick Douglass, "Sound policy, not less than humanity, demands the instant liberation of every slave in the rebel states." Yet Lincoln persisted in appealing to masters' loyalty to the Union, declaring that his objective was "to save the Union, and . . . neither to save or destroy slavery."

Wartime manufacturing and commerce proved to be a boon to enterprising Northerners. Manufacturers made new use of forms of technology (Singer sewing machines to produce uniforms for soldiers, McCormick reapers to harvest grain for soldiers and civilians alike). In Cleveland, a young commission-house operator named John D. Rockefeller was earning enough money to hire a substitute to serve in the army for him. In the middle of the war he shifted his business from trading grain, fish, water, lime, plaster, and salt to refining the crude oil (used in kerosene lamps) recently discovered in western Pennsylvania.

War profiteers were not unique to the North. In 1862 the *Southern Cultivator*, a magazine published in Augusta, Georgia, ran an article titled "Enemies at Home," denouncing the "vile crew of speculators" who were selling everything from corn to cloth at exorbitant prices. However, Republicans saw nothing wrong in enhancing one's fortunes and at the same time contributing to the Union cause. Later recalling his rise to wealth and his effort to bring a bright, clean illuminant to the masses, Rockefeller melded morality with economic self-interest in a revealing and classic Republican way, "Let the good work go on. We must ever remember we are refining oil for the poor man and he must have it cheap and good."

The Republicans' willingness to centralize wartime operations led in 1861 to the formation of the U.S. Sanitary Commission, which recruited physicians, trained nurses, raised money, solicited donations, and conducted inspections of Union camps on the front. During the war, as many as 20,000 white and black women served as nurses, cooks, and laundresses in Union military hospitals. Black women worked primarily in the latter two categories. Appointed superintendent of nurses, Dorothea Dix (an advocate of reform on behalf of the mentally ill during the antebellum period) oversaw a force of 3000 white, mostly middle-class, women nurses. These women served as professional caretakers, often over the objections of skeptical male physicians.

The Republicans believed that the federal government should actively promote economic growth and educational opportunity. Not surprisingly, then, the war deepened the Republicans' determination to enact measures that had previously been thwarted by Democratic presidents and Congresses. In July 1862, the Republicans pushed through an "Act to Secure Homesteads to Actual Settlers on the Public Domain," which granted 160 acres of western land to each settler who lived on and made improvements to the land for five years. Congress also passed the Morrill Act, which created a system of land grant colleges. (Many of these colleges eventually became major public universities, including Colorado State University, Kansas State University, and Utah State University.) Also approved in 1862, the Pacific Railroad Act appropriated to the Union Pacific and the Central Pacific Railroads a 400-foot right-of-way along the Platte River route of the Oregon Trail and lent them $16,000 to $48,000 (depending on the terrain) per mile.

Union military strategy reflected a prewar Republican indifference to the rights and welfare of both northern and southern blacks.

During the first year and a half of war, Union military strategy reflected a prewar Republican indifference to the rights and welfare of both northern and southern blacks. In September 1861 Lincoln revoked a directive released by General John Frémont that would have authorized the seizure of property and the emancipation of slaves owned by Confederates in the state of Missouri. The president feared that such a policy would alienate slaveholders who were considering switching their allegiance to the Union. Later that fall, the capture of Port Royal, South Carolina, gave license to Union soldiers to treat blacks as "contraband of war," the term implying that former southern slaves were now under the control of not southern but northern masters. The policy was an ambiguous one; it denied slaveholders their human property, but failed to recognize blacks as free people with rights.

As Union forces pushed deeper into Confederate territory, U.S. officers devised their own methods for dealing with the institution of slavery. By early 1862, the North had set its sights on the Mississippi River valley, hoping to bisect the Confederacy and cut off supplies and men bound from Texas, Arkansas, and Louisiana to the eastern seaboard. In February General Ulysses S. Grant captured Fort Henry and Fort Donelson on the Tennessee and Cumberland Rivers, the Union's first major victory of the war, and in April New Orleans fell to Admiral David Farragut. In New Orleans, General Benjamin Butler attempted to retain the loyalty of Unionist slaveholders by returning runaway slaves to them. This policy was not always greeted with enthusiasm within Union ranks. A Massachusetts soldier, restless under the command of an officer sympathetic to "slave catching brutes," vowed, "I never will be instrumental in returning a slave to his master in any way shape or manner."

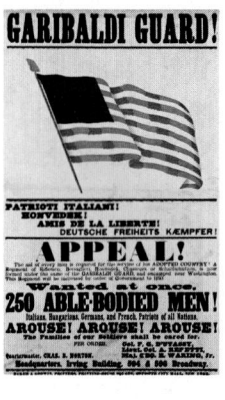

Butler also inflamed local Confederates with his "Woman Order" of May 15, 1862, which held that any woman caught insulting a Union soldier should be considered a prostitute and treated as such. As far away as the British House of Commons, members of Parliament condemned the "infamous" conduct of Butler toward what they considered respectable American ladies.

The Ravages of War: The Summer of 1862

In the summer of 1862, the South suffered a hemorrhaging of its slave population, as the movement of Union troops up and down the eastern seaboard opened the floodgates to runaways. In August a group of Liberty County, Georgia, planters claimed that 20,000 slaves (worth $12 to $15 million) had absconded from coastal plantations, many of them holding "the position of Traitors, since they go over to the enemy & afford him aid and comfort" by providing information and erecting fortifications.

Yet over the course of the summer the Confederacy persevered on the battlefield, aided by the failure of Union armies to press their advantage. In June General George McClellan was turned back on the outskirts of Richmond, convincing Lincoln not only of the incompetence of his chief general but also of the value of a less forgiving approach toward the South. In July, intending to pursue a more aggressive strategy against the massive southern military force, Lincoln brought back the boastful General John Pope from the western campaign ("where we have always seen the backs of our enemies") to command the 50,000-man Army of the Potomac.

The second battle of Manassas in late August pitted Pope and the ridiculed "Tardy" George McClellan against Lee and Jackson. (Among Jackson's footsoldiers in that battle were New Orleans's Pelican Company F, a veritable "congress of nations" including native speakers of German, French, and Spanish.) Within five days the Union force had suffered 16,000 casualties (out of 65,000 men), whereas 10,000 men in Lee's smaller force of 55,000 had been killed or wounded.

The summer of 1862 highlighted the difficulties faced by both sides in fighting a war during warm weather (when roads were passable) in the southern swamps and lowlands. More deadly than bullets and cannon to troops were diseases, especially diarrhea, dysentery, typhoid, pneumonia, and malaria. These killers affected major campaigns, including the failed Union attempt to capture Vicksburg in July. Languishing in the swamps near Richmond, one Union soldier wrote in his diary, "The Army is full of sick men."

In September, Lincoln sent Pope back west to battle on another front. Republican policies related to western homesteads and railroads, combined with a general Union lust for territory, were having a devastating impact on western Indian tribes. The Santee Sioux of Minnesota resented the encroachment of white settlers and the failure of the federal government to make good on pledges of annuity payments and food. Said one white trader, "So far as I am concerned, if they are hungry let them eat grass or their own dung." That particular

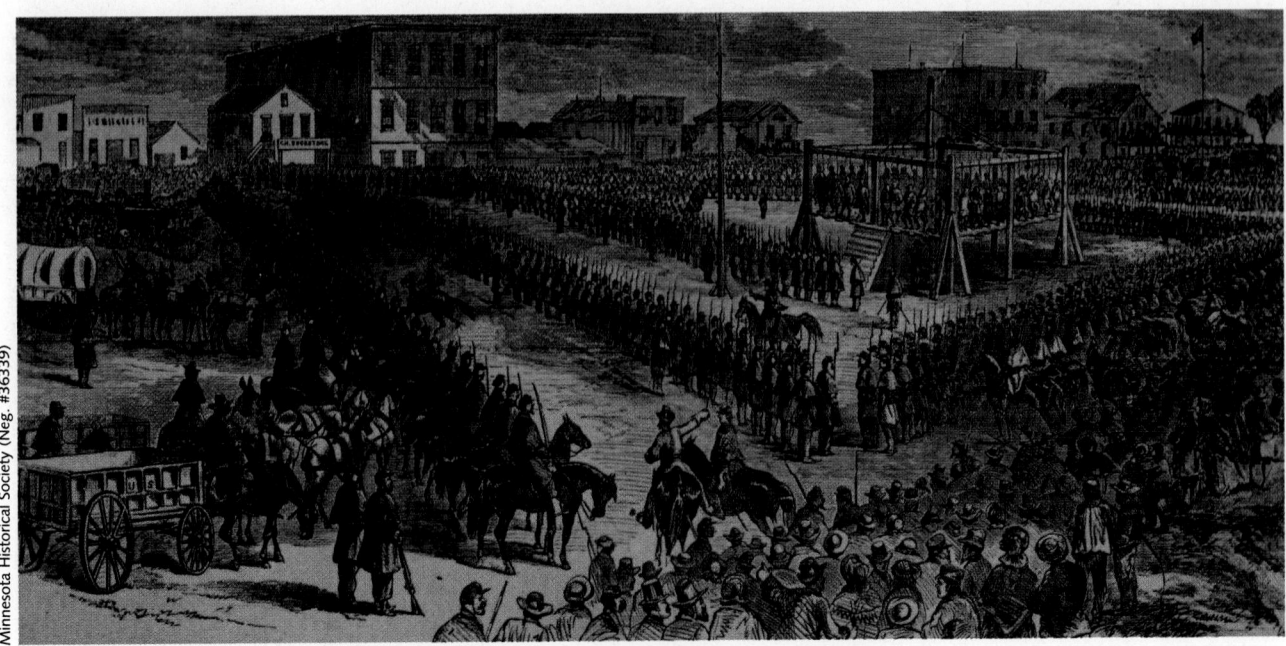

Minnesota Historical Society (Neg. #36339)

■ This lithograph, published in 1883, shows the execution of 38 Minnesota Sioux at Mankato, Minnesota, on December 26, 1862. A crowd of European Americans gathers to watch the hangings. Men with wagons are ready to cart away the corpses. During August 1862, all of southern Minnesota had been engulfed in conflict between the Sioux and rural homesteaders. After the suppression of the uprising, U.S. officials forced the surviving Sioux into reservations in present-day South Dakota.

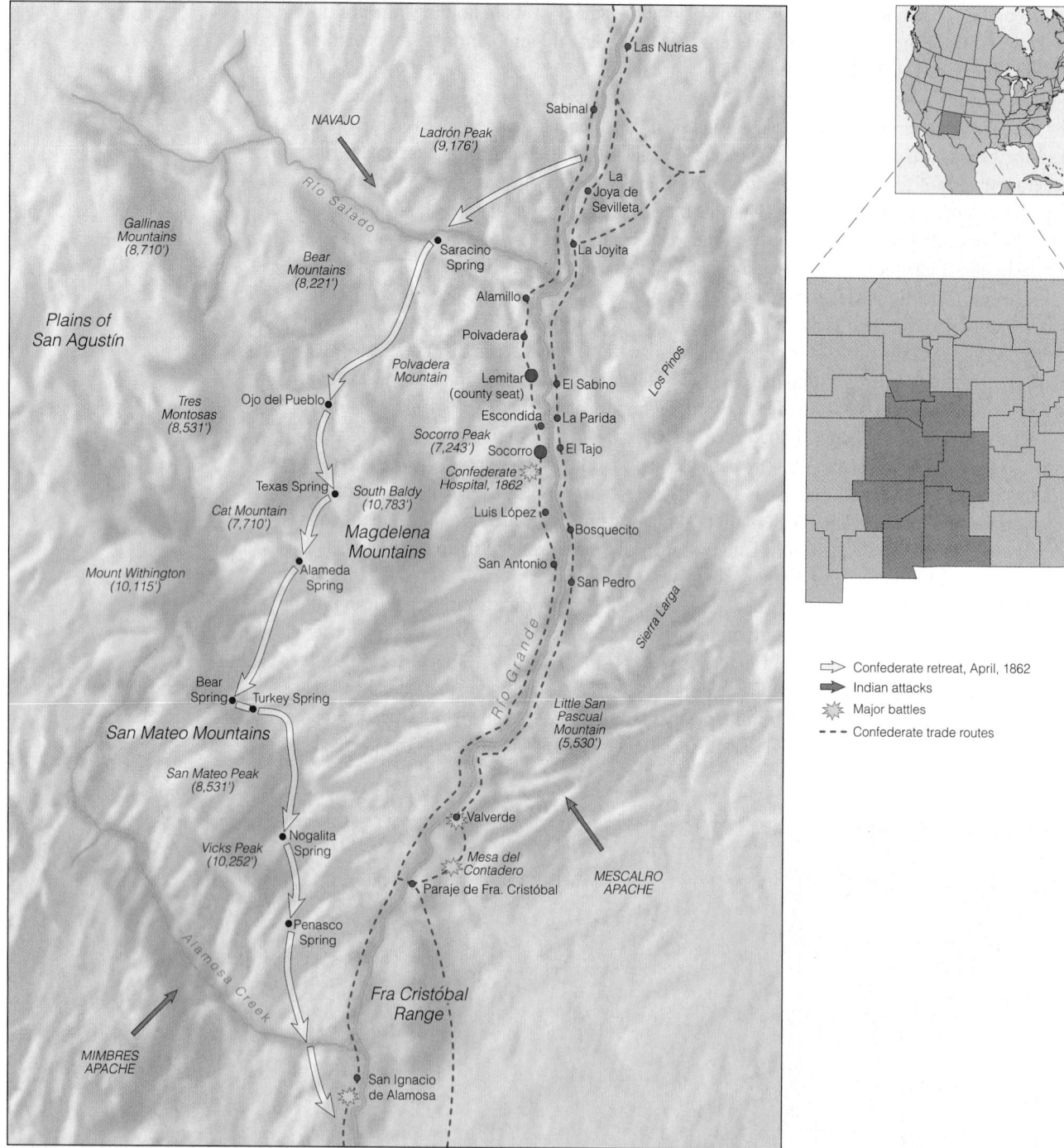

NAVAJO

Ladrón Peak
(9,176')

Las Nutrias

Sabinal

La Joya de Sevilleta

La Joyita

Río Salado

Gallinas
Mountains
(8,710')

Bear
Mountains
(8,221')

Saracino
Spring

Alamillo

Polvadera

*Plains of
San Agustín*

Polvadera
Mountain

Lemitar
(county seat)

El Sabino

Los Pinos

Tres
Montosas
(8,531')

Ojo del Pueblo

Escondida

La Parida

Socorro Peak
(7,243')

Socorro

El Tajo

Confederate
Hospital, 1862

Texas Spring

South Baldy
(10,783')

Luis López

Cat Mountain
(7,710')

*Magdalena
Mountains*

Bosquecito

Mount Withington
(10,115')

Alameda
Spring

San Antonio

San Pedro

Sierra Larga

Bear
Spring

Turkey Spring

San Mateo Mountains

Little San
Pascual
Mountain
(5,530')

San Mateo Peak
(8,531')

Río Grande

Vicks Peak
(10,252')

Nogalita
Spring

Valverde

Mesa del
Contadero

MESCALRO
APACHE

Penasco
Spring

Paraje de Fra. Cristóbal

Alamosa Creek

*Fra Cristóbal
Range*

MIMBRES
APACHE

San Ignacio
de Alamosa

Legend:
⇨ Confederate retreat, April, 1862
➡ Indian attacks
✸ Major battles
--- Confederate trade routes

■ MAP 14.3
MESCALERO APACHES BATTLE CONFEDERATES, CENTRAL NEW MEXICO, 1861   The Confederates hoped to conquer all of the Southwest for slavery. In the summer of 1861, a force led by Colonel John R. Baylor invaded the Mesilla Valley in New Mexico Territory. The Southerners scored a series of notable successes until defeated at La Glorieta Pass, a battle called the Gettysburg of the West, in March 1862. Besieged by Apache and Navajo Indians, the Confederates retreated from New Mexico.

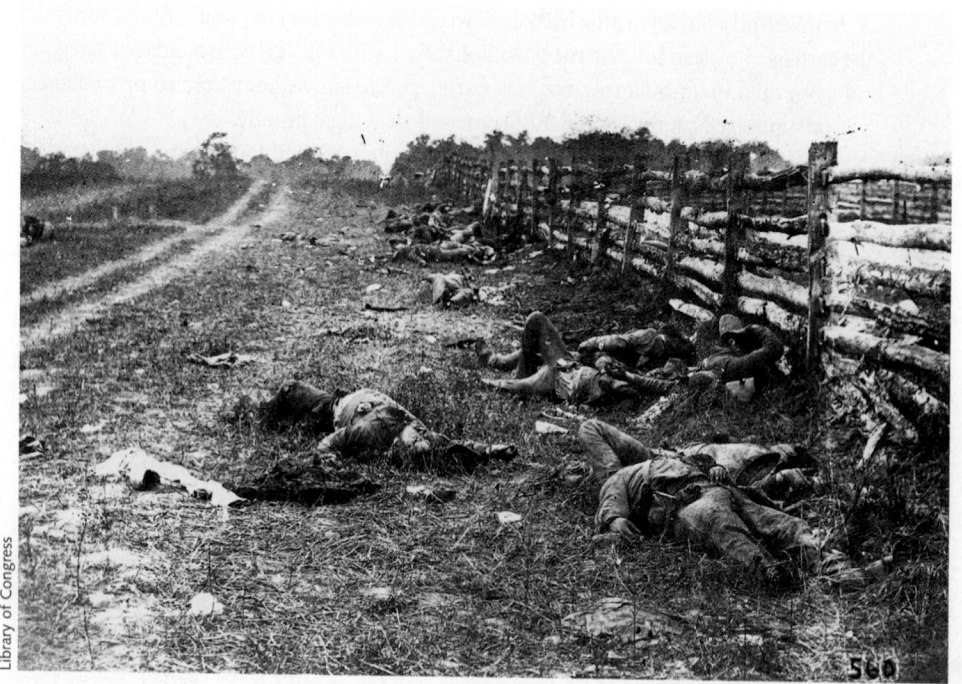

Library of Congress

■ The bodies of soldiers lie where they fell on September 17, 1862, the single day that claimed the largest number of lives in the Civil War. Like many other battles of the war, this one was shaped by the physical features of the battlefield itself, with soldiers on both sides seeking cover in small groves of trees and behind rocks, road ruts, and fences made of stone and wood.

comment helped ignite an uprising among the Sioux, who killed 500 whites before the Minnesota state militia quashed the rebellion at Wood Lake in the fall of 1862. The 38 Indian insurgents hanged by the U.S. Army in December 1862 constituted the largest mass execution in American history.

In other parts of the country the Yankee war against the Confederates spilled over into savage campaigns against Indian tribes. General James H. Carleton routed the Texas Confederates, who had been occupying New Mexico and Arizona, and then provided what he called a "wholesome lesson" to the Mescalero Apache and Navajo who had been menacing Spanish American "placitas" (communities) in the area. Sending his troops out to locate the Mescaleros, Carleton ordered, "The men are to be slain whenever and wherever they can be found. Their women and children are to be taken prisoner." Union soldiers captured Apache leader Mangas Colorado and later murdered him (although he had surrendered under a white flag). The Mescaleros were forced to accept reservation status at Bosque Redondo in the Pecos River Valley. Meanwhile, Colonel Kit Carson conducted a campaign of terrorism against the Navajos, burning *hogans* and seizing crops and livestock, claiming that "wild Indians could be tamed." Many of the survivors undertook the "Long Walk" to Bosque Redondo, a forced march reminiscent of the Cherokees' Trail of Tears a generation before.

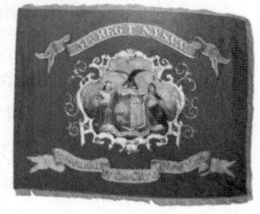

In the East, on the banks of Antietam Creek, in northern Virginia, on September 17, the bloodiest single day of the war claimed 20,000 lives and resulted in a Union victory, although it was a dubious victory indeed. Part of the battle took place in a 30-acre cornfield, where Confederates had hidden themselves. Observing the tips of southerners' bayonets glistening in the sunlight, General Joseph Hooker and his men mowed them down with firepower "as the grass falls before the scythe," in the words of a newspaper reporter present at the slaughter. The corpses mingled among the cornstalks presented a grisly sight. Nevertheless, Hooker recalled of the encounter, "The conduct of my troops was sublime, and the occasion almost lifted me to the skies, and its memories will ever remain near me."

To journalists and soldiers alike, battles could offer stirring sights of long rows of uniformed men arrayed against each other, their arms at the ready, regimental flags unfurled in the wind. Yet for the women of Shepardstown, Maryland, left to clean up after the Antietam slaughter, there was no talk of the glory of war, only a frantic, round-the-clock effort to feed the Confederates and

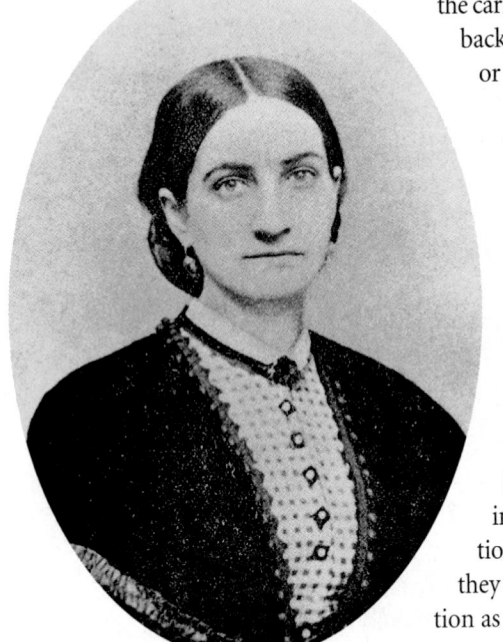

Kate Cumming of Mobile, Alabama, earned the gratitude of the Confederacy for her work as a hospital matron during the war. Before and during the Civil War, many people believed that respectable women should not work in hospitals. Physicians claimed that women were likely to faint at the sight of blood and that they were not strong enough to turn patients over in their beds. Yet as the war progressed, more and more northern and southern women defied these stereotypes and served in hospitals as nurses, administrators, and comforters of the ill and dying. Noted Cumming soon after she first entered a hospital, "The foul air from this mass of human beings at first made me giddy and sick, but I soon got over it." Still, in southern hospitals, soldiers and enslaved workers handled much of the direct patient care.

bind their wounds. Surveying the battlefield wreckage, one observer, Maria Blunt, lamented the carnage: the dead but also men "without arms, with one leg, with bandaged sides and backs; men in ambulances, wagons, carts, wheelbarrows, men carried on stretchers or supported on the shoulder of some self-denying comrade."

Maria Blunt was not alone in challenging gender conventions that decreed that nursing the wounded and comforting the dying in wartime was too gruesome a task for a woman. All over the South white women established temporary hospitals in barns, private homes, and churches and mourned each human sacrifice to the cause: "A mother—a wife—a sister had loved him." In the summer of 1862, Richmond contained 21,000 wounded Confederates, some of them attended by Sally Louisa Tompkins, commissioned a captain in the Confederate army to facilitate the work of her infirmary.

The extraordinarily high casualty rate in the war stemmed from several factors. Confederates and Federals alike fought with new kinds of weapons (rifles and sharpshooters accurate at up to 1000 yards) while troops massed in old-style (that is, close) formation. Soft minie balls punctured and lodged in limbs, leading to high rates of amputation that in turn fostered deadly infections. One Alabama soldier observed in 1862, "I believe the Doctors kills more than they cour [cure]." In fact, twice as many Civil War soldiers died of disease and infection as were killed in combat.

The Emancipation Proclamation

Appalled by the loss of life but heartened by the immediate outcome of Antietam, Lincoln took a bold step. In September he announced that on January 1, 1863, he would proclaim all slaves in Confederate territory free. The wording of the Emancipation Proclamation itself suggested that Lincoln intended to bolster northern morale by infusing the conflict with moral purpose and at the same time to further the Union's interests on the battleground by encouraging Southern blacks to join the U.S. army: "And upon this act, sincerely believed to be an act of justice, warranted by the Constitution, upon military necessity, I invoke the considerate judgment of mankind, and the gracious favor of almighty God." The measure left slavery intact in the loyal Border States and in all territory conquered by the Union. Consequently, nearly 1 million black people were excluded from its provisions. Skeptical of the ability of blacks and whites to live together, Lincoln remained committed to the colonization of freed blacks outside the United States (in Central America or the West Indies).

In the congressional elections of 1862, the Democrats picked up strength in New York, Pennsylvania, and Ohio and carried Illinois. The lower Midwest in general harbored large numbers of Democrats who opposed the war (especially now that it was an "abolition war") and called for peace with the South; these so-called Copperheads disrupted Union enlistments and encouraged military desertions.

As the death toll climbed higher and higher, dissent in the North continued to grow. The Emancipation Proclamation electrified abolitionists, but the war effort was taking its toll among the laboring classes. Especially aggrieved were the working people who paid higher taxes (relative to those paid by the wealthy) to keep the war machine running, and the dockworkers and others who lost their livelihoods when trade with foreign countries ceased. Their resentment boiled over in the summer of 1863.

Persistent Obstacles to the Confederacy's Grand Strategy

From the beginning of the war, the North's effort to blockade 3500 miles of southern coastline met with fierce resistance on the high seas. The South made up in resourcefulness what it lacked in a navy, relying for supplies on swift steamers manned by privateers (British arms smuggled onto remote southern beaches could bring up to 700 percent in profits). Seemingly invincible Confederate ships such as the ironclad *Merrimack* and the well-fortified British-built warships *Alabama* and *Florida* prowled the southeastern seaboard, sinking Union vessels and protecting the blockade runners. Nevertheless, by December 1861, Union forces had established beachheads in Confederate territory up and down the East Coast.

In November 1861 Union naval forces intercepted a British packet ship, the *Trent,* and seized two Confederate diplomats, James Mason and John Slidell, who were en route to London and Paris, where they planned to plead the South's case in a bid to gain diplomatic recognition. To avoid a rift with England, Lincoln and Secretary of State William H. Seward released the two men. In the process Mason and Slidell lost whatever influence they might have had with European governments, and Lincoln enjoyed the praise of the British public for his moderation in handling the so-called *Trent* affair.

More generally, Confederate hopes for diplomatic recognition foundered on the shoals of European politics and economics, in England and in the Western Hemisphere. English textile mills drew on their own immense prewar stockpiles of raw cotton and sought out new sources of fiber in Egypt and elsewhere. Also, English workers flexed their political muscle in a successful effort to forestall recognition of the slaveholders' nation. Textile workers in particular did not want to compete with slave-produced material manufactured in an independent Confederacy.

Early in the war the Confederates recognized the strategic importance of Mexico, both as a trade route for supplies and as a means of access to ports. (Moreover, an estimated 2500 Hispanics fought for the South, among them the Cuban-born Loreta Janeta Velásquez, who disguised herself as a man and joined the Confederate army under the name of Lt. Harry T. Buford.) In approaching Mexican President Benito Juarez for aid in late 1861, Confederate envoy John T. Pickett discovered that, although Mexicans still smarted from their defeat on their own land 13 years before, the Juarez administration remained an ally of the United States. However, another Confederate agent, Juan A. Quintero, did manage to win a trade agreement with the governor of a northern Mexican state, Santiago Vidaurri of Nuevo León.

By the summer of 1862, Britain and France were inclined to mediate peace in favor of Confederate independence, for the two powers assumed that the South's impressive

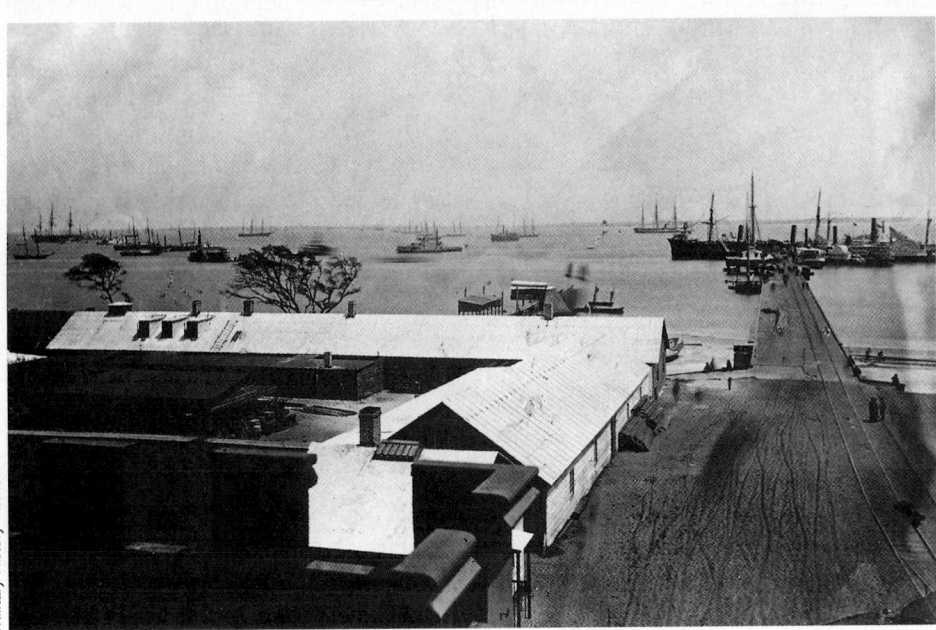

Massachusetts Commandery, Military Order of the Loyal Legion and the U.S. Army Military History Institute

■ Union ships moored at Hilton Head, South Carolina.

victories in Virginia and Tennessee signaled a quick end to the war. Nevertheless, the Confederacy's autumn setbacks of Antietam and Perryville (in Kentucky), combined with ennobling rhetoric of the soon-to-be-announced Emancipation Proclamation, proved that the Union was still very much alive, and the diplomatic recognition the white South so desperately craved remained elusive.

The Other War: African American Struggles for Liberation

From the onset of military hostilities, African Americans, regardless of whether they lived in the North or the South, perceived the Civil War as a fight for freedom. Although they allied themselves with Union forces, they also recognized the limitations of Union policy in ending slavery. Therefore, blacks throughout the northern and southern states were forced to take action to free themselves as individuals, families, and communities. Twenty-year-old Charlie Reason recalled his daring escape from a Maryland slave master and his decision to join the famous 54th Massachusetts Infantry composed of black soldiers: "I came to fight *not* for my country, I never had any, but to gain one." Soon after the 54th's assault on Fort Wagner (outside Charleston Harbor) in July 1863, Reason died of an infection contracted when one of his legs had to be amputated. In countless ways, black people throughout the South fought to gain a country on their own terms.

Enemies Within the Confederacy

In late 1863 a U.S. gunboat picked up 13 black fugitives off the coast of Georgia. Included in the group were the leader, Cain, as well as Bella and her 6-year-old son, Romeo; Lizzie and her four children (ages 5 months to 12 years); and Sallie with four children ranging in age from 7 months to 11 years. Within a few weeks Cain had returned to the mainland to rescue his kinfolk, including Grace and her five children, Grace's son-in-law, Charlie, and her four grandchildren. These groups of self-liberated slaves were like countless others; their ranks were dominated by women and children, for many black men were either "refugeed" farther inland by their masters (to keep them out of the clutches of the Yankees) or fighting in the Union army.

Like the Revolutionaries of 1776, slaveholding whites were shocked when they could not always count on the loyalty of "petted" domestics. Soon after the war began, South Carolina's Mary Boykin Chesnut had expressed unease about the enigmatic behavior of one of her trusted house slaves, Laurence, asking herself of all her slaves, "Are they stolidly stupid or wiser than we are, silent and strong, biding their time?" A few months later Chesnut's cousin was murdered while sleeping, bludgeoned by a candlestick; the cousin's slaves William and Rhody were charged with the crime. Of her own mulatto servant, one of Chesnut's women friends remarked, "For the life of me, I cannot make up my mind. Does she mean to take care of me—or to murder me?" Now rising to the surface, such fears put whites on alert, guarding against enemies in their midst.

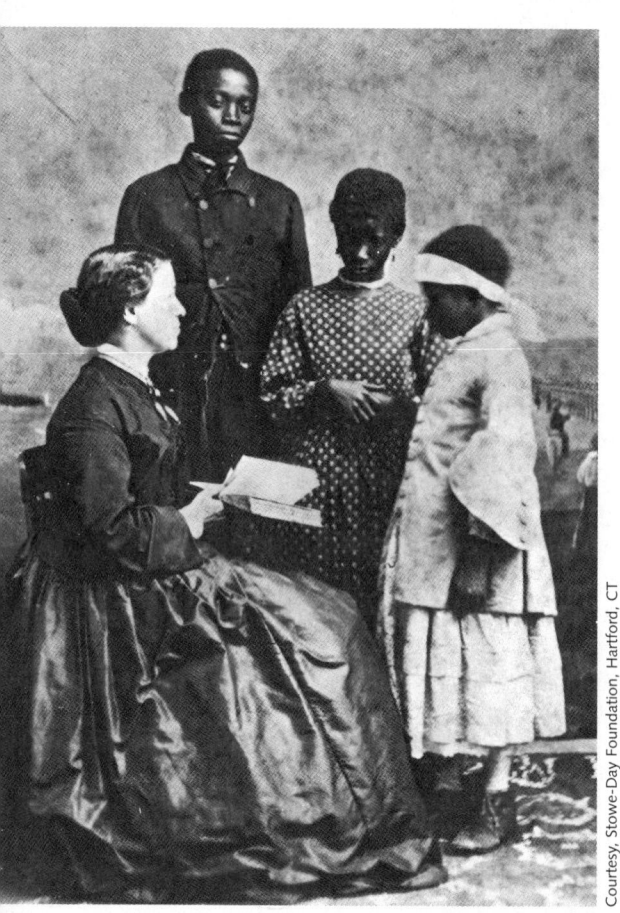

Courtesy, Stowe-Day Foundation, Hartford, CT

■ Laura Towne and three of her pupils pose for a picture on Saint Helena Island, South Carolina, in 1866. A native of Pennsylvania, Towne traveled to the South Carolina Sea Islands in April 1862, soon after they were occupied by Union forces. She and her companion and fellow teacher Ellen Murray represented the hundreds of idealistic northern women who volunteered to teach southern black people of all ages during and after the Civil War. Declared Towne on her arrival in the South, "We've come to do antislavery work, and we think it noble work and mean to do it earnestly."

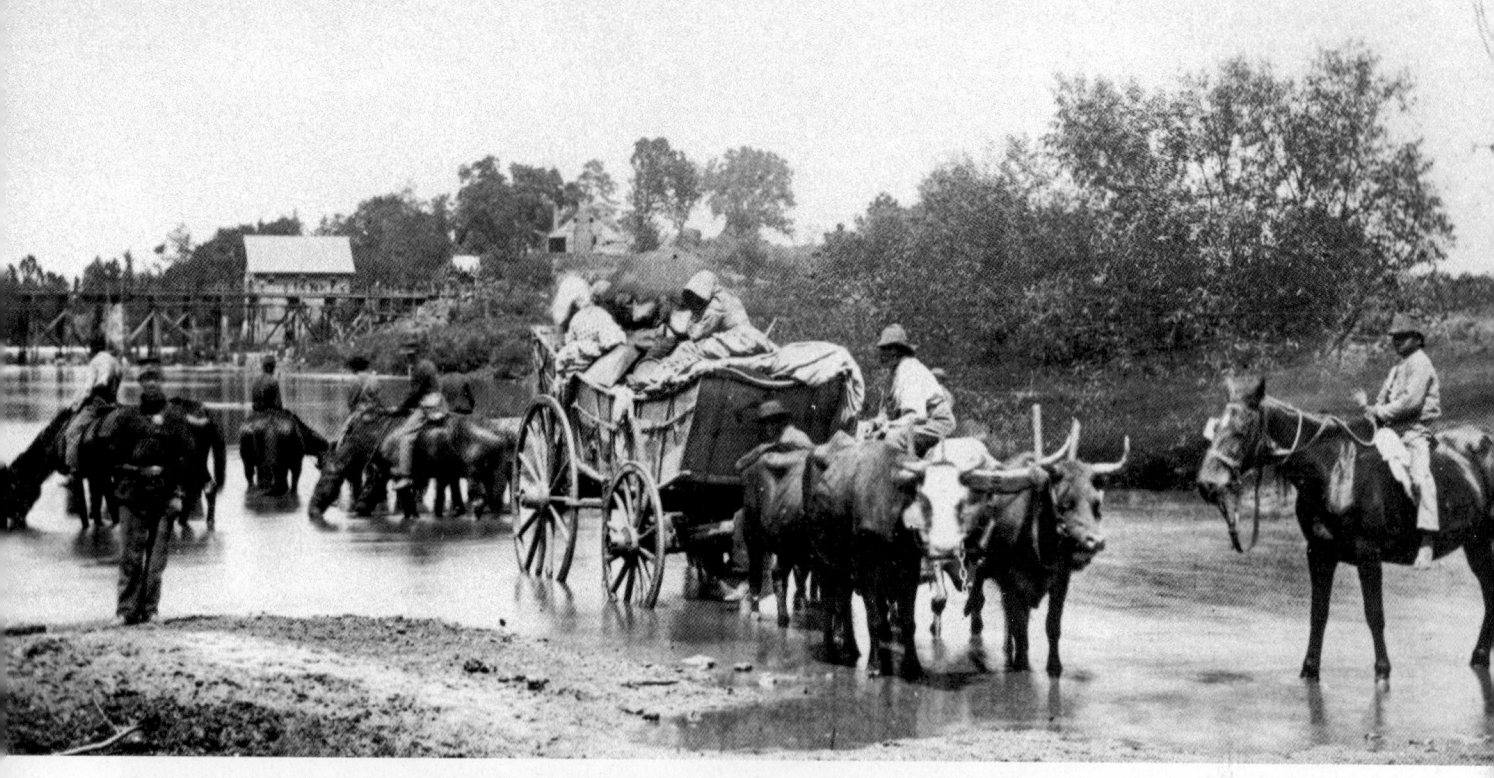

■ All over the South, black people watched and waited for opportunities to claim their own freedom. The movement of Union troops into an area often prompted slaves to flee from the plantation. Individuals and extended families sought safety behind Union lines or in nearby towns or cities or began the quest for long-lost loved ones.

Yet no single white man or woman could halt the tide of freedom. Given the chance to steal away at night or walk away boldly in broad daylight, black men, women, and children left their masters and mistresses, seeking safety and paid labor behind Union lines. Throughout the South, black people waited and watched for an opportunity to flee from plantations, their actions depending on the movement of northern troops and the disarray of the plantations they lived on. In July 1862, the Union's Second Confiscation Act provided that the slaves of rebel masters "shall be deemed captives of war and shall be forever free," prompting Union generals to begin employing runaway male slaves as manual laborers. Consequently, military authorities often turned away women, children, older adults, and the disabled, leaving them vulnerable to spiteful masters and mistresses. For black men pressed into Union military and menial labor service, and for their families still languishing on plantations, "freedom" came at a high price indeed.

The Ongoing Fight Against Prejudice in the North and South

In the North, the Emancipation Proclamation spurred the enlistment of black men in the Union army and navy. The proclamation itself allowed for such recruitment. Furthermore, many black men felt inspired to join U.S. forces since the Lincoln administration had declared the conflict a war for abolition. Eventually, about 33,000 northern blacks enlisted, following the lead of their brothers-in-arms from the South. For example, in October 1862, Massachusetts's Colonel Thomas Wentworth Higginson organized a black regiment on the South Carolina Sea Islands, noting that the First South Carolina Volunteers (unlike their northern white counterparts) were "fighting for their homes and families." The subsequent formation of the famous 54th Massachusetts regiment infuriated southern military leaders, many of whom refused to recognize black men as soldiers at all.

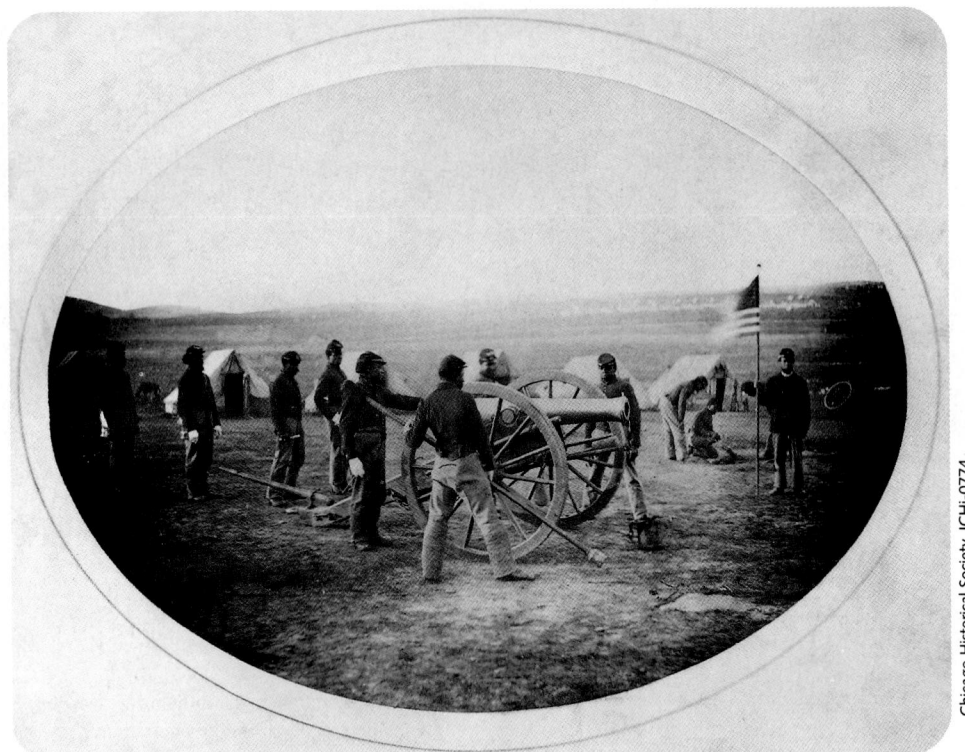

Chicago Historical Society, ICHi-0774

■ An African American regiment stands at attention in Beaufort, South Carolina. Many southern black men first experienced freedom as soldiers for the Union army. They embraced the rituals of Civil War–era manhood, including shouldering arms and participating in military dress parades. The men assigned fatigue work exclusively felt keenly the discriminatory treatment they received at the hands of white officers.

For black northern soldiers, military service opened up a wider world; some learned to read and write in camp, and almost all felt the satisfaction of contributing to a war that they defined in stark terms of freedom versus slavery. They wore their uniforms proudly. However, Northern wartime policies toward black men as enlisted men and toward black people as laborers revealed that the former slaves (as well as free people of color in the North) would continue to fight prejudice on many fronts.

Some northern whites approved recruiting blacks, reasoning that for each black man killed in battle, one white man would be spared. Until late in the war, black soldiers were systematically denied opportunities to advance through the ranks and were paid less than whites. Although they showed loyalty to the cause in disproportionate numbers compared with white men, most blacks found themselves barred from taking up arms at all, relegated to fatigue work deemed dangerous and degrading to whites. They intended to labor for the Union, but, in the words of a black soldier from New York, "Instead of the musket it is the spade and the Whelbarrow and the Axe cuting in one of the horable swamps in Louisiana stinking and misery." For each white Union soldier killed or mortally wounded, two died of disease; the ratio for blacks was one to ten.

Many northern military strategists and ordinary enlisted men showed indifference at best, contempt at worst, for the desire of black fugitives to locate lost loved ones and begin to labor on their own behalf. In the course of the war, Union experiments with free black labor—on the South Carolina Sea Islands under the direction of northern missionaries, and in Louisiana, under the direction of generals Nathaniel Banks and Benjamin Butler—emphasized converting the former slaves into staple crop wage workers under the supervision of Yankees. Some of these whites, in their eagerness to establish "order" in former Confederate territory, saw blacks only as exploitable labor—if not cannon fodder, then hands to dig ditches and grow cotton.

Many southern blacks later recalled grateful first encounters with Yankee soldiers, men who brought them the news of their freedom. But others recalled harsh treatment at the hands of the blue-coated invaders. For example, Union soldiers seized the goods that Nancy Johnson and her husband, Boson Johnson (he was "a good Union man during the war," noted his wife), had spent a lifetime accumulating as slaves on a rice plantation in Canoochie Creek, Georgia: one mare, 625 pounds of bacon, 60 pounds of lard, 12 bushels of corn, 8 bushels of rice, 7 meat hogs, 11 stock hogs, and 25 chickens.

For many blacks, the war brought a mixture of joy and fear. In her book *Reminiscences of My Life in Camp* (published in 1902), former slave Susie King Taylor recalled the heady, dangerous days of 1862, when she fled from Savannah and found refuge behind Union lines off the coast of Georgia. There she met and married Edward Taylor, and together they (along with her uncles and cousins) joined the First South Carolina Volunteers (later known as the 33rd United States Colored Cavalry). The soldiers received no pay for the first 18 months of their service, and even in camp they remained vulnerable to Confederate snipers and bushwhackers. Yet Taylor gained a great deal of satisfaction from conducting a school for black children on St. Simon's Island and performing a whole host of tasks for the fighting men, from cleaning rifles to washing clothes and tending the ill. She understood that her own contributions to the war effort showed "what sacrifices we can make for our liberty and rights."

Battle Fronts and Home Fronts in 1863

In 1863 the North abandoned the strategy of conciliation in favor of an effort to destroy the huge southern armies and deprive the Confederacy of its slave labor force. By this time the war was causing a tremendous hardship among ordinary white folk in the South. Meanwhile, Lincoln found himself caught between African American freedom fighters who resented the poor treatment they received from many white commanders and white Northerners who took their opposition to the war in general and the military draft in particular to the streets. Deprivation at home and the mounting casualty rates on the battlefields were reshaping the fabric of American society, North and South.

Disaffection in the Confederacy

The Civil War assaulted Southerners' senses and their land. Before the war, slave owners and their allies often contrasted the supposed tranquility of their rural society with the rude, boisterous noisiness of the North. According to this view, the South was a peaceful place of contented slaves toiling in the fields, whereas the North was the site of workers striking, women clamoring for the vote, and eccentric reformers delivering streetcorner harangues.

The war exploded on the southern landscape with ferocious force, and the rumble of huge armies on the march shook southern society to its foundations. For the first time many Southerners smelled the acrid odor of gunpowder and the stench of rotting bodies. They heard the booms of near and distant cannon and the mournful sounds of church bells tolling for the dead. They saw giant encampments of soldiers cover what used to be cotton fields and black people where they were not supposed to be: on the road, fleeing from their masters. Some people lived on diets of onions and berries in the absence of harvests of corn and rice. Seemingly overnight, both armies constructed gorge-spanning train trestles and huge riverside docks and warehouses, all in preparation for conflict. As soldiers withdrew from the battlefield, they left behind a scarred and blood-spattered land, cornfields mowed down, fires smoldering in their wake.

These sights and sounds were especially distressing to Southerners who objected to the war as a matter of principle or because of its disastrous effects on their own households. Scattered throughout the South were communities resistant to the policies of what many ordinary whites considered the Richmond elite—the leaders of the Confederacy. In western North Carolina a group calling themselves Heroes of America declared their loyalty to the Union. In northern Alabama, the "Free State of Jones [County]" raised troops for the Yankee army.

Throughout the rural South, army deserters were welcomed home by their impoverished wives and children; it is estimated that during much of the war, as many as one-third of all Confederate soldiers were absent without leave at any particular time.

The antebellum South had celebrated individual households as the foundation of a slaveholders' republic, but now women took the lead in putting the interests of their own families above those of the Confederacy. A letter from "Your Mary" addressed to "Dear Edward" in the service recounted their son's crying the night before: "'O mamma! I am so hungry.' And Lucy, Edward, your darling Lucy; she never complains, but she is growing thinner and thinner every day. And before God, Edward, unless you come home, we must die."

Indeed, all over the South, groups of poor women resisted the dictates of the Davis administration, wealthy men and women who flaunted an extravagant wartime lifestyle of lavish dinners and parties. Women from Virginia to Alabama protested a Confederate 10 percent "tax-in-kind" on produce grown by farmers and the food shortages that reached crisis proportions. In April 1863 several hundred Richmond women, many of them wives of Tredegar Iron Works employees, armed themselves with knives, hatchets, and pistols and ransacked stores in search of food: "Bread! Bread! Our children are starving while the rich roll in wealth." An enraged President Davis told the rioters that he would give them five minutes to disperse before ordering troops to fire on them; the women went home. In their desperation they had highlighted the contradiction between the increasingly efficient process of Confederate industrialization and the increasingly inefficient process of providing basic necessities to people on the home front.

> *During much of the war, as many as one-third of all Confederate soldiers were absent without leave at any particular time.*

Whereas some white women resisted the Confederacy, others leaped to the fore to provide essential goods and services to the beleaguered new nation. Virginia's Belle Boyd kept track of Union troop movements and served as a spy for Confederate armies. Poor women took jobs as textile factory workers, and their better-educated sisters found employment as clerks for the Confederate bureaucracy. Slaveholding women busied themselves running plantations, rolling bandages, and knitting socks for soldiers. In Augusta, Georgia, the Ladies Aid Society sewed garments for the troops, and the Augusta Purveying Association provided subsidized food for the poor. Still, many women felt their labors were in vain. Of the Confederacy's stalled progress, Georgia's Gertrude Thomas noted, "Valuable lives lost and nothing accomplished."

The Tide Turns Against the South

In the fall of 1862 Lincoln replaced General McClellan with General Ambrose E. Burnside. In December, at a major battle at Fredericksburg, Virginia, the general's blundering produced what was called Burnside's Slaughter Pen: 13,000 northern casualties, many fallen in a small area near a stone wall. One survivor described the scene: corpses "swollen to twice their natural size, black as Negroes in most cases." The ground was littered with "one without a head, . . . one without a legs, yonder a head and legs without a trunk . . . with fragments of shell sticking in oozing brain, with bullet holes all over the puffed limbs."

As the northern public tried to come to terms with these losses, Lincoln replaced Burnside with General Joseph ("Fighting Joe") Hooker. In early May 1863, Lee and Jackson encountered Hooker at Chancellorsville, Virginia; the battle left Hooker reeling, but it also claimed the life of Jackson, mistakenly shot by his own men on May 2 in the early evening twilight. The South had lost one of its most ardent champions.

Lee decided to press his advantage by invading Pennsylvania and, it was hoped, encouraging northern Peace Democrats and impressing the foreign powers. The ensuing clash at Gettysburg was a turning point in the war. Drawn by reports of a cache of much-needed shoes, Confederate armies converged on the town, in the south-central part of the state and across the border from Maryland. Union forces pursued. In a three-day battle that began on July 1, the

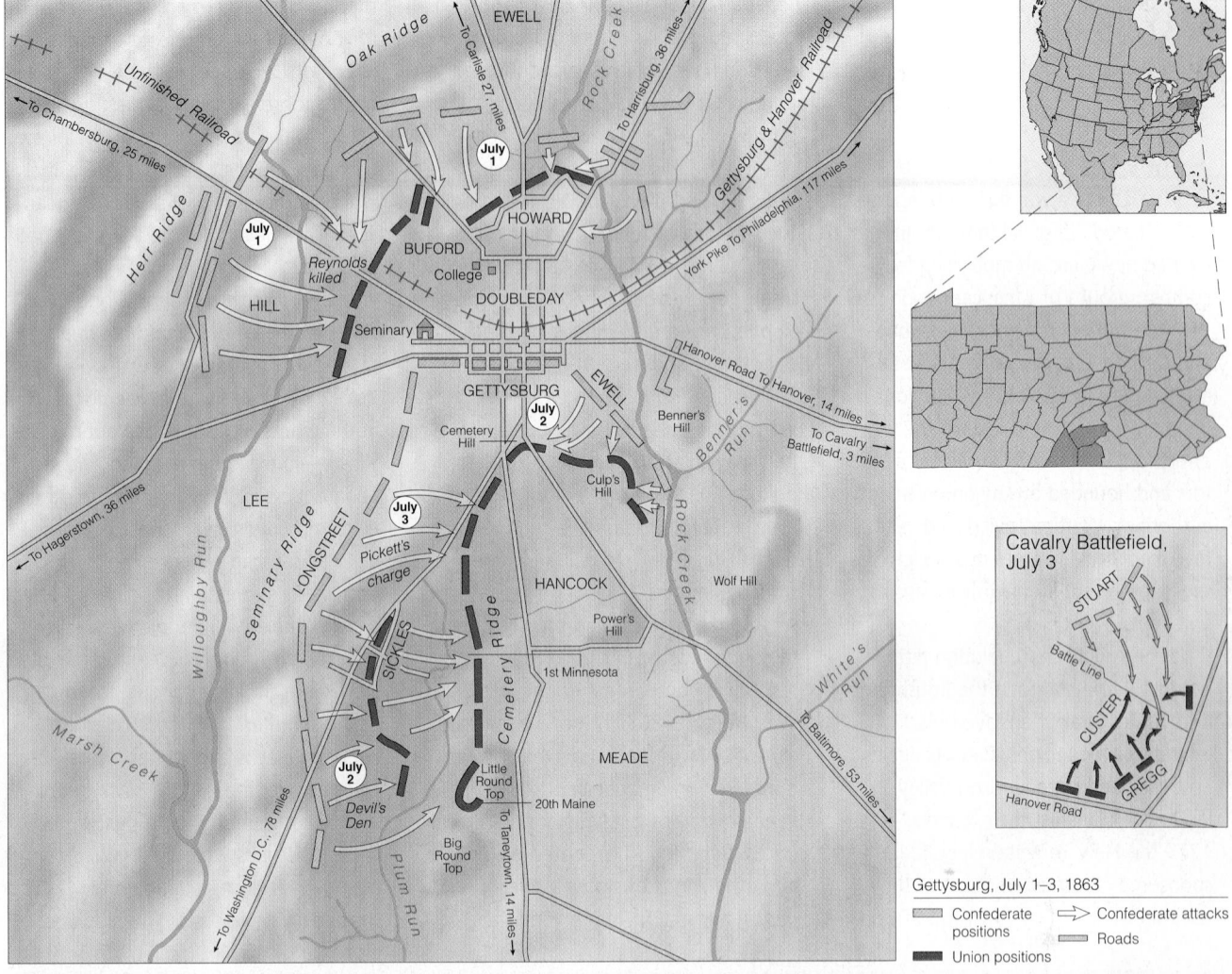

■ MAP 14.4
THE BATTLE OF GETTYSBURG, JULY 1–3, 1863 The three-day battle of Gettysburg was a turning point in the war. This map shows that Confederate soldiers made repeated assaults on Union lines. Lee's confidence in this strategy was misplaced, and some of his own staff recognized it. Recalled General James Longstreet of the third day of fighting, "My heart was heavy. I could see the desperate and hopeless nature of the charge and the hopeless slaughter it would cause. . . . That day at Gettysburg was one of the saddest of my life."

92,000 men under the command of General George G. Meade were arrayed against the 76,000 troops of Robert E. Lee.

Gettysburg later came to represent the bloody consequences of a war fought by men with modern weapons under commanders with a premodern military sensibility. On the last day of the battle, the men under Major General George Pickett moved slowly into formation, passing along the way hastily dug graves and the fragments of bodies blown to bits the day before. At 3 P.M. a mile-wide formation of 15,000 men gave the rebel yell and charged three-quarters of a mile across an open field to do battle with Union troops well fortified behind stone walls. Within half an hour Pickett had lost two-thirds of his soldiers and all 13 of his colonels. The battle's three-day toll was equally staggering: 23,000 Union and 28,000 Confederate soldiers wounded or killed. Fully one-third of Lee's army was dead or wounded.

What made men of both sides fight on under these conditions? Some remained devoted to a cause. Others cared less about the Confederacy or the Union and more about proving their

Civil Disorders During Wartime

Throughout American history, fighting a war has both exacerbated old social tensions and created new ones. In mobilizing for combat, groups of Americans expressed their resentment toward other groups and clashed with each other over the allocation of food, housing, and jobs. People who dissented against the war effort found themselves branded as traitors and hounded by law enforcement authorities. Wartime civil disorders thus reveal political faultlines in a society that seeks to present a united front against an enemy.

The American Revolution pitted not just Patriots against the British but also whites against enslaved blacks, whites against Indians, Patriots against Loyalists, and large Hudson Valley landowners against their tenants. In 1779 the New York state legislature sponsored an armed invasion of the territory occupied by the Iroquois Con-federacy, leading to the destruction of that group's villages and crops. In the Hudson Valley, New England interior, and port towns of Massachusetts, groups of women confronted merchants, demanded an end to price gouging, and then seized the staples they needed to feed their families.

During the War of 1812, political disagreements between Democratic-Republicans and Federalists spilled over into bloodshed. In Baltimore, Republican mobs, enraged by the antiwar policies of a leading Federalist newspaper, attacked several of their political foes, three of whom died. A fourth, Revolutionary War hero Henry (Light Horse Harry) Lee, later died from his injuries.

Both the North and the South had to contend with violence on their respective home fronts during the Civil War. In April 1863, in the Confederate capital of Richmond, a crowd of several hundred women appealed to the Virginia governor for relief from high food prices. Rebuffed, they looted bakeries and other kinds of stores as well. President Jefferson Davis intervened and threatened the women with violence if they did not disperse. A few weeks later, riots broke out in the North as white laborers, many of them Irish immigrants, protested the new Union draft law of July 1. In New York City, workers turned their wrath on African Americans, leaving more than 100 people dead.

Civil disorders during World War I revealed the contradiction between mobilizing for a modern war—a war to "make the world safe for democracy," in the words of President Woodrow Wilson—on the one hand and maintaining racial segregation on the other. At Camp Logan near Houston, Texas, in 1917, African American soldiers protested segregationist policies. In the ensuing melee, 20 people were killed and 100 arrested. Nineteen black soldiers were convicted and later hanged. In the summer of 1919, 26 clashes between blacks and whites broke out in cities all over the nation. Black people sought to exercise their rights as free citizens. Whites were determined to maintain racial segregation and white supremacy at all costs. The bloodiest

manhood and upholding their family's honor. Still others sought to memorialize comrades slain in battle or to conform to standards of discipline drilled into them. A survivor of Pickett's charge downplayed his own courage: "Instead of burning to avenge the insults of our country, families and altars and firesides . . . the thought is . . . *Oh,* if I could just come out of this charge safely how thankful *would I be!*"

The Union victory at Gettysburg on July 3 brought rejoicing in the North. The next day General Ulysses S. Grant captured Vicksburg on the Mississippi River, a move that earned him the rank of lieutenant general (conferred by Congress). Within a year he assumed the position of supreme commander of the Union armies.

Civil Unrest in the North

Yet not all segments of northern society joined in the celebration. Even principled supporters of the Union war effort were growing weary of high taxes and inflated consumer prices, not to mention the sacrifices of thousands of husbands, sons, and brothers. In May, federal soldiers had arrested the defiant and outspoken Copperhead Clement Vallandigham at his home in Dayton, Ohio. Subsequently convicted of treason (he had declared the conflict "a war for the freedom of blacks and the enslavement of whites"), Vallandigham was banished to the South.

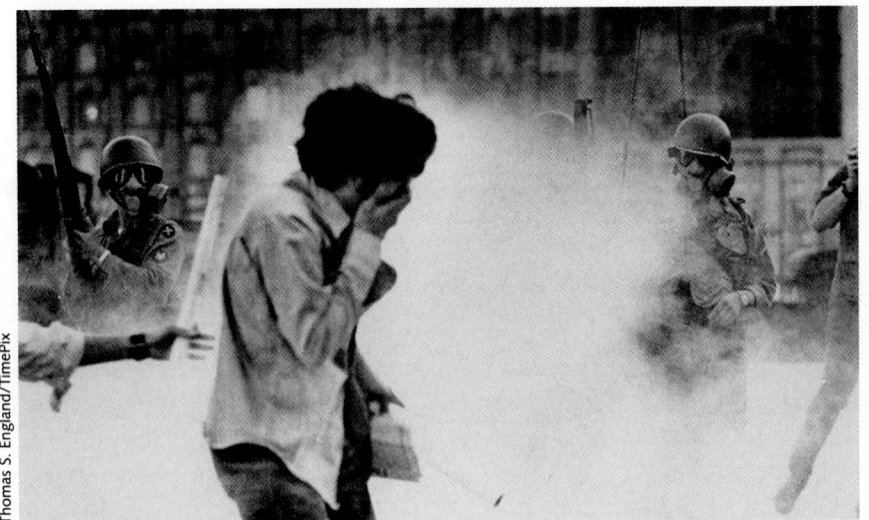

U.S. domestic uprisings during Vietnam war

strators and police. In the summer of 1968 in Chicago, protesters sought to disrupt the Democratic National Convention. Under orders from Mayor Richard Daley, police attacked the demonstrators with tear gas and billy clubs. In the two-year period from 1969 to 1970, radical student groups carried out or attempted 174 campus bombings of Reserve Office Training Corps offices, launching a violent campaign in protest of government war policies.

In the fall of 2001, in response to the attacks on the World Trade Center and the Pentagon, the United States began to wage an aggressive war against terrorists in Afghanistan and elsewhere in the world. Americans overwhelmingly supported this effort and, for the most part, the tactics used to fight it. Protests against specific Bush administration policies, such as the decision to use military tribunals to try certain people accused of terrorism, took the form of legal challenges, candlelight vigils, and newspaper opinion editorial pieces, not bloody riots in the streets. ■

riot was in Chicago, where 38 people were killed.

In World War II, blacks in Harlem launched a civil rebellion in 1943 in response to systematic discrimination in the defense industry. Elsewhere, white mobs attacked people of color who did not conform to traditional standards of submissiveness and deference. In June 1943, white soldiers in Los Angeles beat black and Mexican American

youth, especially those wearing the zoot suits that were fashionable among urban Chicanos then. That same year, Detroit whites and blacks battled each other over limited housing space and job opportunities. The riots left 34 dead and 675 injured and resulted in 1 million hours of lost defense work.

Between 1965 and 1973, opposition to the Vietnam War precipitated violent encounters between demon-

Following a military draft imposed on July 1, the northern white working classes erupted. Enraged at the wealthy who could buy substitutes, resentful of the Lincoln administration's high-handed tactics, and determined not to fight on behalf of their African American competitors in the workplace, laborers in New York City, Hartford, Troy, Newark, and Boston (many of them Irish) went on a rampage. The New York City riot of July 11–15 was especially savage as white men directed their wrath against black men, women, and children. Members of the mob burned the Colored Orphan Asylum to the ground and then mutilated their victims.

A total of 105 people died before five Union troops were brought in to quell the violence. The regiments from Pennsylvania and New York were fresh from the Gettysburg battlefield; now they trained their weapons on citizens of New York City. In response to the rioting and to discourage other men from resisting the draft elsewhere, the federal government deployed 20,000 troops to New York. On August 19, the draft resumed.

The Desperate South

Meanwhile, the South had to contend not only with dissent and disaffection at home but also with the stunning battle and territorial losses it suffered at Gettysburg and Vicksburg. On August 21, Jefferson Davis proclaimed a day of "fasting, humiliation and prayer." Throughout the

Occupation	Failed to Report	Exempted for Cause	Commuted or Hired Substitue	Held to Service
Unskilled Laborer	25%	45%	24%	6%
Skilled Laborer	25%	44%	22%	9%
Farmer and Farm Laborer	16%	34%	31%	19%
Merchant, Manufacturer, Banker, Broker	23%	46%	29%	2%
Clerk	26%	48%	24%	2%
Professional	16%	49%	29%	6%

■ **FIGURE 14.3**
OHIO MEN DRAFTED FOR MILITARY SERVICE WHO REPORTED FOR DUTY OR HIRED SUBSTITUTES

faltering Confederacy white clergy exhorted their congregations to pray for God's mercy. Gone were the confident declarations that "God is on our side"; in their place were the self-doubts of generals and the wails of widows and fatherless children.

Even as Davis was invoking the name of the Almighty, 450 rebels under the command of William Clarke Quantrill were destroying the town of Lawrence, Kansas (long a hotbed of abolitionist sentiment), and killing 150 of its inhabitants. With the exception of Quantrill and John Singleton Mosby (whose squads of men roamed northern Virginia attacking Union posts and troops in 1863), Confederate military leaders shunned guerrilla warfare, preferring to meet the enemy on a field of honor. The desperate Quantrill raid on Lawrence demonstrated that the Confederate cause was, if not lost, then losing in the late summer of 1863.

Before the year was out Davis faced other setbacks as well. In January the French army occupied Mexico City, and the next year Mexican elites, with the aid of the French Emperor Napoleon III, placed Austrian Archduke Maximilian on the throne. With Mexico as part of the French Empire, Napoleon III hoped to use the country as a pawn in his scheme to spread his influence throughout Europe. Still, Grant's successes at Missionary Ridge and Lookout Mountain, in Tennessee, caused both France and England to draw back from offering overt support to the Confederacy in the form of sales of navy warships or diplomatic recognition. The Confederate president had long counted on securing the support of the great European powers; now those hopes were dashed.

Dedicating the national cemetery at Gettysburg on November 19, 1863, Lincoln delivered a short address that affirmed the nation's "new birth of freedom" and its commitment that "the government of the people, by the people, for the people, shall not perish from the earth." Meanwhile, Grant, the hero of Vicksburg, was poised at the border of northern Georgia, ready to push south to the sea and cut in half what was left of the Confederacy.

The Prolonged Defeat of the Confederacy, 1864–1865

By 1864 northern generals, with Lincoln's blessing, had decided to fight a "hard war" against their tenacious enemy. Union troops were authorized to live off the land (denying southern civilians the necessities of life in the process), to seize livestock and other supplies indiscriminately, and to burn everything that the Confederates might find useful. The purposes of this strategy were twofold: to harm irreparably (what was left of) Confederate morale and to facilitate the movement of northern troops through hostile territory. If north-

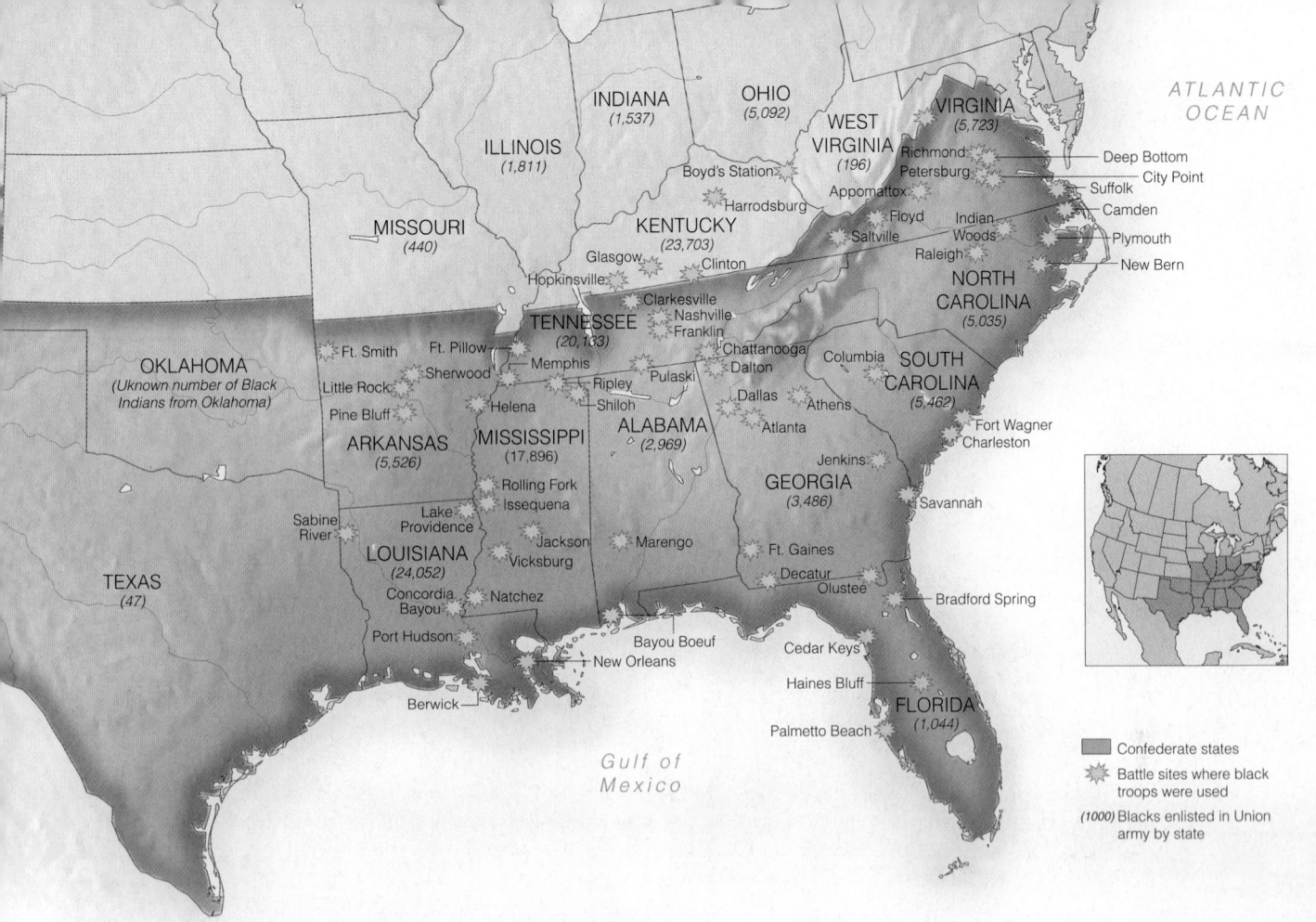

■ **MAP 14.5**

AFRICAN AMERICANS IN CIVIL WAR BATTLES, 1863–1865 Confederates killed African American soldiers captured in battle at Fort Wagner in Charleston Harbor (1863), the Union garrison of Fort Pillow on the Mississippi River (1864), and Petersburg, Virginia (1864), among other battles. By the end of the war, black men had fought in more than 200 battles. Their performance in combat no doubt contributed to the Confederate decision to arm slaves as soldiers in the last few weeks of the war.

ern troops could sever the area west of Georgia from the Confederacy and take Richmond and destroy its surrounding armies, the Union would be safe at last.

White Men's "Hard War" Toward African Americans and Indians

The policy of "hard war" should not be confused with total war, characterized by state-approved terrorism against civilians. However, Confederate policies toward black soldiers and Union policies toward Indian insurgents in the West did show elements of total war against particular segments of the population. In April 1864 Confederate General Nathan Bedford Forrest destroyed Fort Pillow, a Union garrison on the Mississippi River. After surrendering, black soldiers were systematically murdered. Wounded survivors were bayoneted or burned to death. Among southern generals, conventions of war (providing for the detention and exchange of prisoners of war) did not apply to African American soldiers.

Nor were Indian combatants and civilians accorded even the minimal respect shown to most white fighting men. In the early fall of 1864, a group of Cheyenne and Arapaho were camped along Sand Creek in the southeastern corner of Colorado. Black Kettle, a chief of the Cheyenne, had received promises from Union Col. John M. Chivington and others stationed at Camp Weld in Denver that the two sides would remain at peace with each other. Therefore, on the morning of November 29, 1864, when Black Kettle saw Chivington leading a Colorado volunteer militia toward his settlement, he waved a white flag and stood his ground.

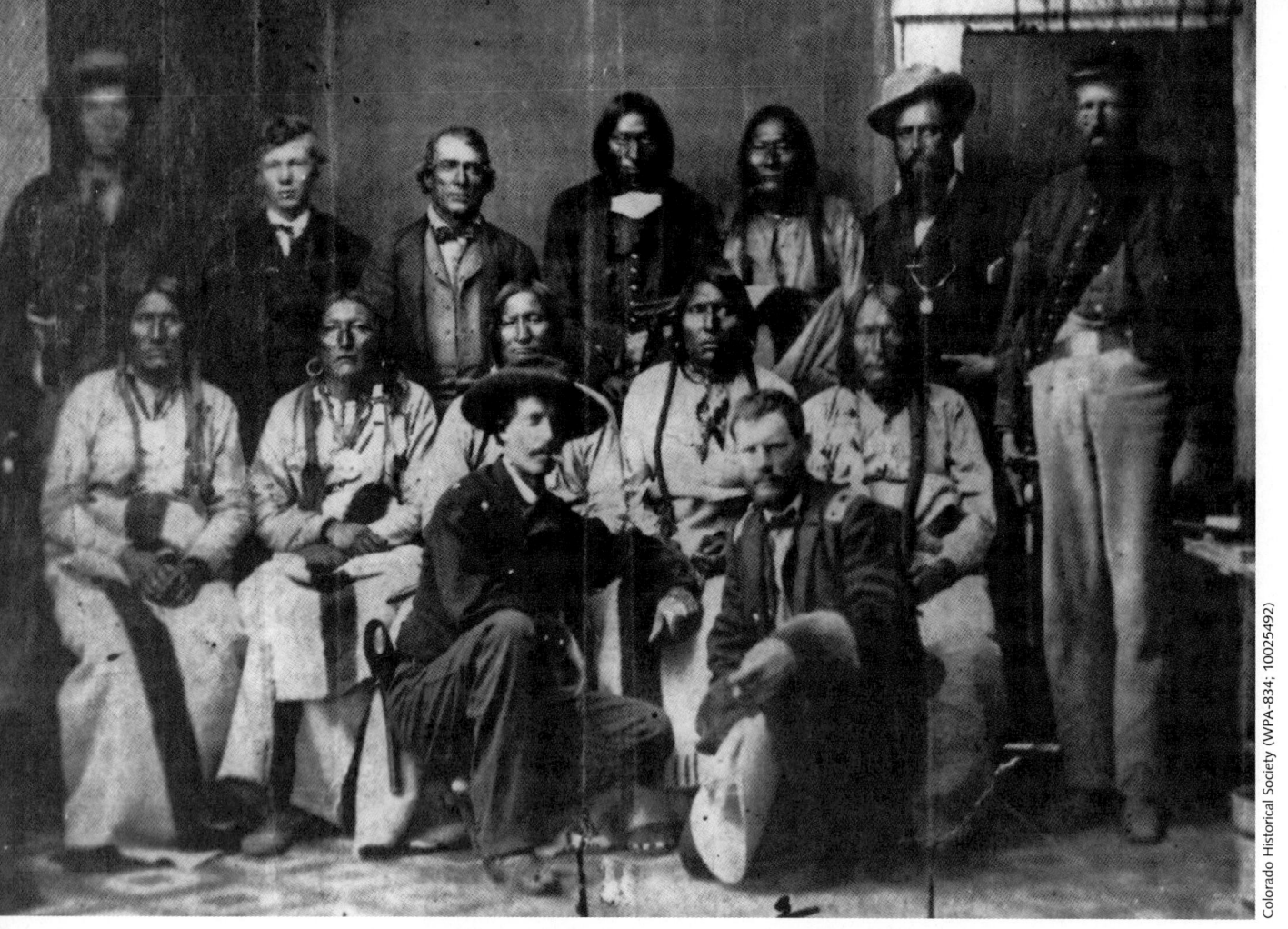

■ In September 1864, the Indian chiefs Black Kettle and White Antelope, with other Cheyenne and Arapaho leaders, met with Colonel John M. Chivington at Camp Weld, Colorado. The purpose of the meeting was to secure a truce between the Indians and European Americans in the area. Two months later, Chivington attacked an encampment of these Indians on the banks of Sand Creek, about 100 miles southeast of Denver.

Chivington did not come in peace. That day he and his men massacred 125 to 160 Indians, mostly women, children, and old people, returning later to mutilate the bodies. In response, the Sioux, Arapaho, and Cheyenne launched their own campaigns on the white migrants traveling the South and North Platte trails. Chivington declared that it was "right and honorable" to use any means to kill Indians, including children ("nits make lice," he said). Captain Silas Soule, who rode with Chivington but refrained from killing innocent civilians on principle, later testified against the colonel during a military investigation in early 1865; walking on the streets of Denver one day, Soule was murdered by a Chivington supporter.

"Father Abraham"

Lincoln's wartime policies consisted of a calculated indifference toward the life and liberties of Native Americans on one hand and a noble defense of the principles of democratic government among white men on the other. The election of 1864 proceeded without major incident, although Lincoln himself faced some opposition within his own party. Together with his new running mate, a former slave owner from Tennessee named Andrew Johnson, Lincoln benefited from a string of preelection victories won for him by Admiral David G. Farragut at Mobile, Alabama, and by General Philip Sheridan in Virginia's Shenandoah Valley. As a result, he defeated the Democratic nominee, his own former general, George McClellan, who managed to garner 45 percent of the popular vote. One of the keys to Lincoln's success was the "peace platform" that the Democrats had drafted at their convention the summer before;

support among Union soldiers for "Little Mac" dropped precipitously as a result, and Lincoln won three-quarters of the army's vote.

Despite his limited military experience, Lincoln possessed a strategic sense superior to that of many of his generals. He played down his own military experience, making light of his minor part in the Black Hawk War of 1832; in that conflict, he reminisced, he had engaged in

TABLE 14-1			
The Election of 1864			
Candidate	Political Party	Popular Vote	Electoral Vote
Abraham Lincoln	Republican	2,213,655	212*
George B. McClellan	Democratic	1,805,237	21

*Eleven secessionist states did not participate.

"charges upon wild onions . . . [and] bloody struggles with the Musquetoes." However, he cared deeply about ordinary soldiers and talked with them whenever he had the opportunity. In return, Union troops gave "Father Abraham" their loyalty on the battlefield and, especially during the election of 1864, at the ballot box.

The Last Days of the Confederacy

Meanwhile, the transformation of the Confederacy—from a loose collection of agrarian states to a centralized war machine—was almost complete, and so the Confederacy itself, as a republic of slaveholders, was doomed. In September 1864 Lee, anxious for troops, had convinced Secretary of War James A. Seddon to impress 20,000 slave men and all free men of color and to organize them into military-like units. By December, only 1200 had been put to work and 800 had run away.

Some slaveholders were acknowledging the "mechanical genius" of their slaves, an argument against pressing them into Confederate service as manual laborers, but an implicit argument in favor of their use as soldiers. If black men were intelligent beings, then they could become disciplined military troops, so this (new) Confederate reasoning held. In January 1865 Lee admitted that the fate of the Confederacy depended on black labor, not only as skilled artisans but as soldiers as well. He noted that the best way to attract men to any "service which imposes peculiar hardships and privations" was to ensure that they had a personal interest in the outcome: "Such an interest we can give our negroes by giving immediate freedom to all who enlist, and freedom at the end of the war to the families of those who discharge their duties faithfully (whether they survive or not), together with the privilege of residing at the South." The South had shifted its cause from the preservation of slavery to the preservation of the Confederacy, with or without slavery.

Union General William Tecumseh Sherman's forces overtook Atlanta in September 1864 and swept southeast toward the coast, living off the land and denying Confederate soldiers and civilians alike food and supplies along the way. En route to Savannah, Sherman's men liberated Andersonville Prison, a 26-square-acre Confederate camp that held 33,000 prisoners in the summer of 1864. Unable to feed their own armies and so unwilling to commit large supplies of food to the prison, the Confederate commander, Henry Wirz, stood by while 13,000 died of starvation, disease, and exposure. (Wirz was the only Confederate officer to be tried, convicted, and executed for war crimes by the U.S. government.) Among the freed prisoners was Payson Wolfe, who had served with Michigan's Company K, an all-Indian company of sharpshooters. Wolfe returned home to Michigan but never fully recovered from the time he spent at Andersonville.

Northerners expressed outrage over Andersonville. However, considering conditions at Bosque Redondo, New Mexico, their denunciations had the ring of hypocrisy. This settlement was an internment camp for Apache and Navajo survivors of the campaign initiated against them in 1862; by spring of 1864 some 10,000 people were confined there, an estimated quarter of whom died before they were allowed to return home in 1868.

After presenting Lincoln with the "Christmas gift" of Savannah in December, Sherman took his 60,000 troops north, slogging through swamps and rain-soaked terrain to confront

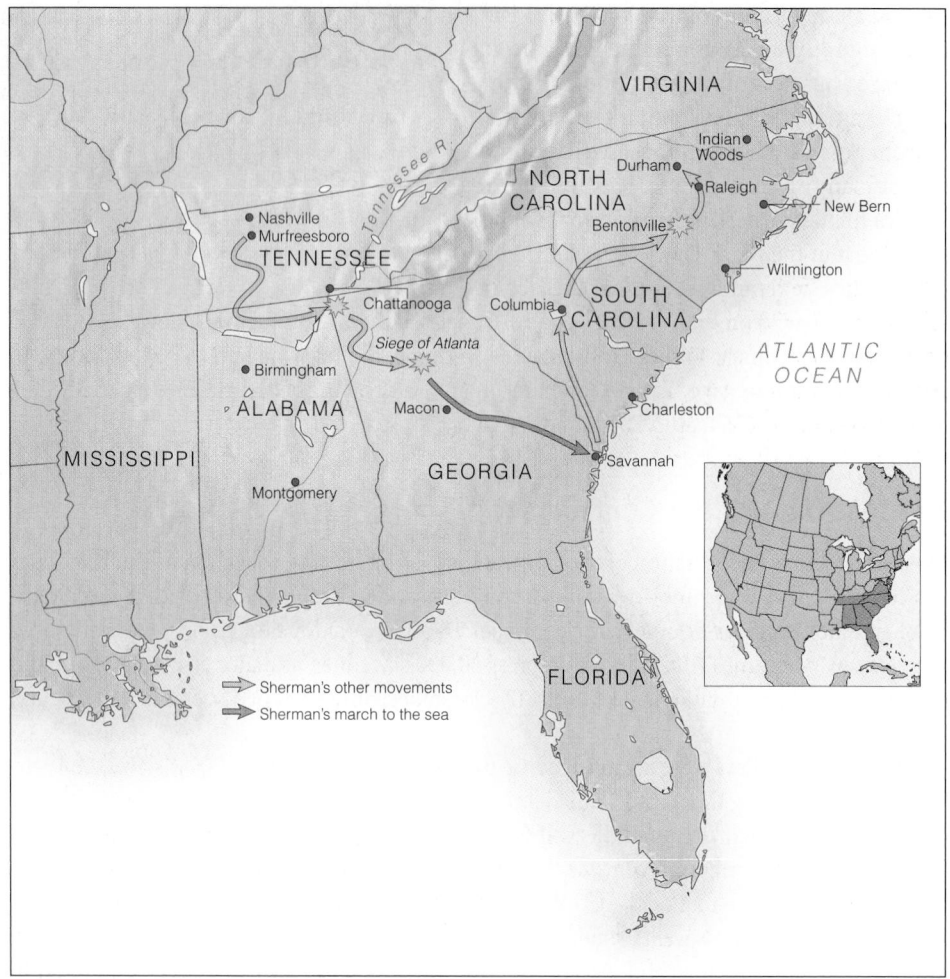

■ MAP 14.6
SHERMAN'S MARCH TO THE SEA, 1864–1865   General William T. Sherman's famous march to the sea marked the final phase of the Union effort to divide and conquer the Confederacy. Sherman's men burned Atlanta to the ground in September 1864. In late December they made their triumphant entry into the city of Savannah. Sherman followed a policy of "hard war" in these final months of the war; he ordered his troops to seize from civilians any food and livestock they could use and to destroy everything else, whether rail lines, houses, or barns. White Southerners expressed outrage over these tactics. Still, Sherman never systematically attacked civilians, a characteristic of the Union's "total war" against Native American peoples in the West.

the original secessionists. Later, he recalled with satisfaction, "My aim then was to whip the rebels, to humble their pride, to follow them to their inmost recesses, and make them fear and dread us." By mid-February, the state capital, Columbia, was in flames. African American troops were among the triumphant occupiers of the charred city.

In his second inaugural address, delivered March 4, 1865, Lincoln declared that the Almighty had rendered final judgment on the abomination that was slavery. The president vowed that the North would persevere "until all the wealth piled by the bondsman's two hundred and fifty years of unrequited toil shall be sunk, and until every drop of blood drawn with the lash shall be paid by another drawn with the sword."

By early April, Grant had overpowered Lee's army in Petersburg, Virginia. Withdrawing, Lee sent a telegram to Davis, who was attending church in Richmond, warning him that the fall of the Confederate capital was imminent. Davis and almost all other whites fled the city. Arriving in Richmond on April 3, only hours after the city had been abandoned, was the commander-in-chief of the Union army, Abraham Lincoln. Lincoln calmly walked the streets of the smoldering city (set afire by departing Confederates), flanked by a group of ten sailors. Throngs of black people greeted the president, exclaiming, "Glory to God! Glory! Glory! Glory!" When a black man kneeled to thank Lincoln, the president said, "Don't kneel to me. That is not right. You must kneel to God only, and thank Him for the liberty you will enjoy hereafter."

On April 9, Lee and his demoralized and depleted army of 35,000 men found themselves outnumbered by Grant and Meade, and Lee surrendered his sword at Appomattox Courthouse in northern Virginia. Lee had rejected a plea by one of his men that the army disband and continue to fight a guerrilla war in the woods and hills. The general predicted that such a force "would become mere bands of marauders," destroying the countryside and with it what was left of the fabric of southern society.

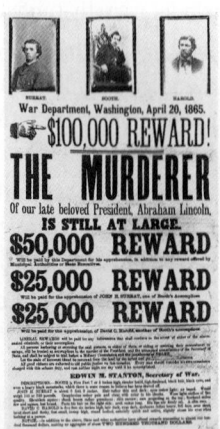

Union officials ensured rebel soldiers protection from future prosecution (for treason) and allowed the cavalry to keep their horses for use in spring planting. These policies were remarkably lenient treatment for traitors. Indeed, a sight on the day of the Confederate surrender suggested that Northerners would pay the defeated Confederates grudging respect. The ragtag members of the so-called Stonewall Brigade, men who had entered the war with Stonewall Jackson four years before, came forward to lay down their arms. In recognition, the Union army gave them a salute of honor, one group of fighting men acknowledging the bravery of another. However, this scene set the stage for the not-too-distant future, when the North and South reaffirmed their ties based on a shared "whiteness" in opposition to African Americans.

Watching a comedy with his wife, Mary, at Ford's Theater in Washington on the night of April 14, Lincoln was one of the last casualties of the war. Shot by John Wilkes Booth, a Confederate loyalist fearful that the president was bent on advancing "nigger citizenship," Lincoln lingered through the night but died the next morning. Booth himself was caught and shot within a matter of days. Of the departed president, Secretary of State Seward said, "Now he belongs to the ages."

Conclusion

Rather than asking why the South lost the Civil War, we might wonder why it took the North four years to win it. Despite all the political dissent and social conflict in the white South, despite the crumbling of the institution of slavery and the lack of support from the European powers, the Confederacy was able to mobilize huge armies under the command of brilliant tacticians such as Lee and Jackson. The war was fought on the battlefield by regiments of soldiers, not on the sea by navies or in the countryside by guerrillas. Therefore, as long as Confederate generals could deploy troops and outwit their foes during brief but monumental clashes, the Confederacy could survive to fight another day. The South had as its immediate goal the slaughter of as many Yankees as possible. Meanwhile, the North staggered under the weight of mobilizing large numbers of men in enemy territory and supplying those men with the necessary resources far from home.

In terms of lives lost (620,000), the Civil War was by far the costliest in the nation's history. (The death toll among American military personnel in the Revolution was 26,000; in World War I, 116,000; in World War II, 400,000; in Vietnam, 58,000.) At the end of the war, the Union was preserved and slavery was destroyed. Yet, in their quest for true freedom, African Americans soon learned that military hostilities were but one phase of a wider war, a war to define the nature of American citizenship and its promise of liberty and equality. Thus April 1865 marked not so much a final judgment as a transition to new battlefields.

Sites to Visit

The Valley of the Shadow: Living the Civil War
Pennsylvania and Virginia
jefferson.village.virginia.edu/vshadow/vshadow.html
> This project tells the histories of two communities on either side of the Mason–Dixon line during the Civil War. It includes narrative and an electronic archive of sources.

The Civil War in Charleston, South Carolina
www.awod.com/gallery/probono/cwchas/cwlayout.html
> This site covers the history of the Civil War in and around Charleston.

Abraham Lincoln Association
www.alincolnassoc.com/
> This site includes digital versions of Lincoln's papers.

United States Civil War Center
www.cwc.lsu.edu/
> Maintained by Louisiana State University, this site aims to promote the study of the Civil War by making available "all appropriate private and public data" related to the conflict.

Civil War Women
scriptorium.lib.duke.edu/collections/civil-war-women.html
> This Duke University library site includes original documents, links, and biographical information about several women and their lives during the Civil War.

Library of Congress Civil War Documents
and Photographs
memory.loc.gov/ammem/
> This Library of Congress site includes a wealth of texts and images related to the history of the Civil War.

Civil War Timeline
www.historyplace.com/civilwar/index.html
> This site offers a comprehensive Civil War timeline that includes photographs.

National Civil War Association
www.ncwa.org/
> This site documents the activities of one of the many Civil War reenactment organizations in the United States.

For Further Reading

General

David Herbert Donald, *Lincoln* (1995).

Edward Hagerman, *The American Civil War and the Origins of Modern Warfare* (1988).

Herman Hattaway and Archer Jones, *How the North Won: A Military History of the Civil War* (1980).

James M. McPherson, *Battle Cry of Freedom: The Civil War Era* (1988).

Reid Mitchell, *Civil War Soldiers: Their Expectations and Experiences* (1988).

Clarence Mohr, *On the Threshold of Freedom: Masters and Slaves in Civil War Georgia* (1986).

Mobilization for War, 1861–1862

Gabor Borit, ed., *Lincoln's Generals* (1994).

Drew Gilpin Faust, *The Creation of Southern Nationalism: Ideology and Identity in the Civil War South* (1988).

Joseph L. Harsh, *Confederate Tide Rising: Robert E. Lee and the Making of Southern Strategy, 1861–62* (1998).

Wilfrid Knight, *Red Fox: Stand Watie and the Confederate Indian Nations During the Civil War Years in Indian Territory* (1988).

Alan Nolan, *Lee Considered: General Robert E. Lee and Civil War History* (1991).

George Rable, *The Confederate Republic: A Revolution Against Politics* (1994).

Ralph Wooster, *The Secession Conventions of the South* (1962).

The Course of War, 1862–1864

Stephen Ash, *When the Invaders Came: Conflict and Chaos in the Occupied South, 1861–1865* (1996).

Howard Jones, *The Union in Peril: The Crisis over British Intervention in the Civil War* (1992).

Elizabeth Leonard, *All the Daring of the Soldier: Women of the Civil War Armies* (1999).

Heather Cox Richardson, *The Greatest Nation on Earth: Republican Economic Policies During the Civil War* (1997).

Stephen Sears, *Landscape Turned Red: The Battle of Antietam* (1983).

Emory Thomas, *The Confederacy as a Revolutionary Experience* (1991).

Lee Ann Whites, *The Civil War as a Crisis in Gender: Augusta, Georgia, 1860–1890* (1995).

The Third War: African American Struggles for Liberation

Ira Berlin et al., *Freedom: A Documentary History of Emancipation: Series 1, Vol. I: The Destruction of Slavery;* Series 2: *The Black Military Experience* (1982).

Ira Berlin and Leslie Rowland, eds., *Families and Freedom: A Documentary History of African-American Kinship in the Civil War Era* (1997).

Robert F. Engs, *Freedom's First Generation: Black Hampton, Virginia, 1861–1890* (1979).

Jacqueline Jones, *Labor of Love, Labor of Sorrow: Black Women, Work, and the Family Since Slavery* (1985).

William S. McFeely, *Frederick Douglass* (1991).

Willie Lee Rose, *Rehearsal for Reconstruction: The Port Royal Experiment* (1964).

Battle Fronts and Home Fronts in 1863

Stephen V. Ash, *Middle Tennessee Society Transformed, 1860–1870: War and Peace in the Upper South* (1988).

Iver Bernstein, *The New York City Draft Riots: Their Significance for American Society and Politics in the Age of the Civil War* (1990).

Paul D. Escott, *Many Excellent People: Power and Privilege in North Carolina, 1850–1900* (1985).

Drew Gilpin Faust, *Mothers of Invention: Women of the Slaveholding South in the American Civil War* (1996).

J. Matthew Gallman, *The North Fights the War: The Home Front* (1994).

Frank Klement, *Dark Lanterns, Secret Political Societies, Conspiracies, and Treason in the Civil War* (1990).

Mark M. Smith, *Listening to Nineteenth-Century America* (2001).

The Prolonged Defeat of the Confederacy, 1864–1865

Michael B. Ballard, *A Long Shadow: Jefferson Davis and the Final Days of the Confederacy* (1997).

Richard Beringer et al., *Why the South Lost the Civil War* (1986).

Ernest Furgurson, *Ashes of Glory: Richmond at War* (1996).

Joseph Glatthaar, *The March to the Sea and Beyond: Sherman's Troops in the Savannah and Carolina Campaigns* (1985).

Mark Grimsley, *The Hard Hand of War: Union Military Policy Toward Southern Civilians, 1861–1865* (1995).

James M. McPherson, *For Cause and Comrades: Why Men Fought in the Civil War* (1997).

J. Tracy Power, *Lee's Miserables: Life in the Army of Northern Virginia from the Wilderness to Appomattox* (1998).

Online Practice Test

Test your understanding of this chapter with interactive review quizzes at

www.ablongman.com/jonescreatedequal/chapter14

Additional Photo Credits

Page 463: Chicago Historical Society, ICHi—22172

Page 465: The Museum of the Confederacy, Richmond, Virginia (CT #495b). Photograph by Katherine Wetzel

Page 475: University of Oklahoma, Western History Collections, Phillips Collection (#1459)

Page 478: Collection of The New-York Historical Society, Acc. #41526

Page 481: (Top) Confederate Memorial Hall, New Orleans, photo by John R. Miller; (bottom) New York Division of Military & Naval Affairs

Page 482: Courtesy, The Museum of the Confederacy, Richmond Virginia

Page 485: Library of Congress

Page 497: The National Park Service

In the Wake of War: Consolidating a Triumphant Union, 1865–1877

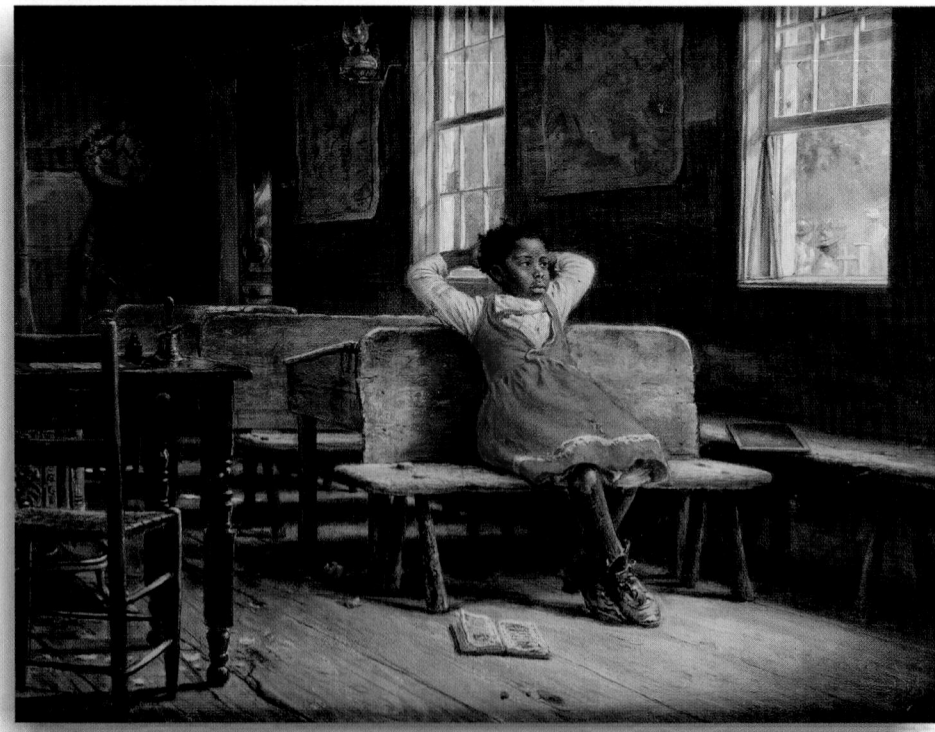

Edward Lamson Henry, *Kept In*, 1889. Fenimore Art Museum, Cooperstown, New York (N-309.61). Photo by Richard Walker

■ The artist Edward L. Henry titled this 1888 painting *Kept In*. A pupil endures her punishment while her classmates frolic outside during recess. Former slaves of all ages eagerly embraced the opportunity to learn to read and write, and many African American communities established their own schools after the war. Some Northerners, mostly young white women, traveled south to teach the freedpeople.

IN SAVANNAH, GEORGIA, IN MID-DECEMBER 1864, AFRICAN AMERICAN MEN, WOMEN, AND children rejoiced when the troops of Union General William Tecumseh Sherman liberated the city: the day of jubilee had come at last! The city's black community immediately formed its own school system under the sponsorship of a new group, the Savannah Education Association (SEA). The association owed its creation to the desire of freedpeople of all ages to learn to read and write. A committee of nine black clergy began by hiring 15 black teachers and acquiring buildings (including the Old Bryan Slave Mart) for use as schools. By January 1, 1865, Savannah blacks had raised $800 to pay teachers' salaries, enabling several hundred black children to attend classes free of charge.

Following hard on the heels of the Union army, a group of northern white missionaries arrived in Savannah to seek black converts for two Protestant denominations, the Presbyterians and the Congregationalists. On the first day of school, in January 1865, these northern newcomers watched a grand procession of children wend its way through the streets of Savannah. The missionaries expressed amazement that the SEA was an entirely black-run organization; these whites had believed the former slaves incapable of creating such an impressive educational system.

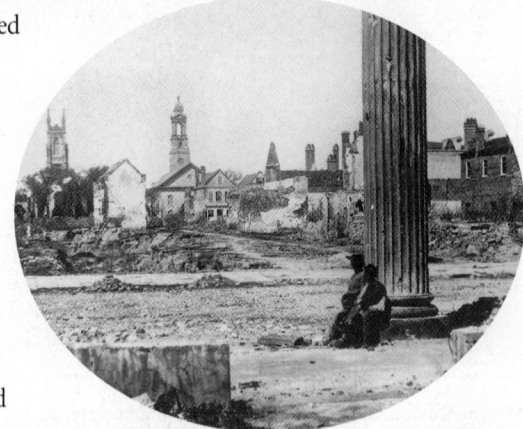

Charleston, South Carolina, after Sherman's 1865 siege.

In March 1865, the federal government, under the auspices of the newly formed Bureau of Refugees, Freedmen, and Abandoned Lands (Freedmen's Bureau), agreed to work with missionaries in opening schools for black children throughout the former Confederate states. In Georgia, missionaries and government officials soon became alarmed that black leaders were willing to accept financial aid from them but not willing to relinquish control of SEA schools to the whites in return. The Northerners were also distressed by the militancy of certain local black leaders. One of these leaders was Aaron Bradley, who, armed with a pistol and bowie knife, was urging other black men to vote as a bloc in all elections.

In an effort to wrest control of the SEA from Savannah blacks, northern missionaries and agents of the Freedmen's Bureau decided to withhold funds from the association. By March 1866, these efforts had paid off: The city's black community, swollen by a refugee population, was no longer able to support its own schools. Northern whites took over SEA operations, and the association ceased to exist.

Postwar political interest in the South unleashed a major conflict between supporters of African American rights and supporters of southern privilege. Republican congressmen hoped to *reconstruct* the South by enabling African Americans to own their own land and to become full citizens. Southern freedpeople sought to free themselves from white employers, landlords, and clergy and to establish control over their own workplaces, families, and churches. In contrast, President Andrew Johnson appeared bent on *restoring* the antebellum

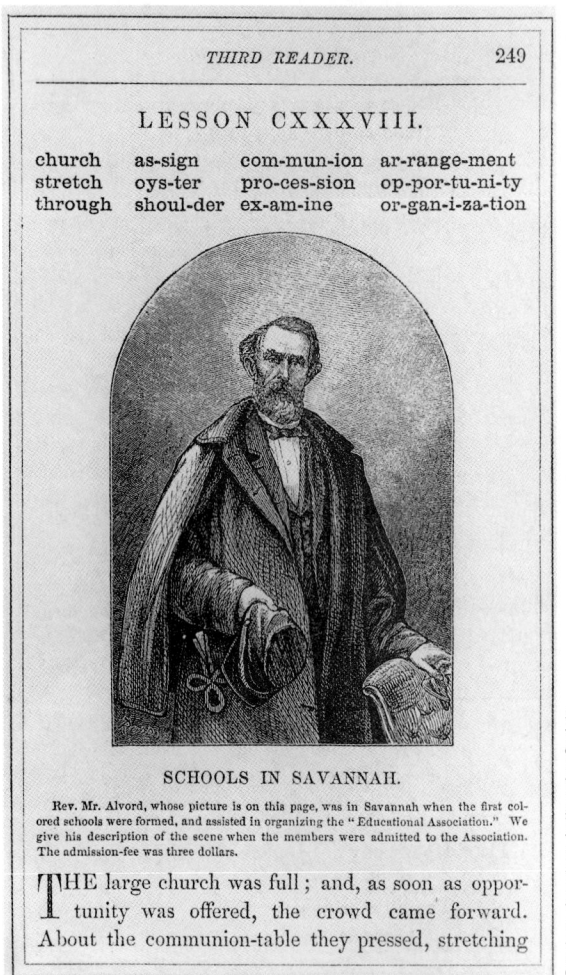

THIRD READER. 249

LESSON CXXXVIII.

church	as-sign	com-mun-ion	ar-range-ment
stretch	oys-ter	pro-ces-sion	op-por-tu-ni-ty
through	shoul-der	ex-am-ine	or-gan-i-za-tion

SCHOOLS IN SAVANNAH.

Rev. Mr. Alvord, whose picture is on this page, was in Savannah when the first colored schools were formed, and assisted in organizing the "Educational Association." We give his description of the scene when the members were admitted to the Association. The admission-fee was three dollars.

THE large church was full; and, as soon as opportunity was offered, the crowd came forward. About the communion-table they pressed, stretching

Courtesy, American Antiquarian Society

■ **The Boston wing of the American Tract Society, an abolitionist group, published a series of reading primers for the newly freed slaves. The primers provided moral lessons as well as reading lessons for the pupils. This page from *The Freedman's Third Reader* focuses on the work of John W. Alvord, the Freedmen's Bureau general superintendent of education. The authors suggest (wrongly) that Alvord played a major role in organizing the Savannah Education Association in Savannah, Georgia, in early 1865.**

power relations that made southern black people field laborers dependent on white landowners. For their part, many southern whites were determined to prevent black people from becoming truly free. Most former rebels remained embittered about the outcome of the war and vengeful toward the freedpeople.

The Civil War hardened the positions of the two major political parties. The Republicans remained in favor of a strong national government, one that promoted economic growth. The Democrats tended to support states' efforts to manage their own affairs, which included regulating relations between employers and employees, whites and blacks.

After the war, western economic development presented new challenges for men who had fought for the Union. In order to open the West to European American miners and homesteaders, the U.S. army clashed repeatedly with Native Americans. On the Plains and in the Northwest, Indians resisted white efforts to force them to abandon their nomadic way of life and take up sedentary farming. William Tecumseh Sherman, Philip H. Sheridan, and George Custer were among the U.S. military officers who had commanded troops in the Civil War and now attempted to subdue the Plains Indians and further white settlement. Sherman declared, "We must act with vindictive earnestness against the Sioux, even to their extermination, men, women and children." The former head of the Freedmen's Bureau, General Oliver O. Howard, oversaw the expulsion of Chief Joseph and his people, the Nez Perce, from their homeland in Washington's Walla Walla Valley in 1877.

U.S. soldiers also contributed to the building of the transcontinental railroad. A former Union military officer, Grenville Dodge, served as chief civil engineer for the Union Pacific Railroad, supervising huge workforces of immigrant laborers. The railroad industry was a potent symbol of postwar U.S. nationalism. It also represented a robust, Republican-sponsored partnership between private enterprise and the federal government. Between 1862 and 1872, the government gave the industry subsidies that included millions of dollars in cash and more than 100 million acres of land. On the Plains, U.S. soldiers protected Union Pacific Railroad land surveyors against the retaliatory raids conducted by Indians who were enraged by this incursion into their territory and by the government's failure to abide by its treaties.

The Civil War, and the economic growth unleashed after the conflict, transformed the physical landscape of the nation. In the South the scars of war were everywhere, in the form of ruined crop fields, pillaged forests, and smoldering cities. Pursuing a strategy of "total war" in the final months of the war, Sherman's troops had destroyed many of the towns and farms that lay in their path on their famous march from Atlanta to Savannah and then north into South Carolina. New train trestles, wharfs, and warehouses stood as monuments to the recent efforts of both rebel and Union forces to move and supply their troops. In the West, construction of new towns and railroad tracks demanded tremendous amounts of lumber. Some observers warned of an impending timber famine, spurring interest in the conservation of natural resources of all kinds.

The Republicans' triumph prompted dissent from diverse people who feared that the victorious Union would serve the interests of specific groups such as men, employers, and white property owners. Some women's rights activists, for example, felt betrayed by the suggestion that this was "the hour of the Negro [man]." These women were not willing to wait indefinitely for their own voting rights. At the same time, in the bustling workshops of the nation's cities, many workers realized that they remained at the mercy of employers bent on using cheap labor. The founding of the National Labor Union in 1866 revealed that members of the laboring classes had a national vision of their own, one that valued the efforts of working people to earn a decent living for their families.

At great cost of human life, the Civil War decisively settled several immediate and long-standing political conflicts. The southern secessionists were defeated, and slavery as a legal institution was destroyed. Nevertheless, the relationship between federal power and group rights remained unresolved, leading to continued bloodshed between whites and Indians on the High Plains, as well as in the former Confederate states between Union supporters and diehard rebels. During the postwar period, federal government officials attempted to complete the political process that the military defeat of the South had only begun: the consolidation of the Union, North and South, East and West. This process encompassed the nation as a whole.

The Struggle over the South

The Civil War had a devastating impact on the South in physical, social, and economic terms. The region had lost an estimated $2 billion in investments in slaves; modest homesteads and grand plantations alike lay in ruins; and gardens, orchards, and cotton fields were barren. Along the seacoast and riverways, fish stocks were depleted. More than three million former slaves eagerly embraced freedom, but the vast majority lacked the land, cash, and credit necessary to build family homesteads for themselves. At the same time, landowning whites considered black people primarily as a source of agricultural labor; these whites resisted the idea that the freedpeople should be granted citizenship rights. This conflict—between blacks as family members determined to control their own lives and whites as landowners determined to reassert authority over blacks—assumed immense proportions.

In the North, Republican lawmakers disagreed among themselves how best to punish the defeated but defiant rebels. President Abraham Lincoln had indicated early that after the war the government should bring the South back into the Union quickly and painlessly. However, his successor wanted to see members of the southern planter elite humiliated, but resisted the notion that freedpeople should become independent of white landowners. In Congress, moderate and radical Republicans argued about how far the government should go in ensuring the former slaves' freedom.

Southern and northern blacks, staunch defenders of the Republican party, hoped to achieve social and economic self-determination. After the war, southern whites condemned what they called the freedpeople's "noxious liberty": their tendency to move around. In fact, all over the South, African American men and women had set out to claim what they believed was rightfully theirs. They traveled great distances, usually on foot, in efforts to locate loved ones and reunite families that had been separated during slavery. They also went to great lengths to resist attempts by white employers to bind them out as apprentices, a new form of bondage. Freed parents turned their energies toward providing for their families, cultivating food crops for their own consumption, and trying to buy land whenever possible. Just as black people had proved to be a military and political force during the war, so they became major actors in the reconstruction of the postwar South.

Wartime Preludes to Postwar Policies

The political and social complications of a northern victory became apparent long before the Confederates laid down their arms at Appomattox Courthouse. Wartime experiments with African American free labor in Union-occupied areas foreshadowed bitter postwar debates. As early as November 1861, Union forces had occupied the Sea Islands off Port Royal Sound in South Carolina. In response, wealthy cotton planters fled to the mainland. As many as 10,000 slaves stayed behind on the islands to fish and to cultivate corn for themselves.

Over the next few months, three groups of northern civilians landed on the Sea Islands with the intention of guiding blacks in the transition from slave to free labor. Teachers arrived intent on creating schools, and missionaries hoped to start churches. A third group, representing Boston investors, had also settled on the Sea Islands to assess economic opporunities; by early 1862, they decided to institute a system of wage labor that would reestablish a staple crop economy and funnel cotton directly into northern textile mills. The freed slaves gave a cautious welcome to the teachers and missionaries, but they resisted growing cotton for the wartime market. They preferred to grow crops for their families to eat rather than cotton to sell, relying on a system of barter and trade among networks of extended families. Their goal was to break free of white landlords, suppliers, and cotton merchants.

Not all Union military men relished the prospect of forcing blacks to work on the plantations where they had been enslaved.

Meanwhile, in southern Louisiana, the Union capture of New Orleans in the spring of 1862 enabled northern military officials to implement their own free (that is, nonslave) labor system. General Nathaniel Banks, the Union officer in charge of occupied New Orleans, outlined the plan. Many blacks had fled from their former owners when the Union army occupied the area. Banks proclaimed that U.S. troops should forcibly relocate blacks to plantations "where they belong"; there they would continue to work for their former owners in the sugar and cotton fields, but now for wages supposedly negotiated annually. The Union army would compel blacks to work if they resisted doing so. Furthermore, said Banks, black men, women, and children must "work diligently and faithfully for one year, respectful of their employers." In defiance of these orders, however, some blacks went on strike for higher wages, and others refused to work at all. Moreover, not all Union military men relished the prospect of forcing blacks to work on the plantations where they had been enslaved. Thus, federal policies returning blacks to plantations remained contested even within the ranks of the army itself. These disputes—between blacks and planters, and among Union officials—would continue throughout the postwar period.

The Port Royal and southern Louisiana precursors to Reconstruction offered variations on two themes: the Republicans' insistence on preserving the southern plantation economy and the former slaves' efforts to achieve freedom from white control.

The Lincoln administration had no hard-and-fast Reconstruction policy to guide congressional lawmakers looking toward the postwar period. In December 1863 the president outlined his Ten Percent Plan. This plan would allow former Confederate states to form new state governments once 10 percent of the men who had voted in the 1860 presidential election had pledged allegiance to the Union and renounced slavery. Congress never acted on Lincoln's plan because many Republicans felt the need for harsher measures.

Instead, at the end of their 1864 session, legislators passed the Wade-Davis Bill, which would have required a majority of southern voters in any state to take a loyalty oath affirming their allegiance to the United States. By refusing to sign the bill before Congress adjourned, Lincoln vetoed the measure (the so-called pocket veto). However, the president approved the creation of the Freedmen's Bureau in March 1865. The Bureau was responsible for coordinating relief efforts on behalf of blacks and poor whites loyal to the Union, for sponsoring schools, and for implementing a labor contract system on southern plantations. Congress also created the Freedman's Savings and Trust Bank in the hope that the former slaves would save a part of their earnings. At the time of his assassination, Lincoln seemed to be leaning toward giving the right to vote the southern black men.

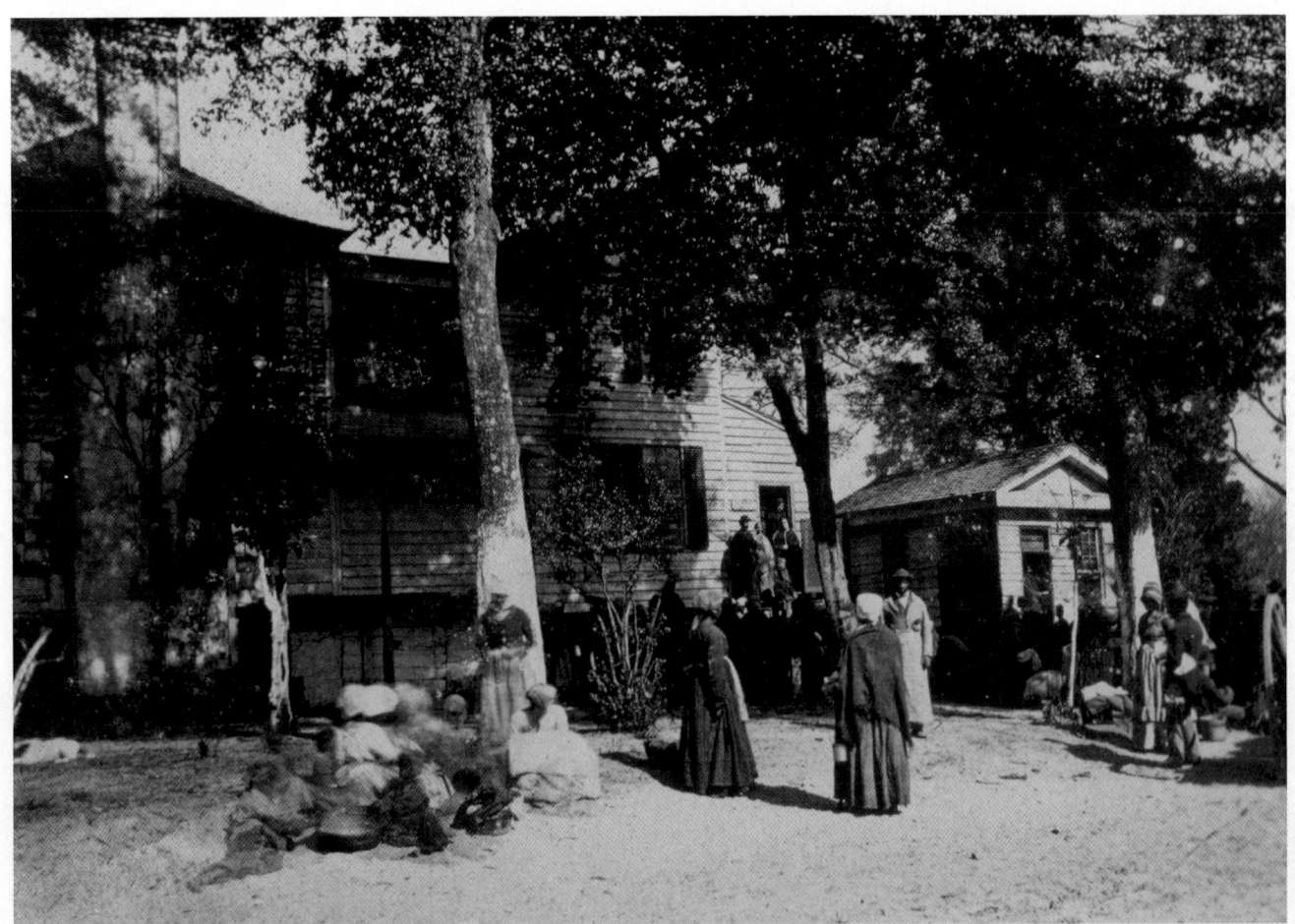

Bettmann/CORBIS

■ Freedmen's Bureau agents distributed rations to former slaves and southern whites who had remained loyal to the Union. Agents also sponsored schools, legalized marriages formed under slavery, arbitrated domestic disputes, and oversaw labor contracts between workers and landowners. This photo shows the bureau office in Petersburg, Virginia.

Presidential Reconstruction, 1865–1867

When Andrew Johnson, the seventeenth president of the United States, assumed office in April 1865, he brought his own agenda for the defeated South. Throughout his political career, Johnson had seen himself as a champion of poor white farmers in opposition to the wealthy planter class. A man of modest background, he had been elected U.S. senator from Tennessee in 1857. He alone among southern senators remained in Congress and loyal to the Union after 1861. Lincoln first appointed Johnson military governor of Tennessee when that state was captured by the Union in 1862 and then tapped him as his running mate for the election of 1864.

Soon after he assumed the presidency, Johnson disappointed congressional Republicans who hoped that he would serve as a champion of the freedpeople. He welcomed back into the Union those states reorganized under Lincoln's 10 percent plan. On May 29, 1865, Johnson announced his own plan for Reconstruction. He advocated denying the vote to wealthy Confederates, though he would allow individuals to come to the White House to beg the president for special pardons. Johnson also outlined a fairly lenient plan for readmitting the other rebel states into the Union. Poor whites would have the right to vote, but they must convene special state conventions that would renounce secession and accept the Thirteenth Amendment abolishing slavery. Further, they must repudiate all Confederate debts—that is, they must default on any loans made by banks or private individuals to finance the southern war effort. The president opposed granting the vote to the former slaves; he believed that they should continue to toil as field workers for white landowners.

Johnson failed to anticipate the speed and vigor with which former Confederate leaders would move to reassert their political authority. In addition, he did not gauge accurately the resentment of congressional Republicans, who thought his policies toward the defeated South were too forgiving. A warning came in December 1865, when Carl Schurz, a German immigrant and former Union brigadier general, issued his "Report on the Condition of the South." In it, he warned that the Freedmen's Bureau was "very unpopular" among white Southerners, who would no doubt fill a power vacuum left by federal weakness and indecision.

> *By January 1865, both houses of Congress had approved the Thirteenth Amendment to the Constitution, abolishing slavery.*

Several developments quickly proved Schurz right. The southern states that took advantage of Johnson's reunification policies passed so-called Black Codes. These state laws were an ill-disguised attempt to institute a system of near-slavery. They aimed to penalize "vagrant" blacks, defined as those who did not work in the fields for whites, and to deny blacks the right to vote, serve on juries, or in some cases even own land. The Black Code of Mississippi barred blacks from marrying whites and from owning land "except in incorporated towns or cities" and restricted the rights of a freedperson to "keep or carry fire-arms," ammunition, and knives and to "quit the service of his or her employer before the expiration of his or her term of service without good cause." The vagueness of this last provision threatened any blacks who happened not to be working under the supervision of whites at any given moment. People arrested under the Black Codes faced imprisonment or forced labor.

At the end of the war, congressional Republicans were divided into two camps. Radicals wanted to use strong federal measures to advance black people's civil rights and economic independence. In contrast, moderates were more concerned with the free market and private property rights; they took a hands-off approach regarding former slaves, arguing that blacks should fend for themselves and avoid dependence on federal aid. But members of both groups reacted with outrage to the Black Codes. Moreover, when the legislators returned to the Capitol in December 1865, they were in for a shock: among their new colleagues were four former Confederate generals, five colonels, and other high-ranking members of the Confederate elite, including former Vice President Alexander Stephens, now under indictment for treason. All of these rebels were duly elected senators and representatives from southern states. In a special session called for December 4, a joint committee of 15 lawmakers (6 senators and 9 members of the House) voted to bar these men from Congress.

By January 1865, both houses of Congress had approved the Thirteenth Amendment to the Constitution, abolishing slavery. The necessary three-fourths of the states ratified the measure by the end of the year. Unlike the Emancipation Proclamation (1863), which freed only slaves in Confederate territory, the Thirteenth Amendment abolished slavery wherever it existed. The federal government now guaranteed freedom for all black people.

However, President Johnson was becoming more openly defiant of his congressional foes who favored aggressive federal protection of black civil rights. He vetoed two crucial pieces of legislation: an extension and expansion of the Freedmen's Bureau and the Civil Rights Bill of 1866. This latter measure, a precursor to the Fourteenth Amendment, was an unprecedented piece of legislation. It called on the federal government—for the first time in history—to protect individual rights against the willful indifference of the states (as manifested, for example, in the Black Codes). Congress managed to override both vetoes by the summer of 1866.

In June of that year, Congress passed the Fourteenth Amendment. This amendment guaranteed the former slaves citizenship rights, punished states that denied citizens the right to vote, declared the former rebels ineligible for federal and state office, and voided Confederate debts. This amendment was the first to use gender-specific language, guarding against denying the vote "to any of the male inhabitants" of any state. The amendment, also, for the first time legally defined the rights of American citizenship and empowered the federal government to protect those rights.

Even before the war ended, Northerners had moved south; and the flow increased in 1865. Black and white teachers volunteered to teach the former slaves to read and write. Some white Northerners journeyed south to invest in land and become planters in the staple crop economy. White southern critics called all these migrants carpetbaggers. This derisive term suggested that the Northerners hastily packed their belongings in rough bags made of carpet scraps and then rushed south to take advantage of the region's devastation and confusion.

Former Confederates were not the only people suspicious of the newcomers. In 1865 a black abolitionist Union officer, Martin R. Delany, condemned the northern white people recently arrived in South Carolina. These Northerners, Delany told a group of freedpeople, had "come down here to drive you as much as ever. It's slavery again: northern, universal U.S. slavery." To many freedpeople, whether they worked for a white Northerner or Southerner, laboring in the cotton fields was but a continuation of slavery.

Freedmen and white Southerners sometimes differed within their own camps about political and economic aims. For example, southern blacks united in their demands for land and the vote but disagreed among themselves over the necessity of political cooperation with whites in general. Some former southern (white) Whigs, who had been reluctant secessionists, now found common ground with northern Republicans who supported government subsidies for railroads, banking institutions, and public improvements. This group consisted of some members of the humbled planter class as well as men of more modest means. Southern Democrats, who sneered at any alliances with the North, scornfully labeled these whites "scalawags" (the term referred to a scrawny, useless type of horse on the Scottish island of Scalloway).

Soon after the war's end, southern white vigilantes launched a campaign of violence and intimidation against freedpeople who dared to resist the demands of white planters and other employers. In 1866 former Confederate General Nathan Bedford Forrest, who had led the massacre of African American soldiers at Fort Pillow, founded a social club composed of Tennessee war veterans. Calling itself the Ku Klux Klan, this group soon became a white supremacist terrorist organization and spread to other states. In May 1866 violence initiated by white terrorists against blacks in Memphis, Tennessee, left 46 freedpeople and 2 whites dead, and in July, a riot in New Orleans claimed the lives of 34 blacks and 3 of their white allies. These bloody encounters demonstrated the lengths to which ex-Confederates would go to reassert their authority and defy the federal government.

Back in Washington, Johnson was not content to veto Republican legislation. In the summer of 1866, he also began to lobby against the Fourteenth Amendment, traveling around the country and urging the states not to ratify it. He argued that policies related to black suffrage should be decided by the states. The time had come for reconciliation between the North and South, maintained the president. (The amendment would not be adopted until 1868.)

Congressional Republicans fought back. In the election of November 1866, they won a two-thirds majority in both houses of Congress. These numbers allowed them to claim a mandate from their constituents and to override any future vetoes by the president. Taking heart from their newfound legislative successes, moderates and radicals together prepared to bypass Johnson to shape their own Reconstruction policies.

The Southern Postwar Labor Problem

Throughout the South, black people aspired to labor for themselves and gain independence from white overseers and landowners. Yet white landowners persisted in regarding blacks as field hands who must be coerced into working. With the creation of the Freedmen's Bureau in 1865, Congress intended to form an agency that would mediate between these two groups. Bureau agents encouraged workers and employers to sign annual labor contracts designed to eliminate the last vestiges of the slave system. All over the South, freed men, women, and children would contract with an employer on January 1 of each year. They would agree to work for either a monthly wage, an annual share of the crop, or some combination of the two.

The Bureau established elementary schools and distributed rations to southerners who had remained loyal to the Union, blacks and whites alike. Agents also conducted wedding ceremonies for the former slaves, who had been denied the right to legalize their unions as marriages. Yet the agency's most formidable challenge was its effort to usher in a new economic order in the South—one that relied on nonslave labor but also returned the region to prewar productivity levels in terms of planting and harvesting cotton.

In April 1866, a white planter in Thomson, Georgia, wrote to a local Freedmen's Bureau official and complained that the black wives and mothers living on his land had refused to sign labor contracts. The planter explained, "Their husbands are at work, while they are nearly idle as it is possible for them to be, pretending to spin—knit or something that really amounts to nothing." These "idle" women posed a threat to plantation order, the white man asserted.

Women who stayed home to care for their families were hardly idle. Yet Freedmen's Bureau agents and white planters alike tended to define productive labor (among blacks) as work carried out under the supervision of a white man in the fields or a white woman in the kitchen. During the postwar period, a struggle ensued. Who should toil in the fields of the South? And under what conditions should they labor?

The physical devastation wrought by the war gave these questions heightened urgency. Most freedpeople understood they must find a way to provide for themselves first and foremost. They thought of freedom in terms of welfare for their family rather than just for themselves as individuals. Men and women embraced the opportunity to live and work together as a unit. For many couples, their first act as free people was to legalize their marriage vows. Black women shunned the advice of Freedmen's Bureau agents and planters that they continue to pick cotton. These women withdrew from field labor whenever they could afford to do so. Enslaved women had been deprived of the opportunity to attend to family life. Now freedwomen sought to devote themselves to caring for their families.

The Freedmen's Bureau's functions in the areas of labor and education represented a new and significant federal role in the realm of social welfare. Yet the agency did not have the staff or money necessary to effect meaningful change.

According to the Northerners, the benefits of this system were clear. Employers would have an incentive to treat their workers fairly—to offer a decent wage and refrain from physical punishment. Disgruntled workers could leave at the end of the year to work for a more reasonable landowner. In the postbellum South, however, labor relations were shaped not by federal decree but by a process of negotiation that pitted white landowners against blacks who possessed little but their own labor.

For instance, blacks along the Georgia and South Carolina coast were determined to cultivate the land on which their forebears had lived and died. They urged General Sherman to confiscate the land owned by rebels in the area. In response, in early 1865, Sherman issued Field Order Number 15, mandating that the Sea Islands and the coastal region south of Charleston be divided into parcels of 40 acres for individual freed families. He also decreed that the army might lend mules to these families to help them begin planting. Given the provisions of this order, many freed families came to expect that the federal government would grant them "40 acres and a mule."

As a result of Sherman's order, 20,000 former slaves proceeded to cultivate the property once owned by Confederates. Within a few months of the war's end, however, the War Department bowed to pressure from the white landowners and revoked the order. The War Department also provided military protection for whites to return and occupy their former lands. In response, a group of black men calling themselves Commissioners from Edisto Island (one of the Sea Islands)

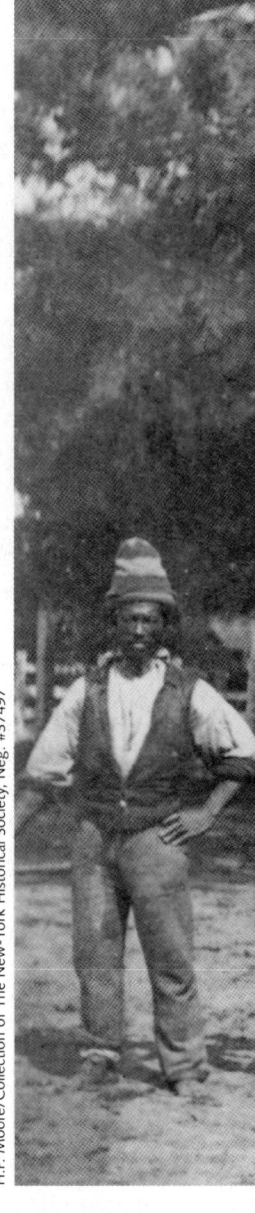

H.P. Moore/Collection of The New-York Historical Society, Neg. #37497

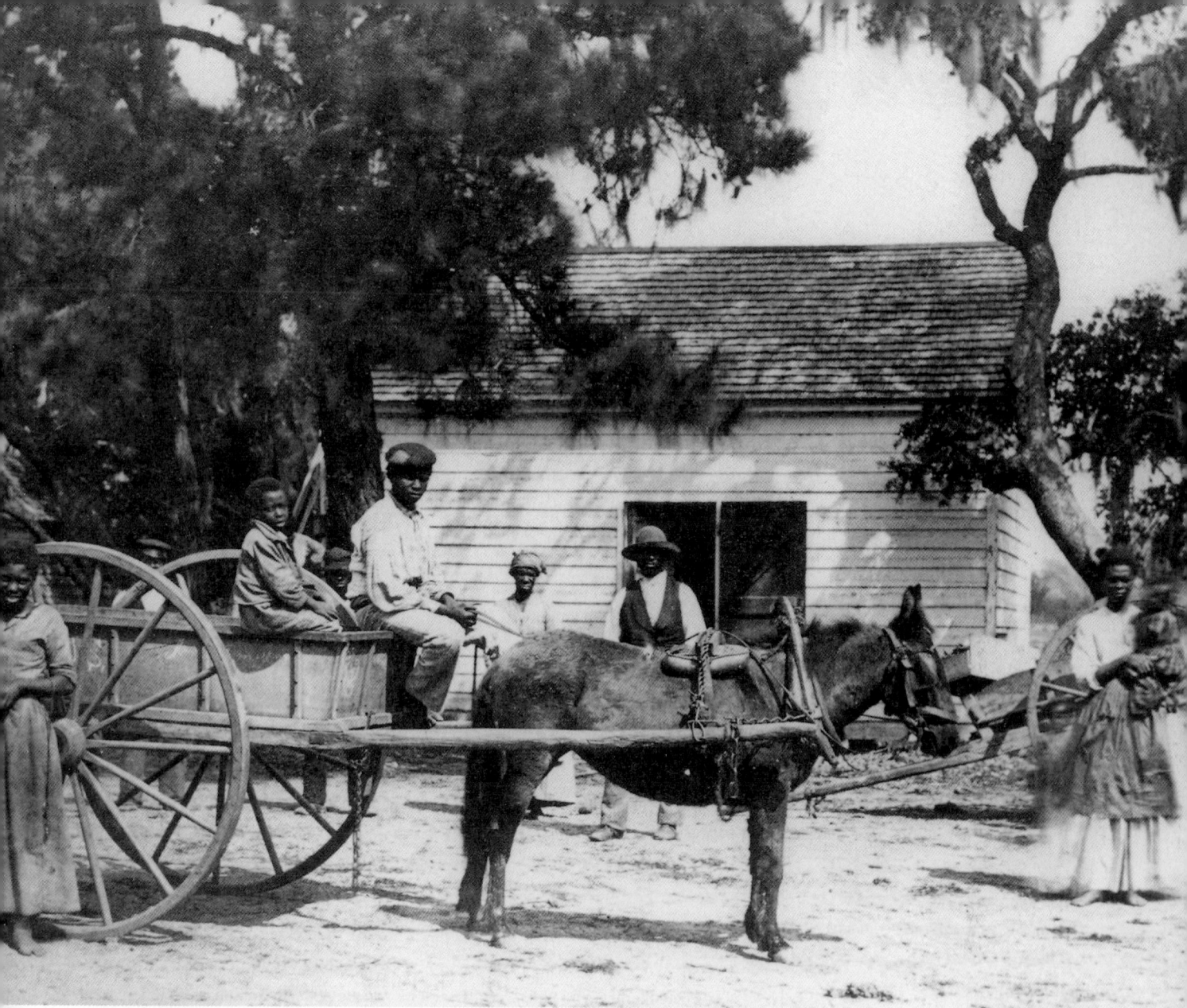

■ Residents of Edisto Island, off the coast of South Carolina, pose with a U.S. government mule cart immediately after the Civil War. U.S. troops captured the island in November 1861. The following March, the government began to distribute to blacks the lands abandoned by their former masters. In October 1865 President Andrew Johnson halted the program. A group of angry and disappointed blacks appealed to the president, claiming, "This is our home, we have made these lands what they are." After meeting with the group, General Oliver O. Howard noted, "I am convinced that something must be done to give these people and others the prospect of homesteads."

met in committee to protest to the Freedmen's Bureau what they considered a betrayal. Writing from the area in January 1866, one Freedmen's Bureau official noted that the new policy must be upheld but regretted that it had brought the freedpeople in "collision" with "U.S. forces."

During its brief life (1865 to 1868), the Freedmen's Bureau compiled a mixed record. The individual agents represented a broad range of backgrounds, temperaments, and political ideas. Some were former abolitionists who considered northern-style free labor to be "the noblest principle on earth." These men tried to ensure safe and fair working arrangements for black men, women, and children. In contrast, some agents had little patience with the freedpeople's drive for self-sufficiency. Some bureau offices became havens for blacks seeking redress against abusive or fraudulent labor practices, but other offices had little impact on the postwar political and economic landscape. For agents without means of transportation (a reliable horse),

A Southern Labor Contract

After the Civil War, many southern agricultural workers signed labor contracts. These contracts sought to control not only the output of laborers but also their lives outside the workplace.

On January 1, 1868, the planter John D. Williams assembled his workers for the coming year and presented them with a contract to sign. Williams owned a plantation in the Lower Piedmont county of Laurens, South Carolina. He agreed to furnish "the said negroes" (that is, the three black men and two black women whose names were listed on the document) with mules and horses to be used for cultivating the land. The workers could receive their food, clothing, and medical care on credit. They were allowed to keep one-third of all the corn, sweet potatoes, wheat, cotton, oats, and molasses they produced. Presumably, they would pay their debts to Williams using proceeds from their share of the crop.

According to the contract, Williams's workers promised to

bind them Selves to be steady & attentive to there work at all times and to work at keeping in repair all the fences on Said plantation and assist in cuting & taking care of—all the grain crops on Said plantation and work by the direction of me [Williams] or my Agent. . . .

And should any of them depart from the farm or from any services at any time with out our approval they shall forfeit one dollar per day, for the first time and for the second time without good cause they shall forfeit all of their interest in the crop their to me the enjured person—they shall not be allowed to keep firearms or deadly wapons or ardent Spirits and they shall obey all lawful orders from me

or my Agent and shall be honest—truthful—sober—civel—diligent in their business & for all wilful Disobedience of any lawful orders from me or my Agent drunkenness moral or legal misconduct want of respects or civility to me or my Agent or to my Family or any elce, I am permitted to discharge them forfeiting any claims upon me for any part of the crop. . . .

Moses Nathan	1 full hand
Jake Chappal	" "
Milly Williams	½ " "
Easter Williams	" "
Mack Williams	" "

At the end of the contract is this addition:

We the white labores now employed by John D. Williams on his white plains plantation have lisened and heard read the foregoing Contract on this sheet of paper assign equal for the black laborers employed by him on said place and we are perfectly Satisfied with it and heare by bind our selves to abide & be Governed & Controwed by it

Wm Wyatte	1 full hand
John Wyatte	1 full hand
Packingham Wyatte	½ " "
Franklin Wyatte	½ " "
R M Hughes	1 full hand
B G Pollard	1 full hand
George Washington Pollard	1 full hand

To sign the contract, all of the blacks and two of the whites "made their marks"; that is, they signed with an "X" because they were illiterate. ■

Source: Rosser H. Taylor, "Postbellum Southern Rental Contracts" [from Furman University library, Greenville, South Carolina], Agricultural History 17 (1943):122–123.

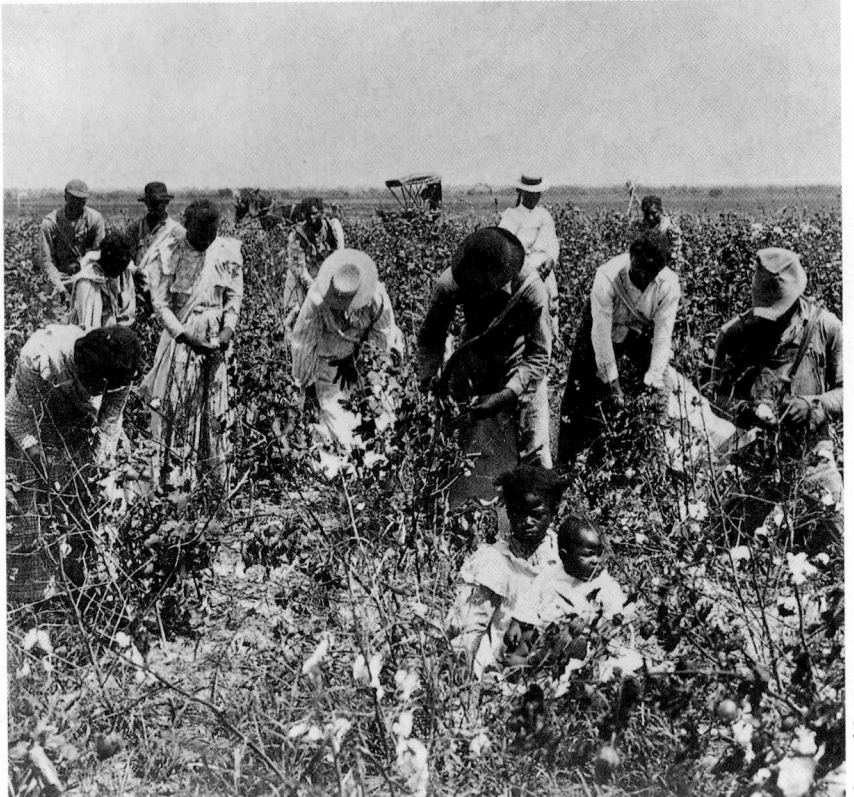

Library of Congress

After the Civil War, many rural southern blacks, such as those shown here, continued to toil in cotton fields owned by whites.

plantations scattered throughout the vast rural South remained outside their control. Because white landowners crafted the wording and specific provisions of labor contracts, the bureau agents who enforced such agreements often served the interests of employers rather than laborers.

In fact, for the most part, postwar freed people pressed for their labor rights independently of the federal government. In the cotton regions of the South, freedpeople resisted the near-slavery system of gang labor that planters tried to enforce right after the war. Instead, extended families came together in groups called squads to negotiate collectively with landowners. Gradually, squads gave way to sharecropping families.

The outlines of sharecropping, a system that defined southern cotton production until well into the twentieth century, were visible just a few years after the Civil War. Poor families, black and white, contracted annually with landlords, who advanced them supplies, such as crop seed, mules, plows, food, and clothing. Fathers directed the labor of their children in the fields. At the end of the year, many families remained indebted to their employer and, thus, entitled to nothing and obliged to work another year in the hope of repaying the debt. If a sharecropper's demeanor or work habits displeased the landlord, the family faced eviction.

Single women with small children were especially vulnerable to the whims of landlords in the postbellum period. Near Greensboro, North Carolina, for example, planter Presley George, Sr., settled accounts with his field worker Polly at the end of 1865. For her year's expenses, Polly was charged a total $69.00 for corn, cloth, thread, and board for a child who did not work. By George's calculations, Polly had earned exactly $69.00 for the labor she and her three children (two sons and a daughter) performed in the course of the year, leaving her no cash of her own. Under these harsh conditions, freedpeople looked to each other for support and strength.

Building Free Communities

Soon after the war's end, southern blacks set about organizing themselves as an effective political force and as free communities devoted to the social and educational welfare of their own people. As early as summer 1865, groups of freedpeople met in convention to press for their rights as U.S. citizens. A group calling itself Colored Citizens of Norfolk, Virginia, issued an address to the people of the United States, warning that the Emancipation Proclamation was insufficient to check the power of diehard rebels. Mass arrests of blacks had been authorized by "the rebel Mayor." Former slaveholders were bent on keeping the blacks "in a state of serfdom," charged the Norfolk petitioners.

Differences among blacks based on income, jobs, culture, and skin color at times inhibited institution-building. Some black communities found themselves divided by class, with blacks who had been free before the war (including many literate and skilled light-skinned men) assuming leadership over illiterate field hands. In New Orleans, a combination of factors contributed to class divisions among people of African heritage. During the antebellum period, light-skinned free people of color, many of whom spoke French, were much more likely to possess property and a formal education compared to enslaved people, who were dark-skinned English speakers. After the Civil War, the more privileged group pressed for public accommodations laws, which would open the city's theaters, opera, and expensive restaurants to all blacks for the first time. However, black churches and social organizations remained segregated according to class. Yet, citywide black conventions held in 1864 and 1867 brought together all groups of African descent in common cause, defined as "the actual liberation from social and political bondage."

For the most part, postbellum black communities united around the principle that freedom from slavery should also mean full citizenship rights: the ability to vote, own land, and educate their children. These rights must be enforced by federal firepower: "a military occupation will be absolutely necessary," declared the blacks of Norfolk, "to protect the white Union men of the South, as well as ourselves." Freedpeople in some states allied themselves with white

TABLE 15-1

Comparison of Black and White Household Structure in 27 Cotton-Belt Counties, 1870, 1880, 1900

1870 (N = 534)

Single Person %	Nuclear %	Ext. %	Aug. %	Ext./Aug. %	Adults %	Total	
3.1	80.7	14.4	1.4	.3	.3	290	Black
2.1	71.3	7.4	17.6	1.2	.4	244	White
2.6	76.4	11.0	8.8	.7	.4	534	

1880 (N = 679)

Single Person %	Nuclear %	Ext. %	Aug. %	Ext./Aug. %	Adults %	Total	
3.7	74.2	13.6	5.9	1.7	.8	353	Black
3.1	62.7	13.5	15.7	5.0	.0	319	White
3.4	68.8	13.5	10.6	3.3	.4	672	

1900 (N = 644)

Single Person %	Nuclear %	Ext. %	Aug. %	Ext./Aug. %	Adults %	Total	
5.7	64.9	22.9	4.0	1.7	.8	353	Black
3.4	65.2	19.0	.7	1.7	.0	290	White
4.7	65.0	21.2	7.0	1.7	.5	643	

Single person: one person living alone.
Nuclear: father, mother, and children.
Ext.: extended family consisting of parents, children, and kin.
Aug.: augmented household consisting of family and nonfamily members (boarders, servants, hired hands).
Ext./aug.: combination of extended and augmented.
Unrelated adults: more than one unrelated adult living together.

Source: Based on information from a sample of households (located in selected cotton staple counties in Alabama, Florida, Georgia, Louisiana, Mississippi, North Carolina, South Carolina, and Texas) listed in the 1870, 1880, and 1900 federal population manuscript censuses.

yeomen who had long resented the political power of the great planters and now saw an opportunity to use state governments as agents of democratization and economic reform.

Networks of freedpeople formed self-help organizations. Like the sponsors of the Savannah Education Association, blacks throughout the South formed committees to raise funds and hire teachers for neighborhood schools. Small Georgia towns, such as Cuthbert, Albany, Cave Spring, and Thomasville, with populations no greater than a few hundred, raised up to $70 per month and contributed as much as $350 each for the construction of school buildings. Funds came from the proceeds of fairs, bazaars, and bake sales; subscriptions raised by local school boards; and tuition fees. In the cash-starved postbellum South, these amounts represented a great personal and group sacrifice for the cause of education.

Black families sought to care for people who could not care for themselves. Freedmen's Bureau agents scoffed at blacks who took in "improvident" and "lazy" elderly kin: how could

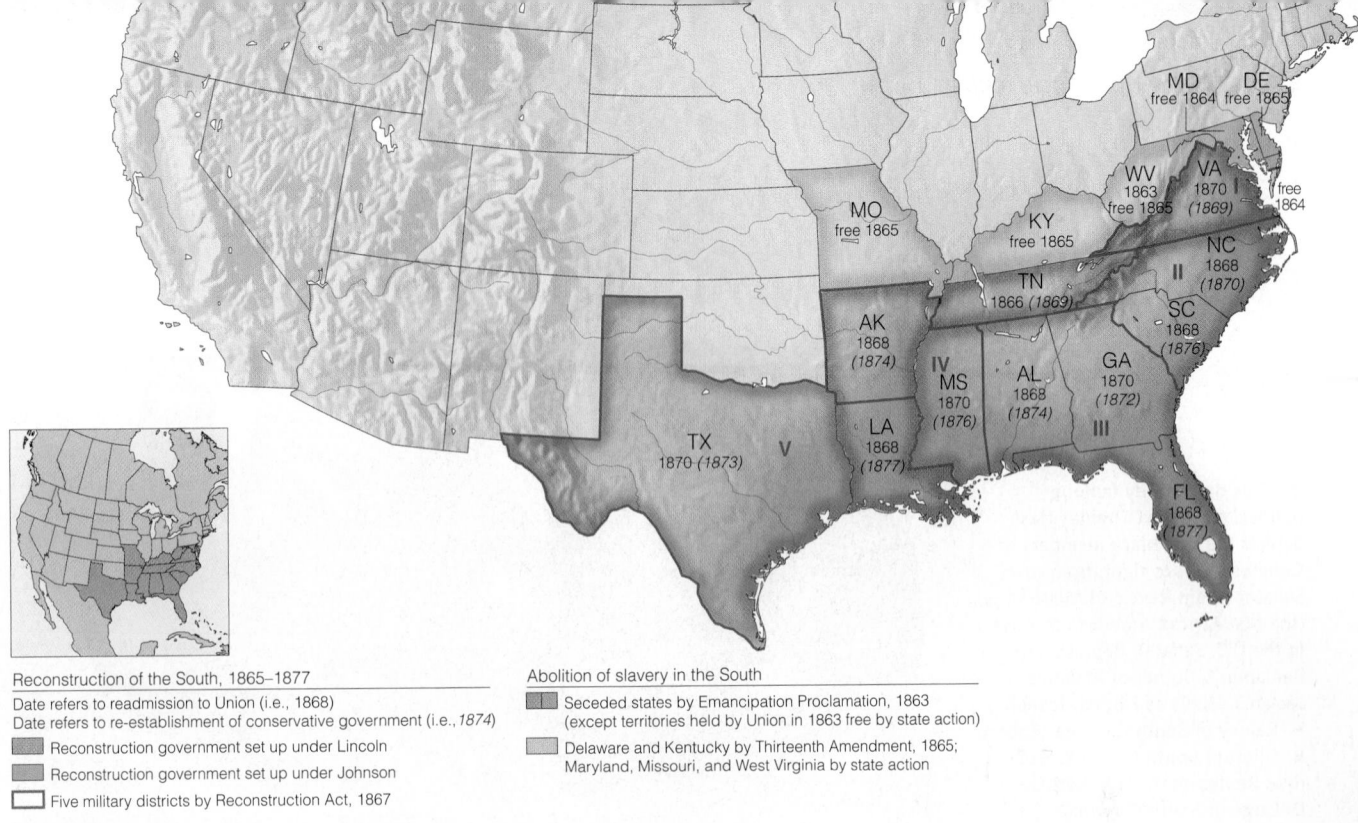

Reconstruction of the South, 1865–1877

Date refers to readmission to Union (i.e., 1868)
Date refers to re-establishment of conservative government (i.e., *1874*)

☐ Reconstruction government set up under Lincoln

☐ Reconstruction government set up under Johnson

☐ Five military districts by Reconstruction Act, 1867

Abolition of slavery in the South

☐ Seceded states by Emancipation Proclamation, 1863
(except territories held by Union in 1863 free by state action)

☐ Delaware and Kentucky by Thirteenth Amendment, 1865;
Maryland, Missouri, and West Virginia by state action

■ **MAP 15.1**

RADICAL RECONSTRUCTION Four of the former Confederate states, Louisiana, Arkansas, Tennessee, and Virginia, were reorganized under President Lincoln's 10 Percent Plan in 1864. Neither this plan nor the proposals of Lincoln's successor, Andrew Johnson, provided for the enfranchisement of the former slaves. In 1867 Congress established five military districts in the South and demanded that newly reconstituted state governments implement universal manhood suffrage. By 1870 all of the former Confederate states had rejoined the Union, and by 1877 all of those states had installed conservative (i.e., Democratic) governments.

the former slaves hope to advance their own interests if they had to support such unproductive people? All over the South, black families charted their own course. They elected to take in orphans, to pool resources with neighbors, and to arrange for mothers to stay home with their children. These choices challenged the power of former slaveholders and the influence of Freedmen's Bureau agents and northern missionaries and teachers. At the same time, in seeking to attend to their families and to provide for themselves, southern blacks resembled members of other mid-nineteenth-century laboring classes who valued family ties over the demands of employers and landlords.

Tangible signs of the new emerging black communities infuriated southern whites. A schoolhouse run by blacks proved threatening in a society where most white children had little opportunity to receive an education. Black communities were also quick to form their own churches, rather than continue to occupy an inferior place in white churches. Other sights proved equally unsettling: on a main street in Charleston, an armed black soldier marching proudly or a black woman wearing a fashionable hat and veil, the kind favored by white women of the planter class. These developments help to account for the speed with which whites organized themselves in the Klan and various other vigilante groups, such as Young Men's Democratic Clubs, White Brotherhood, and Knights of the White Camellia. Members of this last group took an initiation oath that stated, "Our main and fundamental object is the maintenance of the supremacy of the white race in this Republic."

Congressional Reconstruction: The Radicals' Plan

The rise of armed white supremacist groups in the South helped spur congressional Republicans to action. On March 2, 1867, Congress seized the initiative. A coalition led by two

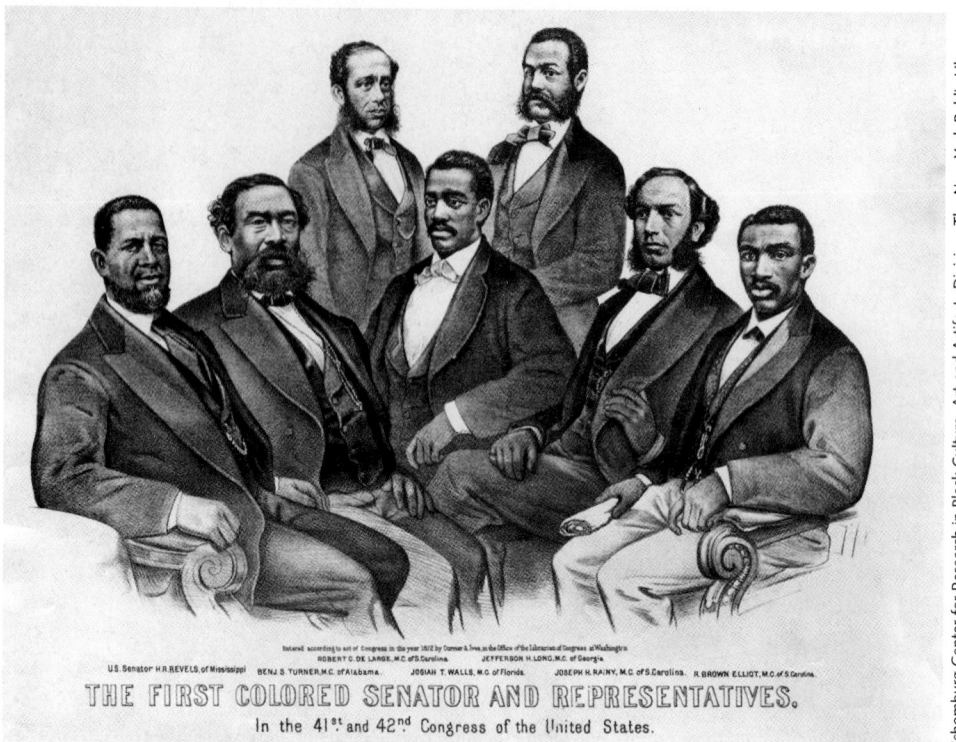

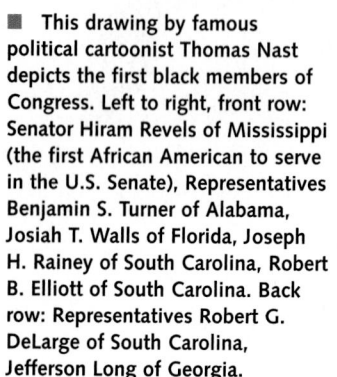

■ This drawing by famous political cartoonist Thomas Nast depicts the first black members of Congress. Left to right, front row: Senator Hiram Revels of Mississippi (the first African American to serve in the U.S. Senate), Representatives Benjamin S. Turner of Alabama, Josiah T. Walls of Florida, Joseph H. Rainey of South Carolina, Robert B. Elliott of South Carolina. Back row: Representatives Robert G. DeLarge of South Carolina, Jefferson Long of Georgia.

radicals, Senator Charles Sumner of Massachusetts and Congressman Thaddeus Stevens of Pennsylvania, prodded Congress to pass the Reconstruction Act of 1867. The purpose of this measure was to purge the South of disloyalty once and for all. The act stripped thousands of former Confederates of voting rights. The former Confederate states would not be readmitted to the Union until they had ratified the Fourteenth Amendment and written new constitutions that guaranteed black men the right to vote. The South (with the exception of Tennessee, which had ratified the Fourteenth Amendment in 1866) was divided into five military districts. Federal troops were stationed throughout the region. These troops were charged with protecting Union personnel and supporters in the South and with restoring order in the midst of regional political and economic upheaval.

Congress passed two additional acts specifically intended to secure congressional power over the president. The intent of the Tenure of Office Act was to prevent the president from dismissing Secretary of War Edwin Stanton, a supporter of the radicals. The other measure, the Command of the Army Act, required the president to seek approval for all military orders from General Ulysses S. Grant, the army's senior officer. Grant also was a supporter of the Republicans. Both of these acts probably violated the separation of powers doctrine as put forth in the Constitution. Together, they would soon precipitate a national crisis.

The radicals' call for the redistribution of land from former slaveholders to freedpeople won few supporters among moderates in Congress. In contrast, both Republican factions threw their support behind an emerging southern Republican party, a move that had a significant impact on postwar politics. Alert to the designs of the "irritated, revengeful South," Thaddeus Stevens, the leading House radical, urged Republicans, black and white, to assume control of the South; otherwise, "all our blood and treasure will have been spent in vain." Giving the vote to black men spurred the growth of southern Republican party organizations, called Union Leagues, that provided a political forum for a host of black leaders.

During Reconstruction, approximately 2000 black men served as local elected officials, sheriffs, justices of the peace, tax collectors, and city councilors. Many of these leaders were of mixed ancestry, and many had been free before the war. They came in disproportionate numbers from the ranks of literate men, such as clergy, teachers, and skilled artisans. In Alabama, Florida, Louisiana, Mississippi, and South Carolina, black men constituted a majority of the voting public. Throughout the South, 600 black men won election to state legislatures. However, nowhere did blacks control a state government, although they did predominate in South Carolina's lower House. Sixteen black Southerners were elected to Congress during Reconstruction. Most of those elected to Congress in the years immediately after the war were freeborn. However, among the nine men elected for the first time after 1872, six were former slaves. All of these politicians exemplified the desire among southern blacks to become active, engaged citizens.

Among this group of black leaders was war hero Robert Smalls of South Carolina, who early in the war had seized a Confederate gunboat and escaped from Charleston Harbor. Other prominent leaders included Tunis G. Campbell, a native of New Jersey who served as a Georgia state senator and justice of the peace; and the Reverend Henry M. Turner of Georgia, who warned against political divisions between dark- and light-skinned blacks. In Mississippi, in February 1870, Hiram Revels became the first black man to serve in the U.S. Senate. Another Mississippi politician, Blanche K. Bruce, dominated the political scene in Bolivar County, where he served as sheriff, tax collector, and superintendent of education all at the same time. In 1875 Bruce was elected to the U.S. Senate.

Newly reconstructed southern state legislatures provided for public school systems, fairer taxation methods, bargaining rights of plantation laborers, racially integrated public transportation and accommodations, and public works projects, especially railroads. Nevertheless, the legislative coalitions forged between Northerners and Southerners, blacks and whites, were uneasy and, in many cases, less than productive. Southern Democrats (and later, historians sympathetic to them) claimed that Reconstruction governments were uniquely corrupt, with some carpetbaggers, scalawags, and freedpeople vying for kickbacks from railroad and construction magnates. In fact, whenever state legislatures sought to promote business interests, they opened the door to the bribery of public officials. In this respect, northern as well as southern politicians were vulnerable to charges of corruption. In the long run, southern Democrats cared less about charges of legislative corruption and more about the growing political power of local black Republican party organizations.

In Washington in early 1868 President Johnson forced a final showdown with Congress. He replaced several high military officials with more conservative men. He also fired Secretary of War Stanton, in apparent violation of the Tenure of Office Act. Shortly thereafter, in February, a newly composed House Reconstruction Committee impeached Johnson for ignoring the act, and the Senate began his trial on March 30. The president and Congress were locked in an extraordinary battle for political power.

During the House debate and the Senate trial, political rhetoric verged on the melodramatic. Representative Stevens condemned Johnson as "the nightmare that crouched on the heaving breast of the nation." Nevertheless, the president managed to avoid conviction. The final vote was 35 senators against Johnson, one vote short of the necessary two-thirds of all senators' votes needed for conviction. Nineteen senators voted to acquit Johnson of the charges. The president celebrated his victory by sharing a round of whiskey with his lawyers. Nevertheless, to win acquittal, he had had to promise moderates that he would not stand in the way of congressional plans for Reconstruction. Johnson essentially withdrew from policymaking in the spring of 1868.

TABLE 15-2
The Election of 1868

Candidate	Political Party	Popular Vote	Electoral Vote
Ulysses S. Grant	Republican	3,013,421	214
Horatio Seymour	Democratic	2,706,829	80

That November, Republicans urged Northerners to "vote as you shot" (that is, to cast ballots against the former Confederates) and elected Ulysses S. Grant to the presidency. Grant defeated the Democratic nominee, Horatio Seymour, a former governor of New York. An estimated half a million former slaves cast their ballots for Grant, whom they hailed as a liberator.

Two Presidents Impeached

The president, a Democrat, had humble roots in the South. He was raised by a hard-working single mother. His tenure as a state governor ill prepared him for the hostility he encountered as chief executive in Washington, where people persisted in gossiping about his personal life. The Republicans, firmly in control of Congress, despised him and managed to impeach him. At the same time, many observers questioned whether his misdeeds rose to the level of "high crimes and misdemeanors." With the aid of skillful lawyers, members of his own party, and a core of Republican moderates, he avoided conviction in the Senate. Nevertheless, the political battle diminished his capacity to lead forcefully for the rest of his term in office.

Andrew Johnson in 1868 or Bill Clinton 130 years later? The answer, of course, is both. Yet these superficial similarities in the careers of the two men mask dramatic differences between them. Andrew Johnson was charged with violating the Tenure of Office Act, a law that probably was unconstitutional in any case. His impeachment took place against the backdrop of a national debate over the course of Reconstruction, a debate that was intensely ideological.

In contrast, Bill Clinton was charged with lying and obstructing justice, charges that stemmed from an

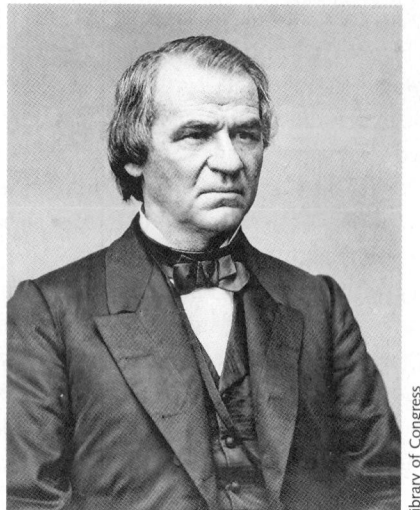

President Andrew Johnson (1865–1868). *Library of Congress*

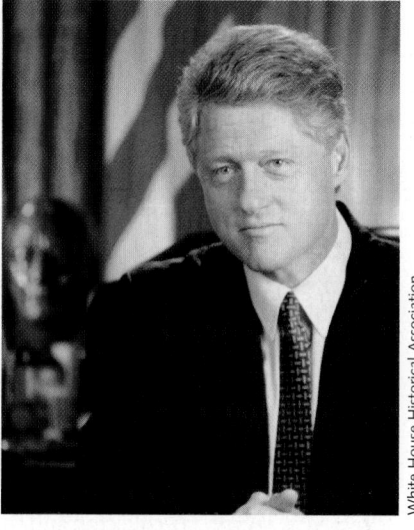

President Bill Clinton (1992–2000). *White House Historical Association*

extramarital affair the president had conducted with a young White House intern, Monica Lewinsky. His impeachment reflected the bitter partisanship and personal animosity between Democrats and Republicans in the 1990s. (See Chapter 29.)

Andrew Johnson was born in Raleigh, North Carolina, in 1808. At age 13, he was apprenticed to a tailor. As a young man, he moved to Tennessee. There he came to identify with the state's yeoman farmers and artisans in opposition to the great planters. Although he served as governor of Tennessee and later U.S. senator, he had little formal education; his wife, the daughter of a Scottish shoemaker, taught him how to write and do arithmetic.

In contrast, Bill Clinton attended Georgetown University and went on to graduate from Yale Law School. Clinton

also appreciated the help and support of his wife, but Hillary Rodham Clinton was a unique First Lady. She possessed impressive skills as a political campaigner and maintained a keen interest in policy issues. In 2000, just as her husband was leaving office, she was elected U.S. senator from the state of New York.

Generations of historians have disagreed about Johnson's case. In the early twentieth century, pro-South scholars sympathized with Lincoln's successor. Yet many scholars later in the century looked more favorably on the radical Republicans; influenced by the Civil Rights movement, these historians focused on Johnson's anti–civil rights stance. Therefore, it is difficult to predict how history will judge Bill Clinton and his battle with congressional Republicans. Historians themselves are an unpredictable lot. ∎

The general had proved himself a brilliant strategist during the war, but he lacked political experience, a shortcoming that soon became abundantly clear.

Political reunion was an uneven process, but one that gradually eroded the newly won rights of former slaves in many southern states. By the end of 1868, Arkansas, North Carolina, South Carolina, Louisiana, Tennessee, Alabama, and Florida had met congressional conditions for readmission to the Union, and two years later, Mississippi, Virginia, Georgia, and Texas followed. The Fifteenth Amendment, passed by Congress in 1869 and ratified by the necessary number of states a year later, granted all black men the right to vote.

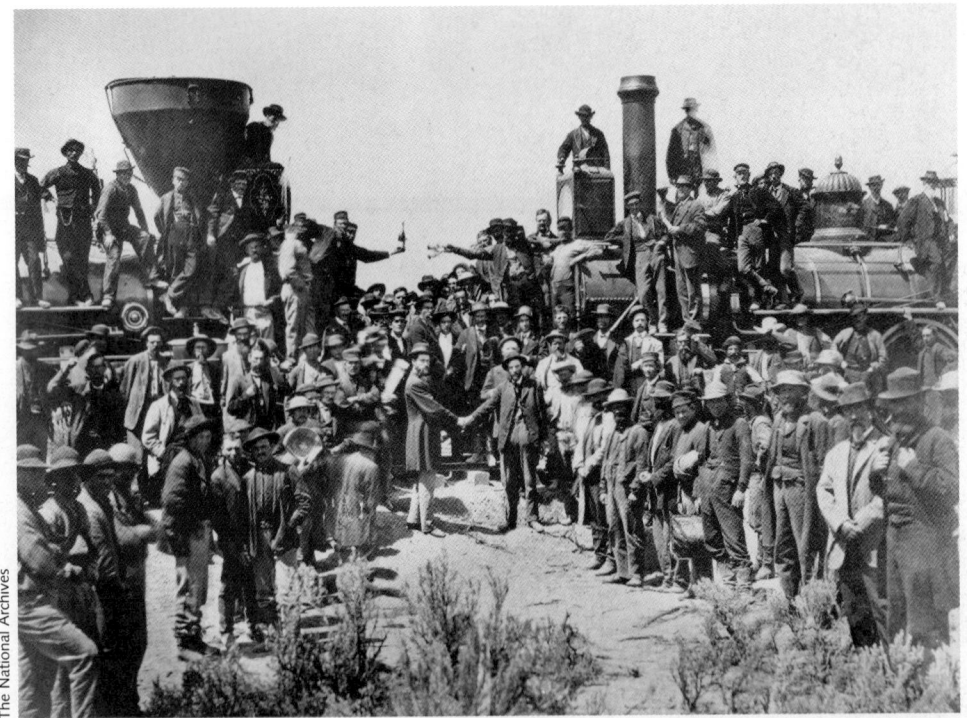

The National Archives

■   At Promontory Point near Ogden, Utah, workers joined the tracks linking the Central Pacific (its wood-burning locomotive, Jupiter, is on the left) with the Union Pacific's coal-burning engine No. 119. This photo was taken during the May 10, 1869, celebration marking the completion of the transcontinental railroad. According to one eyewitness, the crowd included Indians, Chinese and Irish immigrants, European Americans, and Mexicans "grouped in picturesque confusion." Yet this official photo shows little evidence of the Chinese workers who helped to engineer and build the Central Pacific line.

However, in some states, such as Louisiana, reunification gave Democrats license to engage in wholesale election fraud and violence toward freed men and women. In 1870–1871, a congressional inquiry into the Klan exposed pervasive and grisly assaults on Republican schoolteachers, preachers, and prospective voters, black and white. The Klan also targeted men and women who refused to work like slaves in the fields. In April 1871, Congress passed the Ku Klux Klan Act, which punished conspiracies intended to deny rights to citizens. But Klan violence and intimidation had already taken their toll. Republican voting strength began to decline in rural areas where blacks were the majority population and freedmen had attempted to assert their citizenship rights.

Claiming Territory for the Union

In 1871 poet Walt Whitman wrote an essay titled "Democratic Vistas." In it he celebrated the "manly and courageous instincts" that propelled a brave, adventurous people west. Whitman hailed the march across the prairies and over the mountains as a cavalcade of progress. He and other Americans believed that the postbellum migration fulfilled a mission of national regeneration begun by the Civil War. Kansas's population grew by 240 percent in the 1860s, Nebraska's by 355 percent.

To unite the entire country together as a single economic and political unit was the Republican ideal. Achieving this ideal entailed both technological and military means. The railroads in particular served as vehicles of national integration. When the Central Pacific and Union Pacific Railroads met at Promontory Point, Utah, in 1869, the hammering of the spike that joined the two roads produced a telegraphic signal received simultaneously on both coasts, setting off a national celebration. In Philadelphia, the Liberty Bell tolled.

Meanwhile, regular units of United States cavalry, including two regiments of blacks, were launching attacks on Indians on the Plains, in the Northwest, and in the Southwest. Between

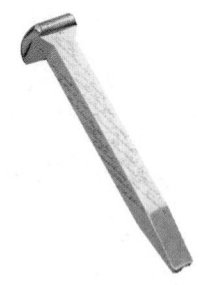

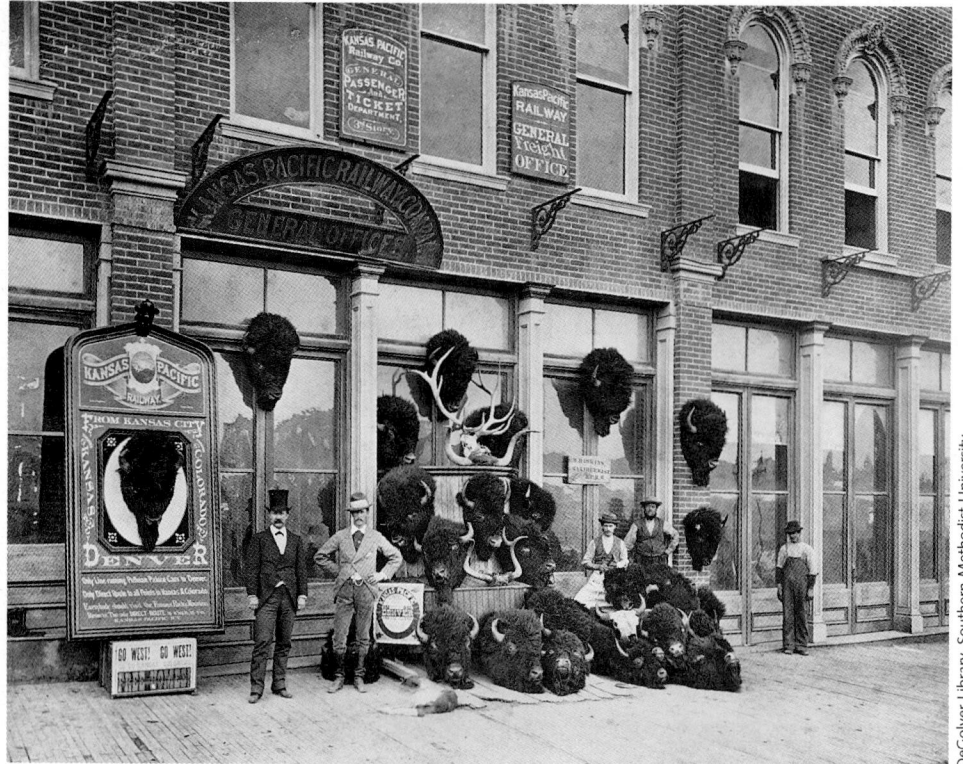

■ With this 1870 photograph, the Kansas Pacific Railroad advertised the opportunity for western travelers to shoot buffalo from the comfort and safety of their railroad car. The company's official taxidermist shows off his handiwork. Railroad expansion facilitated the exploitation of natural resources while promoting tourism.

1865 and 1890, U.S. military forces conducted a dozen separate campaigns against western Indian peoples and met Indian warriors in battle or attacked Indian settlements in more than 1000 engagements. The war for the West pitted agents of American nationalism against Indian groups that battled to maintain their distinctive way of life in a rapidly changing world. In contrast to African Americans, who adamantly demanded their rights as American citizens, defiant western Indians battled a government to which they owed no allegiance.

Federal Military Campaigns Against Western Indians

In 1871 the U.S. government renounced the practice of seeking treaties with various Indian groups. This change in policy opened the way for a more aggressive effort to subdue native populations. It also hastened the expansion of the reservation system, an effort begun in the antebellum period to confine specific Indian groups to specific territories.

In the Southwest, clashes between Indians and U.S. soldiers persisted after the Civil War. In 1867 at Medicine Lodge Creek in southern Kansas the United States signed a treaty with an alliance of Comanche, Kiowa, Cheyenne, Arapaho, and Plains Apache. This treaty could not long withstand the provocation posed by the railroad. The year before, the Seventh U. S. Cavalry, under the command of Lieutenant Colonel George Custer, had been formed to ward off native attacks on the Union Pacific, snaking its way across the central Plains westward from Kansas. In November 1868 Custer destroyed a Cheyenne settlement on the Washita River, in present-day Oklahoma. The settlement's leader was Black Kettle, who had brought his people to reservation territory after the Sand Creek Massacre in Colorado in 1864. Custer's men murdered women and children, burned tepees, and destroyed 800 horses. Sickened by the scene, one army officer later wrote sarcastically of the "daring dash" on the part of "heroes of a bloody day." The soldiers left piles of corpses scattered among the smoldering ruins of the village.

A series of peace delegations to Washington, several led by Red Cloud of the Sioux, produced much curiosity among whites but no end to the slaughter of people or animals in the West.

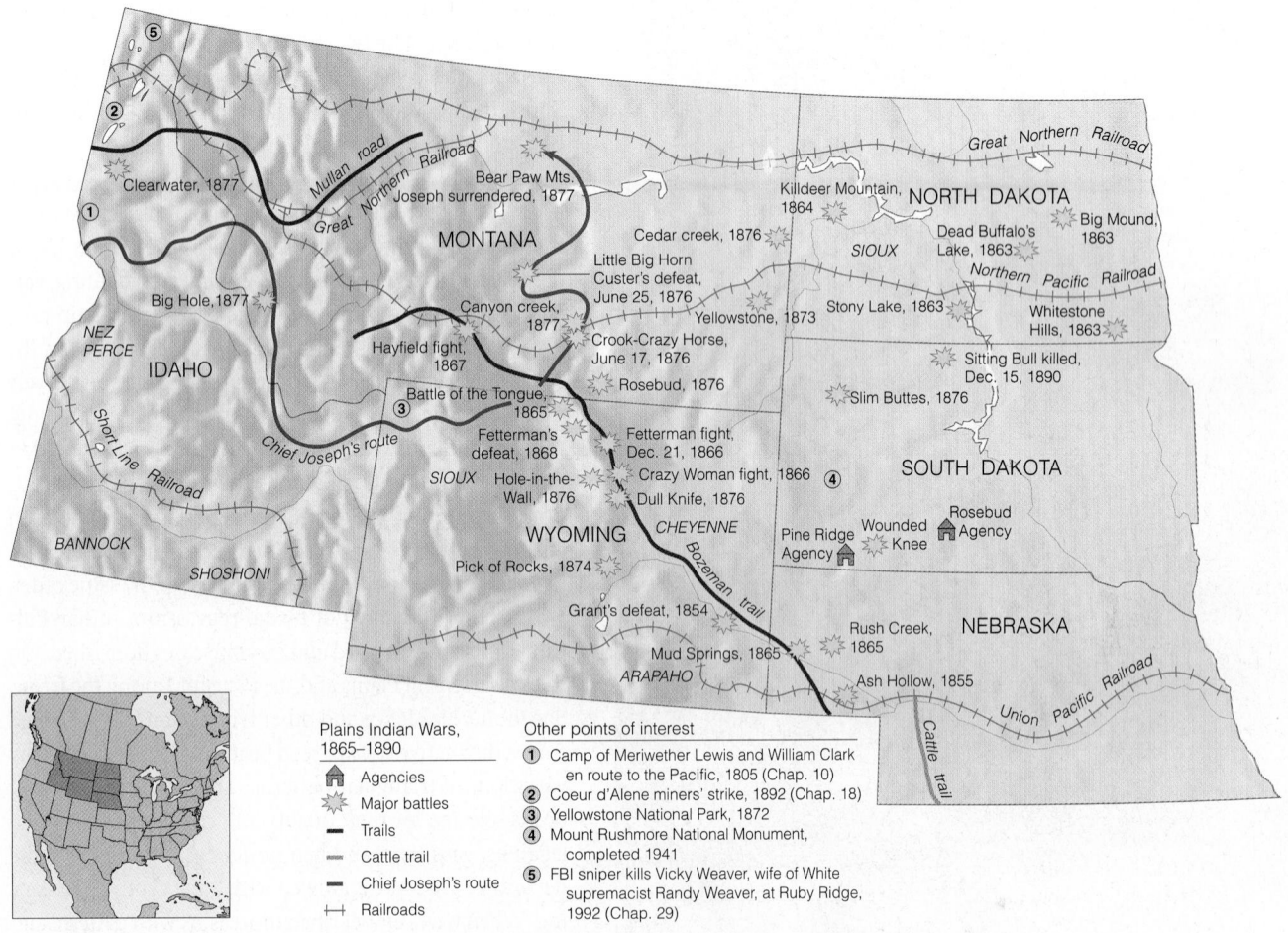

■ **MAP 15.2**

PLAINS INDIAN WARS, 1865–1900 This map reveals that between 1865 and 1890, many of the conflicts between Indians and U.S. troops occurred along either railroad lines or trails used by European American settlers. For example, the Sioux, Cheyenne, and Arapaho fiercely resisted travelers along the Bozeman Trail running from Colorado to Montana.

Indians continued to attack the surveyors, supply caravans, and military escorts that preceded the railroad work crews. Lamenting the loss of his people's hunting grounds to the railroad, Red Cloud said, "The white children have surrounded me and have left me nothing but an island."

The Apache Indians managed to elude General George Crook until 1875. Crook employed some of these Apaches to track down the war chief Geronimo of the Chiricahuas. Like many other Indian leaders, Geronimo offered both religious and military guidance to his people. He believed that a spirit would protect him from the white man's bullets and from the arrows of Indians in league with government troops. Yet Geronimo was tricked into a momentary surrender in 1877. Sorrowfully, he agreed to bring his followers into the San Carlos reservation in eastern Arizona. There he was held in irons for several months before gaining his release and challenging authorities for another nine years.

In 1874 Custer took the Seventh into the Black Hills of the Dakotas, so-called unceded Indian territory. Supposedly, the 1868 Treaty of Fort Laramie had rendered this land off-limits to whites. Custer's mission was to offer protection for the surveyors of the Northern Pacific Railroad and to force Indians onto reservations as stipulated in the 1868 treaty. However, the officer lost no time trumpeting the fact that Indian lands were filled with gold. This report prompted a rush to the Black Hills, lands sacred to the Sioux. Within two years, 15,000 gold

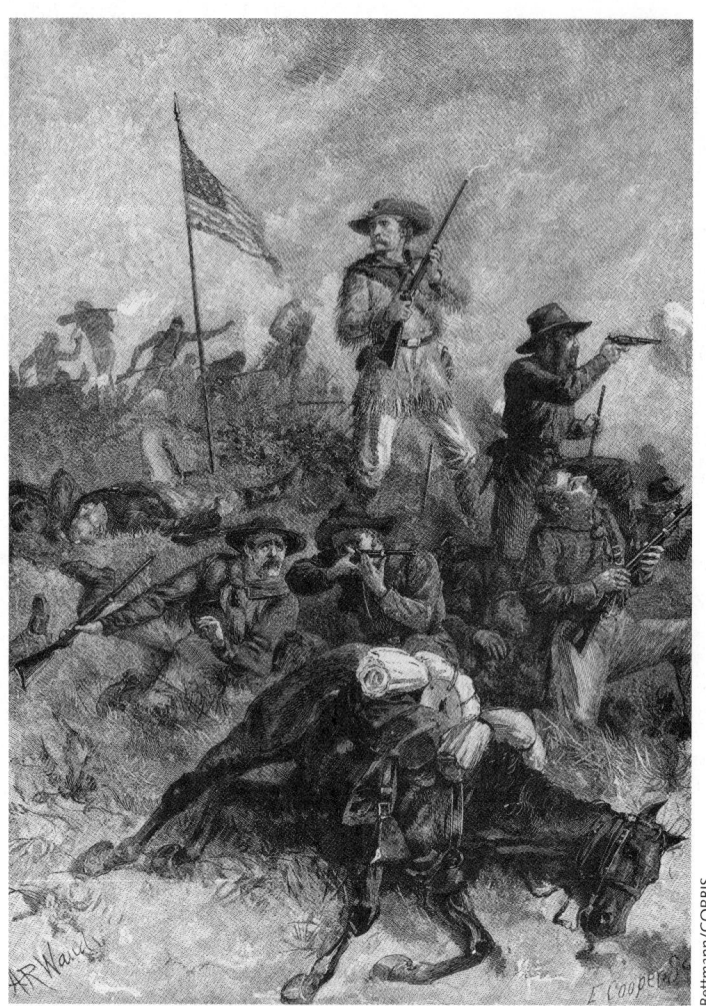

Bettmann/CORBIS

■ During the morning of June 25, 1876, General George Custer and his force of 264 soldiers attacked a Sun Dance gathering of 2500 Sioux and Cheyenne on the banks of the Little Big Horn River in Montana. This European American version of the battle illustrated a book celebrating the life of Custer. The book was published soon after the battle, which took place in June 1876. At the time, the country was in the midst of a celebration marking the centennial of the nation's birth. The engraving portrays Custer and his men making a courageous "last stand."

miners had illegally descended on Indian lands to seek their fortunes. The federal government proposed to buy the land, but leaders of the Sioux, including Red Cloud, Spotted Tail, and Sitting Bull, spurned the offer. "The Black Hills belong to me," declared Sitting Bull. "If the whites try to take them, I will fight."

Indians throughout the West maintained their distinctive ways of life during these turbulent times. Horse holdings, so crucial for hunting, trading, and fighting, varied from group to group, with the Crow wealthy in relation to their Central Plains neighbors the Oglala and the Arikara. Plains and Plateau peoples engaged in a lively trading system. They exchanged horses and their trappings (bridles and blankets) for eastern goods such as kettles, guns, and ammunition. Despite their differences in economy, these groups held similar religious beliefs about an all-powerful life force that governed the natural world. People, plants, and animals were all part of the same order.

Even in the midst of brutal repression, Indian cultural traditions survived and in some cases flourished. On the West Central Plains and the Plateau, among the Crow, Shoshone, Nez Perce and other tribes, women developed a new, distinctive style of seed beadwork characterized by variations of triangular patterns. These designs, made of beads selected for their quality and consistency, adorned leggings, gauntlets, and belt pouches. In these ways, the decorative arts were endowed with great symbolic meaning. When wives embellished moccasins with patterns signifying their husband's military achievements, handicrafts assumed political as well as artistic significance.

The Postwar Western Labor Problem

In the eyes of many European Americans, the West offered vast challenges and opportunities. To construct a railroad across the plains and mountains, to extract rich reserves of timber and minerals, to harvest immense crops of wheat—all of these tasks demanded large numbers of willing workers. But such workers were in short supply. Moreover, available workers wanted employers to pay and treat them fairly.

In 1865 the owners of the Central Pacific Railroad seemed poised for one of the great engineering feats of the nineteenth century. In the race eastward from California, they would construct trestles spanning vast chasms and roadbeds traversing mountains and deserts. Government officials in Washington were eager to subsidize the railroad. What the owners lacked was a dependable labor force. The Irish workers who began the line in California struck for higher wages in compensation for brutal, dangerous work. These immigrants dropped their shovels and hammers at the first word of a gold strike nearby—or far away. As a result, in 1866 the Central Pacific had decided to tap into a vast labor source by importing thousands of Chinese men from their native Guandong province.

The Chinese toiled to extend the railroad tracks eastward from Sacramento, California, up to ten miles a day in the desert, only a few feet a day in the rugged Sierra Nevada Mountains. They alternately loaded and dumped millions of tons of earth and rocks to clear the land and construct the roadbed. In nerve-wracking feats of skill, they lowered themselves in woven baskets to implant nitroglycerine explosives in canyon walls. Chinese

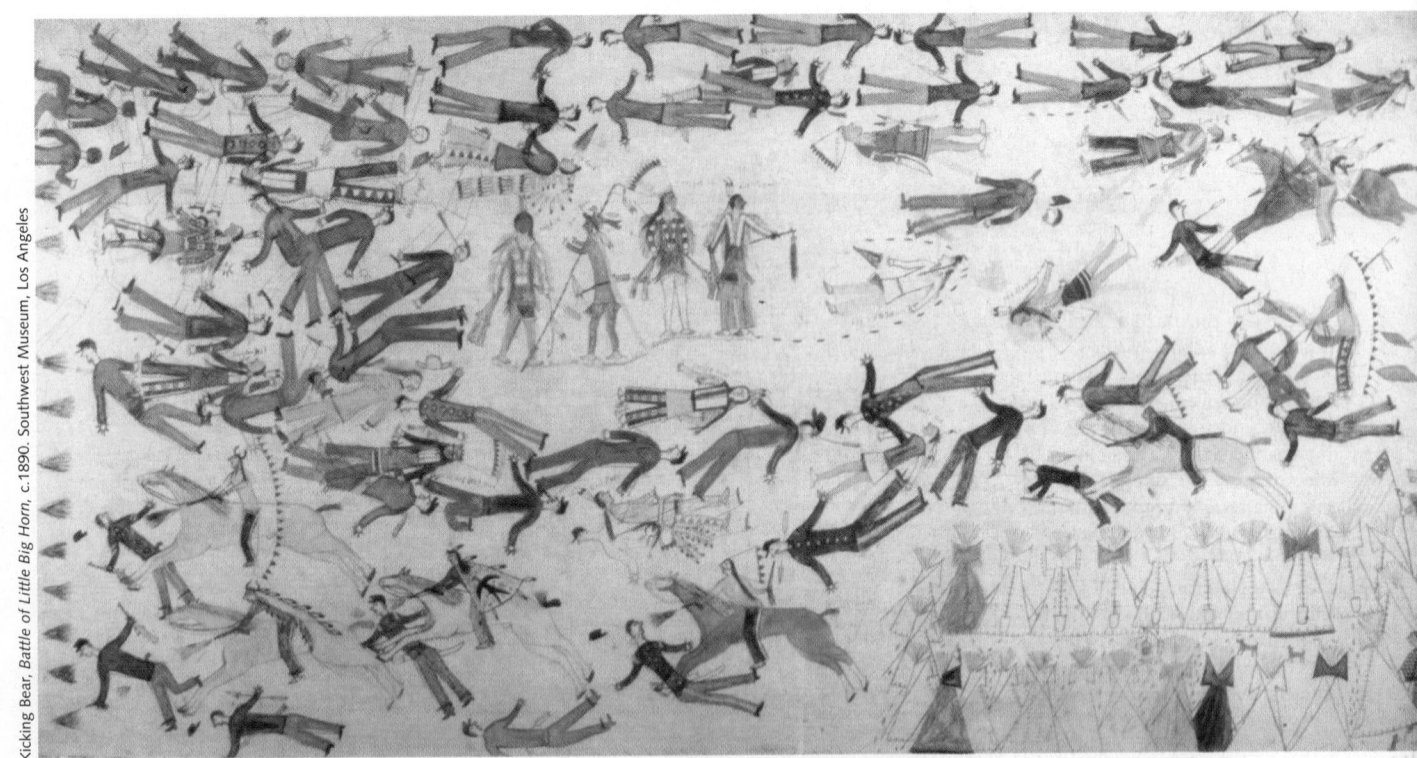

■ Custer foolishly launched his attack without adequate backup, and he and his men were easily overwhelmed and killed by Indian warriors, led by the Oglala Sioux Crazy Horse and others. Reacting to this defeat, U.S. military officials reduced the Lakotas and Cheyennes to wardship status, ending their autonomy. This version of the Battle of the Little Big Horn, by Sioux artist Kicking Bear, highlights the aesthetic and ritualistic elements of the Indian's costume and the decorations attached to his horse. In this picture, warrior and soldier meet face to face. Unarmed and on foot, the soldier is at the mercy of his foe.

laborers toiled through snowstorms and blistering heat to blast tunnels and cut passes through granite mountains. Journalists marveled at the ability of a squad of Chinese to unload 200 tons of iron and 10 tons of spikes from railroad cars in just ten minutes. These reporters also commented on the strange sight of men in their native dress and traditional broad straw hats, taking afternoon tea breaks.

Charles Crocker, the general superintendent of the Central Pacific, observed of the Chinese, "Wherever we put them, we found them good." Paid $1 a day (less than the wage paid to whites), the Chinese had little leverage with which to press for higher compensation. In the spring of 1867, 5000 (out of a workforce of 12,000) walked off the job. They demanded $1.50 a day and an eight-hour day. Crocker responded by withholding rations, and the laborers were forced to return to work within a week. With the final linking of the railroad in Utah in 1869, many Chinese returned to California.

Signed in 1868, the Burlingame Treaty, named for Anson Burlingame, an American envoy to China, had supposedly guaranteed government protection for Chinese immigrants as visitors, traders, or permanent residents. Most immigrants were men. (Six out of ten California Chinese women were listed in the 1870 census as prostitutes, most the victims of their compatriots.) Yet the treaty did not inhibit U.S. employers, landlords, and government officials from discriminating against the Chinese.

By 1870, 40,000 Chinese lived in California and represented fully one-quarter of the state's wage earners. They found work in the cigar, woolen-goods, and boot and shoe factories of San Francisco; in the gold mining towns, now as laundry operators rather than as miners as

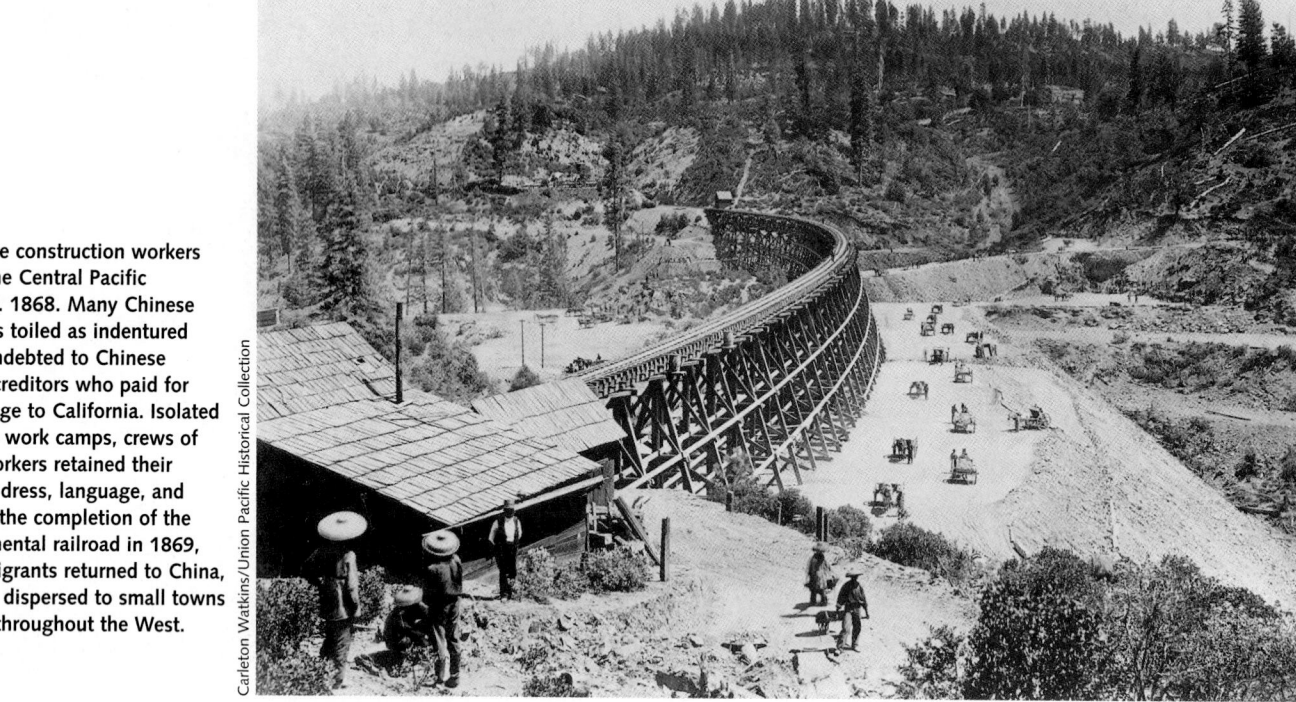

■ Chinese construction workers labor on the Central Pacific Railroad, c. 1868. Many Chinese immigrants toiled as indentured laborers, indebted to Chinese merchant creditors who paid for their passage to California. Isolated in all-male work camps, crews of railroad workers retained their traditional dress, language, and diet. After the completion of the transcontinental railroad in 1869, some immigrants returned to China, and others dispersed to small towns and cities throughout the West.

Carleton Watkins/Union Pacific Historical Collection

they had before the Civil War; and in the fields as agricultural laborers. White workers began to cry unfair competition against this Asian group that was becoming increasingly integrated into the region's economy.

As a group, Chinese men differed from California Indians, who remained trapped in the traditional agricultural economy of unskilled labor. Whites appropriated Indian land and forced many men, women, and children to work as wage earners for large landowners. Deprived of their familiar hunting and gathering lands, and wracked by disease and starvation, California Indians had suffered a drastic decline in their numbers by 1870, from 100,000 to 30,000 in 20 years.

By the early 1870s western manufacturers were faltering under the pressure of cheaper goods imported from the East by rail. At the same time, the growth of fledgling gigantic agricultural businesses opened new avenues of trade and commerce. Located in an arc surrounding the San Francisco Bay, large ("bonanza") wheat farmers grew huge crops and exported the grain to the East Coast and to England. These enterprises stimulated the building of wharves and railroad trunk lines and encouraged technological innovation in threshing and harvesting. Western enterprises showed a growing demand for labor whatever its skin color or nationality.

Land Use in an Expanding Nation

The end of the Civil War prompted new conflicts and deepened long-standing ones over the use of the land in a rich, sprawling country. In the South, staple crop planters began to share political power with an emerging elite, men who owned railroads and textile mills. Despairing of ever achieving antebellum levels of labor efficiency, some landowners turned to mining the earth and the forests for saleable commodities. These products, obtained through extraction, included phosphate (used in producing fertilizer), timber, coal, and turpentine. Labor in extractive industries complemented labor in the plantation economy. Sharecroppers alternated between tilling cotton fields in the spring and harvesting the crop in the fall, while seeking employment in sawmills and coal mines in the winter and summer.

As European Americans settled in the West and Southwest, they displaced natives who had been living there for generations. For example, the U.S. court system determined who could legally claim property. Western courts also decided whether natural resources such as water, land, timber, and fish and game constituted property that could be owned by private interests. In the Southwest, European American settlers, including army soldiers who had come to fight Indians and then stayed, continued to place Hispanic land titles at risk. Citing prewar precedents, American courts favored the claims of recent squatters over those of long-standing residents. In 1869 with the death of her husband (who had served as a general in the Union army), Maria Amparo Ruiz de Burton saw the large ranch they had worked together near San Diego slip out of her control. The first Spanish-speaking woman to be published in English in the United States, de Burton was a member of the Hispanic elite. Nevertheless, she had little political power. California judges backed the squatters who occupied the ranch.

As they controlled more land and assumed public office, some European Americans in the Southwest exploited their political connections and economic power. In the process they managed to wield great influence over people and vast amounts of natural resources. In the 1870s the so-called Santa Fe Ring wrested more than 80 percent of the original Spanish grants of land from Hispanic landholders in New Mexico. An alliance of European American lawyers, businesspeople, and politicians, the Santa Fe Ring defrauded families and kin groups of their land titles and speculated in property to make a profit. Whereas many ordinary Hispanic settlers saw land—with its crops, pasture, fuel, building materials, and game—as a source of livelihood, groups, such as the Santa Fe Ring, saw land primarily as a commodity to be bought and sold.

Seemingly overnight, boom towns sprang up wherever minerals or timber beckoned: southern Arizona and the Rocky Mountains west of Denver, Virginia City in western Nevada, the Idaho–Montana region, and the Black Hills of South Dakota. In all these places, increasing numbers of workers operated sophisticated kinds of machinery, such as rock crushers, and labored for wages. When the vein was exhausted or the forests depleted, the towns went bust.

Railroads facilitated not only the mining of minerals but also the growth of the cattle-ranching industry. By 1869 a quarter of a million cattle were grazing in Colorado Territory. Rail connections between the Midwest and East made it profitable for Texas ranchers to pay cowboys to drive their herds of long-horned steers to Abilene, Ellsworth, Wichita, or Dodge City, Kansas, for shipment to stockyards in Chicago or St. Louis. Large meatpackers, such as Swift and Armour, prepared the carcasses for the eastern market.

Cattle drives were huge; an estimated 10 million animals were herded north from Texas alone between 1865 and 1890. They offered employment to all kinds of men with sufficient skills and endurance. Among the cowhands were African American horsebreakers and gunmen and Mexicans skilled in the use of the *reata* (lasso). Blacks made up about 25 percent and Hispanics about 15 percent of all cowboy outfits. Tracing the evolution of the Chisholm Trail, which

TABLE 15-3

Estimates of Railroad Crossties Used and Acres of Forest Cleared, 1870–1910

Year	Miles of Track	Ties Renewed Annually (millions)	Ties Used on New Construction (millions)	Total Ties Annually (millions)	Acres of Forest Cleared (thousands)
1870	60,000	21	18	39	195
1880	107,000	37	21	58	290
1890	200,000	70	19	89	445
1900	259,000			91	455
1910	357,000			124	620

Source: Michael Williams, Americans and Their Forests (1989), 352.

linked southern Texas to Abilene, from Indian path to commercial route, one observer wrote in 1874, "So many cattle have been driven over the trail in the last few years that a broad highway is tread out, looking much like a national highway." Yet this new "national highway" traversed Indian Territory (present-day Oklahoma), lands supposedly promised to Indians forever.

In knitting regional economies together, federal land policies were crucial to the Republican vision of a developing nation. Yet a series of land use acts had a mixed legacy. The Mineral Act of 1866 granted title to millions of acres of mineral-rich land to mining companies, a gift from the federal government to private interests. In 1866 Congress passed the Southern Homestead Act to help blacks acquire land, but the measure accomplished little and was repealed in 1876. The Timber Culture Act of 1873 allotted 160 acres to individuals in selected western states if they agreed to plant one-fourth of the acreage with trees. Four years later, the Desert Land Act provided cheap land if buyers irrigated at least part of their parcels.

The exploitation of western resources raised many legal questions: Must ranchers pay for the prairies their cattle grazed on and the trails they followed to market? How could one "own" a stampeding buffalo herd or a flowing river? What was the point of holding title to a piece of property if only the timber, oil, water, or minerals on and in it (but not the soil) were of value?

The Apex Mining Act of 1872 sought to address at least some of these issues. This law legalized traditional mining practices in the West by validating titles approved by local courts. According to the law, a person who could locate the apex of a vein (its point closest to the surface) could lay claim to the entire vein beneath the surface. The measure contributed to the wholesale destruction of certain parts of the western landscape as mining companies blasted their way through mountains and left piles of rocks in their wake. It also spurred thousands of lawsuits as claimants argued over what constituted an apex or a vein.

It was during this period that a young Scottish-born naturalist named John Muir began to explore the magnificent canyons and mountains of California. Viewing nature as a means for regenerating the human spirit, Muir emphasized a deep appreciation of the natural world. He contrasted nature's majesty with the artificial landscape created by and for humans. In the wilderness, there is nothing "truly dead or dull, or any trace of

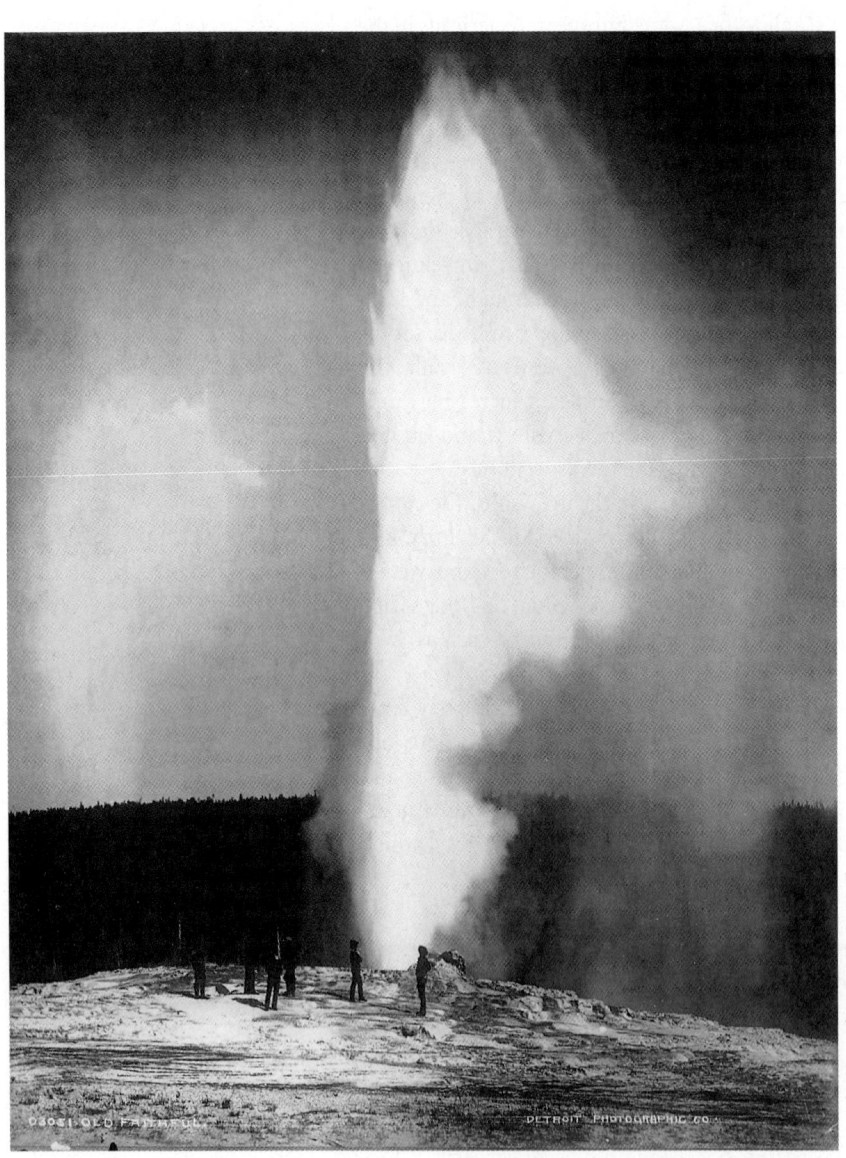

Colorado Historical Society (CHS.J 2067)

■ Chicago photographer Thomas J. Hine titled this stereograph "Old Faithful in Action, Fire Hole Basin." It is the first photograph of the eruption of the famous Yellowstone geyser. Costing 15–25 cents each, stereographs were a popular form of entertainment in middle-class households beginning in the 1860s. The stereoscope merged two identical photos to form a single three-dimensional image. Widely distributed stereographs of scenic natural wonders boosted western tourism.

what in manufactories is called rubbish or waste," he wrote; "everything is perfectly clean and pure and full of divine lessons." Muir believed that the need to protect breathtaking vistas and magnificent stands of giant redwoods compelled the federal government to act as land policy regulator.

Muir was gratified by the creation of the National Park system during the postwar period. By this time, pressure had been building on the federal government to protect vast tracts of undeveloped lands. Painters and geologists were among the first Easterners to appreciate the spectacular vistas of the western landscape. In 1864 Congress set aside a small area within California's Yosemite Valley for public recreation and enjoyment. Soon after the war, railroad promoters forged an alliance with government officials in an effort to block commercial development of particularly beautiful pockets of land. In the late 1860s the invention of the Pullman sleeping car—a luxurious hotel room on wheels—helped spur the drive to protect these areas from farming, lumbering, stock raising, and mining. Northern Pacific railroad financier Jay Cooke lobbied hard for the government to create a two-million-acre park in what is today the northwest corner of Wyoming. As a result, in March 1872, Congress created Yellowstone National Park. Tourism would continue to serve as a key component of the western economy.

Muir and others portrayed the Yosemite and Yellowstone Valleys as wildernesses, empty of human activity. In fact, both areas had long provided hunting and foraging grounds for native peoples. Yellowstone had been occupied by the people now called the Shoshone since the fifteenth century. This group, together with the Bannock, Crow, and Blackfeet, tried to retain access to Yellowstone's meadows, rivers, and forests after it became a national park. However, U.S. policymakers and military officials persisted in their efforts to mark off territory for specific purposes, while Indians were confined to reservations.

Buying Territory for the Union

Before the war, Republicans had opposed any federal expansionist schemes that they feared might benefit slaveholders. However, after 1865 and the outlawing of slavery, some Republican lawmakers and administration officials advocated the acquisition of additional territory. Secretary of State William Seward led the way in 1867 by purchasing Alaska from Russia and trying unsuccessfully to buy the Danish West Indies.

The purchase of Alaska immeasurably enriched the nation's natural resources. For $7.2 million (about 2 cents an acre), the United States gained 591,004 square miles of land. Within the territory were diverse indigenous groups—Eskimos, Aleuts, Tlingit, Tsimshian, Athabaskan, and Haida—and a small number of native Russians. Though derided at the time as "Seward's icebox," Alaska yielded enough fish, timber, minerals, and water power in the years to come to prove that the original purchase price was a tremendous bargain.

The impulse that prompted administration support for the Alaska purchase also spawned other plans for territorial acquisitions. In 1870 some Republicans joined with Democrats in calling for the annexation of the Dominican Republic. These congressmen argued that the tiny Caribbean country would make a fine naval base, provide investment opportunities for American businesspeople, and offer a refuge for southern freedpeople. Frederick Douglass, who had visited the country, claimed that annexing the Dominican Republic would "transplant within her tropical borders the glorious institutions" of the United States.

However, Charles Sumner, chairman of the Senate Foreign Relations Committee, opposed ratification of the annexation treaty. He warned against a takeover without considering the will of the Dominican people, who were currently involved in their own civil war. Some congressmen, in a prelude to foreign policy debates of the 1890s, suggested that the dark-skinned Dominican people were incapable of appreciating the blessings of American citizenship. In 1871 the treaty failed to win Senate approval. A firm supporter of annexation, President Grant felt personally betrayed by the Republicans who opposed him on this issue.

The Republican Vision and Its Limits

After the Civil War, victorious Republicans envisioned a nation united in the pursuit of prosperity. All citizens would be free to follow their individual economic self-interest and to enjoy the fruits of honest toil. In contrast, some increasingly vocal and well-organized groups saw the expansion of legal rights, and gving black men the right to vote in particular, as only initial, tentative steps on the path to an all-inclusive citizenship. Women, industrial workers, farmers, and African Americans made up overlapping constituencies pressing for equal political rights and economic opportunity. Together they challenged the mainstream Republican view that defeat of the rebels and destruction of slavery were sufficient to guarantee all people prosperity.

Government–business partnerships also produced unanticipated consequences for Republicans committed to what they believed was the collective good. Some politicians and business leaders saw these partnerships as opportunities for private gain. Consequently, private greed and public corruption accompanied postwar economic growth. Thus, Republican leaders faced challenges from two very different sources: people agitating for civil rights and people hoping to reap personal gain from political activities.

Postbellum Origins of the Woman Suffrage Movement

After the Civil War, the nation's middle class, which had its origins in the antebellum period, continued to grow. Dedicated to self-improvement and filled with a sense of moral authority, many middle-class Americans (especially Protestants) felt a deep cultural connection to their counterparts in England. Indeed, the United States produced its own "Victorians," so called for the self-conscious middle class that emerged in the England of Queen Victoria during her reign from 1837 to 1901.

At the heart of the Victorian sensibility was the ideal of domesticity: a harmonious family living in a well-appointed home, guided by a pious mother and supported by a father successful in business. Famous Protestant clergyman Henry Ward Beecher and his wife were outspoken proponents of this domestic ideal. According to Eunice Beecher, women had no "higher, nobler, more divine mission than in the conscientious endeavor to create a *true home*." Her husband added, "The laborer ought to be ashamed of himself who in 20 years does not own the ground on which his house stands . . . who has not in that house provided carpets for the rooms, who has not his China plates, who has not his chromos [decorative photographs], who has not some books nestling on the shelf."

Yet the traumatic events of the Civil War only intensified the desire among a growing group of American women to participate fully in the nation's political life. They wanted to extend their moral influence outside the narrow and exclusive sphere of the home. In countless everyday, unsung ways, Union women had supported the Union cause. They had managed farms, raised money for the U.S. Sanitary Commission, and sponsored patriotic rallies. Many women believed that they deserved the vote and that the time was right to demand it.

In 1866 veteran reformers Elizabeth Cady Stanton, Susan B. Anthony, and Lucy Stone founded the Equal Rights Association to link the rights of white women and African Americans. Nevertheless, in 1867, Kansas voters defeated a referendum proposing suffrage for both blacks and white women. This disappointment convinced some former abolitionists that the two causes should be separated—that women should wait patiently until the rights of African American men were firmly secured. Frederick Douglass declined an invitation to a women's suffrage convention in Washington, D.C., in 1868. He explained, "I am now devoting myself to a cause [if] not more sacred, certainly more urgent, because it is one of life and death to the long enslaved people of this country, and that is: negro suffrage."

Douglass left African American women out of his call for "negro suffrage." He implied that the chief advocates of women's suffrage were white and middle class. As a result, Douglass failed to gauge the way in which the issue of universal suffrage connected all black people with all women. African American activist and former slave Sojourner Truth warned white women not to presume to speak for all women, and she also urged black men not to speak for themselves only. At a meeting of the newly formed Equal Rights Association, Truth pointed out, "There is a great stir about colored men getting their rights, but not a word about the colored women; and if colored men get their rights, and not colored women get theirs, there will be a bad time about it."

In 1869 two factions of women parted ways and formed separate organizations devoted to women's rights. The more radical wing, including Cady Stanton and Anthony, bitterly denounced the Fifteenth Amendment because it gave the vote to black men only. In 1868 the two leaders had attempted to organize a Working Women's Party, which they hoped would appeal to female wage earners and serve as the foundation of a new political party dedicated to broad-based reform.

The following year they helped to found the National Woman Suffrage Association (NWSA). Members of NWSA argued for a renewed commitment to the original Declaration of Sentiments passed in Seneca Falls, New York two decades earlier. They favored married women's property rights, liberalization of divorce laws, opening colleges and trade schools to women, a new federal amendment to allow women to vote. In 1869, women's rights proponents Lucy Stone and her husband, Henry Blackwell, founded the rival American Woman Suffrage Association (AWSA). This group downplayed the larger struggle for women's rights and focused on the suffrage question exclusively. Its members supported the Fifteenth Amendment and retained ties to the Republican party. The AWSA focused on state-by-state campaigns for women's suffrage.

New York City newspaper *The Daily Graphic* carried this caricature of Susan B. Anthony on its June 5, 1873, cover. The artist suggests that the drive for women's suffrage has resulted in a reversal of gender roles. Titled "The Woman Who Dared," the cartoon portrays Anthony as a masculine figure. One of her male supporters, on the right, holds a baby, while women activists march and give speeches. On the left, a female police officer keeps watch over the scene.

Library of Congress

In 1871 the NWSA welcomed the daring, flamboyant Victoria Woodhull as a vocal supporter, only to renounce her a few years later. Woodhull's political agenda ranged from free love and dietary reform to legalized prostitution, working men's rights, and women's suffrage. (In the nineteenth century, free love advocates denounced what they called a sexual double standard, one that glorified female chastity while tolerating male promiscuity.) Woodhull's speeches gained her a great deal of publicity; in one political cartoon she was labeled "Mrs. Satan." This was hardly the kind of publicity the NWSA craved. At the group's 1871 convention Woodhull startled many of the old guard with her declaration, "We mean treason! We mean secession. . . . We are plotting Revolution! We will overthrow this bogus republic and plant a government of righteousness in its stead."

In 1872 one of Woodhull's critics successfully challenged her. Woodhull spent a month in jail as a result of the zealous prosecution by vice reformer Anthony Comstock, a clergyman who objected to her public discussions and writings on sexuality. Comstock assumed the role of an outspoken crusader against vice. A federal law passed in 1873, and named after him, equated information related to birth control with pornography, banning this and other "obscene material" from the mails.

Also in 1872, Woodhull formed what she called the Equal Rights Party. This new party nominated its founder for the U.S. presidency. However, Woodhull's proposed vice presidential running mate, Frederick Douglass, declined the honor. He announced that he planned to vote for Grant again.

For her part, Susan B. Anthony used the 1872 presidential election as a test case for women's suffrage. She attempted to vote and was arrested, tried, and convicted as a result. By this time, most women suffragists, and most members of the NWSA for that matter, had become convinced that they should focus on the vote exclusively; they therefore accepted the AWSA's policy on this issue. In the coming years, they would avoid other causes with which they might have allied themselves, including black civil rights and labor reform.

Workers' Organizations

Many Americans benefited from economic changes of the postwar era. Railroading, mining, and heavy industry helped fuel the national economy and in the process boosted the growth of the urban managerial class. In the Midwest, many landowning farmers prospered when they responded to an expanding demand for grain and other staple crops. In Wisconsin, wheat farmers cleared forests, drained swamps, diverted rivers, and profited from the booming world market in grain. Yet the economic developments that allowed factory managers and owners of large wheat farms to make a comfortable living for themselves did not necessarily benefit agricultural and manufacturing workers.

Several organizations offered laborers an alternative vision to the Republicans' brand of individualism and nationalism.

Indeed, during this period growing numbers of working people, in the countryside and in the cities, became caught up in a cycle of indebtedness. In the upcountry South (above the fall line, or Piedmont), formerly self-sufficient family farmers sought loans from banks to repair their war-damaged homesteads. To qualify for these loans, the farmer had to plant cotton as a staple crop, to the neglect of corn and other foodstuffs. Many sharecroppers, black and white, received payment in the form of credit only; for these families, the end-of-the-year reckoning yielded little more than rapidly accumulating debts. Midwestern farmers increasingly relied on expensive threshing and harvesting machinery and on bank loans to purchase the machinery. In cities all over the country, the mass production of shoes and textiles meant that members of the laboring classes depended more than ever on cash to buy such necessities, yet depressed wages and irregular employment put families at risk.

Several organizations founded within five years of the war's end offered laborers an alternative vision to the Republicans' brand of individualism and nationalism. In 1867 Oliver H. Kelly, a former Minnesota farmer now working in a Washington office, organized the National Grange of the Patrons of Husbandry, popularly known as the Grange. This movement sought to address a new, complex marketplace increasingly dominated by railroads, banks, and grain elevator operators. The Grange encouraged farmers to form cooperatives that would market their crops and to challenge discriminatory railroad rates that favored big business.

Founded in Baltimore in 1866, the National Labor Union (NLU) consisted of a collection of craft unions and claimed as many as 600,000 members at its peak in the early 1870s. The group welcomed farmers as well as factory workers and promoted a general program of social reform. The group also favored legislation for an eight-hour workday and the arbitration of industrial disputes.

William Sylvis, a leader of the Iron Molders' International Union in Philadelphia and the second president of the NLU, sounded twin themes that would mark national labor

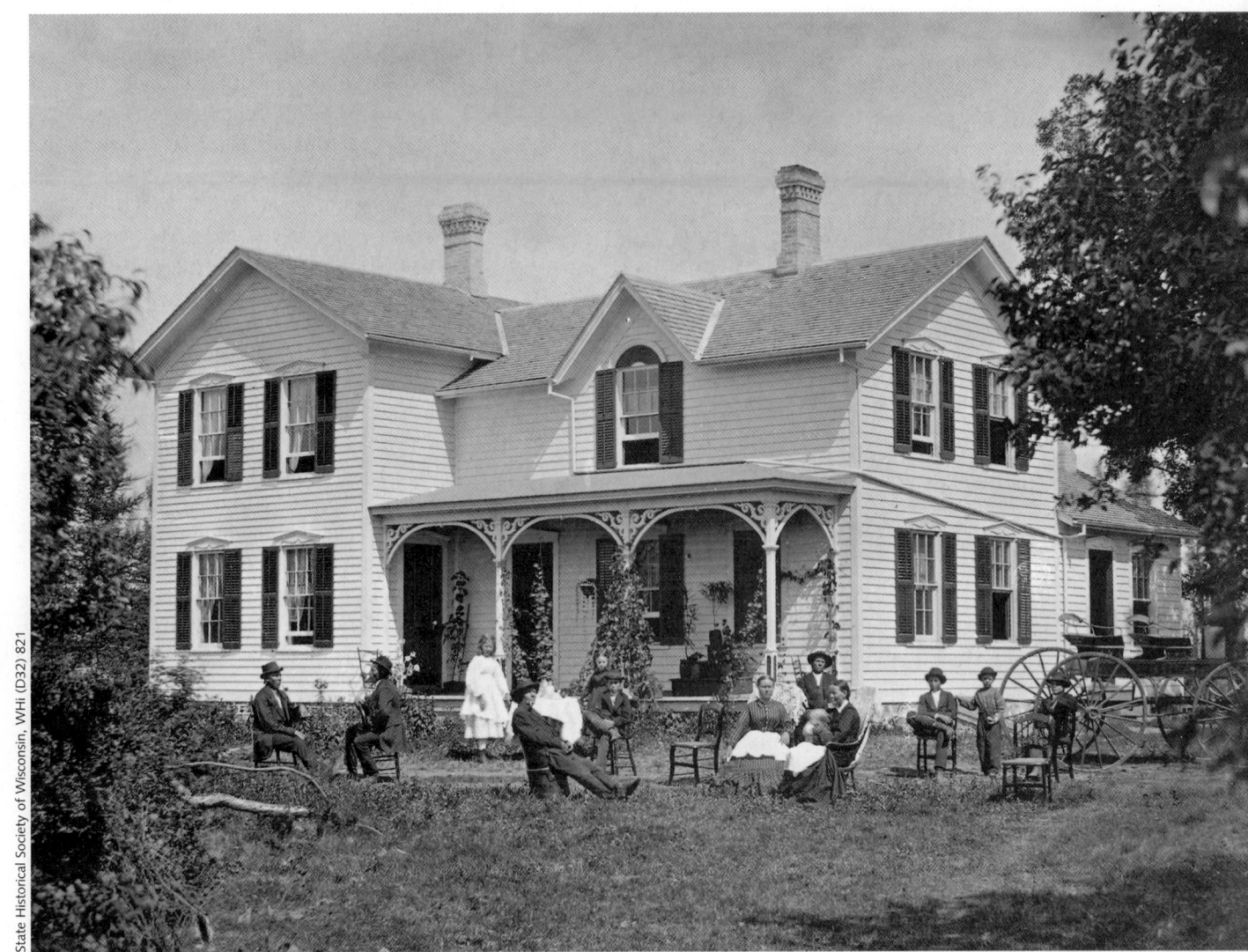

■ A Norwegian immigrant extended family in the town of Norway Grove, Wisconsin, poses in front of their imposing home and up-to-date carriage in this photograph taken in the mid-1870s. Linking their fortunes to the world wheat market, these newcomers to the United States prospered. Wrote one woman to her brother back home in Norway, "We all have cattle, driving oxen, and wagons. We also have children in abundance."

union organizing efforts for generations to come. He called for an alliance of black and white workers. Yet at the same time, Sylvis defended the practice of excluding blacks from positions of leadership on the job and in the union. Impatient with such pronouncements, Isaac Myers, a black ship caulker from Baltimore, helped found the short-lived Colored National Labor Union in Washington, D.C., in 1868. (This association remained small and disbanded within three years.) Myers offered a view of citizenship that differed from white Republicans' exclusive emphasis on the franchise: "If citizenship means anything at all," the black labor leader declared, "it means the freedom of labor, as broad and as universal as freedom of the ballot."

In 1873 a nationwide depression threw thousands out of work and worsened the plight of debtors. Businesspeople in agriculture, mining, the railroad industry, and manufacturing had overexpanded their operations. The free-wheeling loan practices of major banks had

---

TABLE 15-4

**National and International Union Members of the
National Labor Union (with dates of each union's founding)**

National Typographical Union (printers and typesetters) (1850)
Iron Molders' I.U. (1859)
Machinists' and Blacksmiths' I.U. (1859)
American Miners' Association (1861)
  Miners' National Association (1873)
Sons of Vulcan (steel workers) (1862)
National Telegraphic Union (1863)
  Telegraphers' Protective League (1868)
Brotherhood of Locomotive Engineers (1863)
Ship Carpenters' and Caulkers' I.U. (1864)
Cigar Makers' I.U. (1864)
N.U. of Journeyman Curriers (tanners) (1864)
Plasterers' N.U. (1864, again 1871)
Iron and Steel Heaters' I.U. (1865, again 1872)
Coachmakers' I.U. (1865)
Dry Goods Clerks' Early Closing Ass'n. (1865)
Tailors I.U. (1865)
Carpenters' and Joiners' I.U. (1865)
Bricklayers' I.U. (1865)
Journeyman Painters' I.U. (1865, again 1871)
Stationary Engineers' N.U. (1866?)
Mule Spinners' I.U. (textile workers) (1866)
Knights of St. Crispin (shoemakers) (1867)
Conductors' Brotherhood (1868)
Workingmen's Benevolent Association (1868)
Wool Hat Finishers' N.U. (1869)
Daughters of St. Crispin (shoemakers) (1869)
Coopers' I.U. (barrel makers) (1870)
Morocco Dressers' N.U. (hide processors) (1870)
American Bricklayers' N.U. (1871)
N.U. of Woodworking Mechanics (1872)
Sons of Adam (cloth cutters) (1872)
Brotherhood of Locomotive Firemen (1873)
Boilers', Roughers', Catchers', and Hookers', N.U. (1873)

Note: I.U.= International Union; N.U. = National Union.

contributed to this situation. The inability of these businesspeople to repay their loans led to the failure of major banks. With the contraction of credit, thousands of small businesses went bankrupt. The NLU did not survive the crisis.

However, by this time, a new organization had appeared to champion the cause of the laboring classes in opposition to lords of finance. Founded in 1869 by Uriah Stephens and other Philadelphia tailors, the Knights of Labor began as a secret fraternal society. Extending their reach, the Knights aimed to unite industrial and rural workers, the self-employed and the wage earner, blacks and whites, and men and women. The Knights were committed to private property and to the independence of the farmer, the entrepreneur, and the industrial worker. The group banned from its ranks "nonproducers," such as liquor sellers, bankers, professional gamblers, stockbrokers, and lawyers. Both the Knights and the Farmers' Grange would enjoy their greatest successes in the 1880s.

This period of depression also laid the foundation for the Greenback Labor Party, organized in 1878. Debtors feared that government policies were leading to a contraction of the money supply. Within three years after the end of the Civil War, the Treasury had withdrawn from circulation $100 million in wartime, paper currency ("greenbacks"). With less money in circulation, debtors found it more difficult to repay their loans. The government also ceased coining silver dollars in 1873, despite the discovery of rich silver lodes in the West. "Cheap-money men" protested what they called the "Crime of '73." To add insult to injury, the Resumption Act (1875) called for the government to continue to withdraw paper "greenbacks." Thus, hard money became dearer, and debtors became more desperate. In 1878 the new Greenback Labor Party managed to win one million votes and elect 14 candidates to Congress. The party laid the foundation for the Populist Party that emerged in the 1890s.

Federal money policies had a great impact on diverse groups of workers, whether they toiled in the fields, the factory, or the workshop. However, several factors made coalition building among these groups difficult. One was the nation's increasingly multicultural workforce. Unions, such as the typographers, were notorious for excluding women and African Americans, a fact publicized by both Frederick Douglass and Susan B. Anthony, to no avail. In 1869 shoe factory workers (members of the Knights of St. Crispin) went on strike in North Adams, Massachusetts. They were soon shocked to see 75 Chinese strikebreakers arrive by train from California. Their employer praised the new arrivals for their "rare industry." The shoemakers' strike collapsed quickly after the appearance of what the workers called this "Mongolian battery." Employers would continue to manipulate and divide the laboring classes through the use of ethnic, religious, and racial prejudices.

Political Corruption and the Decline of Republican Idealism

Out of the new partnership between politics and business emerged an extensive system of bribes and kickbacks. Greedy politicians of both parties challenged the Republicans' high-minded idealism.

News related to the corrupt intertwining of government power and private economic interests burst upon the headlines in the early 1870s. In New York City, the *New York Times* exposed the schemes of William M. "Boss" Tweed. Tweed headed Tammany Hall, a political organization that courted labor unions and contributed liberally to Catholic schools and charities. Tammany Hall politicians routinely used bribery and extortion to fix elections and bilk taxpayers of millions of dollars. One plasterer employed on a city project received $138,000 in "payment" for two days' work. Political cartoonist Thomas Nast portrayed Tweed with a bulging stomach and a sneering face, taunting the public, "As long as I count the votes, what are you going to do about it?" After the *Times* exposé, Tweed was prosecuted and convicted. His downfall attested to the growing influence of newspaper reporters.

Another piece of investigative journalism rocked the political world in 1872. In 1867 major stockholders of the Union Pacific Railroad had formed a new corporation, called the Crédit Mobilier, to build railroads. Heads of powerful congressional committees received shares of stock in the new company. These gifts of stock were bribes to secure the legislators' support for public land grants favorable to the new corporation. The *New York Sun* exposed a number of the chief beneficiaries in the fall of 1872, findings confirmed by congressional investigation. Among the disgraced politicians was Grant's vice president Schuyler Colfax, who had lied under oath to a Congressional Committee investigating the scandal. Colfax denied accepting Crédit Mobilier stock, although bank records show he had deposited $1200 in cash from one of the finance company's supporters.

The 1872 presidential election pitted incumbent Grant against the Democratic challenger, *New York Tribune* editor Horace Greeley. Republicans, disillusioned with congressional corruption and eager to press forward with civil service reform, endorsed the Democratic candidate. Greeley and his Republican allies decried the patronage (or "spoils")

Harper's Weekly, September 16, 1871

■ In 1871 Thomas Nast drew a series of cartoons exposing the corruption of New York City Democratic boss William M. Tweed and his political organization, Tammany Hall. In this drawing, published in *Harper's Weekly* in 1871, Nast depicts Tweed and his cronies engaging in a "wholesale" looting of the New York City treasury with the assistance of compliant police officers. Those same officers stand ready to crack down on the impoverished father who robs a bakery to feed his family. By portraying Tweed as an enemy of the poor, Nast ignored the fact that the political boss gained a large following among immigrant voters.

TABLE 15-5

The Election of 1872

Candidate	Political Party	Popular Vote	Electoral Vote
Ulysses S. Grant	Republican	3,596,745	286
Horace Greeley	Democratic Liberal		
	Republican	2,843,446	66

system by which politicians rewarded their supporters with government jobs. Nevertheless, Grant won the election.

In an 1872 article titled "The State of the South," a writer for the *Nation* magazine decried northern whites' apparent indifference toward the stalled process of Reconstruction. After four bloody years of war and seven squandered years of postwar opportunity, the federal government seemed prepared to hand the South back to unrepentant rebels. Together, the southern states readmitted to the Union would demonstrate little regard for black people as citizens or as workers. In 1874 the Freedman's Savings Bank failed, taking with it the dreams of many depositors who had saved, on average, $25 out of their hard-won earnings. Neither Congress nor the president attempted to save the bank or reimburse the depositors. Meanwhile, the North showed what one House Republican called "a general apathy among the people concerning the war and the negro." The Civil Rights Act of 1875 guaranteed blacks equal access to public accommodations and transportation. Yet this act represented the final, half-hearted gesture of radical Republicanism. The measure was never enforced, and the Supreme Court declared it unconstitutional in 1883 on the grounds that the government could protect only political and not social rights. White Southerners reasserted their control over the region's political economy.

Grant remained preoccupied by political problems plaguing his administration. In 1875 the so-called Whiskey Ring further tarnished his presidency. The St. Louis–based association consisted of the manufacturers of distilled liquors. Aided by Treasury Department officials and Grant's own private secretary, General Orville E. Babcock, these manufacturers avoided paying sales taxes. With influential friends, members of the ring had eluded detection for years.

The presidential election of 1876 intensified public cynicism about deal making in high places. A dispute over election returns led to what came to be known as the Compromise of 1877. The Republican nominee, Rutherford B. Hayes, a former three-term governor of Ohio, ran against Democrat Samuel J. Tilden. In the popular vote, Tilden outpolled Hayes. However, when the electoral votes were counted, the Democrat had only 184, one short of the necessary number. Nineteen of the 20 votes in dispute came from Louisiana, South Carolina, and Florida, and these three states submitted two new sets of returns, one from each of the two main parties. A specially appointed congressional electoral commission, the Committee of Fifteen, was charged with resolving the dispute. It divided along partisan lines. The eight Republicans outvoted the seven Democrats to accept the Republican set of returns from Florida.

TABLE 15-6

The Election of 1876

Candidate	Political Party	Popular Vote	Electoral Vote
Rutherford B. Hayes	Republican	4,036,572	185
Samuel J. Tilden	Democrat	4,284,020	184

To break the logjam, the Democrats agreed that Hayes could assume office in return for the withdrawal of all remaining federal troops from the South. The Republicans tacitly agreed that their work there was finished and that blacks in the region should fend for themselves. Hayes declined to enforce the Civil Rights Act of 1875. White Southerners were free to uphold the principle of states' rights that had been traditionally invoked to deny blacks their rights in the region.

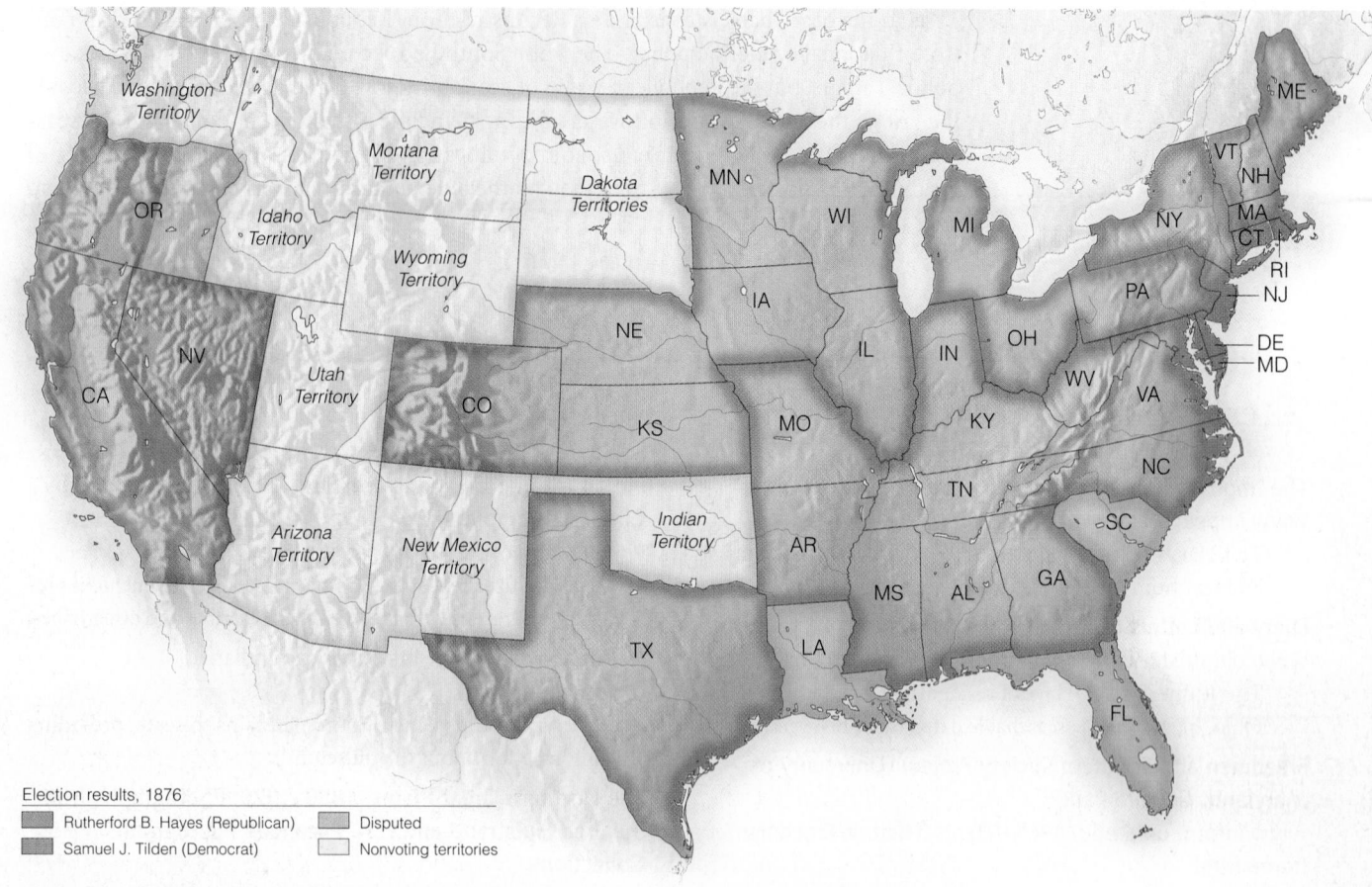

Election results, 1876

■ Rutherford B. Hayes (Republican)   ■ Disputed
■ Samuel J. Tilden (Democrat)   □ Nonvoting territories

■ **MAP 15.3**
THE COMPROMISE OF 1877 During the presidential election of 1876, returns from South Carolina, Florida, and Louisiana (the only states that remained under Republican control) were disputed. Under a compromise reached by Republicans and Democrats in Congress, Republican Rutherford B. Hayes became president, and Congress removed all federal troops from the South. As a result, in many areas of the South, the Republican party all but disappeared.

Conclusion

D uring the dozen or so years after the Civil War, both northern Republicans and southern Democrats registered a series of spectacular wins and crushing losses. Though humiliated by the Union victory, southern white supremacists eventually won for themselves the freedom to control their own local and state governments. As landlords, sheriffs, and merchants, these men defied the postwar federal amendments to the Constitution and deprived African Americans of basic citizenship rights. By the end of Reconstruction, northern Republicans had conceded local power to their former enemies. Apparently, even an aggressive nationalism could accept traditional southern hierarchies: white over nonwhite, rich over poor.

On the other hand, at the end of Reconstruction, Republicans remained in firm control of national economic policy. The white South had secured its right to conduct its own political affairs, but the Republican vision of economic growth and development had become the law of the land. This vision was a guiding principle of historic national and, increasingly, international significance. Economic innovation in particular proved to be a force of great unifying power, stronger even than all the federal military forces deployed during and after the Civil War.

Sites to Visit

The Impeachment of Andrew Johnson
www.impeach-andrewjohnson.com/

This HarpWeek site about the impeachment includes images and text from the Reconstruction period.

Diary and Letters of Rutherford B. Hayes
www.ohiohistory.org/onlinedoc/hayes/index.cfm

The Rutherford B. Hayes Presidential Center in Fremont, Ohio, maintains the searchable database of his writings.

Freedmen and Southern Society Project (University of Maryland, College Park)
www.inform.umd.edu/ARHU/Depts/History/Freedman/home.html

This site contains a chronology and sample documents from several collections or primary sources about emancipation and freedom in the 1860s.

History of the Suffrage Movement
www.rochester.edu/SBA

This site includes a chronology, important texts relating to women's suffrage, and bibliographical information about Susan B. Anthony and Elizabeth Cady Stanton.

Indian Affairs: Laws and Treaties, compiled and edited by Charles J. Kappler (1904)
www.library.okstate.edu/kappler

This digitized text at Oklahoma State University includes pre-removal treaties with the five Civilized Tribes and other tribes.

National Museum of the American Indian
www.si.edu/nmai

The Smithsonian Institution maintains this site, providing information about the museum.

The Northern Great Plains, 1880–1920: Photographs from the Fred Hulstrand and F. A. Pazandak Photograph Collections
www.memory.loc.gov.ammem/award97/ndfahtml/ngphome.html

This American Memory site from the Library of Congress contains two collections from the Institute for Regional Studies at North Dakota State University with 900 photographs of rural and small-town life at the turn of the century. Included are images of sod homes and the people who built them, farms and the machinery that made them prosper, and one-room schools and the children who were educated in them.

For Further Reading

General Works

Ellen Carol DuBois, *Feminism and Suffrage: The Emergence of an Independent Women's Movement in America, 1848–1869* (1978).

Eric Foner, *Reconstruction: America's Unfinished Revolution, 1863–1877* (1988).

David Montgomery, *Beyond Equality: Labor and the Radical Republicans, 1862–1872* (1967).

Amy Dru Stanley, *From Bondage to Contract: Wage Labor, Marriage, and the Market in the Age of Slave Emancipation* (1998).

Ronald Takaki, *A Different Mirror: A History of Multicultural America* (1993).

Robert M. Utley, *The Indian Frontier of the American West, 1846–1890* (1984).

Richard White, *"It's Your Misfortune and None of My Own": A History of the American West* (1991).

The Struggle over the South

Peter Bardaglio, *Reconstructing the Household: Families, Sex and the Law in the Nineteenth-Century South* (1995).

Ira Berlin and Leslie S. Rowland, eds., *Families and Freedom: A Documentary History of African-American Kinship in the Civil War Era* (1997).

Dwight B. Billings, *Planters and the Making of a "New South": Class, Politics, and Development in North Carolina, 1865–1900* (1979).

Lucy M. Cohen, *Chinese in the Post–Civil War South: A People Without a History* (1984).

Frederick Cooper, Thomas C. Holt, and Rebecca J. Scott, eds., *Beyond Slavery: Explorations of Race, Labor, and Citizenship in Post-Emancipation Societies* (2000).

Michael W. Fitzgerald, *The Union League Movement in the Deep South: Politics and Agricultural Change During Reconstruction* (1989).

Michael Golay, *A Ruined Land: The End of the Civil War* (1999).

Thomas C. Holt, *Black over White: Negro Political Leadership in South Carolina During Reconstruction* (1977).

Jacqueline Jones, *Soldiers of Light and Love: Northern Teachers and Georgia Blacks, 1865–1873* (1980).

Leslie Schwalm, *"A Hard Fight for We": Women's Transition from Slavery to Freedom in South Carolina* (1997).

Claiming Territory for the Union

Stephen E. Ambrose, *Nothing Like It in the World: The Men Who Built the Transcontinental Railroad, 1863–1869* (2000).

Orin G. Libby, ed., *The Arikara Narrative of the Campaign Against the Hostile Dakotas, June, 1876* (1998).

Ruth B. Moynihan, Susan Armitage, and Christiane Fischer Dichamp, eds., *So Much to Be Done: Women Settlers on the Mining and Ranching Frontier* (1990).

Richard West Sellars, *Preserving Nature in the National Parks: A History* (1997).

Larry Sklenar, *To Hell with Honor: Custer and the Little Bighorn* (2000).

Robert Wooster, *The Military and United States Indian Policy, 1865–1903* (1988).

Judy Yung, *Unbound Feet: A Social History of Chinese Women in San Francisco* (1995).

The Republican Vision and Its Limits

Leon Fink, *Workingmen's Democracy: The Knights of Labor and American Politics* (1983).

Barbara Goldsmith, *Other Powers: The Age of Suffrage, Spiritualism, and the Scandalous Victoria Woodhull* (1998).

Lyde Cullen Sizer, *The Political Work of Northern Women Writers and the Civil War* (2000).

Irwin Unger, *The Greenback Era: A Social and Political History of American Finance, 1865–1879* (1964).

C. Vann Woodward, *Reunion and Reaction: The Compromise of 1877 and the End of Reconstruction* (1956).

Online Practice Test

Test your understanding of this chapter with interactive review quizzes at

www.ablongman.com/jonescreatedequal/chapter15

Additional Photo Credits

Page 501: Library of Congress

Page 507: Antique Textile Resource, Bethesda MD

Page 517: William T. Garrell Foundry, San Francisco, *The Golden Spike*. The Iris & B. Gerald Cantor Center for Visual Arts at Stanford University (1998.115). Gift of David Hewes

1877	All federal troops withdrawn from the South, ending Reconstruction.
	"Great Uprising" of railroad employees and other workers.
1878	Thomas Edison patents the phonograph.
	San Francisco Workingmen's party stages anti-Chinese protests.
1879	First telephone line connects two American cities (Boston and Lowell, Massachusetts).
1880	New York City streets lit by electricity.

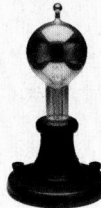

1881	Charles Guiteau assassinates President Garfield.
1882	Standard Oil Trust is created.
	Chinese Exclusion Act.
1883	Pendleton Act (civil service reform).
1884	Mark Twain, *The Adventures of Huckleberry Finn.*
1885	Geronimo leads Apaches to Sierra Madres in Mexico.
1886	Accused Haymarket bombers tried and convicted.
	Geronimo and his followers are sent to Fort Marion, Florida; the children are sent to the government Indian school in Carlisle, Pennsylvania.
1887	Interstate Commerce Act creates Interstate Commerce Commission.
	Dawes Severalty Act.
	United States claims right to Pearl Harbor, leases it as a coaling and repair station.
1888	Edward Bellamy, *Looking Backward.*
1889	First All-American football team, consisting of players from Yale, Harvard, and Princeton.
	National Farmers' Alliance is founded.
1890	Sherman Anti-Trust Act.
	Wyoming admitted to the Union, first state to enfranchise women.
	National American Woman Suffrage Association is formed.
	Wounded Knee Massacre.

PART SIX

The Emergence of Modern America, 1877–1900

THE UNITED STATES BECAME A MODERN NATION DURING THE LAST quarter of the nineteenth century. Vast reserves of coal, timber, and water helped fuel a growing industrial economy. Railroad lines criss-crossed the nation and knit together regional economies. Large numbers of immigrants, many from eastern Europe, arrived in the United States, drawn by America's rising standard of living, high demand for labor, and religious and political freedom.

To raise the money needed to purchase expensive equipment and machinery, coal and oil producers and railroad owners formed modern corporations, businesses that were owned by stockholders rather than individuals. The largest businesses sought to dominate the marketplace by eliminating their competitors. Managers could cut production and operating costs by slashing the wages of workers or by installing labor-saving machinery. Either way, workers paid the price.

The generation that came of age after the Civil War witnessed a series of violent confrontations between workers and employers. Standards of industrial work discipline required workers to labor for long hours at dangerous, disagreeable jobs. Some workers formed new kinds of labor unions to combat the power of big business. Some organizations, such as the Knights of Labor, were national in scope and inclusive in their membership; others represented the interests of specific groups of workers. Employers, local and state law enforcement officials, and judges used a variety of means to suppress strikes and other forms of collective action among workers. Nevertheless, local communities often supported the strikers, who were their friends and neighbors.

During the late nineteenth century, the national economy began to shift to the production of consumer goods. New products gave Americans new ways to spend their money. Manufacturers of everything from toothpaste to bathtubs advertised their goods to a mass market. In cities, department stores offered a dazzling array of goods.

Even as the country was becoming more ethnically diverse, advertisers promoted a single standard of physical beauty and material well-being. At the same time, some scholars and politicians seized on a revolutionary new theory of natural history to argue for the superiority of white, middle-class Americans. Social Darwinism served as the intellectual justification for unfettered economic growth and for the subjugation of darker-skinned peoples, at home and abroad.

Many Americans rejected the trends toward economic standardization and cultural homogeneity. Native Americans in the West continued to resist the railroad and its profound threat to their way of life. By 1890 the U.S. military had forcefully subdued most of these Indians, relegating many to reservations. Together with industrial workers throughout the nation, Hispanic villagers in the Southwest and African American sharecroppers in the South disputed the notion that progress could be defined exclusively in terms of economic growth and development.

Middle-class reformers sought to mediate between what they perceived to be two dangerous groups: arrogant industrialists and discontented workers. These reformers feared that rapid urban and industrial growth would cause rifts in the social fabric. Middle-class women pioneered in the founding of social settlements and other urban institutions to ease the transition of immigrants into modern American society.

The lines between national standards and local cultural interests often blurred. For example, for a short time Sioux chief Sitting Bull (Tatanka Iyotake) appeared with William ("Buffalo Bill") Cody's "Wild West" show, which played to enthusiastic audiences in the United States and Europe. Yet this Indian leader also led the Plains Indians as they attempted to resist U.S. military authorities. Some groups of Americans who sought to preserve their own cultural traditions nonetheless aspired to a middle-class way of life and its material comforts. Elite Hispanic families in the Southwest remained devoted to their Roman Catholic faith and at the same time followed up-to-date clothing fashions marketed by East Coast department stores.

The promise and the conflicts inherent in the emerging modern social order met head on in the 1890s. A new political party called the Populists mounted a brief but potent challenge to entrenched economic and political power. The Populists failed in their attempt to capture the presidency in 1896, but they offered a vision of a new kind of political party, one that would bring black and white farmers and industrial workers together in opposition to landlords, employers, and bankers.

In 1898, in an effort to protect its interests in the Western Hemisphere and to extend those interests into the Pacific, the United States went to war with Spain. This imperialist venture suggested the links among several impulses, including missionary outreach, commercial expansion, and white supremacist racial ideologies. By 1900 the United States was fast becoming a world leader in terms of manufacturing, technological innovation, and the rapid growth of its prosperous middle class.

1891 Populist Party formed.
Eleven Italian immigrants are lynched in New Orleans.

1892 Ellis Island opens as screening site for immigrants.
Miners strike in Coeur d'Alene, Idaho.
Steelworkers strike at Carnegie's Homestead plant near Pittsburgh.

1893 Columbian Exposition opens in Chicago.
Pro-American interests stage a successful coup against Queen Liliuokalani of Hawaii.
Worst nationwide depression to date.

1894 Coxey's Army marches on Washington, D.C.
Pullman workers strike.

1896 Supreme Court decides *Plessy v. Ferguson*, upholds segregation.
W. E. B. DuBois is first black person to receive a Ph.D. from Harvard.

1898 U.S. annexes Hawaii.
Maine blows up in Havana Harbor.

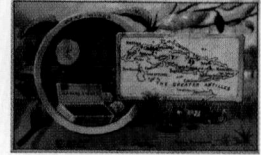

U.S. defeats Spain in Spanish–American–Cuban–Filipino War.
Spain cedes Guam and Puerto Rico to U.S., turns over Philippines in return for $20 million.

1899 Gen. Emilio Aguinaldo leads Filipino revolt against 70,000 U.S. occupying forces.

1900 U.S. troops sent to China to crush Boxer Rebellion.

CHAPTER 16

Standardizing the Nation: Innovations in Technology, Business, and Culture, 1877–1890

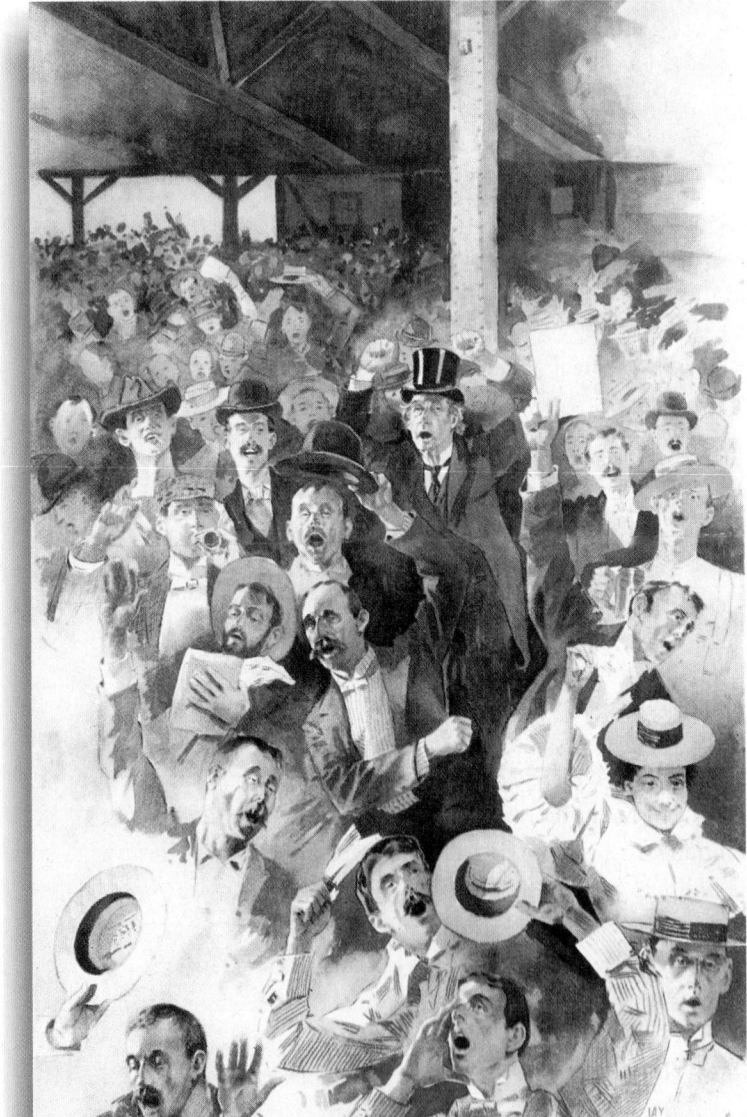

Courtesy, Transcendental Graphics

■ A late nineteenth-century crowd enjoys a baseball game on a summer day. These fans show some of the same characteristics of their twenty-first-century counterparts—men and women cheer lustily for the home team, and at least one spectator is enjoying a mug of beer. During this period, the number of professional baseball teams multiplied. Games such as this one turned athletic competitions into forms of mass entertainment.

THOMAS A. SCOTT'S EARLY LIFE PROVIDED FEW CLUES THAT HE WOULD SOMEDAY BECOME a powerful industrialist. Born in 1823 in a small town in south central Pennsylvania, he was the seventh of 11 children. After his father died in 1835, the youth went to live with relatives. Over the next few years, he worked in country stores, learning and developing bookkeeping skills. His clerking abilities eventually landed him a series of railroad jobs. As an employee of the Pennsylvania Railroad, he supervised the transfer of passengers and freight between trains. In 1858 Scott was promoted to the position of general superintendent of the railroad, and in 1874 he became president of the line.

During his career, Scott gained a reputation as a tenacious defender of the railroad's interests; in the words of one politician, Scott could "engineer" almost any bill through the Pennsylvania state legislature. For example, in 1864, Scott lobbied legislators to repeal the charter of a rival line and to grant a new charter to a trunk line of his own company. After the vote, a lawmaker rose to his feet and asked, "Mr. Speaker, may we now go Scott free?"

In the summer of 1877, Scott and other railroad officials were forced to contend with a workers' strike that spread throughout the country. Trying to cut costs in what had become a bitterly competitive business, many of the railroads had demanded that workers labor for longer hours for 10 percent less pay. Managers instituted the practice of "double-heading"—adding more cars to a train but not hiring more men to tend them, placing added burdens on engineers and other workers. In response, beleaguered rail workers walked off the job. Men and women in other struggling industries—from laundresses and longshoremen in Galveston, Texas, to coal miners in Scranton, Pennsylvania, to packinghouse laborers in Chicago—also went on strike during what came to be known as the Great Labor Uprising of 1877. That July the federal government deployed army troops as a strike-breaking force in Chicago, East St. Louis, and Terre Haute, among other cities.

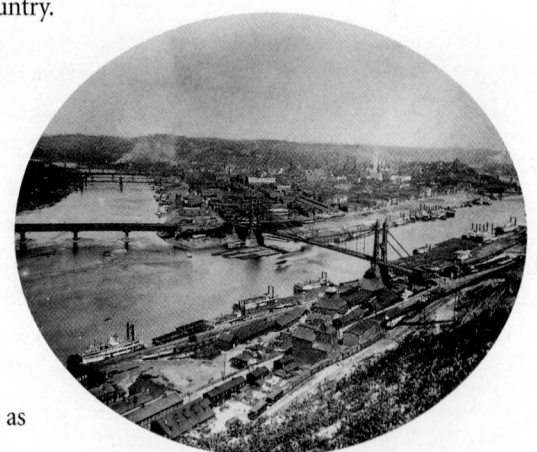

In 1890, commercial establishments lined the riverbanks of Pittsburgh, Pennsylvania.

In a letter to the *North American Review* magazine in August 1877, Thomas Scott justified his railroad's wage cuts and charged that the strikers were under the sway of vicious criminals. Scott hailed the railroads as truly national enterprises, "closely interwoven with the interests not only of our own but other countries." During the Civil War, Union forces had commandeered private rail lines, Scott pointed out. Now it was appropriate that the federal government protect the railroads in this time of crisis. Indeed, according to Scott, "this insurrection," the strike, presented a national emergency "almost as serious as that which prevailed at the outset of the Civil War."

By 1877 the emergence of a national rail system signaled the rise of big business. The railroad industry produced America's first business bureaucracies, employing gigantic workforces to maintain, schedule, operate, and staff trains that traversed 93,000 miles of

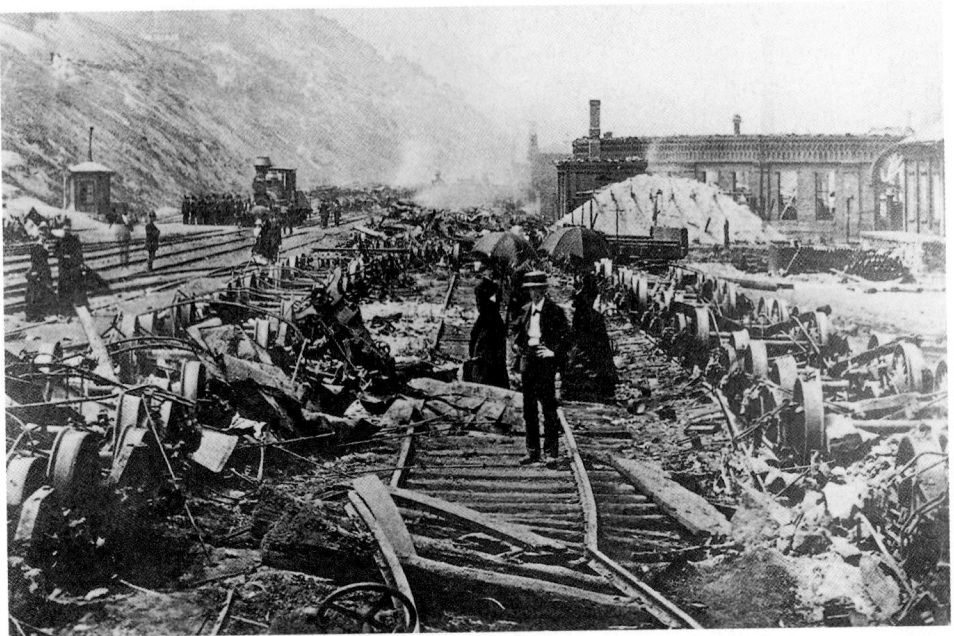

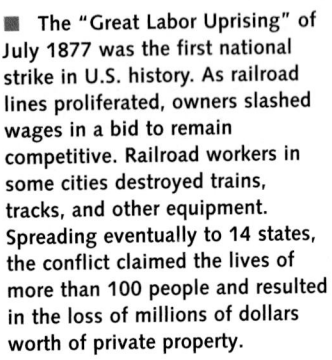

■ The "Great Labor Uprising" of July 1877 was the first national strike in U.S. history. As railroad lines proliferated, owners slashed wages in a bid to remain competitive. Railroad workers in some cities destroyed trains, tracks, and other equipment. Spreading eventually to 14 states, the conflict claimed the lives of more than 100 people and resulted in the loss of millions of dollars worth of private property.

Carnegie Library of Pittsburgh (#P-1987)

track. By 1890 the Pennsylvania Railroad had become the nation's largest employer, with 110,000 workers on its payroll. About one out of seven people worked in the rail industry. The personnel in charge of coordinating these vast operations were among the country's first professional, salaried managers.

Andrew Carnegie, a young Scottish immigrant, absorbed critical lessons about the industry's accounting and managerial procedures. A youthful assistant to Thomas Scott in the 1850s, Carnegie labored as a telegrapher and then as a superintendent for the Pennsylvania Railroad's western division. In 1875 he began building the greatest steel empire in the country, using business principles that he learned while working for the railroad.

The railroad industry was both a great centralizer and a great standardizer. Trains ran on schedules that were set by a central office, and those schedules relied on definitions of actual time that were standard throughout the nation. Moreover, trains broke down regional boundaries by transporting goods to all areas of the counry. For the first time, trains carried brand-name goods and commodities to a national market. A California wheat farmer could purchase replacement parts for his McCormick reaper manufactured in Chicago. An Iowa farm family ordered a new cookstove through a mail-order catalogue. Levi-Strauss, a small clothier in San Francisco, shipped its famous denim pants to cowboys in Texas. Pillsbury Flour of Minnesota distributed its products to bakeries throughout the Midwest. Armour Meatpacking of Chicago sent its sausages to the East Coast. With the introduction of the new refrigerated railroad car, trains also began carrying larger loads of fruits and vegetables over longer distances. The new traffic in produce stimulated commercial agriculture in the South and on the West Coast.

Few Americans amassed the fabulous fortunes of rich industrialists like Scott and Carnegie, yet most people aspired to a better life, even in modest terms. Proprietors, managers, and office workers filled the ranks of the comfortable middle class, men and women freed of the danger and drudgery of manual labor. Between 1880 and 1900, clerical workers tripled in number, and business managers increased from 68,000 to more than 318,000. Enjoying steady work and cash salaries, middle-class employees began to move their families out of the city. Urban areas were becoming increasingly befouled by smokestacks and congested with new factories and workshops.

Providers of goods and services celebrated a "standard" American viewed as white, native-born, middle-class, heterosexual, and Protestant. This image assumed special significance in the marketing of consumer products and in the appeal of new forms of leisure activities. With technical innovations came novel ways for people to spend their money. Athletic contests, traveling road shows, and amusement parks provided exciting sensory experiences for young and old alike. At the same time, the mass marketing of goods gave rise to a consumer culture that valued newness, fashion, and luxury.

Mass advertising techniques heightened distinctions that European Americans drew between themselves and people they considered inferior, exotic, or foreign. Yet the energy and vitality associated with American popular culture served as a magnet for people all over the world. Beginning in the 1880s, eastern European immigrants streamed to the United States. They were also eager to partake of the country's plentiful jobs, material prosperity, and democratic openness. Well into the twentieth century, the nation still showed the ethnic and cultural diversity that was shaped by patterns of immigration during the late nineteenth century.

Economic growth produced contradictory effects. Blessed with abundant and diverse natural resources, American industries became competitive in the world marketplace. However, miners and loggers tended to "cut and run," despoiling streams and forests in the process. Economic growth and development transformed natural landscapes throughout the United States. Citizens in general benefited from the proliferation of new technological marvels, but consumers bore the brunt when big business raised prices and eliminated competition within an industry. Certain workers suffered when new machines displaced them from their jobs.

During the last third of the nineteenth century, the rise of big business, the mass production of consumer goods, and innovations in transportation produced national standards that shaped the economic and social life of the nation. Placing advertisements in newspapers and popular magazines, large companies sought to market their products to all parts of the country. These products, from bathtubs to new fashions in dress, helped to set the standard for middle-class life. In addition, advertising conveyed to the buying public an image of "American" beauty; this standard was narrow by definition but supposedly universal in its appeal. New kinds of commercialized leisure activities, such as shows, athletic competitions, and amusement parks, promoted the idea that all Americans, regardless where they lived or what they did for a living, valued spectacles and thrilling forms of entertainment. At the same time, not all people embraced these standards or the assumption that underlay them—the notion that new kinds of goods and entertainment represented progress in American life.

The New Shape of Business

In 1882 prospectors discovered gold in the creeks of Idaho's Coeur d'Alene region (in Indian territory, about 90 miles east of Spokane, Washington). Multiethnic boomtowns mushroomed in the region, as they had in the California gold fields three decades earlier. Yet this new gold rush differed substantially from its predecessor. First, technology had already powerfully shaped the early history of Coeur d'Alene. The Northern Pacific Railway had promoted settlement, and the primitive techniques that had been used in surface mining soon yielded to far more efficient hydraulic methods of extraction (a process in which powerful water hoses wash the soil away to expose gold deposits).

Second, the mining industry in the region soon emerged as a big business. In 1885 an unemployed carpenter named Noah S. Kellogg set in motion a dramatic chain of events. Kellogg discovered a lode containing not only gold but also zinc and lead. In short order, he sold his mines to a Portland businessman, who paid a whopping $650,000 for them. A group of eastern and

California investors, and finally several large corporations, soon controlled major interests in the mines. Meanwhile, new railroad lines were lacing the area. With the advent of electrification across the region, lamps glowed in saloons and mining shafts. Finally, the miners themselves were not solo prospectors, seeking to make their own fortune, but wage-earning employees paid by the mining corporation. By the mid-twentieth century, mining companies had dug more than a billion dollars' worth of metal out of Noah Kellogg's original stake.

Population growth spurred the growth of industries that expoited nature. Between 1880 and 1890, the U.S. population grew from 50 million people to almost 63 million, and six new states entered the Union: North Dakota, South Dakota, Montana, and Washington (all in 1889) and Idaho and Wyoming (both in 1890). Increased demand in turn hastened large-scale commercial mining, logging, and fishing.

> *Advocates of standardized industrial processes and mass marketing hoped to break down regional barriers and create an integrated national economy.*

Crucial to the process of innovation were engineers, who mastered the technical aspects of construction and design. Many American engineers were trained in Germany, but others attended such schools as the Massachusetts Institute of Technology (MIT) or Cornell University, in New York state, both of which introduced electrical engineering into their curricula in 1882. Engineers were in the forefront of professional associations: civil engineers banded together in 1852, mining engineers in 1871, mechanical engineers in 1880, and electrical engineers in 1884 (chemists formed their own association in 1908). American engineers, such as those who worked in Mexico under the auspices of mining companies and the railroads, served as the vanguard of American capitalism throughout the world. Most engineers were men; however, Ellen Swallow Richards, a graduate of MIT and the first female member of the American Institute of Mining Engineers (in 1875), pioneered in home economics.

Advocates of standardized industrial processes and mass marketing hoped to break down regional barriers and create an integrated national economy. Whether they specialized in railroads or shoes, wheat or steel, business owners and managers who possessed the necessary resources and resourcefulness pursued similar goals: to mine, grow, manufacture, or process large quantities of goods and then market them as widely, cheaply, and quickly as possible. Business put a premium on technological innovation, on the efficient use of workers, and on the reduction of uncertainties that accompanied a competitive marketplace. These guiding principles, formulated during the late 1870s and 1880s, laid the foundations of economic progress in late nineteenth-century America.

Yet not all businesses during this period were big. The entrepreneurial spirit flourished, especially within local markets. In the 1880s, even the newest towns, such as Central City, Colorado, west of Denver, supported a rich mix of financiers, professionals, merchants, storekeepers, and skilled artisans. Central City supplied nearby mining and milling operations, but the trade and service industries patronized by those operations accounted for 52 percent of the city's total wealth and more than a quarter of its population. Thus, the history of American enterprise during this period exhibited two seemingly contradictory impulses: one toward consolidation of industries, the other toward a proliferation of small businesses serving their immediate neighborhoods and regions.

New Systems and Machines—and Their Price

The free enterprise system thrived on innovation. Indeed, during the 1880s, new machines, new technical processes, new engineering feats, and new forms of factory organization fueled the growth and efficiency of U.S. businesses. Many devices that became staples of American life appeared during this period. Alexander Graham Bell invented the telephone in 1876. Thomas A. Edison developed the phonograph in 1877 and the electric light in 1879. Cash registers, stock tickers, and typewriters soon became indispensable tools for American businesses. Beginning in the 1880s, railroad cars installed steam heat and electric lights, boosting the comfort of passengers.

Lesser-known inventions revolutionized specific industries. In 1883 Jan Ernest Matzeliger, a young mechanic who was the son of a Dutch man and a Surinamese woman, developed a successful shoe-lasting machine in Lynn, Massachusetts. (A last was a wooden model of a human foot that shoemakers used to attach and shape the shoe leather.) The prototype of Matzeliger's lasting machine consisted of old cigar boxes wired with pieces of wood. Massachusetts shoe manufacturers embraced the device once he had perfected it, for their highly skilled but poorly paid hand lasters were beginning to form a union. The Yankee lasters' concerns had merit, for patent Number 274,207 ultimately spelled doom for them. Matzeliger's machine had eliminated the need for skilled shoe laborers.

During this period, more and more businesses perfected the so-called American system of manufacturing, which dated back half a century and relied on the mass production of interchangeable parts. Factory workers made large numbers of a particular part, each part exactly the same size and shape. This system enabled manufacturers to assemble products more cheaply and efficiently, to repair products easily with new parts, and to redesign products quickly. In the early 1880s the Singer Sewing Machine Company was selling 500,000 units a year. McCormick was producing 21,600 reapers annually. The American system also spurred technological innovation. For example, in 1884 the twine binder used in wheat harvesting was modified with new parts for use in harvesting rice.

The engineers who designed the modern bicycle (which has wheels of equal size) used the American system to make their product affordable to almost anyone who wanted one. The bicycle craze of the late nineteenth century resulted from the novelty and cheapness of this new form of transportation and recreation, one enjoyed by males and females of all ages. Production techniques used to make bicycles were later adapted to the manufacture of automobiles.

New technical processes also facilitated the manufacture and marketing of foods and other consumer goods. Distributors developed pressure-sealed cans, which enabled them to market agricultural products in far-flung parts of the country. Innovative techniques for sheet metal stamping and electric resistance welding transformed a variety of industries. Eager to satisfy a demand for steel (an alloy that was stronger and harder than iron), U.S. manufacturers stepped up production of the versatile metal. For the first time, they broke free of European suppliers. By 1880, 90 percent of American steel was made by the Bessemer process (named after its English inventor but developed in this country by William Kelly), which injected air into molten iron to yield steel.

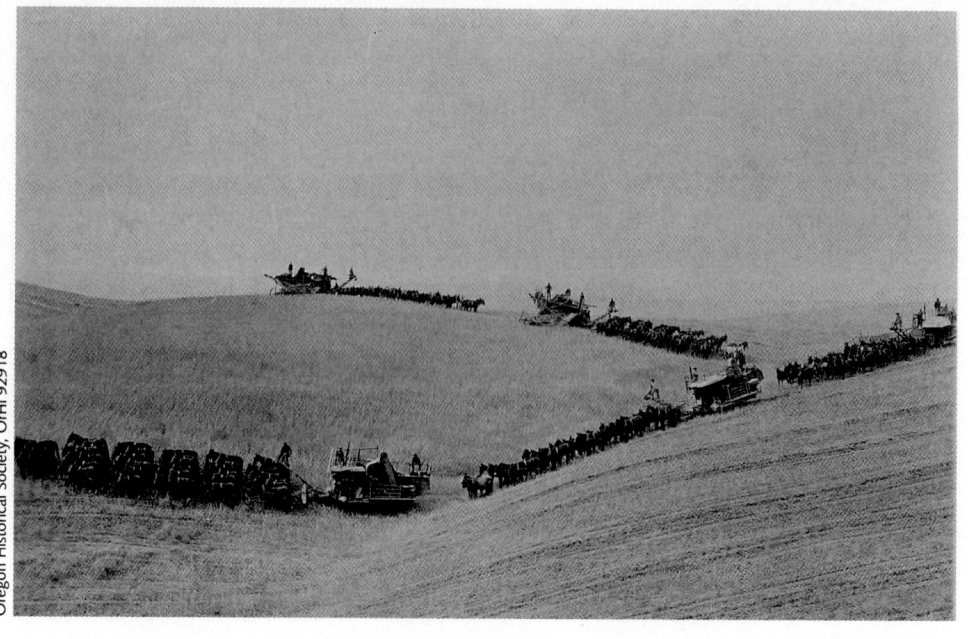

Oregon Historical Society, OrHi 92918

■ Bonanza farms were huge agricultural enterprises, ranging in size from 15,000 to 50,000 acres. This photo shows a bonanza wheat farm in Oregon, c. 1890. Many of these farms relied not only on sophisticated machinery but also on transient labor forces (up to 1000 men at a time) to help plow, plant, harvest, and thresh the crop. Some of the largest landowners abandoned farming when they had an opportunity to sell their vast holdings for a profit.

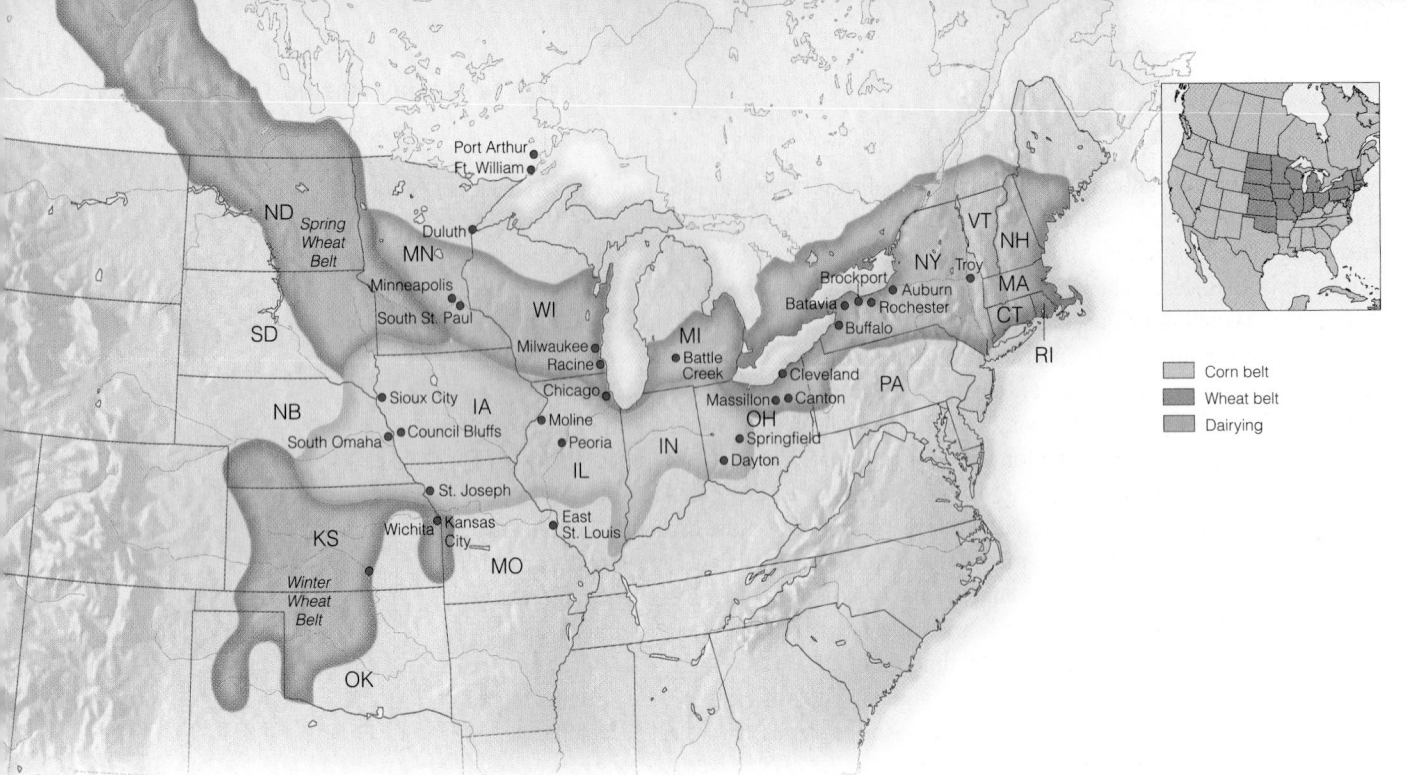

■ MAP 16.1

AGRICULTURAL REGIONS OF THE MIDWEST AND NORTHEAST   By 1890 several Midwestern cities served as shipping centers, getting wheat and corn to the growing metropolitan areas of the Northeast and Mid-Atlantic. Farmers complained that the railroads gave discounts to large shippers, such as Standard Oil, and discriminated against small producers.

The agriculture business benefited from engineering innovations as well. These technological advances included improvements in irrigation and new labor-saving devices, such as the self-binding harvester (1878) and the first self-steering, self-propelled traction engine (1882). These innovations and devices reached across national boundaries. As just one example, the first modern irrigation systems in the Southwest were constructed by Native Americans and *mestizos* (people of both indigenous and Spanish ancestry). And in the 1870s, Japan began importing American farm implements and inviting U.S. engineers to construct dams and canals for new steam- and water-powered gristmills and sawmills. Technology was a universal language, one that many peoples around the globe sought to master.

Long active in territorial exploration and land surveying, the federal government continued to assume a leading role in applied science. In 1879 the U.S. Geological Survey (USGS) was formed, charged with compiling and centralizing data describing the natural landscape, an effort that had originated in 1804 with the Lewis and Clark expedition. In the 1880s, the federal government also began to systematize and disseminate information useful to farmers through the United States Department of Agriculture. Created in 1864, the department originally consisted of several divisions organized around scholarly disciplines, such as chemistry and horticulture. Gradually, administrators looked for ways to solve specific problems faced by farmers. In 1881, for example, the department's Entomology Bureau began to combine current research on insects with practical techniques for pest control.

Like factory machines, new agricultural machinery benefited consumers but also disrupted traditional labor patterns. As farm productivity boomed, the need for hired hands evaporated. Early in the nineteenth century, producing an acre of wheat took 56 hours of labor; in 1880, that number dropped to 20 hours. Machines, such as the self-binding harvester, reduced labor needs by as much as 75 percent. One agricultural worker in Ohio observed, "Of one thing we are convinced, that while improved machinery is gathering our large crops, making our boots and shoes, doing the work of our carpenters, stone sawyers, and builders,

TABLE 16-1

Amount of Forest Clearing Each Decade, by Major Region, 1850–1909 (in thousands of acres)

	1850–1859	1860–1869	1870–1879	1880–1889	1890–1899	1900–1909	Total
Northeast	1,417	619	1,339	62	80	228	3,745
Mid-Atlantic	4,283	2,811	4,278	295	646	87	12,400
Southeast	6,822	1,869	7,612	6,213	5,410	3,712	31,638
Northcentral	8,245	5,566	9,199	2,420	3,804	1,200	30,434
Southcentral	9,025	1,803	9,156	8,168	7,489	5,767	41,408
Lake	5,093	4,188	7,347	3,131	4,575	2,497	26,831
Southwest	3,018	1,422	7,796	7,148	8,020	7,832	35,236
Pacific	1,774	1,188	2,590	1,166	983	1,063	8,764
Total	39,677	19,466	49,317	28,603	31,007	22,386	190,456

Northeast: Maine, New Hampshire, Vermont, Massachusetts, Connecticut, Rhode Island.
Mid-Atlantic: New York, Pennsylvania, New Jersey, Delaware, Maryland.
Southeast: West Virginia, Virginia, North Carolina, South Carolina, Georgia, Florida.
Northcentral: Minnesota, North Dakota, South Dakota, Nebraska, Kansas, Iowa, Montana, Wyoming, Colorado.
Southcentral: Missouri, Arkansas, Louisiana, Mississippi, Alabama, Tennessee, Kentucky, Oklahoma.
Lake: Ohio, Michigan, Indiana, Illinois, Wisconsin.
Southwest: Nevada, Utah, Arizona, New Mexico, Texas.
Pacific: Washington, Oregon, California.

Source: Michael Williams, *Americans and Their Forests* (1989), 36.

thousands of able, willing men are going from place to place seeking employment, and finding none. The question naturally arises, is improved machinery a blessing or a curse?"

Alterations in the Natural Environment

Innovation altered the natural landscape and hastened the depletion of certain natural resources. By the mid-1870s, Texas had new steam-powered lumber mills equipped with saw rigs that could produce up to 30,000 board feet a day. This capacity made Texas lumbering a big business, especially when it was combined with infusions of capital and the expansion of railroad lines into the piney woods region, along the eastern edge of the state. Texas lumber mills were poised to benefit from the exhaustion of the great forests of the eastern and Great Lakes states.

In the Chesapeake Bay, dredge boats were becoming more efficient in harvesting oysters, and shellfish reserves began to decline. In the mid-1880s oyster harvesters took a record 15 million bushels from the bay; the shellfish simply could not replenish themselves. New means of commercial fishing also reduced supplies of salmon in the Northwest.

In 1884 in California, a federal court issued a permanent injunction against hydraulic mining, because it contributed to soil erosion and water pollution. Hydraulic mining had washed an estimated 12 billion tons of earth into San Francisco Bay, raising the floor of the bay several feet. At the same time, mercury flowing into nearby streams from gold mines in the San Jose hills was poisoning fish in the bay, creating pollution that would be felt well into the twentieth century. Similar cases of industrial pollution despoiled other parts of the country. In the absence of any laws to restrain them, Chicago meatpackers befouled the Chicago River with the byproducts of sausage, glue, and fertilizer.

By stimulating manufacturing and extractive enterprises alike, the railroads powered these great environmental transformations, for better or worse. Trains enabled entrepreneurs to develop large-scale copper mines in Arizona, gigantic herds of longhorn cattle in Kansas, and vast textile mills in Georgia. Every western town clamored for a railroad station; they knew that places bypassed by the rails withered and died. The railroads enabled tourists to enjoy the

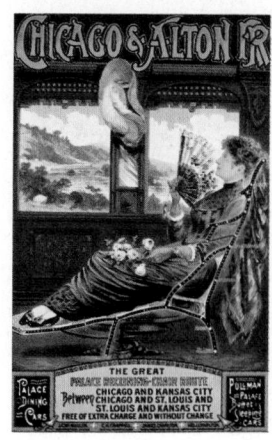

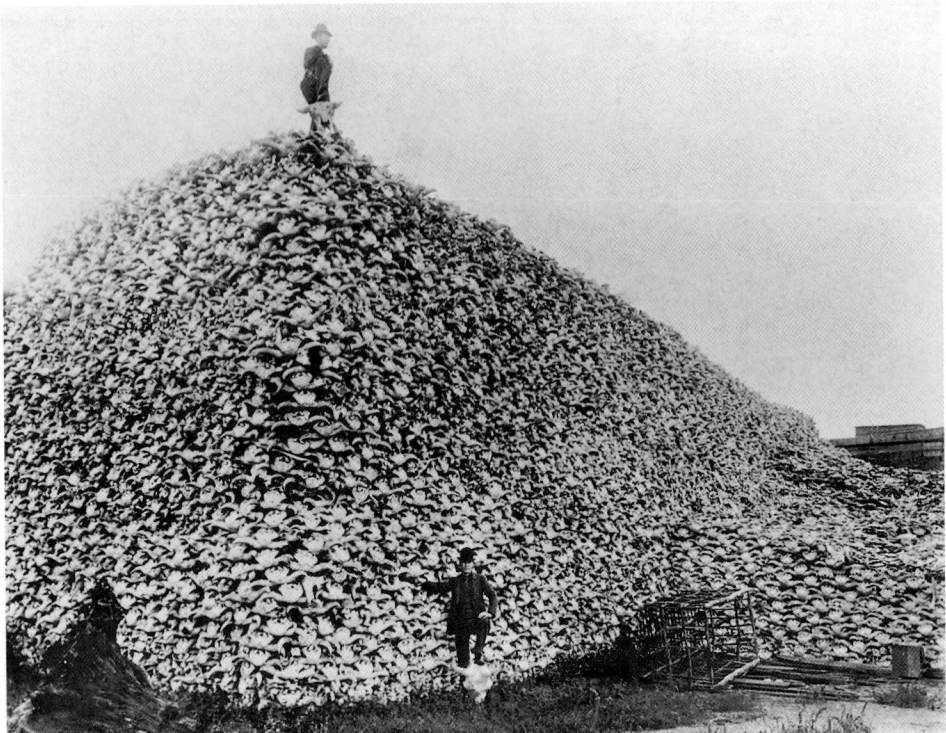

Courtesy, the Burton Historical Collection, Detroit Public Library

■ Following the wholesale slaughter of buffalo on the Great Plains, settlers earned money by gathering the skeletons. "The bones are shipped East by the carloads," reported the Dodge City *Times*, "where they are ground and used for fertilizing and manufactured into numerous useful articles." This mound of buffalo bones at the Michigan Carlson Works in Detroit, c. 1880, suggests the extent of the devastation.

beauty of western wilderness areas. Yet the railroads had an insatiable demand for lumber. Between the late 1870s and 1890, U.S. railroads accounted for 20 to 25 percent of all lumber consumed in the nation. They used wood for fuel, fences, trestles, and stations, along with countless railroad ties. In 1890 scientists estimated that the railroads would need 73 million board feet each year to make new ties to lay beneath expanding lines and to replace ties eaten by pests and decayed with age.

Since buffalo herds impeded rail travel, railroads promoted the shooting of buffalo from trains, a "sport" that almost eradicated the species. By the mid-1880s, the great herds had disappeared, victims of ecological change (the incursion of horses into grazing areas), disease (brucellosis spread by domestic livestock), and commercial enterprise. Eastern consumers prized buffalo-hide coats, and eastern factories used the hides to make steam-engine drive belts. Sioux leader Black Elk decried the slaughter and the "heaps of bones" left to rot in the sun.

Innovations in Financing and Organizing Business

As agents of economic development and cultural change, the railroads knew no peer. As private enterprises, however, they faced the same challenges that all big businesses ultimately must address. The proliferation of independent lines and the high fixed costs associated with the industry made profits slim and competition intense. As a result, railroad companies began to come together in informal pools to share equipment and set prices industrywide. In the 1880s these pools gave way to consolidation, a process by which several companies merged into one large company. Jay Gould's Erie Railroad was a consolidated railroad business.

In these years U.S. businesses grew larger and more quickly compared with their western European counterparts. This difference stemmed in large part from America's astonishing population growth and its rich natural resources. (For example, American coal and iron, the ingredients necessary for making steel, existed in proximity.) Equally significant, the United States possessed a social and legal culture favorable to big business. The absence of an entrenched, conservative elite, along with the spread of state and national laws that protected

TABLE 16-2

How Indians Used the Buffalo

Meat	Food and ceremonial use	Hide	Tipis, robes, dresses, gloves, breech cloth, shirts, leggings, moccasins, bedding, dolls, regalia, cradleboards, implements, drums, tipi furnishings
Fat and marrow	Food, paint, and cosmetics		
Bones	Tools, weapons, knives, pipes, soup, sleds		
Brain	Food, used to tan hides	Skull	Ceremonial use
Intestine	Cord	Horns	Implements, ornaments, ceremonial use, games
Hoofs	Implements, utensils, glue, jewelry, food, ceremonial use		
		Hair	Rope, stuffing, ornaments, ceremonial use
Bladder	Storage pouches	Dung	Fuel
Rawhide	Moccasin soles, shields, containers, ornaments, rattles, snow shoes, mortars, lariats, bridles, boats, luggage, food boiling, medicine bundle, saddles, thongs, stirrups	Sinew and muscle	Thread, cord bow strings
		Tail	Flu brush
		Stomach	Cooking vessel, container for carrying/storing water

Source: Adapted from Arlene Hirschfelder and Martha Kreipe de Montaño, *The Native American Almanac: A Portrait of Native America Today* (New York: Prentice Hall, 1993), p. 18.

private property, stimulated the entrepreneurial spirit. The U.S. government refrained from owning industries, although it heavily subsidized the railroad industry. It taxed business lightly and did not tax individual incomes at all until 1913. Finally, American bankers aggressively promoted growth through their lending practices and bond sales. For example, John Pierpont Morgan, a member of the banking firm of Drexel, Morgan, and Company in the 1880s, reorganized the firm under his own name in 1895 and played a leading role in financing a number of major American businesses.

Several large enterprises began to conquer not just local but also national markets. Examples include Bell Telephone (founded in Boston), the Kroger grocery business (Cincinnati), Marshall Field Department store (Chicago), and Boston Fruit Company. In the South, Midwest, and West, investors rushed to finance gigantic agribusinesses, such as the 1.5 million acres devoted to rice cultivation in southeastern Louisiana and bonanza wheat farms (as large as 38,000 acres) in the Red River Valley of North Dakota. In 1886, a single enterprise, the Calumet and Hecla Mining Company, in Montana, was producing 25,000 tons of copper each year, an amount that exceeded the total national output for every year before 1879.

Owners of these enterprises devised new forms of business organization that helped them grow and survive in a dynamic economy. By combining, or integrating, their operations, manufacturers cut costs and monopolized an entire industry in the process. Unable to withstand the ruthless competition that favored larger enterprises, smaller companies folded. The two icons of American big business in the 1880s—Andrew Carnegie in steel and John D. Rockefeller in petroleum—proved master innovators in both the managerial and technical aspects of business.

In 1875 Carnegie opened the Edgar Thomson Steelworks in Pittsburgh. Within a year, he was producing steel at half the prevailing market price. Carnegie excelled at vertical integration, in which a single firm controls all aspects of production and distribution. Carnegie employed miners in the rich iron and copper deposits in northern Minnesota's Mesabi Range and Michigan's Upper Peninsula (the Lake Superior region) to mine the raw material, and he owned the ships and railroads that brought the ore to the mills in Pittsburgh. Within the mills, he saved money by keeping fuel costs to a minimum (molten steel flowed easily from one processing stage to the next), by maintaining huge outputs, and by cutting labor costs to the bone. His personal connections to his former employer, the Pennsylvania Railroad, ensured a large and stable customer for his steel.

Another form of business consolidation was horizontal integration, in which a number of companies producing the same product merge to reduce competition and control prices. In 1882 John D. Rockefeller, a former bookkeeper, horizontally integrated the petroleum industry by forming Standard Oil Trust. Stockholders in small companies turned over their shares to Standard Oil, which then coordinated operations and eliminated competition from other smaller firms. Standard Oil also practiced vertical integration. Like Carnegie, Rockefeller controlled not only a raw material (in this case, crude oil) but also processing plants, or refineries. He managed to keep transportation costs low by negotiating discount rates from rail shippers. Soon he had positioned himself to buy out his rivals—or ruin them. Trusts placed a premium on efficient production, but they also worked to the disadvantage of consumers, who were hostage to high prices within industries that lacked competition.

For the growing managerial class, trusts helped to eliminate some of the uncertainty associated with an unstable marketplace. They ensured industries' access to raw materials, cheap transportation, expansive markets, and reliable credit institutions. This new form of business cropped up in other industries besides steel and oil. In 1887, the so-called Sugar Trust comprised 17 of the 21 U.S. sugar refiners and monopolized sugar refining east of the Mississippi River.

New Labor Supplies for a New Economy

To operate efficiently, expanding industries needed expanding supplies of workers to grow crops, extract raw materials, and produce manufactured goods. Many of these workers came from abroad. The year 1880 marked the leading edge of a new wave of immigration to the United States. Over the next ten years, 5.2 million newcomers entered the country, almost twice the previous decade's level of 2.8 million.

In the mid-nineteenth century, most immigrants hailed from western Europe and the British Isles—from Germany, Scandinavia, England, and Ireland. Between 1880 and 1890, Germans, Scandinavians, and the English kept coming, but they were joined by numerous Italians, Russians, and Poles. In fact, these last three groups predominated among newcomers for the next 35 years, their arrival rates peaking between 1890 and 1910. At the same time, immigrants from Asia, especially from China, were making their way to the Kingdom of Hawaii, which was annexed by the United States in 1898. Between 1852 and 1887, 26,000 Chinese arrived on the islands. Almost 40 percent of all immigrants to the United States during this period were known as "birds of passage," men who were recruited by American employers and who, after earning some money, migrated back to their native land.

Many of the new European immigrants sought to escape oppressive economic and political conditions in Europe, even as they hoped to make a new life for themselves and their families in the United States. Russian Jews fled discrimination and violent anti-Semitism in the form of pogroms, organized massacres, conducted by their Christian neighbors and Russian authorities. Southern Italians, most of whom were landless farmers, suffered from a combination of declining agricultural prices and high birth rates. Impoverished Poles chafed under cultural restrictions imposed by Germany and Russia. Hungarians, Greeks, Portuguese, and Armenians, among other groups, also participated in this great migration; members of these groups too were seeking political freedom and economic opportunity.

Immigrants replenished America's sense of itself as a haven for the downtrodden, a place where opportunity beckoned to hard-working and

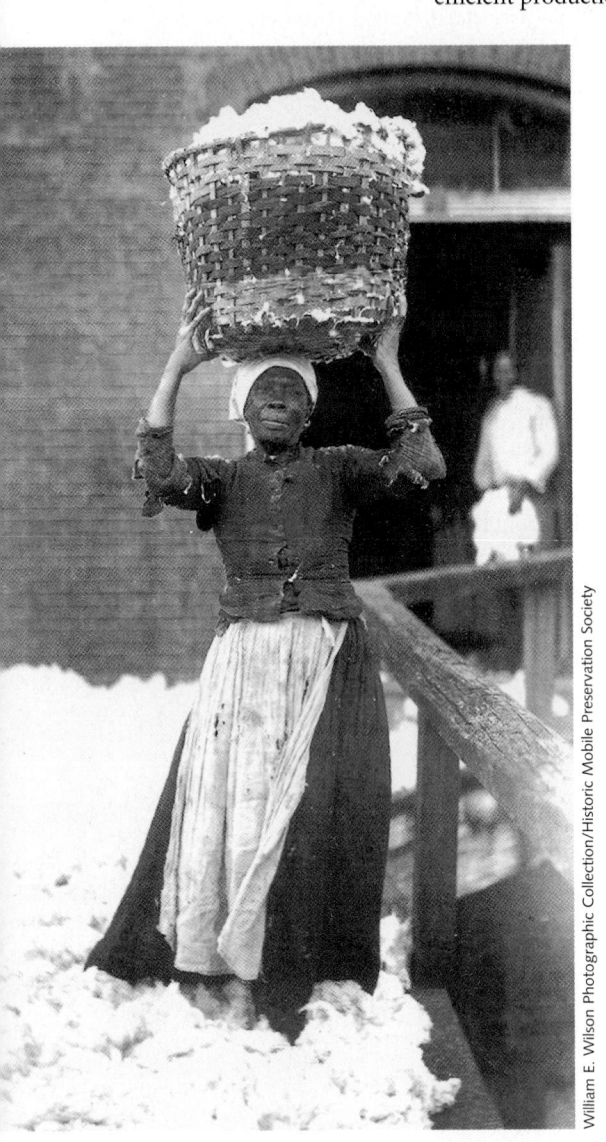

William E. Wilson Photographic Collection/Historic Mobile Preservation Society

■ A burst of technological innovation characterized many American businesses during the last quarter of the nineteenth century. Nevertheless, some, like southern cotton plantations, remained largely unmechanized. Commanding large numbers of (sometimes resistant) black and white workers, southern planters refrained from investing in labor-saving technology. This woman, working at the Savannah Cotton Exchange in 1880, carries a basket of cotton on her head, just as her enslaved foremothers did.

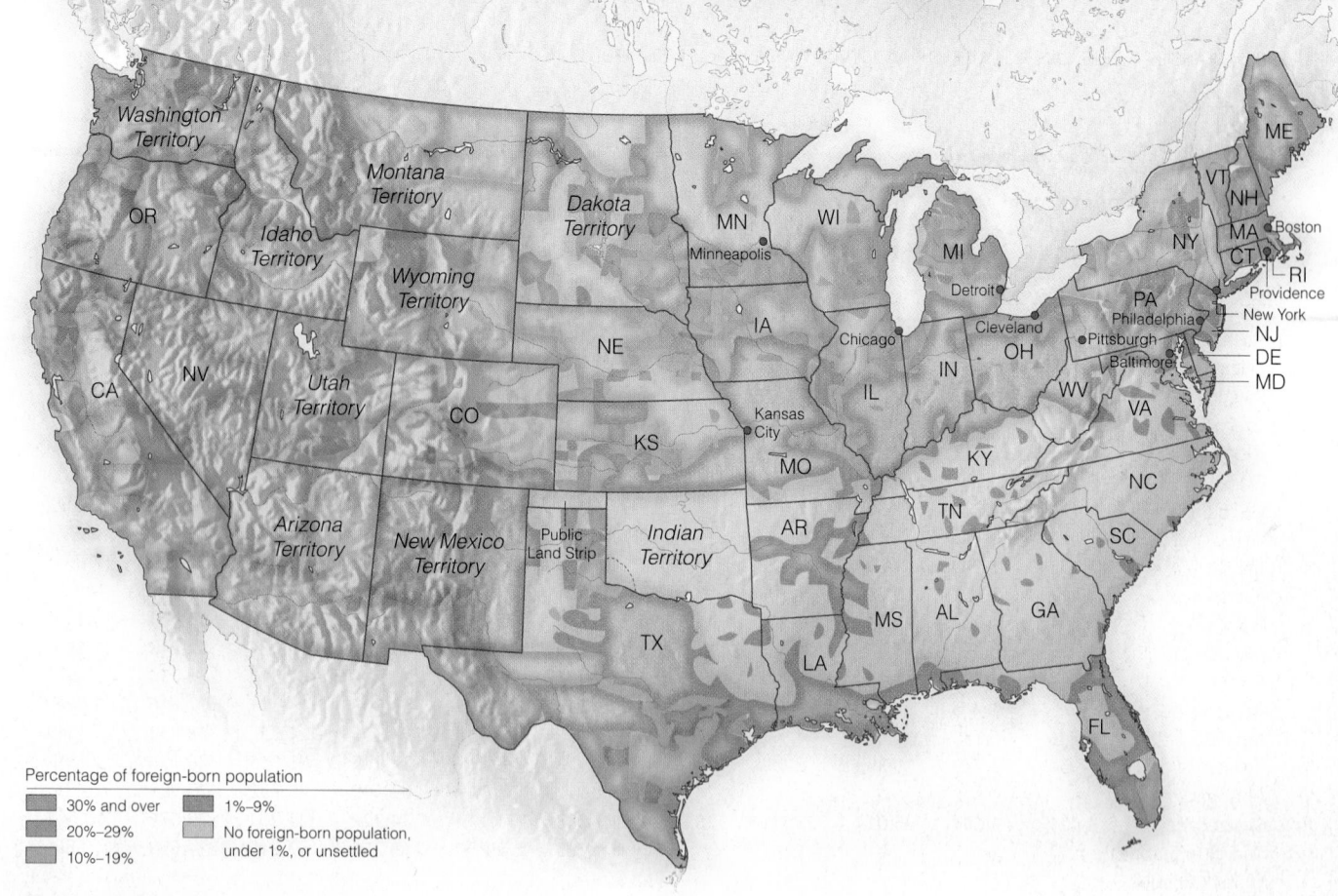

Percentage of foreign-born population

- 30% and over
- 20%–29%
- 10%–19%
- 1%–9%
- No foreign-born population, under 1%, or unsettled

■ **MAP 16.2**

POPULATION OF FOREIGN-BORN, BY REGION, 1880   After the Civil War, large numbers of immigrants settled in northeastern cities. In addition, the Upper Midwest and parts of the western mining frontier drew many newcomers from western Europe. The area along the country's southwestern border was home to immigrants from Mexico. Cuban cigar makers established thriving communities in southern Florida.

ambitious people. "The New Colossus," written by American poet Emma Lazarus in 1883, pays tribute to the "huddled masses yearning to breathe free"—people from all over the world who sought refuge in the United States. The words of her poem are inscribed on the Statue of Liberty at the entrance to New York Harbor. (The people of France presented the statue, called "Liberty Enlightening the World," to America in 1884.)

Most of the newcomers found work in the factories, mills, and sweatshops of New York, Philadelphia, and Chicago. At the same time, large numbers of these fresh arrivals dispersed to other areas of the country to work in a wide variety of enterprises. Scandinavians populated the prairies of Iowa and Minnesota and the High Plains of the Dakotas. Immigrants from Mexico found work in the mines and beet fields of Colorado.

In the South, some planters began to recruit immigrants—especially western Europeans of "hardy peasant stock"—to take the place of blacks who resisted working for whites. Nevertheless, planters' experiments with recruiting immigrants amounted to little. Given the opportunity, many immigrants sought to flee from the back-breaking labor and meager wages of the cotton staple crop economy. A group of Germans brought over to toil in the Louisiana swamps soon after the Civil War quickly slipped away from their employers; they had agreed to the arrangement only to gain free passage to America. Thirty Swedes who arrived in Alabama also deserted at an opportune moment, declaring that they were not slaves. South Carolina planters who sponsored colonies of Germans and Italians gave up in exasperation. The few Chinese who began work in the Louisiana sugar fields soon abandoned the plodding work of the plantations in favor of employment in the trades and shops of New Orleans. Still, in 1890, immigrant worker

TABLE 16-3

Immigration by Country of Origin, 1831–1940

	1831–1840	1841–1850	1851–1860	1861–1870	1871–1880	1881–1890	1891–1900	1901–1910	1911–1920	1921–1930	1931–1940
Austria-Hungary				7,800	72,060	353,722	502,707	2,145,266	806,342	65,548	3,469[a]
Belgium	22	5,094	4,738	6,734	7,221	20,174	18,167	41,635	33,746	15,846	12,189
Bulgaria							160	39,280	22,533	2,945	375
Czechoslovakia								3,426	102,194	8,347	
Denmark	1,063	539	3,749	37,094	31,771	88,132	50,231	65,285	41,083	32,430	5,393
France	45,575	77,202	70,358	35,984	72,201	50,403	30,770	73,730	61,897	49,610	38,800
Germany	152,454	434,626	951,667	787,468	717,182	452,970	505,152	341,498	143,945	412,202	226,578[b]
Greece						2,053	15,079	167,519	184,201	51,084	8,973
Italy	2,253	1,870	9,231	11,728	55,762	307,310	651,893	2,045,877	1,109,524	455,315	57,661
Netherlands	1,412	8,251	10,789	9,102	16,541	53,701	26,758	48,262	43,718	26,946	14,860
Norway	1,201	13,903	20,931	109,298	95,323	176,586	95,012	190,505	66,393	68,531	10,100
Sweden					115,922	391,776	226,266	249,534	95,074	97,249	10,665
Poland[c]	—	—	1,164	2,027	12,970	51,806	96,720	—	4,813	227,734	7,571
Romania						5,938	12,750	53,008	13,311	67,646	1,076
Russia[d]	646	656	1,621	4,536	52,254	265,080	602,011	1,597,306	921,957	78,433	548
Spain	2,954	2,759	10,353	8,493	5,206	4,418	8,731	27,935	68,611	28,958	2,898
Portugal					4,627	11,017	28,323	69,149	89,732	29,994	7,423
Switzerland	4,821	4,644	25,011	23,286	28,293	81,088	31,179	34,922	23,001	29,676	10,547
Turkey in Europe						1,185	3,786	119,256	77,210	14,659	580
United Kingdom											
England	7,611	32,002	247,125	222,277	437,706	644,680	216,726	388,017	249,944	157,420	112,252
Ireland	207,381	780,719	914,119	435,778	456,871	655,482	388,416	339,065	146,181	220,501	25,377
Scotland	2,667	3,712	38,331	38,768	87,564	149,869	44,188	120,469	78,357	159,781	16,131
Wales	183	1,261	6,319	4,313	6,631	12,640	10,557	17,464	13,107	13,012	3,209
Not specified	63,347	229,979	132,199	349,538	16,142	186	67				
Other Europe	96	155	116	210	658	1,346	122	665	18,238	22,983	11,813
Total Europe	495,686	1,597,522	2,453,821	2,074,434	2,274,874	4,783,413	3,655,673	8,175,296	4,407,336	2,427,787	621,704
Canada and Newfoundland[e]			59,304	153,878	383,640	393,304	3,311	179,226	742,515	924,185	171,718
Central America			449	95	157	404	549	8,102	17,159	15,769	21,665
Mexico[e]			3,078	2,191	5,162	1,913	971	49,642	219,004	459,287	60,589
South America			1,224	1,397	1,128	2,304	1,075	17,280	41,899	42,215	21,831
West Indies			10,660	9,046	13,957	29,042	33,066	107,548	123,424	74,899	49,725
Total America			74,715	166,607	404,044	425,967	38,972	361,888	1,143,671	1,516,685	354,804[f]
China	8	35	41,397	64,301	123,200	61,711	14,799	20,005	21,270	29,907	16,709
Japan							25,942	129,797	83,837	33,462	1,555
Turkey in Asia							26,799	77,393	79,389	19,165	218
Other Asia	40	47	61	308	603	6,669	3,696	15,772	8,055	14,866	13,298
Total Asia	48	82	41,458	64,609	123,803	65,380	71,236	243,567	192,559	97,400	31,780
Africa				210	312	358	857	350	7,368	8,443	6,286	7,367
Australia, Tasmania, New Zealand				36	9,886	7,017	2,740	11,975	12,348	8,299	13,805
Pacific Islands					1,028	5,557	1,225	1,049	1,079	427	5,437
All other countries			29,169	17,969	700	789	14,063	33,523[g]	1,147	228	142
Total Immigration	495,736	1,597,604	2,599,373	2,323,967	2,814,793	5,292,980	3,794,259	8,832,666	5,766,593	4,057,112	1,035,039

[a]Hungary only.

[b]Includes Austria 1938–1940.

[c]From 1890–1919, Poland is included with Austria-Hungary, Germany, and Russia.

[d]Including Finland 1831–1920.

[e]No reports from 1886–1893.

[f]Includes other Americas.

[g]Includes 32,897 people returning to their homes in U.S. After 1906, such aliens were considered nonimmigrants.

Source: Lord & Lord, *Historical Atlas of the U.S.* (New York: Henry Holt).

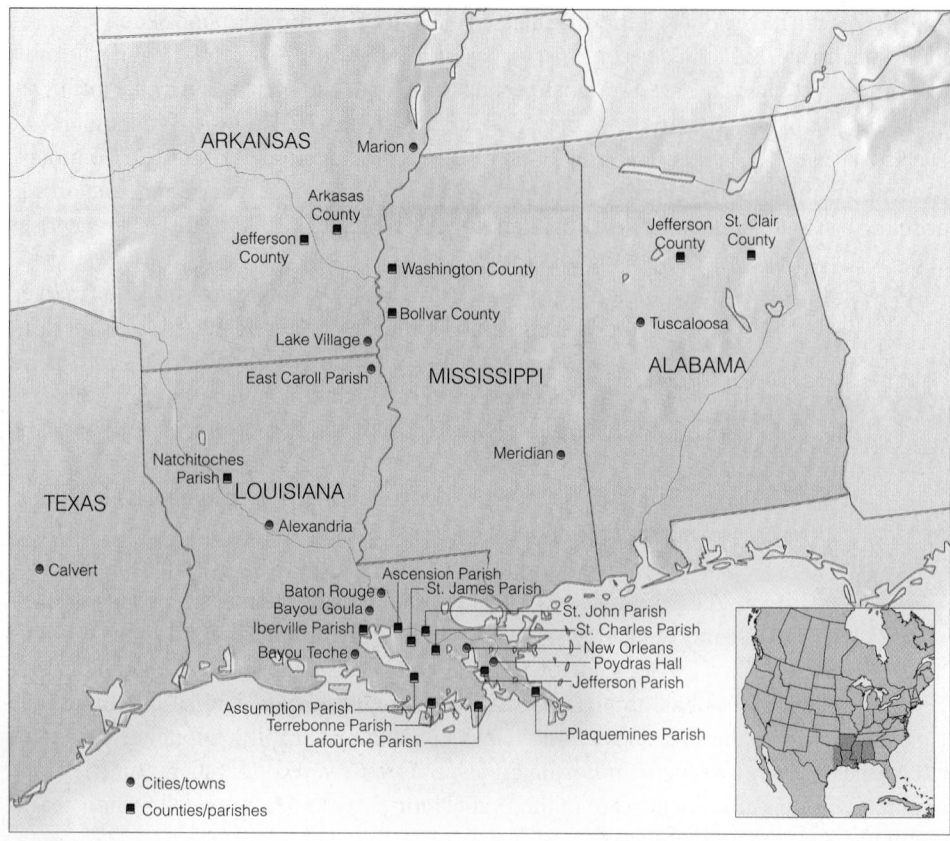

■ MAP 16.3

SOME PLACES WHERE CHINESE LOCATED, 1865–1880 Immediately after the Civil War, some southern whites believed that immigrants would prove to be more reliable and efficient workers than the freedpeople. Planters in Mississippi and Louisiana imported a small number of Chinese from California and others directly from Hong Kong. However, by the early 1870s most of these workers had deserted the fields and moved to nearby towns and cities to work as artisans, grocers, and laundry operators.

enclaves were scattered throughout the South. Irish, Polish, and Italian men were swinging pick-axes in Florida railroad camps. Italian men, women, and children were picking cotton on Louisiana plantations. Hungarian men were digging coal out of mines in West Virginia.

The story of Rosa Cassettari, a young woman who emigrated from northern Italy to the United States in 1884, suggests the challenges that faced many newcomers during this period. Rosa's husband, Santino, had preceded her to America. He had settled in an iron mining camp in Missouri. Leaving her son with relatives, Rosa received the assurances of friends and relatives: "You will get smart in America. And in America you will not be so poor."

In the steerage section of a steamship bound for the United States, Rosa found herself surrounded not only by *paesani* (fellow Italians) but also by Germans, Swedes, Poles, and French— "every kind," she remembered later. After arriving at Castle Garden (an immigration processing center at the tip of Manhattan and a predecessor of Ellis Island), Rosa and her *paesani* were approached by a smooth-talking, well-dressed, Italian-speaking man. Overcharging them for the train trip to Missouri, he left them with no money for food.

Life in the iron camp proved harsh—nothing like what Rosa had expected. Her husband, who was much older than she, neglected her; he preferred the company of prostitutes in the town. The iron was almost depleted, and some workers and their wives had moved on to a new mine in Michigan. Rosa's days centered on caring for her new baby and cooking for 13 of the miners.

Despite these realities, within a couple of years, Rosa grew used to America and considered herself an American. She returned briefly to her hometown in Italy but expressed impatience with the rigid social etiquette that separated the rich from the poor. She also yearned for the hearty meals that had become her staple in the iron camp. Back in Missouri, she mustered enough courage to leave Santino, traveling to Chicago and making a new life for herself in the Italian *colonia* (community) there. She eventually married another Italian man (the two had fallen in love in Missouri) and found work as a cleaning woman at Chicago Commons, a social settlement house. Her new husband alternated between working in construction and peddling bananas and cranberries. Rosa herself gained a reputation as a storyteller; later she said, "Me, I was always crazy for a good story."

The influx of so many foreign-born workers transformed the American labor market. Native-born Protestant men moved up the employment ladder to become members of the white-collar (that is, professional) middle class, while recent immigrants filled the ranks in construction and manufacturing. By 1890 Italian immigrants accounted for 90 percent of New York's public works employees and 99 percent of Chicago's street construction and maintenance crews. Women and children, both native and foreign-born, predominated in the textile, garment-making, and food processing industries.

> *These ethnic niches proved crucial for the well-being of many immigrant communities. They provided newcomers with an entrée into the economy.*

Specific groups of immigrants often gravitated toward particular kinds of jobs. For example, many Poles found work in the vast steel plants of Pittsburgh, and Russian Jews went into the garment industry and street-peddling trade in New York City. California fruit orchards and vegetable farms employed numerous Japanese immigrants. Cuban immigrants rolled cigars in Florida. In Hawaii, the Chinese and Japanese labored in the sugar fields; after they had accumulated a little money, they became rice farmers and shopkeepers. In Boston and New York City, second-generation Irish took advantage of their prominent place in the Democratic party to become public school teachers, firefighters, and police officers.

These ethnic niches proved crucial for the well-being of many immigrant communities. They provided newcomers with an entrée into the economy; indeed, many men and women got their first jobs with the help of kin and other compatriots. Niches also helped immigrants advance within an industry or economic sector. Finally, they enriched immigrant communities by keeping profits and wages within those communities.

The experience of Kinji Ushijima (later known as George Shima) graphically illustrates the power of immigrant niches. Shima arrived in California in 1887 and, like many other Japanese immigrants, he found work as a potato picker in the San Joaquin Valley. Soon, Shima moved up to become a labor contractor, securing Japanese laborers for the valley's white farmers. With the money he made, he bought 15 acres of land and began his own potato farm. Eventually he built a large potato business by expanding his holdings, reclaiming swampland, and investing in a fleet of boats to ship his crops up the coast to San Francisco. Taking advantage of a Japanese niche, Shima had prospered through a combination of good luck and hard work.

Efficient Machines, Efficient People

Just as whole industries consolidated to achieve new milestones in efficiency, productivity, and reliability, so did individual workplaces. Well-oiled machines helped entrepreneurs manufacture mass quantities of uniform parts. Employers now pushed workers to strive for the same level of performance.

By the late nineteenth century, the typical industrial employee labored within an immense, multistory brick structure and operated a machine powered by water or steam. Smoky, smelly kerosene lamps gave way to early forms of electric lighting, first arc and then incandescent light bulbs. Long-standing industries, such as textiles and shoes, were now fully mechanized. The new products flooding the economy—locomotives and bicycles, cash registers and typewriters—streamed from factories designed to ensure maximum efficiency from both machines *and* the people who tended them.

In the 1880s a few factory managers hired efficiency experts. The experts' goal was to cut labor costs in the same way that industry barons had shaved the costs of extracting raw materials or distributing final products. With huge quantities of goods flowing from factories, even modest savings in wages could mean significant profits in the long run. As early as the 1880s, efficiency experts, such as Frederick Winslow Taylor, chief engineer for the Midvale Steel Plant outside Philadelphia, were pioneering in the techniques of "scientific management." These techniques stressed uniform, plantwide procedures for routine machine operation and maintenance and labor organization.

Southern textile mill owners devised their own strategies for shaping a compliant workforce. They employed only white men, women, and children as machine operators, but threatened to hire blacks if the whites protested low wages and poor working conditions. During the prewar period, enslaved workers—males and females, adults and children—had been forced to labor in the small textile mills that dotted the Piedmont region of South Carolina and Georgia. But after the Civil War, employers decided to reserve jobs in the expanding textile industry for whites only in order to preserve and extend divisions within the southern labor force. Poor whites lived in company housing, their children attended company schools, and they received cash wages. In contrast, blacks remained in the countryside, impoverished and without the right to vote. In 1874 the manager of a textile mill in Columbus, Georgia, rationalized his company's exclusive policy: "We do not think the negroes adapted to the labor of cotton-mills. Their lack of quickness, sensitiveness of touch, and general sleepy characteristics disqualify them. . . . Being far better fitted for outdoor labor, they will no doubt always be kept so employed." Prewar textile mill owners, who had used slave labor so profitably, would have been shocked by this later view. In the cities of the North as well as the textile villages of the South, factory workers remained exclusively white until well into the twentieth century.

TABLE 16-4

Number of Firms by Number of Employees per Firm, 1850 and 1880

	Number of Firms							
	1850				1880			
	No. of Employees				No. of Employees			
Industry	0–5	6–50	50+	Total	0–5	6–50	50+	Total
Iron and Steel	6	13	3	22	6	20	17	43
Textiles	46	87	53	186	25	59	8	92
Hardware	76	42	7	125	114	122	27	263
Machines and tools	42	44	6	92	96	113	19	228
Printing	36	60	10	106	105	148	36	289
Building construction	83	59	3	145	588	227	18	833
Clothing	165	294	43	502	301	255	93	649
Furniture	84	66	3	153	185	105	20	310
Metal	83	11	1	95	166	47	5	218
Meat	81	3	0	84	458	23	2	483
Harness	32	15	3	50	96	21	2	119
Baking	384	29	0	413	910	73	8	991
Shoes	339	224	20	583	441	139	34	614
Blacksmith	141	18	1	160	187	12	0	199

Note: Because the census recorded only firms producing more than $500 per year, there may be serious undercounting of firms with one or no employees.

Source: Census of the United States, 1850 and 1880.

The Birth of a National Urban Culture

In the 1880s visitors to the territory of Utah marveled at the capital, Salt Lake City, where Mormon pioneers had made the desert bloom. Situated at the foot of the magnificent snow-covered Wasach Range, this oasis in the Great Salt Basin boasted a built landscape almost as impressive as the natural beauty that surrounded it. In the heart of Salt Lake City lay Temple Square. This broad plaza contained the Mormon Tabernacle, a huge domed structure. Next to it stood the Mormon Temple, a soaring six-spired granite cathedral still under construction. The city had the advantage of rail service (Promontory Point, where the transcontinental railroad was joined, was not far away). Mines in nearby Bingham Canyon yielded rich lodes of silver and large local smelters refined copper ores. Irrigation systems made the city self-sufficient in the production of foodstuffs. A settlement inspired by religious faith, Salt Lake City was at the same time thoroughly modern.

Not just Salt Lake City, but other cities around the country began to assume monumental proportions. In New York, the 1880s marked the completion of Central Park and the Brooklyn Bridge and the arrival of the Statue of Liberty from France. Chicago, rebuilding after a disastrous fire in 1871, became a sprawling rail hub dotted with yards for western cattle, northern timber, and the trains that hauled them. In 1885 Chicago also became the location for a major architectural breakthrough by engineer William LeBaron Jenney. He designed the ten-story Home Insurance Building, the world's first metal frame skyscraper. The steel skeleton weighed only one third as much as the thick stone walls needed to support a similar masonry building, and the design left room for numerous windows. Urban architecture would never be the same again.

Cities in general represented American notions of progress and prosperity; they were places where innovation, consumer culture, and new forms of entertainment grew and flourished. From 1875 to 1900, American cities developed increasingly sophisticated systems of communications and transportation. Streetlights, transportation networks, and sewer lines provided basic services to swelling populations of immigrants and rural in-migrants. Experts in the fields of urban design and architecture and ambitious entrepreneurs in the fields of entertainment and professional sports all left their mark on cities. In a country fascinated with new and bigger and better things, cities set the standard by defining a desirable way of life for a "typical" middle-class American.

In their social and physical configurations, cities also represented a new cultural diversity in American life. At times uneasily, they accommodated immigrants from around the world. San Francisco's Chinatown formed a "city within a city" as hostile European Americans sought to circumscribe its residents. Politics, prejudice, and technology came together to shape the urban landscape.

Economic Sources of Urban Growth

Northeastern and mid-Atlantic cities emerged as centers of concentrated manufacturing activity. Yet, with the aid of eastern capital, western cities also flourished. New York's Wall Street and Boston's State Street, home to the nation's largest investment bankers, financed the Main Streets of the Midwest and West. Some urban areas prospered through milling, mining, or other enterprises, such as lumber and flour milling in Minneapolis and ore smelting in Denver. Others focused on manufacturing to serve a growing western population. Chicago was rivaled only by New York in terms of its industrial economy and the vast territory that it supplied with raw materials, processed food, and manufactured goods. Salt Lake City produced goods for the so-called Mormon Corridor of settlements that stretched west from the city to southern California. By the 1880s San Francisco had a commercial reach that encompassed much of the West as well as Hawaii and Alaska. Writer Henry George noted, "Not a settler in all the Pacific States and Territories but must pay San Francisco tribute. Not an ounce of gold dug, a pound of ore melted, a field gleaned, or a tree felled in all their thousands of square miles, but must add to her wealth."

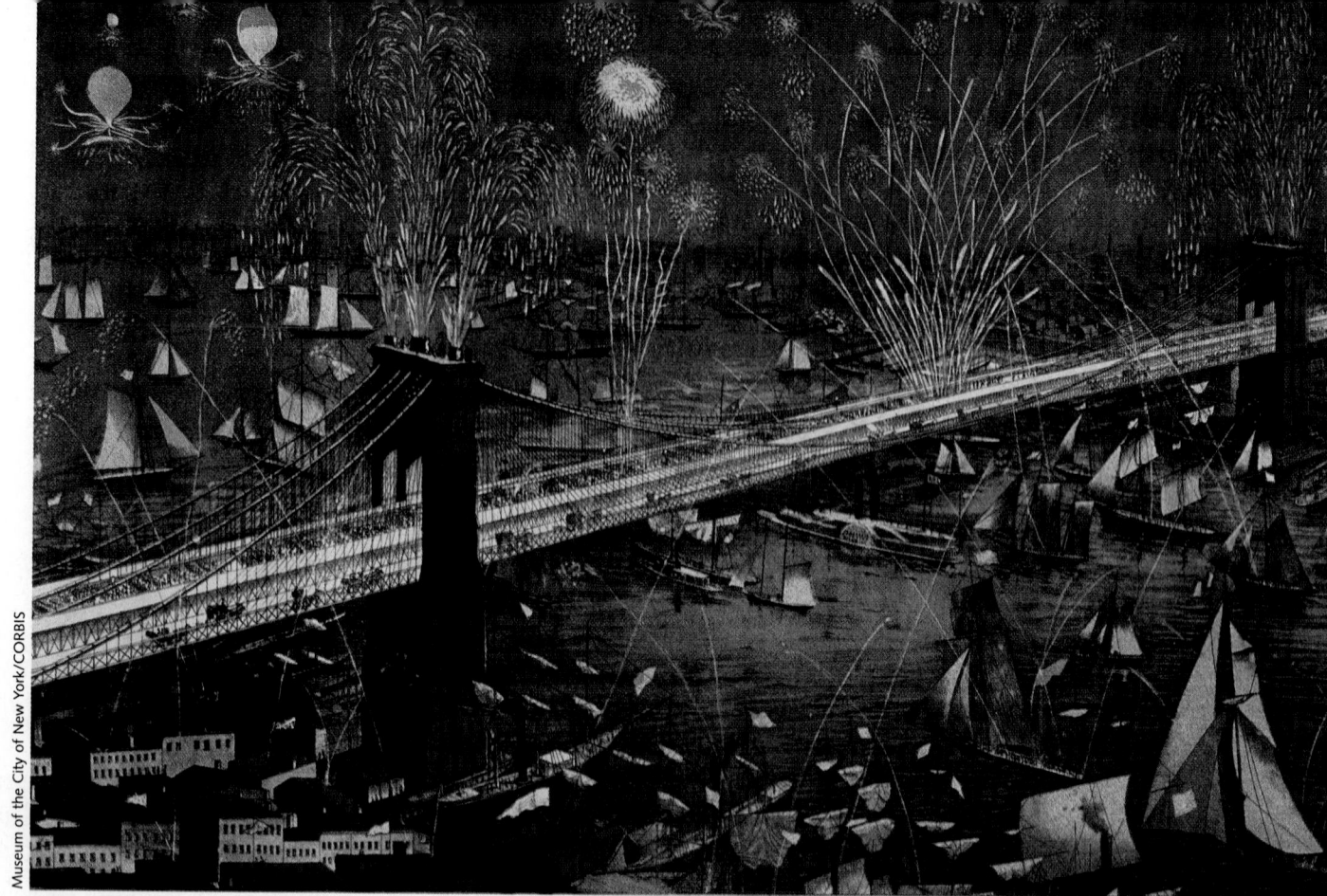

■ Admirers hailed New York City's Brooklyn Bridge as the eighth wonder of the world when it was completed in 1883. With a central span of 1595 feet, it became the largest suspension bridge in the world. Built over 14 years, the bridge linked Brooklyn to Manhattan across the East River, using steel suspension cables that are nearly 16 inches thick. Its total cost was about $18 million.

No trend supported urban growth more than the arrival of newcomers from abroad. To stoke its furnaces, mill its lumber, and slaughter its cattle, Chicago relied on immigrants from Ireland, Slovakia, Germany, Poland, and Bohemia. Of the three cities with the highest percentage of foreign-born residents in 1880, San Francisco (45 percent) ranked higher than both Chicago (42 percent) and New York (40 percent). Yet all large cities also attracted migrants from America's own countryside, as native-born men and women fled the hardship of life on the farm. The use of increasingly efficient agricultural machines meant that rural workers had fewer job opportunities. Most of the immigrants from rural areas to the cities were young women; they included Yankee girls from the hardscrabble homesteads of New England, daughters of Swedish immigrants in Minnesota, and native-born farm tenants in Indiana.

Rural folk sought the steady work and wages afforded by jobs in the city, but they were also drawn to the excitement that had become the hallmark of the urban scene. In the early nineteenth century, Thomas Jefferson had located the heart of America in its sturdy yeoman farmers; by the late nineteenth century, that heart had shifted to the city.

Building the Cities

In 1886 the Reverend Josiah Strong, a proponent of Protestant missionary efforts abroad, condemned the American city as a "menace" to civilization. However, in decrying what he saw the evils of urban life, Strong described its appeal to people of all ages and both sexes: "It is the city where wealth is massed; and here are the tangible evidences of it piled many stories high. . . . Here are luxuries gathered—everything that dazzles the eye or tempts the appetite; here is the most extravagant expenditure." Strong was right that this conspicuous display of wealth would have profound implications for American politics and culture.

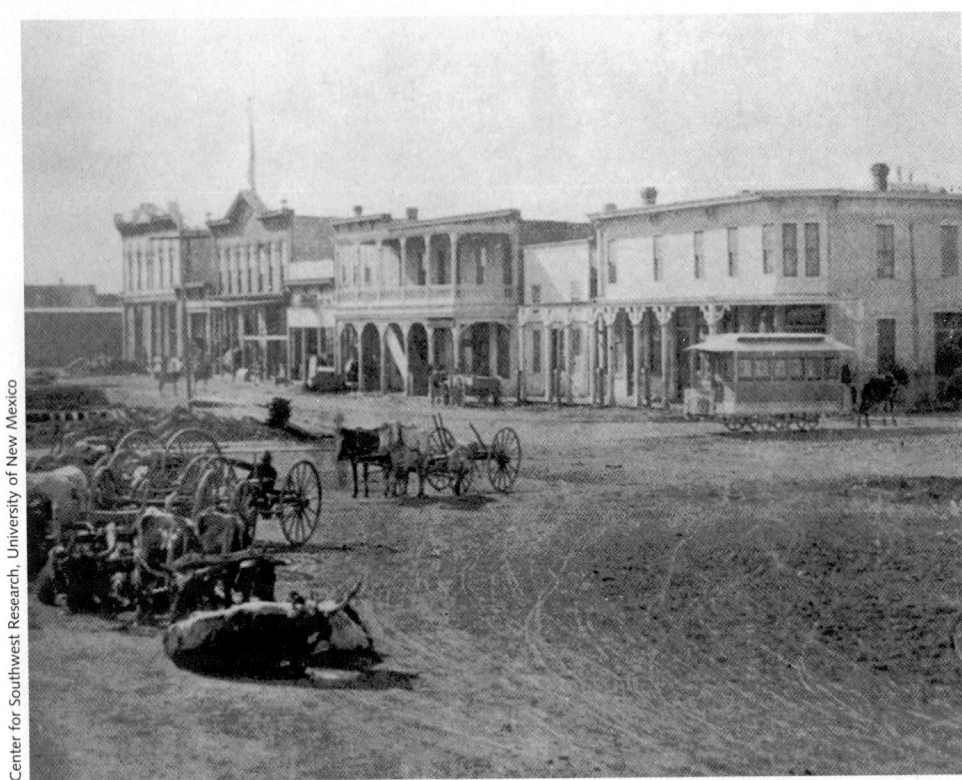

Center for Southwest Research, University of New Mexico

■ Many southwestern cities, such as Albuquerque, were laid out on an Old Town–New Town plan. The original center of settlement, Old Town was characterized by flat-roofed adobe buildings clustered on narrow streets. This photo shows Albuquerque's New Town in the 1880s. Located a mile and a half from Old Town plaza, it consists of Victorian-style buildings. The plan of New Town followed straight lines and right angles, "adapted to the railroad, the regenerator," in the words of one observer.

In these years the American city was emerging as a technological marvel. Through a combination of money and engineering skill, cities managed to provide an adequate water supply for private and commercial purposes, move large numbers of people and goods efficiently, get rid of waste materials, and illuminate thoroughfares at night. Professionals, such as landscape contractors, construction architects, and civil engineers, designed the parks, bridges, public libraries, and museums that made the city so attractive.

Throughout the country, new towns emerged as industrialists and factory owners sought to lure and retain workers. George M. Pullman, who manufactured railroad sleeping cars, built a town outside Chicago and named it after himself. In the South, company towns dotted the Piedmont region (textiles), the steep slopes of the Appalachian Mountains (coal and lumber), the piney woods of Texas (lumber), and the coast of Florida (phosphates). In the West, towns grew up around copper, coal, iron ore, and silver mines. These communities shared a unique characteristic: they directly linked housing, education, and commerce to a particular company.

Cities grew upward and outward as a result of developments in mass production and technology. The availability of factory-assembled building materials accelerated the construction of private dwellings and office buildings. Elevators extended living and office spaces upward (in the Reverend Strong's words, "wealth is massed . . . piled many stories high"). The invention of the electric streetcar in 1888 permitted cities to spread out. Soon, residential suburbs cropped up many miles from urban commercial cores. Wealthy and middle-class urban residents followed the streetcar lines out of the city, hoping to find a green refuge from the grime and noise of downtown while maintaining a manageable commute to work.

As cities expanded, the challenges associated with providing services also grew more complex and expensive. A polluted water supply, for example, meant epidemics of diptheria and cholera, so city taxpayers demanded waterworks that delivered drinkable water through intricate systems of dams, pumps, reservoirs, and pipes. Chicago had long pumped its sewage into Lake Michigan, the source of its drinking water. In the 1880s the city financed the building of a canal and the reversal of the flow of the Chicago River. These changes sent the city's sewage away from Lake Michigan and into the Mississippi River instead. Begun in 1889, the 28-mile Chicago Sanitary and Ship Canal was completed seven years later. One awed observer marveled at the "powerful machinery for digging and hoisting, steam shovels, excavators, inclines, conveyors, derricks, cantilevers, cableways, channelers, steam drills, pumps, etc." The cost: $54 million.

Local Government Gets Bigger

These new systems of services, combined with the mushrooming immigrant neighborhoods, changed both the quality and the quantity of urban problems. Zoning issues—who could build what, where, and when—became flashpoints for conflict as the interests of homeowners, developers, and municipal engineers collided. These controversies called for new forms of local government. Specifically, urban political leaders struggled to improve the city's public works while meeting the needs of multiple ethnic groups. Governing a big city was becoming a big business.

Rising tax rates and ballooning municipal debts told an even larger story. In 1845, the city of Boston spent $8.29 per resident and owed its creditors $748,000. Thirty years later, per capita annual expenditures had risen fivefold, and the city's debt had multiplied several times to more than $27 million. Clearly, running a city was an expensive, full-time enterprise and one that had the potential to be very lucrative to businesspeople and politicians alike.

Although New York's "Boss" Tweed had been convicted on charges of corruption in the early 1870s, the infamous Tammany Hall gang carried on his legacy. The Democratic officials associated with this social and political organization perfected a system of kickbacks linked to municipal construction projects. Under this system contractors paid politicians for city construction contracts. For example, a New York City courthouse that was supposed to cost a quarter of a million dollars ended up costing taxpayers 52 times that amount, or twice as much as the United States paid Russia for Alaska! In the 1880s secretive networks of corruption linking law enforcement personnel, city officials, and construction contractors flourished in many cities. These webs, or "machines," characterized urban life for decades to come.

Local officials went out of their way to support the provision of illegal services demanded by their constituents.

Urban machines existed to secure jobs for their loyal supporters and line the pockets of those at the highest levels of power. Deal-making blurred the lines between private enterprise and public service as everyone from mayors to local ward organizers benefited from the modernization of the American city. In the process, urban bosses ensured that the streets were paved, tenement buildings erected, sewer lines laid, and trolley tracks extended. But taxpayers footed the bill, which included outrageous amounts of money used for bribes and kickbacks.

Local officials went out of their way to support the provision of illegal services, such as prostitution and gambling, demanded by their constituents. Money-grubbing politicians and police extorted "hush money" from brothels, gambling parlors, and unlicensed taverns. In turn, these places became absorbed into the bosses' local empire. Extorted fees greased the palms of the cop on the beat and the judge on the take.

Urban bosses had a vested interest in sponsoring new money-making venues for professional sports and supporting other forms of commercialized leisure activity. Baseball parks, boxing rings, and race tracks yielded huge sums in the form of kickbacks from contractors. Once built, stadiums and boxing rings generated profits indefinitely. Sporting events themselves also gave a city's political, legal, and judicial leaders a chance to meet each other and seal business deals.

Thrills, Chills, and Bathtubs: The Emergence of Consumer Culture

On a hot summer day in 1890, a young mother named Emily Scanlon, with her three-year-old daughter in tow, paid the five-cent admission fee to a popular ride called the Toboggan Slide at the Brandywine Springs Amusement Park near Wilmington, Delaware. The two of them ascended a stairwell to the top of the three-story-high structure and then stepped into a car that ran on a wooden trough. When the attendant released the brakes, the car descended, pulled by gravity. It moved slowly at first, then picked up speed around a curve. Suddenly, Emily Scanlon stood up in the car (perhaps to retrieve her hat, which had blown off), and she and her daughter were thrown from the car. Mrs. Scanlon died instantly of a broken neck, but the youngster survived. Significantly, the tragedy did not provoke a shutdown of the ride or the installation of safety measures. Instead, park managers simply posted a sign that read, "Passengers must keep their seats." Patrons continued to enjoy the thrills of the toboggan.

Brandywine Springs boasted an ornate gateway that proclaimed "Let All Who Enter Here Leave Care Behind." In cities around the country, amusement parks brought men and women, girls and boys together to enjoy merry-go-rounds, prizefights, and circus sideshows. By 1880, railroads and steamships were transporting crowds out of Manhattan to Coney Island, where working-class people mingled with the self-proclaimed "respectable" middle classes.

Late in the century, Americans of all kinds began to sample a new realm of sensual experience—one of physical daring, material luxury, and visual fantasy—either as participants or as observers. The ride at Brandywine Springs was an early prototype of the modern roller coaster. The park afforded patrons not only the thrill of riding the Toboggan Slide but also the sights and sounds of a carnival. The calliope (pipe organ) music and the brightly colored signs beckoned visitors to an exciting world apart from the routine of everyday life.

Ticket holders at Brandywine Springs were participating in an emerging consumer culture. With economic growth and high rates of productivity came the two ingredients necessary to a culture of consumption: industries that catered to the demand for novel experiences, or ready-made goods and people with enough money to buy them. Central to this culture was mass advertising, a form of appeal that sought to instill in consumers the desire for things that were new and visually attractive. Colorful spectacles of all kinds—whether in the form of a department store window or a well-publicized athletic event—became an integral part of American life.

Shows as Spectacles

Public officials, college administrators, and ambitious entrepreneurs alike discovered that Americans craved new and stimulating forms of entertainment and were willing to pay for them. Athletic events began to draw large crowds, revealing their potential as big business. Traveling road shows promoted new products and services by charming their audiences with exotic performances. Though modest by today's standards, such spectacles found a ready market in the United States and other countries.

In the quarter-century after Reconstruction, three major sports began to attract large national audiences. Organized baseball had existed since 1846, when the Knickerbocker Base Ball Club of New York met the New York Nine in Hoboken, New Jersey. (The score was 23 to 1, in favor of the Nine.) The National Baseball League, consisting of eight professional teams, was founded in 1876, the American League in 1900. In the 1880s, several new regulations—those governing the overhand pitch, foul balls, and swingless strikes—helped to standardize the game.

Also in the 1880s, Walter Camp, a former Yale University football player, introduced rules—for instance, the system of downs and the center snap to the quarterback—that made

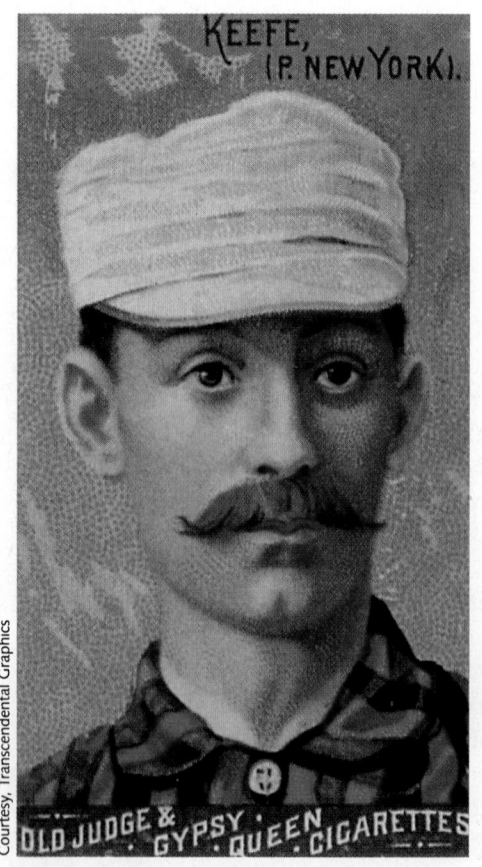

Courtesy, Transcendental Graphics

KEEFE,
(P. NEW YORK).

OLD JUDGE & GYPSY · QUEEN · CIGARETTES

Courtesy, Transcendental Graphics

CHAMPIONS

Base Ball.		Isaac Murphy,	Jockey.
Andrews, (C.F. Philadelphia).		Charles Wood,	do.
Anson, (1st Base, Chicago).		Beeckman,	Lawn Tennis
Brouthers, (1st Base, Detroit).		Dwight,	do.
Caruthers, (P. Brooklyn).		Sears,	do.
Dunlap, (Capt. Pittsburgh).		Taylor,	do.
Glasscock, (S.S. Indianapolis).		Marksman,	
Keefe, (P. New York).		Captain Bogardus.	
Kelly, (C. Boston).		Beach,	Oarsman.
Prince,	Bicyclist.	Jake Gaudaur,	do.
Rowe,	do.	Hanlan,	do.
Stevens,	do.	Teemer,	do.
Wood,	do.	James Albert,	Pedestrian.
Daly,	Billiards.	Pat Fitzgerald,	do
Schaefer,	do.	Rowell,	do
Sexton,	do.	D'oro,	Pool.
Slosson,	do.	Jack Dempsey,	Pugilist
Vignaux,	do.	Jake Kilrain,	do
Broadswordsman,		Mitchell,	do
Duncan C. Ross.		Jem Smith,	do
Capt. Mackenzie,	Chess.	Sullivan,	do.
Steinitz,	do.	Myers,	Runner.
Zukertort,	do.	Strongest Man in the World.	
Foot Ball.		Emil Voss.	
Beecher, (Capt. of Yale Team).		Wild West Hunter,	
W. Byrd Page, High Jumper.		"Buffalo Bill".	
"Snapper" Garrison, Jockey.		Joe Acton,	Wrestler
McLaughlin,	do.	Muldoon,	do.

GOODWIN & CO.
NEW YORK.

CARD COLLECTOR'S CO.
REPRINT

■ Baseball cards, like this one featuring New York Giants player Tim Keefe, were sold at department stores. On the back of the card are listed other national athletes featured in the series. One "Wild West Hunter" is identified as "Buffalo Bill" Cody. This card was also a cigarette advertisement.

that sport quicker and more competitive. Camp was also behind the selection of the first "All America" team (1889) to stimulate fan interest. By this time towns, high schools, and colleges were fielding football teams.

Likewise, boxing emerged as a national, regulated sport. John L. Sullivan, an American, won renown as the world's bare-knuckled champion in 1882, even as more and more fighters had started wearing gloves. Sullivan then joined a traveling theatrical group and demonstrated gloved boxing to enthusiastic crowds all over the country. These exhibitions revealed the fine line between displays of physical prowess and theatrical performances. In 1889, Sullivan defeated an opponent in a 75-round match, the last heavyweight, bare-knuckled championship.

Performances based on skills of all kinds gained national audiences, as the career of William "Buffalo Bill" Cody reveals. Born in Iowa in 1846, Cody parlayed his early years as a Pony Express postal rider, cavalry scout, Indian fighter, and buffalo hunter into a form of mass entertainment. In his "Buffalo Bill Combination" show, cowboy and Indian actors performed skits depicting dramatic events in western history (from a European American point of view, at least). In 1876, Cody briefly left the stage to join a U.S. cavalry skirmish against the Sioux and Cheyenne. Soon he returned to the show to exhibit the dried scalp of the Cheyenne warrior Yellow Hand, whom he claimed he had killed in battle. Cody thus presented the subjugation of the Indians as a form of high drama, a scripted performance that audiences applauded from the comfort of their seats.

In 1882 Cody produced "Buffalo Bill's Wild West," a traveling road show that featured sharpshooter Annie Oakley, cowboy musicians, and Sioux warriors performing authentic Native American dances. Sioux leader Sitting Bull (Tatanka Iyotake), long an admirer of Annie Oakley (he called her "Little Sure Shot"), joined the show in 1885. Like other Indians who

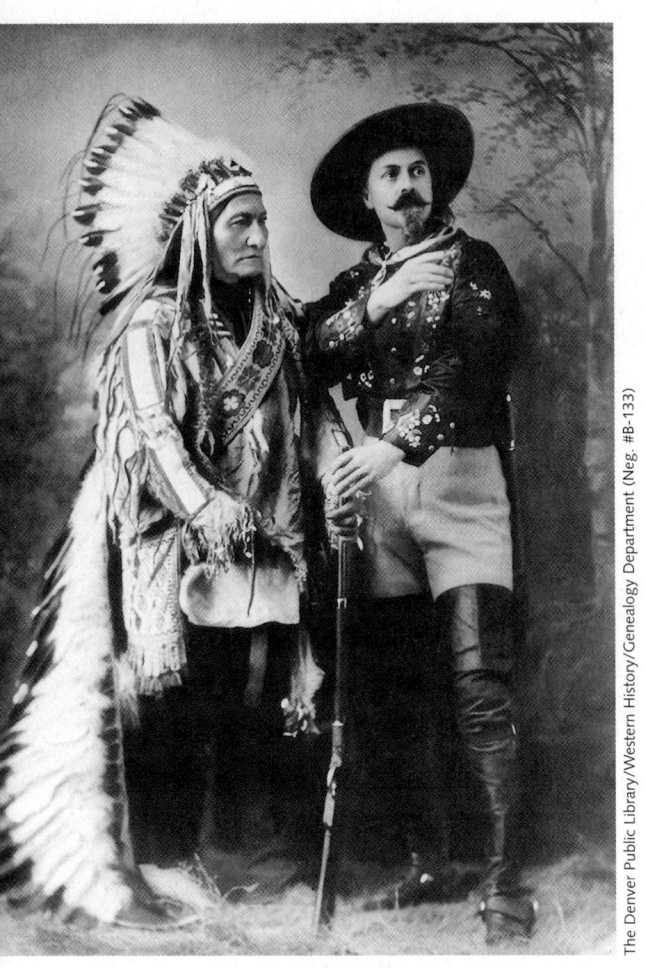

The Denver Public Library/Western History/Genealogy Department (Neg. #B-133)

■ "Buffalo Bill" Cody and Sitting Bull pose for a promotional photo for the 1885 season of the "Wild West." Cody refrained from calling the production a "show," maintaining that it demonstrated frontier skills and recreated historical encounters (such as Custer's Last Stand and stagecoach robberies). The "Wild West" toured Canada and Europe and inspired many imitators.

worked for Cody, Sitting Bull took advantage of the opportunity to escape the confines of the reservation (in his case, Standing Rock in North Dakota). As a member of the "Wild West" troupe, he also enjoyed decent food and accommodations. At a time when whites were denigrating Indian culture, Sitting Bull affirmed that culture by demonstrating his shooting and riding skills. However, white audiences jeered him—they saw him as less an entertainer and more an enemy warrior— and he left after just a year. By the 1890s, Cody was playing to audiences in Europe as well as the United States, dramatizing a West that was fast disappearing. Still, the sight of Annie Oakley shooting glass balls and clay pigeons out of the air, as well as mounted cowboys leading "Custer's last charge," gave customers their money's worth.

One type of traveling road spectacle, the medicine show, had a single purpose: the selling of specific health-related products. In the 1880s N. T. ("Nevada Ned") Oliver hawked an all-purpose remedy called Hindoo Patalka to gullible audiences in New Jersey and Pennsylvania. An ensemble of actors bedecked in Oriental costumes, with a live elephant as a prop, enthralled spectators. Nevada Ned himself testified to the increasing popularity of such presentations, noting that medicine shows were playing in "opera houses, halls, storerooms, ball parks, show boats, and tents, as well as doorways, street corners, and fairs." Increasingly, entrepreneurs saw that many aspects of the American experience— sports, myths about western settlement, anxieties about health and public appearance—could generate profits for shrewd businesspeople.

Mass Merchandising as Spectacle

During the late nineteenth century, the act of shopping in cities for goods, especially luxury goods, became an adventure in itself. A new piece of the cityscape, the department store, welcomed customers into a world of luxury and abundance, a place of color, light, and glamour. These "palaces of consumption" showcased a variety of technological innovations. In Marshall Field's "Grand Emporium" (Chicago), Wanamaker's (Philadelphia), and Lord & Taylor (New York), shoppers glided from story to story on escalators and in elevators. Warmed by central heating, they browsed display cases, racks, and tables laden with enticing goods and illuminated by arc lighting. Their money streamed into cash registers or to a central clerk through cash conveyors.

Thus, department stores not only offered a dazzling array of goods but also made shopping an exciting experience. This appealed particularly to middle-class women, who had the leisure time and the cash to indulge in day-long shopping excursions. In 1880 a New Yorker could arrive at Macy's by taking the Sixth Avenue elevated train and spend the morning exploring any number of specialized departments: ribbons, women's and children's muslin underwear, toys, candy, books, men's furnishings, china and glassware, and so on. Fatigued at noon, she might visit the lunchroom to partake of a modest meal and then devote the rest of her day to examining the colored dress silks, a new department established the year before.

During the 1880s, Macy's expanded its line of goods, introducing items as varied as dog collars and telescopes, mirrors, seeds and garden tools, and Goodyear's rubber boots. The store sold brand names and products manufactured by the company itself, including Red Star silk and Red Star velveteen (a soft, plush fabric). One New York newspaper marveled

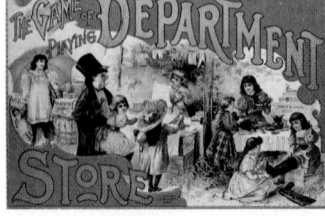

Persuading People to Buy: Advertising in American History

Over the last four centuries, American advertisers have become increasingly creative in using new media to reach potential customers. During the colonial period, inns and taverns identified themselves by hanging sideboards easily recognizable to pedestrians. Early newspapers, such as Benjamin Franklin's *Philadelphia Gazette* (founded in 1728), pioneered in print advertising. Franklin's paper included descriptions of runaway slaves wanted by their owners as well as ads for slaves offered for sale.

In the streets, peddlers called to passersby. Chimney sweeps hawked their services with their distinctive "Sweep O!" refrain. Dry goods merchants distributed cards (handbills) that listed their wares, from corduroy cloth to colorful ostrich feathers. The Stamp Act of 1765 imposed a two-shilling tax on every print advertisement. Colonial merchants rightly feared that this tax would hinder commercial development.

In the antebellum period, mass circulation newspapers featured advertisements as prominently as news stories. In 1833 the *New York Sun* announced that it would provide "ALL THE NEWS OF THE DAY, and at the same time afford an advantageous medium for advertising."

After the Civil War, advertising served as the engine of an emerging consumer economy that depended on the marketing of large quantities of packaged goods. In the 1880s the Proctor & Gamble company initiated an aggressive marketing campaign, touting

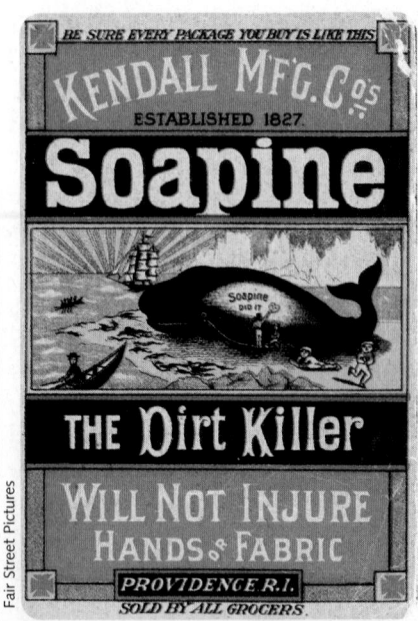

Fair Street Pictures

This ad suggests that the soap Soapine is powerful enough to bleach the black shine out of a whale's hide. Soapine's "scrubbed whale" logo became a familiar sight to late-nineteenth-century consumers.

its brand of Ivory Soap ("99 and 44/100 percent pure") with full-page ads in monthly magazines. (In 1890 the company sold 30 million cakes of the soap.) Traveling road shows advertised patent medicines and at the same time entertained young and old.

The retail sales concerns Montgomery Ward and Sears, Roebuck took advantage of Rural Free Delivery offered by the U.S. Postal Service and sent lavishly illustrated catalogues to households all over the country. In the fall of 1908, Sears distributed 3.7 million copies of its catalogue.

An African American businesswoman, Madame C. J. Walker, built a successful cosmetics company through a variety of modern means; she used print advertising, attractive packaging, endorsements by such celebrities as dancer Josephine Baker, and door-to-door saleswomen called "Walker agents," to enhance her own fame and sell more products.

By the 1920s large advertising agencies were drawing on research in the field of psychology in an effort to create ads that appealed to people's deepest desires as well as their deepest insecurities. In 1957, in *The Hidden Persuaders,* author Vance Packard argued that advertisers used subtle psychological techniques to persuade people to buy goods and services they did not need.

In its 1976 *Virginia State Board of Pharmacy v. Virginia Citizens Council, Inc.* decision, the Supreme Court ruled that advertising was a form of free speech, protected under the Constitution. As a result, professionals such as physicians and lawyers began to advertise their services.

Innovations in communication and transportation opened new channels of advertising. As early as the 1920s, billboards and the sides of barns were used to advertise products to automobile passengers. Radio advertisers specialized in catchy slogans and jingles. In the 1950s television ads became increasingly sophisticated in their use of music and striking visuals. By the late twentieth century, movies and orbiting space capsules provided opportunities for product placement. Airplanes flew advertising banners over crowded summertime beaches and packed football stadiums. Telemarketers pitched their wares over the telephone. Channel One, a closed-circuit television outlet, offered corporate-sponsored educational programming for public school students.

In 1999, U.S. companies, entrepreneurs, and individuals spent more than $200 billion to advertise. By this time, advertising represented a blend of traditional and high-technology methods. The World Wide Web was full of ads, but passersby on city streets were still receiving a barrage of handbills advertising a variety of goods and services. ∎

at the selection and pronounced the store "a bazaar, a museum, a hotel and a great fancy store all combined."

The department store was an exclusively urban phenomenon, but mass merchandising reached far beyond cities. The material riches of American society became accessible to rural people through the mail-order catalogue. This marketing device was pioneered in 1872 by the Chicago company Montgomery Ward, the official supply house for the Farmers' Grange. On homesteads throughout the Midwest, family members gathered to pore over the thousands of items displayed in "The Great Wish Book." The company's motto? "Satisfaction guaranteed or your money back." Farm wives delighted in the latest Parisian fashions, their husbands pondered the intricacies of McCormick threshing machinery, and the children studied the newest line of toys and fishing rods.

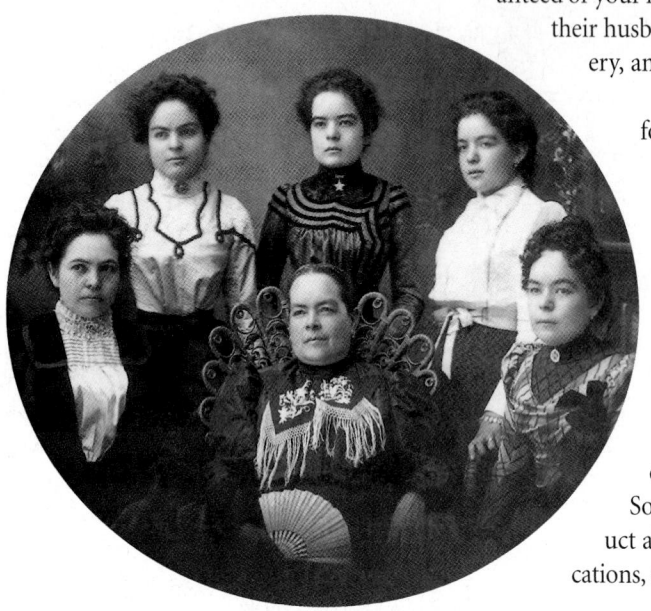

Late in the decade, a competitor appeared on the scene in the form of the Sears, Roebuck Catalogue. A former mail-order watch salesman, Richard Sears soon gained a reputation as a man who could "sell a breath of fresh air." Sears helped pioneer the field of modern advertising hyperbole, claiming, for example, that the sewing machine he offered was the "Best on Earth." Selling was fast becoming a circus sideshow.

The mass production needed to satisfy eager customers itself depended on mass advertising, an enterprise still in its infancy in the 1880s. Yet, some of the principles that would shape the future of this business were in place even at this early date. For instance, soon after the Civil War, the makers of Sozodont dentifrice (toothpaste) plastered the name of their product all over weekly religious magazines and more mainstream publications, such as *Harper's* and *Scribner's*. They labeled the natural landscape as well. Indeed, the word *Sozodont* on Maiden's Rock in Red Wing, Minnesota, was so large that steamboat passengers on the Mississippi River three miles away could plainly read it.

Refugio Amador and her five daughters, Emilia, Maria, Clotilde, Julieta, and Corina, were members of an elite Hispanic family in Las Cruces, New Mexico. Her husband, Martin Amador, was a prominent politician, merchant, hotel owner, and freighter. A subcontractor for the U.S. government, he supplied military troops in the area. The family shopped by mail-order catalogue from Bloomingdale's Department Store in New York City.

The career of L. Frank Baum illustrates the convergence of modern ideas about theatrical performances and sales spectacles. Born to a wealthy German American family in 1856, Baum grew up in upstate New York. His father had made a great deal of money from the oil industry, particularly Pennsylvania gushers that yielded a distinctive emerald green oil. The younger Baum was drawn to what he called the "dream life," with its guilt-free indulgence in pleasure. Together with his wife, he founded a theater troupe that toured the Midwest in the 1880s. He then made a brief foray into merchandising. He marketed Baum's Castorine (axle grease) and opened his own department store, Baum's Bazaar, in Aberdeen, South Dakota, in the northeast corner of the state. There, he also became editor of the town newspaper, the *Aberdeen Saturday Pioneer*.

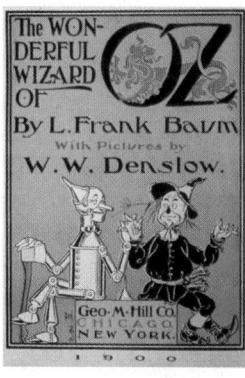

Baum eventually moved his family to Chicago, where he embarked on a career as a department store window designer. He founded the National Association of Window Trimmers in 1898 and started a trade magazine, *The Show Window*. The magazine encouraged designers to strive for a "sumptuous display" of goods and to highlight their rich textures and colors. Baum went on to become a popular writer of children's fiction. His famous book *The Wizard of Oz* (1900), an allegory of late-nineteenth-century life, covered themes as diverse as feminism and rural poverty. An accomplished and successful showman, Baum understood that Americans were eager to buy fantasy wherever they could find it: in a theater, department store, or children's book.

Whether positioned behind a department store display case or in a show window, featured in a magazine advertisement or in a mail-order catalogue, the face of modern mer-

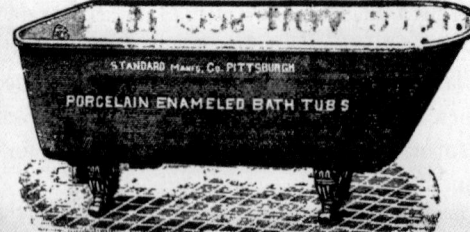

Century Magazine, May 1890

HOUSE FURNISHINGS

ASK YOUR WIFE

If she would not like to bathe in a china dish, like her canary does.

Our Porcelain-lined Bath Tub is a china dish cased in iron.

SANITARY,

DURABLE,

CHEAP.

If you have never tried it, you cannot imagine how delicious a bath can be made by using one of our bath tubs.

The above cut shows tub without rim or fittings. We finish them to suit your taste. This is a luxury you can afford.

Read our advertisement in June CENTURY. Catalogue free.

STANDARD MANUFACTURING CO.
PITTSBURGH, PA.

PIONEER BATHTUB ADVERTISING
(From the Century Magazine for May, 1890.)

■ This advertisement for a Standard bathtub appeared in the May 1890 issue of *Century Magazine*. Early on, advertisers used sophisticated psychological techniques to convince consumers that a wide array of products, formerly considered luxuries, were necessities. This ad suggests that a husband can show his affection for his wife by buying her a new bathtub.

chandising was bound to be young, white, and well-to-do, brimming with health and material well-being. The new consumer culture was marked by a glaring double standard: Although advertisers marketed to the millions, they established a very narrow standard of the "normal" American.

Defending the New Industrial Order

By the late 1870s, intense conflict over fundamental issues had all but evaporated from national politics. Although ethnic and cultural loyalties continued to inflame local and state elections, Republicans and Democrats at the national level disagreed about little except the tariff. Adhering to tradition, Republicans favored a higher tariff that would benefit domestic businesses by making imported goods more expensive. In contrast, Democrats argued that a higher tariff, and resulting higher prices for goods produced in the United States, would harm consumers. Members of the Republican Party called themselves the Grand Army of the Republic; they "waved the bloody shirt"—that is, reminded voters that many of their Democratic opponents, especially those in the South, had supported secession a generation before. Still, the two major parties openly shared a similar goal: to win as many jobs as possible for their respective supporters. Politics served as a vehicle for patronage and favors rather than as a conduit for ideas and alternative visions of the nation's future.

Many politicians also shared a belief in the idea of *laissez-faire* (a French phrase meaning to leave alone, referring to the absence of government interference in the economy). Laissez-faire was actually a flexible concept, invoked to justify government indifference in some areas but government intervention in others. Indeed, politicians tended to favor laissez-faire in social matters more than in the economy. Thus, support for manufacturers and railroads in the form of tariff protection and land grants, for example, was justified. At the same time, however, Congress, the president, and the Supreme Court were reluctant to enact bold measures to redress the growing gap between rich and poor. In fact, certain clergy, businesspeople, and university professors sought to explain and defend the inequality between the captains of industry and the masses of ill-paid laborers. They argued that the system of industrial capitalism was desirable because it was "natural."

Nevertheless, many advocates of laissez-faire in social welfare policy supported government intervention in the economy. These observers argued that the government was justified in providing tangible support (in the form of tariff protection and land grants, for example) to businesses such as manufacturers and railroads.

In 1873 writer Mark Twain (Samuel Clemens) published his first novel, which he cowrote with friend and fellow writer Charles Dudley Warner. Titled *The Gilded Age,* the book satirized the trend toward corruption in public affairs and the wild financial speculation that produced both poverty and great wealth. The growth of large businesses that received economic and political support from government officials served to enrich employers, investors, and politicians at the expense of workers and farmers. The term *Gilded Age* became synonymous with the excess and extravagance on the part of politicians and businessmen alike during the last quarter of the nineteenth century.

The Contradictory Politics of Laissez-Faire

In 1880 the undistinguished President Rutherford B. Hayes chose not to run for office again. That summer the Republicans nominated James A. Garfield of Ohio, a former mule driver who had become a Civil War general. To counter the "bloody-shirt" effect, Democrats put forth their own former Union general: Winfield S. Hancock, who had been wounded at Gettysburg. (Hancock had nevertheless garnered the support of southern whites while presiding over a military Reconstruction district.) The campaign itself was notable for its lack of attention to victims of the recent nationwide depression, such as industrial laborers and southern and midwestern farmers. Garfield won the popular vote by a narrow margin but overwhelmed Hancock in the Electoral College.

TABLE 16-5			
The Election of 1880			
Candidate	Party	Popular Vote	Electoral Vote
James A. Garfield	Republican	4,453,295	214
Winfield S. Hancock	Democratic	4,414,082	155
James B. Weaver	Greenback-Labor	308,578	0

Garfield's arrival in the White House set off a race for patronage jobs among loyal Republicans. Indeed, overwhelmed by office-seekers, the new president remarked, "My God! What is there in this place that a man should ever want to get into it?" Then on July 2, 1881, disaster struck. Charles J. Guiteau, who had unsuccessfully sought the position of U.S. consul in Paris, shot Garfield in a Washington, D.C., train station. Garfield languished for a few months, finally dying on September 19. Guiteau tried to finance his own legal defense by asking for contributions from politicians who might enjoy political gains as a result of the president's death. This audacious strategy did not prevent him from being convicted and executed.

Vice President Chester A. Arthur, a former New York politician, assumed the reins of government. Arthur's administration supported certain forms of government intervention in society, or "social engineering." Arthur and others believed that laissez-faire policies had their limits; strong measures were needed to counter what they and other conservatives considered immoral personal behavior. In 1882 Congress passed the Edmunds Act. Targeting Mormons, the act outlawed polygamy (the practice of having more than one spouse at a time), took the right to vote away from the law's offenders, and sent a five-member commission to Utah to oversee local elections. That same year, Congress responded to pressure from West Coast

European American politicians, the San Francisco's Workingmen's Party in particular, and approved the Chinese Exclusion Act. The act became the first piece of legislation to bar a particular group from entering the United States. Supported by congressmen from other areas of the country as well, this measure was approved after a series of hearings in California and on Capitol Hill. In a petition to Congress, California legislators had charged that Chinese men posed a direct threat to "the most needy and most deserving of our people—those who are engaged, or entitled to be engaged, in industrial pursuits in our midst."

In fact, most Chinese immigrants took jobs that native-born whites shunned. Moreover, unemployment among California white manufacturing workers in the 1870s was caused not by Chinese competitors, but by the flood of cheap eastern-made goods carried into the state by the transcontinental railroad. As eastern goods entered California, manufacturers in the West laid off workers and closed factories. The Chinese, thus, became scapegoats for groups hit hard by larger economic changes. At the national level, then, members of both political parties sought to use congressional power to shape the size and ethnic composition of the domestic workplace.

In 1883 the Supreme Court hurt the cause of blacks' civil rights by declaring the Civil Rights Act of 1875 unconstitutional. (The act had guaranteed blacks equal rights to public accommodations and facilities.) This decision, called the Civil Rights cases, involved five separate cases from Kansas, California, Missouri, New York, and Tennessee. The main issue focused on exclusions of blacks from hotels, railroad cars, and theaters. The court held that state governments could not discriminate on the basis of race but that private individuals could do so. This decision put an official stamp of approval on racist practices of employers, hotels, restaurants, and other providers of jobs and services.

Arthur surprised his critics by embracing the cause of civil service reform. This movement sought to inject professional standards into public service and rid the country of the worst excesses of the corrupt "spoils system," where political victors put loyal supporters into public jobs regardless of their qualifications. In response to Garfield's assassination by Guiteau, the disappointed patronage-seeker, Congress passed the Pendleton Act (1883). This measure established a merit system for federal job applicants and created the Civil Service Commission, which administered competitive examinations to candidates in certain classifications. Within a year, the new regulations covered 10 percent of all federal offices, or about 14,000 jobs.

In 1884 Arthur fell ill (he would die shortly), and the Republicans nominated James G. Blaine of Maine as their candidate for the presidency. Blaine, who had benefited from corrupt deals in the past, offended the sensibilities of a group of reform-minded Republicans, who called themselves Mugwumps. (The term reportedly had its roots in an Indian word that meant "holier than thou.") As a result, Blaine was bested in the national election by the former mayor of Buffalo, Grover Cleveland, who became the first Democratic president in 28 years. Both nominees had avoided making controversial pronouncements on policy issues. Instead, the campaign had a markedly personal tone. Cleveland publicly accepted responsibility for a son born out of wedlock, although apparently there was more than one candidate for paternity of the child. Still, he was unable to avoid the taunts of his rivals, "Ma, ma, where's my pa?" The Democrats countered with a prophetic chant: "Gone to the White House, ha, ha, ha."

Throughout the 1880s, Congress and the chief executive applied the laissez-faire principle selectively—for example, to the status of Indians. Critics of federal Indian policy had come forward to expose, as writer Helen Hunt Jackson put it, the "cheating, robbing, breaking promises" that had devastated the native population since the nation's founding. Published in 1881, Hunt's book *A Century of Dishonor* called for the "protection of the law to the Indian's rights of

TABLE 16-6

The Election of 1884

Candidate	Party	Popular Vote	Electoral Vote
Grover Cleveland	Democratic	4,874,986	219
James G. Blaine	Republican	4,851,981	182

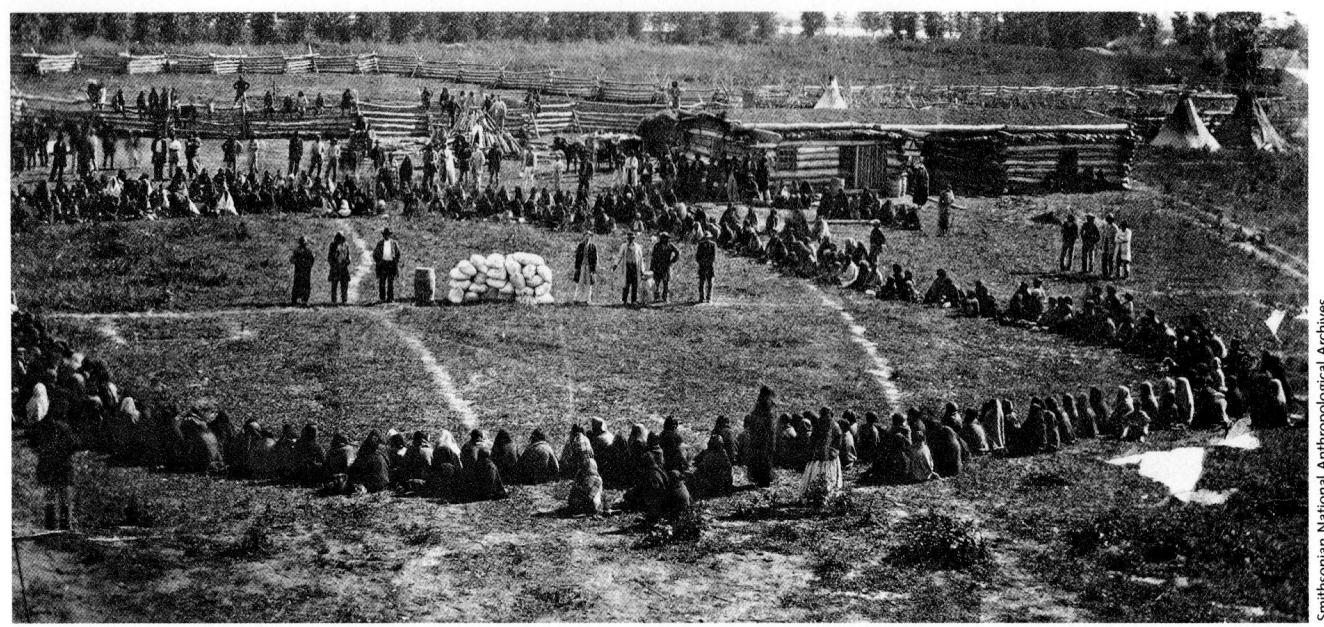

Smithsonian National Anthropological Archives

■ Dakota Indians gather at the Standing Rock Reservation to receive government rations, c. 1880. To counter the Indians' increased dependence on the government for food, Congress passed the Dawes Severalty Act of 1887. U.S. agents cited the act in their efforts to ban crucial aspects of Indian culture, including native practices related to religion, education, language, and even dress and hair styles.

property." Moved to act, Congress passed the Dawes General Allotment (Severalty) Act. The new act was intended to improve the economic condition of Indians by eliminating common ownership of tribal lands in favor of a system of private property. Presumably, the government would withdraw from protecting and supplying Indians (on reservations) and let the free market based on private property run its course. The law distributed plots of land to individual Indians who renounced traditional customs. Such people could gain American citizenship, and their families could receive land grants of up to 160 acres. The law also encouraged these landowners to become sedentary farmers and to adopt "other habits of civilized life." In the end, however, the act amounted to little more than a land-grab on the part of whites; between 1887 and 1900, Indian-held lands decreased from 138 million acres to 78 million acres. The Dawes Act intensified the deep distress of Plains Indians, now deprived of their vast hunting grounds.

By the 1880s, local citizens, through the Grange and their elected public officials, were calling for the states to restrict the monopolistic practices of the railroads. Nevertheless, in *Wabash v. Illinois* (1886), the Supreme Court invalidated a state law regulating railroads, ruling that only Congress, and not the states, could control interstate transportation. The next year Congress took the initiative and passed the Interstate Commerce Act of 1887. This legislation outlawed secretive combinations, such as pools, and mandated that the railroads charge all shippers the same rates and refrain from giving rebates to their largest customers. The act also established the Interstate Commerce Commission to oversee and stabilize the railroad industry. Congress, thus, acknowledged that the public interest demanded some form of business regulation, although enforcement of the act was less than vigorous.

Cleveland invoked laissez-faire principles in 1887 when he vetoed legislation that would have provided seeds for hard-pressed farmers in Texas. As the president put it, "Though the people support the government, the government should not support the people." Furthermore, with his insistence on lower tariff rates, Cleveland alarmed members of his own party, who feared he was handing the Republicans an advantage for the 1888 campaign. As it turned out, most Americans favored government protection of domestic manufacturing in the form of higher tariffs. The Republicans exploited Cleveland's unpopular views on this issue, nominating Benjamin Harrison, grandson of President William Henry ("Tippecanoe") Harrison. The younger Harrison defeated his rival in the electoral college but not in the popular vote.

The principle of government laissez-faire was of little use in addressing a central paradox of the late nineteenth century: The free enterprise system was being undermined by the very

TABLE 16-7

The Election of 1888

Candidate	Party	Popular Vote	Electoral Vote
Benjamin Harrison	Republican	5,447,129	233
Grover Cleveland	Democratic	5,537,857	168
Clinton B. Fisk	Prohibition	249,506	0
Anson J. Streeter	Union Labor	146,935	0

forms of business organization it had spawned and nourished. Trusts and combinations were inherently hostile to competition. In 1890 Congress passed a piece of landmark legislation, the Sherman Anti-Trust Act, designed to outlaw trusts and large business combinations of all kinds. However, the act lacked adequate enforcement mechanisms, and many industrialists simply ignored it. Nevertheless, together with its predecessor, the Interstate Commerce Act, the Sherman Act acknowledged that the largest businesses routinely fixed prices, to the detriment of smaller rival businesses and consumers alike. In the coming years, lawyers and government officials would find the act effective primarily as a tool against another form of "combination": labor unions. The Standard Oil Company, which boldly defied the provisions of the act and continued its trust-building, would not be called to account (and dissolved) until 1911.

Social Darwinism and the "Natural" State of Society

In the late nineteenth century, human-made devices and engineering feats helped create a new social order, one marked by a few very wealthy industrialists, a growing middle class, and an increasingly diverse workforce of ill-paid field and factory hands. Brazenly borrowing from the theories of Charles Darwin, a British naturalist who had pioneered the study of evolution, some prominent clergy, businesspeople, journalists, and university professors sought to defend this new order as God-ordained, or "natural." These observers drew parallels between Darwin's theory of "survival of the fittest" and the workings of modern society. (In his book *Origin of the Species,* Darwin had discussed the study of animals, not people or societies.) In the United States, Social Darwinists warned that "unnatural" forms of intervention—specifically, labor unions or social welfare legislation—were misguided, dangerous, and ultimately doomed to failure. In essence, Social Darwinists distorted a sound scientific theory, misusing it to justify exploitation of the poor and laboring classes.

The ideology of Social Darwinism evolved in response to class conflict and other forms of social turbulence in the 1870s and 1880s. For example, Thomas A. Scott invoked its language when he argued that railroad industry wage cuts were the result of a policy "founded on sound business principles" and that those principles merely reflected "the instincts of humanity."

About the same time, famed Brooklyn minister Henry Ward Beecher cited what he called "the great laws of political economy" to preach the virtues of poverty ("it was fit that man should eat the bread of affliction") and the evils of labor unions. In Beecher's view, unions amounted to "tyrannical opposition to all law and order." Thus, they "could not be defended" and should not be tolerated.

However, Beecher and like-minded thinkers agreed that the government had the right and the obligation to come to the rescue of private companies threatened by angry workers or consumers. These observers also made a distinction between public subsidies to railroads and tariff protection for domestic manufacturers on one hand and public intervention on behalf of workers on the other.

Yale sociologist William Graham Sumner declared that society was like a living organism. For the species to remain healthy, individuals must prosper or decline according to their inherent characteristics. "Society, therefore, does not need any care or supervision,"

Andrew Carnegie and the "Gospel of Wealth"

*I*n an article titled "Wealth," published in the North American Review *in 1889, steel manufacturer Andrew Carnegie defended the amassing of large fortunes on the part of a few. He hailed this trend as a sign of progress.*

"Wealth," *North American Review*

The conditions of human life have not only been changed, but revolutionized, within the past few hundred years. In the former days there was little difference between the dwelling, dress, food, and environment of the chief and those of his retainers. The Indians are to-day where civilized man then was. When visiting the Sioux, I was led to the wigwam of the chief. It was just like the others in external appearance, and even within the difference was trifling between it and those of the poorest of his braves. The contrast between the palace of the millionaire and the cottage of the laborer with us to-day measures the change which has come with civilization.

This change, however, is not to be deplored, but welcomed as highly beneficial. It is well, nay, essential for the progress of the race, that the houses of some

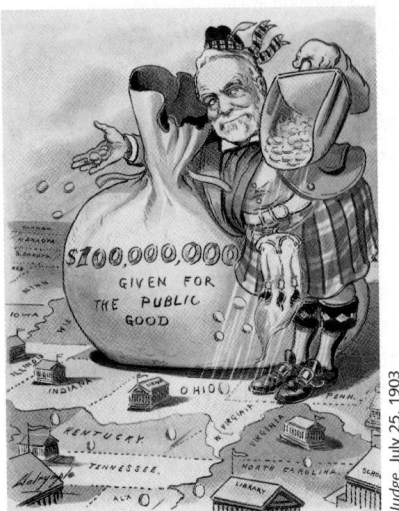

This *Judge* cartoon depicts Andrew Carnegie dispersing his fortune. Many of his donations were used for the establishment of public libraries, a worthy cause according to Carnegie's "gospel of wealth."

should be homes for all that is highest and best in literature and the arts, and for all the refinements of civilization, rather than that none should be so. Much better this great irregularity than universal squalor. . . . Whether the change be for good or ill, it is upon us, beyond our power to alter, and therefore to be accepted and made the best of. It is a waste of time to criticise the inevitable.

Carnegie believed that wealthy people had the responsibility to give away their money before they died, although he had distinct ideas about to whom—or to what—such money should be given. He

elaborated on what came to be called the "gospel of wealth":

There remains, then, only one mode of using great fortunes; but in this we have the true antidote for the temporary unequal distribution of wealth, the reconciliation of the rich and the poor—a reign of harmony—another ideal, differing indeed, from that of the Communist in requiring only the further evolution of existing conditions, not the total overthrow of our civilization. . . . Under its sway we shall have an ideal state, in which the surplus wealth of the few will become, in the best sense, the property of the many, because it is administered for the common good, and this wealth, passing through the hands of the few, can be made a much more potent force for the elevation of our race than if it had been distributed in small sums to the people themselves. Even the poorest can be made to see this, and to agree that the great sums gathered by some of their fellow-citizens and spent for public purposes, from which the masses reap the principal benefit, are more valuable to them than if scattered through the course of many years in trifling amounts.

In 1901, Carnegie sold his steel company to banker J. P. Morgan for $480 million. By the time of his death, Carnegie had given away an estimated $350 million to a variety of causes and institutions. ■

Source: Andrew Carnegie, "Wealth," *North American Review* (1889).

Sumner wrote in his 1883 treatise, *What the Social Classes Owe to Each Other*. These views rationalized not only the hierarchies of the workplace but also the triumph of "Anglo Saxons" on the North American continent and beyond. Editors of the *New York Times* interpreted Darwin's ideas as suggesting that "the red man will be driven out, and the white man will take possession. This is not justice, but it is destiny." In his book *Our Country* (1885), the Reverend Josiah Strong also drew on the ideas of Social Darwinism to claim that just as the fittest plants and animals endure in the natural kingdom, so "civilized" whites would eventually displace "barbarous," dark-skinned peoples, whether on the High Plains of South Dakota or on the savannas of Africa.

Not all Americans studied or debated the theories of Charles Darwin, of course. Nevertheless, middle-class opinion-makers, many of them Victorian Protestants, believed that their own religious and cultural values remained culturally superior to those of other groups of people, at home and abroad. The United States was becoming increasingly diverse in both economic and ethnic terms. At the same time, white, prosperous, native-born Protestants contended that they set the standards for the rest of the nation. These standards revolved around the middle-class domestic ideal, with its rigidly proscribed gender roles, devotion to personal achievement (for men at least), and commitment to moral suasion (that is, regulating a person's behavior by appealing to his or her conscience). Agents of the Victorian middle class included schoolteachers, clergy, magazine editors, business leaders, and other well-educated people able and willing to influence the beliefs of others.

Conclusion

Some historians suggest that the great captains of industry were the chief representatives of widely held values in late-nineteenth-century America. Men such as Carnegie and Rockefeller had the vision and personal ambition necessary to build large corporate enterprises. They became fabulously wealthy by providing the United States with the ingredients necessary to an economic revolution: steel, oil, and other materials. Their ideology of unbridled individualism encouraged many people to aspire to entrepreneurial independence: the tailor's hope that he would someday own his own store, the waiter's dream of opening his own restaurant. The explosion of economic activity during this period—a second American industrial revolution—widened the middle class and lent credence to the notion of widespread upward mobility, modest though it was in most cases.

Nevertheless, a case can be made that engineers were the true representatives of the age. As designers of railroad routes, gravity-defying skyscrapers, and new systems of shop floor management, they oversaw the technical aspects of economic growth and development.

Engineers melded science with mass production to yield a form of capitalism that thrived on consumers' deepest desires and anxieties. That enterprise was not without complications. Throughout the nation, various groups rejected standardization in favor of local tradition or new forms of collective action. Thus, politicians and the Social Darwinists were forced to defend their outlook on life. Some of their critics advanced the idea that society was not a living organism at all. Rather, it was like a machine, a creation of people who had the ability— and the duty—to repair or adjust it. Around the country, in fact, the standardizers met with stiff resistance.

Sites to Visit

Alexander Graham Bell Family Papers at the Library of Congress
www.memory.loc.gov/ammem/bellhtml/bellhome.html

This site contains papers from 1862 to 1839 as well as a chronology, images, selected documents, and interpretive essays about Bell.

John D. Rockefeller and the Standard Oil Company
www.micheloud.com/FXM/SO/

This study with accompanying images by François Micheloud tells of the rise of Rockefeller and his mammoth company.

The Transcontinental Railroad
www.sfmuseum.org/hist1/rail.html

This Museum of the City of San Francisco site has excellent information on the railroad.

Touring Turn-of-the-Century America: Photographs from the Detroit Publishing Company, 1880–1920

www.memory.loc.gov/ammem/detroit/dethome.html

> This Library of Congress collection has thousands of photographs from turn-of-the-century America.

Shadow Ball: The Negro Baseball Leagues

www.negro-league.columbus.oh.us/jimcrow1.htm

> This Harlan William article examines the African American baseball leagues.

African American Perspectives: Pamphlets from the Daniel A. P. Murry Collections, 1818–1907

www.memory.loc.gov/ammem/aap/aaphome.html

> This collection includes writings of famous African Americans, including Frederick Douglass, Booker T. Washington, Ida B. Wells-Barnett, Benjamin W. Arnett, Alexander Crummel, and Emanuel Love.

The Evolution of the Conservation Movement, 1850–1920

www.memory.loc.gov/ammem/amrvhtml/conshome.html

> This American Memory site brings together scores of primary sources and photographs about the historical formations and cultural foundations of the movement to conserve and protect America's natural heritage.

Inside an American Factory: The Westinghouse Works, 1904

www.lcweb2.loc.gov/ammem/papr/west/westhome.html

> Part of the American Memory Project at the Library of Congress, this site provides a glimpse inside a turn-of-the-century factory.

For Further Reading

General Works

Alfred D. Chandler, *The Visible Hand: The Managerial Revolution in American Business* (1977).

Jon Gjerde, *The Minds of the West: Ethnocultural Evolution in the Rural Middle West, 1830–1917* (1997).

Andrew C. Isenberg, *The Destruction of the Bison: An Environmental History, 1750–1920* (2000).

T. Jackson Lears, *Fables of Abundance: A Cultural History of Advertising in America* (1994).

Walter Licht, *Industrializing America: The Nineteenth Century* (1995).

Carroll Pursell, *The Machine in America: A Social History of Technology* (1995).

Alan Trachtenberg, *The Incorporation of America: Culture and Society in the Gilded Age* (1982).

C. Vann Woodward, *Origins of the New South, 1877–1913* (1951).

The New Shape of Business

James R. Barrett, *Work and Community in the Jungle: Chicago's Packinghouse Workers, 1894–1922* (1987).

Ron Chernow, *Titan: The Life of John D. Rockefeller, Sr.* (1998).

Thomas C. Cochran, *Two Hundred Years of American Business* (1977).

Wendy Gamber, *The Female Economy: The Millinery and Dressmaking Trades, 1860–1930* (1997).

Thomas Parke Hughes, *American Genesis: A Century of Invention and Technological Enthusiasm, 1870–1970* (1989).

A. J. Millard, *Edison and the Business of Innovation* (1990).

Daniel Nelson, *Managers and Workers: Origins of the New Factory System in the United States, 1880–1920* (1975).

David E. Nye, *Electrifying America: Social Meanings of a New Technology, 1880–1940* (1990).

Donald J. Pisani, *Water, Land, and Law in the West: The Limits of Public Policy, 1850–1920* (1996).

C. J. Schmitz, *The Growth of Big Business in the United States and Western Europe, 1850–1939* (1993).

George Rogers Taylor and Irene D. Neu, *The American Railroad Network, 1861–1890* (1956).

David O. Whitten, *The Emergence of Giant Enterprise, 1860–1914* (1983).

The Birth of a National Urban Culture

Gunther Paul Barth, *City People: The Rise of Modern City Culture in Nineteenth-Century America* (1980).

Edwin G. Burrows and Mike Wallace, *Gotham: A History of New York City to 1898* (1999).

Howard P. Chudacoff and Judith E. Smith, *The Evolution of American Urban Society,* 5th ed. (2000).

William Cronon, *Nature's Metropolis: Chicago and the Great West* (1991).

Robert V. Hine and John Mack Faragher, *The American West: A New Interpretive History* (2000).

Eric Monkkonen, *America Becomes Urban: The Development of U.S. Cities and Towns, 1780–1980* (1988).

David Nasaw, *Going Out: The Rise and Fall of Public Amusements* (1993).

Steven A. Riess, *City Games: The Evolution of American Urban Society and the Rise of Sports* (1989).

Stanley K. Schultz, *Constructing Urban Culture: American Cities and City Planning, 1800–1920* (1989).

Robert Twombly, *Louis Sullivan: His Life and Work* (1986).

Thrills, Chills, and Bathtubs

Boris Emmet and John E. Jeuck, *Catalogues and Counters: A History of Sears, Roebuck and Company* (1950).

Allen Guttmann, *A Whole New Ball Game: An Interpretation of American Sports* (1988).

John F. Kasson, *Amusing the Million: Coney Island at the Turn of the Century* (1978).

Joy S. Kasson, *Buffalo Bill's Wild West: Celebrity, Memory and Popular History* (2000).

William Leach, *Land of Desire: Merchants, Power, and the Rise of a New American Culture* (1993).

Kathy Lee Peiss, *Cheap Amusements: Working Women and Leisure in New York City, 1880 to 1920* (1986).

Robert C. Toll, *On with the Show! The First Century of Show Business in America* (1976).

Defending the New Industrial Order

Thomas L. Haskell, *The Emergence of Professional Social Science: the American Social Science Association and the Nineteenth-Century Crisis of Authority* (1977).

Richard Hofstadter, *Social Darwinism in American Thought, 1860–1914*, rev. ed. (1955).

Morton Keller, *Affairs of State: Public Life in Late Nineteenth-Century America* (1977).

Valerie S. Mathes, *Helen Hunt Jackson and Her Indian Reform Legacy* (1990).

Louis Menand, *The Metaphysical Club: A Story of Ideas in America* (2001).

Online Practice Test

Test your understanding of this chapter with interactive review quizzes at

www.ablongman.com/jonescreatedequal/chapter16

Additional Photo Credits

CHAPTER

17

Challenges to Government and Corporate Power: Resistance and Reform, 1877–1890

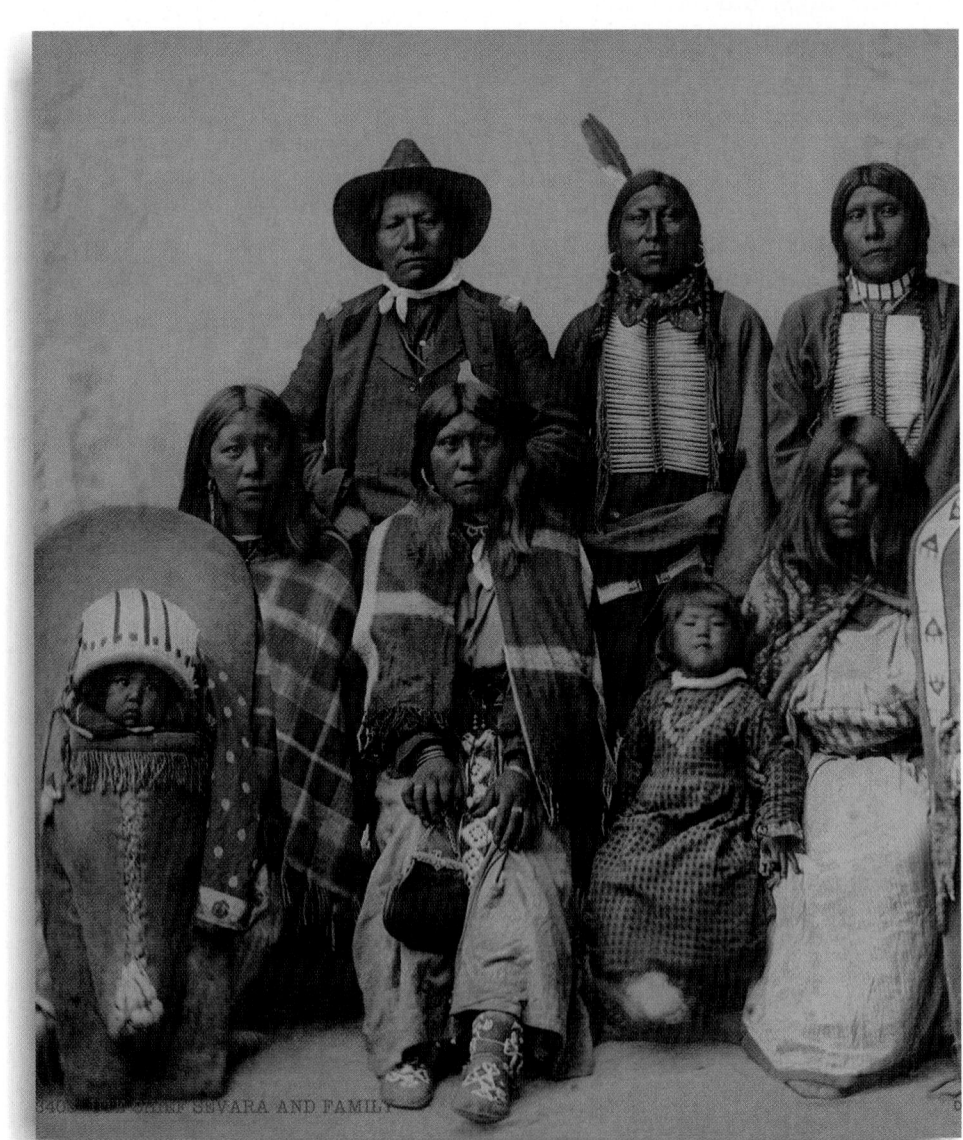

The Collection of Christopher Cardozo, Inc.

■ The Ute chief Sevara poses with his family. In the mid-nineteenth century, European American miners began to push the Utes out of their territory in eastern Utah and western Colorado. Although many Utes resisted government pressure to give up hunting and become farmers, even engaging in gun battles with U.S. troops in 1879, they were gradually forced to yield their remaining lands to whites.

IN THE SPRING OF 1889 MEN IN SAN MIGUEL COUNTY, NORTHERN NEW MEXICO TERRITORY, armed themselves and donned masks. Mounting their horses, they rode out to attack their enemies. As members of a secret organization called *las Gorras Blancas* (the Whitecaps), they banded together in the dead of the night and destroyed the fences of local cattle ranchers, chopping the wooden posts to pieces and scattering the barbed wire. In some of their raids, the rebels shot and wounded ranchers. Over the next year and a half, *las Gorras Blancas* broadened their targets. They burned bridges, haystacks, and piles of lumber; cut telegraph wires; and took axes to electric light poles and to railroad ties belonging to the Atcheson, Topeka, and Santa Fe Railroad. The membership of the group overlapped with that of the Knights of Labor, a national labor union that boasted 20 local assemblies in San Miguel County, east of Santa Fe. On the night of March 11, 1890, *las Gorras Blancas* nailed pieces of paper to the buildings of East Las Vegas, the largest town in the county. These pages, copies of the insurgents' "platform," declared, "Our purpose is to protect the rights and interests of the people in general; especially those of the helpless classes."

Who were these determined nightriders? They consisted of Hispanos—Spanish-speaking natives of the area. Their movement began when Juan Jose Herrera, together with his two brothers, Pablo and Nicanor, organized their neighbors in an effort to block European American ranchers from fencing their land. Labeled *las masas de los hombres pobres* (the masses, the poor people) by a local newspaper, *las Gorras Blancas* were desperately struggling to preserve a traditional way of life that was rapidly disappearing. Fenced lands prevented the area's Hispanic settlers from grazing their stock herds in the customary, open-range manner.

The fence-cutters believed they were upholding American principles of justice and fair play. Released from jail in the town of Las Vegas, New Mexico, a group of them marched down the main street. At the head of their procession, women waved the American flag and sang "John Brown's Body," a song beloved by Union supporters during the Civil War.

Many Hispanos lived in adobe (baked-clay) dwellings in small river valley villages surrounded by breathtaking mesas, ponderosa pine forests, and high dry plains. In addition to raising chickens and grazing sheep, families grew chiles, pinto beans, squash, and wheat. Together, villagers relied on the common lands that had come down to them from their ancestors—land originally bestowed through grants from Spain and then Mexico. After the Civil War, European American interlopers—sheep and cattle ranchers, lawyers, speculators, commercial lumberers, and the railroads—began to encroach on these common lands. Through local courts, the newcomers installed a system of private property that granted exclusive ownership to single individuals. It was these groups, with their fences and their laws governing land title registration, that *las Gorras Blancas* targeted.

By 1889, Santa Fe had seen several centuries of cultural conflict.

Northern New Mexico had long witnessed battles between successive waves of settlers; for example, *Mexicanos* had fought Comanches and Jicarilla Apaches for the land in earlier generations. Yet the upheaval in San Miguel County in 1889 and 1890 did not simply pit Hispanic subsistence farmers against European American "land grabbers." The Spanish-speaking population itself was divided between poor villagers and elite *ricos* (merchants and landowners). Members of *las Gorras Blancas* quarreled among themselves over whose fences to cut and whose barns to burn. They also broke with European American members of the Knights, insisting that, as Hispanos, they had the right and the obligation to protect their common lands, by force if necessary. The insurgents even renounced some of their own Hispanic political leaders. These men, they charged, had become corrupted by greed and were willing to do the bidding of European American interlopers.

Las Gorras Blancas had only mixed success. They managed to discourage new European Americans from settling in the area, and they prevented the railroads from buying more rail ties in northern New Mexico. Yet the nightriders could not stem the tide of land loss throughout the Southwest. The Court of Private Land Claims, established in 1891 by the U.S. government, resolved land disputes between Hispanic and European American claimants. Of the more than 35 million acres of land in dispute in the early 1890s, Hispanic claimants received title to little more than 2 million acres—barely one-twentieth of the land they had held in common.

Las Gorras Blancas represented a unique response to local conditions. But it was also part of a growing, nationwide movement against the standards imposed by industrialization and capitalism. Around the country, a wide variety of individuals and organizations emerged in the late 1870s and the 1880s to challenge employers, landlords, and military and government officials. Members of these latter groups responded with a challenge of their own: Business, they proclaimed, must be allowed to develop fully and freely without "unnatural" intervention in the form of regulatory legislation or grassroots rebellions such as that of *las Gorras Blancas*.

It is difficult to generalize about those who contested the emerging order. Even their own names could be misleading. In the early 1890s, another group called "white caps," this one in Mississippi, consisted of whites who terrorized black landowners and mill workers. And although the Knights of Labor was a national union, it shaped its program in accordance with local issues. In San Miguel County, for instance, the issue was land—who controlled it and under what conditions. In Washington, D.C., the Knights' concern was the welfare of workers in the building trades. The Richmond, Virginia, Knights pioneered interracial organizing, living up to the group's motto, "An injury to one is an injury to all." In contrast, the San Francisco Knights spearheaded the move to bar Chinese laborers from the United States and to limit job opportunities for those who remained. Indeed, groups that challenged the authority of government and large business interests often disagreed among themselves about goals and strategies for change.

Rejecting new business principles that favored aggressive profit-seeking above all else, nightriders, union organizers, machine breakers, visionary prophets, investigative journalists, and settlement house workers all offered alternative visions for America. Members of these groups debated among themselves the changes overtaking American society and the means to control them. Some wielded pens or typewriters to effect change; others took photographs, collected data, or conducted interviews. Still others shouldered arms or torched haystacks. In some cases they sought to preserve local religious and social customs; in others they promoted the health and welfare of factory workers.

> Las Gorras Blancas *had only mixed success. The nightriders could not stem the tide of land loss throughout the Southwest.*

Some proponents of change advocated radical action that challenged the very foundations of American society. Others stressed the need to reform, but not change radically, certain elements of society and politics. Radicals and reformers alike derived both ideas and inspiration from their European counterparts, for the issues confronting a rapidly industrializing society were not unique to the United States during this period. Nevertheless, Americans remained divided in their vision of the good and just society—a vision that would require the commitment of more than any one political party, labor union, reform association, or band of rebels to become reality.

Resistance to Legal and Military Authority

America's march toward national economic centralization and integration was not steady. On the battlefield and in the courts, European Americans pressed their advantage, but these efforts met with stiff resistance from a variety of aggrieved groups. Members of these groups rightly believed they had much to lose from so-called progress. Often the term was used to protect the interests of white men of property and did not result in any real progress for people of color.

Violent prejudice characterized the tactics of elites in expanding and preserving their privileges; vulnerable groups used various strategies to protect themselves and assert their own interests. European Americans repeatedly used the notion of "racial" difference as a justification for depriving darker-skinned peoples of their claims to land, jobs, and even life itself. For example, California lawmakers at both the state and local levels approved legislation that discriminated against the Chinese as workers and as parents of school-aged children. In an effort to seek redress, some Chinese took their claims to court.

In a similar vein, prejudice against African Americans assumed the form of discriminatory legislation and random violence. Blacks chafed under restrictions intended to bar them from good jobs and from associating with white people on an equal basis. Varieties of black resistance to white authority included migration out of the South, creation of community institutions, and violent retaliation.

For their part, during the late 1880s the Plains Indians responded to encroaching railroads, settlers, and military regiments by embracing a movement of spiritual regeneration. On the Plains, whites, and especially U.S. military officers, perceived this movement as more dangerous than an armed uprising, and they reacted accordingly.

Chinese Lawsuits in California

In San Francisco in 1878 Irish-born Denis Kearney founded the Workingmen's Party of California, composed primarily of unemployed whites. Kearney and others agitated for the violent expulsion of Chinese from jobs. They blamed Chinese shoemakers, tailors, and cigarmakers for the distress that native-born factory workers and tradespeople were suffering. One critic remarked that the temperance Kearney "practiced and preached as to liquor and tobacco did not extend to opinions or their expression."

In rural California, job-hungry whites formed anti-Chinese groups such as the American and European Labor Association, founded in Colusa County in 1882. The association also included employers who resented Chinese demands for equal pay. (Most of these immigrants received two-thirds the wages of their white counterparts for the same work.) Yet despite all the personal and legal discrimination, the Chinese resisted.

Opposition to the Chinese hardened in the 1880s. In San Francisco, the Knights of Labor and the Workingmen's Party of California helped to engineer the passage of the Chinese Exclusion Act, approved by Congress in 1882. This measure denied any additional Chinese laborers entry into the country while allowing some Chinese merchants and students to immigrate. (Put to the voters of California in 1879, the possibility of *total* exclusion of Chinese had garnered 150,000 votes for and only 900 against.) In railroad towns and mining camps, vigilantes looted and burned Chinese communities, in some cases murdering or expelling their inhabitants. In 1885 in Rock Springs, Wyoming, white workers massacred 28 Chinese and drove hundreds out of town in the wake of an announcement by Union Pacific officials that the railroad would begin hiring the lower-paid immigrants. While white women cheered from the sidelines, their husbands and brothers burned the Chinese section of the town to the ground. Such attacks erupted more and more frequently throughout the West in the late 1880s and into the 1890s. White men contended that they must present a united front against all Chinese, who, they claimed, threatened the economic well-being of white working-class communities.

Whites held that the Chinese, with their distinctive customs, would never fit into American life. Nevertheless, early on the Chinese demonstrated an understanding and appreciation of American political and legal processes. Beginning in Gold Rush days, Chinese immigrants had taken their grievances to court. Chan Young sued for citizenship in San Francisco's federal district court in 1855. In 1862 in the same city, Ling Sing protested the $2.50 personal tax levied on Chinese exclusively. The California Supreme Court agreed (in *Ling Sing v. Washburn*) that the group could not be singled out for special taxes. In the 1870s Chinese merchants used the provisions of the Civil Rights Act to challenge state and local laws that forbade them from holding certain jobs, living in white neighborhoods, and testifying in court, among other legal liabilities. In the fall of 1885 Chinese residents of Rock Springs, Wyoming, wrote a lengthy appeal to the Chinese consul in San Francisco, relating their story of the massacre and appealing for justice; 559 people signed the document.

In San Francisco in 1885 laundry operator Yick Wo was convicted under an 1880 municipal law prohibiting the construction of wooden laundries without a license. A native of China, Yick Wo had arrived in the United States in 1861. By the time of his arrest, he had operated a legal laundry for 22 years. When he applied for a license, the board of supervisors turned

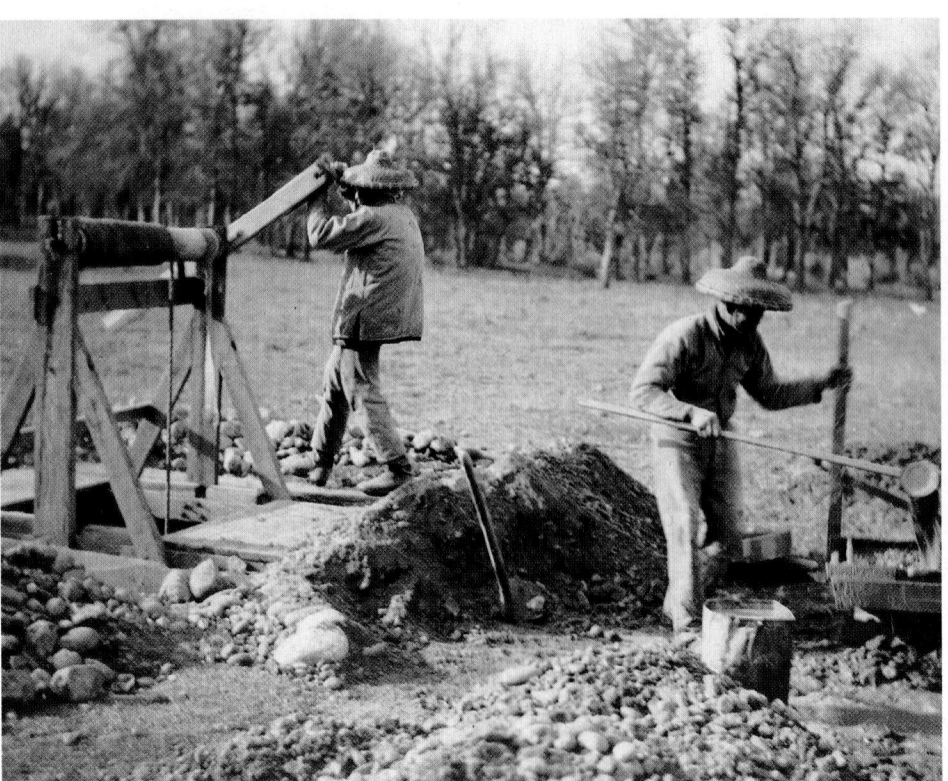

■ In the West, Chinese mining companies used water management techniques based on traditional Chinese machinery such as the waterwheel. This photo shows a Chinese river-mining operation in Siskiyou, California, c. 1890. Chinese workers also constructed flumes, dams, canals, tunnels, and pumps to drain areas efficiently.

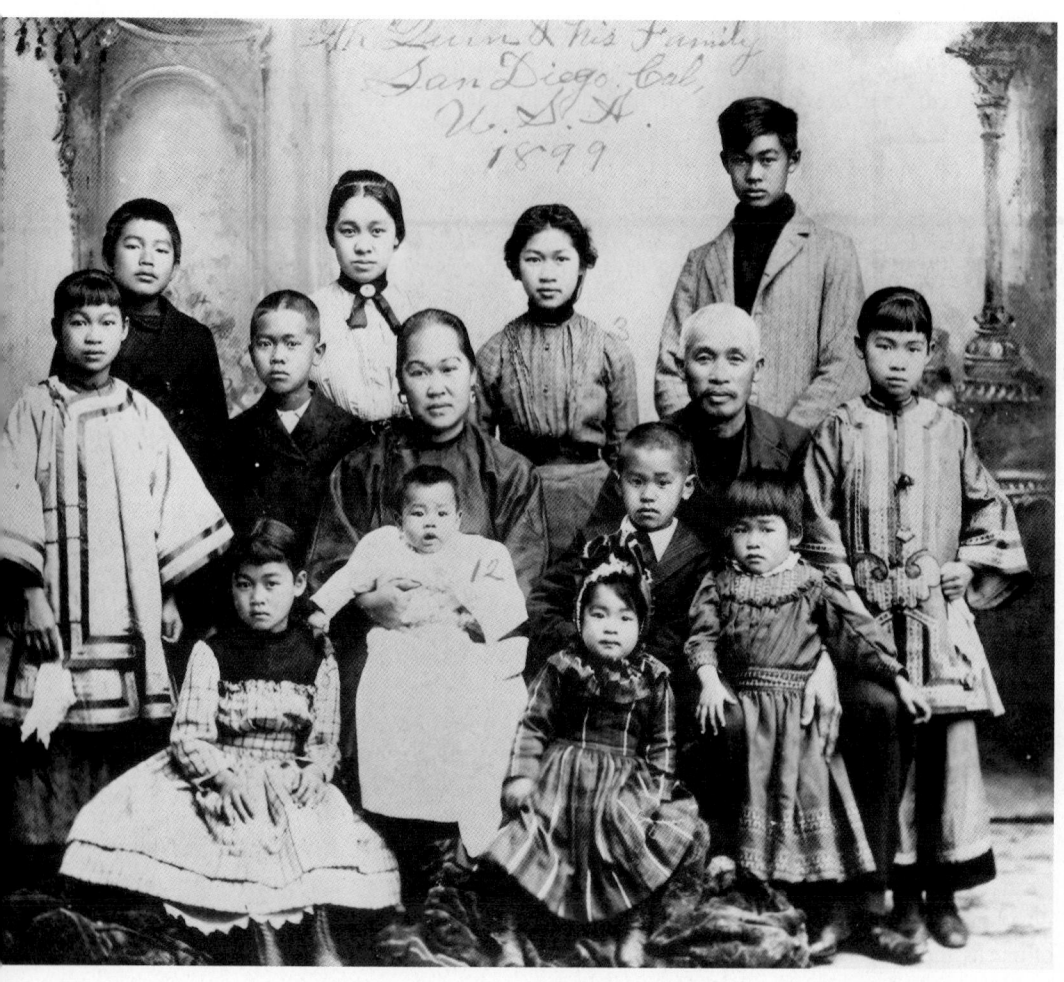

Ah Quin & his family
San Diego, Cal,
U.S.A.
1899

■ Some Chinese made a prosperous life for themselves in the United States. This photo shows Ah Sue, her husband, Ah Quin, and their 12 children. Ah Sue found refuge in the San Francisco Chinese Mission Home in 1879. Two years later she and Ah Quin celebrated their Christian wedding in the Mission Home. Ah Quin rose from the position of cook to become a successful railroad contractor and merchant in San Diego.

him down. His prominent European Americans lawyers soon learned that the board had denied licenses to all Chinese laundry operators who applied. However, it had granted licenses to almost all of their white counterparts. In 1885 the lawyers petitioned the California Supreme Court, which upheld Yick Wo's arrest. The lawyers continued their appeal to the U.S. Supreme Court, maintaining that the board of supervisors intended to bar Chinese from independent laundry work altogether.

In *Yick Wo v. Hopkins* (1886), the Supreme Court reversed the state court's decision. The higher court held that the San Francisco laundry-licensing board had engaged in the discriminatory *application* of a law that on the surface was nondiscriminatory. (The local board had admitted favoritism toward white license applicants but offered no justification for its actions.) The majority opinion noted, "The very idea that one may be compelled to hold his life, or the means of living, or any material right essential to the enjoyment of life, at the mere will of another" has been considered "intolerable in any country where freedom prevails, as being the essence of slavery itself." (In 1954, the Supreme Court cited this case [*Hernandez v. Texas*] when it overturned the criminal conviction of a Mexican American defendant who showed that the county judicial system systematically excluded people of his background from jury service.)

Still, many cases challenging discriminatory laws never made it to the nation's highest court. And state and local courts in general often refused to acknowledge that Chinese immigrants had any civil rights at all. (Chinese immigrants were not granted citizenship until World War II, although their children born in this country qualified as citizens.) In 1885 the California Supreme Court heard the case *Tape v. Hurley,* brought by Joseph and Mary Tape on behalf of their daughter Mamie. Joseph Tape was a Chinese immigrant with some standing in the San

Francisco Chinese community. Mary Tape had been raised in a Shanghai orphanage and had come to the United States with missionaries when she was 11 years old. She grew up to speak English fluently and dressed as a European American. Their daughter Mamie was quite westernized as well.

Even so, Mamie Tape was barred from the city's public school system. The school board claimed that Mamie's presence in the classroom would be "very mentally and morally detrimental" to her classmates. The Tapes sued the city and won (*Tape v. Hurley*), but the school board retaliated by creating a separate school for children of Asian descent within Chinatown. Mary Tape wrote an angry letter to the board: "Dear Sirs, Will you please to tell me! Is it a disgrace to be Born a Chinese? Didn't God make us all!!! What right! have you to bar my children out of the school?" In the end, the Tapes decided to enroll their two children in the segregated school. Yet their legal protest kept alive the ideal of equality under the law.

In other instances, local white prejudice overwhelmed even Chinese who sought legal redress from violence and discrimination. In 1886 the Chinese living in the Wood River mining district in southern Idaho faced down a group of whites who had met and announced that all Chinese had three months to leave town. Members of the Chinese community promptly hired their own lawyers and took out an advertisement in the local paper stating their intention to hold their ground. As a community they managed to survive. Still, their numbers dropped precipitously throughout Idaho as whites managed to hound many of them out of the state.

Blacks in the "New South"

In 1886 Henry Grady, the young editor of the Atlanta *Constitution*, traveled north to deliver a speech to the New England Society of New York. A graduate of the University of Georgia, the 36-year-old Grady had achieved prominence in Georgia politics. In his speech that day Grady hailed what he called the "New South." The former Confederate states, he claimed, were now forward-looking, prepared to embrace industrialization and promote the reconciliation of blacks and whites. According to the journalist, it was time for the South to march forward and join with a larger, modernizing America.

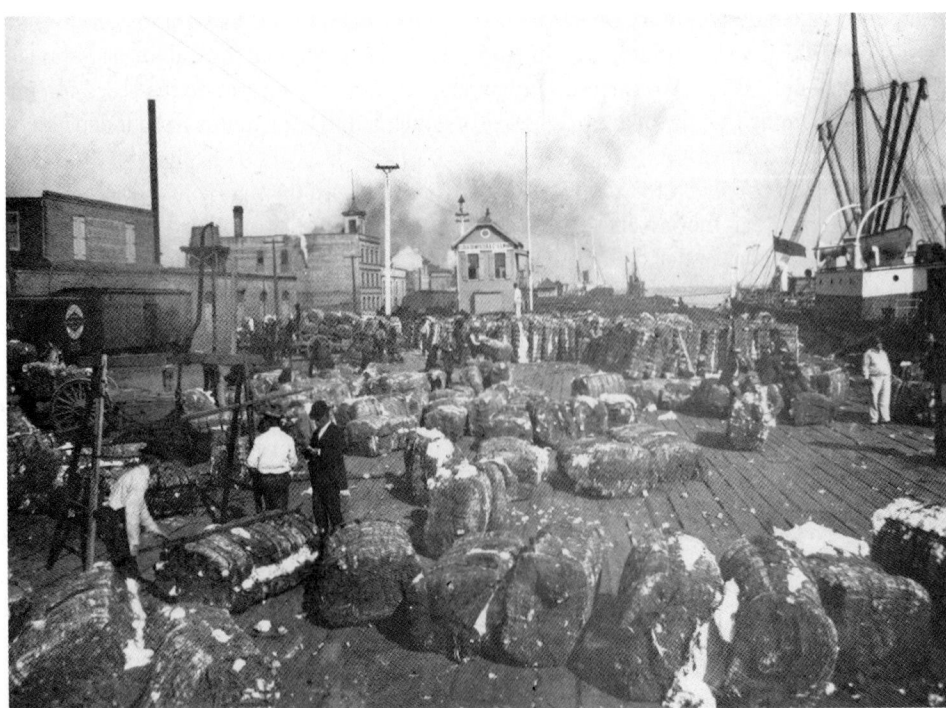

■ This bustling New Orleans waterfront scene, c. 1885, suggests the commercial vitality often associated with the "New South." However, a closer look reveals that all of the activity revolves around loading and unloading bales of cotton. In fact, the so-called New South remained locked in a low-wage, staple crop economy based on the production of cotton.

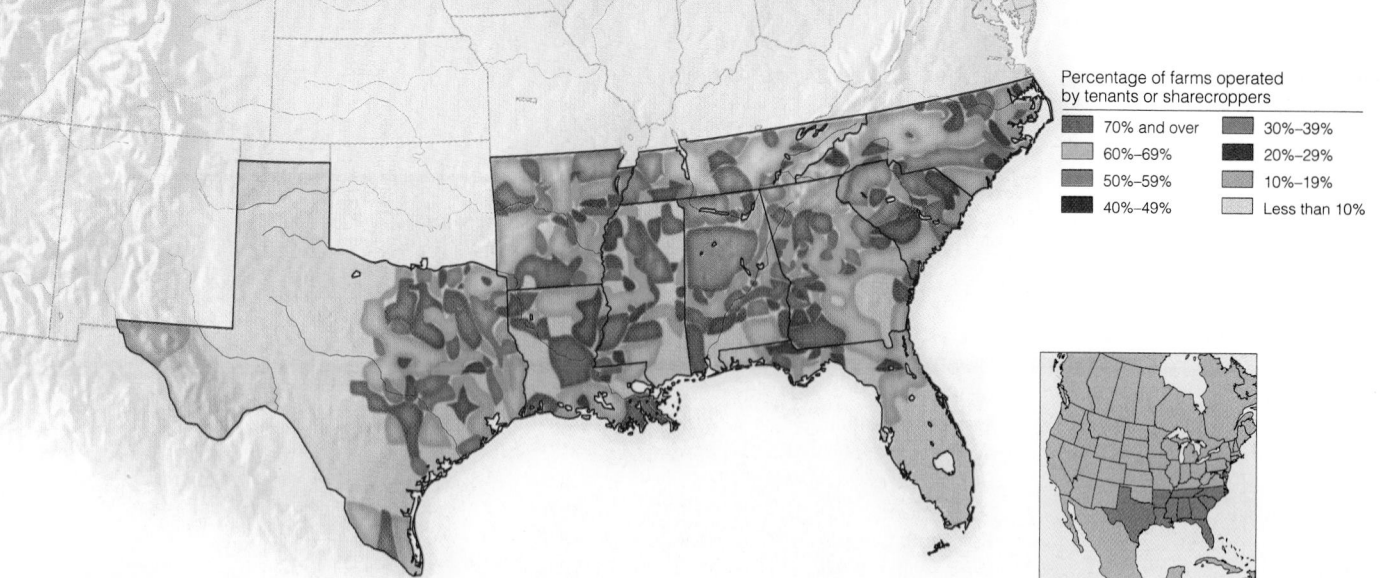

■ **MAP 17.1**

SOUTHERN TENANCY AND SHARECROPPING, 1880 Tenants and sharecroppers were landless families who worked for a landowner. Tenant families usually owned a mule (to pull a plow); sharecropping families depended on their employers for food and farm supplies. This map shows that rates of tenancy and sharecropping were highest in the areas dominated by the cotton staple crop economy, the same areas where slavery prevailed in the antebellum period.

Percentage of farms operated by tenants or sharecroppers

70% and over | 30%–39%
60%–69% | 20%–29%
50%–59% | 10%–19%
40%–49% | Less than 10%

Grady's speech about the "New South" provided a label that stuck. Yet he doubtless spoke too soon and in terms too grandiose. True, he could point with pride to some dramatic industrial developments in the South. The eastern Piedmont (foothills region), for example, was undergoing a fledgling industrial revolution in the 1880s. Soon after James Bonsack invented a cigarette-rolling machine in 1880 James Buchanan Duke pioneered the production of machine-made cigarettes. In 1884 Duke's Durham, North Carolina, company was selling 400,000 of them each day. The southern textile labor force more than doubled between 1880 and 1890, from 17,000 men, women, and children to 36,000, many of them concentrated in the Carolinas and Georgia.

In the mid-1880s, with the backing of the Tennessee Coal, Iron, and Railway Company, the city of Birmingham, Alabama, specialized in pig iron production. Local manufacturers remained at the mercy of high shipping rates imposed by northern-owned railroads, which provided discounts only to raw materials going north and manufactured goods coming south. However, in 1889 even Andrew Carnegie acknowledged the formidable challenge posed by Birmingham blast furnaces to iron and steel producers in the North and abroad.

Factory and professional work in towns and cities offered new opportunities in the South as industry developed. However, these jobs were dominated by white men. Low-paid heavy labor, primarily in rural areas, continued to be the primary source of work for black men. After they finished harvesting cotton in the fall, many black men worked at sawmills or in railroad construction camps during the winter.

The hardest and lowest-paid jobs, such as digging ore out of a hill in northern Alabama or constructing a railroad through the swamps of Florida, often went to convicts whom private employers had leased from the state. Most of these "convict lease" workers were black men who had been arrested on minor charges and then bound out when they could not pay their fines or court costs. In Mississippi a black man could be picked up for "some trifling misdemeanor," in the words of one observer, fined $500, and compelled to work off the fine (at a rate of 5 cents a day) for a local planter. With an almost unlimited supply of such workers, employers had little incentive to ease the brutal living and working conditions endured by these convicts.

Patterns of migration within and outside the South reveal blacks' efforts to resist discrimination. Some blacks fled the countryside and settled in southern cities where good jobs were limited but personal freedom was greater. In 1890, 15 percent of the southern black population lived in towns and cities; they represented a third of the South's total urban population.

TABLE 17-1

Percentage of Farms Operated by Tenants or Sharecroppers

	1880	1890	1900	1910	1920
North	19.2	22.1	26.2	26.5	28.2
New England	8.5	9.3	9.4	8.0	7.4
Middle Atlantic	19.2	22.1	25.3	22.3	20.7
East North Central	20.5	22.8	26.3	27.0	28.1
West North Central	20.5	24.0	29.6	30.9	34.2
South	36.2	38.5	47.0	49.6	46.9
South Atlantic	36.1	38.5	44.2	45.9	46.8
East South Central	36.8	38.3	48.1	50.7	49.7
West South Central	35.2	38.6	49.1	52.8	52.9
West	14.0	12.1	16.6	14.0	17.7
Mountain	7.4	7.1	12.2	10.7	15.4
Pacific	16.8	14.7	19.7	17.2	20.1
U.S.	25.6	28.4	35.3	37.0	38.1

Source: U.S. Special Committee on Farm Tenancy, *Farm Tenancy* (1937), pp. 39, 36.

Gradually, a new black elite arose. These physicians, lawyers, insurance agents, and undertakers reached out to an exclusively black clientele. They also nourished a sense of community. Black men and women continued to sustain their own institutions, such as schools, lodges, benevolent societies, burial organizations, and churches. Black men formed fraternal organizations such as the Colored Masons and the Colored Odd Fellows. Black women created social and service organizations, such as the United Daughters of Ham and the Order of the Eastern Star.

Despite Henry Grady's pronouncements, clearly the South had not abandoned its historical legacy of white supremacist ideologies. In fact, in the late 1880s white Democrats feared the assertiveness of the new black elite. According to whites, this generation of men and women born as free persons and not as slaves must be "put in their place," quite literally. As a result, new state and local laws mandated separate water fountains for blacks and whites, restricted blacks to separate railroad cars and other forms of public transportation, and excluded them altogether from city parks and other public spaces. Long-standing customs barring black people from white-owned theaters, restaurants, and hotels now carried the weight of law. Taxpayers' money went into state school funds, which were then sent back to local districts. There the money was used to support two separate school systems, one white and well funded, one black and starved of cash. Legal discrimination against blacks came to be called the Jim Crow system. The term itself (a reference to a minstrel show character named Jim Crow) had originated during the antebellum period.

Black leaders throughout the country tried to keep a national spotlight on the Jim Crow system, its legal and violent manifestations. A rising tide of lynching (it would crest in the 1890s) engulfed the South, but white officials did little or nothing to halt it. Black men, women, and children were all vulnerable to the fury of the white lynch mob—on the most flimsy pretext. Perpetrators of these atrocities were rarely if ever apprehended and punished. Other blacks throughout the segregated South rightly feared that they too would be targeted if they spoke out against lynching. Yet northern blacks did not hesitate to highlight the hypocrisy of the federal government, which turned a blind eye toward this practice. Frances Ellen Watkins Harper, an educator and writer living in Philadelphia, issued the following challenge to an audience of white club women: "A government which has the power to tax a man in peace, draft him in war, should have the power to defend his life in the hour of peril." Harper condemned "the government which can protect and defend its citizens from wrong and outrage and does not."

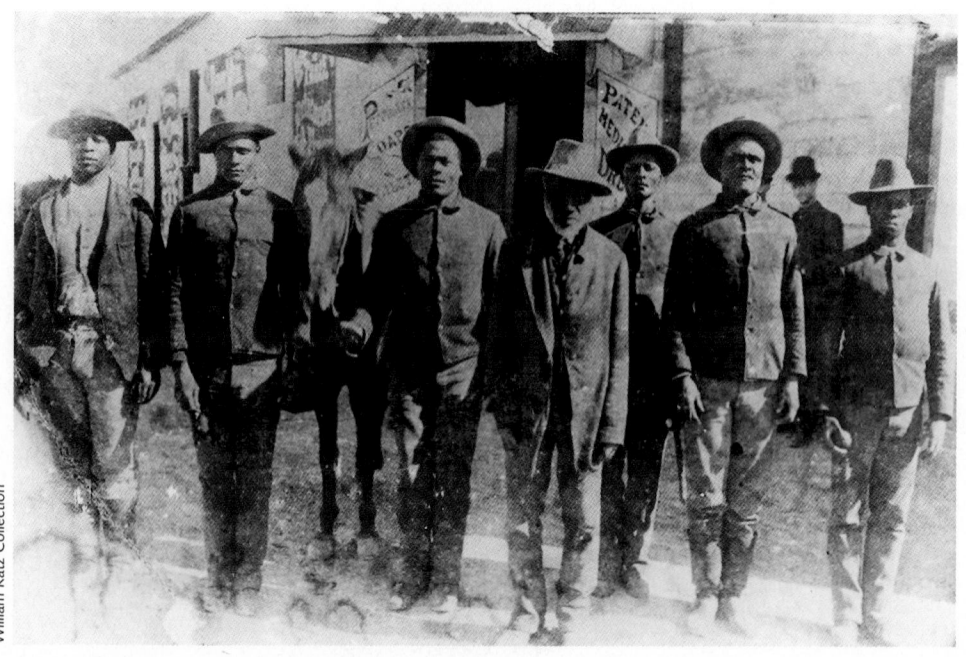

William Katz Collection

■ Among the "buffalo soldiers" who served with the U.S. military were these Seminole scouts. The Seminoles traced their history to the eighteenth century, when Creek Indians and runaway slaves of African descent established communities together in Florida. After the Seminole Wars (1818–1858), many Seminoles were relocated to Indian Territory (present-day Oklahoma). Some fled to Mexico before the Civil War. In 1870 they were recruited by U.S. Army officers to serve as scouts. Their unit was disbanded 11 years later. Racist policies of the military caused some to return to Mexico.

"Jim Crow" in the West

Racial segregation was not limited to the South. The U.S. military enforced its own set of Jim Crow regulations. In 1869 Congress created the 24th and 25th Infantries (Colored) composed of African American soldiers. White officers were appointed to lead these segregated units; consequently, black men who aspired to positions of military leadership found their way blocked. (Before 1900, only three black men received commissions from West Point, and they faced systematic harassment at the academy and after graduation.) Some white officers, such as George Custer, refused to command black troops at all.

Military officials assigned black soldiers to the West, where they became known as buffalo soldiers. (The origins of the term are unclear. It may refer to the buffalo robes worn by many of the soldiers or to Plains Indians' respect for the black men's skills on horseback.) Many of these men were proud to wear a U.S. soldier's uniform, an emblem of their newly won citizenship rights. Organized in two cavalry and two infantry regiments, the soldiers stationed in western outposts found that military duty entailed a combination of new opportunities and old forms of humiliation.

Within their garrisons, they performed a variety of tasks related to everyday military drills and maintenance. Black soldiers helped to construct new roads and forts, protect wagon trains of settlers, and patrol the border between the United States and Mexico. They were an integral part of campaigns to subdue the Cheyenne, Comanche, Sioux, Ute, Kiowa, and Apache Indians. They were among the soldiers deployed to quash strikes among workers (silver miners in Idaho, for example) and to fight forest fires in the Northwest. As members of a novel, all-black regimental musical band, one group played for white audiences from Montana to Texas.

Often the buffalo soldiers encountered hostility from local townspeople, who resented their patronage of local establishments. In 1881 Tenth Cavalry troops stationed at Fort Concho near San Angelo, Texas, reacted angrily when a local white man killed a black soldier in a saloon. Another soldier had died at the hands of a local white within the previous two weeks. In the absence of justice for the murderers, the soldiers blanketed San Angelo with handbills. Signed "U.S. soldiers," the message read, "If we do not receive justice and fair play . . . someone will suffer, if not the guilty, the innocent. It has gone far enough." When some of the soldiers attacked

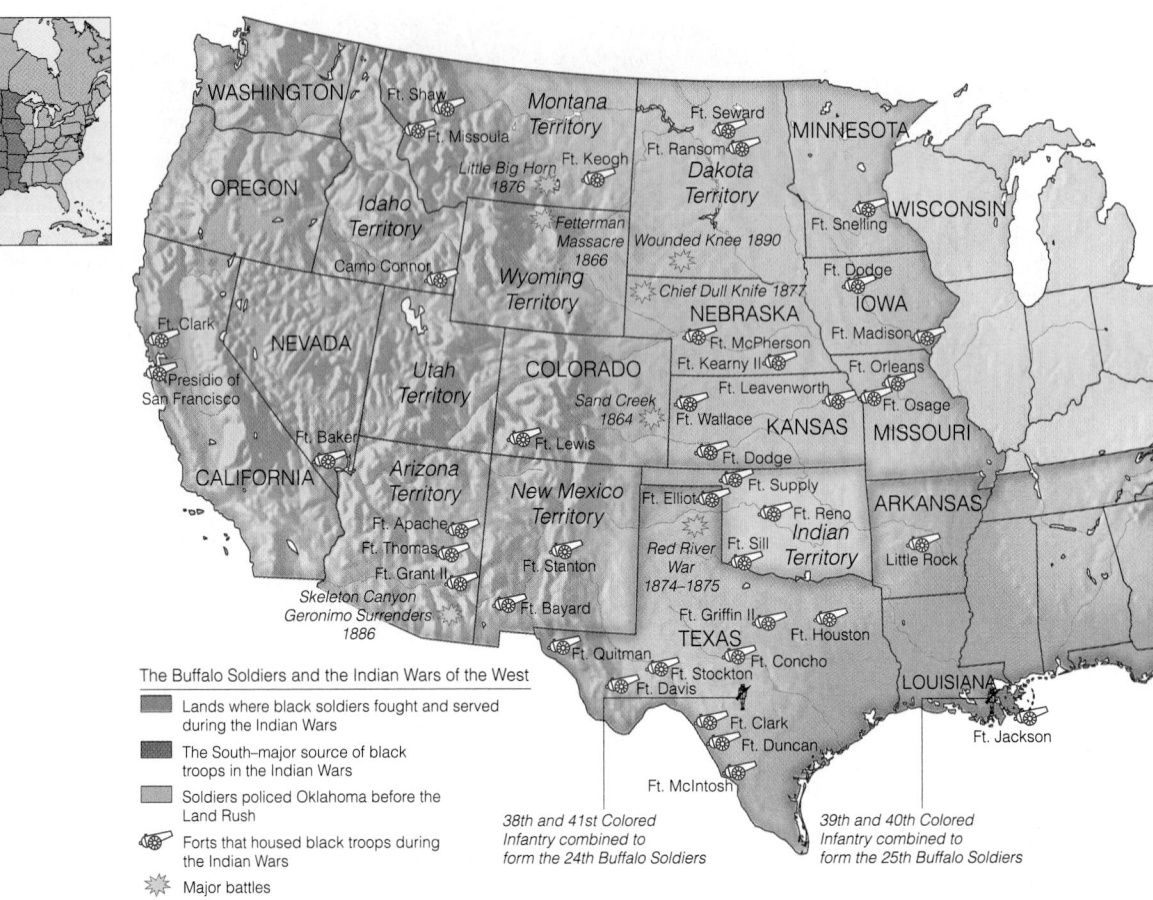

The Buffalo Soldiers and the Indian Wars of the West

- ▮ Lands where black soldiers fought and served during the Indian Wars
- ▮ The South–major source of black troops in the Indian Wars
- ▯ Soldiers policed Oklahoma before the Land Rush
- ⚙ Forts that housed black troops during the Indian Wars
- ✸ Major battles

38th and 41st Colored Infantry combined to form the 24th Buffalo Soldiers

39th and 40th Colored Infantry combined to form the 25th Buffalo Soldiers

■ **MAP 17.2**
BUFFALO SOLDIERS In 1866 Congress authorized the creation of four permanent military units consisting of African American Civil War veterans. These soldiers played a prominent role in the Indian wars of the West from 1866 to 1890. They were stationed in federal forts scattered throughout the western states.

one of the men they believed guilty, the Texas Rangers entered the town to restore order. The army transferred the black companies out of the area and disciplined the leaders of the protest.

Once they were mustered out of the army, some black soldiers decided to settle permanently in the West. There they joined thousands of black migrants who were fleeing the Jim Crow South. In the late 1870s, 20,000 blacks from Tennessee, Mississippi, and Louisiana, called "Exodusters," migrated into western Kansas. The migrants cited the South's convict lease system, poor schools, and pervasive violence and intimidation as reasons for their flight. Henry Adams, a native of Shreveport, Louisiana, and a U.S. army veteran, expanded on the migrants' grievances when he pointed to the failed promise of Reconstruction as the root cause of migration: "The whole South—every State in the South—had got into the hands of the very men that held us as slaves . . . and we thought that the men that held us slaves was holding the reins of government over our heads in every respect almost, even the constable up to the governor."

Some of these migrants established all-black towns in Kansas, Colorado, Nebraska, and New Mexico. Though generally small and poor, such towns were necessarily free of the trappings of Jim Crow. They provided places for blacks to live life on their own terms.

The Ghost Dance on the High Plains

Their lands and way of life threatened by whites, western Indians sought desperately to revitalize their culture and protect themselves. In 1889 an Indian named Wovoka offered the Plains Indians a mystical vision of the future, a vision that promised a return to the beloved past. A leader of the Paiute in Nevada, Wovoka preached what came to be called the Ghost Dance, part religion and part resistance movement. In 1889 a solar eclipse occurred while Wovoka was wracked by fever, and he claimed that the conjunction of the two events enabled him to glimpse the afterworld. The Indians themselves could usher in a new day of peace, Wovoka proclaimed, and this new day would be a time free of disease and armed conflict. The buffalo would return, he promised, and the Indian men and women who had died would come back to replenish depleted villages.

Wovoka's call found its warmest reception among the Plains Indians. In 1890 an anthropologist recorded an exhortation that Wovoka (called Jack Wilson by whites) delivered to the Cheyennes and Arapahos: "When you get home you must make a dance to continue five days. Dance four successive nights, and the last night keep up the dance until the morning of the fifth day, when all must bathe in the river and then disperse to their homes. You must all do in the same way." Some Indians donned so-called ghost shirts, made of white muslin and adorned with images of the sun, moon, stars, and various animals. They believed these garments would provide them with magical powers and protect them from the white men's bullets.

Many of the Indians who performed the Ghost Dance fell into a trance-like state, bringing inspiration to impoverished and disheartened reservation communities. However, as the ritual spread across the Plains, U.S. military officials panicked. In November 1890, E. B. Reynolds, a Special U.S. Indian Agent, described to his superiors in Washington the strange, seemingly dangerous behavior that had gripped the Indians on Pine Ridge Reservation in South Dakota: "The religious excitement aggravated by almost starvation is bearing fruits in this state

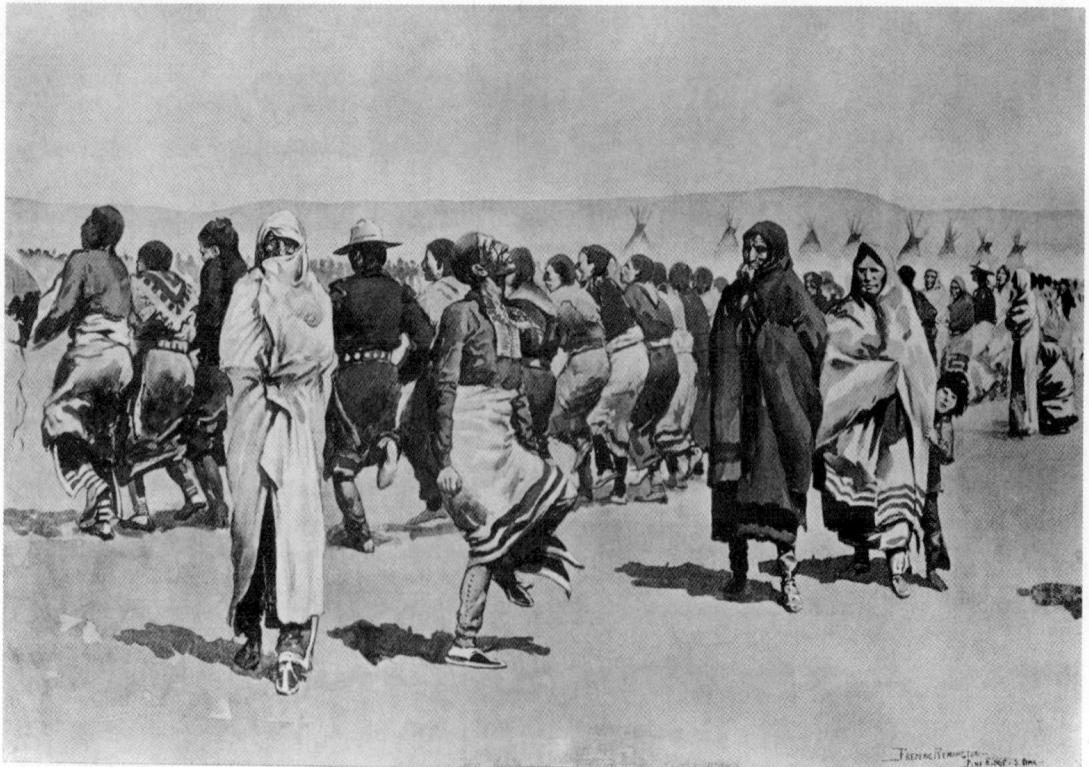

Frederic S. Remington, *The Ghost Dance by the Ogallala Sioux at Pine Ridge Agency, Dakota,* 1890. Amon Carter Museum, Fort Worth, Texas

■ A popular artist featured in leading magazines of his time, Frederic Remington drew a scene from the Oglala Sioux Ghost Dance of 1890. Throughout the Great Plains and the Rocky Mountain region, men, women, and children participated in the ritual dance, moving in a circle and singing. The strange sight frightened many whites. In December 1890 U.S. troops attacked and killed several hundred Indians on the Pine Ridge Reservation in South Dakota. The Wounded Knee Massacre marked the end of the Indian wars of the nineteenth century.

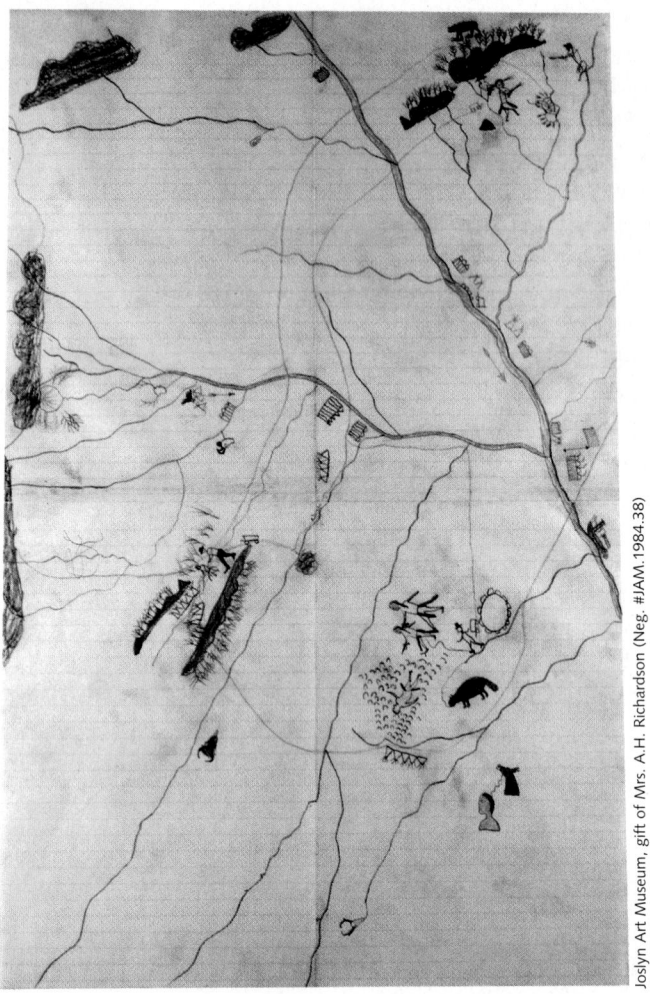

Joslyn Art Museum, gift of Mrs. A.H. Richardson (Neg. #JAM.1984.38)

■ A map drawn by John Crazy Mule, a Cheyenne warrior-turned U.S. Army scout, illustrates several historic encounters between Indians and soldiers. Places and events are designated with pictographs. For example, the Missouri River is marked with a steamboat (center right). Among the events depicted is the capture of Chief Joseph of the Nez Percé in the Bear Paw Mountains in 1877.

of insubordination; Indians say they had better die fighting than to die a slow death of starvation, and as the new religion promises their return to earth, at the coming of the millennium, they have no fear of death."

As tensions between whites and Indians mounted, a Sioux named Sitting Bull emerged as a leader. Born in the early 1830s, he had gained respect among his people as a Wichasa Wakan ("holy man"). At the Battle of the Little Big Horn, he helped protect Indian women and children from Custer's soldiers. Wooden Leg, a Northern Cheyenne, later described Sitting Bull as "altogether brave, but peaceable. He was strong in religion—the Indian religion." After leading his followers into Canada, Sitting Bull returned to the United States in 1881. He surrendered at Fort Buford, Dakota Territory, where he was held prisoner for two years. His brief stint as a performer in Buffalo Bill Cody's "Wild West" show left him disgusted with the ways of white people.

Sitting Bull offered a pointed critique of the sedentary, materialistic way of life promoted by whites:

> White men like to dig in the ground for their food. My people prefer to hunt buffalo as their fathers did. White men like to stay in one place. My people want to move their tepees here and there to different hunting grounds. The life of white men is slavery. They are prisoners in towns or farms. The life my people want is a life of freedom. I have seen nothing that a white man has, houses or railways or clothing or food, that is as good as the right to move in open country, and live in our own fashion.

Sitting Bull rejected white notions of "progress" in favor of his people's traditions.

In mid-December 1890 military officials ordered Indian police to arrest Sitting Bull at his cabin on the Standing Rock Reservation in South Dakota. Alarmed by what they perceived as rising Indian military, white settlers in Nebraska and South Dakota pressured the government to rid the area of the "savages . . . armed to the teeth," men who were "traitors, anarchists, and assassins." While arresting Sitting Bull, his Indian captors killed him. The great man's followers, who had revered him as a prophet, decried the murder.

A week later, on December 28 and 29, soldiers of the 7th Cavalry under Colonel James Forsyth, agitated by the tensions over Sitting Bull's death, attacked and killed 146 Indians at Wounded Knee Creek, South Dakota. More than 60 women and children were among those slain as they fled the oncoming troops. Of the 25 U.S. soldiers who perished, most apparently died from shots fired by their own comrades; according to a government eyewitness, the Indian men were unarmed when the cavalry attacked.

The massacre at Wounded Knee proved the last major violent encounter between Plains Indians and U.S. cavalry forces. By this time, many Indians throughout the Midwest lived on reservations and engaged in farming. In Oklahoma, for example, the Cheyenne learned how to grow cotton and watermelons. Government agents, eager to create independent farmers, instructed Indian men in the use of the plow. But John Stands-in-Timber, a Cheyenne, later recalled how plowing became a collective effort. It engaged the energies of Indian men from Oklahoma to Montana, he noted, as bands would work together until their task was done. Thus some Indian groups attempted to maintain customs of collective endeavor in opposition to the European Americas glorification of ambition and individualism.

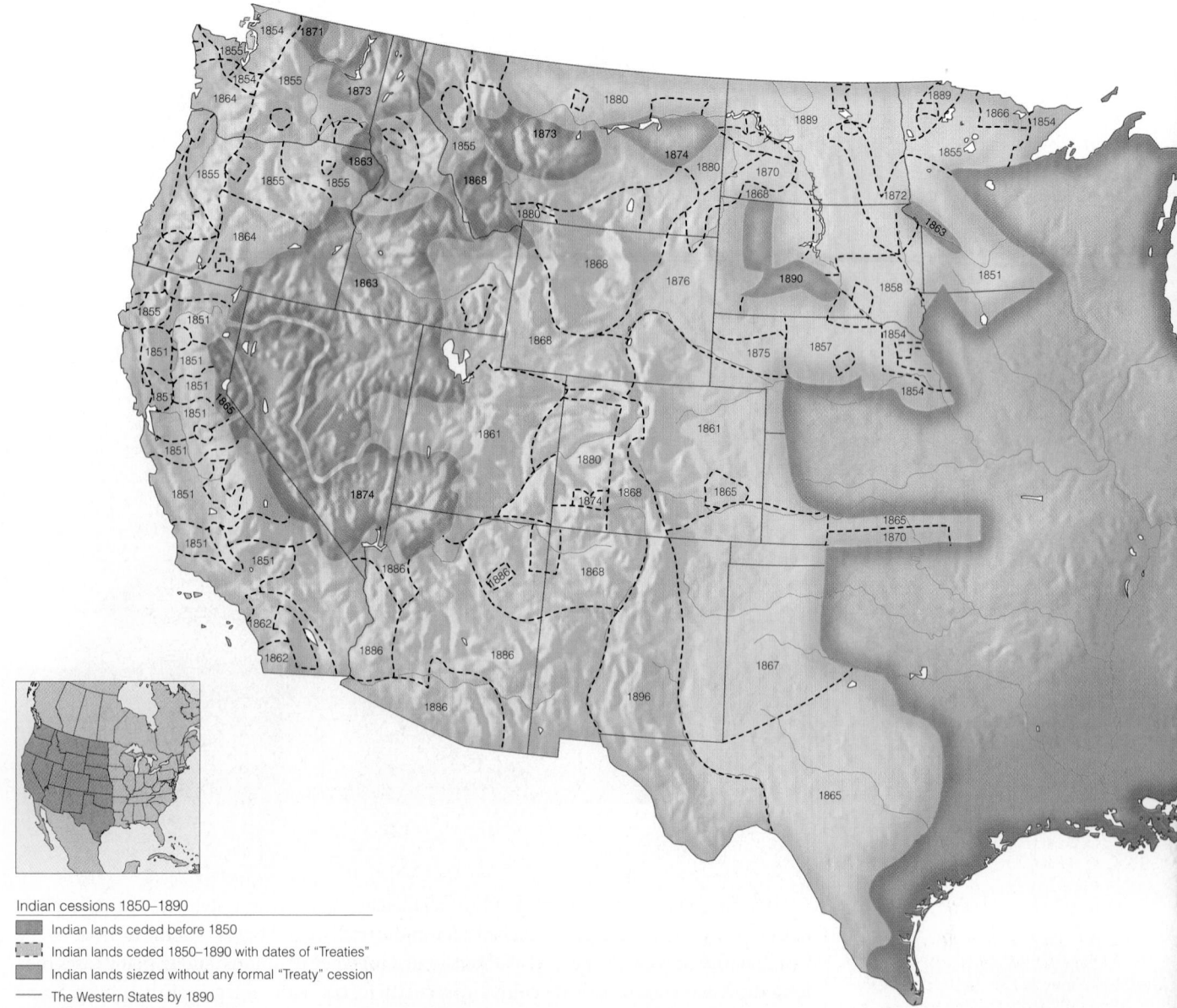

■ **MAP 17.3**
INDIAN LANDS LOST, 1850–1890 Between 1850 and 1890, many "treaties" signed by Indian groups and the U.S. government provided that Indians turn over land in exchange for cash payments. Yet U.S. military forces seized a large portion of western Indian lands by force, without signing any treaty agreements at all. By 1890 many Indians lived on reservations, apart from European American society.

Indian cessions 1850–1890

- Indian lands ceded before 1850
- Indian lands ceded 1850–1890 with dates of "Treaties"
- Indian lands siezed without any formal "Treaty" cession
- The Western States by 1890

Revolt in the Workplace

During the late nineteenth century, workers challenged employers and the new industrial order for many reasons. Factory operatives objected to long hours and to low pay in return for tending dangerous machines. Miners labored daily under hazardous conditions, often without necessary safety equipment or precautions. Field hands worried that they would soon be displaced by machines such as the giant threshers that were far more efficient—quicker and cheaper—than human labor. Small farmers resented their dependence on bankers and owners of grain elevators and railroads. Throughout the country, many different kinds of workers feared that the large influx of immigrants would provide a vast reserve of cheap labor that would serve to depress the wages of and threaten the job security of everyone.

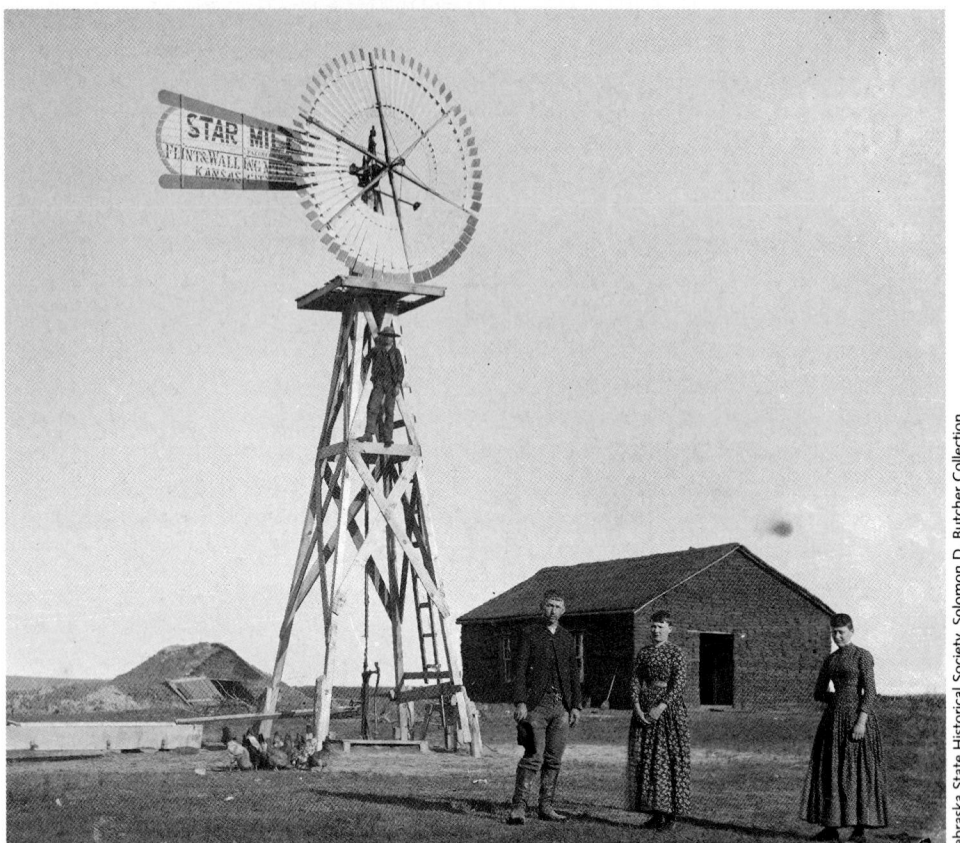

■ A Nebraska farm family poses proudly with their new windmill, c. 1890. Such devices powered water pumps that reached deep into the earth. Though expensive, windmills were necessities for drought-stricken farmers on the Plains, especially during the harsh years of the mid-1880s to the mid-1890s.

Workers launched different kinds of challenges against the system of industrial capitalism, which, many charged, enriched a few industrialists and bankers at the expense of the vast majority of laboring people. Workers joined together in unions, and in many cases they fought the violence of private company security forces with violence of their own. Some men and women destroyed the machinery that threatened to replace them in the workplace. By the early 1890s, critics of the new industrial order—a system driven by technological innovation—had come together in the form of a new political group, the People's Party. This organization aimed to bring together urban and rural, male and female, agricultural and industrial workers to protest the hardships suffered by laborers of all kinds and to demand that the federal government take strong action in rectifying social ills.

Nevertheless, in workplace conflicts, the lines were not always strictly drawn between employees and employers. For example, the late-nineteenth-century laboring classes never achieved the level of unity called for by the Populists. White workers often expressed intense hostility toward their African American and Chinese counterparts. Within small towns, shopkeepers and landlords at times showed solidarity with striking workers; in these cases community ties were stronger than class differences. Also, despite their critique of big business, workers often embraced the emerging consumer culture. In fact, many of them fought for shorter work days and higher wages so that they could enjoy their share of the material blessings of American life—in department stores, movie theaters, and amusement parks.

Trouble on the Farm

In the late summer of 1878 the combined effects of the recent national depression and the loss of jobs to labor-saving technology catalyzed a rash of machine breaking throughout rural

TABLE 17-2

Estimated Membership, by State, of the National Farmers' Alliance, 1890

State	Members	State	Members
Alabama	75,000	New Jersey	500
Arkansas	100,000	New Mexico	5,000
California	1,000	New York	500
Colorado	5,000	North Carolina	100,000
Florida	20,000	North Dakota	40,000
Georgia	100,000	Ohio	300
Illinois	2,000	Pennsylvania	500
Indiana	5,000	South Carolina	50,000
Kansas	100,000	South Dakota	50,000
Kentucky	80,000	Tennessee	100,000
Louisiana	20,000	Texas	150,000
Maryland	5,000	Virginia	50,000
Mississippi	60,000	West Virginia	2,000
Missouri	150,000	Total	1,271,800

Source: Appleton's Annual Cyclopedia and Register of Important Events of the Year 1890 (New York: D. Appleton & Co, 1891), p. 301.

Ohio. The tactics of the machine-breakers bore some resemblance to those of *las Gorras Blancas* in northern New Mexico. In the Midwest, displaced farmhands burned the reapers, mowers, and threshers of their former employers. By autumn the violence had spread to Michigan and Indiana. Scattered reports of torched reapers, mowers, barns, and crops emanated from Illinois, Iowa, Wisconsin, and Minnesota also. Some wealthy farmers responded by abandoning their machinery and rehiring their farmhands. Technology, one noted, "ought to be dispensed with in times like these." Critics charged the machine-breakers with "short-sighted madness." True, seasonal farmhands were fast losing their usefulness in the new machine age. However, the protests revealed that even family farming had become a business. Now farmers needed to secure bank loans, invest in new machinery, and worry about the price of crops in the world market. These changes had profoundly altered labor relations between farm workers and farmers and between farmers and their creditors.

On the Northern Plains, farmers endured extremes of weather and the anxiety of uncertain harvests. This area was home to immigrants from Scandinavia and Russia, drawn to the region by abundant rainfall and cheap land prices in the late 1870s and early 1880s. These men and women concentrated on ranching and farming and built sod houses out of rectangular bricks cut from the hard prairie soil. Warm in winter and cool in summer, the houses nevertheless had roofs that needed shoring up after every rainfall. In Madison County, Nebraska, a family of five lived in a dirt-floor sod house built into the side of a ravine. Their furnishings consisted of a cookstove, a bed, a milk cooler, "and a few other articles."

In the mid-1880s the plight of these Plains farmers worsened when a series of natural disasters highlighted their vulnerability to the elements. No form of modern technology could prevent the drought of 1886, which dragged on for a decade. Combined with declining wheat prices, the prolonged dry weather drove fully half the population of western Kansas and Nebraska back east to Iowa and Illinois during 1888 to 1892. Meanwhile, the bitterly cold winter of 1886–1887 decimated cattle herds throughout the region. The resulting "great die up" ended the days of the huge herds that ranged the Plains. Thereafter, ranchers would concentrate on smaller stock holdings and selective breeding.

Some American writers captured the bleakness of prairie life, highlighting the condition of farmers dependent on predatory institutions and machines, such as banks and railroads.

Writing from first-hand experience of his native Wisconsin, Hamlin Garland portrayed the harsh life endured by men and women who toiled "under the lion's paw" of scheming creditors and landlords. Other chroniclers of life on the Plains portrayed nature as a pitiless adversary that promised bountiful harvests one day but rained plagues of locusts the next.

Things took a radical turn in the 1880s, when a national movement of farmers emerged and tapped into a wellspring of anger and discontent in farming regions throughout the nation. Men and women from the Plains states (organized in the National Farmers' Alliance, or Northern Alliance) joined with their counterparts in Louisiana, Texas, and Arkansas (the National Farmers Alliance and Industrial Union, or Southern Alliance). The Colored Farmers' Alliance was formed in 1886.

The Southern Alliance pressed for an expanded currency, taxation reform, and government ownership of transportation and communication lines. Its members tended to ally with the Democratic party. The Northern Alliance also focused on the expansion of the currency supply—specifically, the coinage of silver—but advocated the formation of a third political party to advance its interests. Both of these large regional groups found adherents in the mountain West. There, miners and farmers joined together to protest the monopolistic powers of the railroads, privately owned water companies, and silver mining interests. These monopolies drove up consumer prices and depressed workers' wages.

Most alliance men and women farmed modest parcels of land. As small producers, they felt powerless to influence the businesspeople and politicians who affected their livelihoods and their life possibilities. Members of the alliance also presented themselves as the last line of defense for the noble yeoman in the face of the corrupting influences of modern capitalism. In rural Alabama, where the Farmers' Alliance had links with local schools and churches, the group's newspapers railed against the "filthy city," a "wicked place" of vice, crime, and dissipation. Farm folk thus distanced themselves from the "New South Creed," which promoted materialism and industrialization.

In many local groups, or suballiances, women stepped forward to claim their due as wives, mothers, and workers. In Tennessee, farm wives who raised chickens and produced milk and butter for market encountered middlemen who set unfair prices for both producers and consumers. Women argued that they were more than their husbands' helpmeets; they were partners in a family enterprise. As such, they demanded respect and a political voice. Wrote one woman to *The Weekly Toiler*, the paper of the state's Farmers' Alliance, "It would be better, methinks, if the men would say, 'come join us in the fight against your enemy' with as bold a front as he says, 'come Betsy, help me hang the meat, and drop the corn and potatoes.'"

Suffering from a recession in the late 1880s, farmers in the Dakotas, Nebraska, Kansas, and Texas began to mobilize into a new political party. Organizing work among Alliance members at the local level laid the foundation for the creation of the People's, or Populist, party. In Johnson County, Wyoming, in 1890, small farmers joined the Populist Party in response to attacks on their property by gunmen hired by the Wyoming Stock Growers Association, a monopoly of large cattle ranchers.

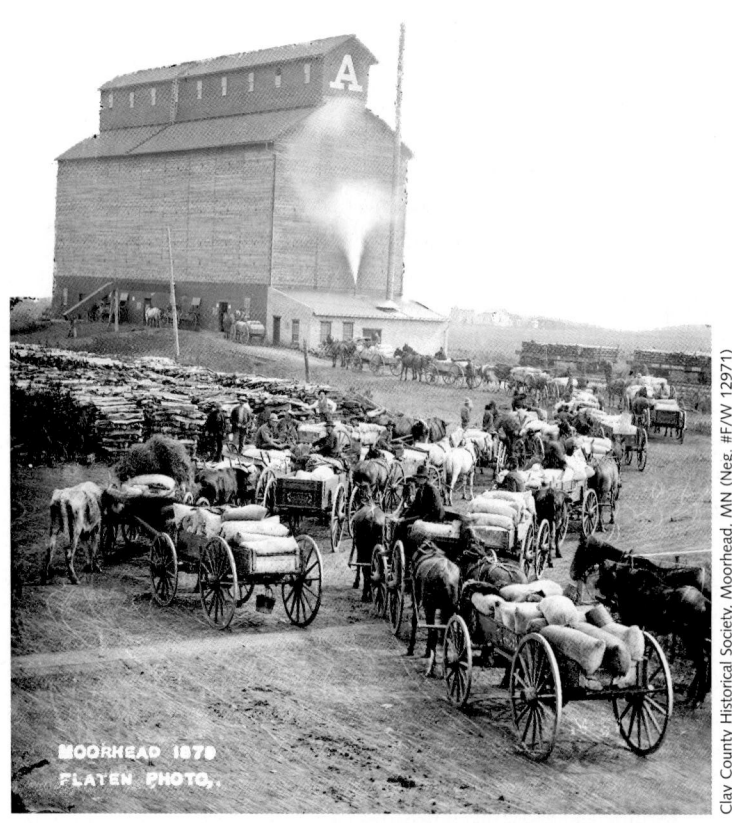

Clay County Historical Society, Moorhead, MN (Neg. #F/W 12971)

■ In the Midwest, farmers had to contend with monopolies that charged high prices for goods and services. Farmers depended on grain elevators (such as this one in Minnesota in 1879) to store their harvests for shipment by rail. In the early 1890s the Populist party exploited the image of the small family farmer at the mercy of powerful industrialists, merchants, banks, and railroads.

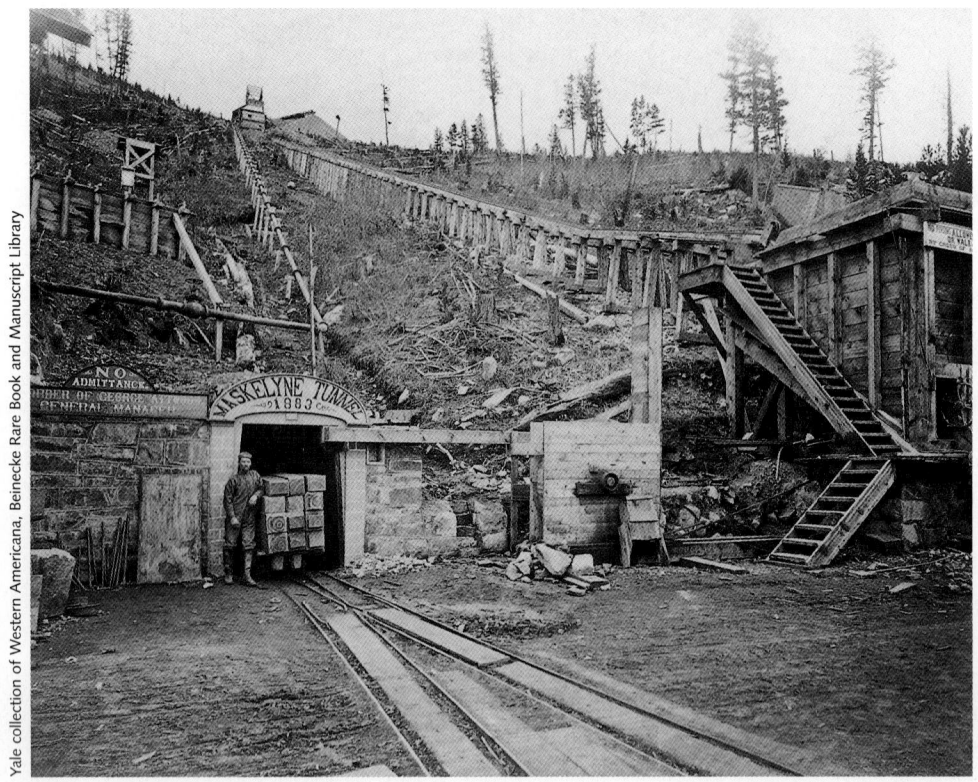

■ Mining was one of the most hazardous occupations in the United States. Below-surface miners worked with explosives and sophisticated kinds of machinery. As a result, the chances of explosions, cave-ins, rockslides, and fires increased. These conditions help to account for the labor militancy of miners throughout the country. This photo shows a mining operation at Marysville, near Helena, Montana, c. 1885.

Although the Farmers' Alliance identified itself primarily with agricultural interests, it made some notable forays into coalition-building. In 1889 the northern and southern groups attempted to combine with the Colored Farmers' Alliance. Together, these groups claimed more than 4 million members. They also sought to join with the Knights of Labor and thus bring all members of the "producing classes" together. By representing the financial interests of all farmers and highlighting the vulnerabilities of debtors, the organization foreshadowed the wider national appeal of the Populist party in the 1890s.

Militancy in the Factories and Mines

The new economy wrought profound hardship on members of the urban laboring classes as well as on small farmers. Many industrial workers faced layoffs and wage cuts during the depressions of the 1870s and 1880s. The great railroad strikes of 1877 (see Chapter 16) foreshadowed an era of bitter industrial conflict. Because no laws regulated private industry, employers could impose 10- to 15-hour workdays, six days a week. (By the 1890s, bakers were working as long as 65 hours a week.) Industrial accidents were all too common, and some industries lacked safety precautions. Steelworkers labored in excessive heat, and miners and textile mill employees alike contracted respiratory diseases. With windows closed and machines speeded up, new forms of technology created new risks for workers. The Chicago meatpackers, who wielded gigantic cleavers in subfreezing lockers, and the California wheat harvesters, who operated complex mechanical binders and threshers, were among those confronting danger on the job.

Women wage-earners also faced dangerous working conditions. In 1884 the Massachusetts Bureau of Statistics of Labor issued a report outlining the occupational hazards for working women in the city of Boston. In button-making establishments, female workers often got their fingers caught under punch and die machines. Employers provided a surgeon to dress an employee's wounds the first three times she was injured; thereafter, she had to pay for her own medical care. Women operated heavy power machinery in the garment industry and

Rural Protests and Rebellions

In New Mexico in the 1880s, *las Gorras Blancas* expressed the grievances of Hispanic farmers against commercial interests. Throughout American history, groups of farmers have protested government policies they considered unfair and harmful to their own interests. Specific farmers' grievances, and the strategies used to express those grievances, have varied through the generations.

In the seventeenth and eighteenth centuries, impoverished backcountry settlers charged that colonial authorities were indifferent to their plight. Some settlers turned their wrath on the Indians in their midst and on government officials located in eastern towns. Sometimes, protest turned into organized uprising as in Bacon's Rebel-

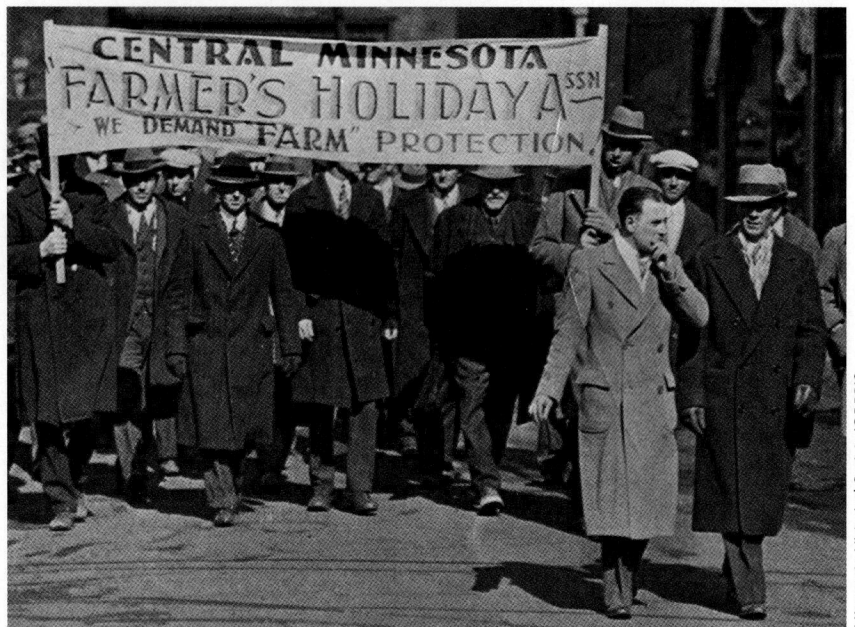

Minnesota Historical Society/CORBIS

■ In Midwestern states during the Depression of the 1930s, some farmers formed "holiday associations" to withhold crops from the market and to prevent creditors from seizing farm homesteads.

lion in Virginia in 1676 and Culpeper's Rebellion in North Carolina the following year.

In 1763 farmers of backcountry Pennsylvania staged a revolt, claiming that the government promoted trade

exposed themselves to dangerous chemicals and food-processing materials in paper-box making, fish packing, and confectionery manufacturing.

Some women workers, especially those who monopolized certain kinds of jobs, organized and struck for higher wages. Three thousand Atlanta washerwomen launched such an effort in 1881 but failed to get their demands met. Most women found it difficult to win the respect not only of employers but also of male unionists. Leonora Barry, an organizer for the Knights of Labor, sought to change all that. Barry visited mills and factories around the country. At each stop, she highlighted women's unique difficulties and condemned the "selfishness of their brothers in toil" who resented women's intrusion into the workplace. Barry was reacting to men such as Edward O'Donnell, a prominent labor official who claimed that wage-earning women threatened the role of men as family breadwinners.

For both men and women workers, the influx of 5.25 million new immigrants in the 1880s stiffened job competition at worksites throughout the country. To make matters worse, vast outlays of capital needed to mechanize and organize manufacturing plants placed pressure on employers to economize. Many of them did so by cutting wages. Like the family farmer who could no longer claim the status of the independent yeoman, industrial workers depended on employers and consumers for their physical well-being and very survival.

Not until 1935 would American workers have the right to organize and bargain collectively with their employers. Until then, laborers who saw strength in numbers and expressed an interest in a union could be summarily fired, blacklisted (their names circulated to other employers), and harassed by private security forces. The Pinkerton National Detective Agency, founded in 1850 by a Scottish immigrant named Allan Pinkerton, initially found eager clients

with Indians over the safety of settlers. The so-called Paxton Boys attacked the nearby Conestoga Indians, although their real grievances lay with the colonial legislature. In 1770 the Green Mountain Boys in Vermont disrupted local courts to protest the proprietary rights of large landowners. In all of these cases, a lack of available land, plus official policies that appeared to favor entrenched political and economic interests, fueled resentment among farmers.

Many farmers believed that the American Revolution failed to go far enough in securing their rights. During the postwar monetary crisis, they faced foreclosures on their property and long sentences in debtors' prison. Shays's Rebellion in the Connecticut River Valley and western Massachusetts in 1786–1787 and the Whiskey Rebellion in western Pennsylvania in 1793–1794 pitted local farmers against militia mobilized by the new national government.

The Civil War represents the country's most dramatic agrarian revolt against the central government. With the election of Abraham Lincoln, wealthy southern planters claimed that Washington was in the hands of Republicans who favored free, as opposed to slave, labor. The Confederates' uprising cost the country more than 600,000 lives and culminated in the abolition of the institution that they were seeking to defend.

Postwar national economic development put family farmers at risk. In the 1890s the Populist Party appealed to farmers in the South, the Midwest, and the Rocky Mountain region. Faced with rising costs and the monopolistic power of railroads and banks, these farmers called for government policies that would be more responsive to the needs of the small landowner. The party achieved some success at the local and state levels.

In the 1930s a number of different farmers' groups protested government policies that drove down crop prices. In the Midwest the Farmers' Holiday Association sought to intimidate local bankers and judges. The Sharecroppers' Union in Alabama and the Southern Tenant Farmers Union in Missouri, like the Populist Party of the 1890s, represented biracial coalitions of farmers.

In 1979, the Nevada state legislature seized 49 million acres of federal land within the state. This measure ushered in the so-called Sagebrush Rebellion, a political coalition of western ranchers who opposed government regulation of the land. Elected to the presidency in 1980, Ronald Reagan served as an advocate of western business interests.

In 1999 the U.S. Department of Agriculture settled a class action suit brought by southern African American farmers, the largest class action civil rights settlement in U.S. history, worth $2 billion. The claimants, most of whom came from Mississippi, Arkansas, Georgia, and Tennessee, successfully charged that for decades the government had engaged in racial discrimination in its farm lending program. ∎

among the railroads. The Pinkertons, as they were called, served as industrial spies and policemen during some of the most bitter and violent strikes of the late nineteenth century.

For example, in 1876 a Pinkerton detective, James McParlan, was hired by railroad operators to infiltrate a local union of Irish immigrant miners in Schuylkill County, Pennsylvania. The miners, members of a secret society called the Molly Maguires, were determined to do battle against the mine owners, who not only suppressed union activity but also controlled local courts and law enforcement agencies. In 1875 the Mollies had called a strike, but their leaders were arrested and charged with waging a guerrilla war against the mines (and their Welsh and English superintendents). In court McParlan offered testimony against the men, evidence that led to the conviction and execution (by hanging) of 20 of them. In the coming years, employers in a number of industries justified their repressive tactics by claiming that all unions represented a threat to law and order.

In small towns where one or two large industries predominated, workers often could count on their middle-class neighbors as allies. In many cases, shopkeepers, tradesmen, clergy, and landlords objected to the arrival of out-of-town strikebreakers, Pinkerton detectives, or federal troops during labor disputes. Local politicians solicited the support of their working-class constituents. As members of churches and voluntary associations, middle-class and working-class people together upheld community values of family welfare in opposition to large industrialists concerned only with profits and worker productivity. During a boycott of antiunion hat factories in Orange, New Jersey, in 1885, the community rallied around the workers. Brewers and bakers refused to supply establishments that opposed the boycott. Service providers of all kinds, from owners of roller-skating rinks to "knights of the razor" (barbers), closed their doors to patrons who expressed sympathy with what was generally called "the foul." In Orange and other towns, then, coalitions of middle-class and working-class residents severely curtailed the industrialists' power.

The Knights of Labor, a secret fraternal order founded in 1869, came under the leadership of Terence V. Powderly a decade later. With this Irish American at the helm (he was called Grand Master Workman), the labor union made impressive gains in the 1880s. Under Powderly, the Knights launched a concerted effort to organize European American, African American, and Hispanic men and women workers.

In the late 1880s the Knights attempted to organize the laboring classes of San Miguel County, New Mexico, and the other parts of the Southwest. The Knights welcomed cowboys into their organization at the same time they were urging railroad workers to join their ranks. One cowhand said, "No class is harder worked, none so poor paid for their services." A cattle drive north from Texas could last for three months and cover more than a thousand miles. On such drives, a single cowboy would be responsible for keeping 250 to 300 head of cattle in line. Wages remained miserable, and unrest spread.

In the spring of 1883, an extensive strike among cowboys enraged the owners of large ranches in the Texas panhandle. To quell the uprising, ranchers paid gunmen to intimidate the strikers and enlisted the support of the state's law enforcement agency, the Texas Rangers. It was a year before the strikers gave up.

According to the Knights, business monopolies and corrupt politicians shared an interest in exploiting the labor of ordinary men and women.

In appealing to many different kinds of workers around the country, the Knights blended a critique of the late-nineteenth-century wage system with a belief in the dignity of labor and a call for collective action. According to the Knights, business monopolies and corrupt politicians everywhere shared a common interest in exploiting the labor of ordinary men and women. The Knights advocated a return to the time when workers controlled their own labor and received a just price for the products they made. "We declare an inevitable and irresistible conflict between the wage system of labor and republican system of government," the Knights proclaimed.

In condemning the concentration of wealth in the hands of a few, the Knights drew on the ideas of popular social critics of the day. In New York City, Henry George, an economist and land reformer, gained the Knights' support when he ran for mayor on the United Labor party ticket in 1886. (He came in second, with 31 percent of the vote, ahead of a young, up-and-coming Republican named Theodore Roosevelt.) George had achieved national prominence with his book *Progress and Poverty* (1879), in which he advocated a single tax on property as a means of distributing wealth more equally.

Journalist-turned-novelist Edward Bellamy echoed these themes. In his popular novel titled *Looking Backward* (1888), Bellamy envisioned a "cooperative commonwealth" in the year 2000, a socialist paradise in which poverty and greed had disappeared and men and women of all classes enjoyed material comfort and harmonious relations with their neighbors. This utopia was within reach, the author argued, if Americans could simply share in the nation's abundance.

The Nationalist movement, a network of clubs inspired by Bellamy's book, included Terence Powderly as a member. Powderly declared, "We work not selfishly for ourselves alone, but extend the hand of fellowship to all mankind." Between 1885 and 1886, the Knights undertook the difficult task of organizing black workers. Many blacks remained suspicious of white-led unions, and for good reason. Historically, the white labor movement had conceived itself as a way to exclude black men and women from stable, well-paying jobs.

In the city of Richmond, Virginia, where workplaces were strictly segregated by race, the Knights made great gains. African American women there found their job opportunities limited to domestic service, laundry work, and unskilled jobs in tobacco factories. Black men were almost entirely excluded from the artisan crafts. By the mid-1880s, the Richmond Knights boasted a total membership of 7000, with a ratio of four blacks to three whites. Yet members were organized into two district assemblies, one for blacks, the other for whites.

In early 1886 a wave of strikes hit Richmond as painters, coopers (barrel makers), typographers, cotton press workers, and foundry workers, among others, all decried their low wages.

A coalition between the Knights and black Republicans posed a formidable threat to the entrenched Democratic leadership. That spring, labor Republican candidates won a majority of seats on the Richmond city council and gained half the board of aldermen slots. Yet the issue of racial equality proved the undoing of the Knights' fragile biracial coalition. Throughout the South, a generation of blacks and whites had allied themselves with different political parties (the Republicans and Democrats, respectively). Moreover, white workers widely perceived blacks as potential strikebreakers. In Richmond, mutual distrust, combined with pressure from white groups such as the local Law and Order League, fragmented the Knights.

Throughout the South, segregation was the norm within biracial unionism. Whites, whether New Orleans dockworkers, Birmingham District coal miners, or lumber workers in East Texas and Louisiana, insisted on separate locals from blacks. Yet African Americans did not necessarily acquiesce to this arrangement. In 1886 Jere A. Brown, a member of the Carpenter and Joiners' Union of Cleveland, wrote to the *New York Freeman,* declaring to readers of the black newspaper, "For years I have been importuned to enter into the formation of an assembly to be composed exclusively of colored men, but have persistently refused, believing as I do in mixing and not in isolating and ostracizing ourselves, thereby fostering and perpetuating the prejudice as existing today."

In 1886 workers around the country began to mobilize on behalf of the eight-hour day. "Eight hours to constitute a day's work" was their slogan. The issue had broad appeal, but the growing diversity of the labor force made unity difficult. For example, among the white workers of the Richmond Knights were leaders with names such as Kaufman, Kaufeldt, Kelly, and Molloy, suggesting the ethnic variety of late-nineteenth-century union leadership. This diversity paralleled the composition of the general population. In 1880, between 78 and 87 percent of all workers in San Francisco, St. Louis, Cleveland, New York, Detroit, Milwaukee, and Chicago were either immigrants or the children of immigrants. Most hailed from England, Germany, or Ireland, although the Chinese made up a significant part of the laboring classes on the West Coast. By 1890 Poles and Slavs were organizing in steel mills, and New York Jews were providing leadership in the garment industry. Italians were prominent in construction and the building trades. In many places, the laboring classes remained vulnerable to divisive social and cultural animosities. The diversity of ethnic groups, coupled with the fact that many newcomers adopted racist ideas to become "Americans," drove wedges between workers.

The Haymarket Bombing

The year 1886 marked the end of an era dominated by the Knights of Labor as the organization experienced first-hand the difficulties of overcoming its members' diverse crafts, racial loyalties, and political allegiances. In 1886 the Knights suffered serious setbacks in their efforts to organize railroad workers. Industrialists dug in their heels and, with the aid of hired detectives, took union leaders to court on charges of sabotage, assault, conspiracy, and murder.

On May 1, 1886, 350,000 workers in 11,562 business establishments went out on a one-day strike as part of the eight-hour workday movement. In Chicago, home to militant labor anarchists (men and women who opposed government authority of any kind), 40,000 workers participated in the strike. Among the Chicago leaders was Albert Parsons. A descendant of New England Puritans and a printer by trade, Parsons had lived in Waco, Texas, where he met his future wife, Lucia Gonzalez, an Afro-Latina (probably born a slave). In 1873 the Parsonses had moved to Chicago to avoid Texas laws against "race mixing," which prohibited interracial marriage. There Albert joined the International Typographical Union, and Lucia took up dressmaking. They were counted among the most famous and feared radicals in the city.

On May 4, things took a bloody turn. Strikers called a rally in Chicago's Haymarket Square to protest the murder of two McCormick Reaper strikers the day before. During the rally, a bomb went off, killing a police officer and wounding seven others, who later died. Although the identity of the culprit was never discovered, eight anarchists, including Albert Parsons, were arrested. All eight (several of whom were German immigrants) were tried and sentenced to death for conspiring to provoke violence. Parsons was not even present when the bomb exploded. Nevertheless, in November 1887, he and three other detainees were hanged. Another committed suicide in his cell, and the rest received pardons years later. After her husband's death, Lucia ("Lucy") Parsons remained active in Chicago anarchist circles. In 1905 she became a founding member of a new, radical labor union called the Industrial Workers of the World.

The Haymarket hangings demoralized the labor movement nationwide. Now associated in the minds of the middle class with wild-eyed bomb throwers, the Knights suffered repercussions from employers and local police forces alike. After reaching a membership high of 700,000 in 1886, the Knights saw their ranks plummet to 100,000 by the end of the decade. Still, the execution of the Haymarket anarchists inspired young radicals, among them a recent Russian immigrant named Emma Goldman, to devote their lives to the cause of working people.

With the demise of the Knights of Labor, the American Federation of Labor (AFL) emerged to become the most powerful national labor movement. Samuel Gompers, an English immigrant cigarmaker, had founded the new group in 1886 partly in response to the Knights' attempts to usurp the Cigar Makers' International Union with a socialist-dominated local. The AFL garnered the allegiance of skilled trade workers (most of them white men) and promoted basic goals such as better wages and working conditions. The AFL emphasized the walkout and boycott as strategies of labor protest. By the mid-1890s, the AFL had embraced a narrow base: skilled trades dominated by white men.

Yet the radical labor tradition persisted. Meeting in Paris in 1889, a congress of world Socialist parties voted to commemorate the American workers who had marched in support of the eight-hour day during the turbulent year of 1886. The congress voted to set aside May 1, 1890, as a day of worldwide celebrations in support of labor and demonstrations in favor of the eight-hour workday. (May 1 became an international labor day, celebrated annually.) In the United States, the United Mine Workers (founded in 1890) and the American Railway Union (1893) followed the radical labor-organizing principles of the Knights of Labor long after the AFL had attained its ascendancy.

Crosscurrents of Reform

In the 1880s a young Danish-born journalist named Jacob Riis prowled New York's East Side slum district in search of stories for the New York *Tribune* and the Associated Press bureau. In this part of the city, more than 37,000 tenement buildings housed more than 1 million people–newcomers from the far reaches of Europe and Asia. As a result of Riis's stories documenting the inhuman living conditions endured by so many men, women, and children, the city formed the Tenement House Commission in 1884. Riis persisted in his exposés. In 1890 he published a collection of his own photographs, along with explanatory notes, under the title *How the Other Half Lives*.

Reformers later called Riis "the most useful citizen of New York." His book galvanized the public in support of slum clearance and housing codes. *How the Other Half Lives* is a powerful indictment of greedy landlords, indifferent city officials, and rapacious sweatshop owners. The photos of sleeping street urchins huddled around sidewalk heating grates, of impoverished English coal heavers and Indian needleworkers, are powerful even today.

During the last decades of the nineteenth century, reformers adopted a range of causes. Some, like Riis, focused on the plight of the urban poor. Others challenged the Indian reservation system, which, they charged, left Indians poor and dependent on the federal government. Settlement house workers aimed to improve the lives of immigrant families. Middle-class women sought to protect and empower women by aiding abused or vulnerable wives and mothers, promoting temperance in alcohol use, and supporting women's suffrage. Many reformers participated in a trans-Atlantic community of ideas, learning about reform strategies and

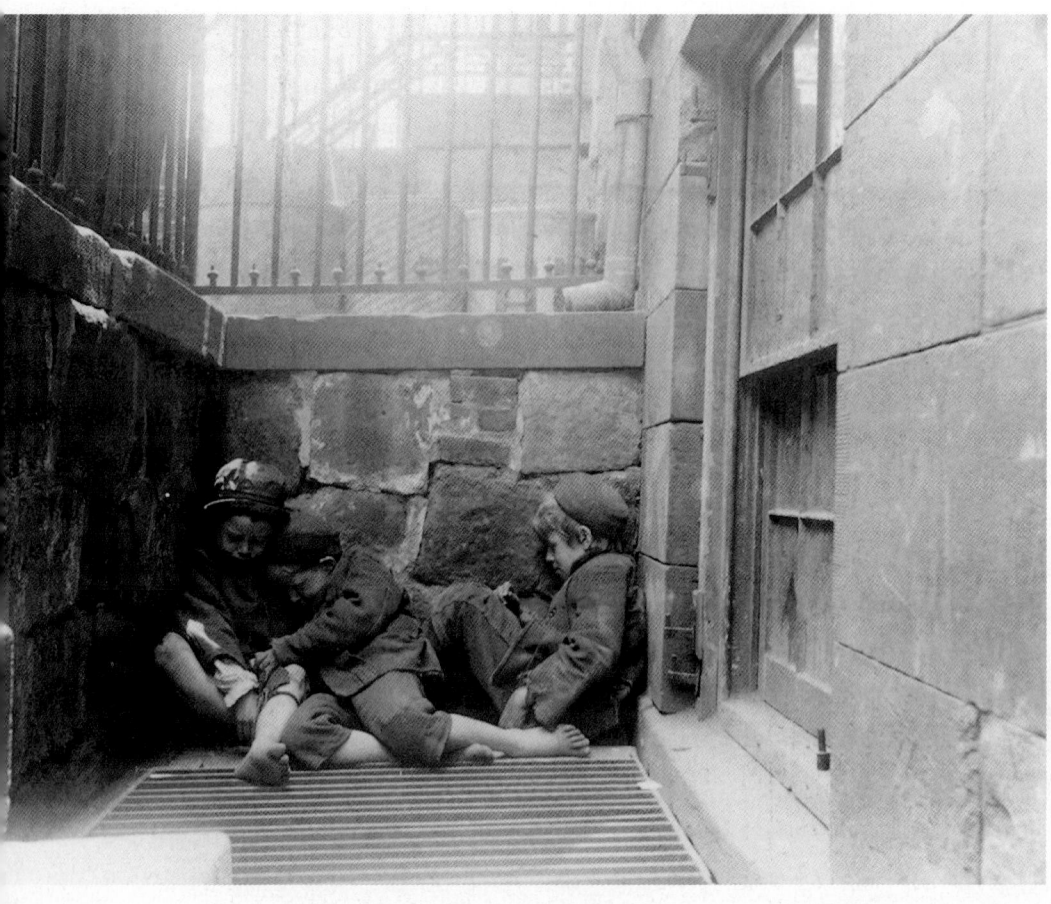

■ Jacob Riis titled this photograph *Street Arabs in Sleeping Quarters [Areaway, Mulberry St.].* Riis's photos, collected in his book *How the Other Half Lives,* exposed the poverty and wretched living conditions endured by many immigrants in New York's Lower East Side. In certain cases, Riis carefully positioned his subjects before photographing them. It is doubtful that these little boys were sleeping while the photographer noisily set up his equipment a few feet away.

institutions from their European counterparts. They stressed legislation, education, and moral rewards over coercion in their efforts to change society.

One factor leading to reform was middle-class Americans' fear that the poor would lash out in angry frustration in order to call attention to social injustice. The reformers reasoned that even modest improvements in the lives of the poor would stave off violent conflict between the classes. Dramatic labor disputes, from the railroad workers' "great uprising" of 1877 to the Haymarket bombing of 1886, frightened many well-to-do people, especially in the nation's largest cities. Yet many reformers were also motivated by a genuine sense of concern for less privileged groups—including American Indians, the country's earliest inhabitants.

Although reformers professed to favor the full integration of various ethnic groups into American life, at times they could hardly help but look down on the people they aimed to help. (*How the Other Half Lives,* for all its sympathetic portrayals of the poor, reinforces negative stereotypes of many immigrants.) Some of the people whom reformers hoped to help rejected part of their benefactors' package of values—Protestantism, for example—while accepting forms of concrete aid, such as shelter from abusive husbands. Thus the history of late-nineteenth-century reform reveals the values and goals of not just middle-class Americans, but the values and goals of a wide variety of other social groups as well.

The Goal of Indian Assimilation

In the mid-nineteenth century many European Americans, including government officials, believed that the reservation system was itself a much-needed reform to protect western Indians. Reservations were tracts of land set aside for the exclusive use of Indians. Whites reasoned that reservation Indians would remain separate from the rest of American society, to the benefit of everyone. Indians could preserve their own culture, and they would remain safe from the attacks of both homesteaders and U.S. army troops. By segregating this group, European Americans were free to settle on rich farmlands, mine for gold and silver, and take advantage of timber resources in the West.

By the 1870s the harsh reality of the reservation system had prompted a group composed of both Native Americans and European Americans to call for reform. The reformers pointed out that most western Indians had previously roamed the Plains in search of buffalo and other sources of food, clothing, and shelter; confining whole tribes to reservations meant that they lost not only their traditional means of feeding and housing themselves but their entire way of life. Reservation lands were often unsuitable for farming, leaving the residents on them without jobs or any other means to make a living. They depended on supplies of food, blankets, and clothing provided by the federal government. Kept apart from the rest of American society, denied the rights of citizenship such as education and the vote, many Indians fell victim to self-destructive behavior, including alcoholism and suicide.

Convinced that the reservation system was a failure, in 1879 reformers began to call for the assimilation of Native Americans into American life. This cause was promoted by some Indians as well as Protestant missionaries. In 1879, Ponca chief Standing Bear toured the East Coast, speaking before large, receptive audiences in Chicago, Boston, New York, Philadelphia, and Washington.

The reformers believed that the values of white middle-class Protestants provided the best guide for Indians.

The chief had already received national attention for his role in the case *Standing Bear v. Crook* (1879). Attempting to leave Indian Territory and return to his homeland in Dakota Territory, to bury his son and daughter who had recently died, the chief and 30 warriors were captured by a U.S. cavalry force commanded by General George Crook. The Indians were imprisoned in Omaha, Nebraska. Two European American lawyers offered to represent the aging Indian. They argued, "In time of peace, no authority, civil or military, exists for transporting Indians from one section of the country to another . . . nor to confine them in any particular reservation against their will." In his decision, the judge ruled that Indians were indeed persons under the law, with inalienable rights. The decision called into question the government's attempts to force Indians onto reservations and to keep them there.

On tour, addressing well-to-do listeners, Standing Bear criticized the federal Indian Office and demanded that Indians be granted full citizenship rights. When he spoke, he was accompanied by two young Omaha Indians who themselves seemed to represent the promise of assimilation. Susette LaFlesche, of French and Indian heritage, assumed the name Bright Eyes for the purpose of the tour. She announced that her people "ask you for their liberty." Her brother Joseph, attired in European American clothing, served as translator for Standing Bear, who appealed to crowds saying, "We are bound, we ask you to set us free."

Standing Bear's appeal helped to galvanize eastern reformers. The Boston Indian Citizenship Committee, the Women's National Indian Association, and the Indian Rights Association, all founded between 1879 and 1882, proclaimed the need to abolish the reservation system, much as their antebellum predecessors had called for the abolition of slavery. Indeed, the campaign for Indian assimilation bore a marked resemblance to the antislavery crusade before the Civil War. Both movements focused on the wrongs perpetrated by the U.S. government (slavery and the Indian reservation system). Both argued that the group in question deserved full citizenship rights. And both promoted the ideal of group self-sufficiency: blacks and Indians tilling the soil, embracing mainstream Christianity, and learning trades.

Beginning in 1883, advocates of Indian assimilation sponsored annual conferences at Lake Mohonk, New York, to plot strategy for the coming year. These conferences brought together scholars, clergy, reformers, and politicians, all of whom considered their cause as part of the tradition of Protestant missionary outreach work.

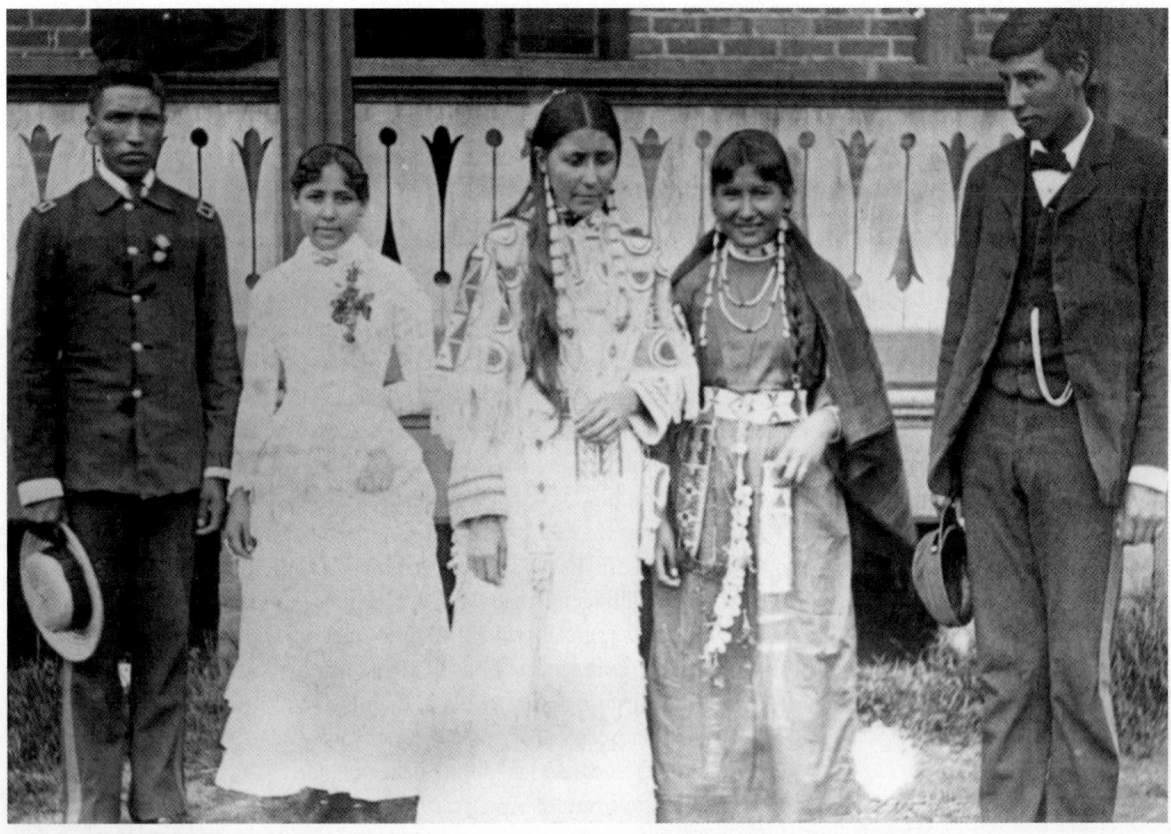

Courtesy, Hampton University Archives

■ Susan LaFlesche was the first Indian woman to become a physician in the United States. Together with her sisters Marguerite and Lucy, Susan attended Hampton Institute in Virginia, a vocational school for African Americans and Indians. This photo, c. 1885, shows Hampton students performing in a pageant at the school. Susan, center, and the woman to her left represented "Indians of the Past." The other students represented "Indians of the Present." Hampton's mission was to prepare its students for farming and the skilled trades.

The reformers believed that the values of white middle-class Protestants provided the best guide for Indians seeking to rid themselves of the hated reservation system. The Women's National Indian Association promoted "civilized home-life" on Indian reservations throughout the West. The Connecticut Branch organized a medical mission to the Omaha tribe in the 1880s. Branch members also paid for the education of another LaFlesche sibling, Susan (a graduate of Hampton Institute) at the Woman's Medical College of Philadelphia. Although LaFlesche's sponsors believed that Indian women could serve as effective agents of civilization, they had less faith in the capacity of Indian men to abandon their traditions and embrace the ways of whites.

Advocates of assimilation received support from people who simply wanted the Plains Indians removed from their land to make way for European American settlers. The *New Orleans Times–Picayune* agreed that the reservation system was flawed, but not because Indians had suffered hardships under the system. The editorialist charged that Indians should not "any longer be permitted to usurp for the purpose of barbarism, the fertile lands, the products of mines, the broad valleys and wooded mountain slopes," which the dominant white society needed.

Out of these conflicting impulses—one on behalf of the Indians' welfare, the other in support of the destruction of Indians' claims to large tracts of land—came two major initiatives that would shape federal Indian policy in the years to come. The first was the Indian boarding school movement, begun in 1879 with the founding of a school near Carlisle, Pennsylvania. The purpose of the movement was to convert Indian children to Christianity, and to force them to abandon their native culture and learn literacy skills. The second was Dawes Severalty Act, passed by Congress in 1887 with the intention of encouraging Indians to farm and apply for citizenship. By allowing reservation land to be divided into separate farms for individual Native American families, the federal act attacked the Indian tribal way of life directly. Moreover, ambitious land speculators and corrupt government officials sought to enrich themselves from the provisions of the act which allowed the sell-off of Indian lands to white buyers.

Trans-Atlantic Networks of Reform

American reformers derived ideas and inspiration from their European counterparts. This trans-Atlantic exchange of ideas was greatly facilitated by improvements in sea transportation. During the 1870s and 1880s, ocean travel became cheaper and safer as well as more efficient and comfortable. The great shipping lines, such as Cunard, began to offer intermediate fares for middle-class passengers who did not want to travel in steerage but could not afford first-class compartments. In 1890 a tourist embarking from New York could cross the Atlantic in just 10 days for about $30.00 (the price of a bicycle) on a well-appointed steamship. Writer Henry James (1843–1916) traveled extensively in Europe before making his home in London in the mid-1870s. In his 1881 novel, *Portrait of a Lady,* the heroine, Isabel Archer, replies to an English gentleman who says he finds her motives for touring Europe "mysterious": "Is there anything mysterious in a purpose entertained and executed every year, in the most public manner, by fifty thousand of my fellow countrymen—the purpose of improving one's mind by foreign travel?"

Contacts between European and American scholars enriched the intellectual life of the United States and bolstered the reform impulse.

Contacts between European and American scholars, students, artists, clergy, writers, and reformers enriched the intellectual life of the United States and bolstered the reform impulse. American women's rights supporters conferred with their counterparts in London. American college students attended classes at German universities. For example, American scholars at German universities absorbed ideas related to "reform Darwinism," the notion that state and private charitable intervention could improve modern social relations. Out of these ideas came the Social Gospel, a moral reform movement that stressed the responsibility of Christians to address the ills of modern urban life. Furthering this exchange of ideas, municipal and federal commissions studied labor unions and prisons on both sides of the Atlantic. Popular journals such as the *Nation* and the *New Republic* reported on social policy initiatives of European governments.

An idealistic graduate of Rockford (Illinois) Female Seminary, Jane Addams journeyed to Europe for the first time in 1883. The sight of large numbers of poor people in London's East End made a lasting impression on her. She returned home, searching for a way to be useful, and for "an outward symbol of fellowship . . . some blessed spot where unity of spirit might claim right of way over all differences." In 1888 she went again to England and visited Toynbee Hall, a social settlement founded to alleviate the problems of the laboring classes. Back in Chicago, she and her friend and fellow classmate Ellen Gates Starr decided to open a settlement house of their own. Called Hull House, it was located in the Nineteenth Ward, home to 5000 Greek, Russian, Italian, and German immigrants.

Social settlement houses—so-called because their goal was to help immigrants with the transition of settling in the United States—provided a variety of services for immigrants, including English language classes, neighborhood health clinics, after-school programs for children, and instruction in personal hygiene and infant care. In 1891, six settlements were in operation, including the Neighborhood Guild of New York City (1886) as well as Addams's Hull House in Chicago (1889). By 1900, the number stood at 200.

Later, Addams recalled that, with the opening of Hull House, she hoped to counter the anarchists and strikers. Like other reformers, Addams believed that social-welfare activities would improve the lot of the poor and thus diffuse their radical, violent impulses. Moreover, she hoped to offer a sphere of useful work for young, well-educated women. Within the settlement house, she believed, these women reformers "might restore a balance of activity along traditional lines and learn of life from life itself." This was a place "where they might try out some of the things they had been taught."

Women Reformers: "Beginning to Burst the Bonds"

Like the Indian assimilation movement, women's reform work in general during this period had a strong missionary strain. In San Francisco, the Occidental Branch of the Women's Foreign Missionary Society enlisted the aid of well-to-do women in sponsoring a rescue home for Chinese prostitutes. Without the protection of traditional kin ties, these immigrants remained vulnerable to sexual and physical abuse. The rescue home enabled the young women to escape the men who exploited them and, in some cases, to reenter society, now as married women or factory wage-earners or small merchants.

In Salt Lake City, a group of women challenged the Mormon practice of plural marriage. In 1886 their Industrial Christian Home Association received a subsidy from Congress to provide shelter for "women who renounce polygamy and their children of a tender age." That same year some Denver women founded the Colorado Cottage Home, a rescue home for pregnant girls and women. Many women sought out by these reformers welcomed services such as job training and shelter from abusive men. However, some women declined to embrace other aspects of these charitable organizations, such as religious lessons.

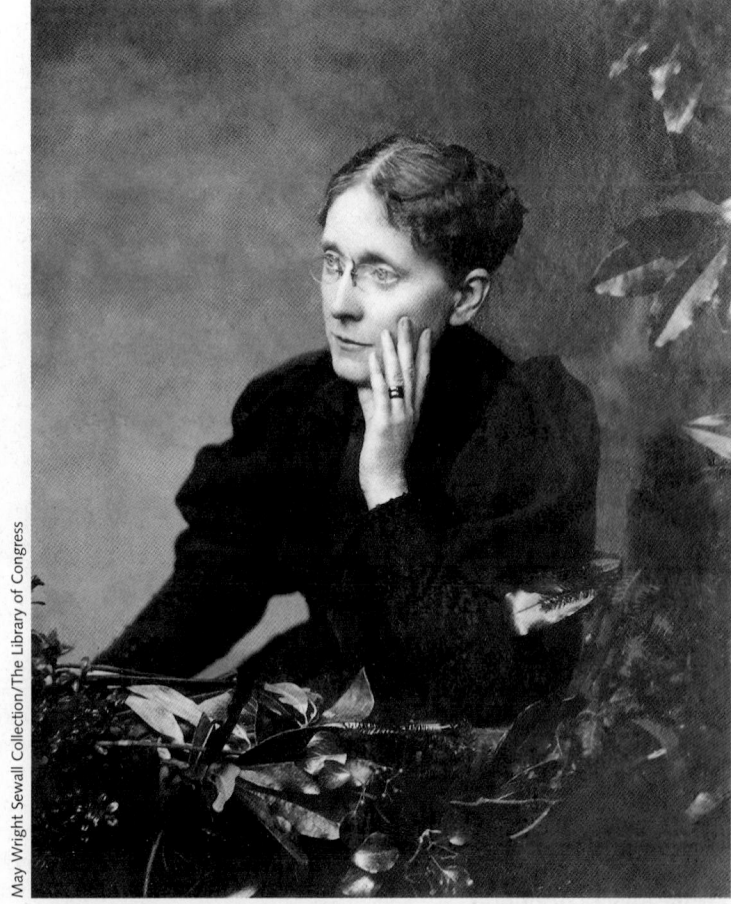

May Wright Sewall Collection/The Library of Congress

■ Frances Willard (1839–1898) grew up on a farm in Wisconsin Territory. She served as the first dean of women at Northwestern University in Illinois. In the mid–1870s, she decided to devote her life to the cause of temperance. From 1879 until her death, she was president of the Woman's Christian Temperance Union. Willard developed what she called a "Do-Everything policy." Under her leadership, the WCTU addressed a range of issues, including woman suffrage and workers' rights.

The Women's Christian Temperance Union (WCTU) is an apt example of the missionary impulse behind late-nineteenth-century reform. Though best known for its antialcohol crusade, the WCTU also sponsored homes for unwed mothers and day and night nurseries for the children of working women. It also stressed the need for women's "purity," claiming that women and children were the chief victims of men's alcohol consumption. But the group went further to denounce women's victimization at the hands of men in general.

Like national labor unions at the time, the WCTU organized African American women into local chapters separate from those of whites. Frances Ellen Watkins Harper served as head of the black division of the organization between 1883 and 1890. Harper, much in demand as a lecturer, also organized Sunday schools for black children and enlisted the aid of black clergy in her campaign against juvenile delinquency in Philadelphia. In 1887 middle-class black women in Atlanta formed the West Atlanta chapter of the WCTU. The group reached out to the students of Atlanta University with talks on topics with titles like "Character Building," "Mother's Influence," and "Unfermented Wine."

Frances Willard proved a popular national speaker from the time she founded the WCTU in 1879 until her death in 1898. She served as the organization's first president during those years and in 1883 formed a world temperance union. Willard believed in the power of direct

Platform Statement of Presidential Candidate Belva Lockwood, 1884

In 1884 a group of women calling themselves the National Equal Rights Party convened in California and nominated Belva Lockwood for president of the United States. Born in Royalton, New York, in 1830, Lockwood was the first woman admitted to practice law before the Supreme Court (in 1879). She was a staunch proponent of woman suffrage and of equal pay for equal work. Lockwood believed that her presidential candidacy would bring much-needed publicity to the cause of women's rights. She accepted the nomination by outlining her platform:

"Two Unpublished Letters from Belva Lockwood"

It will be my earnest effort to promote and maintain equal political privileges to every class of our citizens irrespective of sex, color or nationality, and to make of this great and glorious Country in truth what it has been so long in name, "the land of the free and the home of the brave."

I shall seek to insure a fair distribution of the public offices to women as well as to men, with a scrupulous regard to civil service reform after the women are duly installed in office.

I am also in accord with the platform of the party in the desire

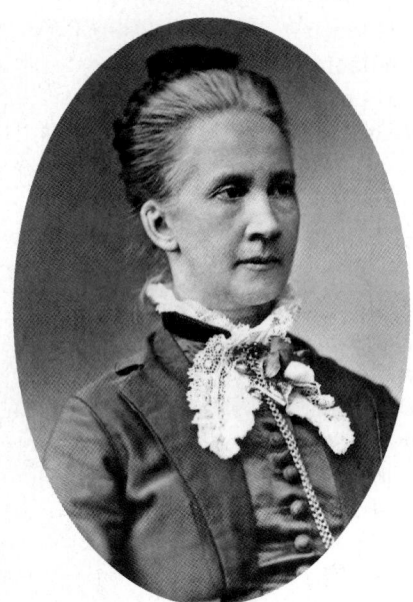

Belva Lockwood.

to protect and foster American industries, and in my sympathy with the working men and women of the country, who are organized against free trade, for the purpose of rendering the laboring classes of our country more comfortable and independent.

I sympathize with the soldier and the soldier's widow; . . . believing that the surplus revenues of the country cannot be better used than in clothing the widows and educating the orphans of our Nation's defenders . . . .

I am opposed to monopoly in the sense of the men of the country monopolizing all of the votes and all of the offices, and at the same time insisting upon having the distribution of all of the money both public and private . . . .

I am in full sympathy with the Temperance advocates of the country, especially the W.C.T.U.,

but believe that Woman Suffrage will have a greater tendency to abolish the liquor traffic, than prohibition will to bring about woman suffrage. If the former is adopted, the latter will be its probable sequence.

If elected, I shall recommend in my Inaugural speech, a uniform system of laws as far as practicable for all the States, and especially for marriage, divorce, and the limitation of contracts, and such a regulation of the laws of descent and distribution of estates as will make the wife equal with the husband in authority and right, and an equal partner in the common business.

I favor an extension of our commercial relations with foreign countries, and especially with the Central and South American States, and the establishment of a high Court of Arbitration to which shall be referred all differences that may arise between these Several States, or between them and the United States.

My Indian policy would be, to break up their tribal relations, distribute to them their lands in severalty, and make them citizens, amenable to the laws of the land as other white and colored persons are . . . .

Again thanking you Ladies for your expression of esteem.

Lockwood received 4149 votes cast in six states in the 1884 election. In the late 1880s and 1890s she devoted her energies to the cause of world peace. Belva Lockwood died in Washington, D.C., in 1917. ■

Source: Madeleine B. Stern, "Two Unpublished Letters from Belva Lockwood," *Signs* 1 (Autumn 1975):274–275.

action. She exhorted groups of women to descend on taverns and rum shops and to shame customers into taking the "cold water pledge." The pledge required its adherents to quench their thirst with cold water, not alcohol.

An enthusiastic advocate of woman suffrage, Willard was instrumental in bringing women's issues into the political realm. In her speeches, she quoted women such as "a

Presbyterian lady" who declared, "For my part, I never wanted to vote until our gentlemen passed a prohibition ordinance . . . and a month later . . . chose a saloon keeper for mayor."

By the 1870s the issue of woman suffrage had captured the attention of men and women throughout the country. And in fact, the issue had special resonance in the West for several reasons. When European American women overcame the hardships associated with the challenge of settling the trans-Mississippi West, they considered themselves worthy of having an equal voice in the polling booth. Reflecting on her hard life as a settler in Circle Valley, Utah, Mrs. L. L. Dalton wrote in 1876 that she was "proud and thankful" to see women "beginning to burst the bonds of iron handed custom" and asserting their "co-heirship" with fathers, brothers, and husbands. Abigail Scott Duniway, who sympathized with the plight of overworked and lonely farm wives, published a women's rights journal, *New Northwest*, in Portland, Oregon, from 1871 to 1887. In 1873 she had helped found the Oregon Equal Suffrage Association and served as its president.

Western politics pitted cattle ranchers against farmers and religious and cultural groups against each other. These conflicts prompted the men of various groups to seek allies wherever they could find them—within their own households if necessary. The territorial legislature of Wyoming granted women the right to vote in 1869. Utah Territory followed suit in 1870, and Washington Territory in 1883. Territorial governments facilitated the enactment of woman suffrage, for they required only that the measure win the approval of a majority of the legislature and the approval of the governor. In contrast, states had to approve a constitutional amendment, which required support of two-thirds of the legislators and a majority of the voters. The states of Wyoming (in 1890), Colorado (1893), and Utah and Idaho (both in 1896) approved suffrage for women. Colorado's victory was the only one resulting from a successful statewide referendum.

The nature of the western suffrage movement points to the need to view women's rights, and women's activism in general, in their historical and regional contexts. For example, African American women also pressed for the right to vote, and their demands assumed special urgency amid violence and terrorism. Ida B. Wells-Barnett would later lead an African American women's suffrage club in Chicago and play a pivotal role in the national suffrage movement. She began her public career as a crusading journalist in Memphis in the 1880s. In the early 1890s she clashed with Frances Willard over the issue of lynching, charging that the WCTU president refused to condemn the barbaric practice. Although Willard had been an active abolitionist and a steadfast campaigner for women's suffrage, according to Wells-Barnett, she was "no better or worse than the great bulk of white Americans on the Negro question." Thus women's political issues reflected tensions between blacks and whites as well as between women and men.

Conclusion

In the 1870s and 1880s the Americans who challenged the power of government and big business represented a wide spectrum of ideologies, tactics, and goals. Some resisted violently, smashing the machines, trains, and telegraph poles that were transforming American society. The Ohio machine-breakers and southwestern *Gorras Blancas* destroyed property in an effort to assert their claims to a traditional way of life. Others formed new institutions such as settlement houses, reform associations, or political parties to advance their agenda on the national scene. Some people hoping to effect social change used the language of evangelical Protestantism, echoing the reform activities of persons who called for the abolition of slavery before the Civil War. Others collected data and interviewed specific groups of workers, women, or immigrants in an effort, first, to expose the conditions under which these groups lived and labored and second, to propose specific legislation to remedy those conditions. Plains Indians embraced religious mysticism in a failed attempt to halt the incursion of European

Americans into their ancient hunting grounds. Thus, powerful groups encountered much resistance from people opposed to their narrow idea of progress—the idea that bigger factories, more efficient farm machinery, and a nationwide network of railroad lines would bring prosperity to all Americans.

As Americans began to think more broadly about their place in the world, some men and women hoped to apply the principles of moral and civic reform to other countries west of the United States. The 1880s thus laid the foundations not only for a trans-Atlantic republic of cultural exchange, but also for a trans-Pacific empire of missionary work and trade. In the process, a new ideology of expansionism emerged, one that blended elements of economic gain, national security, and Christian missionary outreach to peoples in far-off lands.

Sites to Visit

Anarchist Archives at Pitzer University

http://dwardmac.pitzer.edu/Anarchist_Archives/
archivehome.html

This archive includes classic anarchist texts, especially information about and graphics of the Haymarket Riot.

Labor–Management Conflict in American History

www.history.ohio-state.edu/projects/laborconflict/

This Ohio State University site includes primary accounts of some of the major events in the history of the labor–management conflict in the late nineteenth and early twentieth centuries.

Samuel Gompers Papers at the University of Maryland

www.inform.umd.edu/HIST/Gompers/web1.html

This site includes information about the papers project. It also has a photo gallery, selected documents, and a brief history of the first president of the American Federation of Labor.

African American Perspectives: Pamphlets from the Daniel A. P. Murry Collections, 1818–1907

http://lcweb2.loc.gov/ammem/aap/aapone.html

This collection includes writings of famous African Americans, including Frederick Douglass, Booker T. Washington, Ida B. Wells-Barnett, Benjamin W. Arnett, Alexander Crummel, and Emanuel Love.

Coal Mining During the Gilded Age and Progressive Era

www.history.ohio-state.edu/projects/Lessons_US/
Gilded_Age/Coal_Mining/default.htm

This Ohio State University site examines the development of the coal industry, including the sometimes violent labor–management conflict.

African American Women Writers of the Nineteenth Century

digital.nypl.org/schomburg/writers_aa19/

The New York Public Library's Schomburg Center for Research in Black Culture maintains this site, which contains a large number of digital texts by African American women of the nineteenth century.

For Further Reading

General Works

Edward L. Ayers, *The Promise of the New South: Life After Reconstruction* (1992).

Sarah Deutsch, *No Separate Refuge: Culture, Class, and Gender on an Anglo-Hispanic Frontier, 1880–1940* (1987).

Lawrence Goodwyn, *Democratic Promise: The Populist Moment in America* (1976).

Patricia N. Limerick, *The Legacy of Conquest: The Unbroken Past of the American West* (1987).

David Montgomery, *The Fall of the House of Labor: The Workplace, the State, and American Labor Activism, 1865–1925* (1987).

Elizabeth Sanders, *Roots of Reform: Farmers, Workers, and the American State, 1877–1917* (1999).

Resistance to Legal and Military Authority

Tomás Almaguer, *Racial Fault Lines: The Historical Origins of White Supremacy in California* (1994).

Dee Brown, *Bury My Heart at Wounded Knee: An Indian History of the American West* (1970).

Arlen L. Fowler, *The Black Infantry in the West, 1869–1891* (1971).

Alex Lichtenstein, *Twice the Work of Free Labor: The Political Economy of Convict Labor in the New South* (1996).

Leon Litwack, *Trouble in Mind: Black Southerners in the Age of Jim Crow* (1998).

Robert J. Rosenbaum, *Mexicano Resistance in the Southwest: The Sacred Right of Self-Preservation* (1981).

Alexander Saxton, *The Indispensable Enemy: Labor and the Anti-Chinese Movement in California* (1971).

Robert M. Utley, *The Lance and the Shield: The Life and Times of Sitting Bull* (1993).

Revolt in the Workplace

Paul Avrich, *The Haymarket Tragedy* (1984).

Leon Fink, *Workingmen's Democracy: The Knights of Labor and American Politics* (1983).

Philip S. Foner, *The Great Labor Uprising of 1877* (1977).

Jacquelyn Dowd Hall, James Leloudis, Robert Korstad, Mary Murphy, LuAnn Jones, and Christopher B. Daly, *Like a Family: The Making of a Southern Cotton Mill World* (1987).

Stuart B. Kaufman, *Samuel Gompers and the Origins of the American Federation of Labor, 1848–1896* (1973).

Theodore R. Mitchell, *Political Education in the Southern Farmers' Alliance, 1887–1900* (1987).

Bruce Nelson, *Beyond the Martyrs: A Social History of Chicago's Anarchists, 1870–1900* (1988).

Crosscurrents of Reform

Jean Bethke Elshtain, *Jane Addams and the Dream of American Democracy* (2001).

Barbara L. Epstein, *The Politics of Domesticity: Women, Evangelism, and Temperance* (1980).

Paula Giddings, *When and Where I Enter: The Impact of Black Women on Race and Sex and America* (1984).

Frederick E. Hoxie, *A Final Promise: The Campaign to Assimilate the Indians, 1880–1920* (1984).

Jane Taylor Nelsen, ed., *A Prairie Populist: The Memoirs of Luna Kellie* (1992).

Peggy Pascoe, *Relations of Rescue: The Search for Female Moral Authority in the American West, 1874–1939* (1990).

Jacob Riis, *How the Other Half Lives: Studies Among the Tenements of New York* (1971).

Daniel T. Rodgers, *Atlantic Crossings: Social Politics in a Progressive Age* (1998).

Online Practice Test

Test your understanding of this chapter with interactive review quizzes at

www.ablongman.com/jonescreatedequal/chapter17

Additional Photo Credits

Page 573: Ben Wittick, Museum of New Mexico, Palace of the Governors (Neg. #15821 & #58591)
Page 593: Fair Street Pictures
Page 595: Jacob Riis, *Street Arabs at Night*, c. 1890. Museum of the City of New York, The Jacob A. Riis Collection, #123
Page 600: Culver Pictures
Page 601: Courtesy, Janice L. and David Frent

CHAPTER 18

Political and Cultural Conflict in a Decade of Depression and War: The 1890s

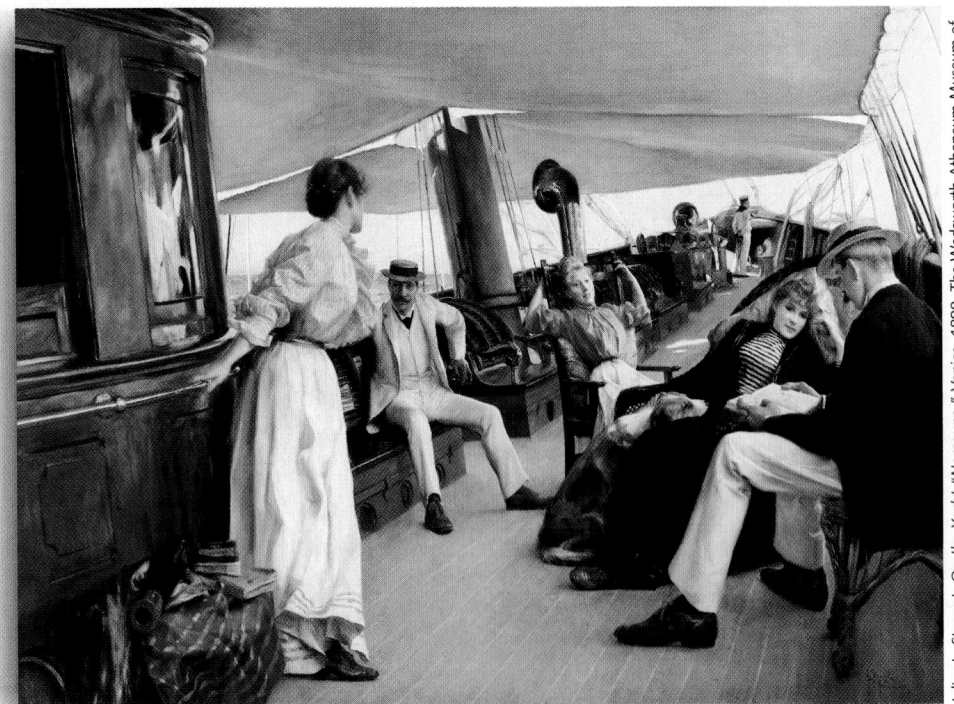

Julius L. Stewart, *On the Yacht "Namouna," Venice*, 1890. The Wadsworth Atheneum Museum of Art, Hartford, CT. The Ella Gallup Sumner and Mary Catlin Sumner Collection Fund, 1965.32

■ Several Americans relax on the yacht *Namouna* as it sails in the waters off the coast of Venice, Italy. By the late nineteenth century, innovations in ocean transportation had made travel cheaper and faster. Wealthy Americans flocked to Europe, contributing to a trans-Atlantic culture of ideas, literature, and fashion.

IN THE EARLY 1890S, LUTHER STANDING BEAR, A YOUNG MAN OF LAKOTA SIOUX ORIGIN, found himself suspended between two worlds. Born in 1868 in South Dakota, he had learned to hunt buffalo in the traditional manner of the Western Sioux. In 1879 he bowed to the wishes of his father, Standing Bear (not to be confused with the Ponca leader of the same name), who insisted that he learn the ways of "Long Knives," or whites. And so the youth was among the first pupils to attend the new federal Indian boarding school in Carlisle, Pennsylvania. En route to Carlisle, the 11-year-old regarding his journey—by boat and train—as an ordeal that he must endure with honor. Once at the school, he discovered that he was to become an "imitation of a white man"—and quickly.

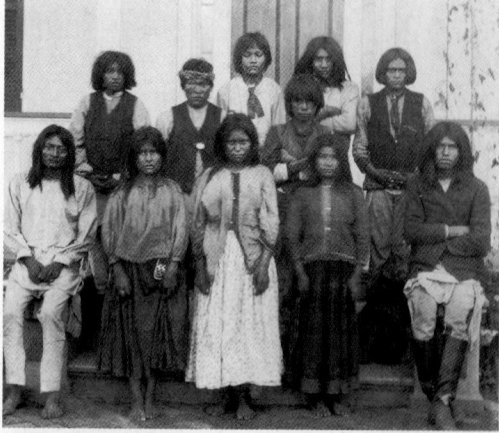

Called Ota Kte, or Plenty Kill, at home, now he was required to pick a new first name from among those listed on a classroom blackboard. He chose Luther. His teachers took away his blanket and moccasins and gave him a coat, pants, and vest to wear. They forbade him to speak his native language, and they cut his long hair. One of his classmates protested, "If I am to learn the ways of the white people, I can do it just as well with my hair on." Like most other youths at Carlisle, Standing Bear learned to read and write English and to practice a craft (in his case, tin-smithing). His teachers encouraged him to embrace Christianity.

In 1884, as part of his government-sponsored training, Luther Standing Bear traveled to Philadelphia to work at the Wanamaker department store. The head of Carlisle, Captain Richard Henry Pratt, had sent the youth on his way with the words, "You are to be an example of what this school can turn out. Go, my boy, and do your best. Die there if necessary, but do not fail." After spending a year stocking shelves and performing other tasks at the famous store, Standing Bear returned to South Dakota. There he taught Sioux children in a school near the place of his birth, now the Rosebud Indian Reservation. He married the daughter of an Indian mother and a white father.

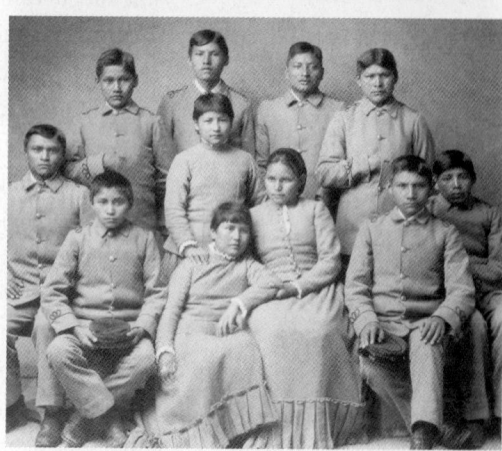

This group of Chiricahua Apache students arrived at the Carlisle Indian boarding school in 1890. Government-sponsored Indian education included dressing them in European American clothing and cutting their hair.

The massacre at Wounded Knee, South Dakota in December 1890, which was not far from his home, left the young man fearful for the safety of his family. He subsequently moved with them to the nearby Pine Ridge Reservation, where he began work as a shopkeeper and postal clerk. In the late 1890s, Luther Standing Bear served as an interpreter for Buffalo Bill's "Wild West" show during its tour in London.

By 1912 he had become an American citizen and settled in southern California, where he began his acting career in the new motion picture industry. He appeared in some of the first movie westerns together with famous actors Douglas Fairbanks and William S. Hart. At the same time, Luther Standing Bear also became an Indian activist, serving as president of the Los Angeles American Indian Progressive Association and speaking out against the "government prison" known as the reservation. Standing Bear died in 1939 while working on a film called *Union Pacific*.

In the 1890s, Luther Standing Bear's journey took place amid the depression, civil strife, and war of the era. Throughout the decade, workers challenged the idea that the United States was immune to the bloody class conflict that had long plagued Europe. Some scholars lamented the closing of the western frontier, prompting fears that America's unique dynamic of growth and social improvement had come to an end.

> *Native-born whites began to seize upon new categories of "racial" difference.*

Domestic developments had a profound effect on American foreign policy. Native-born whites began to seize upon new categories of racial difference to draw distinctions between various groups in the United States and around the world. Faced with declining consumer demand at home, politicians and businesspeople joined forces to expand American markets and American influence abroad. Economic and humanitarian interests often went hand in hand. Reformers claimed that the blessings of American consumer society would "civilize" darker peoples everywhere. In 1896 Merrill Gates, a philanthropist and advocate of Indian boarding-school education, described the goal of such education: "We need to *awaken in him* [the Indian] *wants. . . .* Discontent with the tepee and the starving rations of the Indian camp in winter is needed to get the Indian out of the blanket and into trousers—and trousers with a pocket in them, and with a *pocket that aches to be filled with dollars!*" America's imperialistic ventures would reveal a similar blend of economic interests and missionary outreach.

Thus, the 1890s was a time of stark contrasts. The same year the depression hit, the Chicago World's Fair, called the Columbian Exposition, celebrated American architectural and technological progress. Among the exhibits was an early motion picture camera. This was a decade when bicycling became a craze, and the syncopated rhythms of a new form of music called ragtime became all the rage. But during the same decade, southern lynch mobs burned alive black men and women and American military forces pursued a brutal war in Cuba and the Philippines.

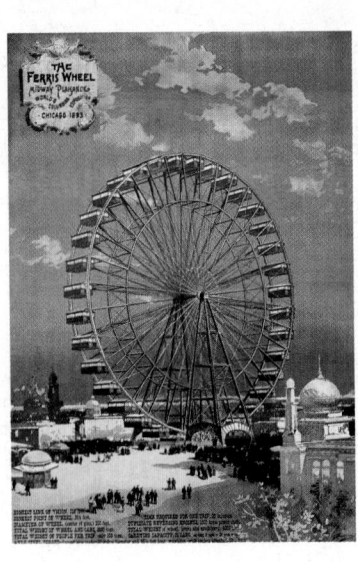

Whereas some Americans tried to define rigid racial and nationalistic boundaries, others sought avenues of connections. A new political party, the Populist, or People's, party, aimed to bring together men and women of all backgrounds and regions. By advocating grassroots democracy as well as government action to regulate the economy, the party paved the way for the Progressive reforms of the early twentieth-century.

Relying on a variety of means, from new legal and educational systems to commercial expansion and the deployment of military might, American elites attempted to consolidate their political power and cultural influence. In the process, the United States confronted not only the domestic challenges of sustaining a modern industrial society but also the worldwide challenges that pitted the enduring ideal of democracy against the emerging reality of colonialism.

Frontiers at Home, Lost and Found

In 1893 historian Frederick Jackson Turner wrote an essay titled "The Significance of the Frontier in American History." Delivered as an address to a group of historians at the Columbian Exposition in Chicago, the essay presented a new way of thinking about American history. According to Turner, the process of settling the West had shaped all of American history. He argued that during the colonial period, the rigors of taming the land had transformed English colonists into more resourceful, more democratic people—in other words, into Americans. With each successive wave of western settlement, American society renewed itself. In his view, the West served as a "safety valve," a place of opportunity that beckoned people out of crowded eastern cities. However, Turner noted, an 1890 Census Report had concluded that the frontier—the unsettled area of the western part of the country—had recently disappeared. The historian sounded an ominous note at the end of his address: "And now, four centuries from the discovery of America, at the end of a hundred years of life under the Constitution, the frontier has gone, and with its going has closed the first period in American history."

Turner's thesis promoted the idea of American "exceptionalism": the idea that its individualism and democratic values made the United States unique among the nations of the world. Yet his association of geography with an "American character" was simplistic at best. In his celebration of the sturdy frontiersman, Turner ignored the bloody legacy of western settlement and its devastating effects on native peoples and Spanish-speaking settlers.

Nevertheless, at the end of the nineteenth century, Turner and others were asking questions. Did America need to conquer new lands and "tame" certain peoples to preserve its distinctive character? Now that the frontier had disappeared, what was to prevent the United States from becoming more like Europe? These urgent concerns led to efforts to assimilate and Americanize certain groups of people and to tighten systems of legal discrimination against others.

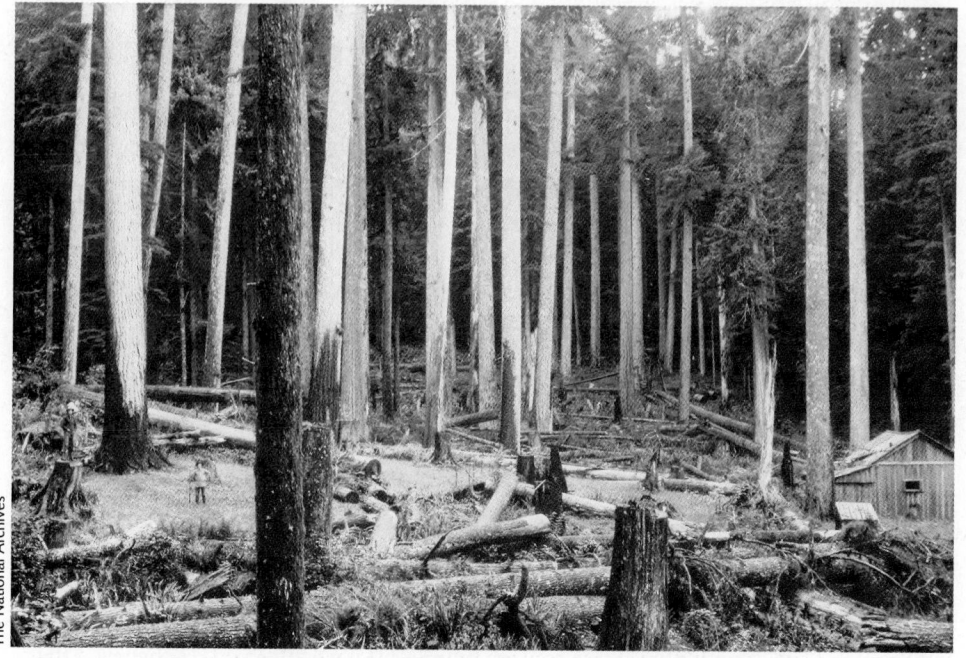

The National Archives

■ Frederick Jackson Turner's 1893 announcement that the western frontier had disappeared was premature. Here, homesteaders in Washington State cut down trees to carve a farm out of the forest, c. 1900. Felling gigantic hardwoods in the Northwest was a formidable challenge to family farmers.

Claiming and Managing the Land

As less and less land was available for cultivation, grazing, and mining, the politics of rural development entered a new phase. In the early 1890s, the last great parcel of Indian land was opened to European American farmers. The Indian Removal Act of 1830 had authorized the federal government to use force in relocating the Five Civilized Tribes from the Southeast to newly designated "Indian Territory." Survivors of the "trail of tears" reestablished native political and cultural institutions in the territory. Between 1830 and 1880, representatives of as many as 50 native groups had settled in this area, including tribes forced out of the Upper Midwest and refugees of the Plains Indian wars.

European American ranchers and farmers in nearby states coveted the fertile lands in Indian Territory. In 1889 President Benjamin Harrison opened to white settlement the unoccupied lands in the present state of Oklahoma. (The name combines two Choctaw words: *okla,* meaning "people," and *humma,* meaning "red.") On April 22 of that year, as many as 60,000 settlers rushed in to claim parcels of land amounting to 2 million acres of the territory.

Congress established the Territory of Oklahoma in 1890, and three years later, the Cherokee Outlet in the north central part of the territory, combined with Tonkawa and Pawnee reservations, was thrown open to settlers and oil developers. On September 16, 1893, 100,000 people claimed 6.5 million newly opened acres in a single day. The "sooners," people who rushed to claim the land, gave the state of Oklahoma its nickname. The "Sooner State" was admitted to the Union in 1907.

Congress took other steps to manage western lands during the 1890s. The Court of Private Land Claims (1891) oversaw land disputes in New Mexico, Colorado, and Arizona. This court favored recent European American claimants over the Hispanic settlers who had received title to the lands from either Spain or Mexico generations earlier. Dispossessed of their land, many Hispanic sheep sharecroppers (*partidarios*) became dependent on European Americans for land and credit. Some were forced to earn a living as wage workers in the mines and beet fields of Colorado.

Land courts were only one example of an expanded federal role in the settlement of the West and management of the land. During the 1890s, the federal government continued to provide information and services for farmers through the U.S. Department of Agriculture (USDA). Among other programs, the USDA encouraged Texas cotton planters to diversify their crops in response to damage caused by the boll weevil, a pest that entered the state from Mexico in 1892. A forerunner of the National Weather Service, the Weather Bureau supplied farmers with forecasts and information related to rainfall and temperatures. The Division of Road Inquiries, formed in 1893 in response to pressure from bicyclists and farmers, aimed to study road building and sponsor pilot projects, including concrete roads. The Division of Biological Survey catalogued and classified species of plants that were disappearing as the population increased and the wilderness disappeared.

Government policymakers argued over the proper balance between conserving natural resources for use by farmers, loggers, and oilmen and preserving the beauty of unspoiled panoramas for the enjoyment of all. In 1890 Congress established a national park in California's spectacular Yosemite Valley. The Yosemite Indians had lived in the valley for hundreds of years, fishing, hunting, and foraging for sustenance. Nevertheless, park officials were determined to create "frontier-like" conditions. These officials stocked local lakes with both native and nonnative fish. The 1891 Forest Reserve Act set aside forest reserves in the public domain; (that is, vast tracts of land still owned by the federal government). Logging companies were allowed to exploit these areas for their timber.

With his appointment as chief of the Division of Forestry in 1898, Gifford Pinchot sought to bring the issue of natural resource conservation to national attention. He believed that a managed forest could provide lumber and then renew itself. His approach suggested that conserving natural resources and using them commercially could be compatible goals.

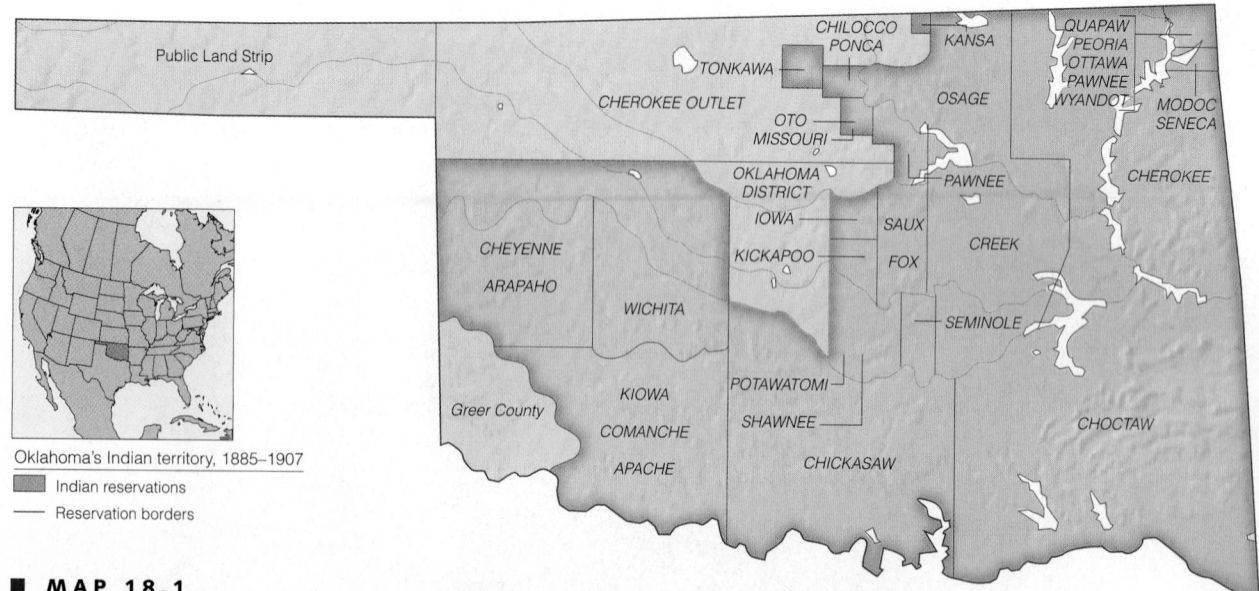

■ MAP 18.1

INDIAN TERRITORY AND THE STATE OF OKLAHOMA, 1885–1907   In the early 1890s, the federal government began to purchase land from the so-called Five Civilized Tribes and other Indian groups to open Indian Territory to European American settlement. The lands of the Potawatomi, Shawnee, Iowa, Sauk, and Fox were opened in 1891; Cheyenne and Arapaho in 1892; the Cherokee Outlet in 1893; Kickapoo in 1895; and Kiowa, Comanche, Apache, and Wichita between 1901 and 1906. In 1907, Indian Territory and Oklahoma Territory merged to become the state of Oklahoma.

Pinchot found his views challenged by John Muir and others who argued that uninhabited regions should be preserved in their natural state, unmarred by dams, mines, or logging operations. In 1892 Muir founded the Sierra Club, a group devoted to preserving wilderness. In 1899 both Muir and the Northern Pacific Railroad lobbied successfully for two new national parks, Mount Rainier in Washington and Glacier in Montana, highlighting the ongoing significance of railroad tourism. The philosophical disagreements between Pinchot and the conservationists on one hand and Muir and the preservationists on the other shaped a wider debate between conservationists and preservationists in the early twentieth century.

"Rusticating," or hiking and enjoying the beauty of nature, became a popular pastime for many Americans in the 1890s. By 1890, tourists from Boston could board a train and, eight hours later, reach the rocky coast of Maine's Frenchman's Bay, where large hotels provided comfortable accomodations and breathtaking views. Throughout northern New England, religious groups and extended families established summer colonies on the coast and in the mountains so that they could live close to "the great outdoors," renewing social ties and refreshing the spirit. Although the frontier of the cattle rancher and farmer was receding, the frontier of recreational tourism was growing by leaps and bounds, as excursion trains provided greater access to beach resorts and mountain retreats.

The Tyranny of Racial Categories

The supposed closing of the western frontier, and with it the disappearance of the "safety valve" for restless Easterners, highlighted urban America's increasing class and cultural diversity. In an effort to categorize social groups, many national opinion-makers—scholars, journalists, and politicians—claimed that people should be distinguished from one another by their inborn, "natural" characteristics, ranging from skin color to facial bone structure and intelligence. Supposedly, these differences defined specific racial categories, such as Caucasoid, Mongoloid, and

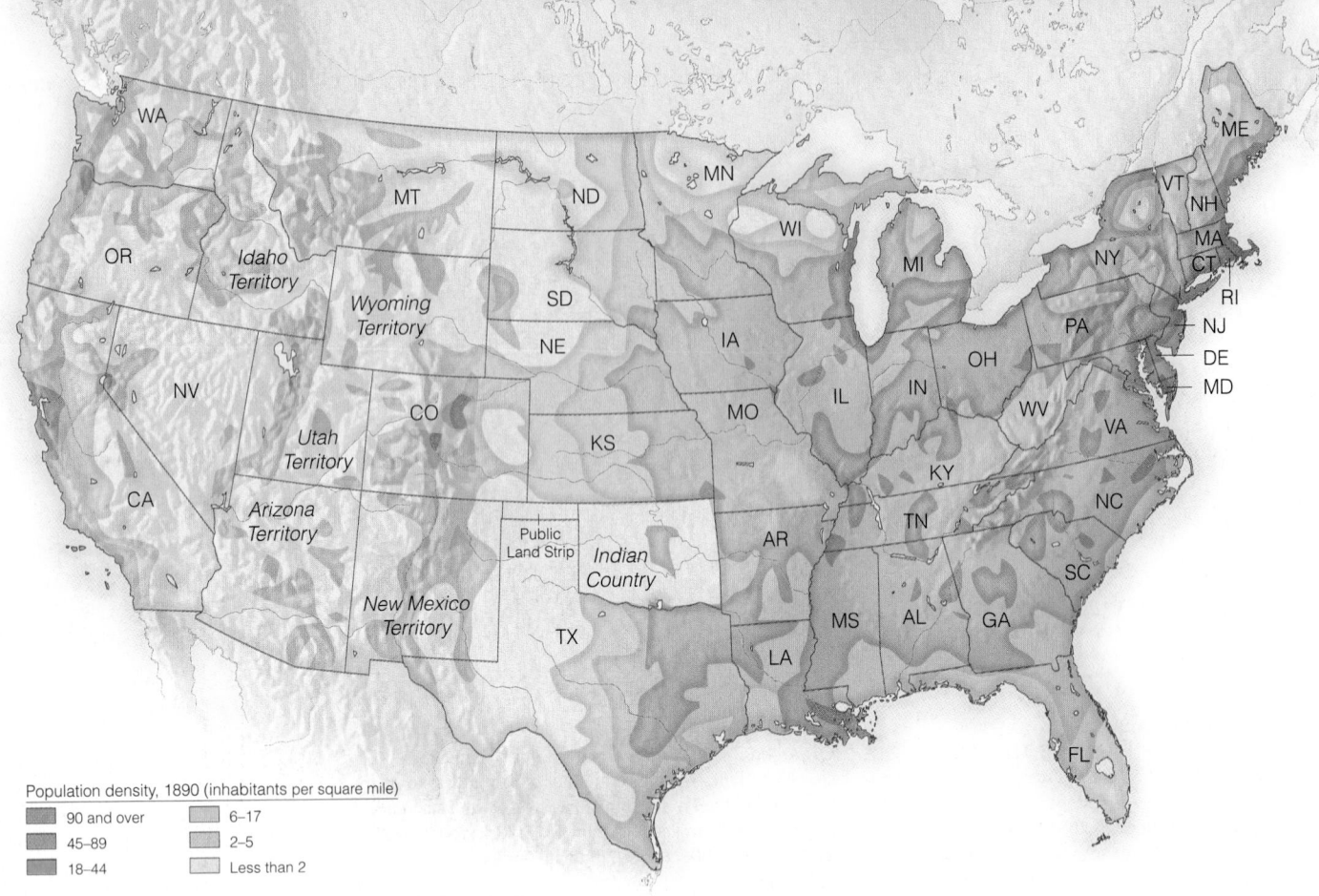

■ MAP 18.2

POPULATION DENSITY, 1890   In 1890 the United States still contained vast tracts of wilderness. Some Americans worried that the Northeast was overpopulated and that, as a result, the country would face the same problems as Europe—class conflict, poverty, and urban ills.

Population density, 1890 (inhabitants per square mile)

- 90 and over
- 45–89
- 18–44
- 6–17
- 2–5
- Less than 2

Negroid. In fact, so-called racial differences between groups were cultural differences. Prewar nativists had opposed foreign immigration because they considered native-born Protestants to be superior to people born in other countries. In contrast, late-nineteenth-century scientific racists ranked "superior" and "inferior" races on an elaborate hierarchy encompassing all groups, native and foreign-born.

Several factors account for this renewed obsession with race in the 1890s. European and American efforts to colonize and explore the far reaches of the globe brought whites face-to-face with darker-skinned peoples, whom scholars in the new discipline of anthropology studied and classified. The "New Immigration" from Eastern Europe raised concerns about conferring citizenship on non-Anglos, such as Russian Jews, Poles, and Italians. Persistent violence along the U.S.–Mexican border, combined with the resistance of Indians and African Americans to the authority of white people, alarmed local and federal officials. Theories of "racial difference" were used to justify attempts to subordinate these groups, by violence if necessary.

Identification of racial categories pervaded the nation's popular, political, and legal cultures. Scientists filled scholarly journals and books with "evidence" of the superiority of the "white race," citing the size and weight of bones of various groups and comparing blacks and Jews in the United States with each other and with Eskimos in Greenland and Tapuyan Indians in Brazil. Based on poor science, this scholarship revealed the researchers' fascination with factors irrelevant to intelligence, such as the size of the skull and jaw projection. First published in 1895, the *Encyclopedia Britannica* listed the physical characteristics that allegedly distinguished the races from each other, including jaw projection and facial angles. Most people did not read these highly technical reports, but images in advertising and other forms of popular culture portrayed blacks and Asians as inferior, servile people.

In the South, the doctrine of white supremacy had disastrous consequences for African Americans. Beginning with Mississippi in 1890, over the next 20 years, white Democrats in all the southern states met in state constitutional conventions and imposed restrictions on the voting rights of African American men, using a variety of means: literacy requirements, poll taxes (fees that people had to pay to vote), and "grandfather clauses." These last measures stipulated that only men whose grandfathers had been eligible to vote before ratification of the Fifteenth Amendment could vote themselves. In some instances, the literacy requirements and poll taxes disenfranchised poor white men as well.

In 1896 the Supreme Court put its stamp of approval on segregated schools, trains, and streetcars in its *Plessy v. Ferguson* opinion. Four years earlier in New Orleans, a black man named Homer Plessy had refused to sit in a segregated railroad car. By a seven-to-one majority, the Supreme Court ruled that states could exercise "reasonable" authority by segregating public accommodations. Such Jim Crow laws, according to the court, did "not necessarily imply the inferiority of either race." Justice John Marshall Harlan dissented from the majority view, pointing out the obvious: "The white race deems itself to be the dominant race," a view that conflicted with the "colorblind" U.S. Constitution.

Between 1882 and 1901, more than 100 people, most of them black men, were lynched every year in the United States; the year 1892 set a record of 230 deaths. In the South, lynch mobs targeted black men and women who refused to subordinate themselves to whites. In 1892 a black woman born in slavery, newspaper editor Ida B. Wells, incurred the wrath of whites in her native Memphis when she condemned the killings of three black men. They had operated a Memphis store, the People's Cooperative Grocery Store, which competed for black customers with a nearby white-owned establishment. While defending their store from a mob of whites, the three men were lynched, their bodies mutilated. In the words of a friend, "They were succeeding too well. They were guilty of no crime but that."

Many black men victimized by lynch mobs were falsely accused of raping white women. In her newspaper *Free Speech,* Wells charged (correctly) that accusations of rape were merely a pretext for the murder of black men. The southern white man, wrote Wells, "had never gotten over his resentment that the Negro was no longer his plaything, his servant, and his source of income." Death threats forced the editor to move north.

In Wilmington, North Carolina, in November 1898 whites again attacked assertive black men and women, those "out of their place," especially professionals and property owners. Alex Manly, an African American newspaper editor, had labeled white men "a lot of carping hypocrites." He charged that white men who exploited black women sexually felt free to call for the murder of alleged black rapists. In retaliation, a mob destroyed Manly's offices and then turned on the city's black residents, driving them into the swamps and chasing them out of town at gunpoint. At least ten blacks were killed in the violence.

Yet even in the South, racial definitions were never as clear-cut or self-evident as racists, scientific or otherwise, claimed. For example, Italians and Jews occupied a middle ground between black and white, as class issues intermingled with racial categories. In 1891 in New Orleans the lynching of a group of 11 Italian prisoners accused of conspiring to murder the city's chief of police met with no public outcry. Instead, a local newspaper condemned the "lawless passions" and "the cutthroat practices" that it claimed were characteristic of all Italian immigrants. However, the Italian government protested loudly against the incident. Armed conflict between the two nations was averted only when the United States agreed to compensate the victims' families.

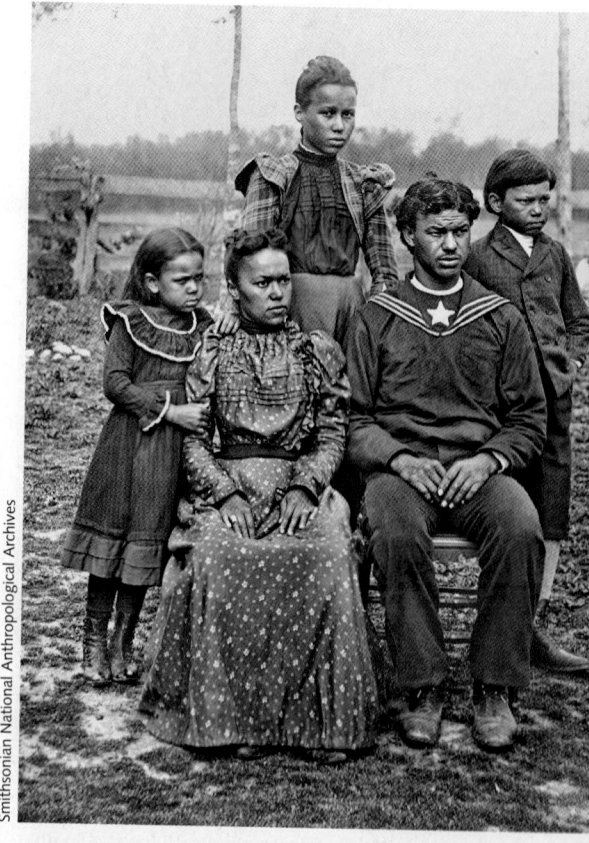

Smithsonian National Anthropological Archives

■ A middle-class Powhatan Indian family in Virginia poses for the camera, c. 1900. Since the seventeenth century, the Powhatans had intermarried with the Nanticokes of Delaware as well as African Americans of the Mid-Atlantic region. Communities such as these defied the efforts of scientists and others to rigidly categorize people according to race.

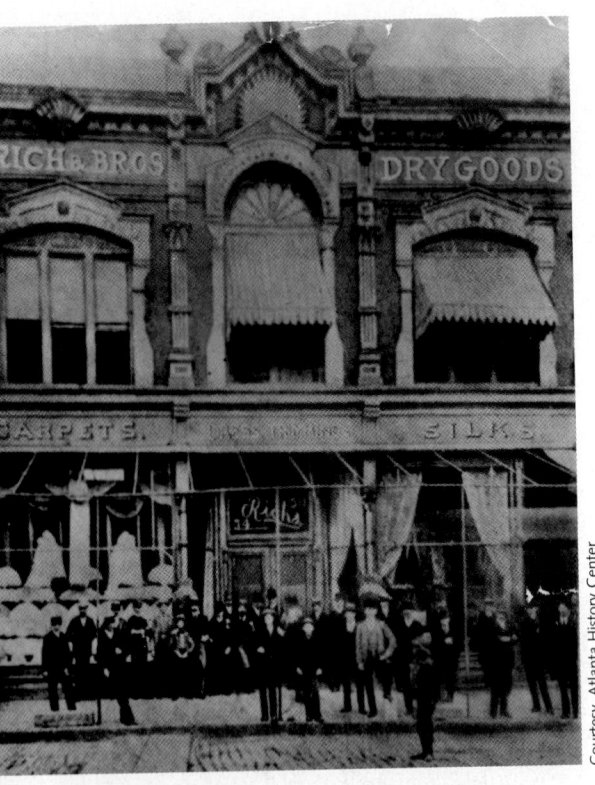

Courtesy, Atlanta History Center

■ As a region, the South lacked the ethnic diversity characteristic of the rest of the country. However, small numbers of Jewish immigrants did settle in the South, and some managed to turn modest dry goods establishments into major urban department stores. Atlanta's Rich & Brothers Dry Goods store, shown here in the 1880s, was founded and owned by Jews.

At the same time, Jewish shopkeepers and merchants in the South gained a conditional entry into the ranks of "whites." In Natchez, Mississippi, the small but prosperous Jewish community owned 45 businesses, about a third of all in the town. Merchant Simon Moses and others like him built grand, Victorian-style houses and worshipped in an imposing synagogue, Temple B'Nai Israel. However, anti-Jewish feeling manifested itself in subtle ways. Living in an overwhelmingly Protestant region of the country, many southern Jews found themselves barred from local social organizations.

A variety of organizations sought to enforce the notion of Anglo superiority in the workplace and in the courts. In 1890 the San Francisco Boot and Shoemakers' White Labor League convinced a shoe manufacturer to fire 15 Japanese workers. The 1891 lynching of the New Orleans Italian workers (deemed nonwhites) was organized by the White League, a terrorist group similar to the Ku Klux Klan. In 1893 the newly formed Immigration Restriction League launched a campaign to impose a literacy test on incoming aliens. Thus definitions of race served as political strategies to limit the power of blacks and other minorities as workers and as voters.

New Roles for Schools

Between 1890 and 1899, nearly 3.7 million immigrants entered the United States, fewer than 1.4 million of them English speakers from the United Kingdom and Ireland, compared to nearly 2.3 million non-English speakers from Germany, Italy, Austria–Hungary, and Russia. During this period, public displays of patriotism became increasingly characteristic of American life. The recitation of the Pledge of Allegiance was introduced into public classrooms and courtrooms in the 1890s.

Victorians (in England and the United States) saw formal education as a great equalizer of social groups. Moreover, many younger immigrants and the children of immigrants eagerly embraced American schooling as a means of upward mobility. However, schools did not always fulfill their promise as agents of equal opportunity for all. Increasingly, schools separated and grouped children according to their culture, religion, and class as well as race.

Reformers, missionaries, philanthropists, and government officials alike extolled the virtues of schooling tailor-made for particular groups. Presbyterian missionary women founded the Presbyterian College of the Southwest to instruct Spanish-speaking girls in both English and Protestantism. European American teachers taught young Indian women at the Cherokee Female Seminary near the Cherokee Nation capital at Tahlequah, Oklahoma.

Whether designed for Indians, Hispanics, or African Americans, boarding schools enabled teachers to exercise authority over pupils day and night. The head of Carlisle, Captain Richard Henry Pratt, expressed the school's principles this way: "I am a Baptist, because I believe in immersing the Indians in our civilization and when we get them under holding them there until they are thoroughly soaked." At the school, boys learned to make harnesses, tin pots and pans, wagons, and carriages, among other products, many of which were sold to local residents to raise money for the school. Girls took in laundry and ironed, also part of the school's money-making effort. The goal of such activities was to enable the pupils to become self-supporting upon graduation.

Indians who taught in Indian schools tried to counter the message that whites had nothing to learn from Indian culture. Born on the Yankton Sioux Reservation in Dakota Territory, Gertrude Bonnin chose the pen name Zitkala-Sa to write about her experiences as a teacher at the Carlisle school. She recounted the shame she felt when one of the white

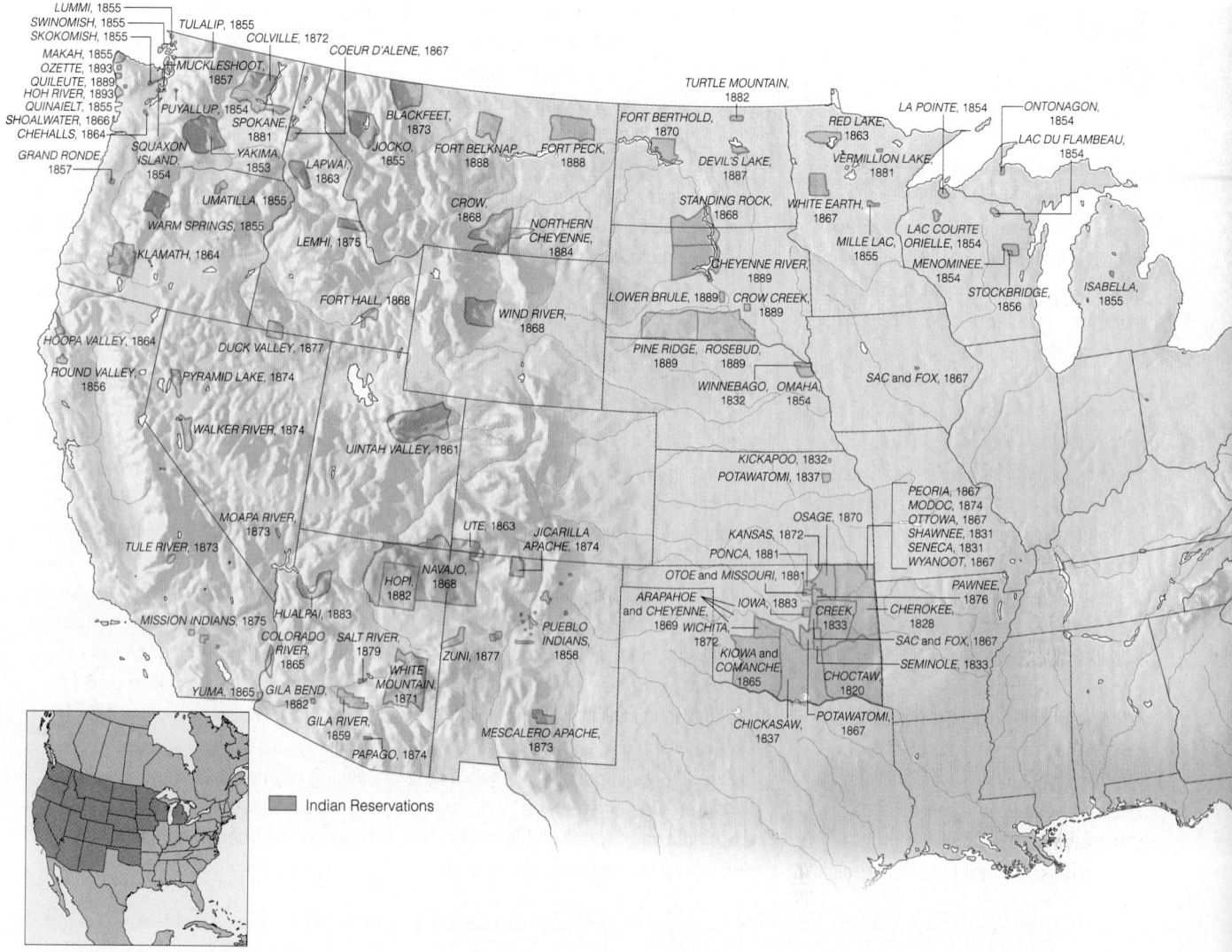

■ **MAP 18.3**

INDIAN RESERVATIONS, 1900 The Dawes Severalty Act, passed by Congress in 1887, intended to abandon the reservation system and integrate Indians into mainstream American society. Nevertheless, many reservations remained intact. As a group, Indians remained apart from European Americans. By the early twentieth century, the Indian as a "vanishing American" had become a stock character in novels and films. Yet Indian activists continued to press the cause of their people: to preserve native cultures and, at the same time, protest persistent poverty.

teachers taunted a young man by reminding him "that he was nothing but a 'government pauper.'" She lamented, "I wished my heart's burdens would turn me to unfeeling stone. But alive, in my tomb, I was destitute!"

The school as a vehicle for vocational instruction also found support among northern philanthropists concerned about education for southern black children and young people. A generation after the Civil War, the persistent poverty of many rural southern blacks convinced northern reformers that this group of Americans should be educated for a distinct form of second-class citizenship. Philanthropists, such as Julius Rosenwald of Chicago, upheld the notion of segregated public education. They created new institutions, or modified existing ones, to stress the trades and "domestic arts" at the expense of such subjects as philosophy, mathematics, and foreign languages. Embracing the "industrial education movement," the white

Systems of Education

Efforts to educate and socialize young people assume many forms. Americans have transmitted skills and moral and religious values to younger generations at home, in the workplace, at school, and through religious institutions.

America's history of religious instruction is as old and as varied as the history of the land itself. In ancient America, in what is now New Mexico, native peoples built kivas, underground ceremonial chambers. There men initiated their sons in the customs and beliefs of their society.

European settlers adhered to and adapted their own distinctive traditions. Catholics and many Protestant denominations offered religious instruction, culminating in a young person's confirmation in the church. Beginning in the 1920s, Jewish girls in reform synagogues celebrated their *bat mitzvah,* a coming-of-age ritual for 13-year-olds.

In Europe, such rituals had been reserved for boys (the *bar mitzvah*).

Much secular instruction took place within the family or workplace. Traditionally, native youth learned from their parents—the boys to hunt and fish; the girls to raise crops, process food and hides, and make garments. In the British colonies, children learned a trade, embraced Christianity, and became responsible community members by participating in a thick web of family, church, and town activities.

In the early nineteenth century, literacy assumed political significance. Southern planters feared that literate blacks would learn of the work of northern abolitionists and communicate among themselves to foment rebellion. Nat Turner's revolt in 1831, in Virginia, led many southern states and towns to crack down on clandestine black schools.

In the North at the same time, Horace Mann and other reformers were promoting tax-supported schools that would provide a "common" (i.e., standard) education for all children. The purpose of the common school system was to educate efficiently the large numbers of immigrants arriving in the United States. The result was the growth of municipal and state educational bureaucracies in the Northeast and Midwest.

Challenges to the reformers came from several quarters. Roman Catholics objected to the use of the King James version (that is, the version favored by Protestants) of the Bible in the public schools. In the early twentieth century, adherents of Progressive education criticized public school instruction as "rigidly prescribed" and "mechanical." The Progressives urged teachers to appeal to their pupils' natural sense of curiosity and love of learning.

Some formal instruction took place outside schools. For example, founded in 1891, the International Correspondence Schools of Scranton, Pennsylvania, boasted more than 2 million students by the 1920s. The schools offered mail-order lessons for land surveyors and mining engineers among others.

Meanwhile, class and racial distinctions had become institutionalized in the public school system. In 1954 trustees of the state-sponsored North Carolina Agricultural and Mechanical College (a segregated black college) voted to exclude women from the school altogether. They reasoned that "neither the girls or boys wanted to engage in the harder kinds of manual labor in the presence of the other sex, but would strive to dress up in fine clothes to impress the other."

This emphasis on vocational training evoked varied reactions from African American leaders. Born a slave in 1858, Booker T. Washington had labored in a West Virginia coal mine before attending Hampton Normal (teacher-training) and Agricultural Institute in Virginia. In 1881 he assumed the leadership of Tuskegee Institute, an Alabama school for blacks founded on the Hampton model. Speaking at the Cotton States Exposition, a fair held in Atlanta in 1895, Washington urged southern blacks to "Cast down your buckets where you are"—in other words, to concentrate on acquiring manual skills that would bring a measure of self-sufficiency to black families and communities. In the same address, Washington proposed that blacks refrain from agitating for civil rights, such as the vote. In return, whites should refrain from attacking innocent men, women, and children. Ignoring this last part of the speech, whites hailed Washington's "Atlanta Compromise" proposal as one that endorsed racial segregation and second-class citizenship for blacks. Nevertheless, in the coming years, Washington worked secretly to undermine the legal foundations of some of the white South's most cherished institutions, including segregated railroad cars and rural forced labor.

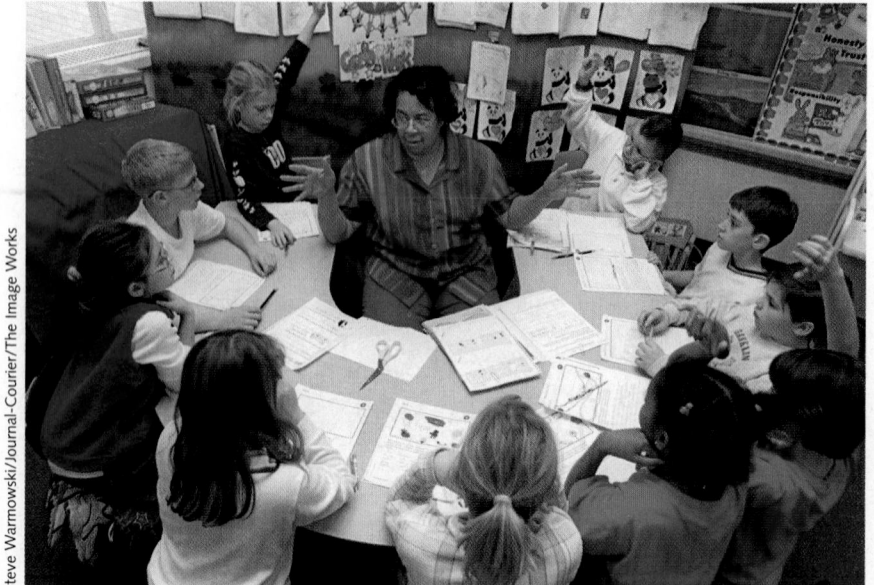

A teacher reviews a story with members of her third-grade class in a Jacksonville, Illinois, school in 2001. Throughout American history, children have received instruction in a variety of settings, not only in formal educational institutions.

the U.S. Supreme Court overturned the 1896 *Plessy v. Ferguson* decision, which had approved the segregation of black children into separate schools. In the 1980s, some poor school districts began to challenge the local property tax as a method of funding public education. Schools in their communities lacked the small class sizes and other advantages enjoyed by their affluent suburban counterparts.

In the early twenty-first century, self-proclaimed education reformers began promoting statewide standardized tests as the key to high-quality instruction. Advocates argued that tests, such as the Massachusetts Comprehensive Assessment System, administered to all fourth, eighth, and tenth graders each year, would monitor pupils' progress and hold teachers and principals accountable for the work they did. By this time, home schooling had undergone a resurgence. Some parents believed that the home was a superior learning environment, especially compared with that of large public schools. ■

Challenging Washington's message, scholar-activist W. E. B. DuBois ridiculed the notion that blacks should be content to become maids, carpenters, and sharecroppers. Similarly, in 1896, John Hope, a young professor at Roger Williams University in Nashville, Tennessee, and future president of Morehouse College and later Atlanta University, renounced Washington's apparent accommodationist stance: "If we are not striving for equality, in heaven's name for what are we living?" he demanded. "Rise, Brothers! Come let us possess this land. Never say, 'Leave well enough alone.'"

Some immigrant groups, responding specifically to the Protestant agenda of most public school systems, preferred to sponsor their own schools. In many urban areas, Roman Catholic nuns founded and staffed parochial (parish) schools that appealed to certain immigrant communities. By 1900 Catholics constituted the largest single denomination in the country, with 9 million members from diverse backgrounds. Catholic newcomers from southern and eastern Europe opposed what they claimed was the attempt by the Irish-dominated church hierarchy to "Americanize" Catholicism. One Chicago Catholic communicant, writing in the Polish-language paper *Zgodat,* charged that the effort to force Polish churchgoers to listen to and speak English was "an insult to all Polish parishes in Chicago as well as in the United States." Catholic churches and schools "built with the hard-earned money of us Polish people" should be kept under community control, he argued.

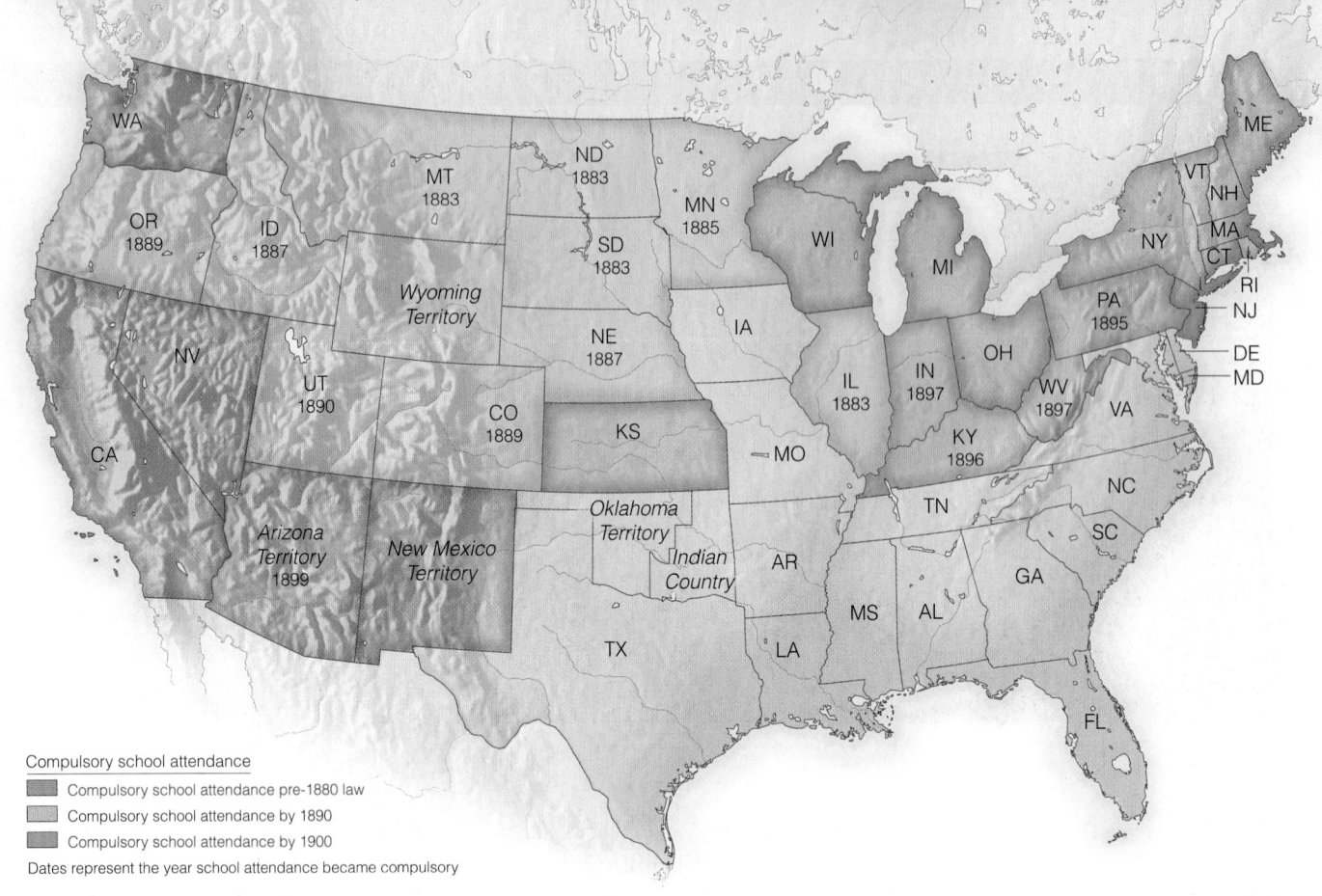

■ MAP 18.4

COMPULSORY SCHOOL ATTENDANCE LAWS, BY STATE Several northeastern, midwestern, and West Coast states enacted compulsory school attendance laws before 1880. A large number of states joined this trend in the 1880s and 1890s. By 1900 the former Confederate and border states, plus Iowa, were the only states not to have laws requiring young children to attend school for part of the year.

New forms of schooling reinforced class and cultural distinctions. No longer dependent on the income their children might earn in the workplace, late nineteenth-century urban middle-class families could allow their sons and daughters to prolong their schooling. High school came to be considered a logical extension of public schooling. Between 1890 and 1900, the number of students graduating from high school doubled, from 43,731 to 94,883.

The spread of private institutions of higher education reflected the wealth of a new industrial owner class and new forms of socialization for young people of privilege. In 1891 Central Pacific Railroad builder Leland Stanford founded Stanford University in California in honor of his recently deceased son. The previous year, Standard Oil's John D. Rockefeller established the University of Chicago.

College life was becoming associated with a particular stage of personal development, a stage marked not only by academic endeavors, but also by uniquely American group activities, such as playing with or cheering for the school football team. In 1893 an editorial in the *Nation* decried "the inordinate attention given to athletics in college" and suggested that "debt, drink, and debauchery" were the natural consequence. The writer singled out athletic scholarships and the recruitment of college baseball players by professional scouts as especially unfortunate developments. College football games had become spectacles, drawing thousands of paying spectators but also costing a great deal of money to produce and staff. The 1892 Yale University athletic budget included funds to pay for transporting the football team and its retinue of doctors, trainers, cooks, and coaches from one game to the next. The game of basketball was invented in 1891, and, soon after, many colleges formed teams that played the new sport.

Connections Between Consciousness and Behavior

In the 1890s some scholars and writers proposed that, although America's geographic frontier was closed, the "interior" frontier (of the human will and imagination) still attracted the curious. In Vienna, professor–physician Sigmund Freud pioneered the study of the human unconscious, the mysterious realm of thought and feeling that lies hidden beneath the mundane activities of everyday life. Freud's *The Interpretation of Dreams* (1900) suggested that dreams reveal the dreamer's unconscious desires and that these desires shape routine behavior.

In the United States, the new discipline of psychology owed much to the work of Harvard University professor William James. In his *Principles of Psychology* (1890), James described the human brain as an organism constantly adjusting itself to its environment; people's surroundings profoundly influence their behavior, he argued. In *The Will to Believe* (1897), he explored the psychology of religious faith. According to James, religion, science, and philosophy all have immediate relevance to the way people live their lives, and these ways of thinking and believing can cast light on social problems and their possible solutions.

Henry James, William's brother, explored the psychological dimensions of class, gender, and national identities in his short stories, plays, and literary criticism. In much of his fiction Henry James probed the consciousness of his subjects and experimented with methods of controlling points of view. Such works as *Daisy Miller* (1878), *The Wings of the Dove* (1902), *The Ambassadors* (1903), and *The Golden Bowl* (1904) reveal his intense interest in encounters between European and American elites and the clash of cultures between the two groups.

Novelist Stephen Crane combined an unflinching look at reality—a blood-soaked Civil War battlefield or the slums of New York City—with a sensitive probing of human psychology. In *The Red Badge of Courage* (1894), Crane explores the fears and self-delusions of a Union soldier, basing his account on first-hand descriptions of the fighting a generation before. By stripping the story of all ideology—northern soldiers are hardly distinguishable from southern soldiers, and political issues are never mentioned—Crane suggests that the real war was that of the combatants battling their own private demons.

> *The new discipline of psychology owed much to the work of Harvard University professor William James.*

Kate Chopin wrote about gender roles in New Orleans Creole, or French-influenced, society. Her novel *The Awakening* (1899) prompted outrage among critics. They objected to the sympathetic portrayal of the wealthy married heroine, Edna Pontellier, who anguishes over her inability to reconcile her artistic, free-spirited temperament with her roles of wife and mother. At the end of the story, she chooses to commit suicide rather than submit to a life of convention. The novel focuses on Edna's reaction to the expectations other people have of her and on her gradual awakening to the idea that she must live life—or die—on her own terms.

Psychologists and novelists were not the only people to explore the uncharted territory of the mind. Some religious leaders saw human consciousness as the key to understanding spiritual growth and development. In the late nineteenth century, the Church of Christ, Scientist, founded by Mary Baker Eddy in 1879, prospered and grew. Eddy held that physical illness was a sign of sin and that such illness could be healed by Christian faith and prayer. By linking religious life to physical health, Eddy affirmed a crucial link between belief and personal well-being. She also suggested that reality was spiritual in nature and not bounded by the material, or physical, realm. In 1892 she reorganized her Christian Science faith around a mother church in Boston. Through branch churches, the American-born sect has now spread to more than 60 countries throughout the world.

The Search for Alliances

In the 1890s, groups of Americans seemed to be estranged from each other as they never had been before. A few were enjoying the fruits of astonishing wealth, building for themselves magnificent, multimillion-dollar "summer cottages" reminiscent of glittering European palaces. In 1899 University of Chicago sociologist Thorstein Veblen coined the term *conspicuous consumption* to describe the expensive tastes of the ostentatious rich. Meanwhile, working men and women toiled long hours under dangerous conditions—when they had jobs. In 1895 the average worker was unemployed for three months of the year. Categories of race pitted various groups, native-born and immigrant, against one another. Self-styled sophisticated city folk derided the "hayseeds" on the farm.

Still, the prosperous middle class believed that certain unifying forces would connect different classes and ethnic groups. Members of the elite, including businessmen, lawyers, and other professionals, placed their faith in public schools, such cultural institutions as public museums and libraries, and the consumer impulse to instill "American" values in newcomers and the poor. The 1890s also witnessed some remarkable alliances between groups of people who had never before found common ground. Some of these alliances were tentative and temporary, others widespread and enduring. The Populist party had a profound impact on the nation's political landscape in the 1890s. And women, through their local and national organizations, helped to blend domestic concerns with politics, offering a new model of civic involvement. Their activities suggested that the boundary separating the household from the wider world had blurred.

Class Conflict

Under President Benjamin Harrison, the Fifty-First, or "Billion-Dollar," Congress earned its nickname by becoming the first body in peacetime to spend that much money on new initiatives. The Pension Act of 1890 provided pensions for all disabled men who had served in the Union army during the Civil War. By the middle of the decade, 970,000 pensioners were receiving a total of more than $135 million in cash annually. The Sherman Silver Purchase Act became law in 1890. This measure received congressional support when western interests agreed to a high tariff (tax) on a wide variety of imported goods (named the McKinley Tariff after Representative William McKinley of Ohio). In return, the federal government promised to buy a total of 4.5 million ounces of silver each month and to issue banknotes for that amount redeemable in gold or silver. As a result, Westerners paid more for home-produced manufactures, but their region benefited from the infusion of federal cash used to purchase silver mined in the West. The northeastern states, more dependent on domestic manufacturing, traditionally supported a high tariff.

The tariff was necessary to pay for the Pension Act, but the pairing of a high tariff with the purchase of silver produced explosive political and economic results. The tax on imported manufactured goods hurt consumers, and when wages did not keep pace with prices, workers revolted. Some employers exploited the vulnerability of workers in this era of rising prices. For example, in 1892 steel magnate Andrew Carnegie and his company chairman Henry Clay Frick launched an all-out assault on the Amalgamated Iron, Steel and Tin Workers, a craft union affiliated with the American Federation of Labor. Called the "aristocrats of labor," members of the Amalgamated took pride in their skills and the strength of their union. Carnegie and Frick initiated a drastic wage cut at the Carnegie Steel Company's Homestead plant, near Pittsburgh. Workers struck in June. They armed themselves with rifles and dynamite and engaged in a pitched battle with some 300 detectives from the Pinkerton agency, men hired by Frick to break the strike. (Homestead town officials had refused Frick's request to subdue the strikers.) Ten people died, and 60 were wounded. In response to the violence, the governor of Pennsylvania mobilized the state's National Guard. The troops escorted strikebreakers to work. The company cut its workforce by 25 percent and reduced the wages of the strikebreakers. All over the country, the Amalgamated Union lay in ruins. Gloated Frick, "Our victory is now complete and most gratifying."

In the West, gold, copper, and silver miners faced daunting barriers to labor organization from within and outside their ranks. Protestants harbored suspicions of Roman Catholics. Ancient hatreds prevented the Irish from cooperating with the English. European Americans disdained Mexicans and the Chinese. However, the workers in Idaho's Coeur d'Alene mines managed to overcome these animosities and strike for union recognition. In March 1892 mine owners in the region formed a "protective association" and slashed wages. When workers walked off the job, the owners imported strikebreakers from other areas of the West. The strikers retaliated by blowing up a mine with dynamite. Fifteen hundred state and federal troops arrived on the scene, and the resulting clash left seven miners dead. The troops confined 300 striking miners in bullpens, where they remained for several weeks before their trials. In this case, too, the strikers met with defeat. However, out of this conflict came a new organization, founded in Butte, Montana, in 1893: the Western Federation of Miners.

Widespread discontent over the tariff and simmering resentment on the part of debtors clamoring for unlimited coinage of silver helped unseat President Harrison in the election of 1892. The victorious Democratic candidate, Grover Cleveland, took office once more in 1893 (the only defeated president to be reelected). A new and noteworthy player in the election of 1892 was the People's (Populist) party, which nominated an old Greenback Labor party man, James B. Weaver. Weaver polled more than 1 million votes, putting both the Republicans and Democrats on notice that the Populists had the potential to swing future national elections.

The first national convention of the Populist party took place in Omaha, Nebraska, in the summer of 1892. The party had emerged from the Farmers' Alliances that had so effectively organized black and white midwestern and southern farmers in the 1880s. In the 1890s the plight of western farmers reflected the state of American agriculture in general. On the Plains, farmers incurred ever deeper debts as they bought more land and invested in expensive machinery to raise pigs, cattle, wheat, and fruit for market. But to put food on their own tables, they had to pay cash for bacon, beef, bread, and canned peaches at the store. The price of wheat had been a dollar a bushel in 1870, but it was only 35 cents 20 years later. Dakota farmers lost 15 cents on every bushel of wheat they sent to market.

As early as 1890 the Populist party was making gains in state legislatures, and a number of Populist orators were making their mark on the political scene. In Nebraska, party activist Luna Kellie explained the fine points of international finance to her listeners, denouncing foreign investors in the state economy and at the same time extolling the opening of foreign markets for the state's crops. "Stand up for Nebraska, so fertile and fair," she urged farmers.

The Populist party platform endorsed at the Omaha convention supported "free and unlimited coinage of silver and gold at the present legal

TABLE 18-1

The Election of 1892

Candidate	Political Party	Popular Vote	Electoral Vote
Grover Cleveland	Democratic	5,555,426	277
Benjamin Harrison	Republican	5,182,690	145
James B. Weaver	Populist	1,029,846	22
John Bidwell	Prohibition	264,133	

TABLE 18-2

Work Hours Needed to Produce Specified Amounts of Wheat, Corn, and Cotton, 1880 and 1900

	1880	1900
Wheat		
Work hours per acre	20	15
Yield per acre (bu)	13.2	13.9
Work hours per 100 bushels	152	108
Corn		
Work hours per acre	46	38
Yield per acre (bu)	25.6	25.9
Work hours per 100 bushels	180	147
Cotton		
Work hours per acre	119	112
Yield of lint per acre (bl)	179	191
Work hours per bale[a]	318	280

[a] Yields are five-year averages, centered on year shown. For statistical purposes, a bale of cotton is 500 pounds gross weight or 480 pounds net weight of lint. Actual bale weights vary widely.

Source: *Historical Statistics of the United States, Colonial Times to 1957* (1961) 281.

ratio of sixteen to one"; a graduated income tax; government ownership of railroad, telegraph, and telephone companies; and an end to land speculation. The delegates also condemned government subsidies to private corporations (for example, land grants to railroads) and called for the direct election of U.S. senators. Populists supported other measures designed to make the political process more open and democratic, such as provisions for voters to recall corrupt elected officials and public referenda on pressing policy issues of the day.

The Populists sought to extend their reach beyond the cotton fields of the South and the plains of the Midwest to working men and women in the nation's cities. Though separated by geography and history, farmers and wage earners could lay claim to certain common interests. The Populists' 1892 platform included resolutions sympathizing "with the efforts of organized workmen to shorten the hours of labor" to an eight-hour work day (many workers were forced to toil 12–14 hours daily) and expressing solidarity with the Knights of Labor in their struggles against "tyrannical" employers. Although the Populist platform sounded radical in comparison to its Democratic and Republican counterparts, it foreshadowed both the substance and spirit of the early-twentieth-century Progressives and the New Deal of the 1930s.

The Populists gained strength when a national depression hit in 1893. This dramatic downturn stemmed from several causes. As debtors clamored for "free silver," foreign investors in the United States became nervous, and European bankers began to call in their loans. A bubble of overbuilding and land speculation burst.

The effects of the depression were widespread. Within six months, 8000 businesses failed, throwing thousands of men and women out of work. As many as 20 percent of all workers lost their jobs. Some took to the road as tramps or hoboes to seek employment; others begged for handouts. In 1894, Jacob S. Coxey, an Ohio quarry owner, dubbed himself a "general" and mobilized his own "army" of 5000 men to march to Washington, D.C. There, the marchers protested the failure of the federal government to provide relief, now that the country was in the midst of the worst depression ever. "Coxey's Army" petitioned Congress to create extensive public works projects at the federal and local levels. However, the "army" met with an abrupt end when Coxey and his men were arrested for trampling the grass on Capitol Hill.

> *Though separated by geography and history, farmers and wage earners could lay claim to certain common interests.*

Also in 1894, Eugene V. Debs, head of the American Railway Union (ARU), inspired the union's 150,000 members to protest conditions at the Pullman Palace Car Company. Employees in the company town of Pullman near Chicago felt squeezed when Pullman cut their wages by one-third but left intact the rents on their company-owned houses. The resulting strike crippled railroads from Chicago to California. The U.S. attorney general, Richard Olney, a former attorney for the railroads, urged President Cleveland to intervene in the strike. Cleveland heeded Olney's advice, declaring that he could not stand by while the strikers interfered with the delivery of the U.S. mail. The president sent troops to quell the uprising, crushing the strike. For the first time, a federal court issued an injunction to force workers to go back to their jobs. Debs and other ARU leaders defied the order and went to jail.

To workers all over the country, the response to the Pullman strike signaled a troublesome alliance between government and big business, two powerful forces that the poor and the unemployed could not hope to counter. That alliance seemed to be solidified in 1895 when federal gold reserves fell to a dangerous low of $41 million (it was widely believed that a minimum of $100 million in gold was necessary to sustain the paper currency in circulation). Cleveland authorized the sale of government bonds for gold, but he also turned to J. P. Morgan, a Wall Street banker, for a loan. Morgan and a group of bankers agreed to lend the government $65 million, earning a $7 million commission for themselves in the process.

Judicial decisions confirmed the belief of many farmers and workers that all branches of the federal government were conspiring to favor the rich at the expense of the poor. In 1895 the Supreme Court rendered two opinions that favored big business and the wealthiest Americans. In *United States v. E.C. Knight,* the court ruled that the Sherman Anti-Trust Act of 1890

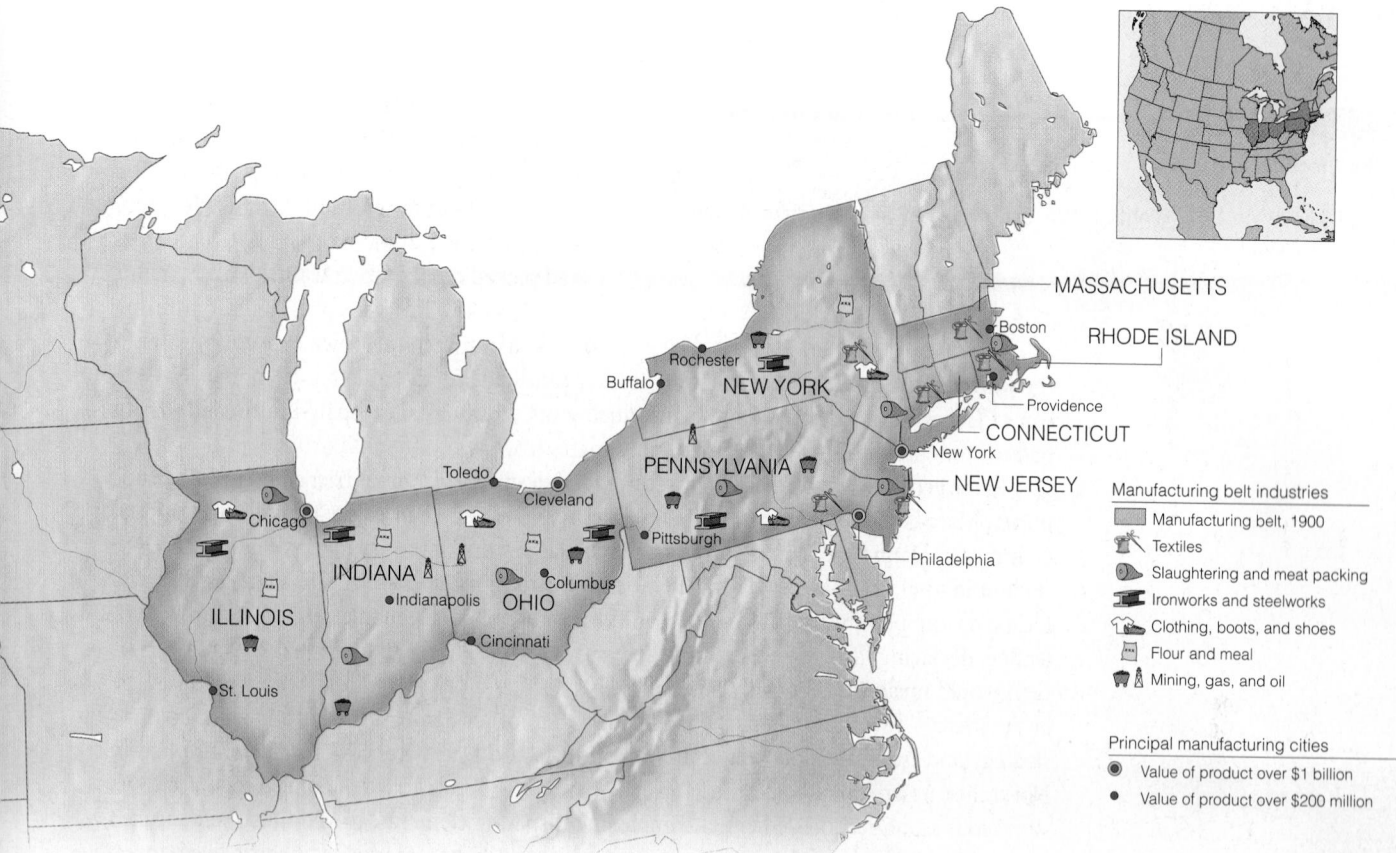

■ MAP 18.5

MANUFACTURING IN THE UNITED STATES, 1900 During the late nineteenth century, most manufacturing took place in the northeastern United States. Exceptions included flour milling in Minneapolis, the growing textile industry in the southern Piedmont, and the emergence of steel production in Birmingham, Alabama, thanks to rich local deposits of iron and coal ore.

applied only to interstate commerce and not to manufacturers. The court had decided in favor of the subject of the suit, the sugar trust that controlled 98 percent of the industry. In *Pollock v. Farmers' Loan and Trust Company,* the court struck down a modest federal income tax (2 percent on incomes over $4,000 per year). These decisions helped set the stage for the showdown between the Populists and the two major parties in 1896.

Demise of the Populists

In 1896 the Republicans nominated Congressman William McKinley of Ohio, whose name had graced the widely unpopular tariff bill of 1890. The Democrats turned their back on Cleveland, regarded as a pariah by members of his own party for his deal with Morgan and his high-handed tactics against the Pullman strikers. Without an obvious presidential candidate at their convention in Chicago in July, the Democrats seemed at loose ends. Then, out of the audience, a young man rose to address the 15,000 delegates. William Jennings Bryan, a 36-year-old Populist from Nebraska, electrified the assembly with his passionate denunciation of arrogant industrialists and indifferent politicians. The country must abandon the gold standard once and for all, he thundered: "You shall not press down upon the brow of labor this crown of thorns, you shall not crucify mankind upon a cross of gold." One awestruck listener, an alternate member of the Nebraska delegation, later said of Bryan's "Cross of Gold" speech, "There are no words in our language to picture the effect it produced upon the vast multitude which heard it." The next day, the Democrats chose Bryan as their candidate for president.

TABLE 18-3

The Election of 1896

Candidate	Political Party	Popular Vote	Electoral Vote
William McKinley	Republican	7,102,246	271
William J. Bryan	Democratic	6,492,559	176

By nominating this eloquent upstart, the Democrats took on the Populist cause of free silver. Conservative Democrats bolted the party or sat out the election. Meanwhile, some Populists were appalled that the Democrats had picked conservative Maine banker Arthur Sewall as Bryan's vice-presidential running mate. Meeting in their own convention later in the summer, the Populists chose Bryan as their candidate for president and Thomas E. Watson of Georgia for vice president. Thus, during his presidential campaign in the fall, Bryan had to contend with two different running mates from two different parties.

In the general election, McKinley received much support from his friend and political supporter, Marcus (Mark) Hanna. A wealthy iron magnate and chair of the Republican National Committee, Hanna coordinated an effort to raise large sums of money for the Republicans ($16 million in total, compared with the Democrats' $1 million). He also fueled a nationwide hysteria over the possibility that Bryan would become president, blanketing the country with leaflets declaring "In God we trust, in Bryan we bust." Hanna charged that Bryan as president would mean disaster for businessmen, bankers, and other creditors, who would now be at the mercy of working people, small farmers, and other debtors. Benefitting from Hanna's strategy and from divisions between the populists and Democrats, McKinley triumphed in November. As a national force, the People's Party rapidly disintegrated after the election of 1896.

Yet as a political movement encompassing disparate elements, the Populists left a mixed legacy. In some areas of the country, the party yielded some remarkable, if short-lived, interracial coalitions. In Grimes County, Texas, in the cotton-growing eastern part of the state, the Populist spirit survived for a few years beyond 1896. Some whites had split from the Democratic party, and some blacks had renounced their traditional allegiance to the Republican party. The alliance brought together blacks, such as school principal Morris Carrington, and whites, such as Garrett Scott, a Populist sheriff.

In the fall of 1899, the White Man's Union (WMU) emerged to oppose this biracial coalition. A member of the WMU tried to put its aims to poetry:

> Twas nature's laws that drew the lines
> Between the Anglo-Saxon and African races,
> And we, the Anglo-Saxons of Grand Old Grimes,
> Must force the African to keep his place.

The WMU made good on its vow to rid the county of "Negro rule." A November 1900 shootout at Anderson, the county seat, left Garrett Scott wounded and his brother Emmett and two other men dead. The gun battle effectively ended the Populist presence in Grimes County.

The Populists were unable to sustain a regionwide biracial coalition in the South. This failure suggests the power of white supremacist beliefs. The threat of cooperation between Republican and Populist voters was powerful, especially in such states as North Carolina. In that state, Republican–Populist fusion had captured the state legislature in 1894 and the governorship in 1896. Throughout the South, the black population was growing—a total of 10 million people in 1890 compared with 4.5 million on the eve of the Civil War. Frightened by this development, white southern Democrats campaigned to disfranchise black men, beginning in the 1890s. Landless blacks and whites would find no common political ground again until the 1930s.

Barriers to a U.S. Workers' Political Movement

In the 1890s, workers in Europe were forging new political parties to represent their interests and, in some cases, to press a bold socialist agenda, in the forum of national politics. Although late-nineteenth-century America showed dramatic evidence of bitter class conflict, it produced no viable workers' party or socialist movement. Why? The answer is not simple. Together, farmers and members of the industrial laboring classes aspired to self-sufficiency, a life free of debt that released their wives and children from unremitting toil and provided some measure of material comfort. Nevertheless, both groups found it difficult to ally with each other.

The large influx of immigrants meant that competition for even low-paying jobs remained fierce among wage-earning men and women. Employers manipulated racial, ethnic, and religious prejudices among workers to keep them estranged. Between 1890 and 1900, at least 29 major strikes—primarily in the iron, steel, coal-mining, meatpacking, railroad, and longshore industries—prompted management to employ African American strikebreakers.

White Protestant workers seized on ethnic and religious distinctions to win for themselves advantages in the workplace. Their unions excluded certain racial and ethnic groups altogether. Even somewhat egalitarian unions fell prey to racial prejudice. For example, the United Mine Workers (UMW) professed to welcome both black and white workers into its ranks. However, an 1892 report from an African American organizer in Jellico, Tennessee, stated that "the whites declare that they won't work" under an African American boss. At best, whites relegated their black and female coworkers to segregated unions and enforced a discriminatory division of labor within the workplace.

Moreover, the pace and processes of mechanization and technological development varied from job to job, making it difficult for workers in one industry to form alliances with workers in another. By 1900 the steel, shoe, and textile industries were fully mechanized. In contrast, skilled craft workers dominated the cigar, garment, and glass-blowing industries, although women machine operatives were beginning to challenge male cigarmakers. Taking pride in their craft and its traditions, skilled workers distanced themselves from those who tended machines.

Many American workers, regardless of ethnicity, religion, or industry, continued to believe that they could eventually own their own businesses; thus, they resisted casting their lot

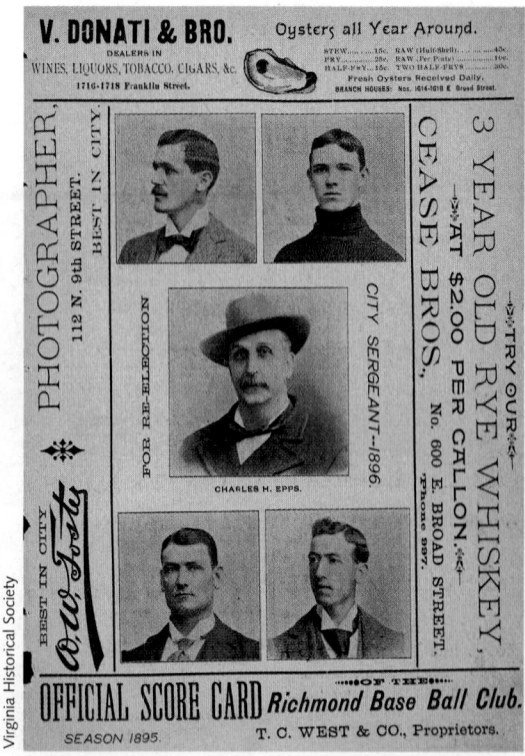

■ In 1896 Charles H. Epps, the city sergeant of Richmond, Virginia, ran for reelection. He distributed these cards to prospective voters. The cards suggest the masculine nature of politics at this time. This one doubled as a scorecard for the city's professional baseball team and carried advertisements for a local whiskey manufacturer and liquor and tobacco store.

TABLE 18-4

Categories of Employment, 1880–1910

Occupation	1880	Percentage	1890	Percentage	1900	Percentage	1910	Percentage
Agriculture, forestry, and fishing	8,705	50.1	10,170	42.8	10,920	37.6	11,590	31.6
Extractive industries	310	1.8	480	2.0	760	2.6	1,050	2.9
Manufacturing	3,170	18.2	4,750	20.0	6,340	21.8	8,230	22.4
Construction	830	4.8	1,440	6.1	1,660	5.7	2,300	6.3
Commerce and finance	1,220	7.0	1,990	8.4	2,760	9.5	3,890	10.6
Transportation and communications	860	4.9	1,530	6.4	2,100	7.2	3,190	8.7
Services	2,100	12.1	3,210	13.5	4,160	14.3	5,880	16.0
Other	195	1.1	170	0.7	370	1.3	600	1.6
Total	17,390	100	23,740	100	29,070	100	36,730	100

Numbers given in thousands.

Source: International Historical Statistics, 154.

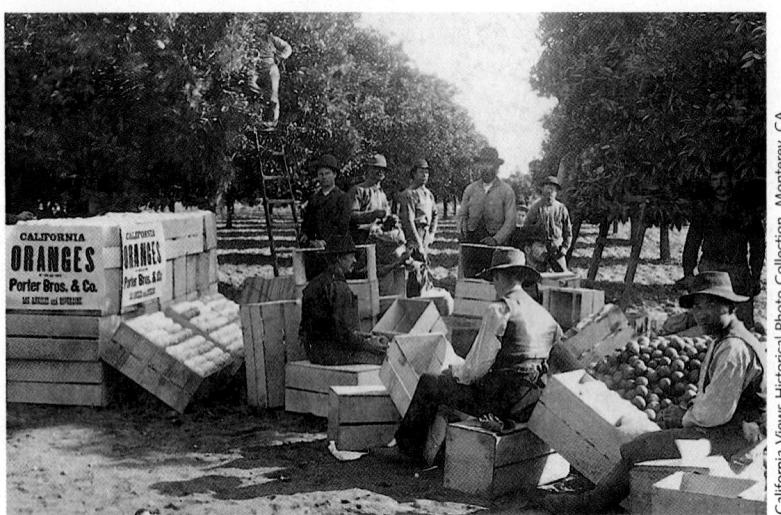

California Views Historical Photo Collection, Monterey, CA

■ The diversity of the American workforce and the American economy inhibited the development of a national workers' political party. By the 1890s, some industries were fully mechanized. Others relied on traditional forms of manual labor. In California, Asian workers faced persistent discrimination from labor unions. These immigrants are picking oranges near Santa Ana, c. 1895.

permanently with unions or other working-class organizations. High rates of geographic mobility also prevented workers from committing themselves to a particular union in a particular place. The power of antistrike forces proved daunting. Private security agencies, such as the Pinkertons, as well as state-deployed National Guard troops, backed up the authority of employers, judges, mayors, and governors. And finally, unlike European parliamentary systems, U.S. politics was based on a "winner-take-all" principle. In America, the two major parties tried to capture the political center, discouraging coalition-building among smaller parties. Such alliances might have pushed the country farther to the left or right.

These factors help to account for the success of the American Federation of Labor (AFL) in attracting and retaining members. By the end of the nineteenth century, the AFL had rejected the rhetoric of radical labor leaders in favor of organizing a select group of workers, mostly skilled white men. Leaders of AFL union affiliates denounced "cheap labor" competitors, whether women workers or Japanese or Chinese immigrants. In the coming years, the AFL would prove that it had staying power, although it represented primarily the interests of white male craftsmen.

Challenges to Traditional Gender Roles

In the 1890s the women's suffrage, club, missionary, and social settlement movements emerged as significant political forces. Nevertheless, for the most part, white women in these movements remained steadfast in their refusal to embrace their nonwhite counterparts.

In 1890 the two major national woman suffrage associations, the National Woman Suffrage Association and the American Woman Suffrage Association, merged to form the National–American Woman Suffrage Association (NAWSA). Elizabeth Cady Stanton served as the new group's first president for two years. The suffrage movement exhibited contradictory impulses. On one hand, it brought together supporters from around the country and yielded striking examples of international cooperation. Beginning in 1890 and every year thereafter until 1920, members of NAWSA branches scattered throughout the United States met in convention to debate strategy. American women consulted with their counterparts in England and western Europe to advance their cause.

On the other hand, in an effort to become "respectable," white native-born Protestant American suffragists sought to distance themselves from the poor, immigrants, African Americans, and the laboring classes within their own country. When NAWSA leaders called for an "educated franchise," they implicitly left out immigrant and poor women. They also refused to admit black women's suffrage clubs into their umbrella organization. In the process, the white women turned their backs on some of the most committed supporters of their own cause.

Identifying themselves primarily as wives and mothers, some women entered the political realm through local women's clubs. They believed that personal intellectual development and group political activity would benefit both their own families and society in general. In the 1880s, the typical club focused on self-improvement through reading history and literature. By the 1890s, many clubs had embraced political activism. They lobbied local politicians for improvements in education and social welfare and raised money for hospitals and playgrounds.

The General Federation of Women's Clubs (GFWC), founded in 1892, united 100,000 women in 500 affiliate clubs throughout the nation.

Yet the GFWC specifically excluded African American clubs. Black women formed their own national federation, the National Association of Colored Women (NACW), in 1896. Through club work, they spoke out against lynch mobs and segregationists and worked to improve their local communities. In 1899 the first president of NACW, Mary Church Terrell, appeared before a mostly white organization, the National Congress of Mothers. She minced no words in contrasting the resources available to white mothers and children with the inferior medical care afforded their African American counterparts. Declared Terrell, "So rough does the way of her infant appear to many a poor black mother that instead of thrilling with the joy which you feel, as you clasp your little ones to your breast, she trembles with apprehension and despair."

In some areas of the country, black and white women did make common cause—to further the goals of temperance, for example—although white women embraced these alliances uneasily. At the end of the century, black women in North Carolina sought to circumvent the sometimes violent political realm dominated by white men. They worked with middle-class white women through voluntary organizations, such as the Young Women's Christian Association and the Women's Christian Temperance Union.

In the West, Protestant-sponsored "mission homes" ministered to women in need. The San Francisco Presbyterian Chinese Mission Home offered a safe haven for Chinese women fleeing abuse and exploitation. In 1898 a young Chinese woman, Lee Yow Chun, appeared before a government official and testified to the poverty of her family in Hong Kong and to the web of deception that had led to her arrival in the United States as a prostitute. Encountering an immigration official in San Francisco, Lee "fell in a lump on the floor and cried loudly, saying I did not want to be landed by those people [who had tricked her]; that I would jump into the sea rather than be taken by them." As a result, she was allowed to go to the mission home. In response to stories such as Lee's, eastern women opened their pocketbooks to further not only the San Francisco mission but also shelters for unwed mothers and abused girls in other cities, in the name of virtuous womanhood.

The daily operations of the settlement house reflected the priorities of its founders.

Religious beliefs inspired some women to go beyond national boundaries in their efforts to reach out to like-minded people. In the 1880s and 1890s, a group of American women participated in an interdenominational, international campaign to support the work of Pandita Ramabai, a native of India who had converted to Christianity and worked to challenge the subordinate role of women in her own country. In 1890 almost 60 "Ramabai Circles" claimed more than 4000 members in the United States and Canada. Ramabai chose not to ally herself with the growing Indian nationalist movement (in opposition to Great Britain, the colonial power that ruled India); in her view, Christianity, not nation-state loyalties, should shape the identities of both men and women.

Social settlements were unique institutions, founded and staffed by well-educated women, many of whom had attended elite women's colleges. The daily operations of the settlement house reflected the priorities of its founders, who often brought activists, public health officials, journalists, and laboring men and women together around the dinner table to discuss problems of the poor. Settlement house workers hoped to instill in poor women the values of domesticity and pride in American citizenship. By 1900 more than 200 social settlement houses were helping to acculturate immigrants by offering classes in a variety of subjects, including English, health, and personal hygiene. In 1893 the women social workers of Hull House successfully lobbied Illinois state legislators for the passage of anti-sweatshop legislation that would protect female employees and prohibit child labor. Florence Kelley, who served for three decades as the general secretary of the National Consumer League, was a resident of Hull House in the early 1890s. In 1899 she moved to New York's Henry Street Settlement (founded by a nurse named Lillian Wald in 1893). The settlement's neighbors included the 500,000 people packed into the Lower East Side, many of them from Italy, Russia, Germany, Greece, and Hungary.

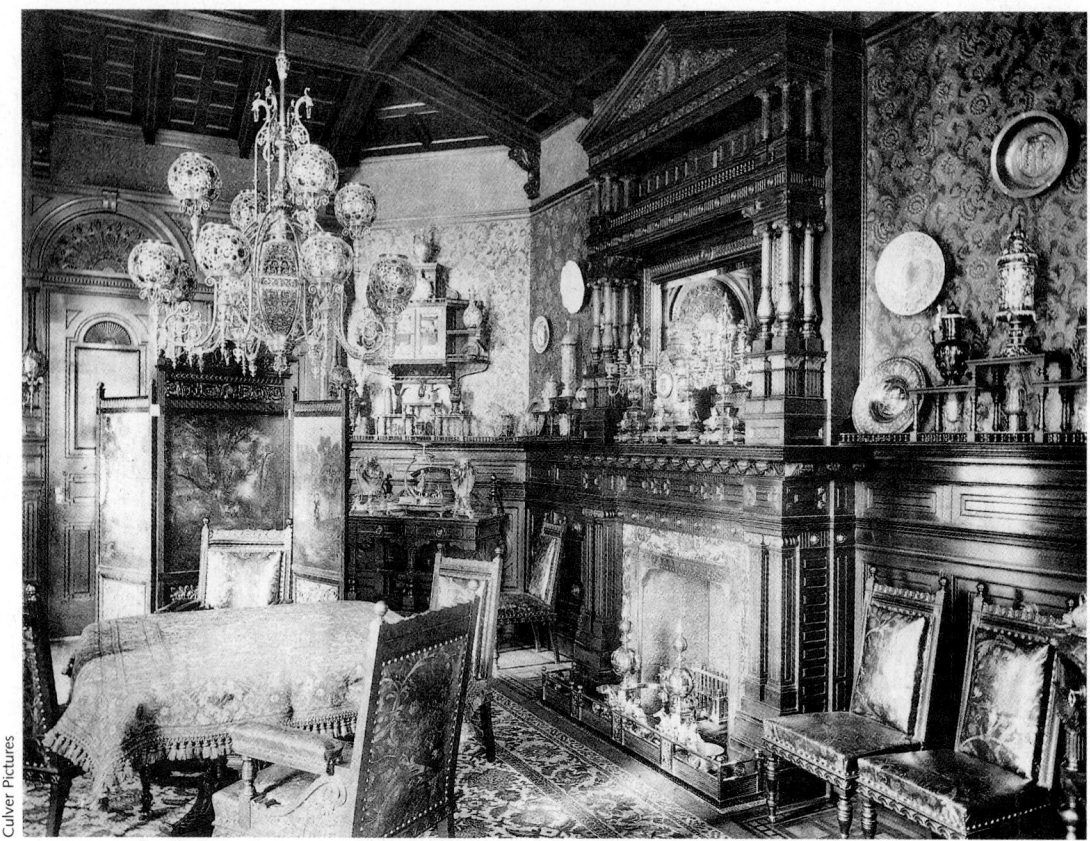

Culver Pictures

■ To the modern eye, the Victorian parlor looks cluttered. Yet to late-nineteenth-century middle-class people, the parlor was a place to display possessions that testified to their comfortable way of life. Books, family photographs, and musical instruments had great social and symbolic value. Families gathered to read aloud, pore over photo albums, and sing old favorites. Some men, worried that their opportunities for "manly" activity were vanishing with the western frontier, considered parlors to be female spaces.

Although often associated with immigrants in the largest cities, settlement houses reached diverse populations. In the late 1890s, a coalition of the Kentucky Federation of Women's Clubs and other organizations sponsored several teachers who organized a summer settlement called Camp Cedar Grove in the eastern part of the state. This venture provided the foundation for the Hindman Settlement School. The school, still in existence, initially aimed to acculturate mountain people to middle-class ways in dress, eating habits, and manners and to preserve traditional mountain music and crafts.

Sensitive to the racial prejudices of their clients and their neighbors, most early settlements failed to reach out to African Americans. This policy stimulated the development of black-led settlements, such as the Phyllis Wheatley Settlement in Minneapolis and the Neighborhood Union in Atlanta. Founded by Lugenia Burns Hope in 1908, the Neighborhood Union aimed "to bring about a better understanding between the races."

In the tradition of Frances Wright and Victoria Woodhull, some women challenged traditional gender relations that relegated women to dependence on men. Emma Goldman, a Russian immigrant and self-proclaimed anarchist, paired the sexual liberation of women with the rights of workers to live a decent life. A radical by any measure, Goldman was, nevertheless, not alone in rejecting the idea that marriage should always be permanent. Between 1890 and 1900, the divorce rate increased from 1 out of every 17 new marriages to 1 out of 12. More and more couples, middle-class and working-class, native-born and immigrant, were seeking means to dissolve marriages that had failed.

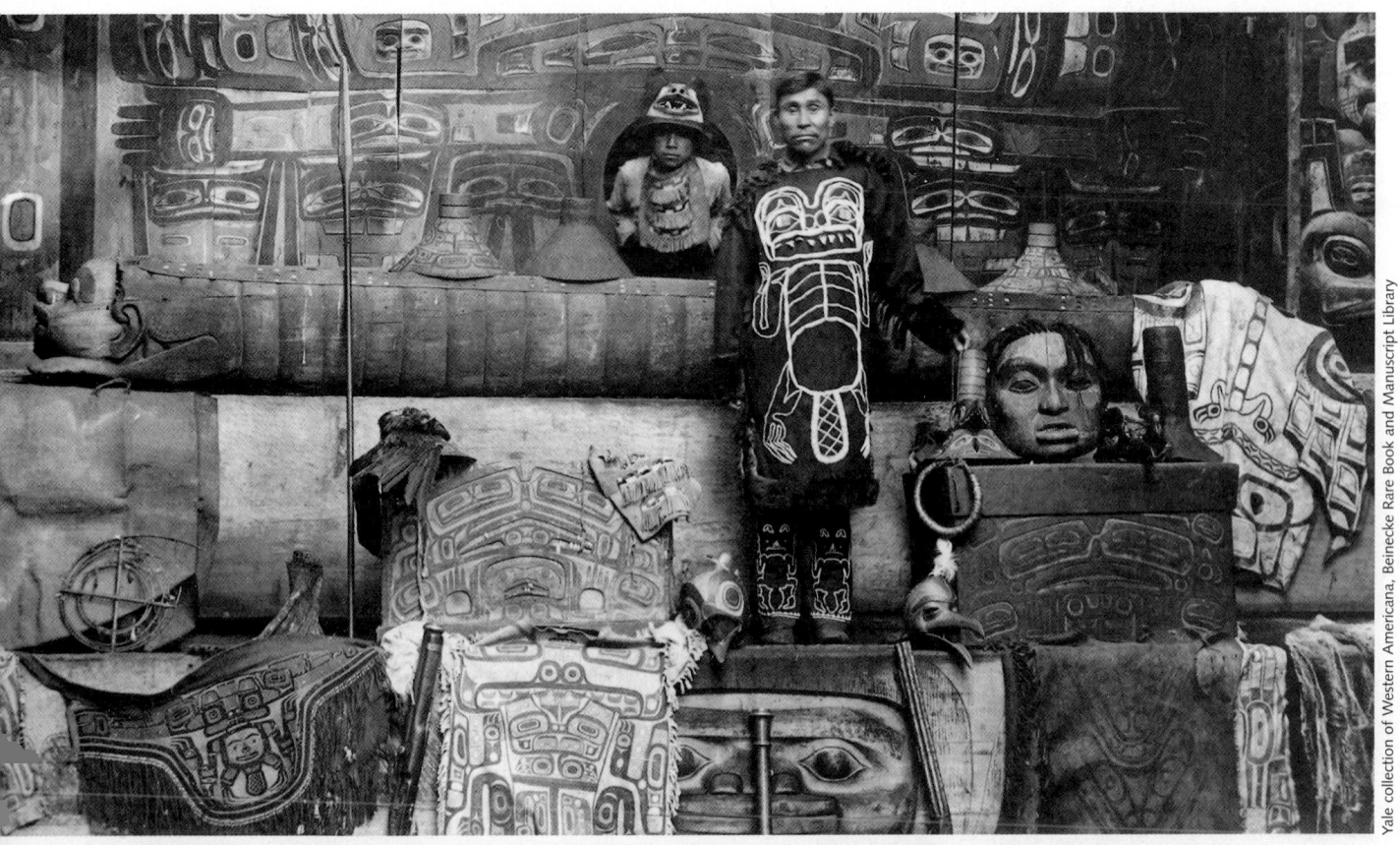

■ This interior of a Tlingit Indian chief's house in Chilkat, Alaska, c. 1900, suggests that the Victorians were not the only group of people to arrange crowded displays of art and other cultural artifacts in central living spaces. Indians of the Northwest coast enjoyed an abundance of marine foods. They had time to devote to making intricate wood carvings in the form of masks and totem poles. Social status was based on inheritable wealth, as revealed by works of art and other material goods.

Charlotte Perkins Gilman was among the most prolific and well-known critics of the conventional division of labor in the home. Through fiction, nonfiction, and poetry, she claimed that humankind had progressed beyond the point where brute strength was the determinant of social status. Gilman proclaimed that women, no longer content to remain dependent on men, must take their rightful place within the economy, working as equals with their brothers and husbands. In *Women and Economics: A Study of the Economic Relations Between Men and Woman as a Factor in Social Evolution* (1898), she proposed that housework be divided into its specialized tasks to be performed by professionals. This system would free women from the unpaid, mind-numbing task of combined "cook–nurse–laundress–chambermaid–housekeeper–waitress–governor." In her critique of gender conventions, Gilman anticipated the feminist movement of the 1960s.

Men also pondered the effects of industrializing society on their own roles. Some elite men revolted against the trappings of Victorian culture. These men worked every day in business offices, not out of doors. Some yearned for "manly" activities such as courageous exploits against nature or other men. They believed that overstuffed parlors represented "feminine" interiors. Life indoors—singing religious hymns around the piano or reading aloud to family members—stifled men's "natural" instincts for bravery and adventure, they claimed. They yearned to embrace the outdoors and prove their masculinity in the process. As assistant secretary of the Navy in the late 1890s, Theodore Roosevelt worried that, in this age of machines, young men lacked the opportunities for "the strenuous life" their grandfathers had enjoyed. He argued that unapologetic masculine bravado provided the key to American strength and rejuvenation on both a national and personal level. In his multivolume history, *The Winning of the West* (1889–96), Roosevelt extolled America's relentless march to the Pacific: "The rude, fierce settler who drives the savage from the land lays all civilized mankind under a debt to him." Imperialism at home and abroad, he declared, was a "race-important work," one that should claim the energies of men as politicians and soldiers.

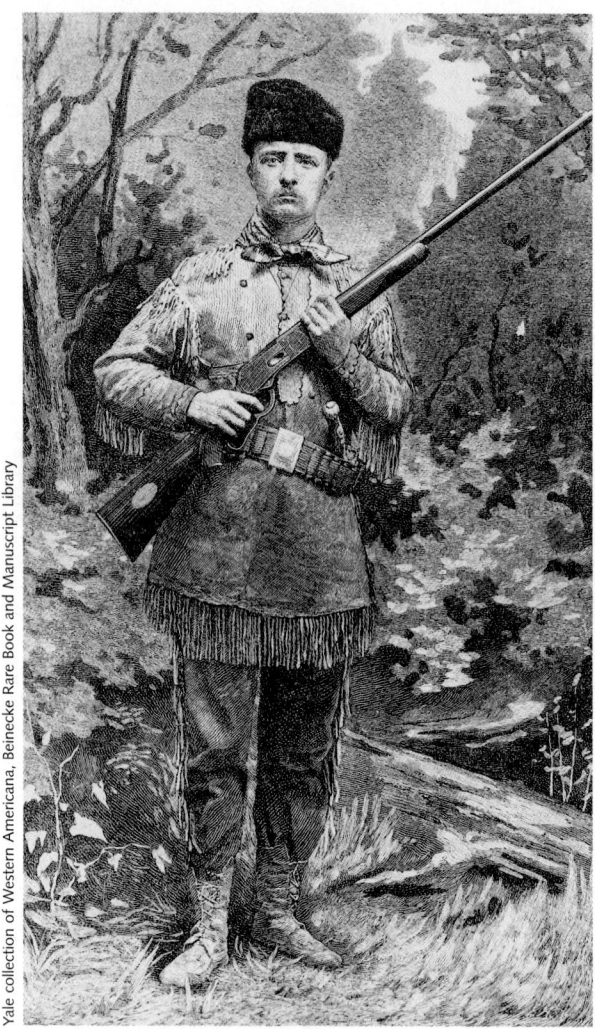

Yale collection of Western Americana, Beinecke Rare Book and Manuscript Library

■ Crushed when his mother and wife both died on the same day in 1884, Theodore Roosevelt abandoned New York politics and spent several years ranching in South Dakota and hunting in Montana. This photo served as the frontispiece for Roosevelt's 1897 book, *Hunting Trips of a Ranchman*. TR believed that the West promoted "the qualities of hardihood, self-reliance, and resolution." In 1886 he returned to New York City and resumed his political career.

American Imperialism

In the 1890s the United States began to extend its political reach and its economic dominance to other parts of the world. Americans looked beyond their borders and saw exotic peoples who represented a variety of opportunities—as consumers of American goods, producers of goods Americans wanted to buy, and objects of American benevolence. This view represented an extension of the reform impulse at home. Indeed, broader thinking about the United States' place in the world reflected a new desire among those who benefited from prosperity to spread American standards—in behavior, productivity, and quality of life—to other peoples.

The country's mighty industrial manufacturing sector demanded new markets and a wider consumer base. The depression of 1893, in particular, raised fears that manufacturers would have to contend with surpluses of goods that Americans could not afford to buy. American businesspeople and state department officials established a partnership that combined private economic self-interest with national military considerations. Some molders of public opinion used the new languages of race and masculine virility to justify an "Anglo-Saxon" mission of conquest of "childlike" peoples. Meanwhile, European countries were carving up Africa and making economic inroads into China. Many Americans believed their own country should join the "race" for riches and "march" to glory as part of the international competition to exploit the natural resources and trade potential of weaker countries.

Cultural Encounters with the Exotic

In early October 1897, 30,000 spectators paid their 25-cent fee to enter New York's Excursion Wharf and observe the strange cargo of the recently arrived steamship *Hope*. Arctic explorer Robert Peary had returned from Greenland, bringing with him six Greenland Eskimos and a 37.5-ton meteorite dislodged from the Cape York region. Among the native Greenlanders were Qisuk and his seven-year old son, Minik. The American public hailed the intrepid explorer Peary as a hero. The American Museum of Natural History put the Eskimos on display, and New Yorkers regarded their odd clothing, language, and eating habits with intense curiosity. But their curiosity was only superficial and did not extend to protection for the young Minik.

Over the next year, four of the Eskimos (including Qisuk) died, and one other returned to his native land. The orphaned Minik survived and remained in the United States. Within a few years, he was abandoned by Peary and museum officials who had initially touted him as a significant scientific discovery. Minik returned to Greenland when he was a young man, but he was restless and unhappy there. He returned to the United States in 1916, eventually finding some peace with a New Hampshire farm family. He died in 1918, a victim of a worldwide flu epidemic.

Minik's short, tragic life reveals certain aspects of Americans' encounter with "exotic" peoples in the late nineteenth century. The Museum of Natural History subjected him and the other members of his group to close study. When Qisuk died, the museum conducted a mock burial for the benefit of his son but then created a public exhibit of Qisuk's bones. (Nearly 100 years later, the passage of the Native American Grave and Burial Protection Act provided an incentive for museum authorities to send the remains of the four Eskimos back to Greenland for burial.)

During the late nineteenth century, Americans were fascinated by artifacts and images dealing with far-away places, especially Africa, the Middle East, and Asia. This impulse, revealed in high art as well as popular culture, stereotyped darker-skinned, non-Christian peoples as primitive, sensual, and inscrutable. Chicago's Columbian Exposition of 1893 featured exhibits depicting harems, spice merchants, and turbaned warriors and performances of "hootchy kootchy dancers," scantily clothed young women writhing to the music of exotic instruments.

Throughout the late nineteenth century, photographers took pictures of Middle Eastern nomads and African villagers. American artists, such as Frederic Edwin Church and John Singer Sargent, traveled abroad to render romantic scenes of deserts, ancient ruins, and mysterious peoples in oils and in watercolors. Painter Eric Pape arranged to have himself tied to a pyramid so that he could partake of an "Egyptian experience"; he produced a painting called *Site of Ancient Memphis* in 1891.

These cultural tendencies could be used to sell products and entertainment. The glassmaker–jeweler Tiffany and Co. evoked Islamic art in its tea services and silver patterns. Tobacco companies marketed mass-produced cigarettes with "Oriental" brand names: "Fatima," "Omar," and "Camel." Thus, a fascination with the exotic encompassed a wide range of impulses in American life and letters, bringing together explorers, scientists, artists, and advertising agents.

Initial Imperialist Ventures

The opening of Asia to American trade, combined with the military challenges posed by the major European imperial powers, stimulated the growth of the U.S. Navy in the 1880s. In 1883, Congress appropriated funds to build 90 small ships, one-third made of wood, the rest out of steel. Seven years later, Captain Alfred Thayer Mahan argued for a modern force of large seagoing battleships. In his book *The Influence of Sea-Power in History, 1660–1763* (1890), Mahan contended that if the United States aspired to be a world power, it must control the seas.

Seeking way stations for its ships, the United States negotiated control over both Pearl Harbor in Hawaii and the harbor at Pago Pago in Samoa in 1887. The state department even achieved a voice in Samoan foreign relations to stave off rivals Great Britain and Germany, which also coveted Pago Pago. In 1889 warships of these three powers gathered in the Samoan harbor. Fortunately, a hurricane thwarted a showdown. The powers, unnerved by their near brush with war, agreed to establish joint control over the islands for the next ten years.

In October 1890, Secretary of State James G. Blaine hosted the first Pan-American Conference in Washington, D.C. a gathering of representatives from 19 independent Latin American republics. Topics included the adaptation of standardized weights and measures for all participants in the conference and a possible intercontinental railroad. These developments suggested the blurring of military, diplomatic, strategic, and economic interests—a mix that characterized American foreign policy for decades to come.

In 1895 the United States signaled to Great Britain that it was prepared to go to war to bar Europeans from colonizing or intervening in the Americas, a policy outlined in the Monroe

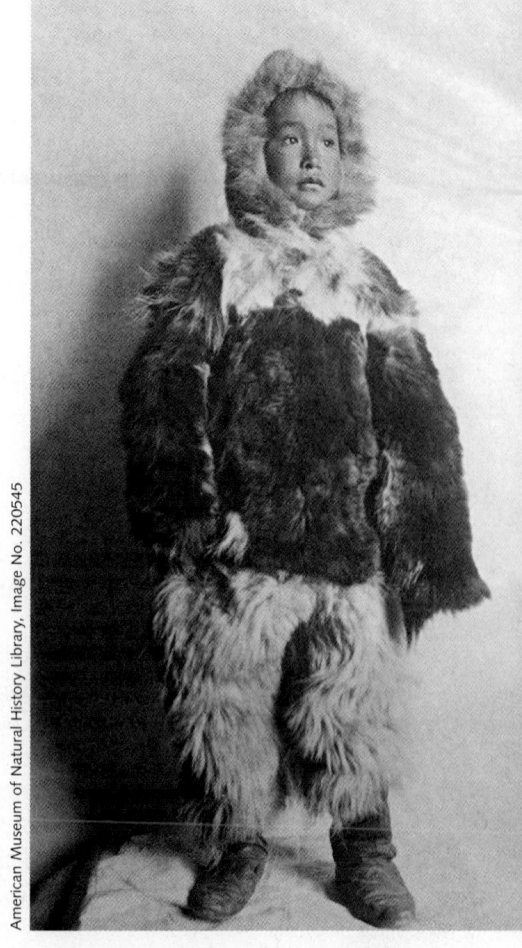

American Museum of Natural History Library, Image No. 220545

■ The Greenland Eskimo Minik is shown here soon after his arrival in New York City in 1897. Minik was devastated by the death of his widowed father, Qisuk; the two were among six Eskimos brought to New York by Arctic explorer Robert E. Peary. Later in his life, Minik spoke of his father to a newspaper reporter, saying, "He was dearer to me than anything else in the world, especially when we were brought to New York, strangers in a strange land."

Doctrine more than 70 years before. Britain had persisted in its long-standing claims to the jungle boundary between its colony of British Guiana and the country of Venezuela on the north central coast of South America. President Cleveland made clear his intention to enforce the Monroe Doctrine. Britain, sensitive to other threats posed by European imperial powers on the far-flung British empire, backed down. Thereafter, Britain began to concentrate on strengthening its diplomatic ties with the United States.

Meanwhile, in the South Pacific, the Hawaiian Islands seemed to pose both a threat and an opportunity for American interests. Located 2000 miles from the California coast, Hawaii had a population of 150,000 in 1890. When English explorer James Cook had landed there in 1778, the islands were inhabited exclusively by the descendants of ancient seafaring Polynesians. Protestant missionaries began to arrive in 1820, and the first sugar plantation appeared 15 years later. In 1875 sugar planters and merchants, many of whom were related to missionaries, negotiated a treaty with the United States that let them ship the crop to the United States duty-free. Production of Hawaiian sugar increased from less than 10,000 tons in 1870 to 300,000 tons 30 years later.

In 1895 the United States signaled to Great Britain that it was prepared to go to war to bar Europeans from colonizing or intervening in the Americas.

By this time, the Chinese, Koreans, Filipinos, Puerto Ricans, the Japanese, and the Portuguese had made their way to the Hawaiian Islands. These groups formed the bulk of the plantation labor force, for disease had decimated the native population. In the fields and in their barracks, immigrant contract workers followed a disciplined regimen under the supervision of mounted, whip-wielding overseers called *lunas*. Indeed, these laborers' workday bore a marked resemblance to that of sharecroppers on the largest cotton plantations of the U.S. South.

Not surprisingly, both clergy and growers were alarmed by the laborers' resistance to regimentation in the fields and in the quarters. Some men and women workers drank on Saturday night, smoked opium, and gambled. Worse, in the eyes of their employers, many grabbed any opportunity to flee the plantation in search of jobs as wage earners or shopkeepers in the city of Honolulu. Some even became rice farmers on their own. Planters were forced to suspend operations to accommodate traditional festivals, such as the Chinese New Year, when workers decorated their barracks and cottages with colorful flags and lanterns. Missionaries and sugar planters alike hoped to transform the workers into more stable, predictable employees.

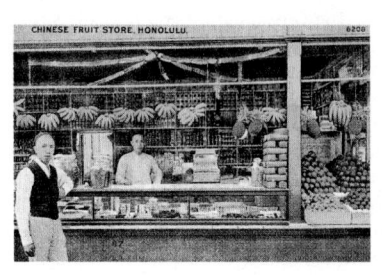

The McKinley Tariff of 1890 raised duties on imports of the islands' sugar. This served to overturn the 1875 pro-planter treaty, causing planters (mostly Americans) to panic about their livelihood. They received no support from the islands' native leader, Queen Liliuokalani, who believed foreigners should be barred from running the country. In 1893 the planters, backed by American Marines, launched a successful revolt that deposed the queen. They then called for the United States to annex the islands as a territory. Upon investigation, President Cleveland discovered that native Hawaiians opposed annexation and so refused to agree to the move. His refusal incurred the wrath of American imperialists, who claimed that the "Hawaiian pear" had been "ripe for the plucking."

The Spanish–American–Cuban–Filipino War of 1898

In the Caribbean, Cuban nationalists staged an uprising against the Spanish in 1895. The leader of the insurrection was José Julian Martí. He had lived in exile in the United States from 1881 to 1895. Rebelling against the repressive Spanish colonialists who had ruled the island for more than 400 years, native *insurrectos* under the leadership of Martí burned crops of sugar cane and attacked passenger trains. American companies with large investments in the Cuban sugar industry (a total of about $50 million) were outraged at the destruction of their property; they had no sympathy for the *insurrectos*. Yet the arrival of Spanish military officials, who herded the rebels into barbed-wire concentration camps, inflamed public opinion in the United States. Both businesspeople and humanitarians urged McKinley to intervene in Cuba.

Two American newspaper publishers, William R. Hearst and Joseph Pulitzer, seized the chance to boost their respective circulations by highlighting Spanish atrocities against Cubans. Pulitzer owned the St. Louis *Post Dispatch* and the *New York World,* and Hearst challenged him with the *San Francisco Examiner* and the *New York Journal.* On February 9, 1898, Hearst published a letter written by the Spanish minister in Washington, D.C. Dupuy de Lôme, in which de Lôme denounced President McKinley as a spineless politician. Six days later, the American battleship *Maine,* which had been sent to Havana harbor to evacuate Americans should the need arise, exploded and sank. Two hundred sixty officers and men were killed. Subsequent investigations concluded that the heat from one of the coal bins had ignited an adjacent powder magazine. But the Hearst papers implied that the Spanish were responsible for the blast.

Attempting to expand their readership, the Hearst and Pulitzer newspapers engaged in "yellow journalism": sensational news reporting that blurred the line between fact and fiction, spontaneous reality and staged theater. War sold papers. During the crisis in Cuba, the *Journal* was selling at a rate of a million copies a day.

McKinley responded to American businesspeople who feared for their interests in Cuba and to other Americans who decried Spain's brutality toward the *insurrectos.* On April 11, 1898, McKinley called on Congress to declare a U.S. war against Spain. His own assistant secretary of the Navy, Theodore Roosevelt, had reportedly called the president a "white-livered" poor excuse for a man. To Roosevelt and other pro-warriors, much was at stake: the large American sugar investment, trade with the island, and American power and influence in the Western Hemisphere. Congress responded to McKinley's message by adopting the Teller Amendment, which declared that the United States would guarantee Cuba its independence once the Spanish were driven from the island. America went to war on April 29.

McKinley hoped to hobble the Spanish navy by making a preemptive attack on the fleet in the Philippines. Commodore George Dewey, stationed with the American Asiatic Squadron in Hong Kong, was dispatched with his ships to Manila Bay, where on May 1, 1898, his force of four battleships sank all ten rickety Spanish vessels, killing 400, with only a few minor American casualties.

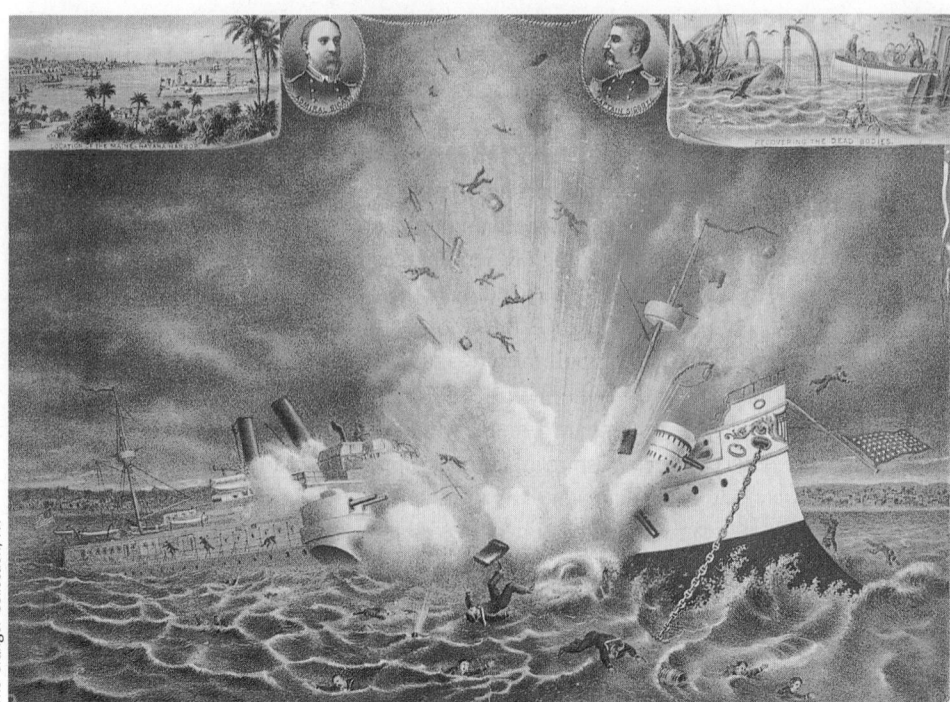

■ The battleship *Maine* exploded and sank in Havana harbor on February 15, 1898.

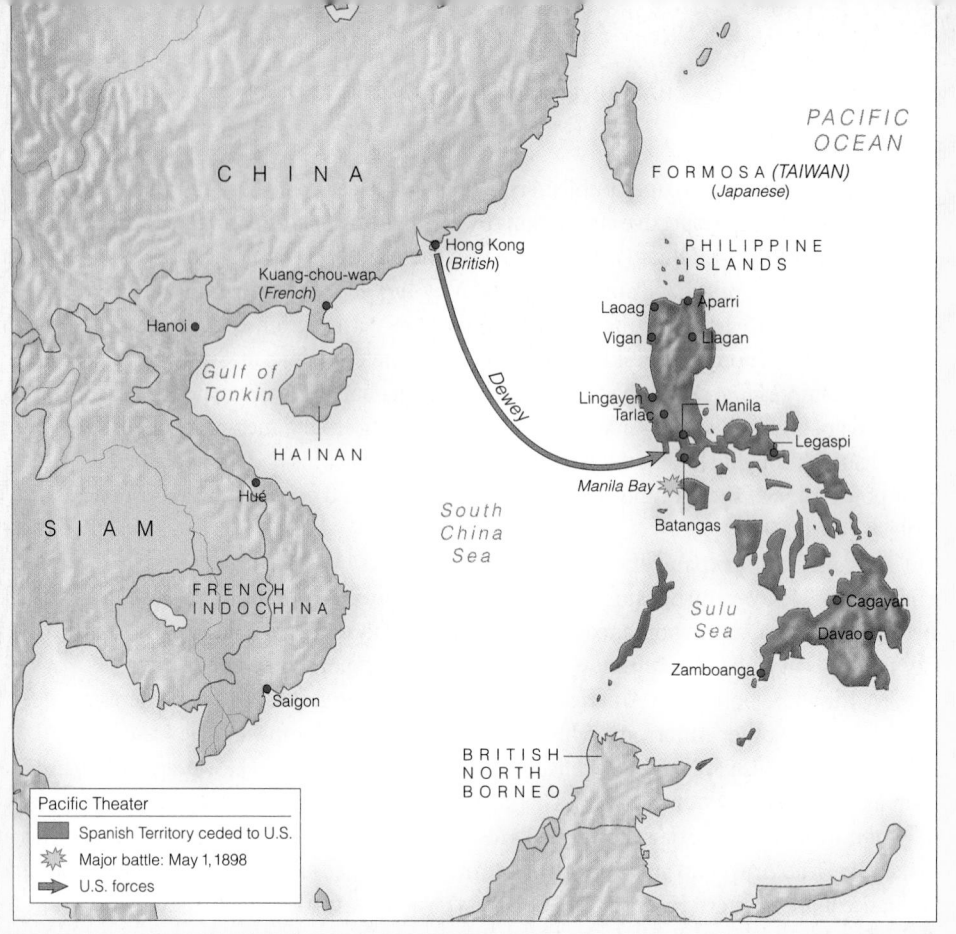

PACIFIC
OCEAN

FORMOSA *(TAIWAN)*
(Japanese)

CHINA

PHILIPPINE
ISLANDS

Hong Kong
(British)

Kuang-chou-wan
(French)

Laoag ● ● Aparri

Hanoi ●

Vigan ● ● Ilagan

Gulf of
Tonkin

Lingayen ●
Tarlac ● ● Manila

HAINAN

Legaspi ●

Hué ●

Manila Bay ✸

SIAM

South
China
Sea

Batangas ●

FRENCH
INDOCHINA

Sulu
Sea

● Cagayan

Davao ●

Zamboanga ●

Saigon ●

BRITISH
NORTH
BORNEO

■ MAP 18.6
THE SPANISH–AMERICAN–
CUBAN–FILIPINO WAR OF 1898
In Cuba, the United States combined
a blockade of the island with an army
invasion to defeat Spanish forces. In
the Philippines, the U.S. triumph over
the Spanish opened a wider war
between American occupying forces
and native Filipinos.

Pacific Theater

▨ Spanish Territory ceded to U.S.

✸ Major battle: May 1, 1898

➡ U.S. forces

Dewey waited in the harbor until American reinforcements arrived in August. Then, with the help of Filipino nationalists led by Emilio Aguinaldo, U.S. forces overran Manila on August 13.

Meanwhile, congressional Republicans had found the necessary votes to annex Hawaii. They claimed that the United States needed the Pacific islands to secure a refueling way station for Dewey's troops. McKinley signed the congressional resolution on July 7, 1898. Hawaiian residents were granted citizenship rights, and the islands became an official U.S. territory in 1900.

Earlier in the summer of 1898, halfway around the globe, 17,000 American troops traveled to Tampa, Florida, in preparation for their incursion into Cuba. Among them were the Rough Riders, a crew of volunteers organized by Lieutenant Colonel Theodore Roosevelt, who had resigned his post as assistant secretary of the Navy to serve as an officer. The troops, woefully unprepared for combat in the tropical heat, landed near Santiago, Cuba, in late June.

On July 1, Roosevelt and his men engaged an unprepared Spanish force of about 2000 men at El Caney and San Juan Hill. The Rough Riders charged up nearby Kettle Hill (they were on foot, not on horses) and into American legend. Later in speeches, Roosevelt boasted of shooting a Spanish soldier at point-blank range. But Roosevelt neglected to mention that he and his men had received crucial backup support from two African American regiments that day. Blacks had formed a skirmish line at the bottom of the hill, and, according to an eyewitness, "with an unearthly yell, charged up it" in company with the white soldiers. Federal military authorities had assigned African American men prominent combat roles in Cuba and the Philippines, believing that blacks were better able than whites to withstand the withering heat of the tropics.

By late July, American warships had destroyed the Spanish fleet in Santiago Bay. Again, Spanish losses were high (500 men killed) and American losses slight (1 man killed). According to Secretary of State John Hay, it had been "a splendid little war," just 113 days long. Battles claimed 385 American lives (although many times that number died from disease—malaria, typhoid, dysentery, and yellow fever—and from the rotten meat the soldiers ate). On August 12, 1898, Spain signed an armistice and later in the year ceded its claim to remnants of its empire, including Cuba and Puerto Rico in the Caribbean and the island of Guam in the Pacific.

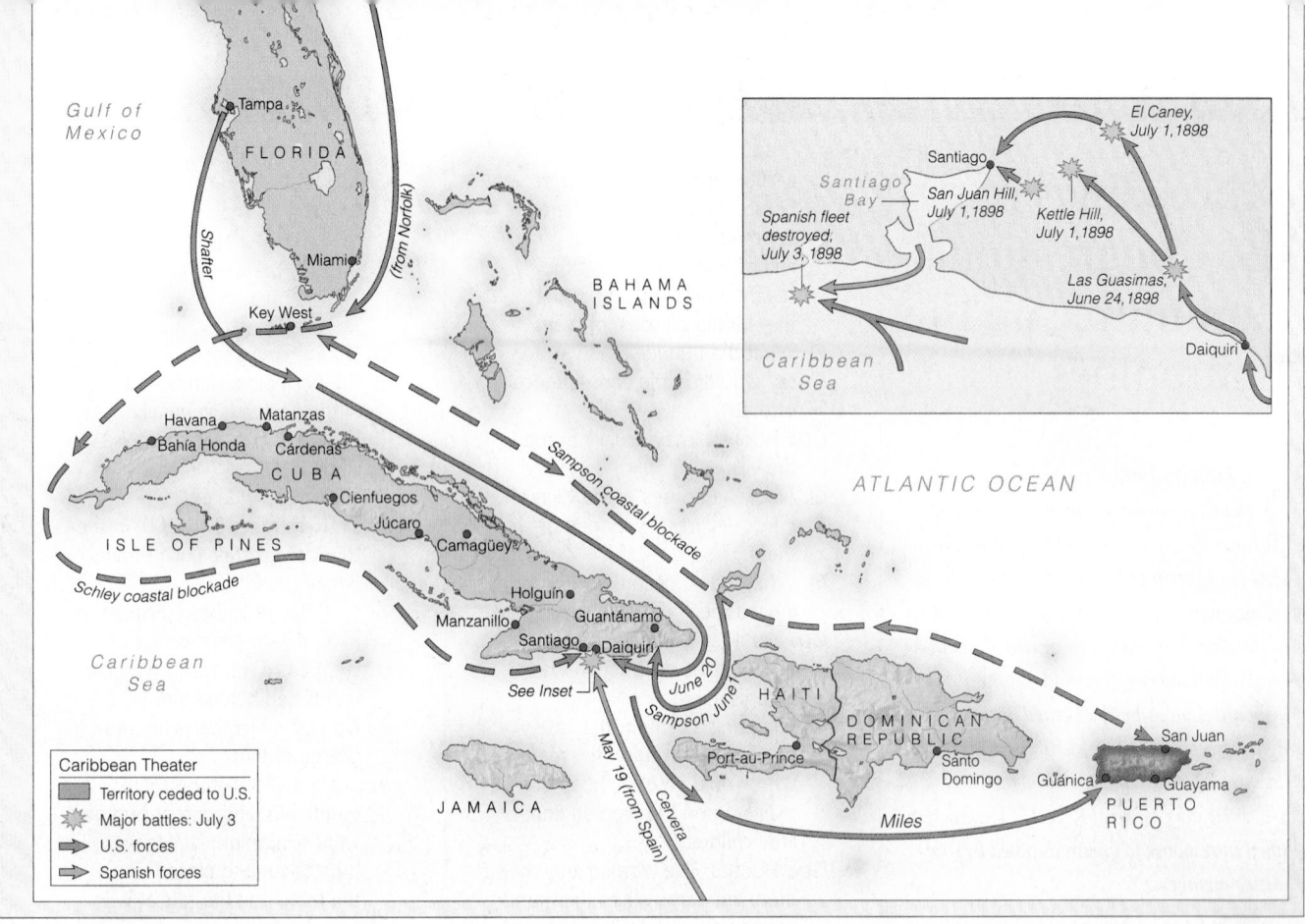

The United States forced Cuba to incorporate into its constitution (written in 1901) the so-called Platt Amendment, which guaranteed continuing U.S. influence over the country, including the stationing of American troops at a naval station on Guantanamo.

Meeting with Spanish negotiators in Paris, the United States agreed to pay $20 million for the Philippines. McKinley's motives in acquiring the islands stemmed from both commercial interests (the Philippines as a gateway to China) and religious concerns (the opportunity for Protestants to convert Spanish-speaking Roman Catholics).

But Filipino rebels were not about to bow to a new colonial power. Over the next two years, the United States committed 100,000 troops to subdue the rebels, using tactics that foreshadowed the U.S. war in Vietnam 70 years later. Hunting down guerrillas hiding in the jungle, American soldiers torched villages and crops. They forced water down the throats of suspected rebel leaders—in a form of torture known as the "water cure"—in an effort to extract information. Four thousand Americans and 20,000 Filipinos died in combat. As many as 600,000 Filipino civilians succumbed to disease and starvation. Not until 1901 could the Americans claim victory over their "little brown brothers," as future president William Howard Taft referred to the Filipino people.

Ownership of the Philippine Islands gave the United States a foothold in Asia. In 1894–1895, Japan had waged a successful war against China, and European traders rushed in to China to monopolize local markets and establish their own spheres of influence. Secretary of State John Hay issued a communication called the Open Door note in the summer of 1899; in it, he urged the imperial powers to respect the trading interests of all nations. The Europeans were reluctant to cede anything to their international competitors, and only Italy agreed to the terms of Hay's policy. But in 1900, the Boxer Uprising in China prompted cooperation between the western powers. The Boxers, Chinese ultranationalists, killed 200 foreign missionaries and other whites in an effort to purge China of outsiders. Together, the Germans, Japanese, British, French, and Americans sent 18,000 troops to quell the revolt. The United States and European nations continued to compete for the China market well into the twentieth century.

Proceedings of the Congressional Committee on the Philippines

In January 1900, Congress established the Committee on the Philippines. Senator Henry Cabot Lodge of Massachusetts was appointed chair of the committee. Its task was to review the American conduct of the war. The testimony of two U.S. officers, which follows, foreshadows the difficulties faced by the United States in fighting a guerilla war in Vietnam six decades later.

Brigadier General Robert P. Hughes testified in response to questions posed by committee members:

Q: In burning towns, what would you do? Would the entire town be destroyed by fire or would only offending portions of the town be burned?

GEN. HUGHES: I do not know that we ever had a case of burning what you would call a town in this country; but probably a *barrio* or a *sitio;* probably a half dozen houses, native shacks, where the *insurrectos* [rebels] would go in and be concealed, and if they caught a detachment passing they would kill some of them.

Q: What did I understand you to say would be the consequence of that?

GEN. HUGHES: They usually burned the village.

Q: All of the houses in the village?

GEN. HUGHES: Yes, every one of them.

Q: What would become of the inhabitants?

GEN. HUGHES: That was their lookout. . . . The destruction was as a punishment.

Q: The punishment in that case would fall, not upon the men, who would go elsewhere, but mainly upon the women and little children.

GEN. HUGHES: The women and children, are part of the family, and where you wish to inflict a punishment you can punish the man probably worse in that way than in any other.

Q: But is that within the ordinary rules of civilized warfare? Of course you could exterminate the family, which would be still worse punishment.

GEN. HUGHES: These people are not civilized. . . .

Sergeant Charles S. Riley also testified in response to the following questions:

Q: During your service there [in the Philippine Islands] did you witness what is generally known as the water cure?

A: I did.

Q: When and where?

A: On November 27, 1900, in the town of Igbaras, Iloilo Province, Panay Island. . . .
[Riley describes a Filipino man, 40–45 years of age, stripped to the waist, with his hands tied behind him.]

Q: Do you remember who had charge of him?

A: Captain Glenn stood there beside him and one or two men were tying him. . . . He was then taken and placed under the tank, and the faucet was opened and a stream of water was forced down or allowed to run down his throat; his throat was held so he could not prevent swallowing the water, so that he had to allow the water to run into his stomach. . . . When he was filled with water it was forced out of him by

Critics of Imperialism

Theodore Roosevelt seemed to personify the late-nineteenth-century idea of American manifest destiny: the notion that the core of the nation's history was a militant mission to expand its territorial reach. However, not all Americans agreed with Roosevelt. New York financier Mark Hanna called him a "madman" and "that damned cowboy." Writer Mark Twain believed him "clearly insane" and "insanest upon war and its supreme glories." Twain and other prominent people founded the Anti-Imperialist League in 1898 in an attempt to stem the rising tide of militarism.

It is difficult to generalize about the politics of anti-imperialists during this period. AFL president Samuel Gompers and industrialist Andrew Carnegie both considered themselves members of the anti-imperialist camp, but clearly that stance did not mean they agreed on much, or even on anti-imperialism. Some critics of imperialism advocated a hands-off policy toward other nations in the belief that all peoples were entitled to self-determination. In contrast, other anti-imperialists used arguments about racial hierarchies to justify their opposition to expansion. Yale sociology professor William Graham Sumner, a proponent of Social Darwinism, argued that "uncivilized and half-civilized peoples" were hostile to democratic self-government and unprepared for its rigors. Thus, Sumner believed that American efforts to "civ-

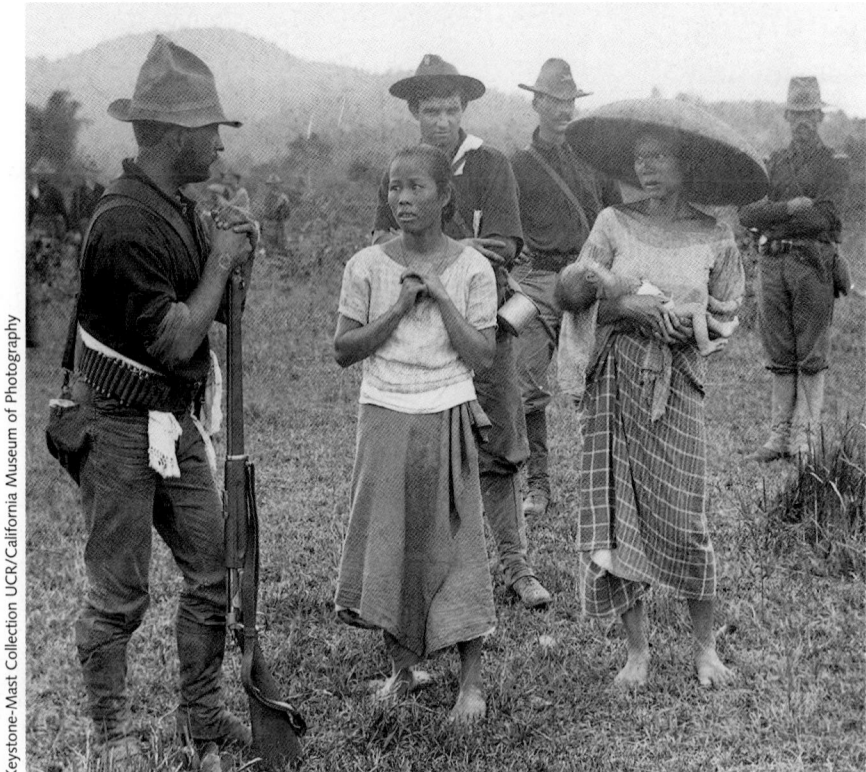

Philippine civilians encounter U.S. army troops during the war of 1898. Resisting attempts to colonize the islands, Filipinos battled American forces in a war that lasted four years. A soldier in the Third Regiment wrote of the indiscriminate killing of civilians, "I am probably growing hard-hearted for I am in my glory when I can sight my gun on some dark-skin and pull the trigger."

pressing a foot on his stomach or else with their hands. . . .

Q: What had been his crime?

A: Information had been obtained from a native source as to his being an insurgent officer. After the treatment he admitted that he held the rank of captain in the insurgent army—an active captain. . . .

Q: His offense was treachery to the American cause?

A: Yes, sir. . . . ■

Source: Proceedings of the Congressional Committee on the Philippines, in Harvey Graff, ed., *American Imperialism and the Philippine Insurrection* (Boston, 1969), pp. 64–79.

ilize" and colonize foreign peoples would inevitably fail because those peoples were incapable of embracing American values.

Recent newcomers to the United States resented the idea that the "march of the flag" was an enterprise to be led by Anglo-Saxons (that is, people of English descent), as some imperialists claimed. German immigrants invoked their heritage of conquest, and the Irish juxtaposed their native culture with what they called the historic "brutal savagery" of the English. Nevertheless, supporting imperialism was one way for immigrants to proclaim their own Americanness and distance themselves from allegedly inferior peoples.

In the summer of 1900, the Democrats and Republicans prepared for the upcoming presidential election. Receiving the Democratic nomination once again, William Jennings Bryan was eager to press the outdated cause of free silver. He also condemned the American presence in the Philippines, although this issue, too, was rapidly losing the attention of the electorate. At the Republican convention, Roosevelt's supporters managed to win for him the slot as McKinley's running mate. That fall, the former Rough Rider waged an exuberant campaign. Accompanied by a retinue of gun-toting cowboys, he wrapped the Republicans in the American flag. When McKinley swept back into office in the fall, few Americans could have anticipated how central Roosevelt's vision would become to the country over the next two decades.

Conclusion

As Americans greeted the twentieth century, they might have marveled at the dramatic changes that had occurred in their country over the last 100 years. In 1800 the United States was home to 5.3 million people who lived in 16 states. One hundred years later, the country included 45 states and boasted a population of 76 million people. Many workplaces, fields as well as factories, were dominated by machines and the people who tended them. The economy was shifting toward the mass production of consumer goods.

In 1900 the United States exerted control over the land and peoples of Alaska, the Hawaiian and Samoan Islands, the Philippines, Guam, Puerto Rico, and (through the Platt Amendment), Cuba as well. These holdings, notable for their strategic significance, illustrated the growing willingness of the United States to extend its influence and economic reach—by armed force if necessary—to the far corners of the earth.

The 1890s foreshadowed many of the major themes of the twentieth century. The Populists looked to the federal government to address social ills, paving the way for Progressives in the early twentieth century and New Dealers in the 1930s. Conversationists provided the foundation for the environmentalist movement of the 1970s. And suffragists were the foremothers of the modern women's movement. Yet for Americans, a generations-old contradiction lingered between prosperity and political equality for some groups and poverty and political subordination for others. On the international stage, the United States was quick to take advantage of weaker nations if such action was deemed crucial to the "national interest." The new drive for worldwide economic and political power was fast eclipsing America's revolutionary heritage, with its values of democracy and self-determination.

Sites to Visit

The Spanish–American War
www.loe.gov/rr/hispanic/1898

This site provides resources and documents about the Spanish-American War, the period before the war, and the people who participated in the fighting or commented on it.

Imperialism Web Page
www.smplanet.com/imperialism/toc.html

Focusing on the late nineteenth and early twentieth centuries, this site includes much information about American imperialism.

Hispanic Voices/Voces Hispanas
www.lib.berkeley.edu/BANC

This interactive site on Latinos in California is maintained by the Bancroft Library in Berkeley. The autobiographical narratives include late-nineteenth-century oral histories with Latinos.

Late Nineteenth-Century Authors
xroads.virginia.edu/~HYPER/hypertex.html

This University of Virginia site includes material on prominent nineteenth-century writers, including William Dan Howells, Mark Twain, and Joel Chandler Harris.

Mary Baker Eddy
www.tfccs.com/GC/MBE/MBEmain.jhtml

This site looks at the founding of Christian Science.

National Arts and Crafts Archives
www.arts-crafts.com/index.html

This site serves as a guide to materials related to the Arts and Crafts movement, which lasted from about 1890 to 1929.

Samuel Gompers Papers
www.inform.umd.edu/HIST/Gompers/page4.html

This site includes information about the Samuel Gompers Papers project at the University of Maryland. It also has a photo gallery, selected documents, and a brief history of the first president of the American Federation of Labor.

The Era of William McKinley
www.history.ohio-state.edu/projects/mckinley/

This Ohio State University site contains a bibliography and numerous images from various periods of McKinley's career. It also includes a section with an excellent collection of McKinley-era cartoons.

For Further Reading

General

Glenda Elizabeth Gilmore, *Gender and Jim Crow: Women and the Politics of White Supremacy in North Carolina, 1896–1920* (1996).

Matthew Frye Jacobson, *Barbarian Virtues: The United States Encounters Foreign Peoples at Home and Abroad, 1876–1917* (2000).

Walter LaFeber, *The New Empire: An Interpretation of American Expansion, 1860–1898* (1963).

Emily S. Rosenberg, *Spreading the American Dream: American Economic and Cultural Expansion, 1890–1945* (1982).

Robert W. Rydell, *All the World's a Fair: Visions of Empire at American International Expositions, 1876–1916* (1984).

Frontiers at Home, Lost and Found

David Wallace Adams, *Education for Extinction: American Indians and the Boarding School Experience, 1875–1928* (1995).

Willard B. Gatewood, Jr., *Black Americans and the White Man's Burden, 1898–1903* (1975).

Matthew Frye Jacobson, *Whiteness of a Different Color: European Immigrants and the Alchemy of Race* (1998).

Neil R. McMillen, *Dark Journey: Black Mississippians in the Age of Jim Crow* (1989).

Donald J. Pisani, *From the Family Farm to Agribusiness: The Irrigation Crusade in California, 1850–1931* (1984).

Barbara M. Solomon, *In the Company of Educated Women: A History of Women and Higher Education in America* (1985).

Mark David Spence, *Dispossessing the Wilderness: Indian Removal and the Making of the National Parks* (1999).

David B. Tyack, *Managers of Virtue: Public School Leadership in America, 1820–1980* (1982).

The Search for Alliances

Paul Buhle, *From the Knights of Labor to the New World Order: Essays on Labor and Culture* (1997).

Sarah Deutsch, *Women and the City: Gender, Space, and Power in Boston, 1870–1940* (2000).

Patricia R. Hill, *The World their Household: The American Woman's Foreign Mission Movement and Cultural Transformation, 1870–1920* (1985).

Elisabeth Lasch-Quinn, *Black Neighbors: Race and the Limits of Reform in the American Settlement House Movement, 1890–1945* (1993).

Seymour Martin Lipset and Gary Marks. *It Didn't Happen Here: Why Socialism Failed in the United States* (2000).

Vicki L. Ruiz and Ellen Carol DuBois, eds., *Unequal Sisters: A Multicultural Reader in U.S. Women's History* (2000).

David E. Whisnant, *All That Is Native and Fine: The Politics of Culture in an American Region* (1983).

American Imperialism

Robert L. Beisner, *Twelve Against Empire: The Anti-Imperialists, 1898–1900* (1968).

H. W. Brands, *Bound to Empire: The United States and the Philippines* (1992).

Paul A. Cohen, *History in Three Keys: The Boxers as Event, Experience, and Myth* (1997).

Kenn Harper, *Give Me My Father's Body: The Life of Minik, the New York Eskimo* (2000).

Thomas J. McCormick, *China Market: America's Quest for Informal Empire, 1893–1901* (1967).

William Appleman Williams, *The Tragedy of American Diplomacy* (1972).

Online Practice Test

Test your understanding of this chapter with interactive review quizzes at

www.ablongman.com/jonescreatedequal/chapter18

Additional Photo Credits

Page 605: (Top) Reproduced by permission of The Huntington Library, San Marino, California, photCL11(52);
(bottom) Reproduced by permission of The Huntington Library, San Marino, California, photCL11(53)
Page 606: Chicago Historical Society, ICHi-02437
Page 630: Fair Street Pictures
Page 631: Fair Street Pictures
Page 635: Courtesy, Janice L. and David Frent

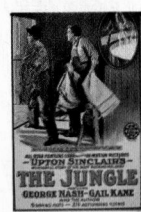
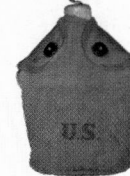
PART SEVEN

Reform at Home, Revolution Abroad, 1900–1929

MANY AMERICANS GREETED THE FIRST YEARS OF THE TWENTIETH century with optimism. Developments at home and abroad seemed to promise a new era of prosperity and progress. The mass manufacturing of automobiles proved a boon to the economy and transformed patterns of travel, leisure, and consumption. The beginning of commercial air flights heralded a revolution in communication and transportation. Moving pictures and new musical forms such as jazz delighted millions.

Focused on the new challenges of urbanization and industrialization, Progressive reformers sought to use science to solve a wide range of problems related to public health and welfare. Some advocated overhauling the system of public education; others pressed for legislation banning the sale and distribution of alcohol. Some lobbied for worker health and safety legislation, and still others sought to exercise social control through eugenics and state-mandated sterilization.

A variety of groups challenged white men's exclusive claim to civil rights. African Americans took the national stage to argue for equality under the law and for freedom from state-sanctioned violence in the form of lynching and debt peonage. Beginning with the Great Migration of World War I, southern blacks abandoned the cotton fields to seek jobs in northern cities.

The changing roles of women bolstered the women's suffrage movement. Growing numbers of women were becoming labor organizers, reformers, and college professors. Rising divorce rates and the emergence of birth control as a political as well as a medical issue signaled challenges to the traditional patriarchal family. At the same time, conflicts among reformers emerged. For example, white middle-class suffragists hoped to maintain their "respectability" in an effort to win the support of reluctant male leaders; in the process, these women distanced themselves from members of the working class and even the African American women active in the suffrage movement. Suffragists' efforts paid off in 1920, with the ratification of the Nineteenth Amendment to the Constitution.

With its lively consumer culture and rising standard of living, the United States continued to attract newcomers from abroad. Immigrants from Mexico and eastern Europe sought refuge from poverty, oppression, and civil strife at home. In 1914, 1.2 million immigrants came to America, the largest number in a single year before or since that date. Between 1900 and 1930, more than 1 million Mexicans migrated north, most settling into existing Mexican American communities in the Southwest or creating new communities there or in the Midwest.

World War I shattered the belief among many Progressives that conflicts could be solved in a rational, peaceful way. The end of the war had permanently entangled U.S. interests in European affairs. Moreover, revolutions in Mexico (1910) and Russia (1917) affected the United States directly, the former by spurring immigration across the country's southwest border, the latter by challenging the nation's system of industrial capitalism. Nevertheless, many Americans remained convinced that the country could and should isolate itself from world affairs.

Natural forces also remained beyond the control of reformers and government officials. The San Francisco earthquake of 1906, the great Mississippi flood of 1927, and the Florida hurricane of 1928 exacted devastating tolls in terms of human life and property damage. The local communities that were directly affected struggled for years to recover from these disasters.

But for many Americans, the 1920s was a period of peace and prosperity. New household appliances and conveniences lightened the burdens of housework. Radios and movies proved to be popular forms of entertainment. Traditional social mores gave way to expressions of sexual freedom. Progressive impulses waned as business values rose to take their place.

The decade after the end of World War I revealed both the persistence of old conflicts and the emergence of new conflicts within American society. Conservatives branded labor union organizers and socialists as unpatriotic and subversive. Asian immigrants on the West Coast and blacks in the rural South and urban North faced continued legal discrimination in the workplace and in the courts. Protestant fundamentalists challenged the move toward secularism and rationalism, claiming that religious faith, not science, set the standard for morality in modern life. Responding to those who feared that foreign immigration represented a threat to American society, Congress imposed immigration restrictions in 1924. Put into effect in 1920, the Eighteenth Amendment to the Constitution prohibited the sale and distribution of alcoholic beverages. The three Republican presidents who served during the 1920s—Harding, Coolidge, and Hoover—retreated from the activist stance favored by their predecessors, including Theodore Roosevelt and Woodrow Wilson.

The stock market crash of 1929 revealed fundamental weaknesses in the American economy. A tide of bank failures engulfed individual American families even as it threatened businesses abroad. As the depression deepened, Americans looked to the federal government to address the crisis.

1916	Jeannette Rankin elected first female member of Congress.
	U.S. Marines occupy Dominican Republic.
1917	U.S. enters World War I. 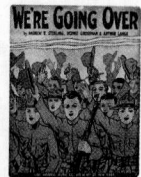
	U.S. Marines occupy Cuba.
	Russian Revolution.
	Residents of Puerto Rico granted U.S. citizenship.
1918	Spanish influenza epidemic kills 20 million worldwide.
	Sedition Act.
	Wilson's "Fourteen Points" speech to Congress.
1919	Versailles Treaty ends World War I. 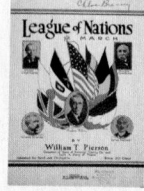
	U.S. Senate rejects League of Nations.
	Eighteenth Amendment (prohibition) ratified.
1920	Nineteenth Amendment (women's suffrage) ratified.
1921	Tulsa whites attack black community.
	Sheppard–Towner Act.
1922	Five-Power Naval Treaty.
1923	Equal Rights Amendment proposed.
1924	Johnson–Reid Act.
	Portable radio introduced. 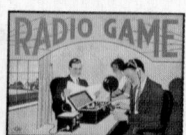
1925	Scopes Trial, Dayton, Tennessee.
	F. Scott Fitzgerald, *The Great Gatsby*.
1926	Gertrude Ederle is first woman to swim across English Channel.
1927	Charles Lindbergh flies nonstop from New York to Paris.
	Al Jolson stars in *The Jazz Singer*, first talking movie.
	Sacco and Vanzetti executed.
	Buck v. Bell upholds compulsory sterilization laws.
1928	Tamiami Trail across Florida Everglades completed.
1929	Stock market crash.

CHAPTER

19

The Promise and Perils of Progressive Reform, 1900–1912

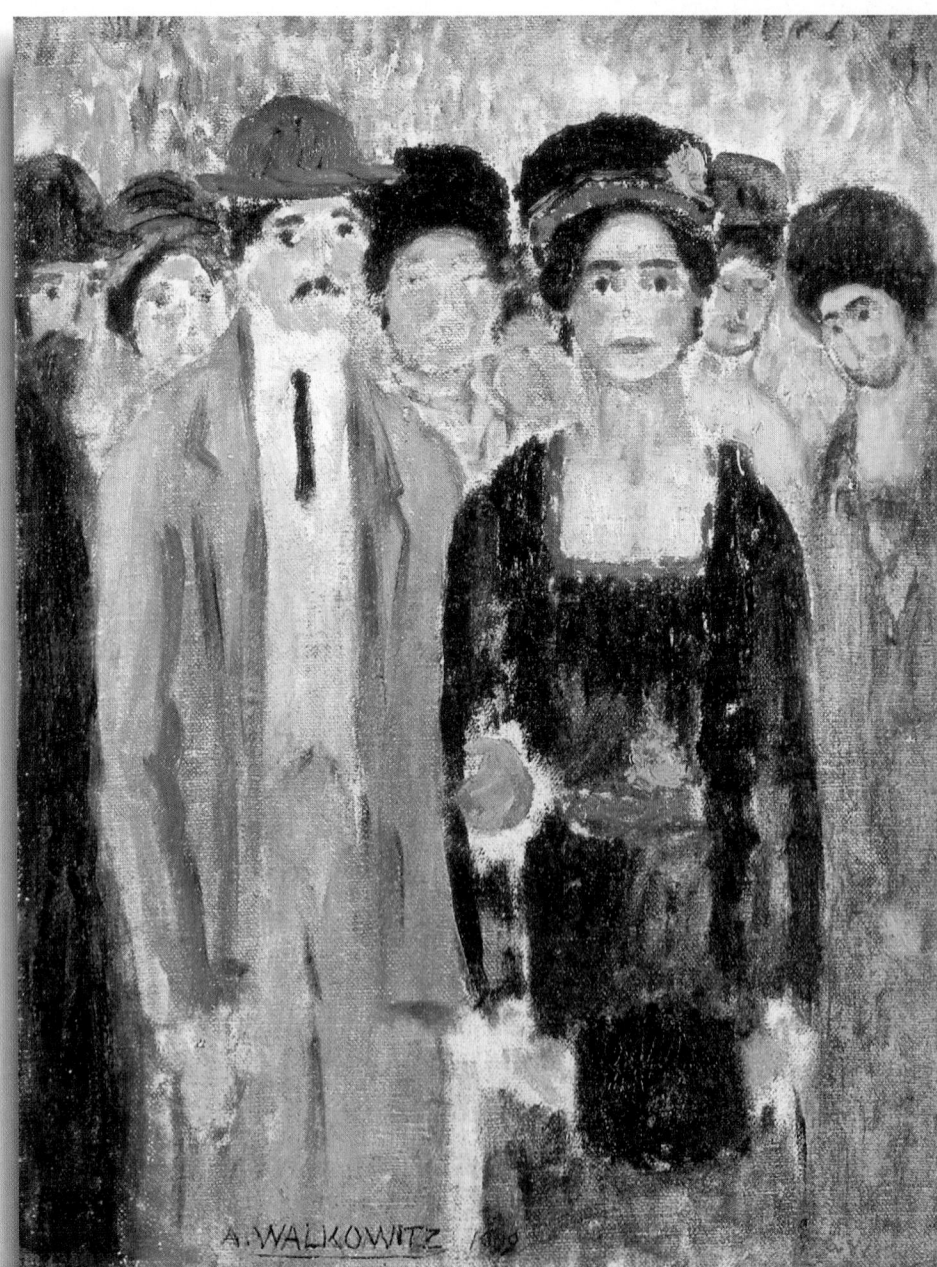

Abraham Walkowitz, "In the Street," 1909. Hirshhorn Museum and Sculpture Garden, Smithsonian Institution, Washington, D.C. (66.5446) Gift of Joseph H. Hirshhorn, 1966. Photograph by Lee Stalsworth

■ Abraham Walkowitz's 1909 painting, *In the Street*, depicts a Jewish immigrant couple on a crowded urban street.

"I AM A WORKING GIRL," DECLARED CLARA LEMLICH IN HER NATIVE YIDDISH, "ONE OF those striking against intolerable conditions." Still in her teens, the petite young woman took the podium on the night of November 22, 1909, in front of thousands of striking workers in New York, and roused them with her passionate, direct call for action: "I am tired of listening to speakers who talk in generalities. What we are here for is to decide whether or not to strike. I offer a resolution that a general strike be declared—now." The next morning, 15,000 garment workers went on strike, demanding that the work week be reduced to 52 hours, with overtime pay and union recognition. Soon, the strikers swelled in number to more than 20,000. Observers at the time were astonished to see lively, fashionably dressed young women filling the picket lines. Ninety percent of the striking workers were women; they were overwhelmingly young Jewish immigrants, with Italian women constituting about 6 percent. Quickly, the strikers drew a wide coalition of support from the International Ladies Garment Workers Union (ILGWU), the Women's Trade Union League (WTUL), and middle-class reformers and activists for women's suffrage.

The strike was a demand for union recognition, reasonable wages and hours, and safe and decent working conditions, including an end to sexual harassment on the job. But at the same time, the strikers insisted that they should be treated as "ladies" and have access to the consumer goods and leisure culture taking shape in American cities. Although the young women were bullied and arrested by police, their high spirits prompted some observers to make light of their struggle. Sarah Comstock, a reporter for *Collier's* magazine, wrote of the strike, "This was a scene of gaiety and flirtation. My preconceived idea of a strike was a somber meeting where somber resolutions were made. . . . But they don't look as if they had any grievances." In response to those who tried to trivialize the women's mobilization and in defense of their desire to be part of the new consumer culture, Lemlich stated, "We like new hats as well as other young women. Why shouldn't we?" Ultimately, the strike ended with a failed compromise when the striking workers overwhelmingly rejected an offer of better wages and working conditions that did not include recognition

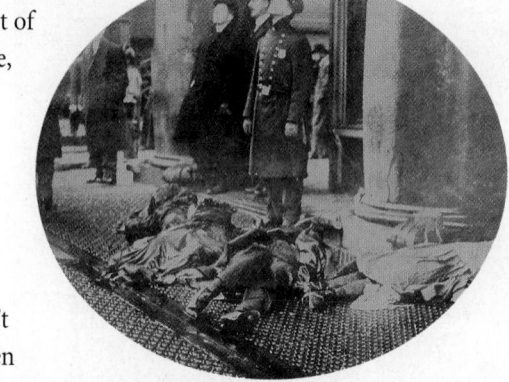

Victims of the Triangle Shirtwaist Company fire.

of their union. Calling the strikers "socialists," their more moderate allies broke from the union and left the young female workers vulnerable to the power of the company owners. The coalition of support fell apart, and most of the strikers eventually went back to work.

Less than two years later, a fire broke out in the top floors of the Triangle Shirtwaist Company, one of the major centers of the 1909 strike. Eight hundred workers, most of them young Jewish and Italian women, were trapped in the inferno because company officials had locked interior doors to prevent the women from taking unauthorized breaks or leaving work early. The flames tore through the building in less than half an hour, leaving 146 young women dead. Those who did not succumb to flames and smoke jumped to their deaths. "One girl after another fell, like shot birds, from above, from the burning floors," remembered one witness. "They hit the pavement just like hail," reported a firefighter. Parents rushed to the scene to find their young daughters dead, dying, or maimed. "My little girl lies dead, shrouds instead of a wedding gown," cried one of the bereaved. One reporter wrote, "I looked upon the dead bodies and I remembered these girls were the shirtwaist makers. I remembered their great strike of last year in which the same girls had demanded more sanitary conditions and more safety precautions in the shops. Their dead bodies were the answer." In the investigation that followed, the owner of the factory was never charged with a crime or held responsible for the tragedy. He claimed that his building was in full compliance with safety laws, but compliance with the laws did not ensure safety for the workers. No laws required sprinklers, adequate fire escapes, or fire drills. Just a few months before the fire, the building had been inspected and declared "fireproof." Defending himself after the fire against accusations of negligence, the building owner pointed to the sturdy brick structure, which, as the *New York Times* noted, "showed hardly any signs of the disaster."

The "uprising of twenty thousand," as the 1909 strike came to be called, and the tragic factory fire that ignited in its aftermath, are two among many dramatic episodes in the early twentieth century that expose the fractures and tensions within the nation at the time. Immigrants and racial minorities demanded the full promise of American life; workers struggled against the exploitation, poor pay, and dangerous conditions that characterized industrial jobs; young women insisted on respect at work and access to the playful environment of urban fashion and popular culture; female voices called for full citizenship and the vote and claimed their right to be heard by male bosses and union leaders; and activists across the political spectrum tried to control and manage the changes taking place around them in accord with their widely differing values.

During the first years of the twentieth century, the nation began to emerge as something profoundly different than it had been in the past. Even the landscape changed as cities continued to grow not only outward but also upward, with the construction of towering skyscrapers, and downward, with the creation of subway systems. But human enterprise continued to be vulnerable to the forces of nature. On April 18, 1906, an earthquake virtually leveled San Francisco. The nation saw in one deadly instant that human technological genius paled in the face of nature's fury. After the quake, fire devoured the city. In the words of writer Jack London, "All the cunning adjustments of a twentieth century city had been smashed by the earthquake. The streets were humped into ridges and depressions, and piled with the debris of fallen walls. The steel rails were twisted into perpendicular and horizontal angles. The telephone and telegraph systems were disrupted. And the great water mains had burst. All the shrewd contrivances and safeguards of man had been thrown out of gear by thirty seconds' twitching of the earth-crust."

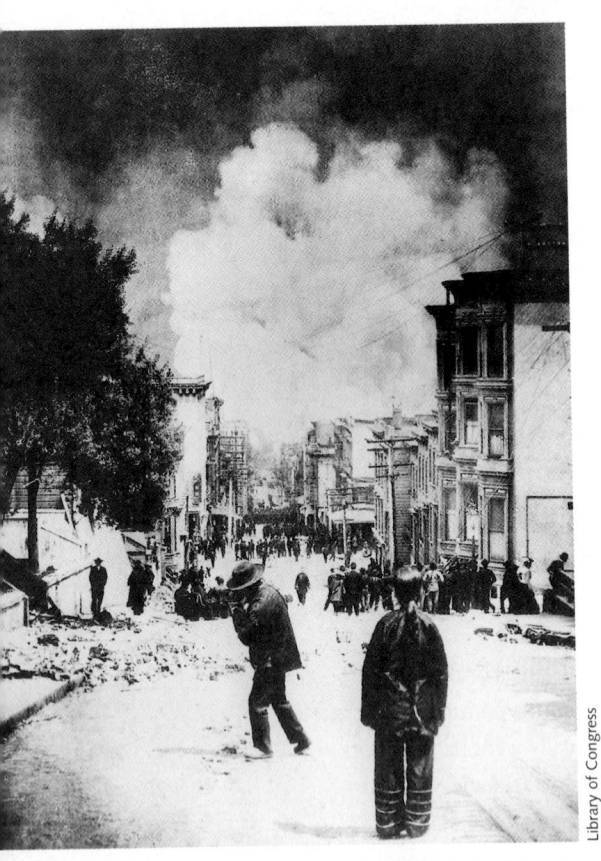

■ An earthquake devastated San Francisco on April 18, 1906. Here a Chinese immigrant watches as the city goes up in flames. Chinatown was destroyed, along with much of the downtown.

Library of Congress

If New York's Triangle Shirtwaist Company building—unscathed after the young women inside perished in flames—was a monument to corporate arrogance, the crumbled buildings of San Francisco offered a lesson in humility. "Never, in all San Francisco's history, were her people so kind and courteous as on this night of terror," noted London. Railroads carried thousands of refugees out of the city, free of

Rose Freedman

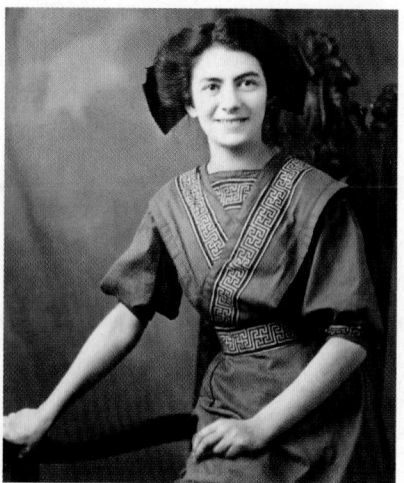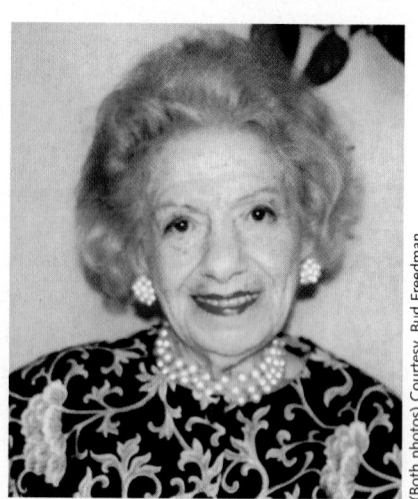

(Both photos) Courtesy, Bud Freedman

Rose Rosenfeld Freedman as a young immigrant, and decades later as a labor activist.

Major historical events sometimes take on a life of their own, locked in a single frame of historical memory. The 1911 Triangle Shirtwaist Company fire is one such event. Rose Rosenfeld Freedman, one of the young women working at the factory on that fateful day, provides a reminder that events are not simply frozen in time. The tragic fire that she survived fueled in her a lifelong committment to the rights of workers.

Rose Rosenfeld was not born into a working class community that might have nurtured her committment to workers' rights. The daughter of a prosperous business owner, she emigrated from Vienna to the United States in 1909 at age 15. She did not need a job, but as a young Jewish immigrant, she recalled, "I wanted to show that I'm [a] real American and I want to work like everybody else. And I went on my own, found a job. . . . And then, I almost paid with my life." She was 16 when she went to work at Triangle, sewing buttons at a wage of $3 for a six-day week.

Rose was working on the ninth floor when the fire alarm sounded at 4:43 P.M. on March 25, 1911. Finding the exit doors locked, she ran up to the tenth floor, where the executives worked, but the bosses were gone. "They saved themselves already." She pulled her dress over her head and followed the bosses to the roof, where firefighters hoisted her to safety on the top of the adjacent building.

The fire inspired her to action. Nearly a century later, her memory of the fire remained vivid: "The executives with a couple steps could have opened the door. But they thought they were better than the working people. . . . What good is a rich man [if] he hasn't

got a heart? I feel it. Still. I feel very bad about it." Outrage over the fire led to the passage of 36 labor and safety laws in the next three years. Rose Rosenfeld left the garment business and went on to college, but she remained a passionate advocate for workers' rights.

In another dramatic brush with history, Rosenfeld demonstrated her willingness to stand up for others whose rights and safety were threatened. She was visiting Austria just as World War I erupted. A Russian Jew who had been spying for Austria arrived at the house where she was staying, begging for protection from Russian soldiers. She hid him in a coal bin in the basement and when the soldiers arrived, she told them to leave. Weeks later, the wife of the man she hid came to the house to thank her for saving the father of their five children.

In 1927, Rose married Harry Freedman, who ran a typewriter business. During World War II, in the midst of a terrifying polio epidemic, she escaped another tragedy. Two of her children were stricken with the disease but recovered. For Freedman, it was another miracle, like her escape from the Triangle fire. Widowed in 1952,

Freedman entered business school at age 59 and got a job with a pen company in New York. At 64, she lied about her age and got a job in customer relations at the Metropolitan Life Insurance Company. She stayed there for 15 years, retiring at age 79.

Still an active crusader, Freedman moved to Los Angeles when she was in her nineties. At age 100, she went to Mexico to study Spanish. Like the shirtwaist workers who wore hats and stylish clothes on the picket line in 1909, Rose Freedman still wore high heels, had her hair done every week, and did her own shopping. Cherishing her independence, she refused to move in with her children, explaining that "young people belong together and I have a life of my own."

In 2000, at age 106, Rose Freedman lectured on sweatshops to enthralled students at Occidental College in Los Angeles. "She loved her career. . . . She believed quite fully in doing things that make you happy," said her granddaughter Dana Walden, head of 20th Century Fox Television. Rose Freedman died in 2001 at age 107, the last survivor of the Triangle Shirtwaist Company fire. ∎

charge. And the national government stepped in immediately, as it would countless times throughout the twentieth century in the face of disaster.

The San Francisco earthquake symbolized American life at the dawn of the twentieth century in one word: upheaval. When the smoke and dust cleared, Chinatown was destroyed, as were the modest homes of laborers, the new houses of the middle class, the palaces of the wealthy, sturdy banks and businesses, and the brick and steel constructions of modernity. But out of death and destruction, the city and its people came back. San Francisco, along with the rest of the country, grappled with upheaval as the nation continued on its path toward the diverse, urban, industrial society that characterized American life in the twentieth century.

The dramatic changes taking place in the nation at the dawn of the new century, from industry and technology down to the most intimate levels of life, sparked equally dramatic efforts to control, tame, and regulate them. Because of the flurry of reform activity during this period, historians call it the Progressive Era. Politicians from all parties participated in the wide range of reform efforts known as Progressivism, fueled by a faith in progress and a belief in the possibility for social improvement.

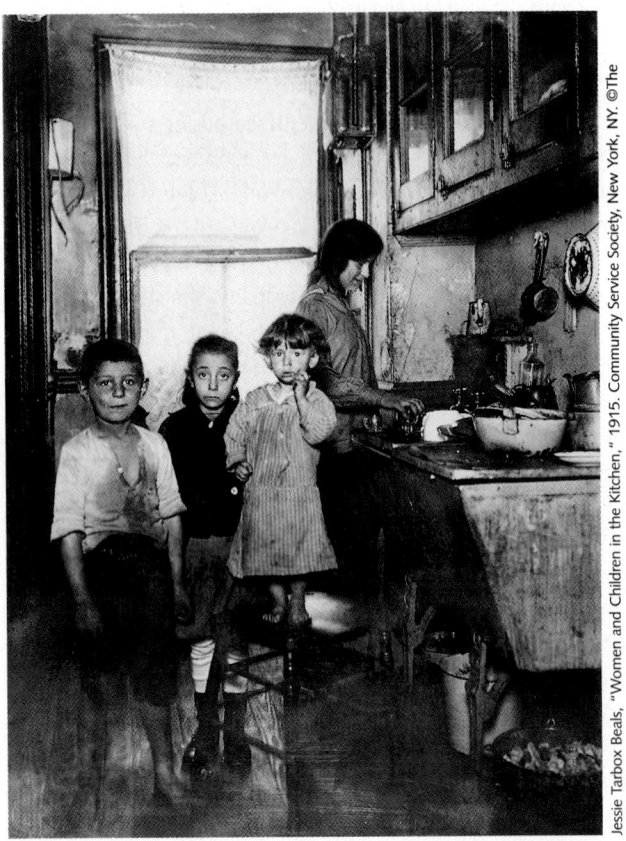

Jessie Tarbox Beals, "Women and Children in the Kitchen," 1915. Community Service Society, New York, NY. ©The Jewish Museum

■ An immigrant family manages the daily routines of life in a tenement flat in 1910. Crowded conditions, poor ventilation, and inadequate plumbing made it impossible for impoverished residents such as these to maintain a clean and healthy environment.

Migration and Immigration: The Changing Face of the Nation

Charismatic young labor leader Clara Lemlich was one of millions of immigrants at the time who were changing the face of the nation. This migration, which began in the latter decades of the nineteenth century, resulted largely from international economic and political upheavals. Facing severe hardships in their home countries, many migrants took the desperate action of departing for foreign lands. Between 1900 and 1910, nearly 9 million immigrants entered the United States, by far the largest number for any single decade in the nation's history before or since. The United States was one of several potential destinations for these courageous and hopeful sojourners. It was particularly appealing because of its often exaggerated, but nonetheless real, opportunities for jobs and economic advancement, its official commitment to freedom of religion and political thought, and its reputation as a nation that welcomed newcomers from abroad.

Many immigrants followed kin or fellow townsfolk who had come in the nineteenth century; others were drawn to the promise of a better life, symbolized by the Statue of Liberty. On arrival, many found that the "promised land" was not the paradise they expected. They faced crowded living conditions in urban tenements, jobs in sweatshops and factories with long hours, low wages, and miserable working conditions, and a hostile reception. Many Americans—including some whose own parents or grandparents had come to the United States as immigrants—looked down on the newcomers as "racially inferior" and morally suspect, feared competition for jobs, and worried that the masses of poor foreigners in their midst would become a burden on taxpayers and public institutions. The Statue of Liberty may have held

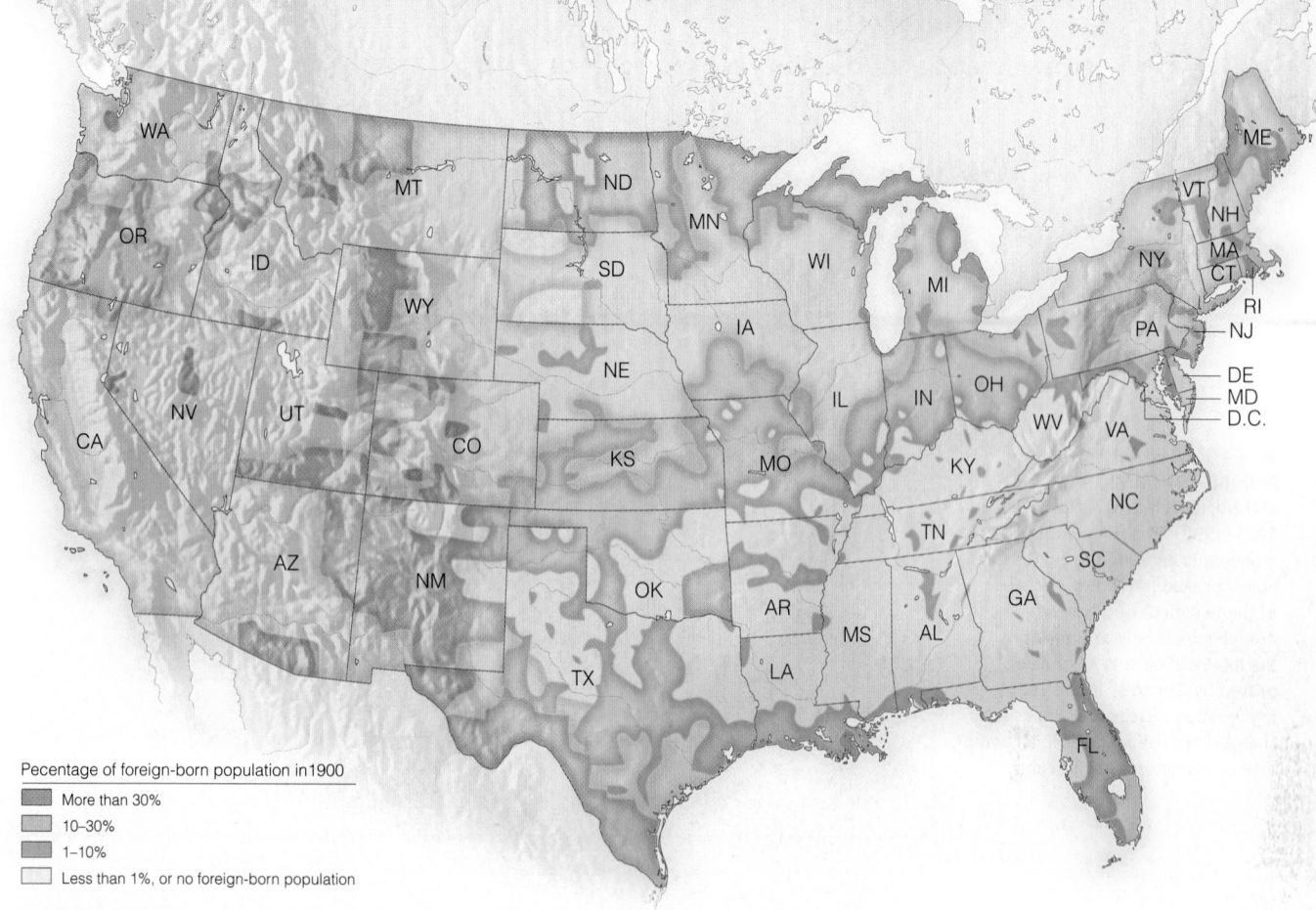

Pecentage of foreign-born population in1900

■ More than 30%
■ 10–30%
■ 1–10%
□ Less than 1%, or no foreign-born population

■ **MAP 19.1**

FOREIGN-BORN POPULATION, 1900 Although the most famous points of entry for immigrants during the turn-of-the-century decades were New York's Ellis Island for people from Europe, and Angel Island off of San Francisco for people from Asia, most immigrants actually settled in the Upper Midwest and the Southwestern region bordering Mexico.

up the torch of welcome, but many citizens, from union halls to legislative chambers, wanted the newcomers to leave.

Many did leave. One-third of immigrants to the United States returned to their home countries. Some came for only a few years and returned to their native lands, including nearly 90 percent of migrants from the Balkans. Other groups, especially those who faced severe hardships in the lands of their birth, were more likely to make the United States their permanent home, settling with their families and building communities. Only 11 percent of the Irish and 5 percent of the Jews returned between 1908 and 1923.

Although some of the newcomers moved to rural areas and worked in agriculture, most settled in the cities, where they were joined by rural Americans leaving farms for new opportunities in the rapidly growing urban centers. In the first decade of the twentieth century, more than four and a half million Americans moved from east to west, and nearly 80,000 migrated from south to north. Each person who took part in this huge global and national migration brought hopes, anxieties, and fears. But over time, these newcomers transformed almost every aspect of American life: political, economic, cultural, and social.

The Heartland: Land of Newcomers

Known as the nation's heartland, the upper Midwest carries associations of small towns dotted with Protestant churches and inhabited by hardy Anglo-Saxon pioneers and their descendants. But at the dawn of the twentieth century, it was not the coastal cities, with their visible

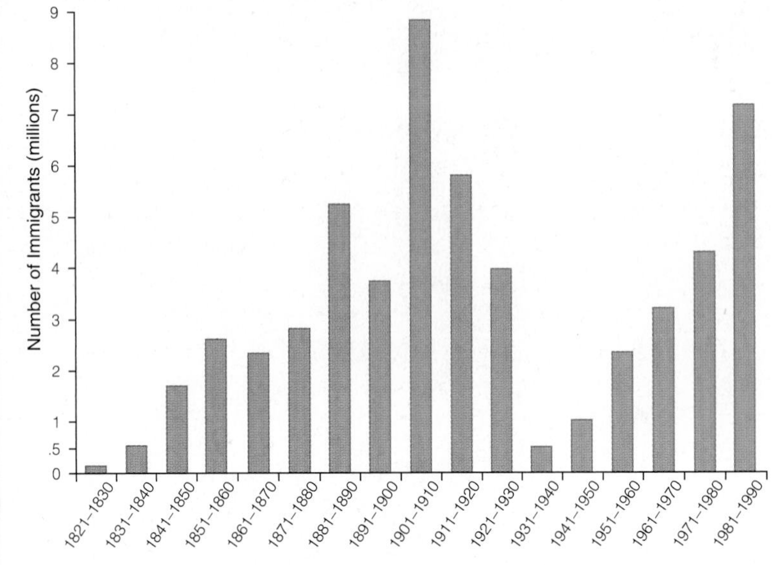

■ **FIGURE 19.1**
NUMBER OF IMMIGRANTS ENTERING THE UNITED STATES, 1821-1990 The number of immigrants entering the United States peaked in the first decade of the twentieth century and dropped drastically as a result of the immigration restriction laws passed by Congress in the 1920s. Immigration increased again as laws changed after World War II, allowing new immigrant groups to enter.

immigrant ghettos, but the settlements in the upper Midwest, along with the lower Southwest, where the greatest concentration of foreign-born residents lived. In the growing towns and cities of the Midwest, newcomers from central Europe and Italy joined the earlier settlers from Germany and Scandinavia to form farming and mining communities on the rich soil and abundant iron deposits of the region.

Immigrants from central and southern Europe settled in the region, which came to be known as the "iron range." In the 1890s, the area was sparsely settled. As a result of the Dawes Act of 1887, which divided tribal lands into individual parcels, much of the land orginally held by Indians had been divided and sold. Most of the Indians who were native to that region were removed to reservations. The iron-rich areas, previously the hunting, fishing, and gathering areas of the Native Americans, were now inhabited by lumberjacks who cut the forests. The harsh climate, ranging from −40°F in the snowy winters to more than 110°F in the sweltering summers, plus aggressive swarms of biting insects made it a difficult place to settle. Nevertheless, mining companies discovered the iron deposits and began recruiting workers, first from northern Europe and then, after 1900, from southern and eastern Europe. By 1910, the iron range was home to 35 European immigrant groups. Gradually, these cohesive working-class communities, like others elsewhere, developed their own brand of ethnic Americanism, complete with elaborate Fourth of July celebrations and other festivities that expressed both their distinctive ethnic identities and their allegiance to their adopted country.

The Southwest: Mexican Borderlands

In 1904 a train carrying Irish orphans from a New York Catholic foundling home chugged westward to deliver its small passengers to waiting Catholic families in Clifton and Morenci in the Arizona territory. Church officials at the New York orphanage had screened the families carefully to be certain that the couples hoping to adopt these children were virtuous churchgoing Catholics, industrious workers, and respectable members of the community. The local parish priest approved these couples, and on the appointed day, they waited eagerly as the orphans, dressed in their best clothes with their pink cheeks scrubbed clean, departed from the train. Along with the expectant couples, the waiting crowd included many women of the town. But when the Anglo-Protestant residents of the town discovered that Mexican Catholic foster parents claimed these fair-skinned children, they were outraged.

That night, the Anglo women gathered to mobilize their husbands into a vigilante posse. In the middle of the night, during a driving rainstorm, the men went to the homes of the Mexican couples, banged on the doors, and kidnapped the children at gunpoint. The next day, the children were distributed to the vigilantes' wives and other Anglo foster parents. Although the Catholic foundling home that had placed the children with the Mexican couples fought a lengthy legal battle to regain custody of the children, the Anglos managed to keep the orphans. The Arizona Supreme Court validated the kidnapping in the name of the "best interests of the children," and the U.S. Supreme Court let the ruling stand.

The struggle over the orphans reflected tensions and divisions in the region along lines of class as well as race. Longtime residents of this borderland region of Arizona included many Mexicans, mainly farmers, ranchers, and miners. In the early twentieth century Mexico's deteriorating economy prompted large numbers of Mexicans to migrate to California and the Southwest, looking for work. The year before the arrival of the orphans, Mexican mine workers had struck for better wages and working conditions against the Anglo owners of the Arizona Copper Company. The owners put down the strike, and the conflict left bitter feelings on both sides. The vigilante kidnapping of the orphans was, in part, retaliation against the Mexican workers who had organized the strike the previous year.

The upheavals of the Mexican Revolution increased migration after 1911. Most of the migrants to the Southwest found work in mining, railroads, and agriculture, usually as unskilled workers earning meager wages. Excluded from most labor unions until the 1920s, they nevertheless organized strikes from time to time to improve wages and working conditions. During the first decade of the century, and especially after the Mexican Revolution, nativist hostility to the Mexicans intensified. Although the orphan abduction was unique, the conditions and tensions that gave rise to it existed across the region.

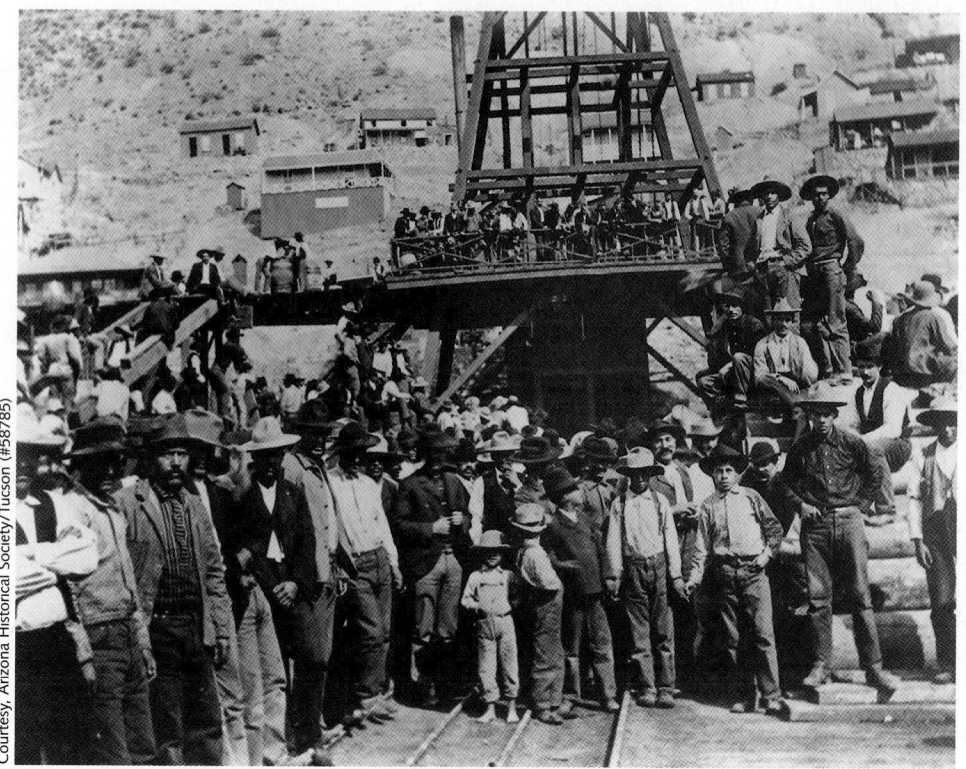

Courtesy, Arizona Historical Society/Tucson (#58785)

■ **Mexican miners in Arizona struck against their Anglo employers in 1903. The mining company paid Mexican workers less than their Anglo counterparts. In addition to the human toll of death and disease caused by the dangerous conditions in the mines, copper mining also caused permanent damage to the environment.**

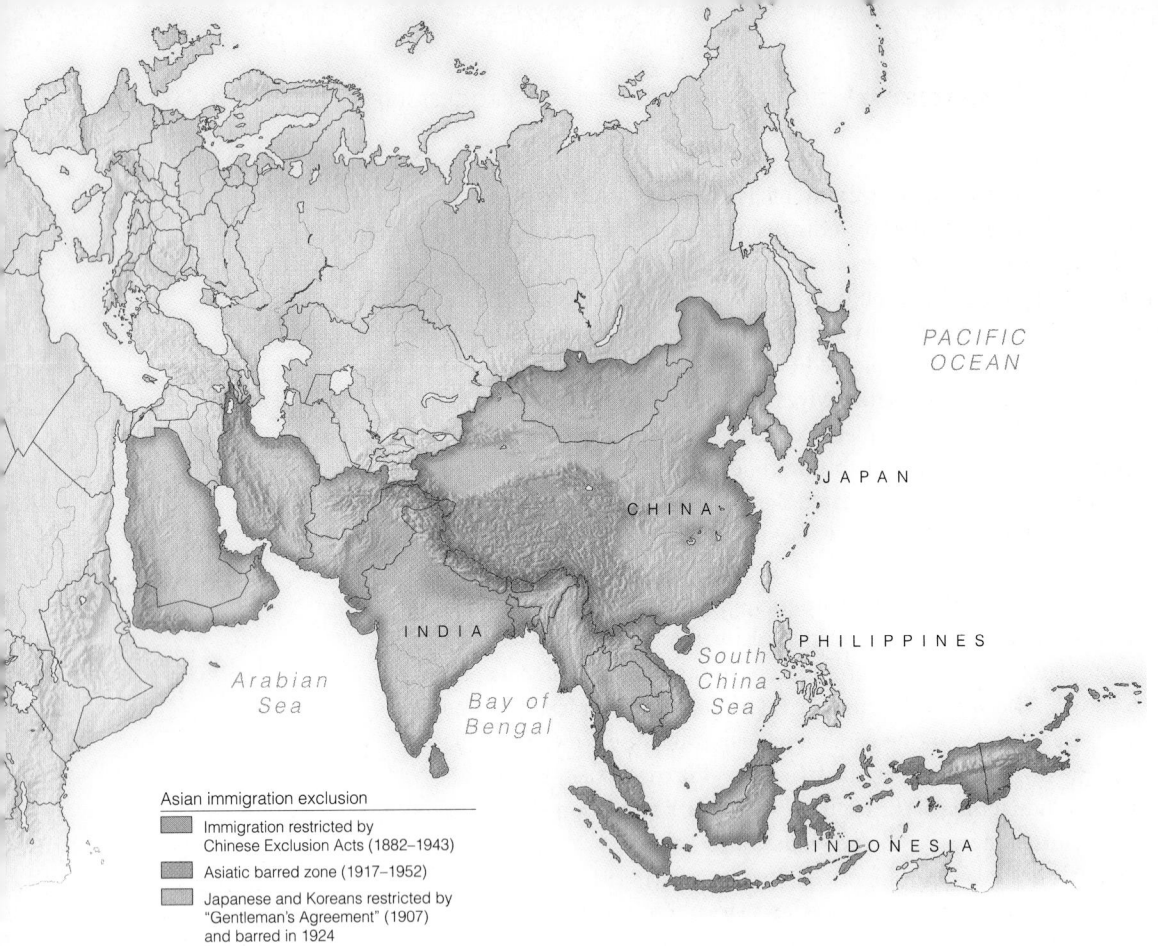

PACIFIC
OCEAN

JAPAN

CHINA

INDIA

PHILIPPINES

*Arabian
Sea*

*Bay of
Bengal*

*South
China
Sea*

INDONESIA

Asian immigration exclusion

▢ Immigration restricted by
Chinese Exclusion Acts (1882–1943)

▢ Asiatic barred zone (1917–1952)

▢ Japanese and Koreans restricted by
"Gentleman's Agreement" (1907)
and barred in 1924

■ **MAP 19.2**

AREAS EXCLUDED FROM IMMIGRATION TO THE UNITED STATES, 1882–1952 In 1882 the United
States barred Chinese immigrants from entering the country; Japanese and Koreans were barred in 1924.
In 1917 the exclusion was extended to people from India, Indonesia, and the Arabian Peninsula. Those laws
remained in effect until 1943 and 1952, respectively.

Asian Immigration and the Impact of Exclusion

Asians continued to face the most severe restrictions on immigration. The Chinese Exclusion Act of 1882, which prohibited most Chinese from immigrating to the United States, was renewed and extended in 1902. As a result, the mostly bachelor Chinese community in the United States declined by nearly half between 1890 and 1920. Many died or returned to China, reducing the numbers from more than 107,000 to about 61,000. The sex ratio remained severely imbalanced, with about 14 men for every woman.

During the exclusion era, certain categories of Chinese immigrants were allowed entry. Wives of Chinese men already in the United States could enter, as could teachers, students, and merchants. These exceptions made it possible for more than 20,000 Chinese to enter the country during the first decade of the new century. One such emigrant was Sieh King King, an 18-year-old student. In 1902, at a meeting of the Protect the Emperor Society, a reform party that advocated restoring the deposed emperor and establishing a constitutional monarchy in China, she addressed a packed hall in San Francisco's Chinatown. The *San Francisco Chronicle* reported that she "boldly condemned the slave girl system, raged at the horrors of foot-binding [a traditonal Chinese practice in which girls' feet were tightly bound to keep them small] and, with all the vehemence of aroused youth, declared that men and women were equal and should enjoy the privileges of equals." Like Clara Lemlich, her eastern European Jewish peer in New York, Sieh King King expressed ideas that were emerging among urban radicals in the United States but also reflected political movements in their home countries. Sieh King

King's sentiments were directly linked to the women's rights and nationalist movements in China, which were central to efforts to modernize China and strengthen it against further foreign encroachments. The radicalism she brought with her from China called for changes in her native land as well as in her adopted country.

Individual Chinese could also immigrate if they had family members in the United States. As a result, American-born Chinese frequently traveled back and forth, claiming on their return that they left a child in China and requesting permission for their offspring to emigrate. In this way they created spaceholders for imaginary kin, allowing other Chinese to enter the country. The American authorities knew of this system of "paper sons" and "paper fathers" and tried to stop the practice with elaborate and lengthy investigations that could last a year or more while hopeful Chinese immigrants waited as virtual prisoners in wretched conditions on Angel Island, the immigrant gateway off the coast of San Francisco.

Not easily thwarted, Chinese Americans on the mainland smuggled information to their fictional relatives, cleverly providing details of their families and communities back home so that their stories would match. Since it was illegal to transmit such information and letters were read and confiscated, these messages often arrived concealed in walnut shells or other camouflages. These subterfuges provided essential information for the hopeful migrants while also contributing to the stereotype that the Chinese were inscrutable and sneaky. The Chinese resisted their exclusion and their unfair treatment in the United States with open and collective action as well. They persuaded China and other Chinese communities overseas to boycott U.S. goods, which led to some improvements in their treatment. Nevertheless, the restrictions remained.

Before the Chinese Exclusion Act in 1882, more than 332,000 Chinese immigrants had entered the United States, most of them unskilled laborers. White Californians, fearing that the Chinese would compete for jobs and drive down the wages, pressured Congress to prohibit Chinese immigration. Only Chinese immigrants were excluded. At the time, there were only about 3000 Japanese immigrants in mainland United States. Japanese immigrants could still enter the country, and nearly 300,000 did so between 1890 and 1920, when opportunities for high-paying jobs in Hawaii and California offered an alternative to the economic crisis they faced in Japan. As one Japanese immigrant wrote in traditional Haiku poetic form,

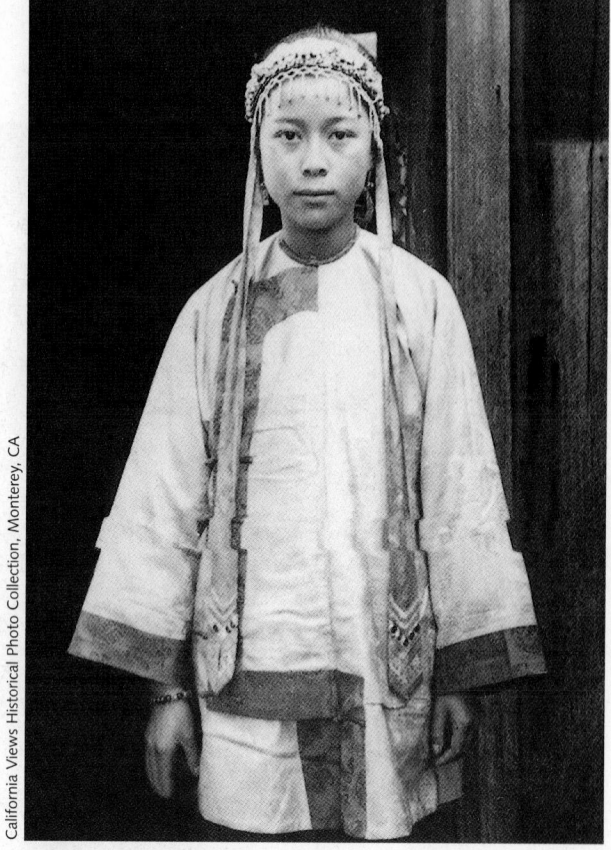

California Views Historical Photo Collection, Monterey, CA

■ This young woman was a "picture bride" whose photograph secured her betrothal to her distant future husband. In this way, many men who emigrated from Asia arranged to marry women they had never met. The young fiancée then left her home to join a strange man in a strange land, hoping for the best.

Huge dreams of fortune
Go with me to foreign lands
Across the ocean.

When the Chinese Exclusion Act was renewed in 1902, nearly as many Japanese immigrants entered the country as had the Chinese during the peak years before their exclusion in 1882. Most of the men came as workers; most of the women arrived as wives. Marriages in Japan generally were arranged by families, and some men returned to Japan to meet and marry their brides. But cost and distance often prevented those meetings. Some women came to the United States as "picture brides" after an exchange of photographs. Although some women were disappointed with their often much older husbands, most accepted their fate as they would have accepted an arranged marriage in Japan. Others were delighted with the opportunity for adventure and life in the new land. As one picture bride explained, many of the people from her village had already gone to the United States, and she wanted to go, too: "I didn't care what the man looked like."

Although the Japanese comprised less than 1 percent of California's population, they faced intense nativist hostility. The Japanese in California protested against the discrimination they faced, and in one case they successfully turned a local case of school segregation into an international incident. In response to the segregation of Japanese children in San Francisco, the Japanese government expressed its extreme displeasure. Hoping to avoid a confrontation with Japan—a significant military power that had just won a war with Russia—President Theodore Roosevelt interceded and convinced the San Francisco school board to rescind its segregation order. This incident led to the "Gentlemen's Agreement" of 1907, in which the Japanese government agreed to limit the number of immigrants to the United States. The numbers of immigrants from Japan dwindled, and Japanese immigrants instead began to settle in Brazil.

Newcomers from Southern and Eastern Europe

Eastern European Jews were among the most numerous of the "new" immigrants in the early twentieth century. In 1880, there were about 250,000 Jews in America; by 1920, there were 4 million, the vast majority from eastern Europe. During those 40 years, a number of factors motivated Jews to leave their small towns, or *shtetls*. Antisemitic policies in Russia and eastern Europe confined them within the Pale of Settlement, an area restricted for Jews. Eco-

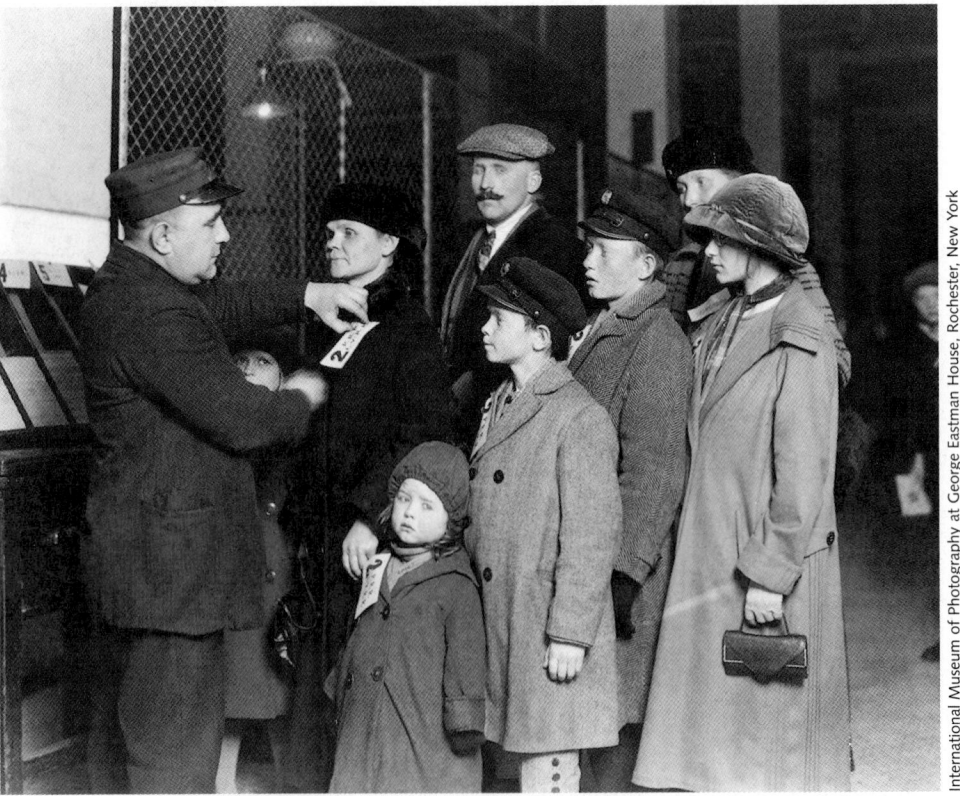

International Museum of Photography at George Eastman House, Rochester, New York

■ **At Ellis Island this immigrant family received identification tags, indicating that they had been examined and declared healthy. Those who were ill, or youngsters without relatives to meet them, were sent to quarantine houses. Some were refused entry and sent back to their home countries.**

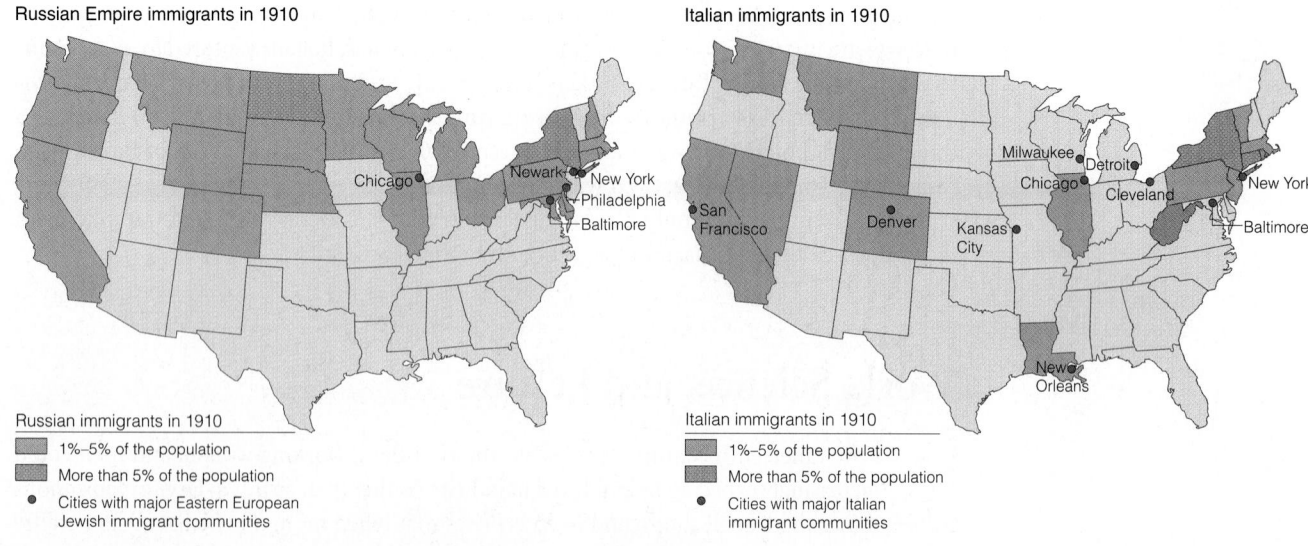

Russian Empire immigrants in 1910

Italian immigrants in 1910

Russian immigrants in 1910
- 1%–5% of the population
- More than 5% of the population
- ● Cities with major Eastern European Jewish immigrant communities

Italian immigrants in 1910
- 1%–5% of the population
- More than 5% of the population
- ● Cities with major Italian immigrant communities

■ **MAP 19.3**
RUSSIAN AND ITALIAN IMMIGRANTS IN THE UNITED STATES, 1910 Immigrants from Russia and Italy settled across the Northeast, Midwest, and West, with concentrations in large cities. Louisiana was the only southern state with a large concentration of Eastern or Southern European immigrants.

nomic turmoil and restrictions on Jewish land ownership, trade, and business left many Jews impoverished. Even more devastating was the increase in anti-Semitic violence in the form of riots, or *pogroms,* in which Jewish towns were attacked and many Jews were beaten and killed. Although Jews were denied civil rights and faced frequent attacks, they were, nevertheless, subject to the draft. Many young boys emigrated to avoid being conscripted into the czar's army.

One such emigrant was young Morris Bass. At age 12 he left his family and ventured alone across the Atlantic. The uncle who was to meet him forgot about his arrival, stranding Morris in the quarantine building on Ellis Island. Although he was among the lucky ones who passed the medical exam and was declared healthy enough to enter the country, he could not be released until a relative came to claim him and guarantee that the boy would be provided with support. After two weeks, just as immigration officials were preparing to send the boy back to Russia, his uncle appeared. He brought Morris home and showed him where to sleep. But as soon as the boy heard his uncle snoring, Morris ran away, furious at this relative who had left him to suffer two miserable weeks in captivity. He did not wander long in the crowded Jewish ghetto before a butcher offered him a job and a place to sleep on a straw mat behind the shop.

Morris did well in the new land. Although he did not live out the rags-to-riches dream, few immigrants did. Like many others, he prospered modestly. After a few years, he was able to strike out on his own as a pushcart peddler. Eventually, he sent home enough money to bring his parents and siblings to America. Some Jewish immigrants struggled to retain the faith and practices of Jewish orthodoxy that had defined their lives in the *shtetl.* But Morris was among those who wanted to assimilate into American life. He retained Jewish cultural practices but abandoned many religious rituals, such as refraining from work on Saturdays (the Jewish Sabbath) and wearing distinctive clothes. Nevertheless, he lived his life as a Jew among Jews, speaking Yiddish, celebrating the religious holidays, and maintaining a kosher home according to Jewish dietary laws, even though he rarely set foot in a synagogue.

Italian immigration also reached its peak between 1900 and 1914. While 90 percent of the Jews who migrated from Russia came to the United States, Italians ventured to many countries around the world. Turmoil in their home country resulting from the political and economic consequences of unification of the Italian peninsula, prompted 27 million Italians—a third of Italy's population—to migrate between 1870 and 1920. The majority of Italians who came to the United States arrived with their families and settled permanently, establishing strong communities and mutual aid societies. Most Italians were committed Catholics, and they preserved their rituals, festivals, and faith in the new country.

Work, Science, and Leisure

As the nineteenth century gave way to the twentieth, working women and men could increasingly expect to be employed in industry rather than farms, in large organizations rather than small shops, and in enterprises that relied more on efficiency than craftsmanship. Towering skyscrapers began to dot the urban landscape, symbolic of the triumph of commerce and corporate power. Science and technology reigned, changing the nature of work as well as the fruits of production. Professional organizations of educators, social workers, physicians, and scientists emerged, while experts with academic credentials became leaders of many public institutions. It seemed as though science could solve virtually any problem. Advances in medical science contributed to improved public health. But in some cases, experts relied on scientific principles to address social problems rather than confronting the underlying structural causes, such as widespread poverty.

The Uses and Abuses of Science

Breakthroughs in science and medicine led to improvements in public health. Reformers exposed the dangers of potions and remedies sold by street vendors, as standards for medications improved. But crowding and lack of sanitation still fostered the spread of disease, especially among the poor. In 1900 the death rate for African Americans was 69 percent higher than the rate for whites. Lack of access to clean water was one of the major causes of disease, along with crowding, lack of medical care, and other chronic problems of poverty. Public sanitation alleviated the problem considerably in the early years of the twentieth century, reducing the incidence of typhoid fever by 70 percent. Among those who contributed to better conditions were community nurses. In 1900 the New York Charity Organization Society hired Jessie Sleet Scales, the first African American public health nurse, to address problems related to tuberculosis. Scales and other public health professionals implemented sanitation standards and provided care for poor communities, helping to control the spread of disease.

Public sanitation remained a problem, however, especially in crowded cities. An outbreak of typhoid among well-to-do New Yorkers led to Mary Mallon, an Irish immigrant, who had worked as a cook for a number of prominent families. When six members of a household where she worked developed typhoid, she was identified as a carrier of the disease. Later, authorities discovered that typhoid outbreaks occurred in seven of eight households that had employed her. Although Mallon had no symptoms, she was forced to remain in a hospital for people with contagious diseases until she sued for her release in 1909 and was released in 1910. She was instructed not to cook for a living, but as she had no other means to support herself, she went back to work as a cook. In 1915, she was arrested again after more typhoid cases were traced to her, and this time she was placed in isolation on an island virtually as a prisoner for 26 years, until her death in 1939.

The local press vilified Mallon, whom they dubbed "Typhoid Mary," and blamed her for the spread of the illness. As a carrier of the disease, she did indeed infect several people.

But she was not the only source of contagion in the city. Typhoid, like many other diseases, was a public health problem. Although Mallon was not the only healthy carrier of typhoid at this time, she was the only healthy person who had never been accused of a crime but was subjected to what amounted to a life sentence of imprisonment. City officials might have pursued other alternatives, such as helping Mallon find a job in which she would not endanger others and developing a broad-based public health approach that would have improved sanitation in the city.

Reflecting a similar impulse to blame social problems on allegedly flawed individuals or groups was the eugenics movement, which advocated scientific breeding to improve the nation's racial stock. The pseudoscience of eugenics emerged in the nineteenth century in England and spread to the United States, where it gained wide support. Drawing on theories of white racial superiority and unscientific notions of genetic inheritance, eugenicists believed that character traits were inherited, including tendencies toward criminality, sexual immorality, and lack of discipline leading to poverty. Eugenicists claimed that social problems resulted from the high birthrate of immigrants and others they considered to be racially inferior to Anglo-Saxon Americans and the low birthrate of educated middle-class whites.

President Theodore Roosevelt was an outspoken advocate of eugenics reform. One of his major concerns was that Americans were shirking their duty to create a robust citizenry for the future. Alarmed by the dramatic decline in the birthrate of native-born Americans and the tendency of college-educated women to remain single and childless, he feared that the immigrants, with their much higher birthrate, would overrun the nation. Roosevelt called upon Anglo-Saxon women to prevent what he called "race suicide," much as male citizens had an obligation to defend the country if called to military duty. In his sixth annual message to Congress in 1903, Roosevelt warned:

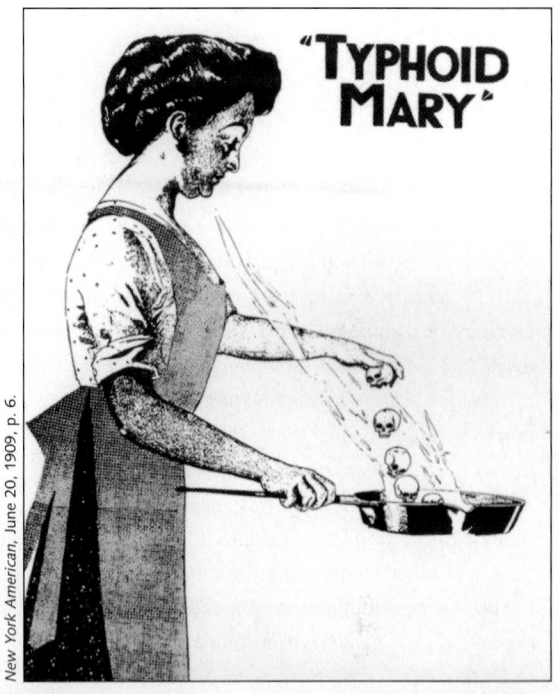

New York American, June 20, 1909, p. 6.

■ "Typhoid Mary" unwittingly mixes death into an omelet in this 1909 poster warning against bad hygiene.

> When home ties are loosened, when men and women cease to regard a worthy family life . . . as the life best worth living, then evil days of the commonwealth are at hand. There are regions in our own land, and classes of our population, where the birth rate has sunk below the death rate. Surely it should need no demonstration to show that willful sterility is, from the standpoint of the nation . . . the one sin for which the penalty is national death, race death. . . . No man, no woman, can shirk the primary duties of life, whether for love of ease and pleasure, or for any other reason, and retain his or her self-respect.

Some eugenics crusaders proposed compulsory sterilization of those they deemed unfit for parenthood. Indiana enacted a eugenic sterilization law in 1907, and other states soon followed. These laws gave legal sanction to the surgical sterilization of thousands of men and even greater numbers of women whom government and medical officials deemed "feebleminded." The criteria for determining "feeblemindedness" were vague at best; often sexual impropriety or out-of-wedlock pregnancy landed young women—generally poor and often foreign-born—in institutions for the feebleminded, where the operations took place. The Supreme Court upheld compulsory sterilization laws in the 1920s. Increasingly, women of color were targeted, and the practice continued well into the 1980s.

Scientific Management and Mass Production

In 1911 Frederick Winslow Taylor wrote *The Principles of Scientific Management,* his guide to increased efficiency in the nation's industries. Taylor began his career as a laborer in the Midvale

Defining Whiteness

Naturalization laws pertaining to immigrants in the early twentieth century were based on racial categories. Asian immigrants, classified racially as "Mongolians," were not allowed to apply for U.S. citizenship. Naturalization was available only "to aliens being free white persons and to aliens of African nativity and to persons of African descent." Because racial theories were imprecise and fluid, and racial identities were not linked to nationality, immigrants occasionally challenged their racial classification to claim that they were "white." John Svan, who was Finnish, petitioned in federal court to contest the labeling of Finns as Mongolians, claiming that he was white

and, therefore, allowed to apply for U.S. citizenship. The petition demonstrates the acceptance of racial definitions based on phenotype—particularly skin color—as well as the imprecise nature of those definitions. The court granted Svan's petition, legally changing his racial identity from Mongolian to white and reclassifying Finns as white people. Here is the court's memorandum, which allowed Svan to become a citizen:

John Svan was born in Finland and calls himself a Finn. . . . According to ethnologists, the Finns in very remote times were of Mongol origin; but the various groupings of the human race into families is arbitrary and, as respects any particular people, is not permanent but is subject to change and modification through the influences of climate, employment, intermarriage and other causes. There are indications that

central and western Europe was at one time overrun by the Finns; some of their stock remained, but their racial characteristics were entirely lost in their remote descendants, who now are in no danger of being classed as Mongols. The Osmanlis, said to be of Mongol extraction, are now among the purest and best types of the Caucasian race. Changes are constantly going on and those occurring in the lapse of a few hundred years with any people may be very great.

The chief physical characteristics of the Mongolians are as follows: They are short of stature, with little hair on their body or face; they have yellow-brown skins, black eyes, black hair, short, flat noses, and oblique eyes. In actual experience we sometimes, though rarely, see natives of Finland whose eyes are slightly oblique. We sometimes see them with sparse beards and

Steel Works near Philadelphia in 1878 and rose through the ranks to become the plant's chief engineer. There he developed a system to improve mass production in factories in order to make more goods more quickly. Taylor's principles included analysis of each job to determine the precise motions and tools needed to maximize each worker's productivity, detailed instructions for workers and guidelines for their supervisors, and wage scales with incentives to motivate workers to achieve high production goals. Over the next decades, industrial managers all over the country drew on Taylor's studies. Business leaders rushed to embrace Taylor's principles, and Taylor himself became a pioneering management consultant.

Henry Ford was among the most successful industrialists to employ Taylor's techniques. Born in 1863 on a farm near Dearborn, Michigan, the mechanically inclined Ford became an apprentice in a Detroit machine shop in 1879. Although he did not invent the automobile—the first motor cars were manufactured in Germany—he developed design and production methods that brought the cost of an automobile within the reach of the average worker. Experimenting with the new internal combustion engine in the 1890s, he built his first automobile in 1896. In 1903 Ford established the Ford Motor Company and began a profitable business. He introduced the popular and relatively inexpensive, mass-produced Model T automobile in 1908, which sold for $850. In 1913 Ford introduced assembly line production, a system in which each worker performed one task repeatedly as each automobile in the process of construction moved along a conveyor. Assembly-line manufacturing increased production while cutting costs. In 1914 Ford increased his workers' wages to $5 per day at a time when industrial laborers averaged only $11 per week. By 1916 the price of the Model T dropped to $360. In this sense Ford was a pioneer not only in production but also in consumption.

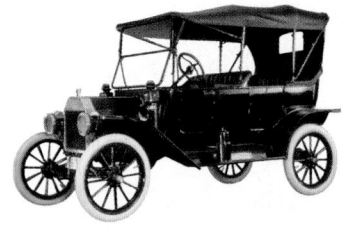

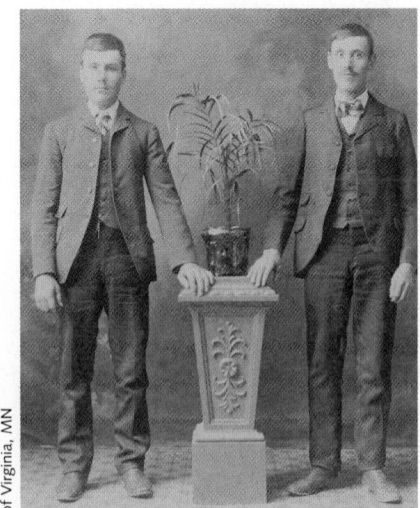
Minnesota Historical Society, Negative #93125. Photo by Maki of Virginia, MN

These Finnish men living in Minnesota were among those whose racial classification was changed from "Mongolian" to "White" as the result of one Finnish immigrant's petition. Along with the Jews, Italians, Irish, and other immigrant groups now considered "white," Finns were classified as nonwhite until the laws and customs changed. Racial categories were fluid and imprecise, but whiteness conferred status and privileges.

sometimes with flat noses; but Finns with a yellow or brown or yellow-brown skin or with black eyes or black hair would be an unusual sight. They are almost universally of light skin, blue or gray eyes, and light hair. No people of foreign births applying in this section of the country for the full rights of citizenship are lighter-skinned than those born in Finland. In stature they are quite up to the average. Confessedly, Finland has often been overrun with Teutons and by other branches of the human family, who, with their descendants, have remained within her borders and are now called Finns. They are in the main indistinguishable in their physical characteristics from those of purer Finnish blood. Intermarriages have been frequent over a very long period of time. If the Finns were originally Mongols, modifying influences have continued until they are now among the whitest people in Europe. It would, therefore, require a most exhaustive tracing of family history to determine whether any particular individual born in Finland had or had not a remote Mongol ancestry. This, of course, cannot be done and was not intended. The question is not whether a person had or had not such ancestry, but whether he is now a "white person" within the meaning of that term as usually understood. This is the practical construction which has uniformly been placed upon the law. . . . Under such law Finns have always been admitted to citizenship, and there is no occasion now to change the construction.

The applicant is without doubt a white person within the true intent and meaning of such law.

The objections, therefore, in my opinion should be overruled and it will be so ordered. ∎

Although an industrial genius, Ford was narrow-minded and bigoted. A ferocious anti-Semite, he later became an active supporter of Adolf Hitler. He fought unionization fiercely with a private police force. But his production methods, as well as the Ford motor car, became fixtures of twentieth-century business and consumer culture. Ford embodied many contradictions: he helped to create modern life, but he was also repulsed by it. He created a nostalgic theme park in Deerfield Village, Michigan, where he brought together old houses and artifacts to recreate a small town of the nineteenth century, where there were no cars or factories. Yet Ford's own life's work had contributed to the disappearance of the way of life represented in Deerfield Village.

New Amusements

As Americans increasingly moved from rural to urban areas, and from farms to factories, new institutions of leisure emerged in the growing cities. Consumer culture was the flipside of business culture in the early twentieth century, and it represented a major change not only in leisure time pursuits but also in cultural values. Newcomers and "outsiders" were largely responsible for those changing values. One of the great ironies of American history in the twentieth century is that its popular culture—which more than anything else identifies the United States to the rest of the world—was largely a creation of immigrants and people of color. During the very years when these groups faced intense discrimination, they developed the cultural products that came to define America itself.

The motion picture industry is a case in point. In 1888 Thomas Edison invented the kinetoscope, the early motion picture camera. The pragmatic Edison thought that his new device might be used in education and industry. But he did not see much commercial potential for the gadget. As he wrote in 1893,

> I have constructed a little instrument which I call a Kinetoscope, with a nickel and slot attachment. Some twenty-five have been made, but I am very doubtful there is any commercial feature in it, and fear that they will not earn their cost. These zeotropic devices are of too sentimental a value to get the public to invest in.

Because of his lack of enthusiasm as well as his lack of investors, Edison did not even bother to take out a foreign patent on the kinetoscope or to seek markets for his invention at home. Not until the early twentieth century, when Jewish immigrant entrepreneurs recognized its potential for mass entertainment, did the moving picture begin to reach a wide audience. Moviemak-

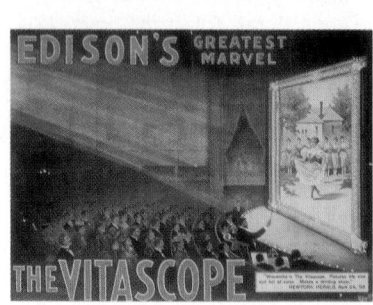

ers left the East Coast and moved to the West, taking advantage of the even climate, cheap land, and nonunion labor. Within a few years, the moviemakers, mostly Jewish immigrants from Europe, established the film industry. By the late teens and twenties, Paramount, Metro-Goldwyn-Mayer, and Fox Studios—all founded by Jews—had become leaders in moviemaking. Hollywood emerged as a major center of American popular culture, sending its products across the nation and abroad.

The first audiences for the motion pictures were in the working-class neighborhoods of the growing cities. New York offers a vivid example of the rapid expansion of the movies as well as other urban amusements. In that city alone, by 1910, there were 1000 small storefront theaters and fun houses known as penny arcades where there had been none 20 years earlier. The numbers of saloons also increased from 7000 to 9000, while the Coney Island amusement park drew thousands to its shimmering lights and thrilling rides. During these same years, the sounds of African American music began to attract audiences among immigrants as well as native-born whites. Youths from all ethnic groups flocked to dance halls where they danced to the lively tunes often played by black musicians who "ragged" the beat with new jazz rhythms.

Working-class youth were not the only ones drawn to the new urban amusements. Glamorous night clubs, known as cabarets, also began to appear, offering dining, dancing, music, and entertainment to the wealthy. Jesse Lasky opened the Follies Bergeres in New York in 1911. Lasky filled his cabaret with lavish furnishings, hired black musicians to play ragtime music, and charged high prices. "Everything about the Follies," Lasky wrote, "was unheard of in New York, including the prices." In an effort to render these upper-class cabarets respectable and distinguish them from the rowdy working-class dance halls, owners tamed the erotic dances to express a more moderate sensuality.

"Sex O'Clock in America"

The sexual mores and behavior of Americans seemed to be changing so dramatically that one observer announced that "sex o'clock" had struck. Indeed, the codes of the past were challenged at every turn. Among the middle class, unchaperoned dating began to replace the previous system of a man "coming to call" at the home of a woman he hoped to court. Automobiles gave young couples more freedom and privacy. Physical intimacy became more acceptable, and even unacceptable sexual behavior became more common.

Immigrants often brought traditional courtship patterns to the new world and extended them into the next generation. One Italian man described his thwarted efforts to woo his fiancée in private. When he visited her home, "She sat on one side of the table, and I at the other. They afraid I touch." Finally, less than a month before their wedding, he got permission to take her to the theater. But the family was unwilling to let them go alone. "We came to the aisles of the theater. My mother-in-law go first, my fiancée next, my little sister, my father in law. I was the last one. I had two in between. . . . I was next to the old man." He tried to steal a kiss a few days before the wedding, but his fiancée rebuffed him: "No, not yet."

In spite of efforts by their elders, native-born as well as immigrant youth challenged the sexual codes of the past. Young working women looked forward to fun in their leisure hours and sometimes exchanged physical intimacies for "treats" from men who took them out to a meal or a dance. These women were known as "charity girls" to distinguish them from prostitutes. Increasing sexual intimacy among unmarried men and women reflected heightened expectations for sexual satisfaction—for women as well as men. These years also witnessed a rise in the proportion of brides who were pregnant at marriage, from a low of 10 percent in the mid-nineteenth century to 23 percent by 1910.

Marriage increasingly held the promise not only of love, intimacy, and mutual obligation, as it had in the nineteenth century, but of sexual fulfillment and shared leisure pursuits. As expectations for marital happiness rose, so did the divorce rate. Liberal divorce laws, combined with expanding opportunities for women to support themselves, prompted increasing numbers of men and women to end unhappy marriages and try again. The rising divorce rate did not signal a decline in the popularity of marriage, however; a greater proportion of Americans married and at increasingly younger ages. Those who divorced were likely to remarry, a pattern that continued through the twentieth century.

> *Marriage increasingly held the promise not only of love, intimacy, and mutual obligation, but of sexual fulfillment and shared leisure pursuits.*

Some women did not marry but instead formed lifelong attachments to other women. Rarely identified as lesbian but often described as "Boston marriages," these unions signified long-term emotional bonds between women who lived together. The widely admired reformer Jane Addams shared her life with Mary Rozet Smith for more than thirty years. Meanwhile, lesbians, as well as gay men, gained greater visibility in the cities. They frequented bars and clubs in such places as Greenwich Village and Harlem, hoping to avoid the attention of police, who were likely to arrest them for indecent conduct. Heterosexual men and women also came to these neighborhoods for entertainment. Drag balls became elaborate annual events that drew thousands of spectators and participants, including large numbers of heterosexuals.

Artists Respond to the New Era

Artists, composers, writers, and architects all contributed to enriching, expressing, interpreting, and transforming the urban industrial landscape. Among the most controversial was a group of painters who focused their attention on portrayals of life in the cities—including urban amusements and diverse working-class subjects. Although these artists did not pioneer new styles of painting, their content was revolutionary. Robert Henri painted scenes of the city including ethnic minorities, William Glackens depicted cabarets and night life, Everett Shinn portrayed prostitutes and other "low-life" characters, and John Sloan evoked New York's Lower East Side, immigrants, and theaters. This art exuded the vitality of urban life and conveyed a gritty reality without moral condemnation; these artists treated their subjects with dignity and humanity. Contemptuous critics referred to them as the "Ashcan School," a label they embraced.

The artistic movement known as realism, characterized by a detached and skeptical approach to subject matter, also infused in the writing of fiction. The novelist Theodore Dreiser wrote in this new style. His 1900 novel *Sister Carrie* narrates the story of an independent young woman who comes to Chicago and uses her sexuality to advance her ambition. Contrary to the morality tales popular at the time, Carrie does not suffer for her sins. Rather, she prospers, while her male lovers are destroyed by their infatuation with her. Because of the novel's scandalous content, Dreiser's publisher did not promote the book, although it was revived and republished in later years.

Photography also began to exhibit a new realism in the work of such documentary photographers as Lewis Hine, who photographed immigrants, industrial work, and urban street

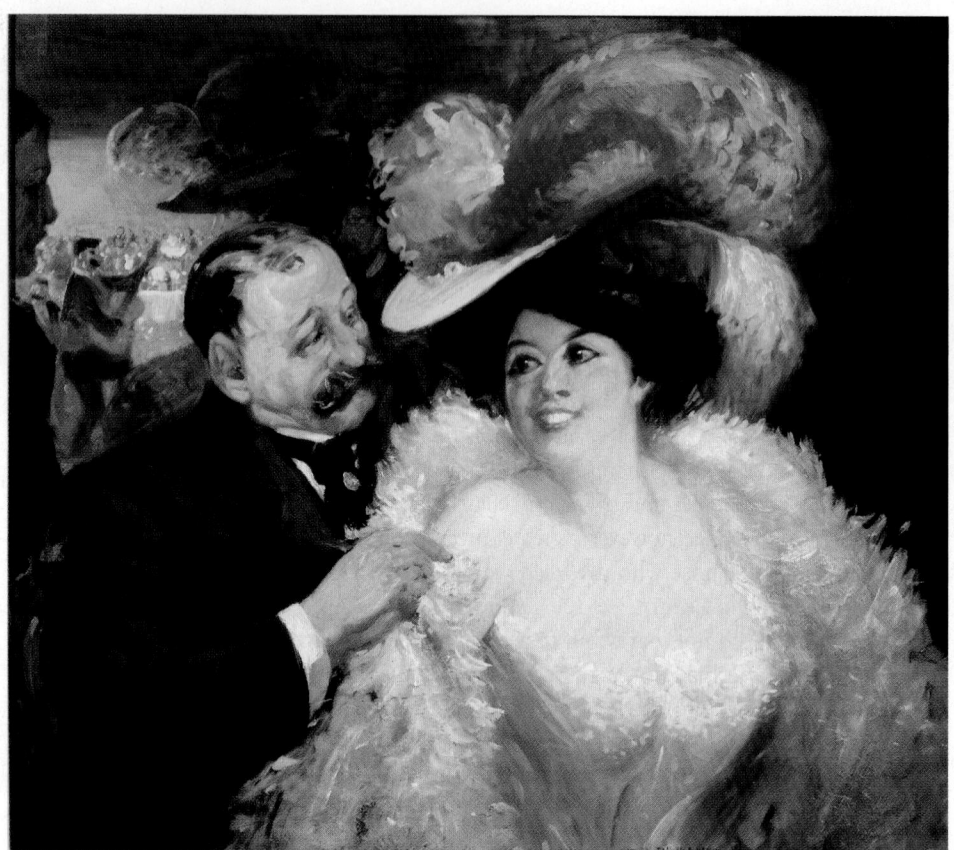

■ *The Café Francis,* by George Luks, c. 1909. Luks was one of the "Ashcan School" artists who celebrated urban street life and popular culture. Their raw and sensual depictions of city entertainments stirred controversy among art critics at the time.

George Luks, *The Cafe Francis*, c. 1909. The Butler Institute of American Art, Youngstown, Ohio

life, and such avant-garde artists as Alfred Stieglitz and Edward Steichen, who drew inspiration from artistic innovations in Europe, such as Cubism. Popular music also flourished in the first decade of the century, especially jazz. From its roots in African musical traditions, slave songs, spirituals, and ragtime, jazz brought together the various strains of African American music and developed new forms. Centered in New Orleans, artists such as pianist Ferdinand "Jelly Roll" Morton and cornet player Charles "Buddy" Bolden played the new syncopated rhythms.

Reformers and Radicals

The broad movement for social reform known as Progressivism included two distinct impulses. On the one hand, many Anglo-Saxon Protestants tried to impose order on a rapidly changing nation. They hoped to stem the tide of immigration, bolster the rapidly eroding sexual codes, and quell the movements for social change. On the other hand, women's rights activists, workers, and African Americans struggled to achieve the rights and privileges available to white men of property and standing. The tensions between these two very different approaches to reform shaped the politics of the era.

Muckrakers, Moral Reform, and Vice Crusades

In the early twentieth century, a group of investigative journalists began to expose the ills of industrial life. President Theodore Roosevelt dubbed them the "muckrakers" in 1906 to signal their tendency to unearth the dirtiest aspects of the nation's political and economic institutions. Although Roosevelt intended the term as an insult, the muckrakers embraced their label. Their best-known works illuminated corruption in business and politics. Ida Tarbell wrote a powerful exposé of ruthless business practices of John D. Rockefeller, who transformed the Standard Oil company into a monopoly. Lincoln Steffens unearthed scandals in city and state politics. By 1912, more than 1000 muckraking articles appeared in widely read and popular magazines such as *McClure's, Everybody's,* and *Collier's.*

One of the best-known muckraking novels was Upton Sinclair's *The Jungle,* published in 1906. A dedicated socialist, Sinclair hoped that his novel would illuminate the exploitation of immigrant workers. *The Jungle* tells the story of Jurgis Rudkus, a Lithuanian immigrant, and his family and friends and provides a grim exposé of horrid living and working conditions. Depiction of the meatpacking plant where Rudkus works includes descriptions of the filth, rats, and even the body parts of workers that end up ground into the packages of meat. The book had a powerful impact, but the effect was not what Sinclair had hoped. Rather than spark interest in socialism or even improved wages and working conditions, the novel aroused consumer indignation and, within months of its publication, led to the passage of the Pure Food and Drug Act and a Meat Inspection Act, which prohibited adulterated or fraudulently labeled food and drugs from interstate commerce. Sinclair later wrote with regret, "I aimed at the public's heart and by accident hit it in the stomach." The Pure Food and Drug Act was the first of a series of consumer protection laws passed in the twentieth century.

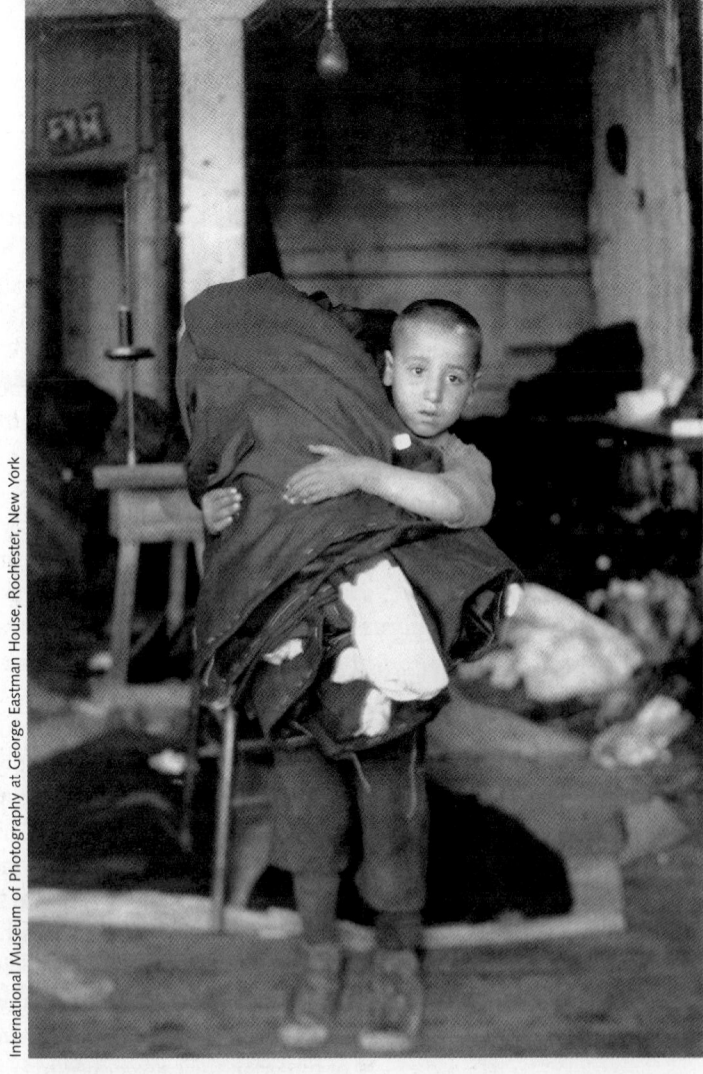

■ In the early twentieth century, many children such as this young boy worked long hours doing hard labor. Photographer Lewis Hine, who took this picture, worked for the National Child Labor Committee. His photographs documented the exploitation of child workers and helped to generate support for child labor laws.

Child labor was another concern of reformers. Children worked in fields and factories across the country, picking cotton in Texas, mining coal in West Virginia, working in the textile mills of North Carolina, and sewing buttons in urban sweatshops. The National Child Labor Committee, organized in 1904, as well as many state committees, endeavored to regulate or eliminate child labor. Children of immigrants and rural migrants often assisted parents on farms or in shops, their labor an accepted part of the household economy. Many parents felt that work also offered children opportunities to learn discipline as well as a trade and to gain a sense of pride and satisfaction as contributors to the family's needs. But the sorts of jobs available to children in the urban industrial world often were dangerous and unhealthy, characterized by long hours, low pay, and miserable working conditions. Reformers attempted to improve the conditions under which children worked and to establish age limits so that children could attend school and spend time in healthful recreation rather than in grim sweatshops and factories. Ultimately, child labor activists succeeded in passing legislation at the state level that restricted child labor, although these efforts were more successful in northern states than in the South.

Protective legislation for women was also controversial. Reformers campaigned for laws that would establish minimum wages, maximum hours, regulations against night work, and restrictions on heavy lifting. When they were unable to secure such safety measures for all workers, they

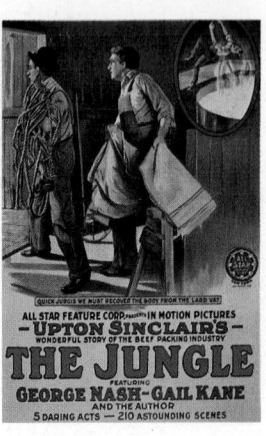

argued that women needed special protections because of their physical frailty and their role as future mothers. Women's rights activists disagreed over these measures. Some argued that they were necessary to protect women from exploitation and dangerous working conditions. Others claimed that women should be treated the same as men, arguing that protective legislation implied that women needed special care and were not suited for particular kinds of work. These debates continued throughout the century.

Women were prominent among Progressive reformers. Jane Addams, founder of Hull House, the immigrant neighborhood center in Chicago, became the most admired woman of her day. But many other influential women left their stamp on the culture and public policies of the era. Florence Kelley, the daughter of a prominent Philadelphia Quaker family, joined Addams's Hull House community and later headed the National Consumers' League (NCL) from 1898 until her death in 1932. Under her leadership, the NCL became the most effective lobbying agency for protective labor legislation for women and children. Kelley was instrumental in the successful defense of the ten-hour working day for women, which was affirmed by the Supreme Court in its 1908 decision, *Muller v. Oregon.*

> *Women were prominent among Progressive reformers and left their stamp on the culture and public policies of the era.*

Another noted reformer was Helen Keller, whose work on behalf of the blind called attention to the needs of the disabled. Keller lost her sight and hearing from an illness at the age of 19 months and learned to communicate through Braille and sign language, which she mastered through touch, with the help of her extraordinary teacher, Anne Sullivan. Keller went on to study at schools for the deaf and graduated with honors from Radcliffe College in 1904. A passionate socialist and advocate of women's rights along with other radical causes, Keller wrote several books and lectured widely all over the world, with the assistance of interpreters.

Most Progressive reformers were prosperous American-born Anglo-Saxon Protestants. Along with their efforts to improve living and working conditions and alleviate the suffering of the poor, they also hoped to eradicate vice from their society. At the level of local government, many reformers promoted zoning laws that would keep commercial entertainments out of residential neighborhoods. Vice crusaders in most of the nation's large cities tried to eliminate prostitution and to patrol dance halls, movie theaters, and saloons. Gay men and lesbians risked arrest if they were discovered mingling in public. At the national level, vice crusading culminated in the passage of the Mann Act in 1910, which made it illegal to transport women across state lines for "immoral purposes." The Mann Act resulted in 1,537 convictions by 1916. Over the years, authorities used the Mann Act not only to police prostitution but also to regulate interracial sex.

One such case garnered national attention. African American boxer Jack Johnson had defeated white fighters in the ring to become the world heavyweight champion in 1910. He was a hero to black Americans but a villain to many whites, who resented not only his athletic success but also his relationships with white women. In 1912, Lucille Cameron, a young white woman from Minnesota, visited Johnson's Chicago nightclub, and the two began an affair. Cameron's mother brought charges of abduction against Johnson, but the young woman refused to testify, so the case was dismissed. The couple later married. Authorities continued their efforts to punish Johnson for his racial and sexual transgressions. When federal agents persuaded one of Johnson's former lovers, a white prostitute, to testify that Johnson had paid for her travel from Pittsburgh to Chicago, he was convicted under the Mann Act and sentenced to one year in prison.

Woman Suffrage

The movement for women's rights, including the effort to gain the vote, was already more than half a century old by 1900. But the movement gained momentum at the dawn of the twentieth century. A new generation of women's rights leaders came together in the suffrage movement. They included working-class women and young college-educated women, some of them with experience in the settlement movement, and others who had participated in socialist and labor circles. They initiated new grassroots strategies, such as door-to-door campaigns, to gather support for woman suffrage. The militance of the suffrage movement in England inspired American activists to develop new tactics and international alliances. These activists achieved legislative success when several western states granted women the right to vote: Washington in 1910, California in 1911, and three more states in 1912. Eventually the movement united around the goal of enacting a federal amendment. The required three-quarters majority of the states ratified the Nineteenth Amendment in 1920, granting women the vote.

The suffrage movement, for all its radicalism, was largely a movement of white middle-class women. White suffrage leaders feared that any alliance with women of color would alienate Southern voters whom they needed for ratification of the Nineteenth Amendment. They also hoped to win over to their cause racist and nativist critics in the North who feared that granting the vote to women would enfranchise "undesirable" voters, specifically immigrant and minority women. Some women's rights leaders argued that granting the vote to women would increase the voting power of white Anglo-Saxons. Belle Kearney, a southern suffragist, saw the ballot for women as a means of keeping African Americans in their place: "The enfranchisement of women would insure immediate and durable white supremacy, honestly attained." The suffrage movement also gained the support of conservatives who believed that women would vote for conservative causes such as prohibition and immigration restriction.

Many minority women, such as Hispana activist Adelina Otero Warren, also supported the suffrage movement even though white leaders kept their distance and refused to embrace the antiracist campaigns of their nonwhite sisters. The African American antilynching activist Ida B. Wells (also known by her married name as Ida B. Wells-Barnett) supported woman suffrage but was unable to convince the white women's rights leaders to denounce lynching. Ultimately, the passage of the suffrage amendment resulted from a combination of factors, including radical activism, strong support of a wide range of reformers, and an alliance with conservative, racist, and anti-immigrant forces.

Radical Politics and the Labor Movement

Progressive reformers believed that American capitalist democracy was a fundamentally sound system that simply needed to be fixed to achieve its full promise. Radicals of the era believed that the system itself was flawed and needed to be fundamentally transformed. Emma Goldman, a Russian Jewish immigrant, was one of many radical activists who gained both fame and notoriety for her outspoken support of radical causes. Like Sieh King King and Clara Lemlich, Goldman was among the growing numbers of women who were leaders in the labor struggles of the day. But women were excluded from most unions. Only 3.3 percent of the 4 million women engaged in nonagricultural jobs in 1900 were members of trade unions. The number doubled in the wake of the successful wave of strikes by young immigrant garment workers in 1909–1910, including the 1909 shirtwaist makers' strike. In 1903 the WTUL brought together elite reformers and female laborers to help working women in their efforts to unionize while also connecting those efforts to the broader movement for women's rights.

Socialism also attracted followers during these years. Socialism was never as strong in the United States as it was in Europe, but it did gain strength at the turn of the century. Socialists promoted labor unions and the rights of women and formed their own political party. Socialist leader Eugene V. Debs gained national fame for his role in the 1894 railroad strike. Radicalized by his involvement in the labor movement, he turned to socialism at the turn of the century as a means for improving the conditions of the working classes. Forging alliances with a number of immigrant socialist groups, he became the spokesperson and leader of the Socialist party. Between 1900 and 1920, he was the party's candidate for president, gaining nearly a million votes, or 6 percent of the electorate, in the 1912 election. Although the socialists never gathered a large enough following to win national elections, they elected hundreds of candidates to local office.

The Industrial Workers of the World (IWW), also known as the Wobblies, offered another possibility for labor radicalism. Organized in 1905 by socialists and labor militants, its founders included Debs, William "Big Bill" Haywood of the Western Federation of Miners, the well-known labor activist Elizabeth Gurley Flynn, and the Tejana of Mexican and African American heritage Lucia Gonzales Parsons, whose husband had been executed as a result of the Haymarket bombing of 1886. The IWW included women, blacks, immigrants, and unskilled and migratory laborers, workers generally shunned by the American Federation of Labor (AFL). The Wobblies organized workers in the mines of the Rocky Mountain states, in the lumber camps of the Pacific Northwest and the South, and in the eastern textile and steel mills. Its membership reached about 3 million people, although no more than 150,000 were members at any one time. Although the Socialist party and the IWW were open to black members, they had no particular interest in combating racism or addressing the unique needs of African American workers. They assumed that labor activism would improve the lives of all workers. To address their unique concerns, black Americans organized on their own behalf.

Resistance to Racism

The Progressive Era was anything but progressive for nonwhite Americans. Although there were notable exceptions, such as Jane Addams, many white Protestant reformers were either indifferent to racial minorities or actively hostile to them. Moreover, most blacks lived in the rural South, not in northern cities where Progressives were most active. Lynching continued into the twentieth century, with nearly 100 lynchings per year between 1900 and 1910. African Americans were the primary targets of lynch mobs, although other minorities were also vulnerable. Black leaders spoke out against lynching and other forms of racial injustice. Ida B. Wells-Barnett, who had launched an international crusade against lynching in the 1890s, worked to establish local and national networks of black women's clubs. As a highly respected national leader, she had a profound impact on black life during these years and formed important alliances with other reformers. Although she was unable to persuade white suffrage leaders to support the cause of racial justice, she worked closely with Jane Addams to prevent the establishment of segregated schools in Chicago.

A number of other black leaders came to prominence in the first decade of the twentieth century as African Americans formed a wide range of organizations that grew and flourished. In 1905 scholar and civil rights leader W. E. B. Du Bois joined with other black leaders to form the Niagara Movement, which called for an end to segregation and discrimination in unions, the courts, and public accommodations, as well as equal economic and educational opportunity. In 1908 black leaders joined with white progressive allies—Hull House founder Jane Addams, philosopher John Dewey, and novelist William Dean Howells, among others—to establish the National Association for the Advancement of Colored People (NAACP). The new organization adopted the platform of the Niagara Movement, and Du Bois became the editor of its journal, *The Crisis.* Wells-Barnett insisted that the organization go on record as opposed to lynching. The NAACP has remained a major voice for African American civil rights and racial justice to this day.

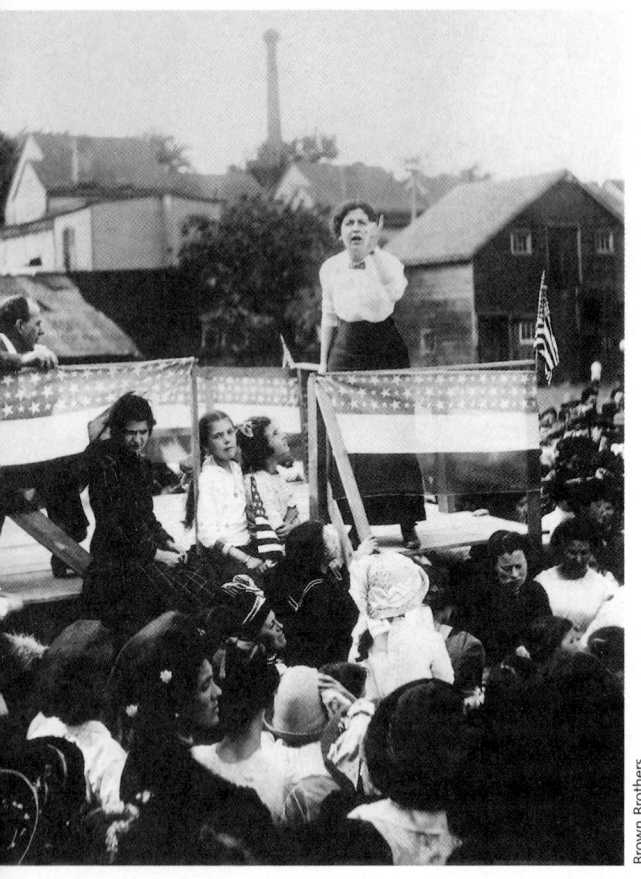

■ Elizabeth Gurley Flynn of the Industrial Workers of the World (IWW) addresses a crowd of women in 1913. Flynn was one of the organizers of the IWW, known as the Wobblies, an organization of workers from diverse backgrounds that enrolled nearly 3 million members.

Brown Brothers

Expanding National Power

Along with flourishing radical and reform movements at the grassroots, the Progressive Era gave rise to a reformist impulse at the national level. The person who most fully embodied the national Progressive movement was Theodore Roosevelt, president from 1901 to 1908. Roosevelt's primary goals as president were to expand the power of the presidency and the federal government and to strengthen American nationalism at home and national power abroad. Roosevelt used his power to regulate big business, intervene in labor disputes, extend the reach of the nation across the world, and control the uses of the natural environment.

Theodore Roosevelt: The "Rough Rider" as President

Theodore Roosevelt rose to prominence in the Republican party in the 1880s and held a number of important political posts, including assistant secretary of the Navy (1897–1898) and governor of New York (1899–1900). In 1900 Republican party leaders selected Roosevelt as William McKinley's running mate, and when McKinley was reelected, Roosevelt became vice president. But in September 1901, McKinley was assassinated, and at age 42, Roosevelt became the youngest person ever to become president.

Roosevelt was a strong proponent of American military and commercial presence in the world. He expanded the power of the federal government both at home and abroad and used the "bully pulpit" of the presidency to exert moral leadership. He favored big government and limitations on corporate power, yet he cooperated with business to foster capitalism and free trade. Using the Sherman Anti-Trust Act of 1890, which gave the federal government the power to break up monopolies, Roosevelt in 1902 ordered the Justice Department to prosecute the Northern Securities Company, a $400-million monopoly that controlled all railroad lines and traffic in the Northwest. Within a year, the company was dissolved. Although this bold act earned Roosevelt the title of "trust-buster," it was not his intention to weaken big business. In fact, he believed that a strong country needed large, powerful industries, and he hoped to regulate them to keep big business strong. His antitrust efforts actually helped big business by fostering competition.

The same year that Roosevelt took on the Northern Securities Company, he also used the powers of the federal government to intervene in a labor dispute. Striking coal miners in eastern Pennsylvania wanted recognition of their union, a 10 to 20 percent increase in wages, and an eight-hour day. But the mine owners refused to negotiate. Roosevelt summoned the mine owners and John Mitchell, president of the United Mine Workers union, to the White House for a meeting. He threatened to send in troops if the mine owners did not agree to the union's request for arbitration. The mine owners backed down, and the arbitrators awarded the miners a 10 percent wage increase and a nine-hour day.

Roosevelt's efforts to strengthen the state and foster American nationalism extended to his attitudes toward immigrants. He believed that discrimination against loyal newcomers harmed the democracy: "It is a base outrage to oppose a man because of his religion or birthplace. . . . A Scandinavian, a German, or an Irishman who has really become an American has the right to stand on exactly the same footing as any native-born citizen in the land, and is just as much entitled to the friendship and support, social and political, of his neighbor." He was proud of appointing a cabinet in which "Catholic and Protestant and Jew sat side by side." But to Roosevelt, becoming an American meant renouncing any loyalties to one's original homeland or culture: "We must Americanize them in every way. . . . [The immigrant]

TABLE 19-1			
The Election of 1900			
Candidate	Political Party	Popular Vote	Electoral Vote
William McKinley	Republican	7,207,923	292
William Jennings Bryan	Democratic-Populist	6,358,133	155

must not bring in his Old-World religious[,] race[,] and national antipathies, but must merge them into love for our common country, and must take pride in the things which we can all take pride in. He must revere our flag; not only must it come first, but no other flag should ever come second. He must learn to celebrate Washington's birthday rather than that of the Queen or Kaiser, and the Fourth of July instead of St. Patrick's Day. . . . Above all, the immigrant must learn to talk and think and be United States." Roosevelt did not believe in cultural pluralism, the idea that the United States could include citizens who retained their ethnic heritage. Rather, he promoted the idea of a melting pot that would blend all diverse cultures into a unique American "race."

Although Roosevelt was a firm believer in Anglo-Saxon superiority, he was the first president to invite an African American leader, Booker T. Washington, to the White House. Roosevelt's meeting with Washington demonstrated his willingness to stand up to southern politicians, but he did not follow that gesture with meaningful policy initiatives such as antilynching or civil rights laws. In the 1904 presidential election, Roosevelt won 57 percent of the popular vote against his Democratic rival, Alton B. Parker.

TABLE 19-2			
The Election of 1904			
Candidate	**Political Party**	**Popular Vote**	**Electoral Vote**
Theodore Roosevelt	Republican	7,623,486	336
Alton B. Parker	Democratic	6,358,133	155
Eugene V. Debs	Socialist	402,283	0

Protecting and Preserving the Natural World

Industrial smoke had long been a problem in both European and American cities, and Progressive Era reformers established organizations in major cities to fight air pollution. At the same time,

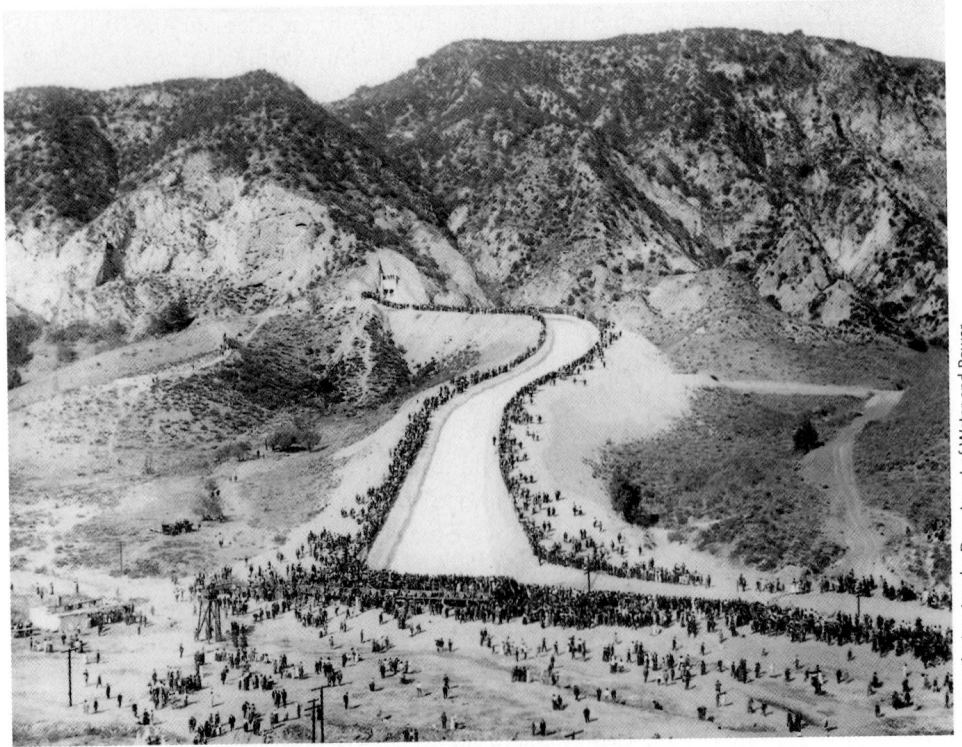

■ The Los Angeles Aqueduct opened at the Cascades on November 5, 1913. The aqueduct brought water from the Owens River, allowing the naturally dry terrain of Los Angeles to flourish and sustain a large population. Residents of the Owens Valley protested the diversion of their water supply, to no avail.

Courtesy, the Los Angeles Department of Water and Power

mining and other industries were depleting natural resources while destroying the natural beauty of the land. More than any previous president, Roosevelt used the federal government to control the natural world. Although his actions did not please everyone on all sides of the debate, Roosevelt's environmental efforts were among his most enduring legacies.

Roosevelt advocated both preservation and conservation (see Chapter 18). His preservation policies doubled the number of national parks, created 16 national monuments, such as Muir Woods in California, and established 51 wildlife refuges. At the same time, he shared the view of conservationists that timberlands, areas for livestock grazing, water, and minerals were at risk of being depleted. He believed the federal government should extend its reach into the management of these resources. Roosevelt transferred 125 million acres of public land into the forest reserves to prevent the depletion of timber, and he set aside land for dam sites, oil and coal reserves, and grazing lands. Some of these efforts faced strong opposition from preservationists because of their negative impact on the natural environment.

Conservationists and preservationists battled frequently, and no issue was more divisive than water. Conservationists favored damming rivers to create reservoirs and aqueducts to provide water and electricity for western settlements. John Muir and the Sierra Club campaigned to protect the Hetch Hetchy Valley in Yosemite National Park, but Congress passed the Raker Act in 1913, allowing the city of San Francisco to build a dam and a reservoir, flooding the valley. Residents of the Owens Valley also protested the building of an aqueduct to divert water to the Los Angeles area. Dams, reservoirs, and aqueducts brought water and electricity to arid regions, allowing such cities as Las Vegas and Los Angeles to flourish in environments that would otherwise be unable to support large populations.

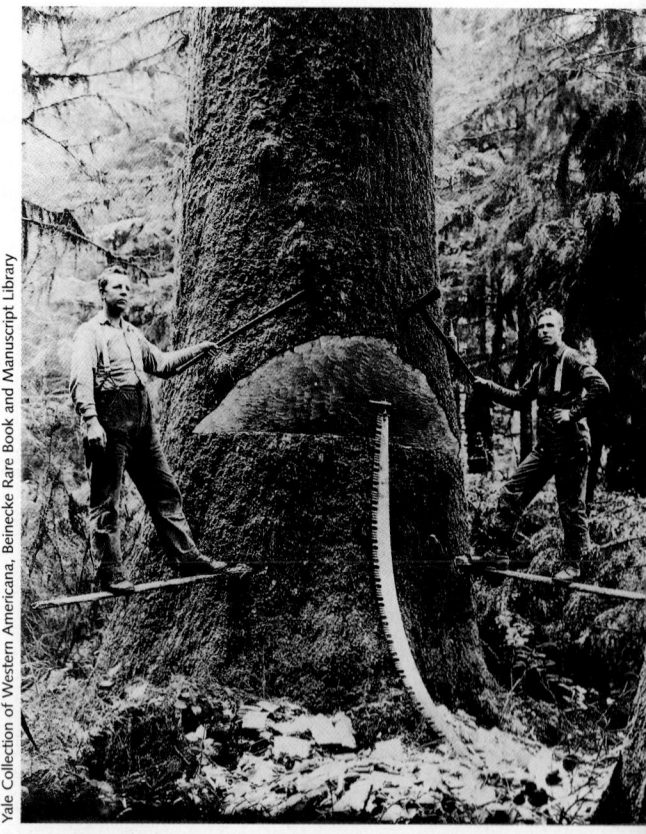

■ Lumberjacks topple a giant spruce tree in a forest in Washington state around 1900. President Theodore Roosevelt believed that the federal government should manage timberlands and other natural resources to prevent depletion while allowing their use. Roosevelt preserved some Pacific Northwest forests in national parks and refuges but allowed others to be cultivated for timber.

Expanding National Power Abroad

The decades surrounding the turn of the twentieth century marked the high point of European and American imperial expansion, bringing 80 percent of the world's land under the control of Europeans or their descendants. Unlike several Western European countries, the United States did not aquire a large colonial empire. Nevertheless, Theodore Roosevelt believed that the United States should be an imperial power with moral and military superiority over what he considered to be less "civilized" lands. He hoped to strengthen the federal government at home, develop the nation's military and commercial might, and extend American power abroad. To further these ends, he sent troops to China as part of the international expedition to crush the Boxer Rebellion in 1900. He also proposed the construction of a canal across the Isthmus of Panama, and Congress approved the Panama Canal project in 1902.

In 1904 Roosevelt increased the authority of the United States to intervene in the affairs of nations in the Western Hemisphere through what came to be known as the Roosevelt Corollary to the Monroe Doctrine. Fearing political uprisings that might threaten American commercial interests, Roosevelt asserted that "chronic wrongdoing" might require the intervention by "some civilized nation" in the affairs of another and that "in the Western Hemisphere the adherence of the United States to the Monroe Doctrine may force the United States, however reluctantly, in flagrant cases of such wrongdoing or impotence, to the exercise of an international police power." The Roosevelt Corollary justified later interventions into the Dominican Republic, Cuba, Nicaragua, Mexico, and Haiti.

Roosevelt also continued the U.S. war against Filipino nationalists that began in 1899. The bloody and costly war lasted four years before the Americans crushed the revolt and established firm colonial rule in the Philippines. William Howard Taft, the future American President, became the colony's first governor-general in 1901. As the war against the rebels continued, Taft developed a program of public works that included an infrastructure of roads, bridges, and schools. He also transferred government functions to those Filipinos who cooperated with American colonial powers. Although the United States promised to grant Philippine independence, that promise was deferred until 1946.

William Howard Taft: The One-Term Progressive

A financial panic in 1907 prompted Roosevelt to increase his efforts to overhaul the banking system and the stock market. But the president's critics among Republican conservatives and the business elite blamed Roosevelt's reform policies for the economic downturn. In the face of increasing rifts within his own party, along with his own earlier pledge to step down, Roosevelt declined to run for reelection in 1908. The Republicans selected Roosevelt's hand-picked successor, William Howard Taft, who won the election with 52 percent of the votes against William Jennings Bryan, the Democratic candidate. Prior to his service in the Philippines, Taft had been a federal circuit judge. In 1904 Roosevelt appointed him sec-

TABLE 19-3			
The Election of 1908			
Candidate	Political Party	Popular Vote	Electoral Vote
William H. Taft	Republican	7,678,908	321
William Jennings Bryan	Democrat-Populist	6,409,104	162
Eugene V. Debs	Socialist	420,793	0

retary of war. Taft was a loyal ally who worked closely with Roosevelt on foreign and domestic policies. Roosevelt assumed that Taft would fulfill his reform agenda.

At first glance, the most obvious difference between Roosevelt and Taft was their appearance. The energetic Roosevelt was a proponent and model of physical fitness, compared with the 300-pound Taft. Political cartoonists never tired of mocking the rotund chief executive. The two presidents also differed in their leadership styles: Roosevelt, relishing the rough-and-tumble of politics; Taft, cautious and averse to taking risks. Taft's respect for the separation of powers spelled out in the U.S. Constitution made him dubious about some of Roosevelt's extensions of the powers of the presidency. Nevertheless, Taft initiated far more antitrust suits than Roosevelt had during his presidency. Despite similar political inclinations, Roosevelt's support for his protégé cooled. Although Roosevelt counted major business leaders among his own advisors, he was displeased when Taft appointed corporate lawyers rather than activist reformers to his cabinet. His displeasure increased when Taft abandoned the fight for an inheritance tax and a reduction in tariffs.

Taft departed from Roosevelt's foreign policy as well. In contrast to Roosevelt, who emphasized military might, Taft claimed that "Dollar Diplomacy" was the best way for the United States to exert influence in the world:

> This policy has been characterized as substituting dollars for bullets. It is one that appeals alike to idealistic humanitarian sentiments, to the dictates of sound policy and strategy, and to legitimate commercial aims. It is an effort frankly directed to the increase of American trade upon the axiomatic principle that the government of the United States shall extend all proper support to every legitimate and beneficial American enterprise abroad.

Taft's relationship with the Philippines illustrates both his policy of Dollar Diplomacy and his reinforcement of American imperialism abroad. Taft took Roosevelt's bloody rule of the islands a step further by establishing U.S. business interests there. As *El Renacimiento,* a Filipino newspaper, put it at the beginning of Taft's administration:

> For [Taft] the present generation is a generation of children, incapable of assuming the responsibilities of self-government; and this point of view we can never accept. Yet we recognize

the power that lies in his hands. . . . President Taft, with the avowed purpose of helping the Filipinos, will encourage the introduction into this country of large capital which will buy up and exploit everything here worth having; and the inevitable result will be the complete domination of American commercial interests. When that day comes, of what benefit will be all this policy of education, this long preparation for self government, except to make servitude more intolerable?

When Taft signed the Payne–Aldrich Tariff in 1909, he disappointed progressive Republicans and aligned himself with the conservative old guard of the party, those who had been most critical of Roosevelt. The breach between Taft and the Progressives widened when Taft's secretary of the interior, Richard A. Ballinger, opened up for commercial development 1 million acres of land that Roosevelt had placed under federal protection. In a further affront to conservationists, Gifford Pinchot, still head of the National Forest Service, discovered that Ballinger had sold Alaskan coal deposits to corporate moguls J. P. Morgan and David Guggenheim. When Taft defended Ballinger, Pinchot leaked the news to the press and called for a congressional investigation. Taft subsequently fired Pinchot, but Roosevelt publicly supported Pinchot and signaled his break from Taft.

Roosevelt returned from big-game hunting in Africa to enter the political spotlight once again. He toured the country in 1910, describing his plan for a "New Nationalism," a far-reaching expansion of the federal government to stabilize the economy and institute social reforms. The election of reformers of both parties to Congress in 1910 indicated that Roosevelt's vision had popular support. With that encouragement, Roosevelt challenged Taft for leadership of the Republican party and announced his intention to run in the Republican presidential primary in 1912. Although Roosevelt had wide public support and easily defeated Taft and the other challenger, Robert La Follette, in the 13 states that held preferential primaries, the old guard still dominated the national party, and they nominated Taft at the Republican National Convention.

The day after Taft's nomination, Roosevelt and his supporters withdrew from the Republican party and formed the Progressive party. They nominated Roosevelt for president and California governor Hiram W. Johnson for vice president. Roosevelt boasted, "I am as strong as a bull moose," inspiring his followers to call themselves the "Bull Moosers." Their reformist platform called for extensive controls on corporations, minimum wage laws, child labor laws, a graduated income tax, and woman suffrage. But the Republican vote split between Taft and Roosevelt, and the victory went to the Democratic candidate, Woodrow Wilson, former president of Princeton University and governor of New Jersey. Wilson also ran on a strong reform platform. Eugene V. Debs, the Socialist party candidate vowed reform as well. The three reform candidates, Wilson, Debs, and Roosevelt, all agreed that the large corporations had too much power. But they disagreed as to what to do about it. Debs argued that the national government should take over the trusts. Roosevelt argued for a "New Nationalism," in which a strong federal government would regulate the trusts and, if necessary, curb their power. Wilson, reluctant to vest so much power in the government, called his approach the "New Freedom," believing that the government should dismantle the trusts and then revert to limited powers. Wilson won the election with 42 percent of the vote, but all three reform candidates together gained 75 percent of the total. Debs won 6 percent, the strongest showing ever for the Socialist party. Wilson took office amid an overwhelming popular mandate for reform.

TABLE 19-4			
The Election of 1912			
Candidate	**Political Party**	**Popular Vote**	**Electoral Vote**
Woodrow Wilson	Democratic	6,293,454	435
Theodore Roosevelt	Progressive	4,119,538	88
William H. Taft	Republican	3,484,980	8
Eugene V. Debs	Socialist	900,672	0

Conclusion

When Woodrow Wilson took office, the nation looked and behaved differently than it had at the turn of the century. Millions of immigrants from Europe, Asia, and Mexico had arrived in the United States and settled in towns and cities across the nation. Growing urban areas with new amusements and increasingly diverse populations emerged as centers of a national mass culture. New developments in science and technology brought the automobile and the motion picture to American consumers. At the same time, industrial production contributed to environmental damage, pollution, and dangerous working conditions.

Progressive reformers and labor activists mounted efforts to curb the ill effects of urban industrial society. Faith in science and expertise gave rise to pervasive optimism that social problems could be solved. Technological changes converged with the widespread belief that society is the sum of interdependent parts that can work together to mitigate the harmful effects of industrial life. At the local level, as well as through state and national institutions, reformers sought to solve society's ills. Muckrakers exposed corruption, women's rights activists pushed for the vote, and African American leaders organized for civil rights and against lynching. In the West and Southwest, Mexicans and Asians challenged discriminatory laws and labor practices. At the same time, moralists and vice crusaders sought to tame what they considered to be dangerous challenges to the social order.

These years also witnessed a major expansion of national power, within the nation as well as abroad. Presidents Roosevelt and Taft strengthened the role of the federal government through new efforts to regulate big business and by extending American military and economic presence abroad. By 1912 most Americans supported a strong reform agenda. But within a few years, the nation became embroiled in a major world war that would challenge the inherent optimism of Progressivism, signaling the end of an era.

Sites to Visit

Touring Turn-of-the-Century America: Photographs from the Detroit Publishing Company, 1880–1920.
memory.loc.gov/ammem/detroit/dethome.html
> This Library of Congress site includes thousands of photographs from turn-of-the-century America.

Coal Mining during the Gilded Age and Progressive Era
www.history.ohio-state.edu/projects/Lessons_US/ Gilded_Age/Coal_Mining/default.htm
> This Ohio State University site examines the development of the coal industry, including experiences of miners and sometimes violent labor-management conflict.

W.E.B. DuBois Resources
www-unix.oit.umass.edu/%7Ecscpo/db.html
> Included here are writings by and about the great African American intellectual and civil rights leader W.E.B. DuBois.

The Triange Shirtwaist Factory Fire, March 25, 1911
www.ilr.cornell.edu/trianglefire/
> Oral histories, cartoons, images, and essays about the fire are included here.

Inside an American Factory: The Westinghouse Works, 1904
lcweb2.loc.gov/ammem/papr/west/westhome.html
> This site provides a glimpse inside a turn-of-the-twentieth-century factory.

Theodore Roosevelt
www.ipl.org/ref/POTUS/troosevelt.html
> This Internet Public Library site contains biographical information about Theodore Roosevelt and his election to the presidency and links to Internet biographies and resources about him.

William Howard Taft
www.ipl.org/ref/POTUS/whtaft.html
> This Internet Public Library site contains biographical information about William Howard Taft and his election to the presidency and links to Internet biographies and resources about him.

The Emma Goldman Papers
sunsite.berkeley.edu/Goldman/
> This site includes information about the famous immigrant radical and selections of writings by and about her.

For Further Reading

General Works

Gail Bederman, *Manliness and Civilization: A Cultural History of Gender and Race in the United States, 1800–1917* (1995).

John R. Borchert, *America's Northern Heartland: An Economic and Historical Geography of the Upper Midwest* (1987).

Herbert Croly, *The Promise of American Life* (1909).

Steven J. Diner, *A Very Different Age: Americans of the Progressive Era* (1998).

Sara Evans, *Born for Liberty: A History of Women in America* (1989).

Gary Gerstle, *American Crucible: Race and Nation in the Twentieth Century* (2001).

Migration and Immigration: The Changing Face of the Nation

Albert Camarillo, *Chicanos in a Changing Society* (1977).

Linda Gordon, *The Great Arizona Orphan Abduction* (1999).

Matthew Frye Jacobson, *Barbarian Virtues: The United States Encounters Foreign Peoples at Home and Abroad* (2000).

Riv-Ellen Prell, *Fighting to Become Americans: Jews, Gender, and the Anxiety of Assimilation* (1999).

Vicki L. Ruiz, *From Out of the Shadows: Mexican Women in Twentieth-Century America* (1998).

Judith Smith, *Family Connections: A History of Italian and Jewish Immigrant Lives in Providence, Rhode Island, 1900–1940* (1985).

Ronald Takaki, *Strangers from a Different Shore: A History of Asian Americans* (1989).

Work, Science, and Leisure

George Chauncey, *Gay New York* (1994).

John D'Emilio and Estelle Freedman, *Intimate Matters: A History of Sexuality in America* (1988).

Elaine Tyler May, *Great Expectations: Marriage and Divorce in Post-Victorian America* (1980).

Lary May, *Screening Out the Past: The Birth of Mass Culture and the Motion Picture Industry* (1980).

Stephen Meyer, III, *The Five Dollar Day: Labor Management and Social Control in the Ford Motor Company, 1908–1921* (1981).

Leon Stein, *The Triangle Fire* (1962).

Reformers and Radicals

Jane Addams, *Twenty Years at Hull House* (1910).

W. E. B. Du Bois, *The Souls of Black Folk* (1903).

Nan Enstad, *Ladies of Labor, Girls of Adventure: Working Women, Popular Culture, and Labor Politics at the Turn of the Twentieth Century* (1999).

Dorothy Herrmann, *Helen Keller: A Life* (1999).

Louise Michelle Newman, *White Women's Rights: The Racial Origins of Feminism in the United States* (1999).

Viviana A. Zelizer, *Pricing the Priceless Child: The Changing Social Value of Children* (1985).

Expanding National Power

Richard Drinnon, *Facing West: The Metaphysics of Indian-Hating and Empire-Building* (1980).

William H. Harbaugh, *The Life and Times of Theodore Roosevelt* (1975).

Richard Hofstadter, *The Age of Reform* (1955).

Hazel M. McFerson, *The Racial Dimension of American Overseas Colonial Policy* (1997).

George Mowry, *Theodore Roosevelt and the Progressive Movement* (1946).

Robert Weibe, *The Search for Order* (1967).

Online Practice Test

Test your understanding of this chapter with interactive review quizzes at

www.ablongman.com/jonescreatedequal/chapter19

Additional Photo Credits

Page 641: Brown Brothers
Page 645: From the HUC Skirball Cultural Center, Museum Collection, Los Angeles, CA. Gift of Brenda Grossman Spivack in memory of Godina Eisenstein Schwartz. Clothes and Textiles: Gift of Harold Brill and Regina Starr Brill. HUCSM 31.194. Photography by Susan Einstein
Page 654: From the Collections of Henry Ford Museum & Greenfield Village
Page 656: The Advertising Archive Ltd
Page 659: Courtesy, The Lilly Library, Indiana University, Bloomington, Indiana
Page 662: Courtesy, Janice L. and David Frent

War and Revolution, 1912–1920

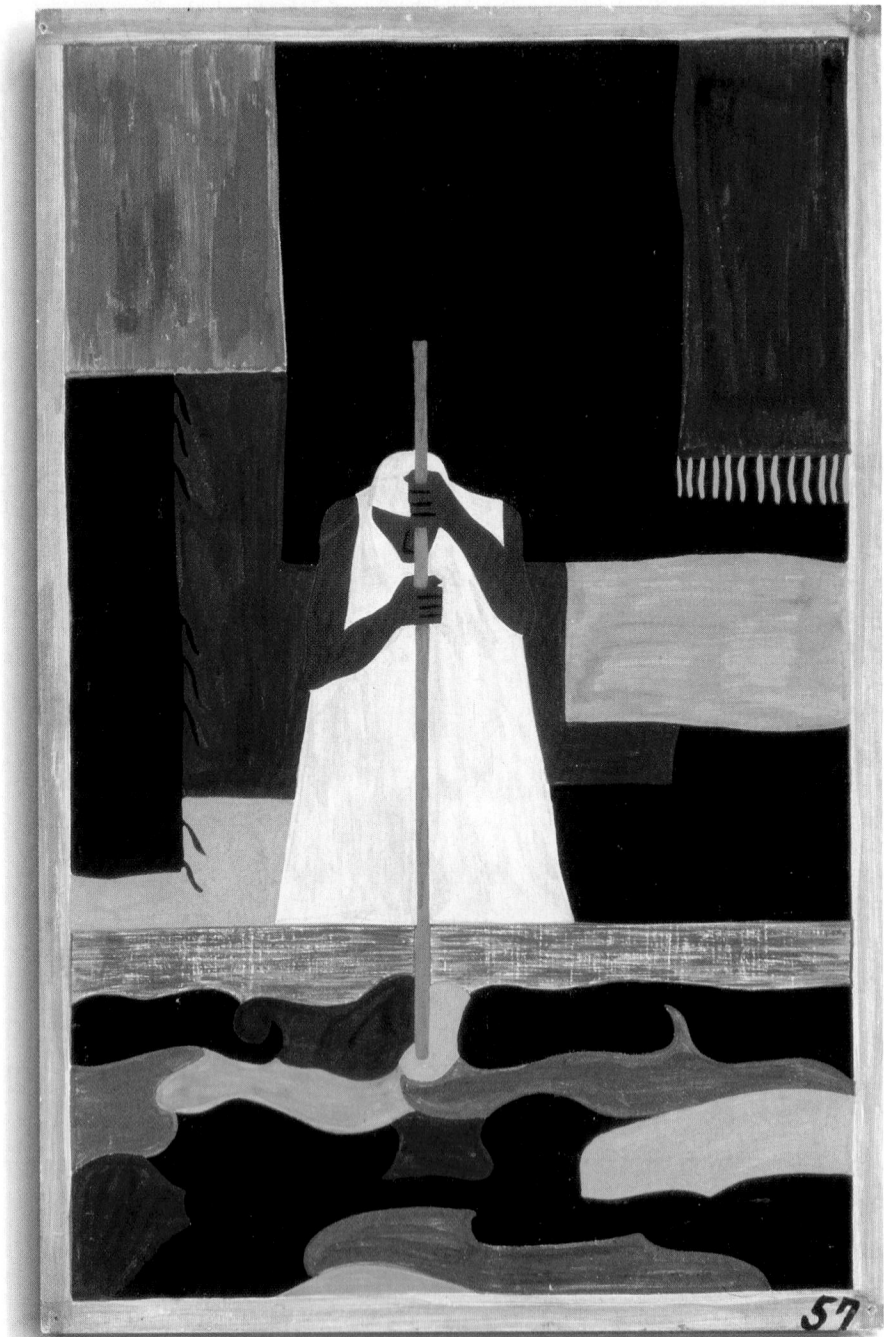

Jacob Lawrence, "The Migration of the Negro Panel no. 57," 1940–41. Acquired 1942, The Phillips Collection, Washington, D.C. Courtesy, Francine Seders Gallery

■ Two million Americans experienced World War I as soldiers serving in France, while all citizens at home felt the impact of that global conflict. *Migration of the Negro* by painter Jacob Lawrence suggests the burdensome toil of Southern African Americans, and why so many moved to Northern cities after 1914 in search of better jobs.

ON THE MORNING OF APRIL 6, 1909, SIX PEOPLE ARRIVED AT THE TOP OF THE WORLD. They had fulfilled at last the dream of two generations of Arctic explorers to reach the North Pole. Exhausted from a month of walking across the treacherous ice of the Arctic Sea, they rested for 30 hours at their polar camp. Then they turned south—the only direction available—and raced for their lives against the brutal cold that threatened to kill them.

Who were these men? Four were Greenland Inuit ("Eskimos"), for whom the Arctic region was home, even if they rarely ventured out on the frozen sea that covered the last 400 miles to the Pole. Two were American. The leader of the party, Bowdoin College graduate and renowned Arctic adventurer Robert Peary, had already built a reputation as a leading figure in the explorations of the Earth's last remote places. The other American to reach the North Pole that day received no such fame. Yet by the accounts of his fellow travelers, Matthew Henson was the indispensable man on the trip. A skilled dogsled driver, a master carpenter who built the expedition's shelters and fixed its sleds, and the only American on the voyage to learn the Inuit language, Henson was the one person Peary said he could not get along without. Henson was also African American. He had grown up during Reconstruction in rural Maryland and Washington, D.C. As a young man he developed a taste for exotic travel by working as a sailor on ships that took him to east Asia, north Africa, and the Black Sea.

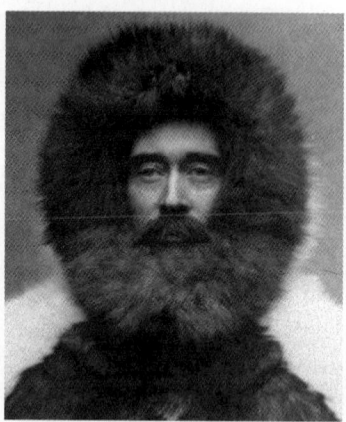

American Robert Peary led the first expedition to reach the North Pole.

Back in Washington, Henson worked as a clerk at an exclusive fur company to which Peary brought furs from his early trips to Greenland. Despite living on opposite sides of the increasingly stark color line of Jim Crow, the two men made strongly positive impressions on each other. Peary, ten years older, hired Henson as his assistant in 1888. Over the next 21 years, as white Americans unleashed a growing torrent of violence against their black fellow citizens, these two men built a relationship of great mutual respect as they pressed northward on several journeys into the icy wilderness of the Arctic. In his intimate working relationship with Henson, Peary acted so much as an equal that he sometimes offended other white Americans on the expeditions.

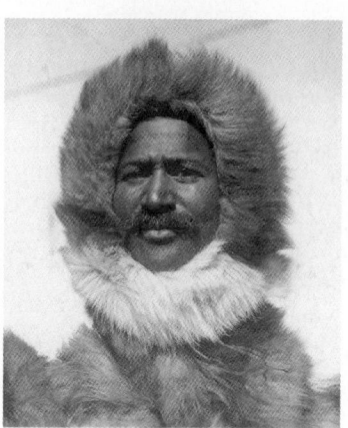

American Matthew Henson accompanied Peary on the epic 1909 expedition.

Twelve years after Henson and Peary stood together to plant the American flag in the Inuit world of the far North, the relations between white and black Americans appeared in a sharply different light in Oklahoma. The former Indian Territory had become a state in 1907 and had more than 50,000 Cherokee and other Native American residents, more than any other state. The discovery at the turn of the century of vast oil reserves along the Arkansas River made Tulsa a boom town, with all the social tensions that accompany rapid growth. The vibrant African American section of the segregated city along Greenwood Avenue offered a strong example of black economic independence.

That entire community was destroyed on the night of May 31, 1921, in the largest American race riot of the twentieth century. In previous years, similar riots had erupted in St. Louis, Chicago, and elsewhere, when white resentment over black mobility and declining deference exploded around a petty pretext. In Tulsa, a false charge against a young black man of attempted rape of a white elevator operator sparked thousands of angry white Tulsans to descend on the county courthouse to seize the suspect from jail. The city's white newspaper spurred them on with an editorial titled "To Lynch Negro Tonight." But many black Tulsans were determined not to let that happen. Veterans just back from World War I insisted that their sacrifices to make the world "safe for democracy" not be marred by terrorism. A group of 75 African Americans drove down to the courthouse to defend it from the mob. Their leader was a former serviceman who, others remembered, "came back from France with exaggerated ideas of equality."

The two groups exchanged words and then gunfire. Several people fell dead. Enraged, the much larger and better-armed white crowd poured across the railroad tracks into Greenwood, shooting and burning. Rather than restraining them, the Tulsa police force deputized hundreds of the marauders with instructions to kill. In the next few hours, the invaders executed as many as 300 African Americans and burned the entire Greenwood district to the ground. Mary E. Jones Parrish, a Greenwood resident, felt as though World War I had come to her town: "The enemy had organized in the night and was invading our district, the same as the Germans invaded France and Belgium." No white Tulsans were ever punished by the law for their actions that night.

The decade that stretched from the discovery of the North Pole to the Tulsa race riot was marked by unusual turbulence in American life. From 1910 to 1914 optimism about solving the nation's social problems rose as reformers attempted to ameliorate some of the worst aspects of modern industrial life. International developments then turned American attentions abroad. Traumatic social revolutions swept through Mexico, China, and Russia, and the conflagration of the Great War—World War I—consumed all of Europe and eventually drew in the United States. What President Woodrow Wilson called the war "to make the world safe for democracy" encouraged people of color, both in the vast European-ruled colonies of Asia and Africa and in the segregated United States, to claim a place of greater equality. But at home the war also created pressures for conformity and an intolerance for dissent. The events in Tulsa were part of a broad pattern of violence against political radicals and people of color that was rampant by 1920. The United States emerged from the war with great prestige and power, but most Americans were not yet convinced of the nation's obligations abroad, and the Versailles Treaty ending World War I failed to create a lasting structure for world peace.

A World in Upheaval

American politics between 1910 and 1920 and the U.S. involvement in World War I must be understood within the context of change and uncertainty in the international system. While world affairs were still dominated by the wealthy nations of western Europe and North America, the first wave of the great revolutions of the twentieth century was beginning to wash away much of the old order. Tensions also sharpened within the United States over traditional hierarchies of color, gender, and class. The struggle between reform and reaction pervaded public life in the United States and much of the rest of the world.

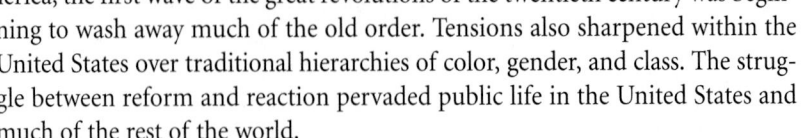

The Apex of European Conquest

On the eve of World War I, all but a quarter of the world's population lived under the rule of Europeans or their descendants. Explorations of the most remote parts of the globe filled in the last blank spaces on world maps, including the North (1909) and South (1911) poles. A 1913 expedition led by Episcopalian missionary Hudson Stuck reached the top of Alaska's Mt. McKinley, at 20,320 feet the highest peak in North America. The granting of statehood to Arizona and New Mexico in 1912 filled out the 48 mainland states. With U.S. control of the continent complete, its native inhabitants began to seem to white Americans less a current threat than a piece of the past to be preserved. The U.S. Treasury issued the first Indian head nickel the following year.

Technological innovations in transportation and communication tied the world more closely together. Just as the Suez Canal (1870) and the trans-Siberian railroad (1904) linked Europe more directly to Asia, the Panama Canal (1914) cut in half the travel time by water between the East and West coasts of the United States. Cables laid on the floor of the Atlantic Ocean in 1914 inaugurated telephone service between Europe and the United States. The first motorized flight by Orville and Wilbur Wright along the Outer Banks of North Carolina in 1903 led to transcontinental airmail service by 1920.

The competition that arose from the expansion of European power sowed the seeds of World War I. Germany, France, Britain, Italy, and Russia raced each other for new colonies and greater influence across Africa and Asia. Conflicts within Europe over disputed borders (Alsace–Lorraine) and nationalist movements (the Balkans) further heightened tensions. The central rivalry emerged between a newly unified Germany (1871) and traditionally dominant Britain. France had been defeated by Germany in the last armed clash in Europe (the Franco-Prussian War of 1870) and feared a renewed conflict with its larger, stronger neighbor. Anticipating trouble, each of the major European powers sought allies to bolster its position. Britain, France, and Russia formed the Triple Entente against the Triple Alliance of Germany, Austria–Hungary, and Italy (when war came in 1914 Italy switched sides and the Ottoman Empire—modern Turkey—joined Germany and Austria–Hungary as the Central Powers). These unprecedented peacetime alliances between global empires meant that a single spark could ignite a worldwide war.

> *The United States had been born in the first successful revolution by colonies against a European empire.*

The United States emerged as a global power in this same period around the turn of the century. Fifteen years after it seized an overseas empire in 1898, the country's economic growth was stunning. U.S. consumption of energy from modern fuels (coal and oil) in 1913 equaled that of Britain, Germany, France, Russia, and Austria–Hungary combined. The United States brought a different history to the world stage. It had been born in 1776 in the first successful revolution by colonies against a European empire. Americans had long understood themselves as a people who opposed empires and supported self-government. The events of 1898 contradicted this legacy, and Americans remained ambivalent about their country's imperial venture. The U.S. Congress promised eventual independence to the Philippines in 1916 and granted U.S. citizenship to residents of Puerto Rico in 1917.

The American rise to world power came just as the major revolutions of the twentieth century began to shatter the structures of imperialism. The United States became the leading status quo power when much of the globe was beginning to reject that status quo. The great example of anticolonial revolution now stood as one of the foremost counterrevolutionary states. Rather than new colonies, however, Americans sought expanded economic opportunities abroad, and they expected their government to help them. While president of Princeton University in 1907, Woodrow Wilson explained that because "the manufacturer insists on having the world as a market, the flag of his nation must follow him . . . even if the sovereignty of unwilling nations be outraged in the process." Wilson's victory in the election of 1912 brought the first native Southerner to the White House since before the Civil War, a

symbol of a reunited majority white population
ready to turn outward.

Confronting Revolutions Abroad

More than most people, Wilson feared social upheaval.
Born in 1856, he had grown up in Augusta, Georgia, amid
the destruction of the Civil War, and he made his career as
a political scientist and as governor of New Jersey (1910–1912)
during a period of labor strife. Whatever Wilson's hopes for a
stable social order at home and abroad, the global process of western capitalist expansion into decentralized, preindustrial societies was
producing a widespread backlash by 1910. The first signs had already
appeared of a broad rejection of the world order dominated by the white
nations of Europe and North America. Ethiopia crushed an invading Italian
army in 1896 in the first victory of an African state over a modern European one.
In 1905 Japan destroyed the Russian army and naval fleet, putting Europeans on notice
that their days of having their way in Asia were over. Harassed across eastern Europe in
brutal pogroms, Jews under the leadership of Theodor Herzl founded the Zionist movement
in 1897 for a national homeland in Palestine. Blacks organized the African National Congress in
1912 to struggle against racial oppression in South Africa, just as African Americans formed
the National Association for the Advancement of Colored People (NAACP) in 1910.

As nationalist movements in China, Russia, and Mexico overturned weak central governments controlled by foreign investors, American economic and security interests seemed to
be at stake on three continents. In Asia, the Chinese deeply resented exclusive foreign enclaves
that dominated their nation's coastal region and exempted foreigners from the constraints of
Chinese laws. Signs in Shanghai reading "No dogs or Chinese" suggested the attitudes that
accompanied European and American control of the bulk of China's wealth. In 1911 nationalist revolutionaries inspired by Sun Yat-sen, a Hawaiian-educated democratic reformer, overthrew the Manchu dynasty that had proven unable to resist western incursions.

The American desire for an open door into China's trade—a door that no other powerful nation could close at will—conflicted with the rising imperial power of the region: Japan.
The Tokyo government, which had annexed Korea in 1910, responded to the outbreak of World
War I by seizing the valuable German-held Shantung Peninsula in northeastern China. In its
famous 21 Demands to China, issued in January 1915, Japan made clear its plans to dominate the development of the Chinese economy. The American relationship with both China
and Japan was undercut at home by continued discrimination and violence against immigrants
from Asia, who remained ineligible for naturalization as U.S. citizens (unlike any children born
on American soil, who were U.S. citizens regardless of their race or ethnicity). In 1913 the
California legislature passed the Alien Land Act to prevent ownership of land in the state by
people "ineligible to citizenship"—people born in Asia, particularly those from Japan.

Revolutionary struggles with implications for America also threatened the monarchs
who ruled eastern Europe. For Russians, defeat at the hands of Japan in 1905 helped precipitate a thwarted revolution in 1905 followed by two years of political turmoil. The Czar survived
to rule another decade, and thousands of political activists—unionists, anarchists, and socialists—joined a growing wave of immigration from Russia to the United States. The wave crested
in 1914 at 1.2 million people, most of them from east or south of the Alps. That same year,
the assassination of the heir to the Austro-Hungarian throne by a Serbian nationalist in Sara-
jevo in June provided the spark that ignited the Great War. Russia's defense of the Serbs put the
alliance system into action as the Entente went to war with the Central Powers.

The most important region of the world for the United States before World War I was Latin
America, especially Central America and the Caribbean islands. This area guarded the nation's

Tijuana

Columbus,
NM

El Paso

MEXICO

Pancho Villa
pursued,
1916–1917

Parral

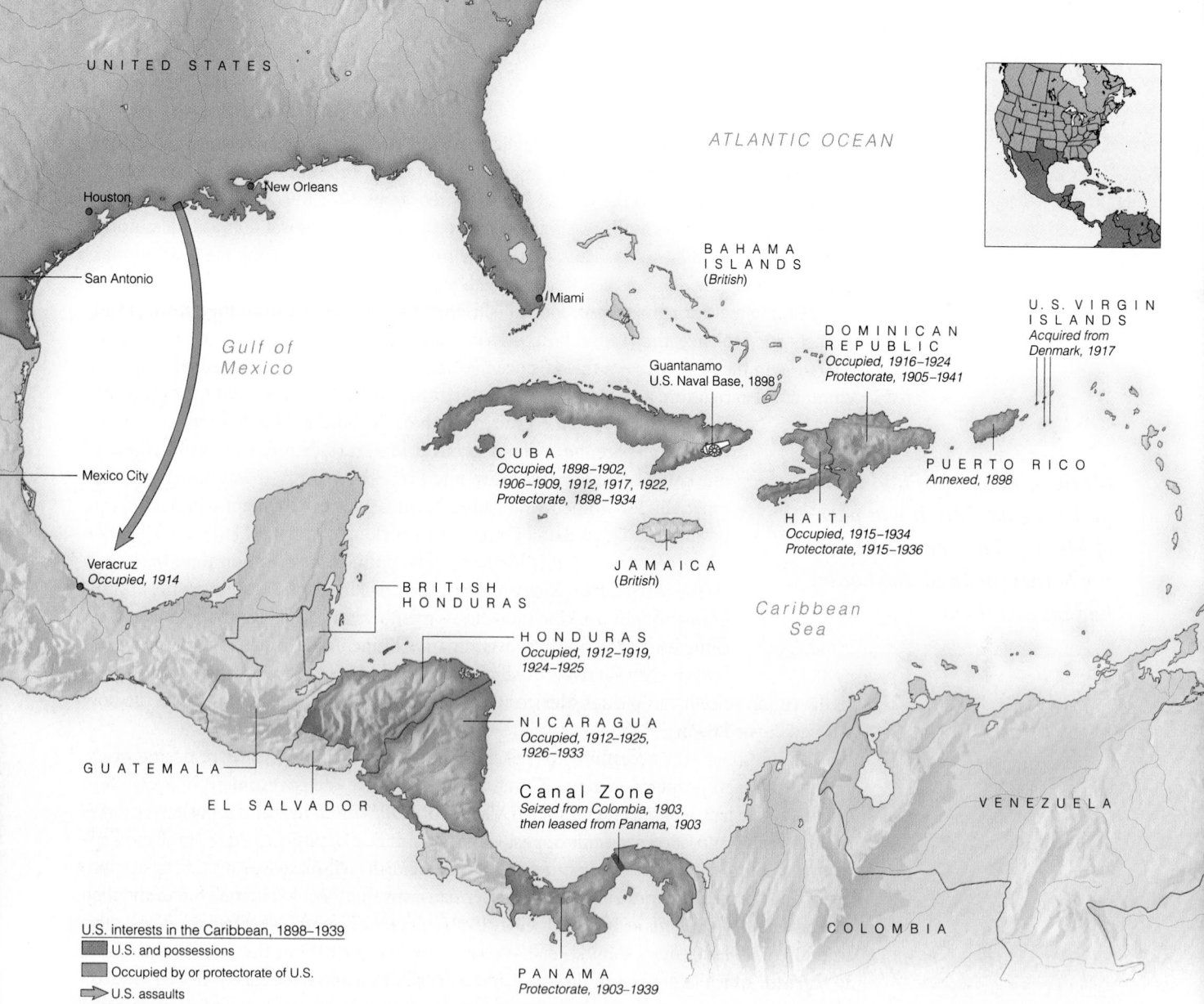

MAP 20.1

U.S. INTERESTS AND INTERVENTIONS IN THE CARIBBEAN REGION, 1898–1939 By its size, wealth, and military power, the United States dominated the Caribbean region to its south. American capitalists invested heavily in Mexico, Central America, and the Caribbean islands, and U.S. troops often intervened to protect those investments. Puerto Rico (by acquisition from Spain) and the Panama Canal Zone (by lease from Panama) became particularly important territories ruled by the United States.

Labels on map:

UNITED STATES

ATLANTIC OCEAN

Houston

New Orleans

San Antonio

Gulf of Mexico

Miami

BAHAMA ISLANDS (British)

DOMINICAN REPUBLIC
Occupied, 1916–1924
Protectorate, 1905–1941

U.S. VIRGIN ISLANDS
Acquired from Denmark, 1917

Mexico City

Guantanamo U.S. Naval Base, 1898

CUBA
Occupied, 1898–1902,
1906–1909, 1912, 1917, 1922,
Protectorate, 1898–1934

PUERTO RICO
Annexed, 1898

HAITI
Occupied, 1915–1934
Protectorate, 1915–1936

Veracruz
Occupied, 1914

JAMAICA (British)

Caribbean Sea

BRITISH HONDURAS

HONDURAS
Occupied, 1912–1919,
1924–1925

NICARAGUA
Occupied, 1912–1925,
1926–1933

GUATEMALA

EL SALVADOR

Canal Zone
Seized from Colombia, 1903,
then leased from Panama, 1903

VENEZUELA

COLOMBIA

PANAMA
Protectorate, 1903–1939

U.S. interests in the Caribbean, 1898–1939
- U.S. and possessions
- Occupied by or protectorate of U.S.
- U.S. assaults

strategic southern flank, and American citizens and corporations invested more money in Latin America than in any other region of the world. President Wilson spoke of the ability of Latin Americans to govern themselves "when properly directed" and proceeded to provide that direction. U.S. Marines occupied Haiti (1915), the Dominican Republic (1916), and Cuba (1917) and maintained their earlier presence in Nicaragua to defend American-owned property and ensure that local debts were paid to American creditors. The Bryan–Chamorro Treaty of 1916 guaranteed that no other nation would build a competitor to the Panama Canal through Nicaragua. The United States purchased the Danish Virgin Islands in 1917 to keep them out of German hands.

American anxieties about stability to the south centered on Mexico. "Land for the landless and Mexico for the Mexicans" became the slogan of revolutionaries there between 1910 and 1920. After troops led by Francisco Madero overthrew the long-standing dictatorship of Porfirio Díaz in 1911, various factions competed to determine the course of the revolution. U.S.

stakes in the Mexican revolution were high. American investors owned 43 percent of all Mexico's wealth (other foreigners owned another 25 percent), and more than half of the country's trade flowed north to the United States. Moreover, by 1921 Mexico became the world's second largest exporter of oil. Washington feared the spread of radical political ideas northward as almost a million Mexicans crossed their northern border during the revolutionary decade, tripling the number of Americans with recent roots south of the Rio Grande.

Many came through El Paso, the "Ellis Island" for immigrants from the south. Fleeing poverty and violence, they found both discrimination and employment. Dam building and irrigation in the American Southwest since the Newlands Act of 1902 had created a boom in commercial agriculture across California and Arizona and a desperate need for farm workers. Employers often recruited south of the border. "I believe that the Mexican laborers are the solution to our common labor problem in this country," one cotton company executive told President Wilson. It was not an easy life, especially for women who had to balance paid employment with taking care of families. Grace Luna remembered picking cotton in Madera, California, where women scaled ladders with 100 pounds of cotton on their backs and "some carried their kids on top of their picking sacks." Whereas most immigrants sought unskilled positions, members of Mexico's professional classes came north for political asylum as well, including teachers, architects, and lawyers. New arrivals of all classes joined Mexican Americans who had lived in the region since it was part of Mexico. They had not crossed the border; in 1848, the border had crossed them.

> *Mexican Americans had lived in the region since it was part of Mexico. They had not crossed the border; in 1848, the border had crossed them.*

Wilson sought unsuccessfully to reestablish in Mexico a political order respectful of the rights of foreign property owners. He refused to recognize the government of Victoriano Huerta, which had deposed and murdered Madero in 1912. Wilson instead supported the forces around Venustiano Carranza while opposing the more radical opposition led by Emiliano Zapata in the south and Francisco ("Pancho") Villa in the north. Wilson twice sent U.S. troops into Mexico, at Veracruz in April 1914 to block a German arms shipment to Huerta's forces and then in pursuit of Villa and his army after their 1916 assault on Columbus, New Mexico. The American forces under General John J. Pershing withdrew in early 1917 as the president prepared to enter the much larger war in Europe. Land redistribution and national control of Mexico's abundant mineral wealth, particularly oil, were written into the new constitution passed a few days later, and the revolutionary upheaval ended by 1920.

Conflicts over Hierarchies at Home

Just as social upheaval threatened monarchies and international investors abroad, less privileged Americans contested traditional lines of hierarchy and control in the United States. For example, racial lines were not always clear. Native-born whites continued to disagree about whether the millions of new immigrants from eastern and southern Europe were also "white." Anthropologists led by Franz Boas at Columbia University began to question the supposed significance of racial differences. Americans of all colors applauded the spectacular successes of Native American athlete Jim Thorpe at the 1912 Olympic Games in Sweden. In 1916 Wilson appointed Louis Brandeis as the first Jewish justice of the Supreme Court, but that same year anxieties about the future of white supremacy found a voice in the popular new book of a conservative New York intellectual named Madison Grant. *The Passing of the Great Race,* a bigoted sociology tract, identified Jesus as "Nordic" to distance the central figure of the Christian faith from the many new Jewish immigrants in America.

The Wilson administration's "New Freedom" slogan did not apply to African Americans, who faced continuing discrimination in employment and housing. The president filled his cabinet with white Southerners who segregated the few federal agencies that had employed

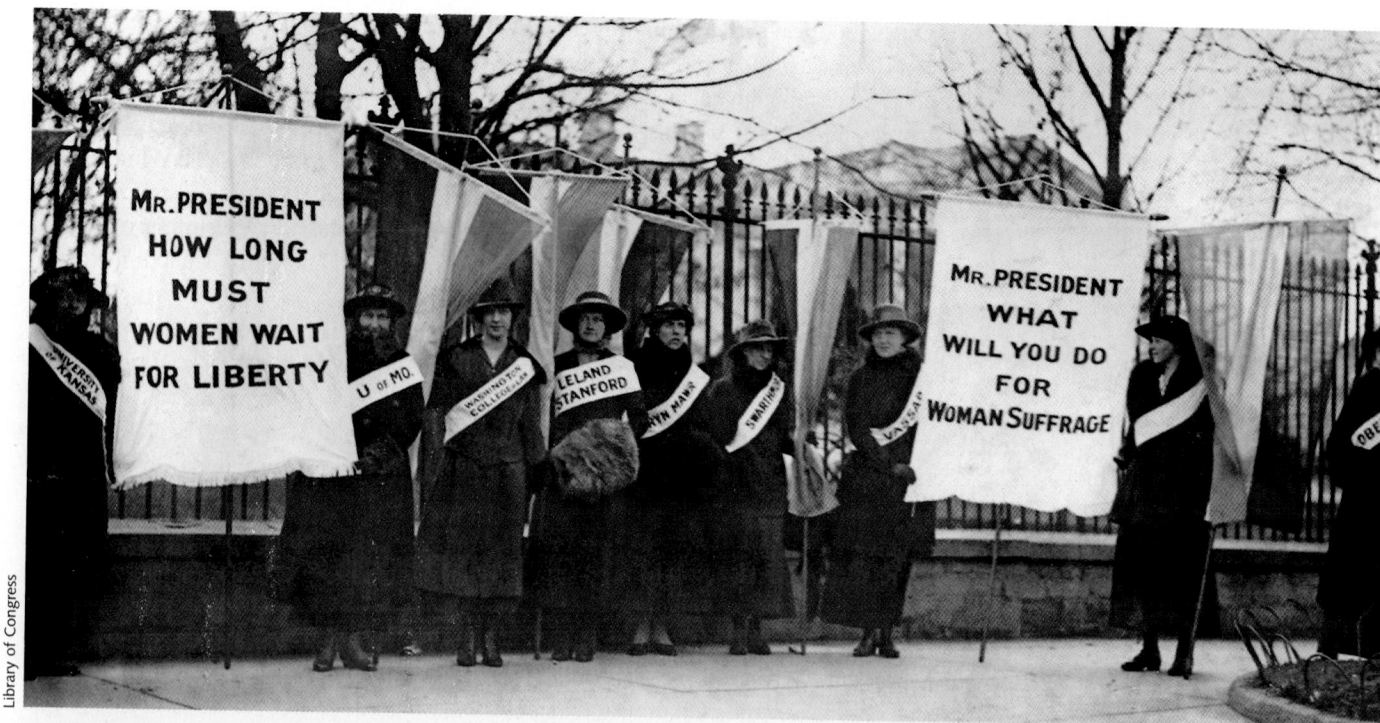

Library of Congress

■ In February 1917, as the United States broke relations with Germany and began to prepare to enter World War I, supporters of woman's suffrage continued to picket on the sidewalk outside the White House. College women joined the effort to ensure that winning liberty at home would go hand in hand with fighting for democracy abroad.

blacks. When Wilson took office African Americans continued to be murdered publicly by vigilante mobs across the South at a rate of more than one person per week. But the president ignored requests from the recently formed NAACP for an antilynching law, and the United States remained one of the few societies in which human beings were burned at the stake. Instead, the historian–president endorsed D. W. Griffith's 1915 film *Birth of a Nation* as "history written with lightning." Griffith, a Kentucky-born champion of the "Lost Cause" of slavery in the South, had created a racist blockbuster that celebrated the Ku Klux Klan of the 1860s and helped inspire the Klan's rebirth that fall at Stone Mountain, Georgia.

Women of all colors lived under particular burdens of discrimination. Their uniquely intimate relationships—as daughters, wives, mothers—to those who did not treat them as equals complicated their efforts at reform. So did their dilemma about women's roles in society: some sought full legal equality with men, and others wanted special protections for women on the grounds that they were fundamentally different. At issue was the nature of women's political identity. Was their primary identification in their attachment to individual men or to the nation? American women lost their U.S. citizenship by marrying a foreigner, whereas American men did not. A growing chorus of female activists rejected this kind of double standard and focused on the key issue of suffrage.

American women's long struggle to vote came to a head in this decade. By 1912, a growing number of European nations and nine American states, all in the West, granted the franchise to citizens of both sexes. Jeannette Rankin, a Republican feminist and pacifist from Montana, won election in 1916 as the nation's first female member of Congress. Suffragists varied in the tactics they believed most effective for winning the vote. The more moderate National American Women Suffrage Association under the leadership of Carrie Chapman Catt worked within the political system, building an alliance with President Wilson after he endorsed women's suffrage in 1916 and supporting the U.S. entry into World War I the next year. Alice Paul and other militants formed the National Women's Party and opposed the war effort as inherently undemocratic because half the adult population could not vote. In 1917 five picketers were imprisoned for seven months for obstructing traffic in front of the White House; despite brutal force-feedings, Paul and Rose Winslow persisted in a hunger strike so "that women fighting for liberty may be considered political prisoners." In 1918 suffragist organizers helped elect a more sympathetic Congress that passed the Nineteenth Amendment, ending sex discrimination in voting two years later.

Contention over women's social roles also divided Americans. Traditionalists promoted the declaration of the first Mother's Day in 1913. The desire to provide special protections for women resulted in the Sheppard–Towner Act of 1921, which expanded the role of the new federal Children's Bureau in providing infant and maternal health services. The struggle over contraception foreshadowed the conflict over abortion that dominated women's politics in the last quarter of the twentieth century. Socialist Margaret Sanger campaigned for women's access to contraception, opening the nation's first birth control clinic in Brooklyn in 1916. Sanger's experiences as a public health nurse with working-class New Yorkers convinced her that controlling pregnancy was the central issue for helping women gain greater autonomy. Unable to separate sexual experience from reproduction and facing poverty and unsanitary living conditions, married women in the lower classes suffered frequent pregnancies and the often debilitating and sometimes fatal consequences of abortions, an illegal but common operation. "The menace of another pregnancy hung like a sword over the head of every poor woman I came in contact with," Sanger recalled. She reached a turning point after hearing the joking response of a physician to the desperate plea of one frail 28-year-old mother of three for help in preventing another pregnancy: "Tell Jake to sleep on the roof!" Sanger was appalled, and the young woman's subsequent death as a result of a botched abortion pushed Sanger to begin her crusade for contraception.

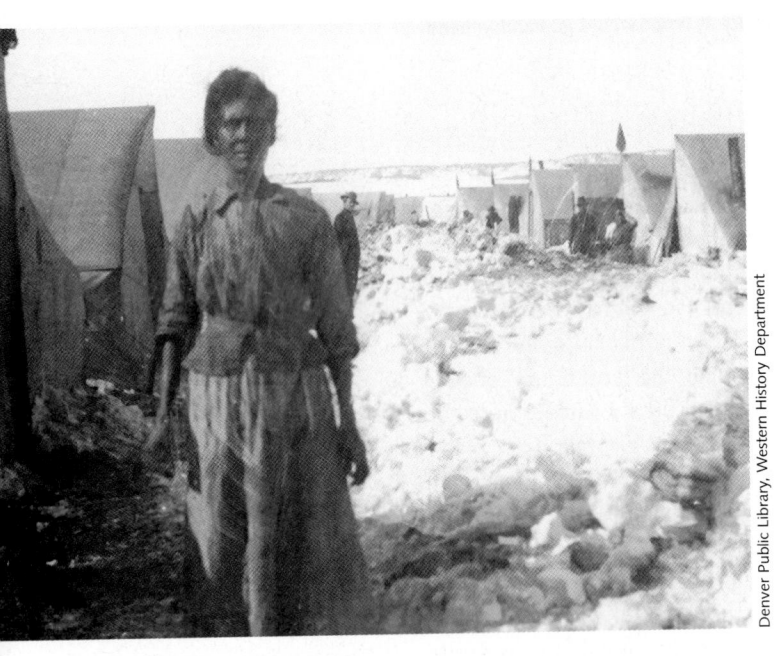

Denver Public Library, Western History Department

■ The coal miners' tent colony outside Ludlow stood on the high plains of south central Colorado, at the base of the mountains of the Front Range. Winter snows and cold temperatures made for a difficult life, as did the grueling and dangerous work of mining coal that was common across the state. Strikers along with their wives and children died in the Ludlow massacre on April 20, 1914.

Most adult Americans—workers—continued to find themselves in frequent conflict with the owners who employed them. Industrial capitalism's efficiency produced great material wealth, but 60 percent of it belonged to 2 percent of the population, whereas two-thirds of Americans owned only 2 percent of the wealth. President Wilson acknowledged that as factories grew larger, "the individual has been submerged." Skills became less necessary in the assembly-line workplace and workers more interchangeable. The anticapitalist aspirations of the Socialist party and the Industrial Workers of the World (IWW) frightened both industrialists and the more conservative labor leaders of the American Federation of Labor (AFL), especially when the western-based IWW led two major strikes in the East, one a success in Lawrence, Massachusetts, in 1912 and the other a failure in Paterson, New Jersey, in 1913. The campaign against a wage cut at the vast Lawrence textile factory was especially impressive in uniting 20,000 workers of 40 different national backgrounds.

Businesses had long opposed workers' efforts to build unions. Some owners sought to undercut union campaigns by providing better working conditions and even company-run "unions." These carrots of concession were accompanied by the stick of force. Bolstered by sympathetic federal courts and state governors, companies usually refused to negotiate with work-

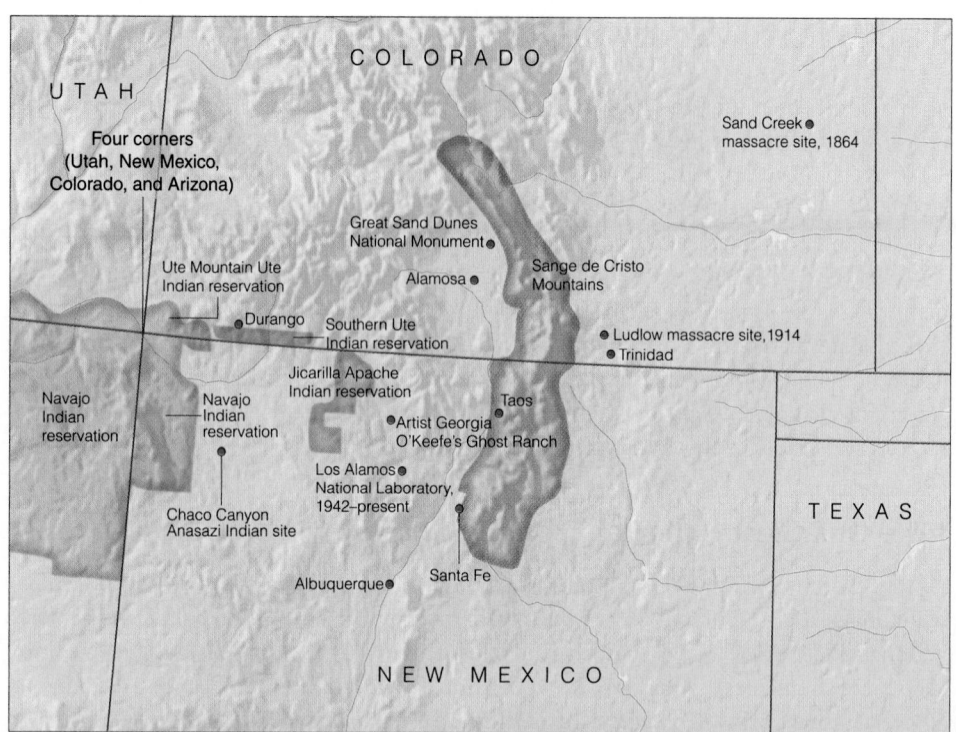
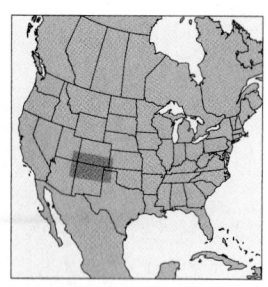

■ **MAP 20.2**

SOUTHERN COLORADO AND NORTHERN NEW MEXICO The mountainous region of southern Colorado and northern New Mexico in the 1910s had an economy based on mining, ranching, and lumbering—like much of the rural West. A large Indian population included Navajos, Apaches, Pueblos, and Utes. Since the 1920s, Santa Fe and Taos supported important communities of artists enchanted by the area's natural beauty. That same beauty attracted growing numbers of visitors later in the twentieth century, as the tourist trade surpassed older extractive industries as the chief source of employment in much of the mountainous West.

ers who went on strike. This pattern reached a shocking climax on Easter night in 1914 outside Ludlow, Colorado, in a mining camp owned by John D. Rockefeller, Jr.'s Colorado Fuel and Iron Company. State militia and company guards broke a strike there with torches and machine guns, burning the miners' tent colony and killing 2 women and 11 children. A total of 66 strikers and strike supporters died before federal troops eventually restored order. Ludlow recalled the actions of the Colorado militia exactly 50 years earlier, when it had destroyed the Cheyenne Indian camp at Sand Creek. Immigrant coal miners and their families had replaced Native Americans as the apparent threat to Colorado's social order.

Such brutality by owners against workers appalled most Americans. The Wilson administration slowly began supporting the right of laborers to organize for collective bargaining with their employers. Wilson's strong backing from Samuel Gompers and the AFL in the 1912 election initiated the modern Democratic–labor alliance. The president named William B. Wilson, a U.S. congressman from Pennsylvania and a former labor activist with the Knights of Labor and the United Mine Workers, to head the new U.S. Department of Labor, the permanent agency established "to foster, promote and develop the welfare of working people" by improving their working conditions and mediating labor disputes. The president appointed labor lawyer Frank Walsh to chair the separate short-term U.S. Committee on Industrial Relations, which for two years explored the causes of industrial violence in public hearings. Walsh even grilled Rockefeller about the events at Ludlow, embarrassing the corporate titan by revealing his close involvement and clear responsibility for what happened.

The Great War and American Neutrality

Most Americans had roots of some kind in Europe and had long defined themselves in relation to life on "the continent." But they also considered themselves part of the New World that was separate from the Old World of kings, castles, and rigid social classes. When Europe stepped off the precipice in August 1914 into a war larger than any previously fought or imagined, few Americans wanted any part of it. Make "no entangling alliances," George Washington had urged his fellow citizens. Europeans must stay out of our hemisphere, the Monroe Doctrine had declared. For generations, the preoccupation of the United States had been constructing the world's "best" society, however Americans might disagree about its proper contours. But migration and commerce had reduced the nation's isolation. International ties proved too important to the well-being of Americans for the country to remain indefinitely on the sidelines of World War I.

"The One Great Nation at Peace"

"It would be an irony of fate," Wilson told a friend, "if my administration had to deal chiefly with foreign affairs." But so it was for the scholar of American history and politics who entered national office with a large domestic agenda. Just a year and a half into his presidency, Americans were stunned as "civilized" Europe slid into savage conflict. "The lamps are going out all over Europe," British Foreign Secretary Edward Grey observed. "We shall not see them lit again in our lifetime." Following traditional U.S. policy, Wilson urged Americans to remain neutral "in fact as well as in name" to promote an eventual "peace without victory."

Neutrality was profitable. Wilson stoutly defended the rights of neutrals to trade with belligerents, the same principle that had led the United States into the War of 1812 against England. American industries depended on overseas trade, he believed, and "they will burst their jackets if they cannot find a free outlet to the markets of the world." After the recession of 1913–1914, war-related demands from abroad for American farm and factory products jump-started the economy. In the course of World War I, American bankers extended $10 billion in loans to the Entente (primarily Britain and France), and the United States changed from a debtor nation to the world's largest creditor.

The nature of the fighting in Europe bolstered the American determination to avoid being drawn into the conflict. Industrialized warfare brought fiendish new ways to kill human beings, including machine guns and poison gas. Gone were the days of bold maneuvers and dashing cavalry charges; now was the time of trench warfare, with its unrelenting misery, terror, and helplessness. Eight and a half million young men lost their lives and another 21 million were wounded, devastating an entire generation of European society. Eight million civilians also died as a result of the fighting, and an international outbreak of influenza in 1918 killed another 20 million around the world. Continuous shelling rendered whole sections of the landscape of northern France a wasteland. Prewar optimism about human progress swiftly disappeared.

In the United States, neutrality also made political sense. Immigrants from every part of Europe lived and voted in the United States, so Americans had blood ties to all the belligerents. Commercial and political elites tended to identify with Britain and France, as did many other Americans. But among two of the largest groups of Americans, those with roots in Germany and Ireland, many took a different view. Few Irish Americans equated England with the cause of democracy after centuries of British rule in Ireland, and London's severe repression of the 1916 Easter Rising in Dublin underscored their case. The sheer scale of the immigrant stream to the United States between 1900 and 1914 reinforced the need to avoid Europe's conflicts. Native-born white Americans were already concerned with preserving unity in their increasingly varied and urban society. Allowing in the hatreds from Europe's battlefields would only exacerbate the ethnic and class tensions that worried social reformers and many politicians, including President Wilson.

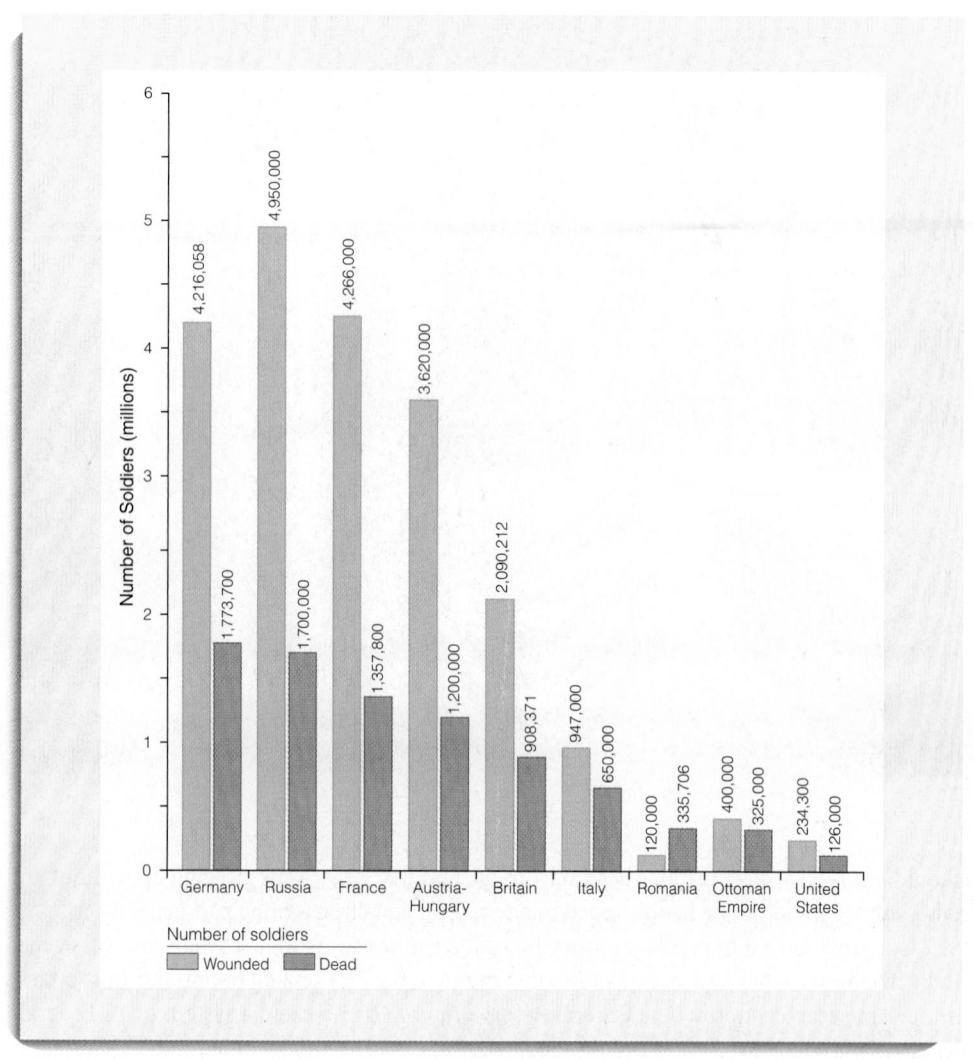

■ **FIGURE 20-1**
CASUALTIES OF THE GREAT WAR,
1914–1918   Compared to the
European combatants who fought
for several years, the United States
suffered far fewer casualties in its
18 months in World War I.

Reform Priorities at Home

Americans traditionally considered powerful government a primary threat to individual liberty, but the rise of mammoth corporations at the start of the twentieth century altered that calculation. Competition was disappearing, particularly in critical sectors of the economy such as oil production and railroads. Laissez-faire policies, by which federal agencies encouraged economic expansion, were no longer adequate; only government could balance the new might of the largest companies. This meant modest regulation of some aspects of the marketplace. Wilson's first term also encouraged such democratic reforms as the ratification of the Seventeenth Amendment for the direct popular election of U.S. senators (1913), previously chosen by state legislatures. Until American entry into the Great War in 1917 turned the nation to a very different task, this period marked the climax of the first chapter of twentieth-century liberalism.

Three areas topped the Wilson administration's reform agenda: taxes, the money system, and monopolies. The Underwood–Simmons Tariff of 1913 cut duties—taxes—on imported goods by almost one-half, helping American consumers and promoting freer trade. The Sixteenth Amendment (1913) allowed a federal income tax, which the 1916 Revenue Act put into effect. This was a progressive tax, one that took a larger percentage of the income of the rich than it took from the poor. The legislation also levied higher taxes on corporate profits and created the first federal estate tax on inheritances. Though small, a tax on inheritances supported the principle of equality of opportunity. It implied that children of the wealthy

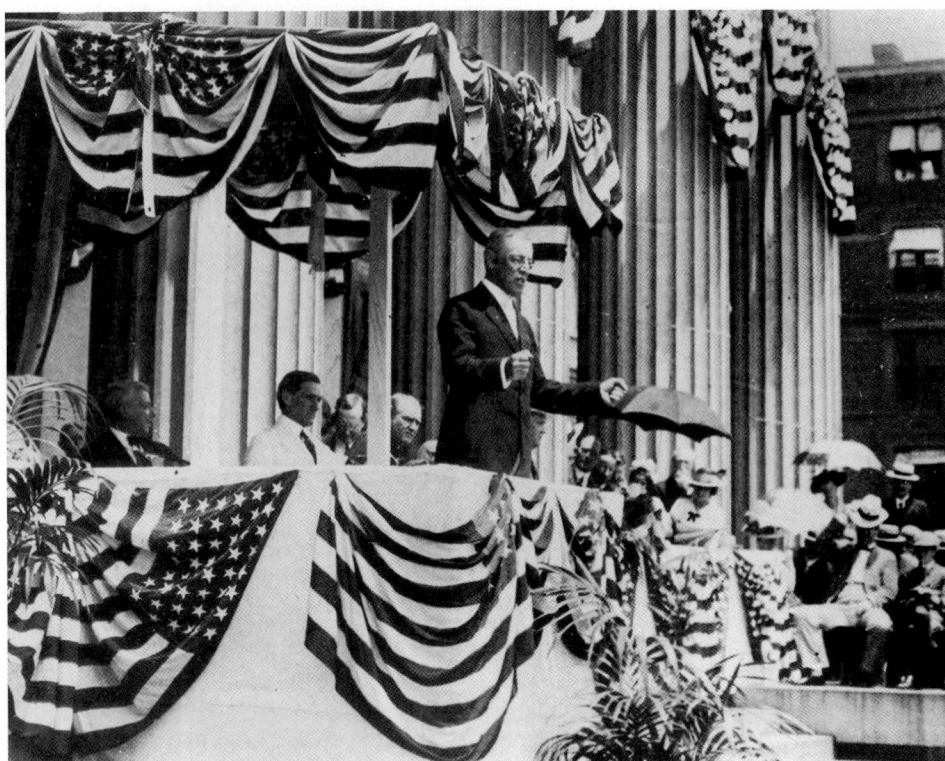

■ A former professor and university president, Woodrow Wilson was the only holder of a Ph.D. to become president of the United States. He was also the first native Southerner elected to the Oval Office since before the Civil War. Wilson's self-confidence and tendency toward self-righteousness alienated some citizens, but a majority found him to be a compelling public speaker.

Hulton Archive/Getty Images

should not receive an enormous head start in life and that Americans growing up without an inheritance should not be handicapped by the large inequalities among past generations.

Congress moved to regulate money in another new way as well. The absence of a centrally managed money system had long contributed to the exaggerated boom-and-bust cycles in the American economy. The Federal Reserve Act of 1913 created a system of 12 Federal Reserve Banks to control the amount of currency in circulation, increasing it in deflationary times and decreasing it when inflation threatened. The system aimed to abolish depressions and prevent bank closures. It did not fully succeed, as the years after 1929 showed, but the Federal Reserve System stabilized the American banking industry and helped position the dollar to become the central global currency.

No issue so dominated American politics between 1913 and 1915 as the tension between huge new corporations and the nation's antimonopoly tradition. The size and market share of companies such as U.S. Steel, American Tobacco, and Du Pont (chemicals) inhibited competition, just as Microsoft dominated computer software at the end of the twentieth century. Investigations by a congressional committee chaired by Arsene Pujo in 1913 revealed the concentration of financial power in the hands of J. P. Morgan and a few other New York bankers, dubbed the Money Trust. Congress created the Federal Trade Commission (1914) to investigate business practices that unfairly prevented competition. The Clayton Antitrust Act of 1914 supplemented the 1890 Sherman Antitrust Act by outlawing specific unfair business practices such as local price cutting and granting rebates to undermine competitors. The Clayton Act also delighted the AFL by declaring that unions should not be "construed to be illegal combinations in restraint of trade." Most federal judges remained unsympathetic to unions, but they could no longer wield the Sherman Act against striking workers rather than against the corporate trusts it had originally intended to target.

The early years after 1910 witnessed the rise of legislation to protect particular groups of citizens, especially women, children, and certain workers. States led the way, with half by 1913 passing workers' compensation laws to provide assistance to workers injured on the job and their

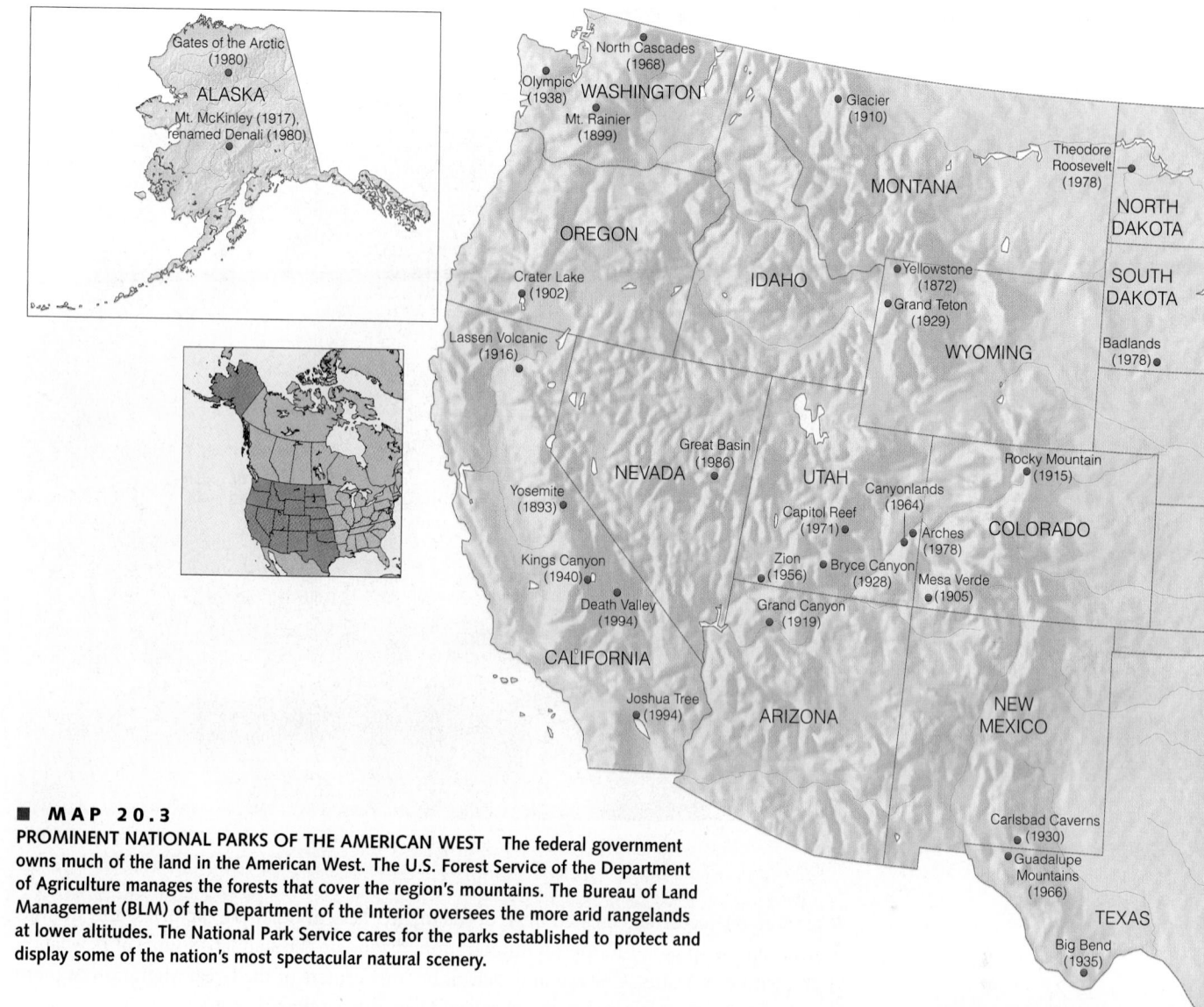

■ **MAP 20.3**

PROMINENT NATIONAL PARKS OF THE AMERICAN WEST The federal government owns much of the land in the American West. The U.S. Forest Service of the Department of Agriculture manages the forests that cover the region's mountains. The Bureau of Land Management (BLM) of the Department of the Interior oversees the more arid rangelands at lower altitudes. The National Park Service cares for the parks established to protect and display some of the nation's most spectacular natural scenery.

families. In 1916 Congress passed the first federal law limiting child labor, the Keating–Owen Act. The Supreme Court later found it to be unconstitutional, but state child labor laws remained in place. The Adamson Act (1916), providing for an eight-hour day for railroad workers, was the first case of the federal government regulating the hours of workers in the private sector.

Another kind of protective legislation focused on conservation through the preservation of natural landscapes. An increasingly urban, industrial society looked to its most beautiful rural places for solace. Local and state governments set aside parklands throughout the Progressive era. Wilson followed in Roosevelt's conservationist footsteps by creating the National Park Service in 1916 to provide unified management of such new national treasures as Glacier National Park in Montana (1910), Rocky Mountain National Park in Colorado (1915), Lassen Volcanic National Park in California (1916), and Acadia National Park in Maine (1919).

The Great Migration

The so-called Progressive era of 1900–1920 was anything but progressive from the viewpoint of African Americans, who experienced little progress. White mob violence reached its apex in these years, with hundreds of lynchings and dozens of race riots. Most African Americans lived in the South, where segregation and discrimination trapped the majority in poverty. Many therefore seized the unprecedented opportunity offered by the outbreak of the Great

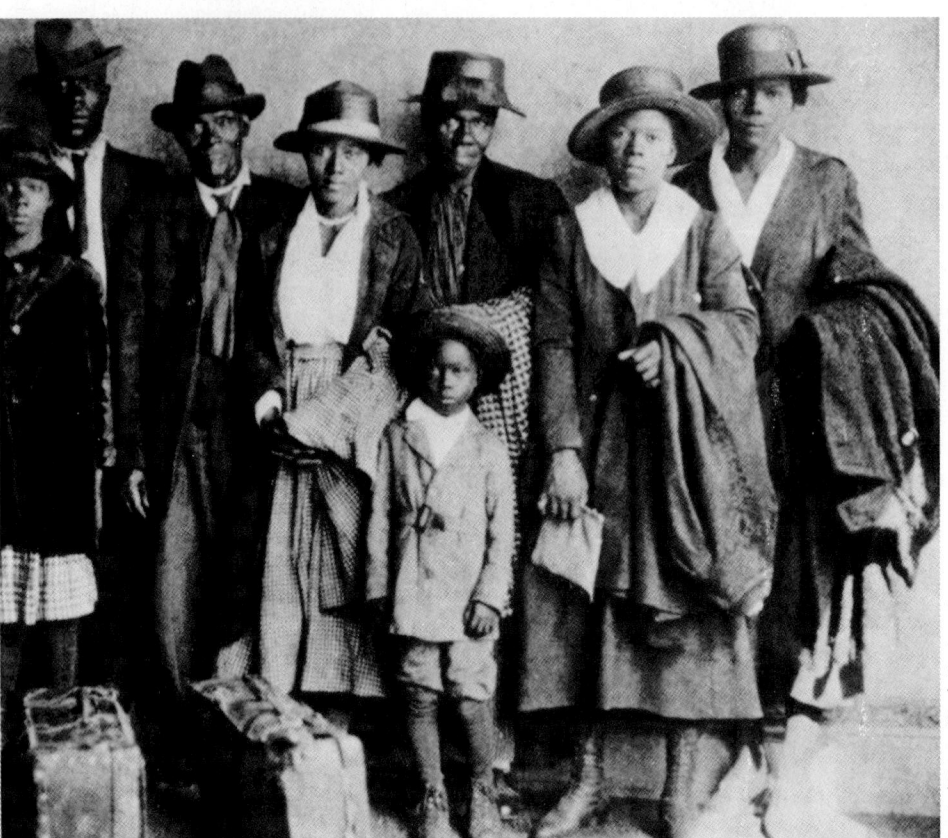

■ A migrant family from the South arriving in Chicago, c. 1916. Southerners of all colors, like Europeans, were drawn by the lure of better jobs to the industrial cities of the American Northeast and Midwest. With immigration from Europe slowed to a trickle by the onset of World War I, industry's demand for southern immigrants increased sharply.

Historical Pictures/Stock Montage, Inc.

War. War-related orders created huge needs for workers in northern factories, and the war also closed the spigot of European immigration, drying up the standard source of new labor. Along with other cities, Chicago and Detroit became centers of the Great Migration of more than half a million African Americans out of Dixie during the war years.

Encouraged by black newspapers such as the *Chicago Defender* and sometimes assisted by northern labor recruiters, black Southerners wanted to go "where a man is a man" regardless of his color. They still found plenty of discrimination in the urban North. But the large black communities of Philadelphia, Cleveland, and New York offered far greater independence than the rural South they left behind. Here "I don't have to humble to no one," one former Southerner wrote home. African Americans could vote, earn higher wages, send their children to better schools, and even sit where they wanted on streetcars. One woman newly arrived in Chicago was stunned the first time she boarded a trolley and saw black people sitting next to whites. "I just held my breath, for I thought any minute they would start something. Then I saw nobody notices it, and I just thought this is a real place for Negroes."

The Great Migration fit in a broader pattern of oppressed peoples seeking greater freedom and opportunity in the industrial workplaces of the American North. African Americans could not change their color and escape from discrimination, as could ethnic Europeans such as Irish, Italians, and Jews who struggled successfully against widespread prejudice to be identified as "white" (while still enduring elements of discrimination). But black Southerners moving north in pursuit of work and liberty acted much as European immigrants had, and they joined other newcomers seeking urban work. The 1920 census showed for the first time a majority of Americans living in towns and cities of at least 2500 people.

When war in Europe shut off most Atlantic immigration after 1914, it opened the door to newcomers who did not have to cross the submarine-infested ocean. Blacks who boarded trains for the North were joined by a similar number of white Southerners leaving rural poverty to look for jobs. A small stream of French Canadians found work in New England factories. A much larger stream of Mexicans and Mexican Americans flowed to jobs across the American Southwest and Midwest. Like African Americans, who had been leaving the South since the Civil War, people of Mexican descent had been moving across the American West for economic reasons since the mid-nineteenth century. World War I and the Mexican Revolution increased their numbers sharply, with the growing cities of Los Angeles, San Antonio, and El Paso remaining particular magnets for new immigrants. The number of Mexican Americans in Los Angeles soared from 6000 in 1910 to nearly 100,000 in 1930.

Limits to American Neutrality

A steady undertow of interests and inclinations pulled against American neutrality after 1914. Most Americans who paid attention to events abroad favored the Entente over the Central Powers. The diversity of Americans' ethnic roots across Europe, Africa, Asia, and Latin America could not mask fundamental cultural and linguistic connections to England, the one-time "mother country." President Wilson deeply admired British political values and institutions, and most influential newspaper editors supported the British cause. Even Americans critical of the British Empire did not want to see the European continent under the autocratic rule of the German Kaiser.

Concrete economic interests also tied the United States to the Allied side. During three years of neutrality, American bankers lent 85 times as much to the Entente nations as to the Central Powers ($2.3 billion versus $27 million). Opponents of American entry into the war later pointed out that bankers and weapon makers had lobbied for joining the British cause, which fattened their wallets. But millions of other Americans also benefited from the nation's trade with Britain and France. Large corporations reaped the bulk of the profits, and agricultural and industrial workers earned decent wages in filling Entente war orders.

Certain powerful Americans, concentrated on the East Coast, tried from the start to prepare the country for entering the war. They emphasized that the U.S. military was much smaller than the forces of European states because of Americans' traditional aversion to large standing armies. Republicans such as Theodore Roosevelt and former Secretary of State Elihu Root led the war preparedness movement, which sought to pressure new immigrants into "100 percent Americanism" and to establish universal military training as "the only way to yank the hyphen out of America."

Progressives themselves split over the war. More radical reformers opposed joining it as a matter of principle. "Let the capitalists do their own fighting and furnish their own corpses," Socialist Eugene Debs wrote in 1914, "and there will never be another war on the face of the earth." Settlement house leader Jane Addams and black labor organizer A. Philip Randolph likewise opposed the war throughout, as did writer Randolph Bourne. They feared, presciently, that going to war would take the wind out of the sails of domestic reform.

TABLE 20-1

The Election of 1916

Candidate	Political Party	Popular Vote	Electoral Vote
Woodrow Wilson	Democratic	9,129,606	277
Charles E. Hughes	Republican	8,538,221	254
A. L. Benson	Socialist	585,113	0

Most Progressives followed President Wilson's leadership, opposing U.S. involvement in Europe at first but gradually shifting to support it. Roosevelt's return to mainstream Republicanism and his enthusiasm for war left Wilson the standard-bearer of Progressivism in the 1916 election. This allowed the president to squeak by conservative Republican nominee Charles Evans Hughes, winning a second term in the White House. "He kept us out of war," his supporters declared, but Wilson himself was less optimistic. He knew where German submarine warfare might lead: "Any little German lieutenant can put us into the war at any time by some calculated outrage."

The United States Goes to War

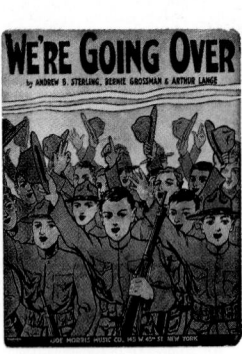

Like Lyndon Johnson in 1964 regarding Vietnam, Wilson won reelection as a liberal reformer and a man of peace, only to go to war within six months. On April 2, 1917, Wilson asked Congress for a declaration of war against Germany "to make the world safe for democracy." Congress agreed by a large majority, and four days later the United States entered the Great War. Mobilization went slowly; it took almost a year before American soldiers in large numbers saw combat in the trenches of northern France. But troops of the Entente took heart from the knowledge that the Yanks were finally coming. American foodstuffs and munitions arrived more quickly, as did American naval ships protecting cargo vessels bound for England. The U.S. entry into the war ultimately provided the narrow margin of victory against the Central Powers.

The Logic of Belligerency

Wilson's insistence on the traditional rights of neutral nations to trade with belligerents clashed with German and British efforts to prevent trade destined for their enemy. The German use of the new submarines or U-boats (from the German *Unterseeboots*) against superior British surface forces pulled Americans into the war. Submarines were extremely vulnerable when not submerged. Before firing on a merchant or passenger ship that might be armed or carrying contraband (war materials), they refused to surface and warn civilian passengers—as required under international law—to evacuate on lifeboats. With Britain arming merchant ships and stowing munitions in the holds of passenger ships, U-boats were the key element in the German campaign to weaken the enemy. The British navy, in turn, seized American goods bound for Germany. But Britain's blockade of the German coastline and neutral ports nearby did not endanger civilians in the same way. "One deals with life; the other with property," Secretary of State Robert Lansing explained.

The deaths of civilians without warning on the high seas shocked and angered the American public, especially the sinking of the magnificent British ocean liner *Lusitania* in May 1915, which killed 128 U.S. citizens and a thousand others. However, some Americans believed Wilson to be less than neutral in negotiating with the British over their offenses while giving ultimatums to Germany. Lansing's predecessor, William Jennings Bryan, resigned in June 1915 to protest the president's manner of defending American trading rights. Bryan found both sides—stalemated and unable to gain victory in the trenches—reprehensible for trying to win by killing "noncombatant men, women, and children." Only their methods differed: Germany drowned innocent civilians; England starved them with its blockade. Hoping not to draw the United States into the war, the German government twice put its unrestricted submarine warfare on hold (the *Arabic* pledge of September 1915 and the *Sussex* pledge of May 1916). By January 1917 the British blockade had reduced German food rations per person to less than half the prewar level. Facing imminent starvation, Berlin decided to take one last chance with unrestricted submarine warfare. The German government calculated that it could force a British and French surrender before enough American assistance arrived. "Not one American will land on the continent," the chief of the German naval staff confidently promised the Kaiser. Two days later, on February 3, the United States broke diplomatic relations with Germany.

Preparing for war with the Americans, German Ambassador Arthur Zimmermann secretly offered German aid to the revolutionary Mexican government "to reconquer the lost territory in Texas, New Mexico, and Arizona" if it joined the Central Powers. Mexico declined, but the Zimmermann telegram leaked to the press on March 1 and outraged Americans. The German threat seemed finally to have reached American soil. One last hindrance to joining the Entente disappeared with the revolution that same month in Russia, which replaced the monarchy with a social democratic government, which Wilson called "a fit partner for a league of

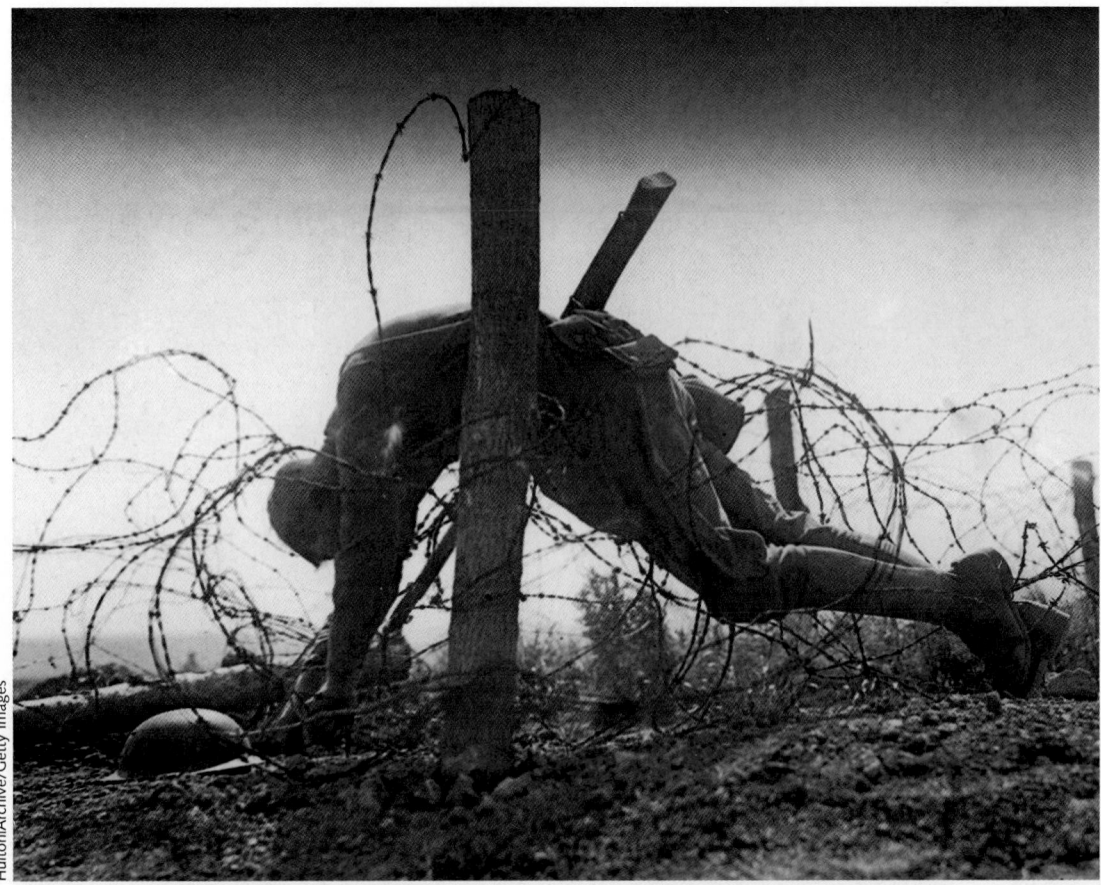

■ The body of a soldier lies caught in barbed wire in the "no-man's-land" between opposing trenches on the western front. Technological advances in weaponry helped make the fighting in World War I vastly more destructive than previous wars. The sheer scale of the slaughter stunned combatants and observers, both in Europe and America, and helped turn many in the postwar generation to deep skepticism regarding the use of military force.

honor." The president could now more genuinely call for a war to make the world "safe for democracy," with France a republic and Britain ruled by Parliament. Politics and economics merged as Lansing underlined the "industrial depression" and "general unrest and suffering among the laboring classes" that an Entente defeat would cause in America.

Still jealous of American autonomy and wary of close identification with the French, British, and Russian empires, however, Wilson took the nation into war as an "Associated" power rather than a full-blown member of the Entente. The president believed that the United States, unique among the belligerents, sought only to defend principles rather than to acquire territory, assuring it of distinctive moral leadership at an eventual postwar peace conference. "We have no quarrel with the German people" themselves but only with the "Prussian autocracy" whose U-boats were engaged in "a warfare against mankind," Wilson declared in calling Americans to a great crusade in Europe. "We desire no conquest, no dominion," but merely to be "one of the champions of the rights of mankind."

Mobilizing the Home Front

Going to war entailed a complete reorientation of the American economy. For the Army and Navy to succeed abroad, mass production of war materials had to be centrally planned, and

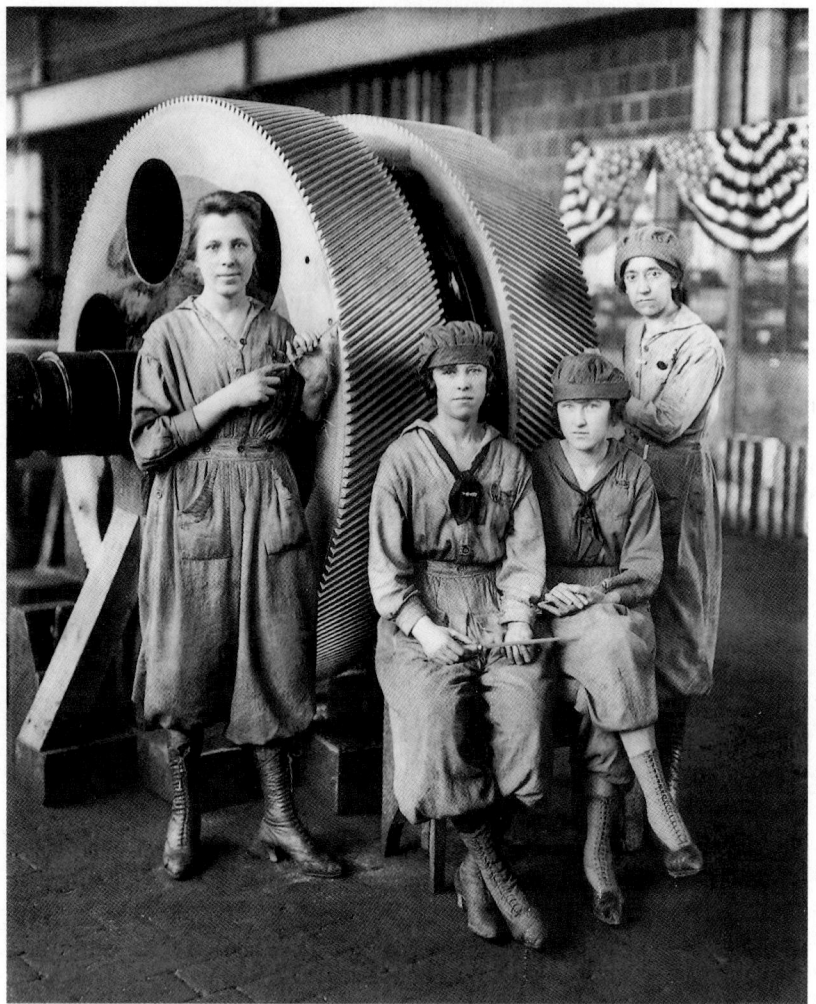

Courtesy, Hagley Museum and Library (Neg. #69.170.13.622)

■ European demand for war-related goods brought the U.S. economy out of the deep recession of 1913–1914 and created hundreds of thousands of new jobs. U.S. entry into the war in April 1917 took several million men into the armed forces, opening better-paying opportunities in manufacturing to many women. Four workers at the Westinghouse Electric Company pause from their labors in 1918.

only the federal government could fulfill this role. Such an expansion of government regulation fit with the broader agenda of Progressive reform. Federal agencies could mediate some of the tensions between capital and labor as they focused on ensuring adequate food, clothing, and weapons for the troops at the front.

The Wilson administration created several new agencies to manage the war effort at home. The Selective Service Act established local boards to draft young men into the military. The U.S. Railroad Administration took control of the nation's primary transportation system to solve railroad tie-ups caused by heavy demands for war materials. The War Industries Board supervised all war-related production, allowing large manufacturers to coordinate their schedules without fear of antitrust action. The War Labor Board resolved disputes between workers and employers, providing the most advanced solution to industrial conflict before the New Deal of the 1930s. The Committee on Public Information (CPI), run by Progressive journalist George Creel, provided the government's version of information about the war. The CPI had the crucial task of inspiring and maintaining public support for Wilson's war policies.

The close cooperation between industry and government, combined with strong demand for American goods from the Allied governments, caused corporate earnings to soar. Cost-plus contracts guaranteed profits by eliminating competition and risk. "We are all making more money out of this war than the average human being ought to," one steel company official admitted privately. And some of the war gains were spread, for a collaborative effort entailed keeping workers productive and content. Taking a position unprecedented in the U.S. government, the War Labor Board promoted an 8-hour workday and the right of workers to form unions. But even as the economy bustled, social unity proved elusive, especially when word of American casualties arrived from Europe.

Ensuring Unity

The deaths of U.S. soldiers and sailors made support for the war an emotional issue, and a pattern of repressing dissent took hold that outlasted the war itself. Everything German was particularly suspect. Several states banned teaching the German language (Nebraska briefly banned teaching any foreign language, even Latin, in a preview of the 1980s "English only" campaign). Sauerkraut became "liberty cabbage," frankfurters became hot dogs, and many German Americans anglicized their names. Temperance reformers cited German beer drinking in their successful campaign for a constitutional prohibition of alcohol production. Congress approved the controversial Eighteenth Amendment in December 1917 as a way to save grain for the war effort, and the states ratified it in 1919. Anti-German sentiment led to sometimes deadly violence against Americans of German descent by the summer of 1918. Congress passed sharply restrictive immigration legislation in 1917 as anti-German feelings fed broader prewar fears of new immigrants.

A wave of discontent among working Americans redoubled anxieties about national unity. The draft and reduced immigration thinned the ranks of labor as the war created a greater need for workers. For the first time in memory laborers could choose between jobs, and corporations were dismayed by rising employee turnover rates. Workers worried about inflation, which doubled between 1914 and 1920. Seeking better wages and more control over the workplace, they joined unions and went out on 6000 strikes during the year and a half in which the United States was in the war. Working-class women and men identified their cause with the war for democracy abroad by calling for the "de-Kaisering of industry" at home.

Industrialists saw the strikers differently. "All they seem to think of is money," one complained, mirroring what workers often said of employers. Anti-unionists tried to tar all of organized labor with the brush of disloyalty. The government passed the Espionage Act (1917) and Sedition Act (1918) to ban written and verbal organizing against the war. Socialists who encouraged draft resistance, such as Eugene Debs and Wisconsin Congressman Victor Berger, went to prison. The Supreme Court in *Schenck v. United States* (1919) upheld restrictions on free speech in the case of a "clear and present danger" to the nation's security. The Justice Department worked closely with private "patriotic" organizations such as the National Security League, which helped spy on potential dissidents.

Hostility to unions mixed with fervent prowar sentiment to produce a devastating campaign against labor activists in the West. Along the Rocky Mountains from Montana to the Mexican border, striking copper miners under IWW leadership found federal, state, and local police forces as well as vigilantes lined up against them. Sheriff Harry Wheeler of Bisbee, Arizona, arrested more than a thousand strikers, many of them Mexican Americans suspected of sympathies with Pancho Villa. Wheeler, a former Rough Rider with Theodore Roosevelt in Cuba, locked the strikers into boxcars in the July heat of 1917 and towed them into the southern New Mexico desert before releasing them. Federal agents eviscerated the antiwar IWW by raiding its offices two months later and putting 166 of its leaders on trial. A visiting British coal-mining executive found "hostility to a quite unbelievable extent against organized labor."

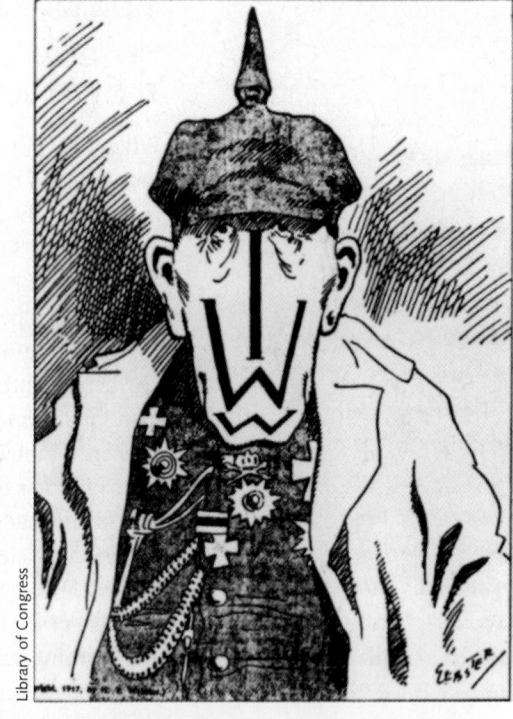

Library of Congress

■ Once the United States joined the Entente side in World War I, dissent against the war became associated for many Americans, including this cartoonist, with aiding the enemy: Germany. Here the antiwar Industrial Workers of the World (IWW) are depicted as allies of the German Kaiser. The IWW's radical politics and fervent opposition to colonialism, capitalism, and monarchy—all features of the German state—made this a particularly ironic portrayal.

Most African Americans agreed with W. E. B. Du Bois's call to "close our ranks shoulder to shoulder" with white fellow citizens in support of the war effort, despite escalating antiblack violence. The arrival of 300,000 to 500,000 black Southerners in northern cities increased competition for jobs and housing, causing resentment among many whites. Employers contributed to tensions by recruiting African Americans as strikebreakers and pitting them against white workers. Whites rioted in East St. Louis on July 1, 1917, causing at least 47 fatalities, most of them black. Black soldiers from the North rebelled against the Jim Crow restrictions they found on southern military bases. On August 23, 1917, African American troops from Camp Logan near Houston intervened to protect a black woman being beaten by police on a downtown street. The resulting gunfire killed 16 whites and 4 African Americans. Swift Army court-martials resulted in executions of 19 of the black soldiers and life imprisonment of 63 others.

The War in Europe

When the United States entered the war in Europe in 1917, crisis gripped the Entente. In the east, much of the war effort collapsed in the confusion of Russia's revolution against the Czar. In the west, 49 divisions of the French army mutinied, refusing orders to make further suicidal advances. And in the South, at Caporetto, Austro-Hungarian forces inflicted a disastrous defeat on the Italian army. It was not clear whether the Americans had joined soon enough to stave off Allied defeat.

No battle-ready American army waited at ports for immediate shipment to the trenches of northern France. U.S. commanders instead had to conscript and train nearly 5 million young men for an American Expeditionary Force (AEF) under General Pershing, and 16,000 young women volunteered for service overseas as nurses and Red Cross workers. U.S. troops participated in their first offensive operations in February 1918, although the veteran French and British lines had to stand largely on their own against the final German spring offensive. American soldiers later engaged in fierce combat at Belleau Wood, Château-Thierry, and St. Mihiel, ultimately losing 114,000 men. As the only army growing stronger in 1918, the AEF contributed crucially to the fall offensive that convinced Germany to surrender on November 11.

Fighting with French and British allies gave many American GIs an appreciation for Europeans that balanced the anti-immigrant sentiments common back home. White U.S. soldiers also bonded with each other across ethnic and religious lines while engaged in the supremely dangerous task of deadly combat. One young captain from Missouri, Harry Truman, returned from the war with a stronger appreciation for Europe that would help alter America's role in the world when he became president in 1945. Truman wrote home to his fiancée, Bess Wallace, from Nice on the south coast of France, "There is no blue like the Mediterranean blue." Almost 400,000 African American soldiers served with particular determination to prove their loyalty and courage, despite being segregated and given the hardest and least inspiring work. The French, delighted to have all who would help defend them, treated black GIs with a respect they had rarely known from whites in America. When acceptance led to growing pride among black troops abroad, U.S. commanders reacted with consternation. "It has gone to their heads," President Wilson worried.

Events in Russia provoked the greatest long-term concerns. On April 8, 1917, just two days after the United States entered the war, Vladimir Lenin and 32 fellow Bolshevik refugees from Czarism left their asylum in Zurich, Switzerland, on a train ride into history. They arrived in the Russian capital of St. Petersburg and in October seized control of the government, building a dictatorship of the Communist party in the name of the working class. The Bolsheviks opposed the Great War, condemning the battle for greater wealth and power as a demonstration of pure greed among rival capitalists. In the Czar's archives, they found and published the secret treaties of the Entente for dividing up their prospective conquests after the war,

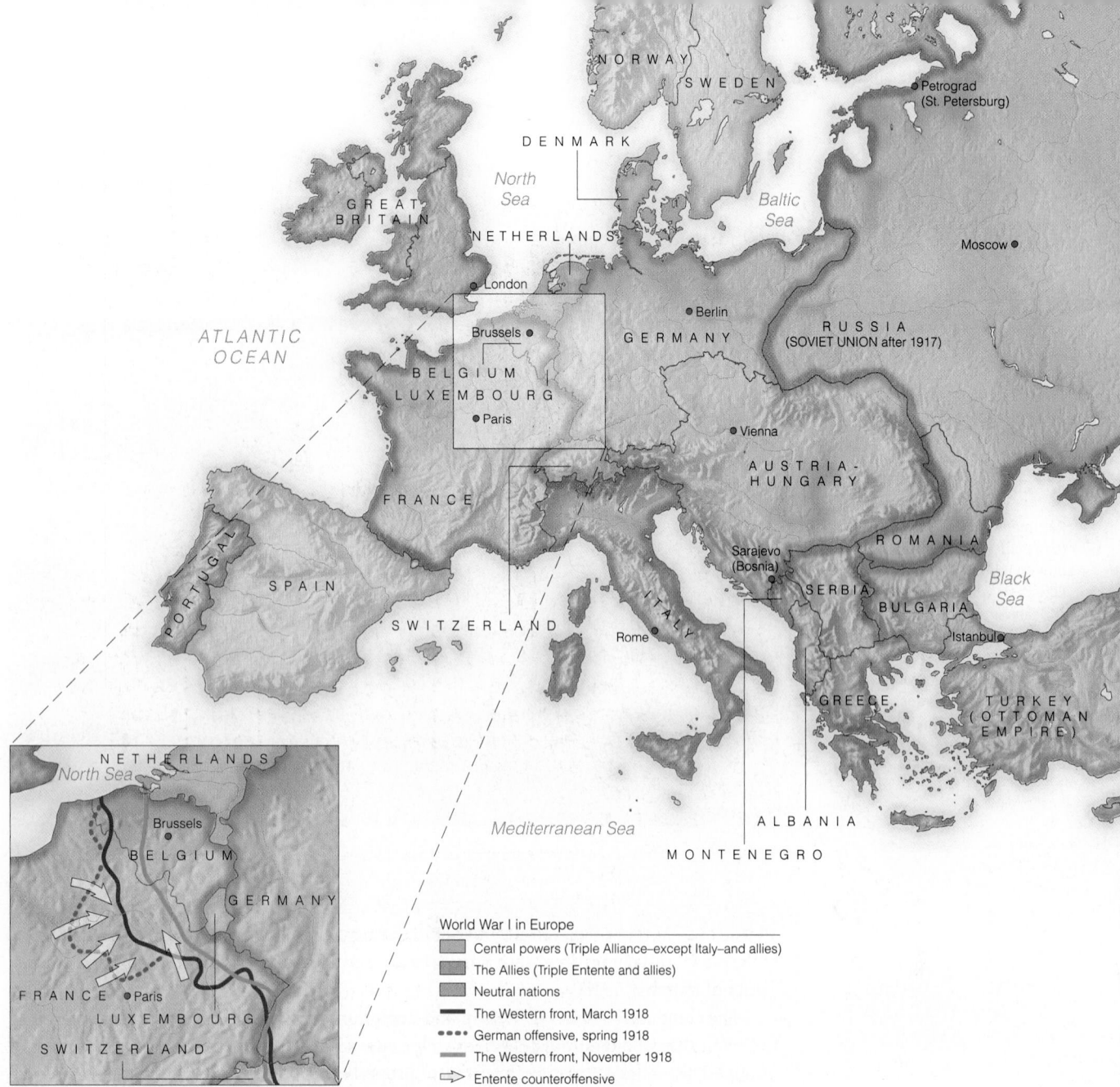

■ MAP 20.4
WORLD WAR I IN EUROPE AND THE WESTERN FRONT, 1918 By the time the U.S. troops arrived in force on the western front in northern France, the new Bolshevik (Communist) government of Russia had made peace with the Germans and withdrawn from the war. Germany now faced enemies only on one front—the western front—and moved all its troops there. In this dire situation for the French and British, American soldiers helped fill the gap in 1918.

both in Europe and in the colonies overseas. While Wilson spoke of a war for democracy, the Bolsheviks asked Russians, "Are you willing to fight for this, that the English capitalists should rob Mesopotamia and Palestine?"

The answer, as Wilson feared, was no. In January 1918 the president gave the famous "14 Points" speech to the U.S. Congress, outlining his aims of a postwar world built not on expansion and revenge but on national self-determination, open diplomacy, and freedom of commerce and travel, to be guaranteed by a new League of Nations. He hoped to dissuade the Bolsheviks from making a separate peace with Germany that would allow Germany to move

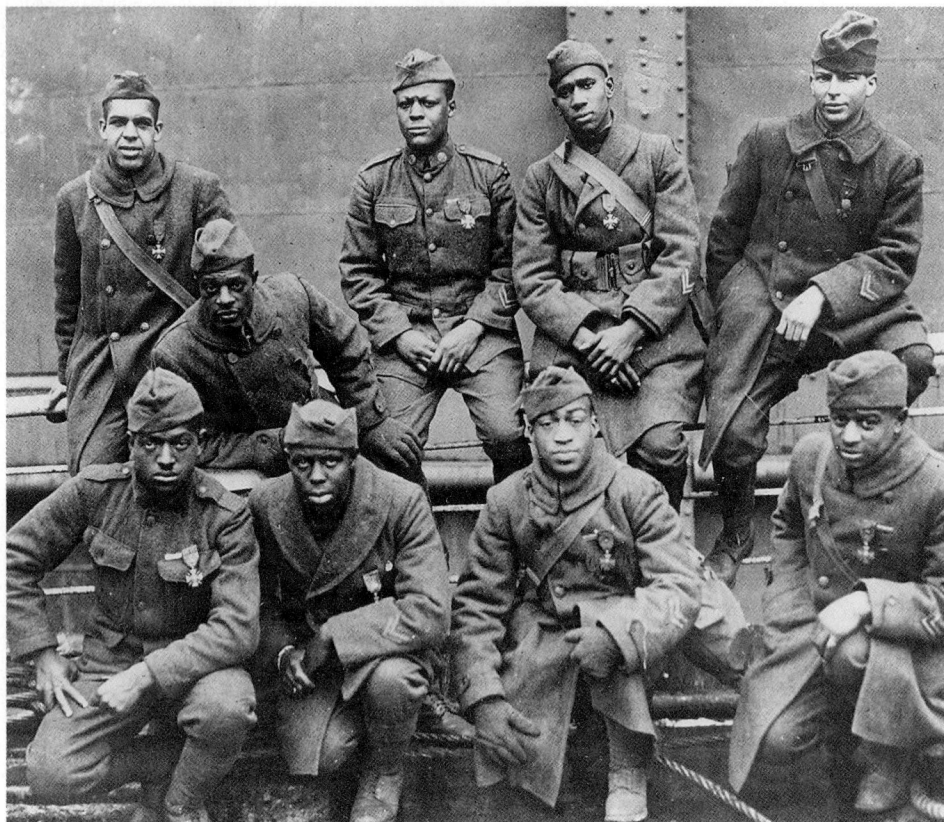

■ Members of the 369th Infantry Regiment wear the Croix de Guerre (Cross of War) awarded to them for bravery by the French government. Like their white fellow soldiers, African American troops often fought bravely and with distinction on the fields of northern France. But they were segregated and given the hardest, most demeaning work by U.S. commanders, following the same pattern at home in the United States.

The National Archives

all its troops to the western front. But Lenin, facing civil war at home, conceded huge swaths of the old Czarist empire in eastern Europe to the Germans to gain peace with the Brest–Litovsk Treaty of March 3, 1918.

The competing visions of Wilson and Lenin for world order contained the roots of the Cold War that would dominate American life after 1945. They agreed that the old diplomacy of imperialist states competing for pieces of property around the globe would no longer work and that only the creation of democratic states would prevent further wars. But they understood democracy very differently. For Wilson, it meant self-governing nations with capitalist economies and republican political practices (at least in Europe and North America, and eventually elsewhere). For Lenin, it meant workers in every land overthrowing the owners of capital and setting up Soviet governments. Whereas Wilson viewed the world as a collection of nations, Lenin saw it as a battleground between two classes.

The Struggle to Win the Peace

World War I killed more than 16 million people and wrought immeasurable physical, social, and psychological damage. Was it worth it? Citizens of the belligerent nations emerged from 1918 convinced that only a guarantee of a future free of war could legitimate such suffering. Some put their hopes in the radical solution unfolding in Russia. Some in the Allied states believed that severe measures against Germany would ensure peace. Most looked to Woodrow Wilson in the winter and spring of 1919 as the world leader whose vision for a more peaceful, democratic postwar order was "all that had made the war

African American Women in the Great War

Just as black American men served in the American Expeditionary Forces in France in 1917–1918, black American women served in auxiliary organizations such as the Red Cross and the Young Men's and Women's Christian Associations (YMCA and YWCA), which worked to boost the soldiers' morale. They staffed canteens set up to provide social and educational support for American troops as an alternative to entertainments such as prostitution and gambling. Addie W. Hunton and Kathryn M. Johnson felt a particular calling to encourage African American soldiers, who suffered from discrimination and segregation even as they fought for democracy. As devout Christians, the two women believed they must model a life of service and compassion, even in the face of persecution. An account of their time in Europe published soon after they returned to the United States suggests some of the complications of a segregated society sending people abroad.

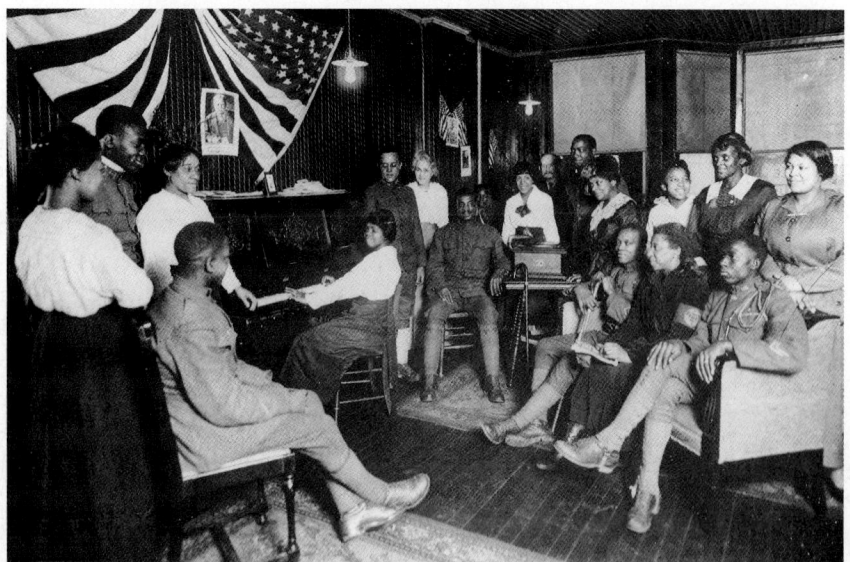

The National Archives

American women supported the war effort in many ways, including working in munitions factories, buying war bonds, single-parenting while husbands were away in the military, and volunteering as nurses for the armed forces in France. Here, African American women entertain black soldiers with music in a service club in Newark, New Jersey, 1918.

Two Colored Women with the American Expeditionary Forces

The relationship between the colored soldiers, the colored welfare workers, and the French people was most cordial and friendly and grew in sympathy and understanding, as their associations brought about a closer acquaintance. It was rather an unusual as well as a most welcome experience to be able to go into places of public accommodation without having any hesitations or misgivings; to be at liberty to take a seat in a common carrier, without fear of inviting some humiliating experience; to go into a home and receive a greeting that carried with it a hospitality and kindliness of spirit that could not be questioned.

These things were at once noticeable upon the arrival of a stranger within the gates of this sister democracy, and the first ten days in France, though filled with duties and harassed with visits from German bombing planes, were nevertheless a delight, in that they furnished to some of us the first full breath of freedom that had ever come into our limited experience.

The first post of duty assigned to us was Brest. Upon arriving there we received our first experience with American prejudices, which had not only been carried across the seas, but had become a part of such an intricate propaganda, that the relationship between the colored soldier and the French people is more or less a story colored by a continued and subtle effort to inject this same prejudice into the heart of the hitherto unprejudiced Frenchman.

[An order posted by white officer of black battalion read:] "Enlisted men of this organization will not talk to or be in company with any white women, regardless of whether the women solicit their company or not."

[Another order read:] "There are two Y.M.C.A.'s, one near the camp, for white troops, and one in town, for the colored troops. All men will be instructed to patronize their own Y."

. . . Quite a bit of unpleasantness was experienced on the boats coming home . . . . On [one] boat there were nineteen colored welfare workers; all the women were placed on a floor below the white women, and the entire colored party was placed in an obscure, poorly ventilated section of the dining-room, entirely separated from the other workers by a long table of Dutch civilians. The writer immediately protested; the reply was made that the southern white workers on board the ship would be insulted if the colored workers ate in the same section of the dining-room with them, and, at any rate, the colored people did not expect any such treatment as had been given them by the French. ■

Source: Addie W. Hunton and Kathryn M. Johnson, *Two Colored Women with American Expeditionary Forces* (New York: Brooklyn Eagle Press, 1920), 28–30, 182–183, 186.

tolerable to many of us," as one admirer put it. The president sailed for Europe in January to lead the conference that would shape the peace. Vast crowds greeted him enthusiastically as he toured England, Italy, and France.

Peacemaking and the Versailles Treaty

War and revolution destroyed the four great empires of Russia, Germany, Austria–Hungary, and the Ottomans (based in modern Turkey). Meeting in Paris from January to June 1919, the "Big Three" of Wilson, French President Georges Clemenceau, and British Prime Minister David Lloyd George took on two major tasks to shape the postwar order. (The Italian prime minister left the conference after failing to get the new territories he had sought.) First, the three leaders redrew the map of eastern and central Europe to create nation-states out of the vanished empires. Second, they had to decide what to do about a defeated Germany. The possible spread of revolution gave the negotiations a particular urgency. Anticolonial revolts broke out in India and China, and pro-Soviet workers' councils seized power briefly in Hungary and southern Germany. "We are running a race with Bolshevism," Wilson warned, "and the world is on fire."

To put out the fire, the Big Three created a string of new nations running from Finland in the north to Yugoslavia in the south. Eastern Europeans were to be self-governing within the new political boundaries. Ultimately, some of the new states—Czechoslovakia and especially Yugoslavia—lacked the sense of nationhood necessary for success and broke apart into smaller ethnic components in the 1990s. But a major purpose of these new nations for the negotiators in Paris was to establish an anticommunist belt keeping Russian communism out of Europe while satisfying their residents' desire for greater self-determination.

How far would "self-determination" go? Secretary of State Lansing worried that the president's language of democracy was "loaded with dynamite." The world's nonwhite majority wondered whether it applied to them. "Security of Life for Poles and Serbs—Why Not for Colored Nations?" asked one black newspaper in New York. A young nationalist from Vietnam named Ho Chi Minh tried but failed to get an audience with Wilson to ask for the 14 Points to apply to his French-ruled country; a generation later, Ho led the Vietnamese people's armed struggle against France and then the United States. The Big Three instead created the mandate system to provide for eventual self-determination for colonies after a period of tutelage under an established power, and they rejected Japan's proposal to include racial equality as a principle of the new League of Nations.

The German question predominated at the Paris conference. To create a long-term peaceful order in Europe, Wilson wanted lenient terms for Germany. But the French and British had lost much more in the war than the Americans, and they believed Germany must pay for that. French security seemed to depend on keeping its powerful and aggressive neighbor down. The Versailles Treaty (named for the famous estate of King Louis XIV outside Paris, where it was signed) reflected compromises that gave each of the Allies what it most wanted. To satisfy France and England, Germany had to admit guilt for causing the war and pay $33 billion in reparations, while losing much of its eastern territory to the new Polish and Czechoslovakian states. For Wilson the League of Nations was the key: this new and unprecedented global organization would keep the peace by ensuring collective security for all nations. Disputes between nations would be mediated before they escalated to armed conflict, and potential aggressors would be deterred by the promise of collective action in defense of any threatened league member.

The absence of certain crucial players from the Paris negotiations undermined the resulting international order. The Soviets and the Germans did not participate. Wilson took in his entourage no representatives of the Republican party. This proved important, for Republicans had won the congressional elections two months earlier, giving them control of the process for ratifying any treaties. Most Republicans objected on principle to one key aspect of the Versailles Treaty: Article 10 of the League of Nations charter, guaranteeing ahead of time a collective response to defend any member's territory from attack. Treaty opponents were deter-

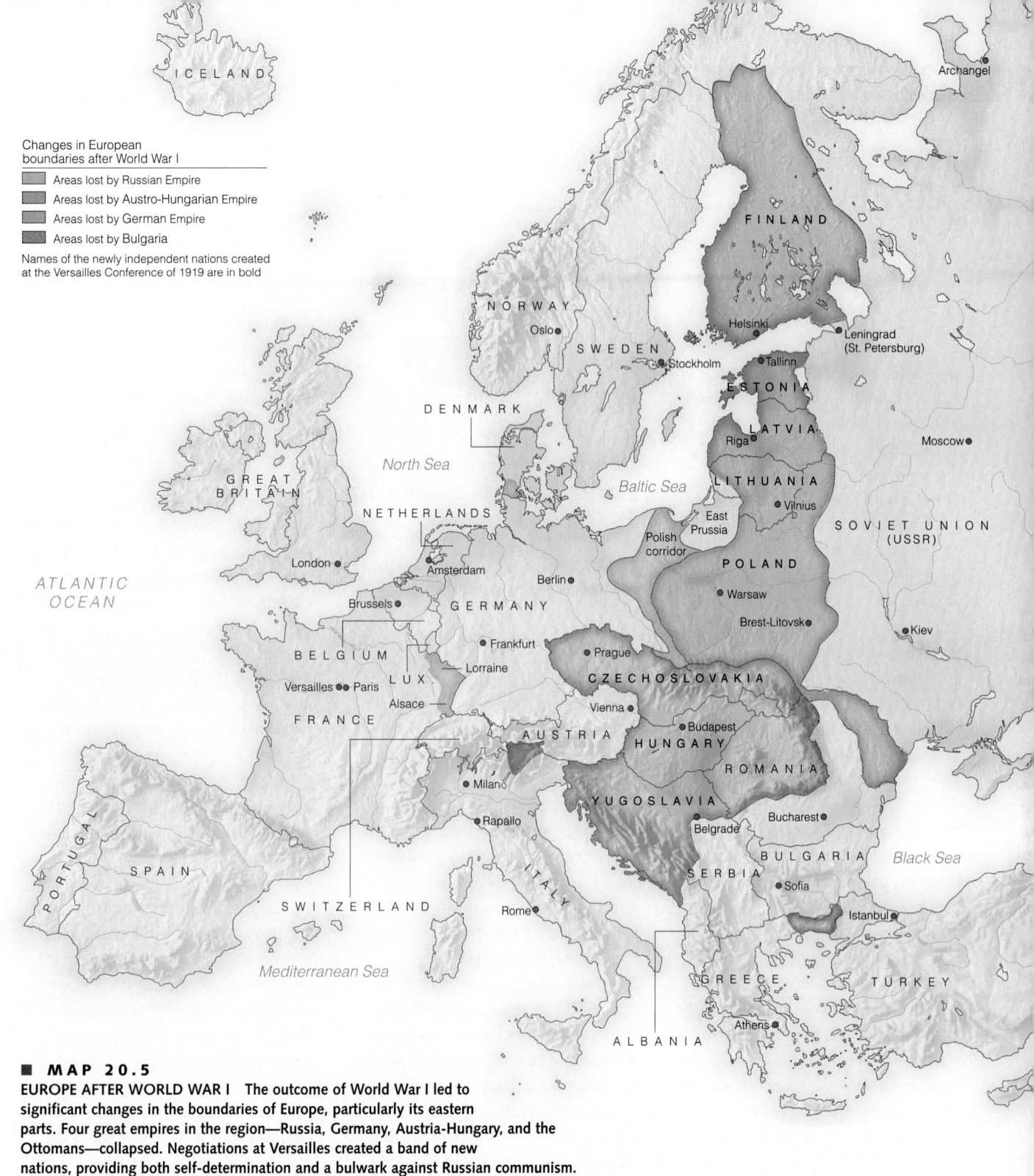

Changes in European
boundaries after World War I

- Areas lost by Russian Empire
- Areas lost by Austro-Hungarian Empire
- Areas lost by German Empire
- Areas lost by Bulgaria

Names of the newly independent nations created
at the Versailles Conference of 1919 are in bold

■ MAP 20.5

EUROPE AFTER WORLD WAR I The outcome of World War I led to
significant changes in the boundaries of Europe, particularly its eastern
parts. Four great empires in the region—Russia, Germany, Austria-Hungary, and the
Ottomans—collapsed. Negotiations at Versailles created a band of new
nations, providing both self-determination and a bulwark against Russian communism.

mined to preserve complete American autonomy, including freedom of action in Latin America. Henry Cabot Lodge, Jr., of Massachusetts, the powerful Republican chair of the Senate Foreign Relations Committee, organized the two Senate votes rejecting American membership
in the league. Hoping to stave off defeat for his idealistic plan, Wilson undertook an ill-advised
national speaking tour to promote the League. His strenuous effort failed to win American participation in the league, and it ultimately broke his fragile health. Wilson suffered a stroke on
October 2, 1919, that left him incapacitated for the rest of his presidency.

The League of Nations and International Security

The experience of World War I stunned Europeans and Americans. Never before had an armed conflict killed and wounded so many people in so brief a time. Observers from outside the Central Powers, like most historians since, placed primary responsibility for the onset of the war on the aggressive actions of German Kaiser Wilhelm II. Other critics noted the expansive empires of every member of the Entente and wondered whether more than just German imperialism was troubling the international system. The sheer scale of the carnage, especially the continuing slaughter of soldiers in indecisive battles on the almost immovable western front for four long years, suggested that something deeper might be wrong with the way nations waged both diplomacy and war.

The intensifying rivalry of the European nations after 1910 created the conditions for the Great War. In the international arena few rules guided how powerful nations behaved, in contrast to the domestic sphere of any particular nation, which had clear guidelines for how its citizens could act. A handful of international conventions created some general expectations for "civilized" actions in peace and war, but no form of effective enforcement backed these up. When a rising power such as Germany (unified in 1871)

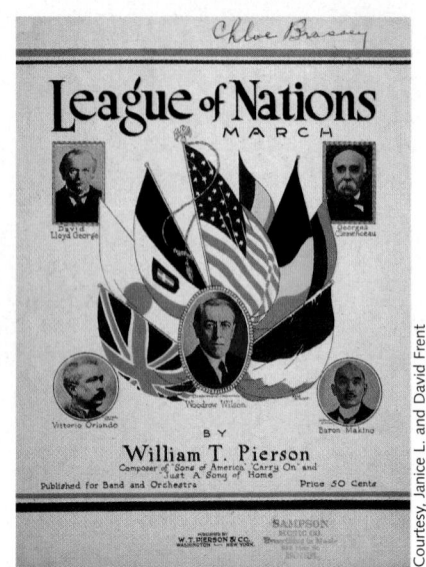

Supporters of the League of Nations even wrote popular sheet music in its honor.

Courtesy, Janice L. and David Frent

chose to upset the existing balance of power between nations, the only recourse available was on the battlefield. The new tools of warfare on display in World War I—machine guns, poison gas, submarines, airplanes—made this a grim prospect.

Woodrow Wilson's original vision for the League of Nations was a bold effort to come to terms with this challenge. Rejecting the amoral old diplomacy of nations strengthening themselves at the cost of weakening others, Wilson called for a new diplomacy of collective security. All nations would agree to protect each other and the status quo, deterring potential aggressors by promising to come to the defense of any nation under attack. Without arms races to destabilize the international order, militarism would subside. The U.S. failure to join the League of Nations undermined its effectiveness, however, as did the competing desire of national leaders to pre-

serve maximum autonomy for pursuing their nations' own interests.

World War II seemed to prove Wilson correct. His vision of substituting collective internationalism for competitive nationalism helped shape the United Nations (UN) in 1945, especially its General Assembly of all nations. However, the UN's powerful Security Council with its five permanent members (Britain, France, Russia, China, and the United States) who each retained the right to veto any action by the organization, limited the degree of collective security that members could depend on. The Cold War (1946–1989) also reduced the UN's effectiveness by dividing the world into two competing collective security systems, one headed by the Soviet Union (Russia) and one by the United States.

In the 1990s the UN gained renewed prominence, first in the international coalition fighting against Iraq in the 1991 Gulf War and subsequently as the source of mediation efforts and peacekeeping forces for civil conflicts around the globe. The growing seriousness of problems that were unarguably international in nature, such as global warming and the proliferation of nuclear weapons, provided a potent argument in favor of collective action. Americans nonetheless remained ambivalent about the UN at the start of the new millennium. As the world's most powerful nation in military and economic terms, the United States expected to lead the UN. But U.S. leaders did not like to be hemmed in by its collective decision-making process. Unilateral freedom of action in the international sphere, like that suggested two centuries earlier by George Washington's warning to avoid "entangling alliances," continued to appeal to many citizens. ∎

Waging Counterrevolution Abroad

Soon after Russia withdrew from the war, the western members of the Entente intervened in the civil war there between the Bolsheviks (the "Reds") and the various counterrevolutionary forces (the "Whites"). The initial military rationale in the summer of 1918 was to reopen the eastern front against Germany. The United States landed 7000 troops in Vladivostock, on Russia's far Pacific coast, to help rescue a large group of former Czech prisoners of war from the Austro-Hungarian army who now wanted to join the Allied side and to deter Japanese expansion into Siberia. In conjunction with the British, 5000 U.S. soldiers went ashore at Archangel in northern Russia to prevent Allied supplies from falling into German hands. They quickly became involved in fighting the Red Army. The Wilson administration meanwhile funneled money and military intelligence to leaders of the White forces.

The Bolsheviks rejected certain values cherished by most Americans: the sanctity of private property and contracts, political liberty, and religious freedom. They liberalized divorce laws and legalized abortion, challenging conservative American attitudes about the relationships between women and men. And they established the Comintern in 1919 to promote similar revolutions around the world. Allied intervention in the Russian civil war failed to overthrow Lenin's government, and American troops pulled out in 1920. They left behind a powerful legacy of anti-American sentiment in Russia, exacerbated by Washington's refusal for the next 13 years to recognize the Soviet government.

Anticommunists used the metaphor of infection to describe Bolshevism. The Kaiser, they said, had allowed Lenin to pass through Germany on a "sealed train," lest the bacillus of revolution leak out and spread through the German population. This image had unusual power in 1918–1919 because of the spread of one of the twentieth century's worst killers. The "Spanish influenza" (named for one of its early victims, the King of Spain) hit the United States much harder than the Great War had, killing six times as many people (675,000). In an era before effective vaccines and antibiotic drugs, little could be done for the 20 million Americans stricken besides comforting them, so nurses were in much greater demand than doctors. Not until the longer-lasting AIDS crisis after 1980 did Americans again live in such fear of a disease.

From Art of the October Revolution, Leningrad, Aurora Art Publishers, 1979

ТОВ. Ленин ОЧИЩАЕТ землю от нечисти.

■ **"Comrade Lenin Sweeps the Globe Clean."** This Bolshevik (Communist) drawing shows Vladimir I. Lenin (1870–1924), the leader of the Russian revolution and founder of the world's first Communist government, ridding the world of capitalists and monarchs. But Lenin also sought western trade and investment, especially from the United States, as a stimulus to reconstructing the devastated postwar economy of the new Union of Soviet Socialist Republics (USSR).

The Red and Black Scares at Home

Four million American workers, one out of every five, went out on strike in 1919—the highest proportion of the workforce ever. They sought improved wages and working conditions as well as recognition of the right to collective bargaining. The scale of industrial unrest provoked fears of a Soviet-style revolution. In Seattle a walkout by shipyard workers mushroomed into a general strike that shut down most of the city for a week. In Pittsburgh, the AFL led a bitter strike against U.S. Steel in pursuit of union recognition. The United Mine Workers led walkouts by hundreds of thousands of coal miners, which evolved into open warfare between miners and coal companies in West Virginia over the next two years. In Boston three quarters of the police force went on strike to protest wages lower than those of common laborers. Traditional May 1 (May Day) parades celebrating the dignity of labor featured violent clashes between socialist marchers and heckling veterans in Cleveland, New York, and other cities. Between April and June, anarchists mailed or delivered bombs to 36 prominent public figures, including Attorney General A. Mitchell Palmer. All were defused except two, one wounding the wife and maid of a U.S. senator from Georgia, the other destroying the front of Palmer's house and dismembering its anarchist deliverer.

Whereas many Americans sympathized with struggles for unionization, others viewed them as dangerous to private property and social order. They associated strikes with radical immigrants and anarchists and considered them "un-American." "Unionism is nothing less than bolshevism," declared the National Association of Manufacturers. The "Red Scare" of 1919 associated reform and social justice of any kind with subversion. To break strikes, employers hired private armies from "detective" agencies such as the Pinkertons and the Baldwin–Felts, often staffed by World War I veterans. Private organizations promoting "100 percent Americanism," such as the Ku Klux Klan and the new American Legion, monitored and harassed potential subversives and the foreign-born. Attorney General Palmer directed the deportation to Russia of 249 foreign-born radicals aboard the *Buford* in December 1919, including anarchist and feminist Emma Goldman. "Palmer raids" led to the arrest of thousands more within a month. U.S. Army troops and state militias brought the ultimate force to bear against union organizers, as at the Battle of Blair Mountain on August 31, 1921, against several thousand striking West Virginia miners.

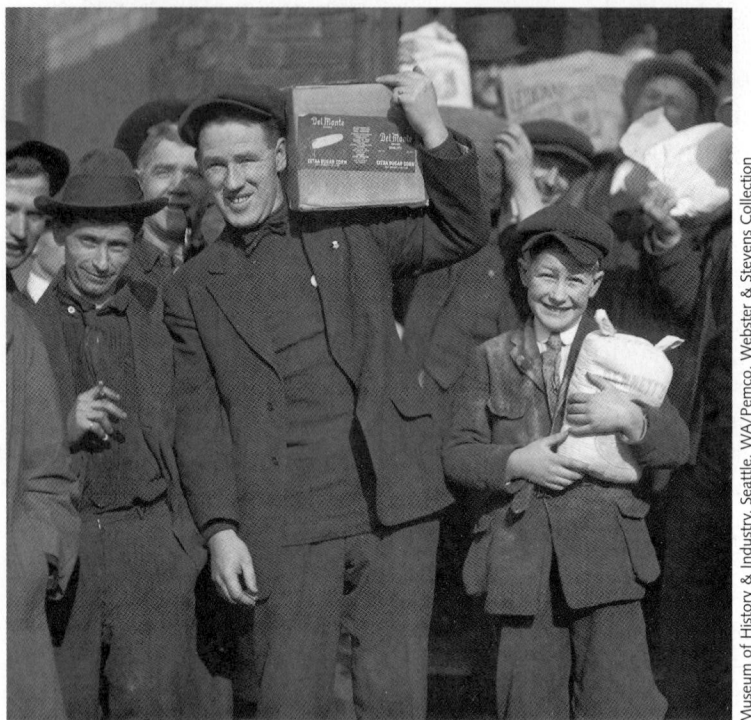

Violence against workers extended to African Americans after World War I. An upsurge in lynching included at least ten black veterans still in uniform and was not limited to the South. In Nebraska white residents of Omaha butchered William Brown with such frenzy that thousands of federal troops had to be called in to restore calm. White mobs burned entire black communities to the ground, including Tulsa's Greenwood neighborhood (1921) and the all-black town of Rosewood, Florida (1923). The Red Scare and the "Black Scare" merged in Phillips County, Arkansas, where black sharecroppers, many of them veterans, formed a union in 1919 to pursue equitable crop settlements from landlords. Fearing insurrection, local white leaders used 2500 federal troops and white vigilantes to massacre more than 200 sharecroppers. But any inclination toward deference in the face of brutality was gone, and African Americans fought back fiercely against white marauders in deadly riots in Washington and Chicago in the summer of 1919. One black woman recalled hearing news that in Washington "our men had stood like men" and crying for joy: "Oh, I thank God, thank God!"

Where was the president during this turmoil? Incapacitated by his stroke, he lay resting in his bed in Washington, the administration managed largely by his wife, Edith, and his secretary, Joseph Tumulty. In any case, Wilson's segregationist policies suggested that he would have been unlikely to provide effective leadership in bridging the nation's racial divides. The only Republican of similar stature, Theodore Roosevelt, had died a few months earlier. "There is no leadership worthy of the name," a veteran reporter lamented. Wilson's breakdown came in the middle of the 1919 baseball World Series, which the heavily favored but poorly paid Chicago White Sox intentionally lost to the Cincinnati Reds, in arrangement with gamblers. Eight "Black Sox" were banned from the sport. With its president out of action and its national pastime corrupted, the nation seemed adrift as the lights dimmed on the Progressive era.

■ The Seattle General Strike Committee took on the responsibility of keeping essential services running in the city. Here its members issue groceries to union families, January 1919. The cooperation necessary among organized workers to keep a strike going offered a different model of community interaction than did the individualism often touted by wealthier Americans.

Museum of History & Industry, Seattle, WA/Pemco, Webster & Stevens Collection

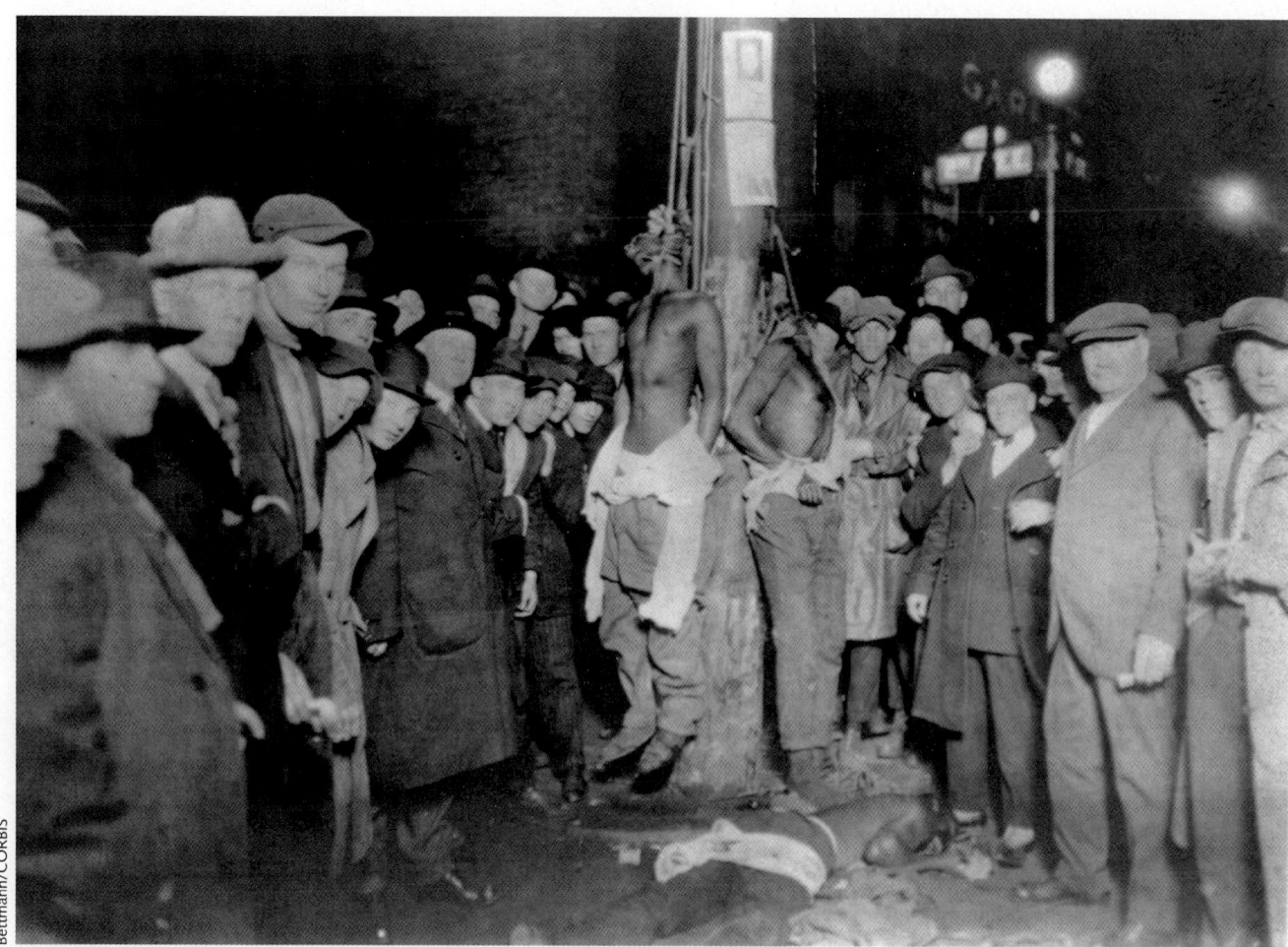

Bettmann/CORBIS

■ Death by hanging or burning, often preceded by torture, at the hands of a white mob constituted one end of a range of tactics of intimidation and coercion used against black Southerners in the early twentieth century. Outnumbered and outgunned, African Americans fought back fiercely when they could. Lynchings sometimes had a festive air for the white participants, with children often present.

Conclusion

How much success could a varied generation of Progressive reformers claim? Women had won the vote with the Nineteenth Amendment, in an expansion of democracy second only to the combination of the Emancipation Proclamation of 1863 and the Fifteenth Amendment, outlawing slavery. African Americans who moved north usually could vote as well, unlike those who stayed in Dixie. On either side of the Mason–Dixon line, however, daily life for Americans of darker hue entailed picking one's way through a maze of discrimination. Most union campaigns stalled by 1920, beaten back by the physical force and cleverness of corporate employers and their government sympathizers. When the Red Scare dissipated, Americans did not return to the reform spirit of Progressivism. Many turned away from politics. Voter turnout in 1920 dipped below 50 percent for the first time in a century. Those who did vote that year gave the Republican party a sweeping victory. Promising "not revolution, but restoration," Ohio Senator Warren G. Harding took the White House. His speeches may have been, as one rival said, "an army of pompous phrases moving over the landscape in search of an idea," but most of the nation sought calm after the upheavals of the previous decade.

American contributions to democracy abroad were similarly ambivalent. Whereas eastern Europeans named streets in their newly independent nations for President Wilson, few Latin Americans believed that U.S. invasions of Caribbean and Central American countries promoted self-government. Russians admired much about American society and the U.S. economy while resenting American troops in their land. Above all hung the problem of Germany, still the most powerful single nation in Europe. The Versailles Treaty imposed harsh terms and embittered a generation of German people. "If I were a German, I think I should not sign it," Wilson admitted privately. The Weimar Republic that replaced the abdicated German Kaiser lasted through the 1920s. But the storms of the Great Depression swamped Germany's republican experiment and gave rise to Adolph Hitler.

Sites to Visit

The Great War, 1914–1918
www.pitt.edu/~pugachev/greatwar/ww1.html

This site offers an array of narratives, photos, documents, statistics, maps, and bibliography, plus links to other useful World War I sites.

Women and Social Movements in the United States, 1775–1940
womhist.binghamton.edu

Maintained by two Binghamton University historians, this site has a rich trove of documents on the history of American women as well as excellent links to others.

The Avalon Project at the Yale Law School: Documents in Law, History, and Diplomacy
www.yale.edu/lawweb/avalon/avalon.htm

Researchers can find here the texts of a large number of the most important primary documents illuminating U.S. relations with other countries, including materials on American responses to the Bolshevik revolution in Russia.

Temperance and Prohibition
prohibition.history.ohio-state.edu/Contents.htm

Cartoons, newspaper articles, and other primary documents available here illuminate in fascinating ways the struggle over whether to prohibit the sale of alcoholic beverages.

The Emma Goldman Papers
sunsite.berkeley.edu/Goldman/

This site has photos and excerpts from the writings and speeches of one of America's most influential radicals and feminists from this era.

Divining America: Religion and the National Culture
scriptorium.lib.duke.edu/wlm/

This site has essays by prominent historians on diverse aspects of the religious history of the United States.

Up South: African-American Migration in the Era of the Great War
www.ashp.cuny.edu/video/south.html

Maintained by the American Social History Project at the Graduate Center of the City University of New York, this site offers details of the mass migration of rural black Southerners to the urban north during World War I.

The Influenza Pandemic of 1918
www.stanford.edu/group/virus/uda/

A variety of information, documents, and photos of the deadly global outbreak of the "Spanish flu" can be found here.

For Further Reading

General

Kendrick A. Clements, *Woodrow Wilson: World Statesman* (1987).

John M. Cooper, *Pivotal Decades: The United States, 1900–1920* (1990).

Alan Dawley, *Struggles for Justice: Social Responsibility and the Liberal State* (1991).

Nell Irvin Painter, *Standing at Armageddon: The United States, 1877–1919* (1987).

Daniel T. Rodgers, *Atlantic Crossings: Social Politics in a Progressive Age* (1998).

A World in Upheaval

Friedrich Katz, *The Secret War in Mexico: Europe, the United States, and the Mexican Revolution* (1981).

Paul Kennedy, *The Rise and Fall of the Great Powers: Economic Change and Military Conflict from 1500 to 2000* (1987).

Arthur Link, ed., *Woodrow Wilson and a Revolutionary World* (1982).

Joseph A. McCartin, *Labor's Great War: The Struggle for Industrial Democracy and the Origins of Modern American Labor Relations, 1912–1921* (1997).

George J. Sánchez, *Becoming Mexican American: Ethnicity, Culture, and Identity in Chicano Los Angeles, 1900–1945* (1993).

The Great War and American Neutrality

John W. Coogan, *The End of Neutrality: The United States, Britain, and Maritime Rights, 1899–1915* (1981).

Steven J. Diner, *A Very Different Age: Americans of the Progressive Era* (1998).

James Grossman, *Land of Hope: Chicago, Black Southerners, and the Great Migration* (1989).

Vicki I. Ruiz, *From Out of the Shadows: Mexican Women in Twentieth-Century America* (1998).

Martin Sklar, *The Corporate Reconstruction of American Capitalism, 1890–1916: The Market, the Law, and Politics* (1988).

The United States Goes to War

Edward M. Coffman, *The War to End All Wars: The American Military Experience in World War I* (1987).

Martin Gilbert, *The First World War: A Complete History* (1994).

David M. Kennedy, *Over Here: The First World War and American Society* (1980).

Kathleen Kennedy, *Disloyal Mothers and Scurrilous Citizens: Women and Subversion During World War I* (1999).

Richard Polenberg, *Fighting Faiths: The Abrams Case, the Supreme Court, and Free Speech* (1987).

Nick Salvatore, *Eugene V. Debs: Citizen and Socialist* (1982).

The Struggle to Win the Peace

Alfred W. Crosby, *America's Forgotten Pandemic: The Influenza of 1918* (1989).

Scott Ellsworth, *Death in a Promised Land: The Tulsa Race Riot of 1921* (1982).

David S. Foglesong, *America's Secret War Against Bolshevism: U.S. Intervention in the Russian Civil War, 1917–1920* (1995).

Thomas J. Knock, *To End All Wars: Woodrow Wilson and the Quest for a New World Order* (1992).

Gordon N. Levin, Jr., *Woodrow Wilson and World Politics: America's Response to War and Revolution* (1968).

William M. Tuttle, Jr., *Race Riot: Chicago in the Red Summer of 1919* (1970).

Betty M. Unterberger, *The United States, Revolutionary Russia, and the Rise of Czechoslovakia* (1989).

Online Practice Test

Test your understanding of this chapter with interactive review quizzes at

www.ablongman.com/jonescreatedequal/chapter20

Additional Photo Credits

Page 671: (Top) Hulton|Archive/Getty Images; (bottom) Culver Pictures

Page 672: National Air and Space Museum, Smithsonian Institution (SI Neg. No. 79-759). Photo by Dane Penland

Page 680: Courtesy, Military Antiques & Museum, Petaluma, CA

Page 686: Fair Street Pictures

CHAPTER 21

The Promise of Consumer Culture: The 1920s

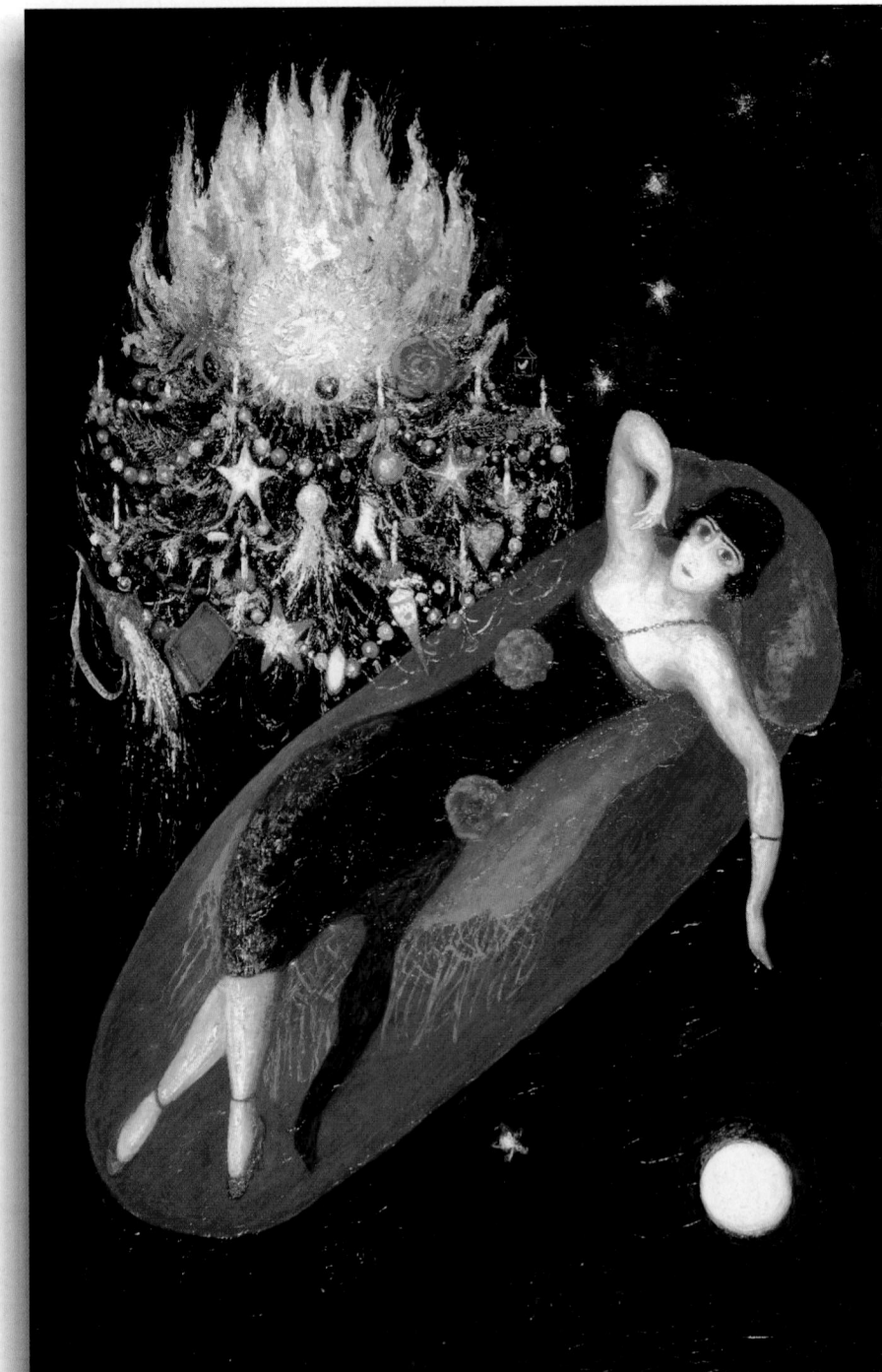

Florine Stettheimer, *Portrait of My Sister Ettie*, 1923. Columbia University in the City of New York, Gift of the Estate of Ettie Stettheimer, 1967 (Neg. #57675)

■ Florine Stettheimer's *Portrait of Ettie* (1923) conveys the glamour and sensuality of the 1920s "flapper."

IN THE SUPERIOR COURT OF LOS ANGELES IN 1920, LORIMER LINGANFIELD, A RESPECTABLE barber, filed for divorce. Although his wife, Marsha, held him in "high regard and esteem as her husband," there were "evidences of indiscretion" in her conduct. She wore a new bathing suit, "designed especially for the purpose of exhibiting to the public the shape and form of her body." To his further humiliation, she was "beset with a desire to sing and dance at cafes and restaurants for the entertainment of the public." When Lorimer complained about her "appetite for beer and whisky" and extravagant tastes for luxury, she replied that he was "not the only pebble on the beach, she had a millionaire 'guy' who would buy her all the clothes, automobiles, diamonds and booze that she wanted." But the ultimate insult was her refusal to have any sexual intercourse, claiming that she did not want any "dirty little brats around her." The judge was sympathetic, and Lorimer Linganfield won his suit.

The Linganfields's difficulties represent a larger struggle as Americans shifted their sensibilities from the producer economy of the nineteenth century, complete with clearly defined gender roles and sexual mores, to the consumer ethic of the twentieth century with its new amusements, changing sexual behavior, and flamboyant "new women." Marsha Linganfield was a "flapper," one of the young women of the 1910s and 1920s who broke from time-honored conventions. With short, "bobbed" hair, knee-length dresses, and boyish styles unencumbered by layers of petticoats, flappers flirted, petted, and danced "wild" dances like the Charleston, an African American dance brought north from South Carolina juke joints. Flappers blurred the line between "good girls" and "bad girls" that had previously defined proper female behavior.

Marsha was fond of fancy clothes and night life. Lorimer undoubtedly was attracted to the lively young flapper whom he wooed and wed. He was surely anticipating conjugal bliss, as experts at the time approved of female sexual pleasure in marriage. New patterns of courtship allowed couples some intimacy now that chaperones were no longer required when a man "came calling." The widespread availability of automobiles offered increased mobility and privacy. So Marsha's sexual refusal, as well as her scandalous rejection of motherhood, must have been intolerable for Lorimer. The "new woman" of the age was allowed more leeway in her dress, demeanor, and behavior, but she was still expected to be virginal at marriage and eager for marital sex and motherhood.

The Linganfields met and married in Los Angeles, home of Hollywood, the beacon of the new culture. The most successful film director of the era, Cecil B. DeMille, made several films in which modern couples seek the right balance between fun and virtue in marriage. The popular DeMille formula offered a blueprint for couples like the

Gertrude Ederle swims the English Channel.

Linganfields. In the typical DeMille plot, either the husband or the wife becomes bored with a spouse who, unable to shed drab old-fashioned virtue, refuses to take part in the leisure-oriented, sexually charged life of the 1920s.

In *Why Change Your Wife* (1920), for example, the heroine loses her husband by refusing to go dancing with him or to wear the sexy lingerie he buys for her. He abandons his wife for a fun-loving flapper, but he leaves the new flame when he finds that she wants only his money and has no interest in settling down to family life. By this time his ex-wife has discovered the error of her ways and transformed herself into an alluring "new woman." The former husband finds her at a beach resort, wearing a revealing swimsuit and surrounded by admiring men. The two renew their love and settle again into marriage, now combining the virtues of domestic life with the excitement of modern consumer culture and sexuality. The final caption of the film warns, "Ladies, if you want to be your husband's sweetheart, you must simply forget [that] you are his wife."

> *The great heroes of the 1920s were celebrities admired for their individual achievements in sports and adventure.*

New forms of popular entertainment that developed in the 1920s, especially Hollywood movies and jazz music, became defining features of the nation itself. The popular arts offered Jews and blacks a space for innovation. At a time when white, Anglo-Saxon, Protestant men had control of nearly all government and business institutions, Jewish moviemakers and African American musicians were creating the culture that would soon represent the nation. During the years when Congress largely closed off immigration, Jewish immigrants built Hollywood into the most American of all industries. In the midst of the Jim Crow era, African Americans created the music that gave the 1920s its identity as the Jazz Age.

The great heroes of the 1920s were celebrities admired for their individual achievements in sports and adventure. In 1927, the same year that Babe Ruth hit a record 60 home runs, Charles Lindbergh flew his small monoplane, *The Spirit of St. Louis,* nonstop from New York to Paris in 33$^1/_2$ hours, a feat that electrified the world and made him an instant hero. Professional sports came of age in the 1920s, giving rise to new heroes such as baseball's Babe Ruth, football's Red Grange, and boxing's Jack Dempsey. It was also a decade of tremendous visibility in women's sports, with such stars as tennis sensation Helen Wills and swimmer Sybil Bauer. In 1926, 19-year-old Olympic gold medalist Gertrude Ederle became the first woman to swim the English Channel. She broke the world's record with her time of 14 hours and 31 minutes, 2 hours shorter than those of the six men who had preceded her. On her return to the United States 2 million cheering fans lined the streets of New York City to welcome her home. The nation idolized this new generation of heroes, who dominated headlines and drew cheering crowds wherever they went.

The glamorous life, however, was available to few. Often characterized as the "roaring twenties" of giddy prosperity and reckless good times, these were also years of widespread poverty, especially in rural areas and urban ghettos. Much of rural America and an estimated 40 percent of the working class remained mired in poverty, with inadequate food and housing. Few Americans were able to afford the new consumer goods that were being mass-produced and were more widely available. At the end of the decade, fewer than half of all households owned a car or a radio; fewer than one in three owned a washing machine or a vacuum cleaner. Only 1 percent of households earned more than $10,000 per year, and two-thirds lived on an annual income of less than $1999.

Conservative politics at the national level prevailed throughout the decade. Disenchantment after World War I prompted national leaders to emphasize economic ties and foreign trade and to shrink from military entanglements. The politics of the era favored big business, but the disparity between rich and poor left the country vulnerable to the downturn of the economy. Business values of material acquisition spread as the expansion of consumer credit weakened the traditions of saving and frugality. For those with money to invest, Wall Street beckoned. The stock market rose to perilous heights, only to collapse at the end of the decade.

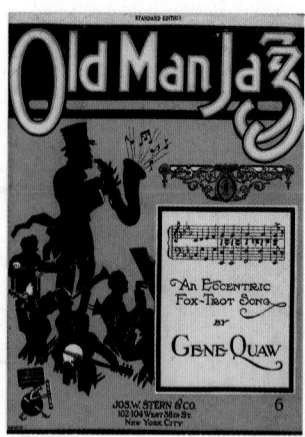

The Decline of Reform

The voices of workers, sharecroppers, and other poor people were muffled in the 1920s, a decade of a booming economy and conservative politics. Reformers who had championed the causes of the marginalized and disadvantaged lost influence. Progressive politics declined precipitously in the wake of World War I. After achieving the vote the women's rights movement splintered as younger women sought new freedoms not through politics but through a social and sexual revolution. Widespread hostility toward immigrants and various ethnic groups were at the root of the outlawing of liquor, new laws restricting immigration, and the rise of the Ku Klux Klan. But progressive political impulses did not entirely disappear, especially among African Americans, who continued to mobilize and organize for civil rights.

Women's Rights in the Aftermath of Suffrage

One indication of the waning of progressive reform was the fragmentation of women's rights activism in the 1920s. The more radical wing of the suffrage movement, the National Women's Party (NWP), under the leadership of Alice Paul, in 1923 launched a campaign for the Equal Rights Amendment (ERA), which was introduced in Congress two decades later with these words: "Equality of rights under the law shall not be denied or abridged by the United States or by any state on account of sex."

The debate over the ERA in the 1920s reflected the fundamental question that would permeate women's rights activism throughout the rest of the twentieth century. On one side were those who believed that women were fundamentally the same as men and deserved equal rights; on the other side were those who argued that women were different and deserved special privileges and protections. Many women's rights activists opposed the ERA because it would undercut efforts to gain special legislative protections for women based on their presumed physical weakness and their potential for childbearing, such as maximum hours, regulations against night work, and limitations on the weights they could lift. These women disapproved of the goals and tactics of the NWP and formed their own nonpartisan organization, the League of Women Voters, which promoted social and political reform.

Legislative gains for women did not entirely disappear in the 1920s. In 1921 Congress passed the Sheppard–Towner bill for maternal and infant health education. The bill provided for public health nurses to educate mothers in prenatal and infant health care to reduce infant mortality. Physicians opposed the legislation because they were consolidating their control over medical practice and did not want nurses functioning as independent health care providers, even though

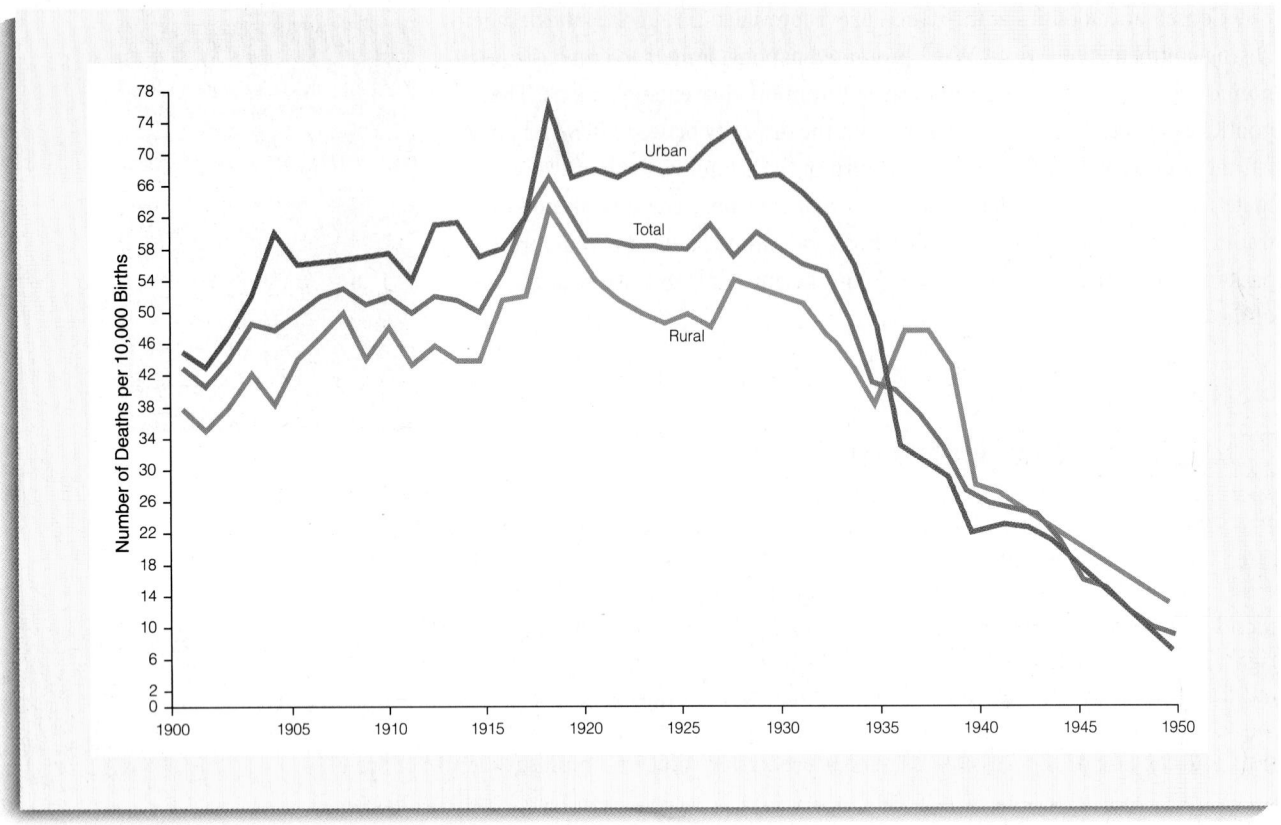

■ **FIGURE 21.1**
MATERNAL DEATH RATES FROM ALL CHILDBIRTH-RELATED CAUSES, UNITED STATES, 1901–1950
During the early decades of the twentieth century, childbirth increasingly took place in hospitals. But the rate of deaths from childbirth actually increased during those years and did not decline until the 1930s.

the nurses offered only preventive health care and advice. Doctors also worried that government-sponsored programs would compete with their private practices. Nevertheless, Sheppard–Towner remained in force until the end of the decade, when its budget was cut, a casualty of the conservative temperament in Congress that saw such forms of government support as socialistic.

One way in which women continued their political influence was by seeking elective office. In 1922, for example, Adelina Otero Warren ran as a Republican candidate for the U.S. House of Representatives, the first New Mexican woman and the first Hispanic woman to run for national office. During the campaign, a cousin publicly revealed that Warren had lied about her marital status, claiming to be widowed when she was really divorced. That revelation dashed her political ambitions. But neither her divorce nor her effort to pass as a widow was unusual at a time when marital breakdown still carried a heavy negative stigma, especially for women. The divorce rate doubled between 1900 and 1920 and continued to rise throughout the 1920s, in part the result of women's increasing independence. As job opportunities for women increased, more women felt able to abandon unhappy marriages.

Prohibition: The Experiment That Failed

The Eighteenth Amendment, prohibiting the manufacture and sale of alcohol, went into effect in January 1920. Several diverse interests came together to promote the ban on liquor. Temperance crusaders in the Anti-Saloon League and the Women's Christian Temperance Union had argued since the late nineteenth century that women and children suffered when men spent their paychecks at the saloon and returned home drunk and violent. World War I prompted others to support a ban on the manufacture of liquor to save grain for the war effort. Anti-immigrant "drys" had political motives for promoting prohibition. They hoped to undercut the power bases of immigrant and ethnic politicians who used local saloons to forge their constituencies and political machines. The "wets" included alienated intellectuals, Jazz Age rebels, and many city dwellers whose social lives revolved around neighborhood pubs, especially in Irish and German communities.

Enforcement was impossible. The 1919 Volstead Act established a Prohibition Bureau within the Treasury Department to allocate funds for enforcement, but budget cuts weakened its effectiveness. Federal agents had responsibility for enforcing the law, but their numbers were inadequate. In order to be effective, federal agents had to work closely with local law enforcement officials. In some urban areas, local officials refused to cooperate with federal agents. New York repealed its prohibition enforcement law in 1923, leaving a small number of federal agents with the daunting task of shutting down illegal clubs where liquor was sold, known as "speakeasies." In sporadic raids, the beleaguered agents closed down some of the speakeasies, only to have them pop up again in new locations. Americans who wanted to drink liquor found many ways to acquire it. Illegal speakeasies abounded where customers could buy drinks delivered by rumrunners who smuggled in liquor from Canada, Mexico, and the West Indies. Many people concocted their own "bathtub gin" or "moonshine whiskey," homemade brews using readily available ingredients and household equipment.

Prohibition was intended to cure society's ills. Instead, it provided vast opportunities for crime and profit, both among criminals and law enforcement agents. Nightclubs and restaurants with an urban middle-class clientele found it difficult to make a profit when they could no longer serve liquor. Many went out of business, opening the way for gangsters and petty criminals to cater to the nightlife crowd. Organized crime received a major boost when violence erupted in the scramble to profit from illegal liquor. Chicago witnessed 550 gangland killings in the 1920s, with few arrests or convictions. Police looked the other way when rival gangs engaged in bloody wars to control the city's liquor business. By 1929 Chicago mob king Al Capone controlled a massive network of speakeasies that raked in $60 million annually.

Those charged with upholding the law often benefited from the illegal trade themselves. Authorities in St. Paul, Minnesota, for example, struck a bargain with gangsters who smuggled in liquor from Canada through the poorly patrolled wilderness in northern Minnesota. After paying a bribe to the local police, the smugglers hid their stash in St. Paul's chalk caves along the banks of the Mississippi River until they were able to transport it down the river.

Prohibition failed to live up to its promise. Within a year of the passage of the amendment, alcohol consumption declined by two thirds. But by 1929 the consumption of alcohol had climbed back up to 70 percent of its pre-Prohibition level. Expenditures for alcoholic beverages actually increased by 50 percent during the Prohibition era, no doubt due in part to higher black-market prices.

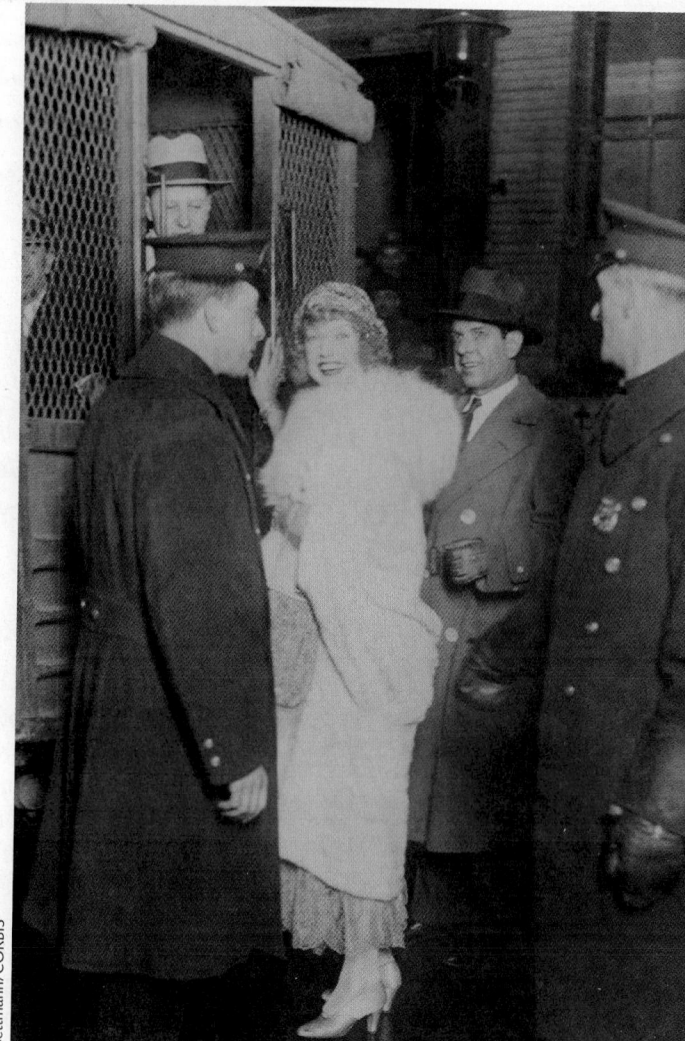

Bettmann/CORBIS

■ Speakeasy hostess Mary Louise Guinan appears unrepentant as she is arrested for selling alcohol during the Prohibition era. Law enforcement was futile because speakeasies that were raided and closed simply reopened in new locations.

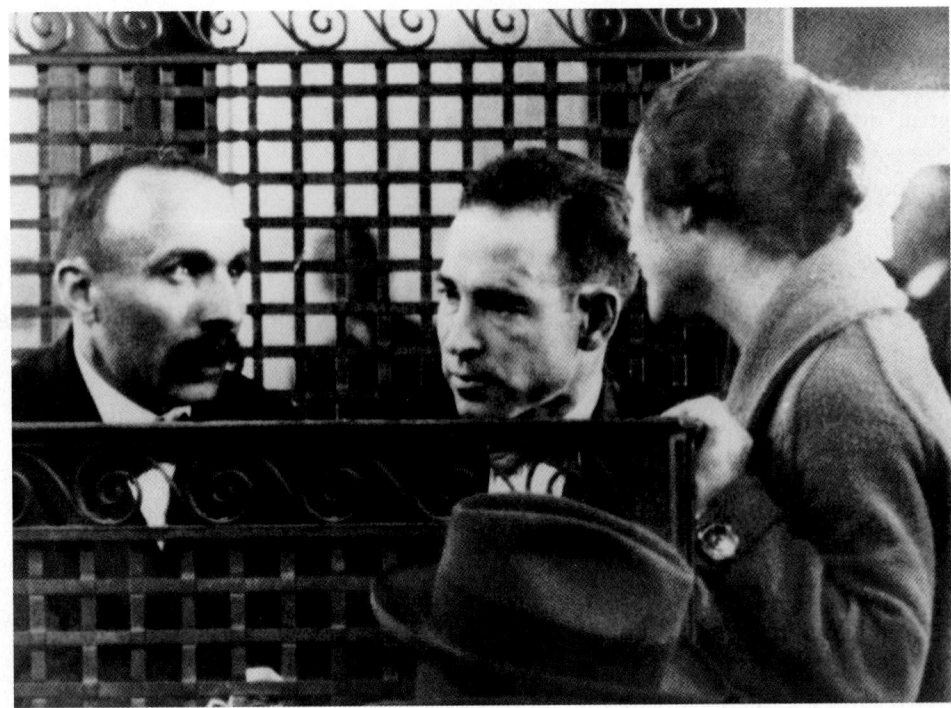

Bettmann/CORBIS

■ Nicola Sacco and Bartolomeo Vanzetti, Italian aliens and self-proclaimed anarchists, were accused of murder in May 1920. The men and their supporters claimed they were on trial not for the crime but for their political beliefs and their immigrant status. After all appeals failed, the two were executed in 1927.

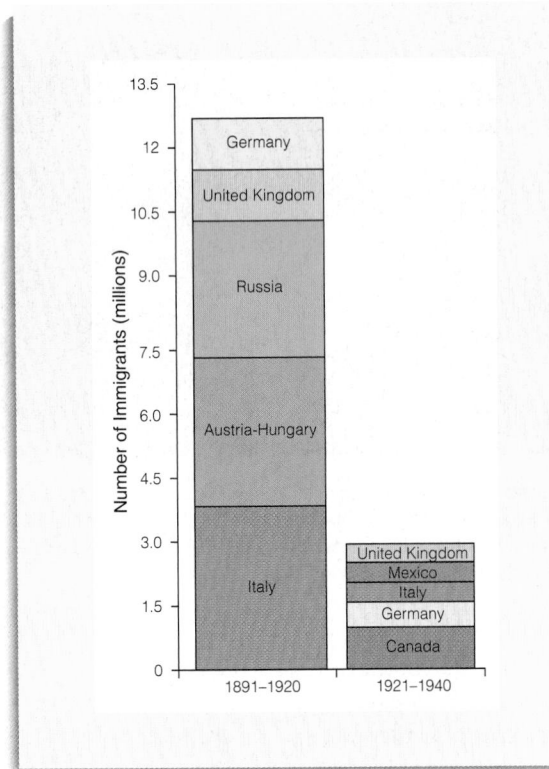

■ **FIGURE 21.2**
NUMBER OF IMMIGRANTS AND COUNTRIES OF ORIGIN, 1891–1920 AND 1921–1940 Before the immigration restriction laws passed in the 1920s, most immigrants came from Russia and southern and eastern Europe. After immigration restriction, most came from Western Europe and Canada.

Reactionary Impulses

The Red Scare after World War I (see Chapter 20) inaugurated a decade of hostility to political radicals and foreigners. Shoemaker Nicola Sacco and fish peddler Bartolomeo Vanzetti were both: Italian aliens and self-proclaimed anarchists. In May 1920 the paymaster and guard of a South Braintree, Massachusetts, shoe company was robbed and murdered, and Sacco and Vanzetti were arrested and charged with the crime. Sacco testified that he was in Boston at the time, applying for a passport, and his alibi was corroborated. Both men proclaimed their innocence and insisted that they were on trial for their political beliefs rather than the crime itself. Their Italian accents and advocacy of anarchism in the courtroom did not help their case with many Americans suspicious of foreign radicals, including the judge presiding at their trial. Despite a weak case against them, Sacco and Vanzetti were convicted of first-degree murder and sentenced to death.

Lawyers for the two anarchists appealed the case several times to no avail. The convictions sparked outrage among Italian Americans, political radicals, labor activists, and liberal intellectuals who believed the two men were falsely convicted. The case soon generated mass demonstrations, appeals for clemency, and petitions from around the world. In response the governor of Massachusetts appointed a commission to review the case, but the commission concluded that there were no grounds for a new trial. Finally, on August 23, 1927, Sacco and Vanzetti were executed by electric chair at Charlestown State Prison.

The case of Sacco and Vanzetti underscored the anti-immigrant sentiment that prevailed in the 1920s. Although efforts to curtail immigration since the late nineteenth century had resulted in numerous federal laws, none were as harsh as those passed in the 1920s, which cut the flow of immigrants down to a tiny trickle. The 1921 immigration restriction act set a limit on the number of European immigrants allowed into the United States. The numbers of immigrants permitted to enter was limited to a percentage of immigrants from each country who lived in the United States in 1910. In that year large numbers of immigrants from southern and eastern European countries lived in the United States, so the quota from each country, while limited, still allowed newcomers from those countries to enter. Then, in 1924, Congress passed the Johnson–Reid Act, imposing a limit of 165,000 immigrants from countries outside the Western Hemisphere and pushing back the quota basis to 1890, a time when British, German, and Scandinavian immigrants dominated the foreign-born population. The Johnson–Reid Act limited entry every year to 2 percent of the total number of immigrants from each country who were present in 1890. This measure effectively barred Jews, Slavs, Greeks, Italians, and Poles because their numbers were so small in 1890. In addition, the 1924 law reaffirmed the exclusion of Chinese immigrants and added Japanese and other Asians to the list, effectively closing the door to all migrants from Asia. Further modification of the immigration laws in 1927 reduced the quota to 150,000 per year, with most slots reserved for northern Europeans. Few Americans objected to these measures, other than the groups whose kin and compatriots were excluded.

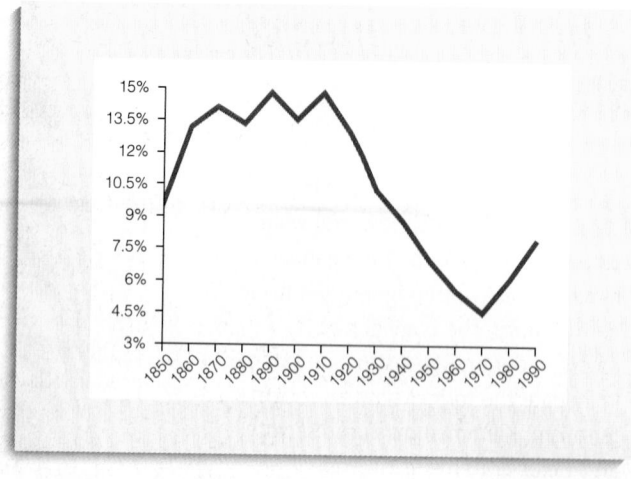

■ **FIGURE 21.3**
PERCENTAGE OF POPULATION FOREIGN BORN, 1850–1990 The immigration restriction laws had a dramatic effect on the foreign-born population, which reached nearly 15 percent of the American population in the first two decades of the century. After immigration restriction, the percentage dropped precipitously until the 1960s, when new laws allowed more immigrants to enter.

Agricultural interests in California and Texas lobbied hard to keep the door open to Mexicans because of the low-waged labor they provided. In the aftermath of the Mexican Revolution, many Mexicans hoped to find stability and jobs in the United States. Between 1910 and 1930, more than 1 million Mexicans, nearly one-tenth of Mexico's population, migrated to the United States, where they found work in the farms, railroads, and mines. Recruiters often stood along the border, waiting to sign up laborers. The U.S. Chamber of Commerce noted in 1930 that Mexican agricultural workers picked more than 80 percent of the perishable goods produced in the Southwest.

Marcus Garvey and the Persistence of Civil Rights Activism

In the midst of a decade of reactionary policies toward outsiders and political activists, African Americans continued their struggle for civil rights. Jamaican-born black nationalist Marcus Garvey moved to New York City's Harlem in 1916 and opened a branch of his Universal Negro Improvement Association (UNIA). By the 1920s, Garvey's organization had 30,000 members in New York, another 6000 each in Philadelphia and Cincinnati, and 4000 in Detroit. Garvey urged black people to establish their own nation-state in Africa: "Africa was peopled with a race of cultured black men, who were masters in art, science, and literature. . . .Africa shall be for the black peoples of the world." The UNIA staged colorful parades, which Garvey led in military uniform. His followers proudly wore the UNIA uniform to express their support for the movement and joined the parades in large numbers. Garvey published a journal, *The Negro World,* and encouraged the establishment of black-owned businesses such as grocery stores and laundries. The UNIA gained nearly 1 million followers and called for political justice and labor rights for black Americans.

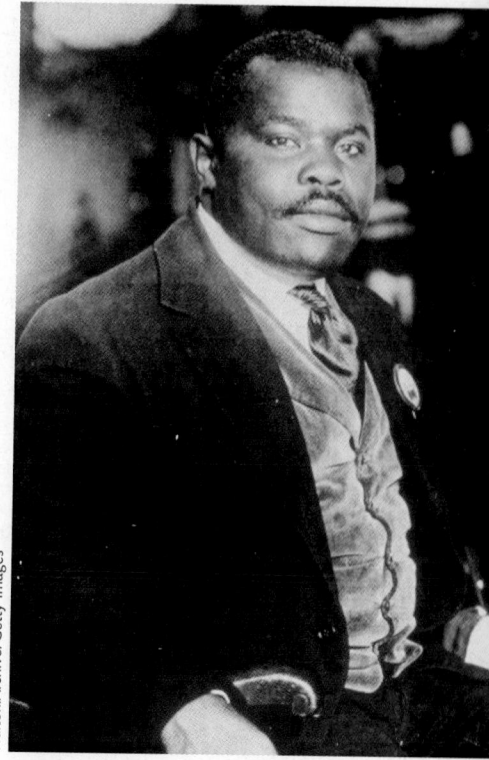

Hulton|Archive/Getty Images

■ Marcus Garvey, founder of the Universal Negro Improvement Association (UNIA), c. 1920. Born in Jamaica, the African American nationalist leader encouraged black people to move to Africa and establish their own nation.

The Persistence of the Ku Klux Klan

In the 1920s the Ku Klux Klan became the most powerful white supremacy group in the nation, remaining active throughout the twentieth century. The original Klan emerged during Reconstruction to intimidate the former slaves through terrorism. Klan members used secrecy and violence to maintain white supremacy in the South. Their vigilante activities included threatening cross-burnings, beatings, and lynchings. The original KKK faded in the 1870s. But the Klan revived in the early twentieth century, moving north and targeting not only blacks but other minorities and immigrants. The new KKK was inspired in part by Thomas Dixon's 1905 novel, *The Clansman,* and its 1915 film version, D. W. Griffith's *The Birth of a Nation,* an epic that portrayed the post–Civil War Klan as a heroic group of vanquished Southerners protecting white womanhood from sexually predatory black men.

The Klan revival remained small until 1920, when its leaders mounted a national membership drive. Under the banner "100 percent Americanism," the Klan promoted itself as a civic organization and claimed to uphold the traditional American values that Klan members believed to be threatened in the new order, harking back to what they considered the true moral and religious virtues of the nation. Klan membership included laborers, businessmen, physicians, judges, social workers, and women who felt that their homogeneous small-town Protestant culture was threatened by the

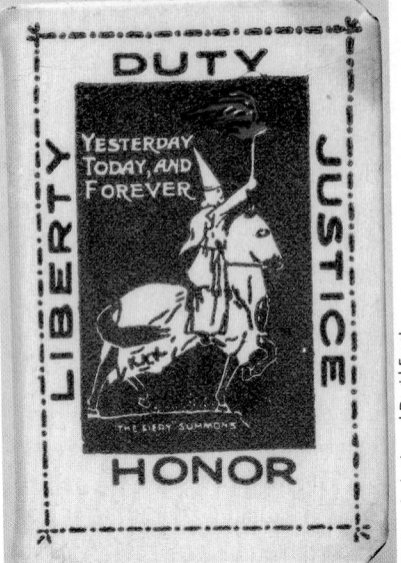

The Ku Klux Klan promoted itself as a patriotic organization dedicated to preserving American values. The white supremacist hate group first emerged in the South after the Civil War to terrorize the newly freed African Americans, was revived in the North during the 1920s, and continues to this day.

evils of modern life, brought on by the influence of morally suspect outsiders.

The women who joined the Klan championed women's rights and worked on behalf of temperance, child welfare measures, public education, good citizenship, morality, and militant Christianity while also supporting white supremacy and initiating whisper campaigns and boycotts against Jewish and Catholic shopkeepers. The Klan used vigilante violence and politically savvy mobilizations to attack African Americans, communists, feminists, Jews, and Catholics who were making economic and social gains in the cities, and divorced or allegedly promiscuous women. The Klan also appealed to voters who were sympathetic to their

views. Growing to 3 million members by the early 1920s, the Klan wielded great power, especially in Texas, Oklahoma, Oregon, and Indiana. Some Klan members continued to engage in vigilante violence, while others held elaborate rallies and parades, burned crosses to intimidate and threaten their foes, and endorsed political candidates. Klan efforts in Oregon persuaded the state's lawmakers to pass a compulsory public schooling bill in 1922 that would have closed private and parochial schools, but the U.S. Supreme Court overturned the law. The Klan-controlled legislature in Oklahoma impeached and removed an anti-Klan governor.

The Klan dwindled and finally disbanded in 1944. But a new Klan emerged barely two years later, once again centered in the South, in reaction to the civil rights movement taking shape after World War II. The membership of this third Klan peaked in the 1960s with about 17,000 members. The Klan's efforts largely backfired as their actions repulsed most white Americans and helped gain support for the civil rights movement. The Klan declined after the 1960s but did not disappear, often joining forces with other white supremacy groups, such as the Aryan Nations and the Skinheads. In 1991 former Klan leader and Nazi sympathizer David Duke ran for governor of Louisiana and garnered 39 percent of the votes. He won 55 percent of the white vote, but Louisiana's African American voters defeated him. At the end of the twentieth century, the Klan still had influence in some localities— running candidates for office, holding rallies and parades, and seeking legitimacy through civic volunteer projects. ■

In keeping with his belief in black-owned businesses, Garvey established the Black Star Line and encouraged his followers to invest in the shipping company: "The Black Star Line Corporation presents to every Black Man, Woman, and Child the opportunity to climb the great ladder of industrial and commercial progress. If you have ten dollars, one hundred dollars, or one or five thousand dollars to invest for profit, then take out shares in the Black Star Line." Nearly 40,000 African Americans invested three quarters of a million dollars to purchase shares of Black Star stock.

But the business ran into problems. Managers purchased ships that needed extensive and costly repairs, and the company ran up huge debts. Garvey claimed that he had paid for a ship that was never delivered. In 1922 Garvey was arrested and charged with mail fraud for advertising and selling stock for a ship that did not exist. Although the government lacked any concrete evidence to prove the case against him, Garvey was convicted and sentenced to five years in prison. Garvey kept up his political activities from prison, sending a message to his followers: "My work is just begun. Be assured that I planted well the seed of Negro or black nationalism which cannot be destroyed even by the foul play that has been meted out to me." Garvey was released after two years and deported to Jamaica as an undesirable alien. Nevertheless, the momentum he sparked continued. The black publication *The Spokesman* declared, "Garvey made thousands think, who had never thought before. Thousands who merely dreamed dreams, now see visions."

Hollywood and Harlem: National Cultures in Black and White

In 1920, for the first time, the majority of Americans lived in towns and cities with populations greater than 2500. Although this shift often is considered a watershed in the transformation from rural to urban America, it is worth noting that because the census defined any town with more than 2500 inhabitants as urban, the majority of Americans still lived in

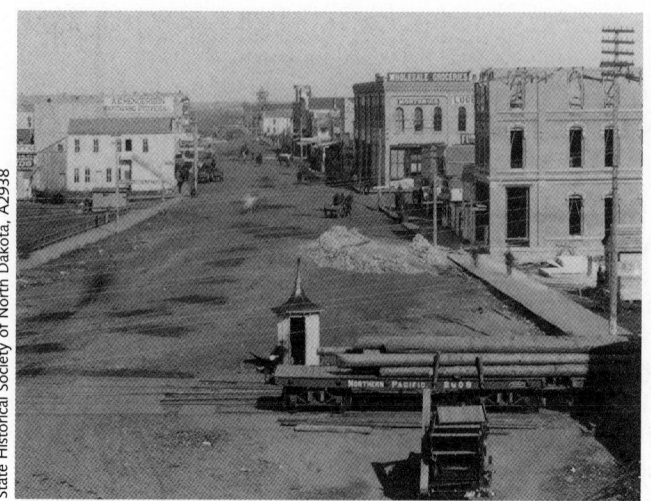
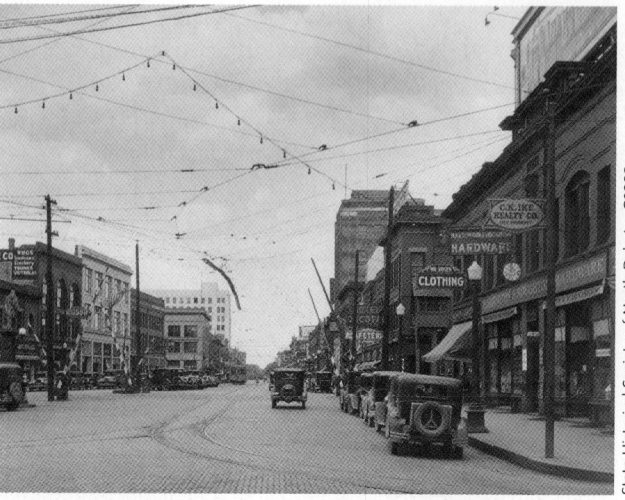

■ Views of Broadway in Fargo, North Dakota, the first taken in 1881, the second in the 1920s. By 1920 Fargo had developed into a bustling town with retail shops, paved roads, automobiles, and a streetcar line.

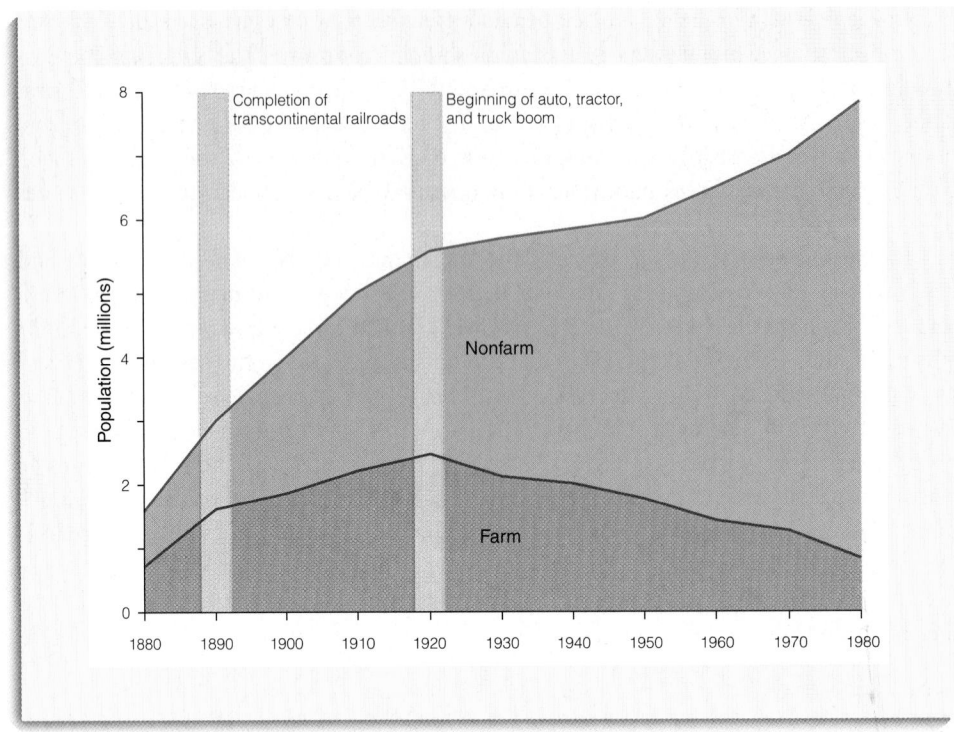

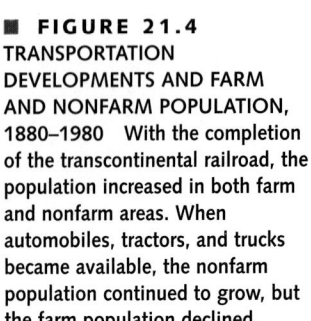

■ **FIGURE 21.4**
TRANSPORTATION
DEVELOPMENTS AND FARM
AND NONFARM POPULATION,
1880–1980   With the completion
of the transcontinental railroad, the
population increased in both farm
and nonfarm areas. When
automobiles, tractors, and trucks
became available, the nonfarm
population continued to grow, but
the farm population declined.

small and ethnically homogeneous towns. Many small-town Americans still viewed big-city life with suspicion. They feared the decline of traditional Protestant American values of hard work, thrift, and discipline. Yet they were drawn to the new urban life. Jewish filmmakers, African American jazz artists, Irish and Italian club owners, and other "outsiders" created new leisure institutions where mainstream Americans shed their daytime routines for nightlife pleasures.

Hollywood on the West Coast and Harlem on the East Coast became centers of cultural innovation that spanned the nation. Both had national reach, and both were the creations of outsiders to the national mainstream. Eventually, the artistic productions of both centers attracted audiences of all racial, class, and regional backgrounds. Increasingly, as Americans moved from place to place, they encountered similar entertainments, music, arts, and consumer products. Movies, automobiles, radios, and advertising all fostered this emerging national culture.

Hollywood Comes of Age

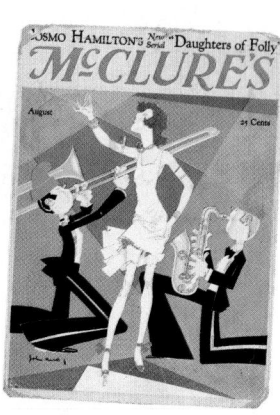

As movie theaters spread into towns and cities across the country, the messages of Hollywood began to reach a mass audience and forge a nationwide popular culture. Movie stars and their films provided models for how to adopt new styles of manhood and womanhood. Douglas Fairbanks showed middle-class men how to break free from the humdrum of white-collar work into the world of leisure. His attire of sports clothes changed the way men dressed in their off-work hours. Female stars, such as Clara Bow, epitomized the flapper and taught female viewers how to be "naughty but nice."

Ironically, as the nation closed its doors to immigrants, foreigners on screen captivated the imagination of a native-born population drawn to the allure of the outsider. Movie stars like Greta Garbo from Sweden, Dolores del Rio, Lupe Velez, and Ramon Navarro from Mexico, and Rudolph Valentino from Italy drew audiences with their foreignness. And yet, because movies were silent until the late 1920s, their accented voices were

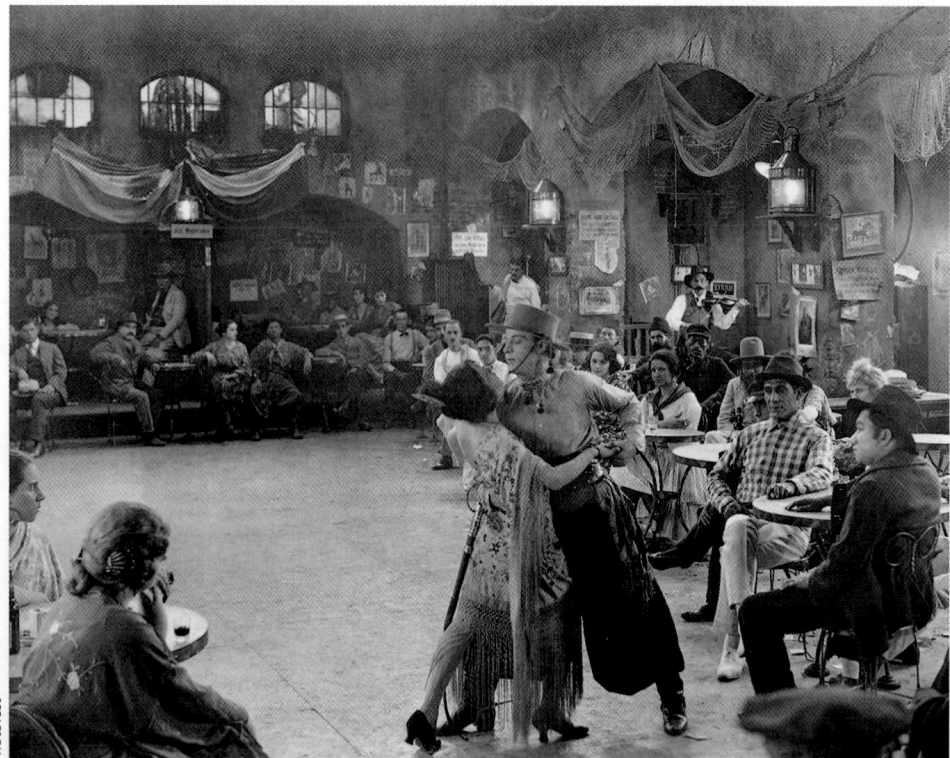

Photofest

■ Rudolph Valentino dances the tango in this famous scene from the 1920 film *The Four Horsemen of the Apocalypse.* Films in the 1920s featured exotic locales with foreign stars such as the Italian-born Valentino. In keeping with the public's taste for grandeur, lavish movie palaces emerged in cities across the country.

not heard. Sound arrived in the late twenties, bringing the voices and dialects of ethnic performers into the movies. For native-born Americans watching films in small towns and cities, sound movies brought the diverse voices of the cities into their communities. For immigrants, sound movies carried their own familiar accents and allowed for a greater sense of identification with the stars on the screen. In 1927 the Jewish performer Al Jolson starred in the first complete talking film, *The Jazz Singer,* about the son of Jewish immigrants who is drawn to jazz music against the wishes of his Orthodox father.

The Harlem Renaissance

While Hollywood in the 1920s developed on the West Coast, a flourishing center of African American culture emerged on the East Coast. The black arts movement known as the Harlem Renaissance drew on European as well as African and African American artistic traditions and gathered white as well as black intellectuals and artists. The young black poet Arna Bontemps was among the many artists drawn to Harlem. In 1924 he described Harlem as "a foretaste of paradise. A blue haze descended at night and with it strings of fairy lights on the broad avenues. From the window of a small room in an apartment on Fifth and 129th Street, I looked over the rooftops of Negrodom and tried to believe my eyes. What a city! What a world!"

Like many other Americans in the 1920s, Bontemps had moved around the country. Born in Louisiana, at age four he moved to Los Angeles with his parents who left the South in the hope of raising their children in an atmosphere less hostile to African Americans. The family settled in Watts, in the center of Los Angeles, and at the time a white neighborhood. He recalled, "We moved into a house in a neighborhood where we were the only colored family. . . . The people next door and up and down the block were friendly and talkative, the weather was perfect, there wasn't a mud puddle anywhere, and my mother seemed to float about on the clean air."

When Bontemps's Uncle Buddy arrived from Louisiana bringing stories of black life in the South, filled with "signs and charms and mumbo-jumbo," the boy was entranced. His father thoroughly disapproved of these stories, but Bontemps was drawn to the earthy sensuality of Uncle Buddy. He did not realize then that life in Jim Crow Louisiana had crushed Buddy's Creole pride and left him ruined and penniless.

When Bontemps finished school, the 21-year-old moved to Harlem. There he looked for the "Negro-ness" he felt his upbringing in California had lacked. In Harlem he found a thriving black community unlike anything he had known before. He landed a teaching job, married, and settled with his family, becoming one of the most prolific writers of the Harlem Renaissance.

Renaissance writers laid claim to their identity as Americans while articulating the culture, aesthetics, and experiences of African Americans. Many of their works contained antiracist political messages. The poet Langston Hughes challenged white America to accept African Americans in his 1925 poem, "I, too, sing America:"

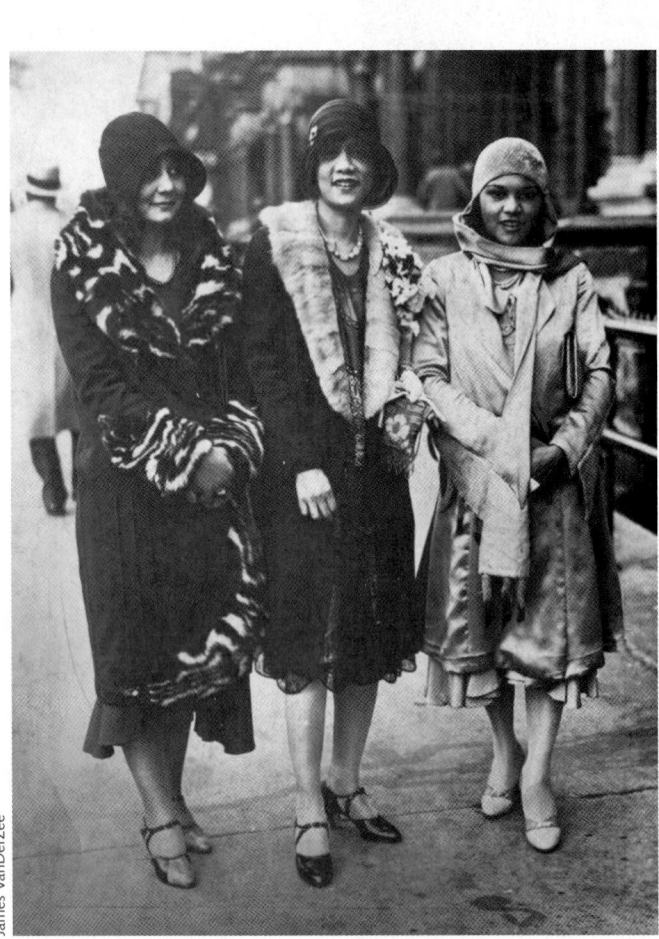

James VanDerZee

■ Women out for a night on the town on a street in Harlem, New York City. During the years of the Harlem Renaissance, Harlem became the center of a flourishing music, literary, and artistic scene as well as home to lively jazz clubs that appealed to blacks and whites alike.

> I, too, sing America
> I am the darker brother
> They send me to eat in the kitchen
> When company comes,
> But I laugh
> And eat well
> And grow strong
> Tomorrow,
> I'll be at the table
> When company comes
> Nobody'll dare
> Say to me,
> "Eat in the kitchen,"
> Then.
> Besides,
> They'll see how beautiful I am
> And be ashamed -
> I, too, am America.

Although portraying the "exotic" and sensual in black culture was controversial among Renaissance critics, some of its greatest artists gained huge followings among black as well as white audiences with unabashed and uninhibited celebrations of sexuality. Josephine Baker gained large audiences dancing to jazz rhythms in her trademark banana skirt. She also used her visibility to criticize American racism and to crusade against lynching. Moving to Paris in 1925, Baker opened her own Paris nightclub, Chez Josephine, where she danced every night. Later, during the Cold War era, she defied anticommunist censors by traveling and performing all over the world and speaking out against American racial discrimination. Baker also adopted 12 children of different races and nationalities.

The music of black America was such an important marker of the era that it provided the decade with its most lasting moniker, *the Jazz Age.* Emanating not from Harlem but from New Orleans, Chicago, and St. Louis, jazz was, nevertheless, central to the black arts movement and the emerging national culture. With the help of the recording industry and radio, jazz and the blues began to reach a wide audience, primarily among blacks but increasingly among whites as well. Blues lyrics expressed themes of working-class protest and resistance to racism. Women who sang the blues, including Bessie Smith, Ma Rainey, and Ethel Waters, asserted their sexuality, their passion for men or for women, their resistance to male domination, their sorrows, and their strength. In "I'm No Man's Mamma Now," Waters sang about divorce not in lament but in celebration:

> You may wonder what's the reason for this crazy smile,
> Say I haven't been so happy in a long while.
> Got a big load off my mind, here's the paper sealed
> and signed,
> And the judge was nice and kind all through the trial.
> This ends a five-year war, I'm sweet Miss Was once more.
> I can come when I please, I can go when I please.
> I can flit, fly and flutter like the birds in the trees.
> Because I'm no man's mamma now. Hey, hey.
> I can smile, I can wink, I can go take a drink,
> And I don't have to worry what my hubby will think.
> Because I'm no man's mamma now.

Black filmmaking flourished during the Harlem Renaissance. Pioneer filmmaker Oscar Micheaux made dozens of films spanning three decades, including *Within Our Gates* (1919) and *Body and Soul* (1924). His films addressed complex themes of class and racial conflict. Known for his style as well as his talent, the six-foot-tall Micheaux wore long Russian coats and wide-brimmed hats and used his charm to raise the necessary funding for his films. As one of his leading actors recalled, he entered meeting halls as if "he were God about to deliver a sermon. . . . Why, he was so impressive and so charming that he could talk the shirt off your back." Micheaux managed to persuade white theater owners in the South to show his films because of the revenues they promised. Southern theater owners showed his films to all-black matinees and at special midnight screenings to white audiences drawn to the allegedly sensual and exotic black experience.

Few people outside the black community took the Harlem Renaissance seriously as a major artistic movement until the Civil Rights era decades later. Nevertheless, the cultural vitality of the black community in the 1920s contributed to the forging of a national mass culture. White patrons who went "slumming" in Harlem or danced to jazz music in clubs across the country incorporated the creativity and vitality of black America into their understanding and experience of modern American life. Still, African Americans continued to face segregation and lynching as well as limited political and economic opportunities.

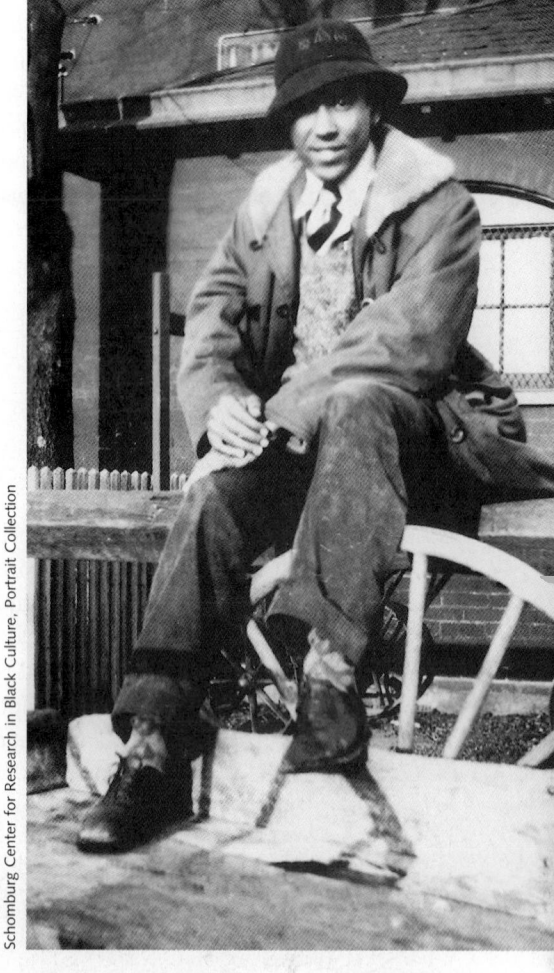

Schomburg Center for Research in Black Culture, Portrait Collection

■ Poet Langston Hughes as a student at Lincoln University, Pennsylvania, in 1927. One of the major literary figures of the Harlem Renaissance, Hughes expressed the hopes, dreams, and sorrows of black Americans.

Radios and Autos: Transforming Leisure at Home

Radio played a major role in linking people across regions through shared information, advertising, and entertainment. Annual radio production increased from 190,000 in 1923 to almost 5 million in 1929. Zenith created the first portable radio in 1924 and added pushbutton tuning three years later. By the end of the decade, more than 6 million radios were in use nationwide. Radios brought jazz and other forms of popular music to the airwaves, transforming the way music was enjoyed in American homes. Americans became more inclined to listen to music on their Victrolas and radios than to make music themselves. By the mid-1920s, sales of records surpassed those of sheet music; production and sales of pianos also dropped precipitously.

The number of radio stations soared from 30 in 1922 to 556 the following year, and national broadcasts began to supersede local ones. Airwaves became so cluttered that by the mid-1920s, the federal government, through the leadership of Secretary of Commerce Herbert

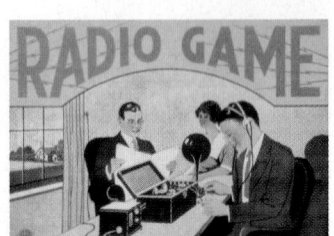

Hoover, created the Federal Radio Commission to regulate and organize access. Meanwhile, American Telephone and Telegraph (AT&T) and the National Broadcasting Company (NBC) combined to form the first national network system, which gave programs and advertisers access to audiences across the country.

As radios entered millions of American homes, automobiles began to extend the mobility of Americans. The automobile offered the possibility of commuting to work without relying on public transportation, encouraging the expansion of suburban communities. The number of passenger cars in the nation more than tripled during the twenties. The Federal Highways Act of 1916 had produced a network of roads all over the country, providing construction jobs and a slew of new roadside businesses, from restaurants to garages. Automobiles also stimulated the tourist industry; Florida, California, and Arizona became vacation destinations in this period. At the same time, tourism disrupted Native American communities in the Southwest as curious motorists intruded into previously isolated reservations.

Automobile production also revolutionized the consumer industry. The pragmatic Henry Ford built inexpensive, functional automobiles that he expected his workers to be able to purchase and keep. But Ford faced serious competition from General Motors' Alfred P. Sloan, Jr., who developed the concept of planned obsolescence and put a new emphasis on auto styling to encourage customers to trade in their old cars for newer and more expensive models. Ford responded to Sloan's low-priced Chevrolet with the Model A in 1927, which had a more stylish look than the Model T and came in a variety of colors.

More than style, however, automobiles offered Americans mobility. Many people mortgaged their homes or did without indoor plumbing to purchase a car. Americans of modest means could expect their car to empty their wallets. In the late 1920s, writer Ernesto Galarza noted that Mexican migrant laborers knew "that the Ford is not a perennial flower . . . far too much of his meager income is left in the tills of gasoline stations and tire shops in his long treks along the Pacific Coast." Cherokee humorist Will Rogers quipped that "America is the only nation in the world that is going to the poor house in an automobile."

The automobile was part of a consumer society increasingly focused on leisure, pleasure, and intimacy. Courtship patterns changed, and sexual activity increased as young couples abandoned the front porch for the back seat. Women gained new freedom and autonomy when they, too, took the wheel. Moralists worried that the automobile would provide youth with too much independence and privacy. One juvenile court judge announced that "the automobile has become a house of prostitution on wheels."

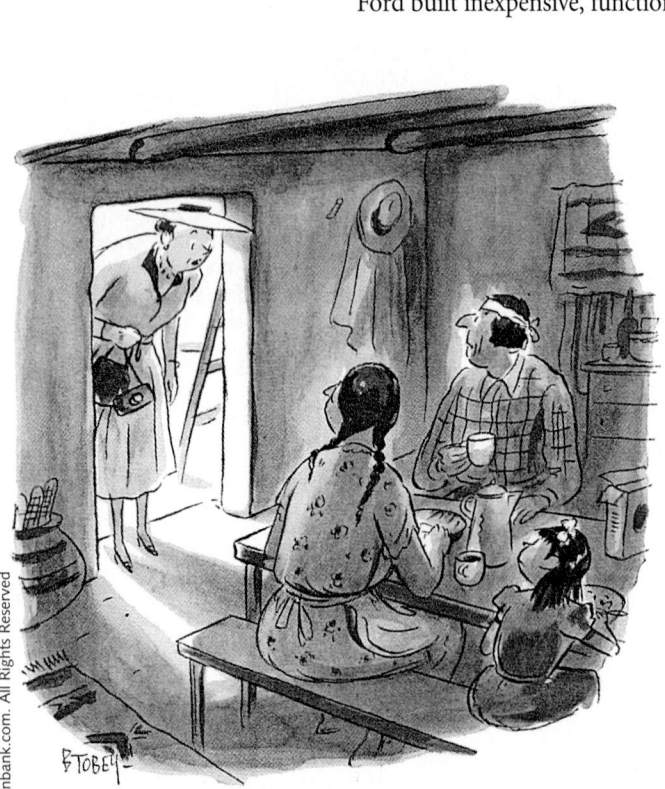

"Oh, I beg your pardon! I thought you were extinct."

■ This cartoon from *The New Yorker* reflects the intrusive aspects of tourism that developed in the Southwest, as well as the widespread erroneous assumption that Native American communities had died out by the twentieth century.

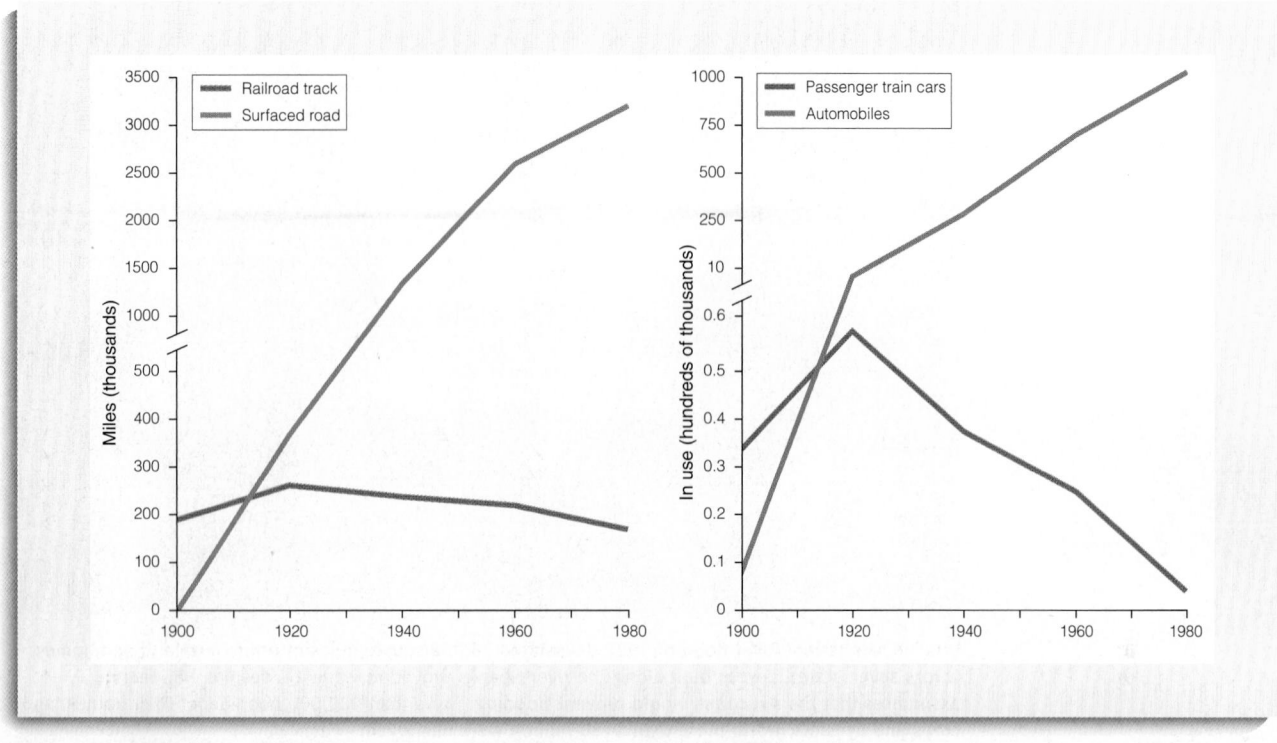

■ FIGURE 21.5
TRAINS AND AUTOMOBILES, 1900–1980 As increasing numbers of Americans acquired automobiles, roads were built to accommodate all the cars. Starting in 1920, passenger trains decreased, along with train tracks.

Science on Trial

Although advances in technology and medicine improved the quality of life for many Americans in the early twentieth century, scientific efforts to alter the natural world did not always lead to expected social benefits. One case in point was the engineering project to build levees along the Mississippi River to prevent flooding. These human-made structures were expected to protect the human-built settlements and agricultural developments in the fertile floodplains where the river would normally expand. As it turned out, the engineers were no match for the river. Scientific ideas were tested not only along the banks of the Mississippi River but also in the nation's courtrooms. Two major cases, the Scopes trial and the Supreme Court's decision in *Buck v. Bell*, subjected scientific ideas to judicial and cultural scrutiny. Although decisions in both cases resolved the immediate legal issues, the questions they raised continued to generate controversy and debate throughout the rest of the century.

The Great Flood of 1927

For half a century the engineers of the Mississippi River Commission had adhered to a policy of building levees, assuming that strong barricades against the river's banks would prevent flooding. Presumably, the levees would allow the rich soil of the floodplains along the river to be settled and farmed rather than leaving the basins empty to provide places for the river to expand and contract. But the levee policy proved to be a disastrous example of human efforts to master the natural contours of the land. In March 1927, the rains came, and the river rose.

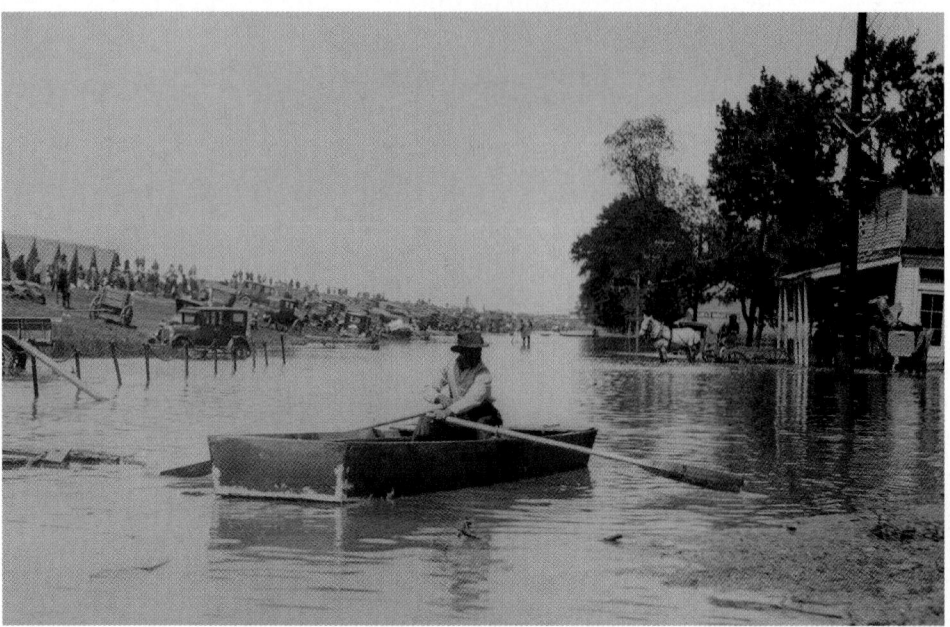

■ The Mississippi River flood of 1927 devastated 26,000 square miles of prime farmland and homes across seven states. Levees built along the river's banks proved inadequate, despite engineers' assurances that the structures would prevent flooding. More than 900,000 people lost their homes, and crops and livestock worth more than $120 million were destroyed.

Public authorities and river experts assured those who watched and worried that the levees would hold. But they were wrong. Torrential rains caused the river to rage across the levees and the land beyond, submerging 26,000 square miles of prime farmland in 170 counties across seven states. More than 900,000 people were forced from their homes. One-third of the refugees found shelter in ill-equipped and understaffed Red Cross camps, and another third received Red Cross rations. The flood caused more than $100 million in crop losses and $23 million in livestock deaths. Journalists at the time called it "America's greatest peacetime disaster."

With the help of the Department of Commerce and the National Guard, the Red Cross set up 154 relief camps for flood victims. The camps were racially segregated. Refugees in the white camps were free to come and go and had more comfortable and generous accommodations and rations than those in the black camps. Armed guards patrolled the camps for black refugees and restricted people attempting to enter or leave. Black laborers had to register and give the names of their employers to receive any shelter or assistance. Only those planters were allowed to enter the camps and reclaim their workers. Relations between plantation owners and share-croppers had been strained across the South before the flood, and many black laborers hoped to leave the plantations and find work elsewhere. But when labor agents came to the camps looking for workers to fill northern jobs, those patrolling the camps denied them entry. Federal authorities, including Secretary of Commerce Herbert Hoover, refused to intervene in local camp management. As a result, southern whites were able to force black sharecroppers back to work on their plantations. Despite the prisonlike conditions, many African American refugees managed to escape and made their way north.

The Triumph of Eugenics: *Buck v. Bell*

In 1924 racial theorist Lothrop Stoddard wrote a best-selling book, *The Rising Tide of Color Against White World Supremacy.* In this polemic, Stoddard predicted a war among the "primary" races of the world and warned of the "weakening" of the white race through immigration and "mongrelization." Stoddard wrote, "The melting pot may mix, but does not melt.

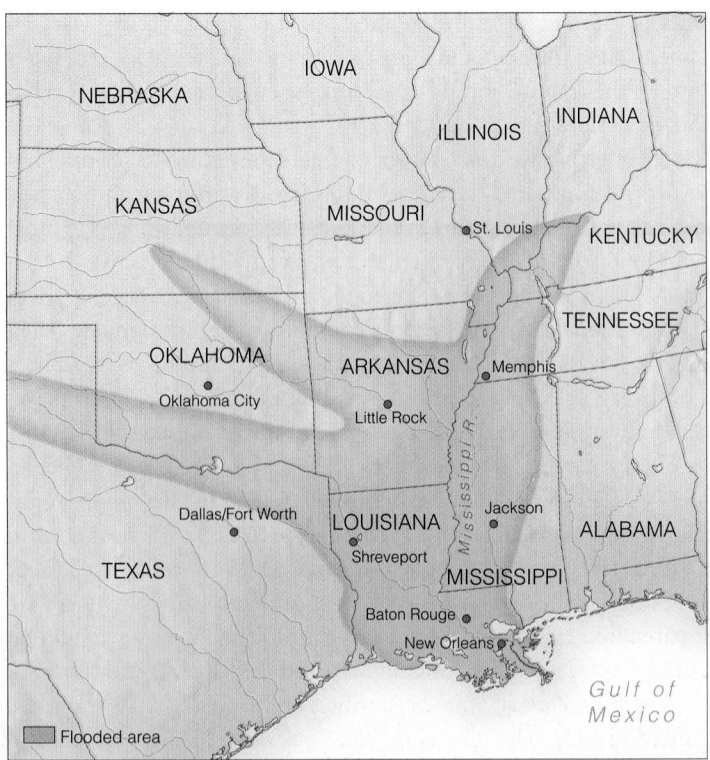

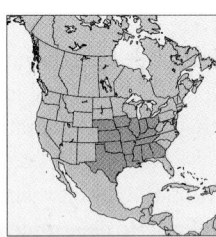

■ **MAP 21.1**
THE MISSISSIPPI RIVER FLOOD OF 1927   The Mississippi River flood in 1927 sent water across a huge area of the South, extending as far west as Texas, covering most of Louisiana, Arkansas, and Mississippi, and reaching north into Kansas, Illinois, and Indiana.

Each race type, formed ages ago . . . is a stubbornly persistent entity. Each type possesses a special set of characters: not merely the physical characters visible to the naked eye, but moral, intellectual, and spiritual characters as well." Stoddard's views were so familiar that F. Scott Fitzgerald placed them in the dialogue of his 1925 novel, *The Great Gatsby*. Fitzgerald's intention was to discredit the theory by showing it to be as ludicrous as other fantasies of his hapless protagonist, Tom Buchanan, who mused, "The idea is if we don't look out the white race will be—will be utterly submerged. It's all scientific stuff; it's been proved."

Fitzgerald may have hoped to discredit Stoddard's ideas, but many Americans, including large numbers of policymakers, believed in white racial superiority. Supposedly scientific theories of race bolstered claims that distinct, biologically based characteristics divided humans into superior and inferior races. These theories had no scientific merit and were later thoroughly discredited. But in the 1920s, these dubious theories of racial superiority supported measures such as immigration restriction and eugenic sterilization laws. Eugenics was a pseudoscience based on notions of racial superiority. Eugenicists claimed that the Anglo-Saxon Protestant "race" was superior to all others, including Jews, Southern Europeans, Catholics, as well as nonwhites. Racial superiority, according to eugenic reformers, might be compromised not only by mixing with inferior groups but also by the propagation of individuals whose mental or moral condition rendered them inferior, and whose offspring would diminish the quality of the Anglo-Saxon "stock."

These ideas were consistent with the theories of social Darwinists, who misused the ideas of Charles Darwin. Darwin's work on evolution focused on the origins of species in the animal world. Darwin found that weaker species died out, while stronger species evolved. Darwin did not study humans. But social Darwinists claimed that Darwin's evolutionary theories were relevant to human society, arguing that only the fittest ought to survive. Social Darwinists argued against government aid to the poor and infirm, claiming that such assistance interfered with "natural selection" of the "fittest." Social Darwinism also supported eugenic theories that provided the rationale for sterilization of the "unfit."

Several states had enacted eugenic laws that allowed the state to sterilize "inferior" individuals without their knowledge or consent. These laws authorized government and medical officials to determine whether or not an individual was inferior, or "feebleminded," and to order that the person be sterilized. Opponents of eugenic sterilization, mostly Catholic activists, challenged these laws in several states. In an effort to put an end to such challenges, eugenic advocates decided to test the constitutionality of the Virginia compulsory sterilization law. Their plan was to bring the case all the way to the U.S. Supreme Court, which they expected to uphold the law. The proponents of the law selected the case of Carrie Buck, in part because she was white. Eugenic advocates did not want race to be at the center of the case, especially because eugenic sterilization laws did not target particular races; they simply targeted the "feebleminded." Feeblemindedness was a loosely defined criterion often used to label poor, immigrant, or minority women who were sexually active. At the age of 17 Carrie Buck was raped and became pregnant; as a result she was sent to a state institution for the feebleminded. Buck was labeled as feebleminded because she had borne a child out of wedlock and was therefore deemed morally unfit for parenthood. The noted eugenicist Harry Laughlin pointed out that Buck herself was born out of wedlock, as was her daughter, and described them as part of the "shiftless, ignorant and worthless class of anti-social whites of the South."

Carrie Buck was sterilized in 1927. The following year, Buck's sister Doris was taken to the Virginia Colony for Epileptics and the Feebleminded and sterilized at age 16. She was told that she had an appendectomy. Later, Doris Buck married and tried to get pregnant. None of the physicians she consulted told her why she could not conceive. She finally learned the truth in 1979. "I broke down and cried. My husband and I wanted children desperately. We were crazy about them. I never knew what they'd done to me."

No evidence established that Carrie Buck, her mother, or her daughter was below normal intelligence. Buck's daughter died as a child, but her teachers described the girl as bright. In writing the majority opinion for the Supreme Court that upheld the law, Justice Oliver Wendell Holmes wrote, "Three generations of imbeciles are enough." Within the next few years, 30 states had compulsory sterilization laws, and the number of operations rose dramatically. In the 1930s the Nazis in Germany modeled their sterilization policies on the California law. Although eugenics in the United States received less publicity during World War II as Nazi sterilization policies became known, the practice continued. Over the next several decades, increasing numbers of coerced sterilizations took place in public clinics and hospitals. Nearly all of these later sterilizations were performed on women of color, including well-known civil rights leader Fanny Lou Hamer in the 1960s. Only the Catholic Church consistently mounted organized opposition to the practice. Finally, in the 1980s, in a rare alliance of traditional Catholics and feminist activists over an issue of reproductive choice, compulsory sterilization laws were repealed.

Science, Religion, and the Scopes Trial

Although there was little organized protest against sterilization laws, many Americans were troubled by eugenics and its corollary, Social Darwinism. The populist leader William Jennings Bryan was among them. Bryan, three times the Democratic candidate for president and Woodrow Wilson's secretary of state, for 30 years had been a powerful voice for reform and social justice. Bryan believed that Social Darwinism was an ill-founded misapplication of scientific theory used to support the subjugation of women, the second-class status of ethnic and racial minorities, the neglect of the poor, and the practice of eugenic sterilization.

In Bryan's last public crusade, he defended his principles in a courtroom in Dayton, Tennessee, in July 1925. Tennessee had recently enacted the Butler Act, which made it illegal to

The Rise and Fall of Man

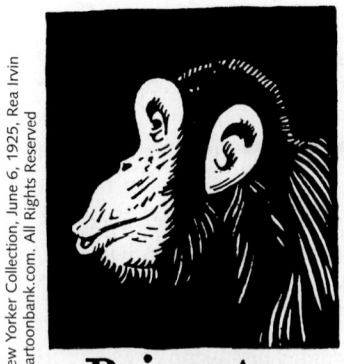 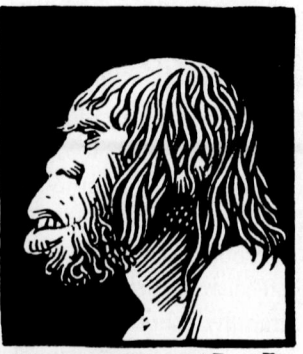 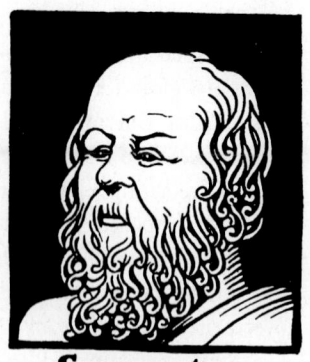 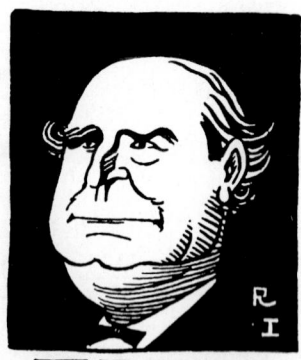

Primate   **Neanderthal Man**   **Socrates**   **W. J. Bryan**

■ This satiric political cartoon, published during the Scopes trial, depicts the theory of evolution as the development of humans from their origins as apes to the "survival of the fittest," portrayed as William Jennings Bryan. Bryan argued the case against evolution in the famous courtroom drama.

teach the theory of evolution in the schools. The American Civil Liberties Union (ACLU) announced that it would defend any teacher charged with violating the Butler Act. A 24-year-old science teacher from the local high school, John Thomas Scopes, agreed to test the law. Using a state-approved textbook, Scopes taught a lesson on evolutionary theory on April 24 to his Rhea County High School science class. He was arrested on May 7 and quickly indicted by a grand jury. Bryan agreed to represent the prosecution; famed Chicago criminal lawyer Clarence Darrow headed the ACLU's team of defense lawyers.

Bryan did not oppose science, but he objected to its misapplication. Darrow did not oppose religion. But he argued that religious fundamentalists—"creationists" who believed in the literal interpretation of the Bible—should not determine the way science was taught in the schools. Reporters at the time, and since, cast the trial as a struggle between religion and science, with rural and small-town Americans on the side of creationism and secular urbanites supporting evolution. But the divide was not so clear-cut. In a poll taken in Arkansas in 1928, city dwellers were more inclined to support creationism than rural residents. Almost all advocates on both sides of the Scopes trial were Christians who disagreed over how to interpret the Bible. They were also believers in science; those opposed to the teaching of evolution considered it to be an unscientific theory.

In the 1920s evangelical religion did not necessarily represent old-fashioned values resisting the new urban consumer culture. To take just one example, evangelist Aimee Semple McPherson regularly filled the 52,000 seats in her elaborate Angelus Temple in Los Angeles and reached many thousands more via radio, preaching the message of her Foursquare Gospel Church with the style and flair of a Hollywood celebrity. McPherson drew followers to 600 branches of her church using the latest techniques of advertising and mass culture. On one occasion, she used a gigantic electric scoreboard to illustrate the triumph of good over evil. Combining show-biz glitz with faith healing, she gathered a wide urban and rural following.

The Scopes trial also contained elements of popular entertainment. Dubbed "the Monkey trial" because Darwin's theory of evolution demonstrated that humans evolved from an earlier primate form that included monkeys and chimpanzees, the trial was one of the first national media events. The judge invited reporters from around the country, including broadcast journalists. The Scopes trial was the first jury trial broadcast on live radio. More than 900 spectators packed into the courtroom, and hundreds more gathered in the streets, where

> *Almost all advocates on both sides of the Scopes trial were Christians who disagreed over how to interpret the Bible.*

a carnival atmosphere prevailed, complete with souvenir stands, food vendors, itinerant preachers, and hucksters, including numerous chimpanzees accompanied by their trainers.

The trial did not deal with the question of the First Amendment, which guaranteed freedom of speech, nor the matter of who should decide the content of classroom education. Rather, religious fundamentalism was on trial. Although rules of evidence cannot apply to matters of faith, Darrow forced Bryan to defend his religious beliefs in a court of law. Darrow fully expected to lose the case so he could appeal it to the U.S. Supreme Court, and the jury obliged, reaching a guilty verdict in just nine minutes. Scopes was fined $100, but the fine was never imposed. Exhausted by the trial and ill with diabetes, Bryan died a week later.

Bryan technically won the case, but most reporters deemed the spectacle a victory for Darrow and the teaching of evolution. That assessment was premature. The Tennessee Supreme Court overturned the verdict on a technicality, robbing Darrow of his chance to take the case to the U.S. Supreme Court. Before the trial, most science textbooks included discussion of evolution; after the trial, material on evolution began to disappear. Laws against the teaching of evolution remained on the books until the U.S. Supreme Court overturned an Arkansas law in 1968.

The Scopes trial did not resolve the debate between creationists and evolutionists, and the controversy continued throughout the century. As late as 2000, the Board of Education in Kansas ruled that creationism and evolution were both unproven theories and that both could be taught in the schools. The Scopes trial may not have resolved anything, but it did have one significant unintended consequence. The trial generated tremendous interest in nonhuman primates. After the trial, attendance at the nation's zoos skyrocketed, boosting their funding and their prestige. So in the end, the real winners in the "Monkey trial" were the monkeys.

The Business of Politics

In 1924, President Calvin Coolidge declared, "The business of America is business." Despite its many critics, with the support of national political leaders, business reigned. After an initial recession following World War I, the economy grew steadily. The Gross National Product (GNP) increased 5.5 percent per year, from $149 billion in 1922 to $227 billion in 1929. Official unemployment remained below 5 percent throughout the decade, and real wages rose 15 percent. These trends fueled the popularity of the conservative, business-friendly presidents of the 1920s. Economic interests also drove foreign policy during the decade. After World War I, with much of Europe in shambles, the United States made loans to foreign countries, becoming the world's leading creditor nation. International markets opened up for American-made products, leading to a tremendous expansion in foreign trade.

Warren G. Harding: The Politics of Scandal

Warren G. Harding, a former newspaper editor and U.S. senator from Ohio, won the 1920 presidential election by the biggest landslide since 1820. Once elected, he released 66-year-old Socialist party leader Eugene V. Debs from prison. He then appointed a strong cabinet, including Herbert Hoover as secretary of commerce, Charles Evans Hughes as secretary of state, and Andrew Mellon as secretary of the treasury.

Harding established the conservative agenda that would last throughout the decade. His administration favored tariff protection, which placed a tax on goods entering the United States from abroad. Tariffs helped American industries by increasing the cost of imported goods. Harding also supported immigration restriction and opposed labor unions. In the wake of World War I, Harding distanced himself from Woodrow Wilson's peace settlement but promoted international treaties. In 1921 and 1922 Secretary of State Charles Evans Hughes achieved the first major disarmament accord, the Five-Power Treaty, signed by Japan, Britain,

France, Italy, and the United States. The five nations agreed to scrap more than 2 million tons of warships in the first such pact of its kind. Instead of an arms buildup, Hughes extended the power of the United States abroad through economic ties, encouraging banks to provide loans to war-ravaged Europe and using the government to protect such investments.

But Harding's presidency was marred by scandal. He had built his political base by handing out favors and deals to his friends, and he continued to do so as president. His buddies used their offices and influence for personal gain, while Harding caroused with them, drinking, despite Prohibition, and engaging in notorious extramarital affairs. At first, the press ignored these obvious abuses, but by 1923, the many scandals finally broke. Harding's cronies were exposed for selling government appointments and providing judicial pardons and police protection for bootleggers.

The most serious scandal of Harding's presidency involved the large government oil reserves at Teapot Dome, Wyoming, and Elk Hills, California. At the urging of Secretary of the Interior Albert Fall, Harding transferred control over the reserves from the Navy to the Department of the Interior. After accepting a bribe of nearly $400,000 from two oil tycoons, Harry F. Sinclair and Edward L. Doheny, Fall secretly issued leases to them without opening up the competition to other oil companies, thereby allowing Sinclair and Doheny to pump oil from the wells in exchange for providing fuel tank reserves to the Navy. Fall went to jail for a year as a result. In another scandal, Charles R. Forbes, head of the Veteran's Bureau, went to prison for swindling the government out of $200 million worth of hospital supplies. Forbes's lawyer committed suicide, as did a close associate of Attorney General Harry Daugherty, who was forced out of the Harding administration in disgrace. When he learned of the scandals that occurred in his close circle, Harding grew deeply worried. The stress probably contributed to the illness that killed him in 1923.

Calvin Coolidge: The Hands-Off President

Harding's vice president, Calvin Coolidge, took over the presidency when Harding died in 1923. Sober, serious, and humorless, Coolidge was not vulnerable to scandal as his predecessor had been. Coolidge believed that the government should meddle as little as possible in the affairs of the nation. He took long naps every day and exerted very little presidential leadership. Known mostly for his hostility to labor unions and his laissez-faire attitude toward business, he was a popular president during the complacent mid-1920s.

Not everyone was pleased with Coolidge's probusiness politics, and opposition mobilized for the 1924 election. Progressive Republicans formed a new Progressive party and nominated Robert M. La Follette for president, with Senator Burton K. Wheeler of Montana for vice president. The Progressive platform promoted conservation measures, higher taxes on the wealthy, doing away with the electoral college in favor of direct election of the president, and the abolition of child labor. The Democrats deadlocked between Catholic candidate Alfred E. Smith, an urban politician from New York, and Protestant William G. McAdoo, who had a base of support in the South and West. On the 103rd ballot, the delegates finally chose a compromise candidate, John W. Davis, a corporation lawyer, with Charles W. Bryan of Nebraska (William Jennings Bryan's brother) as his running mate. The Republicans nominated Coolidge, with Charles G. Dawes of Illinois as

TABLE 21-1

The Election of 1920

Candidate	Political Party	Popular Vote	Electoral Vote
Warren G. Harding	Republican	16,152,200	404
James M. Cox	Democratic	9,147,353	127
Eugene V. Debs	Socialist	919,799	0

TABLE 21-2

The Election of 1924

Candidate	Political Party	Popular Vote	Electoral Vote
Calvin Coolidge	Republican	15,725,016	382
John W. Davis	Democratic	8,386,503	136
Robert M. LaFollette	Progressive	4,822,856	13

his running mate. Coolidge claimed responsibility for the nation's prosperity and won easily, receiving more votes than the other two candidates combined.

Coolidge took pride in measures that prevented the government from interfering in the economy, such as his vetoes of the 1926 and 1928 McNary–Haugen bills, which would have provided government subsidies to farmers if farm prices dropped. The passage of the Revenue Act of 1926, a form of trickle-down economics intended to boost the economy, reduced the high income and estate taxes that Progressive reformers had put into place during World War I. Coolidge also continued Harding's efforts to sustain world peace. In 1928, under the leadership of Secretary of State Frank Kellogg and French Foreign Minister Aristide Briand, delegates from the United States, France, and 13 other nations gathered in Paris to sign the Kellogg–Briand Pact, in which they agreed to resolve conflicts through peaceful means rather than war. Unfortunately, with no means to enforce the agreement, the pact did nothing to alleviate the international hostilities that later erupted into World War II.

Herbert Hoover: The Self-Made President

The 1928 election was a major turning point for the presence of ethnic minorities in politics, for the Democrats broke tradition by selecting an Irish Catholic, Alfred E. Smith, governor of New York, as their candidate. It was the first time a major party had nominated a Catholic for president. Coolidge decided not to run for reelection in 1928, and the Republican party selected Secretary of Commerce Herbert Hoover as its nominee. Prohibition figured prominently in the 1928 presidential campaign. Although the Democratic platform gave lukewarm support to the continuation of Prohibition, Smith made no secret of his support for the repeal of the Eighteenth Amendment. By contrast, Republican Herbert Hoover praised Prohibition as "a great social and economic experiment." The other major issue of the campaign was religion. Anti-Catholic sentiment was strong throughout the country, especially in the South, where Democrats either sat out the election or voted Republican. Smith's opponents attacked his Catholicism, charging that he was more loyal to the Vatican than to the United States. Although Hoover won by a substantial majority, Smith carried the nation's 12 largest cities, indicating the strength of the ethnic vote in urban centers and the political and cultural rift between urban and rural Americans. Smith's candidacy also laid the groundwork for another Irish Catholic, John F. Kennedy, who ran successfully on the Democratic ticket 32 years later.

Herbert Hoover epitomized the values of the self-made man. He was orphaned as a child and raised by relatives of modest means. These early hardships fortified Hoover's ambition to overcome adversity, and he set his sights on business success. After graduating from Stanford University, he went into mining and rose through the ranks to become a wealthy corporate leader. By age 40 he was already a millionaire. Hoover began his career in government during World War I, when he earned widespread admiration for handling the distribution of food relief to European war refugees. He then served ably as secretary of commerce in the Harding and Coolidge administrations. President Hoover believed that his government experience rendered him ideally suited to secure prosperity for the nation's future. Shortly after the election, he predicted, "We in America today are nearer to the final triumph over poverty than ever before in the history of any land." But less than a year into his presidency, his optimism, along with the nation's economy, came crashing down.

TABLE 21-3			
The Election of 1928			
Candidate	Political Party	Popular Vote	Electoral Vote
Herbert Hoover	Republican	21,391,381	444
Alfred E. Smith	Democratic	15,016,443	87
Norman Thomas	Socialist	267,835	0

Consumer Dreams and Nightmares

During the 1920s, spending on recreation nearly doubled. Faith in continuing prosperity promoted the extension of consumer credit to unprecedented heights. Previously, the only major item routinely purchased on credit was a house. But in the twenties, installment buying became the rage for a wide range of consumer goods, from autos and radios to household appliances. Consumer debt rose from $2.6 billion in 1919 to $7.1 billion in 1929. As one official in a midwestern loan company remarked, "People don't think anything nowadays of borrowing sums they'd never have thought of borrowing in the old days. They will assume an obligation for $2000 today as calmly as they would have borrowed $300 or $400 in 1890." This habit of buying on credit boosted the standard of living for many but also left families in a precarious situation and vulnerable to the vagaries of the broader economy.

Marketing the Good Life

Advertising fueled much of the new spending. As one contemporary reporter noted, "Advertising is to business what fertilizer is to a farm." According to advertisers, consumer goods promised health, beauty, success, and the means to eliminate personal and embarrassing flaws, such as bad breath or dandruff. Cigarette companies used advertising to promote smoking as a symbol of independence for women and as a means to achieve beauty. Clever advertising campaigns promised women that if they would "reach for a Lucky Strike" instead of a sweet they would remain slim, healthy, and sexually appealing.

Advertising also fostered a vision of big business as a benevolent force, promoting individual happiness. In his 1925 best-seller, *The Man That Nobody Knows,* advertising executive Bruce Barton portrayed Jesus as a businessman who gathered a group of 12 followers who believed in his enterprise and, through effective public relations and advertising, sold his product to the world. The consumer culture had its temples: movie palaces, department stores, and the 1920s innovation, the shopping center. Kansas City's Country Club Plaza, the first shopping center in the nation, was the brainchild of Jesse Clyde (J. C.) Nichols, who purchased 55 acres of swampland for the project. Like the architects of the movie palaces, Nichols looked to European aristocratic styles for inspiration. He chose a Spanish–Moorish theme for the plaza that included courtyards and stucco buildings with red tile roofs and ornate towers. He adorned the plaza's streets and sidewalks with works of art, columns, wrought iron, and fountains. Most significantly, he designed his shopping center with the car in mind. The shopping center originally boasted eight filling stations and numerous garages and parking lots. Skeptical city leaders called it "Nichols' Folly," but the Country Club Plaza was a commercial success.

A much less successful venture was the Florida land boom, based on fantasies of a consumer paradise. When

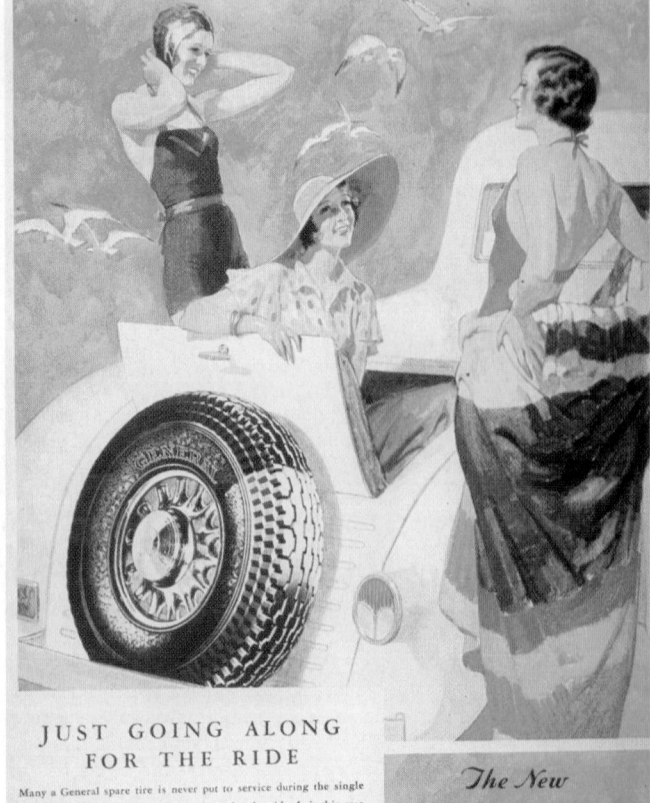

The Advertising Archive Ltd.

JUST GOING ALONG FOR THE RIDE

Many a General spare tire is never put to service during the single ownership of a car—they just go along for the ride. It is this year round freedom from tire worry that has spoiled General Tire users for any other tire. But more important is the factor of safety at today's high speeds. Generals are blowout proof and skid-safe and the exclusive low pressure feature makes comfort a luxurious reality. All of these advantages cost so little when you total up General's almost unheard of big mileage. The General Tire & Rubber Co., Akron, O.

The New **GENERAL** DUAL BALLOON

—goes a long way to make friends

■ In the 1920s advertisers used sexualized images to sell all sorts of products. This advertisement for automobile tires provides very little information about the product itself but evokes images of fun and romance to capture consumers' attention.

World War I closed off routes to the European playgrounds of the American elites, shrewd developers in Florida began to advertise: "Go to Florida, Where enterprise is enthroned. Where you sit and watch at twilight the fronds of the graceful palm, latticed against the fading gold of the sun kissed sky." These promotional efforts sparked a frenzy of investment in Florida real estate. To create "earthly paradises" and resorts, developers rushed to construct roads and find new land on which to build. Forging the Tamiami Trail across 90 miles of Everglades swamp entailed dredging a canal, blowing up the submerged limestone layer with dynamite, piling the broken limestone beside the canal, and then crushing it into a road surface. The dangerous work claimed the lives of many laborers and severely damaged the sensitive ecology of the vast Everglades wetland. When the road was finally completed in 1928, the land boom had collapsed.

Human folly and nature's fury contributed to the Florida land boom and bust. The boom peaked in 1925 and quickly collapsed. In 1926 a Danish ship, being renovated to become a floating cabaret, sank and blocked the entrance to the Miami harbor, stranding dozens of ships filled with building materials necessary for ongoing construction. Then a hurricane hit Miami, killing 130 people and causing millions of dollars of property damage. Another hurricane in 1928 killed more than 1000 people and destroyed several towns. The destruction wrought by the hurricanes, and the exposure of exaggerated promotional advertisements and inflated prices, quickly put an end to land speculation. The collapse of the Florida land boom foreshadowed the collapse of the stock market in 1929.

Writers, Critics, and the "Lost Generation"

Some social critics claimed that consumerism fostered not only economic disasters such as the Florida land boom but also a stifling conformity. Sinclair Lewis was one of several novelists of the twenties whose books expressed biting criticism of the frantic pursuit of material gain and status. George Babbitt, the protagonist of Lewis's novel *Babbitt* (1922), struggles to become accepted and successful in his small town by conforming to the empty materialism and standardized opinions accepted and prized by his neighbors. In *Main Street* (1920), Lewis explores similar themes through the character of a woman, Carol Kennicott. She resides in Gopher Prairie, a thinly disguised version of Lewis's own hometown, Sauk Centre, Minnesota. But unlike Babbitt, Kennicott rebels against the stifling small-town life that traps her.

F. Scott Fitzgerald wrote not about small-town conformity, as Lewis did, but about the modern urban life that was its antithesis. Fitzgerald glamorized, criticized, and in many ways embodied the giddy nightlife and status seeking of the Jazz Age. Born in St. Paul, Minnesota, into a family of modest means, he grew up admiring and emulating the

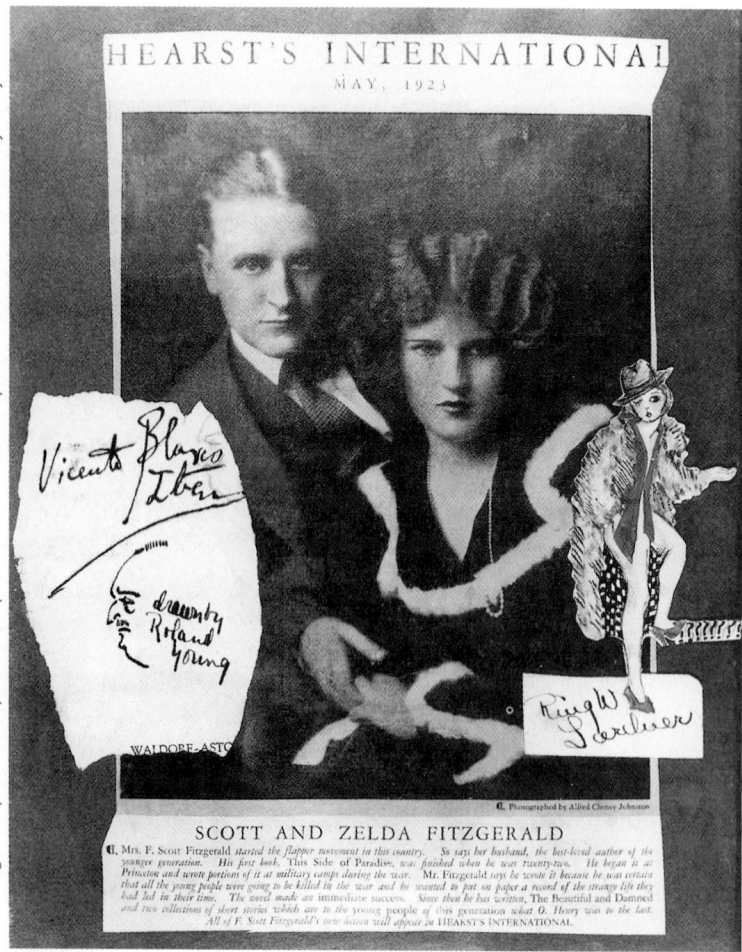

■ Writer F. Scott Fitzgerald and his flapper wife, Zelda, personified the glamorous literati of the Jazz Age. In his writing, Fitzgerald both romanticized and criticized the decadent consumerism of the aspiring and upwardly mobile middle class. In this page from a scrapbook, their photos are adorned with autographs of other famous literary figures.

wealthy. He married glamorous flapper Zelda Sayre, daughter of a prominent Alabama judge, and together they embodied the dizzy, indulgent, free-spirited life of the decade. But Fitzgerald's novels, including *This Side of Paradise* (1920), *The Beautiful and the Damned* (1922), and *The Great Gatsby* (1925), criticized the era's obsessions with success, glamour, consumerism, advertising, and the infatuation with status. The Fitzgeralds, along with other writers who were critical of American superficiality and conformity, moved to Paris. Eventually, the life Fitzgerald both lived and criticized caught up with him. By the end of the decade, he—like the nation—was broken by his excesses. In 1931 he came home to Baltimore an alcoholic; Zelda was diagnosed with schizophrenia and spent the rest of her life in mental institutions.

During their years in Paris, the Fitzgeralds often joined other expatriate writers at the salon of Gertrude Stein, a prolific author of novels, plays, operas, poems, and biographies. Born in 1874 to German Jewish parents in Pennsylvania, she grew up in California and attended Radcliffe College in Massachusetts. In 1903 she moved to France, where she remained for the rest of her life, looking back to America for her subject matter. In Paris she met another American, Alice B. Toklas, who became her lifetime partner. Their openly lesbian relationship gave Stein material for her writing, including *The Autobiography of Alice B. Toklas* (1933). In the 1920s, she dubbed the writers who gathered at her salon the "Lost Generation."

Poverty Amid Plenty

Most Americans in the 1920s were neither investing in Florida real estate nor frequenting Gertrude Stein's Paris salon. Even so, they were not immune to the desires and dreams that the consumer society sparked. The middle class and the more prosperous members of the working class enjoyed many of the comforts, amusements, and appliances that the booming economy made available; the poor struggled just to make ends meet. Throughout the twenties, the nation's poorest people continued to be the most mobile, moving in search of jobs, security, and a place they could settle and call home. Henry Crews, son of a white Georgia sharecropper, longed for "that single house where you were born, where you lived out your childhood . . . your anchor in the world." But he never had such a home. Like that of many other hardworking sharecroppers and factory workers, his family moved frequently in search of a better life, a dream that often proved elusive.

If Zelda Sayre Fitzgerald embodied the Jazz Age, Myrtle Terry Lawrence embodied the experience of the sharecropper. Born in Alabama in 1893, she began chopping and hoeing cotton at age six. She spent two weeks in school in the first grade, which was the full extent of her formal education. She married Ben Lawrence when they were both 13 years old and had her first child at 14. With her husband she worked in the cotton fields for nearly three decades, eventually becoming a major organizer of black and white sharecroppers in the Southern Tenant Farmers' Union (STFU), which fought for the rights of tenant farmers.

Myrtle Lawrence was poor, but she did not consider herself a victim. Her children described her as a "lady," although the tough-talking, tobacco-chewing Lawrence was hardly a southern belle. She took pride in vigorous outdoor work, which she preferred to indoor housework. As her daughter-in-law recalled, "She wasn't no housekeeper. Bless her heart." One of her sons boasted that his mother was paid extra to set the pace for the other workers, including the men, because "she was the best man." In the words of one daughter, "Mama wasn't slow at nothing." Myrtle Lawrence's energy and wits, as well as her refusal to be bullied, won her the admiration of her family and the respect of coworkers and propelled her in the 1930s to leadership in the STFU.

Sharecropping required hard work and careful planning to carve out a meager life, but many did so with pride. Ed Brown, a young black sharecropper, had no formal education but considered himself "pretty schemy." He worked on six different plantations, moving about in

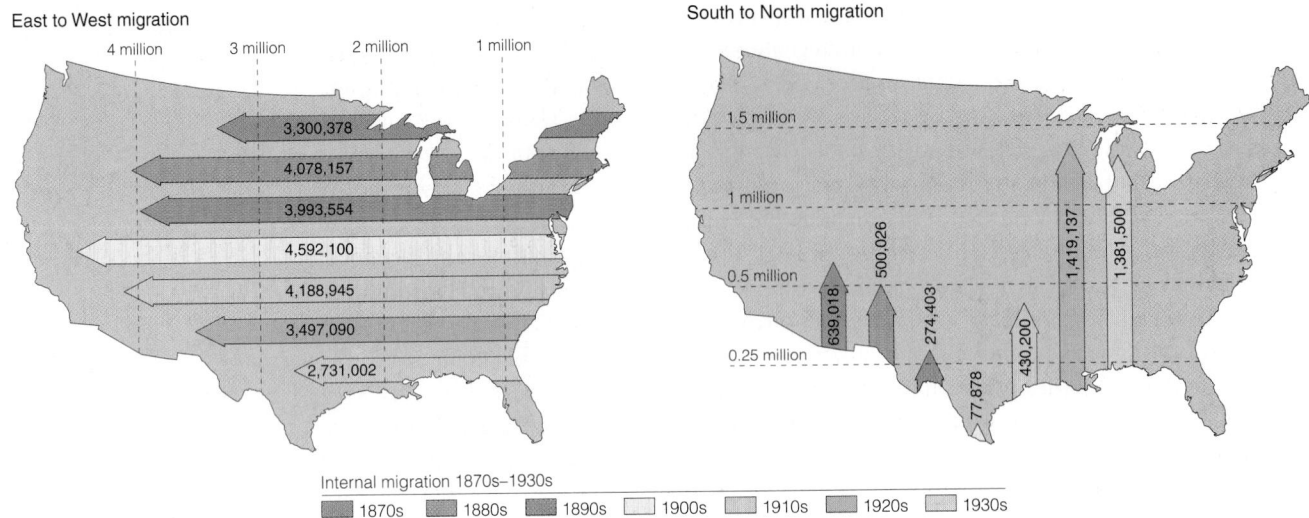

■ MAP 21.2

AMERICANS ON THE MOVE, 1870s–1930s Between the 1870s and the 1930s, millions of Americans moved around the country, mostly from east to west, but also from south to north.

search of better circumstances or to escape from debt or threats of violence. Although he and his wife, Willie Mae, were never able to buy a place of their own, they did improve their circumstances over time. When they finally got out of debt and secured a bit of cash, they used it to adorn their meager cabin. In 1929 they bought an old Model T Ford. But finding it too costly to maintain, they swapped it for a cow and a butter churn and dasher, which provided more practical benefits. Meanwhile, Ed took odd jobs to earn extra money, while Willie Mae took care of the children, picked cotton, took in laundry, and, as Ed noted with appreciation, kept "things . . . lookin very pretty."

Life was a struggle for southern sharecroppers, black and white. But African Americans faced the most difficult jobs and the added insults of racism. Blacks continued to move north in huge numbers in search of improved opportunities. Immigrants had a better chance of moving into semiskilled jobs, while blacks were relegated to unskilled jobs. Many ended up in domestic service, where they worked long hours for low pay. They tried to avoid live-in work, where they had little freedom from the watchful gaze of employers and barely any time with their own families. If they returned to the South, they faced work in the fields or factories for long hours under miserable conditions or in the extracting industries of coal mining, logging, and saw milling, where dangerous working conditions killed thousands of laborers.

Latinos joined African Americans at the bottom of the socioeconomic ladder in the Southwest and Midwest, working in jobs that offered almost no opportunity to save money or acquire property. Plantation owners kept sharecroppers in debt, and mine owners paid their workers in scrip that had to be used in company stores while forcing them to live in company housing.

Immigrants from Asia who arrived on the West Coast also faced difficulty finding stable jobs with decent pay and working conditions. Many ended up in domestic service. A young Japanese woman went to work for a family in Oakland, California, less than a month after arriving in the country. "I had to bring the coal up, all the time I went up and down," she later recalled. "Then I had to wash diapers. Me, I grew up on a farm, so I never had to do that. When I came to America, I didn't know anything. So I just had to cry." Loss of a job also meant loss of housing, creating constant mobility. Nevertheless, the poor maintained strong ties of kinship and community and helped each other survive under difficult conditions.

Industrial workers struggled throughout the decade, especially in a political climate hostile to unions. With the crushing of labor radicalism in the Red Scare after World War I, union organizing and strikes declined. But workers continued to protest low wages and poor working conditions. In March 1929 young women textile workers in Elizabethton, a small town nestled in the Blue Ridge Mountains of eastern Tennessee, closed down the American Glanzstoff plant in protest against low wages, petty rules, and arrogant employers. Soon, the protest spread to textile mills across the region. At Glanzstoff, the strikers returned to work when the company promised better pay and agreed not to discriminate against union members. But the employers broke their promises, so the women struck again. The governor sent in the National Guard, armed with machine guns. More than 1000 people were arrested in confrontations with the troops.

The strikers were young women mostly in their teens and early twenties. They combined labor militance with an air of playfulness. On the picket lines, they expressed their autonomy and independence, but they also found opportunities to flirt and carouse beyond the watchful eyes of parents. Although the strike was ultimately crushed and many of the participants were blacklisted, few expressed regrets. Bessie Edens knew she would not get her job back, but she "didn't care whether they took me back or not. I didn't! If I'd starved I wouldn't of cared, because I knew what I was a'doing when I helped to pull it. And I've never regretted it in any way. . . . And it did help the people, and it's helped the town and the country."

The Stock Market Crash

The symbolic end of the 1920s arrived on "Black Tuesday," October 29, 1929, when the inflated and overextended stock market came crashing down. In one day, stocks fell in value $14 billion. By end of the year, stock prices were down 50 percent; by 1932, they had dropped another 30 percent. In three years, $74 billion of the nation's wealth had vanished. The effect on the economy was catastrophic. Industrial production fell by half. More than 100,000 businesses went bankrupt. Banks failed at alarming rate: more than 2000 banks closed in 1931 alone. Unemployment rose to staggering levels, reaching 25 percent by 1932 and rarely dropping below 17 percent throughout the 1930s.

In keeping with the social policies that had prevailed throughout the 1920s, relief efforts were slim. No federal relief or welfare, no unemployment insurance, no Social Security, no job programs existed to help those who had lost their jobs, their savings, and their homes. Although many wealthy people lost their fortunes, which had been built on speculative investments, the poor suffered the most. People who lost their homes and farms moved into makeshift shelters in shantytowns, which they nicknamed "Hoovervilles" to mock the ineffectual efforts of President Herbert Hoover to respond to their plight.

The causes of the stock market crash and the decade-long depression that followed were complex and varied. Stock prices rose dramatically, especially at the end of the 1920s. Speculators had been purchasing stocks on 10 percent margins, meaning they put down only 10 percent of the cost and borrowed the rest from brokers and banks. The popularity of installment buying in the consumer goods market had devastating effects when applied in this manner to the stock market. Investors expected to get rich quickly by selling their stocks at a higher price and paying back the loans from their huge profits. This system worked for a few years, encouraging investors with limited funds to make risky investments in the hope of gaining large fortunes. When the price of stocks spiraled out of control, far beyond their actual value, creditors demanded repayment of their loans, and investors were unable to pay their debts.

The collapse of the stock market alone would not necessarily have caused such a severe and prolonged depression. Poor decision making by financial and political leaders exacerbated underlying weaknesses in the economy. The Federal Reserve curtailed the amount of money in circulation and raised interest rates, making it more difficult for people to get loans and pay off

Mario Puzo, *The Fortunate Pilgrim*

*I*talians, like most other European immigrants, established households where almost everyone worked to support the family. Fathers earned wages, mothers often took in boarders or did piecework at home to earn extra money, and sons and daughters found jobs in sweatshops and factories. Young Italian women, along with their Jewish peers, often worked for garment manufacturers, such as the Triangle Shirtwaist Company, scene of the strike of 1909 and the tragic fire that followed. Most immigrants married within their own ethnic groups. Often, immigrant families were torn by fierce generational conflicts, as old-world parents tried to maintain traditional ways while their American children struggled to break free. This generational struggle beset nearly every immigrant group.

Mario Puzo, the Italian American novelist best known for The Godfather, was among the many children of immigrants to express the cultures and experiences of newcomers through the arts. His autobiographical novel, The Fortunate Pilgrim, is a portrait of life in the Italian community of New York City in the early years of the century. The book depicts the struggles and triumphs of an Italian immigrant family. The men work long hours for meager wages while the women struggle to maintain the family. Mothers gather on tenement stoops to bemoan the behavior of their Americanized children, yet they dream the American dream of a better life. At the end of the book the mother's dream comes true, and the family moves to a suburban home in Long Island. Yet it is a bittersweet ending, for she and her family realize the loss of the vibrant

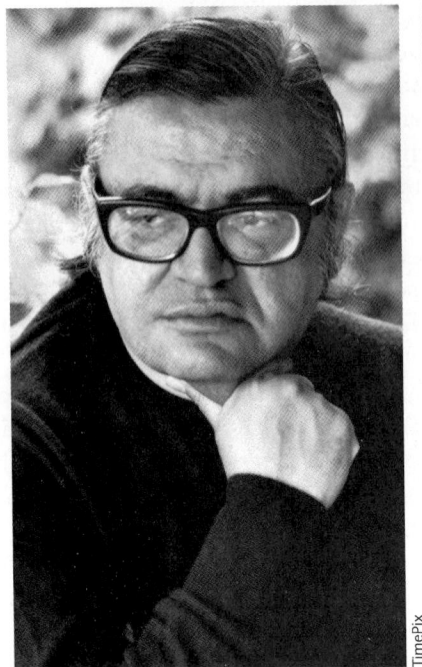

Mario Puzo, author of *The Fortunate Pilgrim* and *The Godfather*.

TimePix

community that, for all its hardship and poverty, had sustained them in the city.

Each tenement was a village square; each had its group of women, all in black, sitting on stools and boxes and doing more than gossip. They recalled ancient history, argued morals and social law, always taking their precedents from the mountain village in southern Italy they had escaped, fled from many years ago. And with what relish their favorite imaginings! Now: What if their stern fathers were transported by some miracle to face the problems *they* faced every day? Or their mothers of the quick and heavy hands? What shrieks if *they* as daughters had dared as these American children dared? If *they* had presumed.

The women talked of their children as they would of strangers. It was a favorite topic, the corruption of the innocent by the new land. Now: Felicia, who lived around the corner of 31st Street. What type of daughter was she who did not cut short her honeymoon on news of her godmother's illness, the summons issued by her own mother? A real whore. No no, they did not mince words. Felicia's mother herself told the story. And a son, poor man, who could not wait another year to marry when his father so commanded? Ahhh, the disrespect. *Figlio disgraziato.* Never could this pass in Italy. The father would kill his arrogant son; yes, kill him. And the daughter? In Italy—Felicia's mother swore in a voice still trembling with passion, though this had all happened three years ago, the godmother recovered, the grandchildren the light of her life—ah, in Italy the mother would pull the whore out of her bridal chamber, drag her to the hospital bed by the hair of her head. Ah, Italia, Italia; how the world changed and for the worse. What madness was it that made them leave such a land? Where fathers commanded and mothers were treated with respect by their children.

Each in turn told a story of insolence and defiance, themselves heroic, long-suffering, the children spitting Lucifers saved by an application of Italian discipline—the razor strap or the *Tackeril*. And at the end of each story each woman recited her requiem. *Mannaggia America!*—Damn America. But in the hot summer night their voices were filled with hope, with a vigor never sounded in their homeland. Here now was money in the bank, children who could read and write, grandchildren who would be professors if all went well. They spoke with guilty loyalty of customs they had themselves trampled into dust. ■

Source: Mario Puzo, *The Fortunate Pilgrim* (New York: Random House, 1997), pp. 10–11.

their debts. These policies had profound worldwide implications and contributed to an international crisis. Banks in Germany and Austria, for example, depended on loans from the United States, and many went bankrupt, causing a ripple effect across Europe. The Tariff Act of 1930, known as the Hawley–Smoot Tariff, also contributed to the downward spiral. The tariff included industrial products as well as agricultural goods and raised duties from 32 to 40 percent. Although industrialists had convinced the Republican-controlled Congress that the tariff would protect American commodities from competition from cheaper foreign goods, they were wrong. Foreign governments retaliated by raising their own tariffs to keep out American goods. These monetary and trade policies backfired, and the economic crisis spread throughout the western industrial world.

Within the United States, the unequal distribution of wealth exacerbated the effects of the economic downturn. The nation may have looked prosperous, but most of the wealth was concentrated in the hands of a small number of people. The gap between the rich and the poor widened during the 1920s, in part because of Coolidge administration policies that lowered taxes on the wealthy. The majority of the population lost purchasing power, resulting in the decline of consumer-oriented industries as the market for their products shrank. Although the wealthy spent money extravagantly, they spent a smaller percentage of their money on consumer goods than wage earners. If average Americans had been able to buy more cars, household appliances, and other products, those industries might have survived, and the economy might have recovered more quickly. Political leaders, and the business-oriented public policies they had promoted throughout the decade, left the country ill prepared to address the crisis and meet the needs of families deprived of their means of livelihood. As the curtain came down on the 1920s, the nation was left suffering.

Conclusion

The stock market collapse, and the prolonged depression that followed, revealed the flaws in the economic system that spurred the apparent prosperity of the 1920s. Beneath the visible affluence was the hidden poverty that prevailed throughout the decade. The aftermath of World War I and the end of Progressive reform led to an era of conservative politics. National leaders promoted business interests and paid little attention to social welfare, the environment, or the need to regulate the economy. By the end of the 1920s, it was clear that Prohibition was a dismal failure and that the federal government was ill equipped to enforce it.

Although political reform withered, cultural vitality flowered. Hollywood emerged as a major industry, and the Jazz Age reflected the widespread appeal of African American music. A black arts movement flourished, centered in Harlem, and writers of the "Lost Generation"—disenchanted with the status quo—gathered in Greenwich Village or moved to France. Across the country, a youth culture challenged the gender and sexual mores of the past. Consumer culture expanded as increasing numbers of families purchased cars, radios, and new fashions.

Few who were involved in the private preoccupations of the decade could have foreseen the disaster ahead. When the stock market crashed and the Depression set in, President Hoover tried to address the crisis by extending the political philosophy that had prevailed throughout the decade: Private enterprise would bring the economy back to health. But Hoover soon discovered that the old formulas would not work in the new reality and that the nation's major economic and political institutions had lost their credibility.

Sites to Visit

Harlem: The Mecca of the New Negro
etext.lib.virginia.edu/harlem/

This site is the on-line text of the March 1925 *Survey Graphic Harlem Number,* which includes writings of many Harlem Renaissance writers.

Calvin Coolidge
www.ipl.org/ref/POTUS/ccoolidge.html

This site contains basic information about Coolidge's election and presidency and online biography.

Warren G. Harding
www.ipl.org/ref/POTUS/wgharding.html

This site contains basic information about Harding's election and presidency and online biography.

Herbert Hoover
www.ipl.org/ref/POTUS/hchoover.html

This site contains basic information about Hoover's election and presidency and online biography.

Harlem 1900–1940: An African American Community
www.si.umich.edu/CHICO/Harlem/

This site of the New York Public Library's Schomburg Center for Research in Black Culture includes information and articles about the history of Harlem as a center of African American cultural life.

The Scopes Trial
xroads.virginia.edu/~UG97/inherit/1925home.html

This site from the University of Virginia's American Studies program includes images, documents, and articles relating to the Scopes Trial.

Temperance and Prohibition
prohibition.history.ohio-state.edu/

This site from Ohio State University covers the history of temperance and prohibition in the United States.

The Flappers
www.geocities.com/flapper_culture/

This site includes images, descriptions, and information on famous "flappers" of the 1920s.

For Further Reading

General

Ann Douglas, *Terrible Honesty: Mongrel Manhattan in the 1920s* (1995).

Lynn Dumenil, *The Modern Temper: American Culture and Society in the 1920s* (1995).

David J. Goldberg, *Discontented America: The United States in the 1920s* (1999).

Robert S. Lynd and Helen Merrell Lynd. *Middletown* (1929).

George Mowry, *The Twenties: Fords, Flappers, and Fanatics* (1963).

The Decline of Reform

Kathleen Blee, *Women of the Klan: Racism and Gender in the 1920s* (1991).

Nancy Cott, *The Grounding of Modern Feminism* (1987).

Kenneth Jackson, *The Ku Klux Klan in the City, 1915–1930* (1967).

Matthew Frye Jacobson, *Whiteness of a Different Color: European Immigrants and the Alchemy of Race* (1998).

Desmond S. King, *Making Americans: Immigration, Race, and the Origins of the Diverse Democracy* (2000).

Nancy MacLean, *Behind the Mask of Chivalry: The Making of the Second Ku Klux Klan* (1994).

Andrew Sinclair, *Prohibition: The Era of Excess* (1962).

Hollywood and Harlem

Beth Bailey, *From Front Porch to Back Seat: Courtship in 20th Century America* (1988).

Ray Batchelor, *Henry Ford, Mass Production, Modernism and Design* (1994).

Nathan Irvin Huggins, *The Harlem Renaissance* (1971).

Angela J. Latham, *Posing a Threat: Flappers, Chorus Girls, and Other Brazen Performers of the American 1920s* (2000).

Virginia Scharff, *Taking the Wheel: Women and the Coming of the Motor Age* (1991).

Science on Trial

John M. Barry, *Rising Tide: The Great Mississippi Flood of 1927 and How It Changed America* (1997).

Richard Hofstadter, *Social Darwinism in American Thought, 1860–1915* (1944).

Daniel Kevles, *In the Name of Eugenics: Genetics and the Uses of Human Heredity* (1985).

Lawrence Levine, *Defender of the Faith: William Jennings Bryan, the Last Decade, 1915–1925* (1987).

Garry Wills, *Under God: Religion and American Politics* (1990).

The Business of Politics

Kendrick A. Clements, *Hoover, Conservation, and Consumerism: Engineering the Good Life* (2000).

John Kenneth Galbraith, *The Great Crash, 1929* (1955).

William E. Leuchtenberg, *The Perils of Prosperity, 1914–1932* (1958, 1993).

Robert K. Murray, *The Politics of Normalcy: Governmental Theory and Practice in the Harding–Coolidge Era* (1973).

Burl Noggle, *Teapot Dome: Oil and Politics in the 1920s* (1962).

Consumer Dreams and Nightmares

William Frazer and John J. Guthrie, Jr., *The Florida Land Boom: Speculation, Money, and the Banks* (1995).

Jacqueline Jones, *The Dispossessed: America's Underclass from the Civil War to the Present* (1992).

Jackson Lears, *Fables of Abundance: A Cultural History of Advertising in America* (1994).

Roland Marchand, *Advertising the American Dream* (1985).

Nancy Milford, *Zelda: A Biography* (1970).

Online Practice Test

Test your understanding of this chapter with interactive review quizzes at

www.ablongman.com/jonescreatedequal/chapter21

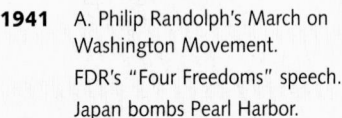

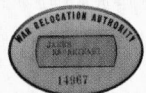

PART EIGHT

From Depression and War to World Power, 1929–1953

THE GREAT DEPRESSION AND WORLD WAR II TESTED AMERICANS' FAITH in their federal government to a degree unmatched in the nation's history. Economic collapse in the 1930s and the threat of Nazi and Japanese aggression from 1941 to 1945 presented challenges beyond the reach of ordinary citizens, local communities, and businesses acting alone. The federal government began to take more responsibility for economic and social well-being at home and for the spread of American values around the world.

The Great Depression resulted in a fundamental reordering of American politics. President Franklin Delano Roosevelt (FDR), who took office in 1933, believed that the federal government must assume an active role in banking, agriculture, and social welfare. He sponsored a large number of federal initiatives, known collectively as the New Deal. The New Deal aimed to put people back to work, restore faith in American businesses, boost purchasing power among consumers, and cushion the effects of economic downturns on industrial workers.

The effects of the New Deal were uneven. Many workers, including domestic servants, agricultural laborers, and part-time and seasonal employees, did not qualify for Social Security and other benefits. In the South government policies that discouraged landowners from planting crops led to the displacement of many black and white sharecropping families. On the other hand, employees of many large companies won higher wages and improved job security as a result of militant labor protests. African American civil rights activists, such local communist organizations as urban Unemployed Councils, and southern sharecroppers' and tenants' unions gave voice to the groups hit hardest by the Depression.

The New Deal did not end the Depression. On the morning of December 7, 1941, the Japanese conducted a surprise air attack on the U.S. Pacific naval fleet stationed in Pearl Harbor, Hawaii. Americans reacted with shock and outrage to what the president called this "day of infamy." The U.S. entry into World War II put large numbers of Americans back to work, many of them in the expanding defense industries.

The conflict brought Americans together in shared hardship, sacrifice, and national purpose. At the same time, the war placed strains on the social fabric. All over the country, family members separated from one another to search for work. In the Midwest blacks and whites competed for scarce wartime resources, such as housing. On the West Coast more than 100,000 Japanese immigrants and U.S. citizens of Japanese descent were forced into internment camps.

Elected to an unprecedented fourth term in 1944, Roosevelt proved to be a commanding leader during wartime as well as depression. In the last stages of the war, the president met several times with his British and Soviet counterparts, Winston Churchill and Josef Stalin, to plan for the postwar reconstruction of Europe and Asia. Roosevelt's death in April 1945 catapulted Vice President Harry S. Truman into the presidency. Germany surrendered to the Allies the next month. In August 1945, the new president authorized the dropping of atomic bombs on the Japanese cities of Hiroshima and Nagasaki, effectively ending the war in the Pacific. Together, the two bombs killed 120,000 Japanese civilians and wounded at least 130,000 more. The Atomic Age ushered in a new chapter in the history of human warfare.

Together with its allies, the United States emerged victorious from the war, but unlike its allies, America escaped physical destruction. Yet in many respects the postwar world was radically different from the world of the 1930s. The Soviet Union, an ally in the war against Germany and Japan, emerged as America's greatest enemy. The development of weapons of mass destruction introduced a new and profound threat to the natural environment, as well as to humans. To secure its supremacy in world affairs, the United States helped to form the North Atlantic Treaty Organization (NATO). For the first time, Americans were part of a multination peacetime alliance, one that required them to defend a member of the alliance even if they themselves were not attacked.

World War II also profoundly altered life in the United States. The perceived communist threat led some Americans to suspect domestic groups of internal subversion: African Americans agitating for their civil rights, labor leaders attempting to organize southern factories, and leftists who expressed support for communism in general and the Soviet Union in particular. Supported by government contracts, the defense industry became an integral part of the nation's economy.

Recovering quickly from the disruptions of war, returning soldiers and their wives hoped to settle down to a normal family life. These couples produced the baby boom, a generation that shaped American culture and society in significant ways. In the new and growing suburbs, many (predominantly white) Americans achieved their dream of home ownership, and businesses found plenty of room to expand in new industrial parks. Yet, not all Americans shared in this new found prosperity and security, and not all were willing to forgo their rights to free speech and free assembly in the struggle against communism.

1943	Smith–Connally Act.
	Zoot-suit riots in Los Angeles.
	Attacks on blacks in Detroit.

| 1944 | Normandy invasion on D-Day (June 6). |
| | Servicemen's Readjustment Act (GI Bill). |

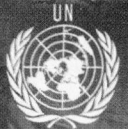

1945	Harry S. Truman becomes president upon death of Roosevelt.
	First test of atomic bomb, Alamagordo, New Mexico.
	Atomic bombs dropped on Hiroshima and Nagasaki.
	V-E Day (May 7); V-J Day (Sept. 2).
	United Nations created.

| 1946 | *Morgan v. West Virginia* outlaws segregation in interstate transportation. |
| | Winston Churchill gives "Iron Curtain" speech, Fulton, Missouri. |

1947	Jackie Robinson joins Brooklyn Dodgers.
	Taft–Hartley Act.
	Truman Doctrine of containing communism announced.

1948	New Mexico and Arizona grant Indians right to vote.
	Modern state of Israel founded.
	Armed Services desegregated.
	Organization of American States (OAS) founded.

1949	Billy Graham launches his first evangelical crusade in Los Angeles.
	Establishment of People's Republic of China.
	USSR acquires nuclear weapons.

1950	North Korean troops invade South Korea.
	Internal Security Act of 1950.
	Sen. Joseph McCarthy accuses State Department of harboring communists.

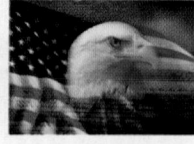

| 1951 | Ethel and Julius Rosenberg convicted of treason. |

| 1952 | McCarran–Walter Act. |
| | Puerto Rico becomes self-governing commonwealth. |

| 1953 | Korean War ends. |
| | Soviet leader Josef Stalin dies. |

Hardship and Hope in the 1930s: The Great Depression

Joe Jones, *We Demand*, 1934. Gift of Sidney Freedman, 1948.
The Butler Institute of American Art, Youngstown, Ohio (948-O-110)

■ This 1934 painting by Joe Jones, *We Demand*, expresses the increasing strength and militance of labor unions in the 1930s.

IN 1934, WILL ROGERS COMMENTED ON THE CAUSES OF THE GREAT DEPRESSION DURING HIS weekly radio broadcast. He noted that it was "not the working classes that brought on the economic crisis, it was the big boys that thought the financial drunk was going to last forever, and overbought, overmerged and overcapitalized." As a result, the "difference between our rich and poor grows greater every year. . . . Our rich are getting richer all the time. . . . There was not a millionaire in the country whose fortune did not come from the labor of others. We need to arrange it so that a man that wants work can get work, and give him a more equal division of the wealth the country produces."

Rogers was a Cherokee, a comedian, a plainspoken critic of the nation's rich and powerful, a movie star, journalist, and advisor to President Franklin Delano Roosevelt (FDR). Rogers articulated a new vision of American national identity that took shape in the 1930s. In contrast to an earlier notion of the United States as an Anglo-Saxon country into which newcomers might assimilate, this new Americanism included ethnic minorities, particularly those of European immigrant background. The Great Depression tarnished the status of the nation's business elite and opened up the political process to party realignments and new leaders. The popular culture expressed and reflected this new Americanism; Will Rogers was its most prominent voice. When the *Wall Street Journal* and the *New York Times* condemned him for his criticism of corporate elites, Rogers responded with a humorous assault on the nation's Anglo-Saxon leaders and their myths:

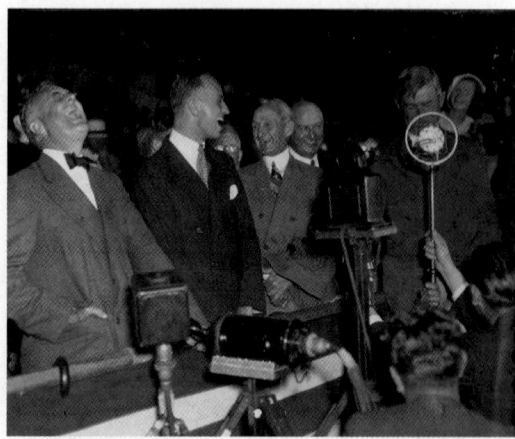

Presidential candidate Franklin Roosevelt (left) delighted in the support of comic Will Rogers (right) in 1932.

> I have a different slant on things, for my ancestors did not come over on the Mayflower. They met the boat. . . . I hope my Cherokee blood is not making me prejudiced, I want to be broad minded, but I am sure it was only the extreme generosity of the Indians that allowed the Pilgrims to land anywhere. Suppose we reverse the case. Do you reckon the Pilgrims would have ever let the Indians land? Yeah, what a chance, what a chance. The Pilgrims wouldn't even allow the Indians to live after the Indians went to the trouble of letting them land, of course, but they'd always pray. . . . You've never in your life . . . seen a picture of one of the old Pilgrims praying when he didn't have a gun right by the side of him. That was to see that he got what he was praying for.

Born in Oolagah in the Indian Territory of Oklahoma in 1879, Rogers got his start as a rope-twirling Indian cowboy on the vaudeville circuit. Like earlier Indian adventurers, including Sitting Bull, he worked his way through Wild West shows, which offered him an opportunity to demonstrate his impressive riding and roping skills, even though he found the spectacles demeaning to Native Americans, who were always defeated in the shows' mock battles. He came to Hollywood in the 1920s, where his Cherokee identity shaped both his humor and his social criticism.

In the 1930s the Great Depression gave rise to a cultural and political upheaval that helped propel Rogers to stardom and political influence. President Franklin Roosevelt coveted his support, and Rogers obliged by promoting the New Deal, the president's program for economic recovery. However, Rogers also pushed the president to the left by advocating such measures as taxing the rich and redistributing wealth. In 1932 Oklahoma nominated Rogers for president as the state's favorite son; three years later, California Democratic leaders urged him to run for the Senate. But in 1935, before any of these possibilities could come to fruition, Rogers died in a plane crash.

The response to Rogers's death illustrates his stature as a national leader and spokesperson for a new multicultural Americanism. Congress adjourned in his memory, President Roosevelt sent a well-publicized letter to Rogers's family, the governor of California proclaimed a day of mourning, flags flew at half mast, bells rang in Rogers's honor in

> *The economic crisis opened the door for a politically radical Cherokee Indian to become one of the most popular figures of the Great Depression.*

more than 100 cities, and nearly 100,000 people filed by his coffin at Forest Lawn Cemetery. Radio stations across the country broadcast his memorial service from the Hollywood Bowl, presided over by a Protestant minister and a Catholic priest, while a Yiddish performer sang a Hebrew mourning chant. Across town, Mexican American citizen groups placed a wreath on Olvera Street that read "Nosotros Lamentamos la Muerte de Will Rogers" ("We Mourn the Death of Will Rogers"). In the predominantly black Los Angeles community of Watts, an African American fraternal group called the Friends of Ethiopia joined black performers from Rogers's films in a parade to honor the Cherokee movie star who had spoken out publicly against Italy's 1935 invasion of Ethiopia. Back in his hometown of Claremore, Oklahoma, the Cherokee Indians performed a death dance in memory of their fallen kinsman.

This massive national grieving reveals not only Rogers's popularity, but also the culture of 1930s America. The economic crisis unleashed changes in society that opened the door for a politically radical Cherokee Indian to become one of the most popular figures of the Great Depression. Millions of Americans experienced poverty—many for the first time. The shared experience of loss and suffering permeated the country.

In the face of widespread hardship, many people felt a common bond and a fresh sense of themselves as Americans. This new type of Americanism was articulated most powerfully by Will Rogers. Those who subscribed to a changing national vision opposed the power of big business, participated actively in the emerging popular culture, and voted Democratic. Many of them came to the polls for the first time to vote for Roosevelt. They included native-born and foreign-born, working class and middle class, Anglo-Saxons and ethnic minorities, and people of color.

Roosevelt drew a new political coalition into the Democratic Party that elected him to the presidency four times. The Depression gave him the opportunity to forge a strong national government and to promote a more representative democracy. His inclusiveness efforts brought citizens of recent immigrant background into the political mainstream but stopped short of the color line. Nevertheless, African American voters abandoned the Republican party to vote for FDR.

The New Deal, a package of remedies put together by Franklin Roosevelt to address the problems of the Depression, provided relief to many Americans in need but did not eradicate poverty or end the Depression. Yet, as American families from every region of the country drew around their radios to hear the president's "fireside chats," as they made heroes of Will Rogers and other outsider celebrities, and as they held onto their faith in the nation's promise in spite of its worst economic crisis, they helped forge a more inclusive nation.

The Great Depression

The Great Depression defined the 1930s in the United States. It shaped the culture, the political life of the nation, the public policies that resulted, and the cultural expressions that reflected the spirit of the people during a time of national crisis. Its effects permeated the lives of Americans from the mansions of the wealthy to the shanties of the poor and from the boardrooms to the bedrooms. But the story is not simply one of despair and hardship. It is also one of strong communities, resourcefulness, and hope.

Causes of the Crisis

The Great Depression of the 1930s was the worst depression in the nation's history. But it was neither the first nor the last. Capitalism, the economic system that forms the basis of the American economy, has cycles of ups and downs. Under capitalism, the free market operates with minimal interference from the government. In the United States, prior to the 1930s, the government stepped in to regulate the economy primarily to protect economic competition. Progressive-era reforms prevented corporations from establishing monopolies, so that competition could flourish and businesses could prosper. In the free market economy, consumers would determine which companies would succeed, based on the quality of their products and services. Because the government did not determine the levels of industrial or agricultural productivity, and did not set the prices, the economy was subject to changing circumstances that led to times of prosperity and times of recession or, in the case of severe economic downturns, depression. The circumstances that affected the up-and-down cycles of the economy included international economic trends, as well as the workings of capitalism itself.

Communism and socialism provide different economic systems, with greater levels of government regulation. Communist countries have state-directed economies in which the government owns and operates the means of production, sets prices, and pays all workers' wages. There is no free market and no competition among businesses. In socialist states, governments own and operate certain industries and services, such as electricity and other utilities, or health care systems. Socialist countries also provide citizens with certain welfare benefits such as medical care, relief from poverty, income for the unemployed, and old age insurance. A number of capitalist countries offer these kinds of benefits to their citizens. These countries operate under a system known as "welfare capitalism," or a "welfare state."

> *The story of the Depression is not simply one of despair and hardship. It is also one of strong communities, resourcefulness, and hope.*

Before the 1930s the United States provided none of these welfare state benefits. Without any policies that would serve as a safety net for workers who lost their jobs, many wage earners and their families fell into poverty during times of economic downturn. In the Great Depression of the 1930s, the economic crisis was so severe that one quarter of the nation's workers, nearly 14 million people, lost their jobs, leaving them and their families—40 million people in all—without any income or security. Many of these people had never known poverty before. Among the newly poor were thousands of middle-class Americans who now faced the loss of their homes and savings. For working-class and poor Americans, the impact of the depression was devastating because they had little economic security to begin with.

The Depression was a global economic catastrophe. Of the major world powers, only the Soviet Union—as a communist society, with state-directed labor, agriculture, and production—was immune to the collapse of the capitalist system after 1929. In fact, its economy grew throughout the 1930s. The relative health of the Soviet economy led many people in troubled capitalist systems to look to communism as an alternative. Socialism gained many converts across Europe, as did communism. The powerful nations of the world all moved toward greater government intervention in their economies. England, France, and the United States moved toward deficit spending to help stimulate the economy and instituted relief programs.

Italy, Germany, and Japan also increased government intervention into the economy, but they used different strategies to address the crisis, particularly military spending. These varied responses to the Depression contributed to the conflicts and alliances that would eventually culminate in World War II.

Within the United States, the business values that had prevailed throughout the 1920s were now suspect. Business practices in every area of the economy, from finance to factories to agriculture, contributed to the disaster. For many Americans the Depression really began in the 1920s. Food production and distribution stumbled along weakly throughout the 1920s, leaving widespread rural poverty in its wake. Large corporations bought up smaller companies, putting many independent shops and manufacturers out of business. During the 1920s, 1200 big corporations absorbed more than 6000 independent businesses. By 1929, 200 corporations controlled nearly half of all industry, which limited competition and made it difficult for new, smaller businesses to flourish.

> *The concentration of wealth among the richest Americans during the 1920s contributed to the persistence of the crisis in the 1930s.*

Although the economy looked healthy on the surface, prosperity rested on an unsound foundation. Many people obtained consumer goods on credit, so when people lost their jobs, they could not pay their debts. Throughout the 1920s, the gap between the rich and poor increased. By 1929 the top 1 percent of Americans earned 14.7 percent of the nation's income, while the poorest 40 percent shared 12.5 percent. Nearly 80 percent of the nation's families had no savings at all. Those with high annual incomes of $10,000 or more—2.3 percent of the people—held two-thirds of all savings. As Will Rogers and many other social critics would later point out, the concentration of wealth among the richest Americans during the 1920s contributed to the persistence of the crisis in the 1930s.

International factors also played a role in the economic collapse. American overseas loans soared in the 1920s, reaching $900 million by 1924 and $1.25 billion by 1928. Germany was a large borrower, for example. Following its defeat in World War I, Germany had been required to make large reparation payments to France and other countries. The United States provided loans to Germany to help the country make its payments; Germany then made debt payments to the United States. When the stock market crashed, foreign economies like that of Germany also weakened and could not repay their debts. To make matters worse, American exports fell $1.5 billion between 1929 and 1933. The United States had established high tariffs to keep foreign goods out of the country so that Americans would buy only American-made goods. This, in turn, encouraged other countries to establish their own tariff barriers. Between 1929 and 1933, the Gross National Product (GNP) fell by $12 billion.

"We Are Not Bums"

In human terms the Depression of the 1930s dealt a devastating blow to large numbers of Americans: crushing poverty, hunger, humiliation, and loss of dignity and self-worth. Many felt a profound shame that they could no longer earn a living and support their families. The few jobs available often went to the young, strong, well-fed, and well-groomed. Thousands of citizens poured out their hearts in letters to the president, hoping that the government could provide some assistance. In 1934 an Oklahoma woman lamented, "The unemployed have been so long without food-clothes-shoes-medical care-dental care etc—we look pretty bad—so when we ask for a job we dont' get it. And we look and feel a little worse each day—when we ask for food they call us bums—it isent our fault . . . no we are not bums." Yet, the shabby appearance of the jobless helped neither their self-respect nor their work prospects. An unemployed worker from Oregon explained the difficult choices: "We do not dare to use even a little soap when it will pay for an extra egg [or] a few more carrots for our children."

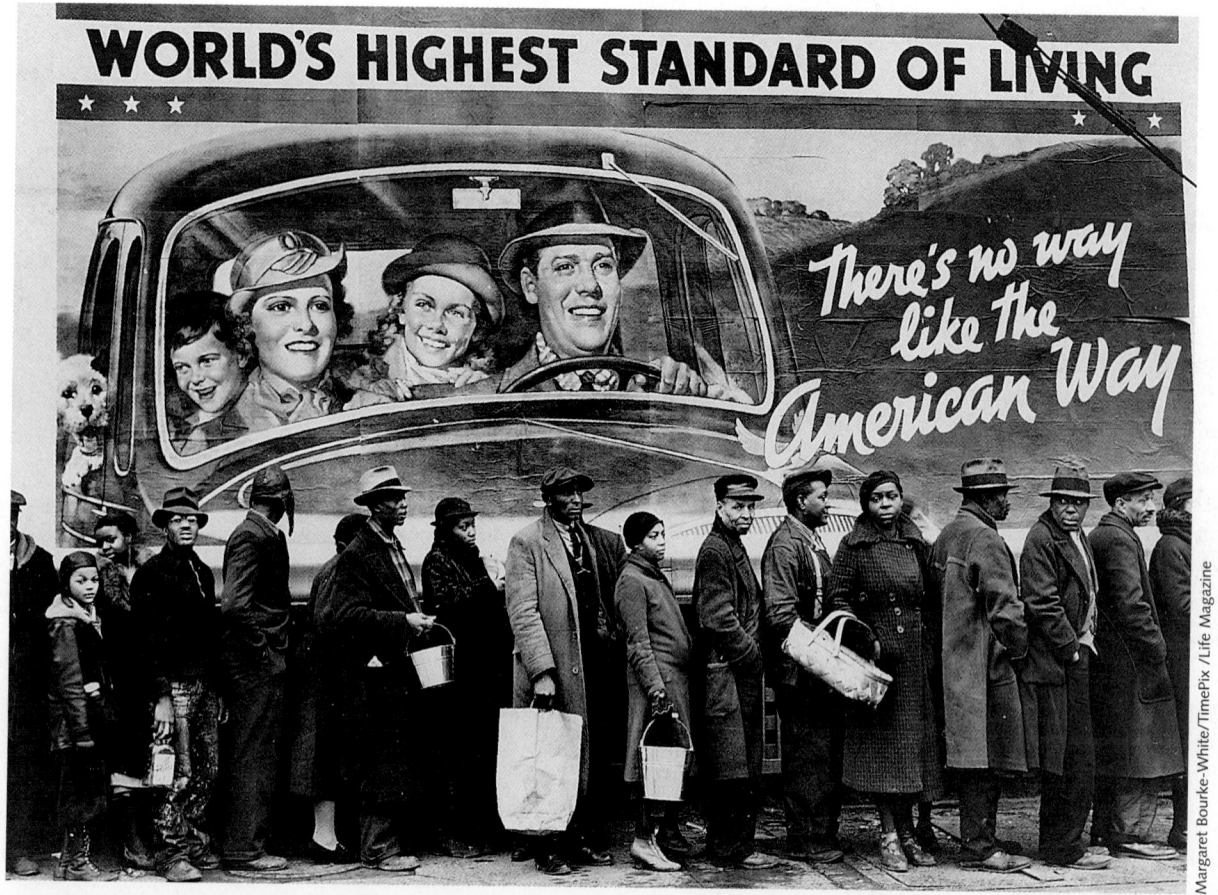

■ Margaret Bourke-White in this 1937 photograph, "At the time of the Louisville Flood," depicts the painful irony of poverty in the midst of affluence. Here, hungry Americans line up at a breadline in front of a billboard proclaiming American prosperity.

Families provided the first line of defense against disaster, especially in the early days of the crisis. Many families adapted to hard times by abandoning time-honored gender roles. As men lost jobs, women went to work. More than 6 million single women held jobs during the Depression. Married women also took jobs to support their families, often providing the only source of income if husbands were out of work. These women often faced hostility from those who assumed that employed wives with husbands to support them took jobs from unemployed men. But, in fact, working women did not take jobs from men; rather, they held jobs defined as "traditional women's work" as secretaries, nurses, and waitresses. These jobs offered lower wages than most jobs held by men. Still, they provided at least a modicum of much-needed income.

Sons and daughters also went to work. For the younger generation, taking on the responsibilities of adulthood provided a sense of independence and self-respect. Marriage rates plummeted as young people delayed or decided against wedlock. As one daughter of Italian immigrants from Providence, Rhode Island, remarked, "It's not that I didn't want to get married, but when you are working and have your own money," there was no hurry to find a husband. Recalled another, "During all the years I worked, I had a boyfriend, but we both had responsibilities at home. . . . Now they say 'career woman' but at the time you wouldn't call yourself that. It's just because you felt you had a responsibility at home, too."

Songs of the Great Depression

Popular songs expressed the spirit, sorrows, and longings of Depression-era Americans. According to folk music historian Alan Lomax, the 12-year-old daughter of a striking Harlan County, Kentucky, mine worker wrote "Which Side Are You On?" in 1937. The song became a popular anthem for labor militancy.

Woody Guthrie (1912–1967) wrote more than a thousand songs about the struggles of common people and the dispossessed. As a teenager, Guthrie left home to hitchhike, ride the rails, live in hobo camps, and follow migrant workers around the country. His song "Union Maid" expresses the hopes and spirit of union workers, and "So Long, It's Been Good to Know Yuh" captures the sorrows of Dust Bowl migrants.

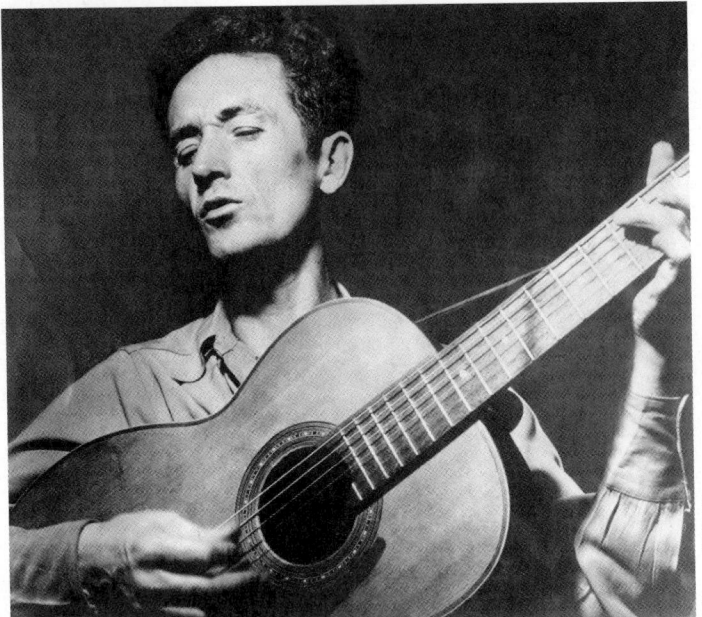

Bettmann/CORBIS

Woody Guthrie, singer and songwriter, immortalized the spirit of ordinary Americans during the struggles of the Great Depression. His songs became anthems of the era and remain classics of American folk music.

"Which Side Are You On?" by Florence Reece (sung to the tune of an old English song, "Jack Munro")

Come all of you good workers
Good news to you I'll tell

Of how the good old union
Has come in here to dwell.

Chorus:

Which side are you on,
Tell me, which side are you on?
My daddy was a miner,
He's now in the air an' sun,

Stick with him, brother miners,
Until this battle's won.

They say in Harlan County
There are no neutrals there
You'll either be a union man,
Or a thug for J. H. Blair.

Many parents struggled to provide for their families under difficult conditions, sometimes risking their health and safety to do so. Erminia Pablita Ruiz Mercer remembered when her father was injured while working in the beet fields in 1933. "He didn't want to live if he couldn't support his family," so he risked experimental back surgery and died on the operating table. Young Erminia then dropped out of school to work as "a doughnut girl" to support her mother and sisters.

Surviving Hard Times

For many poor families, hard times were nothing new. As one black man noted, "The Negro was born in depression. It only became official when it hit the white man." Throughout the 1930s black Americans suffered the impact of economic hard times disproportionately. By 1932 black unemployment reached 50 percent. As increasing numbers of white workers joined the ranks of the unemployed, they began seeking the jobs that were usually held by black workers, even though they would have shunned such work during prosperous times. With local white

O gentlemen, can you stand it,
O tell me if you can,
Will you be a lousy scab,
Or will you be a man?

Don't scab for the bosses,
Don't listen to their lies,
Us poor folks haven't got
a chance,
Unless we organize.

"Union Maid" by Woody Guthrie (first verse and chorus)

There once was a union maid
Who never was afraid
Of goons and ginks and company
finks
And the deputy sheriffs who made
the raids;
She went to the union hall
When a meeting it was called
And when the company boys
came 'round
She always stood her ground.

Chorus:

Oh, you can't scare me.
I'm sticking to the union, (3 times)
Oh, you can't scare me.
I'm sticking to the union, (2 times)
Till the day I die.

"So Long, It's Been Good to Know Yuh (Dusty Old Dust)" by Woody Guthrie (selected verses and chorus)

I've sung this song, but I'll sing
it again,
Of the place that I lived on the wild,
windy plains,
In the month called April, the county
called Gray
And here's what all of the people
there say:

Chorus:

So long, it's been good to know
you; (3 times)
This dusty old dust is a-getting
my home,
And I've got to be driftin' along.

A dust storm hit, and it hit like thunder;
It dusted us over, and it covered
us under;
Blocked out the traffic and blocked
out the sun.
Straight for home all the people
did run.

The sweethearts sat in the dark and
they sparked,
They hugged and they kissed in that
dusty old dark,
They sighed and cried, hugged and
kissed
Instead of marriage, they talked
like this:
Honey, so long, it's been good to
know you. . .

Now, the telephone rang, and it
jumped off the wall;
That was the preacher a-making
his call.
He said, "Kind friend, this may be
the end;
You've got your last chance of salvation of sin."

The churches was jammed, and the
churches was packed,
And that dusty old dust storm blowed
so black;
The preacher could not read a word of
his text,
And he folded his specs and he took
up collection, said:
So long, it's been good to know
you. . . . .

authorities in charge of relief, impoverished Southern blacks had few places to turn for assistance. African Americans also faced increasing violence; the number of lynchings increased from 8 in 1932 to 20 in 1935.

Many poor people joined the growing ranks of hobos, riding the rails from town to town looking for work. But poverty did not erase racial hierarchies or sexual codes, especially for nine young blacks who came to be known as the "Scottsboro Boys." On March 25, 1931, the youths, ranging in age from 13 to 21, were taken from a train in Paint Rock, Alabama, after a fight with a group of white men. Two white women, also on the train, accused the nine of rape. Narrowly avoiding a lynching, the youths were taken to jail in Scottsboro, where they began a long ordeal. Within two weeks an all-white jury convicted them of rape, and they were sentenced to death. The communist-backed International Labor Defense (ILD) took up the case and appealed it to the Alabama Supreme Court. The ILD also organized protests and rallies across the country, calling for justice for the Scottsboro Boys. The National Association for the Advancement of Colored People (NAACP) also tried to get control of the case but withdrew when the defendants committed themselves to the ILD. In spite of the ILD efforts, the

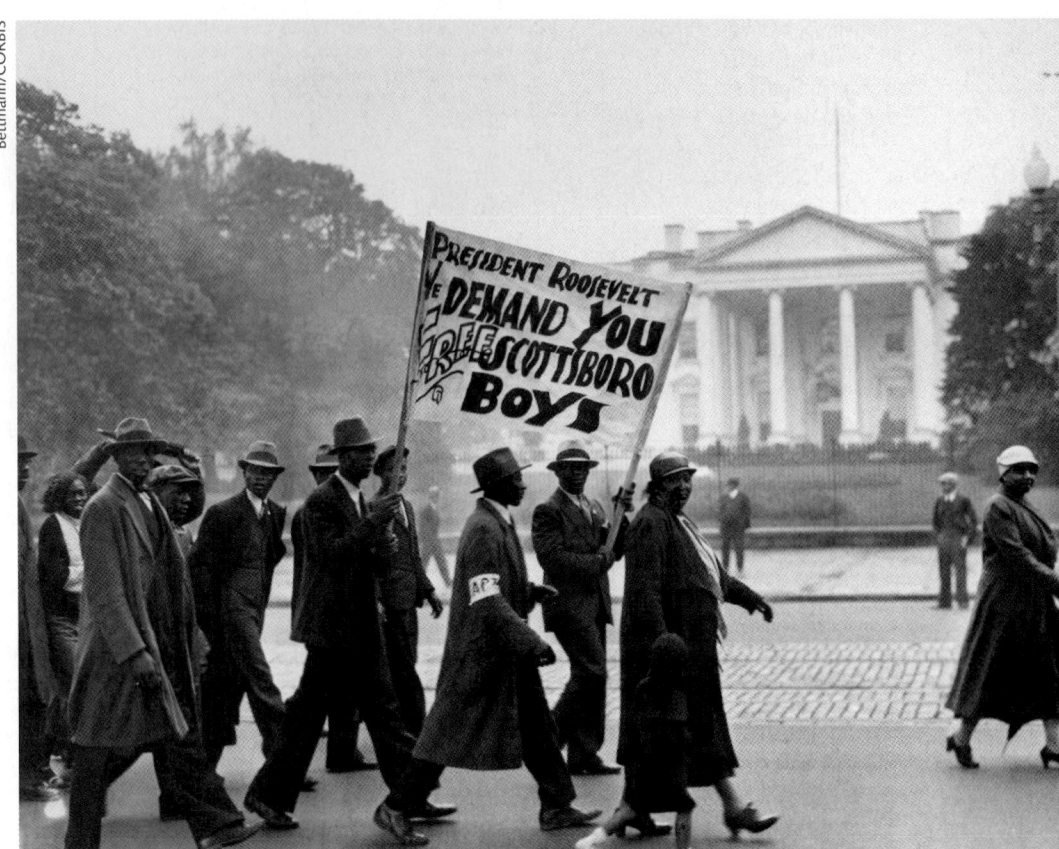

Bettmann/CORBIS

■ In 1933 protesters demonstrated in front of the White House demanding that President Roosevelt release the Scottsboro Boys. The nine black youths were convicted on flimsy evidence of raping a white woman on a hobo train.

Alabama Supreme Court upheld the convictions, but in November 1932 the U.S. Supreme Court ordered a new trial on the grounds that the defendants did not get a fair trial.

The first defendant to be re-tried was quickly convicted again and sentenced to death. At this point, the ILD and the NAACP organized new protests and gained support from across the political spectrum. The case became a major rallying point for civil rights activists, liberals, and radicals throughout the 1930s. Support for the young men came from all over the world, including the British Parliament and the Communist Party. In 1935 the U.S. Supreme Court reversed the second set of convictions on the grounds that excluding blacks from the jury denied the defendants due process. Yet in the next two years, five of the defendants were again tried and found guilty. Although none of the Scottsboro Boys was executed, they all spent long years in prison. The charges against the youngest four were eventually dropped. Although all appeals failed and the five remaining prisoners were never cleared of the crime, several were paroled, and the last of the nine was released from prison in 1950. In 1976 the repentant former segregationist governor of Alabama, George Wallace, pardoned one of the nine, Clarence Norris.

Racial discrimination intensified the suffering of African Americans during the Depression. By 1935, 90 percent of employed black women worked as either domestics or agricultural laborers. As these jobs became scarce, black women's labor-force participation fell from 42 percent to 38 percent over the decade. A white woman working for wages earned, on average, 61 percent of a white man's wages; a black woman earned a mere 23 percent.

Mexican American families could barely survive on the low wages paid to Mexican laborers. According to a 1933 study, working children's earnings constituted more than one-third of their families' total income. The work was often grueling. Julia Luna Mount recalled her first day at a Los Angeles cannery: "I didn't have money for gloves so I peeled chilies all day long

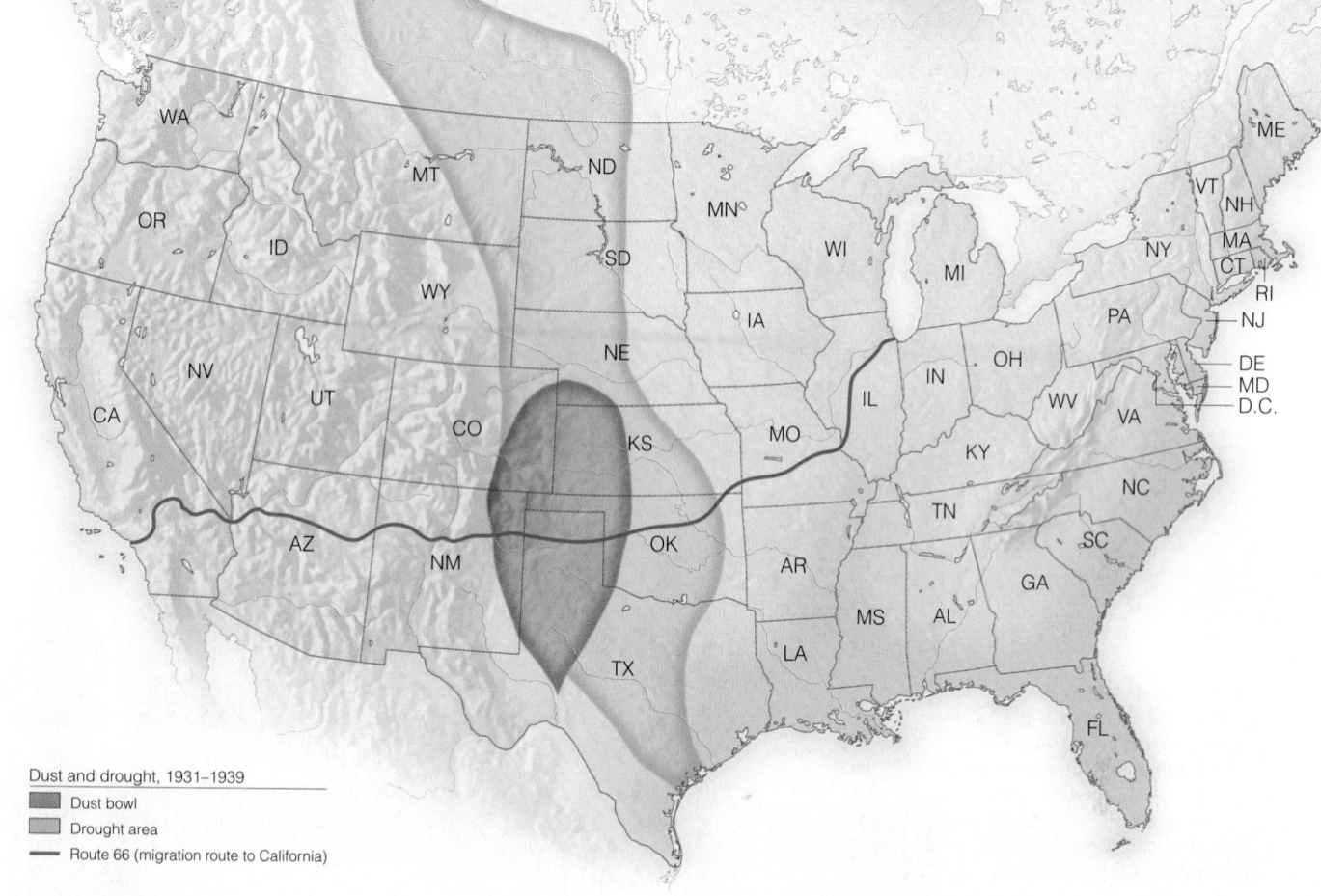

Dust and drought, 1931–1939

- ▬ Dust bowl
- ▬ Drought area
- ▬ Route 66 (migration route to California)

■ MAP 22.1

DUST AND DROUGHT, 1931–1939 Drought cut a giant swath across the middle of America during the years of the Great Depression. The hardest hit region was the Dust Bowl area of Oklahoma, Texas, New Mexico, Colorado, and Kansas. Many people fled the afflicted areas, abandoning farms, piling their belongings on their cars, and driving along Route 66 to California.

by hand. After work, my hands were red, swollen, and I was on fire! On the streetcar going home, I could hardly hold on my hands hurt so much." Young Julia was lucky—her father saw her suffering and did not make her return to the cannery. But Carmen Bernal Escobar's father could not afford to be soft-hearted about work: "My father was a busboy and to keep the family going . . . in order to bring in a little more money . . . my mother, my grandmother, my mother's brother, my sister and I all worked together" at the cannery.

Those with cannery work, hard as it was, were among the fortunate. Many more Mexicans were deported. Between 1931 and 1934, more than 500,000 Mexicans and Mexican Americans—approximately one-third of the Mexican population in the United States—were sent to Mexico. Most were children born in the United States. Throughout the century, the United States opened or closed its doors to Mexican immigrants depending on the need for their labor. They were deported during the Depression when unemployment was high, then recruited again during the labor shortage of World War II. In the 1930s Mexicans who applied for relief were offered assistance only if they agreed to return to Mexico. But deportation brought more sorrows. In Ciudad Juarez 2000 repatriates lived in a large open corral without resources or shelter; dozens died from disease.

The Dust Bowl

Severe drought exacerbated the difficulties of farmers across Oklahoma, Texas, Kansas, Colorado, and New Mexico, an area that came to be known as the Dust Bowl. Farmers had used

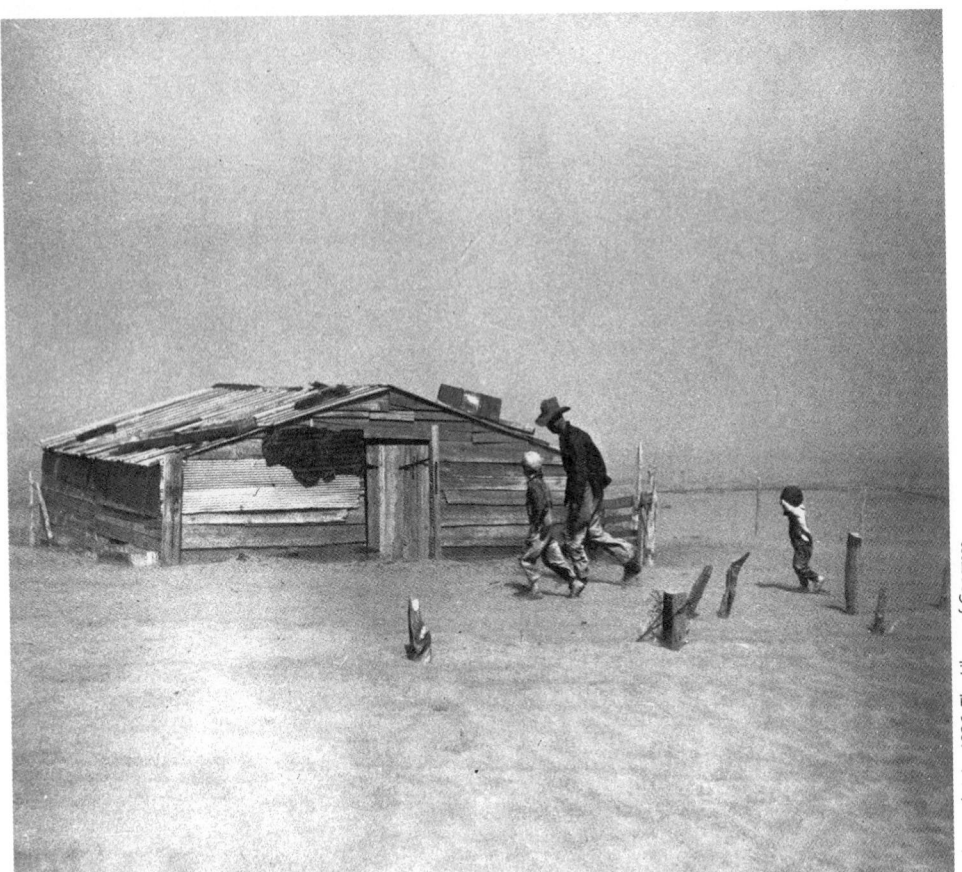

Arthur Rothstein, 1936. The Library of Congress

■ An Oklahoma farmer and his sons try to find shelter from the storm of dust that blew across the plains in 1935. Severe drought after years of excessive plowing created dry loose topsoil that was picked up by high winds. More than half of the residents of the Dust Bowl moved out of the area as a result of the devastation.

the land mainly for grazing until high grain prices during World War I enticed them to plow under millions of acres of natural grasslands to plant wheat. Plowing removed root systems from the soil, and years of little rainfall caused the land to dry up. By the middle of the decade high winds picked up the loose topsoil, creating dust storms across the open plains, as far as 1000 miles. The worst storm occurred on April 14, 1935, when winds up to 70 miles per hour carried clouds of dust that turned the sky black, suffocated livestock, and lodged in people's homes, clothes, hair, and lungs. The ecological disaster drove 60 percent of the population out of the region.

Migrant farm families fleeing the Dust Bowl came to symbolize the suffering wrought by the Depression. The photographs of Dorothea Lange, the songs of Woody Guthrie, and the writings of John Steinbeck all immortalized their plight. Steinbeck's Pulitzer prize–winning novel *The Grapes of Wrath* and its film version have remained classics of American popular art. Writing in *The Nation* three years before the publication of *The Grapes of Wrath* (1939), Steinbeck described the Dust Bowl migrants streaming into California:

> Poverty-stricken after the destruction of their farms, their last reserves used up in making the trip, they have arrived so beaten and destitute that they have been willing at first to work under any conditions and for any wages offered. . . . They are not drawn from a peon class, but have either owned small farms or been farm hands in the early American sense, in which the "hand" is a member of the employing family. They have one fixed idea, and that is to acquire land and settle on it. . . . They are not easily intimidated. They are courageous, intelligent, and resourceful. Having gone through the horrors of the drought and with immense effort having escaped from it, they cannot be herded, attacked, starved, or frightened.

Thousands of "Okies" piled belongings on their cars and made their way to California in hopes of starting over. There they joined Mexican migrant farm workers, African American laborers, and others down on their luck hoping for work.

Presidential Responses to the Depression

U ntil the collapse of the economy, President Herbert Hoover's political achievements had earned wide admiration. He seemed the perfect embodiment of the spirit of the prosperous 1920s. But his ideas about politics and economics were ill suited to the crisis of the 1930s. Dissatisfaction with Hoover's response to the Depression gave Franklin Delano Roosevelt a landslide victory in the 1932 presidential election. Promising to take action to ease the nation's suffering, the optimistic Roosevelt seemed to embody hope for an end to the crisis.

Herbert Hoover: Tackling the Crisis

Hoover's first major political achievement came in Europe during World War I, when he headed the Commission for Relief in Belgium. There he organized a massive effort funded by private and government contributions that fed more than 9 million people for nearly five years. Later, he became the U.S. food administrator and headed the American Relief Administration. He earned praise as a visionary progressive for his ability to mobilize volunteer efforts and to find efficient ways to meet people's needs. President Warren Harding then appointed him Secretary of Commerce.

It is no surprise that the popular Republican won the presidency in 1928. But even Hoover worried about "the exaggerated idea the people have conceived of me. They have a conviction that I am a sort of superman, that no problem is beyond my capacity. . . . If some unprecedented calamity should come upon the nation . . . I would be sacrificed to the unreasoning disappointment of a people who expected too much." The unprecedented calamity arrived, and Hoover's predictions were correct.

Had prosperity continued, Hoover might have left a legacy of outstanding leadership. Declaring that "excessive fortunes are a menace to true liberty," he favored steeply graduated inheritance and income taxes on the wealthy, with no tax burden on the poor. He believed that society had a responsibility to care for those in need and that the prosperous should bear much of the burden. After the stock market crash, Hoover increased spending for public works—programs in which the government created jobs for people who needed employment—to the unprecedented sum of $700 million. He established the Reconstruction Finance Corporation to make government credit available to banks and other financial institutions. Seeking to restore confidence in the economy, he strove for a balanced budget by raising taxes and cutting spending—a strategy that underestimated the depth of the Depression and made the situation worse.

As the Depression set in and brought widespread misery, Hoover fully expected that charitable organizations would step in and provide charity to the poor. He believed that government relief to the needy had demoralizing effects on people. In 1931 he pledged that if voluntary and local efforts were unable "to prevent hunger and suffering in my country, I will ask the aid of every resource of the Federal Government." But he had "faith in the American people that such a day [would] never come." Even when it was clear that the crisis was beyond the help of charitable groups, Hoover remained strongly opposed to direct relief for the poor. Private giving did increase to record levels; unfortunately, it was not sufficient.

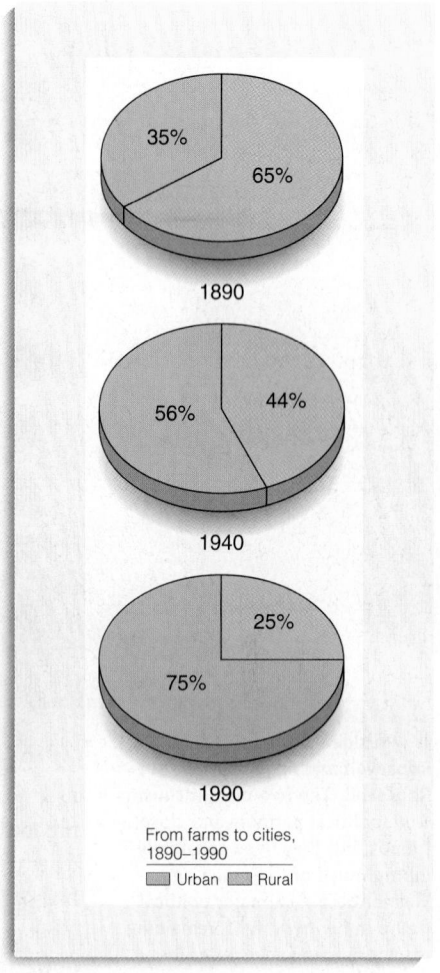

■ **FIGURE 22.1**
URBAN AND RURAL POPULATION, 1890–1990
In the nineteenth century the American population was primarily rural. During the twentieth century, the population became predominantly urban.

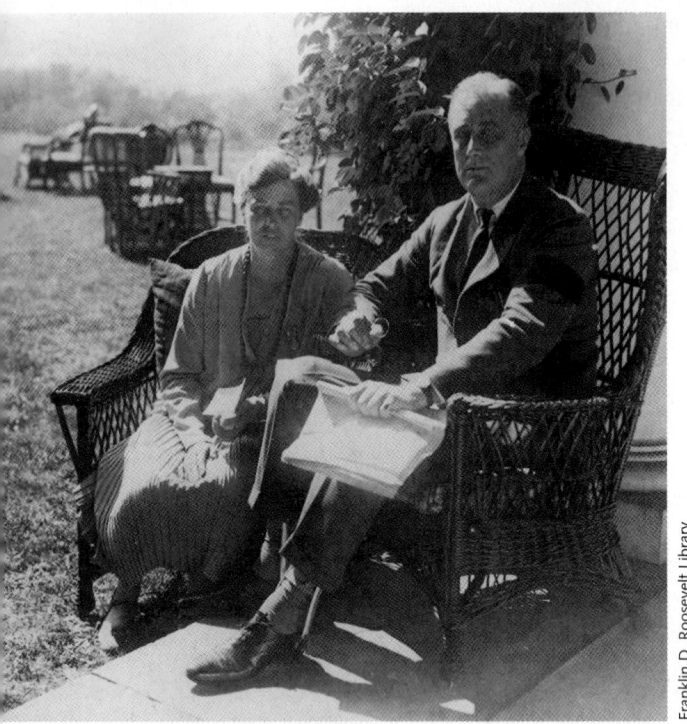

Franklin D. Roosevelt Library

■ **President Franklin Delano Roosevelt and First Lady Eleanor Roosevelt.** The two distant cousins were political partners and close friends, but they lived separately during much of their marriage. Eleanor became a major political figure in her own right, remaining active for many years after the death of her husband.

Hoover felt that giving people the means to make a living was better than offering them direct relief. Thus, for example, he approved a grant of $45 million to feed livestock during the 1930 drought but rejected a proposed grant of $25 million to feed farmers and their families. His logic was consistent: Livestock provided farmers with the means to make a living so they could feed their families. But this philosophy offered little comfort to farmers who watched their families starve as their hogs lapped up food provided by the government.

Hoover's popularity reached its lowest ebb in 1932. A group of World War I veterans in Portland, Oregon, organized a march on Washington D.C. called the Bonus March. The veterans were due to receive a bonus of $1000 each in 1945. The group had asked to have their bonuses early, in 1932, to help ease their suffering during the Depression. But Hoover refused. More than 20,000 veterans traveled to Washington to petition Congress. The House passed a bill to pay the bonus immediately, but the Senate refused to follow suit. The determined veterans set up a tent city and settled in with their families. On the last day of the congressional session, when Hoover again refused to meet with the protesters, the veterans began to leave. But some did not depart quickly enough, and a police officer began shooting at the unarmed demonstrators, killing one person.

Army Chief of Staff Douglas MacArthur stepped in and escalated the violence. His troops used tear gas and bayonets to prod the veterans and their families to vacate the area, then set fire to the tent city. The attack injured more than 100 people and killed one baby. The image of federal troops assaulting a group of peaceful veterans horrified the public. Although MacArthur had ordered the brutality, the public directed its outrage against Hoover. As most people saw it, Hoover had heartlessly spurned the veterans' legitimate request. By the time of the 1932 election, Hoover had lost most of his public support.

Franklin Delano Roosevelt: The Pragmatist

In contrast to Hoover, Franklin Delano Roosevelt was born into a family of wealth and privilege whose ancestors included European aristocrats and passengers on the *Mayflower*. Pampered as a child, at age 14 he went to Groton, the nation's most exclusive boarding school; from there he attended Harvard College and Columbia Law School. In 1905, during his first year at Columbia, he married a distant cousin, Eleanor Roosevelt, the niece of former president Theodore Roosevelt. Like Franklin, Eleanor came from a sheltered, upper-class background. But her early life, unlike his, was filled with sadness. Both her parents died when she was a young child, and at age 10 she went to live with her grandmother, who left her in the care of a harsh governess. The young woman began to flourish when she went abroad to study. The rigorous education developed her strengths and confidence, which would serve her well during her marriage to FDR.

Eleanor bore six children in ten years. A reserved woman raised in the Victorian tradition of sexual reticence, she turned to abstinence to avoid additional pregnancies. In 1918 Eleanor discovered that Franklin was having an affair with her social secretary, Lucy Mercer. Eleanor offered him a divorce, but Franklin promised to end the affair, and the two remained married—although they did not live together. The Roosevelts developed a strong bond of friendship and a deep political alliance. FDR's fondness for Mercer did not end, however. When he was on his deathbed, Eleanor was out of town and Mercer was at his side.

Franklin Roosevelt was elected to the New York State Senate in 1911, and in 1913 he became Assistant Secretary of the Navy. He ran unsuccessfully as the Democratic vice presidential nominee in 1920. His political plans derailed suddenly in 1921 when he was stricken with polio. The painful and incapacitating illness threw the normally ebullient young man into despair. He had always assumed that he would control his own destiny. Now he could no longer use his legs. The formerly athletic Roosevelt depended on braces, crutches, and a wheelchair to move around. But his upbringing had given him extraordinary reserves of self-confidence and optimism, and these qualities helped to sustain him in the face of his paralysis.

FDR's bout with polio and subsequent paralysis did nothing to dampen his political ambitions. He became governor of New York in 1928, following in the footsteps of Theodore Roosevelt. But, unlike his Republican cousin, Franklin was a Democrat. In the 1932 presidential campaign, FDR made few specific proposals, but promised the American people a "New Deal." Although Hoover was intensely unpopular, he had supporters within the Republican party who defended his record and supported his efforts to balance the budget. Along with the Republican incumbent, there were other alternatives on the ballot, notably socialist Norman Thomas and communist William Z. Foster. Polls showed that 5 percent of the electorate favored Thomas, but in the end only half of those, fewer than 1 million voters, actually marked their ballots for Thomas, and a much smaller number for Foster. Many voters on the left cast their ballots for Roosevelt, fearing that a vote for Thomas might throw the election to Hoover. FDR won a landslide victory, the largest electoral margin since 1864.

TABLE 22-1

The Election of 1932

Candidate	Political Party	Popular Vote	Electoral Vote
Franklin D. Roosevelt	Democratic	22,821,857	472
Herbert Hoover	Republican	15,761,841	59
Norman Thomas	Socialist	881,951	0

"Nothing to Fear but Fear Itself"

Like Theodore Roosevelt before him, FDR was committed to strengthening the federal government. But Franklin was less interested in protecting and preserving old-stock Anglo-Saxon Americans from the cultural and demographic impact of immigration than his Republican cousin had been. Lawmakers in the 1920s closed off immigration, silenced dissenters, deported foreign radicals, and suppressed labor insurgency. In contrast, FDR identified the Depression as the nation's enemy rather than particular groups of Americans. His strategy was one of inclusion rather than exclusion; he welcomed the newcomers into his vision of America and cultivated their allegiance. Immigrants from southern and eastern Europe were among FDR's most ardent supporters. Millions of them became naturalized citizens and voted for the first time in the 1930s, overwhelmingly as Democrats.

In his inaugural address, Roosevelt endeavored to ease the nation's anxieties with reassuring words: "Let me assert my firm belief that the only thing we have to fear is fear itself—nameless, unreasoning, unjustified terror which paralyzes needed efforts to convert retreat into advance." Roosevelt launched his advance immediately. Panic had prompted many Americans to pull out their bank savings, causing many banks to fail. To stop the run on banks, FDR called Congress into a special session and announced a "bank holiday," temporarily closing all the nation's banks. He could have nationalized the banking system, a move toward socialism that would likely have received widespread support. But

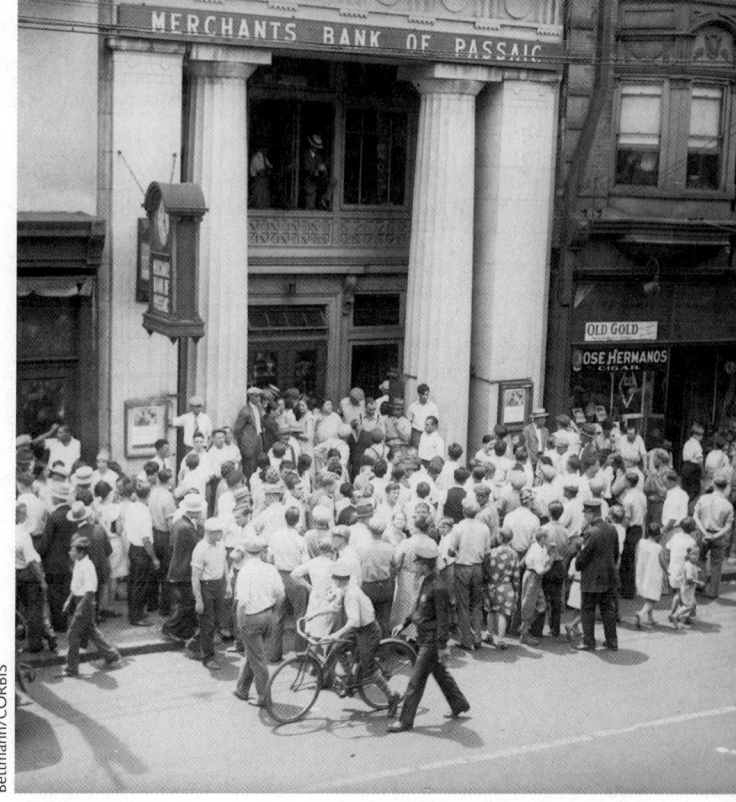

Bettmann/CORBIS

■ Across the country a run on banks depleted cash reserves, so that depositors were unable to withdraw their savings. When a crowd gathered in front of Merchants Bank in Passaic, New Jersey, in 1929, the bank closed its doors.

Presidents and the Media

Franklin Delano Roosevelt was one of several American presidents who used the media and the realm of popular culture to communicate effectively with the public and achieve political goals. Roosevelt broke new media ground with his use of the radio, particularly in his "fireside chats," in which he reassured the people during the Great Depression and explained his New Deal programs in order to gain public support. Before the radio, presidents used their oratorical skills in stump speeches and public declarations. Abraham Lincoln was a gifted orator at a time when political rallies were not only important civic events but also major arenas of popular entertainment. Some of Lincoln's major speeches, including his Gettysburg Address and Second Inaugural, have become part of the national democratic canon.

Theodore Roosevelt used the expanding popular press as a "bully pulpit" to gain public support for his

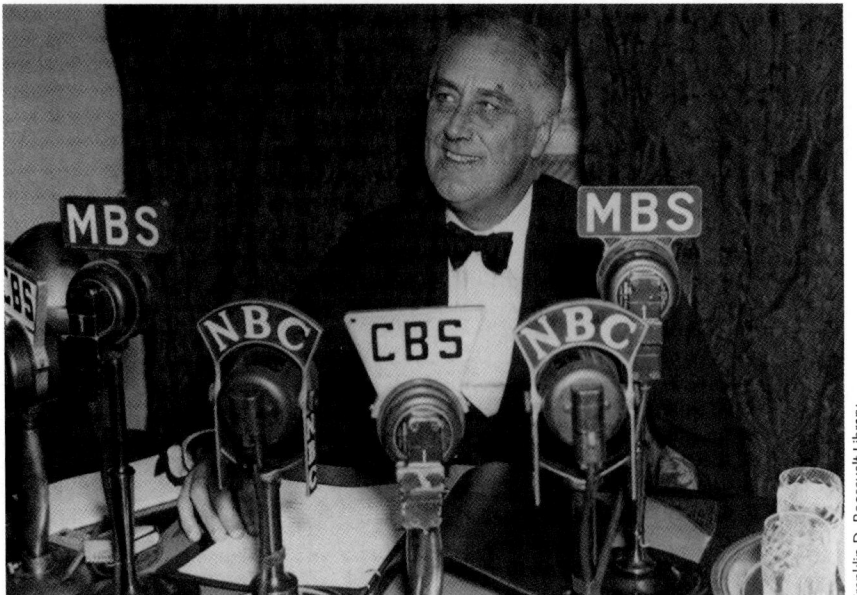

Franklin Delano Roosevelt during a radio broadcast, October 14, 1938. Roosevelt mastered the medium of radio and used it effectively to communicate directly to the people. In what came to be known as "Fireside Chats," Roosevelt addressed his millions of listeners as "my friends."

domestic agenda of progressive reform and "trust busting" of large corporations, as well as for his military exploits abroad. John F. Kennedy took the media presidency to new heights with his effective mastery of television. Kennedy was the first president to inject an element of celebrity stardom into his

media image, projecting an air of charm, grace, and wit. Although some found his media presence arrogant and aggressive, especially in televised debates during the 1960 campaign with his Republican opponent, Richard M. Nixon, he used television effectively throughout his presidency to cast him-

Roosevelt favored government regulation, not government ownership. He proposed the Emergency Banking Bill, providing government support for private banks. Congress passed the bill instantly, to the applause of the bankers who helped draft it.

In the first of his "fireside chats" to millions of radio listeners, whom he addressed as "my friends," Roosevelt assured citizens that the banks that reopened were sound. He used the medium of radio skillfully to explain his policies and to communicate comforting and reassuring messages that reached people in the intimate setting of their homes. The next day, bank deposits exceeded withdrawals as a result of the confidence he inspired.

The New Deal

The New Deal drew on Progressive-era reform impulses to extend the reach of the federal government to solve social problems. It provided assistance to many Americans suffering the effects of the Depression and established the welfare state that would last half a century. Based on pragmatism, experimentation, and shrewd political calculation, FDR's plan began with a flurry of activity in the first 100 days of his administration and developed

self as a tough Cold Warrior, a vigorous athlete (despite serious chronic disabilities), and a devoted family man (despite his adulterous behavior). During tense moments of the Cold War, particularly in the midst of confrontations with the Soviet Union over control of Berlin and missiles in Cuba, he appeared on television to warn the Soviet leadership of his resolve and to rally the nation behind him.

Ronald W. Reagan, known as the "great communicator," was the first professional actor elected to the presidency. His ease in front of the camera and his talent as a communicator allowed him to achieve a personal connection with his audience. Reagan's mastery of the media enabled him to convey his conservative political ideology to the nation and maintain broad-based popular support throughout his presidency. In the 1990s, Bill Clinton went one step further, appearing on talk shows, comedy hours, and MTV, where he played his saxophone, talked about his marital troubles, and answered personal questions about such things as the style of underwear he wore. By the time Clinton became president, the private lives and sexual

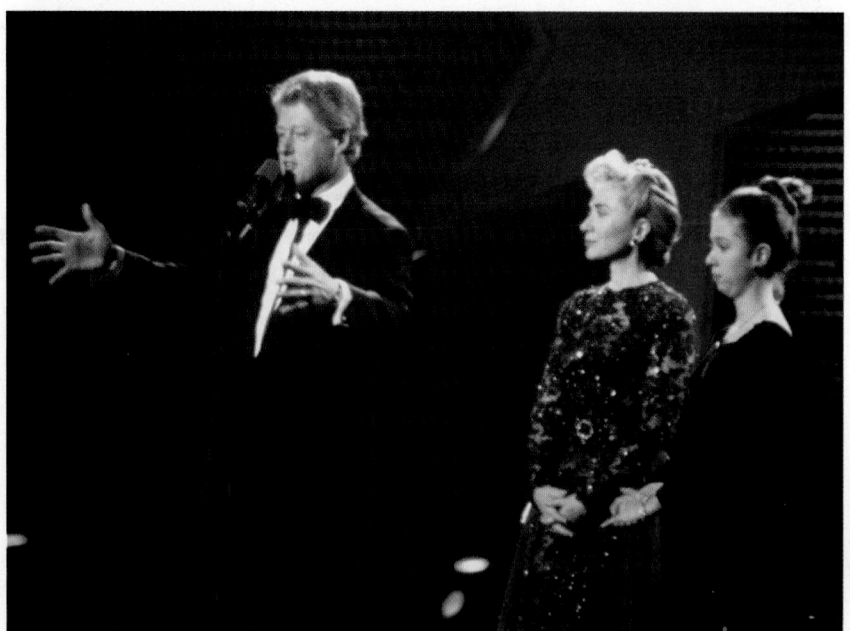

Taking his cues from media celebrities and attempting to appeal to the nation's youth, President Bill Clinton rouses the crowd at the 1993 MTV Rock 'N Roll Inaugural Ball. Political leaders increasingly used the nation's mass media to promote their campaigns and develop a public persona.

behavior of politicians had become fair game for reporters. FDR and JFK had used the media to cultivate their images as strong leaders, while keeping their physical disabilities and their adulterous affairs far from public view. In those years journalistic ethics and etiquette placed the sexual behavior of presidents out of bounds. But all that had changed by the 1990s. The media exposed Clinton's affair with a White House intern, flooding the nation and the world with massive and detailed coverage. ■

into a more progressive agenda by 1935, often called the "second New Deal." New Deal programs countered the cyclical nature of capitalism and offered a safety net for industrial workers. They legitimized labor unions and established a system of regulation and cooperation between industry and labor. Many New Deal programs failed, but those that succeeded created the foundation of the modern American state. The broad-based reform effort, however, did not end the Depression or eradicate poverty.

The First Hundred Days

FDR understood that the people wanted "action, and action now." Roosevelt acted quickly and pragmatically. As one of his first acts, he encouraged Congress to repeal Prohibition. In 1933 the states quickly ratified the Twenty-First Amendment, repealing the Eighteenth. Repeal of Prohibition helped the economy by providing additional tax revenues from liquor sales, since they were now legal, and a market for farmers' corn and wheat, which were used in the production of liquor. Congress created the Securities and Exchange Commission (SEC) to oversee the stock market and the Federal Deposit Insurance Corporation (FDIC) to reform the banking system and provide insurance for deposits.

TABLE 22-2

Key New Deal Legislation, 1933–1938

Year	Act or Agency	Key Provisions
1933	Emergency Banking Act	Reopened banks under government supervision
	Civilian Conservation Corps (CCC)	Employed young men in reforestation, flood control, road construction, and soil erosion control projects
	Federal Emergency Relief Act (FERA)	Provided federal funds for state and local relief efforts
	Agricultural Adjustment Act (AAA)	Granted farmers direct payments for reducing crop production; funds for payment provided by a processing tax, later declared unconstitutional
	Farm Mortgage Act	Provided funds to refinance farm mortgages
	Tennessee Valley Authority (TVA)	Constructed dams and power projects and developed the economy of a seven-state area in the Tennessee River Valley
	Home Owners' Loan Corporation	Provided funds for refinancing home mortgages of nonfarm homeowners
	National Industrial Recovery Act (NIRA)	Established a series of fair competition codes; created National Recovery Administration (NRA) to write, coordinate, and implement these codes; NIRA's Section 7(a) guaranteed labor's right to organize (act later declared unconstitutional)
	Public Works Administration (PWA)	Sought to increase employment and business activity by funding road construction, building construction, and other projects
	Federal Deposit Insurance Corporation (FDIC)	Insured individual bank deposits
	Civil Works Administration (CWA)	Provided federal jobs for the unemployed
1934	Securities and Exchange Act	Created Securities and Exchange Commission (SEC) to regulate trading practices in stocks and bonds according to federal laws
	Indian Reorganization Act	Restored ownership of tribal lands to Native Americans; provided funds for job training and a system of agricultural and industrial credit
	Federal Housing Administration (FHA)	Insured loans provided by banks for the building and repair of houses
1935	Works Progress Administration (WPA)	Employed more than 8 million people to repair roads, build bridges, and work on other projects
	National Youth Administration (NYA)	WPA program that provided job training for unemployed youths and part-time jobs for students in need
	Federal One	WPA program that provided financial assistance for writers, artists, musicians, and actors
	National Labor Relations Act (Wagner Act)	Recognized the right of employees to join labor unions and to bargain collectively, reinstating the provisions of NIRA's Section 7(a); created the National Labor Relations Board (NLRB) to enforce laws against unfair labor practices
	Social Security Act	Created a system of social insurance that included unemployment compensation and old-age survivors' insurance; paid for by a joint tax on employers and employees
1938	Fair Labor Standards Act	Established a minimum wage of 25 cents an hour and a standard work week of 44 hours for businesses engaged in interstate commerce

Roosevelt appointed a cabinet composed of a number of liberals, including Henry A. Wallace of Iowa as Secretary of Agriculture, Harold L. Ickes of Illinois as Secretary of the Interior, and Frances Perkins of New York as Secretary of Labor—the first woman ever appointed to the Cabinet. In addition to his cabinet, FDR appointed several academics to serve as advisors. Known as the Brain Trust, they included Raymond Moley, Adolfe Berle, and Rexford Tugwell of Columbia University; attorney Basil O'Connor; and Felix Frankfurter of Harvard Law School. They helped shape the New Deal into a program of reform that would preserve American capitalism.

One of FDR's most pressing challenges was to prop up prices for producers while keeping them low enough for consumers. Poverty in the midst of plenty was one of the Depression's cruelest ironies. Because farmers could no longer afford to transport their goods to market, food rotted while millions of people went hungry. FDR took action by developing the Farm Relief Act. Included in the Farm Relief Act was the Farm Mortgage Act, which lowered mortgage rates for farmers to help them keep their farms. Also included was the Agricultural Adjustment Act (AAA). In a highly controversial provision of the AAA, the government sought to prop up farm prices by limiting supply. That is, it paid farmers to destroy livestock and take acreage out of production.

Many Americans recoiled at the systematic slaughter of 6 million piglets and the plowing under of 10 million acres of cotton. This policy boosted profits for larger farms but did little to alleviate the problems of smaller, poorer farmers. Sharecroppers and tenant farmers fared even worse. The desperation and pride of rural Americans came through in countless letters to Eleanor Roosevelt. A woman from Winnsboro, Louisiana, pleaded with the First Lady: "I don't want on the relif if I can help it i want to work for my livin byt the last thing we have is gone. . . . Don't you know its aful to have to get out and no place to have a roof over your sick child and nothing to eat I cant tell all my troubles."

Most Americans in need desperately wanted to work. They considered government relief a signal of failure and

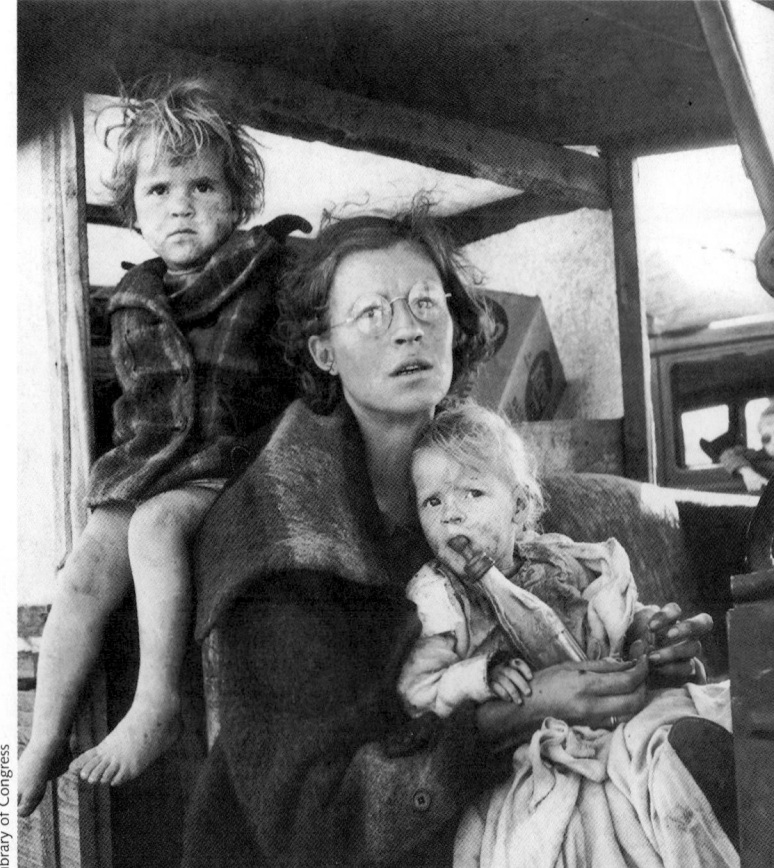

Library of Congress

■ Dorothea Lange took photographs for the Farm Security Administration (FSA) documenting the lives of Depression-era migrants. This 1939 photo, "Mother and Children on the Road, Tulelake, Siskiyou County, California," is one of Lange's many portraits of impoverished families.

a source of deep shame and humiliation. Many citizens searched for ways to preserve their pride. One woman wrote to Eleanor Roosevelt asking to borrow money in order to avoid charity:

> *Please* Mrs. Roosevelt, I do not want charity, only a chance from someone who will trust me. . . . I am sending you two of my dearest possessions to keep as security, a ring my husband gave me before we were married, and a ring my mother used to wear. . . . If you will consider buying the baby clothes, please keep them (rings) until I send you the money you spent. It is very hard to face bearing a baby we cannot afford to have, and the fact that it is due to arrive soon, and still there is no money for the hospital or clothing, does not make it any easier. I have decided to stay home, keeping my 7 year old daughter from school to help with the smaller children when my husband has work. . . . The 7 year old one is a good willing little worker and somehow we must manage—but without charity.

The writer of the letter included a list of items she needed. She concluded with, "If you will get these for me I would rather no one knew about it. I promise to repay the cost . . . as soon as possible."

In March 1933 Congress passed the Federal Emergency Relief Administration (FERA), which provided $500 million in grants to the states for aid to the needy. Roosevelt placed Harry Hopkins in charge. Hopkins, an energetic and brash young reformer, disbursed $2 million during his first two hours on the job. He then persuaded Roosevelt to launch a temporary job program, the Civil Works Administration (CWA). The CWA provided government-sponsored

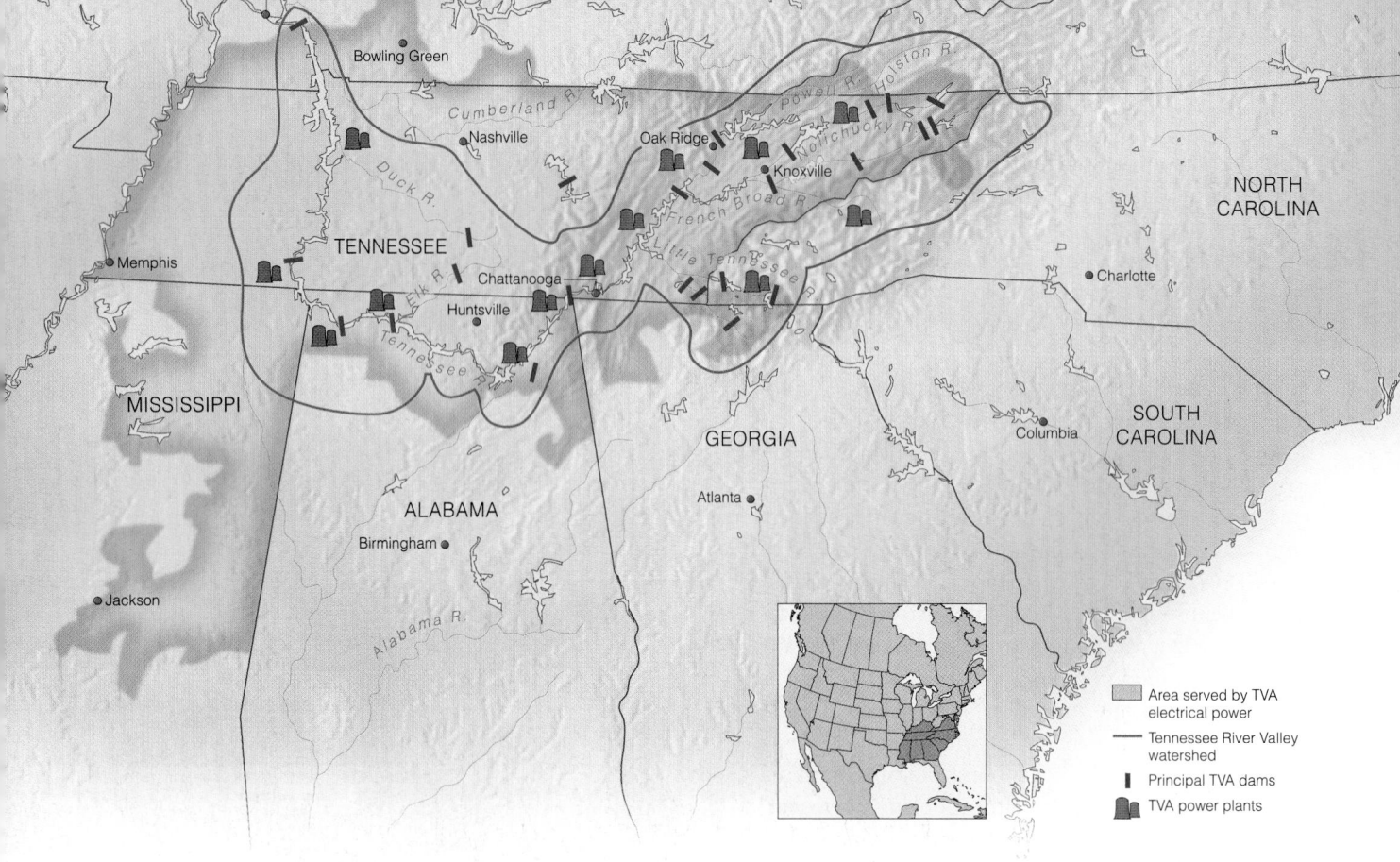

■ **MAP 22.2**
AREAS SERVED BY THE TENNESSEE VALLEY AUTHORITY   The Tennessee Valley Authority (TVA) brought electricity to a large area in western Appalachia, one of the poorest regions in the country. The government-owned project strengthened the economy and improved living conditions in the area.

jobs for more than 4 million workers. But the program came under fire from conservatives, and FDR ended it a few months later.

The New Deal included two major programs that addressed conservation and environmental issues. In 1933, Roosevelt combined his interest in conservation with his goal of providing work for unemployed young men. The Civilian Conservation Corps (CCC) operated under the control of the Army. CCC workers lived in camps, wore uniforms, and conformed to military discipline. They planted millions of trees, dug canals and ditches, built more than 30,000 wilderness shelters, stocked rivers and lakes with nearly 1 billion fish, and preserved historic sites. Their work revived depleted forests and provided flood control. By 1935 the CCC had employed more than 500,000 young men and kept them, in FDR's words, "off the city street corners."

Another measure that linked natural resources to the recovery effort was the Tennessee Valley Authority (TVA). On May 18, 1933, Roosevelt signed into law the Tennessee Valley Authority Act, an experiment in government-owned utilities that brought power to rural areas along the Tennessee River in seven states in western Appalachia—among the poorest areas in the nation. This far-reaching government-owned project offered a radical alternative to American capitalism, based on private enterprise. Under the TVA, the government built five dams, improved twenty others, and constructed power plants; it produced and sold electricity to the valley's farmers and facilitated the development of industry in the region. The TVA also boosted local economies by selling fertilizer and electricity, and by providing flood control, and improving river navigation. Business conservatives and Southern Democratic congressmen opposed the plan because it used government money to provide jobs and electricity to rural African Americans in the Tennessee Valley. Nevertheless, the TVA became one of the largest and cheapest suppliers of power in the nation. Although years later, President Dwight D. Eisenhower condemned the TVA as a New Deal example of "creeping socialism," it was one of Roosevelt's most successful and enduring projects.

The National Industrial Recovery Act (NIRA), passed by Congress in 1933, became the centerpiece of the first New Deal. The NIRA established the National Recovery Administration (NRA) to oversee the regulation of the economy. In his second "fireside chat," Roosevelt called the NRA "a partnership in planning" between business and government. The NRA enabled businesses in each sector of the economy to form trade associations and set their own standards for production, prices, and wages. But in return, businesses had to agree to recognize labor unions. Section 7(a) of the NIRA guaranteed collective bargaining rights to workers, sparking new hope for union organizers.

FDR's first 100 days also included the creation of the Home Owners' Loan Corporation, providing refinancing of home mortgages at low rates. Because the plan helped stem the tide of foreclosures and also guaranteed the repayment of loans, it pleased homeowners, banks, and real-estate interests. It also gained for FDR the support of a large segment of the middle class.

One of the boldest New Dealers was John Collier, whom Roosevelt appointed as Commissioner of Indian Affairs. Collier opposed the policy of land allotment that the Dawes Act of 1887 had enacted. Under allotment, Native American land holdings had dwindled from 130 million acres to 49 million acres—much of it desert. Collier also rejected the assumption that Indians' survival depended on their assimilation into white culture. He altered the government boarding schools' curriculum to include bicultural and bilingual education and eliminated military dress and discipline.

Collier's ideas came to fruition in the 1934 Indian Reorganization Act, which recognized the autonomy of Indian tribes, did away with the allotment program, and appropriated funds to help Indians add to their land holdings. It also provided for job and professional training programs as well as a system of agricultural and industrial credit. In keeping with Collier's goal of Indian self-government, each tribe decided whether to accept the terms of the Indian Reorganization Act. In the end, 181 tribes voted to accept the law, while 77 opted out of it.

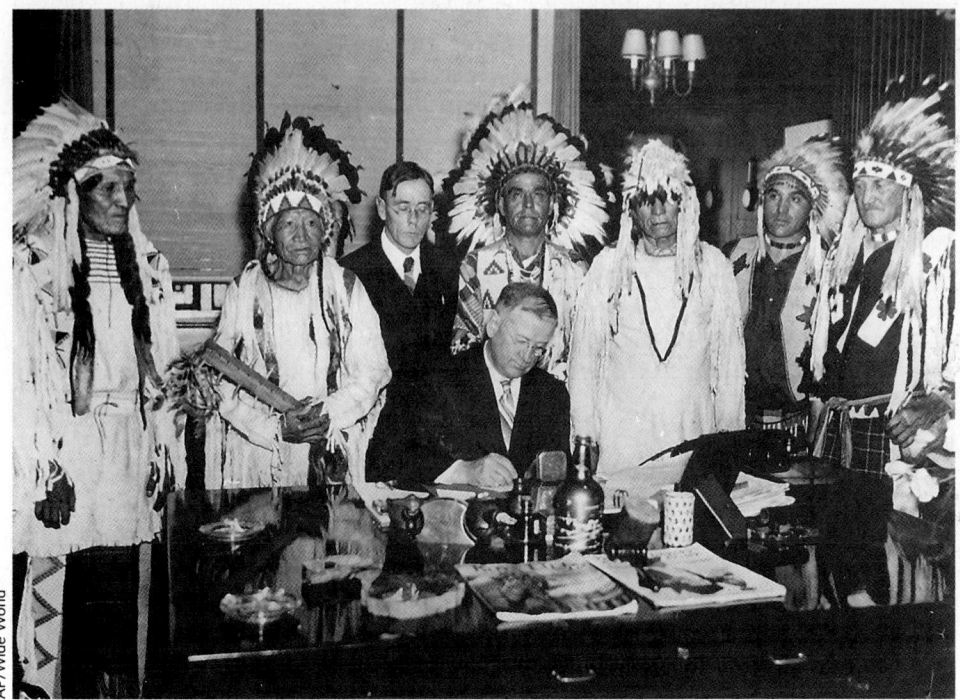

AP/Wide World

■ On October 28, 1935, John Collier, Commissioner of Indian Affairs, stands with a group of Flathead Indian chiefs as Secretary of the Interior Harold L. Ickes signs the first constitution providing for Indian self-rule. Franklin Roosevelt appointed Collier to bring the New Deal to Native Americans.

The Navajos were among the tribes that rejected the Indian Reorganization Act. Many Navajos perceived Collier as yet another heavy-handed government agent. This tension heightened during an environmental conflict over Navajo herding rights. Convinced that the Navajos were herding far more sheep and goats than the fragile desert ecosystem could support, Collier proposed a plan by which the federal government would purchase 400,000 head of Navajo livestock. Although Collier had been more receptive to Indian concerns than almost any other federal authority who had preceded him, he could not reconcile the conflicting interests of tribal autonomy, environmentalism, and development.

Protest and Pressure from the Left and the Right

Challenges to Roosevelt's New Deal took many forms. In spite of FDR's efforts to help businesses survive and remain profitable during the Depression, many business leaders continued to oppose the New Deal, charging that FDR was a dictator and that his program amounted to socialism. At the same time, FDR faced criticism from the left. Many people believed that Roosevelt's policies did not go far enough to ease the suffering caused by the economic crisis. Some thought that New Deal policies aimed at bolstering capitalism were ill-advised, and that capitalism itself was the problem. Disenchantment with capitalism drew many Americans to the cause of socialism and swelled the ranks of the Communist party.

The Communist party drew its inspiration from the Soviet Union and, during the 1930s, developed a strategy known as the Popular Front to build alliances with sympathetic American liberals. Not all liberals belonged to the Popular Front, but many people with progressive political leanings shared with the socialists and the Communist party a commitment to economic justice, unemployment relief, civil rights, and union organizing. The actual membership of the Communist Party remained small—it peaked at 100,000 during World War II when the United States and the Soviet Union were allies—but its influence increased during the Depression.

By 1934 and 1935 much of the pressure on Roosevelt came from workers, whose hopes that the NIRA would guarantee collective bargaining rights were dashed by the intransigence of employers. The 1920s had taken a toll on labor unions. Membership had declined from a high of 5 million in 1920 to 2 million by 1933. But workers continued to strike for improved wages and working conditions. In 1934 nearly 1.5 million workers participated in 1800 strikes. Often, unemployed laborers joined picket lines, refusing to work as strikebreakers.

Many people believed that Roosevelt's policies did not go far enough to ease the suffering caused by the economic crisis.

Workers all over the country organized for better working conditions. Birmingham, Alabama, provides an apt example. The Depression hit Birmingham early and hard. By 1928, unemployment had reached 18 percent. Many impoverished black steelworkers, along with farm laborers in the surrounding countryside, joined the "invisible army" of the Communist party. Together, they fought for better working conditions and racial justice. One young black coal miner, Angelo Herndon, recalled the dangers of organizing and the need for secrecy: "With our few pennies that we collected we ground out leaflets on an old rickety mimeograph machine, which we kept concealed in the home of one of our workers. We were obliged to work very quietly, like the Abolitionists in the South during the Civil War, behind drawn shades and locked doors." Although most African Americans supported FDR and the Democratic party during the Depression, between 3000 and 4000 members of Birmingham's black community joined the Communist party and related organizations during the 1930s.

Mexican laborers in California launched similar efforts. They faced not only persistent exploitation in fields and factories but also the constant threat of deportation. During the Depression, approximately one-third of the Mexican population in the United States—more than half a million people—was deported to Mexico, even though the majority were native-born citizens. Some of those who remained organized unions and struck for better pay and working conditions. During 1933, agricultural workers mounted 37 major strikes in California alone. They scored a number of successes; more than half of the conflicts led to wage increases.

Dorothy Ray was only 16 years old when she began organizing Mexican workers at the grass-roots level in California. She found it particularly rewarding to witness "the diminishing of bigotry . . . watching all those Okies and Arkies . . . all their lives they'd been on a little farm in Oklahoma; probably they had never seen a Black or a Mexicano. And you'd watch in the process of a strike how those white workers soon saw that those white cops were their enemies and that the Black and Chicano workers were their brothers." Another successful effort at biracial organizing occurred in the Arkansas delta in 1934. The Southern Tenant Farmers' Union (STFU) brought together black and white tenants and sharecroppers to fight for better working conditions.

In addition to the communists, socialists, labor unions, and grassroots organizations that sprang up all over the country, a number of individuals proposed alternatives to Roosevelt's program and gained large followings. The most influential of these were Dr. Francis Townsend, Father Charles E. Coughlin, and Senator Huey P. Long. In 1934, Townsend, a retired physician and health commissioner from Long Beach, California, introduced an idea for a pension plan that sparked a nationwide grassroots movement. Townsend proposed a 2 percent national sales tax that would fund a pension of $200 a month for Americans over age 60. The "Townsend Plan" became hugely popular, especially among elderly Americans. In 1936, a national survey indicated that half of all Americans favored the plan. Though the plan was never implemented, the groundswell of support that it generated probably hastened the development and passage of the old age insurance system contained in the 1935 Social Security Act.

Coughlin also inspired a huge following. A Catholic priest from Canada, he served as pastor of a small church outside Detroit, Michigan. He began to broadcast his sermons on the radio, using his magnetic personality to address political as well as religious issues. Soon he became a media phenomenon, broadcasting through 26 radio stations to an audience estimated at 40 million. The "Radio Priest" called for a redistribution of wealth and attacked Wall Street, international bankers, and the evils of capitalism. When a Minnesota radio station polled listeners to see whether they wanted to hear Coughlin's program, 137,000 said yes. Only 400 said no.

Initially, Coughlin strongly supported Franklin Roosevelt and the New Deal. But he soon grew impatient with what he considered the slow pace of New Deal reforms. In 1934, Coughlin launched his own political party, the National Union for Social Justice, which he used to challenge Roosevelt's leadership. The activist priest promoted a populist message that was hostile to both capitalism and communism. He told his radio listeners, "I call upon every one of you who is weary of drinking the bitter vinegar of sordid capitalism and upon everyone who is fearsome of being nailed to the cross of communism to join this Union which, if it is to succeed, must rise above the concept of an audience and become a living, vibrant, united, active organization, superior to politics and politicians in principle, and independent of them in power." Soon, his message turned from social justice populism to right-wing bigotry. His

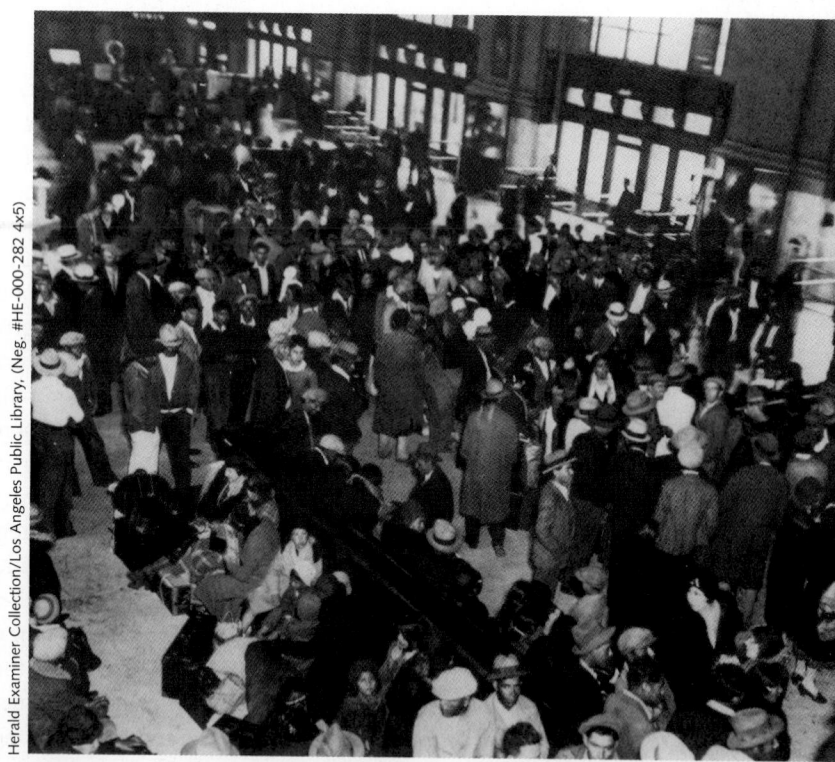

Herald Examiner Collection/Los Angeles Public Library, (Neg. #HE-000-282 4x5)

■ High rates of unemployment and fierce competition for jobs prompted government officials to deport more than half a million people of Mexican descent. In this 1932 photo Mexicans and Mexican Americans line up in Los Angeles for deportation to Mexico.

virulent anti-Semitism and admiration for the fascist regimes of Adolf Hitler in Germany and Benito Mussolini in Italy drove away many of his followers. By 1940, Coughlin had ceased broadcasting and abandoned all political activities, under orders of the Catholic Church.

Huey P. Long was among the most powerful, and colorful, politicians of the era. He rose from modest origins to become a lawyer and a public service commissioner. In 1928, Long won the governorship of Louisiana. His progressive leadership inspired tremendous loyalty, especially among poor workers and farmers. He did more for the underprivileged people of Louisiana than any other governor. He expanded the state's infrastructure; developed social services; built roads, hospitals, and schools; and changed the tax code to place a greater burden on corporations and the wealthy. He proved unique among Southern politicians in that his public statements were free of racial slurs. But he also trampled the democratic process. His ambition had no bounds, and he used any means to accumulate power. Through his tremendous popular appeal, Long developed a massive power base and eventually gained control of Louisiana's legislature, courts, state bureaucracies, and even local governments.

In 1932 Long resigned the governorship and won election to the U.S. Senate. Soon, he gained a huge national following. Initially he supported FDR, but by 1933 he had broken with the president and forged his own political movement based on his Share-Our-Wealth Plan. Giving voice to the resentments many Americans felt toward "wealthy plutocrats," Long advocated a radi-

> *Huey P. Long was among the most powerful, and colorful, politicians of the era.*

cal redistribution of the nation's wealth. He called for new taxes on the wealthy and proposed to use the funds to guarantee a minimum annual income of $2500 for all those in need. As he put it, "How many men ever went to a barbecue and would let one man take off the table what was intended for nine-tenths of the people to eat? The only way you'll ever be able to feed the balance of the people is to make that man come back and bring back some of the grub he ain't got no business with." Long's plainspoken radicalism won the hearts of his followers, including Will Rogers, who publicly urged FDR to back Long's proposals. However, many of his congressional colleagues considered him an agitator. Such skepticism did little to limit Long's ambition, and by 1935 he was planning to challenge FDR in the next presidential election. But he never had the chance. In September 1935 the son-in-law of one of his vanquished political opponents assassinated him.

Other challenges took the form of viable third parties. In Wisconsin, the legacy of Progressive senator Robert M. LaFollette was alive and well, particularly in the political popularity of his two sons, Senator Bob and Governor Phil. In 1934, the brothers formed the Wisconsin Progressive party, which supported the New Deal but pulled it strongly to the left. The state's voters endorsed the radical rhetoric of the LaFollette brothers, reelecting them on the Progressive party ticket with overwhelming victories over their Democratic party rivals.

Meanwhile in neighboring Minnesota, a coalition of workers and farmers formed the Minnesota Farmer–Labor party. In 1930 populist Floyd Olson became the nation's first Farmer–Labor governor. At the party's 1934 convention Olson made his position clear: "I am not a liberal. I enjoy working on a common basis with liberals for their platforms, etc., but I am not a liberal. I am what I want to be—I am a radical. I am a radical in the sense that I want a definite change in the system, I am not satisfied with tinkering, I am not satisfied with patching, I am not satisfied with hanging a laurel wreath upon burglars and thieves and pirates and calling them code authorities or something else." Olson considered the possibility of a third-party bid for the presidency in 1936, but his plans never reached fruition. He contracted cancer and died in August 1936 at age 44.

On the West Coast, discontented voters mounted a similar challenge to party-politics-as-usual. Some Democrats persuaded Upton Sinclair, a veteran socialist and author of the 1906 muckraking novel *The Jungle,* to run for governor on their ticket in 1934. Sinclair ran on his End Poverty in California (EPIC) plan, which would have let the state take over idle land and factories and permit unemployed laborers to use them for their own needs. Sinclair won the

Democratic primary with an overwhelming majority. But Democratic party regulars, including FDR, refused to support his candidacy. Without the support of his own party and facing opposition from wealthy Republicans who spared no expense to defeat him, Sinclair lost the election. Nevertheless, Sinclair's tremendous popularity signaled to Roosevelt that if he hoped to retain the support of his constituents, he would need to move significantly to the left.

Eleanor Roosevelt also pushed FDR to the left, particularly on the issue of civil rights. A political activist in her own right and the most powerful First Lady until Hillary Clinton entered the White House in 1992, Eleanor was among FDR's closest advisors. Although FDR was reluctant to support an anti-lynching bill in Congress for fear of alienating Southern white voters, the First Lady campaigned vigorously against lynching. When the Daughters of the American Revolution (DAR) denied the African American opera star Marian Anderson the right to perform at Constitution Hall in Washington, D.C., Eleanor promptly resigned from the DAR in protest and arranged for Anderson to perform at the Lincoln Memorial on Easter Sunday 1939, where a huge audience stood in the cold to hear her sing.

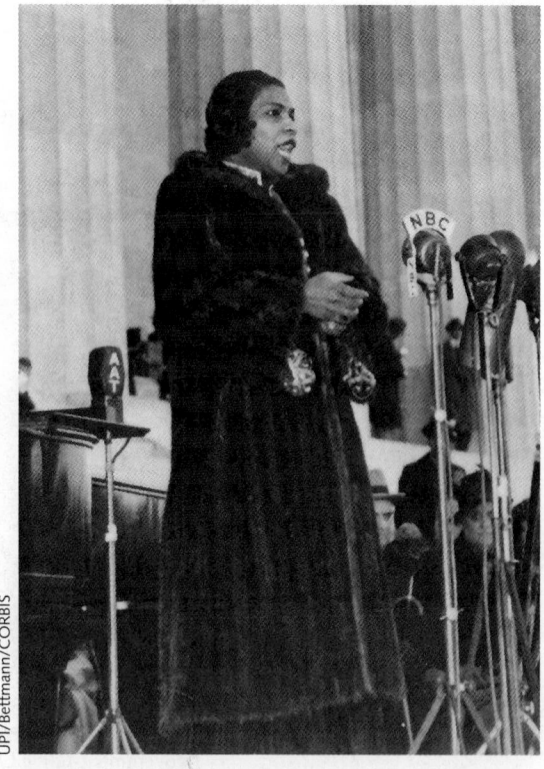

UPI/Bettmann/CORBIS

■ African American contralto Marian Anderson sings on the steps of the Lincoln Memorial on April 9, 1939. Eleanor Roosevelt arranged the concert after the DAR refused to allow Anderson to sing in Constitution Hall. The event attracted an audience of 75,000, and millions listened on the radio.

The Second New Deal

Eleanor Roosevelt's efforts notwithstanding, FDR tread softly on the issue of race. He knew that Southern blacks were disenfranchised, but he depended on Southern white voters to be reelected and to get his New Deal measures through Congress. So he was careful not to alienate Southern Democrats by cultivating African American voters. However, he did reach out to industrial workers. In the spring of 1935, Congress passed the National Labor Relations Act, also known as the Wagner Act, which strengthened and guaranteed collective bargaining and gave a huge boost to labor unions.

Also in 1935, Congress passed the Social Security Act, perhaps the most important and far-reaching of all the New Deal's programs. The Act established a system of old-age pensions, unemployment insurance, and welfare benefits for dependent children and the disabled. The framework of the Social Security Administration shaped the welfare system for the remainder of the century. The welfare state established by the Social Security Act, extensive as it was, did not reach all Americans and left out many of the most needy. It also established a two-track system of welfare. One track provided workers with unemployment insurance and support in their old age. Programs like Social Security, designed primarily for male wage earners, paid retired workers, based on a percentage of the wages they earned while in the workforce. Social Security provided an important safety net for large numbers of workers and the elderly, but it did not cover domestics, seasonal or part-time workers, agricultural laborers, or housewives. The other track made matching funds available to states to provide relief for the needy, mostly dependent women and children with no means of support. Unlike Social Security, which was provided to all retired workers regardless of their circumstances, relief programs, which came to be known as "welfare," were administered according to need.

The architects of this welfare system included top New Deal advisors, many of them women who had been active reformers, such as Eleanor Roosevelt. These advocates hoped to protect women and children from the destitution that almost certainly resulted if a male breadwinner lost his job, deserted his family, or died. The system presumed that a man ordinarily earned a "family wage" that let him support his wife and children and that women were necessarily economically dependent on men. Thus, a deeply entrenched gender system prevailed

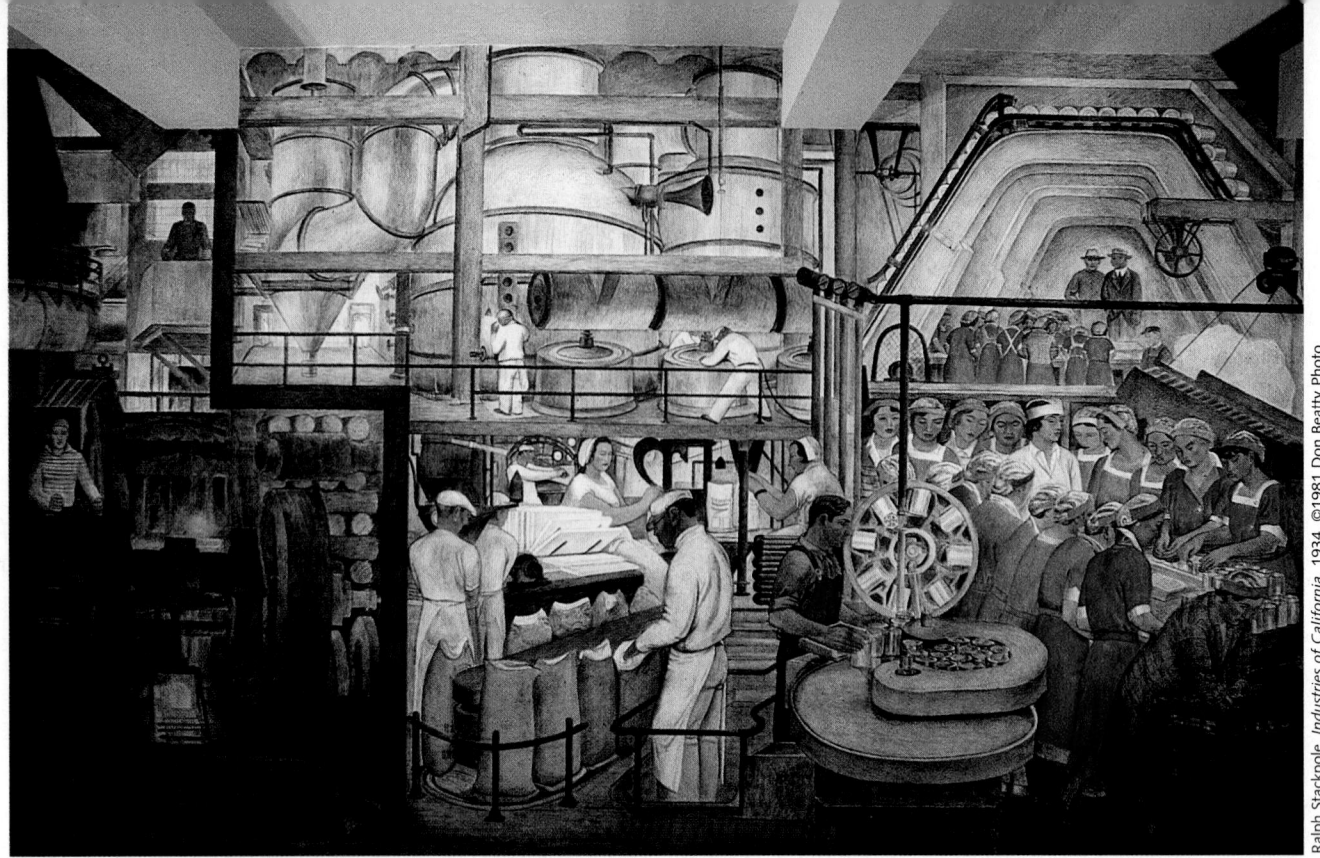

■ In this mural on San Francisco's Coit Tower, "Industries of California," Works Projects Administration (WPA) artist Ralph Stackpole depicts the city's diverse workforce. Across the country, government-funded artists created works of public art that portrayed life in local communities.

through the 1930s. As a result, some—though not all—male breadwinners received benefits like Social Security. Impoverished women and children, on the other hand, received public charity. These payments were usually meager, not enough to lift a woman and her children out of poverty. Inadequate welfare payments never helped the needy become self-sufficient and did nothing to eradicate poverty.

Because there were no nationally established guidelines on how to distribute welfare funds, states could determine who received assistance. As a result, the Social Security Act did little to assist African Americans, especially in the South, where black women were deliberately excluded by local authorities who preferred to maintain a pool of cheap African American labor rather than to provide relief for black families. One Southern public assistance field supervisor, explaining the low numbers of African American families on the welfare rolls, articulated the prevailing attitude: "The number of Negro cases is few due to the unanimous feeling on the part of the staff and board that there are more work opportunities for Negro women and to their intense desire not to interfere with local labor conditions. The attitude that they have always gotten along, and that 'all they'll do is have more children' is definite. . . . There is hesitancy on the part of lay boards to advance too rapidly over the thinking of their own communities, which see no reason why the employable Negro mother should not continue her usually sketchy seasonal labor or indefinite domestic service rather than receive a public assistance grant."

In 1935 Congress allocated the huge sum of nearly $5 billion for the Emergency Relief Appropriation. Roosevelt used a significant portion of the money to expand his public works program. By executive order he established the Works Progress Administration (WPA), which provided millions of jobs for the unemployed. The project mandated that WPA jobs would make a contribution to public life and would not compete with private business. The jobs included building streets, highways, bridges, and public buildings; restoring forests; clearing slums; and extending electricity to rural areas. The WPA National Youth Administration gave work to nearly 1 million students.

The wages paid to WPA workers proved pitifully low. And like most other New Deal programs, the WPA left out the most needy. It provided work only to those already on the relief rolls, and just one person per family could hold a WPA job. This policy ruled out most women as well as older children. It also neglected the vast majority of the unemployed who were not on relief. A 1937 letter to Harry Hopkins from the Workers' Council of Colored People in Raleigh, North Carolina, pointed to the failure of the WPA to provide jobs for black women. The writer explained that the wages paid to domestic and farm laborers were so low that, even if they worked 14-hour days, they could not pay their rent. "If we cannot work on WPA Projects & be compel to take these poor paying jobs; [we request] that food, clothes & rent money be provided for us at once because we are suffering. We the Workers Council understood that no colored women [can] be hired this winter on any of the WPA projects. We wish you to tell us why."

The most effective WPA program was Federal One, which provided financial support for writers, musicians, artists, and actors. The Federal Theater Project, under the direction of Hallie Flanagan, former head of Vassar College's Experimental Theater, shaped the project into an arena for experimental community-based theater. Flanagan focused on contemporary issues and developed such innovations as the "Living Newspaper." The Federal Theater Project included 16 black theater units. Their most notable production was an all-black version of *Macbeth* set in Haiti and staged in Harlem.

Federal One supported thousands of artists and brought the arts to a wide public audience through government-funded murals on public buildings, community-theater productions, local orchestras, and the like. By the late 1930s the program came under political attack for supporting artists who expressed leftist sensibilities, and Congress cut off its funding. In 1943 the WPA was dissolved.

The New Deal did not reach everyone. Programs were geared toward full-time industrial workers, most of whom were white men. Domestic workers, Mexican migrant laborers, black and white sharecroppers, Chinese and Japanese truck farmers—all were among those ineligible for Social Security, minimum wages and maximum hours, unemployment insurance, and other New Deal benefits. But the New Deal established the national welfare state and provided assistance and security to millions of working people along with disabled, dependent, and elderly Americans. Such sweeping programs also solidified Roosevelt's popularity among the poor, workers, and much of the middle class.

FDR's Second Term

In the 1936 campaign FDR claimed that the election was a battle between "the millions who never had a chance" and "organized money." He boasted that the "forces of selfishness and of lust for power" had united against him: "They are unanimous in their *hate* for *me—and I welcome their hatred.*" His strategy paid off. Roosevelt won the election by a landslide of more than 60 percent of the popular vote. Six million more voters cast ballots than had done so in 1932, and 5 million of those new votes went to Roosevelt. His strongest support came from the lower ends of the socioeconomic scale. The election also swept Democrats into Congress, giving them a decisive majority in both the House and the Senate.

With such a powerful mandate, Roosevelt was well positioned to promote a new legislative program. As his first major effort, he took on the Supreme Court. Dominated by conservative justices, the court had invalidated some major legislation of Roosevelt's first term, including the AAA and the NIRA. Roosevelt feared that the justices would unravel the New Deal by striking down its progressive elements. To shift the

TABLE 22-3			
The Election of 1936			
Candidate	Political Party	Popular Vote	Electoral Vote
Franklin D. Roosevelt	Democratic	27,751,597	523
Alfred M. Landon	Republican	16,679,583	8
William Lemke	Union	882,479	0

balance of power on the court, he proposed a measure that would let the president appoint one new justice for every one on the court who had at least 10 years of service and who did not retire within six months after turning 70.

Emboldened by his landslide victory, FDR believed that he could persuade Congress and the nation to go along with any plan he put forward, but he was mistaken. Many viewed his "court packing" plan as a threat to the fundamental separation of powers and feared that it would set a dangerous precedent. Some considered it an affront to the more aged justices, such as the respected liberal Lewis Brandeis, a man in his eighties. Powerful Republicans in Congress forged an alliance with conservative Democrats, mostly from the South, to defeat the plan. This informal alliance dominated Congress for the following two decades. The court blunder cost Roosevelt considerable political capital and empowered his opponents. In the end, his plan proved unnecessary anyway. The court did not undercut the New Deal. Within the next few years Roosevelt succeeded in appointing several new justices who tipped the balance in his favor.

A New Political Culture

FDR continued to face strong opposition from conservatives on the right and radicals, communists, and socialists on the left. But his political fortunes benefited from the emergence of a new and more inclusive national culture. This new Americanism emanated from the working class and found expression in the labor movement, the popular culture, and the political coalition that came together in the Democratic party. These nationalizing forces cut across lines of class and region and occasionally challenged hierarchies of gender and race.

The Labor Movement

The labor insurgency that erupted during the early years of the New Deal demonstrated the need for a new national labor movement. The American Federation of Labor (AFL), restricted to skilled workers, left out most of the nation's less skilled industrial laborers. John L. Lewis of the United Mine Workers (UMW) rose to meet these laborers' need for new leadership. Lewis was one of several union leaders from a number of industries—including mining, steel, rubber, and automobile—who left the AFL to form a new and more broad-based labor organization, the Congress of Industrial Organizations (CIO). Lewis played a key role in the organization's growth into a national force, but the impetus came from the workers themselves.

Sidney Hillman, leader of the Amalgamated Clothing Workers of America, was among the labor leaders who organized the CIO. Hillman had a broad vision of labor unions working with management and government to achieve a strong economy and social justice. Under his leadership, the Amalgamated provided its members with education, subsidized housing, health care, and unemployment insurance long before the New Deal incorporated these programs into national policy. His economic ideas were also in keeping with New Deal efforts to pump money into the hands of consumers. Known as Keynesian economics, named after John Maynard Keynes, this strategy promoted increased spending to stimulate economic recovery.

Hillman argued that higher wages were good for the economy because workers would then be able to purchase consumer products, benefiting industry as well as workers. Although Henry Ford also understood that principle (see Chapter 19), Ford was vehemently anti-union. Hillman argued that powerful unions could help to strengthen and regulate the economy and avoid devastating wage wars. Hillman's leadership in the labor movement brought him into the Roosevelt administration, where he served as Associate Director of the Office of Production Management and became a major political force.

The CIO's first major action came in 1936 in Akron, Ohio, where workers in the rubber industry had organized a "sit-down strike," a new strategy whereby laborers stopped work and simply sat down, shutting down production and occupying plants so that strike-breakers could not enter and take their jobs. Sit-down strikes became a prominent labor tactic during 1936 when 48 strikes broke out across the nation. The numbers shot up the following year to about 500 strikes that lasted more than one day. March 1937 alone witnessed 170 sit-down strikes that affected about 170,000 workers. Striking workers expressed their enthusiasm for the tactic in song:

> When they tie the can to a union man,
>   sit down! Sit down!
> When they give him the sack, they'll
>   take him back, sit down! Sit down!
> When the speed up comes, just twiddle
>   your thumbs, sit down! Sit down!
> When the boss won't talk, don't take a
>   walk, sit down! Sit down!

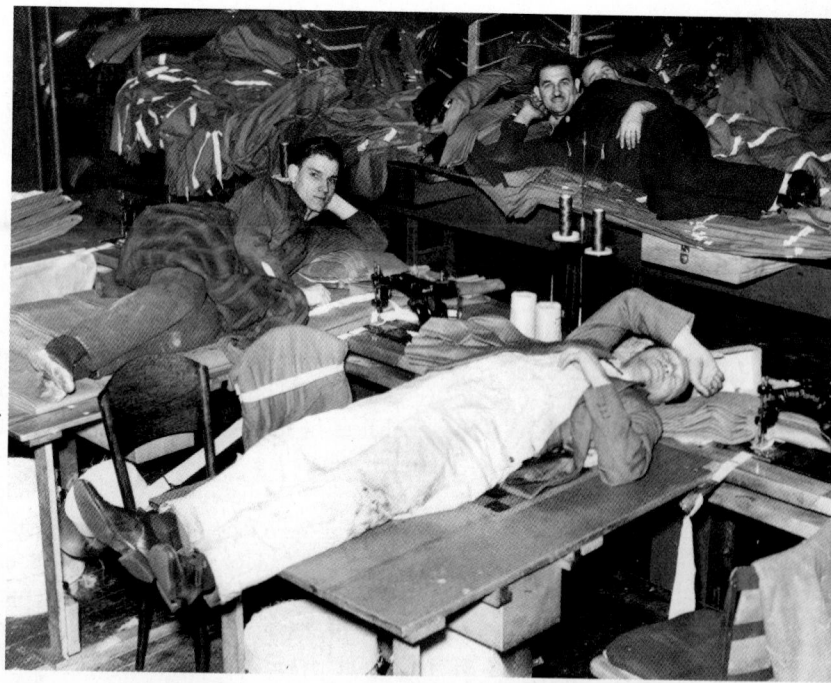

Courtesy, The Wayne State University Archives

■ These sit-down strikers at the Dodge Main plant in Hamtramck, Michigan, slept on their sewing tables while occupying the factory, shutting down production. The sit-down strike became an effective form of labor protest during the 1930s.

The most powerful demonstration of workers' discontent came in the automobile industry, where speed-ups of the assembly line drove workers to rebellion. Charlie Chaplin's poignant film *Modern Times* (1936) expressed workers' frustration at being treated as little more than cogs in machines. "Where you used to be a man," lamented one auto worker, "now you are less than their cheapest tool." In 1936 a spontaneous strike erupted against General Motors in Atlanta; it soon spread to Kansas City, Missouri; Cleveland, Ohio; and the main plants at Flint, Michigan. Two weeks into the strike, workers clashed with police. Frank Murphy, Michigan's prolabor governor, refused to use National Guard troops against the strikers, and Roosevelt declined to send in federal troops. John L. Lewis negotiated on behalf of the workers, who demanded recognition of their union.

Women as well as men participated actively in the Flint strike. Twenty-three-year-old Genora Johnson Dollinger, wife of a striker and mother of two young sons, organized 500 women into the Women's Emergency Brigade, made up primarily of strikers' wives, sisters, and girlfriends. Wearing red berets and armbands, they ran soup kitchens and first-aid stations. They also entered the fray when necessary, as when they broke plant windows so that the company could not use tear gas effectively against the strikers inside. Dollinger arranged a children's picket line as well, in which her two-year-old carried a sign that read, "My daddy strikes for us little tykes." Reflecting on the Women's Emergency Brigade after the strike, Dollinger wrote, "It's a measure of the strength of those women of the Red Berets that they could perform so courageously in an atmosphere that was often hostile to them. We organized on our own without the benefit of professional leadership, and yet, we played a role, second to none, in the birth of a union and in changing working families' lives forever."

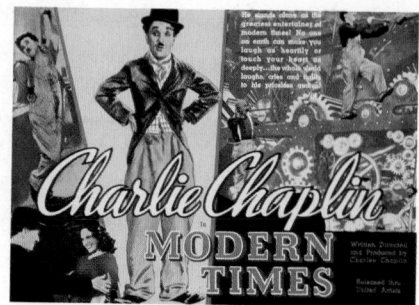

The sit-down strike at Flint lasted 44 days and forced General Motors to recognize the United Auto Workers (UAW), which was a CIO union. The strike scored a clear victory for the workers and boosted the CIO's stature as a national union of industrial workers. Membership in the UAW quadrupled in the next year. Bowing to the formidable power of the national union in the wake of the UAW success, U.S. Steel surrendered to the CIO even without a strike, ending its policy of hiring nonunion workers and signing an agreement with the Steel Workers' Organizing Committee. The CIO brought together workers from all over the country. Most of its member unions were open to racial and ethnic minorities and women.

The New Deal Coalition

FDR's support of labor unions brought workers solidly into the Democratic fold. They joined a coalition that included voters who had never before belonged to the same party, particularly Northern blacks and Southern whites. Although African Americans in the South were disenfranchised, blacks in the North had voted Republican for 60 years, loyal to the party of Lincoln. In a dramatic shift, black voters in Northern cities overwhelmingly backed FDR in 1936 and remained in the Democratic party for the rest of the century.

FDR continued to cater to powerful Southern congressmen and Southern white voters. Nevertheless, he made some gestures on behalf of African Americans and put civil rights measures on the liberal agenda for the first time since Reconstruction. In May 1935 FDR issued Executive Order 7046, banning discrimination in WPA projects. By the late 1930s, 15 to 20 percent of those with WPA jobs were black. Although the pay was meager—$12 a week—it was double what many blacks had been able to earn previously. In spite of FDR's lukewarm support for civil rights, African Americans in the North benefited from New Deal programs. As one black preacher exhorted his congregation prior to the 1936 election, "Let Jesus lead you and Roosevelt feed you."

Other racial and ethnic minorities also joined the New Deal coalition. In 1939, Latinos organized their first national civil rights assembly, El Congreso de Pueblos de Habla Española—the Spanish-Speaking People's Congress, which opened with a congratulatory telegram from Eleanor Roosevelt. Immigrants from Europe and their children also became loyal Democratic voters.

In spite of this diverse coalition, many Americans remained bitterly opposed to FDR. Socialists and communists criticized the New Deal for patching up capitalism rather than transforming the economic system. Conservative business leaders despised Roosevelt for the constraints he placed on business and the intrusion of the government into the economy. Critics from the political right considered the New Deal to be akin to communism. In 1938, Congress created the House Un-American Activities Committee (HUAC), chaired by Martin Dies of Texas. Formed ostensibly to investigate American fascists and Nazis in the United States, the Committee instead pursued liberal and leftist groups throughout World War II and the Cold War.

A New Americanism

The New Deal coalition reflected not only Roosevelt's popularity but also a new and more inclusive American identity. An expanding mass culture fostered this sensibility, spread largely through the national media. It is no accident that Franklin Roosevelt found his way into the homes and hearts of Americans through his "fireside chats" over the radio; his mastery of that technology made him the first media-savvy president. During the 1930s, 70 percent of all households owned a radio—more than owned a telephone. The motion-picture industry also expanded into small towns across the country. Many of the ostentatious movie palaces of the 1920s disappeared, replaced by smaller theaters designed in the sleek modern style of the times, often decorated with murals painted by WPA artists that depicted local scenes and histories. Talking films brought vernacular speech and a variety of accents to diverse audiences who gathered in neighborhood theaters.

Movie plots portrayed the triumph of common people over the rich and powerful and celebrated love across class and ethnic lines. Although racial stereotypes persisted in motion pictures throughout the decade, notable exceptions, such as Will Rogers's films, featured strong minority characters. Popular movies also challenged traditional gender and class hierarchies. Female stars, such as Katharine Hepburn, Rosalind Russell, Bette Davis, and Mae West, portrayed feisty, independent women. Even gangsters appeared as sympathetic characters whose illegal activities seemed somehow justified by the corrupt system they tried to thwart.

New sports celebrities also embodied the nation's diversity. Baseball star Joe DiMaggio, son of an Italian immigrant fisherman, became a national hero. African American boxer Joe Louis, the "Brown Bomber" who was born into a share-cropper family in Alabama, became heavyweight champion of the world at age 23. In 1938, when Louis fought German boxer Max Schmeling at Yankee Stadium, the fight attracted 70,000 fans and grossed more than $1 million. When the black fighter knocked out Schmeling in the first round, he seemed to strike a blow for America against Hitler's Nazi Germany.

A number of women also became heroes in the 1930s for their daring exploits, personal courage, and physical prowess. Unlike earlier national heroines, these female celebrities tran-scended the expected gender role for women. Athletes like tennis champion Helen Wills and Olympic track star and brilliant golfer Babe Didrikson greatly expanded the popularity of women's sports. Renowned aviator Amelia Earhart, the first woman to fly solo across the Atlantic, devoted her life to advancing both fem-inism and commercial aviation. When her plane

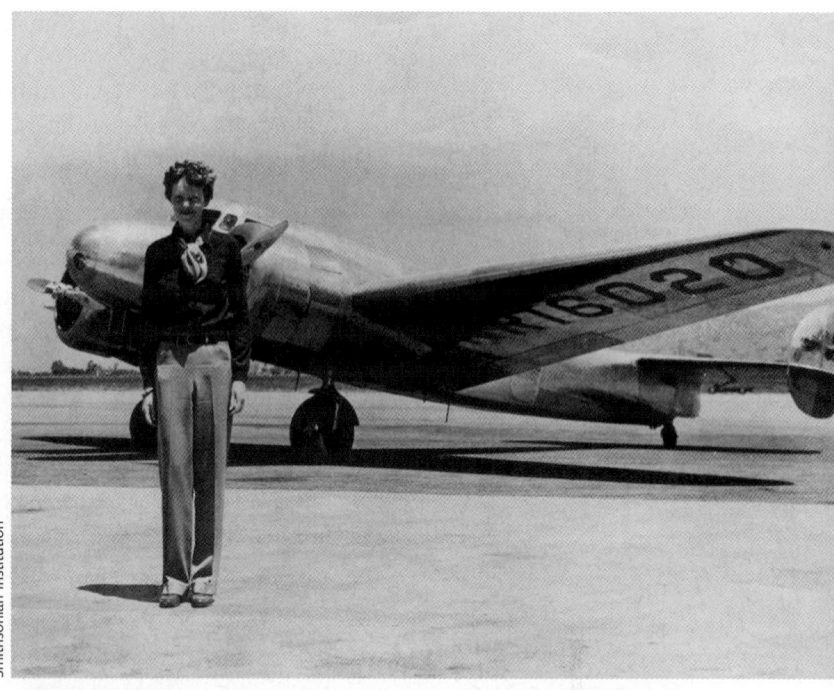

■ Amelia Earhart was the first woman to fly solo across the Atlantic. The legendary aviator gave preliminary flying lessons to her friend Eleanor Roosevelt. FDR convinced his wife not to take up flying, but the First Lady always regretted her decision.

disappeared during an attempted 'round-the-world flight in 1937, many of her admirers were so convinced of her invincibility that they refused to believe she had died. Even today, people still speculate about her fate.

Conclusion

The New Deal set in place a welfare state that established the principle of government responsibility for the well-being of vulnerable citizens. Before the New Deal, people suf-fered the fluctuations of the market economy with no recourse beyond the assistance of kin, communities, and charities. Older Americans who could no longer work had no gov-ernment-guaranteed pensions and often faced poverty in old age. Bank failures could wipe away life savings. Unemployment could mean starvation for a worker's family. The New Deal pro-vided Social Security for the elderly, unemployment compensation for workers who had lost their jobs, minimum hours and wages, and economic aid to women and children who had no means of support. It also established national economic regulations, such as the Federal Deposit Insurance Corporation (FDIC) and the Security and Exchange Commission (SEC), as well as the right of workers to unionize and engage in collective bargaining. These govern-ment protections offered many Americans an unprecedented level of economic security.

The Roosevelt administration addressed many of the nation's problems and used the federal government in innovative ways to intervene in the economy and to mitigate some of the misfortunes caused by the Depression. Most New Deal policies protected factory workers in large companies. The safety net did not extend to many of the neediest Americans, includ-ing Mexican American migrant workers, African American and white sharecroppers, seasonal agricultural laborers, or domestic workers. Although the national government extended its reach considerably, at the local level, many persistent problems remained entrenched. FDR was reluctant to press for anti-lynching legislation for fear of alienating Southern congressmen who still retained enormous power. Efforts to rescue the economy did little to rein in huge corporations like Ford and Standard Oil. Although FDR's conservative opponents accused him of socialist leanings, the New Deal actually rescued and shored up capitalism.

The New Deal was the Roosevelt administration's response to a global economic crisis. With the exception of the communist Soviet Union, which had already abandoned capitalism, almost every industrialized nation responded to the Depression by increasing the role of the state in the economy. Italy, Germany, and Japan moved to fascism and the nearly total state direction of the economy, while Britain and France established welfare states that would become more fully developed after World War II. The United States' system of social welfare was not as extensive and inclusive as those that emerged in some western European democracies. But it was part of a larger trend toward government intervention in the economy and greater protections for citizens. Within the United States, the New Deal neither reached nor satisfied everyone. Some groups thought that it went too far; others believed it did not go far enough. But it eased some of the harshest effects of the Depression and established a national safety net that endured for more than half a century.

Sites to Visit

African American Odyssey: The Depression, New Deal, and World War II

lcweb2.loc.gov/ammem/aaohtml/exhibit/aopart8.html

This Library of Congress site covers the history of African Americans during the years of the Depression and World War II.

Southern Mosaic: The John and Ruby Lomax 1939 Southern States Recording Trip

memory.loc.gov/ammem/lohtml/lohome.html

This site from the American Folklife Center, Library of Congress, provides audio, text, and photos of the Lomax collection of America folk songs collected and recorded across the South.

The 1930s Project

xroads.virginia.edu/~1930s/front.html

This site from the University of Virginia's American Studies program contains materials about the culture and history of the 1930s.

Voices from the Dust Bowl: The Charles L. Todd and Robert Sonkin Migrant Worker Collection, 1940-1941

memory.loc.gov/ammem/afctshtml/tshome.html

This Library of Congress site includes Farm Security Administration studies of migrant work camps in California in 1940 and 1941, with audio, images, manuscripts, and publications.

The New Deal Network

newdeal.feri.org

This site includes images, documents, texts, artifacts, and other materials from the New Deal era.

Franklin Delano Roosevelt

www.ipl.org/ref/POTUS/fdroosevelt.html

This Internet Public Library site contains biographical information about Franklin Delano Roosevelt and his election to the presidency and links to Internet biographies and resources about him.

The Crash of 1929

www.btinternet.com/~dreklind/thecrash.htm

This site includes a discussion of the causes of the 1929 stock market crash, along with audio clips of songs relating to the crash.

Franklin D. Roosevelt Library and Digital Archives

www.fdrlibrary.marist.edu/

This site includes documents, images, audio, and other primary source materials from the Franklin D. Roosevelt Library.

A New Deal for the Arts

www.archives.gov/exhibit_hall/new_deal_for_the_arts/

This site of the National Archives includes artwork, documents, photographs, and information from the New Deal programs that funded artists in the 1930s.

American Life Histories: Manuscripts from the Federal Writers Project, 1936-1940

memory.loc.gov/ammem/wpaintro/wpahome.html

This site from the Library of Congress includes manuscripts written by Federal Writers Project authors who interviewed Americans all over the country and wrote about them.

For Further Reading

General

Steve Fraser and Gary Gerstle, eds., *The Rise and Fall of the New Deal Order, 1930–1980* (1989).

Robert S. Lynd and Helen Merrell Lynd, *Middletown in Transition: A Study in Cultural Conflicts* (1937).

Robert S. McElvaine, *The Great Depression: America, 1929–1941* (1984, 1993).

James R. McGovern, *And a Time for Hope: Americans in the Great Depression* (2000).

Studs Terkel, *Hard Times: An Oral History of the Great Depression* (1986).

The Great Depression

Glen Elder, Jr., *Children of the Great Depression: Social Change in Life Experience* (1974).

Robert S. McElvaine, ed., *Down and Out in the Great Depression: Letters from the Forgotten Man* (1983).

Vicki L. Ruiz, *From Out of the Shadows: Mexican Women in Twentieth-Century America* (1998).

Judith Smith, *Family Connections: A History of Italian and Jewish Immigrant Lives in Providence, Rhode Island, 1900–1940* (1985).

Presidential Responses to the Depression

Edward D. Berkowitz, *America's Welfare State: From Roosevelt to Reagan* (1991).

Blanche Wiesen Cook, *Eleanor Roosevelt.* (1999)

Frank Friedel, *Franklin D. Roosevelt: A Rendezvous with Destiny* (1990).

William E. Leuchtenberg, *Franklin D. Roosevelt and the New Deal* (1963).

Lawrence W. Levine and Cornelia R. Levine, *The People and the President: America's Conversation with FDR* (2002).

Richard Polenberg, ed., *The Era of Franklin D. Roosevelt, 1933–1945: A Brief History with Documents* (2000).

Arthur M. Schlesinger, Jr., *The Age of Roosevelt*, 3 vols. (1957–1960).

The New Deal

Anthony Badger, *The New Deal* (1988).

Alan Brinkley, *Voices of Protest: Huey Long, Father Coughlin and the Great Depression* (1982).

Sidney Fine, *Sit-Down: The General Motors Strike of 1936–37* (1969).

Steven Fraser, *Labor Will Rule: Sidney Hillman and the Rise of American Labor* (1991).

Linda Gordon, *Pitied but Not Entitled: Single Mothers and the History of Welfare* (1994).

Robin D. G. Kelley, *Hammer and Hoe: Alabama Communists During the Great Depression* (1990).

A New Political Culture

Lizabeth Cohen, *Making a New Deal: Industrial Workers in Chicago, 1919–1939* (1992).

Michael Denning, *Cultural Front: The Laboring of American Culture in the Twentieth Century* (1998).

Gary Gerstle, *Working-Class Americanism: The Politics of Labor in a Textile City, 1914–1960* (1989).

Lary May, *The Big Tomorrow: Hollywood and the Politics of the American Way* (2000).

Online Practice Test

Test your understanding of this chapter with interactive review quizzes at

www.ablongman.com/jonescreatedequal/chapter22

Additional Photo Credits

Page 737: Bettmann/CORBIS
Page 751: Courtesy, Janice L. and David Frent
Page 761: Library of Congress
Page 763: Kobal Collection/United Artists

Global Conflict: World War II, 1937–1945

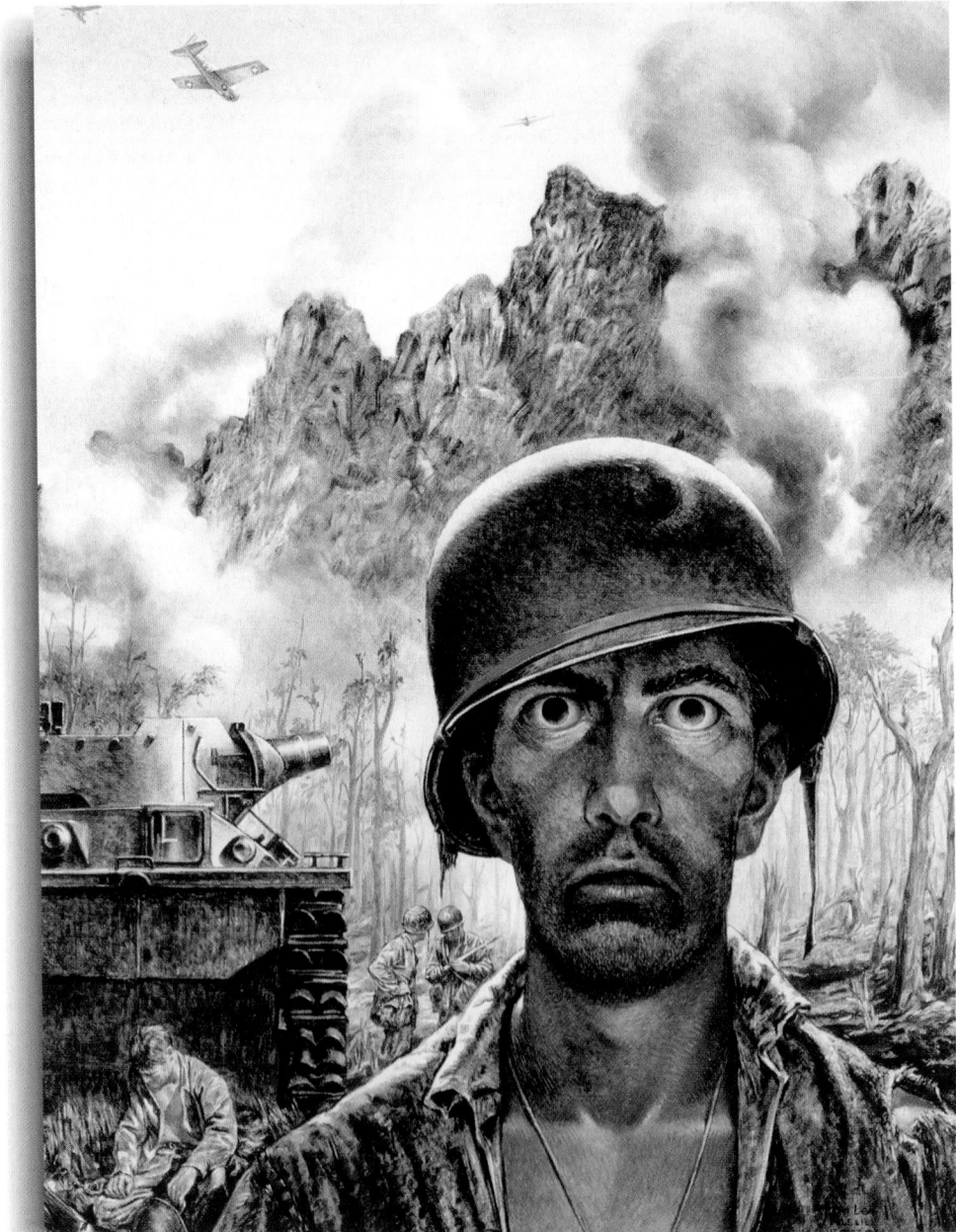

Tom Lea, Marines Call It That Two Thousand Yard Stare, Sept. 16, 1944.
U.S. Army Center of Military History, Army Art Collection

■ Tom Lea's haunting painting of a soldier, *Marines Call It That Two Thousand Yard Stare* (1944), evokes the horrors of World War II.

ON DECEMBER 7, 1941, KEITH LITTLE WAS OUT HUNTING RABBITS WITH FRIENDS AT their boarding school on the Navajo reservation of Ganado, Arizona. When they heard the news that the Japanese had attacked the U.S. naval base in Hawaii at Pearl Harbor, the teenage boys pledged to fight for their country. The next morning, Little and his friends showed up with their hunting rifles at the office of the reservation superintendent, ready to enlist. The previous year, the Tribal Council had voted unanimously to defend the United States against invasion. "There exists no purer concentration of Americanism than among the First Americans," the council declared.

The council vote was no idle gesture, especially given the complex status of Indian tribes within the United States. In some respects the tribes were semiautonomous nations within a nation. Several states, including Arizona, denied Indians the basic rights and obligations of citizenship, such as voting. Moreover, the Navajos were still embroiled in disputes with Commissioner of Indian Affairs John Collier and the Roosevelt administration over Collier's request that they destroy their sheep to reduce soil erosion and overgrazing. So it was by no means obvious that the Navajos would, or even should, fight for a nation they had bitterly fought against only 80 years earlier. Although large numbers of Native American soldiers had fought in earlier wars, especially World War I, the boarding-school boys could not have known that they would soon become part of a Navajo unit of "Code Talkers" that helped win the war.

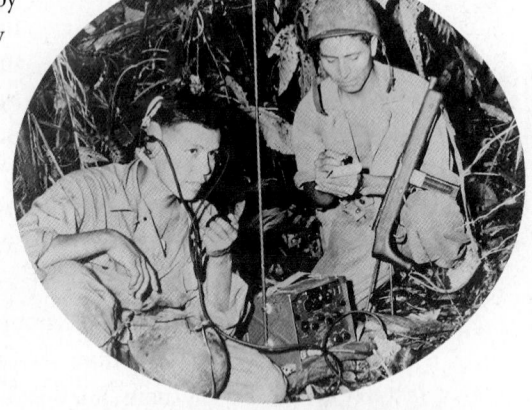

Navajo "Code Talkers" operate a portable radio in the Pacific combat zone in 1943.

Little and about 400 other Navajos became part of a special unit that developed an intricate code, based on the Navajo language, to transmit top-secret information without risk of detection. The Navajo language was particularly well suited to code because very few people besides Navajos knew it. In a process code named "Magic," the all-Navajo 382nd Platoon of the U.S. Marine Corps outperformed the most sophisticated communication technology by encoding and decoding sensitive military information almost instantly and flawlessly. In two days on the Pacific island of Iwo Jima, six "Code Talkers" transmitted more than 800 messages, working around the clock, without a single error. Signal Officer Major Howard Conner recalled, "Without the Navajos the Marines would never have taken Iwo Jima."

The experiences of the Navajo "Code Talkers" echo many larger themes of America's involvement in World War II. Along with numerous other ethnic and racial minorities, the Navajos willingly fought—and many died—for a country that had treated them as second-class citizens. African Americans also joined the war effort, though in segregated units, to fight for the "double V"—victory against fascism abroad and racial discrimination at home. Young Japanese Americans left internment camps where their families had been forcibly detained to join a war against the land from which their parents came.

World War II was a global war, affecting countries and peoples all over the world. The conflict demanded human and technological resources on an unprecedented scale and left massive destruction in its wake. The huge scale of destruction was unlike that of any previous war. At least 55 million people died, including 25 million in the Soviet Union, 10 million in China, and 6 million in Poland. In the Holocaust, Nazi Germany's campaign of genocide, 6 million European Jews perished along with thousands of Romani (Gypsies), Poles, mentally and physically disabled people, homosexuals, and others deemed "racially inferior." The war also had a tremendous impact on countries under colonial rule. France, Holland, Belgium, and Great Britain were major colonial powers, but the war loosened their hold over their colonies. Germany's bombardment of England and occupation of France, Holland, and Belgium weakened all of these countries. Japan's defeat of the American, British, Dutch, and French forces in Southeast Asia from 1940 to 1942 shocked the Western powers and ended white rule in the region, setting in motion a wave of decolonization in Asia and Africa after the war.

The United States was the only major combatant that did not suffer massive destruction on its home territory. It had two powerful advantages: a 3000-mile ocean barrier on its East and West Coasts, plus tremendous natural resources that could provide the materials needed for modern warfare, such as steel and oil. In order to minimize American casualties, President Franklin Delano Roosevelt (FDR) pursued a strategy to make the United States the "arsenal of democracy," providing armaments and supplies to the other Allied powers so that their armies would do most of the fighting. Although the Soviet Union carried the largest burden of fighting the war and suffered the highest losses, millions of Americans also fought, and many died in the conflict. Military service had a leveling effect on social relations, as soldiers came together from all classes and ethnic groups. The vast majority of the troops—more than 85 percent—were white men from a wide variety of backgrounds. Soldiers of color generally fought in segregated units, but their battlefield successes and sacrifices gave them a sense of belonging to the nation and fueled postwar movements for equality and civil rights.

> *The United States was the only major combatant that did not suffer massive destruction on its home territory.*

No bombs dropped on the American mainland, yet the war reached into every aspect of national and personal life. Although wartime brought prosperity, the rationing of essential goods and the scarcity of consumer products brought nearly all Americans into the war effort. As soldiers and war industry workers moved around the country, local and regional sensibilities gave way to a stronger national identity. Factories stopped making consumer items and instead turned out war machines. Scientists developed new weapons of mass destruction. Cities burgeoned as workers flooded into the lucrative war industries. The U.S. military and defense establishment expanded to the formidable scale it would maintain during and after the war, making the United States the most powerful nation in the world.

Most Americans supported the war effort and did their part to stop German and Japanese aggression. Early in 1941, well before the United States entered the war, Roosevelt stressed the need to protect the "Four Freedoms": freedom of speech, freedom of religion, freedom from want, and freedom from fear of armed aggression. For many American GIs, the Four Freedoms translated into intensely personal terms. They fought to stay alive and to return to their sweethearts and families. They fought in hopes of reaping the "good life" that had become the symbol of America. Others, especially soldiers of color, fought not simply to preserve the American way of life, but also to gain access to it.

Mobilizing for War

During the 1930s, the rise of fascism and militarism in Italy, Germany, and Japan created a terrible dilemma for Americans. Disillusioned by World War I and preoccupied with the hardships of the Depression, they disagreed strongly with each other about how to respond to overt aggression in Africa, Europe, and Asia. The ensuing "Great Debate" became a turning point in the nation's relationship with the outside world. Mobilizing for the enormous crusade of World War II gave rise to a unity of purpose that lasted throughout the war and into the postwar era.

The Rise of Fascism

In the 1930s, Depression-era Americans grappled with their problems at home and avoided entanglements abroad. But they found it difficult to ignore events in Europe and Asia. In Italy, Spain, and Germany, where a weak economy and high unemployment created political unrest, fascist leaders rose to power with strong popular support. These new leaders promised economic recovery through strengthening the military and national expansion. They also encouraged intense nationalist sentiments, urging people to identify strongly with the state. Fascist party leader Benito Mussolini had held power in Italy since 1921, suppressing dissident voices and imposing one-party rule. According to Mussolini, "The fascist conception of the state is all-embracing, and outside of the state no human or spiritual values can exist, let alone be desirable." By the early 1930s fascism had gained strength in Germany and Spain. The term *fascist* has since been applied to the various right-wing dictatorships that arose during the period between the two world wars. Fascist governments were antidemocratic, antiparliamentary, and frequently anti-Semitic. Appealing to nationalistic and often racist sentiments, these governments generally ruled by coercion, terrorism, and police surveillance.

Germany emerged as the most powerful fascist state in Europe. After Germany's defeat in World War I and the severe economic depression that Germany experienced in the 1920s, Adolf Hitler's National Socialist (Nazi) party won broad support in the weakened country. On January 30, 1933, five weeks before FDR took the oath as president of the United States, Hitler became chancellor of Germany. Extolling fanatical nationalism and the racial superiority of "Aryan" or "pure" Anglo-Saxon Germans, Hitler blamed Jews for Germany's problems. He began a campaign of terror against Jews, homosexuals, suspected communists, and anyone else he saw as promoting "un-German" ideas. Hitler vowed to unite all German-speaking peoples into a new empire, the "Third Reich."

The fascist governments forged alliances to increase their power and launched campaigns of aggression and expansion. As conflict increased in Europe, hostilities spread into Africa as well. In 1935 Italy invaded Ethiopia, the sole independent African nation. The following year, Nazi troops seized the Rhineland, in the western region of Germany, in violation of the Versailles agreement. Hitler and Mussolini signed the Axis Pact, and Japan forged an alliance with Germany. Soon after that, civil war erupted in Spain. Hitler and Mussolini extended aid to the fascist General Francisco Franco, who was trying to overthrow Spain's republican government.

Although Spanish republicans appealed to antifascist governments for help in the fight against Franco, only the Soviet Union came to their assistance. The United States maintained an official policy of neutrality. Some conservatives believed that the anticommunist Franco would promote social stability. But many on the left, including large numbers of writers and intellectuals, championed the beleaguered Spanish government and denounced the fascists. Cadres of Americans sympathetic to the republican cause, including the "Abraham Lincoln Brigade," joined Soviet-organized international forces to fight against Franco.

In Germany anti-Semitic fervor reached a frenzy on the evening of November 7, 1938. In a spasm of violence known as *Kristallnacht* ("Night of the Broken Glass"), Hitler launched a massive assault against Jews throughout Germany. For three days German mobs attacked synagogues, smashed windows, and vandalized Jewish homes and businesses. Thirty-five Jews were killed, and thousands arrested. The rioters destroyed 7500 shops and 119 synagogues. The Nazi reign of terror against the Jews continued throughout the war, culminating in death camps and genocide.

Aggression in Europe and Asia

In the spring and summer of 1938 Hitler annexed Austria to the Third Reich and then invaded the Sudetenland. In the breakup of the Austro-Hungarian Empire after World War I, this German-speaking area became part of the newly formed Czechoslovakia. The Sudetenland was key to Hitler's goal of uniting all German-speaking Europe into the Third Reich. Josef Stalin, the communist leader of the Soviet Union, offered to join France and Britain to roust Hitler from the Sudetenland and halt his aggression. But the leaders of France and Britain rebuffed Stalin's suggestion. In September they met with Hitler in Munich and agreed to let him keep the Sudetenland in return for his promise that he would seek no more territory. Stalin feared that the anticommunist leaders of France and Britain would try to turn Hitler's aggression toward the Soviet Union. To prevent that possibility, Stalin signed a nonaggression pact with Hitler. Eventually, Hitler broke all his promises. Throughout the war and after, the Munich meeting became the symbol of "appeasement," a warning that compromise with the enemy leads only to disaster.

> *The Nazi reign of terror against the Jews continued throughout the war, culminating in death camps and genocide.*

In the next few years the fascist states expanded their power and territory. In 1939, with the help of the Soviet Union and in violation of the Munich agreement, Germany invaded Poland, which fell quickly, unable to withstand the German *blitzkrieg*, or "lightning war" of land and air strikes. At that point Britain and France declared war on Germany. That same year Madrid finally fell to Franco's forces. Britain, France, and the United States recognized Franco as victor of the Spanish Civil War. The Soviet Union next sent troops into Finland, gaining Finnish territory in 1940.

By 1940 Hitler was sweeping through Europe, invading Denmark, Norway, Holland, Belgium, Luxembourg, and then France. In just six weeks the Nazis had seized most of western Europe. Hitler then turned his forces on Great Britain. In the summer and fall of 1940, German raids on British air bases nearly destroyed the British Royal Air Force (RAF). Hitler then ordered the bombing of London and other English cities, attacking civilians day and night in what came to be called the Battle of Britain.

In the Far East events had taken an equally alarming turn. Nationalistic militarists gained control of the Japanese government in Tokyo and began a course of expansion. In 1931–1932, Japanese troops occupied the large Chinese province of Manchuria, installed a puppet government, and gave the province a Japanese name: Manchukuo. Five years later, the Japanese launched a full-scale war against China. The United States extended aid to China and discontinued trade with Japan. In 1940 Japan joined Germany and Italy in the Axis alliance and invaded the French colony of Indochina. Kazuko Kuramoto remembered the nationalist propaganda she learned as a Japanese child raised in Manchuria:

> I was born into a society of Japanese supremacy and grew up believing in Japan's "divine" mission to save Asia from the "evil" hands of Western imperialism. . . . "You are Japan's only future, a glorious future," adults around us used to say. We believed it with passion. . . . I joined the Red Cross Nurse Corps to help my country win the war. . . . "Asia for the Asians!"

Japan's efforts to rid Asia of white Western imperialism inspired some other Asians who saw Japan as a model of strength. But it was also a cynical ploy of the Japanese leaders, who sought to conquer all of Asia and considered other Asian peoples to be racially inferior to the Japanese. The Japanese treated the people in the countries they occupied with extreme brutality.

The Great Debate: Americans Contemplate War

In the mid–1930s the overwhelming majority of Americans still opposed intervention in foreign conflicts. Congress passed the Neutrality Acts of 1935, 1936, and 1937, outlawing arms sales or loans to nations at war and forbidding Americans from traveling on the ships of belligerent powers. In 1937 a Gallup poll indicated that 70 percent of Americans believed that the United States should have stayed out of World War I. A peace movement spread across university and college campuses. Students marched with banners bearing such slogans as "Scholarships, not Battleships." In a "peace strike" in the spring of 1936, half a million students boycotted classes and attended antiwar events. Nevertheless, President Roosevelt and others believed that the United States would be unable to hold itself aloof from the mounting international crises.

When Japan invaded China in 1937, FDR refused to comply with the provisions of the latest Neutrality Act, on the technicality that neither combatant had officially declared war. By creatively interpreting the law, he was able to offer loans to the embattled Chinese. Roosevelt felt strongly that the United States should actively help to resist the Axis powers. In 1940 he told the nation, "Frankly and definitely there is danger ahead—danger against which we must prepare. But we well know that we cannot escape danger, or the fear of danger, by crawling into bed and pulling the covers over our heads."

U.S. citizens still remained bitterly divided over the question of whether to get involved in the conflict. Those who agreed with Roosevelt believed that the nation should take any action "short of war" to help defeat the aggressors in Europe. By sending supplies, for example, the United States could become the "arsenal of democracy" to fight fascism without sending troops and risking American lives. But opponents to this idea spanned the political spectrum. They included moral or religious pacifists, peace activists of the Communist and Labor parties, and anti-Semites who supported Hitler. The pro-Nazi German American Bund, an organization that supported Germany, complained about Roosevelt's "Jew Deal"—a reference to Jews among FDR's advisors.

The largest organization to resist Roosevelt's effort was the America First Committee. With 450 chapters, the group claimed several hundred thousand members. Centered largely in the Midwest, the America Firsters included some active Nazi supporters. But conservative businesspeople also took part. Committee chair General Robert E. Wood, head of retailer Sears, Roebuck, believed that war would impede American prosperity. Other members had long opposed Roosevelt and the New Deal. They feared that war would give additional power to the already strong federal government. The group's most visible spokesperson was famed aviator Charles Lindbergh, whose anti-Semitism fueled his staunch opposition to any involvement in the conflict. Although Lindbergh's position antagonized many who once admired him, he also attracted followers.

Despite intense nonintervention sentiments, public opinion began to shift. Many Americans were shocked when Hitler swiftly

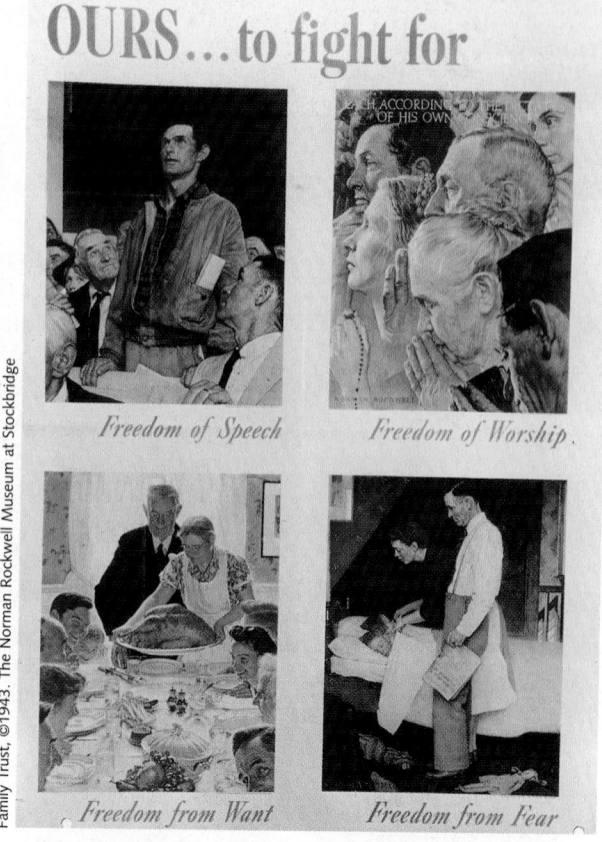

Norman Rockwell, Four Freedoms, War Bond Poster, printed by permission of the Norman Rockwell Family Trust, ©1943. The Norman Rockwell Museum at Stockbridge

■ Norman Rockwell's depiction of the "Four Freedoms" adorned the cover of the *Saturday Evening Post,* inspired the purchase of war bonds, and came to symbolize the democratic values for which the nation was fighting. These four scenes by the popular artist evoked an American ideal of close families and harmonious communities.

conquered much of Europe. Vivid news reports of the German occupation of France, and the intense bombardment of England in the Battle of Britain bolstered FDR's efforts to take action. When Roosevelt made his "Four Freedoms" speech in his annual message to Congress in January 1941, the United States was not yet officially at war. But the president pledged his support for England against the Nazis. A few months later, Congress approved the Lend-Lease agreement to lend rather than sell munitions to the Allied countries.

When Hitler broke his promise to Stalin and attacked the Soviet Union in June 1941, FDR extended Lend-Lease to the Soviets. During the summer, FDR and British Prime Minister Winston Churchill met on a ship off the coast of Newfoundland to develop a joint declaration known as the Atlantic Charter. The two leaders announced that the United States and Britain sought no new territories. Furthermore, they recognized the right of all peoples to choose their own form of government and to approve any territorial changes that might affect them. The charter called for international free trade and navigation as well.

The charter articulated the Allies' war aims, but it also had profound implications for colonial rule around the world. Realizing the possible cost of losing colonies, Churchill retreated from the global implications of the charter. The declaration, he claimed, applied primarily to European nations under Nazi rule. Roosevelt walked a fine line between contradicting Churchill and supporting the idea of empire. However, the words of the charter—along with the Allies' condemnation of racism and territorial expansion by Germany and Japan—emboldened anticolonial activists around the world. Within 15 years after the end of World War II, 800 million previously colonized people won their independence, and 40 new nations would form.

As the United States inched closer to entry into the conflict, FDR still faced political and economic troubles at home. Although Allied munitions orders had already stimulated the economy, as late as 1939, 9.4 million Americans—17.2 percent of the labor force—remained jobless. In the 1940 presidential election Roosevelt defeated Republican challenger Wendell Willkie. FDR began his third term as war loomed and economic hardship at home persisted. But Japan's surprise attack on Pearl Harbor in 1941 ended both the neutrality debate and the Depression.

TABLE 23-1			
The Election of 1940			
Candidate	Political Party	Popular Vote	Electoral Vote
Franklin D. Roosevelt	Democratic	27,244,160	449
Wendell L. Willkie	Republican	22,305,198	82

Pearl Harbor: The United States Enters the War

The Japanese attack on Pearl Harbor shocked the nation and catapulted the United States immediately into World War II. President Roosevelt somberly told millions of Americans gathered around their radios that the day of the attack would "live in infamy." Most former doubters now joined the war effort. The entire nation shifted into high gear to defeat brutal, aggressive regimes intent on conquering much of the world. For some, wartime mobilization offered new opportunities; for others, it brought sacrifice.

December 7, 1941

For nearly a decade, tensions had been mounting between the United States and Japan as American leaders tried to contain Japan's expansion in Asia. Roosevelt assumed that a strong U.S. military presence in the Pacific would persuade Japan's premier, General Hideki Tojo,

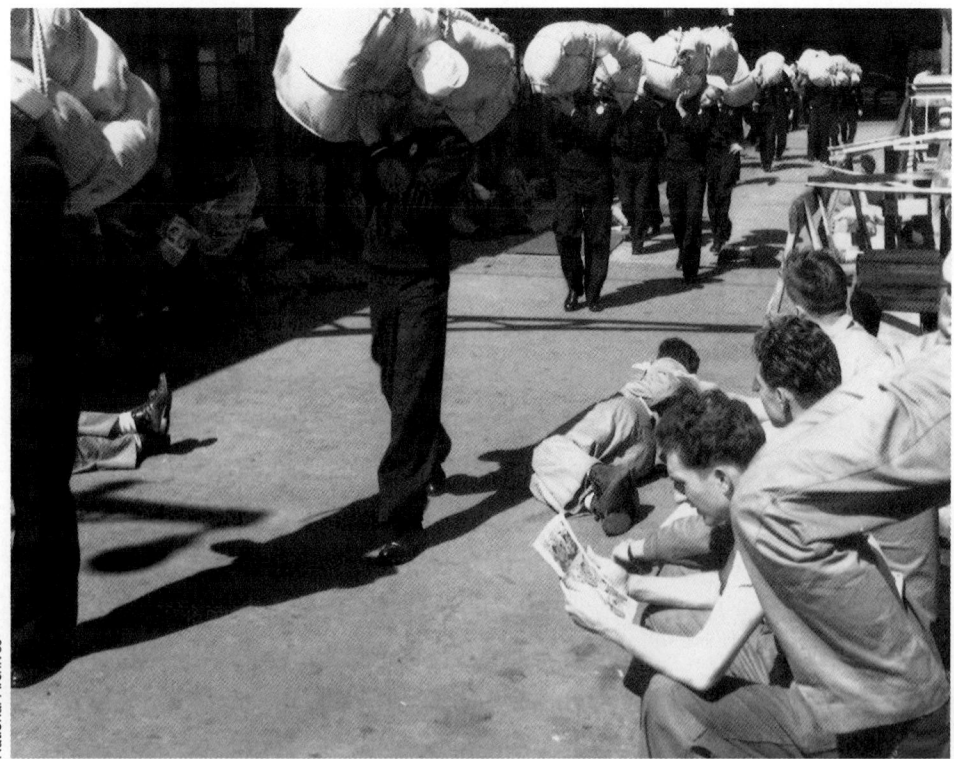

National Archives

■ The attack on Pearl Harbor prompted an immediate mobilization of vast proportions. Within months, thousands of young recruits, such as these sailors boarding ship in San Diego, shouldered their gear and headed overseas. More than 400,000 did not return alive. The government calculated that over four grim years of U.S. involvement, 292,131 Americans died in combat, and there were 115,185 additional service deaths from other causes. Though huge, American losses still proved small in comparison to the destruction suffered in other countries.

to avoid a confrontation with the United States. When Japan continued its aggression in Asia, FDR froze Japanese assets in the United States, putting trade with Japan under presidential control. This move, he hoped, would bring Japan to the bargaining table. Instead, on November 25, the Japanese dispatched aircraft carriers toward Hawaii and sent troops to the border of Malaya in the South Pacific.

Although U.S. intelligence sources had broken the codes with which the Japanese encrypted messages about their war plans, they did not realize that the Japanese intended to strike Hawaii. One memo indicating that the Japanese were heading toward Pearl Harbor lay buried under a pile of intelligence reports. As a result, American military officials failed to warn the U.S. forces stationed in Pearl Harbor. At 7:55 A.M. on December 7, Japanese planes swooped over Pearl Harbor and bombed the naval base. The assault caught the American forces completely off guard and destroyed most of the U.S. Pacific fleet. Only a few aircraft carriers that were out at sea survived. Two hours after the attack on Pearl Harbor, the Japanese also struck the main U.S. base at Clark Field in the Philippines, destroying half of the U.S. Far East Air Force.

At roughly the same time that Keith Little heard the news about Pearl Harbor at his Navajo reservation boarding school, another 16-year-old, John Garcia, watched flames rising at Pearl Harbor from his house four miles away. The young Hawaiian reached the scene in time to witness the second round of bombings. "I spent the rest of the day swimming inside the harbor, along with some other Hawaiians. I brought out I don't know how many bodies, and how many were alive and how many dead. . . . We worked around the clock for three days."

In less than two hours the Japanese had wrecked 188 planes—most of the American aircraft on the island—and sunk 19 ships, including eight battleships, three destroyers, and three cruisers. When the smoke cleared, 2323 American service personnel were dead. Congress immediately declared war against Japan. Representative Jeannette Rankin from Montana cast the only dissenting vote. (The first woman elected to Congress and a lifelong pacifist, Rankin had also voted against the U.S. entry into World War I.) Three days later Germany and Italy declared war against the United States.

Japanese American Relocation

The assault on Pearl Harbor sparked widespread rumors along the U.S. West Coast that Japanese and Japanese Americans living there planned to sabotage the war effort. Although no charges of criminal activity or treason were ever brought against any Japanese Americans, powerful farming interests eager to eradicate Japanese competition pushed for an evacuation. General John L. DeWitt, chief of the Western Defense Command, argued, "The Japanese race is an enemy race, and while many second and third generation Japanese born on United States soil, possessed of United States citizenship, have become 'Americanized,' the racial strains are undiluted. . . . It therefore follows that along the vital Pacific Coast over 112,000 potential enemies, of Japanese extraction, are at large today." People of Japanese descent were the only residents of the United States who were relocated during the war. Although the United States was at war with Germany and Italy, those of German or Italian ancestry were spared internment. Because they were white, nobody claimed that the Germans or Italians belonged to an "enemy race."

Not everyone supported the internment idea. U.S. Attorney General Francis Biddle protested that there was "no reason" for a mass relocation. J. Edgar Hoover, director of the

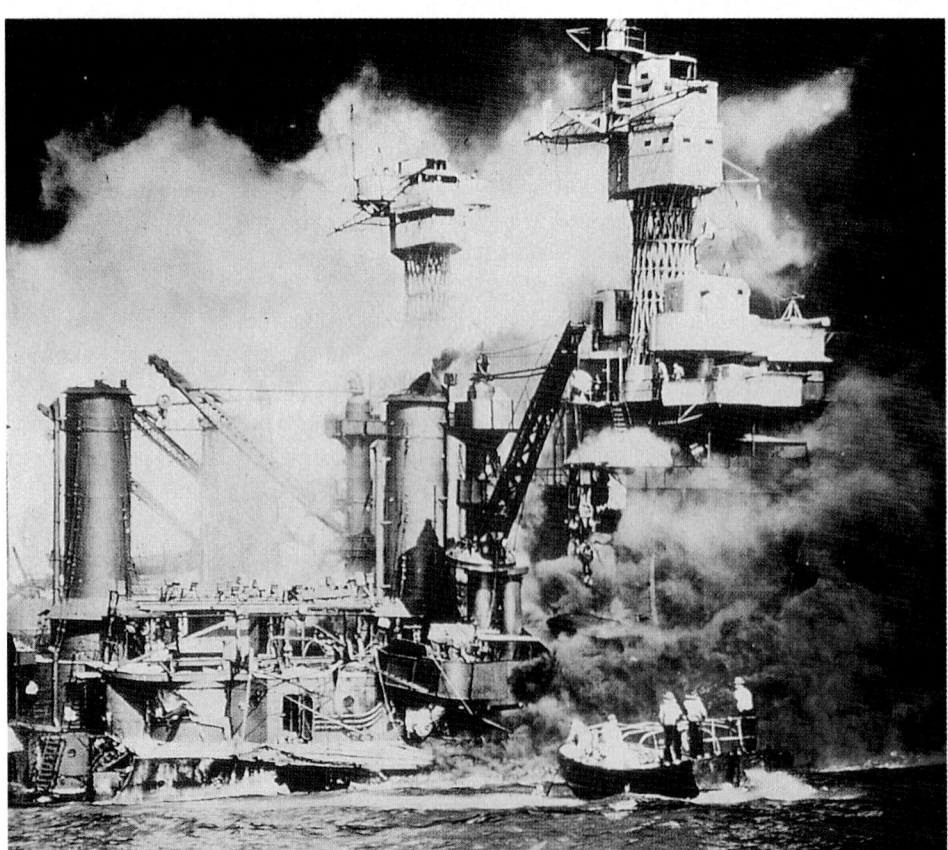

■ On December 7, 1941, the Japanese launched a surprise attack on the U.S. naval base at Pearl Harbor, Hawaii. The attack brought the United States immediately into World War II and was the only time that the war came to American soil.

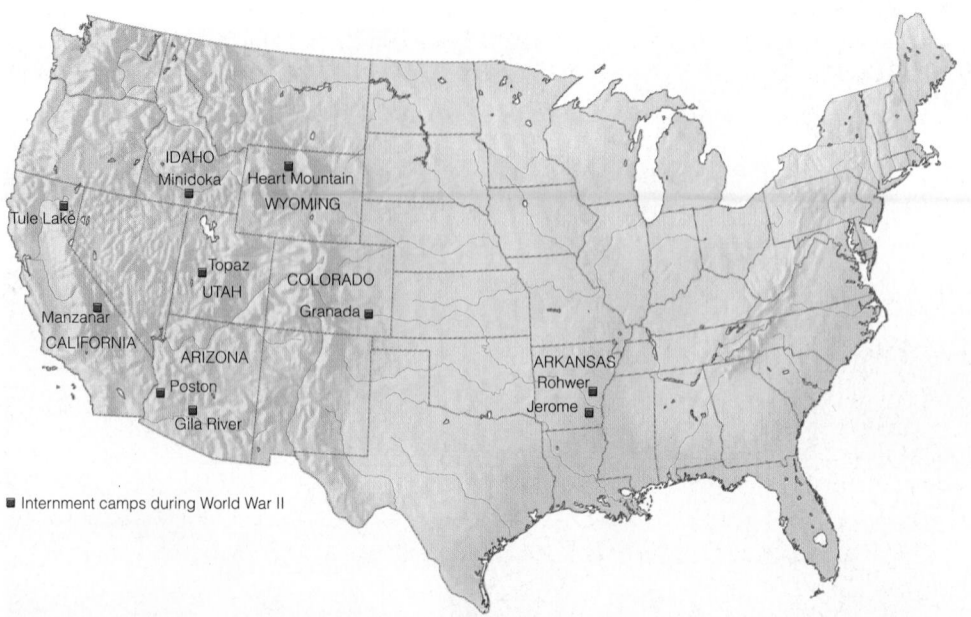

■ MAP 23.1
THE INTERNMENT OF JAPANESE AMERICANS DURING WORLD WAR II After the Japanese attack on
Pearl Harbor, President Franklin Delano Roosevelt signed an order authorizing the removal of people of
Japanese descent from the West Coast. These Japanese Americans were relocated to internment camps built
in arid and isolated areas in the West, as well as in two locations in Arkansas.

FBI, also opposed the plan, arguing that DeWitt's suggestion reflected "hysteria and lack of
judgment." Nevertheless, the Roosevelt administration gave in to the pressure, with the support of California Attorney General Earl Warren. In February 1942, Roosevelt signed Executive Order 9066, which suspended the civil rights of American citizens of Japanese
descent. The order authorized the removal of 110,000 Japanese and Japanese Americans from the West Coast. Of those, 70,000 were *Nisei,* native-born American citizens. Families received one week's notice to evacuate their homes and move to
prisonlike camps surrounded by barbed wire and guarded by armed soldiers. There
were 10 such camps in seven states, all of them located in arid, desolate spots in the
West. At the camps internees lived in makeshift wooden barracks, where entire families
crowded into one room.

Not all Japanese Americans were evacuated. General Delos Emmons, the military governor of Hawaii, insisted that removing the Japanese from those islands would cripple the economy, as well as the defense of Oahu. In Hawaii, Japanese and Japanese Americans made up
more than 90 percent of the skilled workers and agricultural laborers needed to rebuild and
sustain the island. In their defense, Emmons proclaimed, "There have been no known acts of
sabotage committed in Hawaii." Business leaders concurred. But the Japanese living on the West
Coast lacked the broad support that those in Hawaii enjoyed.

The experience of internment proved so devastating that, after the war, 5766 *Nisei* renounced
their American citizenship. One of those was World War I veteran Joseph Y. Kurihara, who
recalled, "It was really cruel and harsh. To pack and evacuate in 48 hours was an impossibil-
ity. Seeing mothers completely bewildered with children crying from want and peddlers taking advantage and offering prices next to robbery made me feel like murdering those
responsible." Kurihara emigrated to Japan—a country he had never seen.

While the internment experience alienated some Japanese Americans, fully 33,000 joined
the armed services—including 1200 who enlisted from the internment camps—and proved
their patriotism on the battlefield. In the Pacific, their knowledge of the Japanese language

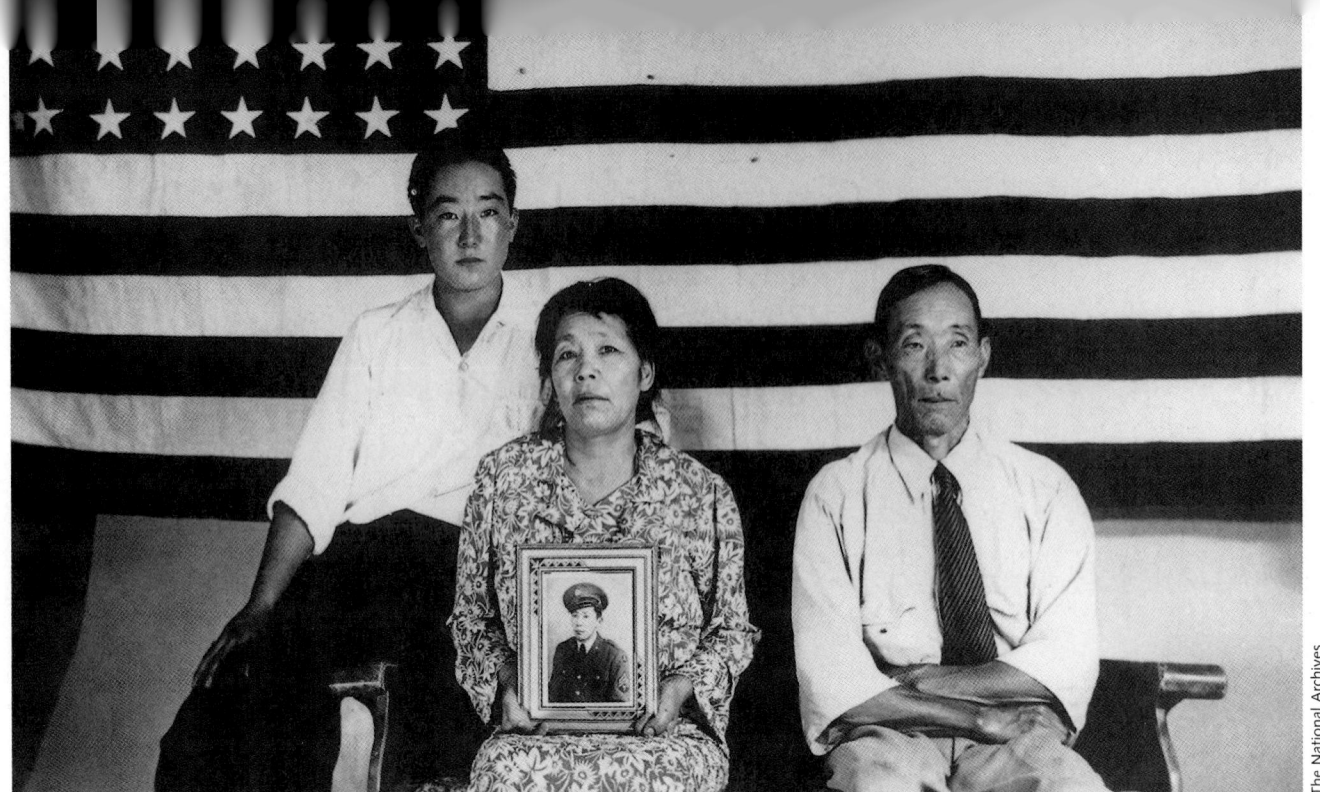

■ The family pictured here was among thousands of loyal citizens of Japanese ancestry removed from their homes on the West Coast and relocated to internment camps. Here, the Hirano family, George, Hisa, and Yasbei (left to right), pose at the Colorado River Relocation Center in Poston, Arizona. Hisa holds a photo of her son, an American soldier, who is off fighting the war.

proved critical in translating intercepted Japanese military documents. General Charles Willoughby, chief of intelligence in the Pacific, estimated that the Japanese American military contributions shortened the war by two years. The Japanese also served ably in Europe, suffering huge casualties. The Japanese Americans of the 442nd Regiment lost one-fourth of their soldiers in battles in North Africa and Italy. They suffered another 800 casualties rescuing the Texan "Lost Battalion," 211 men surrounded by German troops in the Vosges Mountains of France. As one Texan recalled, "We were never so glad to see anyone as those fighting Japanese Americans." The 442nd Regiment won 18,143 individual decorations for distinguished service. Welcoming them home in 1946, President Harry Truman declared, "You fought not only the enemy, you fought prejudice—and you won."

Nevertheless, the U.S. government would take its time acknowledging that the internment had been a grave injustice. The Supreme Court upheld the constitutionality of the policy, and Roosevelt would not rescind the evacuation order until after his reelection in 1944. The camps finally closed in 1945. All told, Japanese Americans lost property valued at $500 million. Not until 1968 would the government reimburse former internees for some of their losses. And not until 1983 would a Special Commission on Wartime Relocation and Internment of Civilians concede that because of "race prejudice, war hysteria and a failure of political leadership," the U.S. government had committed "a grave injustice" to more than 110,000 people of Japanese ancestry. In 1988 Congress would enact legislation awarding restitution payments of $20,000 each to 60,000 surviving internees—a small gesture for Americans whose only "crime" was their Japanese ancestry.

Wartime Migrations

Even before the United States officially entered World War II, the conflict had begun to change the face of the nation. The sleepy town of Richmond, California, perched near the north end of San Francisco Bay, underwent a profound transformation when the nation stepped up war production. The town's mostly white population of 23,000 ballooned to 120,000 after industrialist Henry Kaiser constructed four shipyards there. The yards employed over 150,000 workers, more than one-fourth of them African American. Most were young, married migrants from the South, and there were slightly more women than men. They came to Richmond attracted by the better pay and benefits, along with the opportunity for greater freedom than they had known in the the Jim Crow South.

Margaret Starks, daughter of southern tenant farmers, moved to Richmond. She established a blues club, edited a black newspaper, and played an active role in the National Association for the Advancement of Colored People (NAACP). Her club became a center for African American cultural and political life. Thus, black migrants not only established their own community institutions but also transformed the life of the city. This same process unfolded all over the country, bringing black culture into cities and creating a diverse urban landscape.

Many cities, however, were ill equipped to handle the influx of migrants. An estimated 60,000 African Americans moved into Chicago, for example, causing an enormous housing crisis. Many newcomers lacked even a modicum of privacy as they crowded into basements and rooms rented from total strangers. Huge numbers of whites also came north, many leaving hardscrabble farms hoping to prosper in booming war industries.

Wartime also saw new migration from abroad and a reversal of earlier immigration policies. Because of the alliance with China in the war against Japan, Congress repealed the Chinese Exclusion Act in 1943, and migrants from China became eligible for citizenship for the first time. Few Chinese actually arrived, however, and most immigration restrictions remained in force. The most significant wartime migration from abroad came from Mexico. In 1942, Mexico joined the Allies and provided an air force squadron trained in the United States that fought in the Pacific. An executive agreement between the United States and Mexico created the *bracero* program, which stipulated that the migrants were to be hired on short-term contracts and treated fairly. Under the *bracero* program, 300,000 Mexican laborers, mostly agricultural workers, came to the United States to labor in rural areas like California's San Joaquin Valley, taking the place of "Okies" who migrated to cities for defense work. By the mid–1960s, nearly 5 million Mexicans had migrated north under the program.

The war also prompted large numbers of émigrés to become American citizens. From 1941 to 1945, more immigrants became naturalized citizens than in any previous five-year period. More than 112,000 were naturalized during their service in the armed forces. But the vast majority of those naturalized—1,539,000—were civilians. For the first time, the majority were women. The largest numbers came from countries that were embroiled in the war: the British Empire, Italy, Germany, Poland, and the Soviet Union. Naturalization was a concrete way for newcomers to clarify their status and their loyalty, especially in the wake of the Smith Act of 1940. This law required all foreign-born residents to be registered and fingerprinted, and broadened the grounds for deportation.

The Home Front

Wartime mobilization brought Americans from all regions and backgrounds together in shared service and sacrifice. Industries as well as citizens dedicated themselves to the war effort. Automobile manufacturers stopped making cars and instead turned out tanks, jeeps, and other military vehicles. Citizens made do with government-rationed basic staples, from food to gasoline. As able-bodied men left their jobs to fight the war, new work opportunities opened up for women as well as for disabled Americans. Cities and centers of war production brought together young women and men who found new opportunities for sexual experimentation, while gay men and lesbians discovered newly visible communities in both military and civilian life. Although class, gender, and racial injustices persisted, the war offered new sources of pride and patriotism for women and minorities and raised expectations that they would achieve full inclusion in the American promise.

Many Americans hoped that the liberal spirit of the New Deal would endure during the war; others were eager for an end to what they perceived as Depression-era class conflict and hostility to business interests. To some extent both sides got their wish. Full employment, the increasing strength of unions, and high taxes on the wealthy pleased New Deal liberals. Profit guarantees, freedom from antitrust actions, no-strike pledges, and cheap imported labor gratified pro-business conservatives. Congress dismantled some of the New Deal's most successful agencies, including the Civilian Conservation Corps (CCC), the Works Projects Administration (WPA), and the National Youth Administration. Republicans opposed continued support for those programs, but full employment during the wartime economy made job programs unnecessary.

Building Morale

The United States, like all other major powers involved in the conflict, mounted a propaganda drive to promote support for the war effort. Roosevelt created the Office of War Information (OWI) in 1942 to coordinate morale-boosting and censorship initiatives. Working in partnership with the motion picture industry and other media outlets, the OWI sponsored

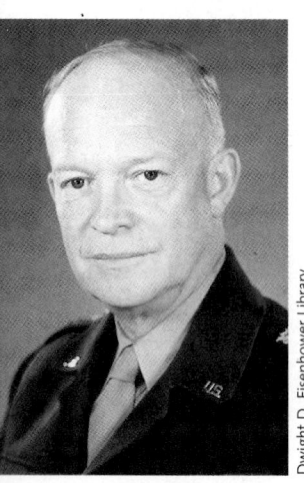
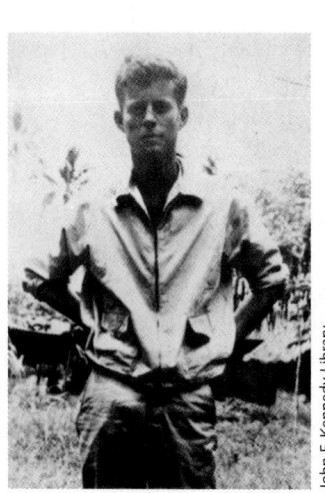
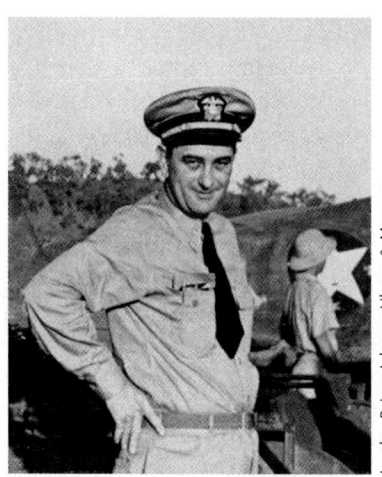
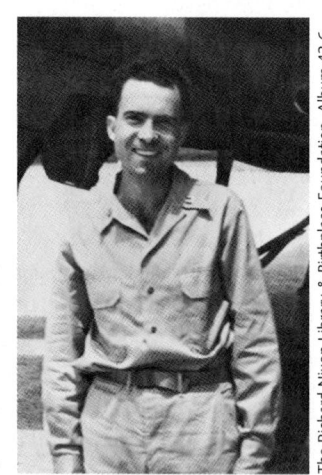

Dwight D. Eisenhower Library
John F. Kennedy Library
Lyndon Baines Johnson Library & Museum
The Richard Nixon Library & Birthplace Foundation, Album 43.6

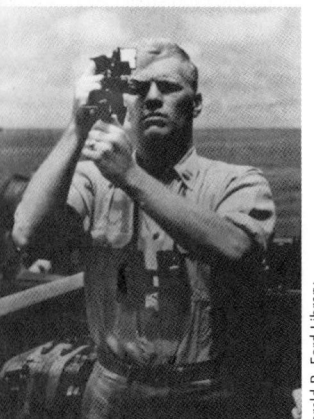
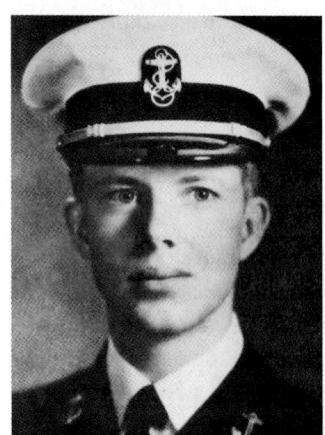
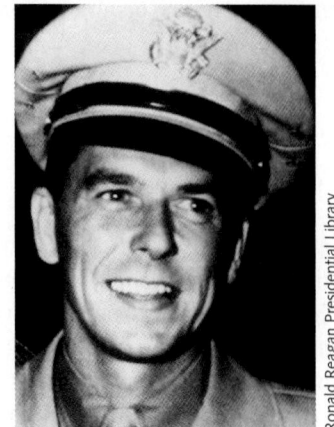
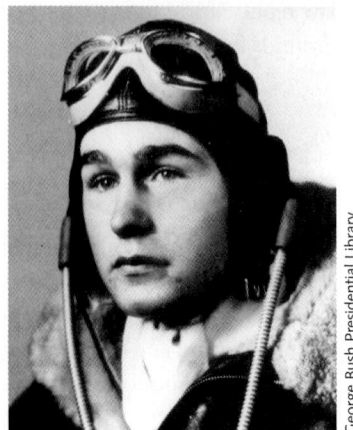

Gerald R. Ford Library
Jimmy Carter Library
Ronald Reagan Presidential Library
George Bush Presidential Library

■ **Eight American presidents elected consecutively following World War II were veterans of that war. Pictured in wartime service, from top left, are: Dwight D. Eisenhower, John F. Kennedy, Lyndon Johnson, Richard Nixon, Gerald Ford, Jimmy Carter, Ronald Reagan, and George Bush.**

movies, radio programs, publications, and posters. These productions portrayed the war as a crusade to preserve the "American way of life" and encouraged American women and men to work in war industries, enlist in the armed forces, and purchase war bonds. Eric Johnston, head of the Motion Picture Producers' Association and FDR's business advisor, insisted that Hollywood remove class conflict from its films: "We'll have no more *Grapes of Wrath*, we'll have no more *Tobacco Roads*, we'll have no more films that deal with the seamy side of American life. We'll have no more films that treat the banker as a villain."

John Ford and Greg Toland heard the message. In the 1930s, they had made movies that carried themes of political dissent. Now they helped to build consensus. In one of their first wartime films, *December 7*, produced for the Navy in 1942, the protagonist is Uncle Sam himself. Visiting Hawaii before the attack on Pearl Harbor, he tolerates labor strikes and lets Japanese Americans speak their own language and practice their Shinto religion. But he learns his lesson when fictional Japanese Americans pass military secrets to the Japanese Imperial Navy, which attacks Pearl Harbor. Uncle Sam then insists that the Japanese shed their distinct traditions, forbids class conflict, and brings all groups together to win the war. Although there was never any evidence of Japanese American sabotage, the film suggested otherwise and warned that ethnic minorities must assimilate into the American mainstream to demonstrate their patriotism.

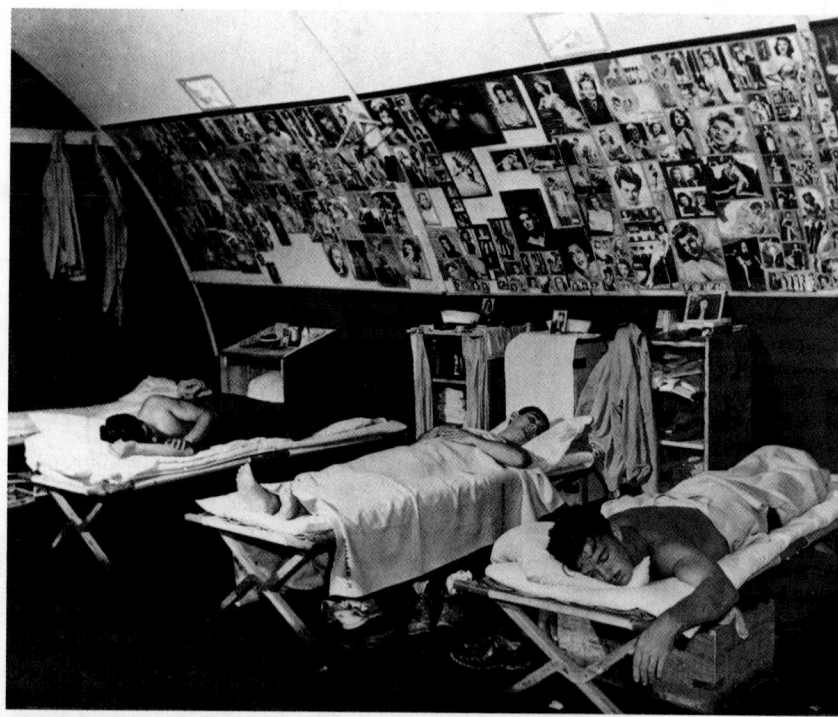

The National Archives

■ Sailors relax in the Aircraft Repair Unit (ARU–145) during their free time at Guadalcanal. The walls above their cots are decorated with "pinups" of young women in alluring poses, reminding the men of the pleasures that await them after the war.

Maintaining morale of the fighting men was critical to sustaining the war effort. Officials tried to ease the hardships of combat by providing cigarettes and beer, entertainment by and for the troops, and live performances by Hollywood celebrities like Bob Hope and Ginger Rogers. Promises of the good life waiting at home—especially images of cozy houses, warm hearths, and sexual fulfillment—reminded the men overseas why they were fighting. "Pinups"—photos of sexy but wholesome-looking women—adorned the walls of barracks, representing the joys that would follow victory.

Under government sponsorship, all the major radio networks aired a series of programs in 1942 to mobilize support for the war. One highly acclaimed segment, "To the Young," included this conversation:

YOUNG MALE VOICE: "That's one of the things this war's about."
YOUNG FEMALE VOICE: "About us?"
YOUNG MALE VOICE: "About *all* young people like us. About love and gettin' hitched, and havin' a home and some kids, and breathin' fresh air out in the suburbs . . . about livin' an' workin' *decent*, like free people."

The enemy drew on the same images in their efforts to persuade American fighting service personnel to surrender. One lurid piece of propaganda that the Japanese scattered among the American troops in the Pacific pictured a young Caucasian man and woman locked in a passionate kiss under the moonlight. The leaflet read:

That unforgettable embrace under the beautiful moon with the warmth of HER shapely body nestled against yours; that blood-tingling kiss; that over-powering sense of passion that sweeps over you—these and many other pleasant memories you'll be able to relive again if you'll throw down your arms, surrender and prepare to get out of this hell-hole.

Inside the card was the grim alternative: the same young man's bloody body with the warning: "BUT if you continue to resist—Then, under the beautiful tropical moon, only DEATH awaits you. Bullet-holes in your guts—agonizing death! You have the two alternatives. Take your choice."

Within the United States, government censors made sure that no photographs showing badly wounded soldiers or mutilated bodies reached the public. The censors also removed any images that might elicit sympathy for the enemy, such as pictures of injured or frightened enemy soldiers suffering at the hands of American soldiers. Photographs that appeared in the American media generally sanitized the horror of war, depicting noble American soldiers and a shadowy, faceless enemy. Rarely, if ever, did those on the home front see the true extent of the war's destructiveness and brutality. When men returned home severely traumatized by what they had seen, even their trauma was censored. As just one example, for more than three decades, the army suppressed John Huston's *Let There Be Light*, a film documentary of World War II veterans in a psychiatric hospital suffering from post-traumatic stress disorder.

Home Front Workers, "Rosie the Riveter," and "Victory Girls"

Wartime opened up new possibilities for jobs, income, and labor organizing, for women as well as for men, and for new groups of workers. Disabled workers entered jobs previously considered beyond their abilities, fulfilling their tasks with skill and competence. Norma Krajczar, a visually impaired teenager from North Carolina, served as a volunteer aircraft warden where her sensitive hearing gave her an advantage over sighted wardens in listening for approaching enemy planes. Deaf people streamed into Akron, Ohio, to work in the tire factories that became defense plants, making more money than they ever made before.

Along with new employment opportunities, workers' earnings rose nearly 70 percent. Income doubled for farmers and then doubled again. Labor union membership grew 50 percent, reaching an all-time high by the end of the war. In spite of no-strike pledges, strikes pressured the aircraft industry in Detroit and elsewhere. A major strike of the United Mine Workers Union erupted in 1943. Congress responded with the Smith-Connally Act of 1943, which gave the president power to seize plants or mines wherever strikes interrupted war production.

Women and minorities joined unions in unprecedented numbers. Some organized unions of their own. Energetic labor organizers like Luisa Moreno and Dorothy Ray Healy organized Mexican women working at the California Sanitary Canning Company into a powerful union that achieved wage increases and union recognition. Unions with white male leadership, however, admitted women and minorities reluctantly and tolerated them only during the war emergency. Some unions required women to quit their jobs after the war.

Nevertheless, World War II ushered in dramatic changes for American women. Wartime scarcities led to increased domestic labor as homemakers made do with rationed goods, mended clothing, collected and saved scraps and metals, and planted "victory gardens" to help feed their families. Employment opportunities for women also increased. As a result of the combined incentives of patriotism and good wages, women streamed into the paid labor force. Many of them took "men's jobs" while the men went off to fight.

"Rosie the Riveter" became the heroic symbol of the woman war worker. Pictures of attractive "Rosies" building planes or constructing ships graced magazine covers and posters. Future Hollywood star Marilyn Monroe first gained attention when her photograph appeared in *Yank*,

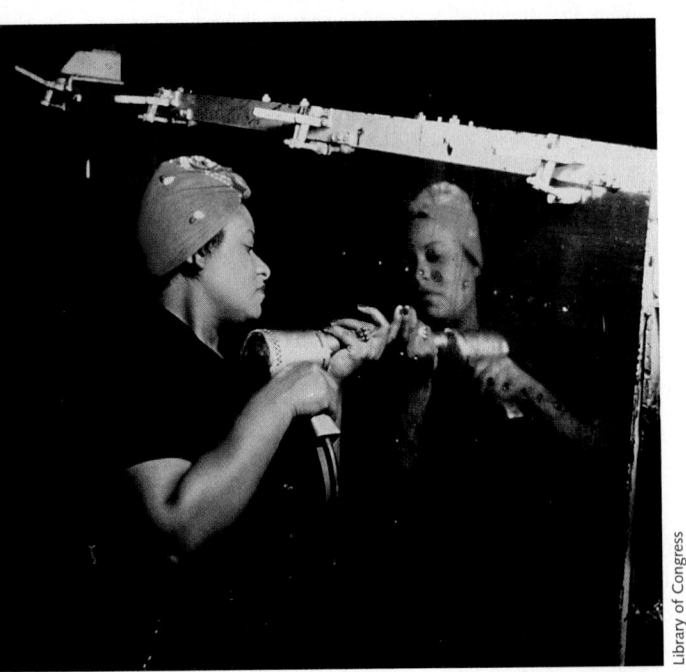

Library of Congress

■ During World War II, "Rosie the Riveter" became an icon of the working woman doing a "man's job" in the war production industries. The "Rosie" pictured here riveting was one of thousands who enjoyed the excitement and high wages of wartime work.

a magazine for soldiers. The magazine pictured her not as the sex goddess she later became, but as a typical "Rosie the Riveter" clad in overalls, working at her job in a defense plant.

Until 1943, black women were barred from work in defense industries. Poet Maya Angelou recalled that African Americans had to fight for the jobs they wanted. She became the first black streetcar conductor in San Francisco during the war, but not without a struggle. She made herself a promise that "made my veins stand out, and my mouth tighten into a prune: I WOULD HAVE THE JOB. I WOULD BE A CONDUCTORETTE AND SLING A FULL MONEY CHANGER FROM MY BELT. I WOULD." And she did.

For the first time, married women joined the paid labor force in droves and public opinion supported them. During the Depression, 80 percent of Americans had objected to the idea of wives working outside the home; by 1942, only 13 percent still objected. However, mothers of young children found very little help. In 1943 the federal government finally responded to the needs of working mothers by funding day-care centers. More than 3000 centers enrolled 130,000 children. Still, the program served only a small proportion of working mothers. Most women relied on family members to care for their children. A Women's Bureau survey in 1944 found that 16 percent of mothers working in war industries had no child-care arrangements at all. Meager to begin with and conceived as an emergency measure, government funding for child care would end after the war.

Before the war, most jobs for women were low-paying, nonunion positions that paid them an average of $24.50 a week. Wartime manufacturing jobs paid almost twice that much—$40.35 a week. During the conflict, 300,000 women worked in the aircraft industry alone. Almira Bondelid recalled that when her husband went overseas, "I decided to stay in San Diego and went to work in a dime store. That was a terrible place to work, and as soon as I could I got a job at Convair [an aircraft manufacturer]. . . . I worked in the tool department as a draftsman, and by the time I left there two years later I was designing long drill jigs for parts of the wing and hull of B–24s."

New opportunities for women also opened up in the armed services. All sectors of the armed forces had dwindled in the years between the two wars and needed to gain size and strength. Along with the 10 million men aged 21 to 35 drafted into the armed services and the 6 million who enlisted, 140,000 women volunteered for the Women's Army Corps (WACs) and 100,000 for the Navy WAVES (Women Accepted for Voluntary Emergency Service).

Most female enlistees and war workers enjoyed their work and wanted to continue after the war. The extra pay, independence, camaraderie, and satisfaction that their jobs provided had opened their eyes to new possibilities. Edith Speert, like many others, was never again content as a full-time housewife and mother. Edith's husband, Victor, was sent overseas in 1944. During the 18 months of their separation, they penned 1300 letters to each other, sometimes two or three times a day. The letters revealed the love and affection they felt for one another, but Edith did not hesitate to tell Victor how she had changed. In a letter from Cleveland, dated November 9, 1945, she wrote:

> Sweetie, I want to make sure I make myself clear about how I've changed. I want you to know *now* that you are not married to a girl that's interested solely in a home—I shall definitely have to work all my life—I get emotional satisfaction out of working; and I don't doubt that many a night you will cook the supper while I'm at a meeting. Also, dearest—I shall never wash and iron—there are laundries for that! Do you think you'll be able to bear living with me?…I love you, Edith

Despite the shifting priorities of women, the war reversed the declining marriage and fertility rates of the 1930s. Between 1941 and 1945 the birthrate climbed from 19.4 to 24.5 per 1000 population. The reversal stemmed, in part, from economic prosperity, as well as the possibility of draft deferments for married men in the early war years. However, the desire to solidify relationships and establish connections to

For the first time, married women joined the paid labor force in droves, and public opinion supported them.

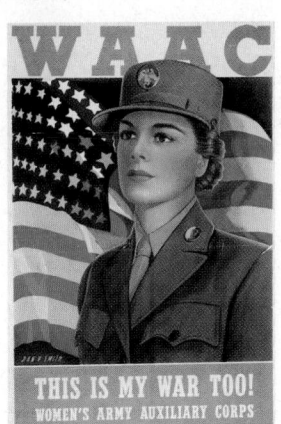

WAAC
THIS IS MY WAR TOO!
WOMEN'S ARMY AUXILIARY CORPS
UNITED · STATES · ARMY

the future during a time of great uncertainty perhaps served as the most powerful motivation. Thus, a curious paradox marked the war years: a widespread disruption of domestic life accompanied by a rush into marriage and parenthood.

At the same time that the war prompted a rush into marriage and parenthood, wartime upheaval sent the sexual order topsy-turvy. For many young women, moving to a new city or taking a wartime job opened up new possibilities for independence, excitement, and sexual adventure. One young worker recalled:

> Chicago was just humming, no matter where I went. The bars were jammed . . . you could pick up anyone you wanted to. . . . There were servicemen of all varieties roaming the streets all the time. There was never, never a shortage of young, healthy bucks. . . . We never thought of getting tired. Two, three hours of sleep was normal. . . . I'd go down to the office every morning half dead, but with a smile on my face, and report for work.

Some young women, known as "victory girls," believed that it was an act of patriotism to have a fling with a man in uniform before he went overseas. The independence of these women raised fears of female sexuality as a dangerous, ungoverned force. The worry extended beyond the traditional concern about prostitutes and "loose women" to include "good girls" whose sexual standards might relax during wartime. Public health campaigns warned enlisted men that "victory girls" would have their fun with a soldier and then leave him with a venereal disease, incapable of fighting for his country.

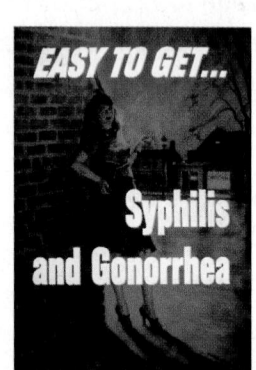

Wartime also intensified concerns about homosexuality. Urban centers and the military provided new opportunities for gay men and lesbians to form relationships and build communities. Although the military officially banned homosexuals from the forces, many served by keeping their orientation secret. If discovered, gay men faced severe punishment, including confinement in cages called "queer stockades" or in psychiatric wards. Lesbians faced similar sanctions, although the women's corps, in an effort to assure the civilian world of their recruits' femininity, often looked the other way.

Antigay crusades and policies sometimes backfired. Nowhere is this more evident than in the 1943 wartime propaganda film *This Is the Army,* starring future U.S. president Ronald Reagan. Sponsored by the Office of War Information and produced by Warner Brothers, the film centers on the romance between a soldier and an army nurse. The two wed just before the hero leaves to fight on foreign shores. The film uses humor to diffuse uneasiness and discomfort with the disrupted gender roles and sexual identities brought about by war. Soldier-comedians joke about their female superior officers. A group of he-men in drag do a clumsy chorus-line routine showing their hairy legs and bulging muscles beneath their skirts. In an ironic twist, *This Is the Army* became a popular wartime cult film among gays and lesbians.

Race and War

The Holocaust, Nazi Germany's campaign to exterminate European Jews, demonstrated the horrors of racial hatred taken to its ultimate extreme. The U.S. government did little to help Jewish refugees or to stem the slaughter of Jews in Europe. Official indifference and widespread anti-Semitism prevailed throughout the war. Nevertheless, Nazi policies against the Jews discredited racial and ethnic prejudice, forcing Americans to confront the reality of racism in their own country. Anthropologist Ruth Benedict, in her 1943 book *The Races of Mankind,* urged the United States to "clean its own house" and "stand unashamed before Nazis and condemn, without confusion, their doctrines of a Master Race." Swedish sociologist Gunnar Myrdal's *American Dilemma: The Negro Problem and Modern Democracy* called on the nation to live up to its democratic promise: "The great reason for hope is that this country has a national experience of uniting racial and cultural diversities and a national theory,

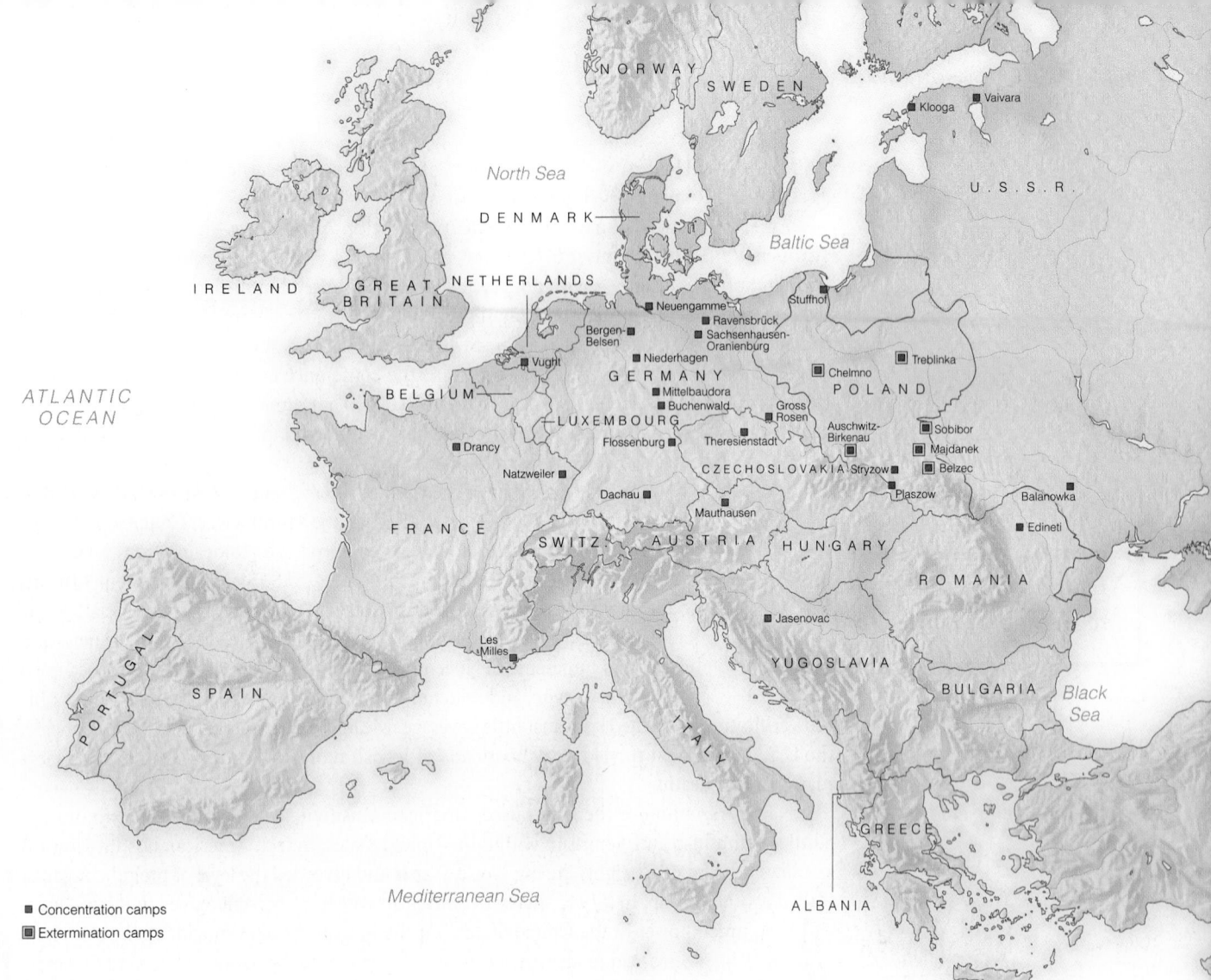

■ MAP 23.2

NAZI CONCENTRATION AND EXTERMINATION CAMPS Under Hitler, the Nazis established dozens of concentration camps where Jews and others whom the Nazis deemed "undesirable" were imprisoned. In addition to these sites, there were hundreds of slave labor camps attached to factories across Germany where Jews were forced to work for Nazi enterprises. After Hitler began his genocidal "final solution," six camps became sites of systematic mass murder, with efficient killing operations, including gas chambers disguised as shower rooms.

if not a consistent practice, of freedom and equality for all." Americans of color responded to the call for unity and demonstrated their patriotism; in return, they expected full inclusion in the democracy. There would be no return to the old racial order. As black leader W. E. B. DuBois noted, World War II was a "War for Racial Equality" and a struggle for "democracy not only for white folks but for yellow, brown, and black."

The Holocaust

Hitler's war aims included conquering all of Europe and destroying European Jewry. Throughout the war, Nazi anti-Jewish policies escalated from persecution and officially sanctioned violence to imprisonment in concentration camps, slave labor, and ultimately Hitler's "Final Solution," genocide. Nazis developed increasingly efficient means of killing Jews. Some Jewish men, women, and children perished by firing squads in mass executions. Others died of disease and malnutrition in concentration camps or at the hands of Nazi doctors in gruesome medical experiments. In the infamous Nazi death camps, guards herded prisoners into "shower rooms" that were actually gas chambers. Out of a prewar European Jewish population of

10 million, the Holocaust claimed the lives of 6 million Jews, along with homosexuals, the disabled, and Romani (also known as Gypsies).

American officials knew of the Nazi persecution of the Jews but did little about it. Throughout the 1930s, American Jewish groups pressured the Roosevelt administration to ease immigration laws to allow Jewish refugees to enter the country. But the United States raised the legal quota of Jewish immigrants only slightly. In 1938, Roosevelt organized an international conference on the refugee crisis in Evian, Switzerland, with 32 nations attending. But no nation agreed to accept large numbers of refugees, so the conference had little practical impact. In 1939, a pro-Nazi rally in New York City drew 20,000. That same year, congressional leaders defeated the Wagner–Rogers bill, which would have amended immigration quotas to allow the entry of 20,000 Jewish children.

> *The U.S. government turned away boatloads of Jewish refugees, sending them back to Germany to their deaths.*

When the Nazis began their policy of extermination in 1941, they tried to keep it a secret. But Dr. Gerhard Riegner, the World Jewish Congress representative in Geneva, Switzerland, learned about the Holocaust from a German source and informed American diplomats. U.S. State Department officials decided not to pass along the information to Washington. Despite official silence, Rabbi Stephen S. Wise, a prominent American Jewish leader, heard the news and held a press conference in November 1942. But the American press, preoccupied with military events and reluctant to publish stories of atrocities without official verification, gave the Holocaust little coverage. Meanwhile, despite news of Nazi genocide, the U.S. government turned away boatloads of Jewish refugees, sending them back to Germany to their deaths.

Nazi persecution of the Jews raised American sensitivity to the issue of racism but did little to diminish anti-Semitism within the United States. In fact, American hostility toward Jews reached new heights during World War II and exceeded the level of prejudice against any other group. In a 1942 survey of American voters, 51 percent agreed that Jews "have too much power in the United States." At the height of Nazi genocide against the Jews in 1944, when asked to identify the greatest "menace" to the nation, 24 percent of Americans polled listed Jews—more than those who listed Germans, Japanese, radicals, Negroes, and foreigners.

In Europe, American military strategists knew of the existence and location of Nazi death camps, but they refused to destroy them or to bomb the railroad lines leading to the camps. Many Europeans under Nazi domination, however, risked their lives to rescue and shelter Jews. While the United States stood by, smaller nations took action. For example, Denmark defied the Nazis even though occupied by them—taking a far greater risk than anything the United States might have done—and managed to save nearly all Danish Jews. And the tiny Dominican Republic took in more Jewish refugees than any other country in the Western Hemisphere. The United States fought a war against the Nazis but did very little to help their victims.

Racial Tensions at Home

Throughout the war years, racial tensions within the United States persisted. Black workers, who were excluded from the best-paying jobs in the defense industry, mobilized against discrimination on the job. Their most powerful advocate was African American Civil rights leader A. Philip Randolph, who had organized the overwhelmingly black Brotherhood of Sleeping Car Porters and won the union a contract with the railroads in 1937. At the beginning of American involvement in the war in 1941, Randolph pressured FDR to ban discrimination in defense industries. He threatened to organize a massive march on Washington if Roosevelt did not respond. Roosevelt got the message and issued Executive Order 8802, which created the Fair Employment Practices Commission (FEPC) to ensure that blacks and women received the same pay as white men for doing the same job. The FEPC narrowed pay gaps somewhat, but it did not solve the problem. The American Federation of Labor, which included the highest-paid workers, still refused to accept blacks as members and fought with the FEPC over the equal-pay policy.

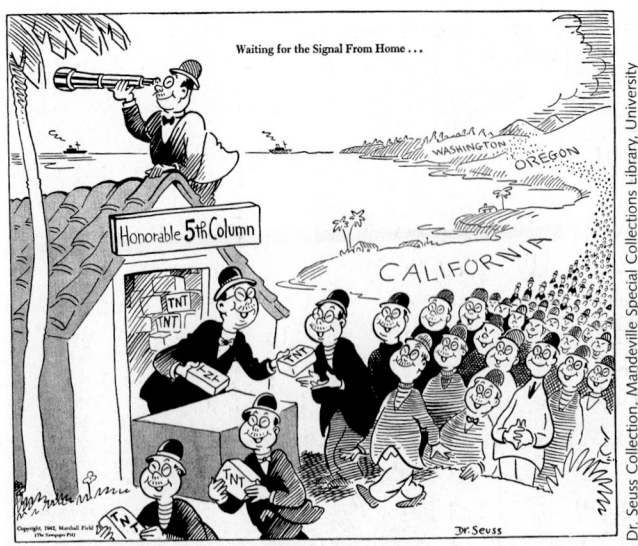

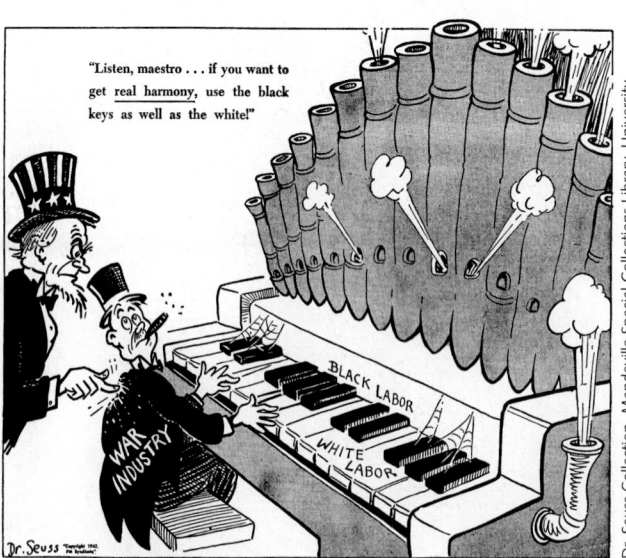

■ These two political cartoons by Dr. Seuss, known for his whimsical children's books and progressive political ideas, demonstrate that even among liberal activists, racial tolerance during World War II did not include Japanese Americans. Dr. Seuss created dozens of cartoons that criticized anti-Semitic and anti-black prejudices, but he also promoted the idea that Japanese American citizens were disloyal and dangerous. Stereotyped images such as these contributed to anti-Japanese sentiment that ultimately resulted in the relocation of Japanese Americans from the West Coast into internment camps.

Sometimes the presence of racial minorities in previously all-white work settings led to hostilities. White men who labored on the home front resented the women and minorities who were filling "men's jobs," as well as the soldiers who earned praise for their heroic manhood. Many worried about losing their jobs to returning veterans.

For example, Montana's copper workers, concerned about their job security and their masculinity, asked the federal government to issue them special certificates equating their wartime contribution with that of soldiers. The government denied their request and in 1942 sent a regiment of black miners from the South to help fill the labor shortage in Montana's copper mines. White miners—many of whom had immigrant parents and had only just begun to enjoy full inclusion in white America—were now being told that black men were their equals. The white miners refused to work next to black men and walked out of the mines en masse.

In 1943 Detroit, white workers at the Packard auto plant also walked off the job when three black employees were promoted. With increasing numbers of white and black Southerners arriving to work in the city's war industries, overcrowding strained the boundaries of traditionally segregated neighborhoods. Clashes at a new housing complex escalated into several days of rioting, resulting in 34 deaths and 1800 arrests.

In Los Angeles, the death of a Mexican American youth, Jose Diaz, at a gravel pit called Sleepy Lagoon sparked sensational news coverage and whipped up anti-Mexican fervor. Although police never determined the cause of Diaz's injuries, they filed first-degree murder charges against 22 Mexican American boys from the neighborhood. The jury found the young men guilty, but an appeals court overturned the convictions. Nevertheless, hostility continued to mount against Mexican American youths, particularly "pachucos" who sported "zoot suits," distinctive attire with flared pants, long coats, and wide-brimmed hats. Pachucos wore the zoot suit as an expression of ethnic pride and rebelliousness, as well as incipient political consciousness. Both boys and girls flaunted their distinctive clothing and enjoyed the sense of unity it inspired. Some zoot-suiters would later become active in the Chicano Movement of the 1960s—including the future leader of the United Farm Workers, Cesar Chávez. Chávez later remembered that it took "a lot of guts to wear those pants, and we had to be rebellious to do it, because the police and a few of the older people would harass us."

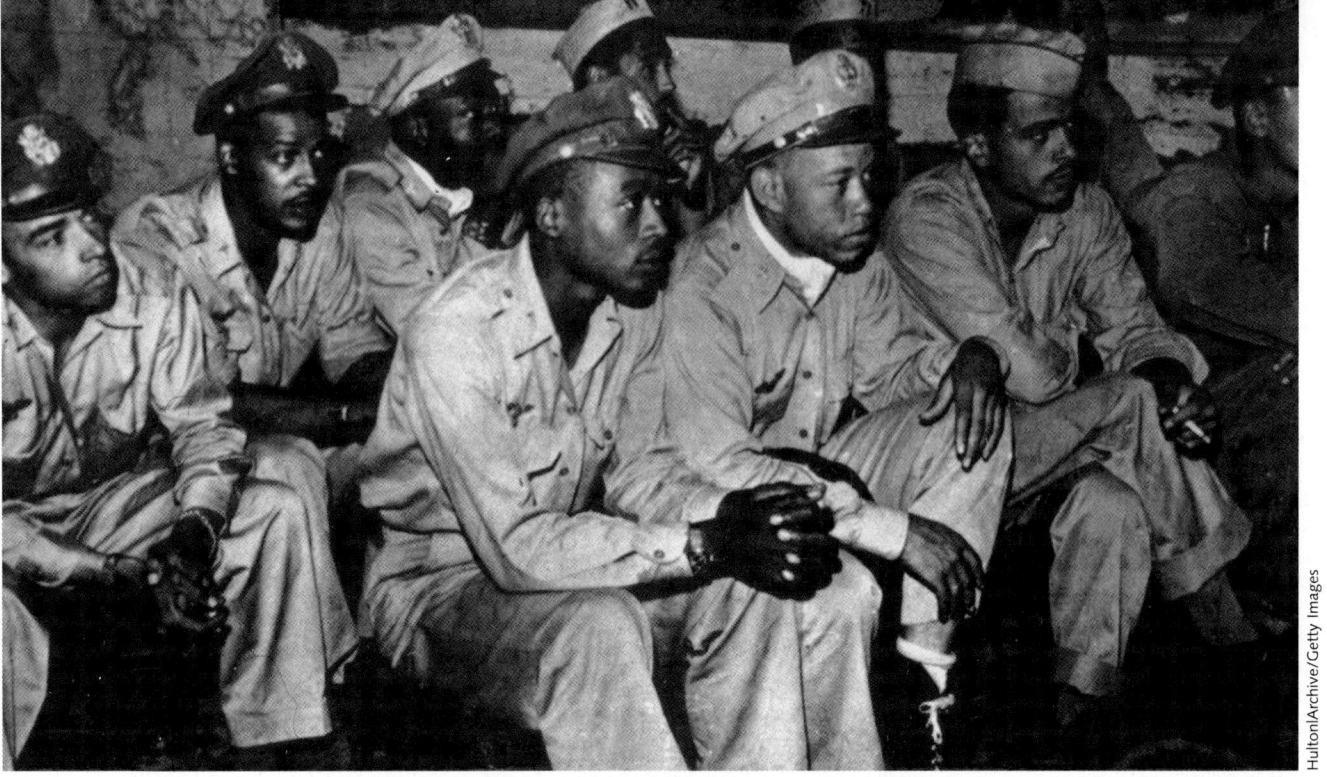

■ African American pilots, known as the Tuskegee Airmen, served in the U.S. army air force. Here members of the Mustang fighter group listen to a mission briefing in Italy in September 1944.

For eight days in June 1943 scores of soldiers hunted zoot-suiters in Los Angeles bars, theaters, dance halls, and even in their homes, pulling off their clothes and beating them. Soon the attacks expanded to all Mexican Americans, and then to African Americans as well, some of whom also wore the zoot-suit style. The Los Angeles police sided with the rioters. They stood by during the beatings and then arrested the naked and bleeding youths and charged them with disturbing the peace. The rioting raged until the War Department made the entire city of Los Angeles off limits to military personnel. Only a handful of soldiers, but more than 600 Mexican Americans, were arrested. President Roosevelt worried that the zoot-suit violence might strain relations with Mexico. He therefore allocated federal funds for job training, educational improvements, and greater access to higher education for Spanish-speaking Americans.

Fighting for the "Double V"

In spite of discrimination at home, members of minority groups responded enthusiastically to the war effort. The numbers of blacks in the Army soared from 5000 in 1940 to 700,000 by 1944, with an additional 187,000 in the Navy, Coast Guard, and Marine Corps. Four thousand black women joined the WACs. Almost all soldiers fought in segregated units, despite protests by the NAACP that "a Jim Crow army cannot fight for a free world." Nearly 1 million blacks also joined the industrial labor force during the war. African Americans fought for the "Double V"—victory over fascism abroad and racial discrimination at home. Wartime experiences and sacrifices would inspire African Americans, along with Mexican Americans and other minority citizens, to mobilize for civil rights after the war.

Like Keith Little and his boarding-school buddies who became Navajo "Code Talkers," American Indians all over the country declared their willingness to fight for the cause. The Iroquois League announced:

> It is the unanimous sentiment among the Indian people that the atrocities of the Axis nations are violently repulsive to all sense of righteousness of our people. This merciless slaughter of mankind upon the part of those enemies of free peoples can no longer be tolerated.

Zelda Webb Anderson, "You Just Met One Who Does Not Know How to Cook"

Zelda Webb Anderson became one of the first black women to enter military service during World War II. She served as an officer in the Women's Army Auxiliary Corps (WAACS), renamed the Women's Army Corps (WACS) in 1942. After the war she earned a doctorate in education at the University of California, Berkeley. Her 42-year career in education included a stint teaching at the University of East Africa in Dar-es-Salaam, Tanzania. She related her wartime experiences to the University of Nevada Oral History Program in 1995.

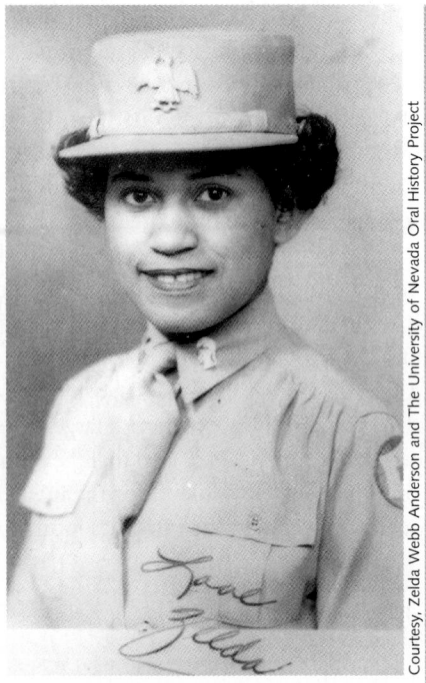

Courtesy, Zelda Webb Anderson and The University of Nevada Oral History Project

Zelda Webb Anderson

I reported for duty in January 1942. . . . This was so exciting to me. We had black officers, and our basic training was the same as for men. They would simply tell us, "You wanted to be in a man's army, so now you got to do what the men do." We learned military courtesy, history, how to shoot an M–1, go on bivouac, bathe in a teacup of water, eat hardtack rations. . . .

Every evening troops of male soldiers would march by our barracks en route to the mess hall. I told the commanding officer that we would like to have some shades at the windows. "Oh, no. You wanted to be in the man's army. Fine—you have to do what the men do." I told all the girls, "Listen, they won't give us any shades. So I want you to get right in front of the windows buck naked." The next day we had shades at all the windows. . . .

They pulled me out of basic training the third week and sent me to officer training in Des Moines. All of the instructors were white, but white and black officers were being trained in the same facility, in the same classes, and we slept in the same barracks. After OCS I was assigned to a laundry unit.

A black enlisted WAAC could either be in the laundry unit or she could be in the hospital unit. In the laundry unit, if she had a college degree, she could work at the front counter. . . . If she had less than that, then she *did* the laundry— very demeaning. And in the hospital unit they let her wash walls, empty basins, wash windows—all that menial work. . . .

I was assigned to duty at Fort Breckenridge, Kentucky. The post commander's name was Colonel Throckmorton. In a pronounced southern accent he told me, "You're going over to that colored WAC company, and you're going to be the mess officer."

I said, "Sir, I have not had any mess training."

"All you nigras know how to cook."

I said, "You just met one who does *not* know how to cook; but if you send me to Fort Eustis, Virginia, for training I will come back and be the best mess officer you have on this post."

"I ain't sending you to no school, and you're going over there to be a mess officer." When I about-faced, I kept on going. I didn't even salute him. . . .

[Much later, after developing a more cordial relationship with Colonel Throckmorton,] I told him that segregation has not allowed white people to know black people: "We know you very intimately, but you don't know how we think, how we react, and so you just try to push your stuff on us, not giving a damn about how *we* feel about this. And then when we rebel, or you meet somebody like me, who decides that you can't do this to me, then you think I'm cantankerous; you think I'm an agitator. I'm just trying to give you an education. . . ."

I lived out the rest of my days very happy in the Army. If I had succumbed to the treatment that they had given other blacks before, and not spoken up for myself, my morale would have been down. . . . In this life, you've got to speak up for yourself. You can't go around shuffling your feet with your head hung down acting apologetic. If you see something you want, you must go after it. One day somebody will recognize it, and it's a victory for you, especially when it's somebody who has denigrated you because of your race. . . .

Our country has not solved all of its problems. You have to live democracy before you can preach democracy. I've got four granddaughters, and I don't want them put in a position where they don't have equal opportunities, equal chances, and then they have to fight the same old battles that I fought again. ∎

The Cheyenne agreed, vowing to defeat an "unholy triangle" determined to "conquer and enslave the bodies, minds and souls of all free people." Fully 25,000 Native Americans, including 800 women, served in the military during the war. By 1945, nearly one-third of all able-bodied Native American men between 18 and 50 had served. Five percent of them were killed or wounded in action. Native Americans enlisted at a higher rate than the general population, prompting the *Saturday Evening Post* to editorialize, "We would not need the Selective Service if all volunteered like the Indians."

In addition to those who enlisted, half of all able-bodied Native American men not in the service and one-fifth of women left reservations for war industry jobs. At the beginning of the war, men on reservations earned a median annual income of $500, less than one-fourth the national average. One-third of all Native American men living off reservations were unemployed. Worse, the average life expectancy for Native Americans in 1940 was just 35 years, compared with 64 years for the population at large. Like others who found new opportunities during the conflict, Native Americans hoped that the economic progress they had made would be permanent. But the boom would end for them when the war ended. Fewer than 10 percent of Native Americans who relocated to cities found long-term employment after the war.

Total War

World War II consisted of two wars, one centered in Europe and the other in the Pacific. Combatants in both conflicts engaged in total war—the bombing of civilian as well as military targets. The advantageous geographic position of the United States enabled it to wage total war without attacks on its own cities.

The war transformed much of the world. By the time it ended, Hitler had killed 6 million Jews and destroyed the Jewish communities in Europe. Large parts of the Soviet Union, Europe, and Asia lay in ruins. The United States had deployed the most powerful weapon ever used in warfare. Of all the combatants, only the United States escaped physical destruction on its own national soil. Coming out of the war physically unscathed, economically sound, and politically strong, the United States became the most prosperous and powerful nation in the world.

The War in Europe

The attack on Pearl Harbor brought the United States immediately into the war in both Europe and the Pacific. The leaders of the Allied Powers, including the United States, Britain, and the Soviet Union, had to develop a strategy to defeat the Nazis. But the Allies did not always agree on how to conduct the war, and relations between the United States and the Soviet Union remained strained. Unable to fully overcome the hostility and suspicion that had marked their earlier encounters, leaders of both countries fought the war with postwar power considerations in mind.

Like the United States at Pearl Harbor, the Soviet Union suffered a shocking blow when the Nazis launched a surprise invasion in June 1941 in violation of the nonaggression pact Hitler had signed with Stalin in 1938. The Soviets suffered huge losses as 200 German divisions advanced across Eastern Europe and into the Soviet Union toward Moscow. With the full might of the Nazi forces concentrated on the front lines against the Russians in Eastern Europe, Soviet premier Joseph Stalin wanted the United States to open a second front in Western Europe to divert the Nazis toward the west and relieve pressure on the Soviet Union. In May 1942 Roosevelt assured Stalin that the United States would support an Allied invasion across the English Channel into France. But the British prime minister, Winston Churchill, persuaded FDR to delay that dangerous maneuver and instead to launch an invasion of French north Africa, which was controlled by the Nazi occupation forces in Vichy, France.

While the Allies turned their attention to north Africa, the Soviets managed single-handedly to force the German army into retreat at Stalingrad, where fierce fighting lasted from August 1942 to January 1943. The Battle of Stalingrad was a major turning point in the war and stopped Nazi aggression on the eastern front. The north Africa campaign, code-named TORCH, also concluded successfully for the Allies. Axis soldiers in north Africa surrendered in May 1943. The following summer the Allied forces overran the island of Sicily and moved into southern Italy. A fascist Grand Council led by Field Marshall Pietro Badoglio had overthrown Mussolini and opened communication with General Dwight D. Eisenhower, commander of the Allied forces in Europe. By 1944 the Allied forces reached Rome and backed the new Italian regime. Roosevelt and Churchill continued to delay the opening of the second front as the Soviets waited for relief.

The long-awaited Allied invasion across the English Channel, Operation OVERLORD, finally began on June 6, 1944, code named D-Day. On D-Day, the force assembled in England crossed the English Channel to France. At dawn, in the largest amphibious landing in history, more than 4000 Allied ships descended on the beaches at Normandy. As the troops splashed onto shore, they met a barrage of German fire. Many thousands died on the beach that day. Over

■ **MAP 23.3**
WORLD WAR II IN EUROPE   Along the eastern front of the war in Europe, Soviet troops did the bulk of the fighting and sustained the highest casualties. The Battle of Stalingrad, in which Soviet troops finally drove back the Nazis after months of brutal fighting, was a major turning point in the war.

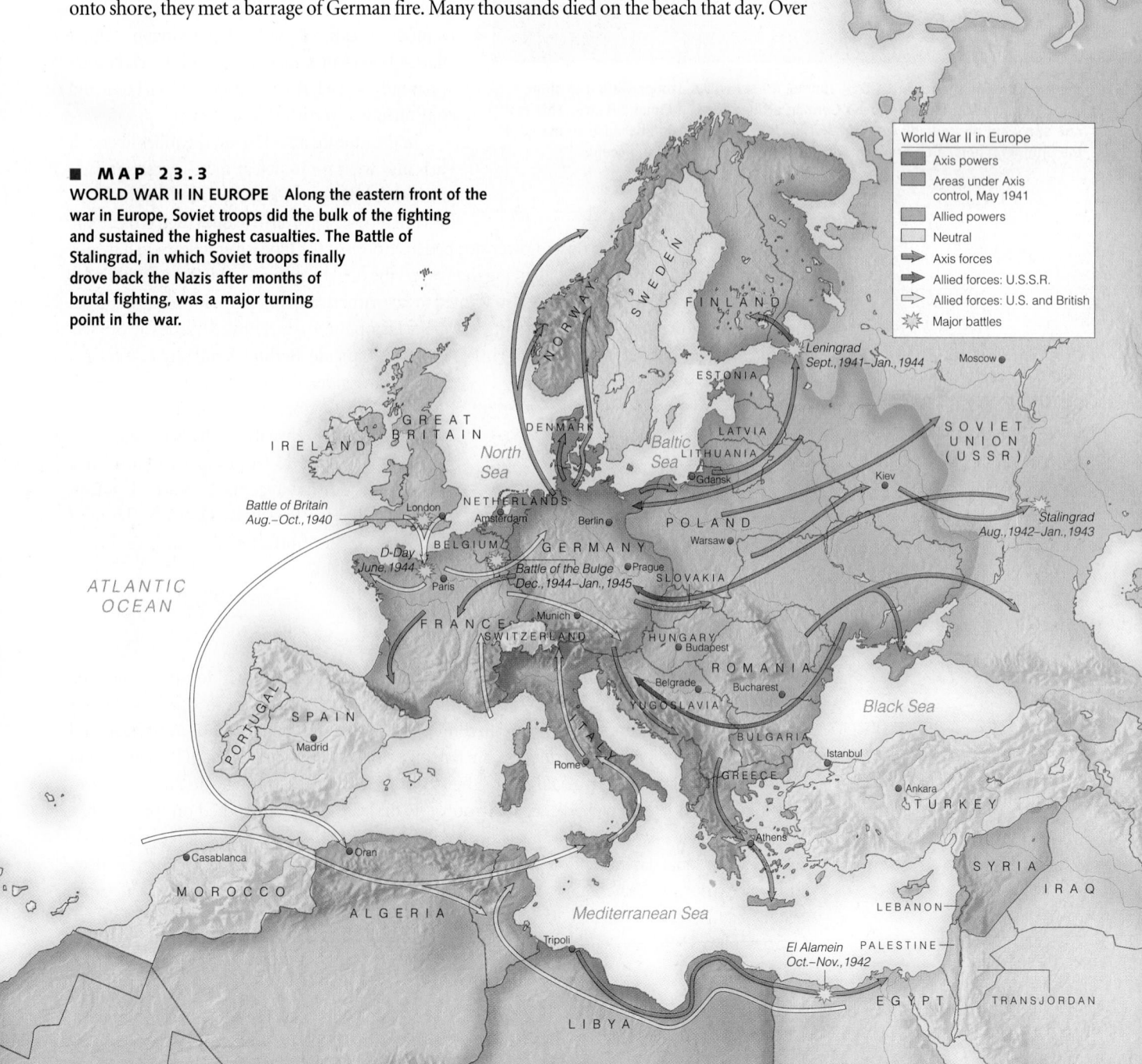

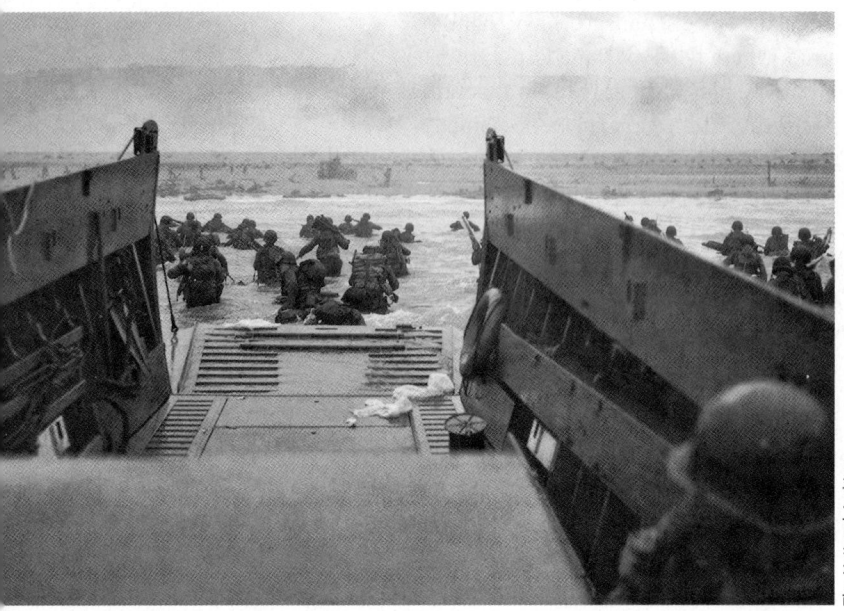

The National Archives

■ A photograph taken on D-Day, June 6, 1944, as U.S. troops waded to shore from their landing craft and faced German artillery fire on Omaha Beach. This is a rare surviving photograph from the initial Normandy invasion because so many of the photographers, along with thousands of soldiers, died at the scene.

the next 10 days, more than 1 million soldiers landed at Normandy, along with 50,000 vehicles and more than 100,000 tons of supplies, opening the way for an advance into Nazi-occupied France.

As the war continued to rage, Roosevelt prepared for the November election. Much of the 1944 campaign swirled around Roosevelt's suitability for reelection: whether he should serve an unprecedented fourth term, and whether his health would hold up—the 62-year-old president suffered from heart disease and high blood pressure. Party regulars persuaded FDR to drop Vice President Henry A. Wallace from the ticket and replace him with Senator Harry S. Truman from Missouri. The Republicans chose Thomas E. Dewey, governor of New York, to run against FDR. Democrats campaigned on the slogan "Don't change horses in midstream," and the electorate apparently agreed. Roosevelt won the election and continued his wartime leadership.

In the months after D-Day, the Allies liberated Paris and went on to defeat the Germans in Belgium at the Battle of the Bulge, sending the Nazis into full retreat. The Allied armies then crossed the Rhine and headed for Berlin. Eisenhower stopped his troops at the Elbe River to let Soviet troops take Berlin. Eisenhower hoped that giving the Soviets the final triumph would ease postwar relations with the Soviet Union—but he also wanted to save American lives. Huge numbers of Soviet troops died in the siege of Berlin, but the war in Europe was nearly over. With the Soviets approaching his bunker in April 1945, Hitler committed suicide. Berlin fell on May 2, and Germany surrendered at Reims, France, on May 7, 1945—V-E (Victory in Europe) Day.

FDR did not live to see the Nazis defeated. On April 12, 1945, he died suddenly of a cerebral hemorrhage. As a stunned nation mourned, Vice President Harry S. Truman took the oath of office as the nation's thirty-third president.

TABLE 23-2			
The Election of 1944			
Candidate	Political Party	Popular Vote	Electoral Vote
Franklin D. Roosevelt	Democratic	25,602,504	432
Thomas E. Dewey	Republican	22,006,285	99

The War in the Pacific

As the conflict in Europe came to an end, the war in the Pacific continued to rage. Following the attack on Pearl Harbor, Japan continued its conquests in the Pacific. In April 1942 General Douglas MacArthur, driven from the Philippines to Australia, left 12,000 American and 64,000 Filipino soldiers to surrender on the Bataan peninsula and the island of Corregidor. On the infamous "Bataan Death March" to the prison at Camp O'Donnell, the Japanese beat, tortured, and shot the sick and starving troops. As many as 10,000 men died on the march.

Now in control of Indochina, Thailand, the Philippines, and the chain of islands from Sumatra to Guadalcanal, Japan's military leaders planned to destroy what remained of the U.S. fleet. But MacArthur marshaled his forces and achieved a major victory in the Battle of the Coral Sea in May 1942. U.S. intelligence sources discovered that the Japanese were planning a massive assault on Midway Island, a naval base key to Hawaii's defense. Under the command of

Admiral Chester Nimitz, the United States launched a surprise air strike on June 4, 1942, sinking four Japanese carriers, destroying 322 planes, preserving the American presence at Midway, and virtually destroying Japanese offensive capabilities. Two months later, Nimitz's forces landed at Guadalcanal in the Solomon Islands, subduing the Japanese in five months of brutal fighting. Having seized the offensive, U.S. troops continued toward Japan. MacArthur's forces took New Guinea, and, by February 1944, Nimitz secured the Marshall Islands and the Marianas.

At about the same time that Allied forces in Europe were landing in Normandy, the United States invaded Saipan, the main island bastion that protected Japan's mainland. In a savage air battle on June 19, the Americans shot down 346 Japanese planes and lost 50 of their own. The attack killed 22,000 Japanese civilians—two-thirds of the island's population. The United States suffered 14,000 casualties. But the grueling battle secured for the United States a strategic base for launching bombing raids on Tokyo. The bloody war in the Pacific continued, with critical Allied victories on the islands of Iwo Jima and Okinawa in the spring of 1945. Crucial to these victories were the sensitive radio communications achieved by the special Marine unit of Navajo "Code Talkers."

In China the struggle against Japanese aggression grew complicated because China was also engaged in a civil war. Initially, the Chinese Nationalists appeared to have the largest military forces to resist the Japanese, so Roosevelt declared support for Jiang Jieshi (Chiang Kai-shek), the corrupt and unpopular Nationalist leader. Jiang continued to demand Allied support as a growing communist movement, led by Mao Zedong (Mao Tsetung), challenged the Japanese and gained support among Chinese peasants. Although the Nationalists failed to stop the Japanese, Roosevelt continued to back Jiang's ineffective leadership, setting the stage for political tensions that persisted after the war.

The war in the Pacific was particularly vicious. Racism on both sides fueled acts of extreme brutality. Japan's leaders believed that their racial superiority gave them a divine mission to conquer Asia. The Japanese tortured prisoners of war and civilians in their conquered lands. They tested biological weapons and conducted medical experiments on live subjects. Japanese troops forced Chinese and Korean women into sexual slavery, euphemistically calling them "comfort women."

Racial hostility also promoted American battlefield savagery. U.S. troops in the Pacific often killed the enemy instead of taking prisoners and desecrated the enemy dead with disrespect equal to that meted out by the Japanese on the bodies of their foes. On the home front, American cultural images and popular sentiments vilified the Japanese not only as a hated enemy but also as a monstrous race. War correspondent Ernie Pyle explained that "in Europe we felt that our enemies, horrible and deadly as they were, were still people. But . . . the Japanese were looked upon as something subhuman and repulsive, the way some people feel about cockroaches or mice." Respectable magazines such as *Science Digest* ran articles titled "Why Americans Hate Japs More Than Nazis."

As American troops closed in on Japan, Roosevelt approved a plan to firebomb Japanese cities. The Allies had already bombed German cities, destroying much of Hamburg and Dresden and killing thousands of civilians. To persuade Americans to accept the bombing strategy with its inevitable civilian casualties, government censors lifted the ban on stories of Japanese treatment

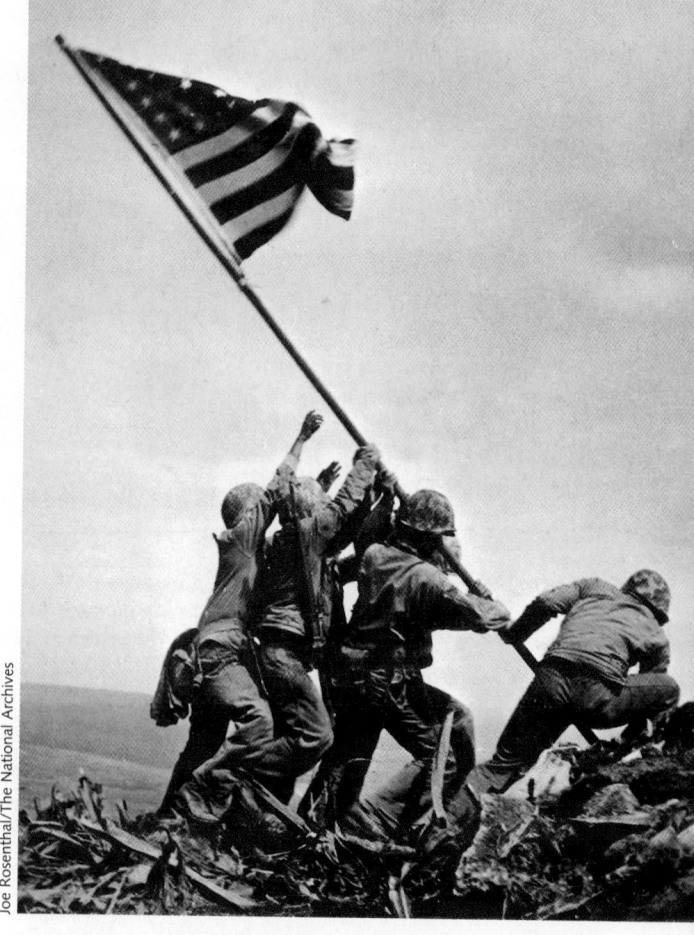

Joe Rosenthal/The National Archives

■ Associated Press photographer Joe Rosenthal took this photo, "Old Glory goes up on Mt. Suribachi, Iwo Jima," and won a Pulitzer Prize for it in 1945. Although controversy surrounded the photo (some witnesses claimed it was staged with a larger flag after the original flag had been planted), it became an icon of American determination and unity in World War II.

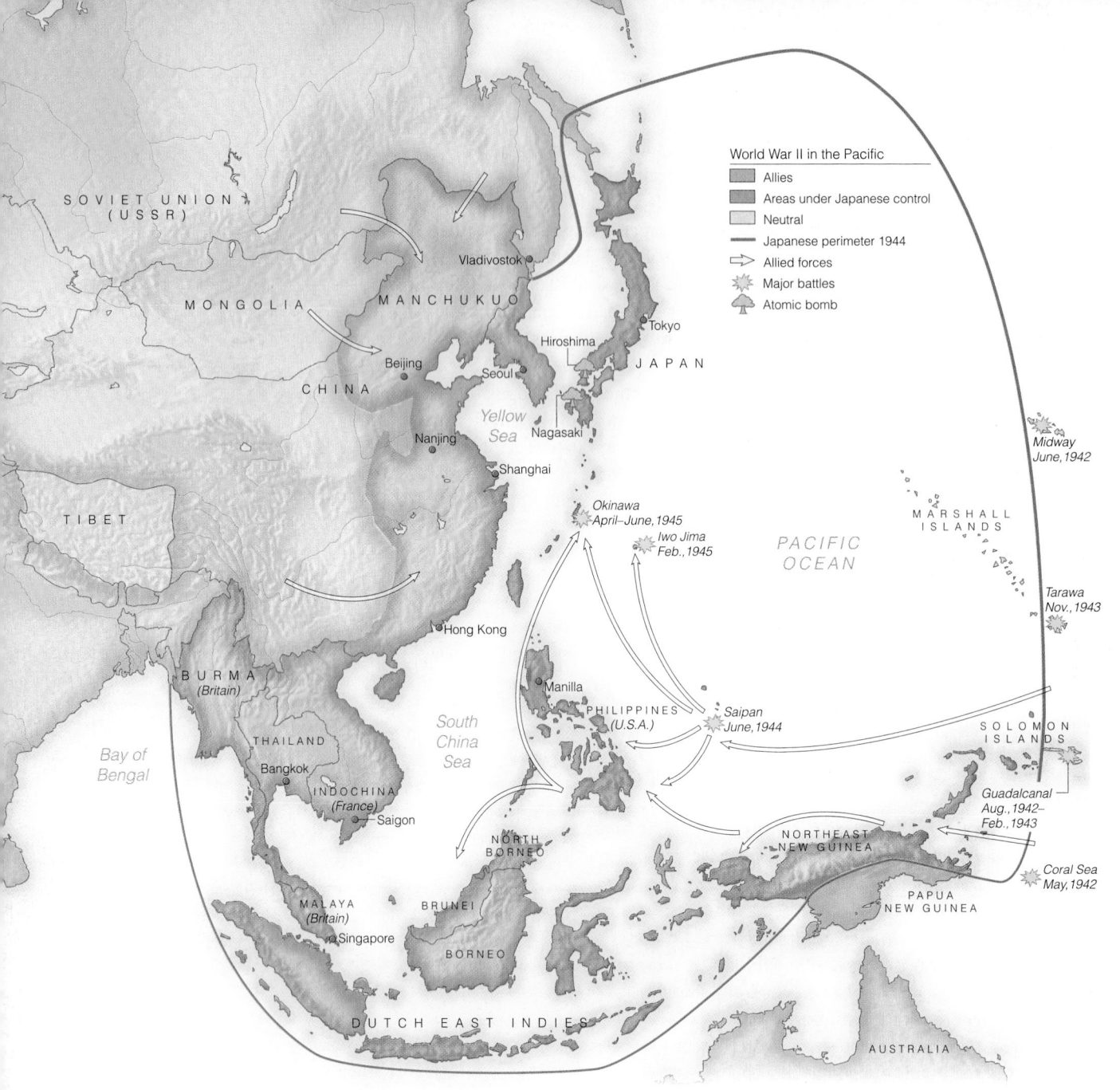

■ MAP 23.4

WORLD WAR II IN THE PACIFIC During World War II, the Japanese occupied vast territories in Asia and the Pacific. The Battle of Midway in 1942 was the first major victory for the United States in the Pacific and helped turn the tide of the war in favor of the Allies.

of American war prisoners. Reports of atrocities, as well as virulently racist images of the Japanese, flooded the media. On March 9 and 10, 1945, bombing raids led by General Curtis LeMay leveled 16 square miles of Tokyo—one-fourth of the city—and left 185,000 dead or wounded. LeMay's bombers then turned to other cities. Firebombs reportedly killed a higher number of civilians than Japanese soldiers who died in battle.

The End of the War

Allied leaders met several times to plan for the postwar era. Roosevelt hoped to ensure American dominance and to limit Soviet power. At a conference in Teheran, Iran, in 1943 Roosevelt insisted that the Eastern European states of Poland, Latvia, Lithuania, and Estonia should be independent after the war. As the war wound down, Churchill, Stalin, and Roosevelt met again at Yalta, in Ukraine, in February 1945. They agreed to demand Germany's unconditional surrender and to divide the conquered nation into four zones to be occupied by Britain, the Soviet Union, the United States, and France. It became obvious at Yalta that separate spheres of influence would prevail after the war. Poland was a source of contention. Although Stalin nominally agreed to allow free elections in Eastern Europe, he intended to make sure that the countries bordering the Soviet Union would be under his control. He also pledged to enter the war against Japan and received assurances that the Soviet Union would regain the lands lost to Japan in the 1904–1905 Russo-Japanese War.

In July 1945 the newly sworn-in American president, Harry Truman, joined Stalin and Churchill (replaced by Clement Attlee after Churchill's election loss) at Potsdam, near Berlin. The three leaders issued a statement demanding "unconditional surrender" from Japan while privately agreeing to let Japan retain its emperor. The rest of the conference focused on postwar Europe. At Potsdam Truman learned of the successful test of the atomic bomb. With the new weapon in his hands, he now knew that Soviet assistance would not be needed to end the war in the Pacific.

As the war ended in Europe, Allied troops liberated the Nazi concentration camps. At that moment, the world finally learned the extent of Hitler's "Final Solution." Among the soldiers who first entered the camps were a number of Japanese Americans. Ichiro Imamura described the sight at Dachau: "When the gates swung open, we got our first good look at the prisoners. . . . They were like skeletons—all skin and bones. . . . They were sick, starving and dying." Some of the survivors saw the Japanese American soldiers and feared that they were Japanese allies of the Germans. A *Nisei* soldier reassured them, "I am an American soldier, and you are free."

As the victors carved up Hitler's Third Reich, the war in the Pacific continued. The United States persisted in demanding "unconditional surrender" and vowed to continue to blockade Japan's ports, firebomb its cities, and possibly launch an invasion if the Japanese refused to surrender. Later, critics of this strategy argued that the demand for unconditional surrender strengthened the Japanese will to resist. They noted that the United States did nothing to assure the Japanese that the victorious Americans would not execute the emperor, nor did American leaders respond to Japanese peace overtures.

The atomic bomb offered Truman a new means to end the war. The secret project to develop the bomb had been under way for several years, initially for possible use against Germany. In 1939 scientists in Berlin had achieved atomic fission by splitting the uranium atom, making it possible to release the tremendous energy stored in the atom. Albert Einstein, the German Jewish physicist who came to the United States after Hitler came to power in 1933, had warned Roosevelt that the Germans might be developing an atomic weapon. Einstein urged the United States to establish a small research program to keep pace. In 1942 American scientists reported that with adequate resources, they could develop an atomic bomb in time to affect the course of the war. Impressed, Roosevelt authorized the Manhattan Project, the

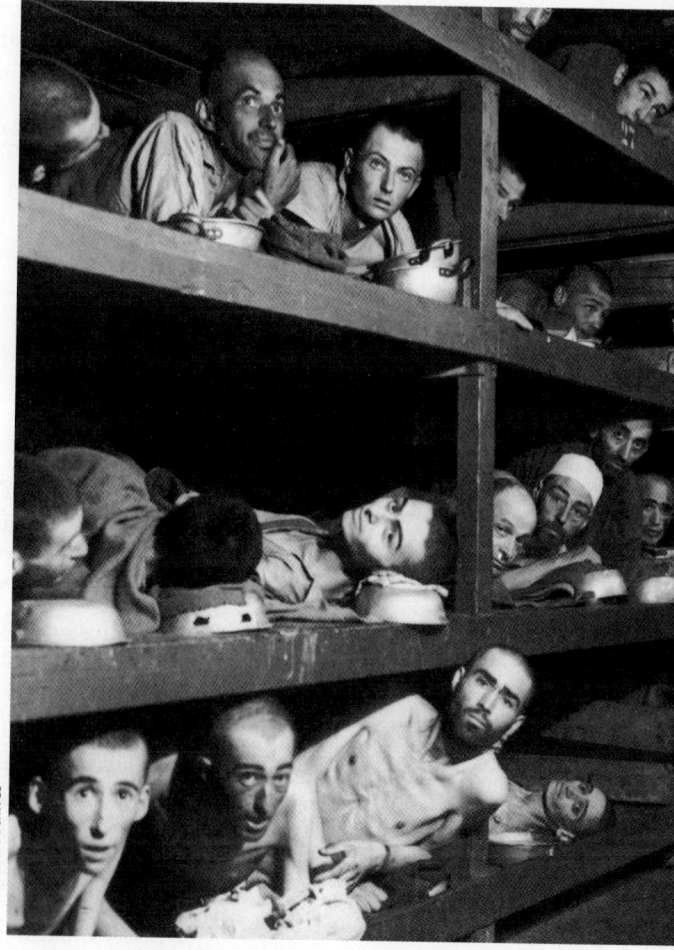

The National Archives

■ Slave laborers rest in the Buchenwald concentration camp near Jena, Germany. These inmates were among those who were still alive when troops of the 80th Division entered the camp on April 16, 1945. At labor camps such as this one, and death camps such as Auschwitz, 6 million Jews, along with thousands of Romani (Gypsies), Poles, mentally and physically handicapped people, and homosexuals, died in the Holocaust.

The Atomic Bomb: Political and Cultural Fallout

Since the dawn of the atomic age, the United States has been the only nation that has actually waged nuclear war. The dropping of the atomic bombs on the Japanese cities of Hiroshima and Nagasaki unleashed not only massive death and destruction but also ongoing controversies over the development and use of nuclear weapons and the nature of modern warfare. The level of destruction inflicted on the Japanese civilian population shocked the nation and the world. But well before the nuclear attacks on Japan, hundreds of thousands of civilians had already perished in the war.

During World War II, bombing of civilian targets became commonplace. The Japanese bombed civilians in Nanjing, China; the Germans did the same in Guernica, Spain. Allied bombing raids nearly demolished the German cities of Berlin and Dresden and the Japanese capitol of Tokyo. One night of conventional bombing in Tokyo in March 1945 killed as many civilians as the atomic bomb dropped on Hiroshima. With its huge Air Force, the United States became the greatest bombing power during the war. But the atomic bombs took civilian casualties to a new level, not only because of the enormous death toll wrought by a single bomb but also because of the deadly radioactive fallout that lingered. Conventional bombing raids did not create fallout to harm survivors, their descendants, or the environment.

With the successful 1952 test of the hydrogen (fusion) bomb—1000 times more powerful than the bombs dropped on Japan—scientists warned that the use of such weapons in warfare could create a "nuclear winter" that would destroy life on Earth. Horror at the impact of the bombs discouraged their use throughout the remainder of the twentieth century.

Civilian casualties, however, remained a fact of warfare. Guerrilla warfare increased the likelihood of civilian casualties in Vietnam, where American troops found it nearly impossible to distinguish combatants from noncombatants. American forces made widespread use of napalm, the antipersonnel weapon that set fire to anyone in its path, civilian or military. Massacres of villagers, such as the infamous killings at My Lai, turned many Americans against the war.

Although the United States and the Soviet Union refrained from using atomic weapons during the many hot wars that erupted during the Cold War, the two superpowers developed tens of thousands of nuclear weapons with sophisticated delivery systems to launch

research program to develop nuclear weapons, under the direction of J. Robert Oppenheimer. The project got under way at a top-secret laboratory in Los Alamos, New Mexico. The building of the bomb was the work of 125,000 people and cost nearly $2 billion. The first test of the device took place on July 16, 1945, at Alamagordo, New Mexico.

When Truman learned of the successful test, he wanted to use the bomb immediately. He hoped to avoid an invasion of Japan that would have cost the lives of many American soldiers, and he wanted to send a message to the Soviet Union that the United States would be the dominant power in the postwar world. But Truman's advisors did not all agree about whether or how the new weapon should be deployed. Some of the scientists who had developed the bomb urged a "demonstration" in a remote, unpopulated area that would impress the Japanese but would not cause loss of life. General George C. Marshall and other military leaders argued in favor of dropping the bomb on military or industrial targets, with ample warning ahead of time to enable civilians to leave target areas. But others agreed with Truman that dropping the bomb on a major city, without warning, would be the only way to persuade the Japanese to surrender unconditionally. Given the death and destruction already inflicted on Japanese cities by fire-bombing, the atomic bomb seemed to some like an escalation of current strategy.

But when the first bomb exploded over Hiroshima on August 6, 1945, and the second on Nagasaki two days later, the horrifying destructiveness of nuclear weapons became apparent. Even though the American public saw few images of the carnage on the ground, the huge mushroom cloud and the descriptions of cities leveled and people instantly incinerated shocked

attacks from land, sea, and air. Proponents argued that the nuclear deterrent prevented the outbreak of World War III. But detractors claimed that the arms race increased international tensions and strained the economies of both nations. In 1962 the Cuban Missile Crisis nearly led to nuclear war.

Fifty years after the end of World War II, the controversy over the use of the weapons remained heated. The Smithsonian Institution planned an exhibit to display the *Enola Gay,* the plane that dropped the atomic bomb over Hiroshima, with an explanation of the arguments on both sides on the issue. Fierce opposition to the proposed exhibit forced the Smithsonian to abandon the plan, prompting the institute's director to resign in protest.

At the dawn of the twenty-first century, the arms race continued to generate policy debates. President George W. Bush revived the "Star Wars" plan of President Ronald Reagan to build a satellite shield against

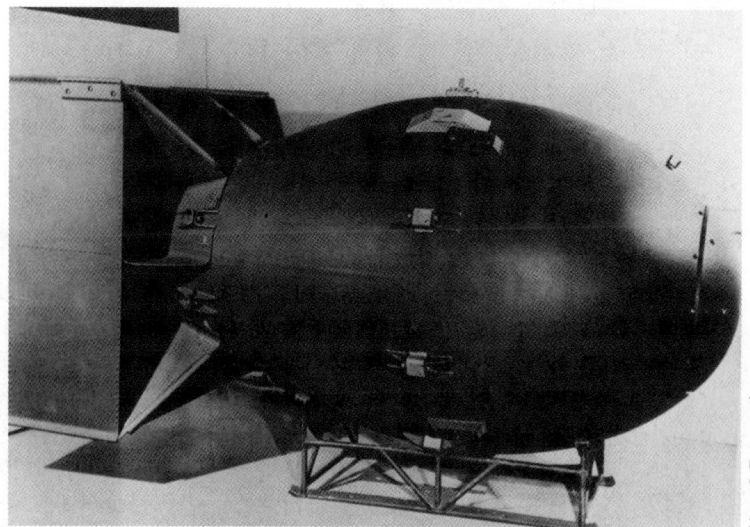

Harry S. Truman Library

This atomic bomb, named "Fat Man," was dropped on Nagasaki, Japan, on August 8, 1945, two days after the first bomb destroyed the city of Hiroshima. The Japanese surrendered soon afterward, bringing World War II to an end. Controversy still surrounds the dropping of these weapons, which killed hundreds of thousands of civilians.

incoming missiles. Advocates of the plan claimed that it would protect the United States from nuclear attack. Critics charged that the system would not work and that it would probably generate a new arms race. As the debate continued, around the world—in missile silos, submarines, and bomber planes—nuclear warheads remained poised to strike. ■

the nation and the world. In addition to the immediate devastation wreaked by the bomb, deadly radioactive fallout remained in the atmosphere, causing illness and death for months and even years after the attack. The Japanese surrendered on September 2, 1945, V-J (Victory in Japan) Day. Many people breathed a sigh of relief that the war was finally over. But doubts and controversies over the use of the weapon, and the nuclear arms race that it sparked, have continued to this day.

Conclusion

World War II left massive devastation in its wake all across the globe. The United States was the only country involved in the war that emerged from it stronger than before the conflict began. With the exception of Pearl Harbor, no fighting took place on American soil. Although thousands of Americans died in the conflict, American casualties were far below those suffered by other countries. The wartime economy provided full employment and brought the nation out of the Depression. At the end of the war, the United States was the most powerful nation in the world.

The war changed life for Americans in profound ways. Although wartime forged a sense of unity as the nation came together to fight against fascism, it also highlighted fissures within American society. Members of minority groups fought in segregated units, but racial tensions

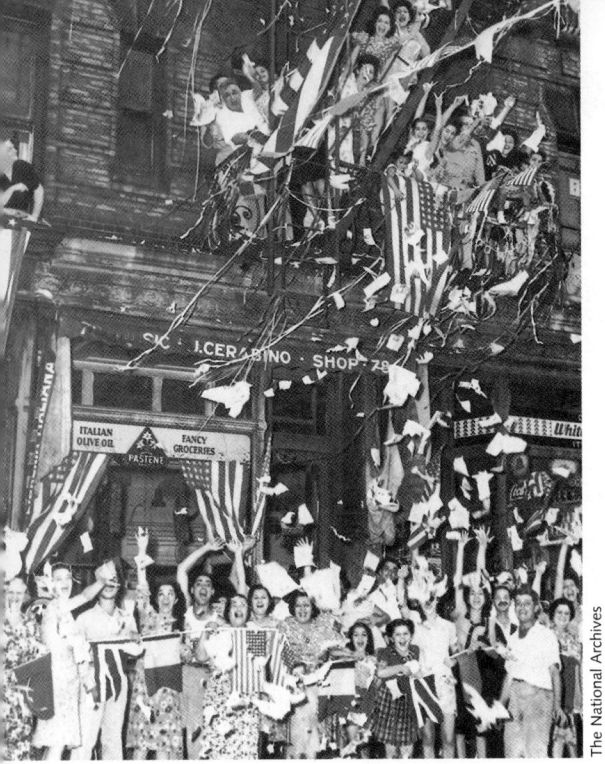

■ On V-J Day, August 14, 1945, New Yorkers of Italian descent celebrate Japan's surrender. Although the United States fought against the country of their ancestors, these Americans showed their spirited support for the Allied cause.

and conflicts erupted at home, even as the country fought against a racist foe. Women joined the paid labor force and the armed services in unprecedented numbers, while at the same time being bombarded by official and cultural messages reminding them that their ultimate service to the nation was as wives and mothers.

At the end of the war, veterans of color returned to fight for the still unfulfilled side of the Double V: victory against racism at home. Women joined returning veterans to form families and have babies in the most dramatic rush into parenthood in the nation's history, but they did not retreat from the paid labor force. World War II marked the beginning of a steady increase in employment for women that continued for the rest of the century.

While life at home changed dramatically, so did the place of the United States in the world. The war's conclusion did not usher in the era of peace Americans expected. European empires staggered on the brink of collapse. Only the United States and the Soviet Union remained as military forces, shifting the international balance of power from a multipolar to a bipolar system. The victors carved up countries in Europe and Asia according to geopolitical considerations, with little regard for national affinities. Soon American troops would fight again in the artificially divided lands of Korea and Vietnam. For the next half century, the fallout from World War II, as well as the power struggle between the United States and the Soviet Union, would shape political relationships across the globe.

Sites to Visit

Powers of Persuasion—Poster Art of World War II
www.archives.gov/exhibit_hall/powers_of_persuasion/powers_of_persuasion_home.html

This Library of Congress site includes posters created during World War II to encourage support for the war and to build morale.

A-Bomb WWW Museum
www.csi.ad.jp/ABOMB/

This site includes information about the impact of the atomic bombs dropped on Japan during World War II as well as materials and images about the development of nuclear weapons.

A People at War
www.archives.gov/exhibit_hall/a_people_at_war/a_people_at_war.html

This National Archives site includes materials and images about the contributions millions of Americans made to the war effort.

The United States Holocaust Memorial Museum
www.ushmm.org/index.html

This official website of the U.S. Holocaust Memorial Museum in Washington, D.C., covers the history and documents of the Holocaust.

Tuskegee Airmen
www.wpafb.af.mil/museum/history/prewwii/ta.htm

This site of the Air Force Museum at Wright-Patterson Air Force Base includes information and photographs of the African American pilots of World War II.

Abraham Lincoln Brigade Archives
www.alba-valb.org/aboutalb.htm

This site has information and articles about the Spanish Civil War and the unit of American volunteers who fought in it.

The Zoot Suit Riots
www.pbs.org/wgbh/amex/zoot/

This website from the Public Broadcasting Service (PBS) documentary series *The American Experience* covers the World War II Zoot Suit Riots in Los Angeles.

William P. Gottlieb Photographs of the Golden Age of Jazz
memory.loc.gov/ammem/wghtml/wghome.html

This Library of Congress site includes images, audio, and articles from *Down Beat* magazine in the 1940s.

America from the Great Depression to World War II: Photographs from the FSA and OWI, c. 1935–1945
memory.loc.gov/ammem/fsahtml/fahome.html

This site from the Library of Congress includes photographs in the Farm Security Administration–Office of War Information Collection taken during the Depression and World War II years.

For Further Reading

General

Paul Fussell, *Wartime: Understanding and Behavior in the Second World War* (1989).

John Keegan, *The Second World War* (1990).

Richard Polenburg, *War and Society: The United States, 1941–1945* (1972).

Studs Terkel, *"The Good War": An Oral History of World War II* (1984).

Mobilizing for War

Michael E. Birdwell, *Celluloid Soldiers: The Warner Brothers Campaign Against Nazism* (1999).

Justus D. Doenecke, *Storm on the Horizon: The Challenge to American Intervention, 1939–1941* (2000).

Thomas J. Fleming, *The New Dealers' War: Franklin D. Roosevelt and the War Within World War II* (2001).

Cecelia Lynch, *Beyond Appeasement: Interpreting Interwar Peace Movements in World Politics* (1999).

Pearl Harbor: The United States Enters the War

Allan Berube, *Coming Out Under Fire: The History of Gay Men and Women in World War Two* (1990).

Allan M. Brandt, *No Magic Bullet: A Social History of Venereal Disease in the United States* (1987).

Akira Iriye, *Pearl Harbor and the Coming of the Pacific War: A Brief History with Documents and Essays* (1999).

Michael S. Sherry, *The Rise of American Air Power: The Creation of Armageddon* (1987).

The Home Front

John Morton Blum, *V Was for Victory: Politics and American Culture During World War II* (1976).

Lewis A. Erenberg and Susan E. Hirsch, *The War in American Culture* (1996).

Susan Hartmann, *The Home Front and Beyond: American Women in the 1940s* (1982).

Elaine Tyler May, *Pushing the Limits: American Women, 1940–1961* (1994).

Race and War

Beth Bailey and David Farber, *The First Strange Place: The Alchemy of Race and Sex in World War II Hawaii* (1992).

Aaron Berman, *Nazism, the Jews and American Zionism, 1933–1948* (1990).

John W. Dower, *War Without Mercy: Race and Power in the Pacific War* (1987).

Barbara Dianne Savage, *Broadcasting Freedom: Radio, War, and the Politics of Race, 1938–1948* (1999).

Davis S. Wyman, *The Abandonment of the Jews: America and the Holocaust, 1941–1945* (1984).

Total War

Ronald Powaski, *March to Armageddon: The United States and the Nuclear Arms Race, 1939 to the Present* (1987).

George H. Roeder, Jr., *The Censored War: American Visual Experience During World War Two* (1993).

Michael S. Sherry, *In the Shadow of War: The United States Since the 1930s* (1995).

Martin J. Sherwin, *A World Destroyed: Hiroshima and the Origins of the Arms Race* (1987).

Online Practice Test

Test your understanding of this chapter with interactive review quizzes at

www.ablongman.com/jonescreatedequal/chapter23

Cold War and Hot War, 1945–1953

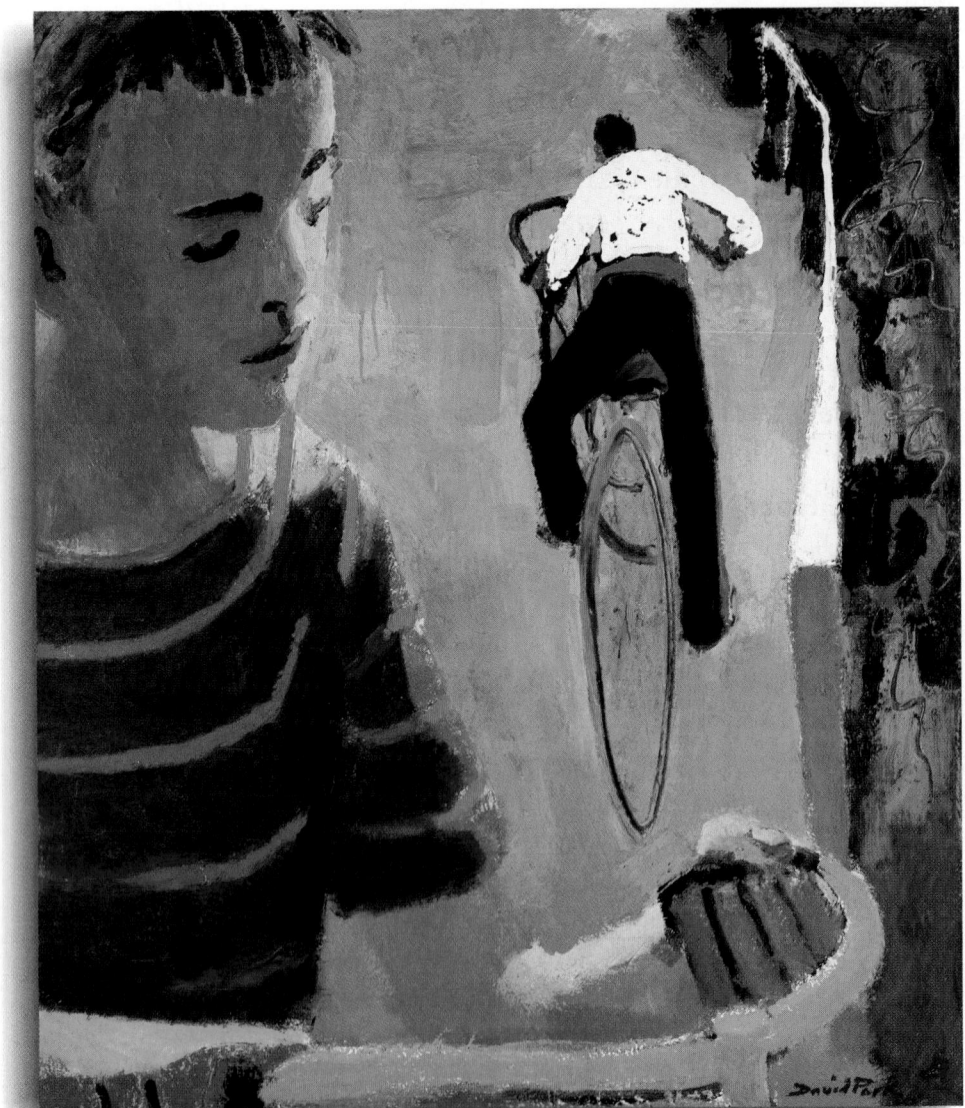

David Parks, "Boys on Bikes," 1950. Curtis Galleries, Minneapolis, MN

■ Robert Park's 1950 painting *Kids on Bikes* reminds viewers that in the midst of the high drama of Cold War international conflicts, most Americans tried to carry on with their normal daily lives. Park himself opted out of the comfortable life of his prominent Boston family, quitting high school and moving to Berkeley, California to work as an artist.

AT 11:30 A.M. ON APRIL 25, 1945, U.S. ARMY PRIVATE JOSEPH POLOWSKY GLIMPSED what looked like the future. The young Chicago native was riding in the lead jeep of an American force along the Elbe River in central Germany when he spotted Russian soldiers on the far side, their medals glistening in the morning sun. Elated, he and five of his comrades found a small boat and paddled across to the eastern bank. Using Polowsky's knowledge of German to communicate, the American soldiers embraced their Soviet allies with laughs and tears. The Russians produced bottles of vodka, and toasts, pledges, singing, and dancing followed. After years of pressing Germany from east and west, the Allies had finally linked up in the heart of Hitler's empire. A reporter wrote of the scene, "You get the feeling of exuberance, a great new world opening up."

Despite his conservative Republican background, Polowsky spent much of his life advocating American–Russian friendship. He could not forget the transforming experience of that April day along the Elbe and the hopes it engendered for a peaceful future. However, what followed the Allied victory turned out not to be a "great new world" of international peace and brotherhood but the Cold War of U.S.–Soviet hostility that lasted for more than four decades. The opposing ideologies—communism and capitalist democracy—joined with conflicting national interests to produce this armed standoff. The American effort to contain the expansion of communist influence entailed a radical reorientation of American involvement abroad in peacetime, including the nation's first peacetime military alliance, the North Atlantic Treaty Organization (NATO). At times the Cold War turned into a hot war of actual shooting, most importantly in the Korean War of 1950–1953.

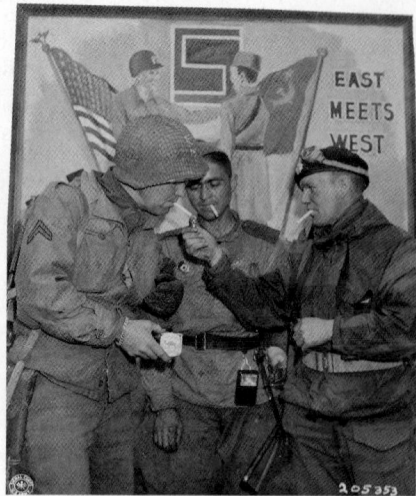

Soviet and American troops meet in central Germany in May 1945.

Soon after the end of World War II, Jim Forman enlisted in the U.S. Air Force. In 1948, he shipped out with his battalion to the huge U.S. base on the island of Okinawa in Japan. There some of the social changes unleashed by World War II caught up with him. President Harry Truman ordered the racial desegregation of the armed forces, and officers chose him to be the first African American to join the 625th Aircraft and Warning Company. Forman reported to his new assignment across the island, expecting trouble from white soldiers: harassment, assaults, and worse. Fearful, he slept only a few hours his first night. When he went to the mess hall for breakfast the next morning, he was stunned. "Fresh eggs. I saw them crack fresh eggs. I did not believe what I saw: fresh eggs. I had been on the Rock [Okinawa] some six months and I had never tasted a fresh egg unless I bought it at the restaurant in town." The white cook asked him how he wanted his eggs cooked and how many. "How many?" Forman asked in amazement. "Do you mean I can have more than two?" It was the same with milk: he could have a whole quart of fresh milk and then come back for more. In his former all-black battalion, he had been served only powdered eggs and powdered milk and only in carefully limited quantities. "I cursed the Air Force for its segregation, but I ate my fresh milk and eggs."

Jim Forman was trying to make sense of the changes and uncertainties that pervaded American society in the late 1940s. Popular support at home was needed for expansive new military commitments abroad, yet Americans had just fought in the largest war in their history, and most were eager to get back to something close to normal peacetime life. For some citizens the war years had provided new opportunities for better work and more independence. Women, workers, and African Americans, for example, did not want to retreat from the advances they had made. Struggles over the place of these groups of citizens helped shape the contours of the immediate postwar years, both in family lives and in the public sphere.

In some ways, the Cold War encouraged efforts at social reform. America's new leading role in world affairs brought its domestic life into the spotlight of world attention. Racial discrimination and violence at home embarrassed American leaders as they spoke of leading the anticommunist "free world" abroad. But in other ways, the Cold War constrained efforts to bring American life more fully into line with its democratic and egalitarian promise. Rising tensions with communist movements and governments overseas stimulated great anxieties about possible subversion within the nation's own borders. Anticommunist fervor put unions on the defensive and encouraged women to shun the workplace in favor of family life and parenting, particularly in the nation's growing suburbs. This second Red Scare—the first had followed World War I in 1919—reached flood tide by 1950 with the rise to prominence of Senator Joseph McCarthy. The young Republican from Wisconsin made a career of blaming supposedly disloyal Americans at home for setbacks to U.S. goals abroad in places such as China and Korea. He left a bitter legacy that long outlasted his political demise in 1954.

The Uncertainties of Victory

It was five in the afternoon when the Senate recessed on April 12, 1945. The Vice President walked through the Capitol building to the private office of his old friend and mentor, Sam Rayburn of Texas, the House majority leader. He had just mixed himself a cocktail when an aide told him that he was to call the White House immediately. Picking up the phone, he was instructed to come to the White House right away. "Jesus Christ and General Jackson," he said as he put down the receiver, his face suddenly pale. Within 15 minutes, Harry Truman was being ushered into the private quarters at 1600 Pennsylvania Avenue. Eleanor Roosevelt greeted him with the somber news: "Harry, the president is dead." Stunned, he finally said, "Is there anything I can do for you?" She replied, "Is there anything *we* can do for *you*? For you are the one in trouble now."

Franklin Roosevelt was dead; it was almost unimaginable. Elected four times to the presidency, he had dominated American politics like no figure before or since. Just as the unprecedented destruction of World War II was finally ending, the leadership of the nation passed into new and less tested hands. Peace brought an array of uncertainties and immediate needs. The victors had to reconstruct a world that had been damaged, physically and psychologically, almost beyond recognition. Spared the destruction visited elsewhere, the United States faced the different challenge of demobilizing its military forces and reconverting to a peacetime economy. Intense conflicts along the color line and in the workplace revealed real differences between Americans about the shape of the democracy they had fought to defend.

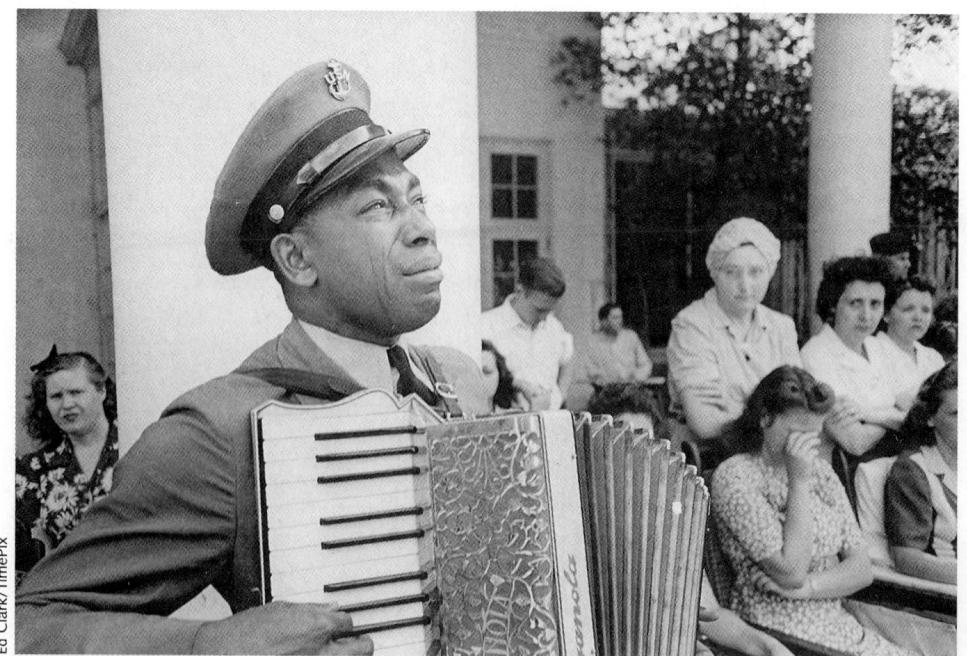

Ed Clark/TimePix

■ Franklin D. Roosevelt's death at his vacation home in Warm Springs, Georgia, stunned a nation and a world that had not known another U.S. president since 1932. Navy bandsman Graham Jackson was one of Roosevelt's favorite musicians. As the procession began to transport the president's body north for burial in Hyde Park, New York, Jackson captured the grief of millions of Americans as he played the sweet, slow strains of "Going Home."

Global Destruction

World War II wrought death on a scale that defies comprehension: 60 million human beings lost their lives. From England in the west to the islands of New Guinea in the east, from Scandinavia in the north to the Sahara Desert in the south, much of Europe and Asia was left in ruins. Soviet and American power had finally crushed the Axis, with Berlin now a "city of the dead" and Japan's urban landscape devastated by firebombing and nuclear attacks. Most of the victors were only marginally better off. China lost 10 million of its citizens to Japanese guns and starvation, and the Soviet victory over Germany came at the cost of more than 20 million Russian lives. Poland, the battleground for the Germans and the Soviets, was a wasteland. And the Nazis had murdered 6 million European Jews, primarily Poles and Germans.

Only one of the major combatants emerged from the war in better shape than at the beginning. With no fighting on their soil after the initial Japanese attack on Pearl Harbor, American civilians spent the war years in safety. Orders for war materials ended the Great Depression in the United States and created full employment as factories worked overtime to supply the Allied armies. The American people, one official remarked in 1945, "are in the pleasant predicament of having to learn to live 50 percent better than they have ever lived before." Many Americans suffered terribly in the war, of course; 400,000 died, leaving behind desolate families, and millions of veterans returned with traumas that colored the remainder of their lives. But such casualties paled in comparison to those of other belligerent nations. With just 6 percent of the world's population and 50 percent of its wealth, the United States enjoyed a position of staggering economic advantage in comparison with the rest of the world.

Americans' overriding fear was that the end of the fighting might return the country to the state it had faced when the war began: economic depression. The nation's awesome industrial productivity depended on government spending, which was now to be cut back sharply. International trade might pick up much of the slack, but the war had destroyed most of the purchasing power of U.S. trading partners in Europe and Asia. Rising tensions between the two primary victors—the United States and the Soviet Union—hampered the process of postwar reconstruction. President Truman showed his frustration with the Soviet military occupation of eastern

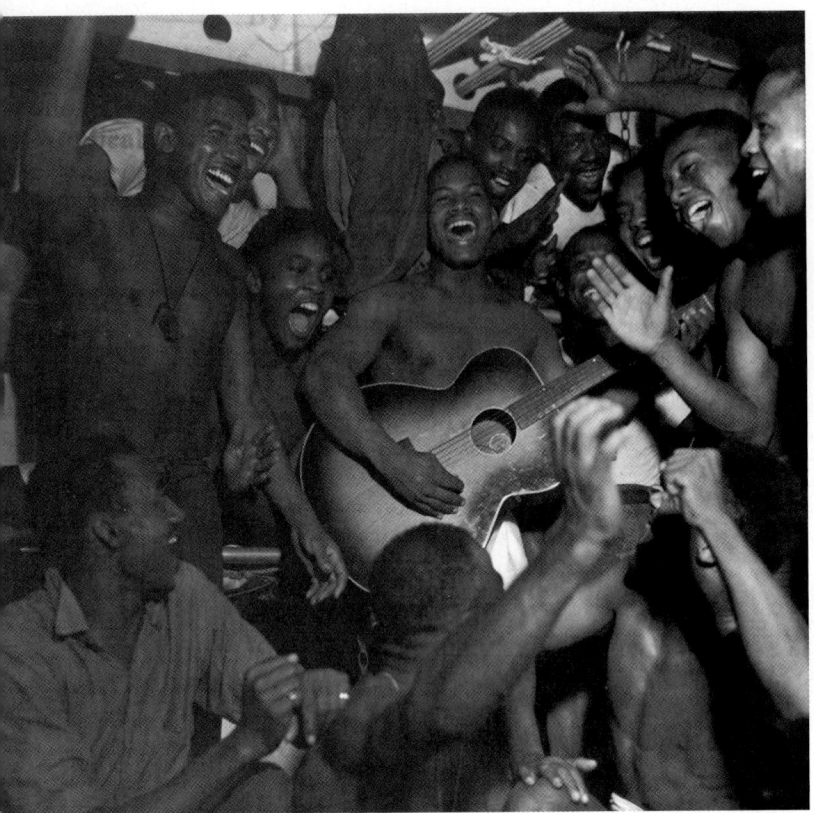

■ American sailors at Pearl Harbor in Hawaii gather around a radio to celebrate the news of Japan's surrender on August 14, 1945. Their lives were suddenly free from the perils of the brutal warfare in the Pacific, where Japanese pilots known as kamikazes had crashed suicide planes into U.S. warships.

Europe by lecturing Soviet diplomats and abruptly cutting off Lend–Lease aid to the USSR. Soviet dictator Joseph Stalin feared America's new global military might, manifest in its monopoly of the atomic bomb, and was determined to secure his European border against future invasion from the West.

Vacuums of Power

World War II altered the world's ideological and physical landscape. Japan and Germany, the centers of prewar power in Asia and continental Europe, were vacuums waiting to be filled and reshaped by their conquerors. In addition to defeating two nations, the Allies had also discredited the ideas on which those governments had been built: fascism and militarism. These were the ideas of the extreme Right: the glorification of the racially defined state and its aggressive military expansion. Fascism's murderous character tarred those who had collaborated with the Axis during the war, primarily conservatives in countries such as France who preferred fascism to socialism. White supremacy and colonialism, two underpinnings of the United States and its western European allies, also lost much of their legitimacy in the war to defend democracy against Hitler's racially genocidal Third Reich.

Into many of the postwar vacuums of power flowed a newly prominent worldwide Left. Socialists, communists, and other radicals espoused communal rather than individualistic values. The Red Army's primary role in defeating the German troops who had overrun Europe evoked admiration for the Soviet Union among antifascists everywhere. The occupying Soviet forces installed communist governments in eastern Europe by force (sometimes called "Red Army socialism"), and Socialist and Communist parties rose sharply in popularity in France, Italy, Belgium, and Scandinavia. The nominally socialist Labor party took power in Great Britain, defeating war leader Winston Churchill and his Conservative party at the polls. Europeans across the continent established welfare states to provide a minimum standard of living for all their citizens.

This turn to the left encompassed most of the globe. Africans began organizing for eventual independence from European rule, and Asians launched the final phase of their anticolonial struggle for liberation. Indonesia fought its way free from the Dutch, and India gained its freedom from Britain. "The sun never sets on the British Empire" had long been a proud colonial refrain, but it was no longer true. In French Indochina, Ho Chi Minh quoted from

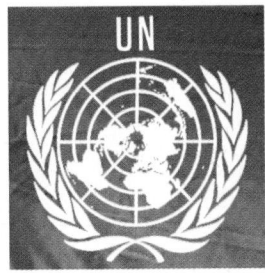

Thomas Jefferson's Declaration of Independence as he announced the creation of an independent Vietnam. (Truman ignored Vietnam's appeal for American recognition, just as Wilson had done 26 years earlier at the Versailles peace conference after World War I; see Chapter 20). Masters of much of the world a few years earlier, the European colonial powers fought desperately to hold onto the last pieces of their escaping empires. The Allies created the new United Nations (UN) in San Francisco in April 1945, just days after Truman succeeded FDR. Eventually housed in New York, it embodied hopes for a more peaceful and democratic world. Its General Assembly gave all nations an equal voice and vote in deliberations, and its small Security Council—responsible for guiding any UN military actions—gave a permanent seat and veto power to five nations: the United States, the USSR, Britain, France, and China. The 1948 UN Human Rights Charter helped put practitioners of colonialism and racial discrimination on the defensive by declaring worldwide support for the principles of national self-determination and equal treatment for all peoples.

Postwar Reconversion

The fundamental task for Americans at home was to reconvert from a wartime society back to a peacetime one. They were especially eager to "bring the boys home." The 12 million men in uniform represented nearly two-thirds of all men between 18 and 34 years old. Despite the worries of U.S. commanders and strategists that rapid demobilization would exacerbate vacuums of power abroad, 9 million American troops came home by mid-1946. Eager to return to civilian life, they walked off ships' gangplanks into a country in transition. Factories were trying to convert from producing war materials to making consumer products. Wartime rationing was lifted on goods such as sugar and gasoline, and the 35-mph speed limit was withdrawn, but unemployment and inflation threatened. Orders for war materials dried up, taking jobs with them, but wartime inflation ("too many dollars chasing too few goods") persisted. Housing remained especially scarce. In the richest country in the world, one-third of the citizens still lived in poverty, with neither running water nor flush toilets.

To ease the transition home, Congress had passed the Servicemen's Readjustment Act of 1944 (the GI Bill) to provide crucial financial aid to veterans. It gave low-cost mortgages that helped create an explosion in home ownership. It created Veterans Administration hospitals to provide lifetime medical care. And it paid tuition and stipends for colleges and vocational training, making higher education broadly available for the first time. The 2 percent of veterans who were women also made use of these benefits. In the postwar era, when American politics generally became more conservative—shifting away from the New Deal reform spirit and toward an anticommunist emphasis—the GI Bill was the one area in which the United States expanded its own welfare state. The $14.5 billion spent on veterans over the next decade marked a public investment that helped propel millions of families into an expanding middle class.

The postwar transition presented particular challenges to American women. Millions of them had gone to work outside the home during the war and found economic independence in doing so. Now they faced powerful pressures to leave the workforce and return to a domestic life of old and new families. Employers fired women, and male veterans expecting jobs did not welcome female competition. The federal government abruptly halted funding for wartime daycare facilities, forcing mothers to quit their jobs. Many women accepted this return to the domestic sphere, content to focus on marriage and family life. But millions felt varying degrees of resentment over their loss of hard-earned compensation and self-esteem. "War jobs have uncovered unsuspected abilities in American women," one argued. "Why lose all these abilities?"

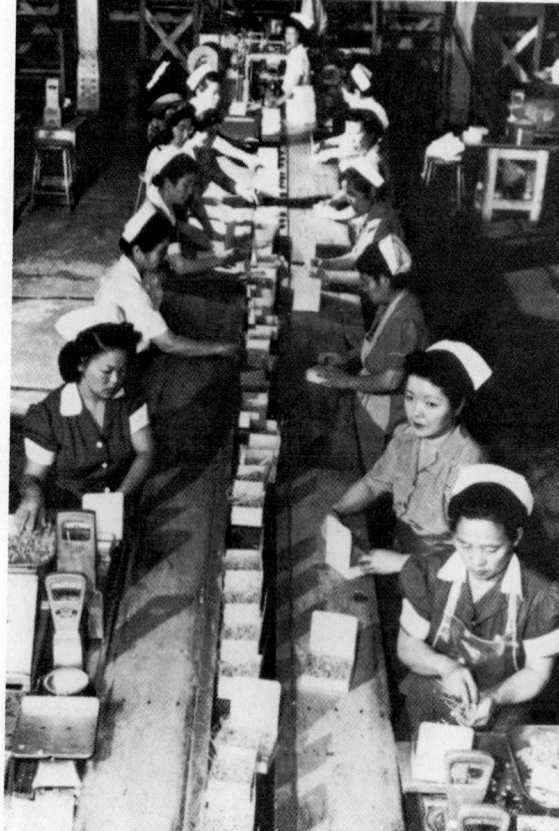

John Vachon

■ Japanese American women pack lima beans into boxes for freezing at Seabrook Farms, near Bridgeton, New Jersey, in 1947. Unlike the northern part of the state, which was closely tied to New York City, rural southern New Jersey was a rich fruit- and vegetable-growing region. After their release from the internment camps of World War II, Americans of Japanese descent joined their fellow citizens in finding work where they could in a peacetime economy no longer shrouded by the Great Depression.

Contesting Racial Hierarchies

African Americans faced a similar problem. After finding new opportunities in industrial employment during the war, they were laid off afterward in favor of returning white veterans. Like women, blacks were expected by others to retreat into deference. Black veterans spearheaded

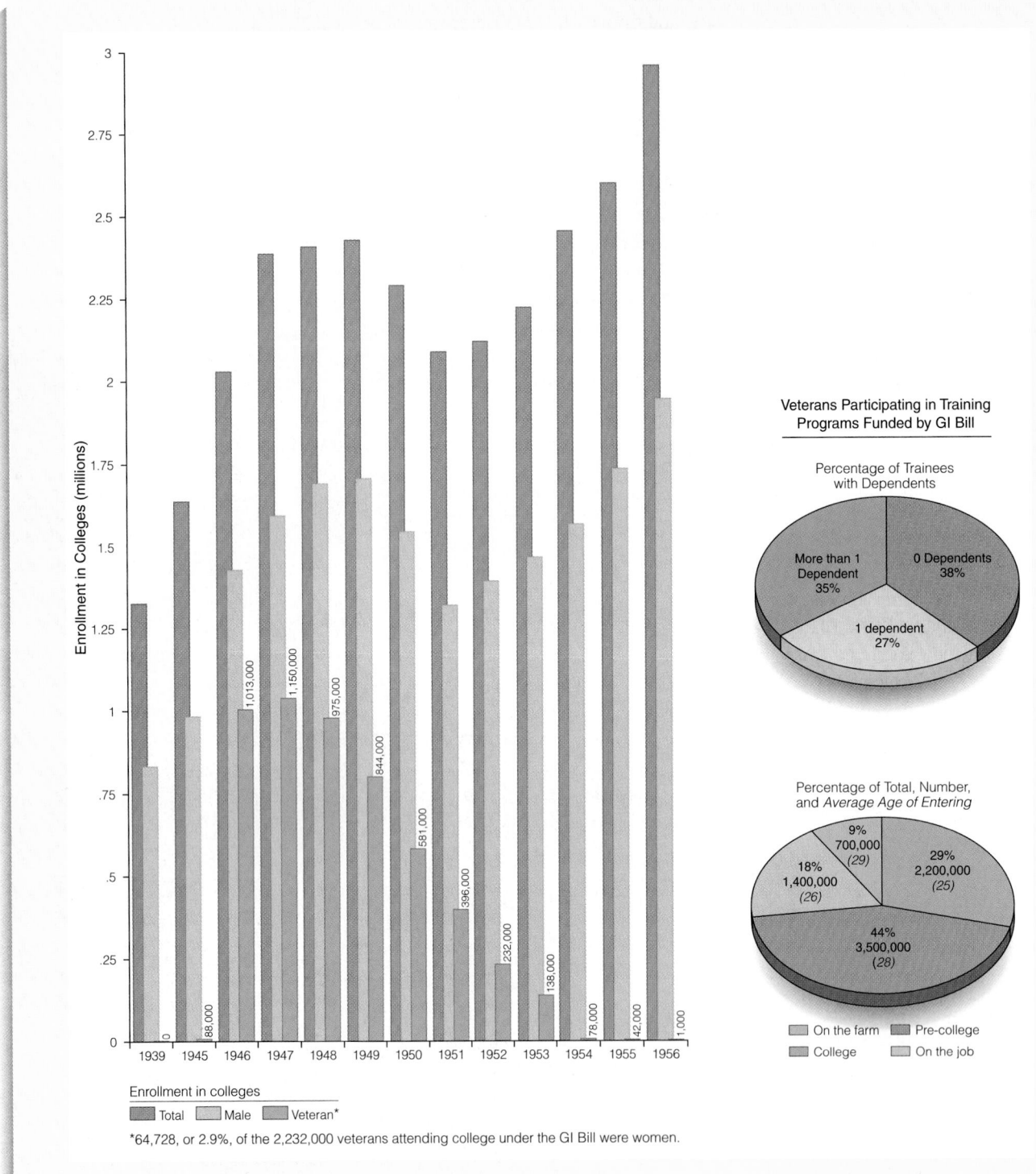

■ FIGURE 24.1

OPPORTUNITIES FOR VETERANS The number of Americans attending college increased sharply after World War II. In the early postwar years, federal government spending through the 1944 GI Bill gave veterans unprecedented opportunities for access to education and other job training programs.

the resistance to this notion. They had fought in disproportionate numbers for their country and for the cause of defeating the world's most murderous racists, the Nazis. They then returned to a nation still deeply segregated, by law in the South and by practice elsewhere. Like Native American, Latino American, and Asian American veterans, they were determined to be full citizens in the country for which they had spilled their blood. "I went into the Army a nigger," one black soldier said about typical white views of him, but "I'm coming out a man."

African American efforts to overcome discrimination met fierce white resistance in 1946 and 1947. In the South, where most black Americans still lived, a wave of beatings and lynchings greeted black veterans in uniform and their attempts to register to vote. White Northerners also used violence to preserve the segregated character of neighborhoods in Chicago, Detroit, and other cities. They destroyed the property and threatened the lives of blacks who dared to move to previously all-white blocks, effectively confining African Americans to impoverished areas. Sometimes local authorities encouraged such extralegal use of force. The police chief of Cicero, Illinois, was indicted for conspiracy to incite a riot in 1951 after several thousand white residents destroyed an all-white apartment building to prevent African American veteran Harvey E. Clark and his family from moving in.

The retreat of European colonialism and American competition with the Soviet Union nonetheless encouraged many white Americans to acknowledge the contradiction between leading the "free world" and limiting the freedoms of Americans of color. A series of Supreme Court decisions validated the long-term strategy of the National Association for the Advancement of Colored People (NAACP) for contesting segregation in the courts. Court rulings outlawed segregation in voting primaries (*Smith v. Allwright*, 1944), interstate transportation (*Morgan v. Virginia*, 1946), contracts for house sales (*Shelley v. Kraemer*, 1948), and graduate schools (*Sweatt v. Painter* and *McLaurin v. Oklahoma*, 1950). The California Supreme Court in 1948 overturned a state law banning interracial marriage, pointing the way toward the elimination two decades later of similar laws in other states in the U.S. Supreme Court's *Loving v. Virginia* decision (1967).

Popular culture moved in the same direction of breaking down racial barriers. *Billboard* magazine in 1949 changed the category of "race music" to "rhythm and blues" as white record producers and radio disc jockeys such as Alan Freed began to bring the early rock 'n' roll of African American musicians to mainstream white audiences. By 1955 young white musicians such as Bill Haley and Elvis Presley joined black stars such as Chuck Berry and Little Richard in creating a wildly popular sound that transcended racial categories. Professional baseball erased its color line when Jackie Robinson, a former four-sport star at the University of California–Los Angeles and lieutenant in the U.S. Army, joined the Brooklyn Dodgers in 1947. In a pretelevision era when professional basketball and football had only minor followings, baseball ruled as the great national pastime. Despite vicious verbal taunting and threats of bodily harm by some fans and players, Robinson refused to lose his temper and remained a model of dignity and excellence as he won the National League's Rookie of the Year honors. Two years later he won the Most Valuable Player award.

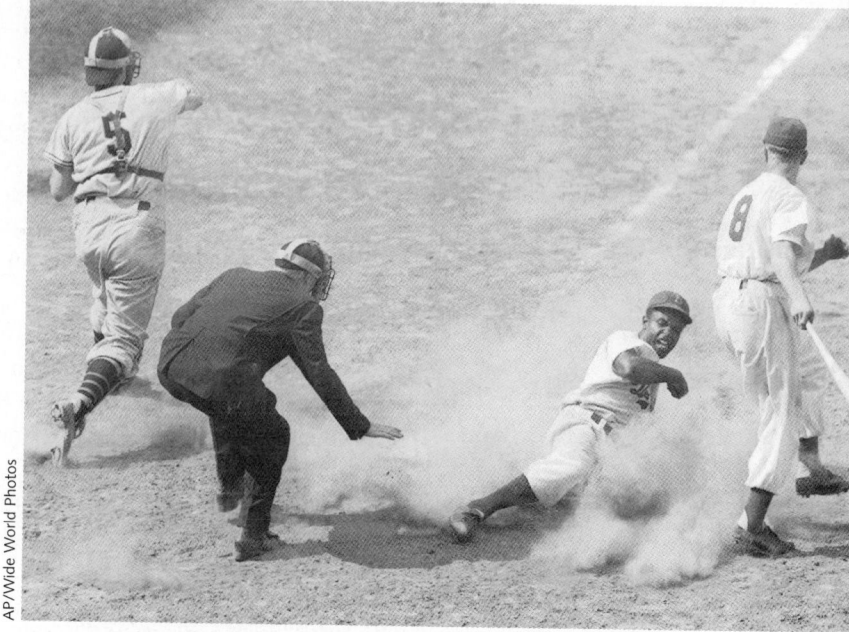

AP/Wide World Photos

■ The first person of color to play major league baseball, Jackie Robinson starred for the Brooklyn Dodgers from 1947 to 1956, helping them win six National League pennants and one world championship. His success opened the way for other black players to follow, eventually bringing the demise of the old professional Negro Leagues. Robinson credited Dodgers general manager Branch Rickey for his willingness to break the color line in what was still the nation's favorite game.

In his ten years with the team, the Dodgers won six National League titles. Millions of white Americans found themselves cheering for their first black hero, and Robinson came in second only to singer Bing Crosby in a national popularity poll.

Native Americans and Mexican Americans faced similar discrimination in the Southwest and elsewhere. With war veterans in the fore, they also organized to contest unfair education and election practices. "If we are good enough to fight, why aren't we good enough to vote?" asked returning Navajo soldiers in New Mexico and Arizona, where the state constitutions prohibited Indian residents from voting until successfully challenged in 1948. When the family of Private Felix Longoria, who died in combat in the Philippines, was denied the right to bury him in the all-white cemetery in Three Rivers, Texas, a new Latino veterans' organization called American GI Forum publicized the injustice. A young Texas senator named Lyndon Johnson, destined for the White House, stepped in and arranged a burial with full military honors in prestigious Arlington National Cemetery instead. The League of United Latin American Citizens (LULAC) followed a strategy similar to that of the NAACP regarding educational discrimination, leading to the Supreme Court's decision in *Mendez v. Westminster* (1946) outlawing segregated schools for Mexican Americans in California. In parallel fashion, indigenous Alaskans organized in the Alaska Native Brotherhood successfully lobbied the territorial legislature in Juneau to pass an antidiscrimination law in 1945.

Class Conflict

In many ways 1946 seemed like 1919. A world war had just ended, in which corporations had made handsome profits. American workers had enjoyed nearly full employment and improving wages and had joined unions in large numbers. In 1946 one-third of the workforce held a union card, the largest portion ever. But the end of war-related orders led to job cuts and the loss of overtime wages. As inflation kicked in, workers felt their marginal economic security slipping away, and by the spring of 1946, 1.8 million of them were out on strike.

Mirroring World War I, the conclusion of hostilities in 1945 revealed rising tensions between the United States and the Soviet Union. The spread of leftist revolutions abroad amplified fears of communist influence in American unions, especially because a few of the most effective Congress of Industrial Organizations (CIO) organizers were Communist party members or at least sympathetic to an emphasis on class conflict between owners and workers. As in 1919, a Red Scare began to develop, egged on by a business community that used the supposed threat of the tiny U.S. Communist party to weaken the much larger and less radical union movement. In contrast to the end of World War I, however, federal law guaranteed the right of workers to bargain collectively, and the strikes of 1946 resulted in some negotiated wage increases.

Organized labor after World War II functioned increasingly as a narrow special interest group rather than as part a broader democratic movement. The tide turned against unions as anticommunism intensified. President Truman, long considered a friend to organized labor, helped crush major strikes by railroad workers and coal miners in 1946 when he saw them as threatening the nation's economy. The CIO's Operation Dixie to organize southern workers of all colors failed, defeated by the skillful appeals of local businesses to white supremacist sentiment in the working class. The Republican party claimed a sweeping victory in the 1946 congressional elections, taking control of both the House and the Senate in a stark rejection of Truman's leadership. Republicans and conservative Democrats then passed the Taft–Hartley Act in 1947 over the president's veto, weakening unions by prohibiting secondary boycotts (against the products of a company whose workers were on strike) and requiring union officials to swear anticommunist oaths. Two years later the increasingly conservative CIO expelled 11 unions that still had leftist and communist leadership. At the same time, the expanding U.S. economy after 1947 pulled many skilled workers up into the middle class and gave them a larger stake in the status quo.

The Quest for Security

On February 21, 1947, a British official in Washington drove to the State Department to inform the U.S. government that Britain could no longer provide financial assistance to the anticommunist governments of Greece and Turkey. This marked a watershed in modern world history. Long the greatest imperial power and the dominant outside force in the Middle East, Britain was beginning a long, slow retreat. Left in its wake were vacuums of power, particularly in the Middle East, South Asia, and Africa. President Truman and his advisers believed that either Soviet or American influence would flow into those regions. In the face of the Soviet Union's eagerness to expand its influence by promoting communist revolutions abroad, American leaders believed they must seize the opportunity for world leadership. The Truman administration formulated a policy to contain communism in the eastern Mediterranean that it quickly expanded to encompass the entire noncommunist world.

Redefining National Security

U.S. policymakers had ended World War II with one primary goal. They were determined to revive the global capitalist economy that had nearly dissolved in the Great Depression of the 1930s and had then been battered by the war. American prosperity and freedom, they believed, depended on a world system of free trade because Americans simply could not consume all the products of their efficient farms and factories. If they could not sell the surplus abroad, the United States would slide back into a depression. The 1930s had shown that closed economic doors led to despair, poverty, and aggression, as in Germany and Japan. "We can't go through the thirties again," President Truman emphasized to his aides. He and other political leaders hoped for a world with greater liberty and more democracy. But Dean Acheson, the powerful undersecretary (1945–1947) and then secretary of state (1949–1953), emphasized that U.S. foreign policy was not primarily concerned with "a lot of abstract notions." Instead, the emphasis with each country was on "what you do—these business transactions."

"National security" was expanding to mean something very different from simply defending the nation's territory against invasion. For the disproportionately powerful United States, national security after 1945 came to be identified with the creation and preservation of a free-trading capitalist world order. American national security was seen to be at stake almost everywhere around the globe—a recipe for riches but also for trouble.

The primary threat to that security came from the Soviet Union. The Red Army's occupation of eastern Europe was part of the problem, as it symbolized the Soviets' military prowess. Even more troubling to the Truman administration was the political influence of the USSR in a world turning leftward. The real danger lay in Soviet encouragement, by example and assistance, of revolutions that rejected market economies and individualist ethics. Demoralized by the war's destruction and by grim postwar economic conditions, western Europeans and others seemed to be considering the paths of socialism and communism. "Hopeless and hungry people," Acheson warned, "often resort to desperate measures."

> *"Hopeless and hungry people,"* Acheson warned, *"often resort to desperate measures."*

Conflict with the Soviet Union

The antifascist alliance of the Soviet Union and the United States dissolved rapidly as their conflicting interests reemerged after the war. Long skeptical of the capitalist world it wanted to replace, the Soviet government viewed expansive U.S. interests as evidence of "striving for world supremacy." Yet Moscow was just as clearly expanding its own sphere of national security, with Soviet troops remaining in areas they had occupied during the war: Manchuria, northern Korea, Iran, and especially eastern and central Europe. These forward military positions, combined with Moscow's rhetoric of encouraging revolution abroad, increased American anxieties about rising communist movements in Asia and Europe. Each side spoke of the other's goal as "world domination."

Contrasting experiences in World War II amplified historical and ideological differences. America and Russia had each entered the war after being attacked by surprise in 1941. But whereas the war brought the United States out of the global capitalist depression (which the Soviets had avoided), it brought the USSR into a depression caused by the invading Germans' destruction of the western portion of the country. With a decimated population, a battered economy, and minimal air and naval forces, the postwar Soviet Union remained a regional power based on its army. The United States was the only truly global power, with a vast naval armada and air force projecting military might on to every continent, undergirded by the most productive economy in world history. The two nations' visions of the postwar world order reflected these relative positions. Americans sought an open world for the free flow of goods and most ideas and proved willing to tolerate and even embrace dictatorial governments as long as they were anticommunist and open to foreign trade and investment. Meanwhile, the Soviets called for a more traditional division into separate spheres of influence for the great powers. The horrific experience of near national extinction at the hands of the Nazis ensured that Stalin would not budge on issues of fundamental Soviet security. At the same time, the exhilarating experience of low-cost victory and unparalleled wealth and might emboldened Truman. The United States "could not, of course, expect to get 100 percent" of what it wanted, he told his advisers, but on important matters "we should be able to get 85 percent."

> *"The reins of world leadership are fast slipping from Britain's . . . hands. These reins will be picked up either by the United States or by Russia."*

Conflicts over specific areas liberated from the Nazis hastened the onset of the Cold War in the first 18 months after the end of World War II. Whereas the Soviets wanted reparations and a deindustrialized Germany that could never threaten it again, the United States considered a rebuilt industrial German state crucial for a healthy, integrated western European economy. Britain and France had gone to war in defense of an independent Poland, and Truman told Stalin bluntly that a free election there, as promised in the Yalta accords, was crucial for 6 million Polish Americans; for Stalin, however, control of Poland was not negotiable because it had been "the corridor for attack on Russia." Moscow and Washington clashed over Iran, on Russia's southern border, where the Soviets briefly encouraged a leftist uprising in the northern part of the oil-rich country to counteract British and American influence in the capital city of Teheran. U.S. policymakers worried about Soviet requests to Turkey for greater control of the Bosporus and Dardanelles, the straits leading out of the Black Sea into the Mediterranean. When the British announced in February 1947 their imminent withdrawal from Greece, where leftists and monarchists were fighting a fierce civil war, the Truman administration believed it was time to respond decisively.

The Policy of Containment

Diplomat George Kennan best articulated the idea of containing Soviet power in an influential telegram sent from his post at the U.S. embassy in Moscow in February 1946. Kennan explained Soviet hostility as a function of traditional Russian insecurity overlaid with newer Marxist justifications. He called for "the adroit and vigilant application of counterforce" against all Soviet efforts at expanding their influence. One month later, on March 5, 1946, former British prime minister Winston Churchill gave a prominent speech in Fulton, Missouri, in which he warned that a Russian "iron curtain" had descended across Europe from the Baltic Sea in the north to the Adriatic Sea in the south, imprisoning all those to the east of it. Kennan and other U.S. policymakers viewed communism as a monolithic movement, directed by Moscow. The metaphor of disease was commonly used, as in references to the Soviets injecting "a hypodermic needle full of Moscow virus" into a vulnerable country. The prominence of local communists, the carriers of that "disease," in the Greek civil war might give Stalin a foothold on the Mediterranean. "The reins of world leadership are fast slipping from Britain's competent but now very weak hands," the State Department argued. "These reins will be picked up either by the United States or by Russia."

Picking up those reins meant a fundamental reorientation for the United States. No longer just the dominant force in the Western Hemisphere, it would have to maintain its wartime projection of military forces around the globe—permanently. To do so would take huge expenditures that Congress had to approve and public support for an unprecedented international role. Critics questioned the virtue of supporting a monarchy in Greece and a dictatorship in Turkey. So Truman and his advisers chose to "scare hell out of the American people," as Senator Arthur Vandenberg put it, to gain their support. In an address to Congress on March 12, 1947, asking for $400 million in aid for Greece and Turkey, the president simplified the world system into two "ways of life," those of "free peoples" and those of "terror and oppression" under communist rule. All nations must choose between them, he declared, and the United States must support "free peoples who are resisting attempted subjugation by armed minorities or outside pressures."

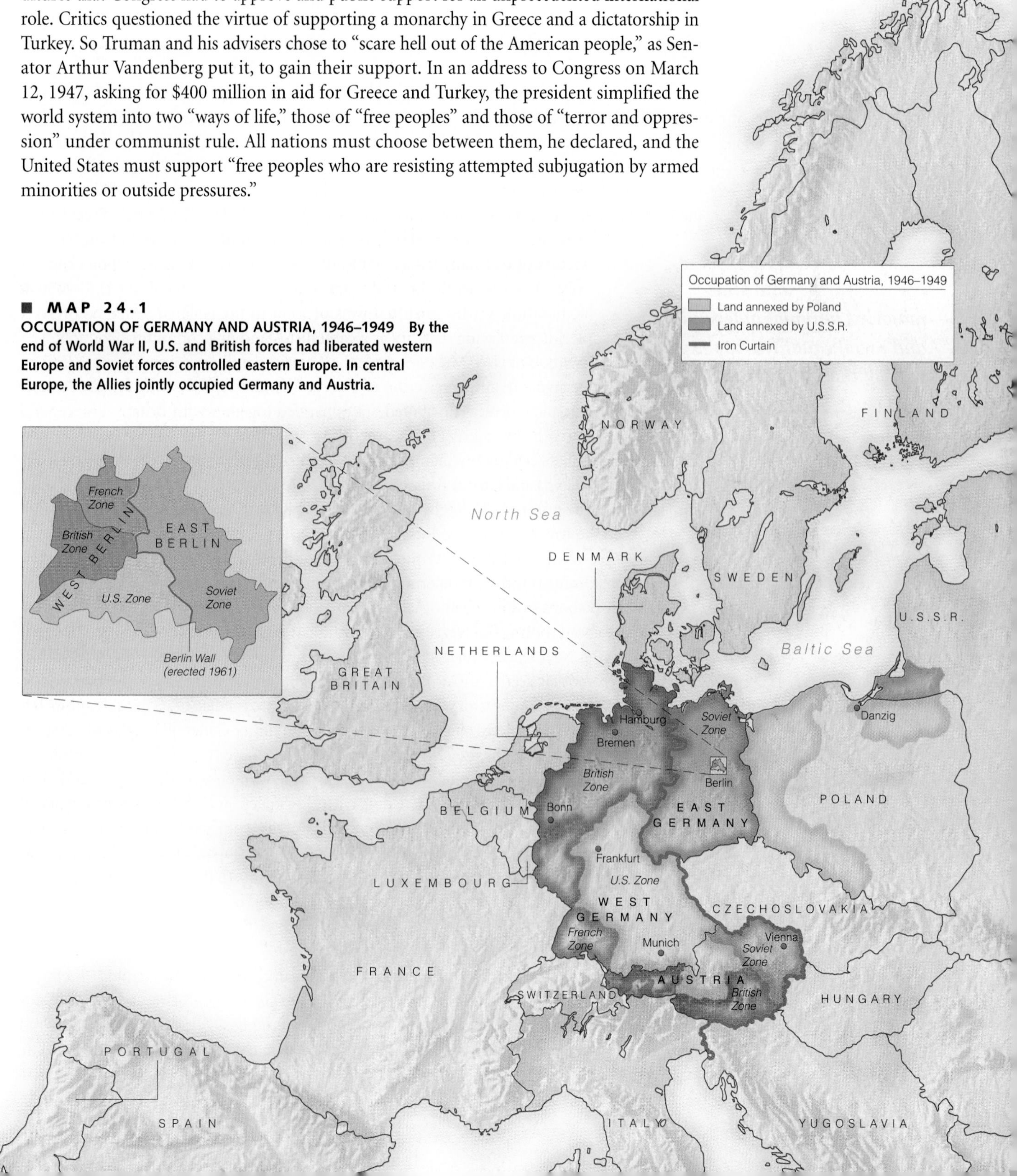

■ **MAP 24.1**
OCCUPATION OF GERMANY AND AUSTRIA, 1946–1949   By the end of World War II, U.S. and British forces had liberated western Europe and Soviet forces controlled eastern Europe. In central Europe, the Allies jointly occupied Germany and Austria.

The Truman Doctrine, as it became known, exaggerated a real problem to win public support for a new international role for the United States. It funded the governments of Turkey and Greece but it framed the new policy broadly, opening the path to supporting anticommunist regimes and opposing revolutions around the world for decades to come. The most important immediate step was the reconstruction of a vibrant, reintegrated western European economy. The United States provided $13 billion between 1948 and 1952 to fund the European Recovery Program, commonly known as the Marshall Plan for its chief architect, Secretary of State George Marshall (1947–1949). His assistant, Dean Acheson, reminded Americans doubtful about such expenditures that western Europe's recovery was "chiefly a matter of national self-interest" for the United States, for European markets were crucial for American economic health.

Ensuring western European security against the Red Army also entailed the first U.S. military alliance in peacetime. The victors of World War II divided a defeated Germany into separate zones of occupation, based on wartime agreements that reflected their respective military positions. The Allies also shared occupation of the capital city of Berlin, although it was deep in the Soviet-controlled eastern sector of the country, in the expectation that a reunified, de-Nazified Germany would be governed from there someday. The British, French, and American decision in March 1948 to create a unified state out of the western sectors of Germany led a few months later to a year-long Soviet blockade of western access to Berlin and fears of a general war. The joint U.S.–British "Operation Vittles" airlifted tons of food to the isolated residents of West Berlin, preserving that city as a capitalist island in a communist country. The creation of NATO in 1949 made the American military commitment to Europe permanent, a firm rejection of George Washington's warning against "entangling alliances." The United States banded together with Britain, France, and the other western European countries to provide for each other's mutual defense against an attack on any member of the alliance, presumably by the Soviets. Headquartered first in Paris and later in Brussels, Belgium, NATO was the first U.S. military alliance in peacetime. The point of NATO for western Europe, its British first secretary general said, was to "keep the Americans in, the Russians out, and the Germans down."

> *For the world's nonwhite majority, national independence and racial equality was the great issue of the late 1940s and 1950s.*

The onset of the Cold War determined the fate of the defeated powers of World War II. The Truman administration was determined to "push ahead with the reconstruction of those two great workshops of Europe and Asia—Germany and Japan." This agenda replaced initial concerns about rooting out Nazism and punishing war criminals, as at the Nuremberg trials of surviving Nazi leaders in 1945–1946. While the Soviets extracted what reparations they could from their sector of Germany, the Americans and British rebuilt the new nation of West Germany. A similar story unfolded in Japan, where the use of atomic weapons left U.S. forces the sole occupiers. The American occupation under General Douglas MacArthur initially (1945–1947) emphasized democratization of Japanese society, including building labor unions, weakening corporate monopolies, ensuring women's political rights, and punishing war criminals. But rising U.S. tensions with the Soviets and the imminent victory of the Communist forces in China's civil war prompted American officials to shift course by 1948. Henceforth, they focused on rebuilding as quickly as possible Japan's industrial economy as the hub of capitalist Asia and reduced efforts at social reforms that might slow that process.

Colonialism and the Cold War

The world's nonwhite majority still lived under European colonial control, and for them the struggle for national independence and racial equality was the great issue of the late 1940s and 1950s. In this North–South conflict, as opposed to the East–West conflict of the Cold War, the United States held an awkward position. Its primary NATO partners included the

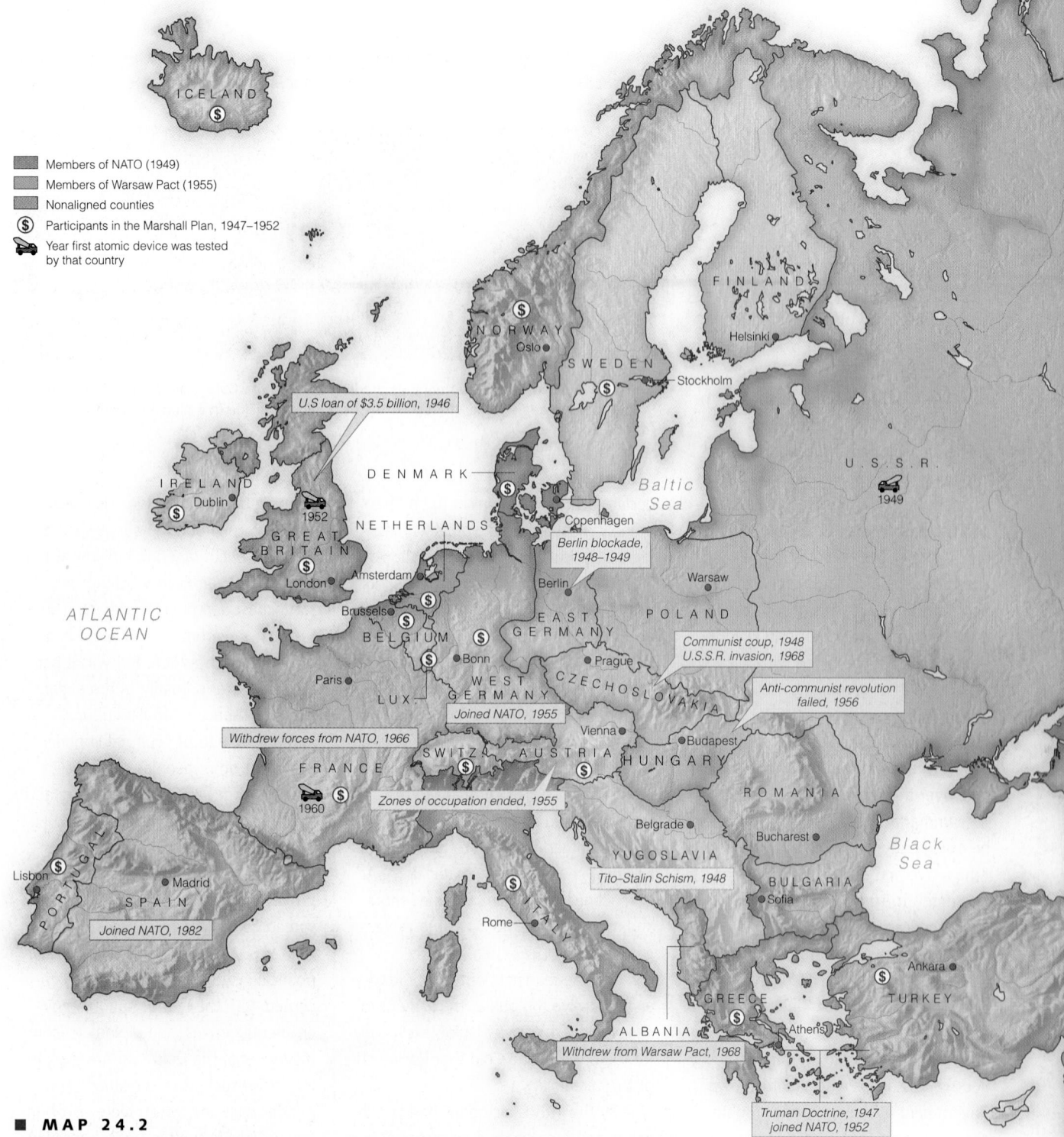

■ MAP 24.2

EUROPE DIVIDED BY THE COLD WAR For centuries Europe had controlled much of the rest of the world. After 1945, Russians occupied the eastern half of the continent and Americans wielded dominant influence in the western half. This division of Europe into Communist and non-Communist blocs lasted until the end of the Cold War in 1989.

greatest colonial powers: Britain, France, Belgium, Holland, and Portugal. Racial segregation in the United States further undercut American leadership of the "free world," as did U.S. support for the anticommunist apartheid (white supremacist) regime that took power in South Africa in 1948. Anticolonial radicals who pointed out these contradictions found their voices drowned out by the rising din of anticommunism.

With European rule in Asia and Africa on the way out, the Truman administration sought a gradual transfer of colonial rule into the hands of local pro-West elites. Violent revolutions—

The Origins of the Cold War

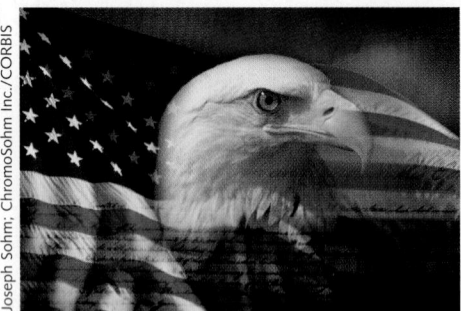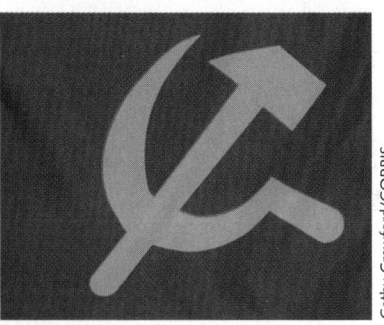

American and Soviet patriotic symbols predominated in the Cold War era. The Stars and Stripes and the eagle faced off against the hammer and sickle in a global competition for influence.

The earliest American accounts of how the Cold War began were written by officials who had participated in the decisions that cemented U.S.–Russian hostility for two generations (1946–1989). Officials such as the State Department's Herbert Feis and academic historians through the 1950s and early 1960s accepted the U.S. government view that Soviet aggression and subversion made the Cold War unavoidable. They pointed to the absence of political and religious freedom and the severe restrictions on the ownership of private property in communist nations, combined with the expansion of communist control into eastern Europe and China. Stalin and his successors in the Kremlin, they believed, were at fault for trying to take over the world. Arthur Schlesinger, Jr., summarized this view in 1967 when he called early U.S. Cold War policies "the brave and essential response of free men" to totalitarian provocations.

America's deepening involvement in the Vietnam War destroyed the Cold War consensus among historians. Schlesinger's "orthodox" interpretation of the events of the late 1940s seemed increasingly suspect to a group of mostly younger historians who saw their own government as the aggressor in southeast Asia in the mid-1960s. They took their lead in part from the iconoclastic William Appleman Williams of the University of Wisconsin, who in 1959 declared U.S. expansionism to be "the tragedy of American diplomacy." Casting a skeptical eye back a generation, these "revisionists" found evidence indicating a greater American than Soviet responsibility in bringing on the Cold War. Gar Alperovitz identified the use of atomic bombs on Japan as unnecessary for the military defeat of Tokyo but useful as "atomic diplomacy" to intimidate Moscow in regard to the postwar world order. Gabriel Kolko emphasized the structural need of U.S. capitalism to expand abroad in search of new markets and new sources of raw materials. As U.S. actions in Vietnam alienated more and more Americans and as the Watergate scandal (1972–1974) starkly revealed the readiness of top U.S. leaders to deceive the public, the early histories blaming the Soviet Union exclusively for the onset of the Cold War lost much of their credibility.

By the 1980s historians had largely exhausted the debate over responsibility for Soviet–American hostilities. Then the fall of the Berlin Wall in 1989 and the dissolution of the USSR in 1991 (turning back into Russia and independent neighboring nations such as Ukraine) encouraged rethinking of the early Cold War. Even Washington's staunchest defenders could admit that the U.S. government had acted in an often imperial fashion. But was it perhaps a matter primarily of the expansion of American popular culture abroad—a kind of "cultural imperialism" that other peoples often welcomed, from Paris to Beijing? Jazz and later rock 'n' roll music, along with Hollywood movies, American consumer goods, and the English language, proved more powerful agents for spreading the American way of life than U.S. Marines or even democratic political institutions. Though still concerned with the role of national governments, armies, and diplomats, some historians of the Cold War are exploring issues such as race relations and gender relations, which were also frontiers of freedom after 1945. Improved U.S.–Russian relations and the release of once-secret documents added interest to Cold War studies. ■

in the spirit of 1776—were to be avoided. The U.S. grant of official independence to the Philippines in 1946, though masking significant continued American influence, was offered as a model, as was the British departure from India a year later. However, America's European priorities included support even for imperialists who did not leave peacefully, such as the French digging in against Communist-led revolutionaries in Vietnam.

The British withdrawal from Palestine in 1948 created a peculiar dilemma for the United States. Jewish settlers—primarily from Europe and often survivors of the Holocaust—proclaimed the new state of Israel against the wishes of the Arab majority. Secretary of State Marshall and others urged Truman not to recognize Israel to avoid imperiling U.S. relations with the Arab oil-producing states. The president sympathized with the Jewish desire for a homeland, however, and understood the importance of American Jews as constituents of the Democratic party in the 1940s. His decision to recognize Israel, which most Middle Easterners viewed as a new colonial state, set the United States on a course of enduring friendship with that nation and enduring conflict with Israel's Arab neighbors and the Palestinians.

The Impact of Nuclear Weapons

Scientists in the 1940s dramatically increased Americans' sense of personal safety by introducing the use of antibiotics. "Miracle drugs" such as penicillin cured common bacterial infections that had previously been debilitating or fatal. Antibiotics suggested a future of personal health and longevity unimaginable to previous generations. What science gave with one hand it threatened to take away with the other, however. The use of atomic weapons on Japan foreshadowed a future of utter insecurity in which instantaneous destruction of entire nations could occur without warning. The ongoing quest for human control over the natural world—over even microorganisms and the insides of the atom—produced mixed results for the American land and people.

Even without being fired again in war after 1945, nuclear weapons altered the American environment. Weapon tests with such code names as "Dirty Harry" released vast quantities of radiation into the atmosphere. The Atomic Energy Commission assured those near the mushroom clouds, "Fallout does not constitute a serious hazard." But local cancer rates spiked upward for Bikini Islanders in the Pacific, where the first tests occurred, and then for farmers

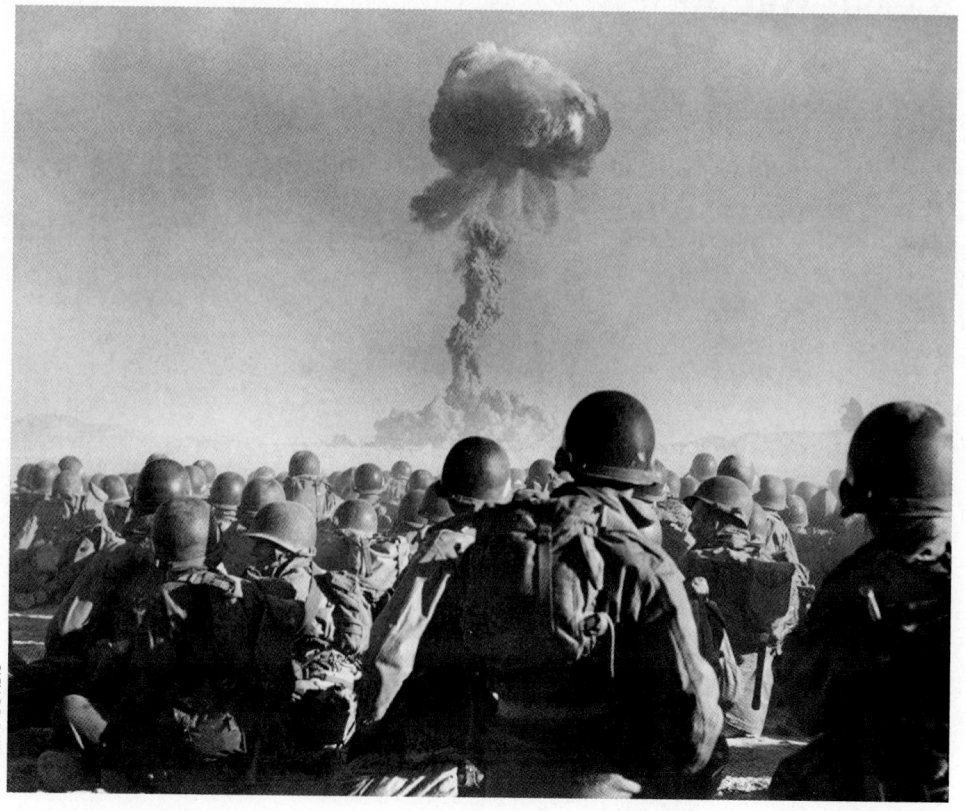

Bettmann/CORBIS

■ Soldiers watch as "Dog," a 21-kiloton nuclear device, is dropped from a bomber at the Nevada Test Site at Yucca Flat, northwest of Las Vegas, in November 1951. U.S. atomic specialists tested nuclear weapons first in the Marshall Islands of the western Pacific Ocean, especially the Bikini atoll, beginning in 1946, and then in Nevada beginning in January 1951. Residents downwind from the test sites suffered various deleterious health effects from radiation exposure, including high cancer rates.

and ranchers in Utah and Nevada, when tests began 65 miles northwest of Las Vegas in 1953. At St. George, Utah, downwind from the test site, radioactive plutonium dusted the citizens, livestock, and a crew shooting a movie in the desert. Of the 220 people from Hollywood who worked on *The Conqueror,* 91 had contracted cancer by 1980 and 40 had died, including film star John Wayne.

Related dangers stalked other parts of the "nuclear West." Navajo Indians mining uranium in the Four Corners region (where Utah, Colorado, Arizona, and New Mexico meet) paid dearly for their intensive exposure to the poisonous material, as did thousands of workers involved

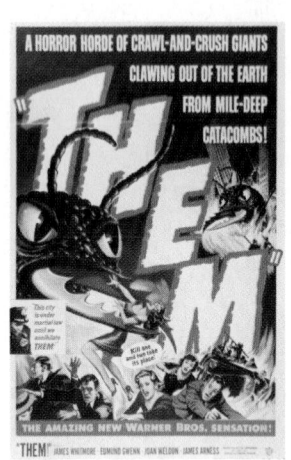

in nuclear weapon production. Weapon assembly plants in Hanford, Washington, and Rocky Flats, Colorado, leaked radioactivity into the groundwater. In combination with the nuclear power industry, atomic weapon development resulted in an enormous supply of radioactive waste—deadly for 10,000 more years—that the U.S. government still does not know how to dispose of safely. The quest for security produced a whole new kind of insecurity.

The government offered reassurances about the safety of the atom, and the Atomic Energy Commission covered up evidence of radioactivity's ill effects. But many Americans were deeply anxious about this destructive new power that loomed over their lives, especially as the Soviet–American arms race intensified. Science fiction stories painted frightening pictures of a future devastated by nuclear war. Movies such as *The Blob* and *The Attack of the Crab Monsters* portrayed a world haunted by exposure to radiation. *Them!* featured mutant ants the size of buses crawling out of a New Mexico atomic test site. Concerns about a nuclear world escalated with the successful 1952 test of an American hydrogen bomb, a thousand times more powerful than the device that destroyed Hiroshima. Always suspicious of centralized power, Americans worried that one person in the Oval Office or the Kremlin could almost instantaneously obliterate entire continents.

A Cold War Society

Expanding economic opportunities and narrowing political freedoms characterized American society in the first decade of the Cold War. A withering fire of anticommunist repression pushed dissident views to the margins of the nation's political life. Americans largely accepted this new conformity for two reasons: their desire to support their government during international crises, especially the Korean War (1950–1953), and a consumer cornucopia that surrounded them with attractive material goods. A generation that had survived the Great Depression embraced the culture of consumption and convenience that emerged after World War II. Factories that had produced jeeps, tanks, and weaponry turned to manufacturing cars and appliances; men who had learned to build roads and barracks for the military now began to erect suburban housing with equal speed.

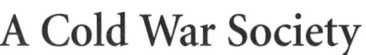

Expanding economic opportunities and narrowing political freedoms characterized American society in the first decade of the Cold War.

By 1947 the United States was launching into an era of extraordinary economic expansion that continued for 25 years. Senator McMahon of Connecticut suggested "mailing millions of mail-order catalogues to the Iron Curtain countries" to turn their inhabitants green with envy over "the consumers' wonderland contained within the pages of a Sears–Roebuck or a Montgomery Ward catalogue." Since Ben Franklin's time, Americans had been known for thrift in their pursuit of wealth, but after 1945 the long-cherished principle of delaying gratification declined steeply. "Buy now, pay later," General Motors urged as it offered an installment plan to customers. Diner's Club introduced the first credit card in 1950. In a formulation breathtaking for its distance from Puritan and immigrant traditions of saving for the future, writer William Whyte observed that "thrift is now un-American."

Family Lives

Many white Americans embraced the opportunity to move to the suburbs after World War II. Seeking larger homes and yards and quieter neighborhoods, they flocked to new developments such as Levittown outside New York City on Long Island. In their first three hours of business in 1949, Levittown's developers sold 1400 houses. In 1944 construction had begun on just 114,000 new houses; in 1950, the number jumped to 1.7 million. Suburbs were not for everyone, however. Even as federal courts struck down segregation laws in some spheres of American life, other federal agencies were encouraging residential separation by race. The Veterans Administration and the Federal Housing Administration distributed billions of dollars in low-cost mortgage loans for suburban homes to white applicants while screening out most people of color. Private banks did the same, and the contracts that developers such as Alfred and William Levitt signed with homebuyers prohibited resale to nonwhites. Other government policies, including highway construction and tax benefits for homeowners, promoted the growth of suburbs at the cost of cities. A third epoch in American residential history began by 1970 when more Americans resided in suburbs than cities, parallel to the 1920 shift from a rural majority to an urban one.

Suburban life encouraged a sharpening of gender roles among the growing middle class. Men commuted to work while women were expected to find fulfillment in marriage and motherhood, including a nearly full-time job of unpaid housework. Most women did so while either feeling isolated in their homes or finding community with other women in their neighborhoods and churches. "We married what we wanted to be," one female college graduate said. "If we wanted to be a lawyer or a doctor we married one." An enormous amount depended on a woman's choice of a husband, including class status and lifelong material well-being. Despite this partial retreat from wartime employment, however, fully one-third of American women continued to work for pay outside the home. The economic circumstances of most black women offered them little choice, and most wound up doing double housework: their own and that of families employing them as domestics. Middle-class women tended to view their paid work as a job rather than a career, a way to increase the family income if they did not have small children at home. Quotas in graduate schools and sex-segregated employment limited the number of female professionals.

Children moved even more firmly to the center of American family lives in these years. After a lengthy decline during the 1930s, marriage and birth rates picked up during the war and then accelerated sharply after 1945. After a brief upward spike in 1946, divorce rates declined for the first time in a century. From 1946 to 1964 women giving birth at a younger age to more children created the demographic bulge known as the baby boom. Large families reinforced the domestic focus of most women, putting the work of child-rearing at the center of their lives. Fatherhood became increasingly a badge of masculinity, with Father's Day emerging as a significant holiday for the first time. Family physician Benjamin Spock published *Baby and Child Care* (1946), a runaway best-seller that helped shift the emphasis in American parenting from strictness to greater nurturance.

Strong feelings about pregnancy hinged on the marital status of the expectant mother. Married mothers were celebrated, but unmarried ones were rebuked. Despite the greater freedom of the war years, the sexual double standard remained in place, with women's virtue linked directly to virginity in a way that men's was not. Birth control devices such as the diaphragm were legal only for married women and only in certain states. Women seeking to terminate unwanted pregnancies had to consider illegal abortions, the only kind available before 1970; millions did so, including one-fifth of all married women and a majority of single women who became pregnant. Two studies of American sexual behavior by Dr. Alfred Kinsey of Indiana University revealed that Americans often did not practice what they preached. The Kinsey reports of 1948 and 1953 shocked the public with their revelation of widespread premarital and extramarital sexual intercourse as well as homosexual liaisons. Rates of sex before marriage actually remained stable from the 1920s to the 1960s, but after World War II rates of teenage sex soared because so many teenagers got married. The average age of couples at the altar dropped as social pressures aimed to contain sex within marriage.

The Growth of the South and the West

Before World War II American cultural, industrial, and financial power had always been centered in the urban North, but federal expenditures during the war began to change this. The U.S. Army built most of its training bases in the South, where land close to the coasts was thinly populated and inexpensive. Military bases and defense industries sprang up along the West Coast to project power into the Pacific against Japan. California alone received 10 percent of all federal dollars spent during the war. The San Francisco Bay area sprawled with shipyards and sailors, and southern California became the center of the nation's aircraft industry. U.S. troops built the Alcan (Alaska–Canada) Highway, and millions of GIs passed through Hawaii en route to the Pacific battlefront. Fighting against the Japanese to defend Pearl Harbor and the Aleutian Islands brought the once-distant territories of Hawaii and Alaska more into Americans' consciousness, setting them on the path to statehood in 1959.

The Sunbelt of the South, the Southwest, and California grew rapidly after the war, whereas older Rustbelt cities of the Northeast and Midwest such as Buffalo and Detroit began to lose manufacturing jobs and population. Like the 440,000 people who moved to Los Angeles during the war, postwar migrants to California and Arizona appreciated the weather and the eco-

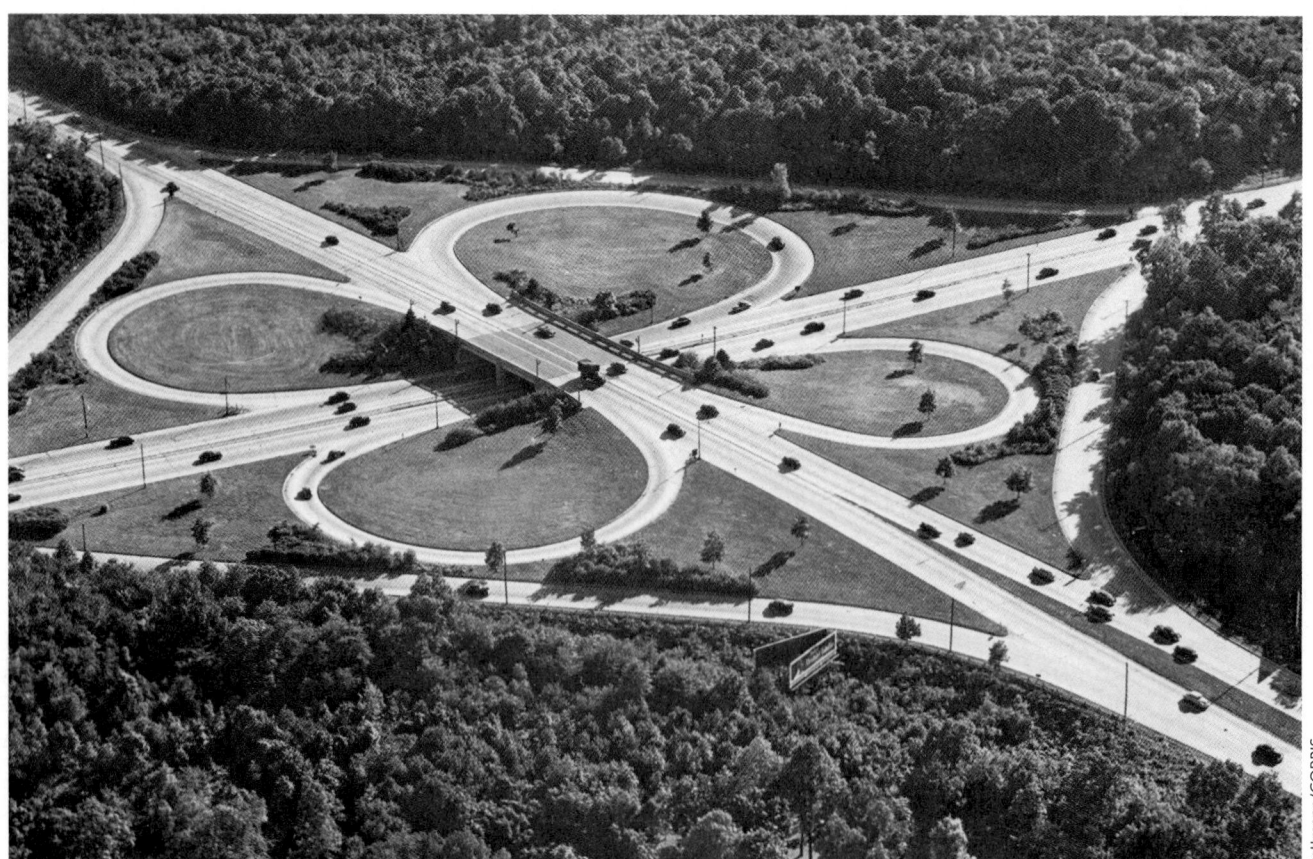

Bettmann/CORBIS

■ A new cloverleaf intersection on a freeway arches across the northern New Jersey suburbs in 1949. Multilane, limited-access highways became common after World War II. A new word, "smog" (neither smoke nor fog), appeared to describe the urban pollution caused by trucks and commuter vehicles.

nomic opportunities. Military spending underwrote half the jobs in California during the first decade of the Cold War. Migrants from south of the border, meanwhile, found work primarily in California's booming agricultural sector. The U.S. government continued to use the Bracero program as an exception to immigration laws for Mexicans willing to do arduous labor in the hot fields of the Golden State, thus encouraging the large influx of Mexicans into the U.S. Southwest. Agriculture in the arid Southwest depended on water management and irrigation, especially from dams on the lower Colorado River for Arizona and on several rivers flowing down from the Sierra Nevada range into California's fertile central valley.

Two industries particularly stimulated the growth of the Sunbelt: cars and air conditioning. Automobiles helped shape the economies of western states, where new cities were built out of sprawling suburbs, and governments erected highways rather than railroads, subways, or other forms of public transportation. New car sales shot up from 70,000 in 1945 to 7.9 million in 1955. Inexpensive gasoline, refined from the abundant crude oil of Texas and Oklahoma, powered this fleet. Automobile exhaust pipes replaced industrial smokestacks as the primary source of air pollution, which by the 1960s shrouded Los Angeles—the "city of angels"—in smog. Air conditioning also became widely available after World War II and contributed to the breakdown of the South's regional distinctiveness. From Miami and Atlanta to Houston and Washington, D.C., the dramatic economic and demographic expansion of the Sunbelt depended on the indoor comfort brought by controlling summertime heat and humidity.

Harry Truman and the Limits of Liberal Reform

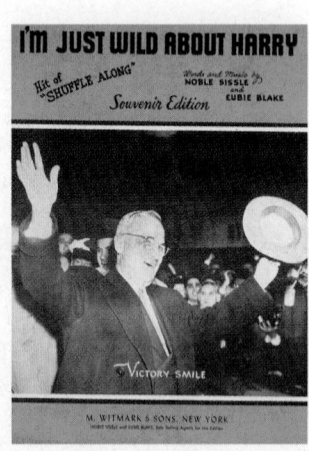

The onset of the Cold War narrowed the range of American political discourse. In seeking to consolidate the New Deal legacy, President Truman found himself boxed in by conservative Republican opponents. Allied governments in western Europe had embraced the idea that access to health care was a right of every citizen in a modern democratic state. But when Truman proposed a system of national health care, conservatives quashed his proposal in Congress, pushed by an American Medical Association lobbying campaign that denounced the idea as a "monstrosity of Bolshevik bureaucracy."

Perhaps the most blatant omission of the New Deal was protection against racial discrimination. Now, as the Cold War intensified, the fact that millions of Americans still lacked basic guarantees for their civil rights was a glaring and embarrassing contradiction amid rhetoric about ensuring rights and liberties throughout the "free world." The President's Committee on Civil Rights called in 1947 for a strong federal commitment to racial equality. Truman campaigned for reelection in 1948 on a platform of support for civil rights that was unprecedented in the White House, including the first presidential address to the NAACP. That summer he ordered the desegregation of the armed forces and the federal civil service. Truman was not a complete egalitarian and did not address underlying structures of segregation in housing and schools. But blatant racial abuses angered him, and he helped set the Democrats on the path to becoming the party of racial equality.

The president's promotion of civil rights also had a political purpose in 1948. Black voters in Chicago, Cleveland, and other northern cities played a key role in swing states; their solid support lifted Truman to a narrow and surprising victory over the heavily favored Republican candidate, New York governor Thomas Dewey. Truman's reelection was all the more impressive because of the fracturing of the Democratic party. Alienated by the civil rights plank, white Southerners walked out of the Democratic convention and ran South Carolina governor Strom Thurmond as an independent candidate. The "Dixiecrats" won four states in

TABLE 24-1			
The Election of 1948			
Candidate	Political Party	Popular Vote	Electoral Vote
Harry S. Truman	Democratic	24,205,695	304
Thomas E. Dewey	Republican	21,969,170	189
J. Strom Thurmond	State-Rights Democratic	1,169,021	38
Henry A. Wallace	Progressive	1,156,103	0

the Deep South, foreshadowing the abandonment by white Southerners of the party of their parents in the 1960s. From the opposite side of the party, many liberals jumped ship for Henry Wallace, Roosevelt's former vice president, running as the Progressive party candidate. Truman won as a man of the moderately liberal center, fierce against communism, usually supportive of the rights of organized labor, and opposed to discrimination.

The Cold War at Home

Anticommunism turned out to be an inadequate shield for liberals and moderates in the partisan warfare pervading American politics in the late 1940s and early 1950s. In a pattern that became known as McCarthyism, mostly Republican conservatives explained communist successes abroad—especially in China and Korea—by "red-baiting" liberal Democrats in the administration, accusing them of sympathizing with and even spying for the Soviet Union. The hunt for domestic subversives to explain international setbacks was grounded in the reality of a handful of actual Soviet spies, most notably Julius Rosenberg (who was executed for treason in 1953 along with his apparently innocent wife, Ethel) and nuclear scientist Klaus Fuchs. But this second Red Scare expressed primarily the frustration of being unable to translate vast U.S. power into greater control of world events. And it served, above all, to cast suspicion on the patriotism of liberals at home. "The fact that a person believes in racial equality doesn't prove he's a Communist," argued the head of one government loyalty board, "but it certainly makes you look twice, doesn't it?"

Despite his general support for civil liberties, Truman helped set the tone for pursuing suspected traitors. In an unsuccessful effort to fortify his right flank against Republican attacks, he established a federal employee loyalty program in March 1947 as the domestic equivalent of the Truman Doctrine. Attorney General Tom Clark drew up a list of supposedly subversive organizations that the FBI and state committees on "un-American activities" then hounded.

The president red-baited the Progressive party in the 1948 campaign, referring to its ticket as "Henry Wallace and his Communists." In a case with sobering implications for free speech, federal courts in 1949 convicted the leaders of the U.S. Communist party of promoting the overthrow of the U.S. government. Words alone, the courts ruled, could be treasonable—the same logic as the wartime Sedition Act of 1918 (see Chapter 20). Conservative congressional Democrats pushed through the Internal Security Act of 1950 to require Communist party members to register with the government and allow emergency incarceration of suspected subversives. Calling it "a long step toward totalitarianism," Truman vetoed the measure, but Congress overrode the veto by a huge margin.

Republicans reaped the benefits of the Red Scare. Most Americans who had sympathized in any way with the Soviet Union in the Depression years were by the late 1940s merely liberal Democrats, but the House Un-American Activities Committee (HUAC) zeroed in on their earlier records. Investigating Hollywood, the television industry, and universities as well as the executive branch of the U.S. government, HUAC destroyed the careers of prominent figures and average Americans. California congressman Richard Nixon made his initial reputation as a young HUAC member by investigating charges that State Department official Alger Hiss had spied for the USSR. Hiss's conviction in 1950

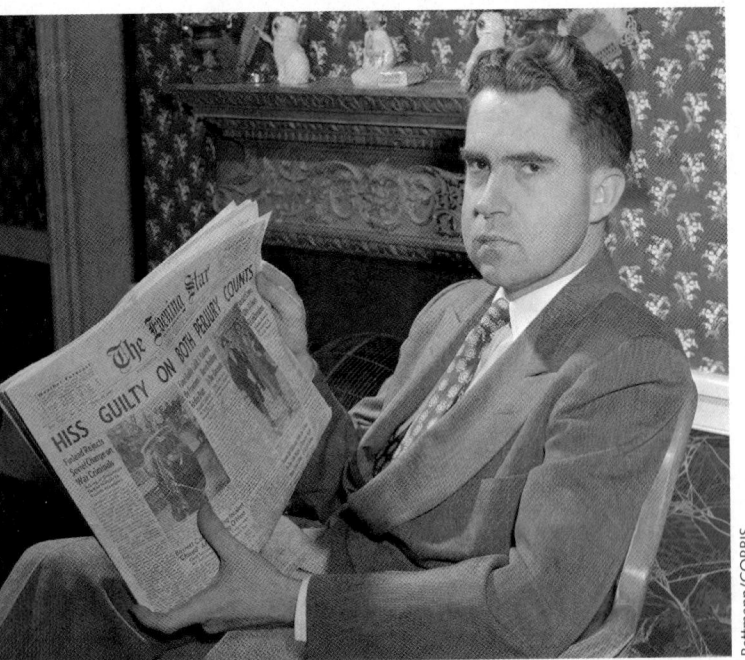

Bettmann/CORBIS

■ Americans later knew Richard M. Nixon as the president who traveled to China in 1972 and brought his administration down in disgrace two years later with the Watergate scandal. Nixon first gained prominence as a young California congressman serving on the House Un-American Activities Committee (HUAC) who led the investigation into accusations that prominent U.S. diplomat Alger Hiss had spied for the USSR in the 1930s.

on charges of perjury (lying under oath) frightened Americans by associating a powerful administration figure with communism.

The era found its name in the previously obscure junior senator from Wisconsin, Republican Joseph McCarthy. With a single speech in Wheeling, West Virginia, on February 9, 1950, this genial but ambitious politician soared to prominence. "I have here in my hand a list of 205" Communist party members working in the State Department, he declared. Over the next four years, the numbers and names changed as McCarthy stayed one step ahead of the evidence while intimidating witnesses before his Senate subcommittee. In reality, one reporter joked, McCarthy "couldn't find a Communist in Red Square" in Moscow. He talked about Communists, but his show was about Democrats. As the war in Korea raged, he mercilessly red-baited the Truman administration. But after the Republican electoral victory in 1952, his excesses lost their partisan utility. With the end of the war in Korea and his ill-advised attacks on the U.S. Army itself as supposedly infiltrated by Communists (the Army–McCarthy hearings), he was at last censured by his Senate colleagues in 1954 and died an early, alcohol-related death in 1957.

Who Is a Loyal American?

The Cold War politics of inclusion and exclusion established a new profile for loyal Americans. Private familial and material concerns were expected to replace public interest in social reform. "No man who owns his own house and lot can be a Communist," real estate developer William Levitt declared. "He has too much to do." He also had a wife, presumably, in an era when anticommunists launched a withering assault on homosexuals as "perverts" and threats to the nation's security. Church membership climbed in tandem with condemnations of "godless Communism," and Congress added the words "under God" to the Pledge of Allegiance. Warning that "God is giving us a desperate choice, a choice of either revival or judgment," revivalist preacher Billy Graham launched his first evangelical crusade in Los Angeles in 1949, en route to becoming the nation's foremost religious figure. Discrimination against Roman Catholics and Jews, though still evident, declined as Catholics such as McCarthy proved intensely anticommunist and as pictures and stories emerged to reveal the horrors of the Nazi Holocaust against the Jews. More inclusive references to the "Judeo-Christian tradition" became common.

American leadership of the global anticommunist cause strengthened the struggle for racial equality at home, within certain limits. The NAACP and most African Americans took an anticommunist position in accord with Truman, in return for his support of civil rights. They downplayed their concern for colonial independence in Africa and Asia to support NATO. The American GI Forum (Latino veterans) and the Japanese American Citizen League also worked within the confines of Cold War politics to end discrimination. More radical black leaders such as scholar W. E. B. Du Bois and actor and singer Paul Robeson refused to make any such accommodation to anticommunism. Offended by the hypocrisy of segregation in the land of liberty, they insisted on full freedom everywhere in the "free world." The government responded by restricting their travel and diminishing their livelihoods. In a move right out of the Soviet playbook, Robeson's name was erased from the list of football All-Americans for 1917 and 1918 (he had starred for Rutgers University), leaving only ten men on those teams.

McCarthy talked about Communists, but his show was about Democrats. As the war in Korea raged, he mercilessly red-baited the Truman administration.

For impoverished Native Americans, the government seemed to give with one hand and take away with the other. In 1946 Truman established the Indian Claims Commission to consider payment for lands taken and treaties broken. But gestures toward compensation led to policies of termination. Developers seeking access to Indian lands joined reformers troubled by reservation poverty in urging Congress—with limited success—to terminate the special status Indian tribes had held with the federal government since its founding. Dillon S. Myer, who had overseen internment camps for Japanese Americans during World War II, became director of the Bureau of Indian Affairs in 1950. He closed reservation schools, withdrew support for traditional cultural

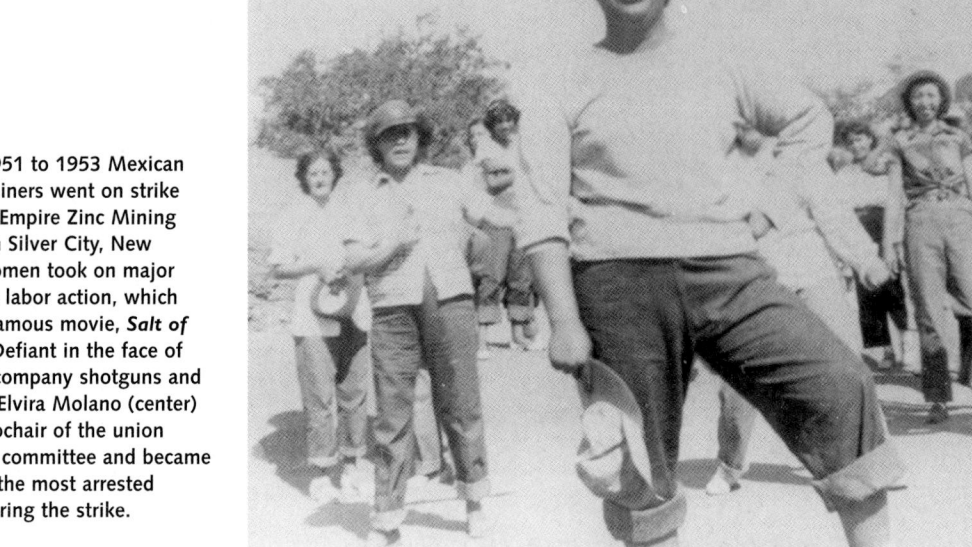

■ From 1951 to 1953 Mexican American miners went on strike against the Empire Zinc Mining Company in Silver City, New Mexico. Women took on major roles in this labor action, which inspired a famous movie, *Salt of the Earth.* Defiant in the face of police and company shotguns and billy clubs, Elvira Molano (center) served as cochair of the union negotiating committee and became known as "the most arrested woman" during the strike.

Courtesy, Los Mineros Collection, Chicano Research Collection, Arizona State University Libraries

activities, and launched an urban relocation program, all intended to move Native Americans into the mainstream and get the government "out of the Indian business."

Immigrants also received mixed messages. The McCarran–Walter Act (1952) ended the long-standing ban on allowing people of Asian descent not born in the United States to become U.S. citizens. But it preserved the discriminatory 1924 system of "national origins" for allocating numbers of immigrants from different countries. The bill also strengthened the attorney general's authority to deport aliens who were suspected of subversive intentions. Like Guatemalan-born leftist Luisa Moreno, a successful labor organizer in California deported in 1950, immigrants learned that their welcome depended on their politics.

The United States and Asia

Japan did not conquer independent nations in its sweep southward at the start of World War II. Tokyo's army defeated imperial powers: the French in Indochina, the Dutch in Indonesia, the British in Singapore and Malaya, and the Americans in the Philippines. In a single swoop, Japanese soldiers demonstrated the absurdity of white supremacy and cleared the way for the end of colonialism in Asia. Japan's retreat in 1945 left vacuums of power throughout the region. Into them flowed two contenders: the returning but gravely weakened European imperialists and Asian nationalists such as Ho Chi Minh in Vietnam (part of French Indochina). Americans were not passive observers of this struggle as they sought to establish a new free-trading order in the region. Less than five years after millions of American citizens had served in the war in the Pacific, hundreds of thousands returned to Asia to fight for an anticommunist regime in South Korea. In Asia, as in much of the Third World, the Cold War quickly turned hot.

The Chinese Civil War

Despite frequent discrimination against Chinese immigrants in the United States, Americans had long felt a special connection to China. Half of the thousands of Christian missionaries sent out by American churches in the early 20th century had been posted there. Entrepreneurs eyed the Chinese market, home to one-fifth of the world's potential consumers. Selling cigarettes to the Chinese brought tobacco baron James B. Duke much of his wealth, which he then used to endow the university in North Carolina that bears his name. During World War II Chinese resistance to Japan's invasion occupied millions of Tokyo's soldiers who would otherwise have been shooting at American GIs. The close U.S. alliance with the government of Jiang Jieshi seemed to confirm American hopes that Asia's largest nation would follow a pro-American path. Republican senator Kenneth Wherry of Nebraska declared that the United States would "lift Shanghai up and up, ever up, until it looks just like Kansas City."

However, many Chinese wanted Shanghai to look just like itself—or perhaps like Moscow. The partisans of the Chinese Communist Party (CCP) under Mao Zedong's leadership fought more effectively against the Japanese than Jiang's soldiers did. Japan's withdrawal in 1945 initiated four years of warfare between the Communists and Jiang's anticommunist Nationalists. Younger American diplomats and journalists in China, many of them missionaries' children who had grown up there, argued that the CCP was more popular than the corrupt Nationalist regime and was independent of the USSR. Rejecting the advice of these "China hands," the Truman administration provided $3 billion in aid to Jiang. The logic of the Truman Doctrine required containment of communism everywhere. Nevertheless, it failed in China. Americans watched in frustration as the CCP defeated the Nationalists, who retreated to the island of Taiwan. On October 1, 1949, addressing a vast crowd in Beijing's Tiananmen Square, Mao announced the establishment of the People's Republic of China (PRC).

Americans were appalled. The most populous nation in the world, the key to Asia, was gone—into the communist camp. More ominously, it was the first communist government created without the presence of Soviet troops. Might the rest of Asia also choose communism? Profound suspicions on both sides prevented any Sino-American accommodation. The U.S. government refused to recognize the People's Republic, just as it had done with the USSR in 1917; instead, Washington for the next 23 years pretended that the

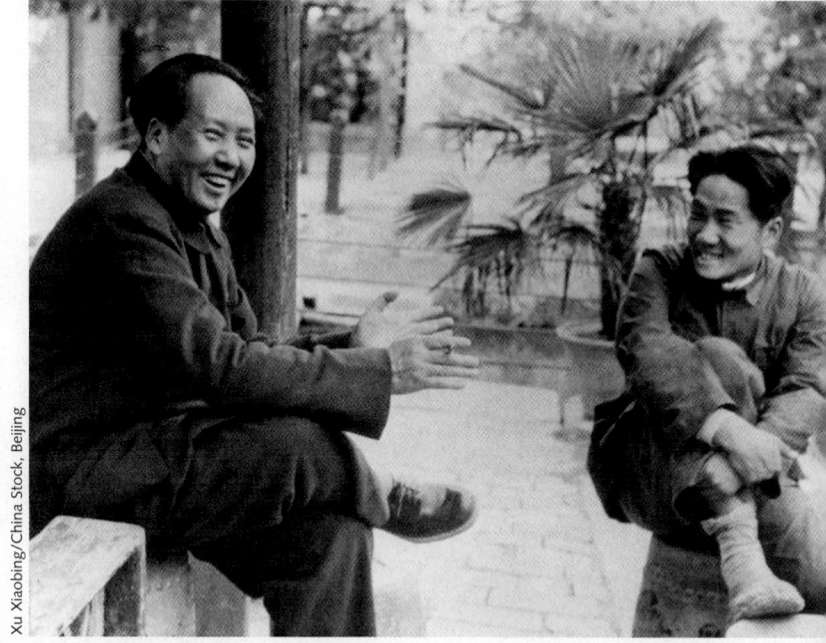

Xu Xiaobing/China Stock, Beijing

■ Mao Zedong led the Communist party that took power in China during the civil war of 1945–1949. Although Americans called this "the fall of China," Mao officially introduced the new government in Beijing by declaring that "China has stood up." Mao (left) talks here with his favorite son, Mao Anying, who was killed in Korea on November 25, 1950, apparently in a U.S. bombing raid.

Nationalists on the tiny island of Taiwan were the real government of China. The CCP had come to power on its own, with minimal help from the Soviets. But faced with U.S. hostility and sharing a common ideology with the Soviet Union, Mao papered over historic Chinese–Russian tensions (which reemerged in the 1960s) and signed a mutual defense pact with Moscow in February 1950. The so-called loss of China increased the importance for American policymakers of building capitalist societies in the rest of Asia, particularly Japan and—fatefully—South Korea and Vietnam. China's revolution also became a major issue in American politics. "Who lost China?" Republicans demanded rhetorically and effectively, presuming that it had once been America's to lose.

The Creation of the National Security State

A week before Mao's announcement that China had become a communist country, President Truman shared some equally grim news with the American public: the Soviet Union had detonated its first nuclear device. The United States had lost the atomic monopoly that for four

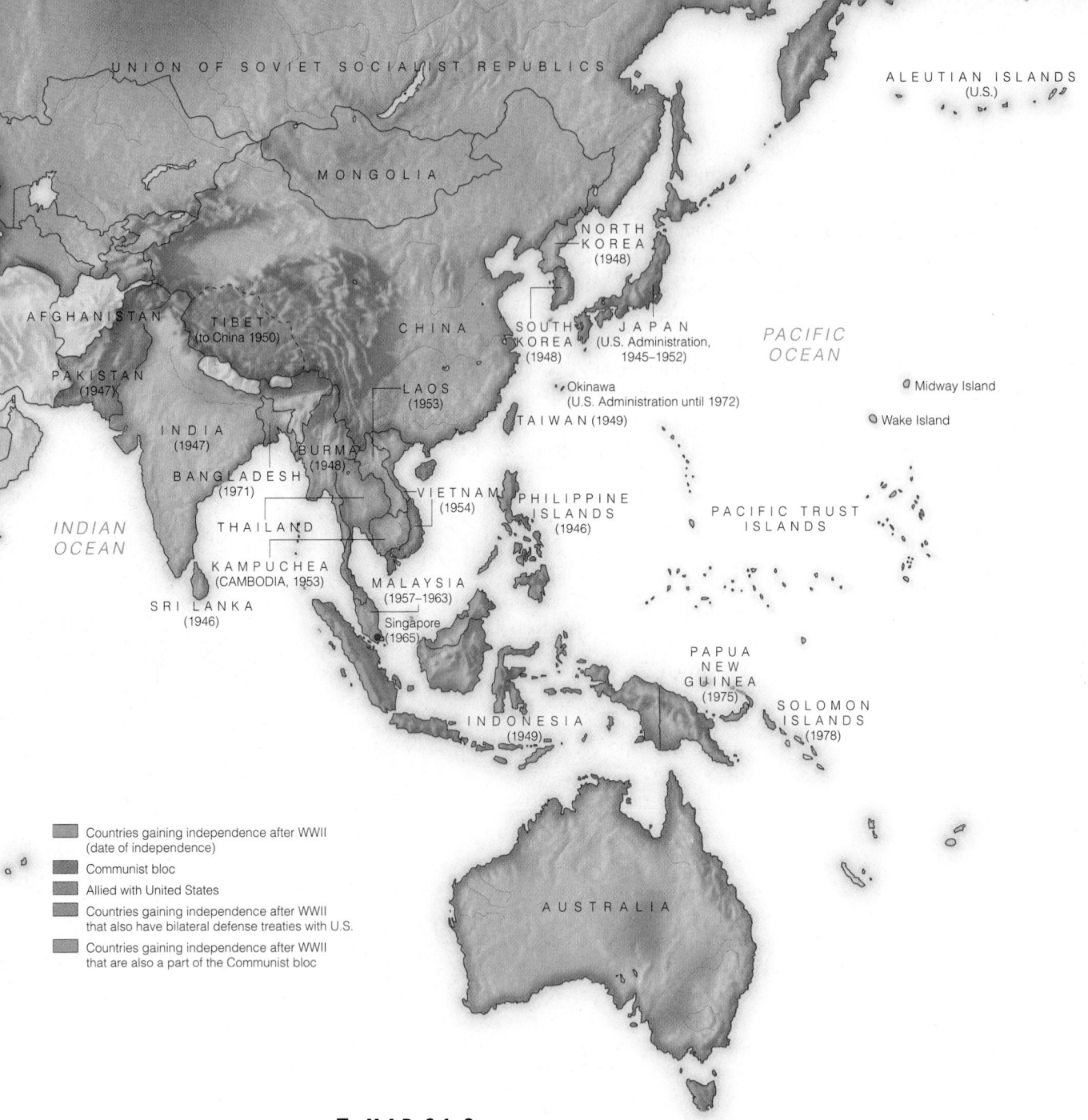

UNION OF SOVIET SOCIALIST REPUBLICS

MONGOLIA

ALEUTIAN ISLANDS
(U.S.)

NORTH
KOREA
(1948)

AFGHANISTAN

TIBET
(to China 1950)

CHINA

SOUTH
KOREA
(1948)

JAPAN
(U.S. Administration,
1945–1952)

PACIFIC
OCEAN

PAKISTAN
(1947)

Okinawa
(U.S. Administration until 1972)

Midway Island

Wake Island

LAOS
(1953)

TAIWAN (1949)

INDIA
(1947)

BURMA
(1948)

BANGLADESH
(1971)

VIETNAM
(1954)

PHILIPPINE
ISLANDS
(1946)

PACIFIC TRUST
ISLANDS

INDIAN
OCEAN

THAILAND

KAMPUCHEA
(CAMBODIA, 1953)

SRI LANKA
(1946)

MALAYSIA
(1957–1963)

Singapore
(1965)

PAPUA
NEW
GUINEA
(1975)

SOLOMON
ISLANDS
(1978)

INDONESIA
(1949)

Countries gaining independence after WWII
(date of independence)

Communist bloc

Allied with United States

Countries gaining independence after WWII
that also have bilateral defense treaties with U.S.

Countries gaining independence after WWII
that are also a part of the Communist bloc

AUSTRALIA

■ MAP 24.3
ASIA AFTER WORLD WAR II   The weakening of Western colonial powers in the war with Japan paved the
way for national independence across Asia after 1945. Some of these newly independent nations chose a
capitalist form of society and others a communist form. The new East–West tensions of the Cold War
complicated the longer North-South struggle for freedom from colonial control.

years had assured Americans of their unique position of military strength. These events in
the fall of 1949 shook the confidence of American political leaders. Truman asked his advisers for a full reevaluation of the nation's foreign policy.

The result was the top-secret National Security Council document 68 (NSC-68), which
articulated the logic of what became the national security state: a government focused on the
imperatives of military power, global involvement, and radically increased defense spending.
NSC-68 argued that there was no longer any such thing as peacetime. The United States had

NSC-68

Concerned about the trend of international events in the wake of the Communist revolution in China and the Soviet Union's acquisition of nuclear weapons, President Truman ordered his National Security Council on January 31, 1950, to conduct "a reexamination of our objectives in peace and war and of the effect of these objectives on our strategic plans." The resulting study, known as NSC-68, called for a military buildup to counter Soviet expansionism. Some specialists on the USSR, such as George Kennan, questioned NSC-68's accuracy regarding Soviet intentions and successes. But the subsequent North Korean invasion of South Korea seemed to confirm the idea of "international communism" on the march.

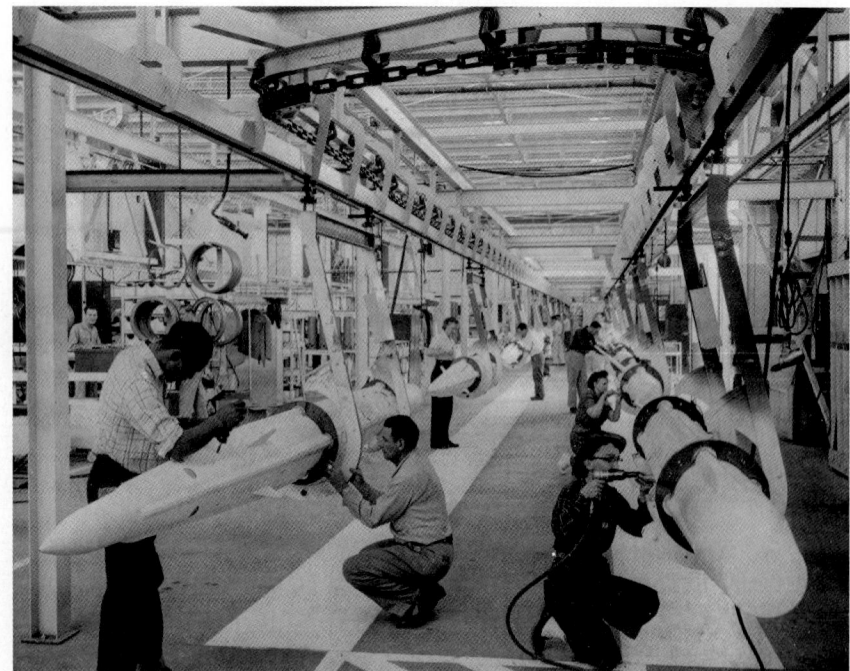

Bettmann/CORBIS

Workers at the Douglas Aircraft Company's Santa Monica factory assemble Nike guided missiles for the U.S. Army in 1955. Large military contracts proliferated during the Cold War and stimulated the growth of Sunbelt states like California.

From NSC-68: U.S. Objectives and Programs for National Security (April 14, 1950)

The Soviet Union, unlike previous aspirants to hegemony, is animated by a new fanatic faith, antithetical to our own, and seeks to impose its absolute authority over the rest of the world. . . .

Any substantial further extension of the area under the domination of the Kremlin would raise the possibility that no coalition adequate to confront the Kremlin with greater strength could be assembled. It is in this context that this Republic and its citizens in the ascendancy of their strength stand in their deepest peril.

The issues that face us are momentous, involving the fulfillment or destruction not only of this Republic but of civilization itself. . . . The assault on free institutions is world-wide now, and in the context of the present polarization of power a defeat of free institutions anywhere is a defeat everywhere. . . .

Our policy and actions must be such as to foster a fundamental change in the nature of the Soviet system. . . . In a shrinking world, which now faces the threat of atomic warfare, it is not an adequate objective merely to seek to check the Kremlin design, for the absence of order among nations is becoming less and less tolerable. . . .

The integrity of our system will not be jeopardized by any measures, covert or overt, violent or non-violent, which serve the purposes of frustrating the Kremlin design, nor does the necessity for conducting ourselves so as to affirm our values in actions as well as words forbid such measures. . . .

The total economic strength of the U.S.S.R. compares with that of the U.S. as roughly one to four. . . . The military budget of the United States represents 6 to 7 percent of its gross national product (as against 13.8 percent for the Soviet Union). . . . This difference in emphasis between the two economies means that the readiness of the free world to support a war effort is tending to decline relative to that of the Soviet Union.

It is true that the United States armed forces are now stronger than ever before in other times of apparent peace; it is also true that there exists a sharp disparity between our actual military strength and our commitments. . . . It is clear that our military strength is becoming dangerously inadequate. . . .

In summary, we must . . . [engage in] a rapid and sustained build-up of the political, economic, and military strength of the free world. ∎

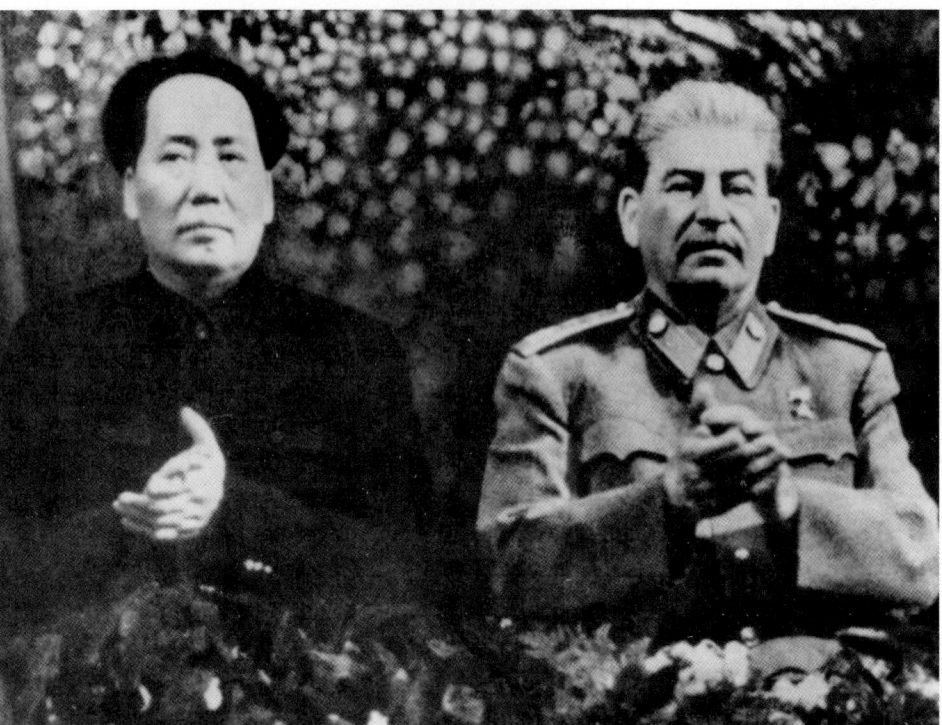

■ Were all Communists conspiring together against the United States and its interests? New Chinese leader Mao Zedong (left) helps Soviet ruler Josef Stalin celebrate his birthday on December 21, 1949. Two months later, the two men signed a mutual defense treaty. But, as their expressions suggest, they shared little personal warmth. Conflicting Chinese and Russian national interests soon strained—and eventually broke—their alliance.

entered an era of permanent crisis because of the expansion of communism and the hostile intentions of the Soviet Union. America's worldwide interests meant that it must oppose revolutions or radical change anywhere on the globe. NSC-68 went beyond the containment policy of the Truman Doctrine to call for fostering "a fundamental change in the nature of the Soviet system." This armed struggle necessitated secrecy and centralization of power in the hands of the federal government.

The National Security Act of 1947 and its 1949 amendments created the institutions of the new national security state. The Central Intelligence Agency (CIA) organized spying and covert operations, the Department of Defense unified the separate branches of the military and the National Security Council (NSC) coordinated foreign policy information for the president. NSC-68 called for permanent military expenditures at a level of war readiness; it argued that this would stimulate rather than bankrupt the U.S. economy. Scores of communities became dependent on military spending—a kind of military welfare state—and many were devastated by its withdrawal at the end of the Cold War in the 1990s. NSC–68's call for secrecy encouraged government deception of the public in the interest of "national security," with a consequent decline in democratic input into the nation's foreign relations.

At War in Korea

Two months after NSC-68 arrived on the president's desk and four months after Senator McCarthy began his attacks on the Democratic administration, troops from Communist North Korea poured across the 38th parallel into South Korea on June 25, 1950. The alarmist recommendations of NSC-68 now seemed fully justified to U.S. policymakers. The origins of the conflict on the Korean peninsula were more complicated than they appeared at first glance, however, and the United States was deeply involved.

Korea had been colonized by Japan since 1910. After Japan's defeat in 1945, Soviet and U.S. forces each occupied half of the peninsula. In the north, the Soviets installed a dictatorial Communist regime under Kim Il-Sung, who had fought with the Chinese Communists in their common struggle against Japan. In the south, the Americans established an authoritarian capitalist regime led by Syngman Rhee, who had taken classes at Princeton University with Woodrow Wilson and had lived in the United States most of the previous four decades. The 38th parallel was an arbitrary dividing line for a nation that had been unified for 1300 years, and both governments sought to reunite Korea under their control. Border skirmishes intensified after the Soviets and Americans withdrew in 1948, and leftist rebellions continued across much of the south. The CIA acknowledged that Rhee was even "unpopular among many—if not a majority—of non-Communist Koreans." Some 100,000 Koreans lost their lives in the fighting between 1945 and 1950, before "the Korean War" officially began with the north's invasion.

U.S. forces arrived in late June 1950, just in time to prevent the South Korean army from being driven off the peninsula, and then slowly pushed the North Koreans backward toward the 38th parallel in hard fighting. Truman received UN approval for this "police action," but he bypassed Congress rather than seek a declaration of war; immediate action, not debate, was needed, and he had support from leaders of both political parties. The precedent of presidential war without public debate facilitated U.S. military involvement in Vietnam a few years later.

Most importantly, Americans believed the North Korean invasion had been orchestrated by Moscow as part of a plan of worldwide communist aggression. The Truman administration considered defense of South Korea crucial to demonstrate the credibility of U.S. power. "Korea is the Greece of the Far East," the president told aides. "If we are tough enough now, if we stand up to them like we did in Greece three years ago, they won't take any next steps." American leaders adhered to the "domino theory," in which a successful communist takeover of one country would supposedly lead to its neighbors falling like dominoes into communist rule. Secretary of State Acheson reminded his colleagues that in Korea "we are fighting the second team, whereas the real enemy is the Soviet Union." The U.S. government took preemptive actions against possible aggression elsewhere. It sent the 7th Fleet to defend Taiwan, which it had previously assumed China would eventually conquer and reabsorb; it increased assistance to anticommunist forces in the Philippines and Vietnam; and it rearmed West Germany as part of NATO. The U.S. annual military budget increased from $13 billion in 1950 before the war to $50 billion in 1953, never to fall again below that level. The United States was fully rearmed.

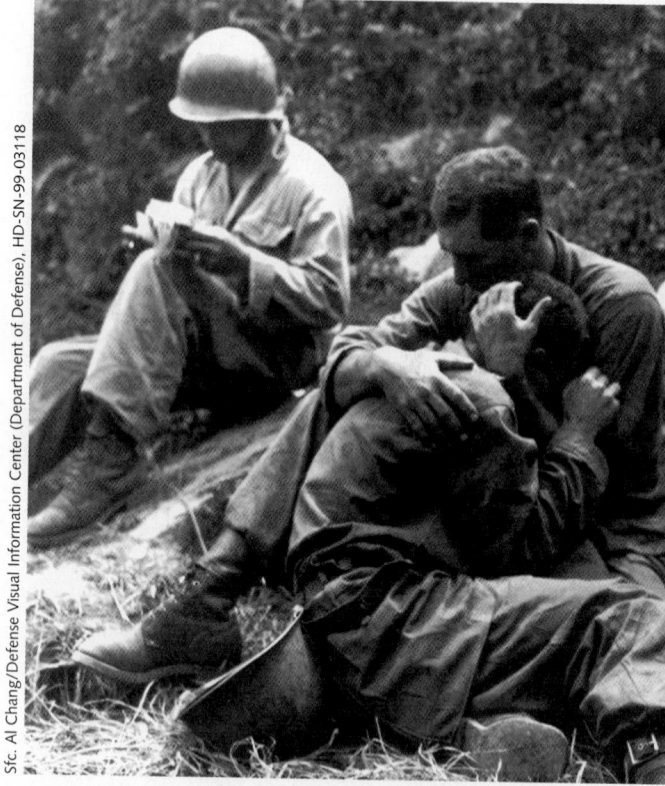

Sfc. Al Chang/Defense Visual Information Center (Department of Defense), HD-SN-99-03118

■ Near Haktong-ni, Korea, on August 28, 1950, an Army corpsman fills out casualty tags, while one American soldier comforts another who has just seen his buddy killed in action. Men who fought together on the front lines in Korea, as in other wars, experienced physical and psychological traumas unparalleled in civilian life. They often developed strong friendships with each other but sometimes had difficulty making the transition back to peacetime routines at home.

General Douglas MacArthur's brilliantly executed landing of fresh U.S. troops at the port of Inchon behind North Korean lines on September 15, 1950, created a turning point in the war. North Korean forces abandoned the South's capital city of Seoul, fleeing northward to avoid being caught between two American armies advancing from different directions. South Korea was retaken; containment had succeeded. Should American commanders now shift to rolling back communism by proceeding north of the 38th parallel? The opportunity was irresistible, despite Truman's determination to keep this a limited war. MacArthur ignored signals that the Chinese would not allow U.S. soldiers to come all the way to their border at the Yalu River—the equivalent for Americans of having the Soviet Army arrive at the Rio Grande. As UN forces—mostly Americans and South Koreans, with a sprinkling of troops from other nations—closed in on the Yalu, 200,000 Chinese soldiers struck hard on November 27. American soldiers were driven all the way south of the 38th parallel again in the longest retreat in U.S. history, some 300 miles.

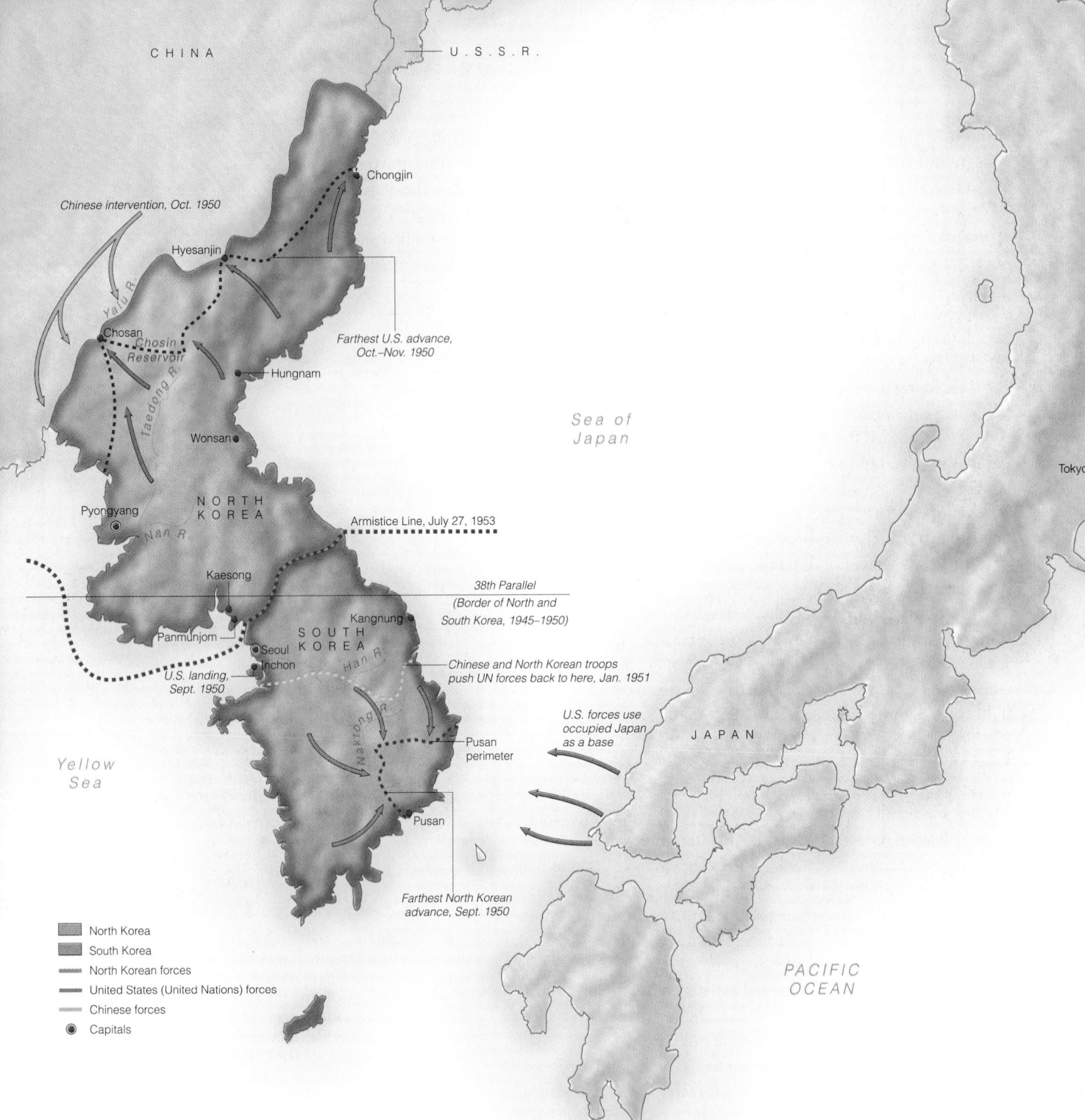

CHINA

U.S.S.R.

Chongjin

Chinese intervention, Oct. 1950

Hyesanjin

Yalu R.

Chosan

Chosin Reservoir

Taedong R.

Farthest U.S. advance, Oct.–Nov. 1950

Hungnam

Sea of Japan

Tokyo

Wonsan

NORTH KOREA

Pyongyang

Nan R.

Armistice Line, July 27, 1953

Kaesong

38th Parallel (Border of North and South Korea, 1945–1950)

Panmunjom

Kangnung

SOUTH KOREA

Seoul

Han R.

Inchon

Chinese and North Korean troops push UN forces back to here, Jan. 1951

U.S. landing, Sept. 1950

Naktong R.

JAPAN

U.S. forces use occupied Japan as a base

Yellow Sea

Pusan perimeter

Pusan

Farthest North Korean advance, Sept. 1950

PACIFIC OCEAN

- North Korea
- South Korea
- North Korean forces
- United States (United Nations) forces
- Chinese forces
- Capitals

■ MAP 24.4
THE KOREAN WAR, 1950–1953

The strategic location of the Korean peninsula enhanced the importance of what had originally been a civil conflict among Koreans. Korea's close proximity to China, the Soviet Union, and U.S.-occupied Japan made the outcome of that conflict very important to all of the great powers. The Americans and Chinese wound up doing the bulk of the fighting against each other in the full-scale war that unfolded in 1950.

MacArthur wanted to take this "entirely new war" directly to the Chinese, using conventional or even nuclear bombing campaigns against the People's Republic. However, Joint Chiefs of Staff chair Omar Bradley called this idea "the wrong war, at the wrong place, at the wrong time, and with the wrong enemy." MacArthur's growing insubordination forced Truman to fire the popular general in April 1951 because the president had no desire to start a larger war

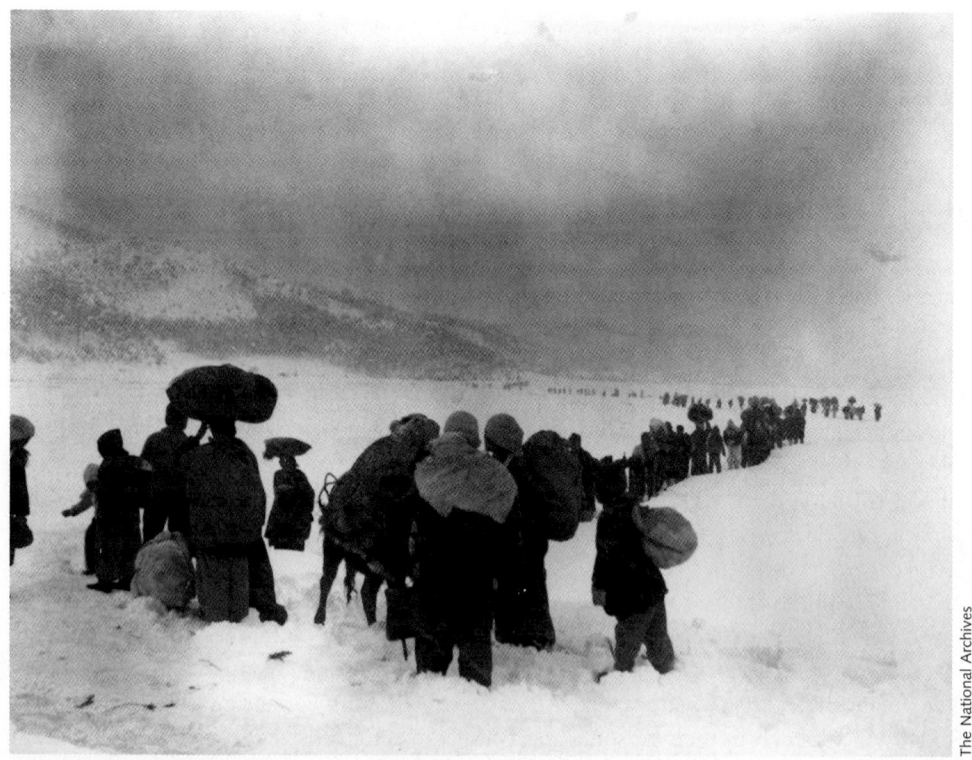

The National Archives

■ Korean refugees carry what they can of their worldly goods through heavy snow near Kangnung, on the east coast just south of the 38th parallel, on January 8, 1951. Wild swings in fortune in the Korean War contributed to the devastation wreaked on the peninsula's civilians who were caught in the fighting, sometimes more than once. First North Korean troops conquered almost all of South Korea, except the Pusan perimeter; then U.S. and UN troops pushed all the way to the Chinese border in the north. At that point, Chinese forces entered the war and hurled the Americans back far south of the 38th parallel. Finally, U.S. and UN troops fought their way back to just north of the 38th, where the ceasefire in 1953 drew the new border between the two Koreas.

that would draw in the USSR. The bloody fighting in Korea stalemated that spring close to the original dividing line, where the front remained as the two sides negotiated for two years before signing a ceasefire in July 1953. All the while, the U.S. Air Force used its supremacy in the skies to rain down extraordinary destruction on the North. "We burned down *every* town in North Korea," boasted General Curtis LeMay. American deaths totaled 37,000, and China lost nearly a million soldiers. Three million Koreans on both sides died—10 percent of the population of the peninsula—and another 5 million were made refugees. Containment succeeded at enormous cost.

Conclusion

The Korean War shaped subsequent American politics and society in critical ways. The stalemate frustrated Americans, who were never very enthusiastic about fighting in a place they knew little about. Having won all previous wars, they agreed with MacArthur that there was "no substitute for victory." But the ominous threat of nuclear weapons meant that wars had to be limited. The fighting in Korea enabled McCarthy and the Red Scare to dominate political life in the United States. The results were sometimes absurd, with the Democratic authors of the containment policy and the national security state being red-baited as "soft on communism." The Republican party rode such charges to electoral victory in November

TABLE 24-2

The Election of 1952

Candidate	Political Party	Popular Vote	Electoral Vote
Dwight D. Eisenhower	Republican	33,936,252	442
Adlai E. Stevenson	Democratic	27,314,992	89

1952. (They also benefitted from evidence of petty corruption among some Truman administration officials, such as the president's appointment secretary accepting bribes). Republican presidential nominee General Dwight Eisenhower was perhaps the most popular American alive because of his leadership of the Allied victory in Europe in World War II, and he swept into the White House over Democrat Adlai Stevenson, the governor of Illinois.

The war in Korea ensured a generation of hostility between the United States and China. It tied the People's Republic more closely to the USSR, strengthening the common belief that international communism was a unified movement. The United States committed itself to defending Taiwan from recapture by the Beijing government. The firing of the "China hands" deprived the State Department of the bulk of its Asian expertise, smoothing the path to an ill-informed war in Vietnam. The Korean War also jump-started the moribund Japanese economy as American dollars poured into Japan, where the U.S. war effort was based. Japanese conservatives called it "a gift from the gods."

Frustrations with the course of war in Korea affirmed the inward focus of American society in the 1950s. The American public largely accepted its own diminished role, and even the smaller role of its elected Congress, in decisions made by national security managers. Despite the organizing efforts of political activists such as civil rights workers, most citizens seemed to look increasingly to their personal and familial lives for satisfaction and meaning. From the powerful U.S. economy flowed an unprecedented river of consumer goods, including the new artificial materials—plastic, vinyl, nylon, polyester, styrofoam—that have pervaded and polluted American life ever since. As peace came to Korea and U.S. soldiers returned from across the Pacific, Americans sought the good life at home.

Sites to Visit

The National Security Archive at George Washington University

www.gwu.edu/~nsarchiv/

This extraordinary site includes the most recent declassified documents on the making of U.S. foreign policy.

Cold War International History Project

cwihp.si.edu/default.htm

The Woodrow Wilson International Center for Scholars maintains this excellent site, which offers newly released documents and up-to-date interpretive essays on the American-Soviet struggle.

The Ad*Access Project of Duke University Library

scriptorium.lib.duke.edu/adaccess/

This site presents fascinating images from over 7,000 advertisements in U.S. and Canadian newspapers and magazines between 1911 and 1955, offering insights into popular culture and consumer life.

Truman Presidential Museum and Library

www.trumanlibrary.org/index.html

The Harry Truman Presidential Library maintains this site, which contains an especially useful collection of docu-

ments regarding crucial foreign policy decisions in the early Cold War.

The Avalon Project at the Yale Law School: Documents in Law, History, and Diplomacy

www.yale.edu/lawweb/avalon/avalon.htm

Researchers can find here the texts of a large number of the most important primary documents illuminating U.S. relations with other countries.

Korea + 50: No Longer Forgotten

www.trumanlibrary.org/korea/

The Truman Library's site on the Korean War has documents, photos, and interpretative essays by prominent historians.

The Bancroft Library Collections

bancroft.berkeley.edu/collections/

The Bancroft Library of the University of California at Berkeley has extensive collections, exhibits, and links revealing the history of California, the nation's most populous state.

For Further Reading

General

William H. Chafe, *The Unfinished Journey: America Since World War II*, 3rd ed. (1995).

Alonzo Hamby, *Man of the People: A Life of Harry S. Truman* (1995).

Godfrey Hodgson, *America in Our Time* (1976).

Walter LaFeber, *America, Russia, and the Cold War, 1945–1996*, 8th ed. (1997).

James T. Patterson, *Grand Expectations: The United States, 1945–1974* (1996).

The Uncertainties of Victory

Thomas Borstelmann, *The Cold War and the Color Line: American Race Relations in the Global Arena* (2001).

Melvyn P. Leffler, *The Specter of Communism: The United States and the Origins of the Cold War, 1917–1953* (1994).

Harvey A. Levenstein, *Communism, Anti-Communism, and the CIO* (1981).

Richard Polenberg, *One Nation Divisible: Class, Race, and Ethnicity in the United States Since 1938* (1980).

Thomas Sugrue, *The Origins of the Urban Crisis: Race and Inequality in Postwar Detroit* (1996).

The Quest for Security

Carolyn Woods Eisenberg, *Drawing the Line: The American Decision to Divide Germany, 1944–1949* (1996).

Michael J. Hogan, *The Marshall Plan: America, Britain, and the Reconstruction of Western Europe, 1947–1952* (1987).

Walter Isaacson and Evan Thomas, *The Wise Men: Six Friends and the World They Made: Acheson, Bohlen, Harriman, Kennan, Lovett, McCloy* (1986).

Melvyn P. Leffler, *A Preponderance of Power: National Security, the Truman Administration, and the Cold War* (1992).

Thomas G. Paterson, *On Every Front: The Making and Unmaking of the Cold War* (1992).

Stewart L. Udall, *The Myths of August: A Personal Exploration of Our Tragic Cold War Affair with the Atom* (1994).

A Cold War Society

Paul S. Boyer, *By the Bomb's Early Light: American Thought and Culture at the Dawn of the Atomic Age* (1985).

Richard M. Fried, *Nightmare in Red: The McCarthy Era in Perspective* (1990).

Kenneth T. Jackson, *Crabgrass Frontier: The Suburbanization of the United States* (1985).

Elaine Tyler May, *Homeward Bound: American Families in the Cold War Era* (1988).

Ellen Schrecker, *Many Are the Crimes: McCarthyism in America* (1998).

Stephen J. Whitfield, *The Culture of the Cold War* (1991).

The United States and Asia

Warren I. Cohen, *America's Response to China: A History of Sino-American Relations*, 4th ed. (2000).

Bruce Cumings, *The Origins of the Korean War*, 2 vols. (1981, 1990).

Jon Halliday and Bruce Cumings, *Korea: The Unknown War* (1988).

Michael J. Hogan, *A Cross of Iron: Harry S. Truman and the Origins of the National Security State, 1945–1954* (1998).

Walter LaFeber, *The Clash: A History of U.S.–Japan Relations* (1997).

Online Practice Test

Test your understanding of this chapter with interactive review quizzes at

www.ablongman.com/jonescreatedequal/chapter24

Additional Photo Credits

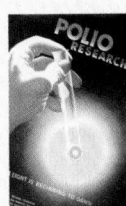

PART NINE

The Cold War at Full Tide, 1953–1979

DURING THE THIRD QUARTER OF THE TWENTIETH CENTURY, THE COLD War cast a long shadow over the United States and the rest of the world. Tensions mounted at home and abroad as the United States and the Soviet Union vied for power among the world's nations. In poor Third World countries, insurgents attempted to throw off the yoke of colonialism and play the two superpowers against each other. The United States used a variety of strategies to counter Soviet influence in Latin America, Africa, the Middle East, and Southeast Asia, including military force in Korea and Vietnam, white-knuckle diplomacy in Cuba, extensive aid to non-aligned countries and covert operations worldwide.

Soviet advances in science and technology spurred the U.S. government to sponsor bold new domestic initiatives in the areas of public education and space exploration. The Cold War even helped to shape a post–World War II domestic ideal: a nuclear family living in a house in the suburbs, with a breadwinner father and a full-time homemaker mother. Many Americans believed that their prosperous, consumer-oriented economy, with its emphasis on individualism and personal choice, was a key weapon in the fight against communism.

In a feverish arms race, both the United States and the USSR rushed to stockpile weapons of mass destruction. Constant innovations in the technology of nuclear weaponry (such as intercontinental ballistic missiles) made the bombers used in World War II obsolete. The hydrogen bomb, tested successfully for the first time in 1953, dwarfed the power of the atomic bomb that had leveled Hiroshima. Nevertheless, citizens who criticized the arms buildup risked being branded unpatriotic. More than ever before, domestic policy was intertwined with foreign policy.

The rise of multinational corporations meant that large, impersonal institutions, whether government or private, were shaping American life. Middle-level managers—men in "grey flannel suits"—represented the corporate ethos of loyalty to the company above all else. At the same time, many Americans sought to work within their local communities for social and political change. In the South, African American men and women launched a dramatic assault on the system of legal segregation known as "Jim Crow." Working at the grassroots level, these activists boycotted buses, marched, sat in at lunch counters, and went to jail. Their efforts provoked the courts and Congress to act, culminating in the Civil Rights Acts of 1964 and 1965. For the first time in American history, the federal government assumed responsibility for eliminating discrimination in the workplace and guaranteeing all its citizens the right to vote.

Other groups also organized and entered the political arena. Indians, disabled Americans, California farm workers, and gay men and lesbians all formed organizations to counter discrimination and advance their civil rights. The women's movement affected all aspects of American society, enabling women to play a fuller role in the political and economic life of the country. A new environmentalist movement secured legislation protecting wilderness areas and endangered species and ensuring that Americans had clean air to breathe and clean water to drink.

Lyndon B. Johnson assumed the presidency after the assassination of John F. Kennedy in 1963. Johnson hoped to revitalize the New Deal legacy by expanding social welfare programs. His program, called the Great Society, sought to address seemingly intractable problems such as poverty, lack of health care for the elderly, and the deterioration of inner-city neighborhoods. But Johnson also expanded the U.S. military presence in Vietnam, an effort that cost an increasing number of American lives. Even constant bombing proved futile to stem the civil war that pitted Americans and anticommunist Vietnamese against the National Liberation Front of South Vietnam and their comrades in the north. Johnson's successor, Richard M. Nixon, also found himself mired in a war that was becoming increasingly unpopular among Americans.

Protests against the war in the late 1960s and early 1970s highlighted an emerging youth culture. The baby boom generation, born in the two decades after World War II, embraced sexual freedom and new forms of music (such as rock 'n' roll) in an apparent attempt to defy their parents and "the Establishment" in general. Many Americans felt betrayed by both Johnson and Nixon, believing that tens of thousands of American soldiers had died in vain in Vietnam. The Watergate break-in at Democratic headquarters, leading eventually to Nixon's resignation, contributed to a growing, widespread disenchantment with government authority.

By the late 1970s, developments abroad had greatly complicated Cold War politics. Middle Eastern oil-producing nations imposed an oil embargo on the United States, highlighting U.S. dependence on fossil fuels. Islamic fundamentalists were beginning to retaliate violently against the spread of American influence and culture in Muslim countries. And at home, a conservative backlash emerged to counter the expansion of the welfare state, the heightened visibility of the feminist movement, and widening civil rights protests.

1968	Martin Luther King, Jr., assassinated. Robert Kennedy assassinated. My Lai massacre. Wild and Scenic Rivers Act. Tet offensive.
1969	Huge antiwar protests in Washington, D.C. Indians occupy Alcatraz, San Francisco Bay. Stonewall raid, New York City. Astronauts Neil Armstrong and Buzz Aldrin walk on the moon.

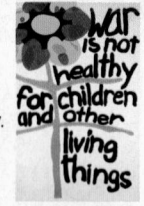

1970	U.S. invades Cambodia. National Guardsmen kill four students, Kent State University.
1971	Pentagon Papers published. Nixon administration creates "plumbers" for illegal activities.
1972	Watergate break-in. Nixon visits China. Founding of *Ms.* magazine.
1973	*Roe v. Wade* legalizes abortion. American Indian Movement members occupy Wounded Knee. Endangered Species Act. OPEC oil embargo. American troops withdrawn from Vietnam.
1974	Nixon resigns presidency; Gerald R. Ford becomes president.
1975	*Mayaguez* incident. Vietnam reunified under communist rule. Congressional investigations of CIA covert operations.
1976	Hyde Amendment prohibits use of Medicaid funds for abortions. Nation celebrates bicentennial.
1977	Carter issues general amnesty for draft evaders. Trans-Alaska pipeline system completed. ABC airs miniseries *Roots,* based on book by Alex Haley.

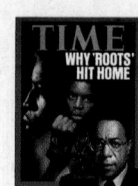

1978	Bakke Supreme Court decision. California Proposition 13.
1979	Camp David peace accords. Partial meltdown of nuclear core at Three Mile Island nuclear plant. Iranian Revolution.

CHAPTER 25

Domestic Dreams and Atomic Nightmares, 1953–1963

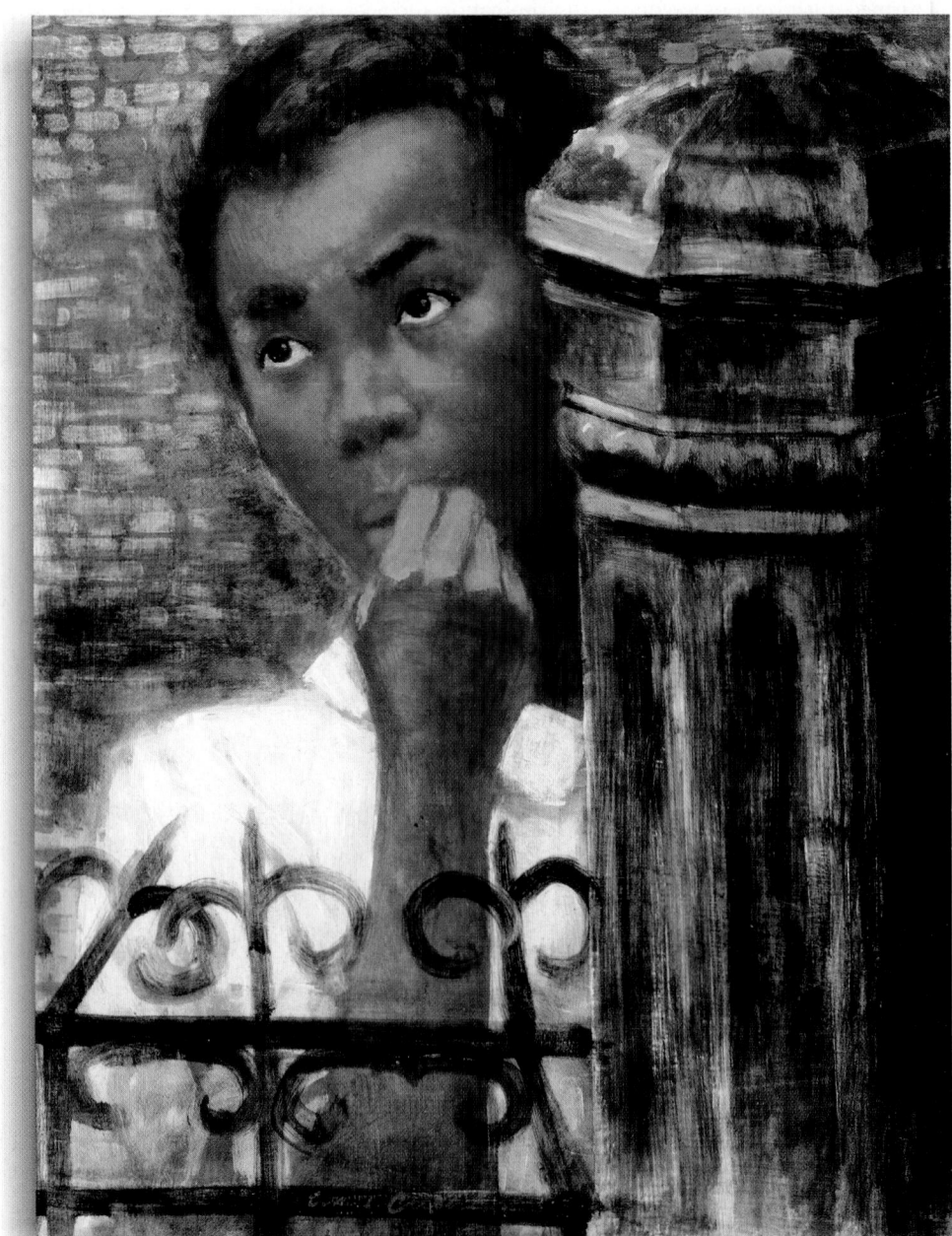

Ernest Crichlow, *By the Gate*, 1953. The Harmon and Harriet Kelley Foundation for the Arts

■ Ernest Chrichlow's 1953 painting *By the Gate* evokes the longings of a young African American.

IN 1959 VICE PRESIDENT RICHARD M. NIXON TRAVELED TO THE SOVIET UNION TO ENGAGE IN what became one of the most noted verbal sparring matches of the century. In a lengthy and often heated debate with Soviet Premier Nikita Khrushchev at the opening of the American National Exhibition in Moscow, Nixon extolled the virtues of the American way of life; his opponent promoted the Communist system. The two leaders did not discuss missiles, bombs, or even modes of government. Rather, they argued over the relative merits of American and Soviet washing machines, televisions, and electric ranges in what came to be known as the "Kitchen Debate."

The Kitchen Debate was a major skirmish on the Cold War's cultural battleground, where the two superpowers struggled for ideological supremacy. For Nixon, American superiority rested on the ability of average Americans to purchase a suburban home, complete with modern appliances. He proclaimed that the home adorned with a wide array of consumer goods represented the essence of American freedom:

> To us, diversity, the right to choose, . . . is the most important thing. We don't have one
> decision made at the top by one government official. . . . We have many different manufac-
> turers and many different kinds of washing machines so that the housewives have a choice.
> . . . Would it not be better to compete in the relative merits of washing machines than in
> the strength of rockets?

Nixon's focus on household appliances was not accidental. After all, arguments over the strength of rockets would only point out the vulnerability of the United States in the event of a nuclear war between the superpowers. Debates over consumer goods provided a reassuring vision of the good life available in the atomic age. So Nixon insisted that American superiority in the Cold War rested not on weapons but on prosperous families living in comfortable suburban homes. Freed by modern appliances from the drudgery of household chores, mothers could spend their time nurturing happy, well-adjusted children. Consumerism provided the means for achieving individuality, leisure, domestic bliss, and upward mobility.

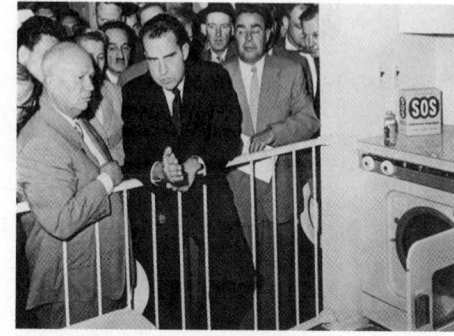

Vice President Richard M. Nixon and Soviet Premier Nikita Khrushchev touring the 1959 American National Exhibition in Moscow.

The American National Exhibition in Moscow was a showcase of American consumer goods and leisure equipment. But the main attraction, which the two leaders toured under international media spotlight, was a full-scale, six-room, ranch-style model house. This model home, filled with labor-saving devices and presumably available to Americans of all classes, offered tangible proof, Nixon claimed, of the superiority of free enterprise over communism.

Nixon called attention to a built-in panel-controlled washing machine. "In America," he said, "these [washing machines] are designed to make things easier for our women." Khrushchev countered Nixon's boast of comfortable American housewives by expressing pride in productive Soviet female workers. The Soviets, he claimed, did not share that "capitalist attitude toward women."

According to American journalists, Nixon's knock-out punch in his verbal bout with the Soviet premier was his articulation of the American postwar domestic dream: successful breadwinners supporting attractive homemakers in well-appointed, comfortable homes. Sharing Nixon's sentiments about politics, consumerism, and gender, most reporters hailed the vice president's trip as a major triumph. The American National Exhibition in Moscow seemed to demonstrate the superiority of the American way of life.

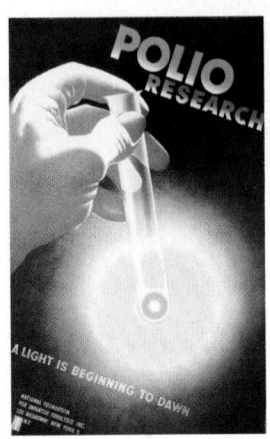

Science and expertise reigned supreme during the Cold War years. Parents turned to Dr. Benjamin Spock's best-selling *Baby and Child Care,* first published in 1946, to guide them in raising their children. Unlike prewar child-rearing experts who encouraged discipline and discouraged coddling, Dr. Spock emphasized nurture and affection. He urged parents to hold and comfort their infants, feed them on demand, and abandon rigid toilet-training routines. Dr. Jonas Salk became a hero for developing a vaccine against polio. Approved for use in 1955 and distributed widely to children in schools and clinics, the Salk vaccine virtually eliminated the dreaded illness within a few years. The oral contraceptive pill, which came on the market in 1960, provided relatively safe and effective birth control. Hailed initially as a boon to family planning, the pill also helped to usher in the sexual revolution of the 1960s.

Scientific discoveries in the 1950s also inaugurated the modern era of exploration beyond the Earth's atmosphere, fueled by the space race between the United States and the Soviet Union. The National Aeronautics and Space Administration (NASA), established in 1958, sent the first American into space in 1961. But science also brought pesticides, smog, and other pollutants. Americans, at the time, rarely considered the environmental effects of consumer goods, cars, petrochemicals, or nuclear power.

The decade from 1953 to 1963 was a time of expansive optimism about the future. The civil rights movement challenged the nation to live up to its promise of democracy for all. The baby boom, generated by young parents from all backgrounds, demonstrated widespread faith in the future for American children. It was also a decade of growth for U.S. influence abroad, the domestic economy, consumer culture, and television. Suburbs, highways, and shopping malls expanded to meet the needs of increasing numbers of families with young children. The nation itself expanded with the addition of Hawaii and Alaska as states.

It was also a decade of anxiety. Americans worried about the perils of the atomic age as the nuclear arsenals of both superpowers continued to grow. The brainwashing of prisoners of war in Korea raised fears about communist propaganda and psychological warfare. Science fiction films about alien invaders reflected concerns about foreign dangers. The Soviet Union's 1957 launching of Sputnik, the first artificial satellite to orbit the earth, alarmed Americans and forced the nation to confront the possibility of Soviet technological superiority. The United States appeared to be at the height of its strength and power, yet, at the same time, more vulnerable than ever before.

Cold War, Warm Hearth

The postwar era was a time of deep divisions in American society, yet in certain ways Americans behaved with remarkable conformity. This is nowhere more evident than in the overwhelming embrace of the nuclear family. The GI Bill, with its provisions for home mortgage loans, enabled veterans of modest means to purchase homes. Although residential segregation prevailed throughout the postwar era, limiting most suburban developments to prosperous white middle- and working-class families, many veterans of color were able to buy their

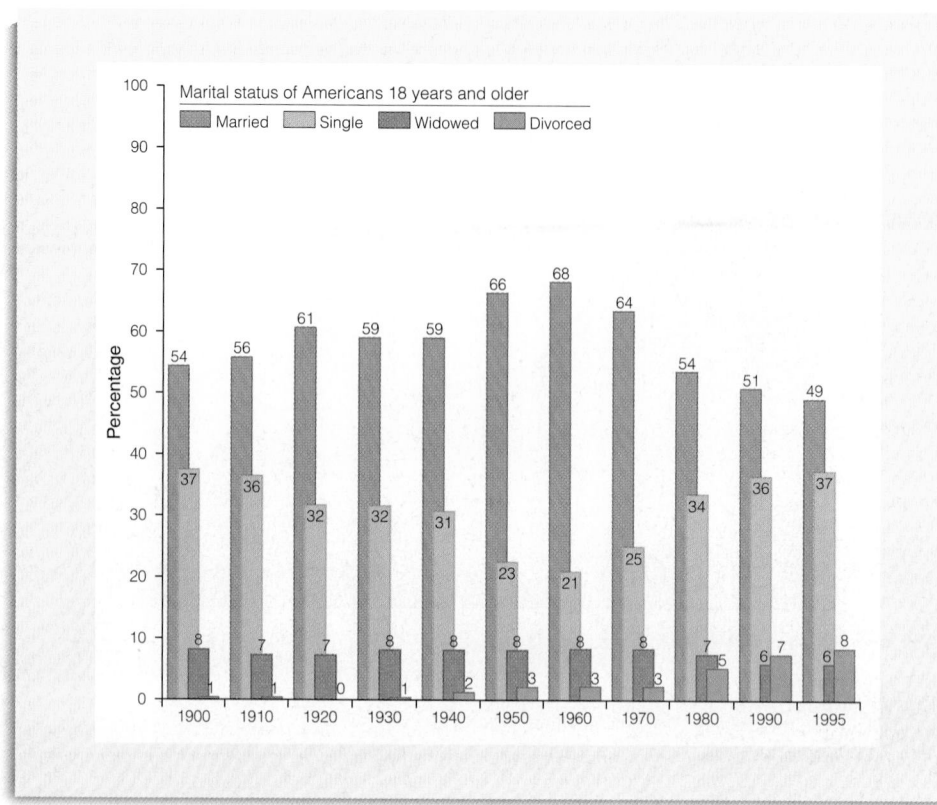

■ **FIGURE 25.1**
MARITAL STATUS OF THE U.S. ADULT POPULATION, 1900–1995
Following World War II, Americans married in record numbers. The high rate of marriage corresponded with a relatively low divorce rate. Beginning in the 1970s, the marriage rate plummeted and the divorce rate rose dramatically.

first homes. Family fever swept the nation and affected all Americans. The trends that began during and immediately after World War II, including the rising rates of marriage and childbirth and the declining age at marriage, continued during the 1950s. Americans of all racial, ethnic, and religious groups, of all socioeconomic classes and educational levels, brought the marriage rate up and the divorce rate down. Popular television shows such as *The Honeymooners,* featuring working-class couples, and *Leave It to Beaver,* depicting middle-class families, placed the consumer-oriented home at the center of attention. So did mainstream *Life* magazine and the African American glossy, *Ebony.* The "American way of life" embodied in the suburban nuclear family, as a cultural ideal if not a universal reality, motivated countless postwar Americans to strive for it, to live by its codes, and—for Americans of color—to demand it.

Consumer Spending and the Suburban Ideal

The postwar years witnessed a huge increase in spending power. Between 1947 and 1961, the number of families rose 28 percent, national income increased more than 60 percent, and the number of Americans with money to spend beyond basic necessities doubled. Rather than putting this money aside for a rainy day, Americans were inclined to spend it. Investing in one's home, along with the trappings that would enhance family life, seemed the best way to plan for a secure future.

Between 1950 and 1970, the suburban population more than doubled, from 36 million to 74 million. Fully 20 percent of the population remained poor during this prosperous time. But most families of ample as well as modest means exhibited a great deal of conformity in their consumer behavior, reflecting widely shared beliefs about the good life. They poured their money into homes, domestic appliances, televisions, automobiles, and family vacations. As prosperity spread throughout the 1950s, expenditures for food and clothing increased modestly, and

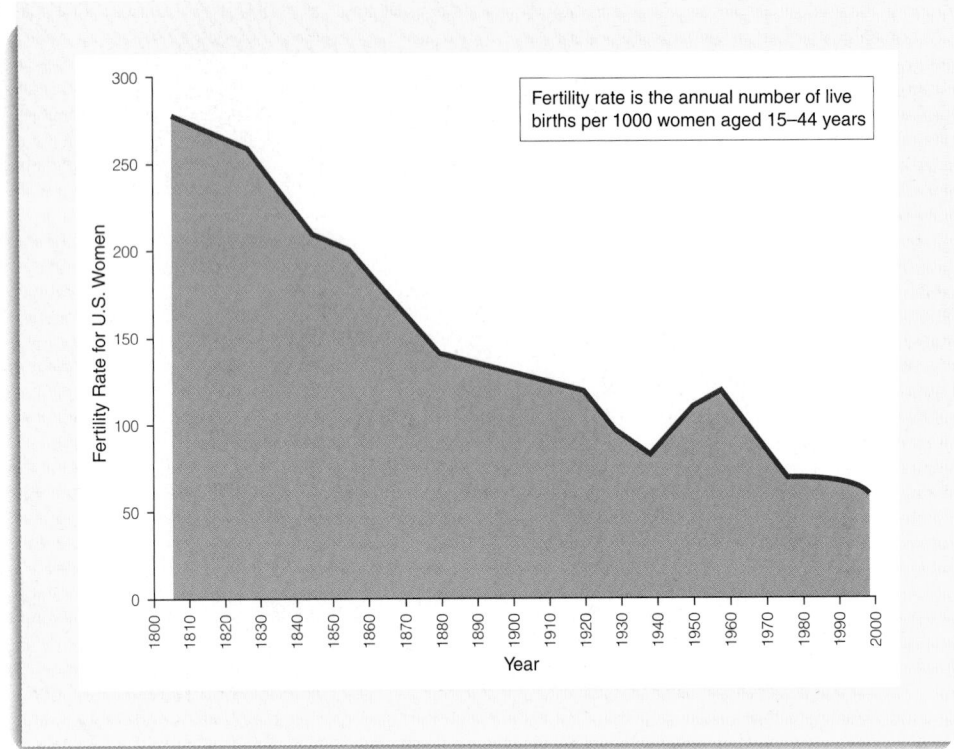

■ FIGURE 25.2
THE BABY BOOM IN HISTORICAL CONTEXT After a decline of nearly a century and a half, the fertility rate of American women surged during and after World War II, producing the baby boom. The boom resulted from the high marriage rate, the lower marriage age, and the rise in the average number of children per couple.

spending on household appliances, recreation, automobiles, and televisions more than doubled. Homeowners moved into more than 1 million new suburban houses each year.

Nuclear families who settled in the suburbs provided the foundation for new types of community life and leisure pursuits, sometimes at the expense of older ones grounded in ethnic neighborhoods and kinship networks. Family-oriented amusement parks such as Disneyland in Anaheim, California, which opened in 1955, catered to middle-class tastes, in contrast to older venues such as Coney Island, known for their thrill rides, class and ethnic mixing, and romantic environments. Religious affiliation rose to an all-time high as Americans built and joined suburban churches and synagogues, complete with youth programs and summer camps. Families piled into the car for outings to local drive-in theaters and weekend excursions or shared leisure time gathered around television sets. In 1949, fewer than 1 million American homes had a television. Within the next four years, the number soared to 20 million.

The house and commodity boom had tremendous propaganda value during the Cold War, as Nixon demonstrated in the Kitchen Debate. Although they may have been unwitting soldiers, consumers who marched off to the nation's shopping centers to equip their new homes joined the ranks of Americans taking part in the Cold War. As early as 1947, newscaster and noted cold warrior George Putnam described shopping centers as "concrete expressions of the practical idealism that built America . . . plenty of free parking for all those cars that we capitalists seem to acquire. Who can help but contrast [them] with what you'd find under communism?"

The Cold War made a profound contribution to suburban sprawl. In 1951 the *Bulletin of Atomic Scientists* devoted an issue to "defense through decentralization" that argued in favor of depopulating the urban core to avoid a concentration of residences or industries in a potential target area for a nuclear attack. Joining this effort was the American Road Builders' Association, a lobbying group second only in power and wealth to the munitions industry. As a result of these pressures, Congress passed the Interstate Highway Act in 1956, which provided $100 billion to cover 90 percent of the cost for 41,000 miles of national highways. When President Dwight D. Eisenhower signed the bill into law, he stated one of the major reasons for the new highway system: "[In] case of atomic attack on our key cities, the road net must permit quick evacuation of target areas." Many people believed that the suburbs also provided protection against labor unrest, which might lead to class warfare.

According to the Cold War ethos of the time, class conflict within the United States would weaken the nation and harm its image abroad, bolstering the Soviet Union and making the United States vulnerable to communism.

The worst-case scenario was communist takeover and the defeat of the United States in the Cold War. Pentagon strategists and foreign policy experts feared that the Soviet Union might gain the military might to allow its territorial expansion and, eventually, world domination. But observers also worried that the real dangers to America were internal: racial strife, emancipated women, class conflict, and familial disruption. To alleviate these fears, Americans turned to the family as a bastion of safety in an insecure world. Most postwar Americans longed for security after years of depression and war and saw family stability as the best bulwark against the new dangers of the Cold War.

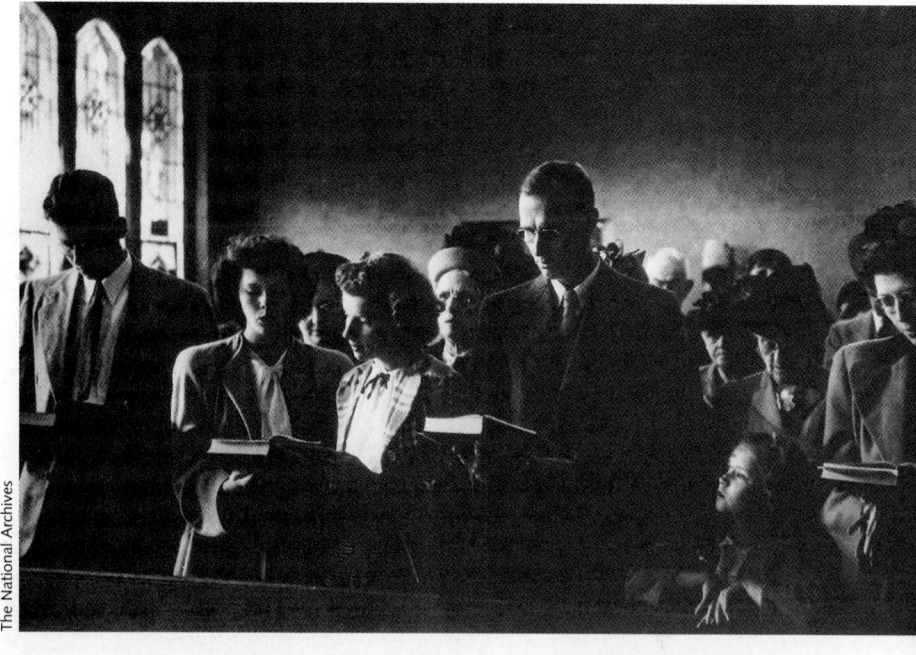

The National Archives

■ During the 1950s, churches and synagogues sprang up in suburban communities across the country, helping to strengthen community ties for newcomers to the suburbs. In the same decade, Congress inserted the phrase "under God" to the Pledge of Allegiance and added "In God We Trust" to U.S. currency.

Race, Class, and Domesticity

Many Americans think of the 1950s as a golden era of economic prosperity and happy families nestled in comfortable suburban homes. But this mythical vision obscures the fact that the government subsidized suburban developments and restricted who could live in them. After World War II, the nation faced a severe housing shortage. The federal government gave developers financial subsidies to build affordable single-family homes and offered Federal Housing Authority (FHA) loans and income tax deductions to homebuyers. These benefits enabled white working-class and middle-class families to purchase houses. Second- and third-generation European immigrants moved out of their neighborhoods in the cities and into the suburbs. Postwar prosperity, government subsidies, and the promise of assimilation made it possible for white-skinned Americans of immigrant background to blend into the suburbs.

In many suburbs, contracts for the sale of houses had included restrictions that prevented Jews and racial minorities from purchasing homes in white neighborhoods. Gradually, these restrictions began to lift. But it remained difficult for people of color to move to the suburbs. Despite the expansion of the black and Latino middle class and the increase in home ownership among racial minorities, most suburban developments excluded nonwhites. The FHA and lending banks maintained policies known as "red lining," which designated certain neighborhoods off limits to racial minorities. They refused mortgage loans to people of color wishing to buy houses in redlined areas, even if the prospective buyers could afford the purchase price. Although Americans of color remained concentrated in urban and rural areas, some did move to the suburbs, usually into segregated communities.

For Americans of color, suburban home ownership offered inclusion in the postwar American dream. In her powerful 1959 play *A Raisin In the Sun,* African American playwright Lorraine Hansberry articulated with great eloquence the importance of a home in the suburbs, not to assimilate into white America but to live as a black family with dignity and pride. Asian Americans also had good reason to celebrate home

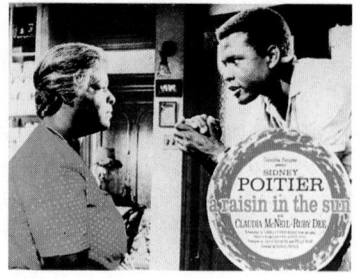

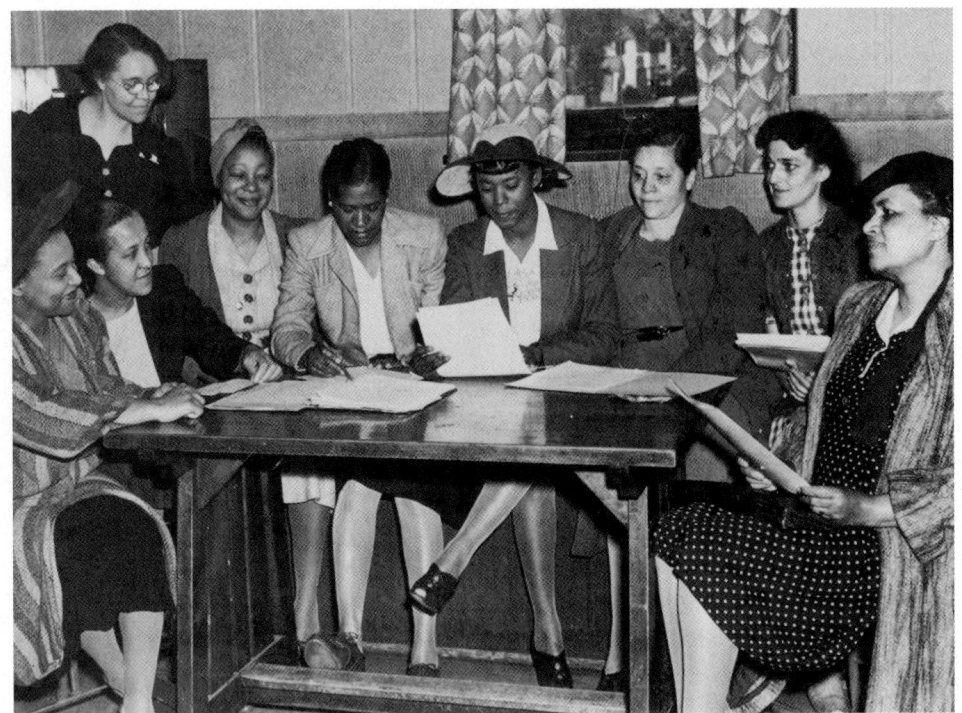

Betty Engle/Minnesota Historical Society, Neg. #64025

■ The Women's Council of St. Paul, Minnesota, was one of many service organizations in which black and white women joined in common projects. Volunteer activities enabled women to serve their communities as well as develop important political and leadership skills.

and family life. With the end of the exclusion of Chinese immigrants during World War II, wives and war brides began to enter the country, helping to build thriving family-oriented communities. After the disruptions and anguish of internment, Japanese Americans were eager to put their families and lives back together. Mexican Americans and Mexican immigrants, including *braceros*, established flourishing communities in the Southwest. Puerto Ricans migrated to New York and other eastern cities, where they could earn four times the average on the island.

Racial segregation did not prevail everywhere. For example, in Shaker Heights, Ohio, a suburb of Cleveland, white residents made a conscious decision, as a community, to integrate their neighborhood. Drawing on postwar liberal ideals of civil rights and racial integration, they welcomed black homeowners. They succeeded in this effort by emphasizing class similarity over racial difference. White residents encouraged other white families to move into Shaker Heights, pointing out that their prosperous black neighbors were "just like us." The city of Claremont, California, established an interracial housing cooperative of Mexican and African American residents along with white married college students at the edge of the Arbol Verde barrio, a Mexican American neighborhood. Desegregation experiments such as these established harmonious racially integrated communities at a time when residential segregation was the norm across the country.

White attitudes toward racial integration began to shift, but only slightly. In the late 1950s, 60 percent of whites outside the South said they would stay in their homes if a black family moved next door, but only 45 percent said they would remain in the neighborhood if large numbers of people of color moved in. In 1964, demonstrating their belief in property rights over civil rights, 89 percent of those polled in the North and 96 percent in the South believed that "an owner of property should not have to sell to a Negro if he doesn't want to." Disapproval of racial integration was strongest in the most intimate realm of life:

the family. During the 1950s, most white Americans—92 percent in the North and 99 percent in the South—approved of laws banning marriage between whites and nonwhites. As late as the mid-1960s, more than half of northern whites and more than three-fourths of southern whites still opposed interracial marriage.

As residents and businesses migrated to the suburbs, slum housing and vacant factories remained in the central cities. With declining tax bases, city governments had few resources to rebuild and revitalize urban neighborhoods. The Housing Acts of 1949 and 1954, promising "a decent home and suitable living environment for every American family," granted funds to municipalities for urban renewal. However, few of those federal dollars provided low-income housing. Mayors, bankers, and real estate interests used the money to bulldoze slums and build gleaming office towers, civic centers, and apartment complexes for affluent citizens, leaving the poor to fend for themselves in the remaining dilapidated corners of the cities.

Although intended to revitalize cities, urban renewal actually accelerated the decay of inner cities and worsened conditions for the urban poor. Federally funded projects often disrupted and destroyed ethnic communities. In St. Paul, Minnesota, the construction of U.S. Highway 94, while enabling suburbanites to commute to the city, obliterated the thriving urban African American neighborhood of Rondo. In Los Angeles, the Dodgers' stadium built in Chávez Ravine offered baseball fans and their families access to the national pastime, but it destroyed the historically rooted Mexican American neighborhood in its path. The $5-million project displaced 7500 people and demolished 900 homes.

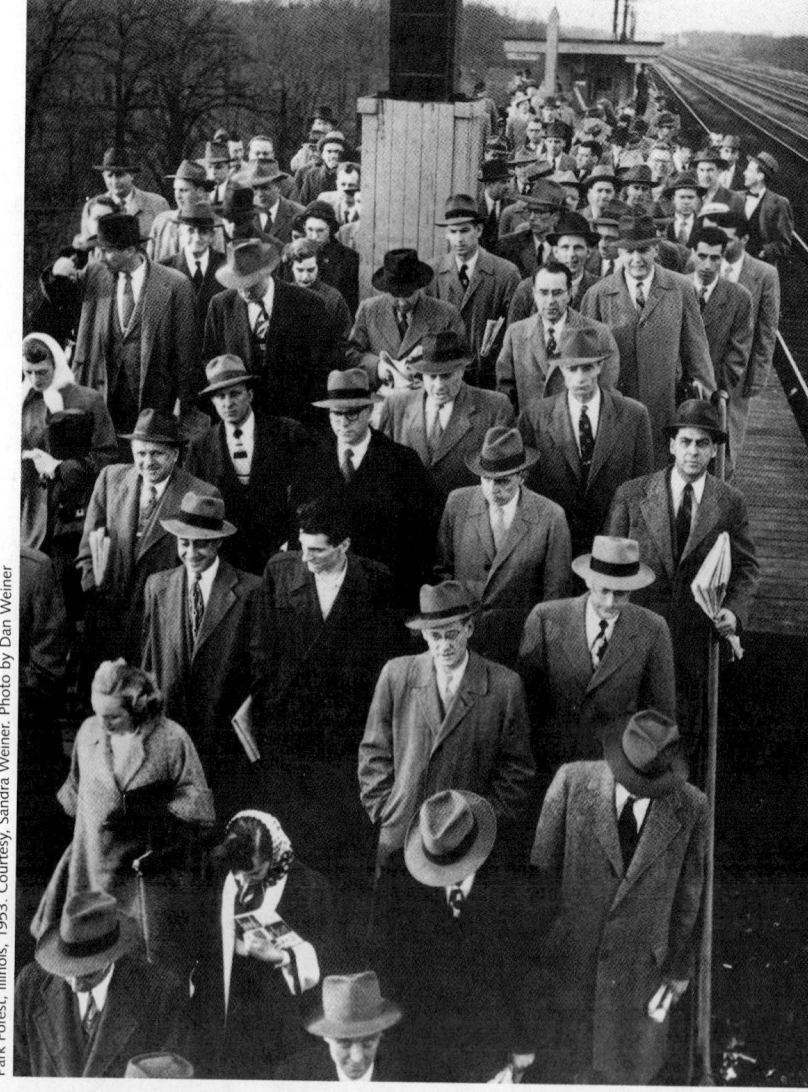

Park Forest, Illinois, 1953. Courtesy, Sandra Weiner. Photo by Dan Weiner.

■ Commuters, mostly men, left their suburban homes each morning to go to jobs in the cities, returning home at night. Suburbs served as "bedroom communities," inhabited mostly by women and children during the day.

Along with the urban poor, rural Americans reaped few benefits of postwar affluence. Many rural residents had no electricity or running water during the 1950s and therefore had no TV sets or washing machines. Much of rural America, especially in the South, remained poor. The 1950s marked the greatest out-migration from the South as the mechanization of farms reduced the number of workers on the land. More than one-fourth of the population left Kentucky and West Virginia, where unemployment in some areas reached 80 percent. For black migrants, the situation was particularly grim. One-tenth of all southern blacks moved north during the decade as the mechanical cotton picker eliminated the need for 80 percent of the sharecroppers. But life in the North did not offer much improvement. Automation in heavy industries reduced the number of available skilled jobs.

Women: Back to the Future

The nuclear family ideal of the 1950s included a full-time wife and mother and a breadwinner husband. This vision of domesticity marked a giant step backward for women, whose opportunities and experiences had expanded dramatically during World War II. The elevation of the housewife as a major cultural icon contrasted sharply with the reality. The proportion of women who fit the mold of full-time homemaker was rapidly shrinking. Although most American women married, had children, and carried the lion's share of responsibility for housework and child-rearing, increasing numbers of married women also held jobs outside the home. The employment of married women began to rise during World War II and kept rising after the war, even though most of the well-paying and highly skilled jobs returned to men at the war's end.

For the majority of white working-class and middle-class women, the end of the war closed off a number of possibilities for occupational training, professional education, and career opportunities. Often a woman's best chance to secure a decent standard of living was to marry a competent breadwinner. But the pressures on blue-collar as well as white-collar men to earn enough money for the trappings of middle-class affluence strained their ability to provide. Married women took jobs to help pay the bills. College-educated women often worked in clerical positions as secretaries or clerks, but these jobs did not make use of their knowledge and skills. Working-class women found work in the "pink collar" service sector of the economy—such jobs as waitress and hairdresser—with low pay and few chances for advancement. But for most Mexican women, pink-collar work was an improvement over migrant labor or factory work. African American women also found these jobs preferable to domestic work in white middle-class homes.

Many women worked part-time while their children were at school, but they considered their primary occupation to be homemaker. With few other opportunities for creative work, women embraced their domestic roles and turned homemaking into a profession. Many fulfilled their role with pride and satisfaction and extended their energies and talents into their

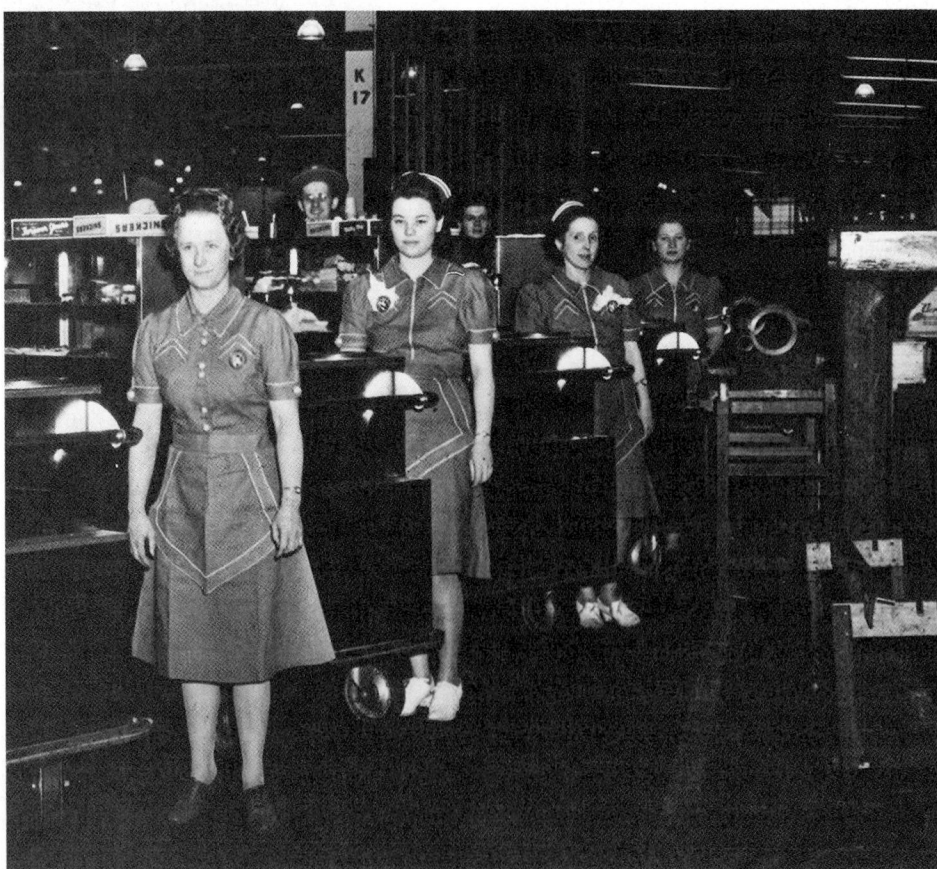

■ After World War II, women were forced out of most of the high-paying skilled jobs that they had occupied during wartime to make room for the returning men. The jobs available to women were mostly so-called pink-collar jobs in the service industry. Here, women operate rolling food carts that enabled a New Jersey factory to feed its workers lunch in a mere 20 minutes.

communities, where they made important contributions as volunteers in local parent–teacher associations (PTAs) and other civic organizations. Most postwar mothers finished childbearing by the time they were 30 and had many years ahead of them when their child-rearing responsibilities ended. Some expanded part-time employment into full-time occupations when their children left the nest. Others felt bored and frustrated and drowned their sorrow with alcohol or tranquilizers. In 1963 author Betty Friedan described the constraints facing women as the "problem that has no name" in her feminist manifesto, *The Feminine Mystique.*

Despite the powerful cultural expectation that women's primary responsibilities were to care for their homes and families, there were many single and married women who followed alternative paths. Women pursued careers in a wide range of fields, including the arts, business, and politics. Harvard Medical School admitted its first female students in 1945, although the medical profession remained heavily male-dominated. Some women managed to buck the prevailing gender role with ease; others found it difficult. Minnesota Democratic Congresswoman Coya Knudson paid a heavy price for her political ideals. While she was in Washington, D.C., working to pass legislation for such causes as college scholarships and school lunches, her husband told *Life* magazine that his wife had abandoned her domestic responsibilities to dally in the male world of politics. The article, titled "Coya Come Home," cast aspersions on the congresswoman's morals and featured a photo of the family having Thanksgiving dinner in a seedy Washington, D.C., cafeteria. Knudson lost her seat in Congress to a Republican challenger who used "Coya Come Home" as a campaign slogan.

Education was one avenue available to women, as students as well as teachers. But higher education did not open its doors fully to women. Because few women gained access to graduate and professional schools and most well-paying jobs were reserved for men, college degrees for white women did not necessarily open up career opportunities or greatly improve their job and earning prospects. By 1956, one-fourth of white female students married while still in college. Many of these women dropped out of school to take jobs in order to support their husbands through college. But the situation was quite different for black women. Like their mothers and grandmothers, most black women had to work to help support their families. Even in the prosperous postwar years, few black families could survive on the meager earnings of a single breadwinner. Job prospects for black women generally were limited to menial, low-paying occupations. Young black women knew that a college degree could mean the difference between working as a maid for a white family and working as a secretary, teacher, or nurse. Although few in number, more than 90 percent of black women who entered college completed their degrees.

Black women also aspired to the role of homemaker, but for very different reasons than white women. Although poverty still plagued large numbers of black citizens, the black middle class expanded during the 1950s. Postwar prosperity enabled some African Americans, for the first time, to strive for family life in which the earnings of men were adequate to allow women to stay home with their own children rather than tending to the houses and children of white families. Celebrating that possibility in 1947, *Ebony* magazine proclaimed, "Goodbye Mammy, Hello Mom." World War II "took Negro mothers out of white kitchens, put them in factories and shipyards. When it was all over, they went back to kitchens—but this time their own. . . . And so today in thousands of Negro homes, the Negro mother has come home, come

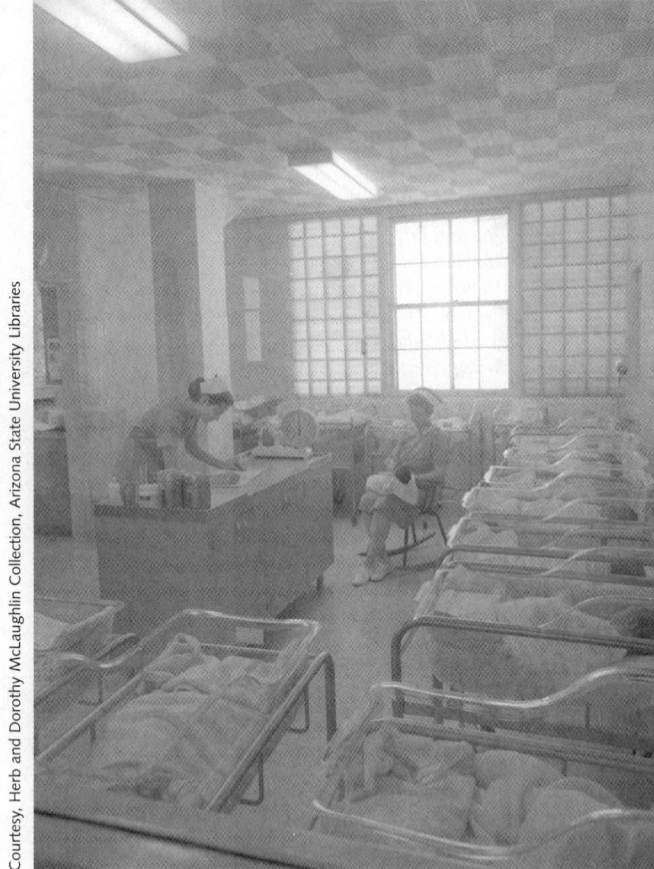

Courtesy, Herb and Dorothy McLaughlin Collection, Arizona State University Libraries

■ Following World War II, hospital nurseries barely had room for all the babies. After a century and a half of steady decline, the birthrate rose dramatically in the 1940s and 1950s. Americans from all backgrounds and socioeconomic levels contributed to the surge in births.

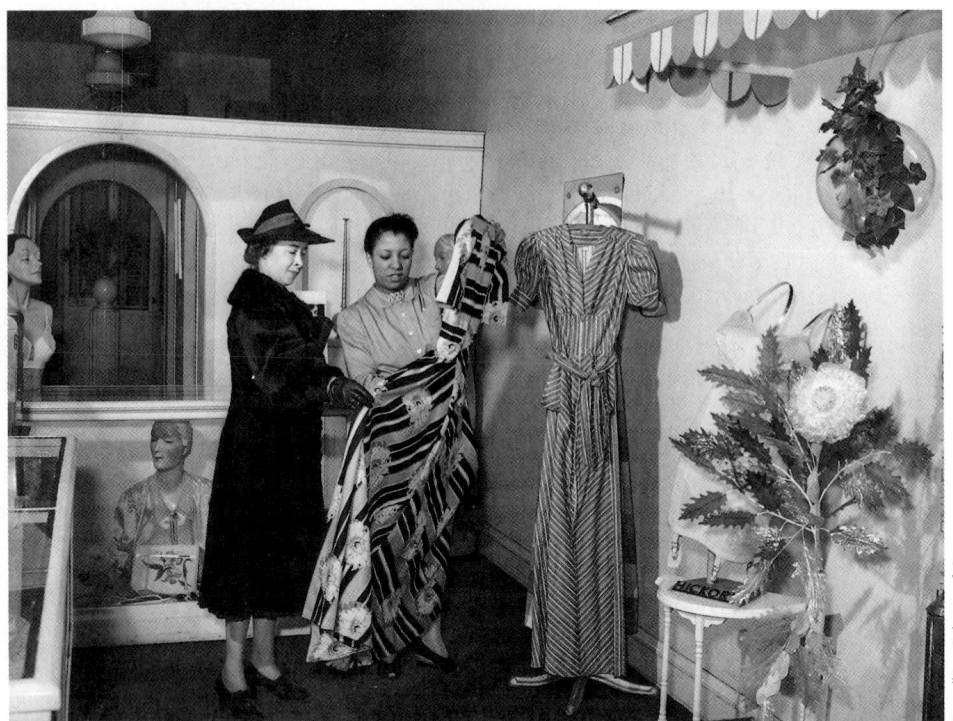

Russell Lee/Library of Congress

■ At a time when many corporations and professions still excluded African Americans, many black entrepreneurs opened their own establishments to serve their own communities. This black-owned dress shop in Chicago catered to middle-class African American women.

home perhaps for the first time since 1619 when the first Negro families landed at Jamestown, Virginia." For black women, domesticity meant "freedom and independence in her own home." It is no wonder that in the early 1960s, women of color bristled when white feminists such as Betty Friedan called upon women to break free from the "chains" of domesticity.

The Civil Rights Movement

As the civil rights movement gained momentum in the South, African American activists faced fierce opposition from local white authorities and contempt from national leaders. Persistent racial discrimination proved to be the nation's worst embarrassment throughout the Cold War. Black leaders and federal officials understood that the national government needed to promote civil rights at home to save face abroad. The Soviet Union and other communist countries pointed to American race relations as an indication of the hypocrisy and failure of the American promise of freedom for all. Yet national leaders paid only lip service to racial justice and failed to provide the strong support necessary to defeat the system of racial segregation in the South known as the "Jim Crow" system. Jim Crow was a legal, or *de jure,* set of institutions that prevailed throughout the South. Although the nation's leaders acknowledged the need to address Southern segregation, they did nothing to address the unofficial, or *de facto,* segregation that prevailed throughout the rest of the country. Nevertheless, at the grassroots level racial minorities continued to work for equal rights. For example, Mexican Americans in the Southwest continued to press for desegregation of schools, residential neighborhoods, and public facilities through organizations such as the League of United Latin American Citizens (LULAC) and the Asociación Nacional México-Americana (ANMA), a civil rights organization that emerged out of the labor movement. It was not until 1963 that the power of the civil rights movement—and the violence of southern white opposition—finally compelled the federal government to take action.

Brown v. Board of Education

The first major success in the struggle to dismantle the Jim Crow system in the South came in the 1954 Supreme Court decision *Brown v. Board of Education*. Civil rights strategists decided to pursue their cause in the courts rather than through Congress. They knew that Southern Democrats in Congress, who held disproportionate power through their seniority and control of major committees, would block any civil rights legislation that came before the House or Senate. They believed that they had a better chance of success through the courts.

Initially, civil rights attorneys worked within the system of segregation. The *Plessy v. Ferguson* decision in 1896 justified Jim Crow laws on the principle of providing "separate but equal" facilities. The attorneys argued that southern school systems violated the segregation laws because the separate, racially segregated schools were far from equal. In Clarendon County, South Carolina, for example, public funds provided $179 per white child compared to $43 per black child. Soon the lawyers shifted their strategy to claim that separate was inherently unequal and began the push to overturn *Plessy v. Ferguson*. Leading the charge was Thurgood Marshall, general counsel of the NAACP and a graduate of Howard University Law School.

The NAACP lawyers filed suit against the Topeka, Kansas, Board of Education, on behalf of Linda Brown, a black child in a segregated school. The case reached the U.S. Supreme Court, where Marshall argued that separate facilities, by definition, denied African Americans their equal rights as citizens. A key argument in the case was the psychological effect of the stigma of segregation on black children. Psychologist Kenneth Clark, testifying as an expert witness, gave evidence showing that black children educated in segregated schools developed a negative self-image and responded more positively to white dolls than to black dolls. Although this argument was persuasive with the Court and helped to bring about school desegregation, some black leaders at the time objected to the use of that psychological argument. Those critics of the strategy argued that black children did not need to interact with white children in order to gain self-esteem and pointed to the positive influence of black teachers who believed in their students' capabilities. They claimed that low self-esteem among black children resulted from widespread discrimination against black Americans, not simply black students' lack of interaction with white students.

In 1953, during the three years that the Supreme Court had the *Brown* case before it, President Eisenhower appointed Earl Warren as chief justice. Warren had been state attorney general and then governor of California during World War II and had approved the internment of Japanese Americans—a decision he later deeply regretted. He now used his political and legal skills to strike a blow for justice. He knew that such a critical case needed a unanimous decision to win broad political support. One by one, he persuaded his Supreme Court colleagues of the importance of striking down segregation. On May 17, 1954, Warren delivered the historic unanimous ruling: "To separate [black children] from others of similar age and

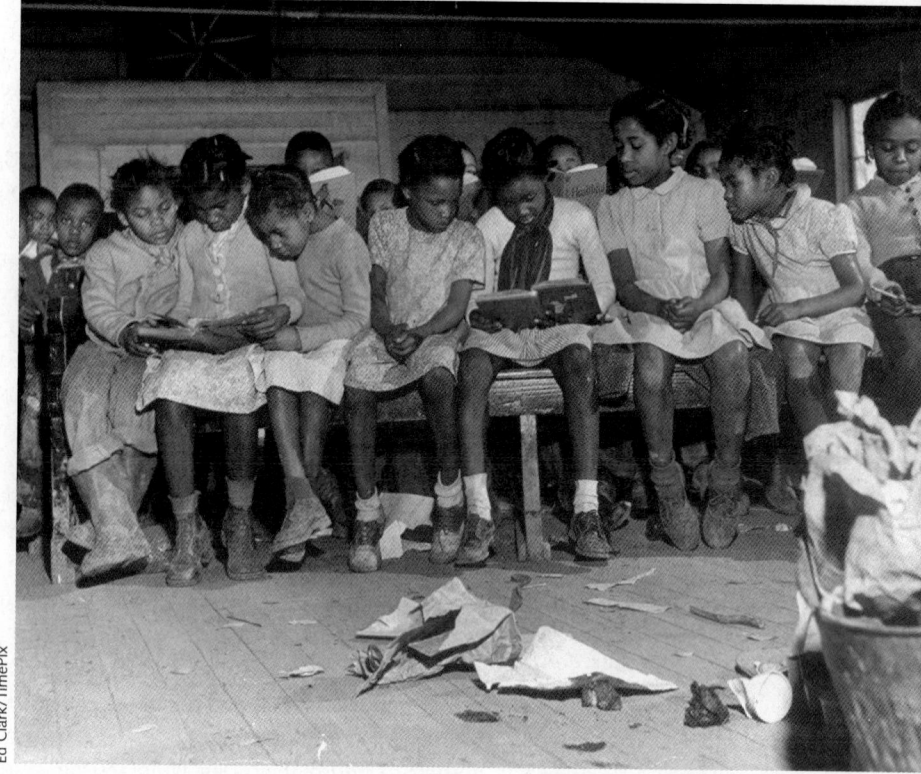

Ed Clark/TimePix

■ Children in segregated schools studied in wretched physical conditions but benefited from dedicated African American teachers. The Supreme Court struck down school segregation in the landmark 1954 case *Brown v. Board of Education,* arguing in its unanimous decision that separate facilities were inherently unequal.

qualifications solely because of their race generates a feeling of inferiority as to their status in the community that may affect their hearts and minds in a way unlikely ever to be undone. . . . We conclude that in the field of public education the doctrine of 'separate but equal' has no place. Separate educational facilities are inherently unequal. . . . Any language in *Plessy v. Ferguson* contrary to these findings is rejected."

White Resistance, Black Persistence

Winning the *Brown* case was a great triumph, but it was only the first step. Desegregation would be meaningful only when it was enforced, and that was another matter entirely. At first, there seemed to be some cause for optimism. Although a few white officials in the South protested vehemently, many others seemed resigned to accept the decision. However, none was willing to take action to implement desegregation. Even the Supreme Court delayed its decision on implementation for a full year and then simply called for the process to begin "with all deliberate speed" but specified no timetable. Political leaders did not come forward to work on the task, leaving sympathetic educators and eager black Americans with no support.

The leader who could have done the most but in fact did the least was President Eisenhower. Instead of calling for immediate desegregation, he made it clear that he strongly disagreed with the Court's decision. Expressing neither "approbation nor disapproval," Eisenhower said, "I don't think you can change the hearts of men with laws or decisions." Just before the Court's ruling, he told Chief Justice Warren that southern white segregationists simply wanted to make sure "that their sweet little girls are not required to sit in schools alongside some big overgrown Negroes." After the decision went against his wishes, Eisenhower remarked that his decision to appoint Warren to the court was the "biggest damn fool mistake" he ever made, claiming that "the Supreme Court decisions set back progress in the South at least fifteen years. . . . The fellow who tries to tell me that you can do these things by force is just plain nuts."

In 1955, the year after the *Brown* decision, several white Mississippians murdered 14-year-old Emmett Till for allegedly whistling at a white woman. The boy had come from Chicago to Mississippi, where he was visiting relatives. His mutilated body was found in the Tallahatchie River. Although Till's killers confessed to the murder, an all-white jury found them not guilty. Eisenhower remained silent about Till's murder and the travesty of justice, even when E. Frederick Morrow, his one black adviser, beseeched him to condemn the lynching.

Eisenhower's hands-off policy emboldened southern segregationists to resist the Supreme Court's desegregation decision. When it became clear that the federal government would do nothing to enforce the ruling, white resistance spread across the South. State legislatures passed resolutions vowing to protect segregation, and most southern congressmen signed the "Southern Manifesto" promising to oppose federal desegregation efforts. To avoid suits by the NAACP, southern states transferred authority over schools to local school boards that assigned students to schools according to concern for the "general welfare," thereby maintaining segregation without specifying race as a criterion.

A crisis at Central High School in Little Rock, Arkansas, finally forced Eisenhower to act. Under a federal district court's order to desegregate, school officials were prepared to comply and had carefully mobilized community support. But Arkansas Governor Orville Faubus, facing reelection, decided to play the race card. Using Central High's integration plan as his target, he created a crisis by instructing National Guard troops to maintain "order" by blocking the entry of black students into the school.

Eisenhower initially refused to intervene in the crisis. Hoping for a compromise, he met with Faubus, who agreed to allow the school to integrate peacefully. But Faubus broke his word, withdrew the National Guard troops, and left Little Rock, leaving the black students unprotected. On September 23, 1957, as nine black students attempted to enter Central High, a huge angry crowd of whites surrounded them. With international news cameras broadcasting pictures of the shrieking and menacing mob, Eisenhower took action to stop the embarrassing fracas. Furious at Faubus for his insubordination, Eisenhower denounced the "disgraceful occurrence," federalized the Arkansas National Guard, and sent 1000 paratroopers to Little Rock. Unwilling to "acquiesce in anarchy and the disillusion of the union," Eisenhower acted to maintain federal authority rather than to support integration. Although the Little Rock Nine, as the courageous students came to be called, finally gained entry to Central High, Governor Faubus closed the schools in Little Rock for the entire next year. Out of 712 school districts that had desegregated after the *Brown* decision, only 49 remained desegregated by the end of Eisenhower's term. Most of the others reverted to segregation.

Boycotts and Sit-Ins

Under Jim Crow laws in the South, black passengers were required to sit in the back section of buses, leaving the front of the bus for whites. If the "white" section at the front of the bus filled up, black passengers were required to give up their seats for white passengers. On December 1, 1955, Rosa Parks and the black community of Montgomery, Alabama, were ready to take on the system. Parks, who worked as a seamstress, was a widely respected leader in Montgomery's black community, active in her church, and secretary of the local NAACP. On her way home from work that day, sitting in the first row of the "colored" section of the bus when the front of the bus filled with passengers, she refused to move when a white man demanded her seat. Parks was arrested, and black Montgomery sprang into action.

> *Eisenhower acted to maintain federal authority rather than to support integration.*

Literally overnight, the Montgomery bus boycott was born. E. D. Dixon, president of the Alabama NAACP and the head of the local chapter of the Brotherhood of Sleeping Car Porters, and Jo Ann Robinson, the leader of the local Women's Political Council (a black alternative to the segregated League of Women Voters), mobilized the boycott. They gathered with 50 community representatives that night at the Dexter Avenue Baptist Church to plan strategy. They mobilized other black churches to spread the word to their congregations on Sunday, and black-owned taxi companies geared up to take the place of buses. By Monday, all of black Montgomery had heard the news of the boycott. The buses that day were empty of black riders. For 381 days, more than 90 percent of Montgomery's black citizens sacrificed their comfort and convenience for the sake of their rights and dignity. As one elderly black woman replied when a white reporter offered her a ride as she walked to work, "No, my feets is tired but my soul is rested."

Martin Luther King, Jr., pastor of the Dexter Avenue Baptist Church, was a newcomer to Montgomery when the bus boycott began. He embraced the opportunity to become the leader of the boycott and, eventually, the most powerful spokesperson for the civil rights movement. His stirring and impassioned words inspired thousands of black citizens to join the cause. As he told the 5000 listeners who gathered in his church on the first night of the boycott, "If you will protest courageously and yet with dignity and Christian love, in the history books that are written in future generations, historians will have to pause and say, 'there lived a great people—a black people—who injected a new meaning and dignity into the veins of civilization.' This is our challenge and our overwhelming responsibility."

The bus boycott ended a year later when the Supreme Court ruled that Montgomery's buses must integrate, but the momentum generated by the boycott galvanized the civil rights movement. King and other leaders formed the Southern Christian Leadership Conference (SCLC), which united black ministers across the South in the cause of civil rights. The boycott tactic spread to other southern cities. As boycotts continued, a new strategy emerged: the sit-in.

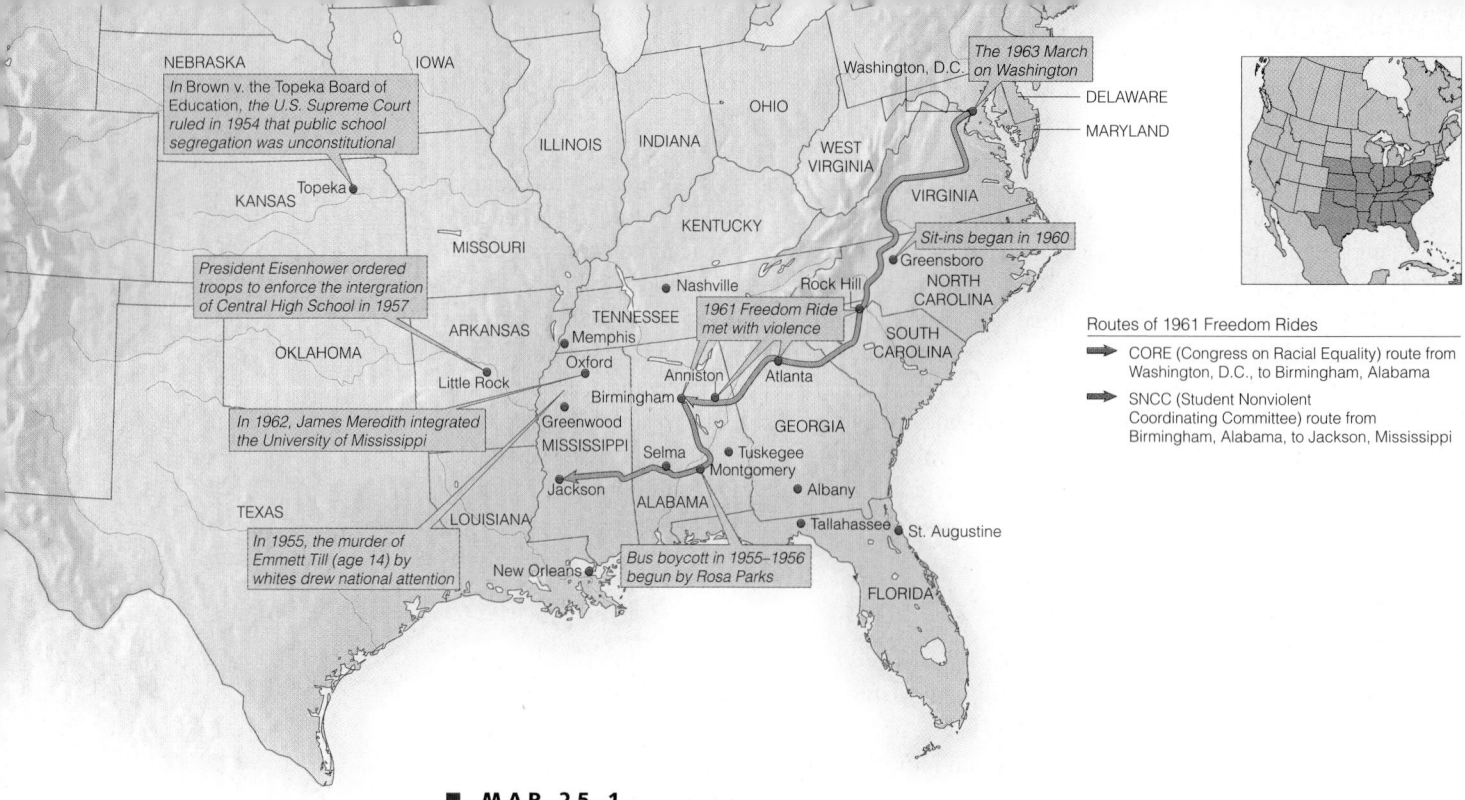

■ MAP 25.1

MAJOR EVENTS OF THE AFRICAN AMERICAN CIVIL RIGHTS MOVEMENT, 1953–1963 Most of the major events of the early stages of the black freedom struggle took place in the South. Black southerners formed the backbone of the movement, but the grass roots protest movement drew participants from all regions of the country, all racial and ethnic groups, cities and rural areas, churches and universities, old and young, lawyers and sharecroppers.

On February 1, 1960, four African American students at North Carolina Agricultural and Technical College in Greensboro, inspired by the example of the bus boycott, entered the local Woolworth store and sat down at the lunch counter. When they were told, "We do not serve Negroes," they refused to leave, forcing the staff at Woolworth's to physically remove the nonviolent protesters. Undaunted, they returned to the lunch counter the next day with 23 classmates. By the end of the week more than a thousand students joined the protest. By this time, white gangs had gathered, waving Confederate flags and menacing the black undergraduates. But the students responded by waving American flags. An expression of their patriotism as well as their political shrewdness, the flag identified the protesters not as subversives acting against social order but as citizens claiming the values and identity of the nation. Black football players kept the angry whites at bay. Taunted with shouts of "Who do you think you are?" they replied, "We are the union army."

In May 1961 members of the Congress of Racial Equality (CORE) organized the Freedom Rides, in which black and white civil rights workers attempted to ride two interstate buses from Washington, D.C., to New Orleans in an effort to challenge segregation at facilities used in interstate travel. Their journey began peacefully, but when they reached Rock Hill, South Carolina, a group of whites beat John Lewis, one of the young black riders, for entering a whites-only rest room. In Anniston, Alabama, a mob slashed the tires of one of the buses, threw a fire bomb through a window, and pummeled the riders with fists and pipes. After the brutal beatings, reinforcements from the Student Non-violent Coordinating Committee (SNCC) arrived to continue the Freedom Rides. They persevered, facing beatings along the way until they reached Jackson, Mississippi, where they were immediately arrested and jailed. By August, 300 additional protesters had been locked in the jail, all refusing bail. The spirit and strength of the civil rights workers inspired many others to join them in the movement. They came from all over the South as well as the North, white as well as black, giving up comfort and safety, risking—and sacrificing—their lives.

The Eisenhower Years

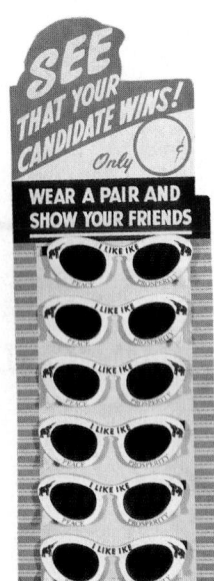

Dwight D. Eisenhower, elected president in 1952, squandered his opportunity to provide strong support for the civil rights movement. A respected and widely admired World War II general, Eisenhower could have used his leadership to bolster the cause, but he did just the opposite. Eisenhower's failure to use his presidential power allowed southern segregationists to block implementation of the *Brown* decision and opened the way for violent resistance to the civil rights movement. His presidency was notable largely for moderation and maintaining the status quo, with very few major new initiatives and a style of leadership that rested more on his personal stature than his actions. Ike, as he was known, presided over the nation during a time of great prosperity, and his policies encouraged business expansion. However, the former general did try to stem the defense buildup. In his farewell address at the end of his second term as president, Eisenhower warned the nation against the growing power of the "military–industrial complex," the term he coined to describe the armed forces and the politically powerful defense industries that supplied arms and equipment to them.

The Middle of the Road

Born in Texas, raised in Kansas, and educated at the U.S. Military Academy at West Point, Eisenhower became a career soldier who served as the supreme commander of the Allied forces in western Europe during World War II. Eisenhower planned and carried out the daring Allied invasion at Normandy on D-Day. As early as 1948, both the Democrats and the Republicans courted Eisenhower as a presidential candidate. But he resisted, believing that military leaders should not get involved in politics; indeed, he had never even registered to vote. In 1952, however, when he was president of Columbia University, he changed his mind and accepted the Republican nomination, choosing California Senator Richard M. Nixon—known as a dogged anticommunist crusader—as his running mate. The Democrats nominated Illinois Governor Adlai E. Stevenson. The cerebral Stevenson, dubbed an "egghead" by the press, was no match for the former general whose supporters donned campaign buttons boasting "I Like Ike." The popular Eisenhower won the election with the largest landslide up to that time and was reelected by an even wider margin in 1956.

As president, Eisenhower pursued a path down the middle of the road. His probusiness legislative agenda and appointments pleased conservatives, and he placated liberals by extending many of the policies of the welfare state enacted during the New Deal. He agreed to the expansion of Social Security and unemployment compensation and an increase in the minimum wage. He also made concerted efforts to reduce defense spending, believing that continued massive military expenditures would hinder the nation's economic growth. In December 1953, with Admiral Arthur Radford, chair of the Joint Chiefs of Staff, Eisenhower announced the New Look, a streamlined military that relied less on expensive conventional ground forces and more on air power and advanced nuclear capabilities.

TABLE 25-1			
The Election of 1952			
Candidate	Political Party	Popular Vote	Electoral Vote
Dwight D. Eisenhower	Republican	33,936,252	442
Adlai E. Stevenson	Democratic	27,314,992	89

TABLE 25-2			
The Election of 1956			
Candidate	Political Party	Popular Vote	Electoral Vote
Dwight D. Eisenhower	Republican	35,575,420	457
Adlai E. Stevenson	Democratic	26,033,066	73

Eisenhower's plans to reduce defense spending derailed on October 4, 1957, when the Soviet Union launched Sputnik, the first artificial Earth satellite. Although Sputnik could not be seen with the naked eye—it was only 22 inches in diameter and weighed only 184 pounds—it emitted a beeping noise that was broadcast by commercial radio stations in the United States, making its presence very real and causing near hysteria among the public. The Soviet's launching of Sputnik II a month later seemed to confirm widespread fears that the United States was behind in the space race and, more significantly, in the arms race. Eisenhower's popularity in the polls suddenly dropped 22 points.

Acquiescing to his critics, the president allotted increased funds for military, scientific, and educational spending. The National Aeronautics and Space Administration (NASA), which developed the program of space exploration, was one result of this increase. But Eisenhower believed that "the most critical problem of all" was the lack of American scientists and engineers. He proposed that the federal government subsidize additional science and math training for both teachers and students. He also called for an improvement in overall education so that the next generation would be "equipped to live in the age of intercontinental ballistic missiles." On September 2, 1958, Eisenhower signed Public Law 85-864, also known as the National Defense Education Act (NDEA), which authorized more than $1 billion in education spending.

"What's Good for General Motors . . ."

Eisenhower's Secretary of Defense, former head of General Motors Charles Wilson, made the memorable comment that "what's good for General Motors business is good for America." But not everyone agreed. Eisenhower's probusiness policies had a devastating impact on the nation's environment. He promoted the passage of the Submerged Land Act, which removed from federal jurisdiction more than $40 billion worth of oil-rich offshore lands. Under the control of state governments, oil companies could—and did—gain access to them. The *New York Times* called the act "one of the greatest and surely the most unjustified give-away program" in the nation's history. The administration's willingness to allow businesses to expand with little regulation, and with virtually no concern for the environment, contributed to increasing pollution of the air, water, and land during the 1950s and sparked the environmental movement of the 1960s and 1970s.

Eisenhower also supported the Interstate Highway Act of 1956, inspired in part by Cold War concerns. An interstate highway system could allow the swift movement of military supplies and, presumably, the evacuation of urban centers in the event of a nuclear attack. The Highway Act had its greatest impact on business and transportation, however. As the largest public works project the nation had ever mounted, this centrally planned transportation system was a boon to the auto, trucking, oil, concrete, and tire industries. In addition, it contributed to the national pastime of family road vacations and tourism. Cheap gas also fueled America's car culture. Cars gave Americans increased mobility, and enabled suburban dwellers to drive to work in the cities. But reliance on the automobile doomed the nation's passenger train system and led to the decline of public transportation. Cars also contributed to suburban sprawl, air pollution, and traffic jams.

Eisenhower's Foreign Policy

The New Look, while containing military spending, also shifted American military priorities from reliance on conventional weapons to nuclear deterrence and covert operations. During Eisenhower's presidency, the United States and the Soviet Union both solidified their separate alliances. The North Atlantic Treaty Organization (NATO), formed in 1949, increased American influence in Western Europe. The 12 NATO nations agreed that an attack on any one of them would be considered an attack on all, and they maintained a force to defend the West against a possible Soviet invasion. NATO expanded in 1952 to include Greece and Turkey, and West Germany joined in 1955. The Soviet Union formed a similar alliance, the Warsaw Pact, with the countries of Eastern Europe. Confrontations between the United States and the Soviet Union over the fate of Europe gave way to more subtle maneuvers regarding the Third World—a term originally referring to unaligned nations in the Middle East, Africa, Asia, and Latin America.

When Joseph Stalin died in 1953, Nikita Khrushchev became the new leader of the Soviet Union and called for peaceful coexistence with the United States. To limit military expenditures and improve relations, the superpowers arranged high-level summit meetings. In 1955 delegates from the United States, the Soviet Union, Britain, and France met in Geneva. Although the meeting achieved little of substance, it set a tone of cooperation. In 1959 Khrushchev came to the United States, met with Eisenhower, and toured the country. But a planned Paris summit in May 1960 was canceled when the Soviets shot down an American U-2 spy plane. U.S. officials initially denied that the plane was on a spy mission until the captured American pilot, Gary Powers, confessed. Powers served two years of a ten-year sentence in a Soviet prison before his release in exchange for a suspected Soviet spy incarcerated in the United States. Despite the U-2 incident, the superpowers began to discuss arms limitation. Both countries agreed to limit aboveground testing of nuclear weapons in light of the health and environmental risks such tests posed.

Anticommunism became the guiding principle behind nearly all U.S. foreign policy, taking precedence over other American ideals.

As the United States and the Soviet Union worked toward greater cooperation, they faced challenges from within their separate "spheres of influence" and vied for the loyalty of newly independent states in the Third World. In 1956 the Soviet Union faced armed uprisings in Poland and Hungary, two "satellite" nations chafing under Soviet domination. In Poland, rebels resisting Moscow's control took to the streets, demanding that the Soviet Union recognize Wladyslaw Gomulka, who had been an opponent of Stalin, as the leader of Poland. After three days of fighting, the Soviet Union capitulated to the rebels' demand. In Hungary, maverick communist Imre Nagy took power and pledged to create a multiparty democracy. As revolution spread across Hungary, Soviet troops brutally crushed the rebellion, killing Nagy and thousands of other Hungarians.

While the United States and the Soviet Union competed with each other to gain influence in Third World countries, leaders from those countries came together to discuss ways to achieve self-determination. In April 1955 in Bandung, Indonesia, representatives from 29 nations—primarily from Asia, Africa, and the Middle East—met in what President Sukarno of Indonesia called "the first international conference of colored peoples in the history of mankind." Nearly all the participants came from countries that had previously been colonized by western European countries. Most were former colonies of Britain, France, Belgium, Holland, or Portugal. Although they shared no specific political ideology, the conference carried an implicit condemnation of western powers and a commitment to eliminating the vestiges of colonialism and racial discrimination worldwide. Suspicious of the motives of the participants and worried about the outcome, Eisenhower sent no greeting to the gathering and tried to ignore or sabotage it. However, Adam Clayton Powell, one of three black members of the U.S. Congress, attended the conference as a "journalist," providing an unofficial U.S. presence.

The Eisenhower administration continued to distrust countries that maintained neutrality in the Cold War, fearing that those not aligned with the United States might turn to communism and become allies of the Soviet Union. In 1956 Secretary of State John Foster Dulles declared that neutrality "is an immoral and shortsighted conception." Anticommunism became the guiding principle behind nearly all U.S. foreign policy, taking precedence over other American ideals, such as support for democratically elected governments and national self-determination. Acting on its anticommunist priority, the United States helped overthrow democratically elected leaders and prop up corrupt and often brutal dictatorships.

The Central Intelligence Agency (CIA) was a major player in this drama, with 15,000 agents working around the world by the end of the 1950s. Congress established the CIA in 1947 to gather strategic intelligence from foreign countries and to engage in covert political activity. Through covert operations, the CIA helped to overthrow the elected government in Iran and to restore the dictatorship of Shah Reza Pahlavi, whose unpopular western-leaning regime was finally overthrown by Muslim fundamentalists in 1979. In 1954 the CIA, working closely

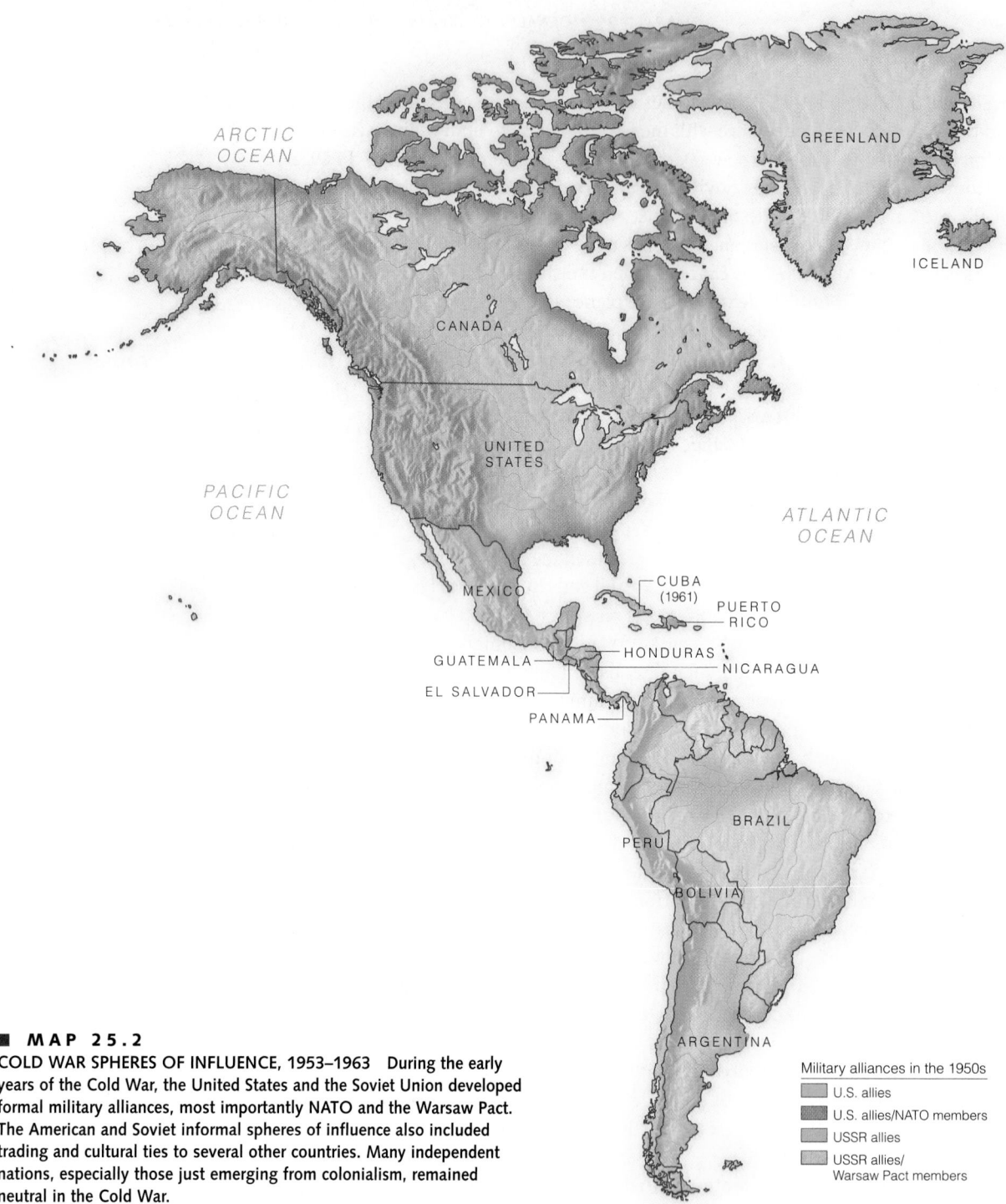

■ MAP 25.2
COLD WAR SPHERES OF INFLUENCE, 1953–1963 During the early years of the Cold War, the United States and the Soviet Union developed formal military alliances, most importantly NATO and the Warsaw Pact. The American and Soviet informal spheres of influence also included trading and cultural ties to several other countries. Many independent nations, especially those just emerging from colonialism, remained neutral in the Cold War.

Military alliances in the 1950s

- U.S. allies
- U.S. allies/NATO members
- USSR allies
- USSR allies/ Warsaw Pact members

with the United Fruit Company, helped overthrow the elected government of Jacobo Arbenz in Guatemala. U.S. and company officials considered Arbenz a communist because he sought to nationalize and redistribute large tracts of land, including some owned by United Fruit. Eisenhower also supported unpopular anticommunist dictators in Peru and Venezuela. In 1958 Latin Americans expressed their displeasure when Vice President Richard M. Nixon, on a good-will tour of South America, faced angry protesters wherever he went. Nixon was nearly killed in Caracas, Venezuela, when demonstrators attacked his motorcade.

In 1959 revolutionary leader Fidel Castro overthrew Cuba's U.S.-friendly dictator Fulgencio Batista. Castro established a regime in Cuba based on principles of socialism. His government took control of foreign-owned companies, including many owned by Americans. Castro's socialist policies alarmed U.S. officials and investors in Cuba. Eisenhower's hostility encouraged Cas-

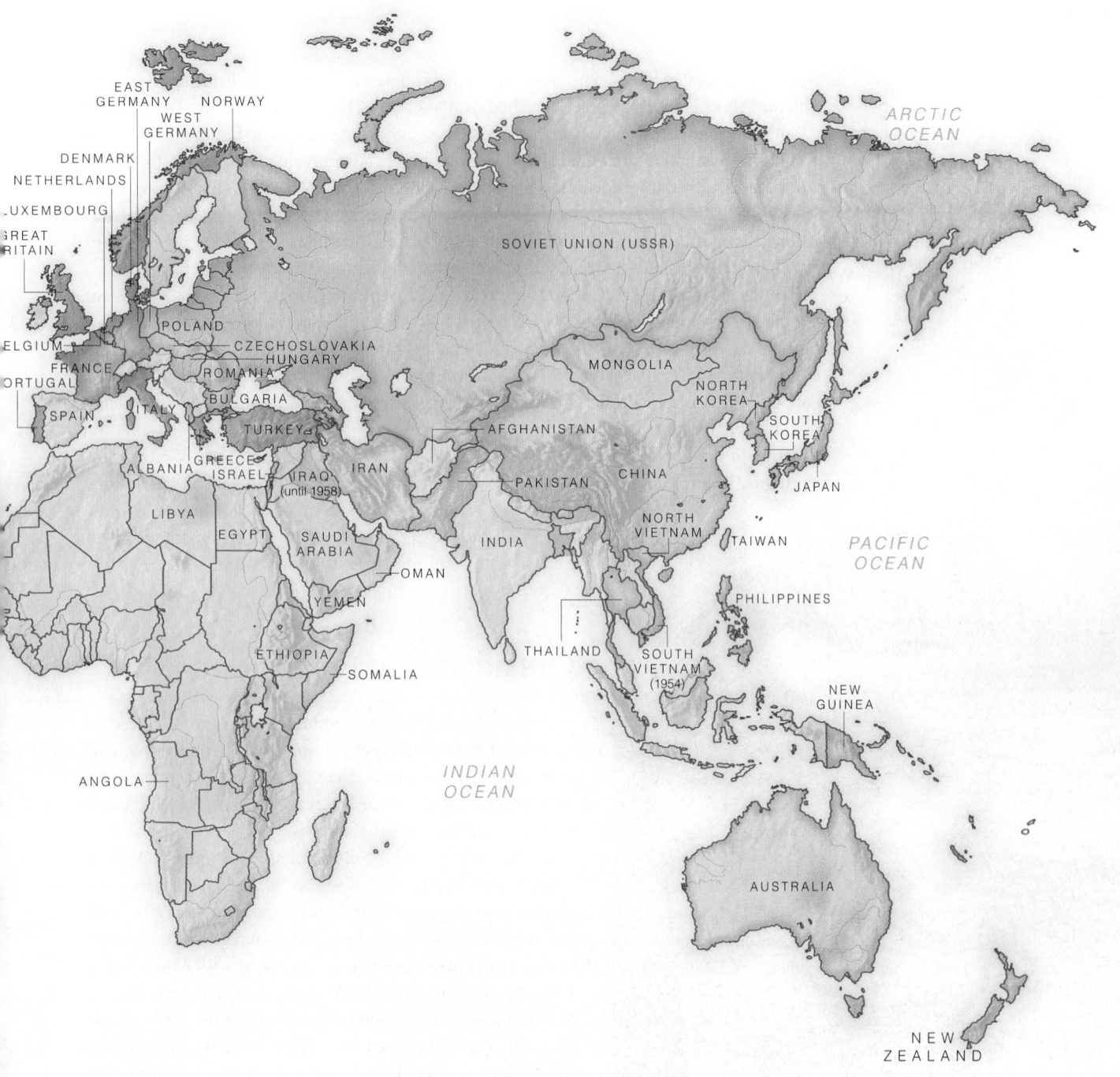

tro to forge an alliance with the Soviet Union. The CIA then launched a plot to overthrow Castro, which would culminate in an ill-fated invasion in 1961. In 1960–1961, the CIA also helped orchestrate the overthrow and assassination of the charismatic left-leaning Patrice Lumumba, the first minister of the Republic of the Congo, soon after its independence from Belgium.

U.S. policymakers, with their anticommunist preoccupations, and people in Third World countries, with their campaigns against colonialism and racism, had little interest in each other's priorities. A case in point was Egypt, where in 1952 Gamal Abdul Nasser overthrew the corrupt monarchy of King Farouk and established a government based on neutrality. In 1954 Nasser declared himself prime minister of the new government and accepted aid from both the United States and the Soviet Union. When Nasser engaged in trade with Soviet-bloc countries and extended diplomatic recognition to communist China, the United States canceled loans that were to support the building of the huge Aswan Dam, a major development project for the Egyptian economy. In response, Nasser nationalized the British-controlled Suez Canal in 1956, arguing that canal tolls would provide alternative funding for the dam. The British government, with the help of France and Israel, launched an attack against Egypt to regain control of the canal.

Although he distrusted Nasser, Eisenhower strongly criticized Britain for its effort to retain its imperial position in the Middle East. To avoid further antagonizing Nasser and other Third World leaders, Eisenhower denounced Britain's Suez attack and threatened economic sanctions, forcing the British to back down. Although leaders in Africa and Asia applauded Eisenhower's actions, the episode weakened U.S. relations with Nasser, who forged ties with the Soviet Union. Eisenhower now feared that "Nasserism" might spread throughout the Middle East.

In the spring of 1957, Congress approved the Eisenhower Doctrine, a pledge to defend Middle Eastern countries "against overt armed aggression from any nation controlled by international communism." However, U.S. policymakers rarely distinguished between nationalist movements and designs by "international communism," which they defined as Soviet aggression. Because American leaders believed that struggles for national self-determination in Third World countries were inspired and supported by the Soviet Union, they used the Eisenhower Doctrine to provide justification for U.S. military intervention to support pro-Western governments. When leaders in Lebanon and Jordan appeared friendly to Nasser, Eisenhower stepped in, sending 14,000 U.S. marines to Lebanon and setting up an anti-Nasser government there. Britain intervened in Jordan, restoring King Hussein to the throne.

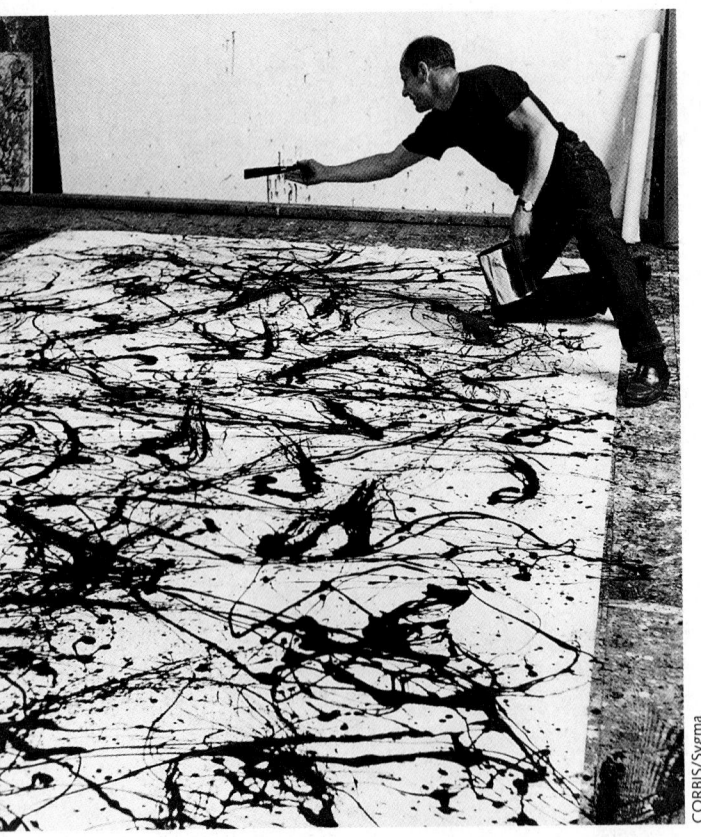

CORBIS/Sygma

■ Jackson Pollock shocked the art world when he began dripping paint on large canvasses. Abstract expressionist painters like Pollock celebrated their break from conventional forms and representations. National leaders embraced abstract expressionism as symbolic of American artistic freedom, and thousands of Americans hung reproductions of abstract art on the walls of their suburban homes.

Outsiders and Opposition

The 1950s often are remembered as a time of political and cultural complacency among white Americans, with most of the opposition to the nation's institutions emanating from people of color. There is a good deal of truth to this picture. But it obscures the many ways in which white Americans also resisted and rebelled against the status quo. Some young whites, in the South as well as North, joined in the struggle for civil rights; their numbers increased in the 1960s. Others were drawn to the music and dance of black America, especially the fusion of rhythm-and-blues with country-and-western, which took the form of early rock 'n' roll. Distinct forms of protest also emerged from within the white middle class: the rebellion of the Beats who rejected staid conformity, the stirrings of discontent among women, and the antinuclear and environmental movements. The arts also reflected a rejection of mainstream values, as Jackson Pollock and other abstract expressionist painters challenged the artistic conventions of the time and shifted the center of the art world from Paris to New York. Even the sexual revolution of the 1960s had its roots in the widespread defiance of the rigid sexual codes of the 1950s. In many ways, the placid surface of white America hid the smoldering cauldron underneath that would erupt in the years ahead.

Youth, Sex, and Rock 'n' Roll

One clue that all was not tranquil was the widespread panic that the nation's young were out of control. Adult authorities worried about an epidemic of juvenile delinquency, blaming everything from parents to comic books. New celebrities such as Marlon Brando and James

Dean portrayed misunderstood youth in rebellion against a corrupt and uncaring adult world. In the classic youth movie *Rebel Without a Cause*, Dean played a good-hearted but angry young man who suffers from a domineering mother and a wimpish apron-clad father who refuses to stand up to her. When asked, "What are you rebelling against, Johnny?" Brando's tough-guy character in *The Wild One* answers, "I dunno; what've you got?" In these films, and in J. D. Salinger's now-classic novel *Catcher in the Rye*, young women and men strain against the authority and expectations of their parents and the adult world, dreaming of freedom and personal fulfillment.

Sexual mores were rigid in the 1950s—and were widely violated. Single young women who became pregnant faced disgrace and ostracism unless they married quickly, which many did. Abortion, which had been illegal since the late nineteenth century but tacitly accepted until after World War II, became increasingly difficult to obtain, with hospitals placing new restrictions on legal therapeutic abortions. Illegal abortionists who had long practiced without interference faced increasing harassment, forcing the practice underground, where it became much more dangerous. A double standard encouraged men to pursue sexual conquest as a mark of manhood and virility but tarnished the reputation of women who engaged in sexual intercourse prior to marriage.

In many ways, the youth of the 1950s were already undermining the constraints that toppled in the next decade. Nowhere is this development more obvious than in the explosion of rock 'n' roll, with its roots in African American rhythm-and-blues, its raw sexuality, and its jubilant rebelliousness. Chuck Berry's hit "School Days" expressed youthful restlessness, and Little Richard's "Long Tall Sally" and "Rip It Up" exulted in sensual pleasure. Bill Haley and his Comets invited youngsters to "Rock Around the Clock."

Rock 'n' roll emerged out of the fusion of musical traditions. Artists from many ethnic backgrounds experimented with a variety of forms. Jewish songwriters Jerry Leiber and Mike Stoller wrote songs such as "Hound Dog" for black artists such as Willie Mae Thornton that were later recorded by white Southerner Elvis Presley. The first Mexican American rock 'n' roll star, Ritchie Valens, sang such romantic ballads as "Donna" along with jazzed-up versions of Mexican folk songs such as "La Bamba." Rosie and the Originals—an all-girl band led by Mexican American Rosie Mendez—sang rock 'n' roll hits such as "Angel Baby."

Performances as well as lyrics carried erotic power. Chuck Berry pumped his electric guitar and shimmied across stages, Little Richard danced on piano tops and tore off his shirts, and James Brown begged "Please, please, please," while collapsing on the floor. Elvis Presley thrust his hips in his trademark style, sending young audiences into a frenzy. Criticism of his sexually charged gyrations persuaded producers to show him only above the waist during his appearance on Ed Sullivan's TV show. Rock 'n' roll music and dancing added powerful elements of sexuality and rebellion to the youth culture of the 1950s. Many of those impulses found political expression in the 1960s.

Rebellious Men

Men, too, were in revolt. According to widely read sociological tracts of the time, such as William Whyte's *The Organization Man*,

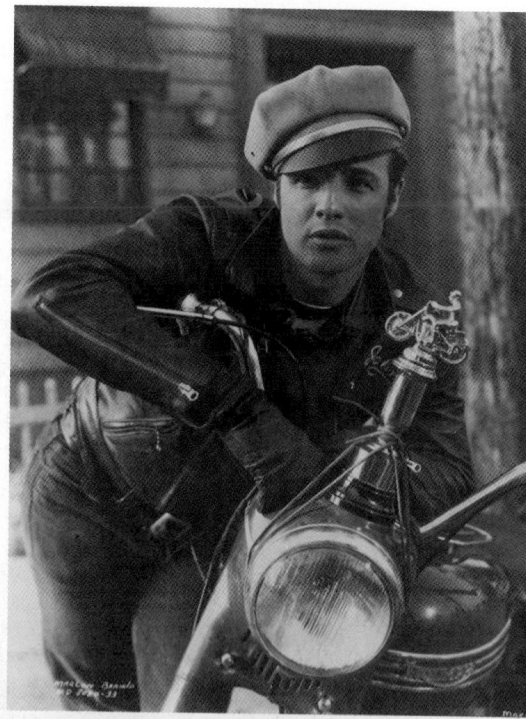

Photofest

■ In *The Wild One* (1954), Marlon Brando portrayed a young man angry at the world. The young actor from Omaha, Nebraska, had already earned acclaim on Broadway. Two decades later he won an Oscar playing the title role in *The Godfather* (1972).

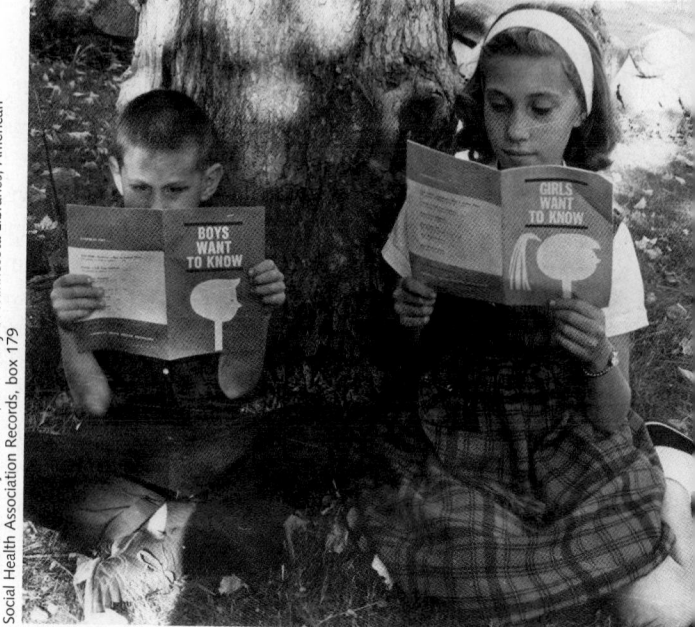

Social Welfare History Archives, University of Minnesota Libraries, American Social Health Association Records, box 179

■ Since sex was rarely discussed in most middle class families, many parents relied on schools to provide elementary sex education, and a generation of suburban children learned the facts of life from nervous teachers and a variety of simplified texts.

C. Wright Mills's *White Collar,* and David Reisman's *The Lonely Crowd,* middle-class men were forced into boring, routinized jobs, groomed to be "outer-directed" at the expense of their inner lives, and saddled with the overwhelming burden of providing for ever-growing families with insatiable consumer desires.

A few highly visible American men provided alternative visions. Hugh Hefner built his Playboy empire by offering men the trappings of the "good life" without its burdensome responsibilities. The Playboy ethic encouraged men to enjoy the sexual pleasures of attractive women without the chains of marriage and to pursue the rewards of consumerism in well-appointed "bachelor flats" rather than appliance-laden homes. *Playboy* magazine celebrated this lifestyle, epitomized in the airbrushed photographs of nearly nude, young, female "bunnies" who seemed to promise sex without commitment.

Beat poets, writers, and artists offered a very different type of escape. In their literary works such as Allen Ginsberg's poem *Howl* and Jack Kerouac's novel *On the Road* and in their highly publicized lives, the Beats celebrated freedom from conformity, eccentric artistic expression, playful obscenity, experimentation with drugs, open homosexuality, and male bonding. While eschewing the sort of luxurious consumerism Hefner extolled, the Beats shared with the Playboy ethic a vision of male rebellion against conformity and responsibility. The mainstream men who indulged in these fantasies were more likely to enjoy them vicariously than to bolt from the breadwinner role. The dads who were honored on the new consumer holiday of Father's Day far outnumbered the freewheeling Beats and bachelors.

Mobilizing for Peace and the Environment

Some women did not wait for the new feminist movement to make their voices heard. Rachel Carson was one such woman. Born in 1907 in Springdale, Pennsylvania, she developed a love of books and nature as a child. She went to college and graduate school during the pre–World War II years before domesticity settled like a fog over women's education. Deeply attached to the sea, she wrote several books and articles about the marine world, most notably her 1951 bestseller, *The Sea Around Us.* Carson became increasingly concerned about the impact of manufactured chemicals on the environment, especially the insecticide DDT, which had been poisoning the earth since World War II. Her last book, *Silent Spring,* published in 1962, brought attention to the worldwide problem of pesticide poisoning. Officially endorsed by President John F. Kennedy's Science Advisory Committee and scorned by the agricultural chemical industry, the book helped launch the environmental movement that has flourished ever since.

Women also led the movement to stop the testing and proliferation of nuclear weapons. On November 1, 1961, 50,000 suburban homemakers in more than 60 communities staged a protest, Women Strike for Peace (WSP). Participants lobbied government officials to "End the Arms Race—Not the Human Race." The strikers were mostly educated, middle-class mothers; 61 percent did not work outside the home. WSP leaders were part of a small group of feminists who had worked on behalf of women's rights throughout the 1940s and 1950s. According to *Newsweek* magazine, the strikers "were perfectly ordinary looking women. . . . They looked like the women you would see driving ranch wagons, or shopping at the village market, or attending PTA meetings. . . . Many [were] wheeling baby buggies or strollers." Within a year their numbers grew to several hundred thousand. The FBI kept the group under surveillance, and in 1962 the leaders were called before the House Un-American Activities Committee (HUAC). Under questioning, these women spoke as mothers, claiming that saving American children from nuclear extinction was the essence of Americanism. They brought their babies to the hearings and refused to be intimidated by their

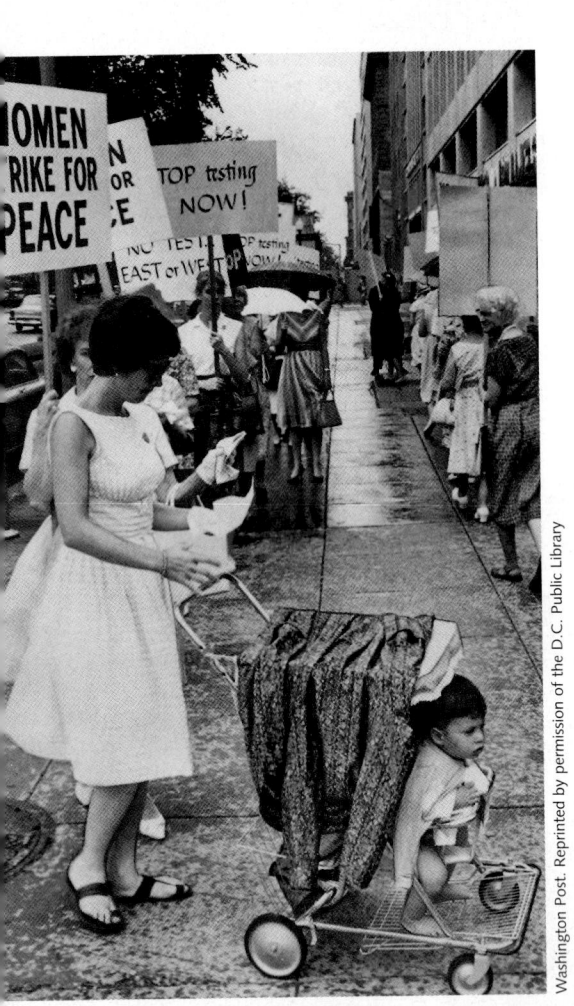

■ On November 1, 1961, 50,000 women in communities across the country took to the streets to protest nuclear testing. Under the sponsorship of Women Strike for Peace, these demonstrators used their authority as mothers, and brought along their children, to highlight their stake in the future.

Washington Post. Reprinted by permission of the D.C. Public Library.

Rachel Carson, *Silent Spring*

In 1962, Silent Spring, Rachel Carson's eloquent exposé of the chemical industry's deadly impact on the health of the planet, landed on the best-seller list, where it stayed for months. The book, which eventually sold 1.5 million copies and remains in print today, galvanized the environmental movement of the 1960s and 1970s. Carson called the chemical industry "a child of the Second World War" and creator of "elixirs of death." She reported that annual pesticide production increased from 124 million pounds in 1947 to 637 million pounds by 1960. Twenty years later it had reached 2.4 billion pounds. "In the course of developing agents of chemical warfare," she noted, "some of the chemicals created in the laboratory were found to be lethal to insects. The discovery did not come by chance: insects were widely used to test chemicals as agents of death for man."

It took hundreds of millions of years to produce the life that now inhabits the earth—eons of time in which that developing and evolving and diversifying life reached a state of adjustment and balance with its surroundings. The environment, rigorously shaping and directing the life it supported, contained elements that were hostile as well as supporting. Certain rocks gave out dangerous radiation; even within the light of the sun, from which all life draws its energy, there were short-wave radiations with power to injure. Given time—time not in years but in millennia—life adjusts, and a balance has been

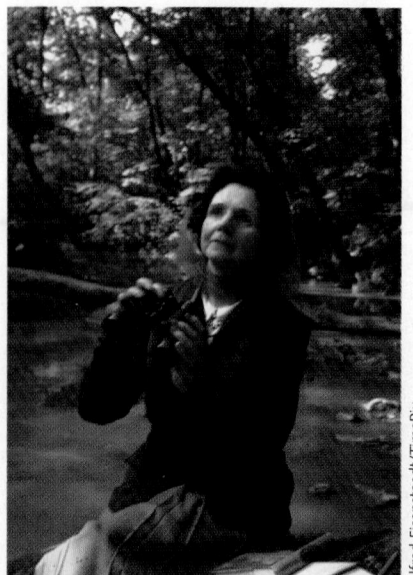

Environmentalist Rachel Carson, author of *Silent Spring.*

Alfred Eisenstaedt/TimePix

reached. For time is the essential ingredient; but in the modern world there is no time.

The rapidity of change and the speed with which new situations are created follow the impetuous and heedless pace of man rather than the deliberate pace of nature. Radiation is no longer merely the background radiation of rocks, the bombardment of cosmic rays, the ultraviolet of the sun that have existed before there was any life on earth; radiation is now the unnatural creation of man's tampering with the atom. The chemicals to which life is asked to make its adjustment are no longer merely the calcium and silica and copper and all the rest of the minerals washed out of the rocks and carried in rivers to the sea; they are the synthetic creations of man's inventive mind, brewed in his labo-

ratories, and having no counterparts in nature.

To adjust to these chemicals would require time on the scale that is nature's; it would require not merely the years of a man's life but the life of generations. And even this, were it by some miracle possible, would be futile, for the new chemicals come from our laboratories in an endless stream; almost five hundred annually find their way into actual use in the United States alone. The figure is staggering and its implications are not easily grasped—500 new chemicals to which the bodies of men and animals are required somehow to adapt each year, chemicals totally outside the limits of biologic experience.

Among them are many that are used in man's war against nature. Since the mid-1940s over 200 basic chemicals have been created for use in killing insects, weeds, rodents, and other organisms described in the modern vernacular as "pests"; and they are sold under several thousand different brand names.

These sprays, dusts, and aerosols are now applied almost universally to farms, gardens, forests, and homes—nonselective chemicals that have the power to kill every insect, the "good" and the "bad," to still the song of the birds and the leaping of fish in the streams, to coat the leaves with a deadly film, and to linger on in the soil—all this though the intended target may be only a few weeds or insects. Can anyone believe it is possible to lay down such a barrage of poisons on the surface of the earth without making it unfit for all life? They should not be called "insecticides" but "biocides." ■

congressional inquisitors as supporters cheered and threw flowers from the gallery. These women carried the banner of motherhood into political activism, much as their nineteenth-century predecessors had done. Their ability to make a mockery of the dreaded congressional committee that had broken the spirits and ruined the careers of so many innocent citizens indicated that the consensus supporting the nuclear arms race was losing its grip.

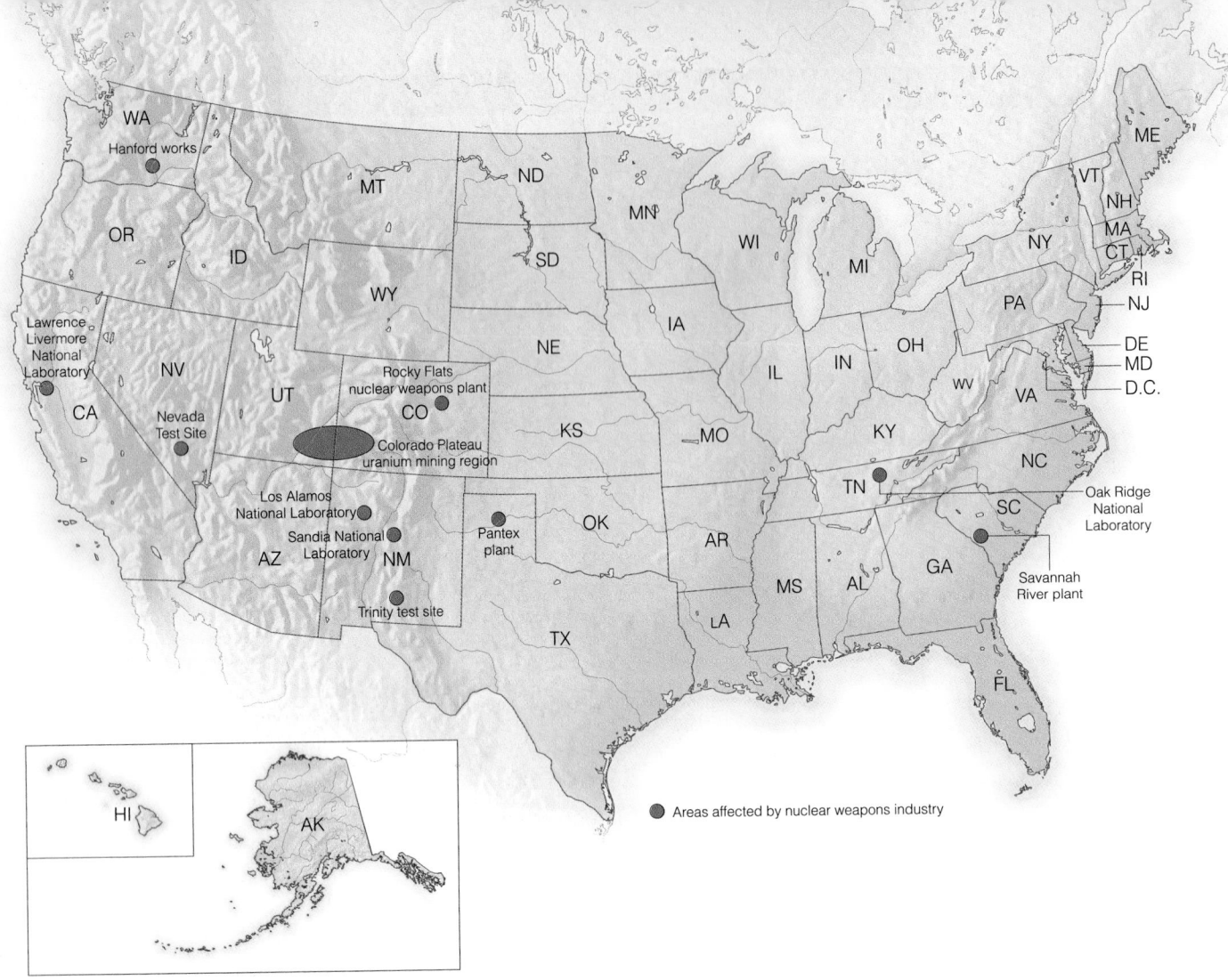

■ MAP 25.3
THE NUCLEAR LANDSCAPE The production and testing of nuclear weapons affected many regions across the country, especially in the West and South. Sites established during World War II remained active during the Cold War, as the nuclear arms race accelerated. The sites included testing grounds, uranium mining areas, laboratories, and plants where weapons were manufactured.

Decades later, the antinuclear protesters were vindicated—unfortunately too late for many people exposed to radiation during the early years of the Cold War. At the time, the real dangers of nuclear testing had not yet come to light. But in the 1980s and 1990s, top-secret documents were declassified, confirming that people living in the path of fallout from nuclear test sites, as well as military personnel working at or near the sites during the 1940s and 1950s, suffered disproportionately from cancer and other illnesses caused by radioactivity.

The Kennedy Era

John Fitzgerald Kennedy was the first American president born in the twentieth century and the first Catholic president. In his inaugural address, he claimed that "the torch has been passed to a new generation." It was a fitting metaphor for a young man who had been reared to compete and to win, whether the contest was athletic, intellectual, or political. But at the time of his election, it was not clear that a new generation had grabbed the torch. The young candidate was largely the creation of his father, Joseph, whose forebears had emigrated from Ireland during the 1840s. Joseph Kennedy rose to power and wealth as a financier, Hollywood executive, and ambassador to England. Ambitious and demanding, the elder Kennedy was known for his ruthlessness in business and politics and for his blatant philandering. He groomed his oldest son, Joseph P. Kennedy, Jr., for greatness, specifically for the presidency. But when young Joe was killed in World War II, the father's ambitions settled on the next in line, John.

John (Jack) Kennedy became a hero during World War II, winning military honors for rescuing his crewmates on his patrol boat, PT-109, when it was rammed by a Japanese destroyer. The rescue left him with a painful back impairment and exacerbated the symptoms of Addison's disease, which plagued him all his life and necessitated daily cortisone injections. His father coached him to bear up under the pain, hide his infirmity, and project an image of health and vitality. "Vigor" was a word Kennedy used often and an aura he projected, inspiring a national craze for physical fitness that survives to this day. Young JFK also emulated his father's brash sexual promiscuity, even after his marriage to Jacqueline Bouvier in 1953.

In 1946 Kennedy won election to the House of Representatives, and in 1952 he defeated the incumbent Republican Henry Cabot Lodge to become the Democratic senator from Massachusetts. JFK's father financed all of his political campaigns, and in 1960 the elderly Kennedy bankrolled and masterminded JFK's run for president. Kennedy selected as his running mate the powerful Senate majority leader, Lyndon B. Johnson of Texas, whom he had battled for the nomination. Concerned that his Catholicism would be a liability in the campaign, Kennedy spoke publicly about his faith, explaining that his religious beliefs would not interfere with his ability to do the job.

TABLE 25-3			
The Election of 1960			
Candidate	Political Party	Popular Vote	Electoral Vote
John F. Kennedy	Democratic	34,227,096	303
Richard M. Nixon	Republican	34,108,546	219

Just before the election, with the help of his brother Robert—whom he later appointed as attorney general—Kennedy arranged to have Martin Luther King, Jr., released from prison in Georgia, where hostile authorities had sentenced him to six months in jail for a minor traffic violation. This intervention secured the African American vote for Kennedy and the support of other minorities: Mexican Americans formed "Viva Kennedy" clubs throughout the Southwest. Voters of color helped Kennedy defeat his Republican foe, Eisenhower's vice president Richard Nixon, by a slim margin.

Domestic Policy

With such a thin margin of victory, Kennedy lacked a popular mandate for change. But he quickly established himself as an eloquent leader. In his inaugural address, the new president inspired the nation with his memorable words, "And so, my fellow Americans, ask not what your country can do for you; ask what you can do for your country." Focusing his address on foreign policy, he declared, "Let every nation know . . . that we shall pay any price, bear any burden, meet any hardship, support any friend, oppose any foe to assure the survival and the success of liberty." In his first two years, he sought mainly to avoid division at home and to wage the Cold War forcefully abroad. He believed that prosperity was the best way to spread the fruits of affluence, rather than government programs that would promote a redistribution of wealth. Accordingly, he supported corporate tax cuts to stimulate the economy, which grew at a rate of 5 percent each year from 1961 to 1966. Kennedy's economic policies continued many of the probusiness initiatives of Eisenhower.

Although Democrats held strong majorities in both houses, powerful southern conservatives often teamed up with Republicans to form a functional majority in Congress to defeat reform legislation. Kennedy knew that it would be futile to champion the cause of civil rights in the face of that alliance. But he did support issues important to his working-class constituents and proposed a number of legislative initiatives, including increasing the minimum wage,

Anticommunism

Throughout the twentieth century, American leaders have felt uneasy about revolutionary movements. On one hand, the United States was the great model of a successful anticolonial rebellion against a European colonial power. But on the other hand, the United States wanted to preserve order and stability in the world. The Russian Revolution of 1917 raised particular concerns because the victorious new communist regime denied Soviet citizens the essential democratic and economic principles that Americans cherished: free speech and elections, freedom of religious expression, private property, and capitalism. The United States officially refused to recognize the Soviet government from 1917 to 1933, as well as the People's Republic of China from 1949 until 1978 and Fidel Castro's Cuba from 1961 until today.

With these national principles and policies providing a foundation, anticommunism tapped widespread political and emotional passions within the United States. At times those passions, whipped up in moments of unsettling international or domestic events, led to extensive domestic repression of the very freedoms Americans have long cherished: free speech and political choice.

The first major wave of anticommunism in the United States came after World War I, in the wake of the founding of the American Communist party. The success of the Bolshevik Revolution and the establishment of the Soviet Union energized a segment of socialists to form a Communist party in the United States in support of Soviet communism. The Red Scare of 1919–1920 was a wave of political repression that targeted not only communists but also left-leaning immigrants, radicals, and labor unions. Immigration officials rounded up thousands of foreign-born

radicals and deported many, including the anarchist Emma Goldman. Many employers also used the rallying cry of anticommunism to break strikes and suppress unions. The Red Scare effectively silenced the Communist party and much of the left throughout the 1920s.

During the Great Depression of the 1930s, as fascism emerged in Europe, the Communist party attracted new members as well as thousands of liberal sympathizers. But enthusiasm for communism diminished in 1939 with the Nazi–Soviet pact and the communist opposition to Roosevelt's foreign policy. Anticommunist sentiment declined in 1941, when Hitler invaded Russia and the Soviet Union became an ally. The alliance was tense, however, as the United States vied with the Soviet Union over power in the postwar world.

The Cold War transformed anticommunism from a right-wing to a mainstream ideology and made it central to American politics and domestic

---

health care for the aged and increased Social Security benefits, and the creation of the Department of Housing and Urban Development (HUD).

When the steel industry challenged Kennedy's authority and threatened his economic policy by announcing a major price increase shortly after he had helped to negotiate a new contract with the steel union that would have kept prices stable, he mobilized all the power of his administration to force the steel magnates to back down. Kennedy also demonstrated strong leadership in the space program, presiding over the first manned space flight and declaring that the United States would land a man on the moon by the end of the 1960s.

Foreign Policy

Kennedy was the first U.S. president to understand and recognize the legitimacy of movements for national self-determination in the Third World. In 1957, while still in the Senate, he gave a speech calling on the French to grant independence to Algeria, which was still under French rule. As President, he endeavored to support movements to end colonial rule while at the same time containing the spread of communism. His efforts earned him a great deal of goodwill among Africans and other non-Europeans. But if nationalist movements appeared friendly to the Soviet Union, Kennedy worked against them. Critical of Eisenhower's defense policies but determined to continue his struggle against the spread of communism, Kennedy sharply increased military spending and nuclear arms build-up as a show of strength and preparedness against possible Soviet aggression.

One of Kennedy's most popular initiatives was the creation of the Peace Corps, a program that sent Americans, especially young people, to nations around the world to work on

culture. Because the United States vied with the Soviet Union for strategic power and territorial influence, the Communist party, with its links to the USSR, was considered a subversive organization. In 1947, the Truman administration barred from government jobs anyone associated with communists, and in 1949 the Justice Department prosecuted the 11 top leaders of the party for violation of the 1940 Smith Act, which made it illegal "to teach and advocate the overthrow and destruction of the United States government by force and violence." They were all convicted and sentenced to prison terms. Under the Smith Act, several hundred communists went to jail, while the House Un-American Activities Committee (HUAC) investigated suspected communist subversives. Hollywood became a primary target of anticommunism in the late 1940s and early 1950s, leading to the blacklisting of dozens of filmmakers

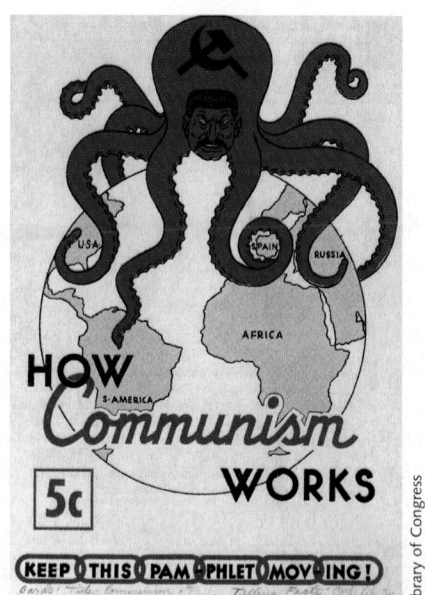

Anticommunist pamphlet published by the Catholic Library Service.

and actors who refused to "name names" before HUAC.

Senator Joseph McCarthy and other zealots used anticommunism to further their own political ambitions at a time when Democrats were on the defensive for being allegedly "soft" on communism. Official anticommunism targeted not only members of left-wing political organizations but also gays, lesbians, and others who allegedly might be vulnerable to blackmail and therefore should not be allowed to work in government offices. The Federal Bureau of Investigation (FBI), under the leadership of J. Edgar Hoover, made anticommunism a high priority. The FBI targeted Martin Luther King, Jr., and other civil rights activists whom Hoover believed were communist agents seeking to destabilize American society. By the late 1950s the anticommunist hysteria had subsided, but it remained part of the political culture throughout the Cold War. During the 1980s, President Ronald W. Reagan revived anticommunist rhetoric when he called the Soviet Union the "evil empire." ■

development projects. In 1961 Kennedy signed the Charter of Punta del Este with several Latin American countries, establishing the Organization of American States (OAS) and the Alliance for Progress, a program designed to prevent the spread of anti-Americanism and communist insurgencies in Latin America. The alliance offered $20 billion in loans to OAS countries for democratic development initiatives.

Kennedy continued the strategies of Truman and Eisenhower to fight communism in South Vietnam by supporting the corrupt regime of Ngo Dingh Diem. But the National Liberation Front (NLF), founded in 1960 and supported by Ho Chi Minh's communist regime in North Vietnam, gained the upper hand in its struggle against Diem. In response, Kennedy increased the number of military advisers there from 800 to 17,000. By 1963 it was obvious that Diem's brutal regime was about to fall to the NLF, and Kennedy allowed U.S. military advisers and diplomats to encourage Diem's dissenting generals to depose and assassinate Diem.

Kennedy also faced a crisis brewing in Cuba. Fidel Castro's revolution initially represented the sort of democratic insurgency that Kennedy wanted to support. But Castro's socialism turned the United States against him, and he established close ties with the Soviet Union. Kennedy now saw the small impoverished island as a major threat where "communist influence . . . festers some 90 miles off the coast of Florida." During the Eisenhower administration, the CIA began planning an invasion of Cuba with the help of Cuban exiles in Florida. Kennedy's national security advisers persuaded Kennedy to allow the invasion to proceed.

On April 17, 1961, U.S.-backed and -trained anticommunist forces, most of them Cuban exiles, landed at the Bahia de Cochinas (Bay of Pigs) on the southern coast of Cuba. Castro expected the invasion—his agents in Florida had infiltrated the Cuban exiles—so his well-prepared troops quickly surrounded and captured the invaders. With no domestic uprising against Castro to support the invasion, Kennedy quickly realized that his only chance of success would be to call in the military with large-scale air support. Unwilling to take that step, Kennedy pulled back in humiliating defeat, telling his adviser Clark Clifford, "I have made a tragic mistake." Nevertheless, Kennedy continued to support covert efforts that tried but failed to destabilize Cuba and assassinate Castro.

Another crisis soon erupted in Berlin. Located 200 miles deep in East Germany, with only two highways connecting it to West Germany, West Berlin was a showcase of western material superiority and an espionage center for the western powers. It was also an important symbolic site, reassuring West Berliners along with western Europeans that the United States would not abandon them. At a summit in Vienna between Kennedy and Khrushchev in June 1961, Khrushchev threatened to end the western presence in Berlin and unite the city with the rest of East Germany. His plan was motivated in part to stop the steady stream of East Germans into West Berlin. Kennedy refused to relinquish West Berlin. On August 13, 1961, the East German government constructed a wall to separate East and West Berlin. Guards patrolled the wall with orders to shoot anyone who tried to cross, and many who tried lost their lives. Two years later, Kennedy stood in front of the wall and pledged to defend the West Berliners, making his memorable statement of solidarity, "*Ich bin ein Berliner*" ("I am a Berliner").

Kennedy put the Strategic Air Command on full alert for possible nuclear war.

The most serious foreign policy crisis of Kennedy's presidency came in 1962, when the Soviet Union, at Castro's invitation, began to install intermediate-range nuclear missiles in Cuba. Kennedy's close advisers presented a series of options for actions that could be taken in response. The most dramatic and dangerous would be a full-scale military invasion of the island, which would topple Castro but would surely have prompted military retaliation by the Soviet Union. Another option was a more limited military intervention, an air strike to destroy the missiles before they became operational. Others proposed a blockade of Cuban ports to prevent the missiles from entering. Another possibility was to negotiate secretly with Castro, Soviet leaders, or both. Kennedy decided against behind-the-scenes negotiations as well as the drastic move of military intervention and instead established a "quarantine" around the island to block Soviet ships from reaching Cuba, hoping that the Soviet Union would back down and withdraw the missiles. A quarantine, unlike a blockade, was not considered an act of war; nevertheless, Kennedy put the Strategic Air Command on full alert for possible nuclear war.

It was a risky move. On national television, Kennedy warned the Soviet Union to remove the missiles or face the military might of the United States: "We will not prematurely or unnecessarily risk the costs of worldwide nuclear war in which even the fruits of victory would be ashes in our mouth, but neither will we shrink from that risk at any time it must be faced." Khrushchev accused Kennedy of bringing the two nations to the brink of nuclear war. For the next five days, tensions mounted as Russian ships hovered in the water beyond the quarantine zone. Finally Khrushchev proposed an agreement, offering to remove the missiles if the United States would agree not to invade Cuba. In secret negotiations, Kennedy also privately promised to remove the Jupiter missiles in Turkey as soon as the crisis was over. The two leaders managed to diffuse the crisis, but they were both sobered by the experience of having come to the brink of nuclear war. They soon established a telephone "hotline" linking the White House and the Kremlin for quicker communication in any future crisis. In 1963 the two leaders signed a nuclear test ban treaty.

A Year of Turning Points

In 1963 the President's Commission on the Status of Women, which Kennedy had appointed under the leadership of Eleanor Roosevelt, published a report that documented widespread discrimination against women in jobs, pay, education, and the professions. In response to the findings, Kennedy issued a presidential order requiring the civil service to hire people "without regard to sex" and supported passage of the Equal Pay Act of 1963. The commission's report, along with the publication the same year of Betty Friedan's call to arms, *The Feminine Mystique,* provided fuel for the feminist movement that burst across the nation in the next few years.

In the spring of that same year, in Birmingham, Alabama, Martin Luther King, Jr., led a silent and peaceful march through the city. Chief of Police Bull Connor unleashed the police, who blasted the demonstrators with fire hoses and attacked them with vicious police dogs. Four black children were later killed when segregationists bombed an African American church.

The Kennedy administration responded by bringing the full force of its authority to bear on the officials in Birmingham. But the crisis intensified. Alabama's segregationist governor, George Wallace, refused to admit two black students to the University of Alabama, threatening to stand in the doorway to block their entrance.

Finally, on June 10, 1963, Kennedy federalized the Alabama National Guard and for the first time went before the American people to declare himself forcefully on the side of the civil rights protesters and to propose a civil rights bill. The violence in the South had raised "a moral issue," he declared, "as old as Scriptures and . . . as clear as the Constitution." A few months later, on August 28, more than 250,000 people gathered at the nation's capitol in front of the Lincoln Memorial for the culmination of the March on Washington, a huge demonstration for jobs as well as freedom, where Martin Luther King, Jr., delivered his inspiring "I Have a Dream" speech, which included these memorable words:

> I say to you today, my friends, that in spite of the difficulties and frustrations of the moment, I still have a dream. It is a dream deeply rooted in the American dream.
>
> I have a dream that one day this nation will rise up and live out the true meaning of its creed: "We hold these truths to be self-evident: that all men are created equal."
>
> I have a dream that one day on the red hills of Georgia the sons of former slaves and the sons of former slave owners will be able to sit down together at a table of brotherhood. I have a dream that one day even the state of Mississippi, a desert state, sweltering with the heat of injustice and oppression, will be transformed into an oasis of freedom and justice. I have a dream that my four children will one day live in a nation where they will not be judged by the color of their skin but by the content of their character. . . . Let freedom ring from every hill and every molehill of Mississippi. From every mountainside, let freedom ring. When we let freedom ring, when we let it ring from every village and every hamlet, from every state and every city, we will be able to speed up that day when all of God's children, black men and white men, Jews and Gentiles, Protestants and Catholics, will be able to join hands and sing in the words of the old Negro spiritual, "Free at last! Free at last! Thank God Almighty, we are free at last!"

In the fall of 1963, a confident Kennedy began planning his reelection campaign for the next year. To mobilize support he visited Texas. "Here we are in Dallas," he said on November 22, 1963, "and it looks like everything in Texas is going to be fine for us." Within an hour of uttering those optimistic words, the president lay dying of an assassin's bullet.

As shock and grief spread across the nation, a bizarre series of events confounded efforts to bring the assassin to justice. Police arrested Lee Harvey Oswald, who had previously lived in the Soviet Union and who had loose ties to organized crime and to political groups interested in Cuba. Oswald claimed that he was innocent. But before he could be brought to trial, Oswald himself was murdered. Jack Ruby, a nightclub owner who also had links to organized crime, shot Oswald while he was in the custody of the Dallas police—an event witnessed by millions on live television. Ruby later died in prison. The newly sworn-in president, Lyndon B. Johnson, appointed a commission to investigate the assassination under the leadership of Supreme Court Chief Justice Earl Warren. The Warren Commission eventually issued a report concluding that Oswald and Ruby had both acted alone. The commission findings created a heated controversy. Many people at the time and since believed that there was evidence of a conspiracy. In 1978 a panel of the House of Representatives suggested that Kennedy may have been the victim of a plot, possibly involving the Mafia. Conspiracy theories continue to circulate to this day, finding expression in dozens of books, articles, and motion pictures.

Conclusion

During the years between the election of Dwight D. Eisenhower and the assassination of John F. Kennedy, the nation experienced unprecedented prosperity as increasing numbers of Americans moved into middle-class suburbs and enjoyed the fruits of a rapidly expanding consumer economy. Men and women rushed into marriage and childbearing, creating the baby boom and a powerful domestic ideology resting on distinct gender roles for women and men. At the same time, fears of nuclear war, intense anticommunism, and pressures to conform to mainstream political and cultural values contributed to anxieties and discontent.

Beneath the apparently tranquil surface, some Americans began to resist the limitations and exclusions of the widely touted "American way of life." African Americans in the South demanded their rightful place as full citizens, challenging the Jim Crow system and accelerating the civil rights movement through nonviolent protests, boycotts, and sit-ins. Young people created a vibrant youth culture to the pulsating rhythms of rock 'n' roll. Beatniks, peace activists, and environmentalists expressed incipient political and cultural dissent. The rumblings of vast social change had already begun and would explode in the years ahead.

Sites to Visit

We Shall Overcome: Historic Places of the Civil Rights Movement
www.cr.nps.gov/NR/travel/civilrights/index.htm
> This site of the National Register of Historic Places provides maps and information about the historic locations of the civil rights movement.

Dwight David Eisenhower
www.ipl.org/ref/POTUS/ddeisenhower.html
> This site contains basic information about Eisenhower's election and presidency, and online biography.

The Literature & Culture of the American 1950s
dept.english.upenn.edu/~afilreis/50s/home.html
> This site by University of Pennsylvania Professor Al Filreis contains a large array of 1950s documents, literature, and images.

Levittown: Documents of an Ideal American Suburb
tigger.uic.edu/~pbhales/Levittown/
> Peter Bacon Hales of the Art History Department at the University of Illinois at Chicago developed this website, which includes images, articles, and information about the post-World War II Levittown suburb.

Hollywood and the Movies during the 1950s
lib.berkeley.edu/MRC/50sbib.html
> This site from the University of California at Berkeley libraries includes information about Hollywood during the 1950s, and links to related sites, such as the Hollywood blacklist and film noir.

Rock and Roll
www.rockhall.com/home/default.asp
> This website of the Rock and Roll Hall of Fame and Museum includes information about the history and major artists of rock and roll.

Little Rock 1959: Pages from History—The Central High Crisis
www.ardemgaz.com/prev/central/
> This site documents the events surrounding the effort to desegregate Central High in Little Rock, Arkansas, in 1959.

From *Plessy v. Ferguson* to *Brown v. Board of Education*: The Supreme Court Rules on School Desegregation
www.yale.edu/ynhti/curriculum/units/1982/3/82.03.06.x.html
> This site includes information about the landmark Supreme Court decision compiled by the Yale-New Haven Teachers Institute.

The Civil Rights Era
lcweb2.loc.gov/ammem/aaohtml/exhibit/aopart9.html
> This Library of Congress site includes information about the people, events, and developments of the civil rights movement.

John F. Kennedy
www.ipl.org/ref/POTUS/jfkennedy.html
> This site contains basic information about Kennedy's election and presidency, and online biography.

For Further Reading

General

Taylor Branch, *Parting the Waters: America in the King Years, 1954–1963* (1988).

William H. Chafe, *The Unfinished Journey: America Since World War II* (1986).

Pete Daniel, *Lost Revolutions: The South in the 1950s* (2000).

Eric Foner, *The Story of American Freedom* (1998).

Godfrey Hodgson, *America in Our Time* (1976).

Cold War, Warm Hearth

Stephanie Coontz, *The Way We Never Were: American Families and the Nostalgia Trap* (1992).

Barbara Ehrenreich, *The Hearts of Men: American Dreams and the Flight from Commitment* (1984).

Ruth Feldstein, *Motherhood in Black and White: Race and Sex in American Liberalism, 1930–1965* (2000).

Kenneth T. Jackson, *Crabgrass Frontier: The Suburbanization of the United States* (1985).

George Katona, *The Mass Consumption Society* (1964).

Elaine Tyler May, *Homeward Bound: American Families in the Cold War Era* (1999).

The Civil Rights Movement

Clayborne Carson, *In Struggle: SNCC and the Black Awakening of the 1960s* (1981).

Mary Dudziak, *Cold War Civil Rights: Equality as Cold War Policy, 1946–1968* (2000).

Hugh Davis Graham, *The Civil Rights Era: Origins and Development of National Policy* (1990).

Steven F. Lawson, *Running for Freedom: Civil Rights and Black Politics in America Since 1941* (1990).

Harvard Sitkoff, *The Struggle for Black Equality, 1954–1992* (1993).

The Eisenhower Years

Stephen E. Ambrose, *Eisenhower* (1983–84).

Thomas Borstelmann, *The Cold War and the Color Line: Race Relations and American Foreign Policy Since 1945* (2001).

Robert F. Burk, *The Eisenhower Administration and Black Civil Rights* (1984).

Robert A. Divine, *The Sputnik Challenge* (1993).

Peter B. Dow, *Schoolhouse Politics: Lessons from the Sputnik Era* (1991).

Dwight D. Eisenhower, *The White House Years: Waging Peace, 1956–1961* (1965).

Fred I. Greenstein, *The Hidden-Hand Presidency: Eisenhower as Leader* (1994).

Outsiders and Opposition

Winifred Breines, *Young, White, and Miserable: Growing Up Female in the Fifties* (1994).

Paul Brooks, *The House of Life: Rachel Carson at Work* (1972).

Rachel Carson, *Silent Spring* (1963).

Betty Friedan, *The Feminine Mystique* (1963).

James Gilbert, *A Cycle of Outrage: America's Reaction to the Juvenile Delinquent in the 1950s* (1986).

Charlie Gillett, *Sound of the City: The Rise of Rock and Roll* (1983).

Serge Guilbaut, *How New York Stole the Idea of Modern Art* (1985).

Joyce Johnson, *Minor Characters: A Young Woman's Coming-of-Age in the Beat Orbit of Jack Kerouac* (1999).

Joanne Meyerowitz, ed., *Not June Cleaver: Women and Gender in Postwar America, 1945–1960* (1994).

Leslie Reagan, *When Abortion Was a Crime: Women, Medicine, and the Law in the United States, 1867–1973* (1997).

Rickie Solinger, *Wake Up Little Susie: Single Pregnancy and Race Before Roe v. Wade* (1992).

The Kennedy Era

Roger Hilsman, *To Move a Nation: The Politics of Foreign Policy in the Administration of John F. Kennedy* (1967).

Elizabeth Cobbs Hoffman, *All You Need Is Love: The Peace Corps and the Spirit of the 1960s* (1998).

Herbert S. Parmet, *J.F.K.: The Presidency of John F. Kennedy* (1983).

Arthur M. Schlesinger, Jr., *A Thousand Days: John F. Kennedy in the White House* (1965).

Online Practice Test

Test your understanding of this chapter with interactive review quizzes at

www.ablongman.com/jonescreatedequal/chapter25

Additional Photo Credits

Page 835: AP/Wide World Photos
Page 836: Library of Congress
Page 839: Photofest
Page 849: Courtesy, Janice L. and David Frent
Page 851: Roger Ressmeyer/CORBIS
Page 863: Fair Street Pictures

CHAPTER

26

The Nation Divides: The Vietnam War and Social Conflict, 1964–1971

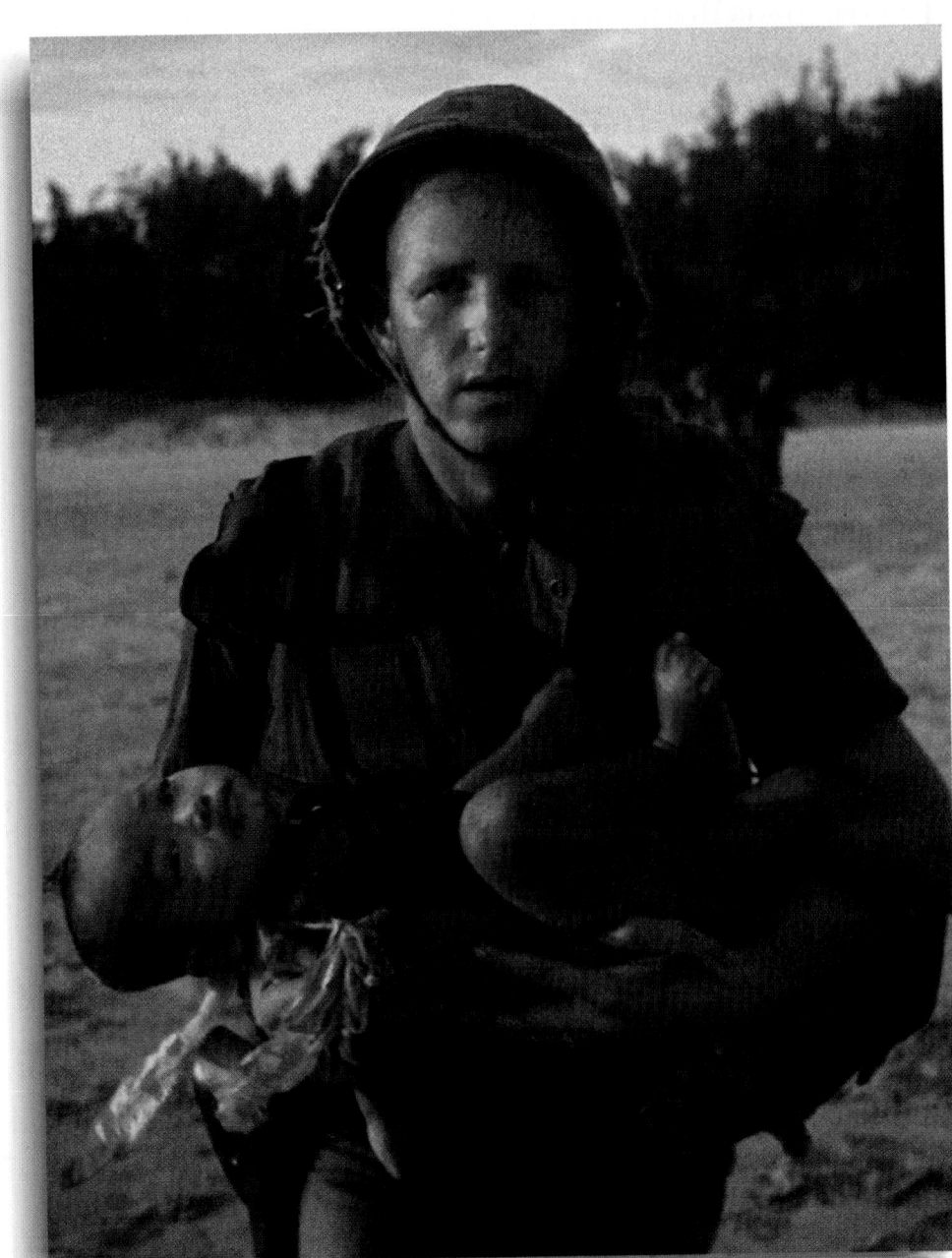

Paul Schutzer/TimePix

■ The deployment of hundreds of thousands of American soldiers in Vietnam intimately affected life there, sometimes in terrible ways and sometimes in helpful ways.

THE SOFT-SPOKEN BLACK MAN WITH THE STRANGE ACCENT FIRST SHOWED UP IN THE small town of McComb, Mississippi, in the summer of 1961. Robert Parris Moses had come on a mission of democracy: he was there to encourage impoverished African Americans to register to vote. He had grown up in Harlem, attended Hamilton College in upstate New York on a scholarship, and was doing graduate work in philosophy at Harvard when his mother's death brought him back to Manhattan to help care for his father. Moses was teaching math at an elite private school when the student sit-in movement against segregation spread across the upper South in the spring of 1960. Deeply impressed by the courage and leadership of those young black southerners, he went south that summer to work with Martin Luther King, Jr.'s Southern Christian Leadership Conference. The following spring, Moses returned to the South as a full-time organizer for the new Student Nonviolent Coordinating Committee (SNCC).

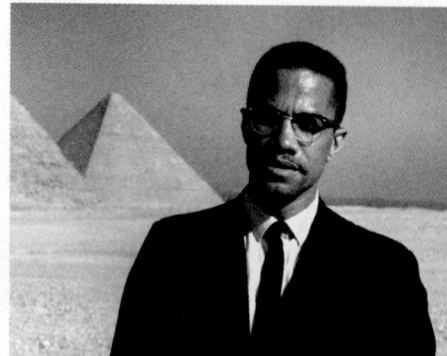

A leading spokesman for the Black Muslims, Malcolm X converted to orthodox Islam and softened his antiwhite rhetoric in the 2 years before his murder in 1965. Like SNCC's Bob Moses, Malcolm increasingly identified with the Third World. Here he is shown in Egypt on a 1964 pilgrimage to Mecca, Saudi Arabia.

Encouraging citizens to vote in the leading nation of the "free world" was a subversive act in 1961, at least when the citizens had dark skin and lived in the southeastern states of the former Confederacy. Over the next 4 years in the Deep South, Bob Moses paid a price for his commitments. Local police imprisoned him, white supremacists beat him severely, and they murdered dozens of his fellow activists in the black freedom movement. But Moses remained committed to nonviolence and racial integration. His quiet courage became legendary in the movement. One summer night in 1962, he returned to a deserted SNCC office in Greenwood, Mississippi, that had just been ransacked by a white mob; three other SNCC workers had barely escaped with their lives. Moses looked around, made up a bed in the corner of the devastated main room, and went to sleep. He refused to be intimidated.

For all his distinctiveness, Moses did not promote himself as a charismatic leader. Like his comrades in SNCC, he did not believe in traditional, top-down leadership. The women and men in SNCC worked instead to get local black communities to organize themselves and to find their leadership among their own members. When others became too dependent on his guidance, Moses even dropped his biblical surname and became simply "Bob Parris" to reduce his public profile. Such rejection of hierarchy put SNCC at odds with other civil rights organizations and with the national Democratic party, which sought black support. By 1964 Moses and other freedom workers grew disillusioned with white liberal leadership, especially after the Democratic convention that August, where President Lyndon Johnson crushed the integrated Mississippi Freedom Democratic party's bid to replace the all-white regular Mississippi delegation. Two trips to Africa expanded Moses' sense of connection to the Third World, and he became increasingly involved with the growing movement against the U.S. war in Vietnam. The federal government responded by drafting him. Moses moved to Canada to avoid being inducted to fight a war he opposed, and then went to east Africa, where he and his wife taught school and raised a family in Tanzania for almost a decade. He returned to the United States only after President Jimmy Carter's general amnesty for draft resisters in 1977.

The trajectory of Bob Moses' life across these years suggests much about the 1960s. An extraordinary number of idealistic young people became involved in public life in an effort to make real their nation's abstract promises of freedom and justice. The civil rights movement inspired the social movements that followed: for ending the war, for preserving the environment, and for liberating women, Latinos, Indians, and gay men and lesbians. But organizing for change inevitably brought activists up against fierce resistance from what they called "the establishment." Disillusionment and radicalization often followed. Whereas Moses went to Africa, other young African Americans moved toward black nationalism at home, a proud cultural identity at odds with the pursuit of integration. Public life became deeply contentious by 1968 as young radicals challenged more conservative citizens on issues of race, war, and gender.

The escalating American war in Southeast Asia loomed over all. Lyndon Johnson brought the nation to its apex of liberal reform with his extensive Great Society legislation. His purpose was to complete and surpass the New Deal promise of his hero, Franklin Roosevelt. However, the high-flying hopes of Democratic liberals crashed to earth with the destructive war that the Johnson administration waged against seasoned communist revolutionaries in far-off Vietnam. Out of the wreckage of 1968 emerged a Republican president, Richard Nixon, and a growing conservative backlash against the social changes advocated by people of color, the counterculture, the antiwar movement, and the rising tide of women's liberation. By the beginning of the 1970s, American politics turned to the right, even as American culture generally remained more tolerant of different lifestyles and values than it had been before the 1960s. This libertarian combination of distrusting government while accepting greater cultural diversity has predominated in American life ever since.

Lyndon Johnson and the Apex of Liberalism

Wealth provided the foundation on which the Great Society was built. American economic expansion since World War II had created history's richest nation by 1960. From 1961 to 1966, the economy accelerated at an annual growth rate of more than 5 percent with very low inflation, stimulated by large tax cuts and extensive military spending. The 41 percent increase in per capita income during the 1960s was not evenly distributed, however. Economist Paul Samuelson explained in 1970, "If we made an income pyramid out of a child's blocks, with each layer portraying $1000 of income, the peak would be far higher than the Eiffel Tower, but almost all of us would be within a yard of the ground." And the distribution of wealth (stocks and real estate) was far more skewed than that of income. U.S. policymakers believed that economic expansion would continue indefinitely and the nation could therefore afford government policies to improve the welfare of less affluent Americans.

The New President

Lyndon Baines Johnson was one of the most remarkable American characters of the twentieth century. Journalist David Halberstam called him "a man of stunning force, drive and intelligence, and of equally stunning insecurity"—both a giant among political leaders and a bully with those who worked for him. Johnson grew up in a family struggling to stay out of

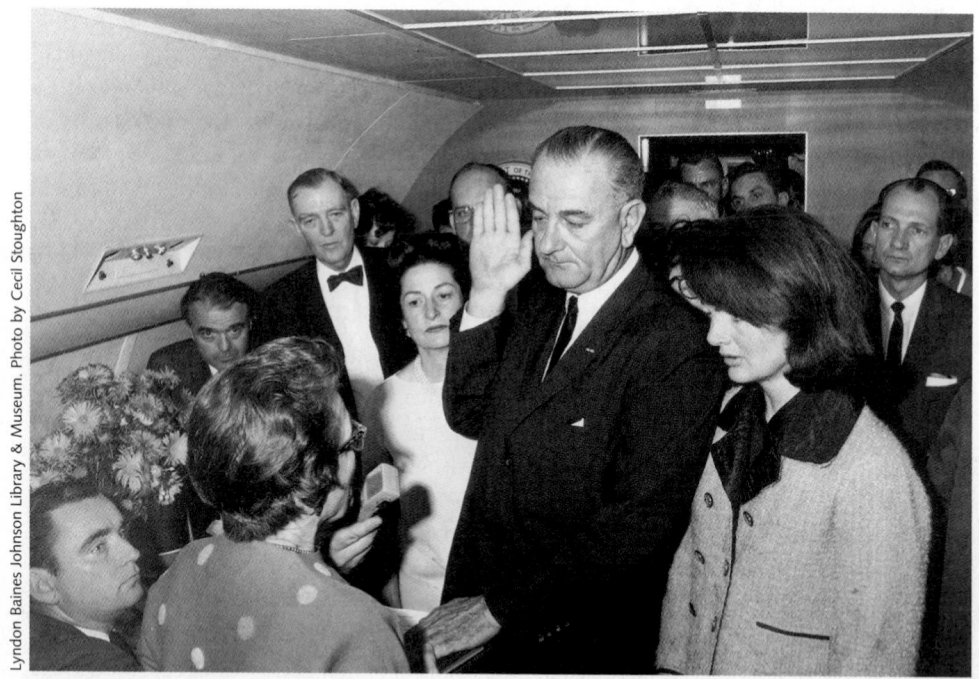

Lyndon Baines Johnson Library & Museum. Photo by Cecil Stoughton

■ Lyndon Johnson took the presidential oath of office on board Air Force One, returning to Washington from Dallas, where John Kennedy had just been assassinated on November 22, 1963. His wife, Lady Bird, is on his right, and Jacqueline Kennedy, still in blood-stained clothes, stands on his left. Johnson adroitly channeled the public outpouring of grief for the murdered young president into support for their shared legislative goals.

poverty in the Texas hill country west of Austin. He entered Democratic politics early as an avid supporter of Franklin Roosevelt and the New Deal, aided by the business savvy and loyalty of his wife, Lady Bird Johnson, who grew wealthy through ownership of TV and radio stations. As First Lady, she became widely known for her leadership in highway beautification. Lyndon Johnson rose like a rocket through Congress to become perhaps the most powerful Senate majority leader ever (1954–1960) and then vice president (1961–1963). Kennedy's assassination catapulted him into the Oval Office as the nation's first Texan president.

Like his home state, Johnson was physically big and at times intimidating. His earthy humor and homely style contrasted sharply with Kennedy's telegenic sophistication. Eastern elites cringed at the idea of Johnson as Kennedy's successor in the White House; the fact that Kennedy was killed in Texas did not help. But Johnson retained Kennedy's cabinet and advisers and used the memory of the fallen young president to rally support for his administration. Johnson turned out to be the more liberal of the two men in part because his early years in Texas had given him a visceral understanding of poverty and discrimination that his predecessor lacked. Johnson's focus was different, too. He retained Kennedy's anticommunist commitments abroad, but his heart remained at home. "I don't want to be the President who built empires, or sought grandeur, or extended dominion," he told the nation. He wanted to perfect American society: to enhance American security by refashioning the central nation of the "free world" into a model for all others.

First he had to win reelection because less than a year remained until voters went to the polls in 1964. The Republicans nominated right-wing Senator Barry Goldwater of Arizona, a sign of the party's sharp swing away from its moderate eastern elements toward its fiercely conservative western and southern constituencies. Conservative organizers such as the Young Americans for Freedom considered such Republican leaders as Dwight Eisenhower and Richard Nixon too much like Democrats. Goldwater instead believed in unrestricted markets and a minimal role for the federal government in every aspect of American life except the

TABLE 26-1

The Election of 1964

Candidate	Political Party	Popular Vote	Electoral Vote
Lyndon B. Johnson	Democratic	43,126,506	486
Barry M. Goldwater	Republican	27,176,799	52

military. He spoke casually about using nuclear weapons against communists abroad. "In your heart you know he's right" his campaign slogan promised. "In your guts you know he's nuts," retorted the Democrats. Goldwater declared that "extremism in the defense of liberty is no vice," but Johnson zeroed in on that extremism and swept to the largest electoral majority of any president (61 percent). Voters also chose the most liberal Congress since the Great Depression. Few realized then that Goldwater, not Johnson, was the better indicator of where American politics would soon be heading.

The Great Society: Fighting Poverty and Discrimination

In pursuit of what he called the Great Society, Johnson first declared a "War on Poverty." No citizen in the richest nation on earth should live in squalor, he believed. The president's sensitivity to this issue, despite his personal rise to wealth, fit with a growing national concern, stimulated in part by political activist Michael Harrington's widely read book *The Other Americans* (1962). The poor were everywhere, from decaying inner cities to rural areas such as Appalachia. More than one out of five Americans lived below the conservatively estimated official poverty line ($3022 for a nonfarm family of four in 1960), and 70 percent of them were white.

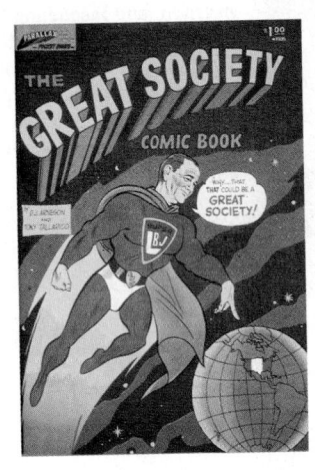

The president and a large congressional majority passed several measures to alleviate poverty. They sharply increased the availability of money and food stamps through the Aid to Families with Dependent Children ("welfare") program, and they raised Social Security payments to older Americans. Several programs focused on improving educational opportunities as an avenue out of poverty: Head Start offered preschool education and meals for youngsters, the Elementary and Secondary Education Act sent federal funds to the least affluent school districts, and an expanded system of student loans facilitated access to college. The Job Corps provided employment training, and Volunteers in Service to America (VISTA) served as a domestic Peace Corps, funneling people with education and skills into poor communities to serve as teachers and providers of other social services.

How well did these programs work? Americans have argued vigorously over this question ever since. Some defended the programs as reducing the number of people living in poverty and giving educational and employment opportunities to many previously deprived of such chances. Critics on the right believed that the programs instead encouraged dependence on government and thus actually worsened the problem. Critics on the left noted that the programs did not go far enough in attacking the root causes of poverty. Three conclusions seem clear about the War on Poverty. First, it did not eliminate poverty. Second, it did help reduce the number of poor people by one-third between 1960 and 1969 (22 percent to 14 percent). Third, the elderly benefited most from the higher payment schedules put into place by the War on Poverty, as the share of Americans over age 65 in the poor population dropped from 40 percent in 1959 to 16 percent by 1974.

No barrier to opportunity in the early 1960s was higher than the color bar. Both opportunist and idealist, Johnson as president shed his segregationist voting record (necessary for election in Texas before 1960) and became the most vocal proponent of racial equality ever to occupy the Oval Office. Two factors facilitated his change in position. Blatant inequalities for American citizens weakened the United States in its competition with the Soviets and Chinese for the loyalty of the nonwhite Third World majority. Moreover, the African American freedom struggle in the South had reached a boiling point. Black frustration was mounting over white brutality and the seeming indifference or even hostility of the national government. "The Negroes are tired of this patient stuff and tired of this piecemeal stuff," the president acknowledged privately. The persistence of local organizers across the South, such as Bob Moses, forced the U.S. government to move.

The Civil Rights Act of 1964 fulfilled the implicit promise of the *Brown v. Board of Education* decision a decade earlier. The 1964 act made desegregation the law of the land as it

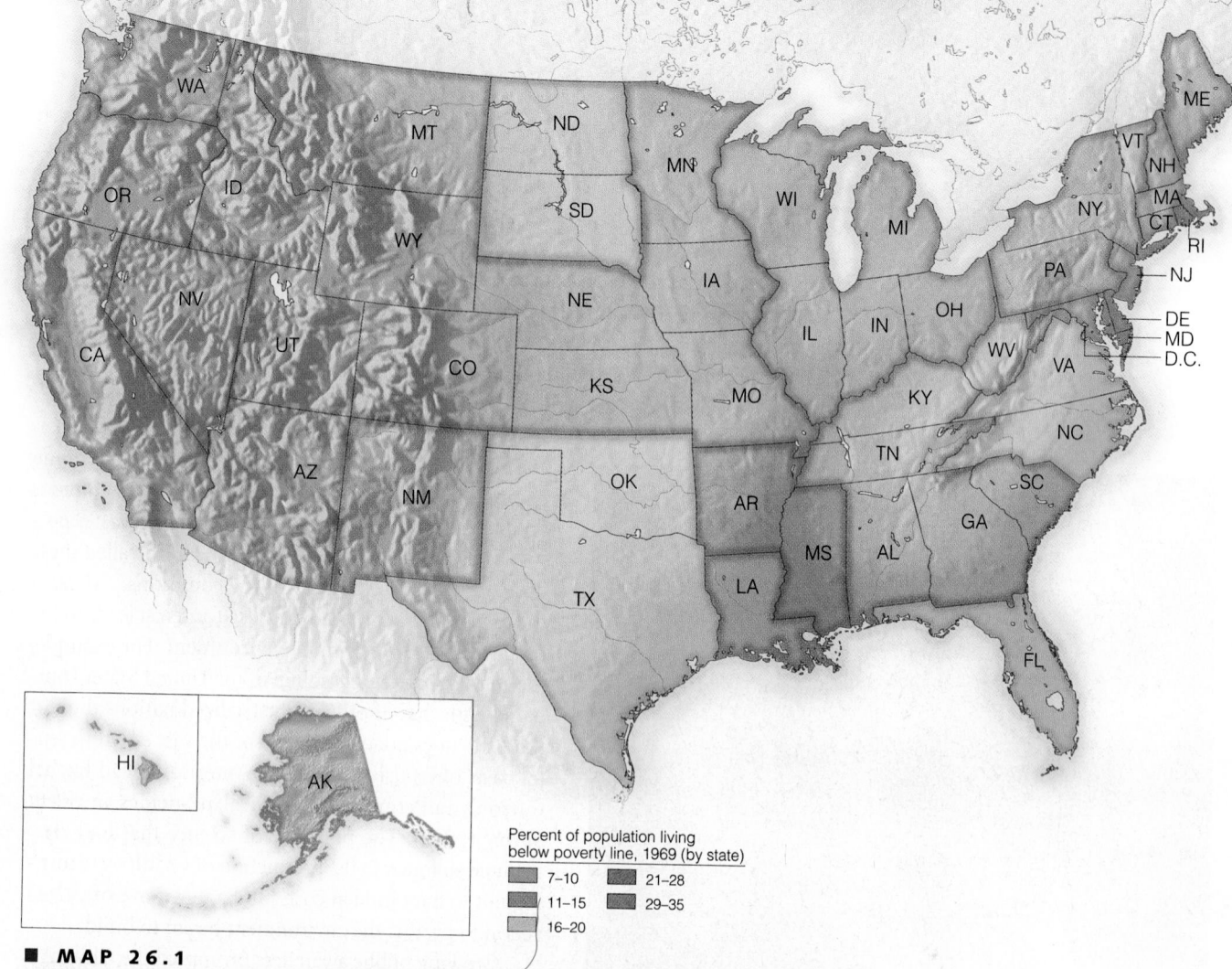

■ MAP 26.1

PERCENTAGE OF POPULATION LIVING BELOW THE POVERTY LINE, 1969 (BY STATE) The United States in the 1960s was a nation of unprecedented wealth and comfort. Yet millions of Americans still lived in poverty. Prodded by other reformers, President Johnson sought to reduce the number of impoverished citizens through the Great Society programs. The southeastern and south central states had the highest poverty rates, a legacy of slavery and limited industrialization.

outlawed discrimination in employment and in public facilities such as restaurants, theaters, and hotels. When Alabama police beat peaceful marchers on the Edmund Pettis Bridge outside Selma on March 7, 1965, horrifying most national television viewers, Johnson seized the opportunity to push through Congress the Voting Rights Act. This legislation outlawed poll taxes and provided federal voting registrars in states that refused the ballot to African Americans. The single most important legislation of the twentieth century for bringing political democracy to the South, the Voting Rights Act increased the percentage of blacks voting in Mississippi from 7 percent to 60 percent in 2 years. Black electoral power began to bring unprecedented change to Dixie's political and racial landscape.

The Great Society: Improving the Quality of Life

Johnson's vision of the Great Society extended to the broader quality of life in the United States. Health care was perhaps the most fundamental issue for citizens' sense of personal security. After 1965, the new Medicare system paid for the medical needs of Americans over 65, and Medicaid underwrote health care services for the indigent. Rising concern about the quality of corporate products led to new federal efforts to protect citizens as consumers. In 1964, when more than half of adults smoked tobacco, the surgeon-general issued the first government report linking smoking to cancer. A year later, consumer advocate Ralph Nader used research studies to show that Chevrolet's sporty new Corvair was "unsafe at any speed." Despite industry resistance, higher federal standards for automotive safety followed. Public pressures also led to the establishment of new requirements for publishing the nutritional values of packaged food. The federally funded Public Broadcasting System (PBS) was established to provide television programs that were more educational than the fare tied to advertising on the three corporate networks (NBC, CBS, and ABC). In fact, most Great Society measures targeted all Americans rather than just the disadvantaged.

Nothing more directly threatened the quality of American life than the degradation of the natural environment. The costs of the unrestrained and much-heralded economic growth since World War II showed up in the nation's air, water, and land. The leaded gasoline that fueled products of the booming auto industry created smog, industrial effluents polluted lakes and rivers, and petrochemical wastes poisoned the ground. Biologist Garrett Hardin called these developments "the tragedy of the commons," wherein the pursuit of narrow individual self-interest leads to the despoiling of the common environment. For example, the very low price of gasoline in the United States compared with that of other industrialized nations did not (and still does not) recoup any of the vast environmental costs of its use. Millions of Americans read Rachel Carson's indictment of chemical pesticides in *Silent Spring* (1962). The products of science that had contributed so much to the production of wealth were turning out to have hidden costs, and a new wave of citizen action to protect the environment began to build.

Growing public awareness prompted the Clean Air Act (1963) and the Clean Waters Act (1966), which set federal guidelines for reducing smog and preserving public drinking sources from bacterial pollution. Even the long dam-building tradition in the American West faced new questions. A quarter century after Hoover Dam blocked the Colorado River, engineers completed the Glen Canyon Dam (1963) upstream at the Arizona–Utah border, drowning one of the nation's most spectacular canyons under the new Lake Powell. Demands for the dam's removal began immediately (they continue to this day) and helped spur passage of the Wild and Scenic

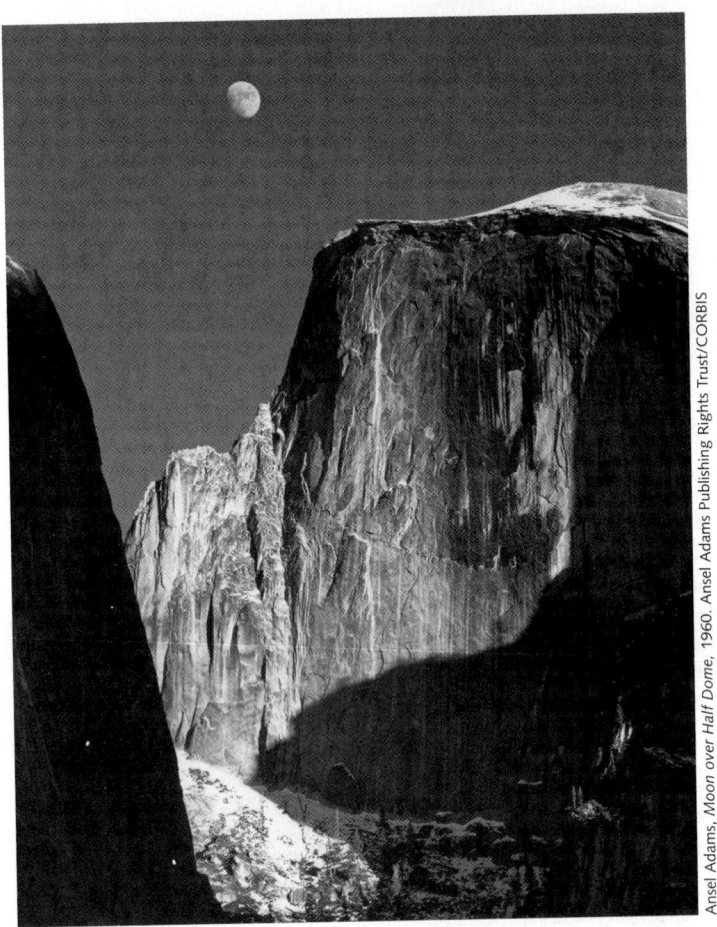

Ansel Adams, *Moon over Half Dome*, 1960. Ansel Adams Publishing Rights Trust/CORBIS

■ The moon rises over Half Dome in Yosemite Valley, Yosemite National Park, California, 1960. With this and other spectacular shots, renowned photographer Ansel Adams contributed to a growing national appreciation for wilderness in the years after World War II.

Rivers Act in 1968. Meanwhile, Congress passed the Wilderness Act in 1964, setting aside 9 million acres of undeveloped public lands as a place "where man is a visitor who does not remain." No longer were wild lands (almost all west of the Mississippi River) targeted solely for economic development and settlement. In a nation growing more urban and more crowded, most Americans began to accept the idea that what little wilderness remained should be preserved. By the year 2000, the wilderness system incorporated 95 million acres of roadless areas.

The Liberal Warren Court

Just as the government's executive branch responded to pressures for reform, so did the judicial branch. Dwight Eisenhower did not expect liberal leadership from Earl Warren when he named him Chief Justice of the U.S. Supreme Court in 1953. As California's secretary of state, Warren had helped implement the internment of Japanese Americans during World War II, but he later came to regret that policy. The Warren Court produced the unanimous 1954 school desegregation case, *Brown v. Board of* Education (see Chapter 25), and steadily expanded the constitutional definition of individual rights. This shift in interpreting the law reached even those deemed to have lost many of their rights: prisoners. *Gideon v. Wainwright* (1963) established the right of indigent prisoners to legal counsel, and *Escobedo v. Illinois* (1964) confirmed the right to counsel during interrogation, a critical hindrance to the use of torture. After *Miranda v. Arizona* (1966), police were required to inform anyone they arrested of their rights to remain silent and to speak to a lawyer. Reading suspects their "Miranda rights" became a touchstone scene for a whole generation of television police shows.

The Warren Court bolstered other rights of individuals against potentially coercive community pressures. Decisions in 1962 and 1963 strictly limited the practice of requiring prayers in public schools. In 1963 the Court narrowed standards for the definition of "obscenity," allowing freer expression in the arts but also in pornography. *Griswold v. Connecticut* (1965) established the use of contraceptive devices as a matter of private choice protected by the Constitution. In 1967 the Court heard the case of Mildred Jeter, a black woman, and Richard Loving, a white man, Virginians who had evaded their state's ban on interracial marriage by traveling to Washington, D.C., for their wedding and then returned to Caroline County to live. In the aptly titled *Loving v. Virginia,* the Court declared marriage one of the "basic civil rights of men" and overturned the laws of the last 16 states restricting interracial unions. Also in 1967 President Johnson appointed the esteemed chief National Association for the Advancement of Colored People (NAACP) legal counsel, Thurgood Marshall—who had mounted the successful argument in *Brown v. Board of Education* 13 years earlier—to the bench, making him the first black Supreme Court justice.

The Supreme Court's interpreting of the Constitution to expand individual rights disturbed many conservative Americans. They saw the Court as another arm of an intrusive national government that was extending its control over matters previously left to local communities. For them, the goal of integration did not justify the busing of school children. Rising crime rates troubled them more than police brutality. Many Roman Catholics were disturbed by the legalization of contraceptives. Incensed by the ban on requiring school prayer, Protestant fundamentalists sought redress through political involvement, which they had previously shunned, initiating a grassroots religious conservative movement that helped bring Ronald Reagan to power in 1980. The Warren Court served as a lightning rod for traditionalists' distress at changes in Americans' private behavior. In the contest between local and national authorities ongoing since the Articles of Confederation of the 1780s, the 1960s represented a high-water mark of Washington's influence in the lives of individual citizens.

Into War in Vietnam

The 1960s also marked the culmination of the U.S. government's efforts to control revolutionary political and social change abroad. The Truman Doctrine's logic of containing communism spanned the entire globe, but few imagined that the United States would overreach itself, tragically, in Vietnam. Johnson's accomplishments at home was forever overshadowed by the war he sent Americans to fight in the quiet rice paddies and beautiful highland forests of Southeast Asia. Putting U.S. combat troops into Vietnam in 1965, where they remained until 1973, drained funds and political will that could have been used to implement the Great Society more fully. The Vietnam War of these years might be better named the "American War": it reflected the beliefs and commitments of Cold Warriors in Washington more than the realities of life on the ground in Southeast Asia. An aggressive U.S. anticommunist policy abroad collided with leftist revolutionaries throughout the Third World, and it was ill fortune for the Vietnamese that this collision struck them hardest of all. "They were just in the intersection when our convertible rolled up," former Stanford University student body president and draft resistance organizer David Harris recalled.

The Vietnamese Revolution and the United States

Americans viewed the conflict in Vietnam as part of a broader struggle between communist and noncommunist nations. It did not start out that way, however. It began as one of many efforts to end European colonialism. Vietnamese nationalists, varying in ideologies but led by Ho Chi Minh and the Indochinese Communist party, sought since the 1930s to liberate their country from French colonial rule. Japanese advances during World War II put the Vietminh (Vietnamese nationalists) on the same side as the Americans, and Ho worked closely with the U.S. Office of Strategic Services (OSS), precursor to the Central Intelligence Agency (CIA). Ho declared the creation of an independent state of Vietnam on September 2, 1945, quoting at length from the American Declaration of Independence with OSS officers looking on.

Independent Vietnam did not last. After the defeat of Germany and Japan, the French wanted to regain control of their colonies in Africa and Asia, including Vietnam. Their British friends provided troop transport ships for French soldiers, and the United States provided most of the funds to support France in its war against the Vietminh (1946–1954). Cold War priorities won out: a weakened France had to be bolstered as the linchpin of a reintegrated, anticommunist western Europe, while the Vietminh were led by Communist party members. Unfortunately for Washington, the Vietnamese defeated the much more heavily armed French, capped by the climactic victory at the battle of Dien Bien Phu in May 1954, which surprised most Western observers. Two months later, the Geneva Accords divided the country temporarily at the seventeenth parallel until national elections could be held within 2 years to reunify Vietnam. Like the thirty-eighth parallel in Korea, the seventeenth parallel was an arbitrary latitude on the map used to divide peoples who did not want to be separated. Ho's forces solidified their control of the north, the French pulled out entirely, and the Eisenhower administration made a fateful decision to intervene directly to preserve the southern part of Vietnam from communism. The United States created a new government led by the Roman Catholic, anticommunist Ngo Dinh Diem in a new country called "South Vietnam." "This is our offspring," Senator John Kennedy observed of the rulers in the capital city of Saigon, but most Americans still knew nothing about South Vietnam.

The Vietnamese Revolution was only half over, however. The French colonialists withdrew, but the Saigon regime ignored the Geneva Accords and the promise of elections to reunify the country. In the north, the internal revolution for the creation of a socialist society proceeded with an extensive program of land redistribution. In the south, Diem ruled for 8 years with increasing repression of communists and other dissenters. U.S. funding kept him in power. One reporter noted that "Diem could not have survived a week without foreign aid." Desperate in the face of Diem's secret police, southern members of the old Vietminh began a sabotage campaign against the Saigon government and formed the National Liberation Front (NLF) in 1960, with the support of the government of North Vietnam in Hanoi. Diem and his American supporters called them Viet Cong or VC, roughly equivalent to the derogatory American term *Commies*. As the struggle to overthrow Diem intensified in the early 1960s, President Kennedy increased the number of U.S. military personnel from the 800 under Eisenhower to 16,000. They made little difference, however, as the unpopular Saigon government continued to lose ground to the NLF guerrillas. Just 3 weeks before Kennedy's murder, several of Diem's own generals assassinated him with the tacit support of U.S. officials in South Vietnam and Washington.

> *As the struggle to overthrow Diem intensified in the early 1960s, President Kennedy increased the number of U.S. military personnel from the 800 under Eisenhower to 16,000.*

Johnson's War

Lyndon Johnson inherited his predecessors' commitment to preserving a noncommunist South Vietnam. Bolstered by Kennedy's hawkish advisers, especially Secretary of Defense Robert McNamara (1961–1968), he believed that American credibility was at stake. But Johnson faced a swiftly deteriorating military situation. The NLF, which the administration portrayed as

Wars and Social Reform in the Twentieth Century

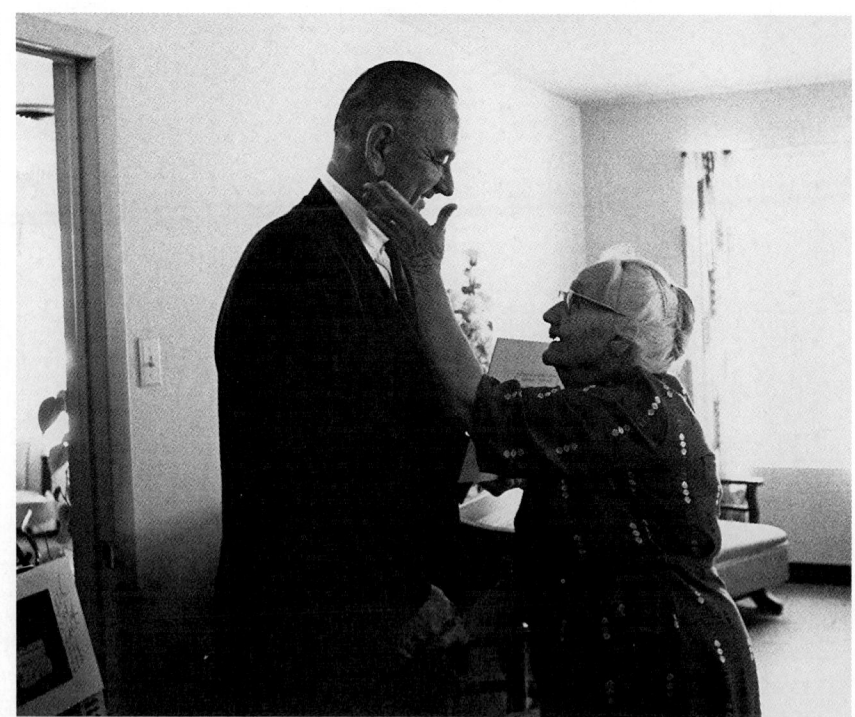

An elderly woman thanks President Johnson for signing the Medicare bill, which provided health care benefits for Americans over age 65 through the Social Security program. The bill, which became effective in July 1966, incorporated parts of the program of national health care proposed by President Truman in 1949.

CORBIS

Lyndon Johnson knew that in going to war in Vietnam, he risked losing public support and congressional funding for his Great Society programs. Yet he felt he had little choice. Facing the growing success of the communist-led insurgency in South Vietnam, the president believed that he had to escalate U.S. involvement there to continue preserving a noncommunist part of Vietnam. That policy had been a commitment of every American president since late in World War II: Franklin Roosevelt, Harry Truman, Dwight Eisenhower, and John Kennedy. Johnson also feared the conservative Republican domestic backlash that he believed would follow a U.S. withdrawal from Southeast Asia and the "fall" of another Asian nation to communist rule. "That bitch of a war" in Vietnam, he said, was forcing him to leave "the woman I really loved—the Great Society."

Johnson's was not the first presidential administration in the twentieth century to find that military conflicts abroad constrained and even derailed domestic efforts at social and political reform. Three other Democratic presidents had encountered similar situations. Woodrow Wilson's Progressive reform agenda was waylaid by the onset of World War I in 1914 and his decision to lead the nation into that conflict 3 years later. Franklin Roosevelt's extensive New Deal programs to restart the ailing economy and improve an array of social ills tapered off as the United States entered World

War II in 1941, as he acknowledged by announcing that "Dr. Win the War" was replacing "Dr. New Deal." Harry Truman's "Fair Deal" reform hopes were more modest than those of Roosevelt, but they included a program of national health care and civil rights legislation. A hostile Congress effectively blocked such initiatives, but Truman's own efforts to promote them declined after he took the nation into the undeclared war in Korea in 1950.

The huge scale of mobilization to fight a major war took a single-mindedness of purpose that left little time for other concerns. Social reformers such as Martin Luther King, Jr., feared military engagements abroad for just this reason (see "Interpreting History" in this chapter). Going to war did sometimes encourage policies that increased social justice if those policies contributed to the war effort. One

example was the War Industries Board in World War I that helped mediate labor disputes and improve workplace conditions; another was the desegregation of the armed forces that happened soon after World War II (in part because of that war's rhetoric about defeating Nazi racism) and was implemented during the Korean War. But having citizens dying in battle abroad more often increased intolerance at home for dissent or diversity. The Alien and Sedition Acts in World War I, the incarceration of Japanese Americans in World War II, and the anticommunist purges led by Joseph McCarthy during the Korean War all undercut civil liberties and discouraged efforts at social reform. Johnson's diminished attention to building the Great Society after he escalated the war in Vietnam in 1965 fit in this broader pattern. ■

merely a tool of North Vietnam, was winning the political war for the south, taking control of the countryside from the demoralized Army of the Republic of Vietnam (ARVN). Faced with the choice of escalating U.S. involvement to prevent an NLF victory or withdrawing entirely from the country, Johnson escalated.

How he did so was crucially important. There was neither a national debate nor a congressional vote to declare war. Johnson did not want to distract Congress from his Great Society agenda, nor did he want to provoke the Soviet Union or China. But he believed he had to preserve a noncommunist South Vietnam or else face a debilitating backlash from Republicans, who would skewer him as McCarthy had done to Truman over the "loss" of China 15 years earlier. So the president used deception, describing offensive American actions as defensive and opening up a credibility gap between a committed government and a skeptical public. This gap widened steadily until it finally drove Johnson not to run for reelection in 1968.

In 1963–1965, while St. Louis was building its famous arch commemorating the city's history as the Gateway to the West, where so many U.S.–Indian wars had been fought, Johnson took the nation through the gateway of the Pacific into a new war in the farther west of Asia. In August 1964, North Vietnamese ships in the Gulf of Tonkin fired on the U.S. destroyer *Maddox,* which was aiding South Vietnamese sabotage operations against the North. The president portrayed the incident as one of unprovoked communist aggression, and Congress expressed almost unanimous support through its Gulf of Tonkin Resolution. With this substitute for a declaration of war, Johnson ordered American planes to begin bombing North Vietnam, and the first American combat troops splashed ashore at Da Nang in South Vietnam on March 8, 1965. In July the administration made the key decision to add 100,000 more soldiers, with more to follow as necessary.

The president also offered a piece of the Great Society to his opponents in Vietnam if they would halt their struggle. He promised a vast economic development program for the Mekong River delta "on a scale even to dwarf our" Tennessee Valley Authority. Like most of his compatriots, the president assumed that foreign peoples fundamentally wanted to be like Americans. Johnson and his advisers tended to believe that, in the words of a U.S. officer in the film *Full Metal Jacket,* "Inside every [Vietcong] there is an American trying to get out."

The carrot of American-style economic development was accompanied by the stick of U.S. military force. American strategy had two goals: to limit the war so as not to draw in neighboring China (to avoid a repeat of the Korean War) and to force the NLF and North Vietnam to give up their struggle to reunify the country under Hanoi's control. The problem was the political nature of the guerrilla war in the South: a contest for the loyalty of the population, in which NLF operatives mingled easily with the citizenry. This kind of war made the enemy difficult to find, as was often true for the British in fighting the American revolutionaries in the 1770s. Because guerrillas were like fish swimming in the sea of citizens who supported them, in Chinese leader Mao Zedong's formulation, U.S. commanders decided to drain the sea. The "strategic hamlet" program uprooted rural peasants and concentrated them in fortified towns, creating "free fire zones" in their wake where anything that moved was a target. The U.S. Air Force pounded the south as well as the north, dropping more bombs on this ancient land (smaller than either Germany or Japan) than had been used in all theaters on all sides in World War II. Under Operation Ranch Hand, American planes used defoliants such as Agent Orange to remove ground cover, rendering one-seventh of the south's land uninhabitable. Their informal slogan was "Only We Can Prevent Forests."

These tactics destabilized and traumatized society in South Vietnam as one-fourth of the population became refugees. The American war urbanized the south by force: from 85 percent rural in 1965, it became 65 percent urban by 1974. The strategy of attrition wielded by General William Westmoreland, the commander of U.S. forces in Vietnam, also alienated the citizenry of the South. Lacking a clear military front in a guerrilla conflict, U.S. commanders used body counts of enemy dead as a primary method of demonstrating progress in the war. This strategy created great pressure on officers to produce bodies. In a war where Americans had difficulty distinguishing the enemy from noncombatants, a new rule became increasingly standard: "If it's dead and Vietnamese, it's VC."

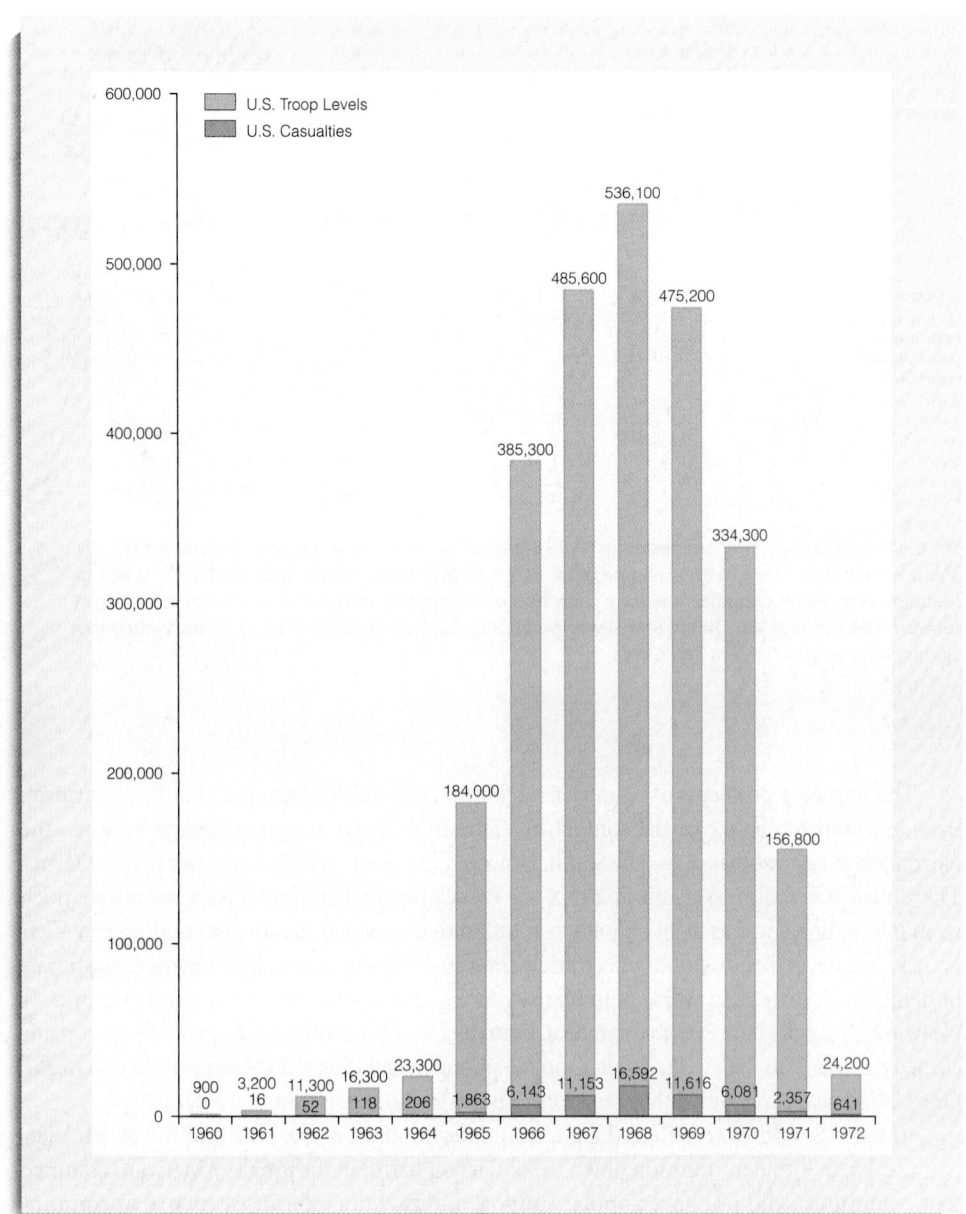

Americans in Southeast Asia

Given America's wealth, size, and superior weaponry, most U.S. soldiers who went to Vietnam in 1965–1966 had no doubt they would win the war. Their confidence reflected generations of American successes on battlefields across Europe and the Pacific Ocean. As emissaries from a culture that valued material wealth and technological sophistication, they tended to dismiss Vietnamese people as primitive and weak. They typically looked down on Asians. Very few knew anything about Vietnamese history or culture, and almost none spoke the Vietnamese language. This war, unlike World War II of their parents' generation, had no D-Day on the beaches of France as in 1944, with a staging across the narrow channel in familiar England. Although a small number of Americans worked closely with their South Vietnamese allies, most GIs encountered Vietnamese in subservient roles as laundry workers, prostitutes, waitresses, and bartenders. Blinkered by anticommunism and far removed from their own revolutionary roots, Americans from the top brass to the lowest "grunts" marched into a country they did not understand but assumed they could control.

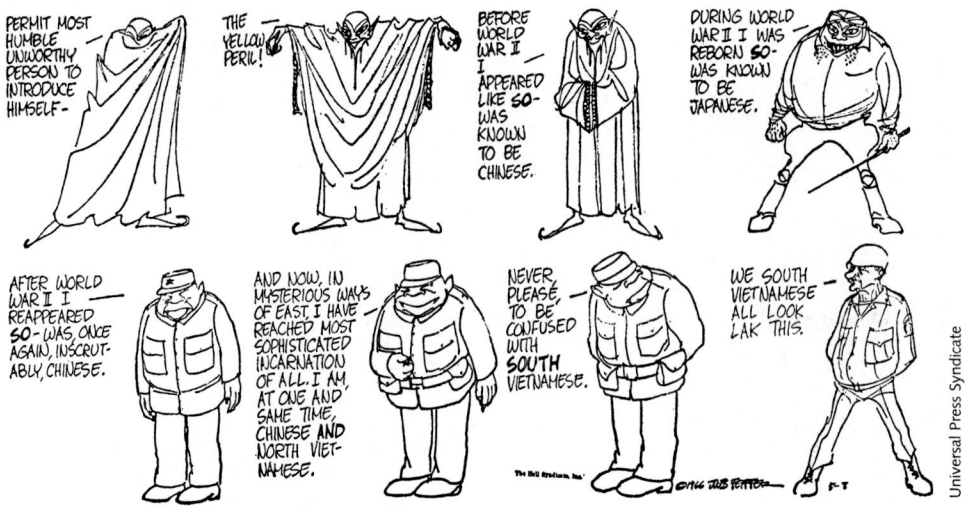

Universal Press Syndicate

■ Cartoonist Jules Fieffer suggested in 1966 some of the ongoing confusion of many Americans about Asia and its many nations and peoples, and why the United States was involved in a war in Vietnam. Anti-Asian prejudice had long contributed to problems in U.S.–Asian relations. President Johnson claimed that the United States was protecting the lives and interests of South Vietnamese against both North Vietnam and China.

The immense problems of counterinsurgent warfare quickly put an end to this optimism. President Johnson spoke of the conflict in Vietnam as a case of one sovereign nation—the North—invading another one—the South. However, few Vietnamese saw the war in those terms. The United States, dismissing the failure of the French before them, had intervened not so much in an international war as in an ongoing revolution that aimed to reunify the country. Few Vietnamese, whatever their opinions of communism, viewed the corrupt Saigon regime as legitimate or democratic. After all, it was kept in place by foreigners, whereas the North was ruled by people who had expelled the French foreigners. Even the U.S. Embassy admitted privately that "if any elected assembly sits in Saigon, it will be on the phone negotiating with Hanoi within one week." One U.S. sergeant concluded that "anticommunism is a lousy substitute for democracy."

Initial U.S. optimism reflected a grave underestimation of the NLF and the North Vietnamese. From President Johnson down to soldiers on patrol in the jungle, Americans assumed that communists did not have popular support and that the inferior weaponry of communist forces could not withstand the firepower of the world's strongest military, which dominated the air and the surrounding sea. These assumptions were fatal miscalculations. Ho Chi Minh was an extremely popular leader, and intervention from the other side of the world only strengthened his position. As the war expanded, NLF recruiting in the south snowballed, and the people of North Vietnam remained loyal to their authoritarian government.

Communist forces proved willing to endure fantastic hardship and sacrifices to prevail, some even living underground in the labyrinthine tunnels of Cu Chi to avoid U.S. bombs. Their morale was much higher than that of the ARVN. Superior organization and commitment enabled them to overcome their technological deficit, and small victories hardened their resolve. The NLF in the south had long armed itself with U.S. weapons captured from the ARVN, declaring that "Ngo Dinh Diem will be our supply sergeant." After Diem's death, American weapons poured into the country at an increasing rate, but the tenacity of the NLF prompted the Soviets and the Chinese to provide antiaircraft guns and other vital military assistance to the north.

Who were the 3 million Americans who went to Vietnam? The initial forces contained experienced soldiers, but as the war escalated this professional army was diluted with hundreds of thousands of young draftees. Student deferments protected more comfortable Americans, so GIs were predominantly those who lacked money and education. Although 70 percent

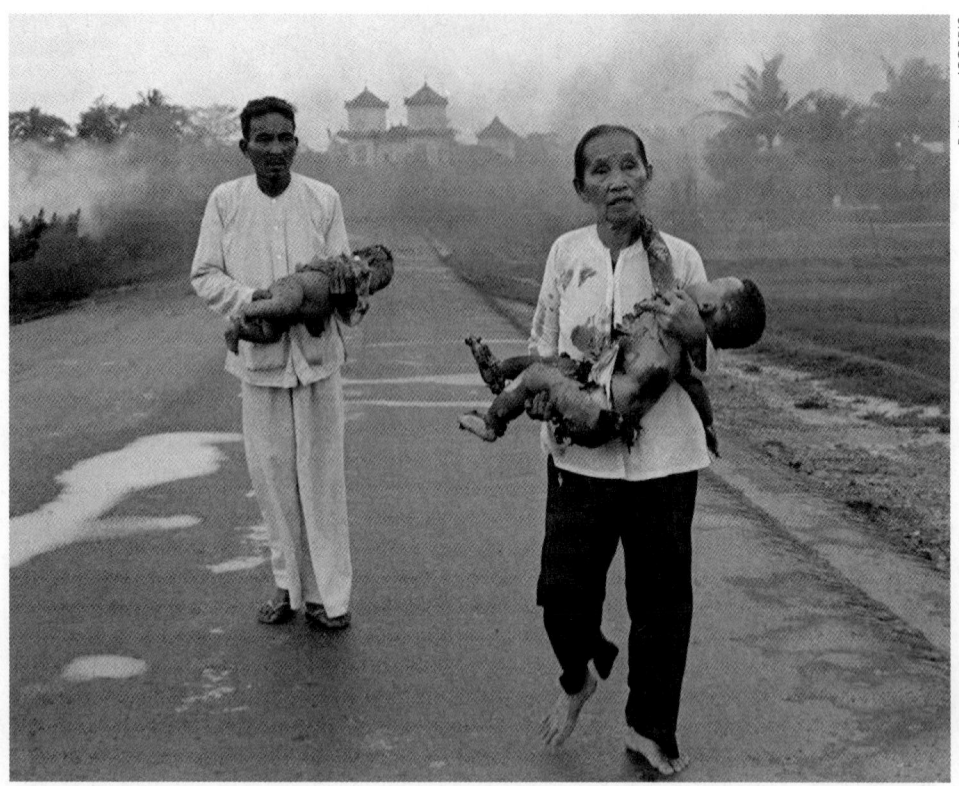

Bettmann/CORBIS

■ Vietnamese villagers flee from an accidental U.S. napalm raid 26 miles southwest of Saigon in the Mekong River delta. U.S. Air Force planes dominated the skies above Vietnam, dropping conventional bombs and antipersonnel weapons such as napalm over both the North and the South. At least 2 million Vietnamese died, many of them civilians caught in the crossfire of a guerrilla war, but sheer destructiveness was unable to win the war for the United States.

were white men, black, Hispanic, and Native American enlistees shipped out in disproportionate numbers. It became a teenaged army, filled with 18-year-olds whose main aim, one ABC correspondent reported, "was to become 19." In sharp contrast to the motives of the NLF and the North Vietnamese army, these young men (along with 10,000 women who volunteered as nurses) were not in Vietnam to win the war regardless of the cost or duration. They had only to survive 12 months before returning home to the safety of a peacetime society. There could hardly have been a sharper contrast between this undeclared war and the total mobilization of the United States in a declared war such as World War II.

Only a small fraction of the American personnel in Southeast Asia experienced actual combat. Most worked in the extensive support systems on bases in rear areas, where daily life was safer and more comfortable. Those who fought in the jungles and rice paddies lived in extreme peril. North Vietnamese regular army units came south to match the growing number of U.S. forces, and they occasionally engaged the Americans in large set battles, as at Ia Drang valley in the fall of 1965. U.S. troops fought well in such firefights, making devastating use of their superior weapons and air power. However, the bulk of the fighting consisted of smaller engagements with deceptive enemies on their home turf who faded in and out of the civilian population with ease. Ambushes and unexpected death haunted Americans on patrol, and relentless heat and humidity wore them down.

American soldiers felt mounting frustration and rage over the nature of the war that they were ordered to fight. Lacking a clear battlefront and an understandable strategy for winning the war, they were commanded simply to kill the often mysterious enemy. Yet distinguishing civilians from combatants in a popular guerrilla war was not always easy, especially when so many civilians evidently supported the NLF and so few Americans spoke Vietnamese. "How can you tell the enemy?" one GI asked. "They all look the same." The U.S. ally, the ARVN, was riddled with NLF infiltrators and rarely fought effectively. Realizing that few of the people they were supposed to be defending actually wanted them there but under orders to produce enemy bodies, U.S. troops on the ground began to slide toward a racial war against

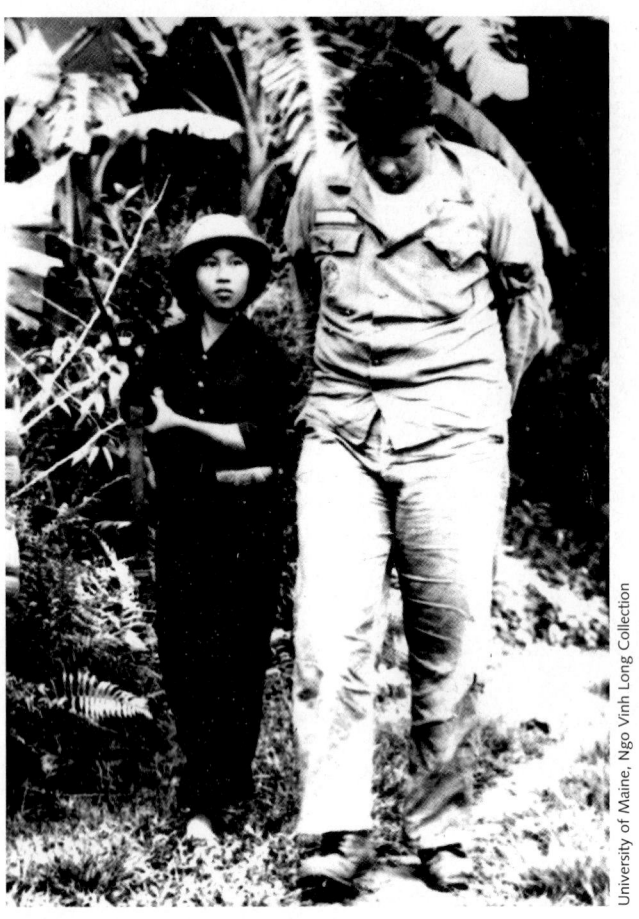

University of Maine, Ngo Vinh Long Collection

■ A North Vietnamese militia fighter named Kim Lai escorts an American pilot whom she captured after his plane crashed over the North. American GIs often were struck by the diminutive size of the average Vietnamese in comparison to the average American. Bigger, better equipped, and much more well armed than their opponents, most U.S. soldiers and officers before 1968 went into the field in Vietnam certain that they would be victorious.

all Vietnamese. "You can't have a feeling of remorse for these people," said one Marine. "I mean, like I say, they are an enemy until proven innocent."

Many GIs resisted this logic, sometimes showing real kindness to Vietnamese civilians. But atrocities on both sides inevitably followed from this kind of war. The worst came in the village of My Lai on March 16, 1968, where 105 soldiers from Charlie Company—enraged by the recent deaths of several comrades in ambushes—slaughtered, often after torturing or raping, more than 400 Vietnamese women, children, and old men. The Army covered up the massacre for a year and a half, and eventually found only Lieutenant William Calley, the leader of Charlie Company's First Platoon, guilty of murdering Vietnamese civilians. Public sympathy for him as a scapegoat for the failings of U.S. military strategy encouraged President Nixon to reduce Calley's sentence of life imprisonment to 3 years. Americans at home were horrified when grim photographs appeared in *Life* magazine, but those who knew the war up close were not surprised. "The people back in the world don't understand this war," one GI in Vietnam bitterly told a reporter. "We are here to kill dinks. How can they convict Calley for killing dinks? That's our job."

1968: The Turning Point

In late 1967 the public face of the war effort remained upbeat, as General Westmoreland declared that he could now see "some light at the end of the tunnel." But other prominent members of the administration, including Secretary of Defense McNamara, were beginning to express doubts privately to the president. Any remaining hopes of an imminent victory were crushed by the startling Tet Offensive (named for the Vietnamese New Year) that began on January 30, 1968. NLF insurgents and North Vietnamese troops attacked U.S. strongholds throughout South Vietnam, even occupying the courtyard of the U.S. Embassy for 6 hours. This risky tactic paid off for the communists with enormous political gains, despite military losses. U.S. troops killed thousands of their enemy as they ended and then reversed the advances of Tet. But the blow to American public confidence in Johnson and his military commanders proved irreversible. Far from being on the verge of defeat, as the administration had been claiming, the communists had shown that they could mount simultaneous attacks around the country. Revered television newscaster Walter Cronkite announced that "we are mired in stalemate" in Vietnam.

The Tet Offensive coincided with two other crises in early 1968 to convince American political and business elites that U.S. international commitments had become larger than the nation could afford. First, a week before Tet began, the North Korean navy seized the U.S. intelligence ship *Pueblo* in the Sea of Japan and temporarily imprisoned its crew. U.S. commanders were left scrambling to find enough forces to respond effectively without weakening American commitments in Europe and elsewhere. Second, a British financial collapse devalued the pound and caused the London government to announce its imminent withdrawal from its historic positions east of the Suez Canal, placing new military burdens on the United States in the Middle East. These events reduced international confidence in the U.S. economy, causing a currency crisis in March 1968 as holders of dollars traded them in for gold. The chairman of the Federal

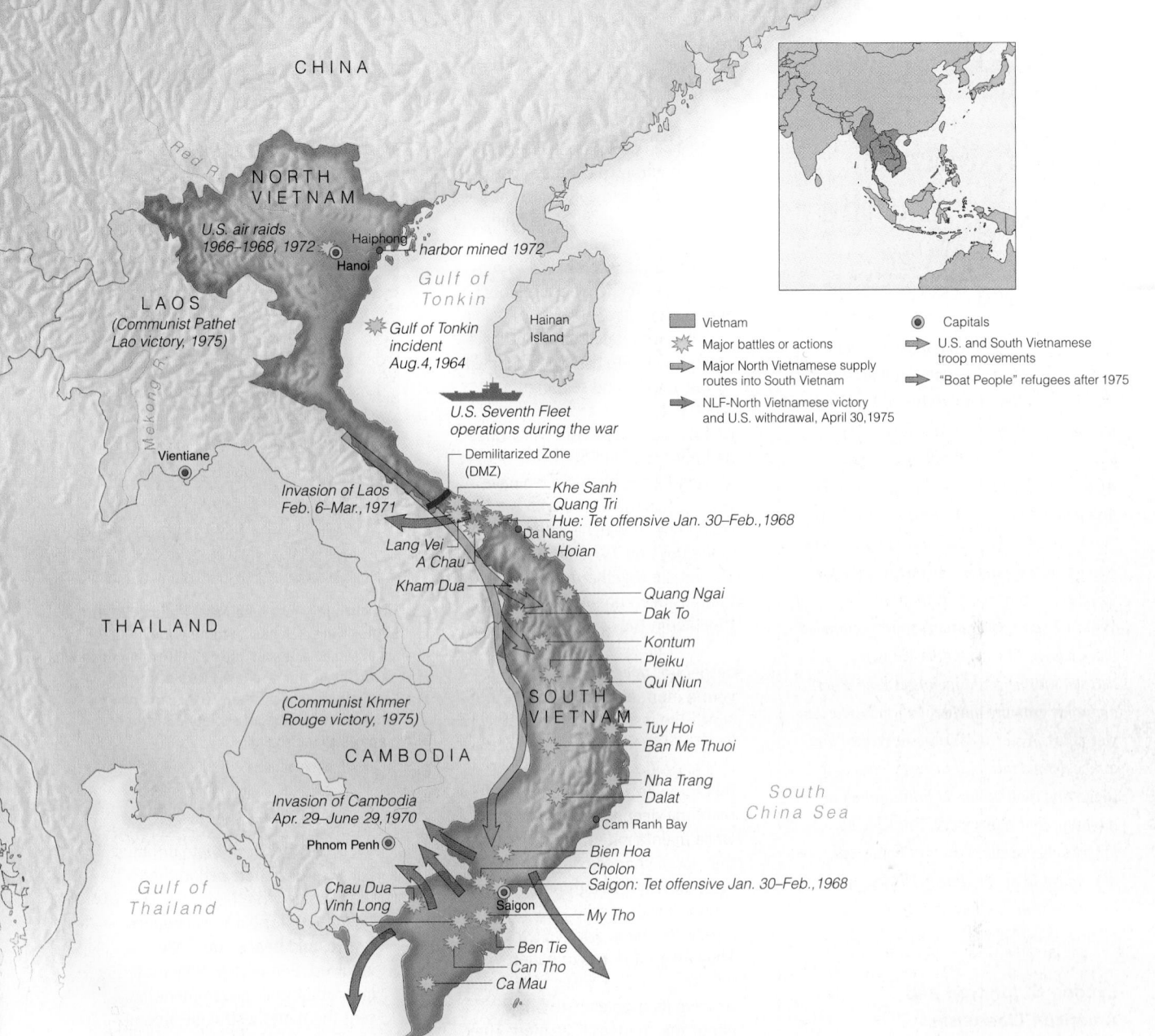

CHINA

NORTH
VIETNAM

*U.S. air raids
1966–1968, 1972*

Haiphong

harbor mined 1972

Hanoi

*Gulf of
Tonkin*

LAOS
*(Communist Pathet
Lao victory, 1975)*

*Gulf of Tonkin
incident
Aug. 4, 1964*

Hainan
Island

Vientiane

*U.S. Seventh Fleet
operations during the war*

— Demilitarized Zone
(DMZ)

*Invasion of Laos
Feb. 6–Mar., 1971*

Khe Sanh
Quang Tri
Hue: Tet offensive Jan. 30–Feb., 1968

Da Nang

*Lang Vei
A Chau*
Hoian

Kham Dua

Quang Ngai
Dak To

THAILAND

Kontum
Pleiku
Qui Niun

SOUTH
VIETNAM

*(Communist Khmer
Rouge victory, 1975)*

Tuy Hoi
Ban Me Thuoi

CAMBODIA

Nha Trang
Dalat

*South
China Sea*

*Invasion of Cambodia
Apr. 29–June 29, 1970*

Cam Ranh Bay

Phnom Penh

Bien Hoa
Cholon
Saigon: Tet offensive Jan. 30–Feb., 1968

*Gulf of
Thailand*

*Chau Dua
Vinh Long*

Saigon

My Tho

Ben Tie
Can Tho
Ca Mau

Legend:
- Vietnam
- ☆ Major battles or actions
- ⇨ Major North Vietnamese supply routes into South Vietnam
- ⇨ NLF–North Vietnamese victory and U.S. withdrawal, April 30, 1975
- ◉ Capitals
- ⇨ U.S. and South Vietnamese troop movements
- ⇨ "Boat People" refugees after 1975

■ MAP 26.2

THE AMERICAN WAR IN VIETNAM Before U.S. combat troops entered Vietnam in 1965, few Americans knew where this Southeast Asian country was. Vietnam's geography and place names quickly became familiar in the United States as hundreds of thousands of young Americans served there and some 58,000 died there. Vietnam's elongated shape, its borders with Cambodia and Laos, and its proximity to China all affected the course of the fighting for Americans between 1965 and 1973.

Reserve Board warned Wall Street leaders of "either an uncontrollable recession or an uncontrollable inflation" as fears rose of another 1929. Financial leaders added their powerful voices to those of other dismayed Americans demanding a deescalation of the war.

The political career of Lyndon Johnson was a final casualty of these events. His support on the left withered as the antiwar and black power movements expanded. Meanwhile, his more centrist supporters were joining the backlash against civil rights, urban violence, and antiwar protesters, peeling off to the Republican party. On March 12 antiwar challenger Senator Eugene McCarthy of Minnesota nearly defeated the incumbent president in the New Hampshire Democratic primary. Johnson's vulnerability was obvious. Senator Robert Kennedy of New York joined the race 2 weeks later. In a televised speech on March 31 that caught the divided nation by surprise, Johnson announced an end to U.S. escalations in the war, the start of negotiations in

Martin Luther King, Jr., and the Vietnam War

Most Americans approved of the war in Vietnam until at least 1968. Appreciative of Lyndon Johnson's commitment to reduce poverty and end racial discrimination at home, African Americans generally supported the president's policies in Southeast Asia. However, younger, more radical civil rights workers were among those who opposed the first insertion of U.S. combat troops in 1965. Within 2 years, the nation's most prominent black leader, Martin Luther King, Jr., decided that he could no longer keep quiet about his growing unease with the American war effort. A storm of criticism greeted his public denunciation of the war, most of it suggesting that he should limit himself to domestic civil rights work. But King no longer believed that events at home and abroad could be separated. The following excerpt is from his speech at Riverside Church, New York City, April 4, 1967:

Lyndon B. Johnson and American Liberalism

A few years ago there was a shining moment in that struggle [against poverty and discrimination]. It seemed as if there was a real promise of hope for the poor—both black and white—through the Poverty Program. There were experiments, hopes, new beginnings. Then came the build-up in Vietnam and I watched the program broken and eviscerated as if it were some idle political plaything of a society gone mad on war. . . . I was increasingly compelled to see the war as an enemy of the poor and to attack it as such . . . .

We were taking the black young men who had been crippled by our society and sending them 8,000 miles away to guarantee liberties in Southeast Asia which they had not found in Southwest Georgia and East Harlem. So we have been repeatedly faced with the cruel irony of watching Negro and white boys on TV screens as they kill and die together for a nation that has been unable to seat them together in the same schools . . . .

As I have walked among the desperate, rejected and angry young men [in the ghettos of the North the last three summers] I have told them that Molotov cocktails and rifles would not solve their problems. I have tried to offer them my deepest compassion while maintaining my convictions that social change comes most meaningfully through non-violent action. But they asked—and rightly so—what about Vietnam? They asked if our own nation wasn't using massive doses of violence to solve its problems, to bring about the changes it wanted. Their questions hit home, and I knew that I would never again raise my voice against the violence of the oppressed in the ghettos without having first spoken clearly to the greatest purveyor of violence in the world today—my own government . . . .

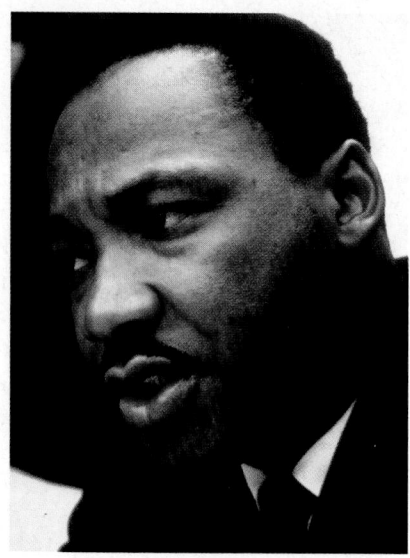

His birthday now a national holiday, Martin Luther King, Jr., has become widely accepted as a heroic figure in the American past. But in the last few years of his life, King's increasingly sharp criticisms of injustice in American society disturbed many fellow citizens.

[Our troops in Vietnam] must know after a short period there that none of the things we claim to be fighting for [such as freedom, justice, and peace] are really involved. Before long they must know that their government has sent them into a struggle among Vietnamese, and the more sophisticated surely realize that we are on the side of the wealthy and the secure while we create a hell for the poor. ∎

Source: Bruce J. Schulman, *Lyndon B. Johnson and American Liberalism* (Boston: Bedford, 1995), 208–212.

Paris with North Vietnam, and an end to his own career: "I shall not seek, and I will not accept, the nomination of my party for another term as your President."

The Movement

While national leaders were defending what they called the "frontiers of freedom" abroad, young Americans in the mid- and late 1960s organized to expand what they considered to be the frontiers of freedom at home. Television for the first time tied

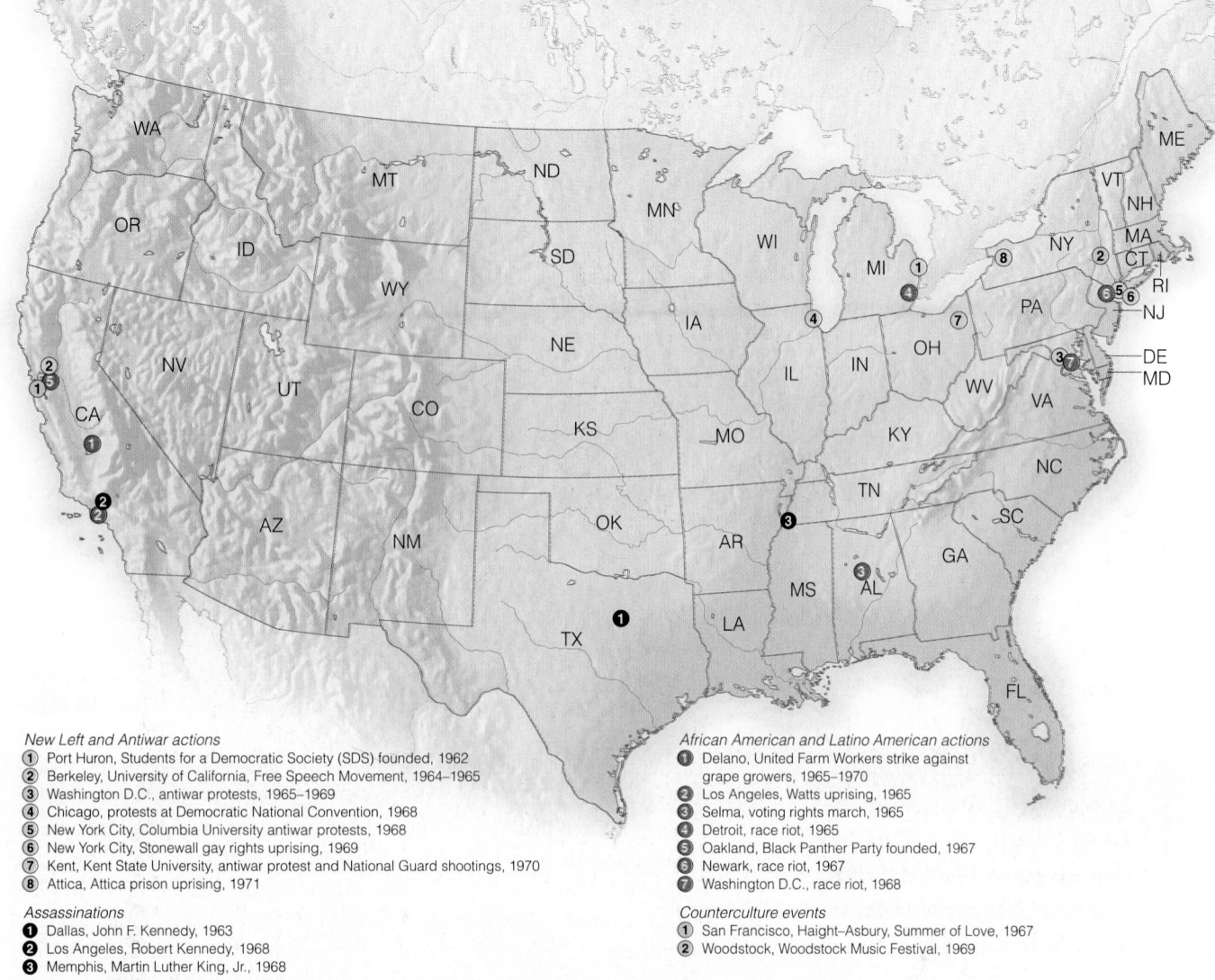

■ **MAP 26.3**

MAJOR SOCIAL AND POLITICAL PROTESTS, 1962–1971   While not the first decade to witness dramatic public protests, the 1960s did become synonymous with large groups of citizens—especially young ones—demanding changes in public policies that they perceived as unjust. Foremost among these groups were civil rights workers, antiwar activists, women's rights supporters, and countercultural youth. Students emerged as important agents of change in the 1960s.

the country together in a common culture whose shared images were transmitted simultaneously around the nation. Over all of the protest movements of the 1960s loomed the expanding war in Vietnam, which radicalized people who had initially been optimistic about reforming American society. Black power, the New Left, the counterculture, women's liberation, and other liberation movements often had quite divergent goals. But participants overlapped extensively and activists spoke of "the Movement" as if it were a unified phenomenon. At the heart of the youth movements of the decade lay a common quest for authenticity—a rejection of hypocrisy and a distrust of traditional authorities—that fused cultural and political protest. Few American households remained untouched.

From Civil Rights to Black Power

The black freedom struggle in the South that broke into the national consciousness so dramatically in the early 1960s inspired other activists. By 1966, however, the civil rights movement fractured as it confronted the limits of its success. It had achieved the goals of ending legal discrimination and putting southern African Americans in the voting booth, but it had not brought about a colorblind society. Racial prejudice among white conservatives remained virulent, and white liberals, such as those in the Kennedy and Johnson administrations, revealed themselves as not always trustworthy allies. Expecting only hostility from conservatives, civil rights workers were more disillusioned with what they saw as liberal betrayals.

The Justice Department and the Federal Bureau of Investigation (FBI) did little to restrain the violence of the Ku Klux Klan until the murders of white organizers Michael Schwerner and Andrew Goodman in the summer of 1964—along with black co-worker James Chaney. Two months later, at the national Democratic party convention in Atlantic City, New Jersey, Johnson crushed the effort of the biracial Mississippi Freedom Democratic party to replace the state's regular, all-white Democratic delegates. The president was determined to avoid further alienating white southern voters as he pursued a huge victory in the November elections. Even the thousand white volunteers from northern and western colleges who courageously came to Mississippi for the 1964 "Freedom Summer" wound up unintentionally alienating many younger black organizers. The confident style and skills of volunteers from Yale, Stanford, and other elite universities highlighted anew the tendency of even well-intentioned whites to try to take over and manage African Americans' lives.

The black freedom struggle for centuries had woven together elements of racial separatism with elements of integration into the larger American culture. For many younger African Americans the pendulum swung toward a need for greater independence from the white majority.

The day after he won the heavyweight boxing title in 1964, Cassius Clay announced that he was a Black Muslim and was changing his name to Muhammad Ali.

They took inspiration from Malcolm X, the fiery and eloquent minister of the Nation of Islam (Black Muslims), who until his murder in 1965 captivated listeners with denunciations of white perfidy and demands for black self-respect. The day after he won the heavyweight boxing title in 1964, Cassius Clay announced that he was a Black Muslim and was changing his name to Muhammad Ali. After fielding hostile questions from journalists at the news conference, Ali declared, "I don't have to be what you want me to be." In 1966 SNCC members began to speak of the need for "black power" rather than for the integrated "beloved community" they had initially sought in 1960.

The issue of violence loomed large in the shift from civil rights to black power. Militant spokesmen Stokely Carmichael and H. Rap Brown called for African Americans to stop turning the other cheek when confronted with white violence—to "stop singing and start swinging," as Malcolm X had put it. The Black Panther party formed in Oakland, California, in response to police brutality. The heavily armed Panthers engaged in several shootouts with police and were eventually decimated by an FBI campaign against them. White Americans were shocked by the uprisings and riots that swept through black urban communities during the summers of 1964–1968. Triggered by the actions of white police, the riots expressed the fierce frustrations of impoverished people whose lives remained largely untouched by the achievements of the civil rights struggle. The most destructive outbreaks occurred in the Watts district of Los Angeles in 1965 and in Detroit and Newark in 1967. The violence in Watts killed 34 people, wounded 1000, and destroyed $45 million of property. Ninety people died, and 4000 were injured across the country in the 1967 riots, most of them African Americans killed by police as fires and looting spread through African American neighborhoods. "Our nation is moving toward two societies, one black, one white—separate and unequal," the National Advisory Commission on Civil Disorders announced in its 1968 report.

SAY IT LOUD I'M BLACK AND I'M PROUD

The greatest significance of black power turned out to be neither its use of mostly rhetorical violence nor its unclear political agenda of black separatism. Rather, black power thrived as a cultural movement that promoted pride in African American and African history and life. The slogan "black is beautiful" captured this spirit: long degraded by their white compatriots as inferior, black Americans in the late 1960s and 1970s reversed this equation to celebrate their cultural heritage. This could be as basic as a hairstyle, the natural Afro replacing hair straightened to look like Caucasian hair. At universities new departments of African

American studies fostered the exploration of black history. Unlearning habits of public deference to whites, most African Americans began referring to themselves as "black" rather than "Negro."

Cultural black power mixed with a different kind of political black power by the late 1960s: the election of black officials. Although militant black power advocates garnered the most media attention, most African Americans supported Lyndon Johnson and used the Voting Rights Act to pursue their goals in the realm of electoral politics. In 1966, Carl Stokes of Cleveland was elected the first black mayor of a major American city. African Americans won local offices across the South, and in 1972 Andrew Young of Georgia and Barbara Jordan of Texas became the first black U.S. representatives elected from the South since Reconstruction. African American public life has blended elements of cultural nationalism with the pursuit of political integration ever since, just as a similar combination has helped define the public engagement of other Americans of color: Latinos, Asians, and Indians.

The New Left and the Struggle Against the War

In the summer of 1962 a group of young liberal college activists met at a labor union summer camp in Michigan. The Students for a Democratic Society (SDS) wrote a charter that became known as the Port Huron Statement, which called for a rejuvenation of American politics and society to replace the complacency that they saw pervading the country. Racial bigotry and poverty particularly troubled these optimistic young reformers, along with the overarching threat of nuclear destruction (highlighted anew by the missile crisis in Cuba a few months later). They hoped to become a kind of "white SNCC," promoting participatory democracy to redeem the promise of Cold War America.

SDS served as the central organization of the New Left. In contrast to the Old Left of the 1940s and 1950s, which had been obsessed with distinguishing itself from communism and the Soviet Union, the New Left considered the Cold War a mask for preserving inequalities in the United States. Communism was simply not important to these activists, nor was conservatism, which was then at its nadir. They focused instead on the behavior of the liberals who ran the U.S. government from 1961 to 1968. They developed a critique of "corporate liberalism" as promoting the interests of the wealthy and the business community far more than providing for the needs of the disadvantaged. From this perspective, communism was a red herring and anticommunism a distraction from the real problems of the nation, especially as the war in Vietnam expanded. New Leftists became, above all, anti-anticommunists.

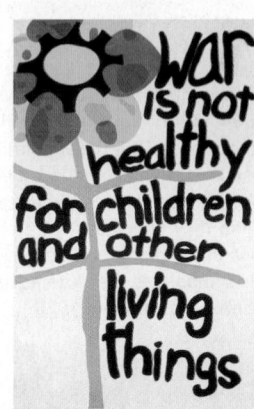

After 1965, SDS's initially broad reform agenda narrowed to stopping the Vietnam War. Protests about other issues also disrupted college campuses, such as the Free Speech Movement at Berkeley in 1964–1965; this successful effort to eliminate restrictions on students' lives set a precedent for campus activists elsewhere. But the escalation of the war moved draft-age opponents to focus on ending it. "Hell no, we won't go!" became their slogan. SDS members organized the first major antiwar protest outside the White House on April 17, 1965, bringing their organization into alliance with the small group of religious and secular pacifists already working against the war. Most importantly, mainstream Democrats began abandoning Johnson over the war as it grew. The president had alienated the powerful chair of the Senate Foreign Relations Committee, J. William Fulbright of Arkansas, with his misleading reports during the brief U.S. military intervention in the Dominican Republic in April 1965 to defeat a left-leaning but not communist coup attempt. Fulbright then held televised hearings on the American war in Southeast Asia in January 1966, raising grave doubts about its wisdom. Within a year prominent African Americans such as Martin Luther King, Jr., and Muhammad Ali joined the growing opposition to the war. Draft resistance increased as young men moved to Canada like SNCC's Bob Moses

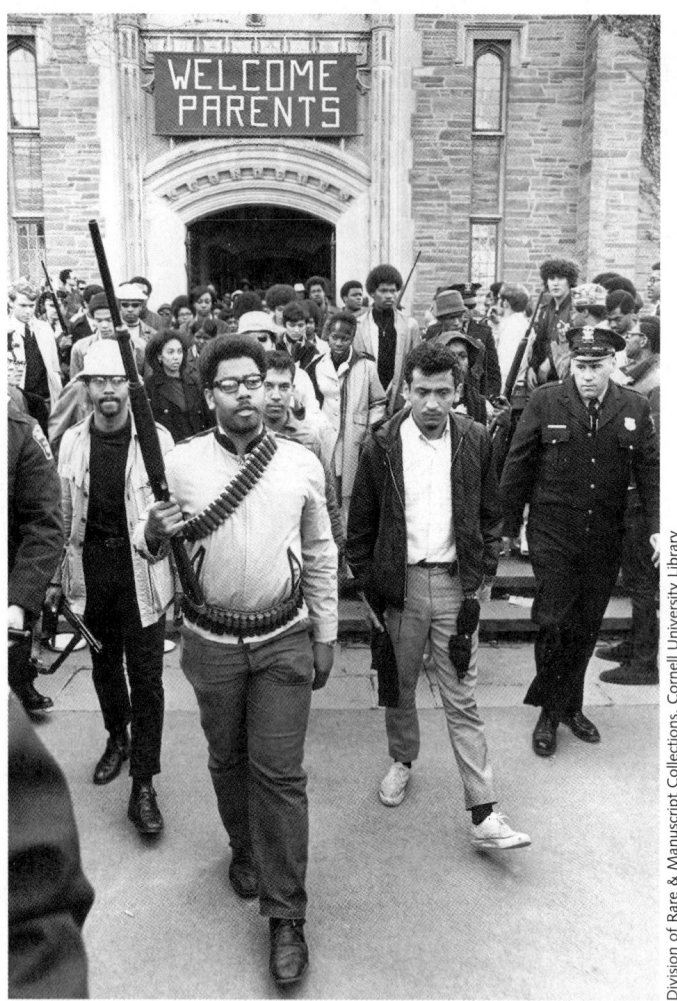

Division of Rare & Manuscript Collections, Cornell University Library

■ **African American students march out of the student union at Cornell University in April 1969** after occupying the building during the annual Parents' Weekend on campus. With the support of radical white students such as those in SDS and some faculty, the black Ivy Leaguers were protesting racial discrimination, racial threats, and a recent cross-burning on campus, and they demanded the creation of a black studies program. The weapons in the picture went unused, but their presence on university grounds symbolized the extreme divisiveness and anger in American society between 1968 and 1970.

or went to jail like Ali. "Man, I ain't got no quarrel with the Vietcong," the boxer explained.

Antiwar protesters followed the same trajectory of radicalization as black power advocates. Their dismay turned to rage as the Johnson administration continued to expand a war that was destroying much of Vietnam while killing tens of thousands of American soldiers for no reason its opponents considered legitimate. Protesters refused to be what they called "good Germans": those who had watched silently as the Nazis killed millions of Jews. Having long admired Castro's revolution in Cuba, SDS began cheering for Ho Chi Minh and imagining itself as "the NLF behind Lyndon Johnson's lines." In combination with or in support of black militants, white radicals took over buildings on university campuses in 1968–1969: Columbia, Cornell, Harvard, San Francisco State, and many others. SDS ultimately broke apart in the confusion and exhilaration of its growing demand for revolution against the larger systemic enemies, imperialism and capitalism, not just corporate liberalism. Such fantasies of violence, as well as real bombings by a splinter group called the Weather Underground, alienated most Americans, including most peaceful antiwar protesters. But radical rage could not be understood apart from the ongoing destruction of Vietnam by a government acting in the name of all Americans.

Cultural Rebellion and the Counterculture

While the New Left moved from wanting to reform American society to wanting to overthrow it, the counterculture sought to create an alternative society. Called "hippies" by those who disliked them, these young people were alienated by the materialism, competition, and conformity of American life in the Cold War. Like utopian idealists in previous centuries, they envisioned an America free from hypocrisy and artificiality. They tried to live out alternative values of gentleness, tolerance, and inclusivity. Sporting headbands, long hair, and beads, many identified with traditional Native Americans, who had repeatedly challenged the greed and deceptions of white culture from the time of Metacom and Popé in the seventeenth century. In place of junk foods, they promoted health foods; in place of profit-seeking businesses, they established co-ops. Referring to themselves as "freaks" for not fitting into "straight" society, they pursued what they saw as an authentic life. "Do your own thing" was the common slogan.

In reaction against the conformity of mainstream society, members of the counterculture explored the limitations of consciousness to expand their self-knowledge. They went beyond the nicotine and alcohol that were the common stimulants of their parents' culture to experiment with such mind-altering drugs as marijuana, peyote, hashish, LSD, cocaine, and even heroin. Spirituality was an important path into consciousness for many in the counterculture. Religious traditions associated with Asia, particularly Buddhism, gained numerous adherents, as did spiritual customs and practices of traditional Native Americans. Others rediscovered the "authentic" Jesus obscured by the institutional structures of the formal Christian church (earning themselves the nickname "Jesus freaks"); Campus Crusade for Christ, Inter-

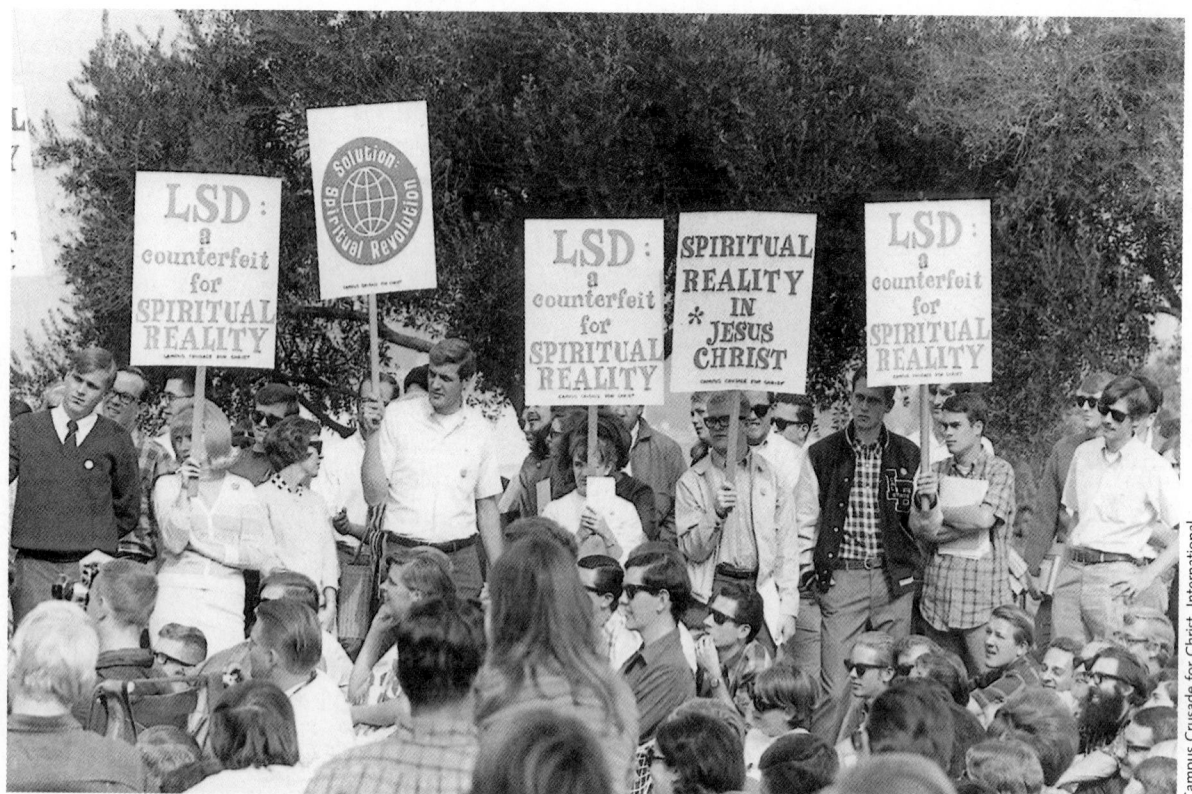

Campus Crusade for Christ, International

■ The search by many young people in the 1960s counterculture for greater consciousness led them to a spiritual path. These young evangelists held a Campus Crusade for Christ rally at the University of Texas at Austin in 1969. The emphasis of evangelical Christians on the person of Jesus rather than on a particular denominational tradition attracted many converts. The sandals, long hair, and gentleness associated with Jesus made a particularly good fit with the style and values of the "hippies," although most evangelicals appeared traditionally clean-cut and held conservative political views.

Varsity, and other evangelical college groups spread across the country. Music served as the most common coin of the countercultural realm, from the political folk sound of Joan Baez and Bob Dylan to the broadly popular Beatles and the more distinctly countercultural rock 'n' roll of the Grateful Dead and Jefferson Airplane.

By its nature the counterculture had no clear membership. Millions of American youth dabbled in it to varying extents, smoking marijuana and listening to rock 'n' roll. A much smaller, more committed group pursued the building of communities—communes—that might coexist with the quest for unrestrained individual expression. These young people were centered in the Haight–Asbury neighborhood of San Francisco until the 1967 Summer of Love, they gathered at the Woodstock music festival in upstate New York in August 1969, and they established 3500 rural communes from Vermont to New Mexico by 1970. With the nation at war against communists in Southeast Asia, critics pointed to communes at home as subversive of the nuclear family and of American capitalist values.

Older Americans experienced the counterculture largely as spectacle. The mainstream media emphasized the alternative aspects of the hippie lifestyle in its coverage. Viewers were varyingly disgusted by, attracted to, and titillated by the hair, clothing, nudity, and blurred gender distinctions. Celebrating the counterculture and its rock 'n' roll sound, the musical show *Hair* took Broadway by storm in 1968. Meanwhile, entrepreneurs realized that they could market the antimaterialist counterculture profitably. Young Americans eagerly bought up records, clothing, jewelry, and natural foods—a revealing demonstration of how consumer values pervaded American life.

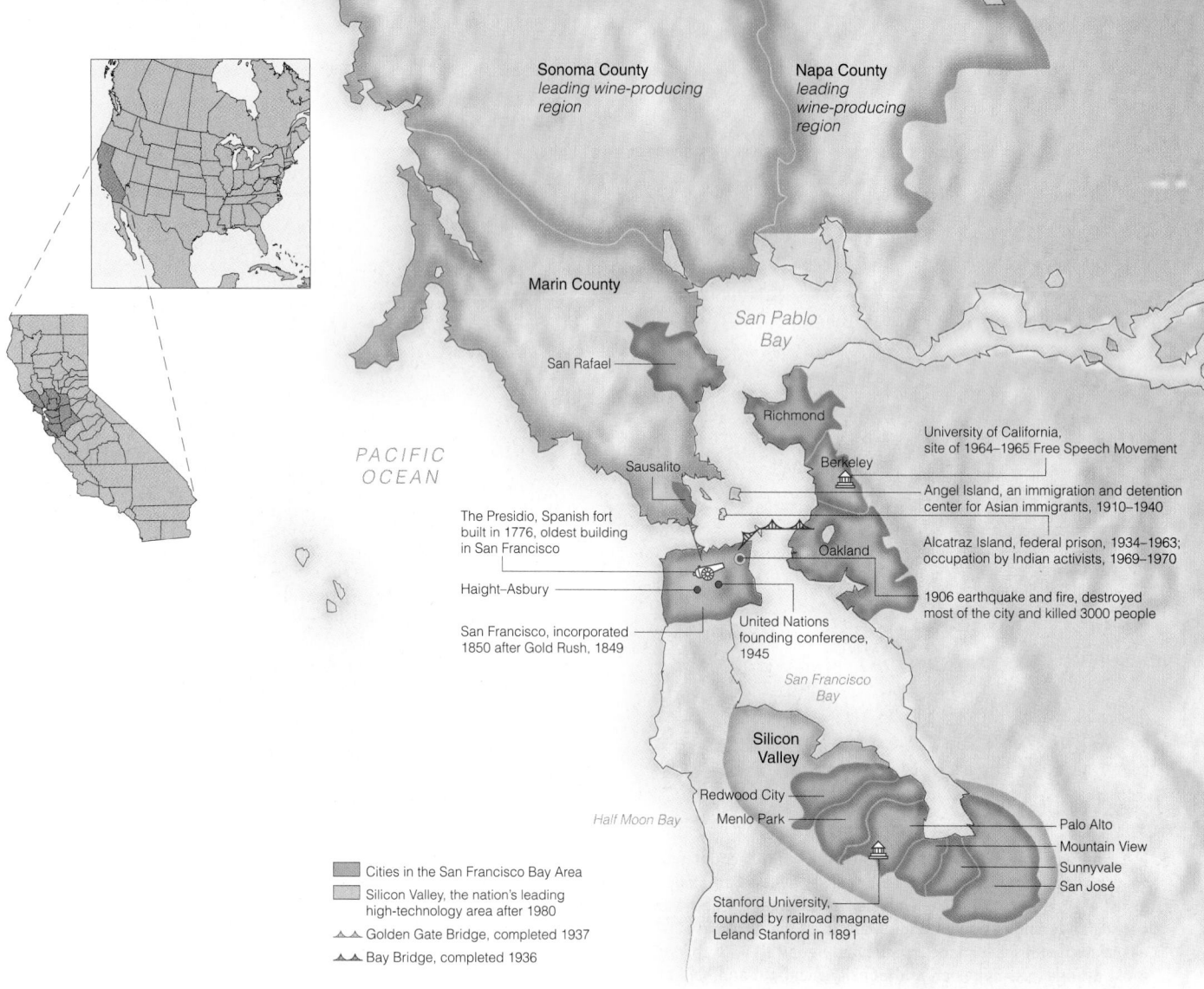

■ MAP 26.4

THE SAN FRANCISCO BAY AREA   In the 1960s California was still a bit exotic for Americans from the East and Mideast. But continuing immigration to the Golden State and the emergence of air travel in this decade as a common means of transportation tied the nation more closely together. San Francisco, or "The City" to locals, became a hub of the counterculture and rock 'n' roll music and a place known for its tolerance and celebration of diversity.

One of the most visible changes of the 1960s was often called the sexual revolution. It had earlier roots, evident in the Kinsey Reports of 1948 and 1953 and in the emergence of *Playboy* magazine's "swinger" style of the 1950s. Changes in Americans' sexual behavior in the 1960s reflected in part the counterculture's goal of living an authentic, honest life in which words matched actions. The sexual revolution removed some of the penalties for the premarital and extramarital sex that had previously been fairly common but unacknowledged. The appearance of the birth control pill in 1960 underpinned the shift to more open sexual relationships by freeing women from the fear of pregnancy. Attitudes toward abortion also became more tolerant. New York passed the first state law legalizing some abortions in 1970, and 3 years later the Supreme Court established a woman's constitutional right to abortion in the landmark case of *Roe v. Wade.* For American women the sexual revolution proved a double-edged sword. It legitimated female sexuality and helped remove the old stereotyping of women as either "madonna" (virginal until married) or "whore" (lustful and degraded). But it also created pressures from men, especially within the counterculture, for women to have sex with many partners lest they be cast as "uptight" and unliberated.

Women's Liberation

The movement for women's liberation arose in the late 1960s as a way to resist these kinds of limitations and expectations. Women's liberation built on developments earlier in the decade. In 1963 writer Betty Friedan, a former labor journalist and then homemaker, published *The Feminine Mystique*, a widely read book that captured the frustrations of many women who had accepted the role of suburban homemaker after World War II. Friedan condemned the middle-class home as a "comfortable concentration camp" for women that limited their growth as individuals with the often monotonous routines of house-work and child-rearing. Friedan and other liberal feminists founded the National Organization for Women (NOW) in 1966 to lobby against sexual discrimination in the public sphere in such areas as employment, wages, education, and jury duty. These challenges had radical implications for women's and men's earnings and thus for responsibilities within families, but NOW did not yet focus on issues inside the private sphere of the home.

The shift to the view that "the personal is political" came from younger, mostly white women who had been active in the civil rights and antiwar struggles. Inspired by the courage and successes of the protest movements in which they figured prominently, these female activists had also learned that traditional gender roles restricted them even in organizations dedicated to participatory democracy. Ironically, radical men could be as patronizing and disrespect-ful of women's abilities as mainstream men. Younger feminists in 1967 and 1968 began to organize themselves to promote their own liberation from the shackles of tra-ditional gender roles. They agreed with NOW's challenge to discrimination in the public sphere, but they focused even more on the personal politics of women's daily lives, on crit-ical issues such as parenting, child care, housework, and abortion. Feminism should liberate men as well as women, they believed, for men also had the contours of their lives unnecessarily constrained by gendered expectations. The women's liberation movement gained visibility at the 1968 Miss America contest in Atlantic City, where feminists denounced the parading of women to be "appraised and judged like animals at a county fair."

The new wave of feminism that washed through Amer-ican culture at the end of the 1960s triggered fierce debates about the nature of gender. Was there a uniquely feminine way of knowing, seeing, and acting, or were women in essence the same as men, distinguishable ultimately by their individuality? Was womanhood biologically or only cultur-ally constructed? Feminists disagreed sharply in their answers. Other differences inevitably divided a broad movement that addressed the lives of 51 percent of the entire American peo-ple. For example, NOW did not support gay rights until 1973, whereas many radical femi-nists believed lesbianism to be critical for women's full independence and autonomy. Women of color often found hierarchies of race and class more significant than those of sex; to them, as to many white working-class women, Friedan's statement that she wanted "something more than my husband and my children and my house" seemed the distant complaint of a woman of the leisure class. One's sex alone did not define one's entire identity.

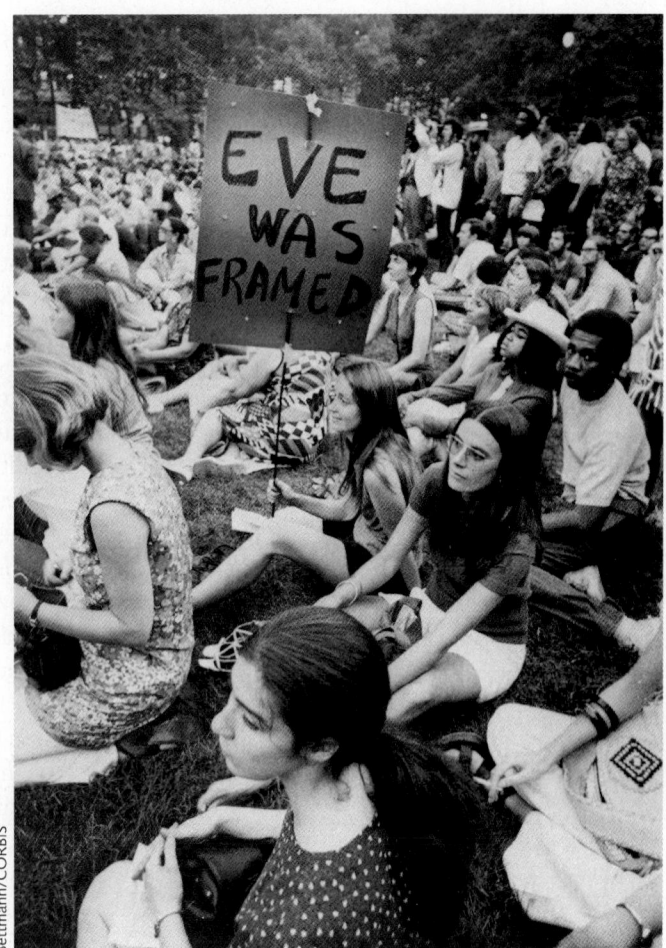

Bettmann/CORBIS

■ The new wave of organizing for women's rights that emerged in the late 1960s had many faces. Some protests against sex discrimination and disrespect for women were angry and others were gentle, as in this 1970 scene. "Raising consciousness" was a central strategy of the movement, as women and men became more aware of the gendered assumptions that had long governed—and channeled—their lives and their thoughts.

However, diversity within the feminist movement did not hide a common commitment to expanding women's possibilities. One critical aspect was the need to unlearn niceness and passivity, just as black power advocates sought to unlearn deference. White men would no longer be the sole proprietors of assertiveness; grown women would no longer be "girls" nor grown black men "boys." The women's movement that emerged out of the 1960s permanently transformed women's lives and gender relations in American society, in areas ranging from job and educational opportunities, sexual harassment, and gender-neutral language to family roles, sexual relations, reproductive rights, and athletic facilities.

The Many Fronts of Liberation

Like the women's movement, the Chicano, pan-Indian, and gay liberation movements of the late 1960s were grounded in older organizing efforts within those communities. The struggles for "brown power," "red power," and "gay power" also reflected the newer influence of black power and its determination to take pride in what the dominant American society had denigrated for so long. Activists on college campuses successfully pressured administrations to establish interdisciplinary ethnic studies programs, such as the first Chicano studies program at California State University at Los Angeles in 1968. Ethnic cultural identity went hand in hand with the pursuit of political and economic integration into mainstream American life.

The most prominent push to organize Latinos was the effort led by Cesar Chávez to build a farm workers' union in California and the Southwest. These primarily Mexican American migrant workers harvested most of the hand-picked produce that Americans ate, but their hard work under severe conditions failed to lift them out of poverty. National consumer support for boycotts of table grapes and iceberg lettuce helped win recognition for the United Farm Workers (UFW) union and better pay by 1970, despite efforts by Republicans such as President Richard Nixon and California governor Ronald Reagan to encourage grape consumption in support of large growers. Younger Mexican Americans organized to oppose the discrimination against them that remained common across the Southwest, especially in schools. They looked with pride on their Mexican heritage, even appropriating the formerly pejorative term *Chicano*. In March 1968, 10,000 youngsters walked out of their East Los Angeles schools to demand curriculum revisions that would include Latino history, recruitment of more Mexican American teachers, and an end to tracking Chicanos into vocational education classes. Two years later 20,000 people attended the Chicano Moratorium in East Los Angeles to protest the U.S. war in Vietnam.

Puerto Ricans, the largest Spanish-speaking ethnic group located primarily on the East Coast, experienced a similar growth in militancy and nationalist sentiment during the late 1960s. Since the United States annexed Puerto Rico after the end of the Spanish–American War in 1898, the Caribbean island had the unusual status of being ruled as a commonwealth of the United States while its residents were U.S. citizens who could not vote in national elections. By the 1960s more than a million islanders had moved to the East Coast, most to the New York City area. The majority came after World War II, and 47,000 served in the Vietnam War. Despite being the only Latino immigrants already holding American citizenship when they arrived, Puerto Ricans experienced similar patterns of both discrimination and opportunity as Mexican Americans. Younger Puerto Ricans formed the Young Lords in 1969 as a more militant and nationalist alternative to established Puerto Rican community organizations, one that combined pride in Puerto Rican identity and the Spanish language with leftist politics and opposition to the Vietnam War.

The most destitute of Americans, Indians also sought to reinvigorate their communities. On the Northwest coast they staged "fish-ins" in the mid-1960s to assert treaty rights, and in 1968 urban activists in Minneapolis formed the American Indian Movement (AIM). On November 20, 1969, just days after the largest antiwar march in Washington, 78 Native Americans seized the island of Alcatraz in San Francisco Bay "in the name of all American

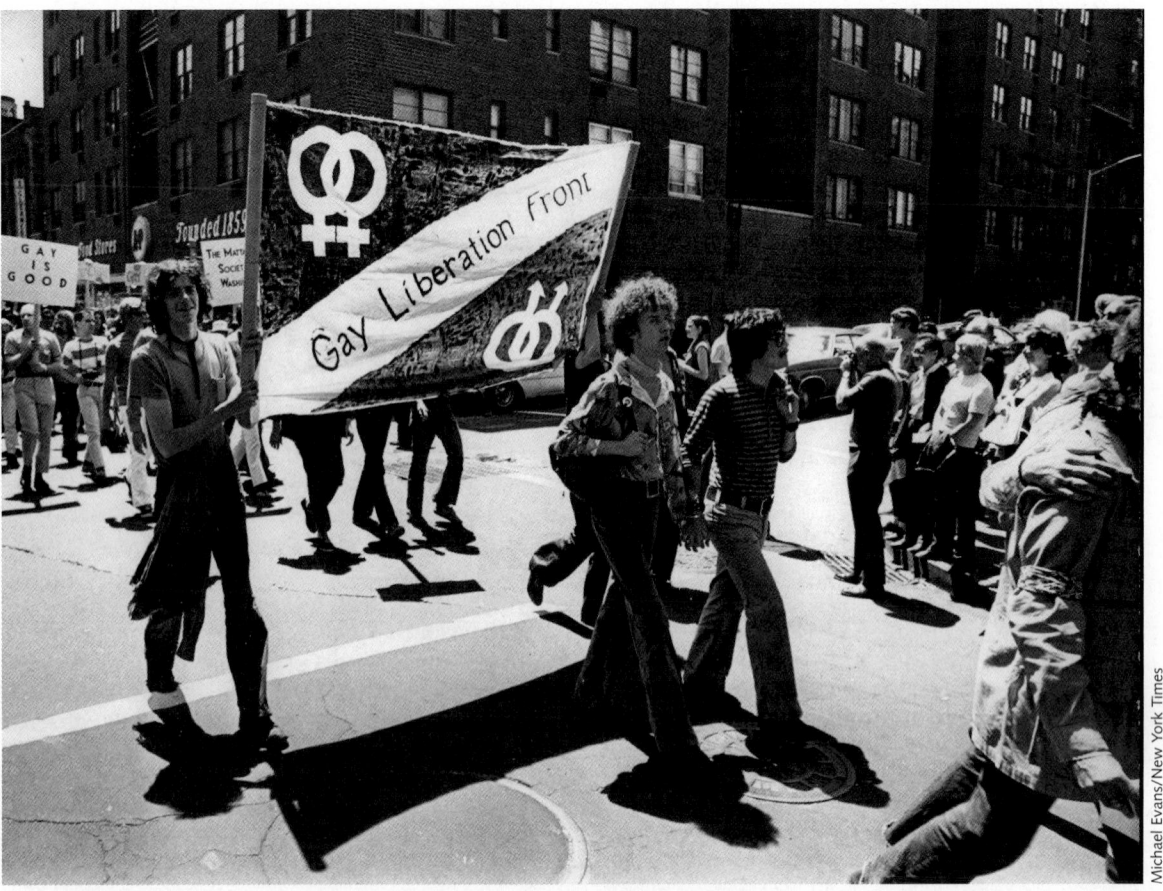

Michael Evans/New York Times

■ The first gay pride parade was a daring and hasty political protest by some 200 men and women, who walked for an hour up the Avenue of the Americas in New York City in 1970. They were taking a public stand against widespread discrimination and violence against homosexuals. Such discrimination and violence did not disappear over the next three decades, but the movement for gay rights dramatically altered the visibility and mainstream acceptance of gays and lesbians in the United States. By 1999 the gay pride parade had become a 6-hour party sponsored by the likes of Budweiser beer and United Airlines and attended by the Democratic first lady of the United States, Hillary Rodham Clinton, and the Republican mayor of New York, Rudolph Giuliani.

Indians by right of discovery." For a year and a half they used their occupation of the former federal prison site to publicize grievances about anti-Indian prejudice and to promote a new pan-Indian identity that reached across traditional tribal divisions. In 1973 armed members of AIM occupied buildings for two months at Wounded Knee near Pine Ridge, South Dakota, site of the infamous 1890 U.S. Army massacre of unarmed Sioux. AIM sought to bring down the conservative tribal government of the Oglala reservation, but the failure of that effort led to internal dissent and FBI harassment that eventually dissolved the organization. Tribal governments sought "red power" in their own quieter way. They asserted greater tribal control of reservation schools across the country. They also regained sovereignty over some lands previously lost, such as Blue Lake in northern New Mexico, which the Taos Indians reacquired.

Although they lacked a unifying ethnic identity, gay men and lesbians also found opportunities to construct coalitions in the more open atmosphere of the late 1960s. Building on the earlier but quieter community organizing of older homosexuals in New York, San Francisco, and Los Angeles, more militant youth began to express openly their anger at the homophobic prejudice and violence prevalent in American society. The demand for tolerance and respect reached the headlines when gay patrons of the Stonewall Bar in New York fought back fiercely against a typically forceful police raid on June 27, 1969. Activists of the new Gay Liberation Front emphasized the importance of "coming out of the closet": proudly acknowledging one's sexual orientation as legitimate and decent. Like "black is beautiful," this tactic represented an effort to recast the terms of one's identity apart from an ongoing tradition of prejudice. The American Psychiatric Association still listed homosexuality as a mental disorder until 1973.

The Conservative Response

The majority of Americans had mixed feelings about the protests that roiled the nation. They were impressed by the courage of many who stood up against discrimination, and by 1968 they wanted to find a way out of the war in Southeast Asia. But they were alienated by the style and values of others who loudly demanded change in American society. Moderate and conservative citizens and generations of recent European immigrants resented what they saw as a lack of appreciation for the nation's virtues and successes. Powerful backlashes developed against the counterculture, antiwar radicals, and changes in race and gender relations. The political and social upheavals of 1968 opened the door to a Republican return to the White House, and Richard Nixon slipped through.

Backlashes

The backlash first developed in response to the increasing assertiveness of people of color. European Americans in every part of the United States had long been accustomed to deference from nonwhites and racial segregation, either by law in the South or by custom elsewhere. Conservatives resented what they considered to be black ingratitude at the civil rights measures enacted by the federal government, including black power's condemnation of whites as "crackers" and "honkies." Urban riots and escalating rates of violent crime, along with the Supreme Court's expansion of the rights of the accused, deepened their anger. They associated crime with urban African Americans, for although whites were still the majority of criminals, blacks (like any other population with less money) were disproportionately represented in prisons. Many in the white working class feared that desegregating schools and neighborhoods would lead to a decline in their property values. While keeping darker-skinned Americans economically and socially subordinated, most whites still expected them to want to emulate mainstream white American society. Leaders such as Cesar Chávez and Martin Luther King, Jr., were devout Christians who emphasized equality and nonviolence, and many whites admired them. But the rise of often angry nonwhite nationalism dismayed most European Americans. They were troubled by the militancy of Chicanos in the Southwest, Puerto Ricans in the Northeast, Indians on reservations and in cities, and African Americans almost everywhere.

The backlash was not only about race. It also represented a defense of traditional hierarchies against the cultural rebellions of the 1960s. Proud of their lives and values, conservatives rejected a whole array of challenges to American society. Raised to believe in respecting one's elders, they resented the disrespect of many youth, who warned, "Don't trust anyone over 30." A generation that had fought and sacrificed in the "good war" against the Nazis found the absence of patriotism among many protesters unfathomable. The United States remained one of the most religious of industrialized societies, and conservative churchgoers emphasized obedience to authorities. They feared the effects of illegal drugs on their children. They resented being told that their assumptions about the roles and behavior of men and women, on which they had built their daily lives, were wrong. They did not want to argue about the behavior of the U.S. government; "America: Love It Or Leave It" became a favorite bumper sticker.

The backlash against the social changes of the 1960s contained elements of class antagonism as well. Working-class whites resented both the often affluent campus rebels and the black

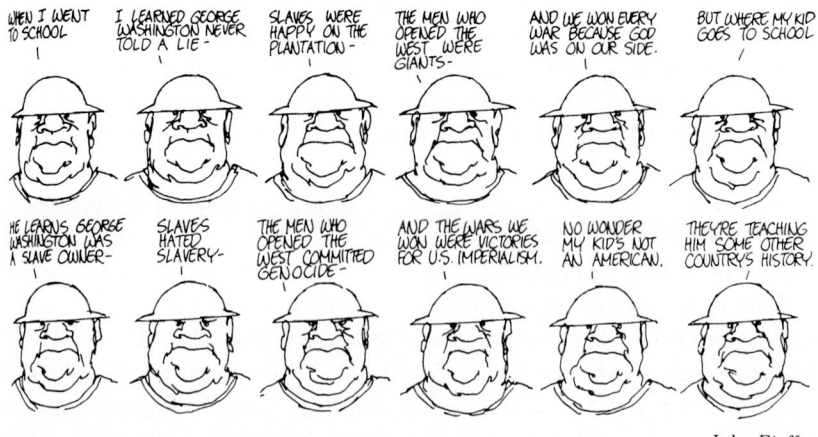

Jules Fieffer

Universal Press Syndicate

■ Cartoonist Jules Fieffer portrayed the generation gap that separated many younger Americans from many older ones by the early 1970s. Movements for black and Native American civil rights and against the U.S. war in Vietnam led to a profound shift in how many citizens, especially younger ones, understood their nation and its politics. A new generation of historians began to cast serious doubts on many long-accepted truisms about the American past.

and Latino poor targeted by some Great Society programs. They believed that their values of hard work, restraint, and respectability were increasingly unappreciated and even mocked. The counterculture's disdain for material comfort and economic security offended many older Americans of all colors who had experienced great deprivation in the 1930s. Politicians seized on these feelings of working-class alienation for political gain. Republican leaders from Goldwater to Nixon to Reagan gave voice to these resentments and drew votes away from Democratic blue-collar strongholds. Democratic governor George Wallace of Alabama also became a spokesperson for the anger of many "forgotten" whites on both sides of the Mason–Dixon line. Even television gave voice to the backlash in the likable character of Archie Bunker on *All in the Family,* a wildly popular program from its first airing in January 1971.

The Turmoil of 1968 at Home

The traumas of 1968 brought the conservative backlash to the critical stage. First came the Tet Offensive in Vietnam, creating fears that the war might become an interminable quagmire. Conservatives, like most other Americans, found it incredible that the mighty United States could not vanquish so small an enemy. Then, on April 4, just 5 days after President Johnson announced his retirement plans, a gunman named James Earl Ray assassinated Martin Luther King, Jr., in Memphis, where he had gone to support a strike by sanitation workers. King had become more openly radical in his final years, opposing the war and working on class-based organizing of poor people. But he remained the nation's leading apostle of nonviolence, and his murder evoked despair among millions of citizens, especially African Americans. Police battled rioters and arsonists in black neighborhoods of 130 cities across the nation, with 46 people dying in the clashes. National Guard troops ringed the White House as smoke from hundreds of fires rose over Washington, D.C.; large parts of the nation's capital looked like a war zone.

Summer brought more shocking news. Robert Kennedy's entry into the presidential campaign inspired renewed hopes among Democratic liberals. The charismatic senator turned against the war in Vietnam, and, unlike Eugene McCarthy, he seemed like a candidate who could attract support from a wide array of Americans, white and nonwhite, young and old. On the night of his victory in the June 5 California primary,

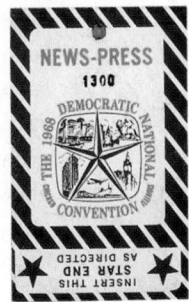

Kennedy was shot by a deranged gunman and died the next morning. Americans were stunned by this second murder of a Kennedy. Vice President Hubert Humphrey seemed assured of the nomination at the Democratic convention in Chicago in August, despite his association with Johnson's war policies. Some 10,000 antiwar activists, including hundreds of FBI *agents provocateurs* (spies seeking to provoke violence), showed up to engage in protests outside the convention. Chicago's Democratic mayor Richard Daley warned that "as long as I am Mayor, there will be law and order in the streets." Instead, he unleashed thousands of police on protesters, bystanders, and photographers in an orgy of beatings that subsequent investigations called a police riot. Ninety million Americans watched on television as a deeply divided Democratic party appeared helpless before the violence.

Into the vacuum of public anger and alienation that accompanied the liberals' self-destruction in Chicago stepped two men. George Wallace had long spoken for white Southerners resentful of the federal government and its growing support for racial equality. The spread of the conservative backlash from 1964 to 1968 gave him a wider constituency for his right-wing populist message of hostility to liberals, blacks, and federal officials. With the national Democratic party committed to racial integration, Wallace ran for president as an independent candidate and won 13.5 percent of the popular vote in November. Republican candidate Richard Nixon, fresh from a unified convention in Miami, campaigned as the candidate of "law and order" and promised that he had a secret plan to end the war in Vietnam. His contacts with the South Vietnamese government helped ensure that no last-minute breakthrough in the Paris peace talks would boost Humphrey's popularity, and the former vice president squeezed past the current one by less than 1 percent of the popular vote.

TABLE 26-2

The Election of 1968

Candidate	Political Party	Popular Vote	Electoral Vote
Richard M. Nixon	Republican	31,770,237	301
Hubert H. Humphrey	Democratic	31,270,533	191
George Wallace	American Independent	9,906,141	46

The Nixon Administration

A lonely, aloof man of great tenacity and ambition, Richard Nixon had worked hard to remake his public image for 1968. Widely viewed as a somewhat unscrupulous partisan since his early career in Congress, he had refashioned himself as a statesman with a broad vision for reducing international tensions between the great powers. Foreign policy fascinated him, and, unlike Johnson, he found domestic governance utterly dull—a matter of "building outhouses in Peoria." He won the Republican presidential nomination primarily because he bridged the gap between the party's conservative Sunbelt wing and its moderate eastern wing. He sounded like a conservative in the campaign against Humphrey, but once in the White House he governed as the most liberal Republican since Theodore Roosevelt, pressed by a Congress still controlled by Democrats.

Nowhere was this clearer than on issues related to natural resources. Much had happened to the environment since the Republican Roosevelt's conservation efforts, none of it for the better. A powerful movement was building to protect natural resources and human health from the effects of air and water pollution. Biologist Paul Ehrlich's best-selling *The Population Bomb* (1968) warned of the dire consequences of the globe's runaway growth in human population. In 1969, the government banned the carcinogenic pesticide DDT, its original usefulness against mosquito-born malaria in World War II now almost forgotten in light of its broadly toxic effects on wildlife and aquatic ecosystems. That same year a huge oil spill off Santa Barbara fouled 200 miles of pristine California beaches, and the Cuyahoga River in Cleveland, its surface coated with waste and oil, caught fire and burned for days. *Apollo 8* astronauts brought home unprecedented pictures of the earth that seemed to dramatize the vulnerability of the small blue-green planet as it hung alone in space. Environmentalists around the country proclaimed April 22, 1970, as "Earth Day."

Congress responded with legislation that mandated the careful management of the nation's natural resources. The Environmental Protection Agency was established in 1970. Amendments to the Clean Air (1970) and Clean Water (1972) acts tightened restrictions on harmful emissions from cars and factories. The Endangered Species Act (1973) created for the first time the legal right of nonhuman animals to survive, a major step toward viewing the quality of human life as inextricable from the earth's broader ecology. Nixon did not take the lead in promoting environmental laws, about which he personally cared little, telling business supporters that "in a flat choice between smoke and jobs, we're for jobs." But the president recognized the bipartisan popularity of actions to limit ecological damage, and he followed Congress's lead.

What Nixon did care deeply about at home was politics, not policy. Antiwar demonstrations reached their height during Nixon's first 2 years in the White House (1969–1970). He and Vice President Spiro Agnew loathed the protesters, whom they saw as weakening the nation. The two men pursued what Agnew called "positive polarization": campaigning to further divide the respectable "silent majority," as the president labeled his supporters, from voluble liberal Democrats in Congress and radical activists on the streets, whom they associated with permissiveness and lawlessness. In this broad cultural battle for political supremacy, the president appealed to conservative white southern and northern ethnic Democrats. His "Southern strategy" centered on opposing the use of court-ordered busing to desegregate public schools. He nominated two very conservative Southerners to the Supreme Court, only to see the Senate vote both of them down.

Early in his administration Nixon began wielding the power of the federal government to harass his political opponents. Johnson had used the FBI, the CIA, and military intelligence agencies to infiltrate and thin the ranks of antiwar demonstrators and nonwhite nationalists. Nixon continued those illegal operations, agreeing with his predecessor that radical activists constituted a threat to national security. Nixon even suggested that the nation's worst enemies were at home: "North Vietnam cannot defeat or humiliate the United States. Only Americans can do that." He went beyond other presidents in assembling an "Enemies List" that included prominent elements of the political mainstream, especially liberals, the press, and his Democratic opponents. The president was particularly concerned about controlling secret information. The Pentagon Papers were a classified Defense Department history of U.S. actions in Vietnam revealing that the government had been deceiving the American public about the course of the war. When disillusioned former Pentagon official Daniel Ellsberg leaked the study to the *New York Times* for publication in 1971, Nixon was enraged. The White House created a team of covert operatives nicknamed the Plumbers to "plug leaks" by whatever means necessary, including breaking into the office of Ellsberg's psychiatrist in search of information they might use to discredit him publicly.

Antiwar demonstrations reached their height during Nixon's first 2 years in the White House (1969–1970).

Escalating and Deescalating in Vietnam

Nixon recognized that in Vietnam the Truman Doctrine (see Chapter 24) had been stretched to the breaking point. The United States simply could not afford to send its troops everywhere abroad to contain the expansion of communism. The president and his national security adviser, Henry Kissinger, had ambitious plans for shifting the relationships of the great powers to America's advantage. To deal with China and the Soviet Union, they first had to reduce the vast U.S. engagement in the small country of Vietnam, which had grown wildly out of proportion to actual U.S. interests there. Their vision became known as the Nixon

Doctrine, in which the United States would provide military hardware rather than U.S. soldiers to allied governments, which would have to do their own fighting against leftist insurgencies. In South Vietnam this doctrine required "Vietnamization," or withdrawing American troops so ARVN could shoulder the bulk of the war.

The key to a successful withdrawal from Vietnam for Nixon was to preserve U.S. "credibility." The perception of power could be as important as its actual exercise, and the president wanted other nations, both friend and foe, to continue to respect and fear American military might. There was no immediate pullout but a gradual process that lasted for 4 years (1969–1973), during which almost half of the total U.S. casualties in Vietnam occurred. To avoid a humiliating collapse of the Saigon regime as soon as Americans left, Nixon did his utmost to weaken the communist forces during the slow withdrawal. The administration escalated in order to deescalate. The president ordered the secret bombing and invasion of neighboring Cambodia and Laos, an intensified aerial assault on North Vietnam, and the mining of Haiphong Harbor near Hanoi. Enormous protests rocked the country after the announcement of the Cambodian invasion on April 30, 1970, including a strike by hundreds of thousands of students that disrupted classes on more than 700 college campuses. National Guard troops killed four students at a demonstration at Kent State University in Ohio and two at Jackson State College in Mississippi, deepening the sense of national division. The hit song "Four Dead in Ohio" by the popular group Crosby, Stills, Nash, and Young quickly became an antiwar anthem.

A majority of Americans now opposed the nation's war effort, a level of dissent unprecedented in U.S. history. Most telling of all was the criticism of some veterans returning from Vietnam. Although most stayed quiet about their traumatic experiences, some organized the Vietnam Veterans Against the War and even held public hearings into atrocities—war crimes—they and others had committed. These dissenters were extremely hard for prowar Americans to discredit. The morale of American soldiers still in Vietnam plummeted as the steady withdrawal of their comrades made clear that they were no longer expected to win the war. Drug abuse and racial conflict increased sharply among GIs. Even "fragging" (killing one's own officers) escalated before the peace accords were signed in Paris and the U.S. evacuated its last combat troops in 1973.

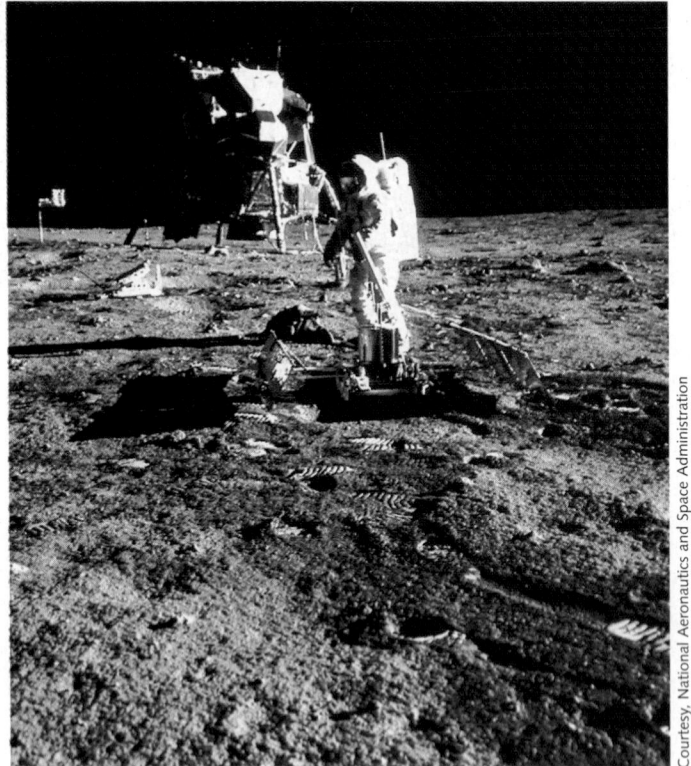

■ On July 20, 1969, astronauts Neil Armstrong and Edwin "Buzz" Aldrin put the first footprints on the moon. The U.S. flag they planted epitomized the sense of national accomplishment in space, even as divisions wracked American society at home. The actual flag here was made of rigid material because no lunar breeze existed to make the flag wave.

Courtesy, National Aeronautics and Space Administration

Conclusion

Between 1964 and 1971 changes shook the foundations of society and altered how Americans understood themselves. Many long-standing hierarchies of age, race, and gender began to break up as young, nonwhite, and female Americans laid claim to greater equality. The ratification of the Twenty-Sixth Amendment in 1971 reduced the voting age from 21 to 18, in acknowledgment of the sacrifices of young people sent to fight in Vietnam. In large numbers, women challenged and overcame traditional limits on their personal and work lives. Racial discrimination and segregation were outlawed. Immigration law for the first time welcomed new Americans equally regardless of nation of origin or color of skin.

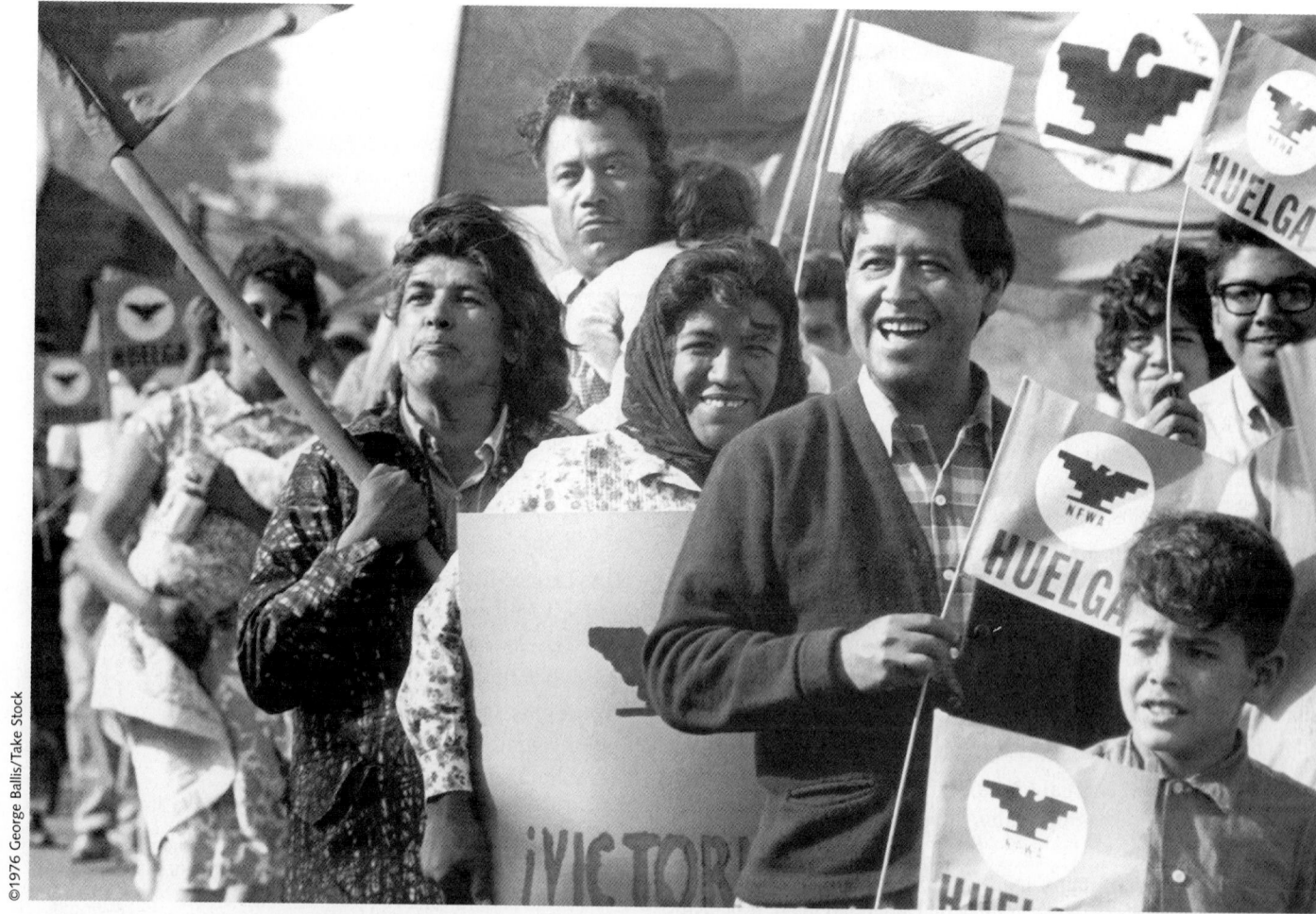

■ Cesar Chávez led a march during the United Farm Workers strike—*huelga*—against large grape growers in Delano, in California's central valley, in 1966. The UFW effort, in which women such as UFW vice-president Dolores Huerta (a mother of 11) figured prominently, included not only union organizing but also building a broader network of community institutions to improve the lives of Mexican American laborers. The Roman Catholic faith and pacifism of Chávez and others in the movement deeply impressed many non-Chicanos who supported the strike, such as Senator Robert F. Kennedy.

These years also witnessed striking disjunctures. The nation accomplished humanity's age-old dream of walking on the surface of the moon when Neil Armstrong stepped out of the *Apollo 11* spacecraft on July 20, 1969, while at home the country sometimes appeared to be coming apart at the seams. Poverty rates dropped to their lowest point ever, yet violence seemed to pervade the land. The slaughter of 43 people (mostly African Americans) by white state police retaking the Attica prison in upstate New York after an inmate insurrection in 1971 was one of the single most deadly confrontations between Americans since the Civil War.

The Vietnam War ended the Cold War consensus about the nation's duty to oppose communism abroad. The loss of this cornerstone of public purpose disoriented many citizens. The deceptive manner in which Johnson and Nixon waged the war eroded Americans' faith in their public officials, a process that the Watergate scandal accelerated between 1972 and 1974. American life also grew more informal as the egalitarian style of the various social movements of the 1960s spread into the broader culture. But the removal of some of the most blatant distinctions of race and gender did not extend to differences of class. In the watershed cases of *San Antonio*

Independent School District v. Rodriguez (1973) and *Milliken v. Bradley* (1974), the Supreme Court, led by Chief Justice Warren Burger, affirmed the autonomy of local school districts. Wealthier districts did not have to share financing with poorer ones, nor did they have to share students by means of busing. The Court ruled that there was no constitutional right to an education of equal quality. The ladder of social mobility remained slippery in a nation whose neighborhoods were still stratified between the affluent and the poor.

Sites to Visit

The Sixties Project
lists.village.virginia.edu/sixties/
> This University of Virginia site has extensive exhibits, primary documents, and personal narratives from the 1960s.

Lyndon B. Johnson Library and Museum
www.lbjlib.utexas.edu/
> This presidential library site has images and online exhibits.

Vietnam War Internet Project
www.vwip.org/vwiphome.html
> This site offers one of the most extensive collections on the Web of useful information on various aspects of the war.

My Lai Court Martial (1970)
www.law.umkc.edu/faculty/projects/ftrials/mylai/mylai.htm
> This site contains images, chronology, and court and official documents maintained by Dr. Doug Linder at the University of Missouri–Kansas City Law School.

The Digger Archives
www.diggers.org
> This site provides information about the San Francisco Diggers, a prominent countercultural group in the Haight–Asbury scene of 1966–1968.

U.S. Latino History and Culture (Smithsonian Institution)
www.si.edu/resource/faq/nmah/latino.htm
> This site offers exhibits, photos, resources, and links to other useful sites on the lives of Latino Americans.

Gay Rights Movement
www.columbia.edu/cu/libraries/events/sw25/casel.html
> This site includes articles from the New York City press as well as first-hand accounts of the 1969 Greenwich Village riots that are commemorated throughout the country during Gay Pride celebrations.

For Further Reading

General

Chafe, William H. *The Unfinished Journey: America Since World War II.* 3rd ed. 1995.

Farber, David. *The Age of Great Dreams: America in the 1960s.* 1994.

Farber, David, ed. *The Sixties: From Memory to History.* 1994.

Isserman, Maurice and Michael Kazin. *America Divided: The Civil War of the 1960s.* 2000.

Patterson, James T. *Grand Expectations: The United States, 1945–1974.* 1996.

Lyndon Johnson and the Apex of Liberalism

Dallek, Robert. *Flawed Giant: Lyndon Johnson and His Times, 1961–1973.* 1998.

Matusow, Allen J. *The Unravelling of America: A History of Liberalism in the 1960s.* 1984.

Powe, Lucas A., Jr. *The Warren Court and American Politics.* 2000.

Schulman, Bruce J. *Lyndon B. Johnson and American Liberalism.* 1995.

The Autobiography of Malcolm X. 1965.

Into War in Vietnam

Gardner, Lloyd C. *Pay Any Price: Lyndon Johnson and the Wars for Vietnam.* 1995.

Herr, Michael. *Dispatches.* 1977.

Herring, George C. *America's Longest War: The United States and Vietnam, 1950–1975.* 3rd ed. 1996.

Rotter, Andrew J., ed. *Light at the End of the Tunnel: A Vietnam War Anthology.* Revised ed. 1999.

Schulzinger, Robert D. *A Time for War: The United States and Vietnam, 1941–1975.* 1997.

Young, Marilyn B. *The Vietnam Wars, 1945–1990.* 1991.

The Movement

Anderson, Terry H. *The Movement and the Sixties: Protest in America from Greensboro to Wounded Knee.* 1995.

Echols, Alice. *Daring to Be Bad: Radical Feminism in America, 1967–1975.* 1989.

Evans, Sara. *Personal Politics: The Roots of Women's Liberation in the Civil Rights Movement and the New Left.* 1979.

Gitlin, Todd. *The Sixties: Years of Hope, Days of Rage.* 1987.

Miller, Timothy. *The '60s Communes: Hippies and Beyond.* 1999.

Van Deburg, William L. *New Day in Babylon: The Black Power Movement and American Culture, 1965–1975.* 1992.

Wells, Tom. *The War Within: America's Battle over Vietnam.* 1994.

The Conservative Response

Carter, Dan T. *The Politics of Rage: George Wallace, the Origins of the New Conservatism, and the Transformation of American Politics.* 2nd ed. 2000.

Kimball, Jeffrey. *Nixon's Vietnam War.* 1998.

McGirr, Lisa. *Suburban Warriors: The Origins of the New American Right.* 2001.

Rothman, Hal K. *The Greening of a Nation? Environmentalism in the United States since 1945.* 1998.

Small, Melvin. *The Presidency of Richard Nixon.* 1999.

Online Practice Test

Test your understanding of this chapter with interactive review quizzes at

www.ablongman.com/jonescreatedequal/chapter26

CHAPTER

27

Reconsidering National Priorities, 1972–1979

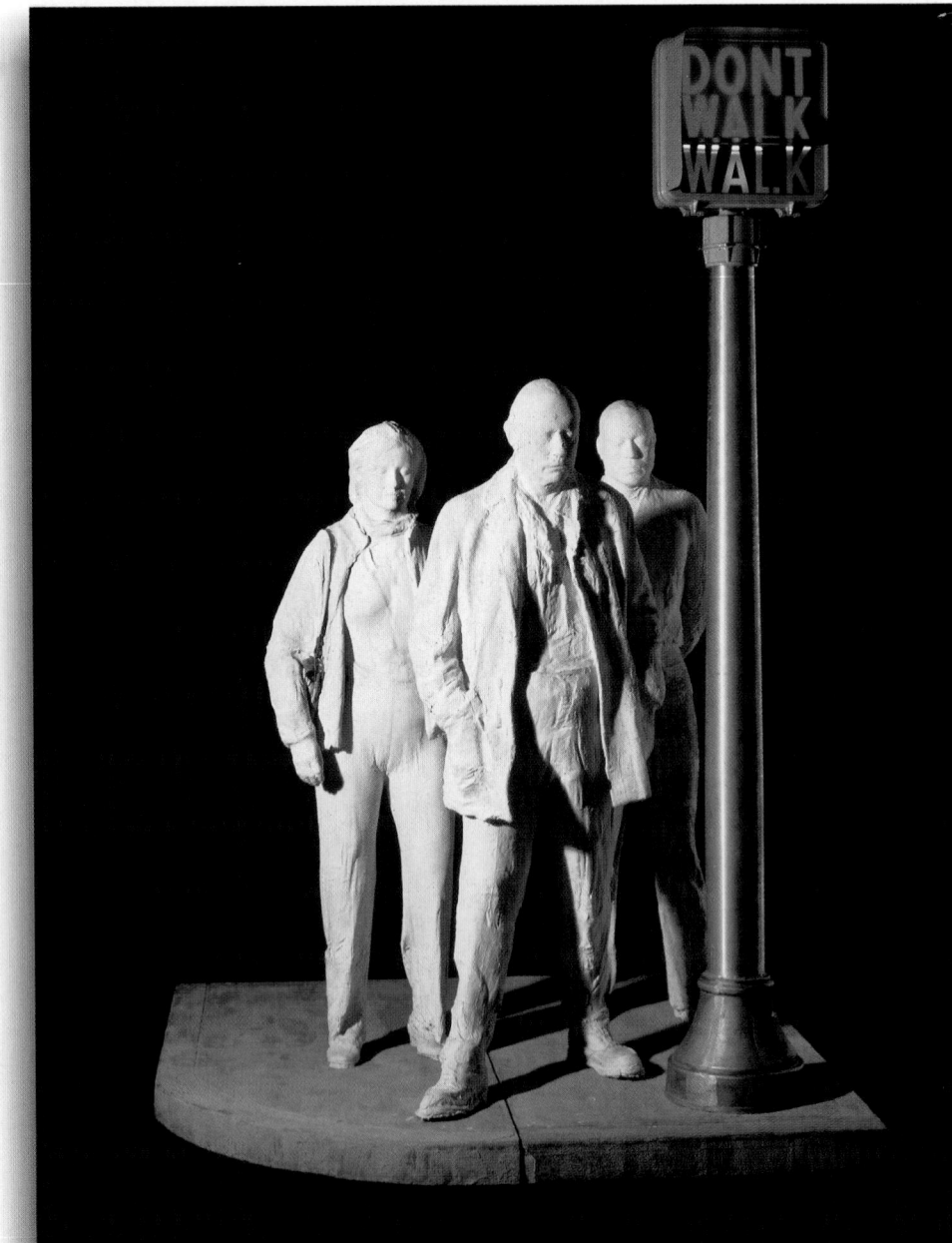

George Segal, "Walk, Don't Walk," 1976. ©The George and Helen Segal Foundation/Licensed by VAGA, New York, NY. Purchase, with funds from the Louis and Bessie Adler Foundation, Inc., Seymour M. Klein, President, the Gilman Foundation, Inc., the Howard and Jean Lipman Foundation, Inc. and the National Endowment for the Arts. Photograph ©1996: Whitney Museum of American Art, New York (79.4)

■ This 1976 sculpture by George Segal hinted at the uncertainties that pervaded American society in the mid-1970s.

KAREN SILKWOOD GREW UP IN AN UNASSUMING MIDDLE-CLASS FAMILY IN NEDERLAND, Texas, near the Gulf Coast. She baby-sat at her church nursery, earned straight A's through high school, and went to Lamar College on a full scholarship to study medical technology. Marriage, three children, and a divorce intervened, and in 1972 she began working as a laboratory analyst at Kerr–McGee's plutonium processing plant in Crescent, Oklahoma. There the highly poisonous radioactive material was made into fuel rods for nuclear power plants.

In the summer of 1974, at age 28, Silkwood was elected a local official of the union that represented many Kerr–McGee workers and began organizing for greater worker safety. She learned of numerous incidents of radioactive contamination at the plant. She also uncovered evidence of significant quantities of missing plutonium and of doctored quality assurance records for defective fuel rods. On November 5, she was mysteriously contaminated with potentially lethal levels of plutonium. On November 13 Silkwood set out for Oklahoma City to meet a national representative of her union and a *New York Times* reporter, intending to give them documents proving that Kerr–McGee was knowingly manufacturing defective nuclear products. She never made it. Her car was forced off the road and she died instantly when it crashed into a concrete culvert.

Karen Silkwood challenged the power of one of the nation's largest energy corporations and paid with her life. Her brief career as a whistleblower brought together major issues of the 1970s: labor organizing, environmental damage, the safety record of nuclear energy, and the power of corporations over individual citizens. Her dismissive treatment by some fellow workers, her employers, and the media also suggested the lack of respect that women had long endured, especially when they moved out of the traditional homemaker role. ABC television news anchor Howard K. Smith began his coverage of a women's rights march in New York City in 1970 by quoting with approval the words of Vice President Spiro Agnew: "Three things have been difficult to tame. The ocean, fools, and women. We may soon be able to tame the ocean, but fools and women will take a little longer."

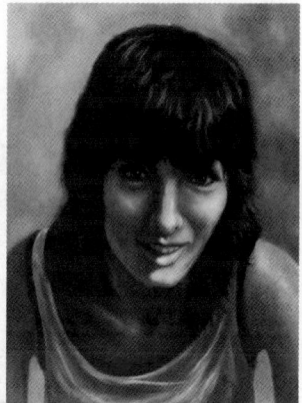

Karen Silkwood became a symbol of courage to many.

Condescension toward women still pervaded American society, and few men even noticed it. The political upheavals of the 1960s had barely touched the relationships between most women and men by the start of the new decade. But all this changed as the 1970s unfolded. The spread of ideas about women's liberation in the 1970s transformed the personal lives of almost every American, female and male alike. Feminism challenged the most basic and intimate assumptions about relationships, family, work, and power. It also sharply expanded women's opportunities. At the end of the decade, Dr. Martha Hurley of Kansas City recalled, "In the middle of an operation today, I looked around the room—to the first assistant, my scrub nurse, and circulating nurse, the anesthesia doctor, nurse anesthetist, and the patient—and suddenly realized that we were performing major surgery and there was not a man in the room!"

Who were the feminists? They were mothers and wives, college students, professional women, and working-class women. Their growing awareness of gender discrimination had made them angry but also optimistic about change. And some feminists were men who realized that the movement could liberate them from their own narrowly defined masculine roles. Feminists of all stripes could be both deadly serious and disarmingly funny. Journalist Gloria Steinem, who founded *Ms.* magazine in 1972, became one of the prominent faces of the movement. Steinem's appearance enabled her to finagle a job as a cocktail waitress at the New York Playboy Club in 1963. Her goal: to write an exposé of the decidedly unsexy working conditions of the famous Playboy "bunnies." Steinem later lampooned men's common sense of entitlement and privilege and their often competitive attitudes toward their bodies in an essay called "If Men Could Menstruate": "Clearly, menstruation would become an enviable, boastworthy, masculine event: Men would brag about how much and how long. Young boys would talk about it as the envied beginning of manhood. Gifts, religious ceremonies, family dinners, and stag parties would mark the day."

Not all Americans were amused by challenges to long-standing beliefs about men's and women's proper roles. J. Edgar Hoover, director of the Federal Bureau of Investigation (FBI), exemplified the resistance that could catalyze against demands for fair treatment of women. Well known for his dislike of leftists, African Americans, homosexuals, and anyone else who questioned the existing social order—including labor organizers such as Karen Silkwood—Hoover ordered his agents to infiltrate the women's liberation movement. (Ironically, Hoover was a cross-dresser in private and perhaps also gay, an apparent case of self-loathing.) Feminists, he warned FBI regional directors, "should be viewed as part of the enemy, a challenge to American values." At one point, the director instructed an FBI field office to "identify the officers and aims and objectives of this organization." But despite determined digging for information, a paid informant could report only that "this movement has no leaders, dues or organizations." Women's liberation was both nowhere and everywhere. No one could trace it to a specific group of conspirators.

> *The feminist wave called traditional values and hierarchies into question as it washed over the United States in the 1970s.*

In a certain sense, Hoover was right: the feminist wave did call traditional values and hierarchies into question as it washed over the United States in the 1970s. It joined with other developments of the decade to force Americans to reexamine much that they had taken for granted. Elected on the promise to end the war in Southeast Asia "with honor," President Nixon escalated the fighting before eventually withdrawing U.S. forces from Vietnam. At the same time, he repaired relations with both China and the Soviet Union as those two communist powers drew apart. Americans thus suffered their first clear defeat in war while also seeing the Cold War splinter. Scandal in the White House then forced the first resignation of a U.S. president and deepened public distrust of political authorities. American economic growth—the foundation of the country's power—stumbled because of spending on the Vietnam War and oil shortages. High-paying manufacturing jobs declined as factories began to move overseas in pursuit of cheaper labor, and skilled blue-collar workers saw their status as middle-class Americans start to slip. Unemployment grew sharply. And a growing environmental movement raised disturbing questions about whether an expanding economy and exploitation of natural resources should continue to top the country's list of priorities.

The nation celebrated its two-hundredth birthday in 1976 amid these uncertainties. That year, one-term Georgia governor Jimmy Carter won election to the White House by promising to restore honesty and trust to the federal government. In his first two years in office, Carter shifted the nation's foreign policy focus away from fighting communism toward building warmer relations with the Third World. He saw Americans' dependence on imported oil as a primary national security problem and implored citizens to scale back their lavish consumption of fossil fuels. But his presidency eventually foundered on persistent economic stagnation and inflation at home, upheavals abroad, and Carter's own limitations as chief executive.

Journalist Tom Wolfe dubbed the 1970s the "Me Decade," a phrase that proved even more appropriate for the 1980s. The label did have some merit: many Americans turned away from the public sphere after the exhilarating but divisive politics of the 1960s and pursued self-exploration and self-fulfillment instead. Crime, divorce, premarital and extramarital sex, and drug use all increased while the nation's economic health and international status declined. But the 1970s also witnessed a rethinking of long-standing assumptions: about how democracy should work at home, what role the nation should play in international affairs, how people ought to treat the environment, and how men and women should relate to each other. The decade offered a window of opportunity for Americans to reimagine their values and priorities for the future.

Twin Shocks: Détente and Watergate

Richard Nixon had long been the nation's leading anticommunist. No one had more fiercely opposed leftists at home and communists in China and the Soviet Union. However, the president was more a savvy political opportunist than an ideologue. He and his national security adviser, Henry Kissinger, saw a chance to use mounting Chinese–Soviet tensions to the advantage of the United States as they withdrew American armed forces from Vietnam. Nixon and Kissinger recognized that the United States had entered an era of new limits to its power. They cleverly tapped into the rivalry dividing the communist world to preserve U.S. influence overseas. Their efforts ultimately eased Cold War tensions.

At the same time that Nixon manipulated the Cold War abroad, the Republican president initiated a campaign of illegal actions at home to destroy his political opponents in the Democratic party. This strategy backfired in a scandal that drove him from office in 1974. Having undercut the logic of anticommunism abroad by warming relations with communist leaders in Beijing and Moscow, Nixon eroded the bipartisan consensus at home that had long supported the Cold War. Wearied by the deceptions and debates of Vietnam, Americans found themselves questioning anew their political assumptions and the trustworthiness of their leaders.

Triangular Diplomacy

Nixon and Kissinger prided themselves on their "realpolitik" approach to foreign policy: their pragmatic assessment of other powers' security needs, regardless of ideology, and their collaboration with those powers on issues of common concern. In 1969, China and the USSR gave Nixon and Kissinger an ideal opportunity to exercise their realpolitik skills. That year, tensions that had

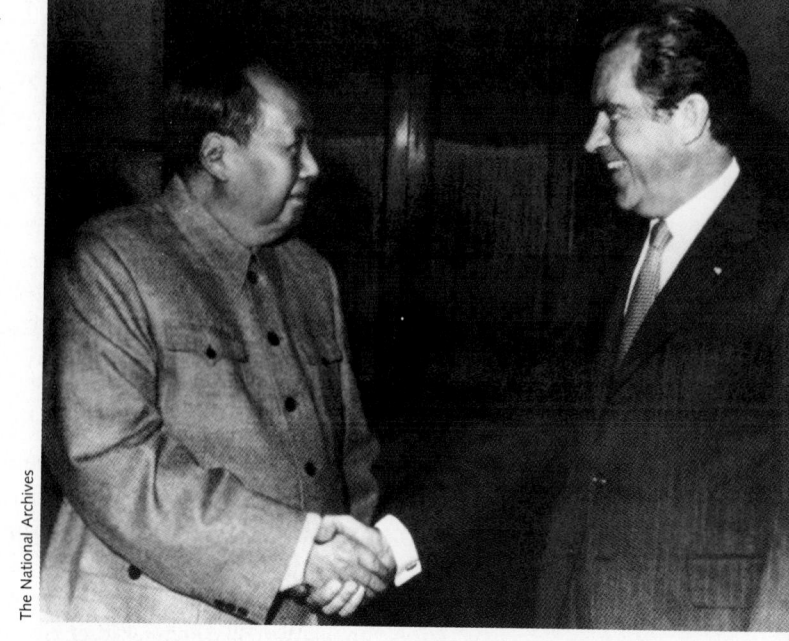

The National Archives

■ President Nixon met the premier of the People's Republic of China, Mao Zedong, in Beijing on February 29, 1972. The U.S. government had shunned China since its communist revolution in 1949. Richard Nixon's amiable visit there stunned observers and altered the dynamics of the Cold War.

■ **MAP 27.1**
NUCLEAR WEAPONS BEFORE DÉTENTE   The massive nuclear arsenals of the United States and the Soviet Union utterly surpassed those of the other nuclear powers. During the 1970s the Soviets achieved rough parity with the Americans in total nuclear warheads. The numbers for both sides were sufficient to destroy the entire populated world many times over.

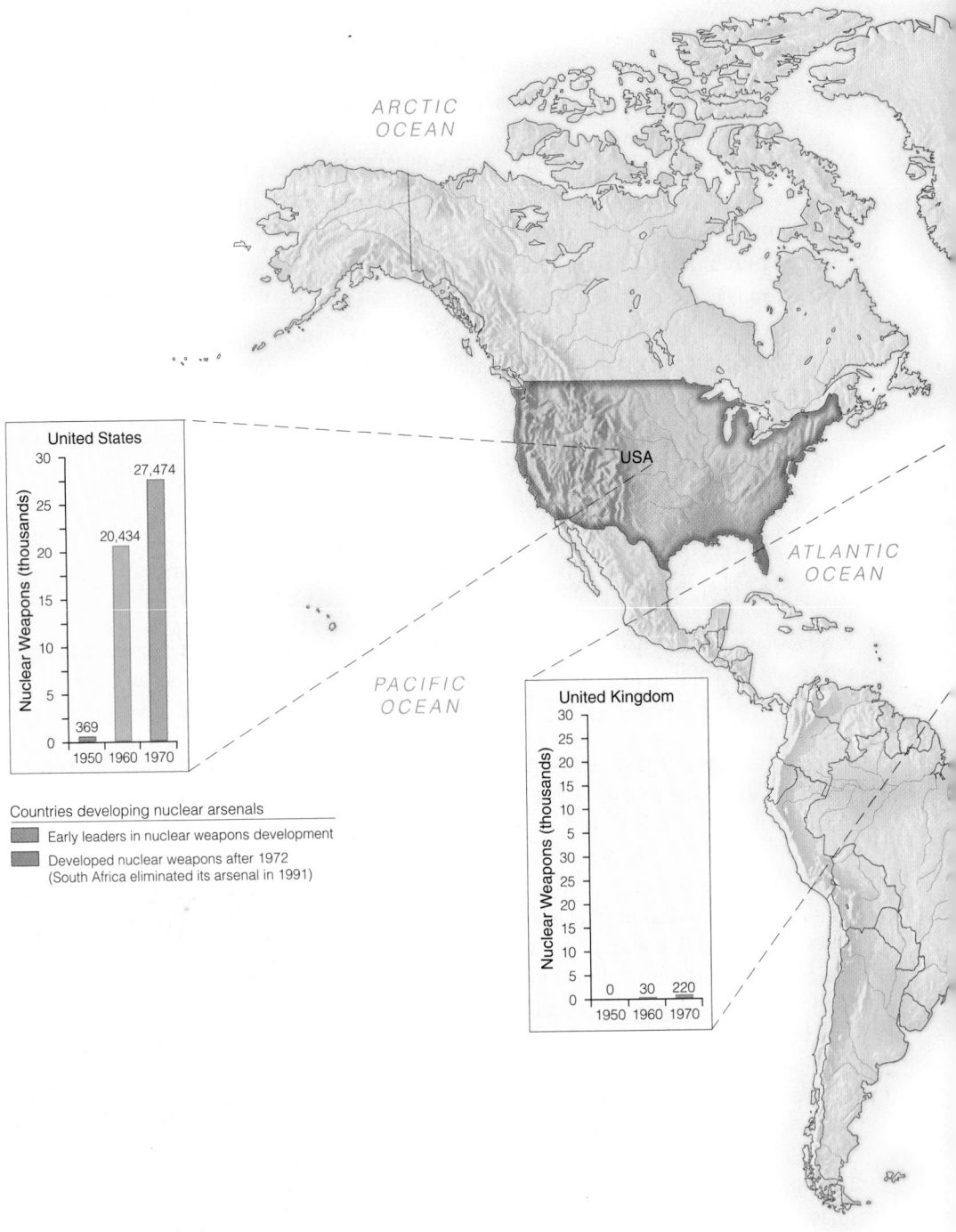

been building between the two communist states erupted in brief skirmishing between Chinese and Soviet troops on their shared border. For two decades, Americans had seen the Communist bloc as impenetrable. Nixon realized he could play China and the USSR against each other, and he seized the chance. That is, he saw a way to make both Soviet leader Leonid Brezhnev and Chinese leader Mao Zedong into another "Tito," an independent communist with ties to the West, like Premier Josef Tito of Yugoslavia. He thus envisioned a "triangular diplomacy" that he hoped would divide the communist world.

The president and Kissinger, a former Harvard professor with an intriguing German accent, also shared a commitment to secrecy. Any fundamental revision of the nation's for-

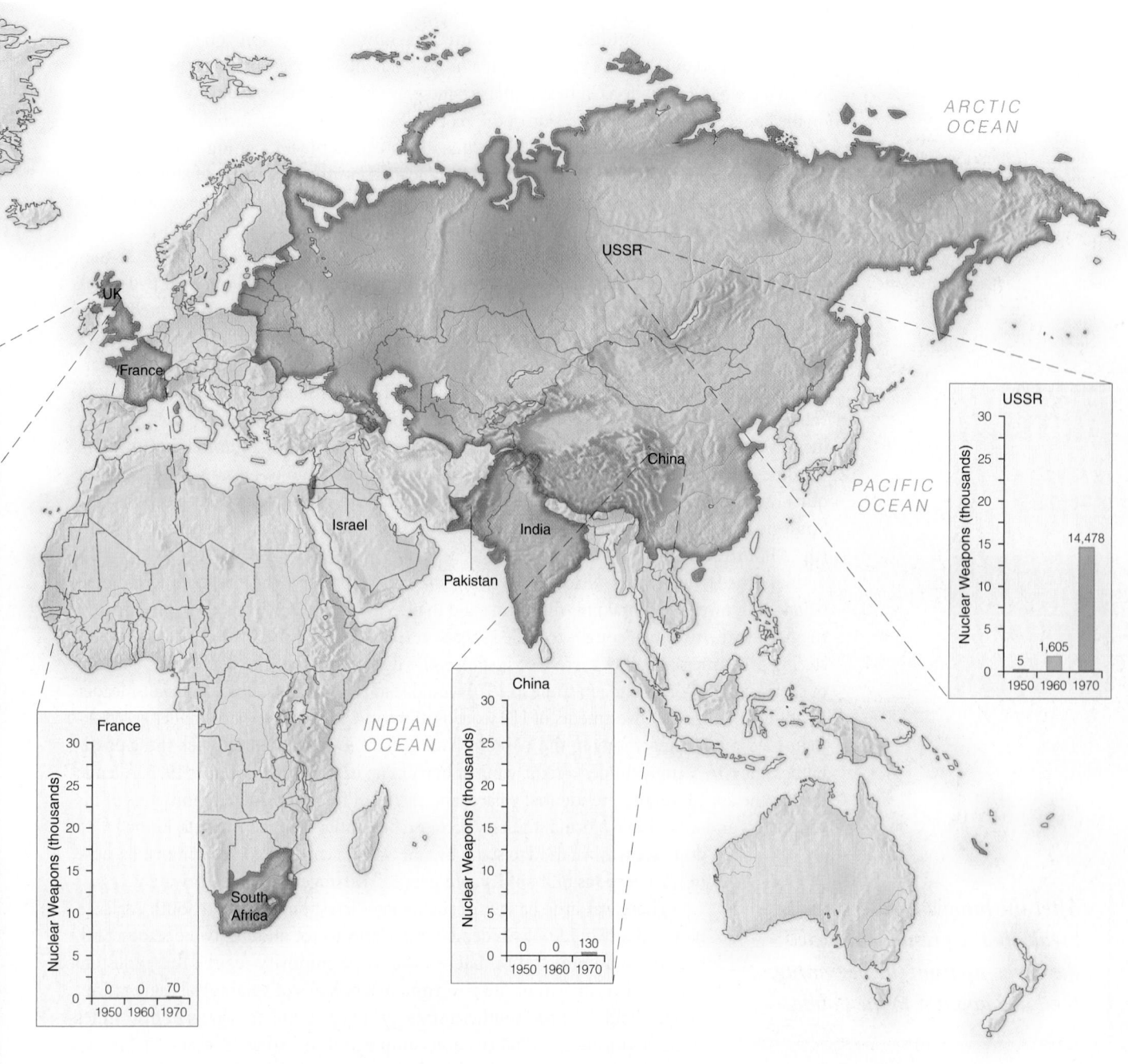

eign policy, they believed, could happen only if they concentrated all decision-making in the White House. They set out to keep Congress, the press, and even their own State Department in the dark. Diplomatic innovation thus went hand in hand with an unprecedented extension of the secretive national security state.

In February 1972, after a secret foray by Kissinger to Beijing, Nixon stunned Americans and the world by announcing that he would be the first U.S. president to visit China. The Soviets and the Vietnamese expressed dismay at the news, and liberal Democrats at home could only gape, speechless, at their opponent's diplomatic coup: how could Nixon, a dyed-in-the-wool anticommunist, go to China? But that was precisely the point: as Democratic party insider

Clark Clifford explained, Nixon was "the first president since the [Second World] War who didn't have to worry about Richard Nixon" attacking him for being "soft" on communism.

As it turned out, Nixon's visit brought a host of benefits. Live television coverage showed Nixon toasting Mao while a Chinese military band played "America the Beautiful" and "Home on the Range." Americans' impression of the People's Republic as a grim, forbidding land began to give way to a renewed interest in China as an exotic but intriguing place. Cultural exchanges soon proliferated: first ping-pong teams, eventually legions of students. U.S. businesses also cast a covetous eye at the immense China market. Trade between the two nations rose dramatically over the next three decades.

Nixon and Kissinger now constructed the other leg of their diplomatic triangle. As they anticipated, the Soviets had taken alarm at the warming of relations between their two greatest rivals. They signaled their concern to Washington and suggested that the United States include them in the new arrangements. Nixon and Kissinger understood that behind Moscow's veneer of revolutionary dogma stood a powerful nation increasingly committed to the international status quo. Moreover, the Russians and the Americans shared similar concerns. Both wanted to reduce the costliness of maintaining enormous nuclear arsenals, and each side saw lucrative trading possibilities with the other. Nixon flew to Moscow for a summit meeting with Brezhnev in May 1972 that initiated a policy of détente (relaxation of tensions). A trade pact quickly followed. The two superpowers also agreed to limit offensive nuclear weapons (the Strategic Arms Limitations Treaty, or SALT I) and to ban antiballistic missile defense systems (the ABM treaty).

Like the Soviet leaders, Nixon and Kissinger sought to preserve the existing international balance of power. Deal-making with China and the USSR constituted one step in this process. In another, the two men sought to stifle socialist revolutions in Third World nations by bolstering pro-American allies there. For instance, the duo feared that the democratic election of socialist Salvador Allende in Chile in 1970 would lead to "another Cuba." A socialist leader might nationalize the investments of U.S. corporations in Chile and perhaps challenge Washington's capitalist hegemony in the Western Hemisphere. Determined to block these possibilities, the CIA secretly funded a right-wing military coup in Chile in September 1973. Allende died in the assault on the presidential palace, and the rebel forces murdered thousands of his supporters and established a brutal military dictatorship under General Augusto Pinochet. "I don't see why we need to stand by and watch a country go Communist because of the irresponsibility of its own people," Kissinger explained privately.

After the bungled Watergate break-in, the president directed the cover-up from the beginning, then lied about it to the public.

There was little danger of such voter "irresponsibility" in South Africa, a nation that would not see democratic elections for another two decades. Still, the Nixon administration backed the white minority regime there, despite worldwide criticism of the government's policies of total racial segregation, or apartheid. Nixon's "southern strategy" of appealing to segregationist whites at home during the 1968 election campaign thus had an international parallel. In South Africa, "the whites are here to stay," a key National Security Council study declared. The study affirmed the president's goal of preserving a pro-American order in South Africa, the southern tip of a continent rife with political instability.

Nixon and Kissinger reached beyond Latin America and Africa. They also bolstered the autocratic regime of Shah Reza Pahlavi of Iran. They sold him unlimited arms in return for Iranian oil shipments and political support in the strategic Middle East, where the United States had few allies. The president could not know it at the time, but preserving the Shah's oppressive rule carried a high price—one that the United States would pay later.

Scandal in the White House

On June 17, 1972, Washington police caught agents of Nixon's reelection campaign breaking into the Democratic National Committee headquarters in the Watergate hotel and office complex. The burglars' goal was to put in place secretive listening devices, or "bugs." Later, the White House tried to cover up its connections to the caper. Ironically, the Republicans hardly needed to resort to illegal actions to hold onto the White House in 1972. The New Deal coalition that had kept the Democrats as the majority party since the 1930s was fast unraveling. White Southerners and many ethnic European Northerners were abandoning the party amid its increasing identification with black civil rights, feminism, and cultural liberalism. Middle- and upper-middle-class liberal activists had helped nominate South Dakota senator George McGovern, a former World War II pilot and college professor, as the Democratic presidential candidate, primarily on the basis of his principled and long-standing opposition to the war in Vietnam. Playing upon voter anxiety about cultural changes, the Republicans tarred McGovern's supporters with favoring "the 3 A's": acid (the drug LSD), abortion, and amnesty for draft evaders. McGovern's campaign never overcame that image of radicalism, and in November Nixon won 61 percent of the popular vote. He also swept the electoral votes of every state but one. Bumper stickers reading "Don't blame me, I'm from Massachusetts" proliferated as the Watergate scandal deepened.

TABLE 27-1			
The Election of 1972			
Candidate	**Political Party**	**Popular Vote**	**Electoral Vote**
Richard M. Nixon	Republican	47,169,911	520
George S. McGovern	Democratic	29,170,383	17

But the Watergate break-in was only one step in Nixon's broader campaign of illegal warfare against his political opponents. An insecure and unhappy loner, Nixon harbored an almost paranoid suspicion when he took office in early 1969. The conflict still raging in Vietnam had polarized Americans more than at any time since the Civil War, and the president compiled a lengthy and secret "enemies list." "This is a war. . . . They are asking for it and they are going to get it," he told aides. The president continued his predecessor's harassment of antiwar dissidents. He also agreed with Johnson's advice that "leaks can kill you" and sought tighter control over all executive agencies of the federal government.

Nixon and Kissinger took things one step further in May 1969, when they established the first in a long series of wiretaps without court warrants on their own staffs and reporters. They were determined to discover the source of a newspaper story that had mentioned secret American bombing of neutral Cambodia. Several wartime presidents in the past had successfully silenced dissenters, but Nixon overreached still further. The president ultimately poisoned the very heart of American politics by his clandestine use of the government's powerful executive branch to undermine the mainstream opposition party and others who seemed to challenge his policies.

The president and his aides regularly discussed "how we can use the available federal machinery to screw our political enemies," in the words of White House counsel John Dean. They persuaded the FBI and the CIA to monitor and harass antiwar activists and pushed the Internal Revenue Service to investigate prominent Democrats. They extorted large contributions to the Republican party from corporate executives by making it clear that federal agencies would otherwise impede the pursuit of their business interests. The *New York Times*'s publication of the classified Pentagon Papers in 1971 stiffened the resolve of the Committee to Reelect the President (CREEP) to stop any further leaks. The committee assembled a group of undercover operatives (the "plumbers") to engineer "dirty tricks" against the Democrats. Their activities included smearing the reputation of one leading presidential candidate, Senator Edmund Muskie of Maine, and sowing dissent and distrust among Democratic voters. For example, during the New Hampshire primary, Democrats in that nearly all-white state received late-night phone calls from a mysterious "Harlem for Muskie" committee. Callers urged them to vote for the senator because of his supposed support for African Americans' interests—a devious ploy to arouse potential racism.

After the bungled Watergate break-in, the president directed the cover-up from the beginning, then lied about it to the public. He also used the CIA to hinder the FBI's investigation

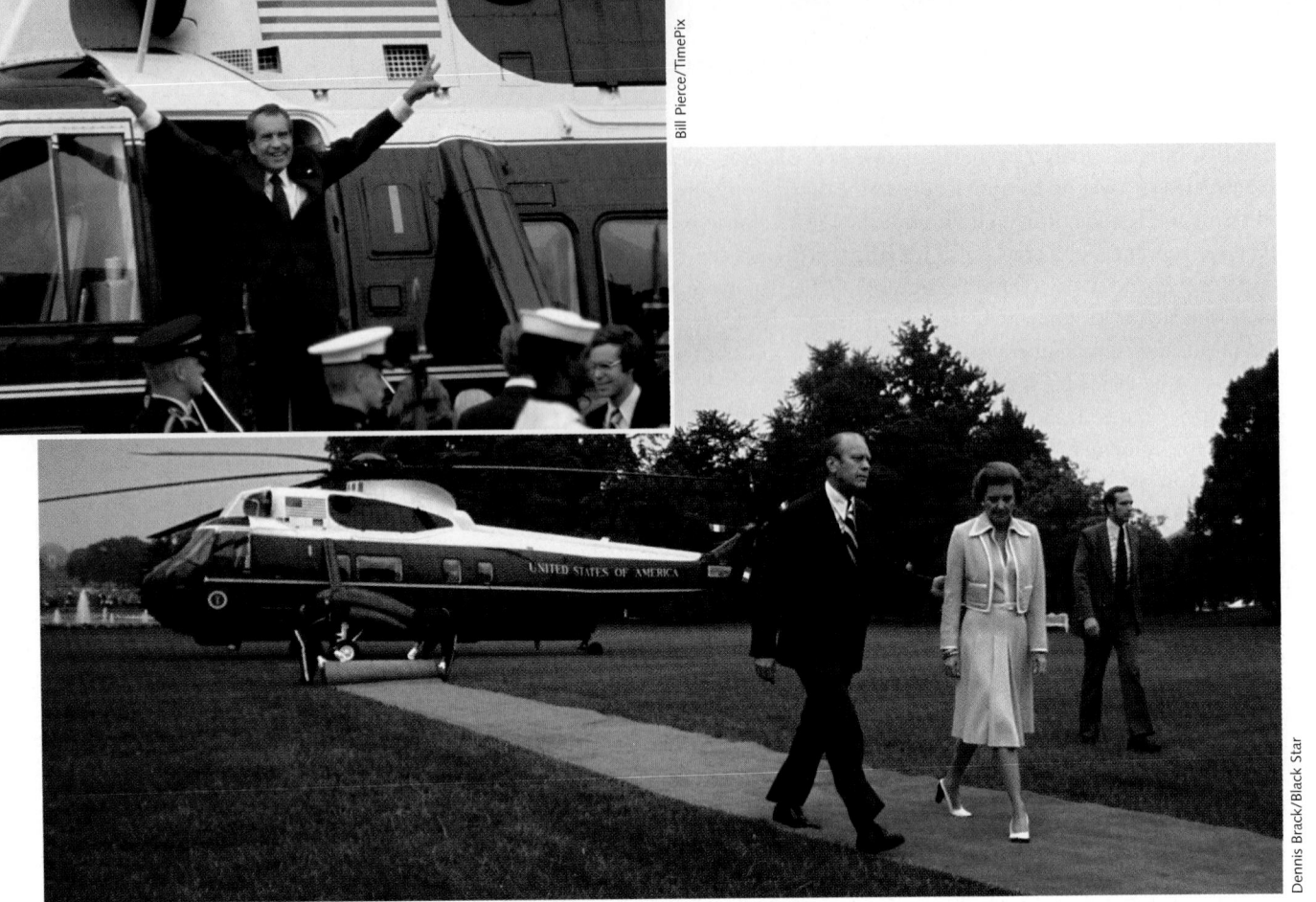

■ On August 9, 1974, Richard Nixon became the only U.S. president to resign from office. As he left by helicopter one last time from the South Lawn of the White House, he offered a defiant victory gesture rather than a presidential salute (inset). Vice President Gerald Ford and his wife, Betty, then walked back to the White House for him to be sworn in as the nation's 38th president.

into the matter. He approved payments of hush money to the burglars to keep them quiet about their ties to the White House. Nixon's abuse of power escalated as he pressured his subordinates to perjure themselves in court. For most of a year the cover-up held, and Nixon won reelection in 1972.

But the persistent investigations by *Washington Post* journalists Bob Woodward and Carl Bernstein kept the heat on. In early 1973, the administration began to crack due to a grand jury probe in the federal court of Judge John Sirica. The president's men lost confidence that the cover-up would hold and began looking for ways to save their own skins. Convicted Watergate burglar James McCord wrote Judge Sirica that the White House had indeed been involved in the break-in. White House counsel Dean and former Attorney General John Mitchell refused Nixon's requests to absorb full blame and become scapegoats. Congress initiated its own televised investigations that mesmerized a national audience. The Senate Watergate committee, chaired by eloquent conservative North Carolina Democrat Sam Ervin, methodically exposed the criminal actions in the White House with growing bipartisan support. The key issue, as framed by Republican committee member Howard Baker of Tennessee becam, "What did the president know, and when did he know it?"

On July 16, 1973, White House aide Alexander Butterfield told the Ervin Committee that a built-in recorder taped all conversations in the Oval Office. Almost certainly, these tapes would provide answers to questions about the president's role. Both Congress and Justice Department special prosecutor Archibald Cox subpoenaed the White House tapes, but Nixon refused to hand them over. Instead, he fired Cox on October 20 in what became known as the Saturday Night Massacre. Outraged, Congress initiated impeachment proceedings against the president.

In the spring of 1974, the House of Representatives passed bills of impeachment for his specific abuses of power. Before the Senate could vote on whether to find Nixon guilty of the House charges, the Supreme Court ruled that the White House had to turn over the subpoenaed tapes. The content of the tapes revealed the extent of the president's involvement in the cover-up and his personal crudeness, vindictiveness, and ethnic and racial prejudices. Facing a certain guilty verdict, Nixon resigned on August 9, 1974, less than halfway through his second term.

A President Laid Low

Never before had a U.S. president been driven from office. Many citizens celebrated the outcome of the Watergate investigations as evidence of democracy's resilience and power to uncover criminal activity in the White House and bring down a corrupt president. But the affair also discredited political institutions Americans had long respected. If you can't trust the president, U.S. citizens lamented, whom *can* you trust? Indeed, the Nixon administration proved quite corrupt. A whole raft of senior officials, including the president's closest aides, H. R. Haldeman and John Ehrlichman, went to prison. Even Vice President Spiro Agnew was forced to resign amid the Watergate investigations when a Maryland jury found him guilty of tax evasion dating back to his years as governor there. The actions of Nixon and those who served him permanently tarnished the reputation of politicians, and citizens responded by disengaging from the political process. The percentage of eligible voters actually casting ballots sank from 61 percent in 1968 to 53 percent in 1980, diminishing the practice of democracy: rule by the people.

Unlike the impeachment of President Bill Clinton 26 years later, which centered on executive lying about a sexual affair in the Oval Office, the Watergate scandal involved larger issues of presidential power in the public realm. It also raised questions about the balance of power throughout the U.S. political system. Since 1945, the executive branch had grown increasingly powerful during the international crises of the Cold War, but Nixon's fall crippled the "imperial presidency." After Watergate, Congress began to reclaim its constitutional responsibilities in international affairs. As the bicentennial of American independence approached, citizens' suspicion of corruption in high places recalled the Whiggish attitudes of the country's revolutionary leaders two centuries before. Most immediately, Congress swung strongly to the Democrats in the 1974 elections, slowing the Republicans' rise to the status of majority party.

The man who replaced Nixon in the White House faced a daunting situation. Gerald Ford, longtime Republican congressman and House minority leader from Grand Rapids, Michigan, had been tapped by Nixon to replace Agnew as vice president. Well liked by members of both parties, Ford seemed to embody the antidote to the extreme styles of both Nixon and Agnew. To restore decency and trust in the government, Ford saw his role as healing what he called "the wounds of the past." Within a month, he granted a "full, free, and absolute pardon" to Nixon for any crimes he may have committed as president, precluding any trial and punishment within a court of law. However, most Americans believed that Nixon should have faced justice for his actions, just as the people did who carried out his orders. Ford's popularity plummeted overnight from 72 percent to 49 percent and never fully recovered.

If Ford inherited the fallout from Watergate at home, abroad he inherited the pending defeat in Vietnam. Few Americans wanted to dwell on the meaning of the disastrous U.S. involvement in Southeast Asia. Military veterans returned to a nation determined to ignore or demean their sacrifices, and they quickly learned to keep their combat-induced traumas to themselves (and sometimes even from their families). When Saigon finally fell to the combined invasion of National Liberation Front and North Vietnamese fighters on April 30, 1975, Americans watched the televised images with both bitterness and relief. Two weeks later, Cambodian communist forces briefly seized the U.S. container ship *Mayaguez,* provoking Ford to demonstrate

> *As the bicentennial approached, suspicion of corruption in high places recalled the attitudes of the country's revolutionary leaders two centuries before.*

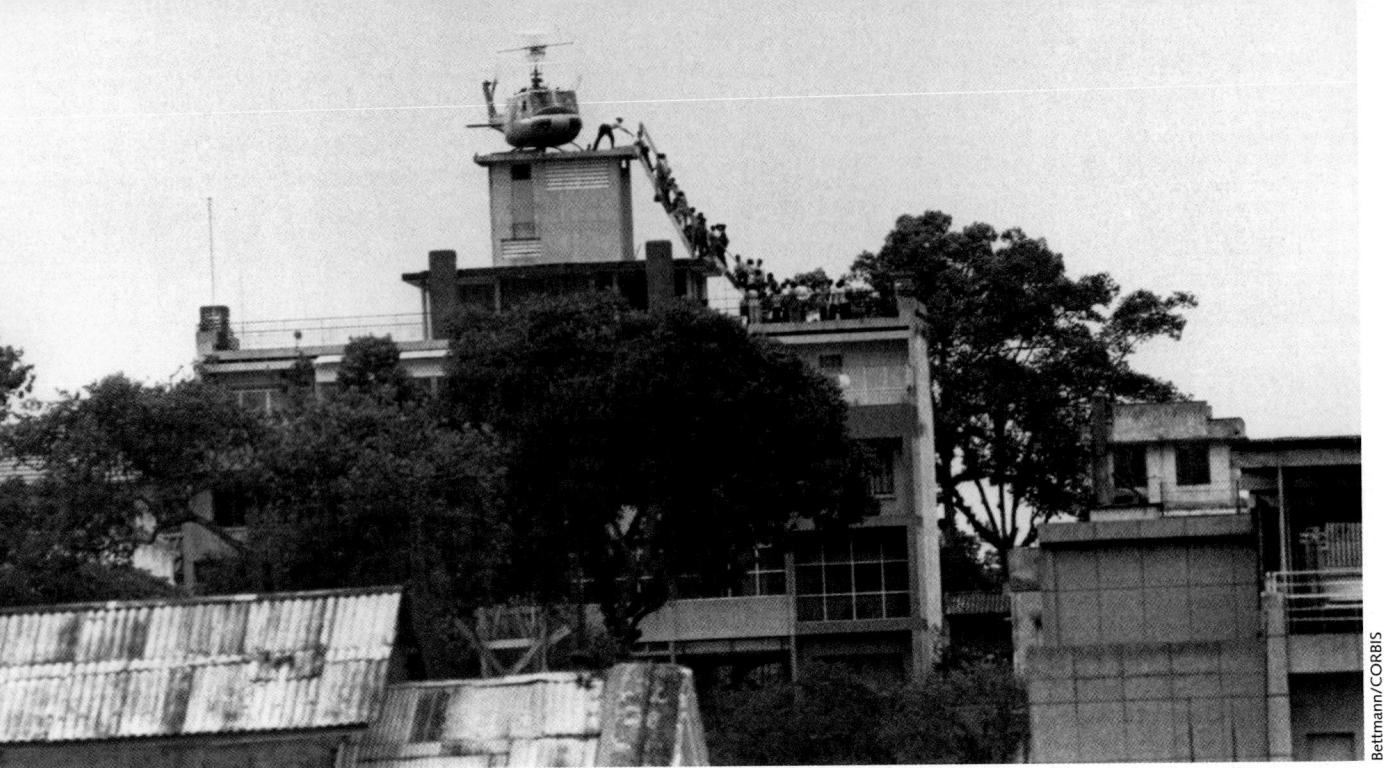

■ The last U.S. combat troops left Vietnam in 1973. Forces of the National Liberation Front and North Vietnam swept into the capital of South Vietnam, Saigon, on April 30, 1975. Here, one day earlier, a Marine helicopter on the roof of the U.S. embassy loads Americans and a few Vietnamese allies onto one of the last flights out.

that the United States was still ready and willing to flex its military muscle. But 41 U.S. soldiers died in the rescue mission to save 39 sailors whom, it turned out, Cambodia had already released. Ford and Kissinger, serving as the new president's secretary of state, continued to pursue détente with the Soviets at summit meetings in Vladivostock (1974) and Helsinki (1975). At the same time, they supported anticommunist forces in various Third World conflicts, such as the civil war that erupted in Angola after that country achieved its independence in 1975.

Discovering the Limits of the U.S. Economy

If money makes the world go around, the United States began to lose some of its ability to spin the globe in the early 1970s. Generation after generation of Americans had watched their incomes rise, and most children expected to be wealthier than their parents had been. Since World War II had pulled the U.S. economy out of the Great Depression, median family income had doubled. Most Americans saw themselves as citizens of the world's richest country and prized the status that came with this privilege. But by 1973, the famous American standard of living began to decline. The three pillars of postwar prosperity—cheap energy, rising wages, and low inflation—simultaneously crumbled. The costs of the Vietnam War struck home at the same time that an oil embargo spawned by conflict in the Middle East gripped the country. Moreover, a widening environmental movement raised questions about the pursuit of endless economic growth on a planet that more and more people realized had limited natural resources. For the first time since the 1930s, Americans started to doubt what the economic future had in store for them.

The End of the Long Boom

Stagnation and inflation typically do not strike an economy at the same time. With stagnation, prices and wages stay level or even decline; with inflation, prices rise and jobs grow. During the 1970s, however, a terrible new economic scourge dubbed "stagflation" hit the United States. For the first time, employment and wages stagnated while prices climbed. What explained this phenomenon? Spending on the Vietnam War had pulled prices upward. The government had never raised enough taxes to cover the expense of the war, so it paid the bills by simply printing more dollars—a sure-fire way to create inflation. In 1971, annual inflation stood at 4.5 percent, more than twice the pre-Vietnam rate; two years later it reached 10 percent, and by 1980 it topped out at 18 percent.

These figures devastated Americans' sense of economic security. Average real wages (income adjusted for inflation) dropped by 2 percent a year from 1973 to the 1990s. Unemployment rose to 9 percent in 1975, driven in part by continued automation of the workplace. Only the continued flow of women into the workforce, seen by most families as an economic necessity, kept the majority of U.S. families afloat financially. The number of citizens living in poverty, which had dropped sharply through the 1960s to 11 percent in 1973, rose again, hitting 15 percent by 1982. The gap between rich and poor began widening, a process that persisted into the next millennium.

So ended the long boom of economic growth that had buoyed American life since 1945. But perhaps the most important evidence of the weakening economy came with the drop in the growth of productivity: output per worker-hour had risen at an annual average of more than 3 percent during the boom. From 1974 to 1992, it rose at less than half that rate.

This decline stemmed in part from competition from abroad, particularly West Germany and Japan. With U.S. assistance (and without the military expenditures that so burdened the United States), those countries had finally rebuilt their economies after World War II and boasted new, more efficient industrial facilities. Imported cars, for example, grew from just 8 percent of the U.S. market in 1970 to 22 percent in 1979 as Hondas, Toyotas, Volkswagens, and Mercedes streamed onto American highways. And the trade surplus that had long symbolized global U.S. economic superiority evaporated in 1971. That year, U.S. imports overtook exports for the first time in the twentieth century. Worried international investors traded in dollars for gold, forcing Nixon to end the 27-year-old Bretton Woods monetary system that had linked all other currencies to the dollar at fixed exchange rates. Freed from the fixed rate of $35 per ounce of gold, the dollar dropped like a stone; by the end of the decade, it took $800 to buy an ounce of gold.

Only the continued flow of women into the workforce, seen by most families as an economic necessity, kept the majority of U.S. families afloat financially.

In this competitive environment, the *Wall Street Journal* reported, American companies "seek places where labor, land, electricity, and taxes are cheap." Corporations found those places in the American South and Southwest, regions characterized by scarce unions, low wage rates, minimal taxes, and negligible local government regulations. Many more such places were in neighboring Mexico. The long-term decline of the Rustbelt—the series of urban industrial centers strung across the Northeast and Midwest—accelerated in the 1970s. As one example, RCA (the Radio Corporation of America) moved its production facilities from Camden, New Jersey, to Bloomington, Indiana, in the 1940s, and eventually to Ciudad Juarez, just over the border from El Paso, Texas, in the 1970s.

Workers lost positions on assembly lines and found jobs at lower wages in the expanding and less unionized service sector. There were exceptions. For instance, when the mostly female Mexican workers at the Farah slacks company in El Paso and other Southwestern cities went on strike from 1972 to 1974, they won the sympathy of a national consumer boycott. Eventually they received some concessions from the company. But the logic of what would soon be called globalization kept most workers at a disadvantage as owners of capital moved production lines to wherever costs were lowest.

Increasingly, U.S. companies shifted their manufacturing to Mexico, where they established *maquiladoras* as early as 1965. These assembly plants, often just a few hundred yards across

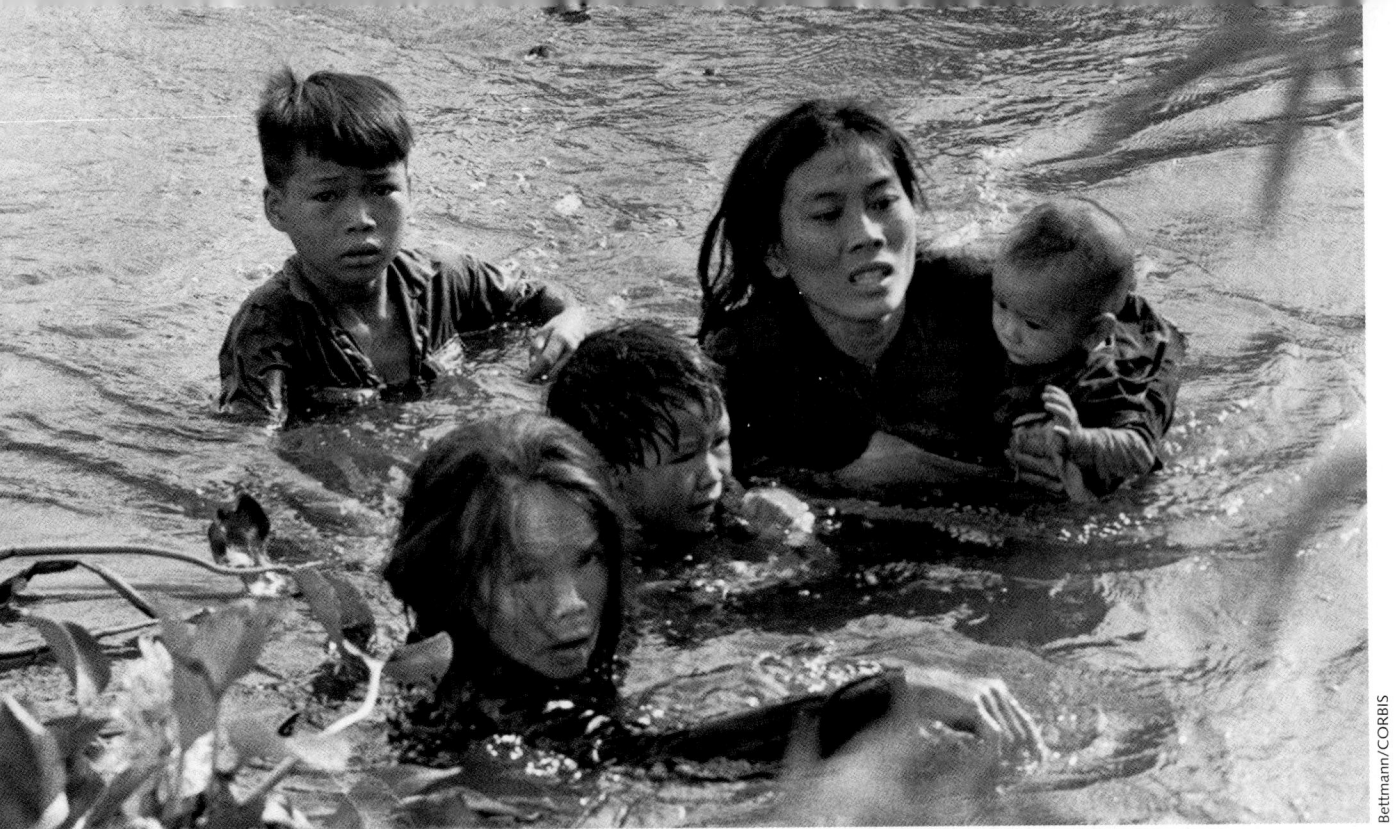

■ Many South Vietnamese fled the communist victory in their country in 1975, including this woman and her children crossing the Mekong River. Most of the refugees undertook extremely perilous journeys by boat to other Southeast Asian nations, and hundreds of thousands eventually made their way to the United States.

the Mexican–U.S. border, gave corporations an opportunity to hire primarily female workers at low wages and avoid strict U.S. environmental, labor, and safety laws. "The worst drawback of maquiladora work is all the damage we do to our health" by working with toxic chemicals and solvents, one employee reported. The wages, cheap by U.S. standards, were nonetheless higher than elsewhere in Mexico and drew laborers from central Mexico north to the border region. And few Americans noticed the damage that the factories south of the border were causing to the environment and to the health of workers.

High unemployment and shrinking real wages contributed to rising anti-immigrant sentiment. Two white autoworkers in Detroit in 1982 got into an altercation in a bar with Vincent Chin, a Chinese American (and son of a World War II veteran) whom they called a "Jap." Angered that Japanese auto sales were undercutting jobs in Detroit, they made Chin a scapegoat for their rage, chasing him down the street and beating him to death with a baseball bat. At the same time, Vietnamese refugees who had fled the communist victory in their homeland in 1975 to make a life as shrimp fishers on the Gulf Coast of Texas found their equipment sabotaged by some white competitors.

From Texas to California, Latinos also suffered violence at the hands of both officials and private citizens. For example, three members of the Ku Klux Klan abducted a Latino hitchhiker outside San Diego and delivered him to the U.S. Immigration Service for deportation to Mexico even though he was an American citizen. A wave of police brutality against Latinos alarmed even the White House by 1978, thanks to the lobbying of outraged Latino citizen organizations.

Black Americans also faced an increasing backlash against hard-won civil rights gains. While court-ordered busing to integrate schools in segregated neighborhoods proceeded slowly but peacefully in the South, northern urban whites dug in their heels. In Boston, violence erupted in the school hallways and the streets from 1975 to 1978 as economically vulnerable working-class whites harassed African Americans attending schools in white ethnic neighborhoods of South Boston, and blacks defended themselves.

The Oil Embargo

Nothing revealed Americans' newfound economic vulnerability more than the 1973–1974 boycott initiated by the Oil Producing and Exporting Countries (OPEC). The United States and the Soviet Union, along with Mexico and Venezuela, retained large oil reserves. But the largest producers were the Arab countries around the Persian Gulf, especially Saudi Arabia. These nations had resented the creation of Israel in 1948 and the resulting displacement of the Palestinians. Hostility intensified with the events of 1967. That year, Israel seized control of the West Bank of the Jordan River and the Gaza Strip. Six years later, Egypt and Syria struck back, attacking jointly on Yom Kippur, the holiest day of the Jewish year. The Arab armies threatened to overrun Israel until the United States gave the Israeli army a critical resupply of weapons, which helped turn the tide of battle.

Henry Kissinger then shuttled between Tel Aviv and Cairo to negotiate a ceasefire. His diplomatic skills won him the Nobel peace prize and laid the groundwork for a warming of U.S. relations with Egypt (the most populous Arab nation but not an oil producer). However, the other Arab states expressed outrage at this demonstration of America's close links with the

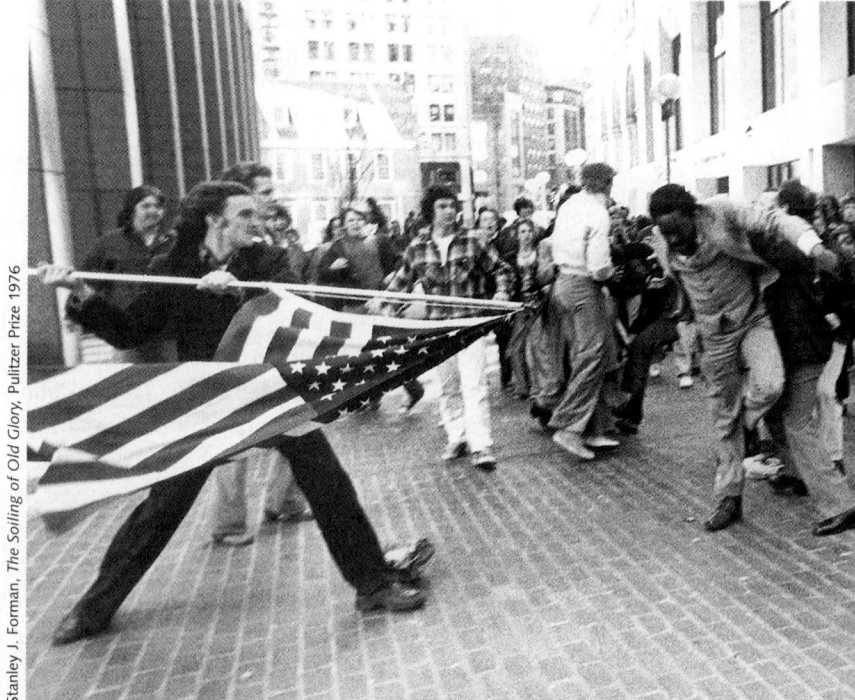

Stanley J. Forman, The Soiling of Old Glory, Pulitzer Prize 1976

■ White resistance to school busing in Boston sometimes turned violent in the mid–1970s. On April 5, 1976, white high school students from South Boston and Charlestown met with a city councilwoman who supported their boycott of classes. Outside City Hall, they chanced upon lawyer Theodore Landsmark and assaulted him. Photographer Stanley J. Forman won the Pulitzer Prize for this photo.

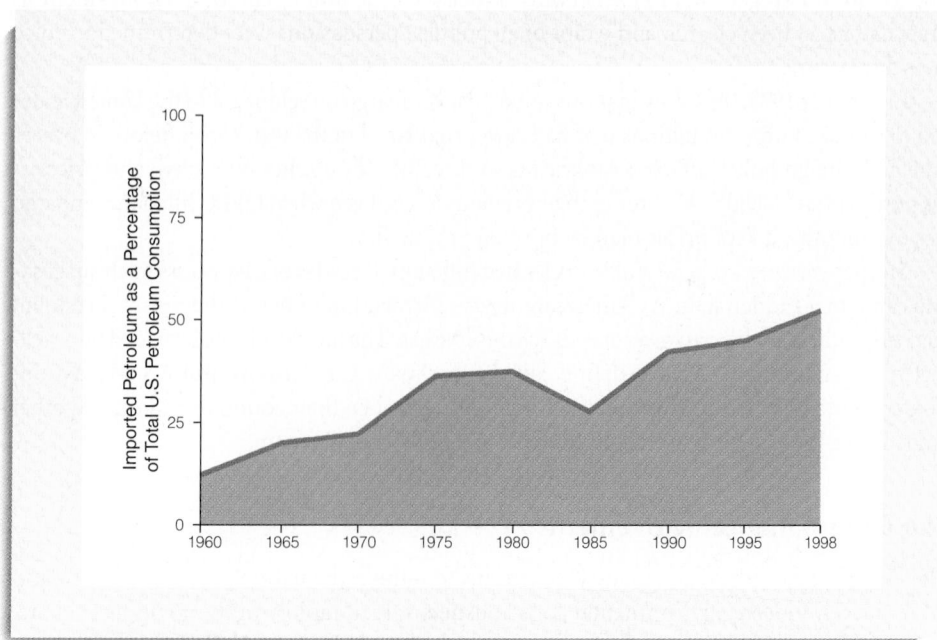

■ **FIGURE 27.1**
IIMPORTED PETROLEUM AS SHARE OF U.S. CONSUMPTION
Abundant natural resources, especially coal and oil, encouraged Americans' long-standing feeling of national strength and autonomy. After World War II, however, the United States switched from exporting oil to importing oil. Conservation measures in the 1970s temporarily reversed America's growing dependence on oil from abroad.

Energy Use in the United States

Most Americans who lived through the 1970s remember gasoline shortages and price hikes as one of the decade's most distinctive features. No previous generation had experienced so steep a decline in the availability of a primary source of energy that was the key to its transportation system. In World War II the government had rationed gasoline to conserve it for military use. But never before had international market forces confronted Americans with their growing dependence on imported petroleum.

The Arab oil embargo of 1973–1974 and the decline in oil supplies after the Iranian revolution of 1979 battered a U.S. economy already weakened by spending on the Vietnam War. The oil shocks drove inflation sharply upward. They raised fundamental questions—not asked since the

Great Depression of the 1930s—about whether the world's largest economy could continue to grow. And the oil price rise suggested that energy independence might be a crucial component of real national security.

Rich natural resources had long satisfied Americans' needs for energy sources. During the colonial period, wood from abundant forests and coal deposits provided heat. Whale oil powered lamps. Transportation came from the work of domesticated animals as well as sailing vessels that captured the force of the wind. In the era of the American Revolution, manufacturers built the first factories on riverbanks next to falls, where waterwheels produced the power to drive mechanical equipment.

In the 1800s, the spread of the Industrial Revolution increased the demand for energy, particularly coal. By the 1830s, coal fired the steam engines that pushed ships across the Atlantic Ocean and the railroads that would one day tie the growing nation together.

In 1859, on the eve of the Civil War, drillers near Titusville in northwestern Pennsylvania made a momentous discovery: oil. Refined into kerosene, oil lighted many American homes and city streets for more than a generation. Then Thomas Edison designed the first electricity-generating station in New York City in 1892, beginning the era of coal-fired electric utilities that spread rapidly over the next two decades.

Oil's real significance emerged in the twentieth century. Refined into gasoline, oil powered the new internal combustion engines that revolutionized transportation. Gasoline allowed the Wright brothers' airplane to leave the ground in 1903 and fueled the automobiles that began to pour off Henry Ford's assembly line with the first Model T in 1908. Inexpensive gasoline enabled cars to become Americans' foremost means of transportation. U.S. military forces depended on oil in all their wars of the twentieth century. Indeed, the United States fought in the Persian Gulf

Israelis, and Kissinger's being Jewish only underlined the point. The U.S. commitment to Israel had never been clearer, and Arabs of all political persuasions were determined to voice their displeasure.

In October 1973, the OPEC nations initiated an embargo on selling oil to the United States and to western European nations that had supported Israel in the war. Never before in peacetime had foreign policy affected Americans so directly. Oil supplies dwindled, and prices at gas pumps skyrocketed to four times their previous levels. Even when OPEC lifted the embargo afer five months, it kept prices high by limiting production.

Steeper energy costs powerfully accelerated inflation. Decades of easy access to cheap gasoline came to a sudden halt. As American drivers formed long lines at the pump, President Ford urged them to drive at lower speeds to conserve gas. The independence provided by a well-fueled automobile had come to define daily life for many U.S. citizens. But Americans confronted new and sobering limits on their mobility, just when their country encountered other limits in the form of Nixon's failed presidency and defeat in Vietnam.

The Environmental Movement

The oil embargo encouraged many U.S. citizens to rethink the nation's cavalier use of natural resources. Indeed, environmental consciousness spread rapidly in the 1970s as evidence revealed the impact of industrial growth on the quality of life in the United States. Environ-

War of 1991 primarily to preserve western access to oil from the Gulf region.

In the 1970s, the oil shocks and the growing environmental movement encouraged both energy conservation and the development of alternative, renewable sources. Many citizens paid increasing attention to solar, wind, water, and geothermal power. But corporations, encouraged by the federal government, paid far more attention to another alternative: nuclear energy. (The first American nuclear power plant had been built at Shippingport, Pennsylvania, in 1957.) Despite creating radioactive waste, nuclear power generated one-fifth of the nation's electricity by the twenty-first century.

In 2001, fossil fuels continued to provide 85 percent of the total energy used in the United States: oil, 40 percent; natural gas, 25 percent; and coal, 20 percent. Coal-burning plants created just over half the nation's electricity, and the United States had one-fourth of the world's coal supplies. However, unlike renewable energy sources, fossil

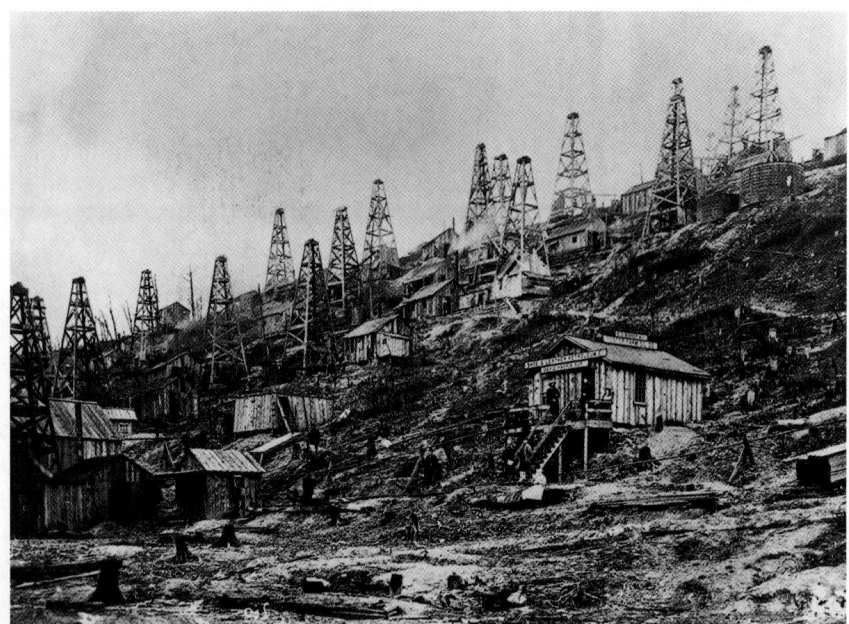

Oil derricks cover a hillside near Titusville, Pennsylvania in the era of the Civil War. Unlike renewable energy sources such as falling water or the sun, fossil fuels like oil and coal have to be burned and create serious air pollution in the process. The extraction of fossil fuels—so basic to the modern American economy—often involves damaging natural landscapes as well.

fuels are a finite resource that eventually will be used up. Burning them also contributes to air pollution, atmospheric ozone depletion, and global warming.

Nonetheless, at the turn of the century fossil fuels remained the cheapest source of power, a temptation too strong to resist. ■

mental organizations such as the Sierra Club, the National Wildlife Federation, and the Audubon Society saw their memberships soar. And for the first time, the media began to examine the daunting range of environmental problems plaguing the United States and the rest of the world: acid rain, groundwater contamination, smog, rainforest destruction, oil spills, nuclear waste disposal, species extinction, ozone depletion, and global warming. A growing interest in ecology—human interaction with the wider web of life—expanded the efforts of conservationists to preserve parklands. Residents of an urbanized mass society began to contemplate the wider consequences of small private acts such as watering the lawn, flushing the toilet, or leaving the lights on.

Environmentalism had perhaps even more radical implications than women's liberation or the counterculture had. "*Indefinite* growth of whatever kind cannot be sustained by *finite* resources," a prominent group of ecologists pointed out in 1972. Yet indefinite economic growth had been Americans' credo since the earliest days of European colonization. "Growth is the ideology of the cancer cell," writer Edward Abbey declared, helping to inspire the formation of the radical environmental group *Earth First!* in 1979. Yet even the nation's fiercest ideological opponents abroad agreed that the creation of wealth entailed the exploitation of natural resources. "Growth of industrial and agricultural production," Soviet leader Nikita Khrushchev had announced a decade earlier, "is the battering ram with which we shall smash the capitalist system." Now environmentalists were questioning an idea that even Communists had taken for granted.

A new generation of Americans, unable to remember Depression scarcities and wartime rationing, was wasteful, sometimes extravagantly so. U.S. soldiers had expressed surprise when displaced Vietnamese civilians built shelters out of the aluminum cans the troops threw away so casually. Home to only 6 percent of the global population, the United States consumed as much as a third of the world's energy from nonrenewable fossil fuels such as oil and coal. Polluted air hung over the largest U.S. cities. The first evidence of global warming began to appear in the 1970s. Scientists also noticed the rapid thinning of the ozone layer in the earth's atmosphere in 1973. They attributed the problem in part to the widespread use of aerosol spray cans—especially by Americans, the world's wealthiest people. The production of inexpensive plastics from oil had also soared since World War II. Styrofoam cups and plastic containers littered the roadsides. Disposable diapers and other nonbiodegradable products accumulated in landfills in what became known as the throwaway culture.

Environmentalists argued that the idea of unlimited consumption of natural resources was fundamentally irresponsible, both to future human generations and to other species. They urged Congress and the Environmental Protection Agency (EPA) to require fuel-efficient engines from carmakers and to promote renewable energy sources such as water, solar, and wind power. Citizen groups such as the Clamshell Alliance in New England and the Abalone Alliance in California protested the construction of new nuclear power plants. These operations, they pointed out, had no reliable method in place for disposing of nuclear waste. What if the public were exposed to radiation? Their warnings had merit: cancer rates began to rise in populations that had close contact with radioactive materials from the early Cold War years forward, such as communities near the Hanford nuclear facility in south central Washington state and towns downwind from the Atomic Test Site in Nevada. One Utah mother who lost a daughter to cancer felt "disappointed and hurt" by the "horrific neglect and indifference" of a government that would permit such contamination and then deny that there was any danger. "We were used. We were conned," another woman testified to Congress about government secrecy regarding the impact of radiation. "They knew and they didn't tell us."

A broad critique of the chemical industry's impact on public health also emerged in the 1970s. As it turned out, pesticides worked their way up the food chain into people's bodies. Some artificial sweeteners proved carcinogenic, and the lead that manufacturers had added to gasoline and house paint for generations caused brain damage. Long-standing industrial dumping of toxic chemicals made headlines. In 1975, for example, investigations revealed that tons of cancer-causing polychlorinated biphenyls (PCBs) from General Electric plants lined the bottom of the Hudson River north of New York City. Four years later, the EPA announced that the nation had 32,000 to 50,000 major sites containing hazardous waste.

Environmentalists argued that the idea of unlimited consumption of natural resources was fundamentally irresponsible, both to future human generations and to other species.

But it was the crisis at Love Canal in New York that helped bring the issue of toxic waste home to Americans. The Hooker Chemical Company had buried tons of poisonous waste in a dry canal in the town of Niagara Falls between 1947 and 1952 and then covered it over with dirt. The company gave the land to the town, which promptly built a school on it. A middle-class neighborhood soon grew up around the site. But the ground smelled odd and oozed mysterious substances. Sometimes it even caught on fire for no apparent reason. By the 1970s local rates of cancer and other severe illnesses had soared. The chemical and industrial plant workers who lived in the neighborhood began to suspect that their quiet loyalty to their employers was no longer worth the risk to the health of their families. Persistent activism by community members, led by Lois Gibbs and publicized by reporter Michael Brown, finally overcame local, state, and company officials' efforts to keep the contents of the buried canal secret. In August 1978, New York governor Hugh Carey at last agreed to buy out the entire neighborhood, seal it off, and move residents elsewhere. An early public revelation of the cost of industrial progress, the Love Canal debacle accelerated American workers' loss of faith in the

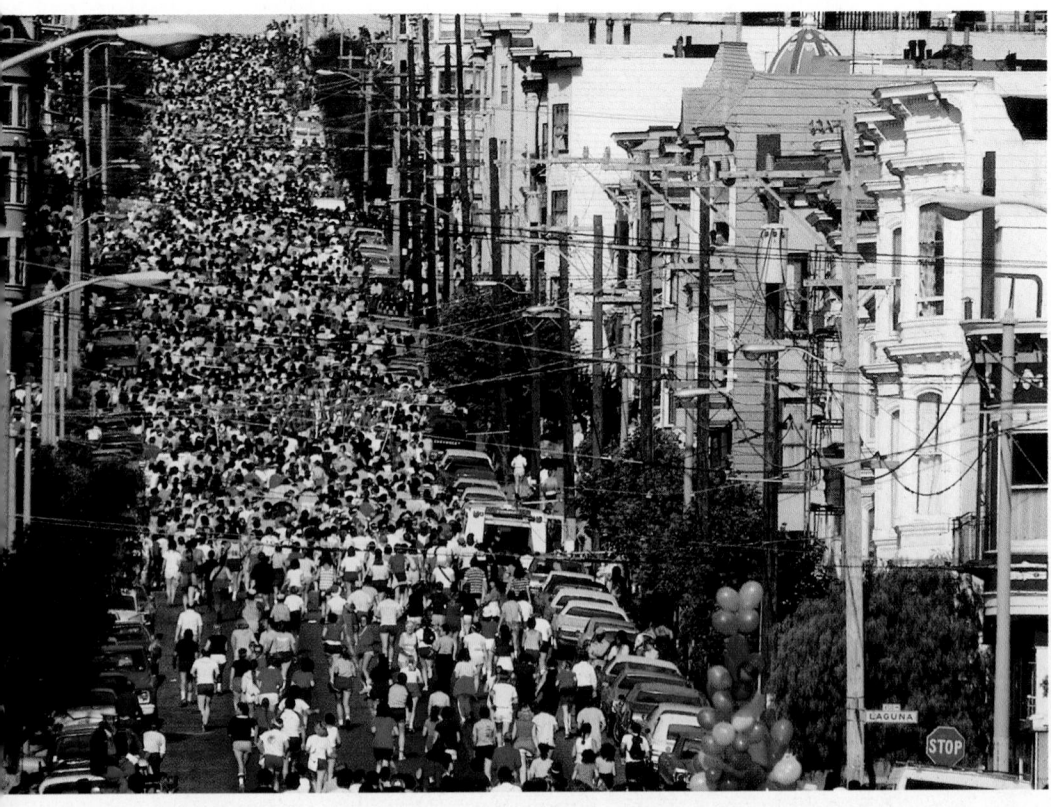

Peter Menzel/StockBoston

■ Thousands of runners surge up the Hayes Street hill in San Francisco in the annual 7-mile Bay-to-Breakers race across the city. In the 1970s regular exercise began to become a common part of daily life for many Americans. At the same time, fast food and higher-fat diets contributed to a growing pattern of Americans being overweight and even obese.

corporations and governments they had once trusted. "There are ticking time bombs all over," an EPA official concluded. "We just don't know how many potential Love Canals there are."

Discovering the limits of the U.S. economy so soon after the Vietnam War and the Watergate scandal spawned a crisis of confidence throughout the United States. Some Americans resented the idea of limits: on how much gas they could buy, how much the economy could grow, how much influence the United States could have abroad. At the same time, others began to embrace the idea of creating a healthier lifestyle that focused less on material consumption. Cigarette smoking started to decline. Organic food sales picked up. Exercise, especially running, began to become an increasingly common activity for middle-class adults. The wildly successful Nike athletic shoe company was founded in 1972, and entrants in the New York City Marathon ballooned from 126 in 1970 to 10,000 by 1978. Interest in outdoor recreation—hiking, camping, and bicycling—grew exponentially. Recycling also started its climb from a fringe activity to common practice in a few parts of the country. The government began to get the message, too. Federal agencies banned the use of hazardous products such as the pesticide DDT and the artificial sweetener sodium cyclamate in the original Gatorade formula. And in January 1974, Congress reduced the national speed limit to 55 miles per hour to conserve fuel.

Reshuffling Politics

The skepticism toward authority and tradition spawned by the counterculture, the Vietnam War, and the Watergate scandal spread through American culture in the 1970s. The use of illegal drugs, especially marijuana, was widespread. Casual sexual relationships proliferated in a decade when contraceptive pills had become widely available and the AIDS virus had not yet been identified. Popular and critically acclaimed films featured tales of

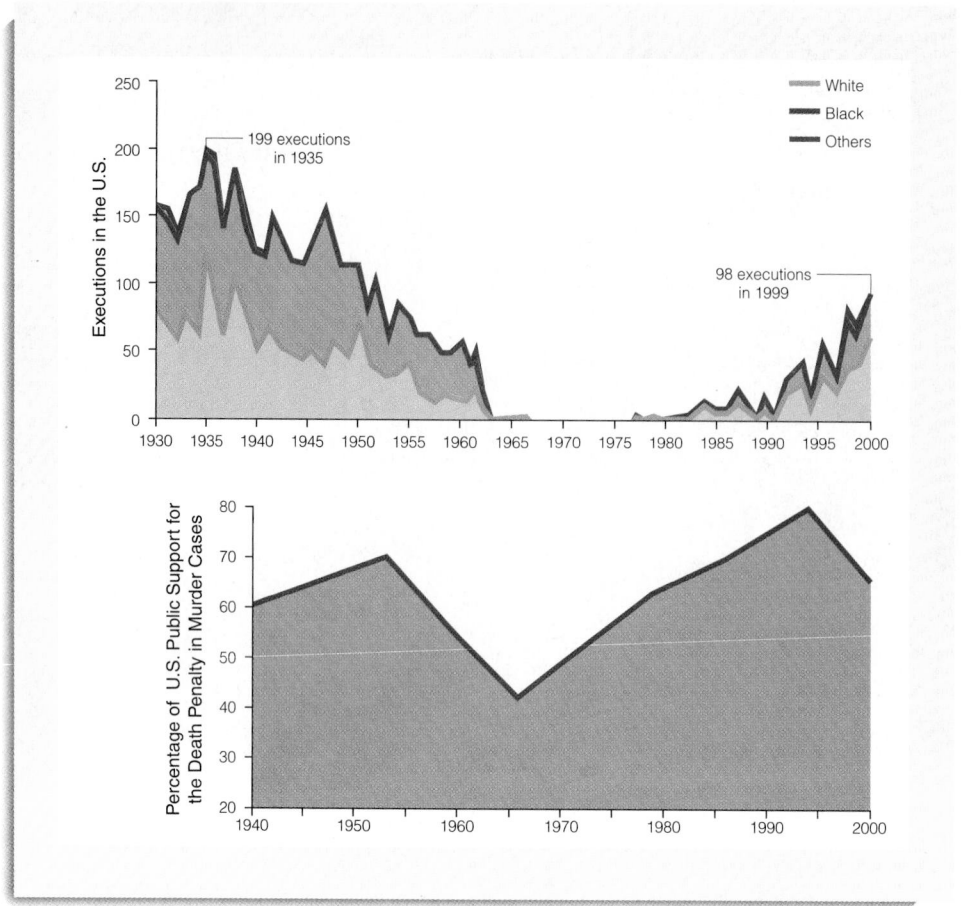

■ **FIGURE 27.2**
THE DEATH PENALTY: PRACTICES AND OPINIONS   The use of the death penalty distinguished the United States from most other industrialized nations, which had banned it. In 1972, The Supreme Court struck down existing capital punishment statutes as "arbitrary and capricious." Four years later, the Court upheld rewritten state and federal laws that provided clearer guidance for the imposition of the death penalty.

malfeasance in high places. *All the President's Men* (1976) told the story of the Nixon administration's Watergate crimes. *Apocalypse Now* (1975) revealed the madness of the American war in Vietnam. *Three Days of the Condor* (1975) portrayed the CIA as a rogue agency beyond democratic control. *Chinatown* (1975) suggested the vast corruption marring the early-twentieth-century growth of Los Angeles. *Blazing Saddles* (1974) hilariously spoofed the heroic Westerns that had long served as the staple of American moviegoers' diet. And *One Flew over the Cuckoo's Nest* (1975) used novelist Ken Kesey's story of an insane asylum to imply that those in charge were more dangerous than the inmates. In this atmosphere Congress began to reassert its authority against the "imperial presidency," and in 1976 voters put an obscure, devout Georgia peanut farmer and former one-term governor in the White House.

Congressional Power Reasserted

Before the twentieth century, the U.S. legislative branch had been the most powerful wing of the federal government. This emphasis on the authority of Congress as the closest representatives of the people had a long history. In the 1770s, Americans had fought their way free from a British empire whose powerful sovereign inspired deep and abiding distrust of executive authority. But the U.S. acquisition of its own overseas empire beginning in 1898 and its growing international prominence had slowly assuaged such anxieties. Many Americans came to believe that the country needed a strong president to direct the assertion of U.S. power abroad. World War II and the Cold War had dramatically accelerated this process. The balance of terror that came with the nuclear age seemed to demand secrecy and centralized decision-making. Americans had rejected this leadership style in their own revolution two centuries before. Yet the tide had turned, and the national security state and imperial presidency from Truman to Nixon emerged as the result.

The double shock of defeat in Vietnam and the Watergate scandal reawakened a Congress that had grown accustomed to deferring to the White House in foreign affairs. Tellingly, Congress had never formally declared war on North Korea or North Vietnam, although such declaration is its constitutional duty. Angered by the illegalities and deception in both the Johnson and Nixon administrations, Congress passed the War Powers Act in 1973 to limit the president's capacity to wage undeclared wars. The bill required the chief executive to obtain explicit congressional approval for keeping U.S. troops in an overseas conflict longer than 90 days. In 1976 Congress reinforced the message. It passed the Clark Amendment to cut off U.S. aid to anticommunist forces in the civil war in newly independent Angola, on the southwest coast of Africa. The House and Senate had resolved not to get drawn into "another Vietnam."

Congress did not limit its muscle-flexing to keeping Americans out of conflicts with Third World leftists. It also promoted human rights within the Communist bloc, cutting against the grain of Secretary of State Kissinger's realpolitik approach to Moscow. The Jackson–Vanik Amendment of 1974 sought to make the Soviet Union pay for its repression of Jewish dissidents by linking détente directly to human rights, much to Kissinger's dismay. To acquire most-favored-nation trading status with the United States, Moscow would have to let Jews emigrate.

With encouragement from voters and journalists, Congress also uncovered its eyes and began to investigate the covert side of American foreign policy that had gathered momentum since 1945. After Watergate popped the cork on the bottled-up secret abuses of the executive branch, other troubling news spilled out about the nation's intelligence agencies. Dissident former CIA agents such as Philip Agee began revealing "dirty tricks" that the agency had long used. And investigative reporter Seymour Hersh, author of the My Lai massacre exposé a few years earlier, uncovered the CIA's Operation Chaos. This program of illegal domestic espionage against antiwar dissidents paralleled FBI abuses such as the COINTELPRO campaigns to defame Martin Luther King, Jr., and destroy the Black Panthers and the American Indian Movement. Congressional committees led by Otis Pike of New York in the House and Frank Church of Idaho in the Senate initiated their own investigations of the national security state's tactics. Their documentation of CIA involvement in assassination attempts against foreign leaders such as Fidel Castro of Cuba and Patrice Lumumba of the Congo suggested that United States government agencies would secretly go to any lengths to prevail in the Cold War.

Defeat in Vietnam and the Watergate scandal reawakened a Congress that had grown accustomed to deferring to the White House in foreign affairs.

These revelations stirred fierce controversy among those who took an interest in national and international politics. The United States apparently had been almost as devious in its covert actions abroad as the reviled Soviet Union had been. Many citizens decried what their government had done in their names and without their knowledge. However, officials claimed that the extreme conditions of the Cold War and the duplicity of the Soviets necessitated secrecy. Convinced that information gathered by the Church and Pike committees threatened to undermine public trust in U.S. foreign policy officials, congressional leaders stopped official publication of the Pike report (although the *Village Voice* published a leaked copy). Nonetheless, in combination with the Freedom of Information Act of 1974—which forced the public release of most federal documents after 25 years—these congressional reports created a paper trail that altered Americans' perceptions of what their government did abroad.

At the core of this controversy were two burning questions. How transparent could a democratic society and its government afford to be when they also had global interests to protect? And when democratic openness and imperial self-interest conflicted, which should win out?

The Church Committee and CIA Covert Operations

In 1975–1976 the U.S. Senate Select Committee to Study Governmental Operations with Respect to Intelligence Activities engaged in the first comprehensive review by Congress of the actions of the Central Intelligence Agency. Under the leadership of Frank Church (D-Idaho), the committee investigated both intelligence gathering ("spying") and covert operations, the secret side of American foreign policy during the Cold War. One of the most controversial issues that the Church Committee examined was evidence of the CIA's attempted use of assassination as a means of dealing with key figures in Cuba, the Congo, the Dominican Republic, South Vietnam, and Chile.

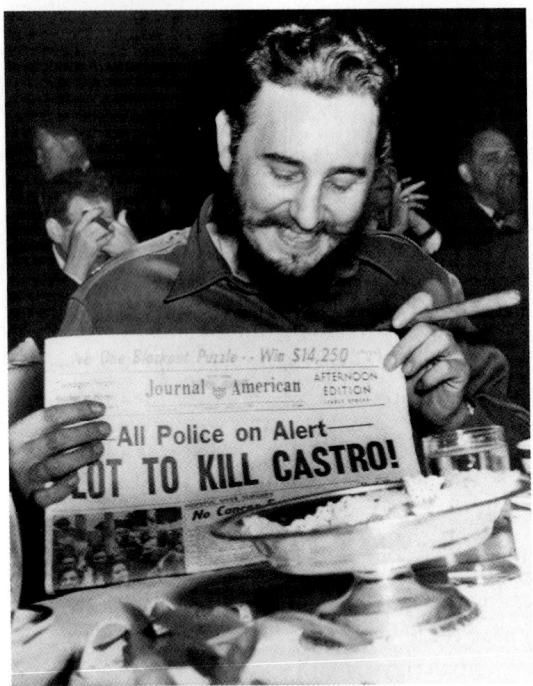

A star baseball pitcher who once turned down an offer to sign with the New York Yankees, Fidel Castro led a leftist, anti-American revolution in Cuba in 1959. U.S. hostility and Castro's evolving politics led him to declare Cuba a Communist state in 1961. The CIA tried unsuccessfully to arrange for Castro's assassination.

Bettmann/CORBIS

Alleged Assassination Plots Involving Foreign Leaders (Interim Report, November 20, 1975)

The Committee has received evidence that ranking Government officials discussed, and may have authorized, the establishment with the CIA of a generalized assassination capability. . . .

The evidence establishes that the United States was implicated in several assassination plots. . . . Our inquiry also reveals serious problems with respect to United States involvement in coups directed against foreign governments. . . .

Once methods of coercion and violence are chosen, the probability of loss of life is always present. There is, however, a significant difference between a coldblooded, targeted, intentional killing of an individual foreign leader and other forms of intervening in the affairs of foreign nations. . . .

Non-attribution to the United States for covert operations was the original and principal purpose

of the so-called doctrine of "plausible denial."

Evidence before the Committee clearly demonstrates that this concept, designed to protect the United States and its operatives from the consequences of disclosures, has been expanded to mask decisions of the President and his senior staff members. . . .

"Plausible denial" can also lead to the use of euphemism and circumlocution, which are designed to allow the President and other senior officials to deny knowledge of an operation should it be disclosed. . . .

It is possible that there was a failure of communication between policymakers and the agency personnel who were experienced in secret, and often violent, action. Although policymakers testified that assassination was not intended by such words as "get rid of Castro," some of their subordinates in the Agency testified that they perceived that assassination was desired and that they should proceed without troubling their superiors. . . .

Running throughout the cases considered in this report

was the expectation of American officials that they could control the actions of dissident groups which they were supporting in foreign countries. Events demonstrated that the United States had no such power. This point is graphically demonstrated by cables exchanged shortly before the coup in Vietnam. Ambassador Lodge cabled Washington on October 30, 1963, that he was unable to halt a coup; a cable from William Bundy in response stated that "we cannot accept conclusion that we have no power to delay or discourage a coup." The coup took place three days later. . . .

Officials of the CIA made use of persons associated with the criminal underworld in attempting to achieve the assassination of Fidel Castro. These underworld figures were relied upon because it was believed that they had expertise and contacts that were not available to law-abiding citizens. . . .

It may well be ourselves that we injure most if we adopt tactics "more ruthless than the enemy." ∎

"I Will Never Lie to You"

These same questions underlay the presidential election in the bicentennial year of 1976. As the nation celebrated the two-hundredth anniversary of its Declaration of Independence, some commentators could not help noting that the U.S. withdrawal from Vietnam in some ways echoed the British surrender at Yorktown in 1781. In each case, a determined nationalist army seeking freedom from foreign control had forced the world's strongest military power to withdraw in defeat.

In the backwash of Watergate, two presidential candidates—both outsiders to national politics—became advocates for opposing sides in the power and openness debate. Former California governor Ronald Reagan made a strong run at the Republican nomination, falling just short at the Kansas City convention as incumbent Gerald Ford held on to head the GOP ticket. Reagan articulated conservative Americans' anger at seeing U.S. autonomy and power abroad hemmed in. He opposed détente with the Soviets, supported anticommunists everywhere, and warned against a treaty that would return control of the Panama Canal to the Panamanians. Ford found himself burdened by the faltering economy, weakened by Reagan's criticisms from the right, and hampered by widespread resentment of his pardon for Nixon. He struggled back from a 33-point deficit in opinion polls to fall just short with 49 percent of the votes in the general election. The hopes of moderate Republicans faded as the party moved to the right after 1976.

TABLE 27-2			
The Election of 1976			
Candidate	Political Party	Popular Vote	Electoral Vote
Jimmy Carter	Democratic	40,828,587	297
Gerald R. Ford	Republican	39,147,613	241

Jimmy Carter was the winner. The former Georgia governor had worked relentlessly to gain the Democratic nomination after starting out as the choice of just 4 percent of primary voters. He based his candidacy on moral uplift. Contrasting himself to the Nixon administration, he told audiences, "I will never lie to you." Instead, Carter promised openness, accountability, and a government "as good and decent as the American people." He pledged to heal a nation exhausted by conflict. The emphasis on morality came naturally to the born-again Christian who taught Sunday school. His campaign manager admitted wryly that Carter's religious bent was a "weirdo factor" in national politics. The Georgian was also the first president to hail from the Deep South in more than a century. His open faith and cultural conservatism won him support from less liberal Democrats whom the McGovern campaign had alienated in 1972.

Carter was also a Naval Academy graduate, a former nuclear engineer, and a successful peanut farmer and businessperson. Yet the unusual green color of his campaign buttons and posters conveyed a subtle conservationist message, and liberals appreciated his attention to issues of poverty. Moreover, his support for civil rights during his governorship in Georgia had made him a symbol for a pragmatic new generation of white and black southerners. Americans were not sure who their new president really was. Carter kept his diminutive first name: Jimmy, not James or even Jim. He wore denim, and he carried his own bags. At his inaugural parade, he and his wife Rosalynn chose to walk down Pennsylvania Avenue rather than ride in a limousine.

The new president entered the White House at a time of unusual resistance to executive authority. He encountered an assertive and suspicious Congress. He served an alienated and isolationist public that had given him a slim victory with no clear mandate. He had to grapple with an alert and skeptical media that had dropped most vestiges of its traditional deference to the Oval Office. And he faced an economy still mired in stagflation as unemployment and prices kept rising and interest rates reached 21 percent.

Politics and ideology also hamstrung the new president, limiting his ability to lead his own party in governing the nation. The New Deal coalition of the working class,

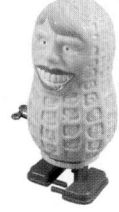

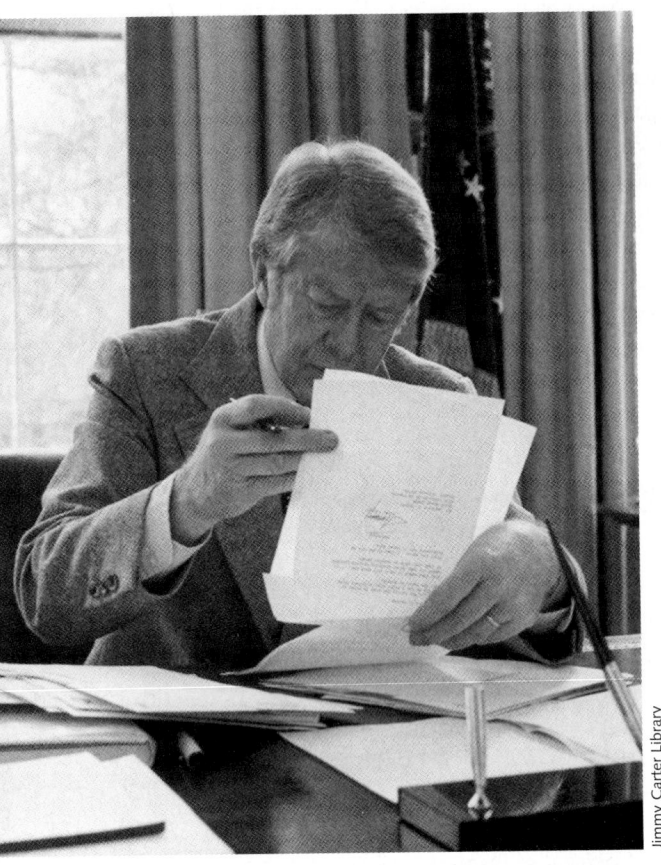

Jimmy Carter Library

■ After his inauguration as president, Jimmy Carter got down to work in the Oval Office. Serious, conscientious, and extremely hard-working, Carter immersed himself in many of the details of his administration's policies. The image of him sequestered and industrious at his desk came to symbolize, for many, both the strengths and weaknesses of his presidency.

people of color, and liberals had been unraveling for more than a decade. Carter had campaigned almost as an independent and developed few ties to the main Democratic constituencies. Thus he enjoyed little loyalty from his own party. The Georgian was also the first Democratic president since the 1930s who did not fully subscribe to the New Deal principle of government regulation of the economy. As a social moderate but an economic conservative, Carter had a strong desire to balance the federal budget. This vision placed him closer to the Republicans than to many in his own party. A businessperson, he also considered fiscal responsibility a primary virtue. Powerful liberal Democrats in Congress, by contrast, remained committed to government spending on programs such as Social Security and welfare, which Carter supported with less enthusiasm.

Carter's tendency to take moralistic stands did not mesh well with the horse-trading style of compromise that characterized Congress. In this sense, he was the opposite of Lyndon Johnson. Carter relied on a small circle of advisers from his days as governor in Atlanta. The northeastern-based media dubbed them the "Georgia Mafia." The president and his aides tried to govern as outsiders to the federal government. They viewed insiders as selfish and narrow-minded. They failed to cultivate relationships with Democratic leaders in Congress such as powerful House Speaker Thomas ("Tip") O'Neill of Massachusetts. Meanwhile, seasoned legislators of both parties looked down on the new administration as inexperienced and naive. With suspicion and condescension flowing in both directions between the White House and Capitol Hill, one senior Democratic congressman complained that Carter's popularity with the legislature was so low that he "couldn't get the Pledge of Allegiance through Congress" if he needed to.

Rise of a Peacemaker

Carter's idealism proved more effective, at least during his first two years, in refashioning U.S. foreign policy. The president started the national healing process with his first official act in office: he granted a "full, complete, and unconditional pardon" to those who had evaded the draft during the Vietnam War. He also tried to replace indiscriminate anticommunism with the promotion of human rights as the main theme in international affairs. "We are now free of that inordinate fear of Communism which once led us to embrace any dictator who joined us in that fear," he told an audience at Notre Dame University.

All presidents since 1945 had loudly supported human rights in the Soviet bloc. Carter defended dissidents in authoritarian countries friendly to the United States as well. His commitment to ending racial discrimination at home and his promotion of human rights abroad led to his administration's strong support for an end to white minority rule in southern Africa, including the establishment of Zimbabwe out of the old white-ruled Rhodesia in 1980. In a highly symbolic move, Carter appointed black civil rights leader and fellow Georgian Andrew Young as UN ambassador and point man on Africa policy.

Upon taking office, Carter fired the director of the CIA, George H. W. Bush. In the wake of the congressional investigations of the CIA, he reined in the agency's covert operations. Carter wanted to shift Americans' attention away from East–West Cold War tensions. Instead, he encouraged the public to acknowledge the burgeoning problems between industrialized nations of the North and mostly poor countries of the Southern Hemisphere. The president made control over the Panama Canal a test case for this reorientation. The huge canal sym-

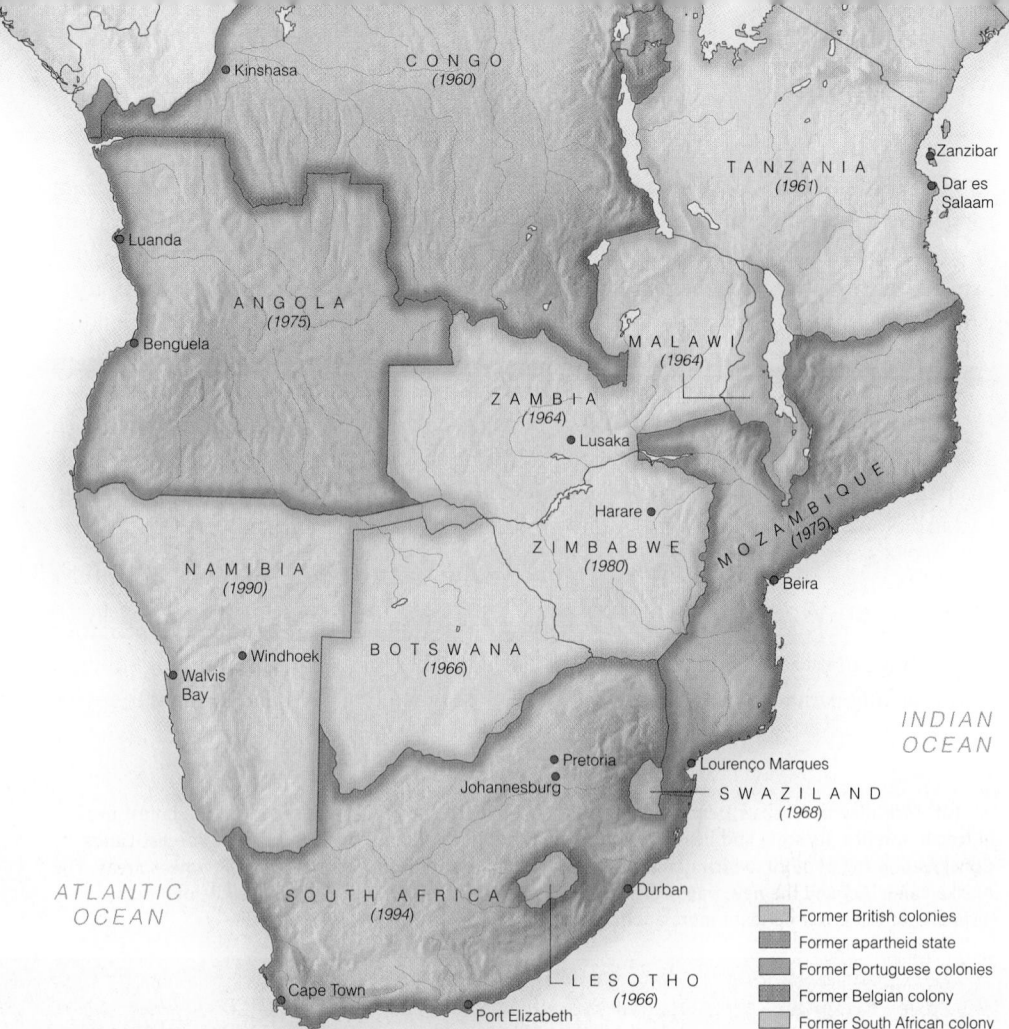

CONGO *(1960)*

Kinshasa

TANZANIA *(1961)*

Zanzibar

Dar es Salaam

Luanda

ANGOLA *(1975)*

Benguela

MALAWI *(1964)*

ZAMBIA *(1964)*

Lusaka

MOZAMBIQUE *(1975)*

Harare

ZIMBABWE *(1980)*

Beira

NAMIBIA *(1990)*

Windhoek

BOTSWANA *(1966)*

INDIAN OCEAN

Walvis Bay

Pretoria

Johannesburg

Lourenço Marques

SWAZILAND *(1968)*

ATLANTIC OCEAN

SOUTH AFRICA *(1994)*

Durban

Cape Town

LESOTHO *(1966)*

Port Elizabeth

Former British colonies

Former apartheid state

Former Portuguese colonies

Former Belgian colony

Former South African colony

■ **MAP 27.2**
THE GRADUAL LIBERATION OF SOUTHERN AFRICA FROM WHITE MINORITY RULE The Carter administration supported the ending of white minority rule in Southern Africa. The last redoubts of "white supremacy" included Rhodesia, which became Zimbabwe in 1980, and South Africa, which granted independence to Namibia in 1990 and ended apartheid in 1994.

bolized U.S. dominance of the hemisphere and served as a focus of resentment among many Latin Americans. Since 1903, the United States had ruled the 10-mile-wide Canal Zone as its own colony. Acknowledging this colonialist past, Carter signed treaties on September 7, 1977, to return sovereignty of the canal to Panama.

Defenders of U.S. control of the canal, led by prominent Republican Ronald Reagan, fought the treaties fiercely. They saw them as irresponsibly giving away an American asset. "We built it, we paid for it, and we're going to keep it," Reagan insisted. But other prominent conservatives, including Henry Kissinger and movie star John Wayne, acknowledged the symbolic importance of the canal for strengthening U.S. relations with Latin America. They supported the president. Carter threw all his political weight into the campaign, and the Senate approved the treaties by a thin margin in the spring of 1978.

The Carter administration's other great diplomatic achievement came with the Camp David accord, an agreement between Egypt's president Anwar Sadat and Israel's prime minister Menachem Begin. The Arab–Israeli conflict had remained one of the most intractable problems in modern diplomacy, yet Carter had unusual credibility in tackling the issue. His concern as a Christian for the "Holy Land" claimed by both Jewish Israelis and mostly Muslim Palestinians gave him sympathy for both sides. Sadat himself created an opening for diplomacy in 1977 by becoming the first Arab leader to visit Israel. But as the leading outside power in the region and Israel's closest ally, only the United States could move the peace process further along.

Carter took action. He invited Sadat and Begin to Camp David, the presidential retreat in rural western Maryland. There his persistence, plus promises of American aid to all parties, kept the marathon negotiations on track. In March 1979, the Egyptian and Israeli leaders signed two accords: Egypt became the first Arab state to grant official recognition to Israel. In turn, Israel agreed to withdraw its troops from the Sinai peninsula and apparently to stop building additional settlements on the Palestinian West Bank of the Jordan River. The framework for peace implied eventual autonomy for the Palestinians in the West Bank and the Gaza strip.

Though promising, the Camp David accords failed to bring peace to the Middle East. Israeli settlements in the West Bank continued to proliferate, and anti-Israeli terrorism by Palestinians persisted. But Carter had persuaded two major players in the region to take a big step back from open hostility. The world rightly proclaimed him a peacemaker.

The War on Waste

Within three months of taking office, Carter called for the "moral equivalent of war" to meet the deepening national energy crisis. The OPEC oil embargo of 1973 and his own thought-

■ Mt. McKinley in Alaska's Denali National Park rises to 20,320 feet above sea level, the tallest peak in North America. Its scale and beauty inspired many supporters of the Alaska National Interest Lands Conservation Act of 1980, which dramatically expanded the nation's parklands and wilderness areas. The Alaska Lands Act and the new trans-Alaska oil pipeline, completed three years earlier, helped many residents of the lower 48 learn more about the nation's largest and most remote state.

Danny Lehman/CORBIS

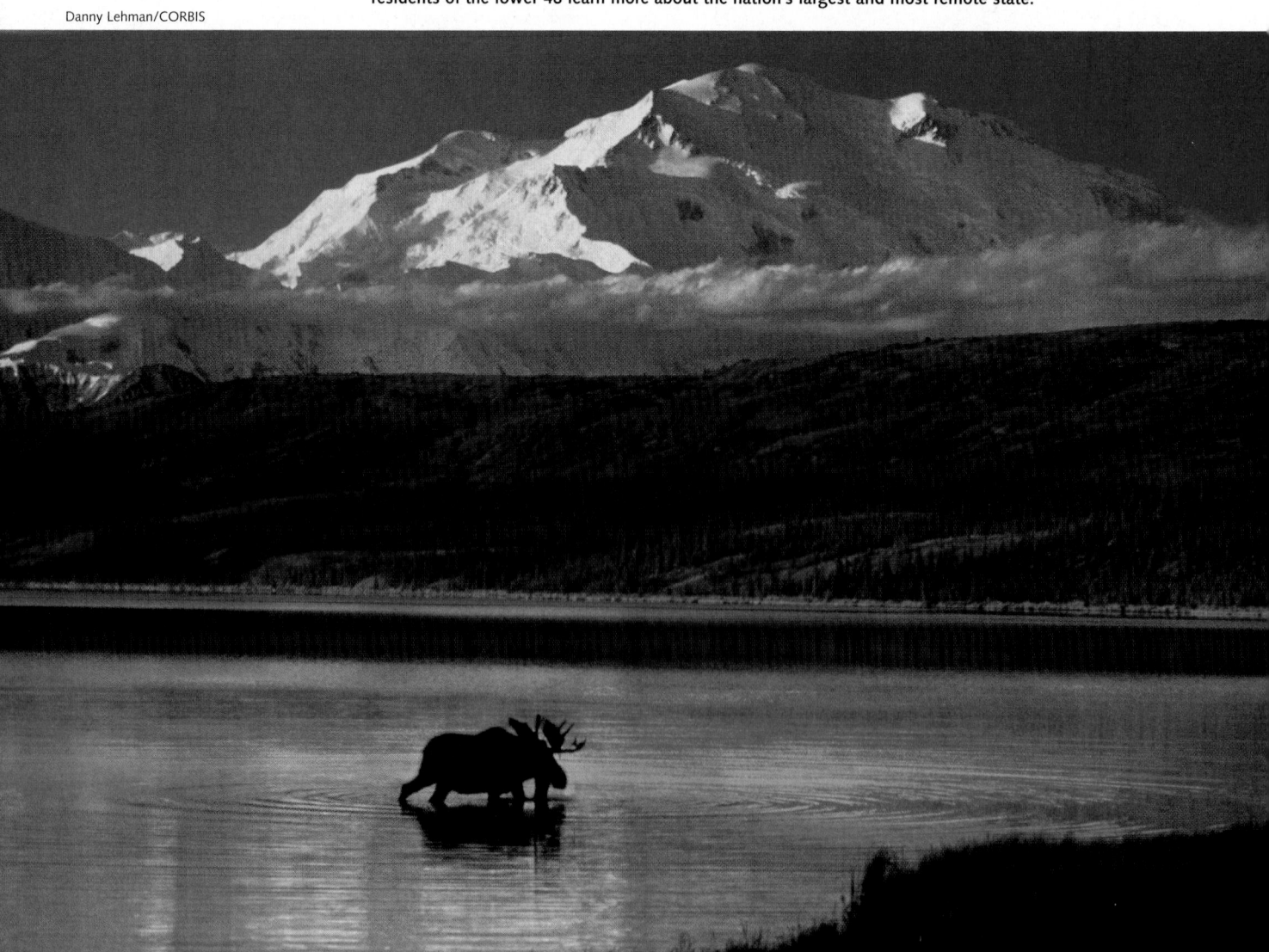

fulness allowed the president to understand better than his immediate predecessors that the country's addiction to imported oil put Americans at the mercy of other oil-producing nations. He exhorted his fellow citizens to stop being "the most wasteful nation on Earth." Conserve energy, he implored them. Switch off lights and turn down thermostats.

The administration created the Department of Energy and granted tax incentives to promote development of alternative sources such as solar energy. The EPA required U.S. automakers to meet stricter fuel efficiency standards for their engines. High prices encouraged a renewed search for domestic sources of oil. In 1977 workers completed the 800-mile-long, 48-inch-wide Trans-Alaska Pipeline System. The system linked the state's northern oil fields at Prudhoe Bay on the Arctic Ocean with a tanker terminal in Valdez, on Alaska's southern coast on the Pacific Ocean. With new oil now flowing freely, Carter worked with Congress to pass the 1980 Alaska National Interest Lands Conservation Act. This legislation created the single largest addition ever to the nation's wilderness system, 47 million acres, and the new Wrangell–St. Elias National Park.

The most controversial power alternative came in the form of nuclear energy. Obtained by harnessing the force of splitting atoms, nuclear energy seemed to promise unlimited pollution-free power. But it entailed the use of a deadly radioactive fuel, uranium. Was it the clean solution to the nation's energy needs or a lethal nightmare waiting to overtake an unsuspecting public? *The China Syndrome,* a popular 1978 film, suggested the latter. A few months later, life imitated art. In March 1979, a partial meltdown of the nuclear core of the Three Mile Island reactor near Harrisburg, Pennsylvania, leaked radiation and forced a major evacuation. Government officials tried to reassure a panicked public. However, in July, a dam burst near Church Rock, New Mexico, flooding the Rio Puerco valley with radioactive wastewater.

Despite these obstacles, existing nuclear power plants continued to generate 11 percent of the nation's electricity in 1979, a figure that climbed to 22 percent by 1992 as other plants under construction came on line. Nonetheless, because of negative public opinion and the high cost per unit of nuclear power, no new plants ordered by utility companies after 1974 were ever completed.

In 1979, a revolution in Iran cut off the United States from the world's second-largest oil producer. The event initiated a new round of energy price increases, escalated inflation, and further intensified public anxieties. In an unusual display of frankness for a country's leader, President Carter acknowledged that the

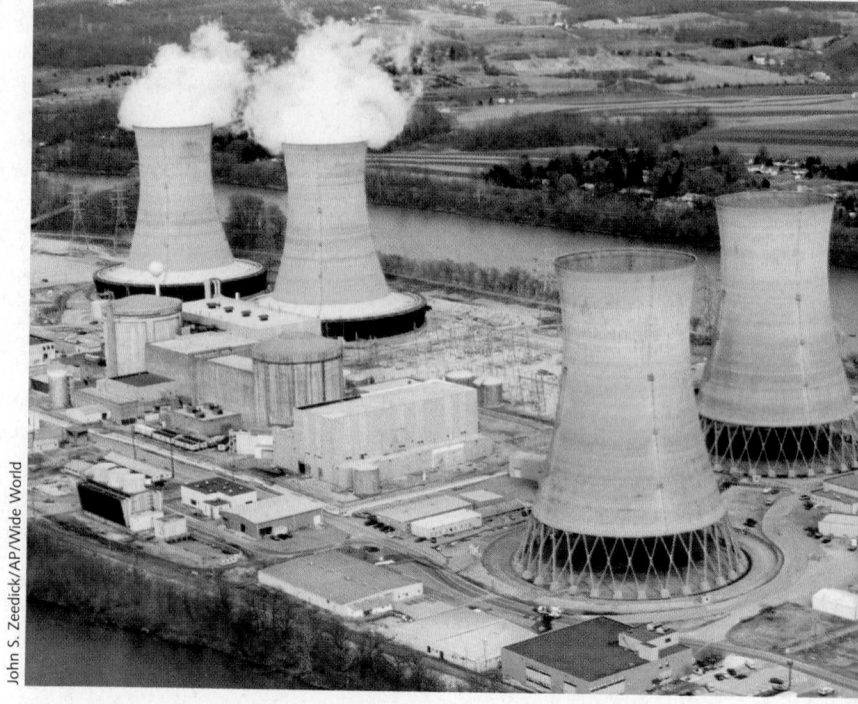

John S. Zeedick/AP/Wide World

■ The cooling towers of the Three Mile Island nuclear power plant loom over the Susquehanna River just south of Harrisburg, Pennsylvania. Nuclear energy epitomized the centralization of power: citizens benefited from the electricity produced but had little knowledge or control of a technology that could go astray more easily than authorities liked to admit.

nation seemed adrift. He gathered an array of advisers at Camp David for extended reflection on how the nation might set a new direction for itself. He emerged to give a major speech on July 15, 1979. In it, he linked America's energy problems to a broader national "crisis of confidence." "In a nation that was proud of hard work, strong families, close knit communities and our faith in God," he explained, "too many of us now tend to worship self-indulgence and consumption."

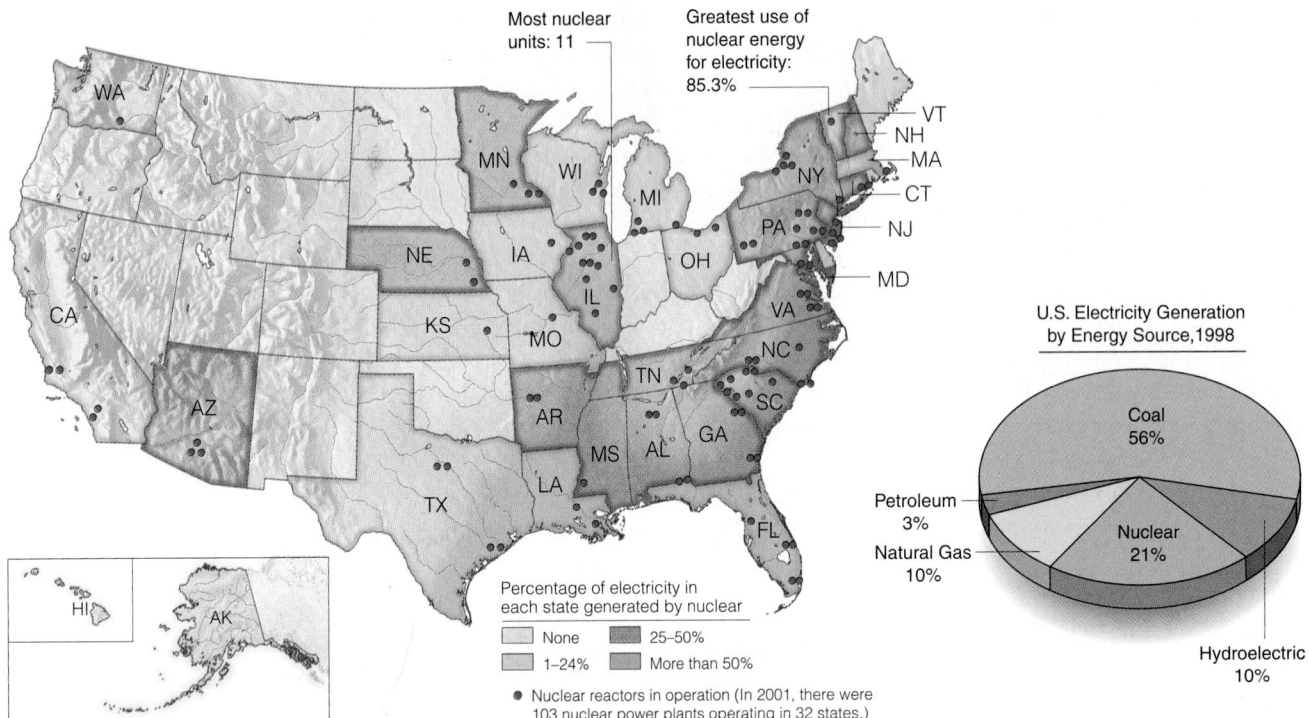

■ **MAP 27.3**
BUILDING NUCLEAR POWER PLANTS Between 1969 and 1980, all of the nation's 103 commercial
nuclear power reactors either came on line (56) or were in the process of being planned or built (47). The
United States has roughly one-quarter of the 434 commercial nuclear power reactors in the world. Despite
nuclear energy's important role in U.S. electricity production, there is still no system in place for the
permanent disposal of radioactive waste.

But Carter proved more effective at identifying the problem of America's insatiable appetite
for energy than he was at offering a remedy. His call for sacrifice and unity made for courageous but ultimately self-defeating politics in a society accustomed to unrestrained consumption. Other politicians, such as Ronald Reagan, moved swiftly to smooth Americans' ruffled
feathers with a cheerful message: U.S. citizens were fine just as they were. As one supporter
of the oil and gas industry claimed, "This country did not conserve its way to greatness. It
produced its way to greatness."

Diffusing the Women's Movement

"Good morning, boys and girls!" This standard classroom greeting reveals the central
place of gender in how Americans identify people from a young age. Few people consider the phrase offensive, even though they probably would protest if a teacher
addressed class members as "blacks and whites" or "tall people and short people." Should one's
sex (a biological characteristic) or gender (the social assumptions associated with sex) constitute the fundamental dividing line among human beings? The spread of feminism through
U.S. society from the 1970s onward raised this question.

The Meanings of Women's Liberation

In a decade marked by hard rethinking of major issues, feminists provided one of the most profound challenges of all. Few American households avoided at least some reconsideration of the

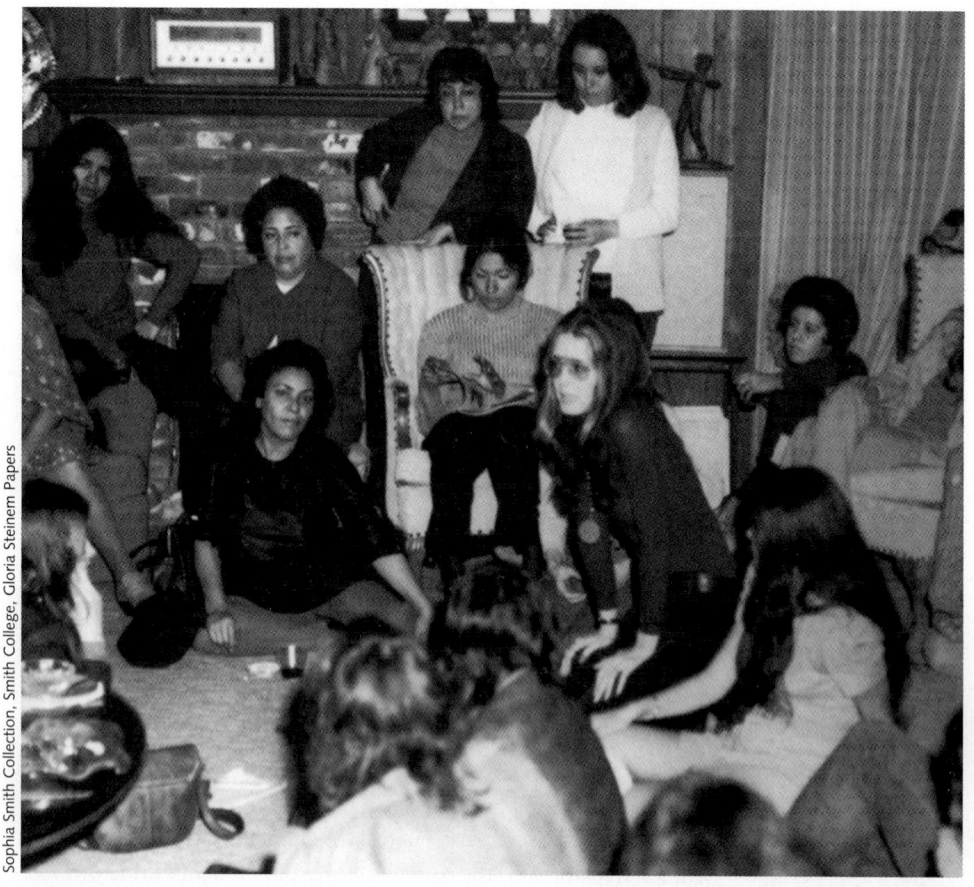

Sophia Smith Collection, Smith College, Gloria Steinem Papers

■ Gloria Steinem, on her knees, speaks at a meeting of a women's consciousness-raising group in the early 1970s. Similar groups gathered informally in homes around the country and helped women articulate their common struggles against discrimination.

roles of men and women. Just as the nation reimagined its foreign policy in less assertive terms and with greater concern for human rights, feminists called for equality between the sexes while honoring their differences. This call resonated with a growing number of Americans. The women's movement cast a spotlight on the need for justice in both the private sphere of personal relationships and the public sphere of the workplace and the law.

Between 1968 and 1973 some 500 new feminist publications cropped up in the United States. Gloria Steinem's *Ms.* magazine became the most prominent, selling out the 250,000 copies of its first issue in January 1972 within eight days. Its then-revolutionary name symbolized women's desire not to have their marital status revealed through the title of "Miss" or "Mrs." After all, the title "Mr." said nothing about a man's marital status, so why should not a woman's title be similarly neutral? Thousands of consciousness-raising meetings also made women aware that their own experiences with discrimination were part of a broader pattern of injustice toward women.

The millions of American women who found their lives changing in the 1970s did not agree on all issues. African American and Latino American women balanced identities as women with identities as people of color, which aligned them closely with men of their communities. Like Karen Silkwood, working-class women of all colors often focused on issues common to all workers, including wages, workplace conditions, and union representation. Community organizers such as Lois Gibbs of Love Canal zeroed in on neighborhoods and families. The educated white women who tended to form the most visible part of the movement for equality differed among themselves on such issues as pornography: some found it inherently exploitive of women, while others considered it primarily a matter of free expression.

However, all women shared certain concerns. Even as many female Americans remained wary of the label *feminist*—fearing associations with anger, militancy, and dislike of men—they nonetheless tended to side with feminist positions on issues from equal pay for equal work, to abortion rights, to more egalitarian distribution of household chores within families. Even women who still chose to wear makeup and dress in traditionally feminine fashion shared a desire for men to take women more seriously for their ideas and beliefs than for their appearance. The women's movement also sought to unmask the violence constraining all women's lives: sexual harassment, domestic abuse, and rape. Whereas some men joked about rape, women called it what it was: a form of torture that kept many reluctant to venture out of their homes alone. And even a woman's home was not safe at times. Until the mid-1970s, a husband could force himself sexually on his wife and not be considered a rapist by the law.

New Opportunities in Education, the Workplace, and Family Life

In the 1970s, educated women gained access to a host of new opportunities in the workplace. Young women in college, unlike their mothers, expected to choose and develop a career after graduation even more than they anticipated getting married. The number of women entering graduate and professional schools soared. The percentage of female students in law school shot up from 5 percent to 40 percent between 1970 and 1980. In addition, most single-sex private colleges and universities, such as Yale and Vassar, went coeducational. Many dormitories housed both men and women, allowing young people from the middle and upper classes to live in close physical proximity for the first time.

A similar process unfolded in the workplace. Employment in the United States, formerly divided into "men's" and "women's" work, saw a blurring of those lines. Help-wanted advertisements stopped categorizing jobs as male and female, and women joined the ranks of police officers and construction workers. The post-1950 pattern of women flocking into the paid workforce passed a milestone in 1980. That year, more than half of women with children under six years old had paying jobs outside the home. However, most of these jobs were lower-wage service positions that offered neither union support nor much upward mobility. Women fared better in the professions; the percentage of female lawyers and Ph.D.s tripled in the 1970s, and that of female physicians doubled.

Despite these gains, professional women still averaged only 73 percent of the pay of their male colleagues. They also encountered stubborn traditional gender expectations. Late in the decade, one New York City judge ordered a female attorney—dressed in a tailored designer pantsuit and silk blouse—to leave his courtroom and not return unless she showed up in a skirted suit that demonstrated "proper respect" for the court.

Not surprisingly, family life also changed shape in these years. In the 1950s more than 70 percent of American families with children had had a father who worked outside the home and a mother who stayed at home. In 1980, only 15 percent of families were configured that way. Yet society's growing acceptance of mothers in the workforce did not necessarily mean that these women enjoyed a lighter domestic load. Most working mothers still had primary responsibility for parenting. For example, President Nixon vetoed a 1970 bill to establish a federally funded daycare system. Such a program, he declared, "would lead to the Sovietization of American children." Although many fathers accommodated their wives' work lives, working mothers continued to bear the brunt of the "second shift": child-rearing and housework in addition to a full-time paid job.

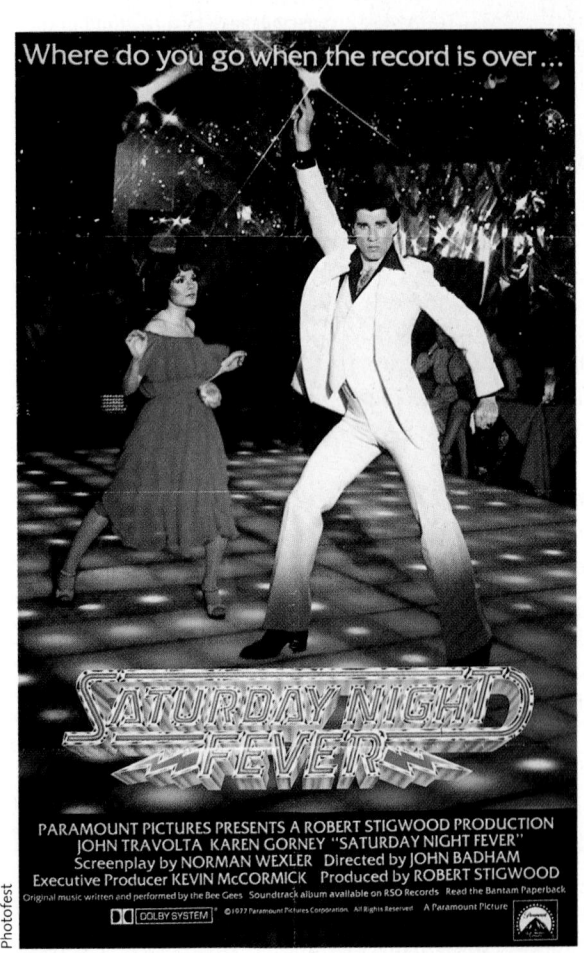

■ The hit 1977 film *Saturday Night Fever* starred John Travolta, Karen Gorney, and the popular disco music of the late 1970s. Disco's many critics granted its success as dance music but condemned it as banal and uncreative. Punk was an angrier and edgier musical style that evolved in the same years out of the rock 'n' roll of the late 1960s and early 1970s.

Changing roles brought new marital stresses, and divorce rates climbed in this decade. In 1970, one-third as many divorces as marriages occurred annually; in 1980, the figure was one-half. No-fault divorce laws, beginning with California's in 1970, eased the process and the stigma attached to divorce, although its emotional impact on adults and children remained hard to measure. Men benefited financially when marriages split up. Their average living standard rose sharply, whereas that of women and their children plummeted. Children living with both parents had a 1-in-19 chance of growing up poor. The likelihood rose to 1 in 10 for kids living with just a father; for those living with just a mother, the odds reached 1 in 3.

Equality Under the Law

Paralleling the logic of the black civil rights movement, the modern women's movement pressured lawmakers to eliminate the legal underpinnings of sex-based discrimination. Title IX of the Educational Amendments of 1972 required schools to spend comparable amounts on women's and men's sports programs. This critical step symbolized women's shift away from spectatorship and cheerleading to the female athleticism that helped define American popular culture by the end of the twentieth century. Mia Hamm and her teammates—members of the wildly popular U.S. women's soccer team that won the world championship in 1999—represented the first generation of women to grow up with strong institutional support for girls' sports.

After languishing for decades among failed proposals in Congress, the proposed Equal Rights Amendment to the Constitution finally rode to an overwhelming victory among senators and representatives in 1972. The legislature then sent it to the states for possible ratification by 1980. Simple in its language, the ERA declared, "Equality of rights under law shall not be denied or abridged by the United States or by any State on account of sex." On January 22, 1973, in the landmark case of *Roe v. Wade*, the Supreme Court ruled (by a 7–2 vote) that constitutional privacy rights were "broad enough to encompass a woman's decision whether or not to terminate her pregnancy" in its first six months. This decision established women's constitutional right to determine the course of their own pregnancies. Feminists had pointed out that the question was never *whether* women would have abortions but *how:* they would have them at the hands of illegal and often dangerous practitioners or in the offices of skilled physicians.

Finally, women's battle for equality under the law raised questions about military service. The Selective Service Act of 1980 still required only men to register for the draft on their eighteenth birthdays. But women's exemption from one of the highest duties of national citizenship was slipping fast. Within ten years, some 35,000 American women in the volunteer armed forces served in the 1991 Persian Gulf War, mostly in rear support positions but also as pilots flying reconnaissance and search-and-rescue missions. Fifteen died, and enemy forces captured two others. Even though many of these female service personnel in the war had small children, their assignments close to the line of fire generated little public outcry. American women could now be warriors.

Backlash

Even as the majority of Americans accepted the fundamental tenets of feminism, some fiercely defended existing gender roles. The mainstream media often painted women's rights activists as angry man-haters. Indeed, the media seized the opportunity to associate feminism with "bra-burning," a titillating way to blend women's rights with the sexual revolution and thus avoid the serious issues that women were raising. One Chicana worker involved in the strike against the Farah slacks company in Texas responded, "I don't believe in burning your bra, but I do believe in having our rights."

The women's movement posed a daunting challenge to traditional ideas about masculinity. "We have new men as well as a new society to build," feminist Kathie Amatniek (who later changed her surname to Sarachild) wrote in 1968. Men wondered what equality for women really meant and how it might change their intimate and professional relationships with them. Should men still open doors for women? Should they begin to do half (or more) of housework and parenting? Should they not comment on a female colleague's appearance?

To be sure, women's growing economic independence and educational opportunities often altered the dynamics of power in male–female relationships. Many men from all classes and ethnicities, feeling defensive about assumptions and behaviors that were increasingly labeled sexist, resisted these changes. One Latino graduate student at Stanford University resolved never to date "college girls." "When I want a real woman, I go to the barrio in East San Jose and pick up a high school girl." Many men also found the increasingly open acknowledgment of lesbianism threatening because it implied their potential irrelevance to women. The challenge to machismo took the form of public spectacle in 1973. That year, women's tennis champion Billie Jean King agreed to play 55-year-old former Wimbledon champion Bobby Riggs in a nationally televised "Battle of the Sexes" in the Houston Astrodome. More than 45 million Americans watched King crush her self-proclaimed "male chauvinist pig" opponent in straight sets.

> *Should men still open doors for women? Should they begin to do half (or more) of housework and parenting?*

That men would have mixed feelings about women's liberation surprised no one. But some of the stiffest resistance came from certain women. Those who had built their identities on motherhood and homemaking fiercely defended that tradition. Led by Illinois lawyer Phyllis Schlafly, antifeminists sought to uphold an established family structure that they believed divorce, gay rights, abortion, and daycare would destroy. In their view, femininity meant service to one's family. "Feminists praise self-centeredness," Schlafly declared, "and call it liberation." In addition to defending their own choices, female antifeminists also worried about the impact of dual-career families on children.

Opponents of women's liberation made two major legislative gains in the late 1970s. First, Congress passed the Hyde Amendment in 1976, which forbade the use of Medicaid funds for abortions. In practice, the amendment limited access to abortion to those women who could afford to pay for it themselves. Second, Schlafly's Stop-ERA campaign helped defeat the Equal Rights Amendment by limiting its ratification to only 35 of the required 38 states. Schlafly claimed that the amendment would "destroy the family, foster homosexuality, and hurt women." ERA opponents condemned "unisex toilets" and the drafting of women into combat that they believed the amendment would bring. In these women's views, the ERA would also draw out the worst in men, letting husbands opt out of supporting their wives and freeing divorced men from paying alimony. Antifeminists resented the disrespect for motherhood that they felt from some feminists. Still, they agreed with feminists that tens of millions of American women were just one man removed from welfare. At the heart of the controversy, the two sides differed on the best way to protect women's interests. Should their economic independence be enhanced, or should men be tied more tightly to their families?

Though discouraging for some, the narrow defeat of the ERA could not mask feminism's growing influence throughout American culture. The "first woman" stories that began showing up in the media during the 1970s marked the entrance of women into previously all-male roles. Like physicians, lawyers, and other figures of cultural authority, religious leaders now increasingly consisted of women, including the first Lutheran pastor (1970), the first Jewish rabbi (1972), and the first Episcopal priest (1974). In 1981 Sandra Day O'Connor became the first female Supreme Court justice. And mainstream organizations such as churches and municipalities ran feminist-created community institutions, including rape crisis centers, women's health clinics, and battered women's shelters. In 1978 the National Weather Service began using male as well as female names for hurricanes. By the 1980s, the movement had made major inroads into gender discrimination, although subtle forms of it remained. Younger women, confident that their fair treatment under the law was secure, began shying away from the term *feminism* and its lingering associations with rejection of men.

Conclusion

In 1978 a divided U.S. Supreme Court handed down a ruling on the contentious policy of affirmative action. The justices decided by a 5–4 vote in the *Bakke* case that strict racial quotas were unconstitutional but that universities could consider race as one of several factors in determining a candidate's qualifications for admission. The Court, like the American public, was wrestling with the broader 1970s problem of how to reform American society in ways that would preserve its historic strengths while removing the ills that the previous decade's political activism had laid bare. Traditional hierarchies of gender, race, and even presidential privilege were fraying badly, even as differences in wealth and income between citizens remained dramatic.

A central problem was the tension between the ideal of colorblind integration and new expressions of pride in distinctive racial and ethnic identities. In 1973 the armed American Indian Movement activists who for two months occupied buildings in Wounded Knee, South Dakota—site of the infamous 1890 U.S. Army massacre of defenseless Sioux—promoted a pan-Indian nationalist consciousness. In 1977 ABC's enormously popular eight-part television miniseries, *Roots*, dramatized the human pathos contained in the long saga of African American slavery. Many white ethnic Americans in these years leavened their long-standing cultural assimilation with renewed attention to their own roots in particular European countries, especially Ireland and Italy. The debates over the roles of women and men likewise reflected reconsideration of some fundamental matters of identity in the United States.

Americans' self-confidence and pride as a nation had been deeply shaken by the combination of the Vietnam War, the Watergate scandal, and the economic downturn after 1973. Disillusioned by the corruptions of public life, many citizens turned inward and heeded the advice of Robert J. Ringer in his 1977 bestseller, *Looking Out for Number One*. But others found motivation in the decade's events—especially the revelation that presidents, corporate executives, and other authorities had lied to them. They learned what earlier Americans had discovered in the 1760s about imperious British officials and the corrupting effects of managing a global empire. Like the revolutionaries of George Washington's generation, they sought to strengthen democracy. They pressed Congress to investigate the executive branch, and they elected an unusual outsider as president in 1976. Historians in this decade began to write more skeptically about those in power and more sympathetically about average Americans whom the history books had long ignored. The resurgence of conservatism in the 1980s recast many public policies, but it could not erase the vision of gender equality, environmental responsibility, and egalitarian governance that had taken hold among many citizens.

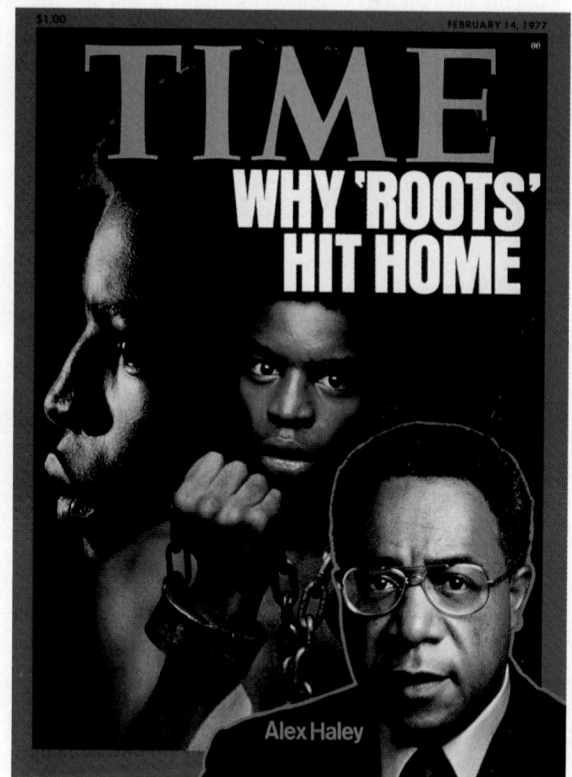

■ The 1977 miniseries version of Alex Haley's *Roots* captured the largest television audience ever to that time. The powerful drama about Haley's ancestors offered tens of millions of Americans an intimate and sympathetic understanding of the horrific story of black slavery and survival. *Roots* also represented the post-1960s emphasis on preserving and respecting group histories and identities rather than emphasizing only individual success and assimilation into the mainstream.

Sites to Visit

Divining America: Religion and the National Culture

www.nhc.rtp.nc.us:8080/tserve/divam.htm

> This site has essays by prominent historians on diverse aspects of the religious history of the United States.

Documents from the Women's Liberation Movement

scriptorium.lib.duke.edu/wlm/

> Provocative and fascinating articles from feminists of the late 1960s and 1970s make this site worthy of a visit.

The National Security Archive at George Washington University

www.gwu.edu/~nsarchiv/

> This extraordinary site includes the most recent declassified documents on the making of U.S. foreign policy.

The Natural Resources Defense Council

www.nrdc.org/

> This site contains considerable information and links about environmental issues, particularly those that emerged into public consciousness in the 1970s.

The Oyez Project of Northwestern University

oyez.nwu.edu/

> Arguments from important Supreme Court cases plus information about Supreme Court justices make this a most useful site for legal history.

Gerald R. Ford Library and Museum

www.ford.utexas.edu/

> The Ford presidential library maintains this site, with documents and photographs from the mid-1970s.

Watergate 25

www.washingtonpost.com/wp-srv/national/longterm/watergate/front.htm

> The *Washington Post* created this informative site about the Watergate scandal 25 years after the events took place.

For Further Reading

General

William C. Berman, *America's Right Turn: From Nixon to Bush* (1994).

Peter N. Carroll, *It Seemed Like Nothing Happened: America in the 1970s* (1990).

William H. Chafe, *The Unfinished Journey: America Since World War II*, 3rd ed. (1995).

E. J. Dionne, Jr., *Why Americans Hate Politics* (1991).

Bruce J. Schulman, *The Seventies: The Great Shift in American Culture, Society, and Politics* (2001).

Twin Shocks: Détente and Watergate

Stephen E. Ambrose, *Nixon*, 3 vols. (1987, 1989, 1991).

Walter Isaacson, *Kissinger* (1992).

Jeffrey Kimball, *Nixon's Vietnam War* (1998).

Stanley I. Kutler, *The Wars of Watergate: The Last Crisis of Richard Nixon* (1992).

Melvin Small, *The Presidency of Richard M. Nixon* (1999).

Discovering the Limits of the U.S. Economy

J. Anthony Lukas, *Common Ground: A Turbulent Decade in the Lives of Three American Families* (1985).

Allen J. Matusow, *Nixon's Economy: Booms, Busts, Dollars, and Votes* (1998).

Thomas J. McCormick, *America's Half-Century: United States Foreign Policy in the Cold War and After*, 2nd ed. (1995).

Hal K. Rothman, *The Greening of a Nation? Environmentalism in the United States Since 1945* (1998).

Daniel Yergin, *The Prize: The Epic Quest for Oil, Money, and Power* (1991).

Susan Zakin, *Coyotes and Town Dogs: Earth First! and the Environmental Movement* (1993).

Reshuffling Politics

Samuel P. Hays, *Beauty, Health, and Permanence: Environmental Politics in the United States, 1955–1985* (1987).

Burton I. Kaufman, *The Presidency of James Earl Carter, Jr.* (1993).

John Ranelagh, *The Agency: The Rise and Decline of the CIA* (1986).

Gaddis Smith, *Morality, Reason, and Power: American Diplomacy in the Carter Years* (1986).

U.S. Congress, Church Committee, *Alleged Assassination Plots Involving Foreign Leaders: Interim Report of the Select Committee to Study Governmental Operations with Respect to Intelligence Activities* (1976).

Diffusing the Women's Movement

Susan J. Douglas, *Where the Girls Are: Growing Up Female with the Mass Media* (1994).

Alice Echols, *Daring to Be Bad: Radical Feminism in America, 1967–75* (1989).

Arlie Russell Hochschild, *The Second Shift: Working Parents and the Revolution at Home* (1997).

Ruth Rosen, *The World Split Open: How the Modern Women's Movement Changed America* (2000).

Gloria Steinem, *Outrageous Acts and Everyday Rebellions* (1983).

Online Practice Test

Test your understanding of this chapter with interactive review quizzes at

www.ablongman.com/jonescreatedequal/chapter27

Additional Photo Credits

Page 901: Sean Sweeney
Page 906: Courtesy, Janice L. and David Frent
Page 916: Courtesy, Sharp Electronics Corporation
Page 921: Courtesy, Janice L. and David Frent
Page 929: Courtesy, Inkworks Publishers

1979 Iranian Revolution; militants take American hostages.

Soviet Union invades Afghanistan.

Sandinista rebels seize control of Nicaragua.

1980 Failed attempt to rescue American hostages in Iran.

Ronald Reagan elected president.

1981 President Anwar Sadat of Egypt assassinated.

Iran releases American hostages.

U.S. funds "Contras" to try to overthrow Nicaraguan government.

1982 Recession hits U.S.

Nuclear freeze movement holds large protests in the U.S. and western Europe.

1983 HIV identified as virus that causes AIDS.

First compact discs (CDs) marketed.

241 Marines killed in bombing of Beirut barracks.

Strategic Defense Initiative proposed.

Martin Luther King, Jr.'s birthday designated a national holiday.

1984 Russia boycotts summer Olympic Games in Los Angeles.

1985 First Reagan–Gorbachev summit in Geneva.

1986 Chernobyl nuclear power plant disaster (Ukraine).

Iran–Contra scandal revealed.

Fall of Ferdinand Marcos in the Philippines.

Congress passes sanctions against South African apartheid government.

1987 Intermediate Nuclear Force Treaty.

Stock market crash.

1988 Indian Gaming Regulatory Act.

Libyan terrorist bomb downs Pan Am Flight 103 over Lockerbie, Scotland.

U.S. invades Panama to seize Manuel Noriega.

1989 Grounding of oil tanker *Exxon Valdez* off Alaska coast.

Last Soviet troops withdraw from Afghanistan.

Berlin Wall falls.

1990 Radiation Exposure Act.

Nelson Mandela freed from prison in South Africa.

Iraq invades and occupies Kuwait.

PART TEN

A Nation of Immigrants, a Global Economy, 1979–2001

SOON AFTER THE BEGINNING OF THE TWENTY-FIRST CENTURY, AMERICANS confronted a frightening paradox: the defeat of old enemies gave rise to new ones. The Cold War had ended with the demise of the Soviet Union. And yet the post–Cold War world continued to be a violent, and in certain respects even more terrifying, place. As colonial and totalitarian political systems collapsed around the globe, local ethnic and religious conflicts rose to the surface. To some extent, those conflicts remained confined within regions: the Balkans, Indonesia, the former Soviet Union, and parts of Africa. However, the spread of worldwide terrorist networks threatened all parts of the globe. Instances of mass murder on American soil, especially the attacks on the World Trade Center and the Pentagon in 2001, proved that the United States was vulnerable to horrific acts of violence initiated from home and abroad.

In the 1980s, President Ronald Reagan left his imprint on both domestic and foreign affairs. Reagan gave voice to conservatives, including those who favored a federal retreat from social welfare programs. Bolstered by the Moral Majority and other fundamentalist Christian groups, conservatives engaged in the so-called culture wars with liberals. Conservatives disapproved of feminists, black power advocates, gay rights activists, and environmentalists. Reagan and Congress implemented policies that shrank the federal government's commitment to social welfare programs. Reagan also reinvigorated Cold War rhetoric—he denounced the Soviet Union as an "evil empire"—and pushed military spending to unprecedented levels. Yet Reagan welcomed the initiatives of Soviet leader Mikhail Gorbachev, who sought to ease tensions with the West.

Unable to meet the basic needs of its own people and bogged down in an unwinnable war in Afghanistan, the Soviet Union disintegrated in 1991. Simultaneously, the United States embarked on a remarkable period of economic growth and expansion. President Bill Clinton favored free trade policies, such as the North American Free Trade Agreement (NAFTA), which he and others hoped would knit the world's nations together in pursuit of political and economic progress.

Nevertheless, domestic and foreign conflicts thwarted much of this hopeful vision. At home, the AIDS epidemic and drug addiction claimed many lives. Clashes among African Americans, Latinos, and Koreans in Los Angeles in 1992; the bombing of an Oklahoma City federal building by domestic antigovernment terrorists in 1995; attacks on abortion clinics; and a series of shootings by high school students revealed persistent faultlines in American society. Backed by the Supreme Court, a number of state and local governments passed anti-immigrant and anti–affirmative action laws. The culture wars were hot and, in some cases, deadly.

The most violent assault on the United States came from forces outside as well as within it. The Middle East had become a tinderbox of fears and resentments. In Iran, Islamic militants overthrew the U.S.-backed Shah in 1979. Throughout the region, many Islamic fundamentalists expressed their resentment over the military and political presence of the United States in Israel and Saudi Arabia. During the 1991 Gulf War, the United States successfully reversed Iraq's seizure of oil fields in Kuwait. Yet U.S. attempts to protect its economic and political interests in the Middle East continued to outrage Islamic militants.

By the end of the 1990s, some Americans were able to focus inward and enjoy prosperity. The stock market was booming. Cheap gas prices encouraged affluent Americans to purchase huge sport utility vehicles with little regard for their environmental impact. However, ten years of high employment masked the hidden effects of a transformed economy, one characterized by a decline in labor union membership and the rise of an ill-paid service sector. A substantial proportion of Americans lived from paycheck to paycheck.

On September 11, 2001, Americans were forced to confront their own vulnerabilities. Anti-U.S. terrorists hijacked commercial airliners and flew them into the Twin Towers of the World Trade Center in New York City and into the Pentagon outside Washington, D.C. Some 3000 people were killed. Within a month, anthrax-laced letters caused death and havoc in the offices where they were delivered and the postal centers that processed them, heightening pervasive fear and insecurity among Americans.

The events of September 11 highlighted a grim reality: certain foreign groups despised such cherished American values as democracy, liberalism, and consumerism. Moreover, U.S. foreign policies in the Middle East fanned the fires of anti-western extremism. Terrorists were becoming more successful in enlisting people who were willing to die in attacks on the United States and more resourceful in using modern technology in those attacks. These terrorists were stateless, freed from the political tasks of protecting their own citizens, monitoring national borders, or dealing with internal dissidents. In contrast to the cold warriors, fighters against terrorism faced an elusive, dispersed, and, in some cases, suicidal enemy.

1991	Clarence Thomas–Anita Hill congressional hearings.
	Persian Gulf War against Iraq.
	Los Angeles police beat, arrest Rodney King.
	Soviet Union dissolves into Russia and other component states.
1992	South Central Los Angeles riots follow acquittal of police in King case.
	FBI shootout at Ruby Ridge, Idaho.
1993	FBI storms compound of the Branch Davidian cult in Waco, Texas.
	Congress approves North American Free Trade Agreement (NAFTA).
	Arab–Israeli peace talks.
	18 American soldiers die in Somalia; U.S. withdraws.
1994	House leadership announces "Contract with America."
	Republicans win majority in House of Representatives.
	O. J. Simpson murder trial.
	Freedom of Access to Clinic Entrances Act.
1995	Truck bomb destroys federal building in Oklahoma City.
	Congress revokes 55-mph speed limit.
	U.S. intervenes against Serbs in war in Bosnia.
	Dayton peace accords signed.
1996	Welfare Reform Act.
1997	Dow Jones average passes 8000.
1998	Lewinsky–Clinton affair revealed.
	Clinton impeached by House of Representatives.
1999	Senate acquits Clinton.
	Dow Jones passes 10,000.
	U.S. bombing campaign frees province of Kosovo from Serbian rule.
	Preparations for "Y2K."
	Elian Gonzales affair.
2000	Supreme Court decides contested election; George W. Bush (R) becomes president.
	Scientists map human genome.
2001	Democrats regain control of Senate after Sen. James Jeffords leaves Republican party.
	Terrorists attack World Trade Center and Pentagon.
	Anthrax in letters causes illness and death in Florida, Washington, D.C., and New York City.

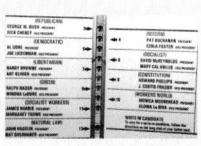

CHAPTER
28

The Cold War Returns— and Ends, 1979–1991

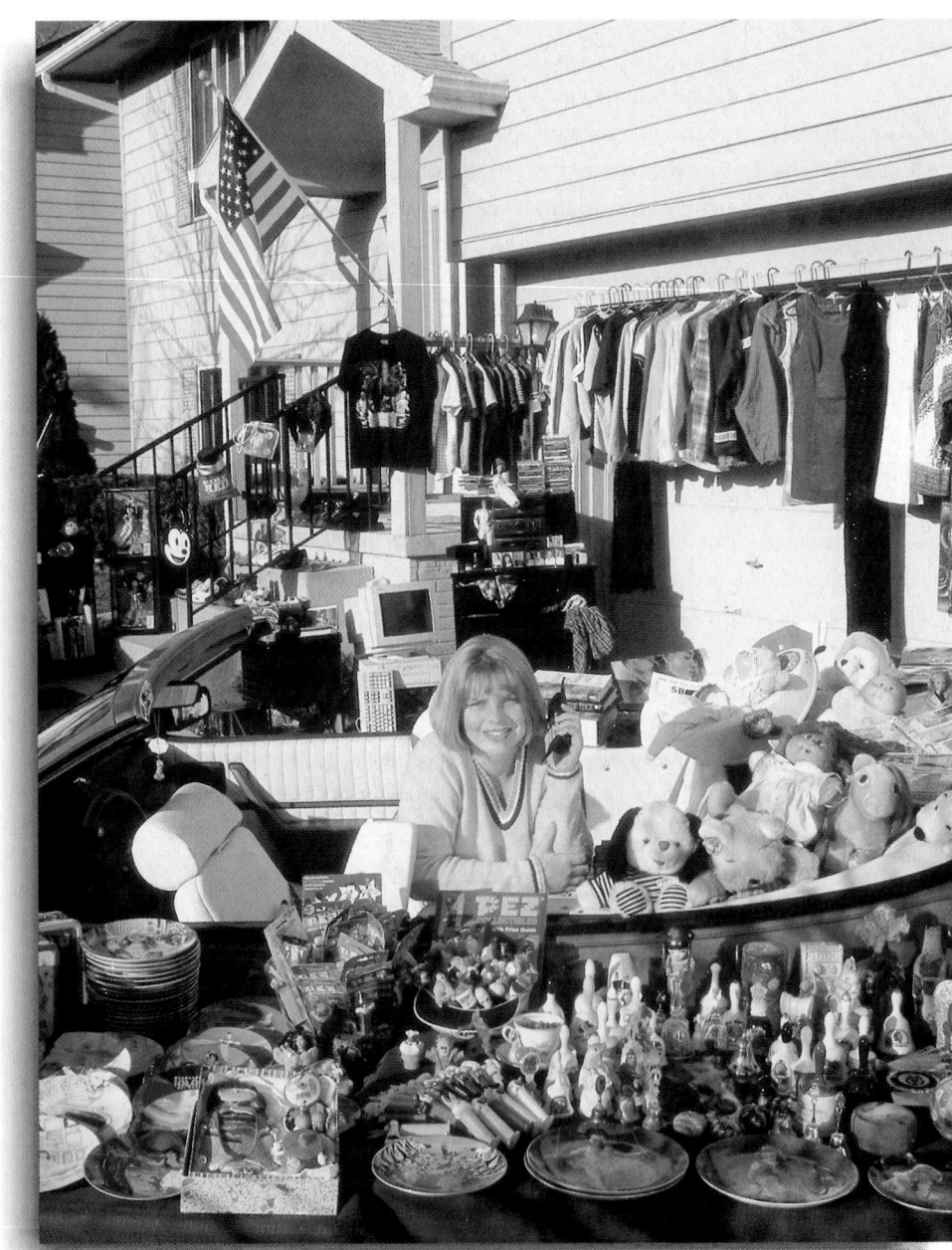

©1999 Peter Menzel

■ After the economic and international uncertainties of the 1970s, the 1980s brought a renewed sense of patriotism and a concentration on material acquisitions for many Americans.

O N JULY 16, 1979, JUST WEST OF ALBUQUERQUE, NEW MEXICO, A DAM HOLDING wastewater and residue from a uranium mine broke. Some 94 million gallons of radioactive water flooded into the Rio Puerco, giving it what one resident called "a terrible odor and a dark chocolatey color" as it flowed toward the Rio Grande. One of the worst nuclear accidents in U.S. history, the flooding proved far graver than the well-publicized meltdown of the Three Mile Island reactor in Pennsylvania a few months earlier. Yet few Americans heard about it for it affected mostly Navajo and Laguna Indians.

Nearby, the Anaconda Copper Company operated the nation's largest uranium mine, which closed in the early 1980s. At public hearings in 1986 concerning the future of the mine and its small mountain of poisonous tailings, Anaconda's scientists argued that the mine did not threaten human health in the area. Thus, they said, the tailing piles and the polluted ponds did not need to be cleaned up. Herman Garcia, a Laguna Indian who lived in the adjoining village of Paguate, listened carefully but remained unconvinced. "We lost five people from cancer" last year in tiny Paguate alone, he explained. "I'm no expert," he concluded, but "I'd like for some of these experts to go out there and swim in those ponds. Then when I see them swim, then maybe I feel more secure."

Uranium fuels nuclear power. The largest deposits of the element in the United States lie underground in the Four Corners region, where New Mexico, Arizona, Colorado, and Utah meet. Known on American Automobile Association maps as "Indian Country," this region is also home to the vast Navajo, Hopi, Laguna, and other Native American reservations.

The Native American West and the nuclear West have overlapped to a remarkable extent ever since participants in the Manhattan Project began building the first atomic bomb in 1942. Repeatedly, the U.S. government constructed major nuclear sites in the West on lands surrounded by Indian settlements. These included the laboratories of Los Alamos, New Mexico; bomb factories and nuclear waste dumps of Hanford, Washington; the Nevada Test Site for atomic weapons north of Las Vegas; and uranium mines in the Black Hills of South Dakota. Some of this overlap resulted from geological coincidence: almost 90 percent of the nation's uranium lay on or adjacent to Indian lands. Some of it stemmed from politics. The sparse populations of Pueblos, Western Shoshones, and Yakimas lacked the political clout to prevent their lands from becoming what the National Academy of Science called "national sacrifice areas." Raymond Yowell, chief of the Western Shoshones living immediately downwind from the Nevada Test Site, observed, "We are now the most bombed nation in the world."

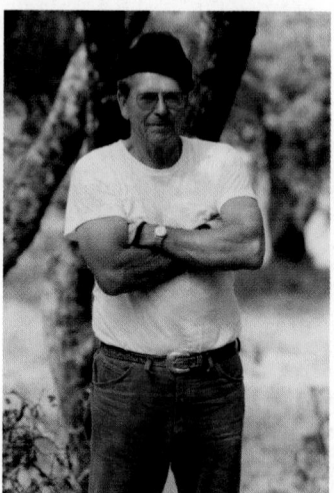

Ronald Reagan loved spending time at his ranch near Santa Barbara, California.

In the 1980s, nuclear weapons and waste once again sparked controversy in the United States. President Ronald Reagan expanded the nation's nuclear arsenal, and his administration publicly discussed fighting and winning a nuclear war against the Soviet Union. An accident in 1986 at the Chernobyl nuclear power plant outside the Soviet city of Kiev only heightened public concerns. The disaster killed more than 100 people and irradiated hundreds of thousands more. Frightened by rising U.S.–Soviet tensions, citizens in western Europe and the United States organized an international movement to freeze further development of nuclear weapons.

In these same years, non-Indians grew more aware of Native Americans, in part because of economic growth in the southwestern Sunbelt. Indians made up a larger percentage of the population there than in the rest of the country. White emigration from urban California to the Rocky Mountain states also contributed to this process. So did the growing popularity of "New Age" spiritualism, with its appropriation of many Indian religious symbols. And writer Tony Hillerman achieved great commercial success with his crime novels set on the Navajo reservation in Arizona and New Mexico and populated by interesting Indian characters.

Native Americans themselves responded to the renewed focus on nuclear weaponry with a combination of resistance and accommodation. Along with their non-Indian supporters, some protested at the Nevada Test Site. At the same time, former Navajo uranium miners—many of them now stricken with cancer—sued the government for failing to inform them of the risks in handling radioactive materials. Other Indians, such as the Mescalero Apaches in New Mexico and the Goshutes in Utah, allowed nuclear waste storage facilities on their land. In their view, this move would gain them both money and control over radioactive materials that were within their borders anyway. In 1990, the U.S. Congress finally passed the Radiation Exposure Act. The law designated funds to provide some compensation for those damaged by the nation's quest for nuclear supremacy during the Cold War.

At its root, what did the Iranian challenge mean for American power? Khomeini and his followers despised the values they associated with modern U.S. culture.

The controversies over nuclear power, weapons, and radioactive waste revealed several key themes characterizing the 1980s, especially U.S. military standing, government deregulation, and renewed anticommunism. In 1979, two international incidents raised questions about U.S. military effectiveness. That year, a revolution in Iran led to the taking of American hostages and a dramatic rejection of American cultural values, and the Soviet Union sent troops into Afghanistan to prop up a Soviet-allied but weakening government. Humiliated, Americans put tough-talking Republicans in the White House for 12 years. These leaders' emphasis on military might challenged the Soviet leadership, while changes in eastern Europe and the USSR brought an end to the Cold War and the breakup of the Soviet Union.

The Reagan administration also avidly promoted free markets. Its policies produced astounding wealth at the top of the socioeconomic ladder, increasing the distance between the daily experiences of the rich and the poor. And these policies catalyzed bitter struggles over natural resources, particularly those on western public lands.

Finally, the newly organized religious right clashed with liberal opponents over such issues as abortion and homosexuality. In these years, Christian fundamentalists and their allies sought to reverse cultural liberties that had emerged since the late 1960s. This conservatism paralleled a political shift to the right. After nearly half a century, the New Deal order that had relied on Washington to get things done gave way to a diminished faith in government. The turning tide renewed the hopes of some Americans—disillusioned by the persistence of poverty and crime—that a self-governed marketplace might solve the nation's most pressing social problems.

Anticommunism Revived

"We're going down!" cried U.S. political officer Elizabeth Swift on the phone to the State Department. These were her last words as a crowd of young Iranians poured into the U.S. embassy in Teheran on the morning of November 4, 1979, and cut telephone lines. In a move that shocked Americans, Islamic militants next seized 52 embassy personnel. They held the hostages for over a year.

In the late 1970s, revolutionaries of a different political bent—that of socialism and the left—took the offensive against authoritarian regimes in Central America. Indeed, the Third World seemed to be turning away from U.S. leadership in the wake of the American defeat in Vietnam. To make matters worse, the Soviet Union stepped up its support for leftists abroad. In December 1979, the Red Army invaded Afghanistan. Fed up with these humiliating events overseas and with relentless inflation at home, American voters elected Ronald Reagan as president—the most conservative chief executive since Calvin Coolidge. Reagan promised to resurrect the Cold War, and he delivered.

Iran and Afghanistan

In January 1979, the Iranian people overthrew the longtime authoritarian government of Shah Reza Pahlavi. Under the Shah's rule, the nation's enormous oil wealth had flowed into the hands of a small elite. Meanwhile, the impoverished majority of devout Shi'ite Muslims grew increasingly resentful of the Shah's closeness with his American allies. His secret police had detained 50,000 political prisoners; in the Shah's time, his critics said, "only the cemeteries prospered." The revolution found its leader in the austere religious figure Ruhollah Khomeini, who shouldered aside more moderate opposition groups. Returning from exile in Iraq and then Paris, Ayatollah Khomeini created a popular theocratic state grounded in a strict interpretation of Islamic law.

For the United States, connections with both Iran and Saudi Arabia since the 1940s had formed the two pillars of American policy toward the oil-rich Persian Gulf. Indeed, the CIA had engineered the 1953 coup that overthrew the short-lived Iranian nationalist government of Muhammad Mussadiq and restored the young Shah to power. American officials maintained close ties with the Shah thereafter.

The drop in Iran's oil production that accompanied the 1979 revolution unleashed the United States' second oil shock of the 1970s. By that time, the nation depended on imports for as much as 42 percent of its oil. American gas prices soared by 60 percent amid shortages, sending another wave of inflation rolling through the U.S. economy.

Hunted by the rebels, the Shah took his money and fled Iran. Several months later, the Carter administration let him fly to New York to seek treatment for cancer. Enraged that the United States harbored their nation's most wanted criminal, Iranians demanded the Shah's extradition to Teheran to stand trial. Washington refused. Within a month, militants stormed the U.S. Embassy—"that nest of spies," Khomeini called it, referring to the CIA's presence in Iran.

The hostages' captors paraded them before television cameras to force Washington to return the Shah. Carter refused to give in, but he focused the rest of his presidency on engineering the hostages' release. He thus had little energy and few resources to devote to his campaign for reelection. ABC television created the news show *Nightline* to provide daily reports on the crisis. In April 1980, Carter finally approved a military rescue effort. But mechanical failures forced the mission to abort, and the collision of two helicopters during the attempt killed several U.S. soldiers. Secretary of State Cyrus Vance resigned in protest against the attempted use of force. He was the first State Department head to quit over a matter of principle since William Jennings Bryan resigned in 1915 to express his desire to stay out of World War I. Americans' frustration deepened, and their resentment of anti-American radicals in the Third World intensified. Not until after the Shah's death in 1980 did the two governments finally negotiate the hostages' release. Even then, the Iranian leaders delayed the Americans' departure until moments after Carter left office in January 1981.

At its root, what did the Iranian challenge mean for American power? Khomeini and his followers despised the values they associated with modern U.S. culture: secularism,

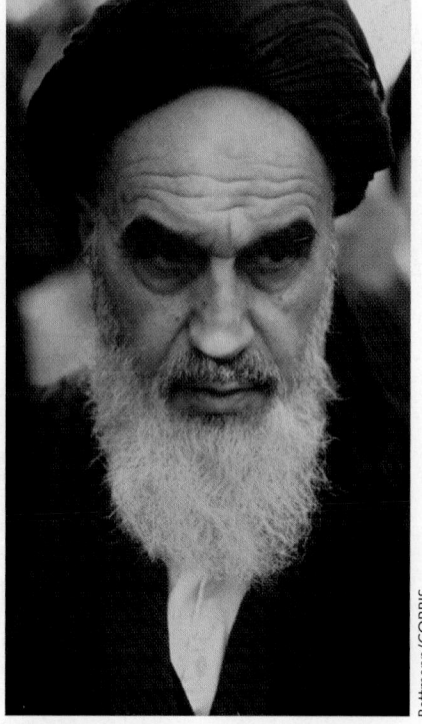

■ Ruhollah Khomeini led the 1979 revolution in Iran that established the modern world's first Islamic theocratic state. The events in Iran encouraged Islamic revolutionaries across the Middle East, Asia, and North Africa. For Americans, the closest analogy was the Bolshevik revolution of 1917 in Russia, which provided a model for other Communist revolutions abroad.

Bettmann/CORBIS

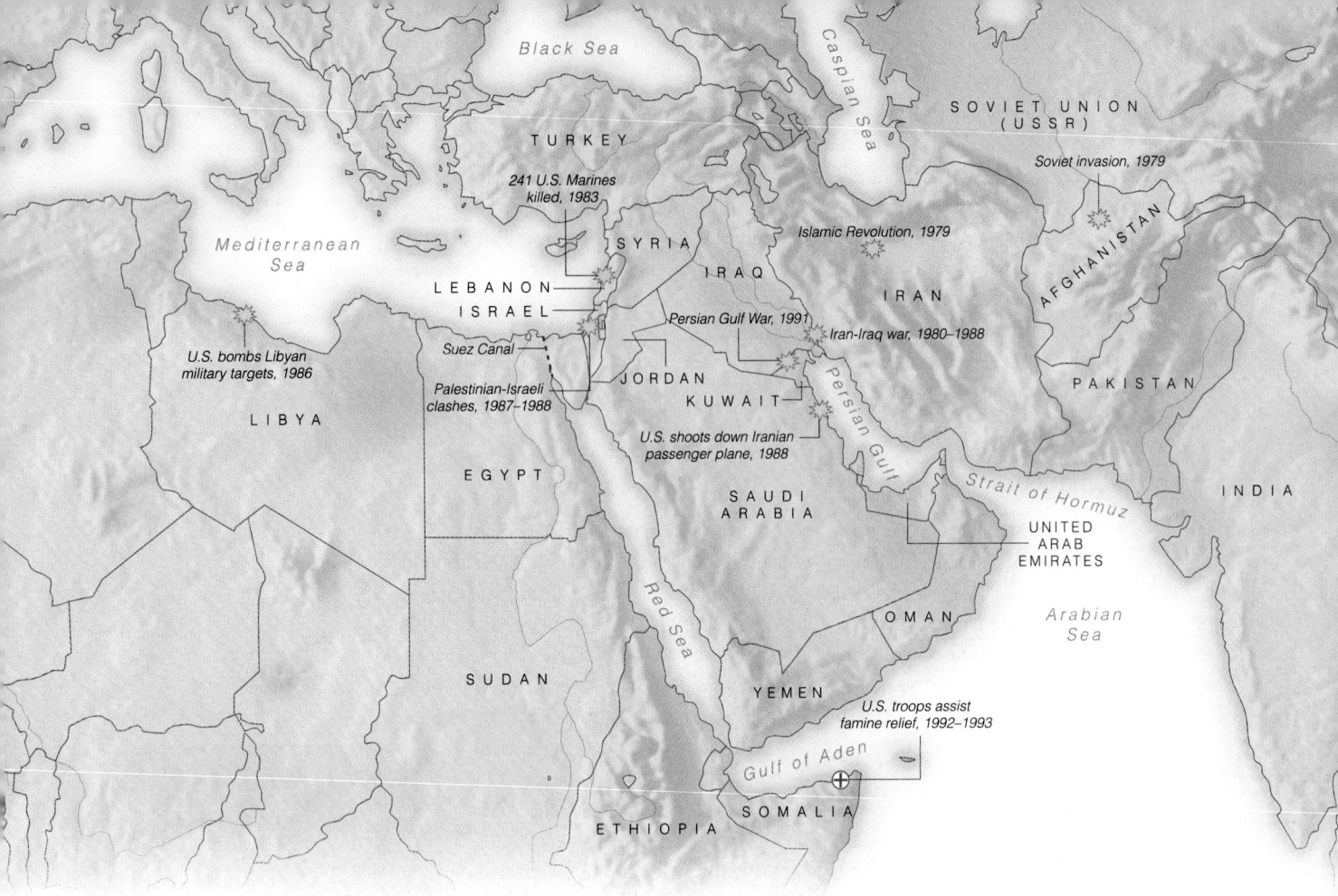

■ MAP 28.1

TROUBLE SPOTS IN THE MIDDLE EAST, 1979–1993 Oil production around the Persian Gulf and the close American relationship with Israel made political instability in the Middle East a central concern of the U.S. government. American leaders particularly feared the spread of either Soviet influence or Islamic revolution, both of which opposed American cultural values and U.S. strategic interests.

materialism, gender equality, alcohol consumption, and sexual titillation. Back in the 1630s, John Winthrop and other members of the new Massachusetts Bay colony might well have understood this perspective. But the modern Iranian radicals sought to export the cleansing power of a puritanical Islamic faith throughout the Middle East and beyond. Indeed, the revolutionaries condemned the atheistic Soviets just as fiercely as they did the materialistic Americans. Khomeini applauded all movements that sought "to gain liberation from the superpowers of the left and the right." U.S. policymakers had feared that instability in Iran might lead to a communist takeover of that country. Instead, the creation of the world's first revolutionary Islamic state in 1979 presented an entirely different challenge to American interests overseas.

Just seven weeks after the outbreak of the hostage crisis in Teheran, the first of 110,000 Russian troops rolled south across the USSR's border into neighboring Afghanistan. Their goal: To stabilize the pro-Soviet government there against anticommunist Islamic guerrilla fighters. Moscow had resolved to prevent the spread of Islamic revolution into the heavily Muslim southern regions of the USSR.

But few Americans saw this invasion as a defensive operation. Rather, they feared a push toward vulnerable Iran as Red Army troops marched beyond eastern Europe for the first time in more than 30 years. The Carter administration halted most trade with the Soviets and withdrew the Strategic Arms Limitation Treaty (SALT II) nuclear arms control treaty from Senate consideration. In addition, the president organized a western boycott of the 1980 Olympics in Moscow and increased military spending. The "Carter Doctrine" proclaimed the U.S. commitment to preserve the status quo in the Persian Gulf region, even if it meant the use of military force. And the CIA began funding the Afghan guerrillas. Détente was dead; containment was back. Next came efforts to roll back the Soviets.

The Conservative Victory of 1980

By mid–1980, Carter's public approval rating had dropped to the lowest level of any modern president. Interest rates surpassed 20 percent, and inflation reached 17 percent. Even the president acknowledged a "crisis stage." With their dollars no longer buying what they used to, Americans wondered what the future would bring. For many voters, Carter's inability to free the hostages in Teheran or reverse the Soviet occupation of Afghanistan symbolized the limitations of his presidency. Even his own party threatened to abandon him, as the vigorous challenge in the Democratic primaries by liberal Senator Edward Kennedy of Massachusetts revealed. Many moderate Democrats and unaffiliated voters backed the independent candidacy of John Anderson. The moderate Republican congressman from Illinois managed to win 7 percent of the popular vote that November.

Onto this stage strode Ronald Reagan. Long considered too conservative to win the presidency, the former California governor projected the confidence and strength that many Americans wanted, even if they did not share all of his views. The 69-year-old one-time actor sailed through the Republican primaries. For his main tactic, he appealed to nostalgia, particularly among white men, for a rosier past—a time of rising wages and U.S. military might. While Carter spoke of learning to live within limits, Reagan insisted that "we are too great a nation to limit ourselves to small dreams." He painted a compelling picture of military pride and power abroad, of unlimited consumption of energy, and of infinite economic growth. Reagan located Carter's "crisis of confidence" in the U.S. government, not in the American people. The "truth is," he contended, "there are simple answers—just not easy ones." Still, his answers looked both simpler and easier than Carter's, and Reagan crushed the incumbent in the November election.

Reagan's victory symbolized the meshing of politics and entertainment. An actor on the ultimate stage, he understood the presidency as a matter of public performance more than substantive policies. With little interest in the actual process of governing, he gave his advisers minimal guidance. He focused his own efforts on selling an idealized version of America to the public. He deeply believed in this version, even when his stories about it derived from film plots. For example, he claimed to have filmed the liberation of Nazi death camps in Europe in World War II, when in fact he did not leave the United States during the war. Nevertheless, with his sunny disposition and ease before the camera, Reagan projected the image of an attractive, competent leader.

The media loved Reagan. Indeed, his presidency fit with the new emphasis on constant entertainment, as cable television, VCRs (1976), MTV (1981), and CDs (1983) swept the culture. Daily newspaper readership plummeted from 73 percent to 50 percent during the 1980s. Equally telling, the average length of an uninterrupted "sound bite" on the evening news dropped from 42 seconds in 1968 to fewer than 10 seconds in 1988. Anything longer, the networks believed, would bore viewers. And no one projected simplicity with greater warmth or sincerity than Reagan. Even his fiercest opponents admired his irrepressible humor when, after being shot by would-be assassin John Hinkley in 1981, the president surveyed the surgeons standing around his operating table and announced, "I hope you're all Republicans."

TABLE 28-1

The Election of 1980

Candidate	Political Party	Popular Vote	Electoral Vote
Ronald Reagan	Republican	43,901,812	489
Jimmy Carter	Democratic	35,483,820	49
John B. Anderson	Independent	5,719,722	0

Yet the 1980 election was about more than just Reagan's likable personality. It revealed the nation's renewed infatuation with conservative ideas. Republicans won control of the Senate for the first time since 1952. They managed to defeat several of the chamber's most respected liberal Democratic members, such as Frank Church of Idaho, who had led the investigation of CIA spying practices. The Grand Old Party had repositioned itself to be more ideologically consistent. It now had fewer traditionally moderate northeastern members and millions of new conservative white southern members.

Several basic values united the party: an unhindered private sector and entrepreneurial initiative to create affluence plus free markets and individual responsibility to solve the nation's social problems. Republicans, like most Democrats, also believed that the United States had a moral obligation to preserve world order and halt further expansion of communist influence. Reagan proclaimed that "government was the problem, not the solution." For conservatives, government had two specific roles: to prevent disorder—crime at home, revolution abroad—and to support the business community. The United States' key European allies also moved to the right in the 1980s, especially Great Britain under the leadership of Margaret Thatcher.

Renewing the Cold War

"Sometimes in our administration," Reagan once joked, "the right hand doesn't know what the far-right hand is doing." But all hands in the White House agreed on the importance of restoring confidence in the nation's engagements abroad, particularly in the Third World. In the 1970s, leftist insurgencies in Asia, Africa, and Latin America—especially Vietnam, Cambodia, Angola, Ethiopia, El Salvador, and Nicaragua—had suggested the retreat of U.S. power. Equally troubling to many, when the U.S. government did assert its power, it often seemed to support anti-democratic or racist governments—as long as they were anticommunist and open to foreign investment. Never much concerned with foreign affairs in the best of times, most Americans now felt disillusioned.

Reagan set out to heal the public's bruised pride, using the logic of his new UN ambassador, Jeane Kirkpatrick. A former Georgetown University professor, Kirkpatrick distinguished between nondemocratic nations on the right ("authoritarian") and the left ("totalitarian"). They were not morally equivalent, she argued. In her view, "authoritarian" regimes were friendly to the United States and could be reformed, but "totalitarian" communist governments had close ties to the Soviet Union and could be changed only by force. The peaceful fall of the Berlin Wall in 1989 disproved her theory.

Reagan blamed the Soviet Union for "all the unrest that is going on." He rejected the 1970s policy of détente that had emerged during the Nixon administration and had taken further shape under Ford and Carter. Often, Reagan spoke as though the Chinese–Soviet split had never happened. His was "a kind of 1952 world," one aide recalled. "He sees the world in black and white terms." Pointing to the Soviet occupation of Afghanistan and its 1983 shoot-down of a Korean Air Lines civilian jet that had strayed into Soviet airspace, the president denounced the USSR as "an evil empire." His pronouncement echoed the language of the wildly popular film *Star Wars* (1977) and its two sequels. The three movies cast the plucky heroes—like Americans and their allies—as righteous rebels against a malignant imperial power. The Vietnam War, Reagan insisted, was not a destructive imperial cause but a "noble effort" on the part of dedicated American patriots. Indeed, as governor of California in the late 1960s, Reagan had declared that the United States should "level Vietnam, pave it, paint stripes on it, and make a parking lot of it." Americans, Reagan vowed, must overcome their post–1973 "Vietnam syndrome" and stand ready once again to use force abroad.

The Reagan administration backed up the president's words by launching the largest peacetime military build-up in American history. The Pentagon's budget ballooned 40 percent between 1980 and 1984. The new president also revived covert operations. He gave CIA

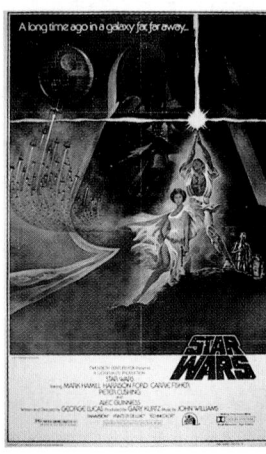

director William Casey the green light to provide secret assistance to anticommunist governments and insurgencies throughout the Third World, despite their often gruesome human rights records.

However, the administration's aggressive rhetoric about rolling back communism masked an unwillingness to put U.S. soldiers in harm's way abroad. The one exception came during the civil war in Lebanon in 1983. U.S. forces initially deployed as peacekeepers there began siding with the Israeli-backed Christian government troops against Syrian-supported Muslim rebels. Within weeks, a Muslim suicide bomber—one of the first of many to come in the Middle East—drove a truck full of explosives into the American barracks at the Beirut airport, killing 241 marines. The administration quietly backed off from mediating further Middle East conflicts. It covered its retreat with an invasion two days later of the tiny Caribbean island of Grenada. There, thousands of U.S. troops quickly overthrew a Marxist government and a small contingent of Cuban supporters.

Reagan was the only Cold War president to take almost no interest in the details of foreign policy. International issues "weren't terribly important to the president," national security adviser Robert McFarlane explained. Reagan delegated most foreign policy planning to his advisers—except for the rising tide of leftist revolution in Central America. In that region, extreme inequalities between landowning elites and vast peasant majorities had fueled insurgencies against the authoritarian governments of El Salvador, Guatemala, and Nicaragua. Moreover, some small assistance from Cuba and the Soviet Union had found its way to the rebels. Reagan passionately opposed these insurgents. He authorized the CIA to work hand in hand with the regimes, even though they used death squads to torture and murder dissidents and slaughtered whole villages and towns to wipe out possible resistance.

In Nicaragua, the Sandinista rebels had managed to overthrow the pro-American dictatorship of Antonio Somoza in 1979. Their name reflected loyalty to a long-standing left-leaning effort in Nicaragua to eliminate U.S. dominance of the country; in the 1920s and early 1930s, General Augusto Sandino had led rebel troops against the U.S.-supported dictatorial regime of Somoza's father. Forty years later, the Sandinistas set about building a more egalitarian and socialistic state while still preserving 60 percent of the nation's wealth in private hands. Carter had adopted a wait-and-see attitude. But after Reagan took office in 1981, the CIA created the counterrevolutionary "Contras," recruited primarily from Somoza's murderous former National Guard. The Contras waged an undeclared war on the new government in the Nicaraguan capital of Managua. By 1987, 40,000 Nicaraguans had died in the fighting, most of them civilians. Reagan called the Contras "freedom fighters" and declared them "the moral equal of our Founding Fathers."

Nevertheless, several European and Latin American allies considered the Contras an illegitimate force of terrorists. A large coalition of church and university groups in the United States agreed. They organized fact-finding visits to Nicaragua and lobbying trips to Washington. Christian activists formed the "Sanctuary" movement to aid refugees from the right-wing dictatorships in Central America that sympathized with the Contras. The Pentagon, for its part, had no interest in sending troops to fight a popular government abroad. The opposition finally prevailed; Congress passed the Boland Amendments of 1982 and 1984 to restrict U.S. assistance to the Contras.

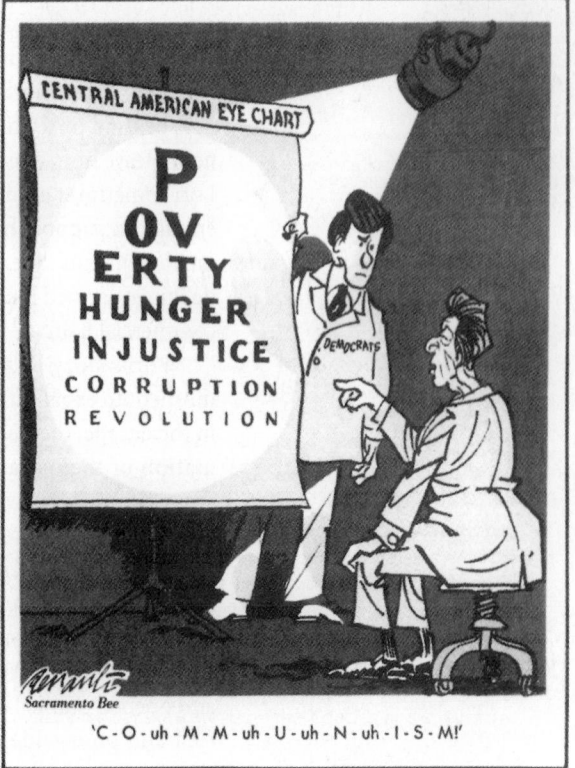

■ Critics of Reagan's policies toward Central America believed that he ignored the indigenous problems encouraging revolutions there, blaming instead the USSR and Cuba. The cartoon suggests that the Democratic party took a different view than the president. Many Democrats in the Congress did, and they were responsible for limiting Reagan's promotion of the Nicaraguan Contras. But many others went along with the popular president in defending the Contras and supporting right-wing regimes in the region.

The plight of refugees fleeing the civil wars in Central America exposed the politicized thinking that had influenced U.S. immigration policies for decades. Officials distinguished between "political" refugees and "economic" refugees. The former, they felt, had a well-founded fear of persecution. The latter were supposedly looking only for better economic opportunities. The Reagan administration used this distinction to justify supporting certain foreign governments while opposing others. For example, the U.S. government had warmly welcomed and financially assisted people fleeing communist regimes, such as Hungary in the 1950s and Cuba since the 1960s. Likewise, Nicaraguan immigrants were treated well because their choice to leave Nicaragua provided ammunition in the propaganda war against the Sandinistas. However, Salvadorans and Guatemalans, deemed "economic" refugees, were turned away. In 1984, U.S. officials admitted only 328 Salvadorans into the country while refusing 13,045—a ratio opposite that for Nicaraguans.

These policies encouraged the emergence of militantly anticommunist expatriate communities in the United States. These groups then lobbied to sustain U.S. hostility toward leftist regimes in their homelands. The anti-Castro Cuban community in Miami offered the most dramatic example. Immigrants who left Vietnam and Cambodia after the communist victories there in 1975 brought a similar perspective.

Republican Rule at Home

Lori was what the president called a "welfare cheat." Writer Barbara Ehrenreich told the story of a young neighbor in New York City representative of welfare recipients: a single white mother with one child. Lori had been married for two years to a man who beat her and once chased her around the house with a gun. Welfare had made it possible for her to leave him, a move she described as like being born again, "as a human being this time." Lori sometimes earned close to $100 a week from cleaning houses and waiting tables—not enough to support herself and her daughter, but a useful supplement to the small government payments. She chose not to report this to the welfare office, spending it instead on little things deemed inessential by welfare regulations: deodorant, hand lotion, and an occasional commercial haircut.

Lori's story helps illuminate some of the major trends of the 1980s. Just as its commitment to expanding U.S. economic opportunities abroad helped renew the Cold War early in the decade, the Reagan administration's beliefs in free markets and scant government regulation of the private sector shaped politics at home during this decade. In some ways, the economy's behavior seemed to affirm the wisdom of these beliefs: inflation finally eased and the stock market perked up. Congress and the White House slashed taxes. However, annual budget deficits and the national debt (the accumulation of previous deficits) soon soared as tax revenues decreased and military spending increased. The administration shrank government programs for the poor and portrayed welfare recipients like Lori as lazy and irresponsible. Washington turned a cold shoulder to concerns over the environment and opened public lands in the West to new commercial uses. By the 1990s, the gap between rich and poor widened so much that the vaunted American middle class threatened to shrink beyond recognition.

"Reaganomics" and the Assault on Welfare

Taxes played a crucial role in the Reagan administration's efforts to reduce government involvement in the economy. Compared with America's closest allies in Europe, U.S. tax rates were already low because of the country's smaller welfare provisions. But a tax revolt had begun brewing in the 1970s, exemplified by California's Proposition 13 (1978), which cut property taxes by more than half. In 1981, Reagan proposed a new tax law to lower federal income tax rates by 25 percent over three years. Congress passed the legislation, and the top individual rate—paid only by the wealthiest Americans—dropped from 70 percent to 28 percent. Congress also slashed taxes on corporations, capital gains, and inheritances, further benefiting the most affluent Americans.

As taxes shrank, federal spending on the military soared. The Pentagon bolstered its conventional and nuclear arsenals and gave service personnel a morale-boosting salary increase. After 1983, billions of dollars poured from the U.S. Treasury into the president's proposed Strategic Defense Initiative (SDI). An immense project, SDI sought to create a national missile defense system involving lasers that could shoot down incoming nuclear missiles. Most scientists considered the concept technically unfeasible, and critics dubbed it "Star Wars" for its resemblance to some of the fantasy weapons in the popular science fiction film of the same name. Still, the jump in military spending created new jobs, just as earlier boosts had done under Truman and Kennedy.

With less money coming in from taxes but more money flowing out to the military, the government did not seem to be on the path to fiscal responsibility touted by the Republican party. The funds for the weapons build-up could come from only one source: social programs at home. However, most domestic spending went to popular programs, such as Social Security and Medicare, which primarily benefited the middle class. Leaving those in place, Reagan instead reduced funding for welfare programs, including food stamps, school lunches, job training, and low-income housing. His administration derided impoverished single mothers as "welfare queens." The welfare state, the administration contended, was only encouraging dependence and stifling individual responsibility. Frustrated by the persistence of poverty, many well-off Americans found this view persuasive. Numerous people, such as conservative writer George Gilder, found it much easier to assume that the poor "are refusing to work hard" than to examine the more complicated roots of poverty.

Congress slashed taxes on corporations, capital gains, and inheritances, further benefiting the most affluent Americans.

The assault on welfare had links to racial issues as well. Reagan portrayed welfare recipients—most of whom were white and lived in rural areas—as primarily urban and African American. The president had made a blunt appeal to white southern voters in 1980. He had campaigned in Philadelphia, Mississippi, a tiny town but a national symbol of antiblack violence since three civil rights workers had been murdered nearby in 1964. There, Reagan spoke of his support for "states' rights"—the same language that those who supported the killers had used.

The Republican desire to transfer the responsibility for citizens' well-being from the national government to the states resonated with opponents of the civil rights movement. In 1978, the Supreme Court's *Bakke* decision had supported this goal by banning the use of actual racial quotas in college admissions, although the Court did allow the affirmative action principle of considering race as merely one of many factors in admission decisions. The Reagan administration opposed any form of affirmative action, calling instead for the "colorblind" application of law. The president and his supporters argued that prejudice no longer had any effect on the decisions that employers and others made. Ironically, Reagan's own Justice Department demonstrated the opposite: it sought unsuccessfully to win tax-free status for Bob Jones University in Greenville, South Carolina, and other schools and colleges that discriminated against people of color.

Reducing welfare spending did not close the budgetary gaps that lower taxes and higher military outlays had opened. "Supply-side" economists had promised that tax cuts would encourage investment and thereby generate wealth and eventually more tax revenues, even with lowered rates. But Reagan's own vice president and former challenger in the Republican primaries, George H.W. Bush, had dismissed these assumptions as "voodoo economics." Bush's perspective had merit. To close the budget gaps, the government resorted to borrowing money. Formerly the world's largest creditor nation, the United States became its largest debtor nation. Between 1981 and 1989, the national debt ballooned to almost $3 trillion. Moreover, during 12 years of Republican rule, annual budget deficits jumped from $59 billion to $300 billion. Paying the interest on the new debt pushed interest rates higher and siphoned off funds that could have been used for any number of productive purposes.

Despite these problems, "Reaganomics" helped the national economy recover somewhat from the traumas of the 1970s. The tight money policies of the Federal Reserve Board after 1979 eventually tamed inflation, which dropped from 14 percent in 1980 to less than 2 percent in 1983. The Fed's high interest rates also choked off the nation's cash flow and provoked a severe recession in 1981–1982, with unemployment reaching above 10 percent. However, the economy revived again in 1983 and was growing at a robust annual rate of 6.8 percent by 1984.

In that year, rising confidence in the economy helped Reagan crush his opponent, Carter's former Vice President Walter Mondale. Even the novelty of placing a woman, Geraldine Ferraro, on a major ticket as the vice presidential candidate could not bolster the Democratic challenge. Reagan, now 73 and limiting his campaign appearances to well-orchestrated photo oportunities, won re-election handily and continued his economic course. After several years of excellent returns on Wall Street, the stock market crash of October 1987 caught investors by surprise. Nevertheless, it did not provoke a broader economic downturn, as the 1929 crash had done.

TABLE 28-2			
The Election of 1984			
Candidate	Political Party	Popular Vote	Electoral Vote
Ronald Reagan	Republican	54,455,075	525
Walter Mondale	Democratic	37,577,185	13

An Embattled Environment

The 1980 election marked the sharpest turn ever in American environmental politics. The new administration reversed two decades of growing bipartisan consensus on the need for greater protection of the environment. Reagan instead supported corporations' demands for fewer environmental regulations and easier access to natural resources on public lands. The president ridiculed the idea of preserving wilderness for its own sake. Noting that plants emit carbon dioxide, he even claimed that "trees cause more pollution than automobiles do." A

■ James Watt, Reagan's first Secretary of the Interior, became one of the most polarizing figures in a polarized decade. He made clear that he considered environmentalists to be his opponents as he worked to promote the interests of mining and timbering companies as well as ranchers. The Department of the Interior manages the national parks, monuments, and wildlife refuges, as well as the Bureau of Land Management's extensive lands (national forests fall under the Department of Agriculture's jurisdiction).

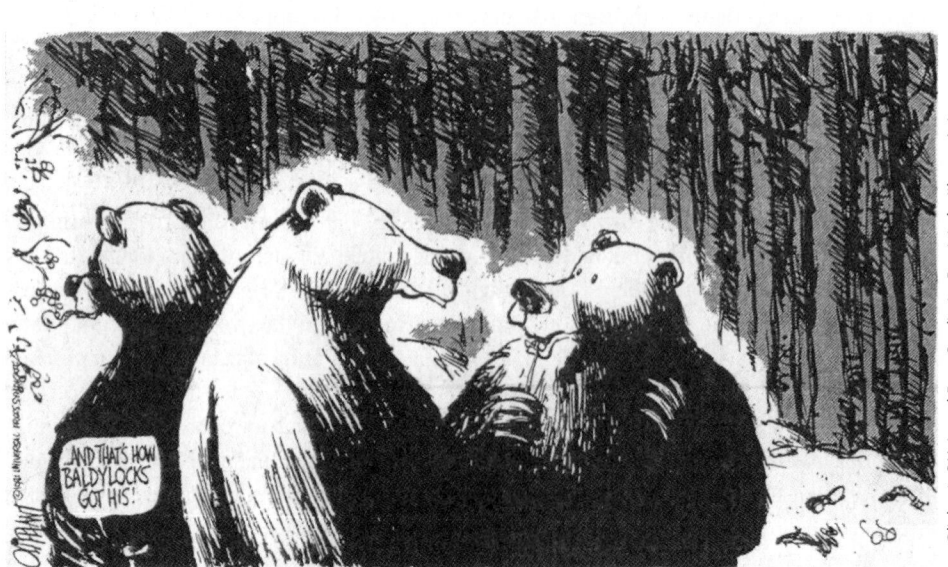

'SURELY,' SAYS I, 'NOT THE JAMES WATT, FOLK-HERO AND FAMOUS WILDERNESS RAPIST!' 'THAT'S ME,' SAYS HE. AND I SAYS, 'NOT THE RENOWNED DESPOILER OF OUR PRECIOUS NATIONAL HERITAGE!' 'RIGHT,' SAYS HE. SO I ATE HIM.'

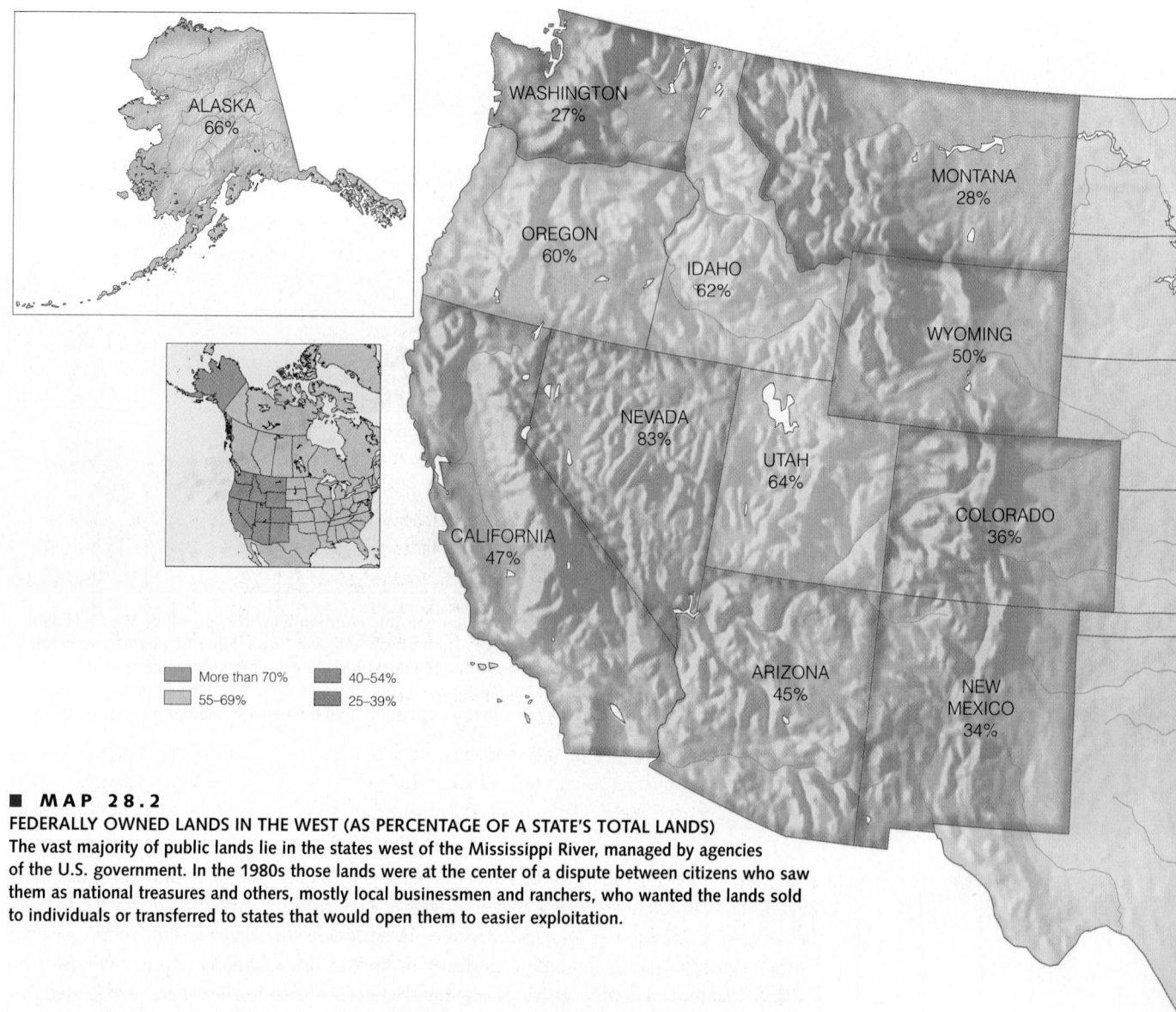

■ MAP 28.2
FEDERALLY OWNED LANDS IN THE WEST (AS PERCENTAGE OF A STATE'S TOTAL LANDS)
The vast majority of public lands lie in the states west of the Mississippi River, managed by agencies
of the U.S. government. In the 1980s those lands were at the center of a dispute between citizens who saw
them as national treasures and others, mostly local businessmen and ranchers, who wanted the lands sold
to individuals or transferred to states that would open them to easier exploitation.

coalition of powerful western land users and politicians known as the "Sagebrush Rebel-lion" had an ally in the White House. Emboldened, they launched a quest to turn federal lands over to the states and open them to commercial use. These lands, most of them in the West, were administered by the U.S. Forest Service and the Bureau of Land Management (BLM). They had ended up in federal hands primarily because successive waves of settlers had deemed them undesirable. They included snowy mountains in the Rockies and Sierras and vast deserts in the Great Basin of Nevada and Utah. By the 1980s, different groups desired them for two mutually exclusive purposes: corporations and ranchers wanted to harvest timber and min-erals from them and use them for grazing, and environmentalists and outdoor enthusiasts sought to designate them for recreational and scenic use.

The officials Reagan appointed to oversee these lands and assume responsibility for pro-tecting them had little respect for the agencies they ran. Critics described the situation as "foxes guarding the chicken house." The officials openly disdained environmentalists, including those in the moderate wing of the Republican party. Anne Gorsuch at the Environmental Protec-tion Agency (EPA), Robert Burford at the BLM, and John Crowell in charge of the Forest Service explicitly rewrote regulations to favor private enterprise. They sold grazing, logging, and mining rights on public lands at prices far below market value, despite their stated com-mitment to market economics.

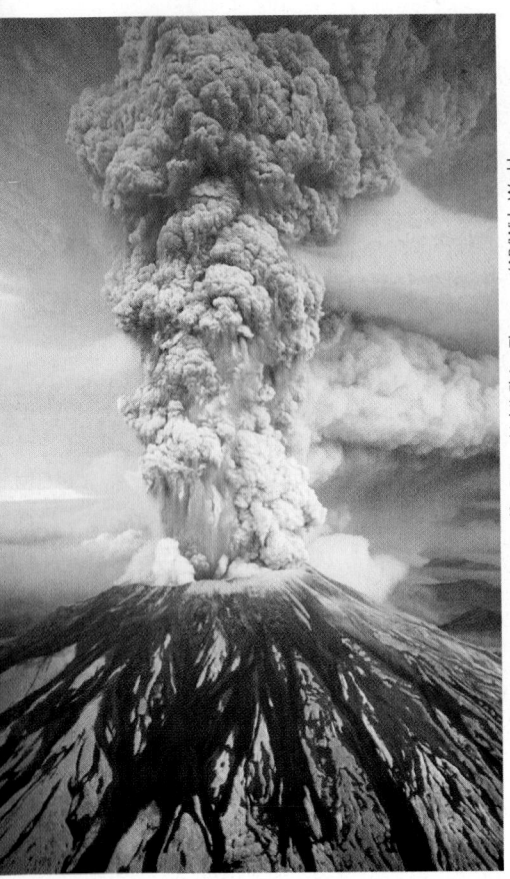

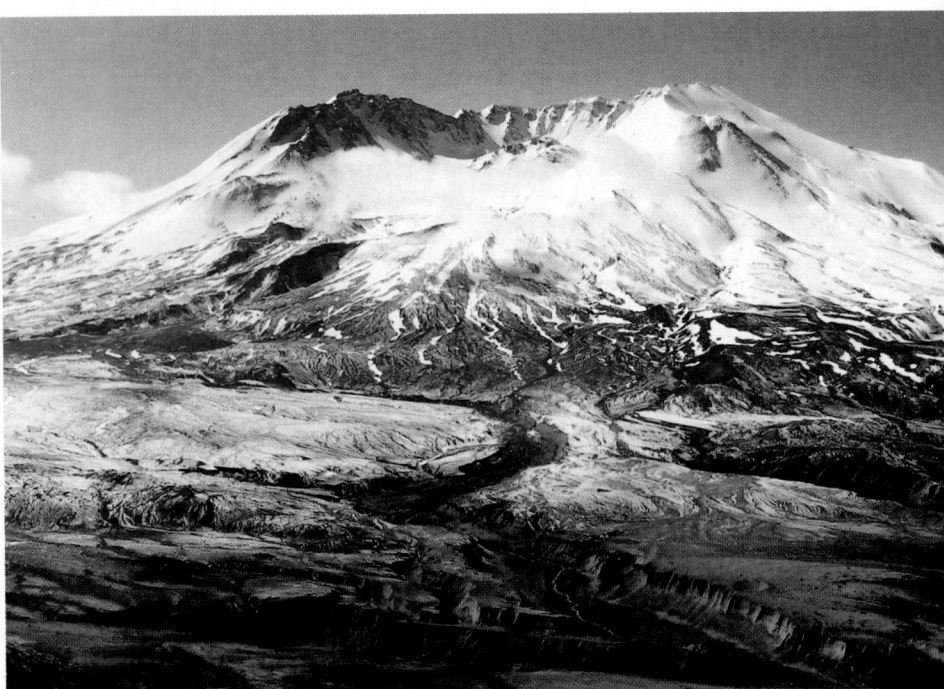

(Left) Roger Worth/Woodfin Camp; (right) Elaine Thompson/AP/Wide World

■ On May 18, 1980, a spectacular volcanic eruption blew the top off of Mt. St. Helens in Washington's Cascade Range. The hot ash and lava flows killed 57 people and created an ash-covered landscape out of a previously lush forest. The eruption reminded Americans of all political persuasions of the power and unpredictability of nature, just months before the Reagan administration initiated new environmental policies opening up natural resources to easier exploitation.

Gorsuch, Burford, and Crowell were moderates in comparison to James Watt, the new Secretary of the Interior who controlled national parks and wildlife refuges. A native of Wheatland, Wyoming, Watt had worked as a lawyer in Denver for a private foundation dedicated to businesses seeking access to public lands. An ideologue, he declared that only two kinds of people lived in the United States: "liberals and Americans." Watt was also a Christian fundamentalist who believed that the end of time was very near. In his Senate confirmation hearings, he suggested that the nation had little need for long-term public land management because Christ would soon be returning and the known world would pass away—an interpretation of stewardship that not even all fundamentalists shared, much less the broader American public. Watt's abrasive personal style eventually alienated even the White House, and he resigned in 1983.

The administration's reversal of federal environmental policies alarmed a wide range of citizens and stimulated a powerful backlash. In particular, Watt's smug extremism made him a lighting rod for criticism. Membership in environmental organizations soared, in such traditional groups as the Sierra Club and the Audubon Society, as well as in more radical ones, such as Greenpeace. Most Americans wanted to breathe cleaner air, drink safe water, and make recreational use of national forests, national parks, and BLM lands. Even Americans sympathetic to extractive industries such as timbering lamented the scars that clearcutting and strip mining left. In much of the rural West, jobs in the recreation industry

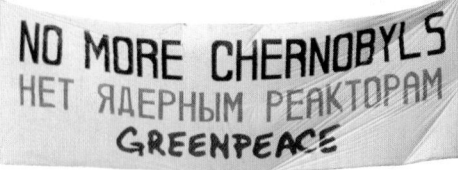

outnumbered those in the logging, mining, and ranching businesses. The public also took alarm at the 1986 Chernobyl nuclear accident in the USSR. Three years later, concerns intensified when the oil tanker *Exxon Valdez* ran aground in Prince William Sound in Alaska, coating 1000 miles of pristine coastline with crude oil. Reagan's Republican successor in the White House, George Bush, caught on and tried to portray himself as an environmentalist.

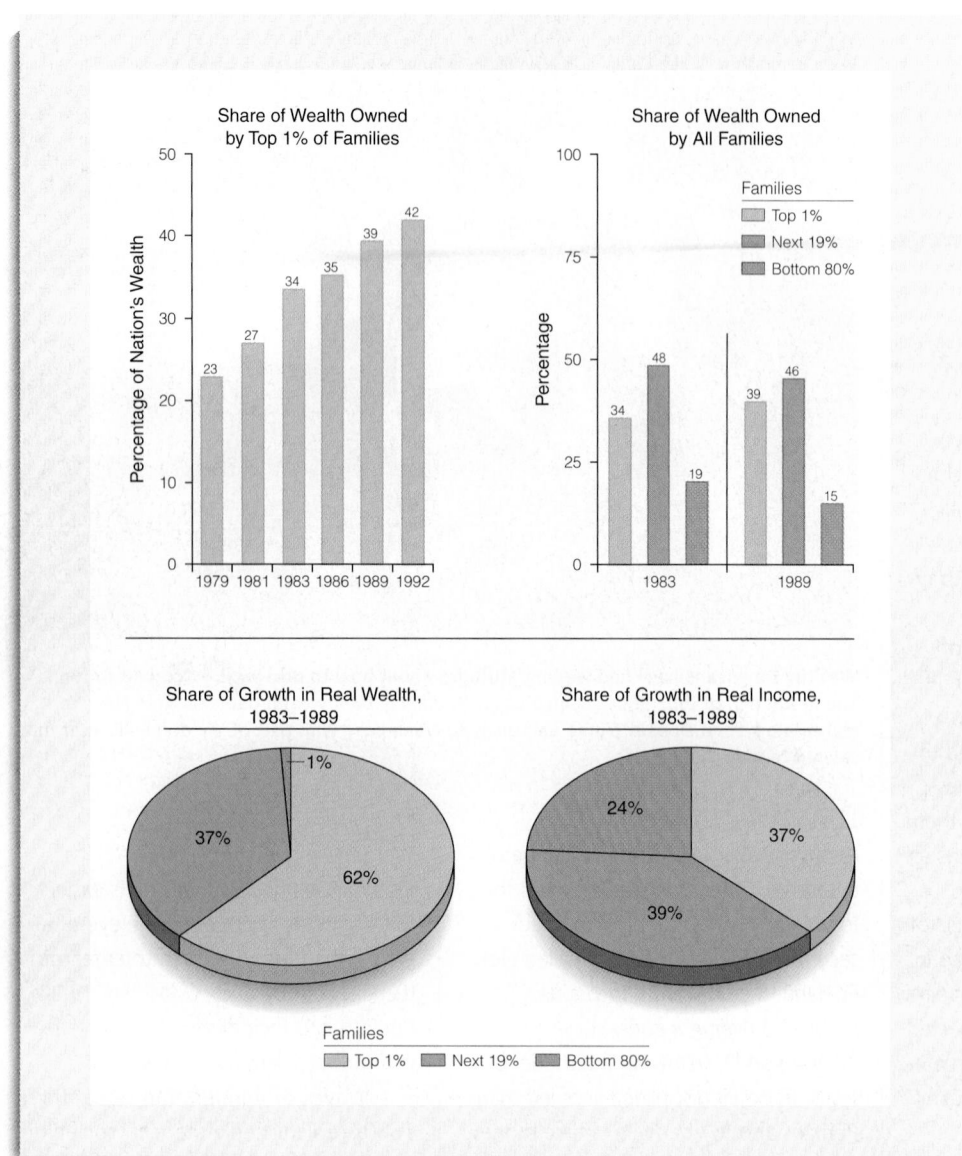

■ FIGURE 28.1
**DISTRIBUTION OF WEALTH AND
INCOME**   The 1980s were excellent
years for wealthy Americans.
The "trickle-down" effect touted
by some Reagan administration
officials—predicting that greater
wealth accumulation among the
rich would trickle down to the less
affluent—had little impact.

A Society Divided

As the Reagan administration eased corporate access to the nation's natural resources, the disparity between rich and poor expanded further. This gap was already more prominent than that of other industrialized democracies, including Japan and West Germany. But the distribution of income became even more skewed, and wealth flowed increasingly to already affluent Americans.

Whereas most Americans' real wages (wages after inflation is factored in) declined, the professional classes fared well, and the wealthiest citizens gained enormously. For example, the salary of an average corporate chief executive officer was 40 times greater than that of a typical factory worker in 1980; by 1989, it was 93 times greater. The net worth of the 400 richest Americans tripled. The wealthiest 1 percent of citizens received 60 percent of the after-tax income gain during the decade. By 1989, the top 1 percent of American families possessed more assets than the bottom 90 percent—a ratio typical of Third World nations.

A series of corporate mergers and consolidations further enriched well-off Americans, as did financial speculation and manipulation on Wall Street. *Business Week* wrote of a "Casino

Is Material Success Corrupting?

"Will you tell me," former president John Adams asked former president Thomas Jefferson in 1819, "how to prevent riches from becoming the effects of temperance and industry? Will you tell me how to prevent riches from producing luxury? Will you tell me how to prevent luxury from producing effeminacy, intoxication, extravagance, vice and folly?"

Adams had his finger on one of the enduring dilemmas in American life. Discipline and hard work—"temperance and industry"—tended to lead to material success. But acquiring riches tended to change people. It made them more self-indulgent and less virtuous as citizens of a republic, Adams feared.

Adams's concerns mirrored those of his Puritan ancestors who had arrived in Massachusetts almost two centuries earlier. So strongly had the Puritans rejected what they saw as the spiritual and material corruptions of life in England that they left to start anew across the

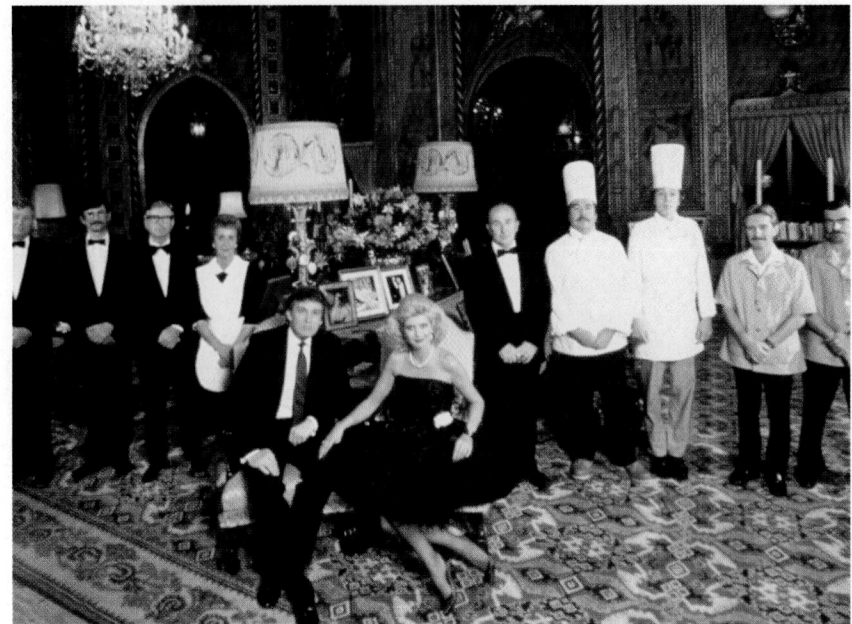

Wealthy Americans have had varying attitudes about how to deal with their good fortune. The newly rich of the 1980s seemed eager to display their wealth publicly. Here New York real estate tycoon Donald Trump and his wife Ivana pose with part of the domestic staff that catered to their daily needs.

Ted Thai/CORBIS/Sygma

Atlantic Ocean, a profoundly dangerous enterprise. Once they had survived the terrible first winters and established secure colonies in what they called New England, they began to face a new problem. Building a godly society meant "doing good": following the model of Jesus. But their disciplined lives led many Puritans also to "do well": make money.

Were these two compatible? After all, Jesus himself had warned, "It is easier for a camel to go through the eye of a needle than for a rich man to enter into the kingdom of God" (*Matthew* 19:24). Puritans and their descendants wrestled with this problem for generations.

Waves of immigration since the 1600s replenished American society

Economy" in which insider trading and leveraged buyouts (business takeovers financed by debt) created paper wealth rather than actual products. Defenders of the aggressive new tactics on Wall Street argued that those taking great risks deserved great rewards and that new wealth trickled down to the broader American citizenry. "Greed is all right," fabulously wealthy financier and corporate takeover specialist Ivan Boesky assured the 1986 graduating class of the business school of the University of California at Berkeley. "I want you to know that. I think greed is healthy. You can be greedy and still feel good about yourself." Six months later, however, Boesky began a three-year prison term for illegal insider trading.

The explosion of wealth at the top fueled an emerging culture of extravagance, reminiscent of similar trends in the late nineteenth century and the 1920s. Newly identified "yuppies" (young urban professionals) embodied the drive for material acquisition, in contrast to the anticonsumerist inclinations of the late 1960s and early 1970s. Jerry Rubin had made a reputation as a member of the anarchist "yippies" in the 1960s. He and comrade Abbie Hoffman once dropped dollar bills onto the floor of the New York Stock Exchange—which traders

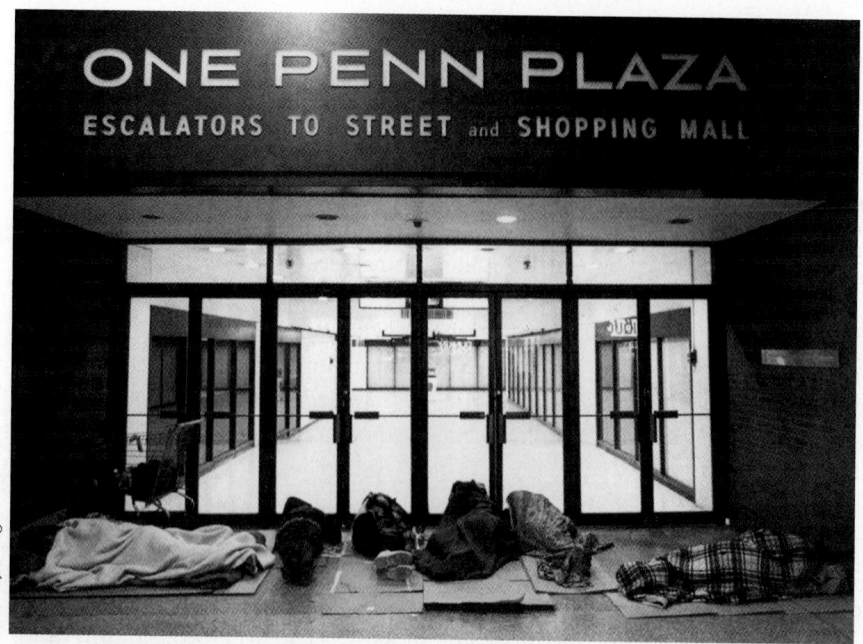

Photo by George Cohen

Neither homelessness nor poverty in general was new in American society in the 1980s. But the numbers of Americans living on the streets increased sharply. They were especially visible in the centers of large cities, such as these sleeping in New York City's Pennsylvania station in January 1990.

with people seeking opportunity. The hardships that attend moving to a new country ensured that new Americans tended to be strivers and risk-takers. Some came for religious and political freedom, but many others were drawn by the possibility of "doing well" economically. With effort, most fared much better than they had previously. The United States remained, in the old words of nineteenth-century Chinese immigrants, "the Golden Mountain."

Despite their enthusiasm for pursuing private material success, Americans in the twentieth century at times indicated public ambivalence about great wealth. During the trauma of the Great Depression and the national unity of World War II, displays of extravagance drew scorn, and government policies became somewhat more redistributive of the national wealth. The communes of the 1960s, like earlier utopian communities, sought to create a life free from what their members saw as the corruptions of materialism. In the Cold War competition for influence abroad, U.S. officials sent diplomats and aid workers to Africa but worried that Soviet and especially Chinese personnel, accustomed to fewer material comforts at home than Americans, were fitting much better into poor African societies and making more positive impressions on their hosts.

In other periods of modern American history, however, public life celebrated the success of the nation's richest citizens. During the Gilded Age of the late 1800s and the Jazz Age of the 1920s, political and cultural leaders admired and shared the affluence associated with names such as Rockefeller, Carnegie, and Ford. The 1980s became another era for ostentatious displays of wealth. "If you've got it, flaunt it," became a familiar expression. The proliferation of stretch limousines epitomized a decade marked by "conspicuous consumption." ■

scurried madly to grab—to dramatize the stock market's pursuit of profit. By the 1980s, however, Rubin was working as an investment banker. Ronald and Nancy Reagan were older but shared similar values. They relished lavish amenities like those made popular on the television shows *Dynasty, Dallas,* and *Lifestyles of the Rich and Famous.* The contrast to the austere Jimmy Carter could hardly have been more stark.

As the affluence gap widened, the broad middle class watched its job security slip. Early in the decade, the recession had prompted factory shutdowns and mass layoffs. More than a million industrial jobs disappeared in 1982 alone. Manufacturers' decisions to keep moving plants abroad for cheaper labor only worsened the situation. Although the 1980s saw the creation of 20 million new jobs, most of these were in the nonunionized service sector. Thus they offered low pay and few benefits. By 1990, 8 million Americans had tried the unskilled work available at McDonald's fast-food restaurants. "To work at McDonald's you don't need a face, you don't need a brain," one of them recalled. "You need to have two hands and two legs and move 'em as fast as you can. That's the whole system. I wouldn't go back there for anything."

Organized labor suffered during these years as well, losing 3 million members as the manufacturing sector of the economy shrank and the government encouraged corporate opposition to unions. In his first year in office, Reagan broke a strike by the nation's 12,000 air traffic controllers by firing the protesting public employees and hiring permanent replacements. Worried about the disappearance of high-wage industrial jobs, American families tried to preserve their living standards by putting more of their members in the workforce, especially women and teenagers. They also put off paying for their lifestyles by charging more purchases to credit cards, taking out larger home mortgages, and signing on for longer car loans. As their government carried more debt, so did private citizens.

The poorest Americans fared badly in the 1980s. The bottom tenth saw their already meager incomes decline by another 10 percent. In 1986, a full-time worker at minimum wage earned $6700 per year—almost $4000 short of the poverty level for a family of four. Homelessness worsened in the cities as the government cut funding for welfare and institutional care for the mentally ill while housing costs rose. More than 1 million people lived on the streets, one-fifth of them still employed. One out of eight children went hungry, and 20 percent lived in poverty, including 50 percent of black children.

These Americans received minimal sympathy from the nation's political leaders. By contrast, Congress and the White House provided huge federal subsidies to "needy" businesses such as the Chrysler Corporation. The collapse of the savings and loan (S&L) industry provides the most striking example. Deregulation in the late 1970s had reduced oversight of the formerly sedate financial practices of S&Ls by federal regulators. But S&Ls remained insured by the U.S. government. As a result, some S&L executives, such as Charles Keating, engaged in rampant speculation and fraud. A decline in real estate prices bankrupted 600 shaky S&Ls by 1991, leaving taxpayers with a bill for nearly $500 billion. Federal Deposit Insurance Corporation chairman William Seidman described the U.S. government as "a full partner in a nationwide casino."

Despite Reagan's record, many working-class and middle-class Americans voted for him twice. Forty percent of union household members and 50 percent of all blue-collar workers cast their ballots for this staunch opponent of unions. Why? Part of the explanation lies in the decline of working-class voting during the 1970s. Disillusioned with a political process they saw as corrupt, numerous workers neglected to go to the polls on voting day. Many of those who did vote decided that the Democratic party had become increasingly co-opted by cultural liberalism and no longer spoke for the working class. They cast their ballots for the Republicans for the first time. Reagan had great personal charisma, and his staff brilliantly managed his image in the media. The former actor's effective appeal to patriotism also attracted many citizens who might once have voted for their economic interests instead. Finally, white Americans increasingly defined their political loyalties on the basis of social and cultural issues—such as opposition to abortion, homosexuality, and affirmative action—rather than economic interests. Conservative Christians, in particular, strongly supported the Republican cause.

Cultural Conflict

One of the nation's foremost religious figures, Reverend Pat Robertson controlled the Christian Broadcasting Network and ran unsuccessfully for the 1988 Republican presidential nomination. Like other social conservatives of this era, he promoted "family values" and traditional gender roles. Robertson went so far as to declare that feminism "encourages women to leave their husbands, kill their children [and] practice witchcraft." In contrast, author Susan Faludi wrote the 1991 best-seller *Backlash* about opposition to the women's movement. She became an important critic of gender roles in American society and how they limit people's life experiences and possibilities. In completely opposite fashion from Robertson, Faludi concluded, "All women are feminists. It's just a matter of time and encouragement."

Throughout the 1980s, Americans embroiled themselves in a contentious debate about values. Their society had changed in the previous generation in ways that some citizens disdained but others applauded. Americans argued primarily about issues that had come to the fore during the social movements of the 1960s and 1970s: sexuality, gender roles, the place of religion in public life, and multiculturalism. These often bitter "culture wars" dominated talk shows and newspaper editorial pages throughout much of the last two decades of the twentieth century.

The Rise of the Religious Right

Some of the Americans most troubled by the state of American society were conservative white Protestants. Disproportionately from the South, they had long avoided political involvement and sought to keep church and state separate. They had particularly distrusted Roman Catholicism and state aid for religious education that would include parochial schools. But anti-Catholicism declined sharply among these conservative Christians after the Supreme Court banned organized school prayer in 1962 and legalized abortion in 1973. Increasingly, conservative white Protestants saw secularism as their real enemy and conservative Catholics as allies.

Together these groups bemoaned the post–1960s shift in mainstream values away from respect for traditional authorities—the church, political leaders, and the military—and toward freer sexual expression and general self-indulgence. What the nation needed, they believed, was a return to reverence for God. The growth of this Christian fundamentalism also paralleled rising religious fundamentalism around the globe, whether among Jews in Israel, Hindus in India, or Muslims in Iran and the Arab Middle East. For all their differences, religious people in these cultures shared a common quest: preserving spiritual purity and cultural traditions in an increasingly secular, integrated world.

Conservative Protestants were not a fringe group. As many as 45 million Americans—20 percent of the population—considered themselves fundamentalist Christians in 1980. In combination with a similar number of Catholics, they represented a vast potential force in American politics. And their ranks were growing. While membership in the more liberal mainline Protestant denominations, such as the Presbyterians and Episcopalians, declined steadily after the 1960s, the fundamentalist Assemblies of God grew 37 percent and the Southern Baptists 18 percent between 1965 and 1975. Rather than emphasizing theological doctrine, these groups focused on individuals' emotional connection with a forgiving God. They built church schools, Bible colleges, and publishing houses to reinforce their message. Evangelism on secular college campuses expanded through such organizations as Intervarsity and Campus Crusade for Christ. Hal Lindsey's apocalyptic story about the second coming of Christ, *The Late Great Planet Earth*, sold more than 10 million copies in the 1970s.

> *Americans argued primarily about issues that had come to the fore during the social movements of the 1960s and 1970s.*

Conservative Christians mobilized in the 1980 campaign to support Reagan's candidacy. Critics noted that Reagan himself attended church only occasionally and seemed an indifferent father. They contrasted the divorced candidate with his born-again, Sunday-school–teaching opponent, Jimmy Carter. But Reagan's conservative views on abortion and gay rights and his support for school prayer resonated with fundamentalists. They flocked to the Republican party and to new right-wing religious organizations, such as the Moral Majority, founded in 1979 in Lynchburg, Virginia, by Reverend Jerry Falwell. More than 60 million people each week watched—and many sent money to—"televangelists," including Falwell, Robertson, and Jim Bakker.

Suffusing the GOP with a distinctly southern, grassroots flavor, the religious right also highlighted a major faultline in the modern Republican party: the tension between social conservatives, who emphasized community and tradition, and free marketeers, who promoted

Religion and Politics in the 1980s

In 1979, Baptist minister Jerry Falwell founded the Moral Majority in Lynchburg, Virginia. The organization represented the growing engagement of conservative evangelical Christians in American politics, and Falwell emerged as the most prominent figure of the new religious right. However, not all Christians were conservative. Robert McAfee Brown, a Presbyterian minister and theologian, represented more liberal elements of the church that understood both the Bible and the problems of American society differently than Falwell.

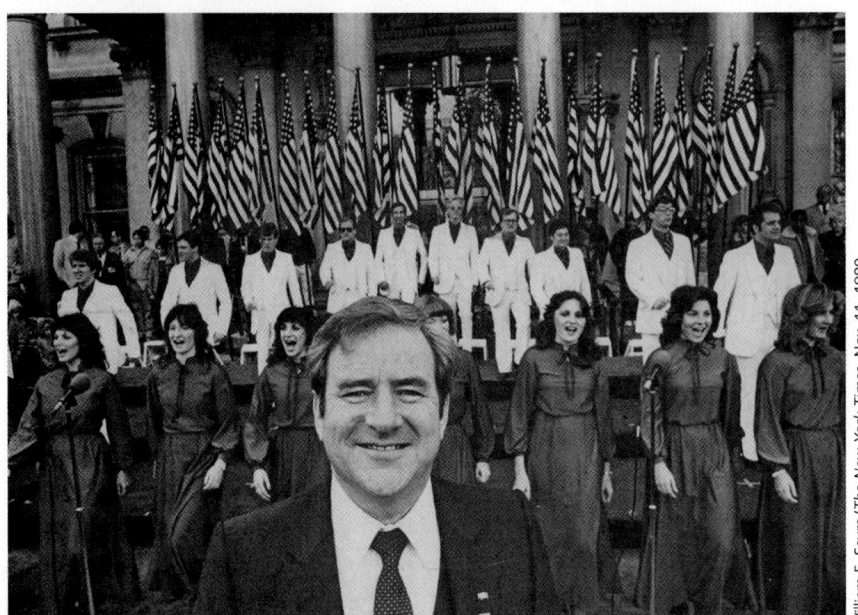

William E. Savro/*The New York Times*, Nov. 11, 1980

Before he became involved in politics, Jerry Falwell had already made a name for himself as a prominent preacher in his hometown of Lynchburg, Virginia, as the senior minister of the large Thomas Road Baptist Church and the founder of Liberty University. His organization, the Moral Majority, became the most well-known conservative evangelical Christian organization of the 1980s.

The Goals of the Moral Majority (1980) by Jerry Falwell

We must reverse the trend America finds herself in today. Young people . . . have learned to disrespect the family as God established it. They have been educated in a public-school system that is permeated with secular humanism. They have been taught that the Bible is just another book of literature. They have been taught that

entrepreneurial capitalism. In its quest for profits, unrestrained capitalism had no inherent respect for tradition. Indeed, it could bring unwelcome changes, as Rustbelt industrial workers had discovered when their employers moved south and overseas. Marrying Jesus to the market proved difficult: should the state play a minimal role in the economy and society, as free-market libertarians believed, or should it monitor personal behavior, as social conservatives implied?

Reagan managed to keep the two wings of the party together, often referring to his "11th Commandment" to "speak no ill of another Republican." But tensions persisted. When Falwell called on "all good Christians" to oppose the 1981 Supreme Court nomination of Arizona's conservative Sandra Day O'Connor on the grounds that she was insufficiently hostile to abortion, Arizona senator and party elder Barry Goldwater—a staunch proponent of small government and personal privacy—retorted that "every good Christian ought to kick Jerry Falwell right in the ass."

Gender and sexuality issues particularly aroused the ire of religious conservatives. They blamed feminism for weakening male authority in the family and for increasing divorce rates. A growing anti-abortion movement gained national visibility by 1980; "Operation Rescue" even borrowed the tactics of civil disobedience from the civil rights movement. During the 1970s, 22 states repealed their sodomy laws, reflecting a slowly increasing acceptance of gays and lesbians. But the religious right, which viewed homosexuality as an abomination, fiercely resisted this trend. Dismayed by the prevalence of casual sexual relationships in the 1970s, church conservatives urged abstinence on young Americans.

there are no absolutes in our world today. . . . These same young people have been reared under the influence of a government that has taught them socialism and welfarism. . . .

I personally feel that the home and the family are still held in reverence by the vast majority of the American public. I believe there is still a vast number of Americans who love their country, are patriotic, and are willing to sacrifice for her. I remember that time when it was positive to be patriotic. . . . I remember as a boy . . . when the band struck up "The Stars and Stripes Forever," we stood and goose pimples would run all over me. . . .

It is now time to take a stand on certain moral issues. . . . We must stand against the Equal Rights Amendment, the feminist revolution, and the homosexual revolution. . . .

Americans have been silent much too long. We have stood by and watched as American power and influence have been systematically weakened in every sphere of the world. . . .

The hope of reversing the trends of decay in our republic now lies with the Christian public in America. We cannot expect help from the liberals. They certainly are not going to call our nation back to righteousness and neither are the pornographers, the smut peddlers, and those who are corrupting our youth.

The Politics of the Bible (1982) by Robert McAfee Brown

In Christian terms, and I think in terms with which all Jews could also agree, my real complaint about the Moral Majority's intrusion of the Bible into American politics, is that they are not biblical enough. . . .

The Moral Majority's biblically inspired political agenda involves a very selective, very partial, and therefore very distorted use of the Bible. They have isolated a set of concerns that they say get to the heart of what is wrong with America—homosexuality, abortion, and pornography. . . .

Take the issue of homosexuality. If one turns to the scriptures as a whole, to try to come up with their central concerns, homosexuality is going to be very low on such a list even if indeed it makes the list at all. There are perhaps seven very ambiguous verses in the whole biblical canon that even allude to it. . . . [But there are] hundreds and hundreds of places where the scriptures are dealing over and over again with question of social justice, the tendency of the rich to exploit the poor, the need for all of us to have a commitment to the hungry, . . . [and] the dangers of national idolatry, that is to say, making the nation into God, accepting uncritically whatever we have to do as a nation against other nations. . . .

When one looks over the agenda of the Moral Majority there is absolutely no mention of such things. . . . We seem to be living in two different worlds, reading two different books. ■

Source: Irwin Unger and Robert R. Tomes, *American Issues,* 2nd edition (Prentice-Hall, 1999), vol. 2, pp. 362–364, 375–377.

The heyday of the sexual revolution ended in 1983, when researchers identified the human immunodeficiency virus (HIV), which causes acquired immunodeficiency syndrome (AIDS). The deadly epidemic spread swiftly through the gay male communities of San Francisco and New York as a result of unprotected sex. Many fundamentalists viewed AIDS as a divine punishment for homosexual activity. "The poor homosexuals," Reagan aide Pat Buchanan wrote. "They have declared war on nature and now nature is exacting an awful retribution." The Reagan administration refused to help mobilize a campaign against the new plague. AIDS continued to spread during the 1990s and beyond, among gays and heterosexuals, both in the United States and abroad—especially in such places as China, southern Africa, and Russia. New drugs slowed the onset of actual AIDS in many HIV-infected Americans while scientists continued the frustrating quest for a cure for the disease.

Yet another epidemic swept through the United States during the 1980s, striking impoverished urban neighborhoods especially hard. The culprit was crack cocaine. Powerfully addictive, it contributed to gang violence and record homicide rates in several cities. Drug-related convictions skyrocketed, stimulating a boom in prison building and a doubling of the nation's inmate population. Conservatives strongly supported the "war on drugs" touted by the White House, and police departments created special weapons and tactics (SWAT) teams to deal with heavily armed drug operators.

This effort tended to ignore the real forces behind drug dealing, which included persistent poverty and a consumer culture obsessed with immediate gratification. Dealing crack offered a rare avenue to wealth to the poorest communities. On the wall of one Detroit crack house, a dealer posted this notice for employees: "[With] hard work and dedication we will all be rich within 12 months." Yet for all the mayhem they caused, crack and other illicit drugs killed less than 1 percent as many Americans per year as the 500,000 felled by tobacco and alcohol. Clearly, addiction to legal as well as illegal substances remained a pervasive problem.

Dissenters Push Back

The liberal and radical reform energies that had percolated in the late 1960s and early 1970s did not evaporate entirely in the conservative 1980s. To be sure, some former activists converted to Republican orthodoxies, investing on Wall Street and enjoying the material comforts of affluence. However, many activists continued to work for social justice in their communities. Numerous activists focused on environmental issues. In combination with younger organizers, many from college campuses, they kept alive a national resistance to conservative politics. Some coined the term "politically correct" or "PC" as an inside joke about fellow leftists who were overly concerned with ideological purity in an era of pervasive conservatism. Right-wingers soon turned "PC" into a derogatory term for those deemed too supportive of multiculturalism or egalitarian causes.

Nuclear threats engaged activists from both the peace and environmental movements. The accidents at Three Mile Island (1979) and Chernobyl (1986) intensified public anxieties about the dangers of nuclear energy. Nuclear weapons were even deadlier: after all, their very purpose was to wreak destruction on a scale that would create what scientists called "nuclear winter," a depopulated planet shrouded in radioactivity. The sharp increases in both Soviet and U.S. nuclear arsenals alarmed residents in those countries and across Europe, where many of the missiles were located. Americans and others who remembered Hiroshima expressed shock when Reagan administration officials spoke of winning a nuclear war and the president wrongly claimed that commanders could recall submarine-based missiles after firing them. The broad-based nuclear freeze movement that emerged in the United States and western Europe in the early 1980s instead encouraged arms control negotiations that would bear fruit a few years later.

Gays and lesbians remained the only Americans against whom tens of millions of their fellow citizens openly believed it acceptable to discriminate

Racial justice remained a primary concern for Americans of color and liberal and leftist activists, particularly in light of the Republican administration's opposition to affirmative action. Determined to honor the foremost leader of the civil rights movement, antiracists convinced Congress in 1983 to designate Martin Luther King, Jr.'s birthday a national holiday. By 1985, a robust antiapartheid movement—inspired by South African church leader and Nobel peace prize winner Desmond Tutu—successfully campaigned to reduce U.S. investments in racially segregated South Africa. A year later, Congress passed the Comprehensive Anti-Apartheid Act over the president's veto, enacting economic sanctions against South Africa—despite opposition from conservatives, such as Congressman Dick Cheney of Wyoming and Senator Jesse Helms of North Carolina. Such international pressure played a central role in the South African government's decision four years later to end apartheid and release African National Congress leader Nelson Mandela from jail. The long era of explicit white supremacy, embodied in international colonialism and American segregation as well as South African apartheid, finally ended.

Perhaps the most prominent face of left-leaning politics in the decade was that of Reverend Jesse Jackson, a former aide to Martin Luther King, Jr. Jackson sought the Democratic nomination for president in 1984 and 1988, winning a handful of primaries in 1988 with his multiracial Rainbow Coalition. Jackson's candidacy encouraged several million African Americans to register to vote for the first time. They, in turn, helped pressure southern Democratic senators to provide the crucial votes in 1987 to reject Robert Bork, a right-wing ideologue (and former Solicitor General in the Nixon administration) nominated by Reagan for a seat on the Supreme Court.

Gay rights advocates also raised their voices in the 1980s. Faced with the twin scourge of AIDS and homophobic violence, homosexuals and their heterosexual supporters lobbied for the inclusion of sexual orientation as a category of discrimination in civil rights laws. Others took to the streets, organized by the militant organization AIDS Coalition to Unleash Power (ACT-UP). In October 1987, nearly half a million Americans marched in Washington in support of gay rights. A few widely admired figures, such as tennis champion Martina Navratilova, publicly acknowledged their homosexuality, helping others to view this sexual orientation as acceptable rather than deviant. By the end of the 1980s, the record was mixed. Gays and lesbians remained the only Americans against whom tens of millions of their fellow citizens openly believed it acceptable to discriminate, but the rights of homosexuals, nonetheless, had much wider support than ever before.

The New Immigration

For two decades after the restrictive immigration law of 1924, the flow of newcomers from abroad had slowed to a trickle. The trickle became a stream again after World War II, and then legislation in 1965 opened the gates even wider. As a result, a wave of new immigrants, 3.5 million in the 1960s and 4.5 million in the 1970s, hit the United States. The 1980s set the record as 6 million people entered the country legally, along with a similar number without documentation.

These newcomers brought an unprecedented cultural and ethnic diversity. Communist rule in eastern Europe and prosperity in western Europe had reduced the emigration from that continent; only 10 percent of the most recent arrivals in the United States were Europeans. Forty percent came instead from Asia—particularly China, the Philippines, and South Korea—and 50 percent from Latin America and the Caribbean, particularly Mexico. From 1965 to 1995, 7 million Latinos and 5 million Asians moved to the United States. Mexicans had been journeying north in smaller numbers since that country's 1910 revolution. But between 1970 and 1990, the Mexican American population of the southwestern states tripled, and the Asian American population of the western states increased sixfold.

The new immigrants came for the same reasons their predecessors had. Many were fleeing political and religious persecution in their home countries, but most sought new economic opportunity. A small number, primarily from South Korea and Hong Kong, arrived with some assets that helped them get started in business. However, most came with few resources and took what work they could find. Although Canada and Australia attracted them as well, no country matched the United States in its reputation for the sheer creation of wealth. The immense difficulties facing new immigrants often induced homesickness. Maria Salas told of crossing the U.S.–Mexican border with her children to join her husband, who was working as a migrant farm laborer in North Carolina: "We walked six days. We suffered a lot. And there were so many snakes. . . . Now that we are here, I ask the girls if they want to go back to Mexico. They say they wish to return, but not if they have to walk back."

Like other new arrivals of earlier eras, the most recent immigrants were more willing than U.S. residents to work for low wages in poor conditions. An employer's dream, they quickly

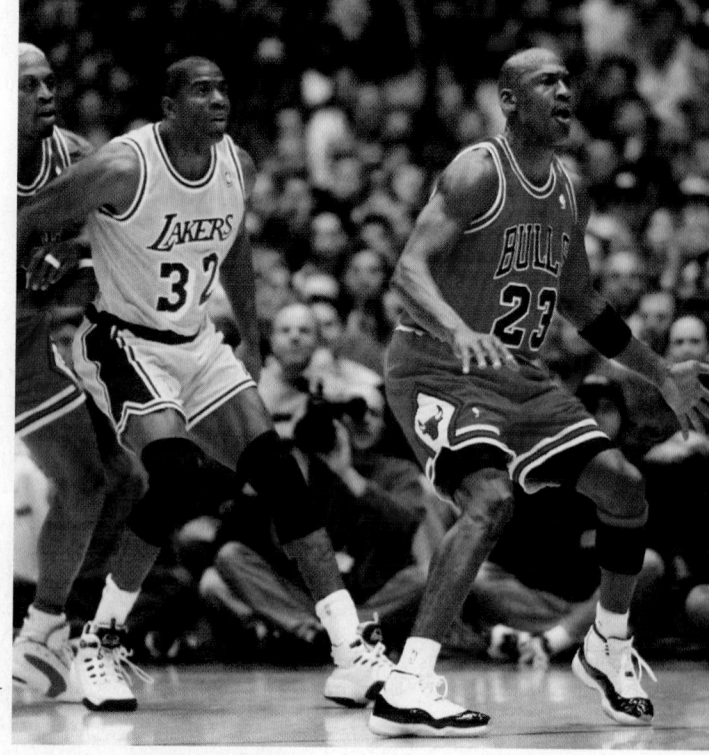

Eric Draper/AP /Wide World

■ While immigrants brought their own distinctive cultures to the United States, American popular culture spread abroad. The broadcast of National Basketball Association (NBA) games in dozens of other countries helped basketball climb to being the world's second most popular game (after soccer). Personable stars like Earvin "Magic" Johnson of the Los Angeles Lakers and particularly Michael Jordan of the Chicago Bulls became popular icons around the world.

found work in garment sweatshops, on farms, as domestic servants and janitors, and as gardeners. Hailing from countries with dramatically lower standards of living than in the United States, they willingly endured profound hardship to build better lives for their families. They also rekindled the nation's long-standing cultural diversity, especially in Sunbelt cities from Miami, Florida, to San Diego, California. The historic Mexican majority in El Paso, Texas, grew larger. In 1981, citizens of San Antonio elected Henry Cisneros as the first Mexican American mayor of a major city. In Los Angeles, one-third of residents were foreign born by 1990, and the city had more Spanish speakers than anywhere else in North America besides Mexico City.

Most Americans had foreign-born ancestors who had come to the United States with the same dreams that motivated the newest arrivals. Still, the non-European origins of the latest immigrants troubled some white citizens. Conservatives, in particular, worried about the growing diversity of American society and feared a decline of the Eurocentric culture they had grown up with. They were also anxious that poor immigrants might drain taxpayers' dollars by winding up on welfare. The Immigration and Naturalization Service (INS) stepped up patrols of the 2000-mile U.S. border with Mexico to limit the rising number of undocumented Mexican workers heading north. By the early 1990s, the INS was apprehending and expelling 1.7 million undocumented workers every year. The desperate efforts of migrants to elude Border Patrol officers and cross into the United States led to deaths from thirst and exposure in the deserts that stretched across much of the region. A sign on one California freeway near the border showed the silhouette of a fleeing family as a warning to drivers to watch for pedestrians.

Despite the distaste that some Americans of European heritage felt for the new immigrants, the Latin American and especially Asian origins of the recent arrivals mirrored the rising economic significance of the Pacific Rim countries to the United States. In 1979, U.S. trade across the Pacific surpassed trade across the Atlantic for the first time. By 1996, the value of American trade with Asia was more than twice that with Europe. And Latin Americans, particularly Mexicans, provided a convenient supply of workers for the U.S. economy. They were available when companies needed them, and they could be shut out when that need evaporated.

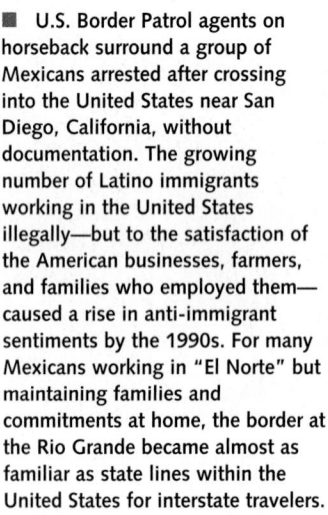

■ U.S. Border Patrol agents on horseback surround a group of Mexicans arrested after crossing into the United States near San Diego, California, without documentation. The growing number of Latino immigrants working in the United States illegally—but to the satisfaction of the American businesses, farmers, and families who employed them—caused a rise in anti-immigrant sentiments by the 1990s. For many Mexicans working in "El Norte" but maintaining families and commitments at home, the border at the Rio Grande became almost as familiar as state lines within the United States for interstate travelers.

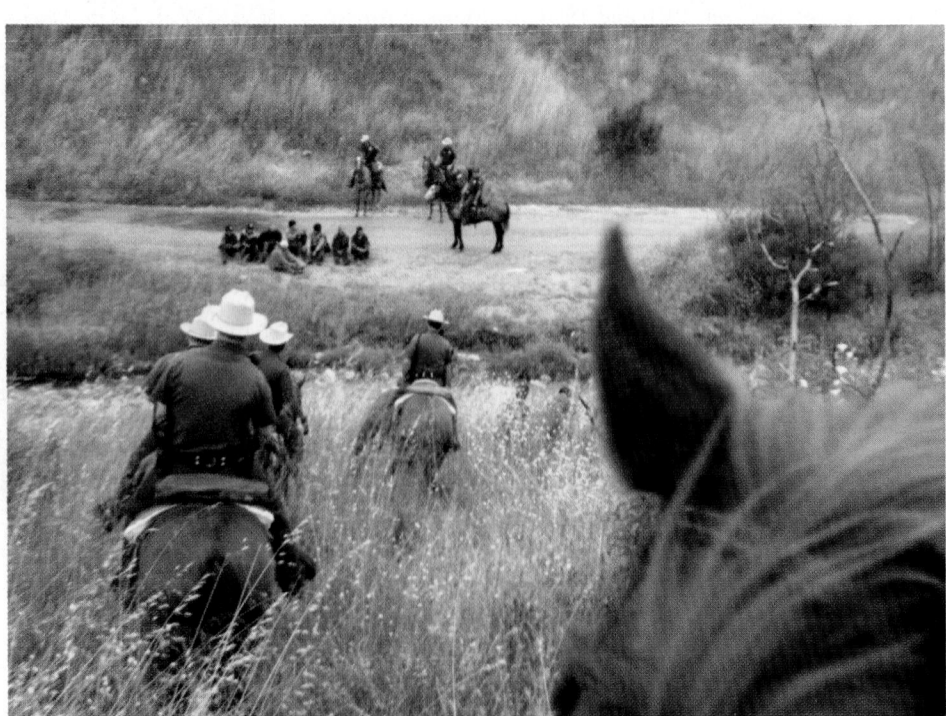

U.S. Border Patrol, San Diego HQ, Public Information Office

The End of the Cold War

"M y fellow Americans, I'm pleased to tell you today that I've signed legislation that will outlaw Russia forever. We begin bombing in five minutes." Ronald Reagan, in 1984, thought he was telling a joke at a microphone that was not turned on. He was wrong. Indeed, after three years of the president's military build-up and confrontational rhetoric toward the Soviet Union ("the focus of evil in the world")—including talk of fighting and winning a nuclear war—many Americans found his attempted humor appalling. However, by the end of his presidency four years later, a stunning reversal had occurred. Reagan had traveled to Moscow, embraced Soviet leader Mikhail Gorbachev in front of Lenin's tomb, and announced that the Soviets had changed.

For Americans, the greatest surprise of the 1980s came with this warming of U.S.–Soviet relations after 1985. Few had imagined such a scenario during Reagan's first two years in office. During that period, his administration became the first in four decades not to collaborate on nuclear arms control with the USSR. In the Soviet Union, the rise to power of Communist Party reformer Gorbachev permanently changed the face of international politics. The American president finally agreed to work toward the common goal of reducing tensions between the two superpowers.

At the same time, the Reagan administration stumbled badly at home when a scandal involving Iran and the Nicaraguan Contras came to light in 1986. The disaster revealed a secret foreign policy apparatus and a president out of touch with the daily governance process. Dramatic events in Europe then unfolded with little input from the administrations of either Reagan or George H.W. Bush, his successor in the White House. In 1989, Eastern Europeans tore down the Berlin Wall and ended Soviet rule in their countries. Two years later, the Soviet Union itself unraveled into its separate components, Russia being the largest. The end of the Cold War enabled Bush to focus on the Middle East, where an international force drove Iraq out of occupied Kuwait and reestablished the status quo in that oil-rich region.

From Cold War to Détente

In the 1980s, internal Soviet politics finally ended the Cold War. Gorbachev was the key figure. He and other reformers had grown up during the post–1956 campaign to reinterpret the leadership of former General Secretary Josef Stalin. Like Americans in the 1960s, Gorbachev's generation boldly questioned orthodox thinking. They could see that the vast military expenditures of the 1960s and 1970s, along with efforts after 1980 to keep up with skyrocketing U.S. military spending, had devastated the Soviet economy. By the 1980s, the USSR's state-run economy was creaking to a halt. It simply could not provide the consumer products that Soviet citizens had learned about from the world outside their borders. Gorbachev warned of the danger of Russia becoming merely "an Upper Volta with missiles"—an impoverished nation that had sqaundered its wealth to build a nuclear arsenal.

As the 1980s unfolded, events further weakened the authority of the Soviet government. The USSR's occupation of Afghanistan became a quagmire resembling the United States' disastrous involvement in Vietnam. The brutality and illegitimacy of the occupation disillusioned Red Army soldiers on the front lines and their families at home. Moreover, the Afghan resistance proved tougher than the USSR expected. The last Soviet troops finally withdrew in 1989. Initial government efforts to cover up the nuclear accident at Chernobyl only worsened matters, revealing the costs of corrupt communist rule. And nationalist movements for independence in the Baltic states, the Caucasus region, and central Asia gathered momentum. In his six years in power (1985–1991), Gorbachev tried to preserve the Soviet system by reforming it through *glasnost* (greater political liberty) and *perestroika* (economic restructuring

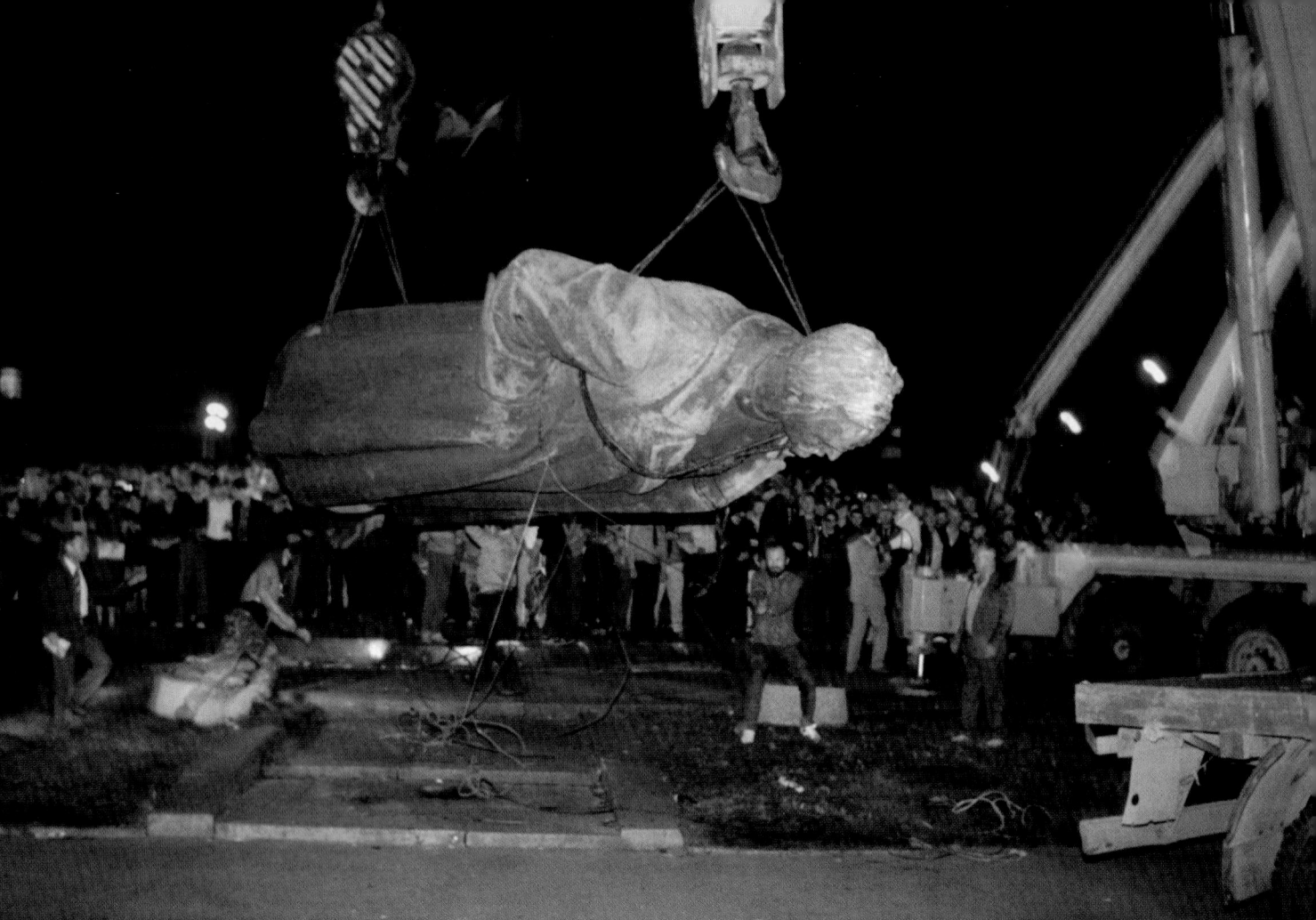

■ Workers in Prague, Czechoslovakia, haul away a bust of Josef Stalin after the peaceful "Velvet Revolution" that overthrew communist rule there in 1989. Similar scenes unfolded across eastern Europe as Czechs, Poles, Hungarians, and others removed symbols of four and a half decades of Soviet domination. Accustomed to often extravagant accounts of the strength of the Soviet Union, Americans were stunned by the swiftness with which the Soviet empire and then the USSR itself unraveled.

allowing some private enterprise). However, his government proved unable to control the forces for change that it had helped unleash.

Reagan's primary role in ending the Cold War was to support Gorbachev's quest for change within the Soviet Union. To that end, Reagan moved from confrontational rhetoric to pursuing a policy of détente. His trajectory contrasted directly with that of Jimmy Carter, who had shifted from an initial period of détente to helping renew U.S.–Soviet tensions.

Reagan's timing was now crucial. Gorbachev became head of the Soviet Communist party in 1985, at the start of Reagan's second term. The American president had already built up the U.S. military and was now thinking about his place in history. He wanted to leave office having earned a reputation as a peacemaker. His influential wife, Nancy, helped promote this idea, and the two received additional support from the less hawkish members of the administration, particularly Secretary of State George Schultz.

Beneath Reagan's strident rhetoric about national military strength ran a streak of radical idealism, including a desire to eliminate the threat of nuclear warfare. This desire prompted him to launch the Strategic Defense Initiative. He expected the United States to eventually share the technology with the Soviets. Despite his Cold War posturing during his first term, the U.S. president had been troubled by the 1983 television drama *The Day After*. The movie conveyed sobering images of the aftermath of a nuclear war on American soil. The Soviet downing of a

Korean Air Lines civilian jet that fall reminded him and others of the tragic costs of making mistakes with weapons.

Once he felt convinced of Gorbachev's seriousness about internal reform and rapprochement with the United States, Reagan took action. At a summit conference in Reykjavik, Iceland, in 1986, the two leaders came within a whisker of agreeing to eliminate nearly all of their nations' nuclear arsenals. The next year, they signed the more limited but still symbolically important Intermediate Nuclear Force (INF) treaty. The agreement removed short-range and intermediate-range missiles from Europe and enabled each side to conduct on-site verification of the other side's compliance. INF marked the first actual reduction in the total number of nuclear weapons stored in the two nations' arsenals.

The Iran–Contra Scandal

Failures elsewhere offset Reagan's success with the Russians. His administration suffered its worst damage when it tried through illegal means to solve two foreign policy challenges with one stroke. Its main strategy consisted of linking a problem in the Middle East with one in Central America. Since the 1940s, the U.S. government had struggled to balance three often conflicting goals in the Middle East: maintaining access to the region's oil, preserving a strong Israel, and excluding communist influence. But a new problem emerged when the pro-Iranian, anti-American, and anti-Israeli Islamic revolution began to spread after the 1979 overthrow of the Shah.

As revolutionary fervor intensified in the region, hostage taking and terrorism—the "poor man's nuclear bomb"—proliferated. In 1981, U.S. warplanes shot down two Libyan fighter jets when the jets tried to restrict American pilots' movements over the Mediterranean Sea. In 1986, Americans bombed the Libyan capital of Tripoli in retaliation for apparent Libyan involvement in the killing of two U.S. soldiers in Germany. In 1988, things took an even nastier turn when an American warship in the Persian Gulf killed 290 civilians by shooting down an Iranian airliner, apparently by mistake. In revenge, pro-Iranian agents exploded a bomb on Pan Am Flight 109 over Lockerbie, Scotland, before the end of the year, killing 11 on the ground and 259 aboard the plane, including 35 students from Syracuse University.

Bettmann/CORBIS

■ U.S. Lieutenant Woody Lee guards the briefcase (known as "the football") containing the codes to be used by President Reagan if he were to decide to launch nuclear weapons. Lee's job was to remain close to the president at all times and to protect "the football" with his life. Ironically, Lee stands here in Moscow's Red Square in 1988, where Reagan was holding a summit meeting with Soviet leader Mikhail Gorbachev, so many of those U.S. nuclear missiles, presumably, were aimed at them.

Islamic revolutionaries also threatened moderate Arab leaders and assassinated Egyptian president Anwar Sadat in 1981. Lebanon became the center of a radical anti-Israeli campaign to seize Americans as hostages, especially after the United States' 1983 engagement against Muslim forces in the civil war there. Despite his 1980 campaign promise never to negotiate with terrorists, Reagan approved the illegal sale of U.S. arms to Iran in return for the freeing of a handful of hostages held by pro-Iranian radicals in Lebanon.

Events were heating up in Central America as well. The CIA-created Contras failed to overturn the new Sandinista government in Nicaragua. Even though the Contras lacked public support in Nicaragua and the United States, the president and his advisers were determined to keep them afloat. But they had a problem: how to fund the effort. Most Americans did not share Reagan's enthusiasm for the Contras and feared greater U.S. military involvement in Central America. Beginning in 1982, Congress passed the Boland Amendments, restricting aid to the

Nicaraguan counterrevolutionaries. These restrictions culminated in a 1984 ban on helping them "directly or indirectly" beyond a token dose of humanitarian assistance. Faced with their chief's expressed desire to shore up the Contra cause, the president's men found an alternative solution.

The National Security Council (NSC) established a secret operation run by staff member Lieutenant Colonel Oliver North. Free from public or congressional oversight, North worked closely with CIA director William Casey. North and his colleagues solicited funds for the Contras from wealthy, conservative Americans and from sympathetic foreign governments, including Saudi Arabia and Taiwan. Then North hit on what he called the "neat idea" of "using the Ayatollah Khomeini's money to support the Nicaraguan freedom fighters." Iran desperately needed weapons for its war against neighboring Iraq (1980–1988), so North and his colleagues started diverting profits to the Contras from new sales of U.S. Army property to Teheran. One operative joked about the "Contra-bution," although some of the funds wound up in the private accounts of North and others involved in the diversion.

The NSC's action was illegal: it sold U.S. government property without authorization from the Pentagon, and it broke U.S. laws banning aid to the Contras. When news of the operation finally leaked out in November 1986, it shocked the nation. Details emerged from separate investigations by a presidential commission, a Justice Department independent prosecutor, and a congressional committee.

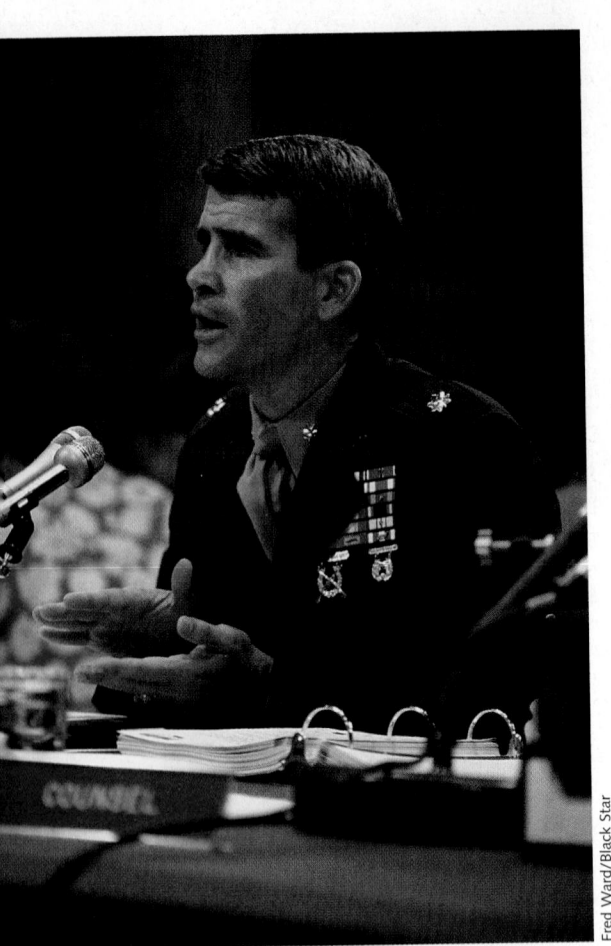

Fred Ward/Black Star

■ Lieutenant Colonel Oliver North of the National Security Council became the public face of the Iran-Contra scandal. North displayed his medals from the Vietnam War in testimony before Congress, but his smug version of patriotism and his deceitfulness alienated many senators and congressmen.

North's televised testimony before Congress made him a hero to some. He indicted Congress for its failure to support the president's policies in Central America, and he painted his own actions as patriotic. Others thought him a scoundrel. After all, he had run a private foreign policy that subverted the legislature's constitutional responsibilities and then had shredded documents that detailed his role. He later admitted, "I tried to avoid telling outright lies [before Congress], but I certainly wasn't telling the truth." His celebrity status among conservatives almost won him a victory as the Republican candidate for the U.S. Senate from Virginia in 1992.

What did the president know, and when did he know it? The old Watergate question about Richard Nixon came to the fore again. Reagan called North a "national hero" but claimed ignorance of any illegal activities, including the diversion of funds from Iranian arms sales to the Nicaraguan rebels. When some of Reagan's aides testified that he had approved negotiating with terrorists for the release of hostages, the president denied it. Questioned by investigators, the president said he could not remember details about his decisions and policies. This possibility gained credence a few years later when the public learned of his affliction with Alzheimer's disease.

But in early 1987, 90 percent of Americans did not believe Reagan was telling all he knew. His reputation for candor suffered permanent damage. People could not decide which scenario was worse: that Reagan knew about the Iran–Contra deal and approved it or that he did not know what his own administration was doing in his name. It was hard even to imagine the latter situation occurring under any other president.

Reagan's job approval ratings dropped from 67 percent to 46 percent within a month as the Iran–Contra revelations came on the heels of the failed Reykjavik summit and the Democrats' victory in the 1986 congressional elections. The first round of memoirs by former aides also appeared in the final years of his administration. These books revealed an isolated president out of touch with the government he nominally headed. For example, the former actor breezily admitted that he was happiest when "each morning I get a piece of paper that tells me what I do all day long." The leaking of news that an astrologer—hired by First Lady Nancy Reagan—had helped set the president's schedule for years did not help either. Nonetheless, Reagan held onto much of his personal popularity to the end of his term. In the phrase of Representative Pat Schroeder of Colorado, he was the "Teflon president" to whom no bad news could stick.

A Global Policeman?

Although George H. W. Bush had made his career in the Texas oil business and then in that state's Republican party, his roots lay in the party's moderate northeastern elite. His father, Prescott Bush, had been a U.S. senator from Connecticut, and he himself ran the CIA in 1975–1976. After losing in the 1980 party primaries, Bush agreed to run as Reagan's vice-presidential candidate. He then moved to the political right throughout the 1980s.

When Bush's turn at the presidency finally came in 1988, he ran a bruising campaign that made a caricature of his Democratic opponent, Governor Michael Dukakis of Massachusetts. Even more than previous presidential campaigns, this one turned on symbols rather than issues. Three proved particularly important. First, Bush repeatedly led audiences in reciting the Pledge of Allegiance in response to a wave of flag-burning demonstrations. (A year later, the Supreme Court affirmed the act as a form of free speech guaranteed by the Constitution.)

Second, Bush skewered his opponent as a liberal and a "card-carrying member" of the American Civil Liberties Union, an organization dedicated to defending the Bill of Rights. Senator Joseph McCarthy had used precisely this phrase to describe members of the American Communist party four decades earlier. Thus, Bush implied that liberals were subversives.

Third, Bush accused Dukakis of coddling criminals. His campaign ads focused on Willie Horton, a black man convicted of murder. While on parole from a Massachusetts prison during Dukakis's governorship, Horton raped a white woman and killed her husband. Republicans appealed to whites' anxieties about race, sex, and safety. "If I can make Willie Horton a household name," Bush's campaign strategist Lee Atwater promised, "we'll win the election." He succeeded on both fronts.

TABLE 28-3			
The Election of 1988			
Candidate	Political Party	Popular Vote	Electoral Vote
George H. W. Bush	Republican	48,886,000	426
Michael S. Dukakis	Democratic	41,809,000	111

As president, however, Bush proved cautious. Hemmed in by a Democrat-controlled Congress, he had what his chief of staff called a "limited agenda" at home. His most enduring domestic action came with his 1991 appointment of archconservative Clarence Thomas, an African American lawyer from Georgia, to fill the seat of retiring Supreme Court justice Thurgood Marshall. Only 43 years old and with little experience as a judge, Thomas was chosen because of his conservative views and his race. The Senate narrowly confirmed him, 52–48, after contentious hearings in which a former aide, Anita Hill, accused Thomas of sexual harassment.

"I much prefer foreign affairs," the president once confided in his diary. Yet he proceeded just as carefully in this realm as he did with domestic policy. Some of the most dramatic events of the twentieth century unfolded during his presidency. Poles, Czechs, and Hungarians—encouraged by Gorbachev's promise not to intervene militarily in other Warsaw Pact nations—peacefully overthrew their communist rulers in 1989. East Germans did the same. The Berlin Wall—the 28-year-old symbol of Cold War tensions—finally toppled on November 8. Three months later, Nelson Mandela walked out of the South African prison where he had been held for 27 years. The white supremacist government there agreed to hold the first elections in which all South Africans could vote. The Baltic states of Lithuania, Latvia, and Estonia also seceded from the USSR in 1990 and 1991. Rather than rejoicing at the shrinking of Soviet power, Bush urged Soviet citizens to move cautiously. The president feared that too much change too fast might create unrest across Russia and eastern Europe. But after a failed coup attempt by Communist hard-liners in August 1991, the Soviet Union broke into its 16 constituent states. Russian president Boris Yeltsin replaced Gorbachev as the major figure in Moscow.

The Bush administration acted more boldly in its own hemisphere. In Panama, under the brutal leadership of Manuel Noriega, tensions grew between the Panamanian Defense Forces (PDF) and U.S. soldiers based in the Canal Zone. Bush and Noriega had known each other since the mid–1970s, when each had headed his country's intelligence agency. They had worked together in the early 1980s when Noriega provided logistical support for the Contras' war in nearby Nicaragua. But the Panamanian strongman had since parted ways with the Americans and had deepened his lucrative role as an intermediary in smuggling Colombian cocaine into the United States. Meanwhile, the crack cocaine epidemic tightened its grip in

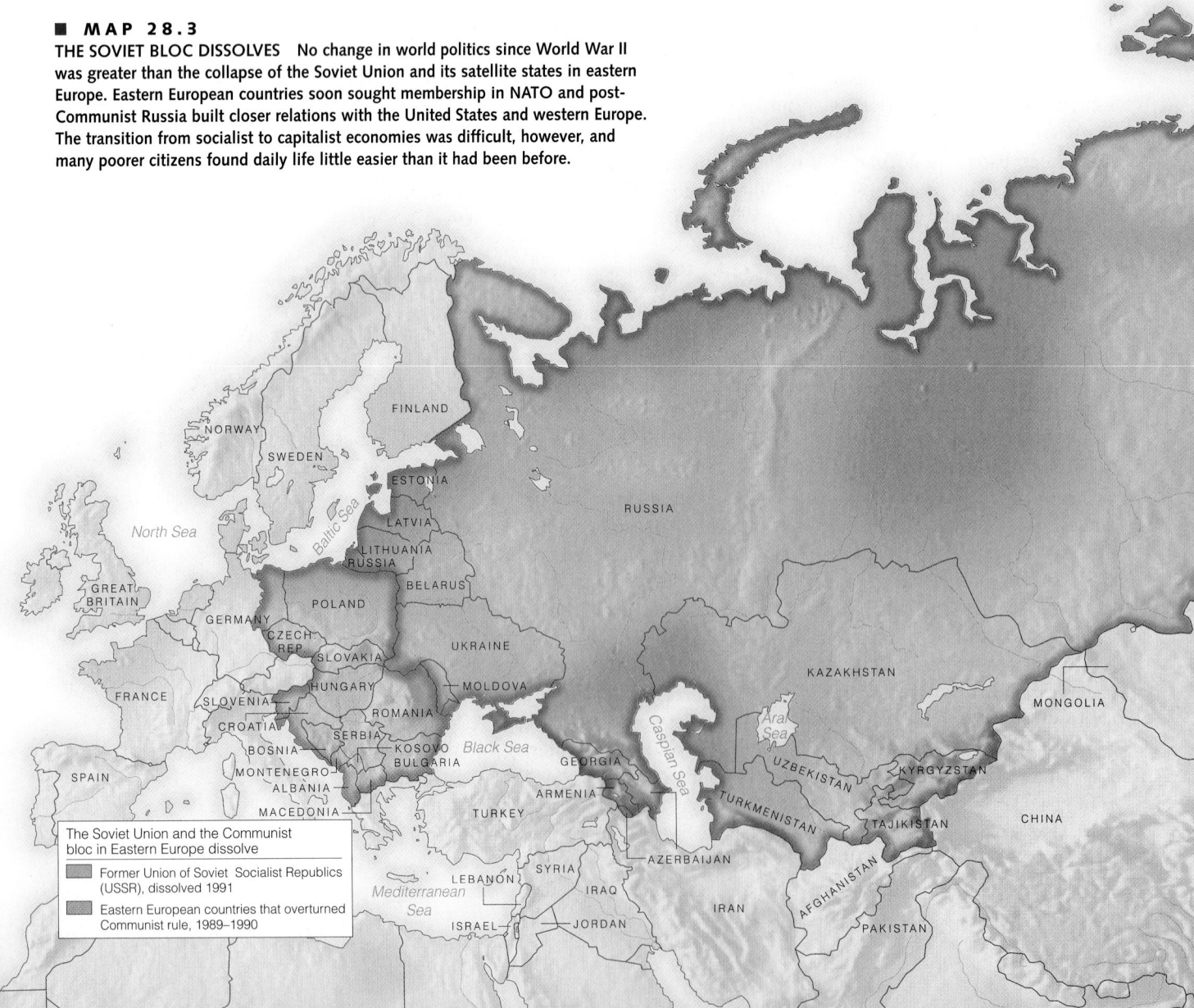

■ **MAP 28.3**
THE SOVIET BLOC DISSOLVES   No change in world politics since World War II was greater than the collapse of the Soviet Union and its satellite states in eastern Europe. Eastern European countries soon sought membership in NATO and post-Communist Russia built closer relations with the United States and western Europe. The transition from socialist to capitalist economies was difficult, however, and many poorer citizens found daily life little easier than it had been before.

poor American neighborhoods. Rising popular concern about crack-related violence increased Americans' willingness to take action against Noriega. When the dictator overturned Panamanian election results that went against him and further confrontations erupted between American and Panamanian soldiers, Bush decided to step in.

In December 1989, 24,000 U.S. troops invaded the small Central American nation. They crushed the PDF, and thousands of civilians died in the crossfire. Noriega took refuge in the home of the Vatican emissary in Panama City. U.S. commanders applied psychological pressure. Knowing Noriega's distaste for rock 'n' roll music, they set up enormous speakers and floodlights outside the residence. At a deafening volume, they blared such songs as Linda Ronstadt's "You're No Good" and Sonny Curtis's "I Fought the Law (and the Law Won)." Noriega eventually surrendered and was brought to Miami, where he was convicted of drug trafficking and imprisoned.

Developments in the Middle East provoked the most important move of the Bush administration: the initiation of the Gulf War of 1991. After the Iranian revolution, Iraq and Iran had clashed over disputed border territories. The Reagan administration had provided weapons to both sides at different points. The president wanted neither combatant to win a decisive victory that would destabilize the area. With two-thirds of the world's known oil reserves in the states surrounding the Persian Gulf, the U.S. government especially dreaded seeing control of the region's oil prices and supplies shift from Saudi Arabia to revolutionary Iran.

Iraq ended the war in a strong position in 1988, and two years later, it invaded tiny, neighboring oil-rich Kuwait, annexing it as Iraq's "19th province." With Americans and their Japanese and European allies dependent on Middle Eastern oil, Bush declared the invasion unacceptable. He rushed more than 200,000 troops to Saudi Arabia in "Operation Desert Shield" to discourage further aggression by Iraqi leader Saddam Hussein. At the same time, the United Nations slapped economic sanctions on Iraq.

Three months later, Bush shifted his attention to liberating Kuwait. He doubled the number of U.S. troops in the region to 430,000. He also gained the support of the UN, which demanded Iraqi withdrawal by January 15, 1991. The U.S. Congress backed him as well, voting to support any actions necessary to drive Iraq out of Kuwait. Bush went on the offensive because he faced a shrinking window of opportunity. He had wide international support, including troops from several Arab nations, but growing clashes in Jerusalem between Israelis and Palestinians threatened to break up this alliance by rekindling Arab anger at Israel. Meanwhile, Saddam Hussein loudly supported the Palestinians and denounced the Americans as Israeli allies.

Bush believed that the brief war helped Americans to finally "kick the Vietnam syndrome": no longer would they hesitate to use force abroad.

On January 16, 1991, Allied planes began five and a half weeks of bombing against Iraq. Then, on February 25, Allied forces poured across the border from Saudi Arabia in "Operation Desert Storm." The offensive freed Kuwait and sent Iraqi troops in headlong retreat toward Baghdad. The Iraqis burned oil wells as they fell back, blanketing the battlefield in smoke. Four days later, Bush halted the U.S. advance, having restored Kuwaiti sovereignty. Saddam Hussein remained in power and later crushed uprisings by Iraqi dissidents. The politics of coalition warfare helped prohibit further U.S. action, for no Arabs wanted Americans ruling Iraq.

What did the Gulf War reveal? It showed Bush at his most successful, managing an international coalition few would have thought possible a few years earlier. The withdrawal of Soviet power from the region had played a crucial role, after decades of Moscow's support for Iraq. In its first major post–Cold War engagement, the United States demonstrated its military supremacy. Still, the opposition had proven surprisingly weak. One U.S. soldier later described himself as participating in "the biggest firing squad in history." Bush nonetheless believed that the brief war helped Americans to finally "kick the Vietnam syndrome": no longer would they hesitate to use force abroad.

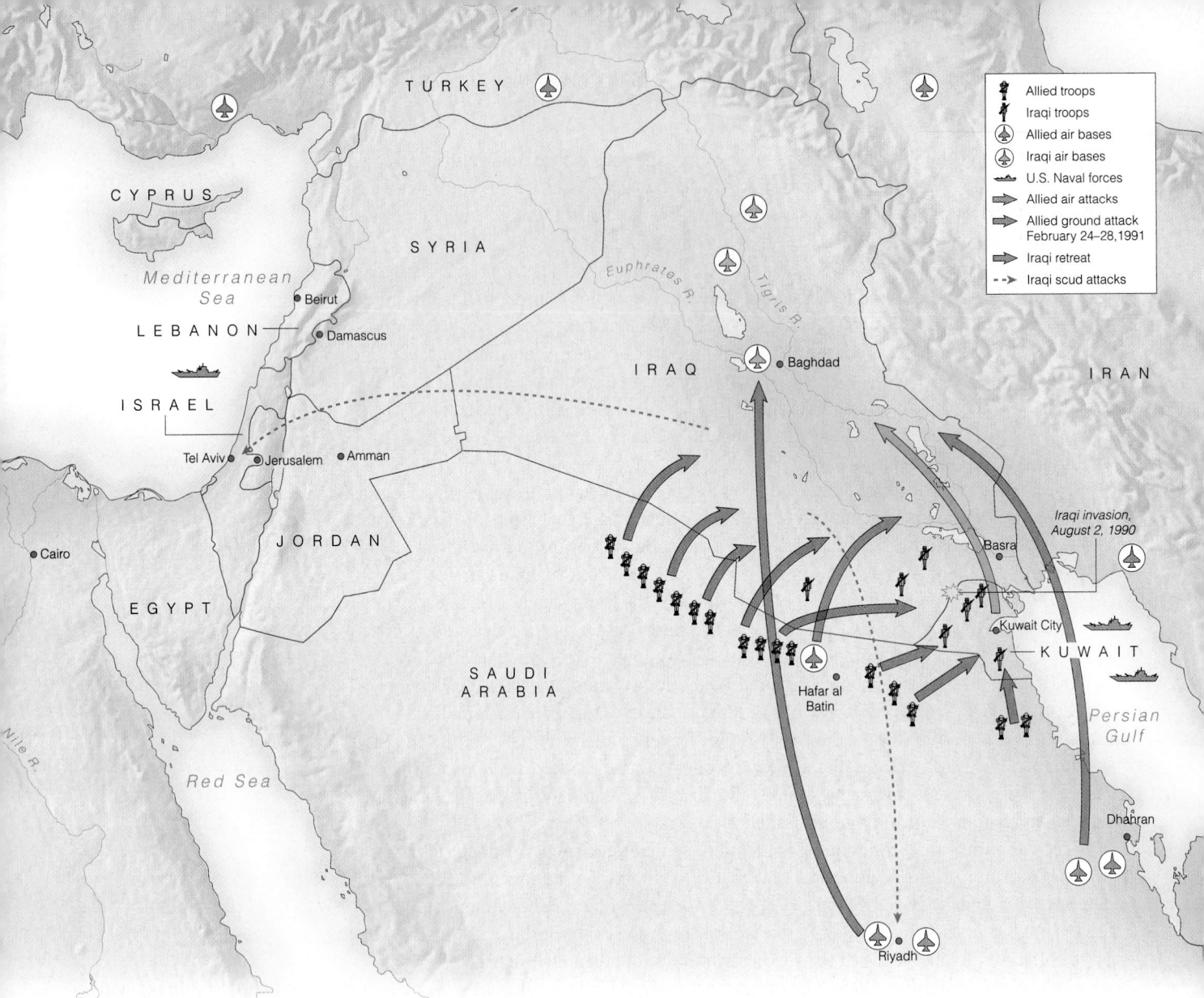

■ **MAP 28.4**

THE GULF WAR, 1990–1991 Rarely had U.S. strategic and economic interests been so openly the motivation for war. Oil brought American soldiers to defend Saudi Arabia and drive Iraqi troops out of Kuwait. But many Arab states supported the U.S.-led coalition because they opposed Iraqi President Saddam Hussein's occupation of Kuwait.

The war's outcome seemed to validate two strategic lessons that U.S. commanders had learned during the Vietnam War. The first was the importance of preserving absolute control of the media. During the Persian Gulf conflict, the Pentagon kept journalists away from most of the action to control the images that Americans saw of the fighting. The public viewed endless videos of "smart" bombs hitting their targets in Baghdad but none of the tens of thousands of Iraqi soldiers being slaughtered during their retreat from Kuwait. Second, General Colin Powell, the African American chair of the Joint Chiefs of Staff who emerged from the war as a national hero, insisted on marshaling overwhelmingly superior forces before going into battle, thus ensuring the success of the operation.

The Gulf War raised the question of whether the U.S. military had become a mercenary force, with allies chipping in more than seven times what Washington spent to fund U.S. soldiers. "Why should I fight?" one wealthy Kuwaiti sitting out the war in comfort in Cairo asked. "We can pay other countries to fight for us." The conflict seemed to demonstrate a

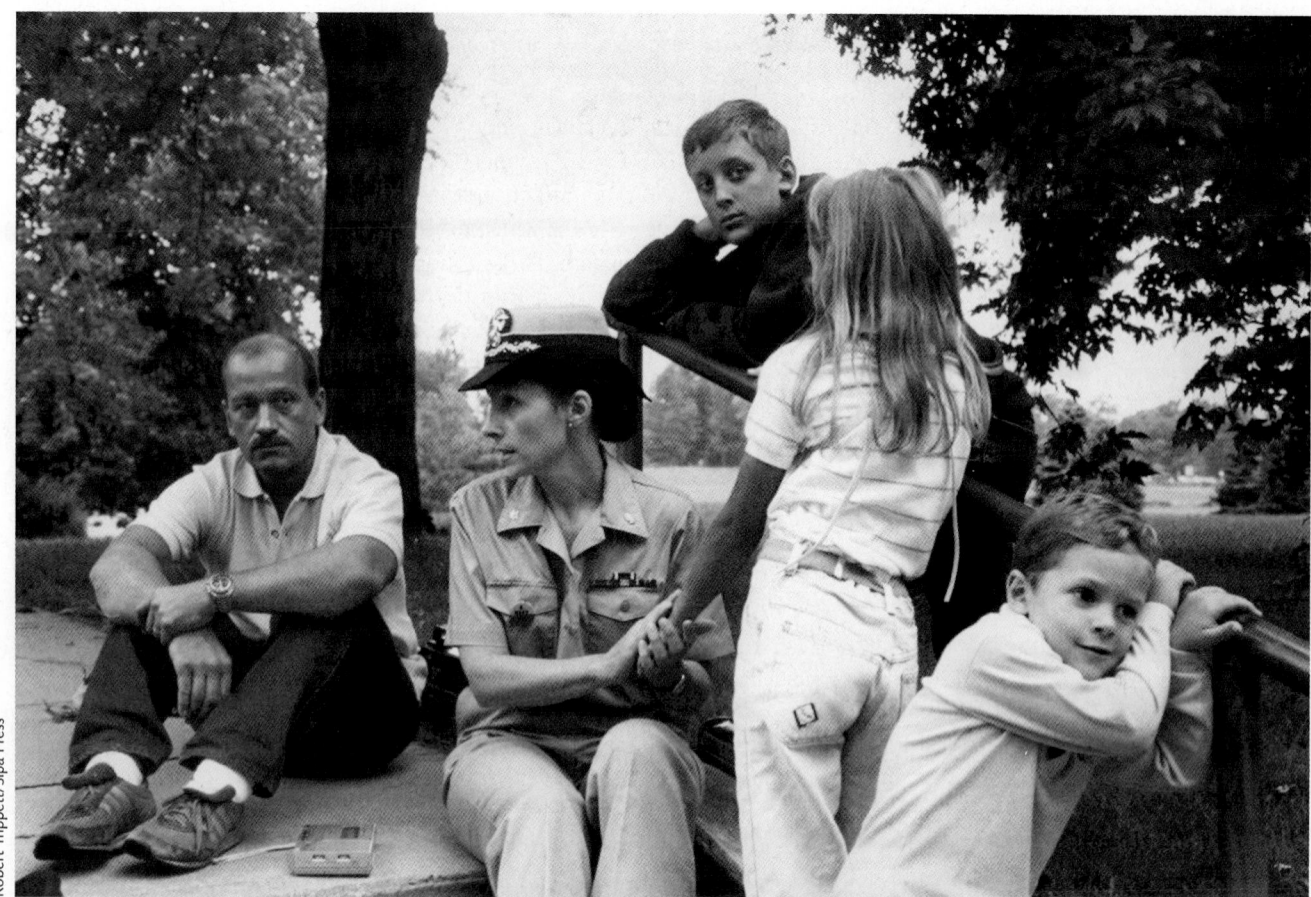

■ In the 1970s anti-feminists defeated the Equal Rights Amendment in part by opposing the idea of American women in combat. Attitudes about women had changed enough by 1991 that thousands of female service personnel participated in the Gulf War—including a few being captured and killed—with no public outcry. In Bethesda, Maryland, one soldier says goodbye to her family before shipping out to the Persian Gulf in September 1990.

U.S. willingness to act as a global police force in the post–Cold War era. But the war also stimulated the further growth of anti-Americanism among Islamic revolutionaries, including Saudi-born Osama bin Laden; they considered it sacrilege for non-Muslim American soldiers to operate bases in Saudi Arabia, home to Mecca, Islam's holiest site. Finally, the war foreshadowed Bush's defiant claim at a 1992 international environmental conference that, when it came to oil, "the American lifestyle is not negotiable."

Conclusion

The Republican era of Ronald Reagan and George H.W. Bush reshaped American relations with the rest of the world, as well as politics and economics in the United States. Both sets of changes hinged on the elevation of individualism and market forces above communal values and government planning. At home, the Republican ascendancy successfully challenged five decades of New Deal assumptions about government's role in economic regulation and its responsibilities toward the poor. A booming stock market underwrote a culture increasingly focused on the individual acquisition of wealth. Popular television shows of the

1980s, such as *Dynasty* and *Lifestyles of the Rich and Famous,* reflected a widespread admiration for affluence and conspicuous consumption.

The collective dreams represented by the Soviet experiment evaporated into history in these years, leaving capitalism unchallenged as a system of economic organization across most of the globe. U.S. military power stepped into the vacuum left by the Soviet demise, most visibly in the Gulf War. But that military revival came at the cost of vast deficit spending and a sharp recession in 1991–1992, which paved the way for Bill Clinton's victory over Bush in the 1992 presidential campaign. The assertion of military strength also demonstrated anew America's overriding Middle Eastern priorities of preserving access to the region's oil and defending Israel. This combination helped motivate the eventual attack on the United States by Islamic extremists on September 11, 2001.

Sites to Visit

Digital Atlas of the United States, 1990

130.166.124.2/USpage1.html

This site offers an overview of the geography and demography of the U.S. population in 1990.

Immigrant Fact Sheet, 1996

www.ins.usdoj.gov/graphics/aboutins/statistics/110.htm

The U.S. Immigration and Naturalization Service posted this site with historical statistics about immigration into the United States, especially from 1981 to 1996.

Divining America: Religion and the National Culture

www.nhc.rtp.nc.us:8080/tserve/divam.htm

This site has essays by prominent historians on diverse aspects of the religious history of the United States.

Ronald Wilson Reagan

www.ipl.org/ref/POTUS/rwreagan.html

The Internet Public Library maintains this site, which has essential information about Reagan and his presidential administrations as well as his most important speeches.

The National Security Archive at George Washington University

www.gwu.edu/~nsarchiv/

This extraordinary site includes the most recent declassified documents on the making of U.S. foreign policy.

Cold War International History Project

cwihp.si.edu/default.htm

The Woodrow Wilson International Center for Scholars maintains this excellent site, which offers newly released documents and up-to-date interpretive essays on the American-Soviet struggle.

The Gulf War

www.pbs.org/wgbh/pages/frontline/gulf/

The Public Broadcasting System's "Frontline" series created this site with information about the Persian Gulf War, including oral histories of U.S. commanders and of Americans taken as prisoners of war.

For Further Reading

General

E. J. Dionne, Jr. *Why Americans Hate Politics* (1991).

Frances FitzGerald, *Way Out There in the Blue: Reagan, Star Wars, and the End of the Cold War* (2000).

Neil Postman, *Amusing Ourselves to Death: Public Discourse in the Age of Show Business* (1985).

Michael Schaller, *Reckoning with Reagan: America and Its President in the 1980s* (1992).

Anticommunism Revived

James A. Bill, *The Eagle and the Lion: The Tragedy of American–Iranian Relations* (1988).

Thomas Ferguson and Joel Rogers, eds., *The Hidden Election: Politics and Economics in the 1980 Presidential Campaign* (1981).

Michael T. Klare and Peter Kornbluh, *Low-Intensity Warfare: Counterinsurgency, Proinsurgency, and Antiterrorism in the Eighties* (1988).

Walter LaFeber, *Inevitable Revolutions: The United States in Central America*, 2nd ed. (1993).

William E. Pemberton, *Exit with Honor: The Life and Presidency of Ronald Reagan* (1998).

Republican Rule at Home

Thomas Byrne Edsall and Mary D. Edsall, *Chain Reaction: The Impact of Race, Rights and Taxes on American Politics* (1991).

Barbara Ehrenreich, *The Worst Years of Our Lives: Irreverent Notes from a Decade of Greed* (1990).

J. R. McNeill, *Something New Under the Sun: An Environmental History of the Twentieth-Century World* (2000).

Kevin Phillips, *The Politics of Rich and Poor: Wealth and the American Electorate in the Reagan Aftermath* (1990).

Mark Robert Rank, *Living on the Edge: The Realities of Welfare in America* (1994).

Cultural Conflict

Susan J. Douglas, *Where the Girls Are: Growing Up Female with the Mass Media* (1994).

Todd Gitlin, *The Twilight of Common Dreams: Why America Is Wracked by Culture Wars* (1995).

Martin E. Marty and R. Scott Appleby, *The Glory and the Power: The Fundamentalist Challenge to the Modern World* (1992).

Nicolaus Mills, ed., *Culture in an Age of Money: The Legacy of the 1980s in America* (1990).

David M. Reimers, *Still the Golden Door: The Third World Comes to America*, 2nd ed. (1992).

Randy Shilts, *And the Band Played On: Politics, People and the AIDS Epidemic* (1987).

The End of the Cold War

Theodore Draper, *A Very Thin Line: The Iran–Contra Affairs* (1991).

John Robert Greene, *The Presidency of George Bush* (2000).

Dilip Hiro, *Desert Shield to Desert Storm: The Second Gulf War* (1992).

Michael J. Hogan, ed., *The End of the Cold War: Its Meanings and Implications* (1992).

Jane Mayer and Doyle McManus, *Landslide: The Unmaking of the President, 1984–1988* (1989).

David Remnick, *Lenin's Tomb: The Last Days of the Soviet Empire* (1993).

Online Practice Test

Test your understanding of this chapter with interactive review quizzes at

www.ablongman.com/jonescreatedequal/chapter28

Additional Photo Credits

Page 937: Ronald Reagan Presidential Library
Page 941: Courtesy, Janice L and David Frent
Page 942: Photofest
Page 948: Vladimir Sichov/Sipa Press
Page 957: AFP/CORBIS

CHAPTER 29

Post–Cold War America, 1991–2000

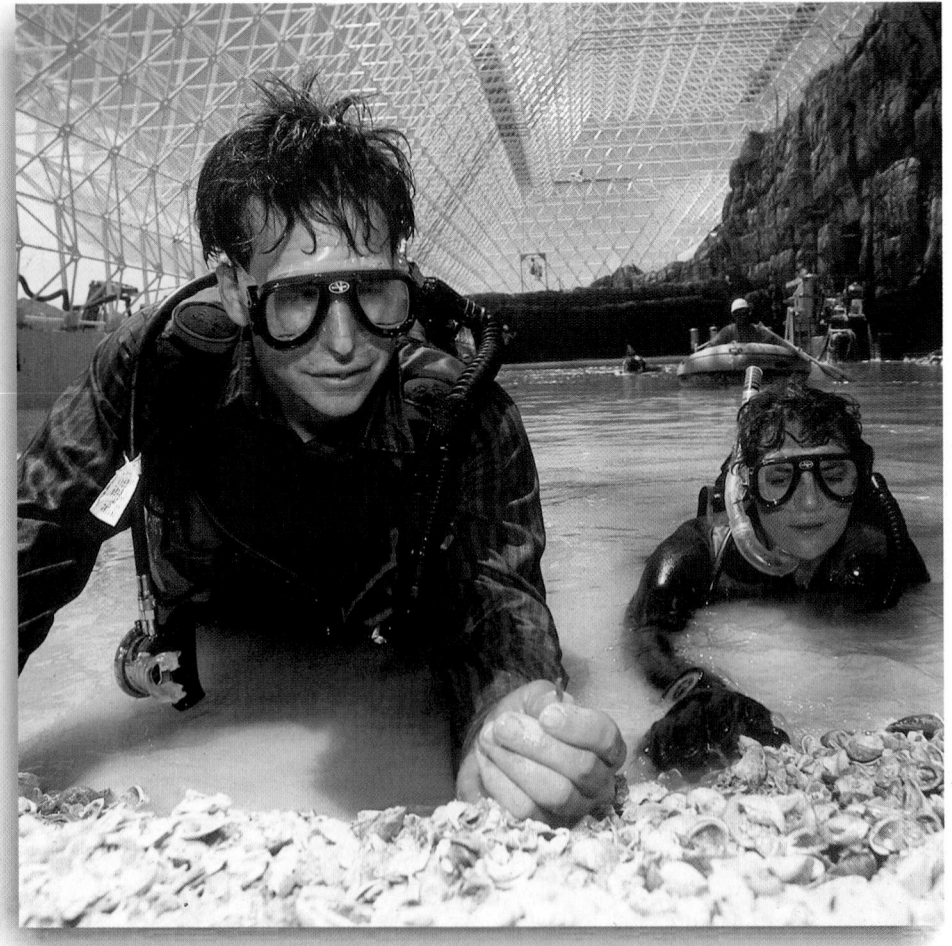

©1990 Peter Menzel

■ Underwater explorers examine shells at the manufactured beach in Biosphere 2, an artificially created ecosystem in the Arizona desert inhabited by eight "biospherians" from 1991 to 1993. The attempt to create a self-sustaining "mini-earth" failed within two years.

ON A COLD DECEMBER NIGHT IN 1997, 23-YEAR-OLD JULIA BUTTERFLY HILL CLIMBED onto a small platform that had been constructed 180 feet above ground in a giant redwood tree in a forest in Humboldt County, California. She remained there for two years, trespassing in an act of civil disobedience on the property of the Pacific Lumber Company, which was threatening to cut down the 1000-year-old tree as part of its logging operations. Julia Hill had not planned to become an internationally famous environmental activist. She grew up in Arkansas, the daughter of an itinerant preacher. When friends invited the restless young woman to join them on a drive to California, she eagerly went along. "I had been on a journey, searching for my purpose in life," she recalled, "I ended up finding it in the redwoods." When she first saw the giant redwoods, "Gripped by the spirit of the forest, I dropped to my knees and began to sob. . . . I could feel my whole being bursting forth into new life in this majestic cathedral."

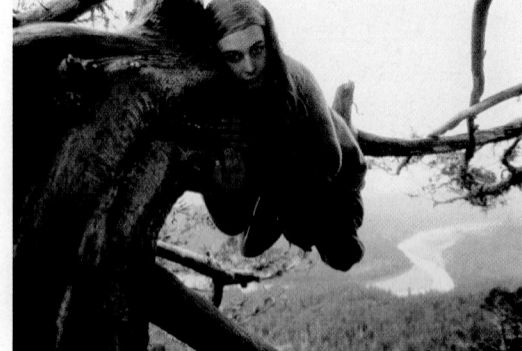

Julia "Butterfly" Hill in the giant redwood tree she named "Luna."

Hill's spiritual connection to the forest drew her to political activism, and she joined Earth First!, an environmental group that was working to save the redwoods from the logging industry. She discovered that 97 percent of the old-growth redwoods had already been destroyed and that the rest were threatened by clearcutting, toxins, and diesel fuel. Tree sitting was a strategy the Earth First! activists developed to protest the destruction of the trees. They had named this particular tree Luna, after the goddess of the moon, because they had built the small platform in it by moonlight. Julia Hill took a forest name—Butterfly—and settled in for her turn at tree sitting. Although the strategy usually involved tree-sitting for a week at a time, Butterfly Hill decided that to have an impact the protest needed to be taken to "a different level." "I realized I had to give more. I needed to give my word that my feet would not touch the ground" until the tree was safe from destruction.

Those two years were rough. The young woman survived rain and hail storms, 90-mile-per-hour winds that tossed the tiny platform into the air, and bone-chilling cold that turned her feet black. Friends and supporters provided her with food and other supplies using a rope pulley. She ate mostly raw fruits and vegetables, slept in a hammock, took sponge baths, and used a bucket for a toilet. She faced harassment from the logging company and derision from some skeptics. But she also had a powerful network of supporters and celebrities who raised money, brought her food, and publicized her protest.

Hill's effort to save an ancient tree as old as the last millennium was conducted using the global technology of the new millennium. Critical to the success of her protest was her ability to communicate with the entire world from her treetop perch. She set up a Web site on the Internet visited by people from all across the globe. Schoolchildren in Germany sent her pictures of themselves in front of their favorite trees. People responded to her from as far away as Turkey and Australia. She used a solar-powered cell phone to speak with radio stations, schools, rallies, religious groups, reporters, and talk show hosts.

The lumber company also used state-of-the-art technology in its efforts to stymie her protest, cutting down trees to make them fall in her direction, flying helicopters to hover noisily over her head, and using air horns to keep her awake at night.

The president of Pacific Lumber, John Campbell, eventually came to the tree to negotiate with Hill, and they made a deal. The company agreed never to cut down the tree or other trees in a 2.9-acre buffer zone. Hill agreed to come down. For her civil disobedience, she paid a $50,000 fine, contributed by supporters, which the court designated to Humboldt State University for forestry research. Although her success was modest in terms of saving endangered forests, her actions raised environmental awareness across the globe.

Activists such as Julia Butterfly Hill addressed political concerns through personal beliefs and direct action as part of social movements that evolved out of a century of such protests. But the issues had reached a global scale. Internationally, Cold War power struggles gave way to other issues: regional and civil wars, ethnic strife, the environment and global warming, trade and labor relations, and terrorism. Domestically, concerns of environmentalists ranged from the protection of a single tree to climate change affecting the entire planet. The labor movement turned much of its attention to service workers and the global economy, with problems ranging from the export of jobs to the existence of sweatshops at home and abroad.

> *Throughout most of the 1990s, one party controlled the White House while the other controlled the Congress.*

In the United States the economy expanded throughout the 1990s. Increasing numbers of Americans invested in the soaring stock market, many for the first time. The crime rate declined. Yet the strong economy also emboldened consumers to buy and use products and resources, such as huge gas-guzzling sport utility vehicles, with little concern for the environmental impact. Moreover, as the economy grew, so did the gap between the wealthy and the poor. As the new millennium dawned, the economy began to falter. The stock market fell, and there were signs of an impending recession.

The 2000 U.S. Census revealed a number of striking changes in the nation's population during the 1990s. Among the most dramatic was the 60 percent growth in the Latino population, from 22.4 million to 35.3 million, making the number of Latinos—most of them Mexican American—nearly equal to that of African Americans. In certain states the increase was even larger. The Latino population in California grew 35 percent during the decade and became a powerful economic and political force in the state. In Nevada the Latino population doubled, to become 20 percent of the state's residents. Immigrants from Asia and Latin America also added increasing linguistic diversity, fueling controversies over bilingual education and "English-only" political initiatives.

In national politics the rifts between liberals and conservatives that had opened up in the 1960s persisted. Struggles over cultural issues such as abortion and gay rights polarized the political climate. Throughout most of the 1990s, one party controlled the White House while the other controlled the Congress. A Democratic Congress during the Republican administration of George H. W. Bush passed the 1990 Americans with Disabilities Act, requiring reasonable accommodation for disabled persons in employment and access to public places. The Clean Air Act, passed in the same year, reduced smokestack and auto emissions. New legislation also increased funding for Head Start and boosted the minimum wage.

After a number of scandals in Congress over misuse of congressional bank accounts and votes to raise their own pay, the 27th Amendment to the Constitution, ratified in 1992, prohibited midterm congressional pay raises. In 1992 Democrats took back the White House, but in 1994 Republicans swept into control of Congress with a conservative agenda, hemming in President Bill Clinton, a Democrat of liberal social inclinations who, nonetheless, presided over the final destruction of the Aid to Families with Dependent Children (AFDC) program, which had been the central feature of the national welfare system since the New Deal of the 1930s.

Throughout the decade, racial hostilities flared, intensified by such events as the beating of motorist Rodney King and the murder trial of media celebrity O. J. Simpson. Anti-immigrant sentiments increased in response to recent immigration from Asia, Latin America, and especially Mexico. Nevertheless, studies showed that Americans had become more accepting of people whose racial or national backgrounds were different from their own. Americans' faith in political leadership, at a low ebb since Watergate, sank even farther as Republicans doggedly pursued Clinton's unseemly sexual behavior, leading to his impeachment by the House of Representatives, although he remained in office.

Money continued to pour into politics, even as voters called for campaign finance reform. New third-party candidates tapped widespread eagerness for a new type of politics. A Supreme Court dominated by conservatives nevertheless upheld liberal decisions, including abortion rights in *Planned Parenthood of Southeastern Pennsylvania v. Casey* (1992), gender equality in *U.S. v. Virginia* (1996) stating that the Virginia Military Institute could not exclude women, and the rights of gays and lesbians in *Romer v. Evans* (1996), which declared unconstitutional a Colorado amendment that nullified civil rights protections for homosexuals. In 2000, however, the Supreme Court decided one of the closest and most divisive elections in the nation's history, handing the White House to the Republican candidate, George W. Bush, son of the former president.

With the end of the Cold War, American foreign and domestic politics no longer revolved around the old, familiar enemies. Global power relations shifted with the dissolution of the Soviet Union, reviving long-dormant ethnic conflicts. Violence erupted in the Balkan countries of central Europe. In the Middle East, conflict between Israelis and Palestinians escalated, even as efforts at a peace process continued. Military confrontations flared elsewhere in the region as well. The post–Cold War era raised new questions about the role of the United States in the world. Americans no longer looked to Russia as a threat but to new international foes, especially terrorist networks operating outside the authority of particular countries. Within the nation, episodes of domestic terrorism, such as the bombing of a federal building in Oklahoma City and a series of school shootings by children made Americans feel that dangers lurked within their previously safe havens.

The Economy: Global and Domestic

After the sharp recession of 1991–1992, by nearly all measures, the economy expanded in the 1990s. The stock market boomed, unemployment declined, and most Americans appeared to be better off financially at the end of the decade than at the beginning. But the overall growth of the economy did not benefit everyone, and many actually lost ground—especially those who lost jobs to mechanization, nonunionized workers who toiled for low wages under grim working conditions, and the nation's most vulnerable workers: poor single mothers, new immigrants, and unskilled people of color.

The Post–Cold War Economy

The end of the Cold War had a profound effect on the nation's economy. The demise of the Soviet Union put a final end to the arms race against a superpower foe and made cutting the defense budget politically acceptable. But the closing of defense-related plants in southern

California, once the center of the nation's Cold War defense contracts that absorbed nearly a fifth of all federal defense dollars, devastated the regional economy. By the mid-1990s, half the workers in the southern California aerospace industry had been laid off, part of a national trend that resulted in the loss of more than half a million jobs, half of them in the manufacturing sector. Many workers lost not only their jobs but also their homes, their economic security, and their sense of community. Louis Rodriguez, president of the International Federation of Professional and Technical Engineers Local 174, explained how he felt when his Long Beach, California, shipyard closed: "The shipyard has been a second family to me. When I get out of here, I'm really going to be lost as a whole. I will have lost my family."

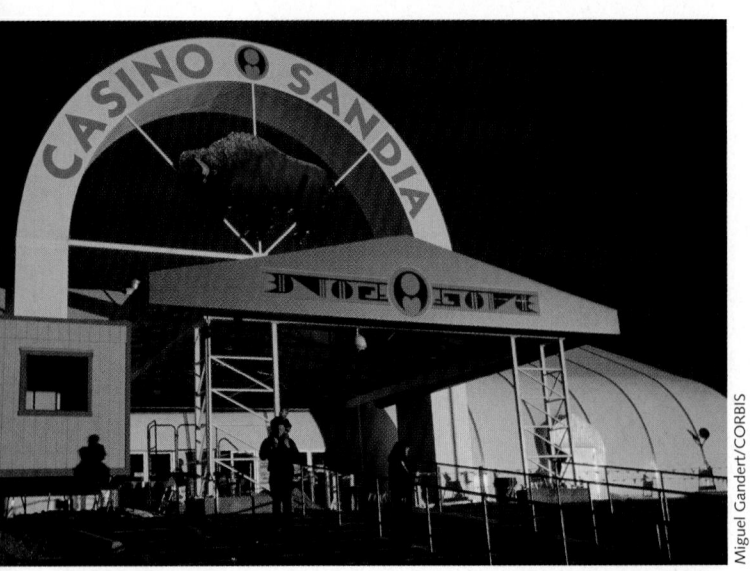

While defense industries shrank, the technology sector of the economy expanded, opening up new opportunities for young computer experts and entrepreneurs and generating fortunes for corporate executives. At the same time, mergers of giant multinational companies concentrated wealth and power in an ever-smaller number of ever-larger corporations. In the last three years of the decade, mergers totaled $5 trillion. Media giants America Online and Time–Warner merged in 2000. In 2001 Nestlé bought Ralston–Purina for $10 billion. Many of the largest mergers crossed national boundaries, such as German automobile maker Daimler–Benz and U.S. Chrysler. American companies were the largest target of global buyouts. In 1999 alone, foreigners paid $233 billion to buy American companies.

While corporations expanded, so did efforts to control their power. Microsoft initially lost an antitrust suit that ordered the computer software giant to be split into two companies. Microsoft appealed the ruling in 2001, and ultimately the Justice Department settled the suit with minor sanctions against the company. The controversial settlement generated opposition. Nine states that participated in the original suit refused to endorse the agreement, and calls for tougher penalties continued. In several states, civil suits against huge tobacco companies limited cigarette advertising and marketing and levied fines on tobacco companies totaling in the billions. Although the publicity surrounding these cases exposed the tobacco companies' efforts to deceive the public about the health risks of cigarettes, the lawsuits did not lead to a decline in cigarette smoking, and tobacco companies continued to advertise and market their product at home as well as abroad.

The nation's elite were not the only ones to capitalize on new entrepreneurial opportunities. The 1988 Indian Gaming Regulatory Act enabled Native Americans to build lucrative Las Vegas–style casinos on tribal lands, bringing new jobs and an estimated $4 billion a year to formerly impoverished communities. The Mashantucket Pequots east of Hartford, Connecticut, opened Foxwoods in 1992, and it quickly became the largest casino in the Western Hemisphere. The Oneidas followed suit a few years later with the Turning Stone casino near Utica, New York. In Arizona casinos brought in $830 million a year. Some Indian casinos failed, however, and gambling always took a largely hidden toll in the losses of already poor local residents. Native Americans remained divided about the wisdom of trying to profit from America's growing inclination to take risks in hopes of winning big. Jose Lucero of New Mexico's Santa Clara tribe near Santa Fe feared that rebuilding Indian life around gambling was "like a leisure virus—we're trading our souls for money (when) we are supposed to be stewards of this land."

However, the advantages for the tribes were substantial. The Oneida tribe of Wisconsin, for example, used the profits from its 2000-slot-machine complex outside Green Bay for an electronic component factory, an industrial park, a printing firm, a bank, a hotel, and four convenience stores. Tribal

■ **Casino Sandia on the Sandia Pueblo in New Mexico. Many Native American communities across the country built gambling facilities on tribal lands. Although casinos brought needed income, they remained controversial.**

Miguel Gandert/CORBIS

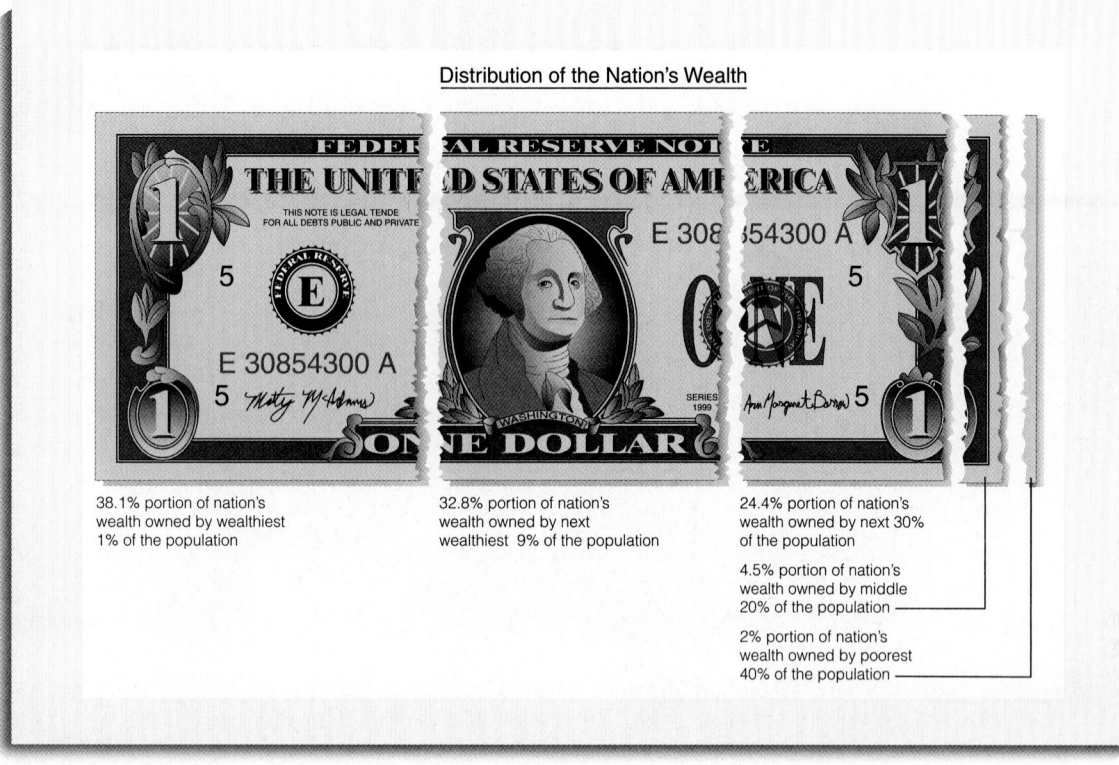

Distribution of the Nation's Wealth

38.1% portion of nation's wealth owned by wealthiest 1% of the population

32.8% portion of nation's wealth owned by next wealthiest 9% of the population

24.4% portion of nation's wealth owned by next 30% of the population

4.5% portion of nation's wealth owned by middle 20% of the population

2% portion of nation's wealth owned by poorest 40% of the population

■ **FIGURE 29.1**
CONCENTRATION OF WEALTH, 1990s During the final decades of the twentieth century, the gap between the wealthy and the poor increased as the nation's wealth became concentrated in the hands of a small number of very wealthy people. By the end of the century, the richest 1 percent of Americans owned 38 percent of all the nation's wealth while the poorest 40 percent shared a mere 0.2 percent of the nation's wealth. The figure also demonstrates that more than 70 percent of the nation's total wealth was in the hands of the most affluent 10 percent of the population, while the majority of Americans—60 percent—was left sharing a mere 5 percent of the nation's wealth.

government outlays increased from $40 million to $250 million over the decade, providing subsidized housing, health care, student counseling, a new daycare center, and a new elementary school built in the shape of a turtle, a sacred creature in Oneida mythology. The money also helped to revive the Oneida language, with a new written form and a CD of ancestral tales told by tribal elders. The tribe also spent $11 million in 1995 recovering property it once owned, bringing it into the tax-free zone of the reservation. In addition to this communal spending, the tribe paid out $225 a year to all its members. By comparison, the tiny band of Minnesota Shakopees, just south of Minneapolis and St. Paul, used much of the profits from its bustling casino to provide annual bonuses of $400,000 to each of its members.

The Widening Gap Between Rich and Poor

Commenting on the state of the economy in the mid–1990s, two economists noted, "The tide of economic growth no longer lifts all boats. We see the recent period as one in which the large yachts, moored in the safe harbors, rose with the tide, while the small boats ran aground. The notion that we can 'grow our way out' of the economic problems facing so many families is now obsolete." In the last decade of the century, the bottom 60 percent of the population saw their income decline, even as the economy boomed. Accumulated wealth—property and investments—was an even better measure of security and influence, and the top 1 percent of Americans owned more wealth than the bottom 90 percent combined. Microsoft chair Bill Gates alone

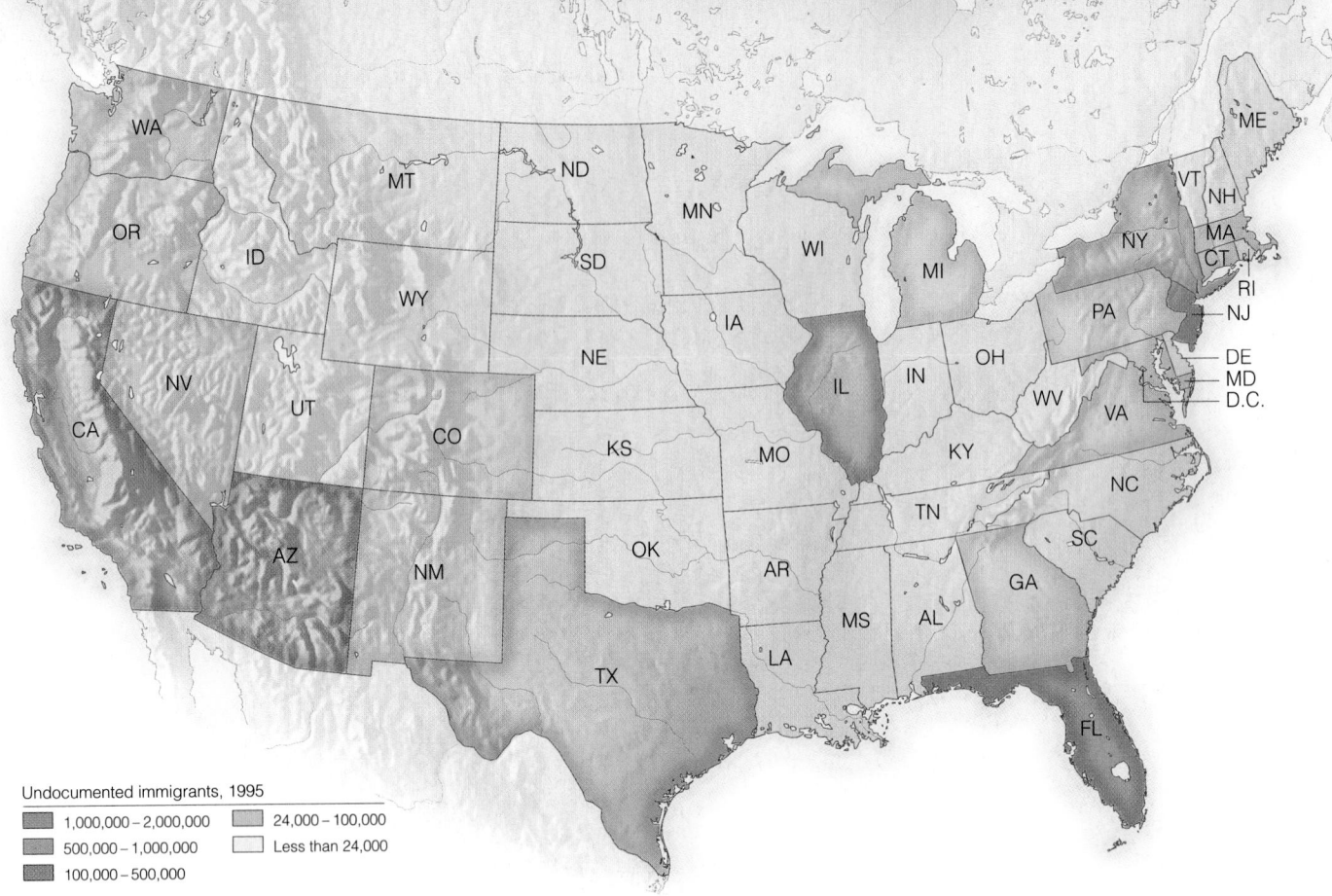

■ MAP 29.1

STATES WITH LARGE NUMBERS OF UNDOCUMENTED IMMIGRANTS, 1995 Fully 77 percent of all undocumented immigrants entered the country legally, with visas in hand. During the 1990s, the total proportion of the foreign born in the United States, including those with and without legal status, was about half what it had been in 1900 (8 percent compared to 15 percent). Immigrants payed $133 billion dollars annually in local, state, and federal taxes, and generated an annual contribution to the American economy in the range of $25 to $30 billion.

was wealthier than the bottom 45 percent of all U.S. households together. Famed capitalist J. P. Morgan maintained a century earlier that no corporate chieftain should earn more than 20 times what his workers were paid, but by 1980 a typical chief executive of a large U.S. company took home 40 times the earnings of an average factory worker; by 1990 the ratio had grown to 85 times, and by 1998 it reached 419 times.

Although one-third of the nation's African Americans were part of the middle class, black families had fewer assets and resources, making their hold on middle-class status more precarious than that of their white peers. The poorest African Americans were concentrated in low-paying jobs, lacking the quality health care and education that would make social and economic mobility possible. Full-time employment did not necessarily mean an escape from poverty. Among fully employed black heads of households without a high school education, 40 percent of the women and 25 percent of the men did not earn enough to achieve economic self-sufficiency. Almost 50 percent of all black children lived in households below the poverty line, compared to 16 percent of white children. The rate of unemployment was more than twice as high for blacks as for whites.

Recent immigrants from Asia, Africa, and Latin America joined African Americans in jobs at the bottom of the economy. Despite the controversy over illegal immigration, a quarter of a million undocumented workers toiled in the fields of agribusiness. At the same time, 2 percent of able-bodied citizens were in jail, nearly half of them black, because of the arrest and incarceration policies of the "war on drugs" that hit minority communities particularly hard. Prisoners were often required to work while incarcerated. Convicts provided data entry, packed

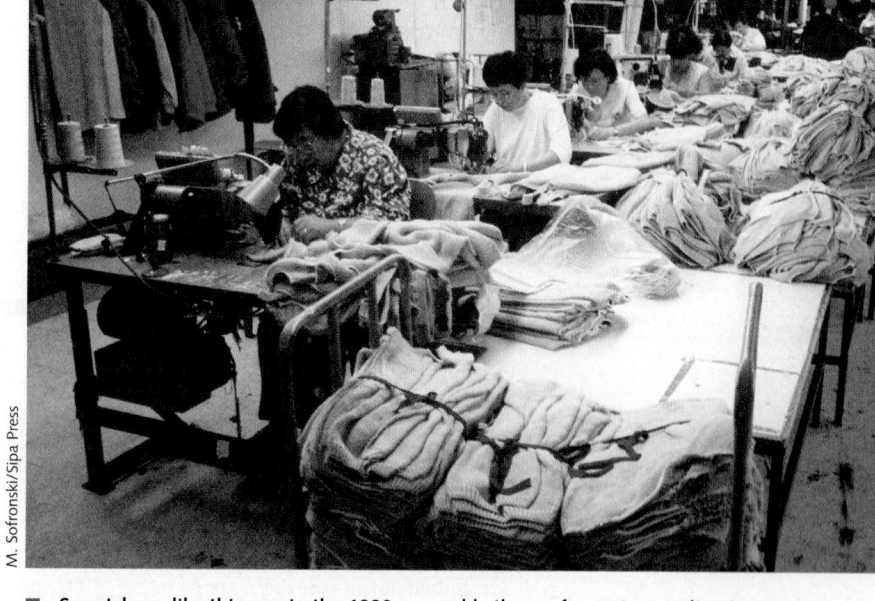

golf balls, and filled a wide array of jobs for less than minimum wage, and most of their earnings went back to the government. These and other workers at the bottom of the labor force gained little or nothing from the economic boom of the 1990s.

Labor Unions

Low-wage workers in the service industries had one advantage over laborers working for multinational corporations: their jobs could not be exported. Many service workers organized successfully for better wages and working conditions. In April 2000, for example, striking janitors of Service Employees International Union (SEIU) Local 1877 in Los Angeles marched 8 miles past cheering

■ Sweatshops like this one in the 1990s resemble those of a century earlier. Immigrant women labor in garment factories, working long hours in miserable conditions for meager wages.

crowds to the upscale business center of Century City. A few weeks later, the janitors had achieved a wage increase of 26 percent, raising their hourly pay from less than $8 to more than $10. This was a tremendous triumph for a union whose membership was 98 percent immigrant: 80 percent Central Americans, more than half women, and all of them poor.

Other service workers also won improved contracts. Unionized hotel workers in San Francisco negotiated a five-year contract that increased pay for the lowest-paid workers, room cleaners and dishwashers, by 25 percent, from $12 to $15 an hour. In Las Vegas, African American hotel worker Hattie Canty, who helped organized 40,000 employees of large casino hotels, said of her efforts, "It has not been a picnic for me, but I don't think I'd like to go on a picnic every day. I have enjoyed the struggle. I'm not the only Hattie. There's lots of Hatties out there." Yatta Staples went out on the picket line in front of the Minneapolis hotel where she worked as a waitress, telling reporters, "I'll stay here as long as it takes." In the summer of 1997, 185,000 Teamsters went on strike against the United Parcel Service and won an improved contract with higher wages and benefits for part-time as well as full-time workers.

Strikes did little to benefit nonunionized workers, especially undocumented immigrants, and sweatshop laborers both inside and outside the United States. There were some attempts to improve working conditions for those most exploited by the global economy. In April 1997 representatives from clothing manufacturers, human rights groups, and labor organizations drafted an agreement that tried to improve conditions for garment workers around the world. Companies that agreed to the voluntary pact would limit work weeks to 60 hours, with a maximum of 12 hours of overtime. The companies had to pay "at least the minimum wage required by local law or the prevailing industry wage, whichever is higher." The pact forbade children under 15 to work and contained policies protecting workers from harassment and unsafe working environments. Even full compliance with such minimal standards would leave workers in the global garment industry subject to much longer hours, lower wages, and worse working conditions than legally permitted in the United States. Critics also raised questions about how enforceable such voluntary standards would be. Nevertheless, the pact was a small step in the right direction that at least called attention to widespread exploitation in the global economy.

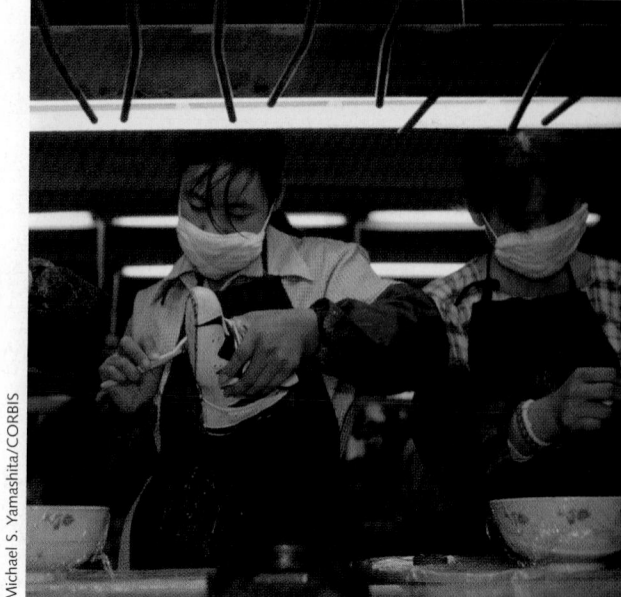

■ U.S.-owned multinational corporations exported jobs to take advantage of cheap labor in developing countries. Here, workers in a Reebok factory in China wear masks as they apply glue to sport shoes.

Tolerance and Its Limits

Racial discrimination had eased over the course of the twentieth century, but persistent inequalities of power and economic opportunity continued to disadvantage Americans of color, who remained disproportionately poor, in prison, and on welfare. The economic downturn of the early 1990s widened the chasm between affluent white and poor non-white Americans. Highly publicized incidents of police brutality directed against Americans of color generated protests and, occasionally, violence. Nevertheless, there were signs that Americans were becoming more tolerant of one another and more willing to accept and even appreciate their diversity.

"We Can All Get Along"

Shortly after midnight on March 3, 1991, police pulled over Rodney King, an African American motorist, after a high-speed chase on a Los Angeles freeway. The four officers dragged the unarmed black man from his car and kicked and beat him with their batons for 15 minutes. The beating left King with a fractured cheekbone, broken bones at the base of his skull, and a broken leg. A bystander recorded the beating on videotape, which was broadcast repeatedly on national television, sparking outrage among Americans of all races. A year later, in April 1992, the four police officers went on trial for use of excessive force.

At the highly publicized trial, defense lawyers for the police officers argued that King, who was clearly cowering on the videotape, was resisting arrest and that the police responded appropriately. The jury of ten whites, one Asian, and one Latino acquitted the officers. The acquittal ignited five days of rioting in the African American community of South Central Los Angeles, leaving 58 people dead and $1 billion in property destroyed. Community leaders called for calm; even Rodney King spoke publicly: "I mean, please, we can get along here," he implored, "We can all get along. We've just got to." Months later, a federal court in Los Angeles convicted two of the officers involved in the beating of violating King's civil rights–too late to avert the violence that erupted after the initial verdict.

Of the 58 people who died in the violence, 18 were Latino, 26 were black, 10 were white, and 2 were Asian. Of the 4000 businesses that were destroyed, most belonged to Latinos and Koreans. Perpetrators of the violence, as well as the victims, came from all racial groups. Antonia Hernandez, president of the Mexican American Legal Defense and Educational Fund, noted, "The hardest part is rebuilding the spirit of the city—what holds us together as Angelinos. It's the rebuilding of trust. . . . It's connecting communities that have never been connected." Several community groups came together in an effort to ease tensions. The Japanese American Citizens League, Chinese for Affirmative Action, and the Asian Pacific Legal Center released statements denouncing the verdict and calling for a federal investigation. "I think that much of the cause of the race relations problem comes down to economics—who has jobs, who has businesses, where is the money going," said Los Angeles City Council member Michael Woo. Jimmy Franco, director of the League of United Latin American Citizens, concurred: "These areas are the poorest areas of the city. If it weren't Rodney King, it would have been something else. It just took something like this to set off the anger."

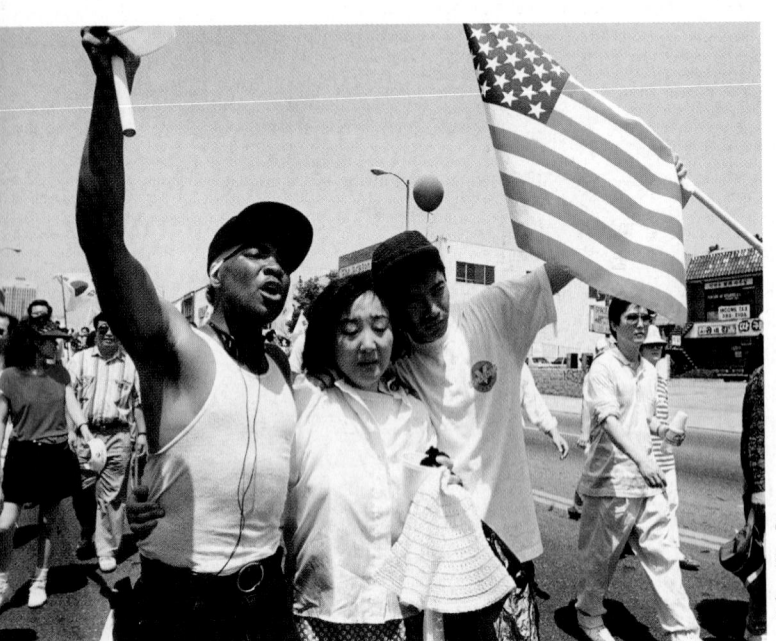

Lee Celano/Sipa Press

■ In the aftermath of the violent uprising that followed the acquittal of police officers in the beating of motorist Rodney King, Koreans and African Americans in Los Angeles express their solidarity, hoping to heal the wounds and divisions that had torn apart their city.

Values in Conflict

In 1991 former University of Colorado football coach Bill McCartney formed the Promise Keepers, a fundamentalist Christian group dedicated to restoring the traditional privileges and responsibilities of husbands and fathers in the home. The Promise Keepers held evangelical revivals that drew tens of thousands of mostly working-class white and some black men to rallies across the country. They believed that men should be good providers for their families, strong role models for their children, and committed spouses. The Promise Keepers were not alone in their concern for what they perceived to be the declining status of fathers. New groups and initiatives appeared that appealed to men across the political spectrum: the National Fatherhood Initiative, Father to Father (launched by Vice President Al Gore in 1995), the Fatherhood Project, the Institute for Responsible Fatherhood and Family Revitalization, and Fathers' Education Network.

Although white men continued to control nearly all the major economic and political institutions in the nation, a 1993 poll found that a majority of white men believed that their advantage in terms of jobs and income, along with their influence over American culture, was declining. African American men also felt the need to bolster manhood and fatherhood. Efforts geared specifically toward African American men included M.A.D. D.A.D.S. (Men Against Destruction—Defending Against Drugs and Social Disorder) and the 1995 Million Man March, organized by Nation of Islam Reverend Louis Farrakhan, which drew hundreds of thousands of black men to demonstrate their solidarity at a rally in Washington, D.C.

At the same time, gay men and lesbians mobilized to gain acceptance and legitimacy for the families that they formed. Many gay and lesbian activists pushed for legalization of same-sex marriage. Although a 1994 poll showed that 52 percent of respondents "claimed to consider gay lifestyle acceptable," 64 percent were opposed to legalizing gay marriage or allowing gay couples to adopt children. Vermont became the first state to grant legal status to civil unions between same-sex couples, although a fierce backlash threatened to overturn the legislation.

Values also collided around the rights and traditions of Native Americans as tribal communities came into conflict with non-Native environmentalists, sports enthusiasts, and

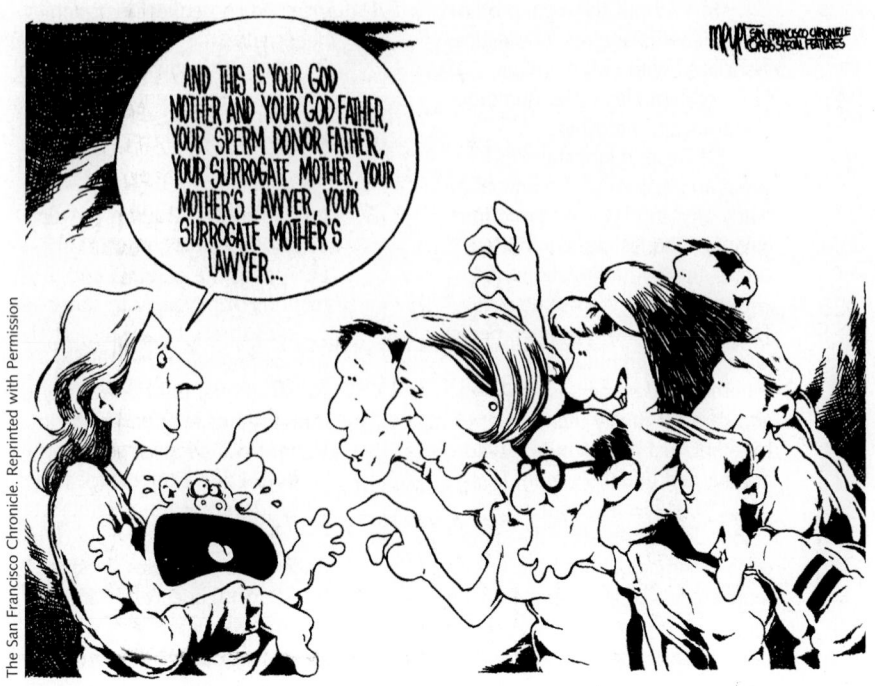

The San Francisco Chronicle. Reprinted with Permission

■ New reproductive technologies confounded definitions of mothers, fathers, and family members. It was now possible to create embryos in laboratories, and to have children with as many as five "real" parents: genetic mother, genetic father, gestational mother, social mother, and social father. This 1986 cartoon is by Tom Meyer of the *San Francisco Chronicle*.

Vermont Civil Union Law

On April 26, 2000, Vermont became the first state to grant legal recognition to same-sex couples, affording them all the legal protections, privileges, and responsibilities of married couples. The law unleashed a storm of controversy and raised questions about the legal status in other states of civil unions contracted in Vermont. Nevertheless, in the first year after its enactment, 2479 same-sex couples forged civil unions in Vermont, 478 of them among Vermonters, and the rest from other states. Two-thirds were lesbian unions. Several states began to consider similar bills, but others moved to prohibit such unions. Nebraska amended its state constitution to outlaw same-sex marriage and civil unions. On the national level, conservative lawmakers endeavored to introduce a constitutional amendment that would ban civil unions and restrict marriage to heterosexual couples. Among other provisions, the Vermont Civil Union Law stipulated that

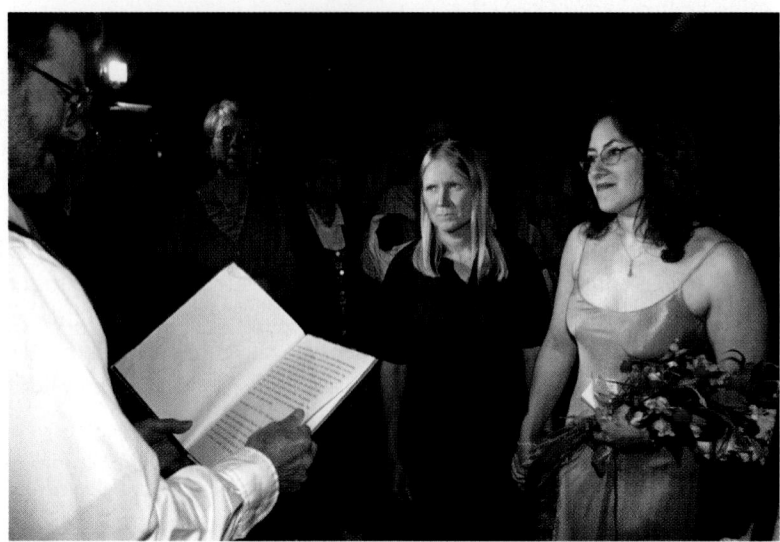

Kathleen Peterson and Carolyn Conrad exchange vows in front of Justice of the Peace T. Hunter Wilson. The ceremony in Brattleboro, Vermont, on July 1, 2000, marked the first legal union under Vermont's Civil Union law. Vermont was the first state to provide recognition and legal status to gay and lesbian couples.

(1) Civil marriage under Vermont's marriage statutes consists of a union between a man and a woman. . . .

(2) Vermont's history as an independent republic and as a state is one of equal treatment and respect for all Vermonters. . . .

(3) The state's interest in civil marriage is to encourage close and caring families, and to protect all family members from the economic and social consequences of abandonment and divorce, focusing on those who have been especially at risk.

(4) Legal recognition of civil marriage by the state is the primary and, in a number of instances, the exclusive source of numerous benefits, responsibilities and protections under the laws of the state for married persons and their children.

(5) Based on the state's tradition of equality under the law and strong families, for at least 25 years, Vermont Probate Courts have qualified gay and lesbian individuals as adoptive parents.

(6) Vermont was one of the first states to adopt comprehensive legislation prohibiting discrimination on the basis of sexual orientation. . . .

(7) The state has a strong interest in promoting stable and lasting families, including families based upon a same-sex couple.

(8) Without the legal protections, benefits and responsibilities associated with civil marriage, same-sex couples suffer numerous obstacles and hardships.

(9) Despite longstanding social and economic discrimination, many gay and lesbian Vermonters have formed lasting, committed, caring and faithful relationships with persons of their same sex. These couples live together, participate in their communities together, and some raise children and care for family members together, just as do couples who are married under Vermont law.

(10) While a system of civil unions does not bestow the status of civil marriage, it does satisfy the requirements of the Common Benefits Clause. Changes in the way significant legal relationships are established under the constitution should be approached carefully, combining respect for the community and cultural institutions most affected with a commitment to the constitutional rights involved. Granting benefits and protections to same-sex couples through a system of civil unions will provide due respect for tradition and long-standing social institutions, and will permit adjustment as unanticipated consequences or unmet needs arise.

(11) The constitutional principle of equality embodied in the Common Benefits Clause is compatible with the freedom of religious belief and worship guaranteed in Chapter I, Article 3rd of the state constitution. Extending the benefits and protections of marriage to same-sex couples through a system of civil unions preserves the fundamental constitutional right of each of the multitude of religious faiths in Vermont to choose freely and without state interference to whom to grant the religious status, sacrament or blessing of marriage under the rules, practices or traditions of such faith. ■

scientists. In the upper Midwest, treaties with the government in 1837 and 1842 granted the Chippewa hunting, fishing, and gathering rights in the territories ceded to the United States. Federal courts have consistently upheld these treaties, which include rights to take up to half of the fish and game allowed by state conservation requirements and to use methods such as spear fishing that are illegal for non-Indians. In the 1980s and 1990s, non-Indians challenged these policies and accosted Native Americans in fishing boats with rocks and insults.

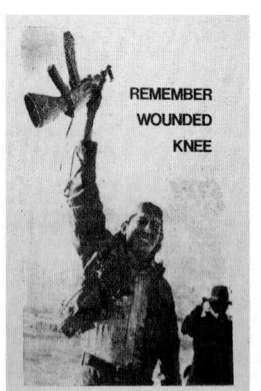

Native American cultural practices also clashed with environmentalist sensibilities over religious practices involving the gathering and sacrificing of golden eaglets. The Department of the Interior, weighing laws protecting Indian religious freedoms against those protecting national parks and wildlife, allowed the Hopis to gather up to 40 young eagles a year. The Hopi usually took about 15 birds for a ceremony that culminated in their sacrifice. The Interior Department's policy is consistent with long-standing treaties as well as recent law, including the American Indian Religious Freedom Act of 1978. But many environmentalists agreed with the news columnist who wrote, "When native peoples, no matter how badly abused by us in the past, seek to perpetrate equally senseless barbarities on helpless creatures, we should stand on principle and use our awesome power to stop, not to enable them." Animal rights activists raised similar arguments against mainstream institutions, including scientific laboratories that used animals for research, and the meat industry, which engaged in inhumane practices.

Courtroom Dramas

Two of the most controversial legal spectacles of the decade centered on accusations against successful black men and exposed deep chasms along class and gender as well as racial lines. The first of these episodes was the Senate hearing of October 1991 to confirm the appointment of Judge Clarence Thomas to the U.S. Supreme Court. President George H. W. Bush nominated the conservative Clarence Thomas to replace retiring liberal Justice Thurgood Marshall. Both jurists were black but otherwise had little in common; they occupied opposite ends of the political and judicial spectrum. Although Bush claimed that Thomas was the "best man for the job," the American Bar Association gave him the lowest rating of any justice confirmed in the previous three decades. Many people became skeptical during the confirmation hearings when Thomas claimed that he had not formed any opinion on the highly charged issue of abortion. Support for Thomas among the Senators on the Senate Judiciary Committee fell largely along party lines. But when University of Oklahoma law professor Anita Hill accused Thomas of sexual harassment when she worked for him at the Equal Opportunity Employment Commission in the early 1980s, the question of Thomas's professional qualifications faded to the background and the hearings focused exclusively on Hill's accusations.

In live televised hearings, the African American law professor testified that Thomas had made crude and lurid remarks to her as well as unwanted sexual overtures. Several of the all-white-male panel of senators questioned Hill's credibility, wondering why she continued to work for Thomas after the alleged harassment. Thomas drew on the long history of black men being falsely accused of sexual aggression to counter the charge of sexual harassment, accusing his Democratic opponents of conducting a "high-tech lynching." In the end Thomas was confirmed. But Hill's testimony, and what appeared to her supporters as the insensitive behavior of the senators, brought the issue of sexual harassment to a high level of national consciousness. The hearings also highlighted the fact that Congress was overwhelmingly white and male, motivating female candidates and their supporters to alter that reality the following year. As a result of the 1992 elections, the number of female senators tripled from two to six, including the first black female senator, Carol Moseley Braun, Democrat from Illinois. The number of congresswomen rose from 28 to 47.

In 1994 television viewers were again riveted by a media spectacle, this time a sensational murder case. On the night of June 12, Nicole Brown Simpson and her friend Ronald Goldman were stabbed to death outside Simpson's West Los Angeles apartment. The murdered white woman was the ex-wife of black celebrity O. J. Simpson, former football star and film actor. O. J. Simpson's blood was found at the scene, hair and other forensic and DNA evidence linked him to the crime, he had no reliable alibi, and a motive was evident in his pattern of jealous rage and brutality against the murdered woman. No other suspects in the case were ever identified. But Simpson's team of lawyers unearthed evidence that before the Simpson case, white police detective Mark Fuhrman had boasted of planting evidence and had made racist comments. The mostly black and female jury was sympathetic to the possibility that Fuhrman had framed Simpson. In Los Angeles, in the wake of the Rodney King beatings, African Americans had good reason to distrust the police.

Finally, in early October 1996, after a trial that lasted nearly a year, it took the jury only two hours to acquit Simpson of all charges. Pundits focused on the racial divide: blacks were more inclined to believe Simpson was innocent, and whites more likely to consider him guilty. The families of Ronald Goldman and Nicole Brown Simpson filed a wrongful death civil suit, in which the standards for conviction require merely a preponderance of evidence rather than guilt beyond a reasonable doubt. Simpson was convicted in the civil suit, which found him responsible for the deaths, and ordered to pay damages.

The Changing Face of Diversity

These highly charged events illuminated racial tensions, but there was also evidence that Americans were starting to accept the nation's diversity and adopt a more inclusive vision. The number of immigrants living in the United States tripled in three decades, to nearly 27 million, representing 10 percent of the population—the highest proportion of foreign-born residents since the 1930s. The numbers of Asians and Pacific Islanders increased by 45.9 percent, with those of Chinese ancestry comprising the largest group, followed by those with origins in the Philippines. The Latino population grew by 39.7 percent. Among the nation's Latinos, nearly two-thirds were of Mexican ancestry.

Not everyone celebrated these developments. In California, with one-third of the nation's Latino population, voters responded with Proposition 187 to deny public education and most other public social services to undocumented immigrants, and Proposition 227 to end bilingual education. Large numbers of Latino voters opposed these measures. In subsequent elections many young Latinos and new citizens marshaled their political power and voted for the first time. Evidence of the growing political power of Latinos was the mounting support in California for a bill that would require the U.S. government to return back pay that was taken from the wages of Mexican agricultural workers who came to the United States during World War II under the *Bracero* program. In Los Angeles during the 1990s, Latinos became the largest single ethnic group. By 2000 whites no longer constituted a majority of California's multiethnic population, dropping from 57 percent in 1990 to 47 percent in 2000.

At the same time, politics and ideas based on distinct and rigid racial lines gave way to a growing recognition of intermixing. Artists actively explored this hybridity. Dramatist Anna Deveare

Jack Smith/AP/Wide World

■ **Golf superstar Tiger Woods celebrates his triumph at the U.S. Amateur Championships in North Plains, Oregon, August 25, 1996. Woods, the son of an African American father and a Thai mother, was one of several mixed-race celebrities in the 1990s.**

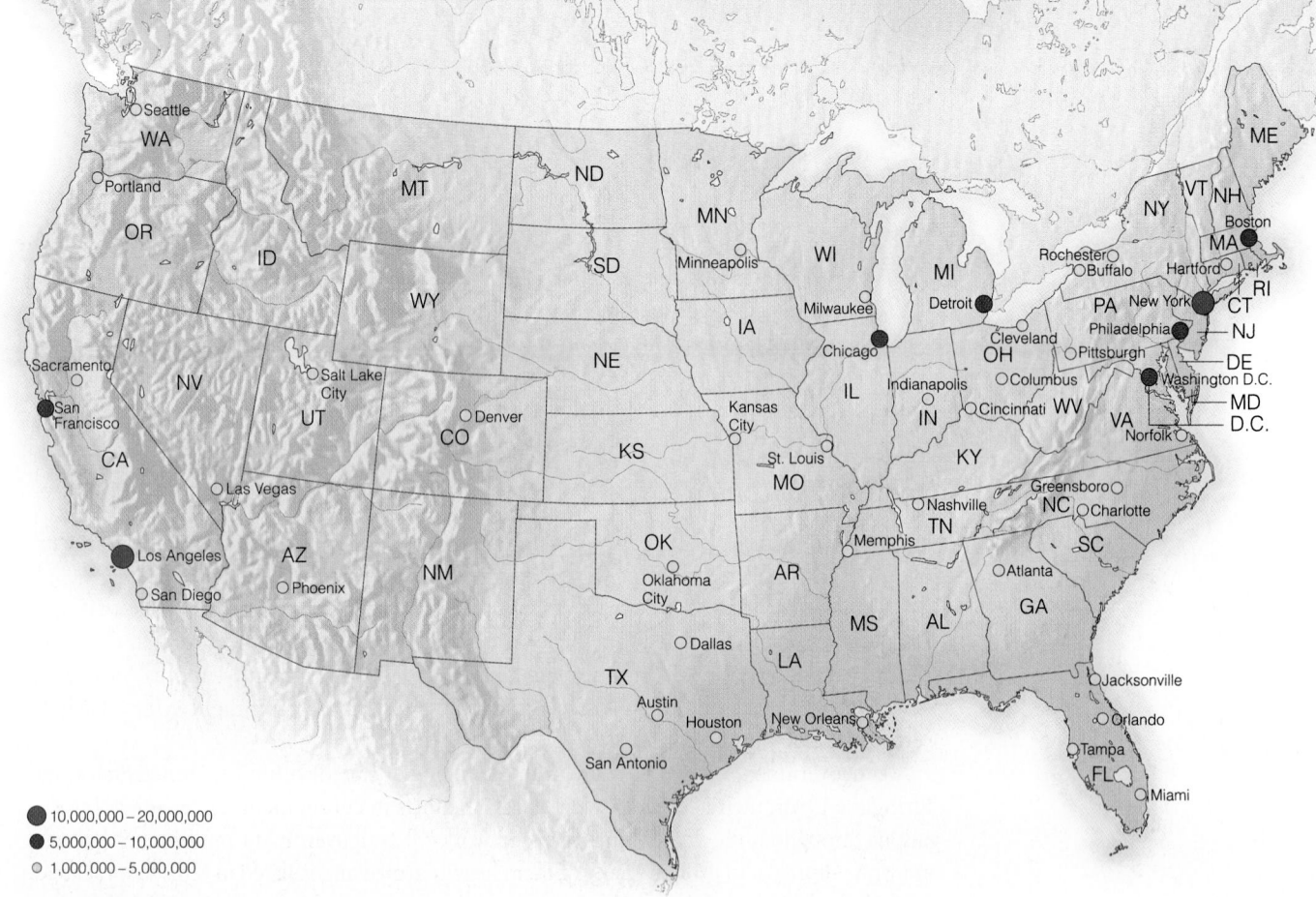

■ MAP 29.2

POPULATION OF MAJOR METROPOLITAN AREAS, 1990 By 1990 the nation's population was concentrated in large metropolitan areas, most of them along the East and West coasts, the Sun Belt, and the Upper Midwest. One hundred and twenty million Americans, about half of the population, lived in suburbs.

Legend:
- 10,000,000 – 20,000,000
- 5,000,000 – 10,000,000
- 1,000,000 – 5,000,000

Smith, for example, wrote and performed a theatrical production in which she interviewed and studied many people involved in the uprising in South Central Los Angeles, from the white chief of police to a Korean woman whose family business was destroyed in the riots. In her widely acclaimed one-woman play *Twilight, Los Angeles,* the mixed-race Smith took on the many identities of the white, black, Asian, Latino, male, female, young, and old people she represented. By transforming herself on stage into each of those people, she suggested that we, as a society, were all of those people as well. In his 1996 film *Lone Star,* John Sayles examined a Texas border town where white, black, Latino, and Indian peoples were all interwoven and connected in their lives, communities, and families. From cross-racial love to debates over the local school's history curriculum, the film explored in microcosm the challenges and rewards of an inclusive American identity.

Racial intermixing was evident in other areas as well. In the world of sports, young golfer Tiger Woods, son of a black Vietnam veteran father and a Thai mother, became the reigning superstar of the sport most closely identified with the world of the white elite. Pop star Prince was one of many artists who crafted a persona that highlighted both racial and gender ambiguity. On job and college application forms, a growing number of mixed-race Americans refused to be identified as belonging to one particular racial group. Reflecting this development, the U.S. Census of 2000 allowed people to check more than one box to indicate their racial identity. In California, where nearly 5 percent of the population checked more than one box, nearly all of those who checked white and another box were Latinos.

Violence and Danger

Violence was nothing new in American society, but new types of mayhem in the 1990s—including domestic terrorism and school shootings–sparked national soul-searching and wide-ranging debate over the causes of violence and what to do about them. Meanwhile, ordinary Americans inflicted various harms on themselves, often in class-distinct ways. Eating disorders and obesity reached epidemic proportions, and Americans continued to turn to drugs, most of them legal, to make them feel better.

Domestic Terrorism

On the morning of April 19, 1995, a 2-ton homemade bomb exploded at the Alfred P. Murrah Federal Building in Oklahoma City. The huge building crumbled, killing 168 people, including 19 children. The attack was the worst act of terrorism in the nation's history to that date. Initial news reports speculated that the terrorists were Arabs, but it turned out that the attack was carried out by American citizens with a hatred for the government. Timothy McVeigh, a Persian Gulf War veteran turned antigovernment terrorist, and his accomplice, Terry Nichols, were found guilty of the bombing.

Antigovernment individuals and groups had long operated within the United States, and during the 1990s, their activities—as well as FBI efforts to curtail them—intensified. Investigations throughout the decade uncovered networks of antigovernment militias, tax resisters, and white supremacist groups, many of them heavily armed and isolated in remote rural areas. Some antigovernment extremists acted alone, like former mathematics professor Theodore Kaczynski, known as the "Unabomber," who for two decades sent bombs through the mail, killing 3 people and injuring 29. His demand to have his antigovernment manifesto published in major national newspapers led to his identification and arrest.

The FBI tried to prevent these extremists from causing harm, but some of their efforts went awry. In 1992 an FBI agent shot and killed the wife and son of Randall Weaver, a former Green Beret and antigovernment militia supporter who had failed to appear for trial on weapons charges, in a shootout at their Idaho home. The following year in Waco, Texas, the FBI stormed the heavily armed compound of an antigovernment religious sect known as the Branch Davidians. The leader of the group, David Koresh, had barricaded the compound. The FBI, acting on reports of abuse of members, particularly women and children, tried to force Koresh and his group out of the building. But a fire broke out, killing 80 men, women, and children inside. The FBI came under intense criticism for its aggressive tactics in these cases. For antigovernment extremists, these actions prompted revenge. The Oklahoma City bombing, apparently, was intended in part as retaliation for the FBI assault against the Branch Davidians precisely two years earlier.

Timothy McVeigh was sentenced to death for the Oklahoma City bombing. But shortly before the scheduled execution in May 2001, more than 4000 pages of FBI documents relating to the case that had not been seen by McVeigh's attorneys suddenly surfaced. The discovery raised new questions about the competence of the FBI and delayed McVeigh's execution for a month. The execution by lethal injection took place on June 11. The case revived a debate about the death penalty, particularly in light of recent evidence of many botched legal defenses in capital cases. Opponents pointed to the preponderance of convicts of color on death row, representation by incompetent attorneys, and the execution of mentally retarded offenders to argue that the death penalty should be abolished. The governor of Illinois declared a moratorium on executions when a study revealed that many death row inmates were cleared of charges as a result of new DNA evidence. Public opinion began to shift, but the majority—including the U.S. presidents from both parties throughout the decade—continued to support the death penalty.

The Oklahoma City bombing was the worst but not the only example of domestic terrorist attacks. After the Supreme Court's 1973 decision in *Roe* v. *Wade* legalized abortion, antiabortion activists worked to have the decision reversed. Most antiabortion protesters were peaceful and law-abiding. But a small militant fringe of antiabortion crusaders switched their targets of protest from elected officials to abortion providers and turned to violence. In 1993 half of all abortion clinics reported hostile actions, including death threats, fires, bombs, invasions, blockades, and shootings. In 1993 and 1994 vigilantes shot and killed one abortion provider, tried to kill another, and shot employees at two clinics in Brookline, Massachusetts.

The violence spurred Congress to pass the Freedom of Access to Clinic Entrances Act in 1994, making it a federal crime to block access to clinics. But ultimately, the intimidation and violence were effective. Although abortion remained legal, the procedure became increasingly difficult to obtain. Few medical residency programs in obstetrics and gynecology routinely taught the procedure, and considering the dangers posed by antiabortion terrorists, few physicians were willing to perform abortions. By the end of the decade, there were no abortion providers in 86 percent of largely rural counties in the country. Abortions continued to be available in cities, mostly in specialized abortion clinics. Between 1990 and 1997, the number of abortions declined by 17.4 percent. But the political battles continued. After years of controversy and debate, the French abortion pill RU–486 received FDA approval for use in the United States, making it possible for individual doctors to prescribe the pill and for women to avoid surgery.

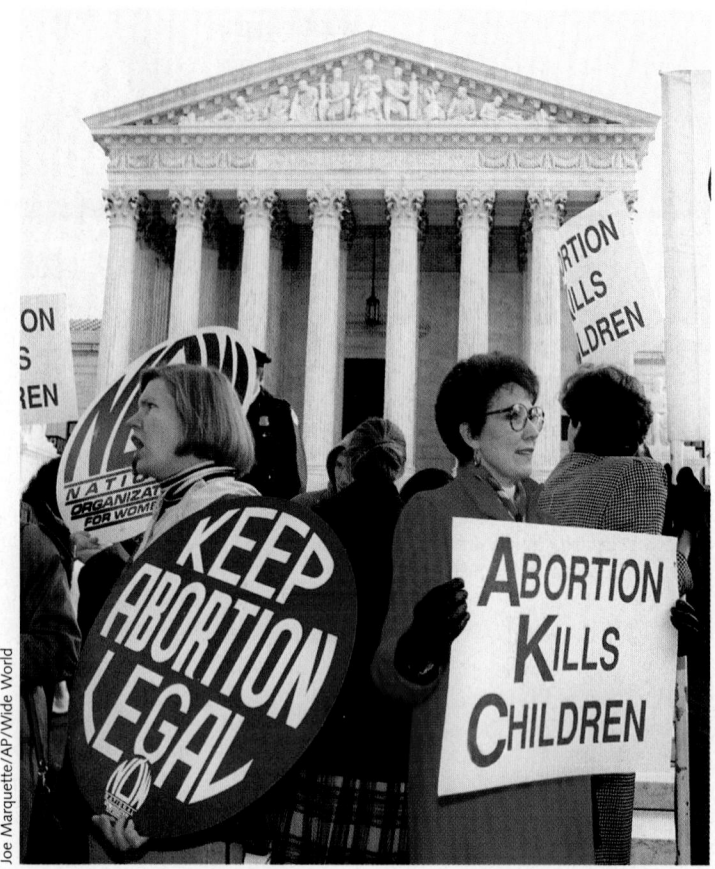

Joe Marquette/AP/Wide World

■ Abortion remained one of the most controversial political issues throughout the 1990s. Here abortion rights advocate Inga Coulter of Harrisburg, Pennsylvania, and antiabortion crusader Elizabeth McGee of Washington, D.C., take opposing sides in a demonstration outside the Supreme Court building on December 8, 1993.

Kids Who Kill

Although violent crime declined throughout the decade, especially crimes committed by youths, a spate of school shootings in which children murdered other children sparked national soul searching and finger pointing as Americans wondered whom and what to blame. The murderers were mostly white middle-class boys who appeared to be "normal kids." The worst of these shootings occurred on April 20, 1999, at Columbine High School in a suburb of Denver, Colorado, where two boys opened fire and killed 12 of their schoolmates and a teacher before killing themselves.

These shootings happened in middle-class suburbs where families believed they were safe from the perceived dangers of the inner cities. But such havens could not keep dangerous elements out if the dangers came from within. Some commentators blamed inattentive parents; others pointed to the violence-saturated popular culture. A few noted that when youth of color were victims or perpetrators of violence, the media devoted little attention to the tragedies, suggesting that such crimes were shocking only if committed by white middle-class youths.

The common factors in all of these killings were that the children used guns and that they got the weapons easily, often from their own homes. Gun control advocates noted that the easy access to firearms in the United States was unique among western industrial nations. In 1992, 367 people were killed by handguns in Great Britain, Sweden, Switzerland, Japan, Australia, and Canada combined. The total population of those countries equaled that of the United States, where in that same year, handguns killed 13,220 people. Public opinion polls showed that most Americans favored gun control, but the powerful gun lobby and the National Rifle Association argued that the Second Amendment to the Constitution guaranteed individuals

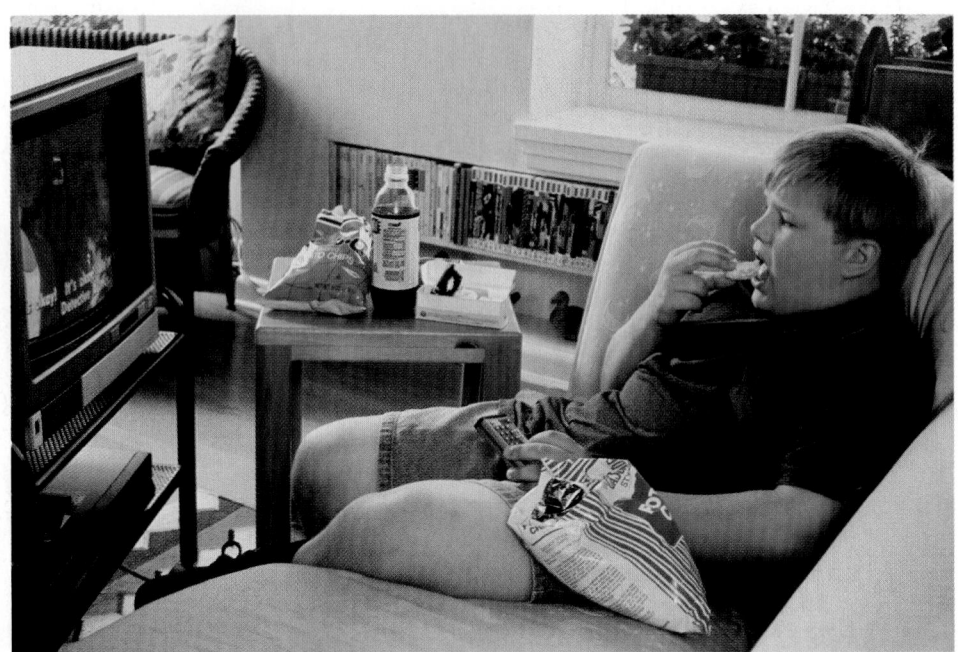

Getty Images

■ Childhood obesity reached epidemic proportions in the 1990s. Too little exercise, too much TV, and the proliferation of fast food outlets, especially in low-income areas, contributed to the problem.

the right to bear arms. Congress enacted the Brady Bill, a gun control measure named for James Brady, the White House press secretary who was gravely wounded in the 1981 assassination attempt on President Ronald W. Reagan. The bill required a waiting period for handgun purchases and banned assault rifles. Nevertheless, access to firearms remained easy. In the 2000 election, only two states, Oregon and Colorado—where two of the worst school shootings occurred—voted to establish some controls on the purchase of guns.

A Healthy Nation?

Despite the nation's near obsession with fitness, both the wealthy and the poor suffered from a number of afflictions. Eating disorders plagued millions of Americans. Among the affluent, anorexia nervosa (self-starvation) and bulimia (frequent binging and purging) affected an estimated 5 million Americans, especially young women, fed in part by a fashion fad that glamorized emaciated bodies. Men also strove for the fashionable body, sometimes with the aid of drugs to enhance athletic performance or muscle build-up. In 2000 the Mayo Clinic reported a 30 percent increase in eating disorders per year, mostly among young women, but in a growing number of men as well. The opposite problem plagued the lower end of the class ladder, where obesity increased dramatically, especially among children. Fast-food chains targeted low-income areas with franchises and promotions offering "supersized" high-fat meals. Childhood obesity jumped from 5 percent in 1964 to 20 percent in 2000.

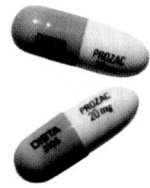

Illegal drugs, including marijuana, cocaine, and heroin, remained popular in spite of official efforts to curb the trade. However, illegal drugs represented only one dimension of Americans' desire to solve their problems through the use of substances. Some mind-altering drugs were legal and available by prescription, such as Prozac and other antidepressants. These psychopharmaceuticals saturated the prescription drug market. Some mental health experts worried that these drugs were being overprescribed, especially for children, as life's normal ups and downs were increasingly diagnosed as maladies such as depression and attention deficit disorder. Aging baby boomers also boosted the profits of pharmaceutical companies. Women turned to hormone replacement therapies to offset the effects of menopause. Skyrocketing sales of Viagra, a drug for treating male impotence, reflected middle-aged men's concerns about waning sexual potency.

Medical developments brought new worries in the wake of new cures. Antibiotics were so widely prescribed that forms of drug-resistant bacteria began to proliferate. Tuberculosis appeared in new deadly forms that did not respond to treatment with available antibiotics. In 1997 researchers in Scotland cloned a sheep, raising hopes that cloning could lead to new medical breakthroughs and fears that human cloning might be next. In 2000 scientists charted the entire human genome, or genetic code, offering the hope of finding causes and cures for genetically linked diseases. Advances in reproductive medicine provoked controversies over the benefits and dangers of such procedures as embryo selection, in vitro fertilization for postmenopausal women, and the long-term implications of egg and sperm donation. In one 1999 case that sparked a debate among medical ethicists, a couple advertised for an egg donor in the student newspapers of prestigious colleges, offering $50,000 to a donor who was athletic and tall, had no major family medical problems, and had scored at least 1400 on the Scholastic Achievement Test. Like the eugenic campaigns of earlier decades, these sorts of cases raised concerns about efforts to create "superior" children.

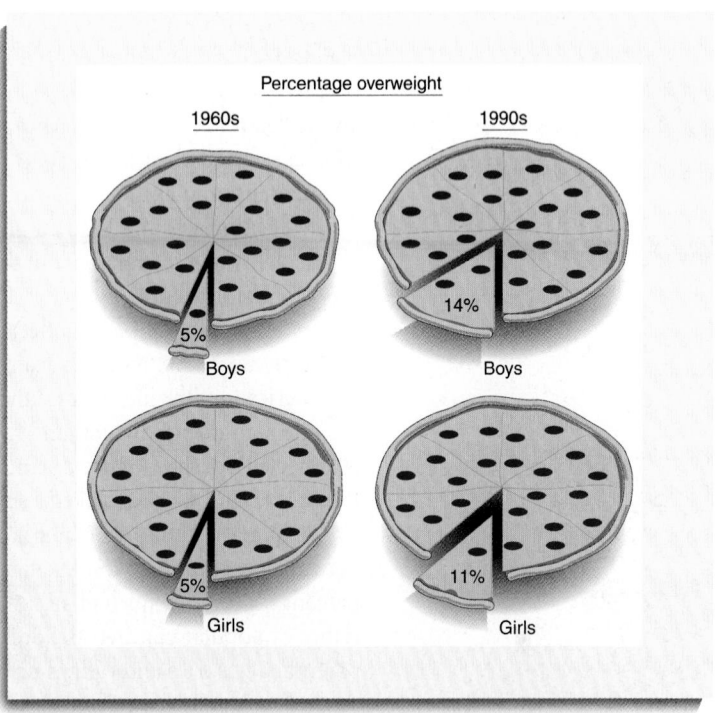

■ **FIGURE 29.2**
CHILDHOOD OBESITY RATES FOR BOYS AND GIRLS AGED 6–17, 1960s AND 1990s During the last half century, obesity rates among children rose dramatically, especially in the 1990s. Childhood obesity is associated with a wide range of medical problems that can affect the health of overweight children throughout their lives. In the 1960s, boys and girls were equally likely to be overweight. But by the 1990s, obesity had become more prevalent among boys.

The Clinton Presidency

William Jefferson Clinton was the first American president born after World War II. Raised in Arkansas in a working-class family, Clinton attended Georgetown University and studied at Oxford University in England as a Rhodes Scholar. Like many college students of his generation, he opposed the Vietnam War and avoided the draft. He attended Yale Law School, where he met Hillary Rodham from Illinois, whom he married in 1975. In 1978, at the young age of 33, he was elected governor of Arkansas. After one term he was defeated in his bid for reelection. He made a comeback by defining himself as a New Democrat with centrist political inclinations and reclaimed his job as governor. When he ran for president in 1992, Clinton received the support of the Democratic Leadership Council, a group of New Democrats who shifted the national party to the right of its previous New Deal liberal position.

Clinton was a brilliant campaigner and a charismatic leader with a disarming personal style that contributed to his victory over the incumbent George H. W. Bush. The sluggish economy also helped Clinton win the election. Throughout his presidency, despite political failures and scandals, Clinton achieved consistently high presidential job performance ratings in national polls. He also benefited from the recovery of the economy during his administration. But accusations of corruption and sexual impropriety plagued him throughout his two terms. Ultimately, during his second term as president, an affair with a young White House intern led to his impeachment by the House of Representatives. Although he was not removed from office, the incident cast a cloud over his presidency.

Clinton: The New Democrat

In 1992 the incumbent president, George H. W. Bush, faced an uphill battle. The recession of 1991–1992 hit white-collar as well as blue-collar workers as unemployment climbed above

8 percent. During the 12 years of Republican rule, the national debt had more than quadrupled to $4.4 trillion. The Republican party platform, reflecting pressures from the right wing of the party, attacked permissiveness in American society, opposed abortion and gay rights, and called for a smaller government. The Democrats nominated 46-year-old Bill Clinton, who selected as his running mate Al Gore, senator from Tennessee, known as a strong environmentalist and author of *Earth in the Balance: Ecology and the Human Spirit*. A wildcard in the election was the Reform party candidacy of H. Ross Perot, a Texas billionaire who financed his own campaign and used the national media to tap into voter discontent with the two major parties.

Much of the campaign reflected the culture wars, pitting what many saw as the socially permissive legacy of the 1960s against conservative efforts to restore traditional "family values" to American public life. Many Americans worried that the prevalence of single-parent families, the high rate of divorce, and the pervasiveness of sex and violence in the popular culture all reflected a decline in moral standards and an erosion of American society. In May 1992 Vice President Dan Quayle delivered a speech criticizing the popular television show *Murphy Brown*, whose unmarried title character had given birth to a child. Quayle's attack on *Murphy Brown* may have backfired; a poll taken after the Republican national convention showed that 57 percent of respondents had an unfavorable view of him. But Republicans were not the only critics of popular culture. Al Gore's wife, Tipper, for example, had long been an advocate of parental advisories and ratings of popular music. Despite their criticisms, all the candidates made full use of the media in their campaigns.

Clinton won the election by a comfortable margin, but Perot garnered 19 percent of the popular vote, the largest showing for a third-party candidate since Theodore Roosevelt ran on the Progressive party ticket in 1912. Clinton began his term with a solid Democratic House and Senate, which included a new infusion of women, along with the nation's first senator of American Indian descent, Ben Nighthorse Campbell of Colorado. Saying that he wanted his cabinet to "look like America," Clinton appointed two Latinos, three blacks, and three women to the 14-member cabinet. Among his first executive orders were lifting Bush's restrictions on abortion counseling, allowing fetal tissue research, and permitting a review of the prohibited French abortion pill RU-486, which finally gained FDA approval in 2000.

TABLE 29-1			
The Election of 1992			
Candidate	Political Party	Popular Vote	Electoral Vote
William J. Clinton	Democratic	43,728,375	370
George H. W. Bush	Republican	38,167,416	168
H. Ross Perot	Independent	19,237,247	0

Clinton's Domestic Agenda and the "Republican Revolution"

Clinton ran into trouble early in his administration when he tried to fulfill his campaign promise to allow gays and lesbians to serve openly in the military, reversing a policy that dated back half a century. Top military officials, already unhappy with having a new commander-in-chief who had avoided military service during the Vietnam War, vehemently opposed lifting the ban against gays. Ultimately, Clinton compromised and established a new policy of "don't ask, don't tell," which allowed homosexuals to serve as long as they did not make their sexual orientation known. The compromise proved to be unworkable and left many gays and lesbians feeling betrayed.

Clinton's effort to reform the health care system was equally unsuccessful. With rising health care costs and millions of uninsured citizens, Clinton's campaign promises to provide national health insurance and reduce the cost of health care had wide public support but fierce opposition from the medical establishment and the pharmaceutical industry. Clinton appointed his wife, Hillary Rodham Clinton, an attorney and longtime advocate on behalf of children and families, to head a task force to develop a plan. But the task force, deliberating behind closed doors, failed to come up with a workable strategy acceptable to all sides. After a year of hearings and no action in Congress on the complicated task force proposal, the Clintons abandoned the effort.

Clinton achieved a major success when he pushed through Congress a budget that raised taxes on the wealthiest Americans, cut spending to reduce the deficit, and expanded tax credits for low-income families. Vice President Gore cast the tie-breaking vote in the Senate, with no Republican voting in favor. In the next three years the economy markedly improved. Other legislative successes included passage of the "motor voter" act, which allowed eligible voters to register when applying for drivers' licenses, and the Family and Medical Leave Act, which required employers to grant unpaid medical leave for up to 12 weeks. Clinton appointed two new Supreme Court Justices, Ruth Bader Ginsburg in 1993 and Stephen Breyer in 1994, whose liberal perspectives contrasted with the largely conservative bent of the court.

The 1994 congressional elections dealt a devastating blow to Clinton's legislative agenda. In the midst of the campaign, about 300 Republican congressional candidates, under the leadership of Speaker of the House Newt Gingrich, stood on the Capitol steps and endorsed a "Contract with America," calling for welfare reform, a balanced budget, more prisons and longer sentences, increased defense spending, an end to legal abortion, and other conservative measures. Only 39 percent of the electorate voted, and a whisker-thin majority of those voted Republican. Nevertheless, the Republicans declared a "Republican Revolution" as they took control of both the House and Senate for the first time in 40 years and pushed Congress to the right of center.

The new Congress passed a large tax cut and a tough anticrime bill, increased military spending, and reduced federal regulatory power over the environment. Clinton used his veto power to limit the Republican agenda, but he also undercut the conservative momentum by taking on some of their issues as his own, such as free trade and welfare reform. The "Republican

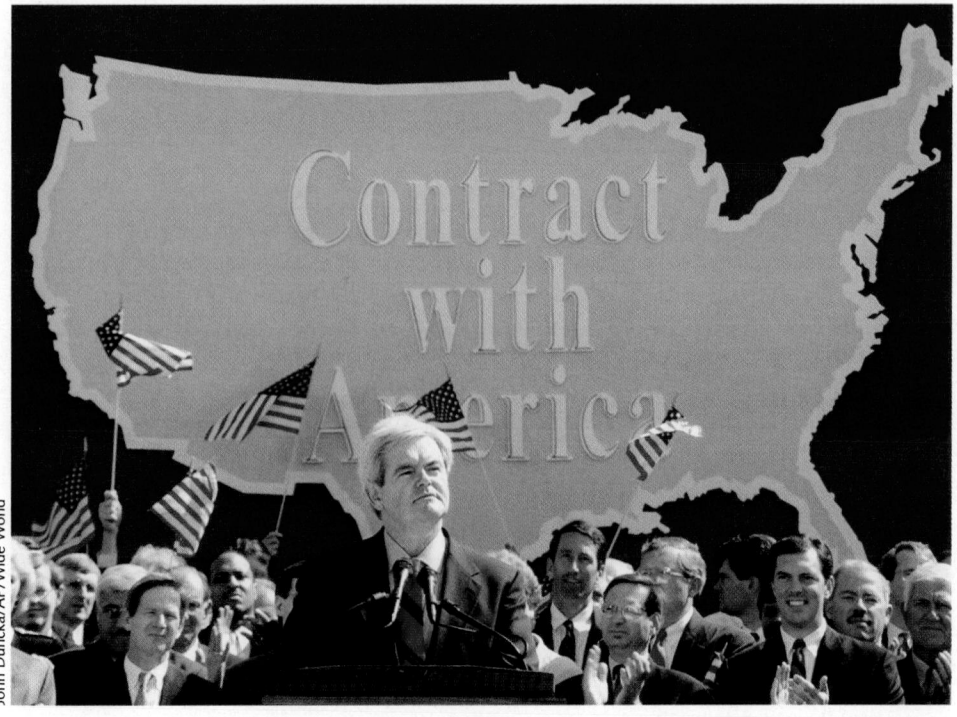

John Duricka/AP/Wide World

■ On September 27, 1994, Congressman Newt Gingrich, a Republican from Georgia, stood on Capitol Hill with Republican congressional candidates and pledged a "Contract with America." Republicans took control of both houses of Congress and declared a "Republican Revolution."

Revolution" did not last long. In 1995 and again in 1996, Congress forced a shutdown of the federal government rather than agreeing to Clinton's proposed budget, leading to widespread frustration and anger as Democrats and Republicans blamed each other for the stalemate. Support for the "Contract with America" wore thin, and the public was quickly disenchanted with the gridlock in Washington. In his 1996 State of the Union address, Clinton announced that the "era of big government is over." In August of that year, after vetoing two earlier versions, Clinton finally agreed to a compromise measure and signed the Welfare Reform Act, abolishing the 60-year-old program Aid to Families with Dependent Children (AFDC).

Clinton won reelection easily in 1996, defeating the 73-year-old Senate Majority Leader, Republican Bob Dole of Kansas. Republicans lost some seats but stayed in control of both houses of Congress. The 1996 campaign was the most expensive in history, with Democrats spending $250 million and Republicans $400 million. Billionaire H. Ross Perot ran again, although his showing at the polls was much weaker than in 1992. Public opinion polls showed a growing concern over the vast amounts of money poured into elections, but campaign finance reform remained a difficult issue for lawmakers, whose own success at the polls depended on large financial contributions.

TABLE 29-2

The Election of 1996

Candidate	Political Party	Popular Vote	Electoral Vote
William J. Clinton	Democratic	45,590,703	379
Robert Dole	Republican	37,816,307	159
H. Ross Perot	Reform	7,866,284	0

The Impeachment Crisis

Clinton's personal behavior left him vulnerable to political enemies, who took full advantage of every opportunity to discredit him. In 1993 the Clintons were investigated for possible complicity in a failed Arkansas investment scheme known as Whitewater. Although a few of the Clintons' close associates were found guilty of conspiracy, tax evasion, and mail fraud in the deal, four years of persistent investigation cleared the Clintons of any wrongdoing. Nevertheless, the Whitewater scandal activated the Office of the Independent Counsel, an independent investigative unit put into place during the Nixon administration to investigate the Watergate break-in. The independent counsel, former judge Kenneth Starr, with the help of the congressional Republicans, pursued Clinton throughout his two terms and nearly brought down his presidency. In the end, however, it was not Clinton's financial dealings but rather his sexual behavior that led to his impeachment.

Clinton's sexual behavior became an issue well before he entered the White House. During the 1992 campaign, Gennifer Flowers, a former nightclub singer, told a tabloid that she and Clinton had an affair when he was governor. Early in his presidency, Paula Jones, a former Arkansas state employee, filed a sexual harassment suit against Clinton, claiming that he had propositioned her when he was governor of Arkansas. Eventually, the case was dismissed, but it came back to haunt him later.

In 1998, Kenneth Starr reported to the House Judiciary Committee that he had evidence that Clinton had an extramarital affair with a young White House intern, Monica Lewinsky. Starr claimed that Clinton had broken the law in an effort to cover up the affair. Lewinsky and Clinton had both been called to testify in the Paula Jones case, and both denied having had a sexual relationship. Starr claimed that Clinton had lied under oath and had instructed his close advisor and friend, Vernon Jordan, to find Lewinsky a job to keep her quiet. Starr charged Clinton with perjury, witness tampering, and obstruction of justice. As proof of the affair, Starr produced 20 hours of taped phone conversations recorded by Lewinsky's co-worker and confidante, Linda Tripp. Clinton vehemently denied the charges, but Lewinsky had saved a dress with a stain containing the president's DNA, providing the investigation with the "smoking gun" it needed.

As Starr and congressional Republicans pressed the investigation with relentless determination, the media saturated the nation and the world with sordid and graphic details of the president's sexual encounters with the young intern. Polls showed that Americans disapproved of Clinton's personal behavior, but they did not want him removed from office. With the economy booming and the country running smoothly, Clinton garnered high job performance ratings, rising to 79 percent at the height of the scandal. Negative sentiment against Kenneth Starr and congressional Republicans mounted as the investigation dragged on for four years at a cost to taxpayers of $40 million.

Public opinion notwithstanding, the House of Representatives impeached Clinton on December 19, 1998, charging him with perjury and obstruction of justice, based on Clinton's false testimony in the Paula Jones case. Removal from office requires two steps: the House of Representatives brings formal charges known as "articles of impeachment," and the Senate tries the impeached official on these articles. A two-thirds vote of the Senate is required for conviction. The vote in the House of Representatives fell strictly along party lines. The Bill of Impeachment was then sent to the Senate, where the majority of senators determined that Clinton's misdeeds did not meet the standard for "high crimes and misdemeanors" required to remove a president from office.

The Nation and the World

C linton tried to prevent the scandals that plagued him at home from interfering with his foreign policy. He hoped to maintain a focus on peacekeeping and peacemaking while expanding trade and diplomatic relations, especially to countries that had been considered unfriendly during the Cold War. Clinton took on the role of peace broker by facilitating negotiations in long-standing conflicts in Northern Ireland and the Middle East. But hostilities in those areas proved too deep to be fully resolved. Military interventions in Somalia, Haiti, and Kosovo yielded mixed results, and trade agreements generated heated controversy. Episodes of international terrorism against U.S. embassies and military personnel killed hundreds of people and highlighted the strength of extremist groups whose members were deeply hostile to the United States and its interventions around the world.

Trade Agreements

In 1993, with President Clinton's strong encouragement, Congress approved the North American Free Trade Agreement (NAFTA), eliminating tariffs and trade barriers among the United States, Mexico, and Canada and thus creating the largest free trade zone in the world. In 1994 Congress approved the General Agreement on Tariffs and Trade (GATT), which reduced tariffs on thousands of goods and phased out import quotas imposed by the United States and other industrialized nations. Supporters argued that these measures would increase global competition and improve the U.S. economy. Businesses would benefit from the easing of trade barriers, and consumers would have access to lower-priced goods.

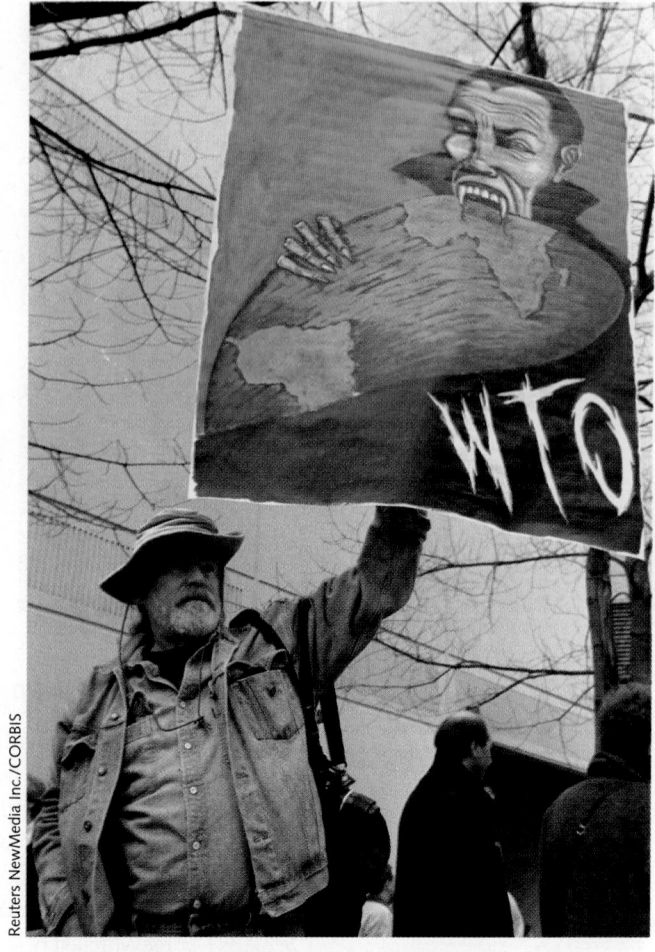

Reuters NewMedia Inc./CORBIS

■ **Activists protest at the opening of the meeting of the World Trade Organization (WTO) in Seattle, Washington, on November 1, 1999. During the four days of the meeting, hundreds of demonstrators took to the streets in opposition to the organization's environmental and labor policies.**

But NAFTA and GATT barely passed Congress. Clinton faced strong opposition from liberal Democrats in industrial areas and from labor unions, who feared that these measures would result in jobs going abroad, declining American wages, and a relaxation of environmental controls over companies moving outside the U.S. borders. In the first few years of NAFTA and GATT, these fears seemed justified. Some jobs went abroad, and threats of moving gave employers a negotiating edge over workers. In Mexico the impact of NAFTA was even worse. The peso collapsed as money and goods flowed across the border, and the average wages for workers fell from $1.45 to $.78 per hour.

Equally controversial were Clinton's efforts to grant China most-favored-nation status, which would designate China as a full trading partner with the United States. Human rights activists argued that China's dismal record of violent suppression and imprisonment of political dissenters should preclude such favorable trading terms. But with an eye to China's huge potential market for American goods and favorable site for U.S.-owned factories, Congress approved Clinton's proposal.

Despite this new alliance with a former foe, Cold War politics did not entirely disappear from foreign policy. The tiny communist nation of Cuba, suffering severe economic hardship since the collapse of its benefactor, the Soviet Union, remained off limits to U.S. trade

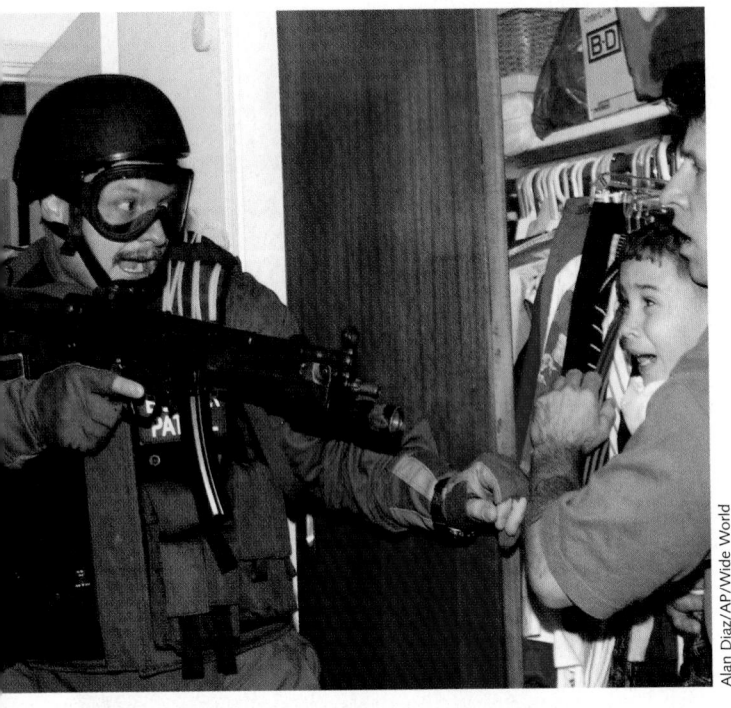

Alan Diaz/AP/Wide World

and tourism. Cuban Americans in southern Florida, who had fled Cuba after Fidel Castro's successful revolution, blocked any efforts to ease relations between the two countries. Democrats as well as Republicans were reluctant to alienate these voters; their numbers and political clout in the most populous part of the nation's fourth largest state gave them power.

Cuban–American relations were strained anew in November 1999 when a small boat carrying a group of Cubans trying to escape to Florida capsized, drowning everyone aboard except a six-year-old boy, Elian Gonzales, who was found floating on an inner tube off the coast of Florida. Elian's relatives in Miami argued that Elian should stay in the United States, where he could grow up in a democratic society—a goal his mother died trying to achieve. However, his father wanted him back in Cuba, and the Clinton administration determined that the boy should be returned to his remaining parent. After months of intense media coverage in both countries and futile efforts at negotiation, in April 2000 U.S. government agents stormed the small house where Elian was staying and seized the boy, who eventually returned to Cuba with his father.

■ On the morning of April 22, 2000, federal agents stormed the house where relatives were holding 6-year-old Elian Gonzales. The boy was the sole survivor of a boat carrying a group of Cubans escaping to the United States. His mother was among those who perished. Elian was eventually reunited with his father and returned to Cuba.

Efforts at Peacemaking

Less controversial than relations with China and Cuba were Clinton's peacemaking efforts. Northern Ireland had been fraught with violent conflict for 30 years. Irish Catholic nationalists wanted to break ties with England and join the Republic of Ireland; Protestants loyal to Great Britain wanted to remain part of the United Kingdom. The United States, with political and diplomatic connections to London as well as strong ties to the Irish, wanted to help resolve the crisis. Clinton made several trips to Ireland to promote peace. He appointed former Senator George Mitchell of Maine as negotiator, who spent months working on a settlement. Despite dissent and violence by extremists on both sides, by the time Clinton left office, an agreement had been reached that established a shared coalition government.

In the Middle East, Clinton brought Yasser Arafat, leader of the Palestinian Liberation Organization (PLO), and Yitzak Rabin, Israeli Prime Minister, to Washington for talks that led to a historic 1993 handshake and pledges to pursue a peace agreement. As in Northern Ireland, those efforts were hampered by violent extremists on both sides. Rabin was assassinated by a fanatical right-wing Israeli, leading to the election of a hawkish new prime minister, Benjamin Netanyahu. The peace process fell apart for several years until negotiations finally resumed in the late 1990s. But just when an agreement seemed to be within reach, large-scale violence between Palestinians and Israelis erupted again in the summer of 2000. Clinton left office with no agreement in sight.

In the final weeks of Clinton's presidency in 2000, he made a historic visit to Vietnam—the first by an American president since the war. Because Clinton had protested against the war decades earlier, his visit held great symbolic power. Although the United States lost the war, westernization had taken hold in Vietnam, with investment beginning to flow in from Europe, the United States, and Japan, as well as American popular culture and technology. Cheering crowds welcomed the president of the superpower that had been vanquished 25 years earlier.

Military Interventions and International Terrorism

The end of the Cold War raised new questions about how and when to use American military force. Most of the overseas crises stemmed from problems of national disintegration, ethnic conflict, and humanitarian disasters resulting from political chaos and civil wars. These sorts of problems would have challenged even the most internationally focused president, but Clinton was concerned mainly with domestic matters. Aside from his interest in expanding U.S. trade, he had few guiding principles in foreign policy other than his desire to broker peace agreements in tenacious hot spots.

On the Caribbean island of Haiti, a military coup in 1991 had ousted the democratically elected President Jean Bertrand Aristide. In a striking departure from former Cold War policies, Clinton backed the black populist Aristide against the coup leaders, who had strong ties to the CIA. In 1994, the United States received UN support for an invasion to restore Aristide to power. To avert a large-scale military conflict, Clinton sent former President Jimmy Carter to Haiti to negotiate a settlement. The resulting agreement allowed the coup members to leave the country, and Aristide returned. Six years later, however, the United States criticized Aristide for corruption and fraud in his 2000 reelection.

In 1992 President Bush had sent U.S. marines to Somalia in east Africa as part of a UN effort to provide famine relief and to restore peace in the war-torn nation. After Clinton took office, Somali warlord Mohammed Farah Aidid killed 50 Pakistani UN peacekeepers. The UN forces then mobilized against Aidid, shifting the peacekeeping mission to military engagement. As part of the effort to hunt down Aidid, U.S. soldiers killed hundreds of Somali citizens, creating intense anti-American sentiment among the population. Amid that hostile atmosphere, in September 1993, Aidid's forces killed 18 American soldiers under the UN command in a firefight and dragged one of their bodies through the streets. The outraged American public viewed the grim spectacle on TV, and the experience left Clinton with no clear guidelines on humanitarian intervention abroad. Largely as a result of the disaster in Somalia, when ethnic conflict led to genocide in Rwanda in central Africa in 1994, the United States and other western nations refused to intervene.

Ethnic conflict was also the cause of trouble in the Balkans. From 1945 to 1980 Marshal Josip Broz Tito ruled over a unified communist Yugoslavia, maintaining stability by suppressing ethnic rivalries. But after Tito's death in 1980, ethnic nationalism pulled Yugoslavia apart, with Slovenia and Croatia breaking away, and then Bosnia and Serbia. The region erupted in bloody conflicts, escalating into full-scale war after the breakup of Yugoslavia in 1991. After sustained

Serbian attacks on Muslims in Bosnia between 1992 and 1995, Clinton reluctantly agreed to air strikes against the Serbs, leading to the 1995 Dayton Accords, which brought an end to the war. But Serbian president Slobodan Milosevic continued to foment anti-Muslim and anti-Croat fervor. Soon the Serbs embarked on a murderous campaign to drive the Muslim ethnic Albanians out of Serbia's southern province of Kosovo. The United States was reluctant to intervene despite the brutality, but the situation reached such drastic proportions that Clinton finally decided to send troops to Kosovo in 1999. The action had the unintended effect of weakening the Serbian opposition against Milosevic as Serbs closed ranks against the foreign troops. Eventually, a tenuous peace was restored, and Milosevic was voted out of office in 2000. The following year, Serbian authorities arrested Milosevic and turned him over to the War Crimes Tribunal in The Hague, which had indicted Milosevic for crimes against humanity.

U.S. interventions around the world failed to quell ethnic tensions or eradicate poverty. Although some military actions achieved their immediate goals, the presence of the United States abroad also fueled anti-American sentiment. In some regions of the world, resentment against the United States found expression in violence and terrorism. In June 1996 a truck bomb killed 19 U.S. airmen in Dhahran, Saudi Arabia. Two years later, bombs exploded at two U.S. embassies in east Africa, killing 224 people in Nairobi, Kenya, and Dar es Salaam, Tanzania.

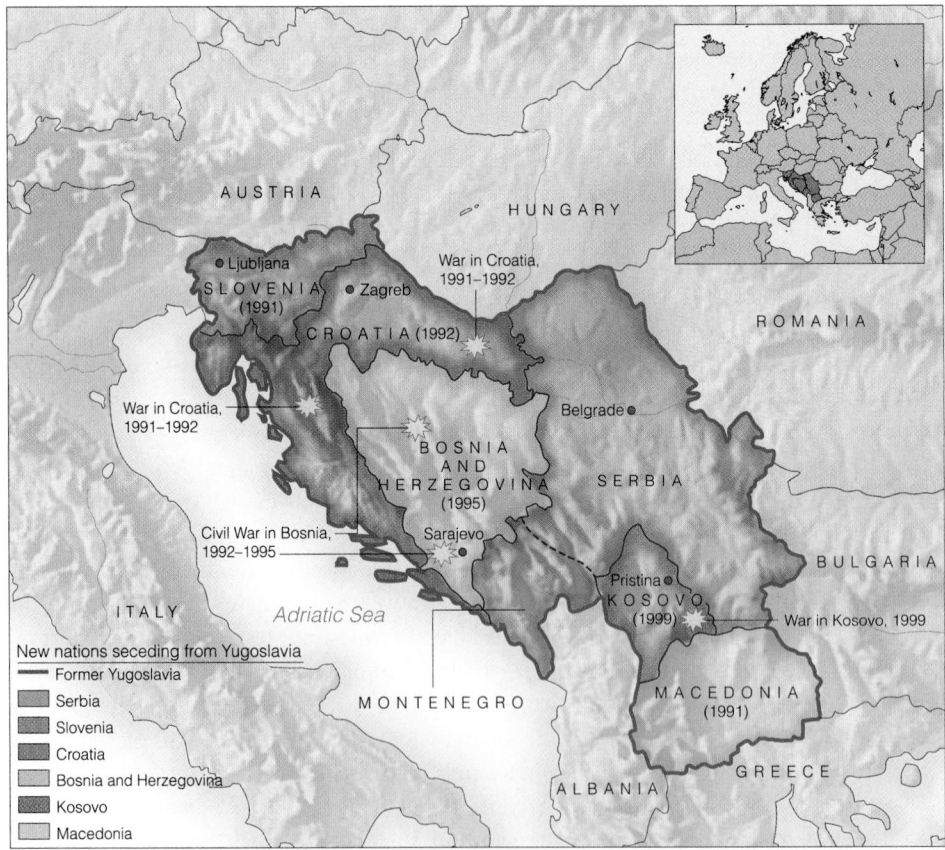

■ **MAP 29.3**

THE BREAKUP OF THE FORMER YUGOSLAVIA Created in 1919 as a multiethnic nation, Yugoslavia split apart in 1991–1992. After Slovenia and Croatia gained their independence swiftly, Bosnia deteriorated into fierce ethnic fighting dominated by Serb atrocities and encouraged by the Serbian government of Slobodan Milosevic. A brief U.S. bombing campaign in 1995 finally brought the Serbs to peace negotiations. Similar ethnic fighting in the province of Kosovo in 1999 led to another U.S. bombing campaign and Kosovo's current quasi-independence under NATO guidance.

Four men were convicted of conspiracy in the terrorist attacks. They were identified as followers of Islamic militant Osama bin Laden, who was also indicted in connection with the embassy bombings. Bin Laden, originally from Saudi Arabia, was living in Afghanistan under the protection of the fundamentalist Taliban regime and remained a fugitive. He was known to be the leader of the al Qaeda terrorist network operating in several countries throughout the Middle East. On October 12, 2000, a small boat pulled up next to the destroyer USS *Cole* in Yemen's port of Aden. A bomb exploded and ripped a hole in the destroyer, killing 17 Americans and wounding 39 others. Two suicide bombers carried out the attack. U.S. officials believed that they, too, were associated with Osama bin Laden.

On February 26, 1993, a bomb exploded in the parking garage underneath the World Trade Center, the skyscrapers dominating the New York skyline in Lower Manhattan. Five people were killed and more than a thousand were injured. The *New York Times* reported that the explosion "destroyed a multistoried parking garage under the trade center, knocked out power to the center and touched off fires that sent smoke billowing up through its 110-story twin towers and forced 50,000 people into a nightmarish evacuation that took all day and half the night." President Clinton tried to quell the fears of the nation in the face of what appeared to be an act of international terrorism. "Working together, we'll find out who was involved and why this happened," the president declared. "Americans should know we'll do everything in our power to keep them safe in their streets, their offices and their homes." However, international terrorists proved difficult to identify and bring to justice. Eight years later the same twin towers were attacked again, with far more devastating consequences.

The Contested Election of 2000

The first presidential election of the new millennium was the most bitterly contested in more than a century. The Democratic candidate won the national popular vote, but with ballot counts incomplete in the key state of Florida, the Supreme Court ultimately declared the Republican candidate the victor. The election exposed defects in the election process, from faulty ballots and voting machines to the role of the media, and raised serious questions about the value of the Electoral College. The election also revealed that flaws in the system disfranchised large numbers of poor and minority voters. But in the end, the transfer of power took place smoothly, and the nation accepted the outcome.

The Campaign, the Vote, and the Courts

The 2000 campaign was fairly lackluster. The Democrats nominated Vice President Al Gore, who hoped to benefit from Clinton's high approval rating and the healthy economy. The Republicans nominated George W. Bush, governor of Texas and son of the former president. Bush chose as his running mate Dick Cheney, who had been the elder Bush's secretary of state. Gore chose Senator Joe Lieberman from Connecticut as his running mate, the first Jew to run on a presidential ticket. Gore's popularity peaked after the Democratic National Convention, where he delivered a rousing speech filled with populist themes and gave a passionate kiss to his wife, Tipper, which garnered more media attention than the speech itself. But he distanced himself from the popular master campaigner Clinton. Bush gained the upper hand during the televised debates, where he portrayed himself as a "compassionate conservative" and promised to restore "dignity to the White House." As the election neared, Gore's lead in the polls narrowed.

Only half of the nation's eligible voters turned out to vote. But African Americans went to the polls in unusually high numbers and voted overwhelmingly for Gore, largely out of loyalty to Clinton. Even before all the polls had closed, the national media began to report

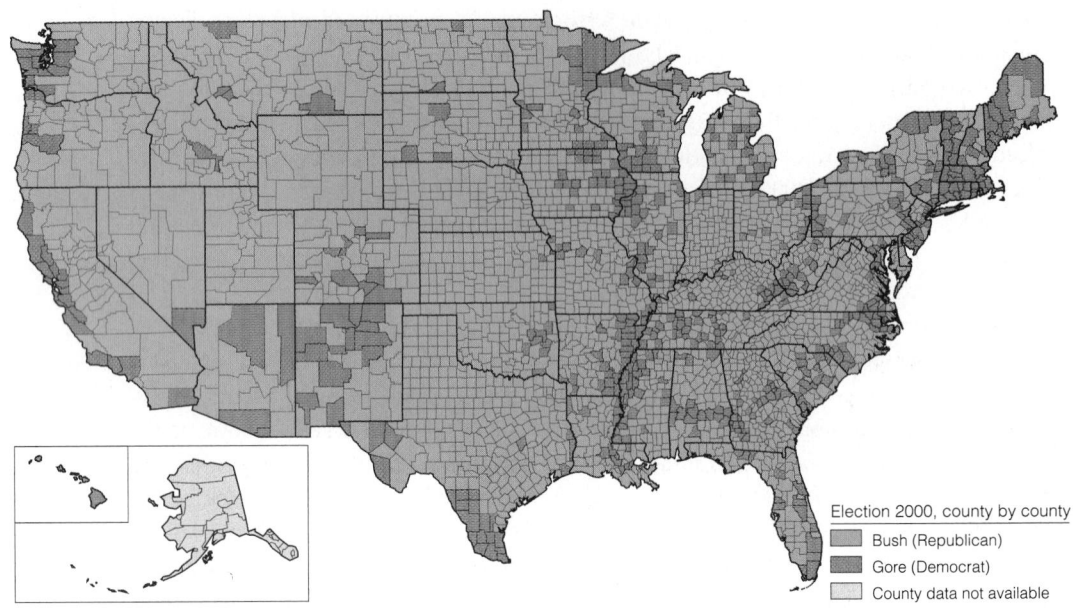

Election 2000, county by county
■ Bush (Republican)
■ Gore (Democrat)
□ County data not available

■ **MAP 29.4**

THE CONTESTED ELECTION OF 2000   The 2000 election was so close, and so fraught with problems, that it was ultimately decided by a 5–4 vote of the Supreme Court. As this map shows, Democratic votes were concentrated in the densely populated urban areas and Republican votes in the sparsely populated rural areas.

the results. Early in the evening, they declared that Florida, a key state with 25 electoral votes, had gone to Gore. But soon after that announcement, they changed their projection and put Florida back into the "undecided" group of states. As the hours dragged on, it became clear that whoever took Florida, where Bush's brother Jeb Bush was governor, would win the election. By the next day, Gore had won the national popular vote by half a million votes, but Bush was ahead in Florida. Bush's lead was so narrow that it triggered an automatic recount.

With all eyes on Florida, a number of serious irregularities surfaced. Voters in Palm Beach County were given a confusing "butterfly" ballot, resulting in more than 20,000 mismarked ballots. In other counties, registered voters were turned away at the polls because of inaccurate and incomplete voter registration lists. Some voter lists inaccurately listed eligible voters as felons. Most of these disfranchised voters were African American. In several largely minority counties, old voting machines that used a punched-ballot system failed to count thousands of ballots.

For weeks after the election, the outcome was still unknown. Democrats insisted that because Bush's lead had narrowed to a few hundred votes, tallied by inaccurate voting machines, ballots in four Florida counties should be recounted by hand. Republicans pointed out that it would be unfair to recount votes in only four heavily Democratic counties, especially with no standard way of determining voter intent on punch-card ballots with ambiguous marks on them. Florida's secretary of state, Katherine Harris, a Republican who headed Florida's campaign for George W. Bush, refused to extend the deadline to allow the recounts to take place and declared Bush the winner by 537 votes out of 6 million cast statewide.

TABLE 29-3

The Election of 2000

Candidate	Political Party	Popular Vote	Electoral Vote
George W. Bush	Republican	50,456,167	271
Al Gore	Democratic	50,996,064	266*
Ralph Nader	Green	2,864,810	0

*One District of Columbia Gore elector abstained.

Gore contested the results, and the Florida Supreme Court ordered that the recount proceed. Bush then appealed to the U.S. Supreme Court to reverse the decision of the Florida Supreme Court. After 36 days of partial vote counting and court battles, the U.S. Supreme Court declared Bush the winner in a sharply divided 5–4 decision. The four dissenting judges issued a stinging rebuke of their five colleagues responsible for the decision. In his dissenting opinion, Justice Stephen Breyer wrote that the majority ruling "can only lend confidence to the most cynical appraisal of the work of judges throughout the land."

The Aftermath

After the election, reporters continued the hand-counting process in Florida in an effort to discover who would have won if all the votes had been counted. The results can never be absolutely conclusive, given the many irregularities in the process. What did become clear in the months after the election were the widespread flaws in the election system in Florida and elsewhere. Across the country outdated voting machines yielded inaccurate vote counts, and long lines at polling places prevented voters from casting ballots. Low-income and minority voters were more likely to be disfranchised because they lived in precincts with faulty voting machines or overcrowded polling places. The U.S. Civil Rights Commission estimated that in Florida black voters were nine times more likely than white voters to have had their votes rejected.

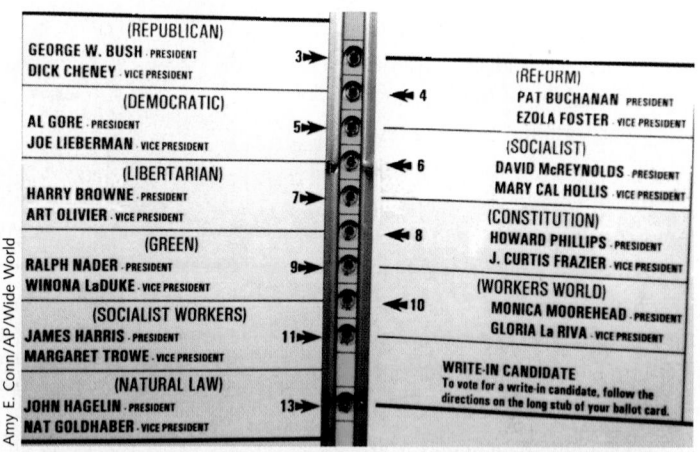

■ In Palm Beach, Florida, voters received this confusing "butterfly ballot." Thousands of voters in this predominantly Democratic county accidentally voted for Reform candidate Pat Buchanan instead of Democrat Al Gore. With only a few hundred votes separating Bush and Gore in Florida, it is quite possible that the butterfly ballot may have cost Gore the election.

In addition to those whose votes did not count, many others were prevented from voting altogether. In Florida, "suspected felons" were removed from voter registration lists without being informed and without the opportunity to demonstrate that they were law-abiding citizens eligible to vote. An estimated 15 percent of the list was inaccurate, and more than half of those voters were African American. According to the U.S. Civil Rights Commission, "Perhaps the most dramatic undercount in Florida's election was the nonexistent ballots of countless unknown eligible voters, who were turned away, or wrongfully purged from the voter registration rolls . . . and were prevented from exercising the franchise." As a result, hundreds of African American citizens with no criminal record arrived at the polls, only to discover that they had been disfranchised. An investigation by scholars of constitutional law concluded that the disfranchisement of African American voters in Florida constituted a violation of the 1965 Voting Rights Act. They determined that if those African American voters had been able to cast ballots, they would have provided more than the 537 votes Gore needed to win.

The election also renewed a national debate over the value of the Electoral College. Opponents argued that Gore was the rightful winner because he won a majority of the popular vote. Advocates claimed that the Electoral College protected the interests of less populous states and that Bush was fairly elected because he won the majority of states. Congress and state legislatures began discussions of various forms of electoral reform, but abolishing the Electoral College was not among them. Representatives of small states probably would block any such measures.

Policymakers and media moguls also debated the role of the media in reporting election returns. Some argued for a blackout on early returns until all polls across the country were closed to avoid the possibility that early results might influence voters who had not yet voted. Others proposed that only official results be announced to avoid the problem of erroneous reporting that occurred on election night 2000. But media representatives countered that a free press should be able to report the news as it happens, although they agreed on the need to ensure accuracy.

Voting

One of the most troubling revelations to surface in the wake of the 2000 election was the news that millions of citizens, in Florida and elsewhere, were thwarted in their effort to vote or to have their votes count. Studies conducted after the election showed that 4 to 6 million Americans were disfranchised as a result of faulty equipment, confusing ballots, erroneous voter registration lists, long lines at polling places, and problems with absentee ballots. Voters in low-income precincts with a large percentage of citizens of color were much more likely to have their votes discarded, or to be turned away at the polls, than voters in more affluent and whiter districts. These revelations sparked outrage among Americans who believe that voting is one of the fundamental rights of democratic citizenship. But the disfranchisement of potential voters has a long history in the United States, beginning with the founding of the nation.

The Constitution does not guarantee anyone the right to vote. After the American Revolution, the majority of Americans—including women, slaves, most free black men, propertyless white men, apprentices, indentured laborers, felons, and those considered mentally incompetent—were denied the right to vote. New Jersey was the only state to allow women the vote.

Debates over who should vote, and efforts both to expand and to restrict suffrage, continued for most of the nation's history. During the first half of the nineteenth century, Democrats viewed the vote as a right of all white men, whereas Whigs argued that voting was a privilege to be reserved for the elite. Although the United States was the first western nation to expand the electorate by lowering economic

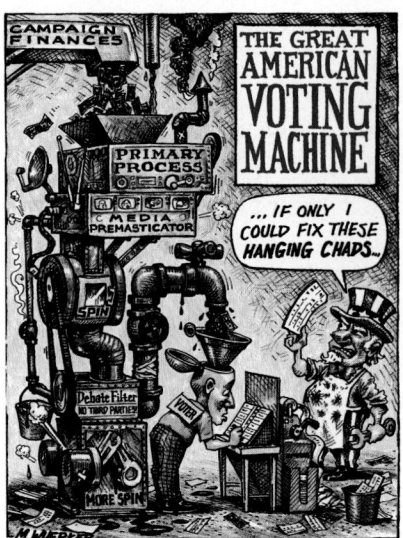

The 2000 election exposed many problems in the voting process. This political cartoon suggests that the controversial Florida ballots and methods of counting them were only the final symptoms of an electoral system that was flawed at many levels.

barriers to voting, for a long time after that, the laws governing the right to vote actually limited rather than broadened access to the polls.

Between the Revolution and the Civil War, race and gender replaced property as the primary criteria for voting. Nearly every state disfranchised free blacks while dropping the property requirements for white men. States in the West tended toward more inclusive voting rolls. Several gave the vote to aliens who had established permanent residence and to Native Americans who had relinquished tribal citizenship. Some politicians were eager to expand suffrage to portray themselves as champions of the common people and win the votes of the newly enfranchised.

But several states restricted voting well into the twentieth century. Rhode Island required foreign-born citizens to meet a property requirement to vote, and California prevented Asians from voting. In 1921 New York adopted English literacy tests to prevent immigrants from voting, disfranchising hundreds of thousands of citizens as late as the 1960s. As a result of these restrictions, voter turnout began to decline in the late nineteenth century. This shrinking of the electorate was not accidental. In 1907 the voter registration board of Pittsburgh boasted that in only two years the Pennsylvania registration law had cut the number of registered voters in half. Women achieved the right to vote in 1920, but most women of color and many immigrant women remained disfranchised for decades.

African Americans officially gained the right to vote in 1870 with the ratification of the Fifteenth Amendment. But by 1900, almost all blacks as well as poor whites in the South had been disfranchised through poll taxes and literacy and property requirements. Not until passage of the 1965 Voting Rights Act were African Americans in the South able to vote. Suffrage expanded again in 1971 when the Twenty-Sixth Amendment lowered the voting age from 21 to 18. The Vietnam War revived claims made since the Revolution that citizens old enough to fight and die for their country were old enough to vote.

By the time of the 2000 election, universal suffrage was the law of the land. Although only half of all eligible voters went to the polls that year, the number of voters had increased tenfold since 1888. Still, questions remained about the fairness of the process, whether intentional or not. When the winner of the popular vote lost the election to a candidate without a clear victory in the Electoral College, critics of the system called for direct election of the president. In the end, however, it was neither the voters nor the Electoral College, but the justices of the U.S. Supreme Court, who elected the president by a vote of 5–4. ■

Hightower Lowdown, Vol. 2, No. 12, Dec. 2000, pg. 1

Legacies of Election 2000

In addition to the unprecedented Supreme Court decision, the 2000 election was remarkable in other ways. For the first time, a First Lady was elected to public office: Hillary Rodham Clinton became a Democratic senator from New York. In another Senate race, a deceased candidate was elected. Mel Carnahan, Democratic governor of Missouri, had run against Republican incumbent John Ashcroft. But Carnahan died in a plane crash a few weeks before the election, too late to have his name removed from the ballot. The acting governor pledged to appoint Carnahan's widow if he won the election, and she picked up the campaign. Carnahan was elected and his widow went to the Senate. (The defeated candidate, John Ashcroft, became George W. Bush's attorney general.)

Third-party politics also influenced the outcome of the election. Several third-party candidates had achieved national visibility during the 1990s and won elections at the state and local levels, including professional wrestler Jesse Ventura, elected governor of Minnesota in 1998 on the Reform party ticket. In 2000 Ralph Nader wreaked havoc for the Democrats with his Green party candidacy for president. Although Nader gained fewer than 3 percent of the votes, his candidacy drew off some of the left-leaning elements of the Democratic party—enough votes to cost Al Gore the election.

The election results left the Congress almost evenly divided, with a thin Republican majority in the House and a 50–50 split in the Senate. But within a year, Senator James M. Jeffords from Vermont bolted the Republican party and became an Independent, giving the Democrats a majority in the Senate. The closely divided Congress began to take up issues raised by the contested election, including various measures to improve the voting process, and campaign finance reform.

President George W. Bush immediately began to reverse several Clinton-era policies, including a number of environmental protections. His first major legislative success was the passage of a major tax cut. During his first year in office, the economy went from boom to bust and headed into a recession. The robust stock market of the 1990s wilted in early 2001. Nevertheless, as the new millennium dawned, the United States remained the wealthiest and most powerful nation in the world. Bush retreated from international treaties on issues ranging from global warming to nuclear test ban agreements, and revived the Reagan-era proposal for a nuclear missile shield. But the place of the nation in the global community was yet to be defined. Soon, monumental events shattered the nation's sense of security and forced Bush to abandon his retreat from international alliances and to engage in the world in unprecedented ways.

Conclusion

In the 1990s the role of the nation in the world shifted and a half-century of political certainties evaporated. The end of the Cold War meant that the United States had to develop a new international mission. The struggle against the Soviet Union and the communist foe had come to an end. Russia was our friend; China was our trading partner. Conflicts around the globe, many of them grounded in ancient ethnic hostilities, posed challenges for the world's most powerful nation. The United States had new international concerns, including desires for markets and trade, the nation's supply of oil, the need for political order to maintain international stability, and the danger of "rogue nations" developing nuclear arms. President Clinton tried to be a peacemaker in hot spots around the world while attempting to respond to violent episodes of international terrorism.

At home, Americans demonstrated increasing tolerance for people who looked and acted differently from themselves. Polls showed declining levels of racial, ethnic, and religious hostility and greater acceptance of homosexuality, single parenthood, and family arrangements that deviated from the nuclear family model. But episodes of racial discrimination—by police, courts, and voting officials—continued. Politics remained an arena in which culture wars flared over abortion, gun control, and welfare reform. A Democratic president faced impeachment by his Republican foes in Congress while maintaining high approval ratings from the public.

At the dawn of the new century, several crises challenged Americans' sense of security. A deeply flawed presidential election revealed profound problems in the nation's voting system. A sharp and sudden downturn in the economy shattered the optimism many middle-class people felt during the booming Clinton years and forced many of the working poor into desperate circumstances. Already reeling from these disturbing developments, the nation was soon shaken to its core by a terrorist attack that forced a new reckoning at home and abroad.

Sites to Visit

William Jefferson Clinton
www.ipl.org/ref/POTUS/wjclinton.html
This site contains basic information about Clinton's election and presidency and an online biography.

Distribution of Wealth and Income
www.inequality.org/factsfr.html
This site provides facts and figures about the distribution of wealth and income in the 1990s.

American Identities
xroads.virginia.edu/~YP/ethnic.html
This site of the American Studies program at the University of Virginia includes information and resources for studying America's multiple ethnic identities.

The O.J. Simpson Trial
www.cnn.com/US/OJ/index.html
This CNN site provides basic facts and interpretive essays, plus additional links about the O. J. Simpson trial.

Investigating the President: The Trial
www.cnn.com/ALLPOLITICS/resources/1998/lewinsky/
This CNN site provides information and documents about the scandals surrounding President Clinton's impeachment.

Focus on Kosovo
www.cnn.com/SPECIALS/1998/10/kosovo/
This in-depth CNN interactive site looks at the development and current resolution to the turmoil in Kosovo.

Oklahoma City Bombing
www.cnn.com/US/9703/okc.trial/
This CNN interactive site has information about the domestic terrorist bombing in Oklahoma City and the trial that followed.

Why Do Campaign Polls Zigzag So Much?
www.psych.purdue.edu/%7Ecodelab/Invalid.Polls.html
This site, created by Gerald S. Wasserman of the Psychological Sciences Department at Purdue University, examines polling data from the 1996 presidential campaign.

For Further Reading

General

Stephanie Coontz, *The Way We Really Are: Coming to Terms with America's Changing Families* (1997).

Thomas L. Friedman, *The Lexus and the Olive Tree: Understanding Globalization* (2000).

Clara E. Rodriguez, *Changing Race: Latinos, the Census and the History of Ethnicity in the United States* (2000).

Leland T. Saito and Roger Daniels, *Race and Politics: Asian Americans, Latinos, and Whites in a Los Angeles Suburb* (1998).

The Economy: Global and Domestic

Sheldon Danziger and Peter Gottschalk, *America Unequal* (1995).

Julia Butterfly Hill, *The Legacy of Luna: The Story of a Tree, A Woman, and the Struggle to Save the Redwoods* (2000).

Jacqueline Jones, *American Work: Four Centuries of Black and White Labor* (1998).

William A. Orme, *Understanding NAFTA: Mexico, Free Trade, and the New North America* (1996).

Tolerance and Its Limits

Jeffrey Abramson, ed., *Postmortem: The O. J. Simpson Case: Justice Confronts Race, Domestic Violence, Lawyers, Money, and the Media* (1996).

Robin D. G. Kelley, *Yo' Mama's Disfunktional!: Fighting the Culture Wars in Urban America* (1998).

Jane Mayer and Jill Abramson, *Strange Justice: The Selling of Clarence Thomas* (1994).

Michael Omi and Howard Winant, *Racial Formation in the United States: From the 1960s to the 1990s* (1994).

Alan Wolfe, *One Nation, After All: What Americans Really Think About God, Country, Family, Racism, Welfare, Immigration, Homosexuality, Work, the Right, the Left and Each Other* (1998).

Violence and Danger

Joan Jacobs Brumberg, *The Body Project: An Intimate History of American Girls* (2000).

Joan Jacobs Brumberg, *Fasting Girls: The History of Anorexia Nervosa* (2000).

Susan Faludi, *Stiffed: The Betrayal of the American Man* (1999).

Peter D. Kramer, *Listening to Prozac* (1997).

Rickie Solinger, ed., *Abortion Wars: A Half Century of Struggle, 1950–2000* (1998).

Judith Stacey, *In the Name of the Family: Rethinking Family Values in the Postmodern Age* (1996).

Steven Wisotsky and Thomas Szasz, *Beyond the War on Drugs: Overcoming a Failed Public Policy* (1999).

The Clinton Presidency

William C. Berman, *From the Center to the Edge: The Politics and Policies of the Clinton Presidency* (2001).

James MacGregor Burns and Georgia J. Sorenson, *Dead Center: Clinton–Gore Leadership and the Perils of Moderation* (1999).

Steven E. Schier, ed., *The Postmodern Presidency: Bill Clinton's Legacy in U.S. Politics* (2000).

The Nation and the World

John Dumbrell and David M. Barrett, *The Making of U.S. Foreign Policy* (1998).

Thomas H. Henriksen, *Clinton's Foreign Policy in Somalia, Bosnia, Haiti, and North Korea* (1996).

Richard A. Melanson, *American Foreign Policy Since the Vietnam War: The Search for Consensus from Nixon to Clinton* (2001).

The Contested Election of 2000

Alan M. Dershowitz, *Supreme Injustice: How the High Court Hijacked Election 2000* (2001).

E. J. Dionne and William Kristol, eds., *Bush v. Gore: The Court Cases and the Commentary* (2001).

Samuel Issacharoff, Pamela Karlan, and Richard H. Pildes, *When Elections Go Bad: The Law of Democracy and the Presidential Election of 2000* (2001).

Alexander Keyssar, *The Right to Vote: The Contested History of Democracy in the United States* (2000).

Charles Lewis, *The Buying of the President 2000* (2001).

Richard A. Posner, *Breaking the Deadlock: The 2000 Election, the Constitution, and the Courts* (2001).

Bill Sammon, *At Any Cost: How Al Gore Tried to Steal the Election* (2001).

Jeffrey Toobin, *Too Close to Call: The Thirty-Six-Day Battle to Decide the 2000 Election* (2001).

Online Practice Test

Test your understanding of this chapter with interactive review quizzes at

www.ablongman.com/jonescreatedequal/chapter29

Additional Photo Credits

Page 971: Walker Shaun/SIPA Press
Page 974: Courtesy, Casio Corporation
Page 981: Tamiment/Wagner Poster and Broadside Collection, Tamiment Library, New York University
Page 986: James Keyser/TimePix

CHAPTER

30

A Global Nation for the New Millennium

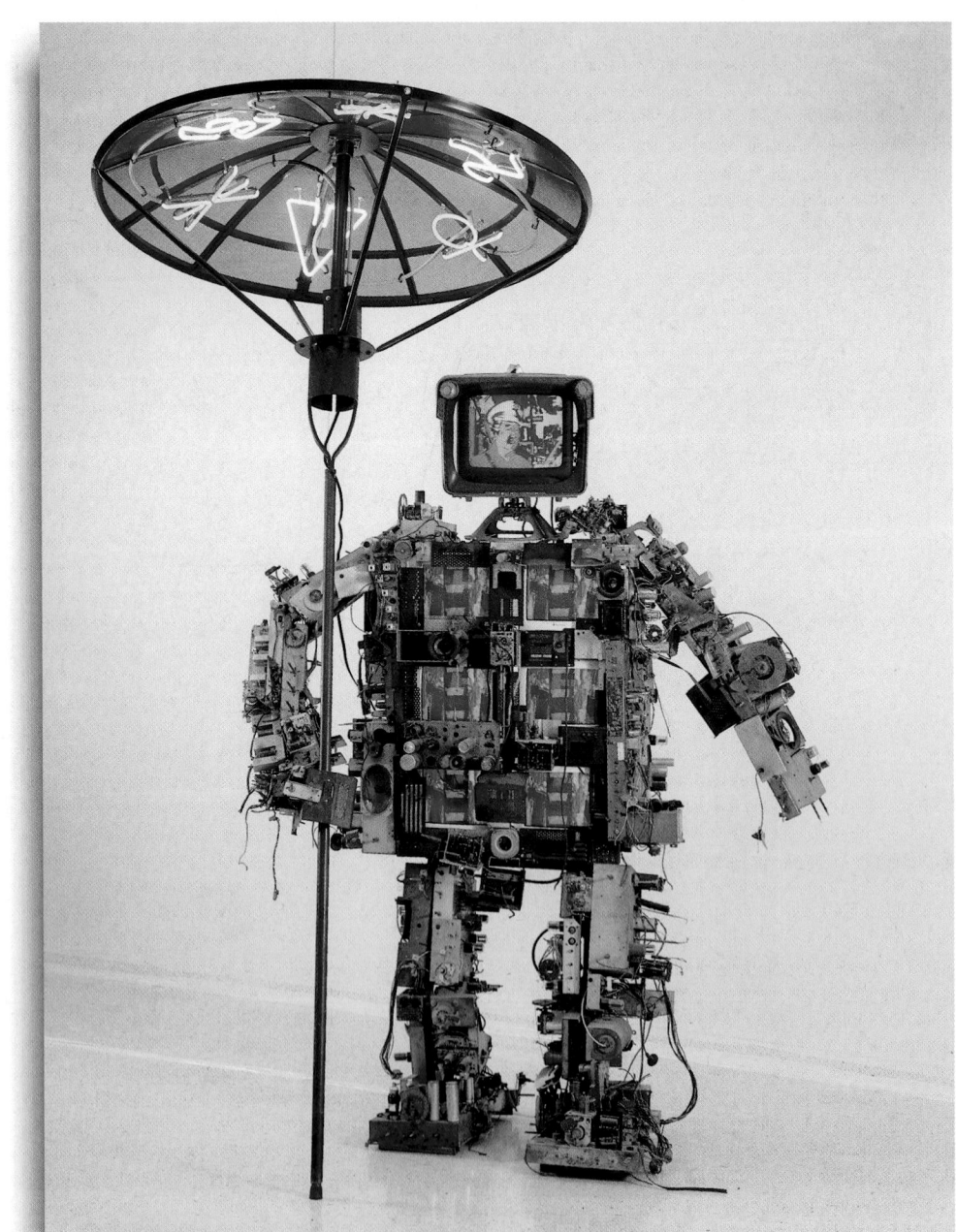

Nam June Paik, *Global Encoder*, 1994. Courtesy of Nam June Paik and Carl Solway Gallery, Cincinnati, Ohio. Photo by Tom Allison and Chris Gomien.

■ At the beginning of the new millennium, computer technology and the Internet linked Americans closely to each other and to events around the globe. Electronic circuitry enabled information to flow at a pace unimaginable to previous generations.

"THOSE MEXICAN GUYS WORK, THEY REALLY WORK," THE FORMER OWNER OF A carpet-cleaning business in Las Vegas observed in a sentiment widely shared among employers in southern Nevada's booming desert city. Mostly young Latinos, along with a smattering of whites and blacks, workers lined up on D Street in North Las Vegas every morning waiting for employers to drive up. "Drive past the white guys; they're all derelicts," explained a young white tree-cutter just out of drug rehabilitation and looking for help at the day labor market. He bluntly stereotyped native-born workers of any color in comparison to immigrants. "Drive past the black guys, too. Get the Mexicans. They work." For $8 an hour, he hired a man to work with him trimming palm trees, hard, nasty work made tougher by desert temperatures of more than 100 degrees. At the end of the day, $64 changed hands, and the Latino went his own way, leaving the tree-cutter satisfied. In Las Vegas and across the country, immigrant labor is prized: undocumented immigrants work hard for low wages and cause few problems for those who hire them.

Latinos were not always easily distinguished from other workers in southern Nevada. In 1991, the Frontier Hotel and Casino on the famous Las Vegas Strip slashed employees' wages and benefits, prompting hundreds of unionized workers to walk out and begin the longest strike of the decade in the United States. For more than six years, union members of different races and ethnicities walked the picket line together outside the Frontier. Twelve of them even walked the 300 miles across the Mojave Desert to Los Angeles to pro-mote public awareness of their cause. Gloria Hernandez was a Mexican-born mother of two, a restaurant hostess, and a union activist who stayed out on strike until the Frontier was sold in 1998, and the new owner reinstated wages and benefits similar to those at the other large casinos. In the final year of the strike, Hernandez quali-fied for naturalization and became an American citizen, just in time to return to her old job.

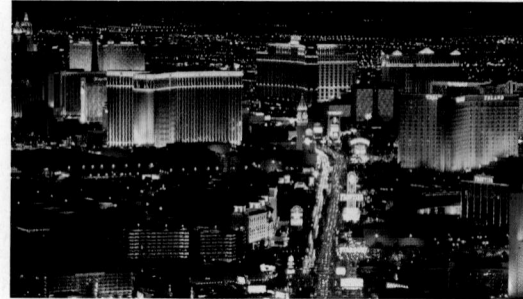

Vast power plants allow Las Vegas to glitter at night.

This was an old story in America, of determined newcomers often making great sacrifices to create a life of better opportunities and greater freedoms for them-selves and their families. But like most old stories, it was also more complicated than it first appeared. Latino or Hispanic Americans did not form a single, coherent community, despite the prominence of people of Mexican extraction. Their roots ranged from the southern tip of Chile in South America to the Rio Grande, from the Caribbean islands to the Pacific coast. They were not all in the working class: the first Spanish-speaking people drawn to modern Las Vegas for its economic opportunities were middle-class Cuban refugees from Fidel Castro's 1959 revolution, which eliminated Havana's gambling palaces and put skilled casino operators out of work. Nor were they all immigrants. The area that is now southern Nevada was part of Mexico for more than two centuries after the Pilgrims sailed into Massachusetts Bay in 1620, and many of its current

Latino residents were born in the United States. Latinos represented a large part of the future of Las Vegas, where their numbers more than doubled in the 1990s to constitute 18 percent of the population, and they made up the fastest-growing ethnic group in the United States. Las Vegas was on track to join Miami and Los Angeles as major American cities where Spanish was spoken as commonly as English.

For most of the twentieth century, Nevada seemed to outsiders a distant desert state where the rules that governed most American lives could be bent. Prostitution was legal, as was gambling— "gaming," as industry spokespeople called it—and divorce could be easily obtained. A reputation as a mecca for pleasure tourism drew visitors to Las Vegas, especially with the advent of jet airline service in the 1960s and an expansion of the city's McCarran Airport. With its population more than quadrupling since 1970, the fastest-growing metropolitan area in the nation had one and a half million residents in 2000. Even as the city drew migrants to it, its values seemed to spread outward: a nation that had long condemned gambling as a vice now embraced the gaming business as a partial replacement for declining industrial employment. By 2000, most states had lotteries or some other form of legalized betting, and casinos spread from Atlantic City, New Jersey, to riverboats on the Mississippi River and Indian reservations across the country. The early nickname for Las Vegas—"Sin City"—no longer fit a place that had become a model of the new service economy and the American demographic shift to the Sunbelt of the West and South.

Las Vegas resident and historian Hal Rothman has called his city "the last Detroit." Like the famous hub of the auto industry for earlier generations, Las Vegas offered unskilled but industrious workers an opportunity for real upward mobility. Inexpensive housing and a low cost of living were important, and a mostly unionized work force provided the linchpin, just as it had in Detroit's auto plants. The organized housekeepers and other service employees in the city's vast hotels and casinos, whose large Culinary Workers Union was led in 2000 by an African American woman, Hattie Canty, earned decent wages and crucial benefits, such as health insurance and pension plans that could pull them into the middle class. The traditional American dream of improving one's socioeconomic status through sheer hard work was a more viable option here than in most places in the United States, after three decades of declining real wages for those without a college education and two generations of shrinking union membership.

These economic dreams and successes were built on a slim and imperiled natural resource base, however. Unplanned and largely unregulated urban sprawl spread like an environmental cancer across Las Vegas and surrounding Clark County as roads, housing developments, and shopping malls swallowed thousands

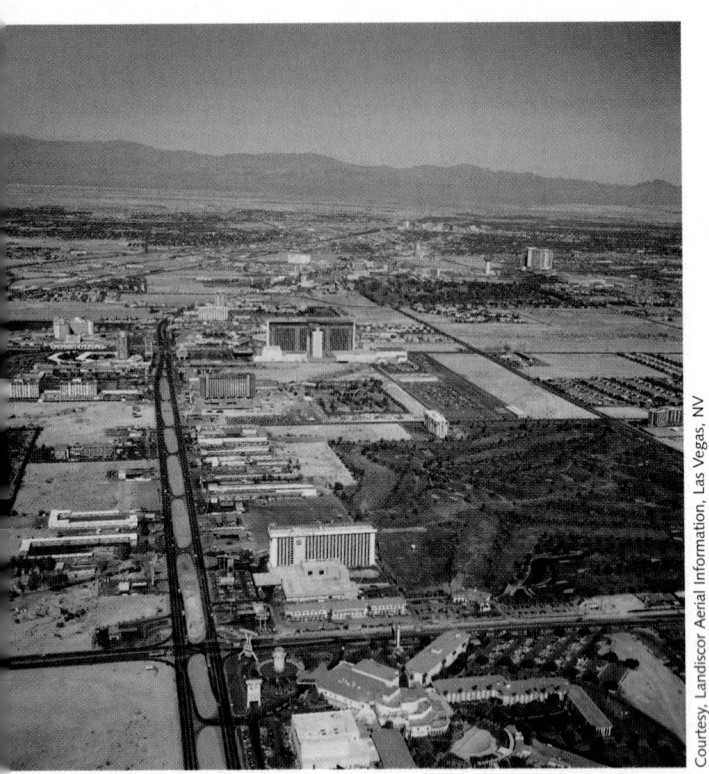

■ Aerial view of Las Vegas, c. 1970.

Courtesy, Landiscor Aerial Information, Las Vegas, NV

of acres of fragile desert landscape, bringing congestion, smog, and other pollutants to a harsh but once pristine climate. Like its spectacular casinos built to resemble New York City or the Egyptian pyramids, Las Vegas was in many ways an artificial city. Everything was imported from elsewhere: people, food, capital, grass, and especially water. Annual rainfall was less than 5 inches, yet vast fountains and swimming pools graced the grounds of the large casinos. Limited in the share of water it could divert from the nearby Colorado River, the city pumped groundwater to quench its growing thirst—the same process that was drying up underground aquifers across much of the arid West. "There is no lack of water here," essayist Edward Abbey warned about the parched Great Basin country of Nevada and Utah, "unless you try to establish a city where no city should be."

In southern Nevada, the four primary themes of this story of the American past come into focus in the present. It remains a story about the distribution of wealth and power, the identities Americans construct for themselves in a multicultural society, the international ties that help shape American life, and the natural environment in which the United States builds its future.

The American Place in a Global Economy

Mollie Brown grew up in the small Virginia town of Cartersville, 45 miles west of Richmond. In 1950, at age 19, she moved to Paterson, New Jersey, joining the broad river of black Southerners who sought better economic opportunities and greater personal freedom in the North. There she married Sam James, another migrant from Virginia who worked at a foundry in Paterson, and together they raised four children. An employed mother like most African American women, Mollie James took a job in 1955 with the Universal Manufacturing Company in Paterson with wages and decent treatment unlike what had been available to her in Virginia. She stayed with Universal for 34 years, becoming its first female union steward and one of its first black union stewards. With union-negotiated wages, overtime work, and company-paid health insurance, she helped pull her family into the middle-class world of owning their own home and car and saving for retirement. But the peace of mind that came from a secure job vanished in 1989 when Universal closed the Paterson plant and moved its manufacturing operations to Matamoros, Mexico, just across the Rio Grande River from Brownsville, Texas.

James's job did not disappear. It moved and was inherited by 20-year-old Balbina Duque Granados. She, too, had grown up in a small town located in an agricultural area, in the Mexican province of San Luis Potosí, and she, too, had moved 400 miles north to find better-paying work in a booming manufacturing city. She was thrilled to land the difficult, repetitive job—her "answered prayer"—at a *maquiladora,* one of the foreign-owned assembly plants along Mexico's border with the United States that wed First World engineering with Third World working conditions. Her employer was also satisfied, paying her $.65/hour to do what James had been paid $7.91/hour for. But Granados's job was no more secure than James's had been. The beginnings of successful worker organizing in Matamoros encouraged the company to shift many of its operations 60 miles upriver to Reynosa, where the union movement was weaker. A journalist asked whether she would move there if her job did. "And what if they were to move again?" she replied. "Maybe to Juarez or Tijuana? What then? Do I have to chase my job all over the world?"

The Logic and Technology of Globalization

Like many other workers in the United States and abroad, Mollie James and Balbina Duque Granados learned first-hand the relentlessly international logic of the economic system known as capitalism. Those who had capital—extra money—invested it in corporations, whose purpose

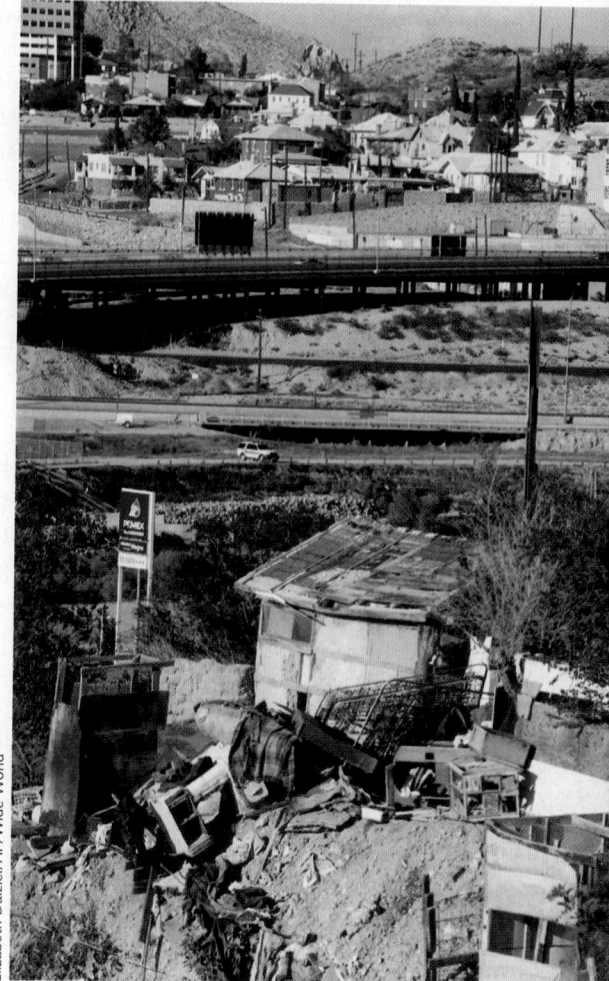

Elizabeth Dalziel/AP/Wide World

■ The U.S.–Mexico border divides a great deal of wealth from stark poverty. Here a shack in Ciudad Juarez contrasts with El Paso in the background. But the border region from Texas to California is also a vibrant economy where the languages and cultures of the two countries mix in fascinating ways.

The Internet and the World Wide Web

For students entering college after the mid-1990s, the Internet and the World Wide Web were an integral part of daily life. Electronic mail (e-mail) made communicating with friends and relatives easy and nearly instantaneous, whether they were on the same college campus or on the other side of the world. The Web transformed the availability of information about nearly all subjects. The foremost symbol of the process of globalization, it linked people everywhere who had access to computers, reducing the importance of a person's geographic location.

The Web had limitations: Internet access remained disproportionately available to people with higher incomes, and there were no controls on the accuracy or usefulness of the information it carried. Risks accompanied

the Web as well, including the dissemination of pornography to children, the emergence of sexual predators via e-mail, and the rise in the theft of personal information. But the Web did connect students and other researchers to vast resources for knowledge that seemed destined to grow indefinitely. For a society and an economy increasingly centered on the management of information, the establishment of the Internet and the Web appeared to mark the beginning of a new era.

Yet the Internet and the Web were only the most recent in a long line of developments in telecommunications linking distant parts of the globe more closely together. In the 1830s, the telegraph first enabled instantaneous communication on the same continent. The first undersea cable laid across the floor of the Atlantic Ocean in 1866 enabled Americans to get news directly from Europe. Ten years later, Alexander Graham Bell added the human voice to the technology of the telegraph by creating the telephone. In 1895, Italian inventor

Guglielmo Marconi freed long-distance communications from the earthly constraints of copper wires by sending the first radio ("wireless") transmission; in 1901, he established the first radio link from North America to Europe. By 1940 the ability to transmit images enabled television broadcasts in the United States and England, and in the 1950s TV became widely popular and available.

The ENIAC computer, built at the University of Pennsylvania in 1945, and its successors were vast machines that filled entire rooms. Altair offered the first microcomputer, or personal computer (PC), as a kit in 1975. Apple followed with the fully assembled Apple I in 1977 and the Macintosh in 1984, the latter initiating the use of a mouse to point and click at items on a screen. The entry of powerful International Business Machines (IBM) into the PC market in 1981 marked the movement of computers into the mainstream of American society.

The search by the U.S. Department of Defense for a communication net-

was to produce a profit for their shareholders. A corporation's profitability depended on keeping costs—labor and materials—down and expanding into new markets. Those markets were not limited by nationality; a manufacturer tried to sell not just to Americans but to customers wherever they might be found. The technological innovations facilitating the integration of the U.S. economy into the world economy in the late 1900s were not so much a new force as an acceleration of an older trend. Just as the telegraph and telephone had helped create a nation unified by rapid communication, the spread of personal computers and the Internet linked Americans even more closely to other nations. In the 1920s, the head of General Electric, Owen Young, spoke of his ambition to "obliterate the eastern, western, northern and southern boundaries of the United States," for "the sphere of our activities is the world." Capitalists were rarely nationalists but rather internationalists.

At the close of the twentieth century, engineering breakthroughs sped up the process of globalization. Bill Gates of Seattle became the world's wealthiest person in the 1990s, with assets at one point worth $100 billion as the company he headed, Microsoft, provided the software for operating most personal computers. At just 34 years old, Michael Dell of Austin leapt to fifth place on the list of wealthiest Americans in 1999 by selling computers through a mail-order business, Dell Computers. The integration of computers into every aspect of commerce and private life increased the efficiency with which businesses could operate. Retailers, for example, could monitor their inventory much more closely and eliminate unnecessary expenses. The dependence of the entire infrastructure of modern American life on computers generated fears

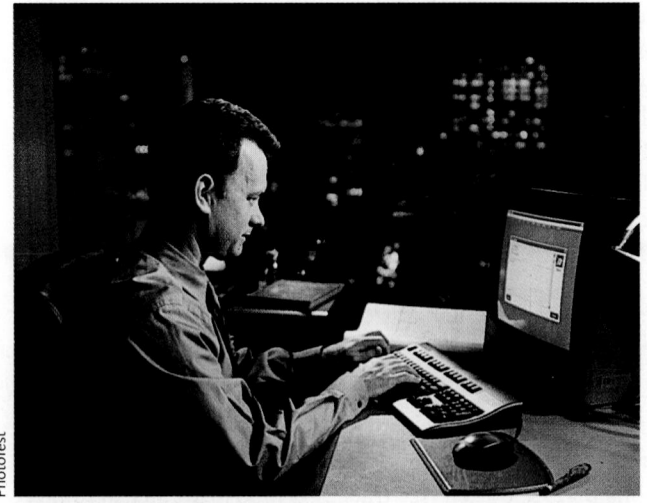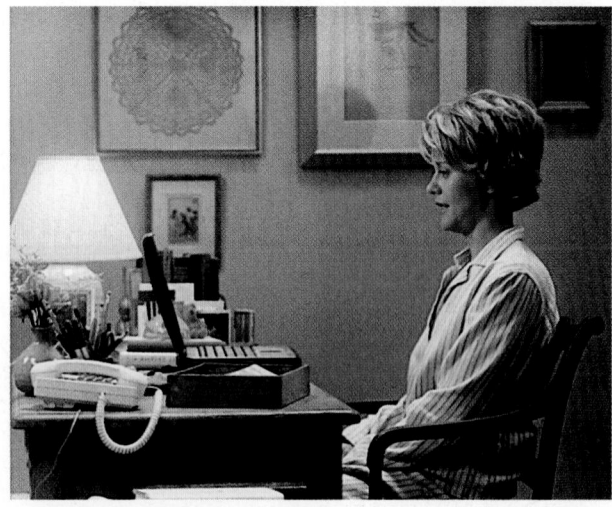

The popular 1998 film *You've Got Mail* starred Tom Hanks and Meg Ryan as bitter New York business rivals by day who unknowingly fall in love through an anonymous computer chat room. Since the mid-1990s, e-mail provided a quick and convenient form of communication that fell somewhere between a telephone call and a traditional letter. Many American workers found that the efficiency of e-mail was somewhat offset by the need to spend more time reading and sending it.

work invulnerable to nuclear attack led to the creation of ARPANET in 1969, a forerunner of the Internet, which began to function in 1983. These systems transmitted only text—words—between computers that were connected to each other by telephone links. In 1990, software researchers created the World Wide Web, which used the Internet to send graphic and multimedia information as well as text. Audio and visual capacity now joined words on the growing web of connected networks. In 1993, the White House joined the rush of users establishing sites on the Web, and by 1995, public access to the World Wide Web was widely available in the United States. ■

that aging software might be unable to handle the "Y2K" (year 2000) problem of changing more than two digits from 1999 to 2000, but the first hours of the new year came and went without incident. Computers boosted American productivity (the amount of work performed by a person in a given time period), which had declined between 1973 and 1996, and the U.S. economy enjoyed its longest-ever expansion during the presidency of Bill Clinton. Americans were plugged in: since the 1980s the spread of cable television and videocassette recorders (VCRs) provided constant entertainment, and Cable News Network (CNN) offered a standardized package of world news available 24 hours a day around the globe. Atlanta-based CNN was so international in its aims that its founder, Ted Turner, banned the word *foreign* from its broadcasts.

Americans were also speeding up their daily routines as the new millennium approached. The desire for immediate gratification and efficiency that had nurtured fast food and microwave ovens encouraged the spread of cell phones, beepers, fax machines, overnight package delivery, and constant news headlines scrolling across TV screens. Computers processed more information faster on ever-smaller silicon chips. Cell phones proliferated among businesspeople, students, and drivers. As prices dropped, they even reached into poorer areas, such as the vast Navajo nation on the Arizona–New Mexico border, where traditional phones were scarce. International air travel for business and pleasure quadrupled between 1980 and 1998, and international tourism vied with oil as the world's largest industry. The spread of the Internet and the use of electronic mail (e-mail) after the early 1990s best represented the shift toward

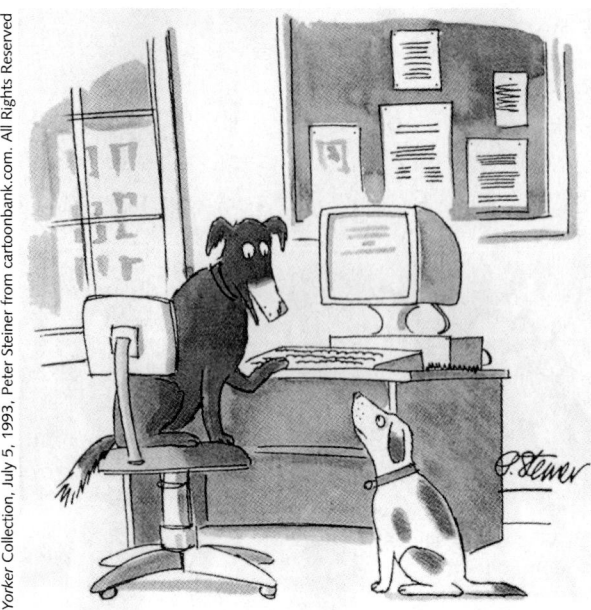

"On the Internet, nobody knows you're a dog."

■ The Internet provided both immediate connections with other people around the world and the safety of personal anonymity. Internet users could not be judged by their appearance or material possessions, only by the words they typed. Americans debated whether the popularity of the Internet represented a new kind of virtual community that would strengthen their connections to each other or merely another way for citizens to remain isolated in their own homes rather than engaged with each other in civic organizations.

instant global communication. Though still in its infancy, the Internet was already shaping patterns of personal and commercial interactions, even as access to the Internet remained disproportionately available to those with greater wealth and education. Just as the Berlin Wall had long symbolized the divided world of the Cold War, the Internet became the emblem of the post–Cold War era of an increasingly unified global economy.

Free Trade and the Global Assembly Line

The ideology of free trade underpinned the tighter meshing of Americans' lives with the world economy. Free trade meant the reduction of tariffs, or taxes on imported and exported goods. Nations that supported free trade had industries that were eager to expand and were strong enough to compete successfully in a global market; nations with less competitive industries used tariffs to protect those industries from less expensive and higher-quality imports. As a new nation in the late 1700s and 1800s, the United States had enacted high tariffs to protect its domestic producers, but England, the world's leading economic power at the time, had sought to reduce tariffs and increase trade with America. When the United States emerged after World War II as the new leading economic nation and U.S. manufacturers and farmers looked increasingly to foreign markets, U.S. tariff rates plummeted. From averages of 30–50 percent before 1945, they dropped to 5 percent by 1990. The minimal tariffs associated with most-favored-nation status became standard for almost all U.S. trading partners. In 1965, the sum of all exports and imports amounted to 10 percent of the U.S. gross national product (GNP); by 1990, it had surpassed 25 percent and continued to climb.

Advocates of free trade argued that global markets unhindered by national tariffs benefited consumers everywhere by giving them access to the best goods at the lowest prices. America's NAFTA treaty with Canada and Mexico reflected this belief (see Chapter 29), as did the European Union with its newly unified currency, the Euro. In the United States, by the start of the new millennium most leaders of both major political parties, corporate executives, bankers, and most other elites supported free trade. But others objected to this internationalist economic ideology. Post-1945 British leaders, sensitive to their country's decline relative to American power, called the U.S. promotion of free trade "freedom of American trade" to emphasize that greater international exchanges of goods disproportionately benefit the more powerful of the trading partners. Larger, more efficient manufacturers could undersell smaller, more labor-intensive local producers. By 2000, environmentalists and labor unions led the forces opposing unregulated globalization of the U.S. economy. Environmentalists warned of the pollution costs to the world's environment of U.S. factories relocating to poorer and less regulated nations, such as Mexico and China. Labor organizers decried the flight of American jobs as manufacturers sought less expensive and more compliant—often desperate—workers abroad. Human rights activists spotlighted the grim working conditions in many overseas plants, including the prevalence of child labor. In 1999, in Seattle, and in 2001, in Genoa, Italy, thousands of antiglobalization protesters disrupted meetings of the World Trade Organization and the leaders of the largest industrialized nations.

A "race to the bottom" for labor and environmental standards resulted from the development of a global assembly line. With capital able to move swiftly around the world and take its factories with it, nations and localities felt that they had little choice but to compete in offering multinational corporations the most advantageous terms possible. Such terms meant minimal government regulation, little protection for workers, nonexistent pollution standards, and even local subsidies in place of corporate taxes. Just as in the 1890s, industries had formed national trusts to evade state regulations on commerce, a century later, multinational corporations escaped the reach of national governments. This trend also represented an extension of the same logic that created the American Sunbelt over the previous half-century: businesses from the Northeast and Midwest relocating to states (that happened to be warmer) with lower wage rates, fewer unions, weaker environmental standards, and minimal taxes. Corporate income taxes, which had been dropping since the 1950s, shrank by another third between 1986 and 2000. The *maquiladoras* on the Mexican border were part of a broader pattern of the corporate search for efficiency and profit, as companies, like Mollie James's Universal Manufacturing Company and RCA, took their production lines first to the American South and then abroad.

As a result, corporations and their products became less identifiable by nationality. Boeing Aircraft had long been the largest employer in the Seattle area, but was its new Boeing 777, manufactured piece by piece in 12 different countries, an "American" airplane? Japanese companies also moved many manufacturing plants overseas, including to the United States, to be closer to important markets. Was a Toyota made by American workers in Georgetown, Kentucky, a "foreign" car? A worker sewing the "American" company label on a trendy piece of clothing might be in Malaysia or Taiwan. Or she might be a Mexican American working in a southern California garment factory—and have a sister across the border in Mexico sewing for the same company at still lower wages. In an age of globalization and international commerce, insistence on purity of product lineage—"Buy American" campaigns—seemed to make little more sense than discredited notions of "racial purity."

> *Was a Toyota made by American workers in Georgetown, Kentucky, a "foreign" car?*

Who Benefits from Globalization?

The increasing globalization of the U.S. economy at the end of the twentieth century created enormous wealth while sharpening class inequalities. The stock market skyrocketed. The Dow Jones average of the value of 30 top companies' stocks rose steadily from 500 in 1956, to 1000 in 1972, and to 3000 in 1991. Then it more than tripled in value in just eight years, surpassing 10,000 in 1999. Wealthy Americans who owned the bulk of corporate stock reaped the most gain, but middle- and even working-class Americans with retirement funds invested in the market also benefited handsomely. However, the process of globalization and the steady expansion of the U.S. economy after 1992 also encouraged a growing belief among Americans, especially affluent ones, that markets alone offered the best solution to social problems. For example, more Americans believed that welfare recipients should be forced to find work in the job market to regain independence and pride. Only the unfettered laws of supply and demand could sustain prosperity, many believed, and government regulation—already gravely weakened by capital's ability to move across national borders—should be kept to a bare minimum. But markets and their strict dependence on the profit motive proved unable to preserve the quality of the environment, to pull the 36 million officially poor Americans above the poverty line ($17,000 for a family of four in 1999), or to preserve the security of the vast middle class that had stabilized American politics since World War II. Inequalities within the United States reflected growing global inequality as 20 percent of the world's people (mostly in Europe and North America) consumed 86 percent of its goods and services. The $8 billion Americans spent annually on cosmetics, for example, could instead provide running water and sanitation for almost all of the 2 billion people worldwide who lack these basic amenities.

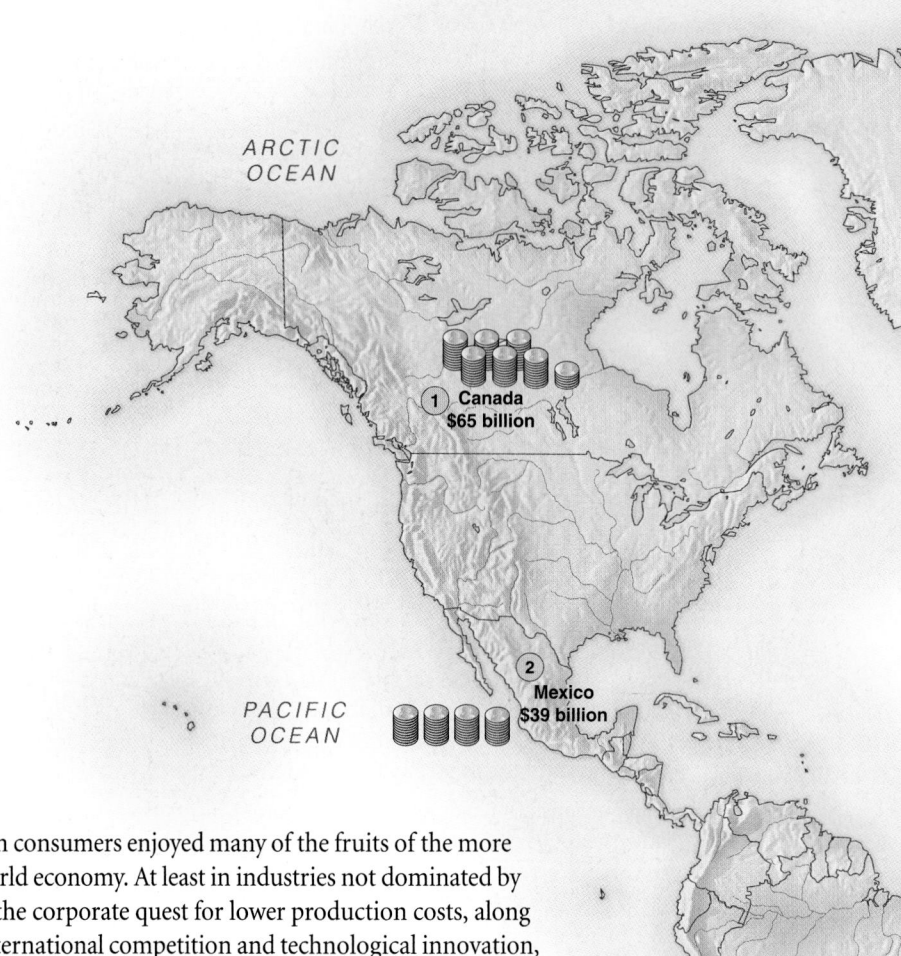

■ **MAP 30.1**

TOP TEN U.S. TRADING PARTNERS (RANKED, WITH TOTAL VALUE OF IMPORTS AND EXPORTS COMBINED FOR JANUARY–FEBRUARY 2001)
Americans do the most business with Canada and Mexico, followed by east Asia and then western Europe. U.S. economic vitality has always depended to some extent on foreign trade, but that dependence grew steadily in the past generation.

American consumers enjoyed many of the fruits of the more integrated world economy. At least in industries not dominated by monopolies, the corporate quest for lower production costs, along with fierce international competition and technological innovation, reduced prices of many goods and services. Computers, airline travel, and gasoline were all significantly less expensive in real dollars (adjusted for inflation) than they had been a generation earlier. Competition abounded in the robust retail sector of the U.S. economy, including catalog and Internet shopping. Wal-Mart represented the epitome of how the globalized economy could benefit consumers. By 2000, the discount store that Sam Walton had opened in Arkansas in 1962 surpassed General Motors as the largest American company, responsible for 6 percent of all U.S. retail sales. It sold 20,000 pairs of shoes an hour. Wal-Mart's success resulted from relentlessly cutting costs through sharp management, using cheaper imported goods and employing a nonunion workforce, and passing its savings along to customers in the form of lower prices. In towns across the United States, Wal-Mart put smaller local competitors out of business, and its efficiency became the standard to which other retailers aspired.

The benefits that the working-class majority of Americans experienced as consumers in the global economy were offset by their declining status as workers. As manufacturers moved to the Sunbelt and then overseas, high-wage, unionized jobs providing health insurance and pension benefits disappeared. Average real wages declined steadily after 1973, and union membership slid from one-third of the workforce in the early 1950s to one-tenth in 2000. Family incomes were maintained only by the addition of second and third wage earners, especially women. Americans spent more than they earned. The average household had 11 credit cards and carried $7000 in debt on them, in addition to owing car and home mortgage payments. In a nation of debtors, more than 1 million citizens filed for bankruptcy each year. A growing divide separated the experiences of well-educated Americans, who were able to seize

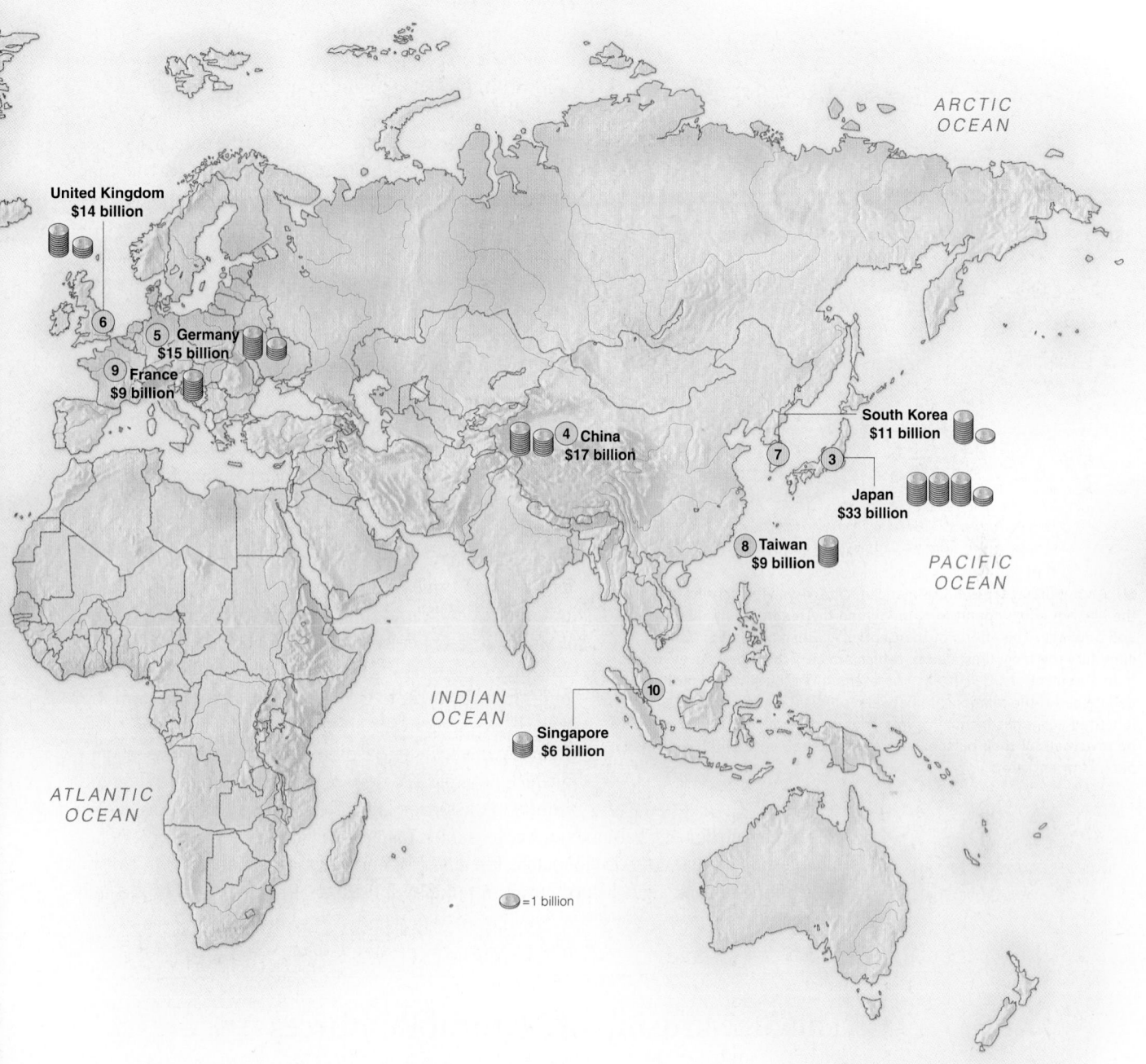

United Kingdom
$14 billion

6

5 Germany
$15 billion

9 France
$9 billion

4 China
$17 billion

South Korea
$11 billion

7

3

Japan
$33 billion

8 Taiwan
$9 billion

10

Singapore
$6 billion

ARCTIC OCEAN

PACIFIC OCEAN

INDIAN OCEAN

ATLANTIC OCEAN

= 1 billion

opportunities in the new economy involving high technology and information management, and their fellow citizens with at most a high school education.

Already wider in the United States than in any other industrialized nation, the distance between rich and poor continued to grow, whittling away at Americans' self-image as a middle-class society. The share of the national income going to the richest 1 percent nearly doubled in the last quarter of the twentieth century, while the share going to the bottom 80 percent shrank. Three million Americans lived in gated communities in extremely affluent suburbs, but one of five American children grew up in poverty and 21 million citizens sought emergency food assistance each year. One of the nation's leading newspapers unknowingly captured this disparity with two articles a few pages apart, headlined "As Closets Bulge, Americans' Taste in Gifts Often Turns Toward the Taste Buds" and "Food Drives Find Cupboard Is Nearly Bare."

The political system, which helps determine how wealth and opportunity are distributed in a society, seemed to offer little respite from the widening gap between haves and

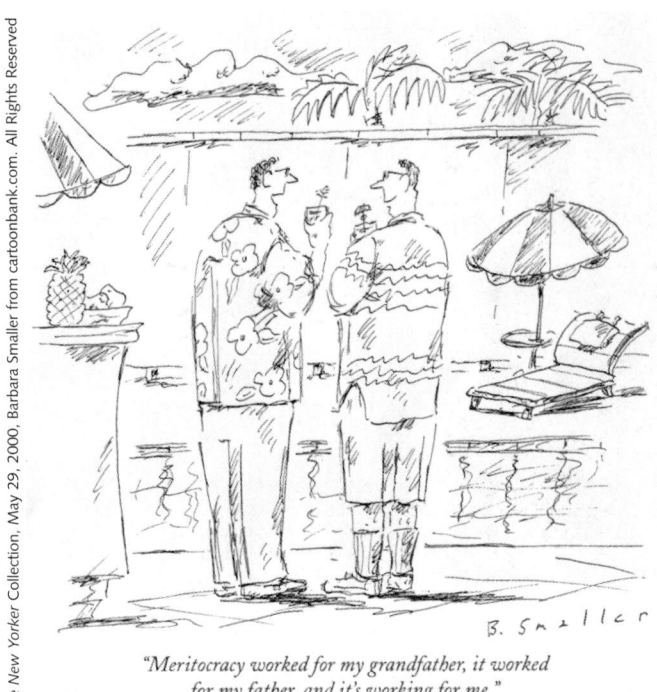

"Meritocracy worked for my grandfather, it worked for my father, and it's working for me."

■ An important tension in American history was the conflict between the ideal of equal opportunity for all and the reality of inherited wealth and privilege. The efforts of the George W. Bush administration to eliminate the federal estate tax, which affected the inheritances of less than 1 percent of U.S. citizens, represented the latest round in the debate about the relationship between political democracy and inherited economic inequality. In a pure meritocracy, all citizens would be rewarded for their personal achievements rather than those of their parents or ancestors.

have-nots. The fraction of eligible citizens who make the effort to vote in presidential elections declined to just half in 2000 and in off-year congressional elections to a mere third, with the likelihood of voting closely correlated to a person's affluence. The hardships of daily survival deterred some potential voters, especially among the poor. The fierce partisanship, personal attacks, and culture of scandal that came to dominate American politics in the past two decades alienated others. Some saw little difference between the two major parties during the Clinton presidency, as many Democrats moved closer to Republicans on such issues as welfare, crime, and the budget.

Many citizens were also disillusioned by the blatant manner in which money came to dominate the political process. In the 1990s, President Bill Clinton regularly invited large contributors to the Democratic party to spend a night in the Lincoln Bedroom of the White House. Able to raise millions of dollars, George W. Bush declined federal funding for his 2000 presidential campaign to avoid the spending limits that accompanied such aid. With the average cost of a successful Senate campaign at $5 million and a House campaign approaching $1 million, few but the wealthy could campaign for Congress, and elected members spent inordinate amounts of time raising money from wealthy donors. Democratic Senator Richard Durbin of Illinois admitted that the system of fund-raising is corrupting: "It forces you into compromising yourself." Republican Senator John McCain of Arizona called campaign financing "an elaborate influence-peddling scheme in which both parties conspire to stay in office by selling the country to the highest bidder." For average Americans, exclusive fundraising dinners that sometimes reaped more than $30 million signaled a kind of political access they could not hope to match. The ability of business to outspend labor 15 to 1 in contributing to campaigns helped ensure minimal publicity to any discussions of the gulf between rich and poor.

The Stewardship of Natural Resources

No issue was more global than the environment. Winds and waters did not respect political boundaries, nor did the materials borne on them. The condition of the natural environment affected all living creatures, yet the prevailing calculus of the market and private ownership did not apportion responsibility for its care. The free market system had no mechanism for offsetting, or even measuring, the costs of depleted natural resources. A generation ago, biologist Garrett Hardin had warned of the tragedy of the commons: that individuals' incentives to preserve the quality of their own property did not carry over to resources held in common. The pursuit of narrow self-interest too often resulted in the spoiling of common grounds, such as parks and national forests. Litter was an obvious example, and air, water, and ground pollution were the more serious cases. American culture had long celebrated human domination of the natural world and the benefits it brought, especially the growth in productivity that permitted living standards to rise dramatically across decades and centuries. At the same time, the rise of environmentalism and ecological understanding since 1960 offered a different way of imagining people's place on the earth. A tension existed between exploiting finite natural resources to create wealth and managing them for long-term sustainability. This dilema reached an acute stage by the turn of the new millennium.

Ecological Transformation in the Twentieth Century

Ecosystems are always dynamic, and changes in weather and Native American land use had reshaped the North American environment long before the followers of Christopher Columbus arrived on the continent. But European settlement and industrialization altered the face of the land in ways that would dumbfound a time traveler from the 1500s. Even a visitor from 1900 would be astonished by the intensity of human development of the land: vast cities with their sprawling suburbs and roads and highways everywhere. The key factor was population growth. Just as the number of people in the world quadrupled from 1.5 billion to 6 billion during the twentieth century, the population of the United States almost quadrupled from 75 million to 281 million, with the largest increase for a single decade (33 million) coming in the 1990s. Immigration and natural reproduction accounted for much of this, but so did the much-longer average lifespan ushered in by antibiotics and antiviral vaccines, which sharply diminished the often fatal impact of infectious diseases and allowed noncommunicable maladies, such as cancer and heart disease, to become leading causes of death instead. The various drug-resistant bacteria that began to develop by the 1970s and the emergence of HIV infection and AIDS in the United States by 1980 brought an end to the brief post-1945 golden age of disease containment, locking researchers into a seemingly permanent arms race against virulent microbes. HIV's apparent origins in central Africa suggested the problems of easy introduction of exotic species in an age of frequent international travel.

The most dramatic changes in the land in the twentieth century resulted from the exploitation of wood, minerals, and water, particularly in the majority of the country lying west of the Mississippi River. Commercial logging destroyed all but 3 percent of the old-growth forests of the 50 states, both on private lands and on lands managed by the U.S. Forest Service, which as part of the Department of Agriculture traditionally emphasized the harvesting of wood products. The clearcuts scarring the mountainsides and hillsides of the Pacific Northwest and Alaska told the tale, as did the erosion caused by the overgrazing by cattle of public lands managed by the Interior Department's Bureau of Land Management in Utah, New Mexico, and other western states. The Mining Act of 1872 still granted to private corporations the rights to such valuable minerals as gold and copper on public land for the remarkable nineteenth-century price of $2.50 per acre. Mining companies took full advantage of the opportunity, and resulting rock and chemical wastes piled in vast slagheaps and dumped in toxic holding ponds from Arizona to Montana. In the arid but increasingly populated western states, water was the most critical resource for population growth. The U.S. Army Corps of Engineers and the Bureau of Reclamation built huge dams from the 1930s to the 1980s, providing irrigation, flood control, and hydropower but also destroying wild rivers and causing silt to begin filling up the reservoirs. Increasing diversions of the Rio Grande left that now misnamed river so dry that, by 2001, it failed to reach the Gulf of Mexico, trickling to a halt 50 feet short. Groundwater pumping for agricultural irrigation in the plains

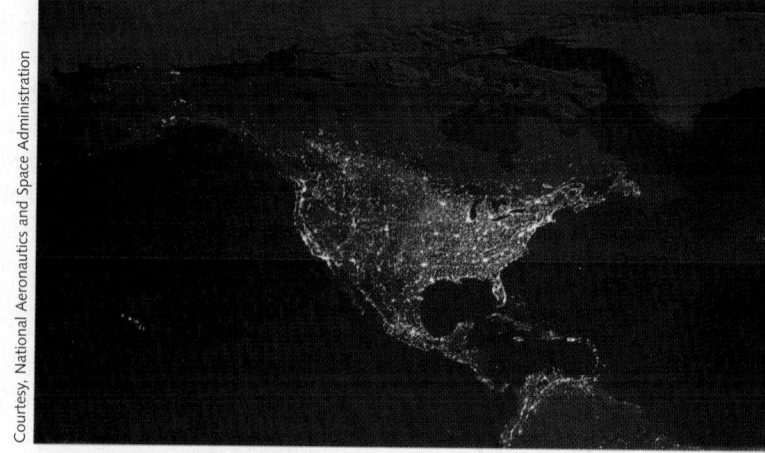

Courtesy, National Aeronautics and Space Administration

■ A nighttime photograph taken from a satellite above the south Pacific Ocean reveals the use of electricity in North America. Only Alaska and some parts of the inland western states (Nevada, Idaho, eastern Oregon) appear mostly unlit. The growth of the Sunbelt states of the South and West after 1970 was dramatic, but the bulk of the U.S. population remained east of the Mississippi River, especially in the Northeast and Midwest. The demand for electrical power even with most citizens in bed was enormous.

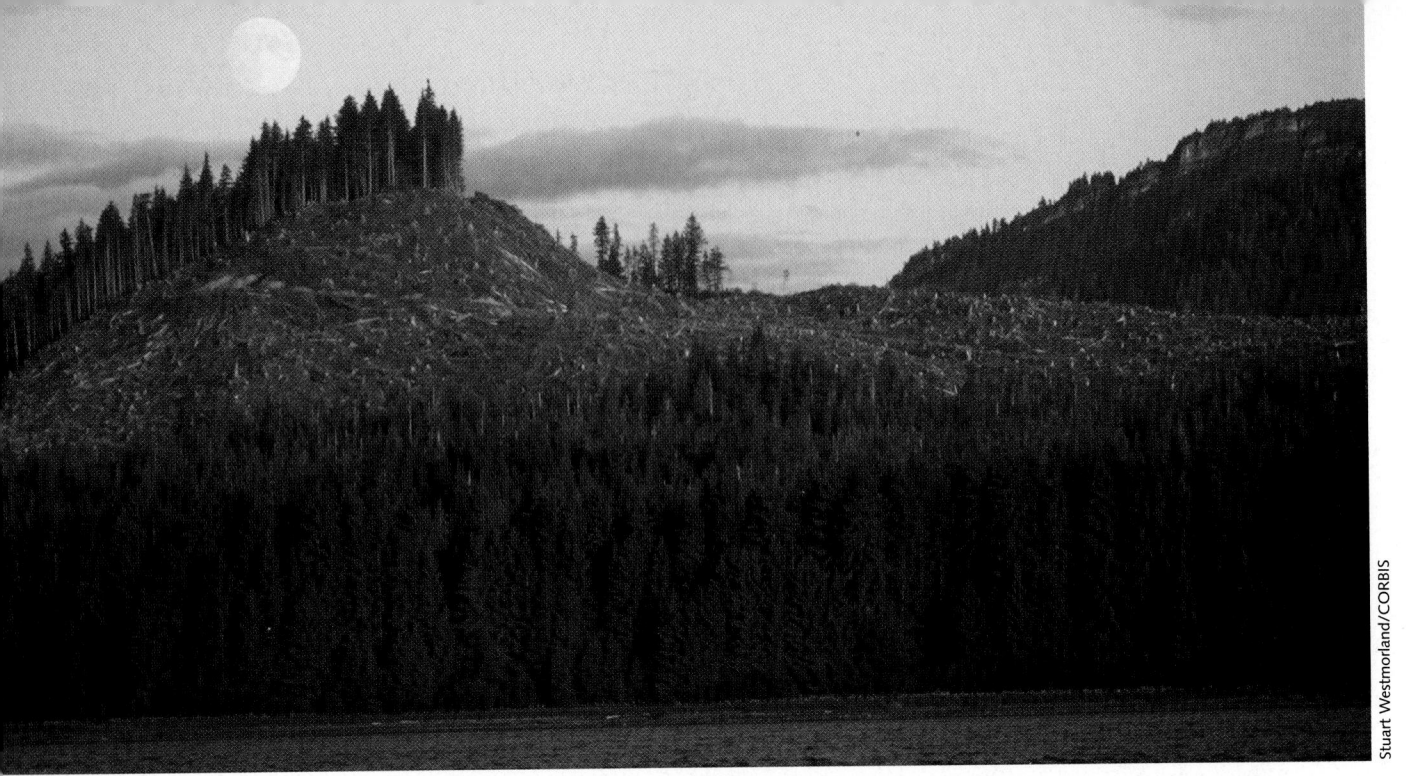

■ Clearcutting scars mountainsides on both private and public lands, especially in the Pacific Northwest and here on Kupreanof Island in the Tongass National Forest of southeastern Alaska. Clearcutting is a more efficient method of timber harvesting than selective tree thinning, but it encourages soil erosion, mudslides, and flooding.

states and on the eastern slope of the Rocky Mountains was draining the vast underground Ogallala Aquifer at a rate that will empty it within a few more decades.

American prosperity came at a price. The prodigious growth of the U.S. economy in the twentieth century depended on the consumption of ever-increasing amounts of energy. Some came from renewable sources, such as hydropower and nuclear power and smaller amounts from solar and wind power, but the bulk of the nation's energy was derived from coal, oil, and natural gas. Though making up less than 5 percent of the world's population, Americans accounted for a quarter of the globe's energy consumption. They depended on other countries to provide much of it for them: the United States imported 22 percent of its total energy needs and 69 percent of its oil, primarily from Saudi Arabia, Venezuela, Canada, and Mexico. Fossil fuels, such as coal and oil, could not be renewed; once burned, they were gone, and the world had a finite supply of such fuels. Americans' unquenchable thirst for gasoline and electricity helped them build history's largest and richest industrial economy, but they did so by constructing a lifestyle that was unsustainable in the long run. The energy crisis that began in California in early 2001 after the state ended its regulation of electricity production, and the rolling blackouts it caused, suggested that the long run might come sooner than expected.

Pollution

The world's growing population was consuming five times as much fossil fuel in 2000 as in 1950, helping to stimulate a steady rise in the earth's average temperatures. Americans caused 36 percent of such carbon-based emissions, the largest contribution to the foremost environmental problem, global warming. The release of large amounts of carbon dioxide from burning coal, oil, and other fossil fuels helped trap extra heat within the earth's atmosphere—the greenhouse effect—and melt ice in high-altitude and polar regions. In the summer of 2000, startled scientists found open water at the North Pole, a sight humans had never before seen. Greenhouse gases also contributed to a thinning of the ozone layer of the atmosphere, which

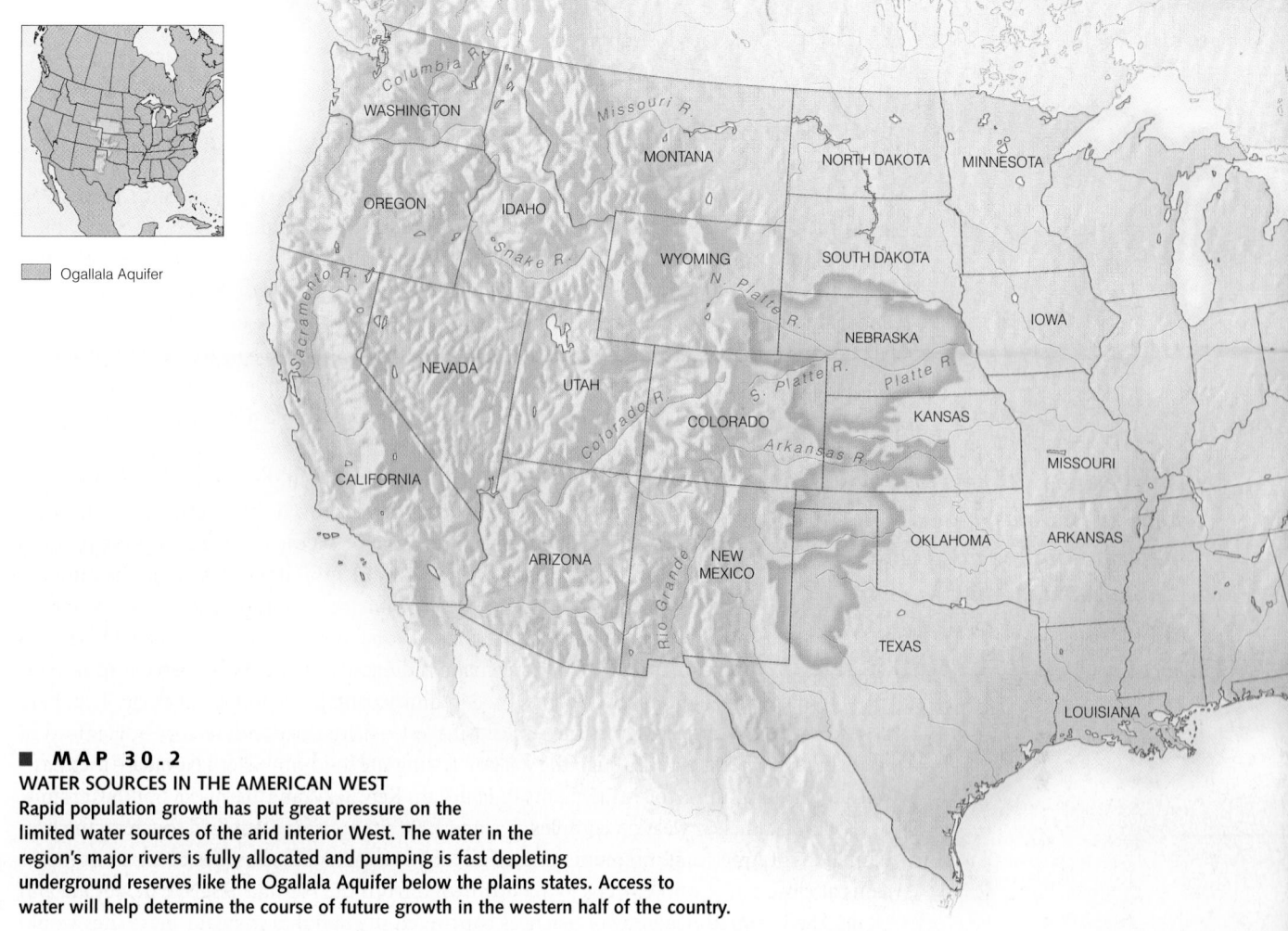

■ **MAP 30.2**

WATER SOURCES IN THE AMERICAN WEST
Rapid population growth has put great pressure on the
limited water sources of the arid interior West. The water in the
region's major rivers is fully allocated and pumping is fast depleting
underground reserves like the Ogallala Aquifer below the plains states. Access to
water will help determine the course of future growth in the western half of the country.

enabled more of the sun's ultraviolet rays to reach the earth's surface. As a result, skin cancer rates soared, particularly in the Southern Hemisphere, where the ozone hole was largest.

Industrial manufacturing still figured importantly in the human assault on the air and the atmosphere, but the internal combustion engine had long since surpassed coal burning as the leading cause of pollution. The United States produced and used more cars and trucks than any other nation. The automobile and its symbolism of convenience and personal freedom defined much of American culture, and citizens who could not drive or did not have access to a car were at a real disadvantage in a nation of freeways, shopping malls, and suburban housing. With minimal public transportation outside a handful of major cities, Americans were deeply committed to a car-dependent lifestyle. As a price, they quietly accepted an annual death toll of more than 40,000 people from accidents on the road, two-thirds the number each year of all U.S. deaths in the Vietnam War. The highway infrastructure strained under the pressure of a 60 percent rise in the number of licensed drivers from 1970 to 2000 but only a 6 percent growth in total miles of roads. Negotiating traffic jams became a standard part of the daily lives of the majority of Americans who lived in the suburbs created by urban sprawl, especially around such cities as Los Angeles and Atlanta. Citizens spent three times as many hours stalled in traffic in 1999 as they did in 1982. Smog increasingly obscured the once-sublime vistas of Arizona's Grand Canyon. Yosemite National Park in the Sierra Nevada mountains of California, a spectacular natural wonder drawing millions of visitors each year in the nation's most populous state, embodied the problems of an automotive society. Thousands of cars jammed Yosemite Valley every day, making it an almost urban setting with air quality on the verge of violating federal standards. Yet park managers' efforts to limit car access to the valley were repeatedly defeated by popular opposition.

Daily life in the United States came to depend in countless ways on the use of synthetic chemicals, production of which was 350 times greater in 1982 than in 1940. Only 3 percent of the 75,000 new chemicals had been tested for safety, but 40 of those examined proved to be human carcinogens. More than 50,000 known toxic waste dumps in the United States leached poisonous chemicals and heavy metals into the soil and water, such as the polychlorinated biphenyls that lined the bottom of the Hudson River north of Albany and the arsenic and cadmium that clogged the Milltown Dam on Montana's scenic Clark Fork River 6 miles upstream from Missoula. Cancer rates among Americans grew sharply in the twentieth century, partly because people lived significantly longer lives (giving more time for cancers to appear) and partly because they were exposed to a much larger array of carcinogenic materials in the environment.

No one knew yet how to dispose safely of millions of tons of materials impregnated with plutonium and other human-made radioactive elements.

No synthetic product was more pervasive in the United States than plastic, a post-1945 product made from petroleum. Its prevalence and extraordinary durability helped it become a major factor in loading up the nation's landfills. But the most deadly and durable pollutants remained the radioactive wastes created by five decades of nuclear development. No one knew yet how to dispose safely of millions of tons of materials impregnated with plutonium and other human-made radioactive elements, 30 percent of it casually poured into dirt or stored in flimsy containers prone to leakage. The chain of nuclear poison arched across the American West—from the bomb factory at Hanford in south central Washington through the weapon testing site in southwestern Nevada—then eastward to the uranium-processing plants in Paducah, Kentucky, and Barnwell, South Carolina.

The U.S. nuclear weapon complex of some 3000 sites put its often fatal touch on the lives of millions of Americans: uranium miners, military workers, soldiers used to observe test explosions at close range, and citizens living downwind from the Nevada Test Site in Nevada and Utah. The National Academy of Sciences concluded in 2000 that many of these sites would be permanent national sacrifice zones, toxic to humans for at least tens of thousands of years. The dissolution of the Soviet Union in 1991 relaxed some of the secrecy surrounding nuclear weapons on both sides. In 1993, the U.S. Department of Energy admitted that it had conducted radiation experiments for years on largely unsuspecting populations, both in the United States and on remote Pacific islands where some early nuclear bombs were tested. Russian sources revealed that Soviet leaders had been even more cavalier in their handling of nuclear wastes, simply dumping many of them in the Arctic Ocean. The environmental costs to Americans and others of the Cold War are yet to be fully calculated.

Environmentalism and Its Limitations

The ideas of most Americans about how to manage natural resources changed in the twentieth century. Environmental consciousness blossomed since the 1960s, rediscovering a tradition that linked eighteenth-century naturalist William Bartram with nineteenth-century transcendentalist Henry David Thoreau and twentieth-century conservationists of both major political parties. Awareness of humans' connections with their broader ecological context led to significant reforms, such as the banning of carcinogenic pesticides and leaded gasoline, the cleaning up of polluted water in the Great Lakes, and the introduction of catalytic converters to reduce harmful emissions from automobile exhaust pipes and factory smokestacks. Recycling became common, and some dams were destroyed, freeing long-constricted rivers, such as the Penobscot in Maine. Yet issues of public land management and pollution control remained among the most controversial problems in American public life. Since 1980, the Republican party has supported the exploitation of natural resources to produce wealth and raise standards of living, departing at least in tone from the party's earlier conservationist bent.

Meanwhile, the Democratic party became associated with environmental protection. This contrast was dramatically displayed in January 2001 when President Clinton rushed to provide new protections to a swath of federal lands in the West before his term ended, while president-elect George W. Bush was appointing as secretary of the interior Colorado attorney Gale Norton, who strongly opposed such protections. Both Bush and his vice president, Dick Cheney, had personal ties to the energy idustry, and their administration promoted new oil and gas drilling in wilderness locations that included Alaska's Arctic National Wildlife Refuge.

Beyond partisan differences and the broad tendency of even the most well-known corporate polluters to pose as friendly to the environment, the relationship of Americans to their natural environment continued to be paradoxical. By large majorities in public opinion polls, they supported strong antipollution laws and the preservation of public lands from economic development. They flocked to such films as *Erin Brockovich* and *A Civil Action,* in which average citizens and lawyers won court cases against large corporate polluters. And they no longer agreed with the slogan common in Houston in the 1960s about the odoriferous smog created by the booming city's petrochemical industries and cars: "Smell that—that's prosperity."

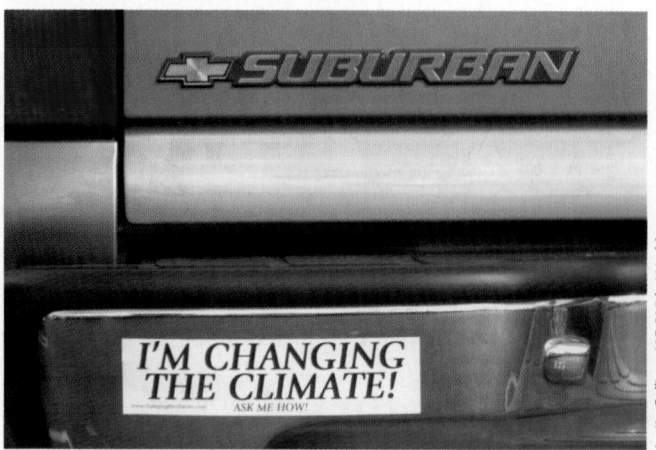

The oil crises of the 1970s led automobile manufacturers to improve the efficiency of gas mileage in their cars. By the 1990s, however, gasoline was once again inexpensive and growing numbers of Americans were buying large new sport utility vehicles (SUVs) such as the Chevrolet Suburban, despite their low gas mileage. A few environmentalists placed bumper stickers on other people's SUVs to highlight the key role of auto emissions in the accelerating process of global warming.

But in their daily lives, Americans consumed natural resources, especially gasoline, electricity, and water, at a rate unmatched by other societies. Measures that had reduced some of the nation's energy consumption since the 1970s were reversed by 2000: Congress revoked the national 55-mph speed limit in 1995, and ever-larger cars, trucks, and especially sport utility vehicles steadily reduced the average gas mileage of passenger vehicles. While scientists and some utilities urged a reduction in the nation's expanding use of fossil fuels, Vice President Cheney dismissed conservation as merely "a sign of personal virtue" rather than a basis for a sound energy policy. Many residents across the arid Southwest, most of them newcomers, remained determined to recreate the green lawns they had left behind in the East and Midwest. When an investigator for the Las Vegas city water district confronted one resident about his wasteful sprinkler, the man responded, "Man, with all these new rules, you people are trying to turn this place into a desert."

The Expansion of American Popular Culture Abroad

Just as the U.S. economy and American environmental problems could not be separated from the outside world, the nation's cultural life grew more closely tied to that of other nations at the dawn of the new millennium. During the Cold War, from the 1940s through the 1980s, American foreign relations hinged on problems of national security and the projection of military might abroad. The dissolution of the Soviet Union in 1991 and the retreat of communism ended the bipolar division of the world and left the United States the sole remaining superpower. But by 2000, American popular culture rather than armed strength had emerged as the leading edge of U.S. influence around the world.

Over the first half of the twentieth century, the United States slowly replaced Great Britain as the dominant force in international affairs. The economic and military aspects of this shift of influence were clear by the end of World War II, and its cultural elements soon followed. American power extended the preeminence of English as the global language of commerce and diplomacy, and ambitious and privileged youth from beyond Europe aimed no longer for an education at England's Oxford and Cambridge but rather at prestigious U.S. universities. American culture had become less regionally distinctive and more nationally homogeneous in the twentieth century because of improvements in transportation and communication. By the end of the century, this same process of homogenization of popular consumer culture was at work on a worldwide scale. American themes and products stood out in an increasingly global popular culture, although they were resisted by some abroad who preferred more local identities and traditions, often rooted in ethnicity or religious conviction.

A Culture of Diversity and Entertainment

Known for its informality and diversity, American culture proved powerfully attractive to peoples all over the world, partly because racial and ethnic diversity was more pronounced in the United States than in any other major power. African Americans, Latino Americans, and Asian Americans all figured prominently in the popular realms of sports, music, and films. Television was the leading medium for this culture of entertainment, beaming CNN, MTV, and "reality" shows, such as *Survivor,* around the world. From jazz to rock 'n' roll to rap, American popular music spread across the globe, as did such clothing of American youth as jeans and sneakers, symbols of informality and comfort. Hollywood's movies dominated cinemas and VCRs everywhere, providing 85 percent of films screened in Europe and projecting the alluring entertainment values of sexuality, violence, and wealth. Overseas markets grew so large that producers edited different versions of popular films for specific cultures, just as American magazines tailored separate editions to expand sales in diverse countries.

From jazz to rock 'n' roll to rap, American popular music spread across the globe, as did such clothing of American youth as jeans and sneakers.

The idea of individual choice pervaded American culture, backed by constitutional guarantees of freedom of expression. Freedom to choose included matters of religion, politics, and other weighty areas, which had long made the United States a beacon of liberty to people oppressed for their beliefs. But freedom of choice came increasingly by the end of the twentieth century to refer to options for consumption in the marketplace. The United States was the largest market in the world, and its affluent citizens had unparalleled choices of what to buy. In 1960, Americans already had 3000 shopping centers and 4 square feet of retail space per person. By 2000, those numbers had soared to 40,000 and 19, respectively, for their children and grandchildren. The premium placed on acquiring material goods seemed to many foreign observers the primary American value, visible anew in the rapid rise of legalized gambling in the last generation and the nation's declining savings rate. Indeed, *saving* had been largely redefined to mean buying at a discount rather than putting money away for the future.

Advertising grew in prominence as the central link between popular culture and the selling of products, and sports became steadily more commercialized. Postseason college football games began in 1985 to include the names of their corporate sponsors, creating such events as the Chick-Fil-A Peach Bowl and the Weed Eater Independence Bowl. By 2000, newspapers ranked bowl games—once hallowed for their own traditions—by the simple criterion of how much money sponsors paid to participating teams. In the 1990s "hoops" joined baseball as a popular U.S. export. Led by such talented and flashy stars as Michael Jordan, an American "Dream Team" won the Olympic basketball competition in Spain amid worldwide fanfare.

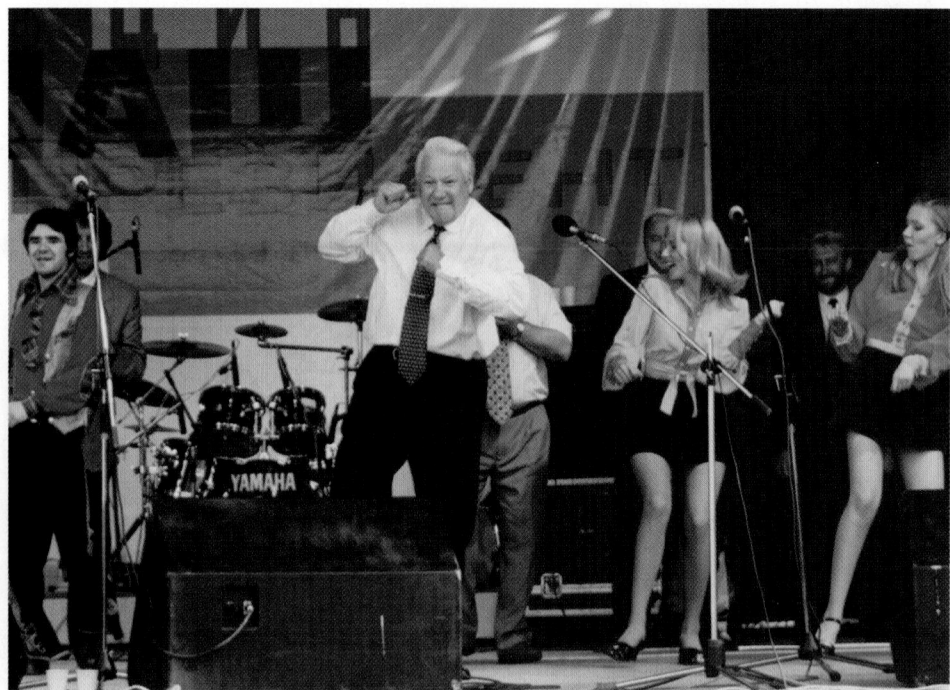

AP/Wide World Photos

■ Perhaps no other element of American popular culture spread abroad as quickly as rock 'n' roll music. Like jazz after the 1920s, rock 'n' roll after the 1950s captured a vast listening audience overseas. Most Russian leaders during the Soviet era before 1991 appeared publicly as stiff, serious figures, but by 1996, Russian president Boris Yeltsin joined Russian rock 'n' rollers on stage in an event during his successful campaign for reelection.

Swiftly, the National Basketball Association (NBA) made the leap from an American league to a global phenomenon, its games telecast to more than 190 countries in 41 languages. Sports also brought foreigners to the United States as professional baseball and basketball teams began recruiting Latin American, European, African, and Asian athletes.

U.S. Influence Abroad Since the Cold War

Cultural influences flowed both ways for Americans, with immigrants in particular bringing with them traditions and perspectives that refreshed the cultural mix of life in the United States. Japanese Pokémon trading cards, Thai cuisine, and Cuban salsa music pervaded daily routines for many Americans. The rapidly growing popularity of American-style pizza outside the United States suggested the complexity of cultural exchange, as fast-food chains Domino's and Pizza Hut sold from Hong Kong to the Congo a food originally brought to New York by Italian immigrants. But increased trade and communication since the end of the Cold War above all enabled the further spread of American popular culture. American-accented English straddled the globe, the language of international commerce and of 80 percent of listings on the World Wide Web. The informality and individualism of the Internet made it feel quintessentially American in style. The U.S. dollar remained the world's primary trading currency and became the de facto and even the de jure currency of many other nations. Mickey Mouse's empire expanded to EuroDisney outside Paris and Tokyo Disneyland; Kodak even sold film in Antarctica. American studies became a major field of scholarship at universities around the world.

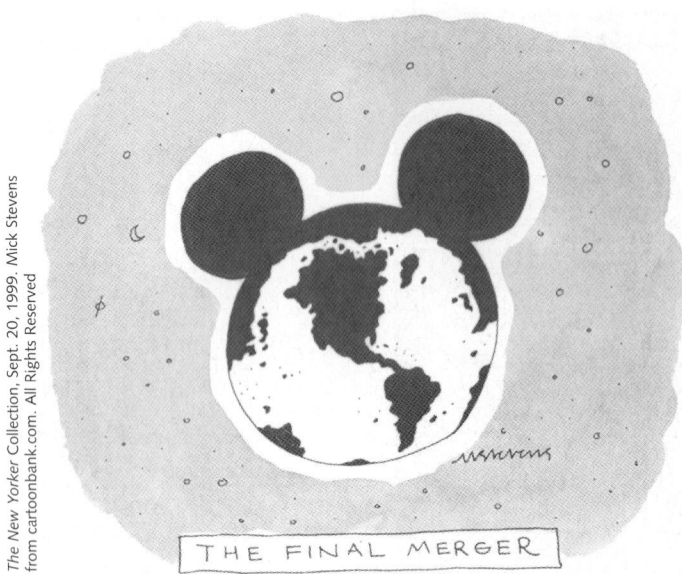

THE FINAL MERGER

■ By 2000, the process of globalization tied the world more closely together than ever before. Increasing trade, tourism, and communication encouraged the mixing of different cultures. American popular culture was a powerful influence around the globe, including American music, fast food, television, clothing, and movies. Mickey Mouse's ears famously symbolized the Disney Company, American television and films, and their worldwide prominence in popular entertainment.

America's most popular eatery served 20 million customers a day at its 23,000 franchises across the globe. McDonald's Golden Arches appeared everywhere, from Japan and France to Russia and China. Even Mecca in Saudi Arabia, the holiest site in Islam and the destination of millions of Muslim pilgrims, had a McDonald's. The company generated half of its revenues from non-U.S. operations.

Nor did only U.S. material interests spread abroad swiftly in recent years. American religious missionaries worked in poor countries around the world, combining their spiritual mission with a commitment to improving daily life in concrete ways involving health care, education, and agriculture. Pentecostalists gained millions of converts in Latin America since the 1970s, and mainstream denominations, such as the Lutherans, Episcopalians, and Roman Catholics, saw their numbers rise sharply in Africa. The most fully home-grown American religion was especially active in proselytizing abroad. As a result, the Church of Jesus Christ of Latter Day Saints (Mormons), headquartered in Salt Lake City, had 5 million members in the United States and another 5 million worldwide. Such international growth and Utah's hosting of the 2002 Winter Olympics symbolized how fully integrated into the outside world even America's most remote parts and once-reclusive peoples had become. (Salt Lake City's rapid growth made its population half non-Mormon by 2000.)

The United States retained its military superiority, with a defense budget larger than that of the next ten biggest military powers combined. The country's size, technological sophistication, and bipartisan commitment to a vast armed force ensured that its power on the battlefield was unlikely to diminish any time soon. But the difficulties of unconventional warfare, from Vietnam in the 1960s to Somalia in 1993, combined with the apparent disappearance of a major threat to the nation's security after the demise of the Soviet Union, made U.S. policymakers and citizens reluctant to put American troops in harm's way abroad, at least until after the terrorist attacks of September 11, 2001. Instead, the expansion of American culture abroad seemed a safer and more effective way to influence other nations. A generation earlier, Soviet leader Nikita Khrushchev had threatened to "bury the West," but in 1999 his son Sergei became an American citizen. His decision epitomized the continued allure of life in the United States.

Resistance to American Popular Culture

In the 1920s, Hasan al-Banna, founder of the Muslim Brotherhood, railed against "the wave of atheism and lewdness" engulfing Egypt, a wave that "started the devastation of religion and morality on the pretext of individual and intellectual freedom." Freer western and especially American standards of behavior offended the sensibilities of traditionalists across the Muslim world throughout the twentieth century, especially in matters of gender roles. Referring to tourists and their swimsuits, al-Banna blamed Westerners for importing "their half-naked women into these regions, together with their liquors" and other vices. The Iranian revolution of 1979 gave such complaints a new force by producing a theocratic government in one of the largest Muslim nations.

Like Christian, Jewish, and Hindu fundamentalists, all of whom grew prominent in the final decades of the twentieth century, Muslim fundamentalists rejected the radical egalitarianism and the unbridled pursuit of pleasure—especially the sexual titillation—so prevalent in American popular culture. The relative equality of women and the lack of respect for traditional social and religious hierarchies seemed to them emblems of American decadence, as the Islamic rulers of Afghanistan (known as the Taliban) demonstrated in the 1990s in their brutal repression of women's rights. Osama bin Laden and his followers resented U.S. policies of supporting Israel and certain oil-producing Arab nations, but they also fiercely condemned the secular, egalitarian character of American society, which they considered anti-Islamic. During the 1991 Gulf War, Saudi Arabian officials tried to isolate U.S. troops from Saudi citizens, fearing the effects of contact with such diverse forces as female soldiers, bawdiness, Christianity, and American music and television. An Indian official reflected his government's anxiety about the new availability of MTV in India: "Our own social ethos, our cultural values—we would not like them to be subverted."

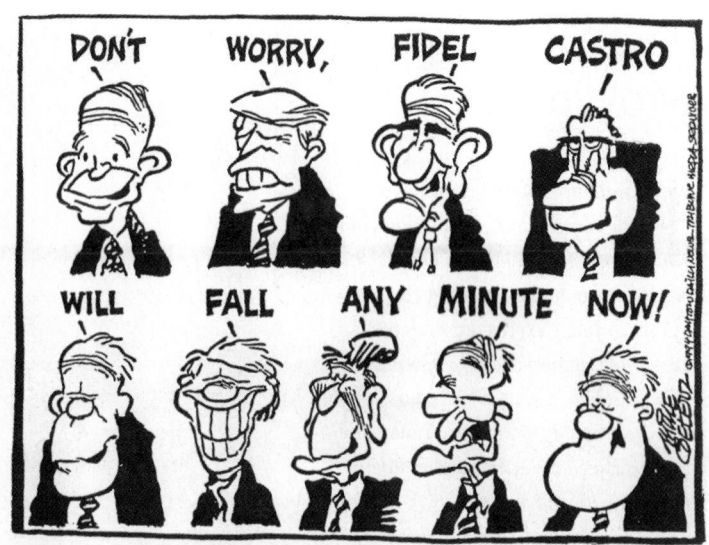

■ By the start of the new century, the hopes of nine U.S. presidents that the communist leader of Cuba would be swept out of power had been dashed. Four decades after leading the leftist revolution of 1959 and ten years after the collapse of communism in Russia and eastern Europe, Castro remained defiant toward the United States. He continued to denounce free market capitalism, whose price, he claimed, was paid in human misery, child labor, prostitution, and vast social inequalities.

©1994 Mike Peters/Dayton Daily News

The demise of Communist regimes in Russia and eastern Europe opened the gates to a flood of western influences and brought the opportunities and inequalities of a suddenly privatized economy. State-provided safety nets disappeared, class differences widened, women's economic status declined, and the old Communist parties regained some popularity among voters scared by the instabilities of American-style capitalism. Western Europeans also remained ambivalent about the spread of American values and lifestyles. Although many of them, especially among the young, found American culture attractive and learned English in record numbers, traditionalists who were proud of their own national culture took a dim view of such innovations as fast food. A "slow food" movement emerged in France, celebrating traditional home and café meals, and protesters against McDonald's became national celebrities.

Other nations sometimes found the U.S. government overbearing and resented its unparalleled military power. Bin Laden and many other Middle Easterners blamed American arms for bolstering the governments of Israel and the Arab states whose moderate stance toward the West they abhorred. Rapidly modernizing China, the world's most populous country, seemed a growing rival to the United States in Asia, even as the two nations became major trading partners. In April 2001, a U.S. surveillance plane collided over the South China Sea with a Chinese fighter jet that had been following it. The Chinese pilot died, but the American plane managed to crash-land safely at a Chinese military airport on Hainan Island. China detained the crew of 24 men and women for ten days. Public and congressional anger in the United States paralleled the outrage in China, but the two governments, mindful of their growing economic interdependence, resolved the crisis after a brief standoff. Americans who had assumed that China's greater political openness of recent years, including widening access to the Internet, would reveal a people eager to be like Americans were surprised by the intensity of anti-American nationalism within Chinese society.

Two opposing trends characterized world affairs. One consisted of the unifying forces of economic internationalism and globalization, carrying with them a tide of American-dominated

The Slow Food Movement

For many people in countries other than the United States, as for many Americans, McDonald's and other U.S.-based fast food restaurants offered an attractive dining experience. Customers everywhere appreciated the efficient and friendly service, clean surroundings, and the consistent quality of the food. Their enthusiasm explained the extraordinary international growth and profitability of such chains as Burger King and Kentucky Fried Chicken at the end of the twentieth century.

For other people, the rapid spread of fast-food franchises around the globe threatened cherished values and lifestyles. The Slow Food Movement emerged in western Europe in the late 1980s as a loose-knit organization, head-quartered in the northern Italian town of Bra. The movement sought to preserve and celebrate traditional cuisines and methods of food production in Europe and around the world. Slow Food's 60,000 members objected not only to the specific taste of fast food, but also to broader cultural changes symbolized by McDonald's and its competitors: the speeding up of daily life, including the loss of sociability around more leisurely meals; the gradual replacement of family farming and food production by corporate agriculture; and the erosion of distinctive local cooking and dining traditions.

The Slow Food Manifesto (November 9, 1989)

Our century, which began and has developed under the insignia of industrial civilization, first invented the machine and then took it as its life model.

We are enslaved by speed and have all succumbed to the same insidious virus: *Fast Life,* which disrupts our habits, pervades the privacy of our homes and forces us to eat *Fast Foods.*

To be worthy of the name, *Homo sapiens* should rid himself of

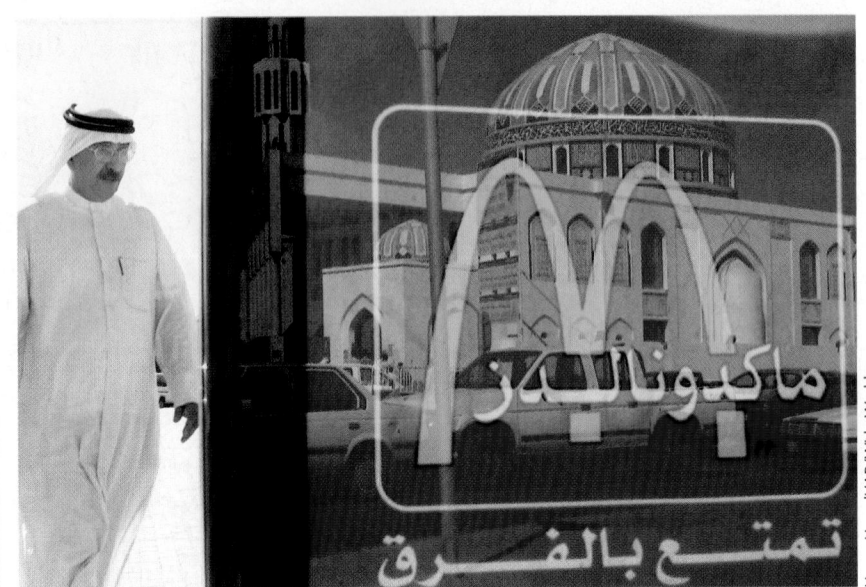

Hasan Hamali/AP/Wide World

The spread of American fast food chains around the globe suggested that American culture may be a more powerful influence abroad than U.S. military might. The end of the Cold War led to McDonald's restaurants proliferating in downtown Moscow and Beijing, the capital cities of America's greatest opponents since World War II. The Golden Arches even invaded Mecca, Saudi Arabia, the holiest city of Islam.

speed before it reduces him to a species in danger of extinction.

A firm defense of quiet material pleasure is the only way to oppose the universal folly of *Fast Life.*

May suitable doses of guaranteed sensual pleasure and slow, long-lasting enjoyment preserve us from the contagion of the multitude who mistake frenzy for efficiency.

Our defense should begin at the table with *Slow Food.* Let us rediscover the flavors and savors of regional cooking and banish the degrading effects of *Fast Food.*

In the name of productivity, *Fast Life* has changed our way of being and threatens our environment and our landscapes. So *Slow Food* is now the only truly progressive answer.

That is what real culture is all about: developing taste rather than demeaning it. And what better way to set about this than an international exchange of experiences, knowledge, projects?

Slow Food guarantees a better future.

Slow Food is an idea that needs plenty of qualified supporters who can help turn this (slow) motion into an international movement, with the little snail as its symbol.

Slow Food operates to protect the right to pleasure, the respect of the rhythms of life and a harmonious relationship with nature. It also seeks to explore, describe and improve the culture of food, to develop a proper education of taste and smell from childhood and to safeguard and defend the agroindustrial heritage while respecting the cuisines of each single country.

The Slow food Manifesto *was ratified in Paris at the Founding Congress of the International Slow Food Movement on December 9, 1989.*

Source: http://www.slowfood.com.

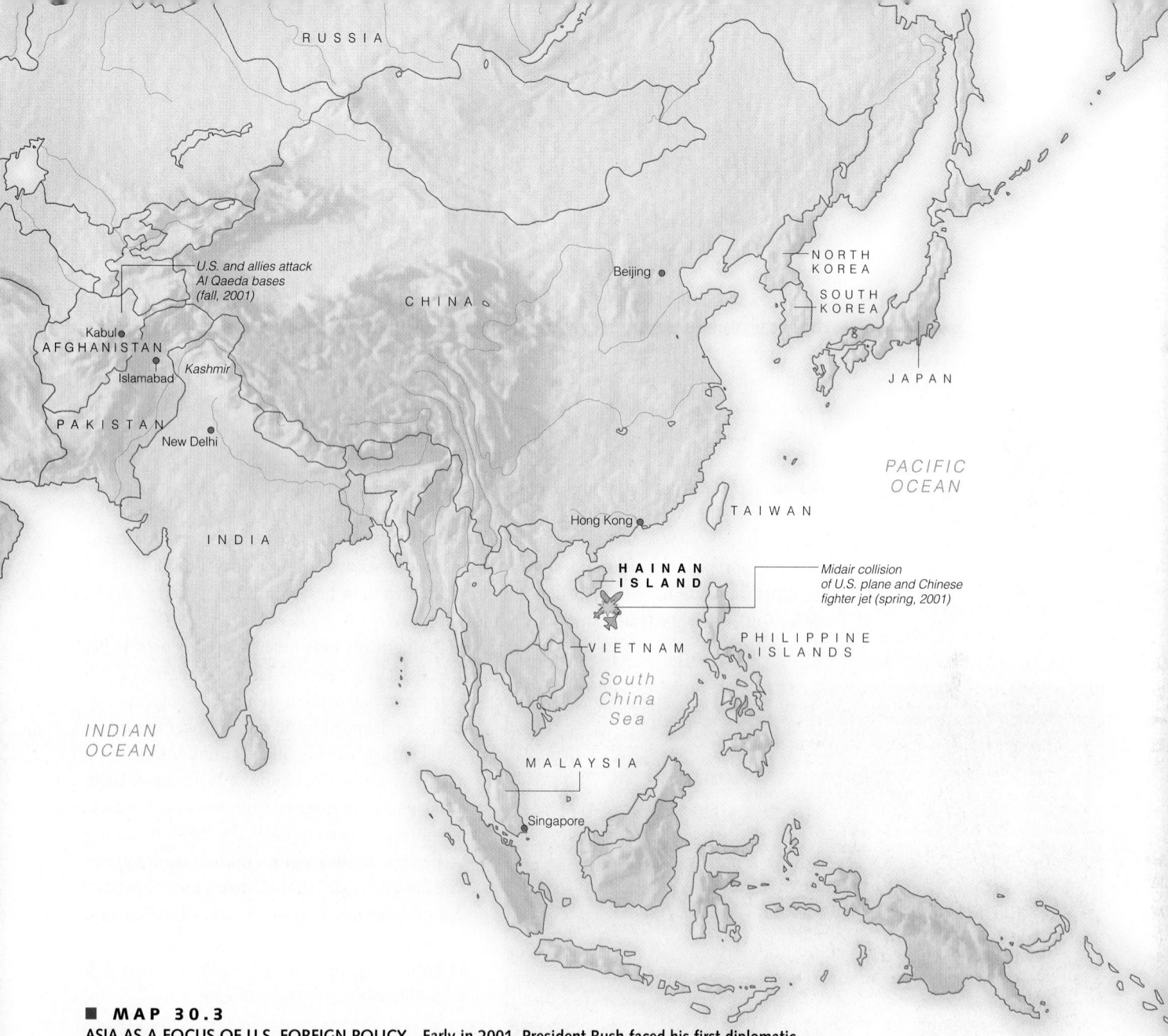

■ MAP 30.3
ASIA AS A FOCUS OF U.S. FOREIGN POLICY Early in 2001, President Bush faced his first diplomatic crisis when a Chinese fighter jet collided with a U.S. spy plane near Hainan Island. Tensions rose between the United States and China, suggesting that their renewed rivalry might dominate international politics in the new millenium. But the September 11 terrorist attacks from the Afghanistan-based Al Qaeda network shifted diplomatic attention to a different part of Asia. The United States and China, along with Russia, worked to oppose radical Islamic revolutionaries and to prevent a nuclear war between India and Pakistan over the disputed region of Kashmir.

cultural styles. The other was made up of the resisting forces of political and ethnic nationalism. A world more tightly integrated in economic ways was at the same time divided by ethnic conflicts, revealed in wars in the Balkans in southeastern Europe, the Caucasus region on Russia's southern border, and central Africa. As people around the world felt themselves increasingly sucked into the vortex of a powerful global economy that they could not control, many of them responded by renewing their allegiances to older, more local traditions. Ethnic, religious, and national identities often offered more meaningful alternatives to a purely economic identity as consumers. "I don't find foreign countries foreign," Gillette Corporation chair Alfred M. Zeien said, and many people in other nations felt the same way about the United States. But for others, as the terrorist attacks of 2001 made all too clear, American life seemed fundamentally alien and increasingly threatening.

Identity in Contemporary America

The 2000 U.S. census revealed a society in the midst of change. Americans have long been known as a particularly restless and mobile people, and one out of five changed residences every year. The post-1965 wave of immigrants continued to rise (and foreign adoptions rose dramatically), bringing in millions of new Americans of Asian heritage. Latino Americans came to equal African Americans as the nation's two largest minorities with 35 million people each. This latest surge in immigration boosted the number of Roman Catholics and Buddhists as American society remained the most openly religious—still primarily Protestant— of the industrialized nations. Geographically, Americans lived farther south and west than earlier generations. Of the ten largest cities 100 years ago, only New York, Chicago, and Philadelphia remained on the list, while cities such as Atlanta, Houston, and San Diego replaced Boston, Cleveland, and St. Louis. None of the 20 fastest-growing states were in the Northeast or Midwest. The West Coast housed the country's two largest philanthropic foundations: the Gates Foundation of Seattle and the Packard Foundation of Los Altos, California. Rooted in the new money of the computer and high-technology sectors, these institutions surpassed the older foundations in the Northeast built on the wealth of heavy industries, such as Rockefeller (oil), Carnegie (steel), and Ford (automobiles).

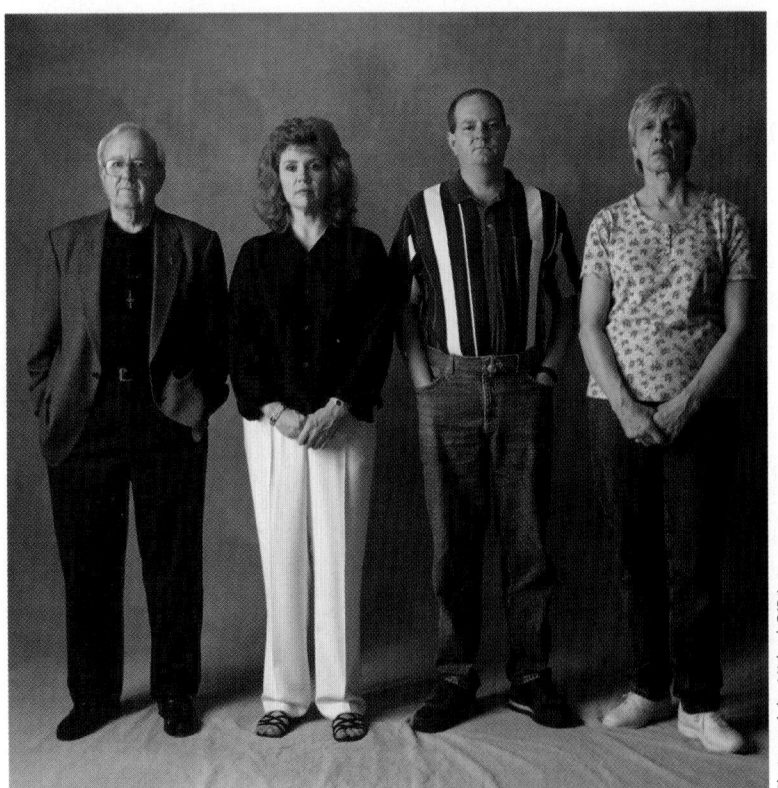

Photograph by Michael O'Brien

■ One aspect of American identity that continued to distinguish the United States from the industrialized countries of western Europe was enthusiastic support for the death penalty. Most surviving victims and relatives of victims of the 1995 Oklahoma City federal building bombing were eager for the execution of the confessed and unrepentant perpetrator, Timothy McVeigh, in 2001. However, a few overcame their grief and rage to oppose having the government kill the killer, including Bud Welch, Kathy Wilburn, Patrick Reeder, and Rosemary Koelsch (L to R), each of whom lost loved ones in the mass murder.

Americans were older than they used to be: life expectancy rose to 77 from 45 years in 1900. More than half lived in suburbs. Average household size dropped by 50 percent over the twentieth century, as only one in four consisted of a married couple with children. Whereas in 1900, just 6 percent of married women worked outside the home, 61 percent did so by 2000, including 64 percent of those with children under age 6. The "family wage" that so many men earned in the mid-twentieth century was disappearing, helping bring in its wake changes in gender roles as women became crucial breadwinners, as well as homemakers and child-raisers.

Negotiating Multiple Identities

Americans derived their sense of identity from myriad sources, including nationality, work, socioeconomic status, religion, race, ethnicity, family, gender, region, and sexual orientation. Since the struggles for equality that emerged dramatically in the 1960s, individual identities and group identities have often been in tension. The black civil rights movement, along with the struggles of women, Latinos, Native Americans, and homosexuals, sought an end to unequal treatment and full inclusion in American life for all individual citizens, regardless of race, sex, sexual orientation, or disability. However, the achievement of legal equality and the outlawing of

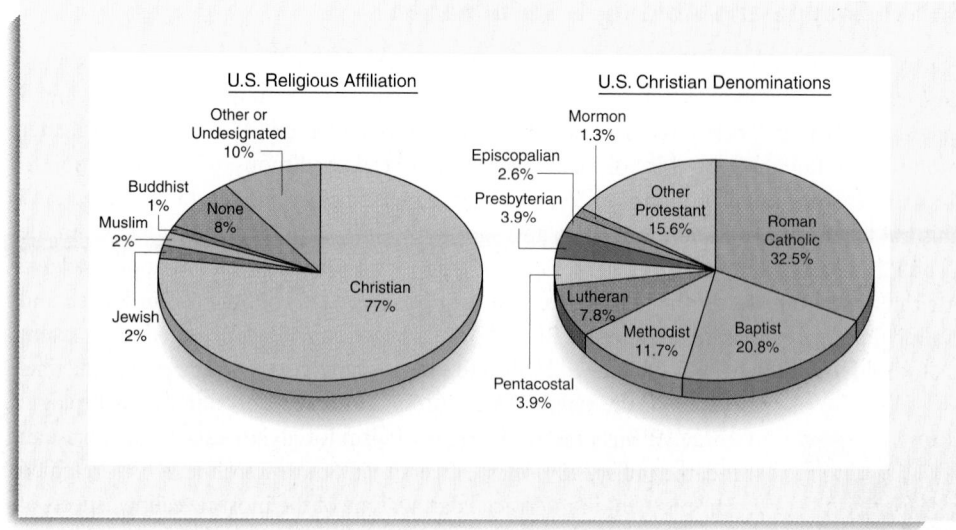

■ **FIGURE 30.1**
SELF-DESCRIBED RELIGIOUS AFFILIATION IN THE UNITED STATES, 2000   The most noticeable change of the last 30 years in American religious life has been the growth of evangelical and fundamentalist Protestant congregations (shown here as Pentacostals and "Other Protestants") and the shrinking of mainline Protestant denominations.

explicit discrimination did not immediately change deeply embedded patterns of exclusionary behavior. The policy of affirmative action had developed as a preference in hiring or admission for members of an underrepresented group who were roughly comparable to others in qualifications. It aimed to balance some of the effects of existing but little-noticed habits of "affirmative action" for white Americans and men, as when colleges used lower admission standards for children of alumni or powerful white men tended to hire other white men. Opponents of affirmative action called it "reverse discrimination" and argued that race and sex should no longer be criteria for success in a colorblind society that promoted individual achievement. By 2000, these opponents had succeeded in eliminating affirmative action from the admission process of the large state university systems of Texas and California. Supporters of the policy, including President Bill Clinton, observed that employers and others were certainly not colorblind yet, so that a group remedy, such as affirmative action, remained essential for the advancement of more than a token few from groups that had faced discrimination in the past.

Ideas about racial identity remained at the heart of controversy over affirmative action. Those who used the term *race* to group people according to skin color and other visible features, such as eye shape, commonly assumed that race had an important biological meaning as a way of distinguishing one human population from another. However, biologists noted that the genetic differences between races are miniscule compared with differences between individuals of the same race; they suggested that categorizing people by skin color made as much sense as organizing library books by the size and color of their covers rather than their internal contents. The mapping of the entire human genome by 2001 further clarified the biological insignificance of race. Indeed, the racial category "white" had changed over time to encompass such formerly excluded groups as Irish Americans and Jewish Americans. Despite its lack of scientific basis, the use of race as a primary marker of identity long served to preserve a higher status for Americans of European heritage. One could be mostly white yet still be "black," thanks to the one-drop tradition regarding African heritage (that any observable percentage of African "blood" defined a person as black). Thus, a white woman could have a black child in the United States, for example, but a black woman could not have a white child. The U.S. government's decision in the 2000 census to allow citizens to identify themselves as belonging to more than one racial group reflected the complications and occasional absurdities of racial categorization.

Social Change and Abiding Discrimination

One of the most striking changes in American society over the past five decades has been the desegregation of public life. Latinos and Asians became much more numerous in the United States, and African Americans emerged from the enforced separation of Jim Crow into greater prominence. Roughly one-third of blacks were middle-class and thousands won election to local, state, and national political offices, and black Americans became central in the nation's cultural life in music, literature, theater, and sports. By 2001, even a new president from the Republican party—known since 1964 for its lack of support from black voters—appointed two African Americans to run the nation's foreign relations: Secretary of State Colin Powell and National Security Adviser Condoleezza Rice. Workplaces were racially integrated to an extent that would have been hard to imagine in 1950, and interacial marriages rose steeply in the final decades of the twentieth century. In the 2000 presidential campaign, George W. Bush received sharp criticism for giving a speech at Christian fundamentalist Bob Jones University in South Carolina, which retained a campus ban on interracial dating. One of the most revealing aspects of the controversy was the response of conservative and even reactionary religious and political leaders: none supported the ban. "The fact is you have an indefensible policy," declared U.S. Representative and Bob Jones alumnus Asa Hutchinson of Arkansas. The sexual fears that had so long underpinned white racial violence in the past had dramatically receded in the nation's public life.

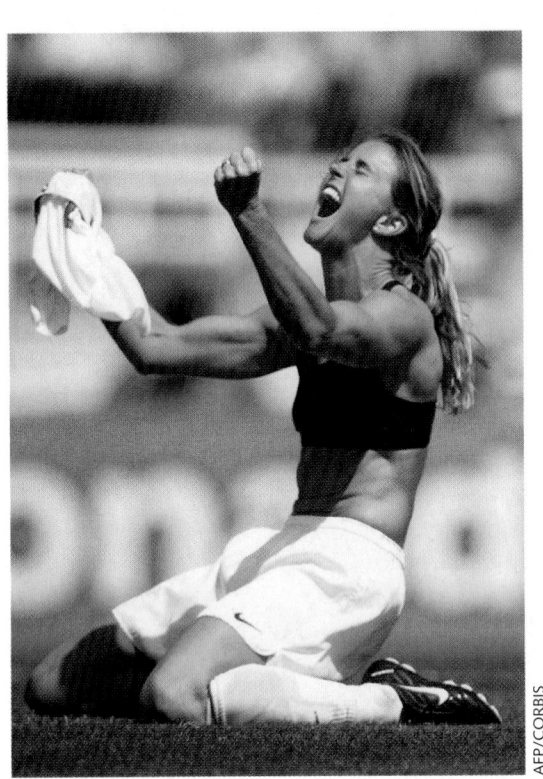

AFP/CORBIS

■ **Defender Brandi Chastain celebrates after her decisive penalty kick against China gave the U.S. women's soccer team the 1999 World Cup title. Ripping off her shirt just as male soccer players often did (to reveal a not very revealing sports bra), Chastain shocked some viewers but impressed others who saw muscular athleticism rather than the sexual suggestiveness of bikini swimsuits.**

The lives of women in the United States also changed dramatically during the last half of the twentieth century. Most worked outside the home, from jobs in the service and manufacturing sectors to careers in the professions and politics. In 2000, women made up a third of the students in the nation's medical schools and a half in law schools. Their presence in leading political positions ranged from local officials to more than a dozen U.S. senators, two U.S. Supreme Court justices, a U.S. attorney general, and a U.S. secretary of state. The passage of Title IX in 1972, prohibiting gender discrimination in school programs that received federal money, created a tidal wave of social change for American girls. In 1971, 1 in 27 girls played high school sports; by 1998, the ratio was 1 in 3. Sports programs and teams for girls comparable to those for boys nourished a new generation of American women for whom athletic competition and achievement were the norm rather than the exception. The U.S. national women's soccer team won the World Cup in 1999 and became a popular sensation, with players like Mia Hamm emerging as household names. Anti-homosexual attitudes persisted as one of the nation's fiercest prejudices but nonetheless declined in mainstream American society during the 1980s and 1990s. Gay men and lesbians became more open and prominent in such public venues as television and politics, helping millions of other Americans to shed some of the homophobia they had unknowingly learned during childhood.

These improvements for the majority of Americans who were not heterosexual white men jostled against abiding forms of discrimination and inequality. Violence and the threat of violence against homosexuals, people of color, and particularly women (primarily domestic violence at the hands of husbands and lovers) remained very real, but most prejudices found more subtle avenues of expression. Working women continued to average less than three-quarters the wages of working men. Many employers, police officers, store owners, bank loan officers, and others in positions of authority treated African Americans and Latino Americans with greater suspicion than they did other citizens, a practice that became known as racial profiling. Poverty and unemployment disproportionately affected black communities and families. Given the powerful legacy of the past, white individuals on average possessed ten times more real wealth (much of it inherited) than their African American counterparts. Residential neighborhoods and public schools remained largely segregated by race, and the deeply symbolic Confederate flag still occupied a place of public honor in several southern states. Popular black comedian Chris Rock reminded mostly white audiences of the enduring but unstated advantage of being white in the United States: "Ain't no white man here willing to trade places with me—and I'm rich!"

Native Americans shared this combination of improving status and continuing discrimination. Their numbers were reviving, from a mere 250,000 in 1900 to 2 million in 2000, and a new National Museum of the American Indian arose on the mall in the nation's capital. A series of federal court decisions in the 1970s and 1980s strengthened Indians' "unique and limited" sovereignty over the tribal reservations, which constituted 2 percent of U.S. land. Starting with the Iroquois of upstate New York in 1970, several eastern Indian nations sued state and federal governments for the return of parts of lands that had been illegally seized from them in the past. From Florida to Maine, these nations won a combination of small portions of public land and millions of dollars in compensation in cases from the 1970s through the 1990s. Casino revenues in the 1990s brought much-needed resources to a number of Indian nations. At the same time, the process of assimilation continued as a majority of Indians lived in urban areas and were married to non-Indians. Reservations suffered from severe unemployment rates and remained some of the poorest communities in the country, dependent on federal assistance for food and other basic necessities. Anti-Indian sentiments occasionally surfaced in states as diverse as Montana, Wisconsin, Arizona, and New York.

> *Chris Rock reminded mostly white audiences of the enduring but unstated advantage of being white in the United States.*

Still an Immigrant Society

Economic opportunity and individual liberty continued to lure millions of people from other nations to the United States at the start of the new millennium. From its peak in the first decade of the twentieth century, the annual number of immigrants declined steadily after the restrictive immigration laws of the early 1920s, the Great Depression of the 1930s, and World War II in the 1940s. After the war, the number began to rise slowly again until the 1965 reforms encouraged a new period of immigration as large, by the 1990s, as that of a century earlier. Some 800,000 now came legally each year, and another 300,000 entered without official papers. For the first time since the 1930s, 1 in 10 Americans had been born abroad; in New York City the ratio was 1 in 4. Fifteen percent came from Europe, 26 percent arrived from Asia, and 51 percent moved north from Latin America and the Caribbean. Like Italy in 1900, Mexico in 2000 became the most important single source of new Americans, highlighting the importance of the nation's 2000-mile southern border as a conduit. The cultural exchange from Europe to the American East and Midwest 100 years earlier was replaced by a new exchange from Asia and Latin America centered in the Sunbelt states from Florida to California. The demographic transition of California in 2000 from a white majority to a more diverse ethnic and racial mix like that of Hawaii symbolized the nation's turn to the South and West, even as the motives and work habits of the newcomers remained very much the same as those of their European predecessors.

Only the hardiest and most motivated people made the difficult, emotionally wrenching, and often dangerous move to the United States. Many fled political persecution in countries like Guatemala, Haiti, Vietnam, and Cuba. In contrast to the left-leaning and often socialist

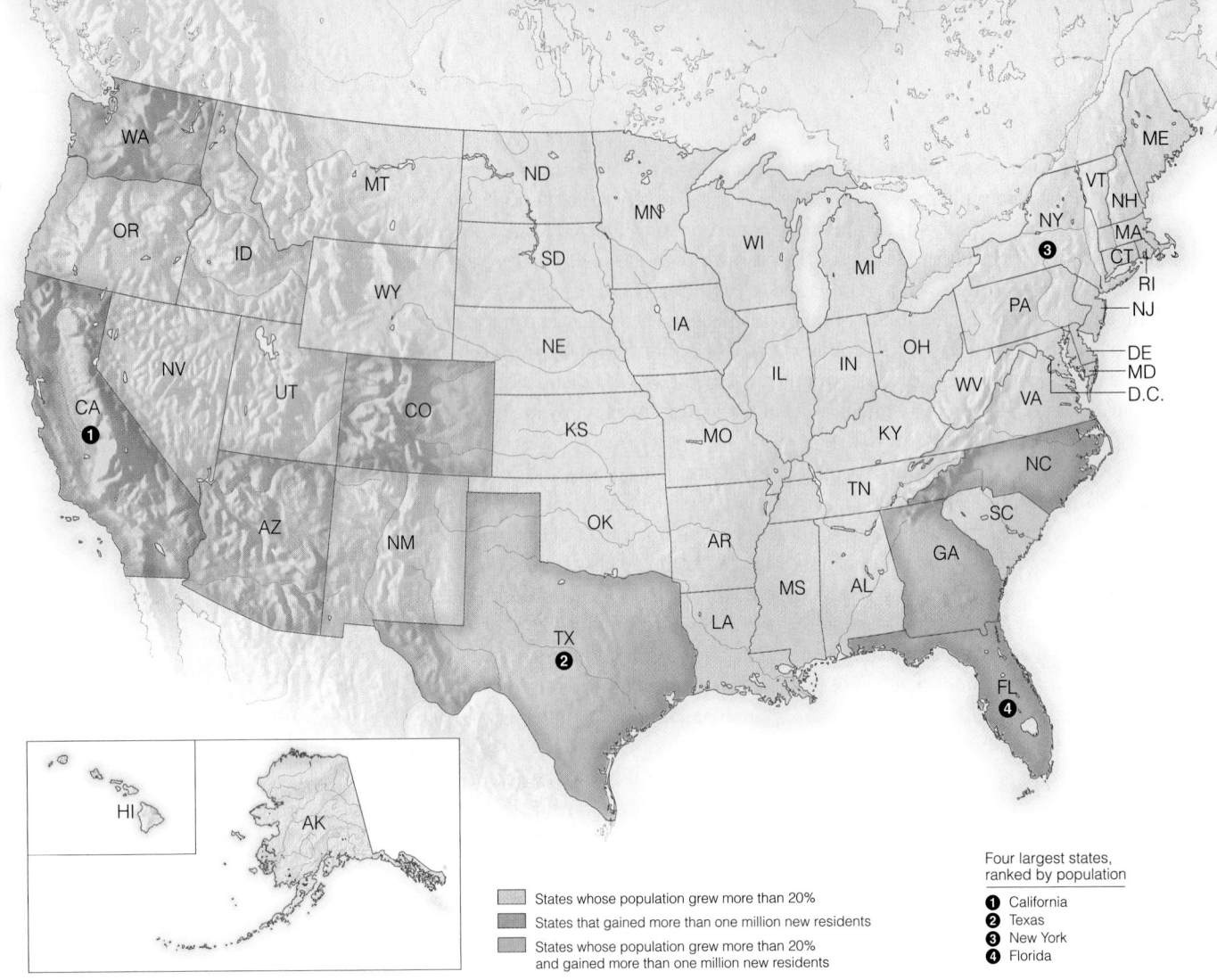

States whose population grew more than 20%

States that gained more than one million new residents

States whose population grew more than 20% and gained more than one million new residents

Four largest states, ranked by population

❶ California
❷ Texas
❸ New York
❹ Florida

■ **MAP 30.4**

STATE POPULATION GROWTH, 1990–2000   The population of the United States continued to shift slowly out of the long-urbanized Northeast to the Sunbelt of the South and West. Los Angeles replaced Chicago as the nation's second largest city, after New York. Retirees and workers alike seemed to prefer sunnier, warmer climates.

attitudes of immigrants in 1900, political refugees in 2000 were sometimes fierce anticommunists who helped pressure the U.S. government to take an even harder line toward regimes in Havana and Hanoi. Most newcomers sought greater economic security, like the 80 percent of young men of the village of Ting Jiang in China's Fujian province who made the perilous voyage by sea to find work in American restaurants or construction. "Sure, work is hard" in the United States, one of their wives at home in China explained, "but with tips you can make more than $2000 a month," compared with $40 a month at home in Ting Jiang. "So now no one in the village works before they go to America. There's no point." Most immigrants came to stay, but some worked to save money and return home to their families, carrying with them not only money, but also bits of American culture. Other people flowed outward too, as American students and tourists traveled all over the globe. Some Americans worked abroad, usually for U.S.-based multinationals such as oil companies, to earn better wages and then return home. Others served in the military, worked for aid agencies and church groups, or joined in the resurgence of the Peace Corps.

Despite increasing contacts overseas, Americans responded to the wave of newcomers with an ambivalence common in previous periods of high immigration. For a society made up of people from elsewhere and their descendants, there was no obvious answer to the question of when to close the door to new arrivals. Many in the working class feared competition from highly motivated laborers accustomed to much lower wages. Many elites worried whether cultural diversity might weaken national unity. Conservative political leaders promoted new restrictions and stronger border patrols. One Arizona resident wrote to *The Arizona Republic* to defend controversial police harassment of Latinos in the Phoenix suburb of Chandler in 1997: "If your skin is brown, this is a probable cause [for arrest as an illegal alien] and a police officer may assume you are breaking the law until proved differently." Some U.S. Congressmen ridiculed the idea of there being value in traveling abroad by boasting that they did not even have passports. In 1998, Republican House majority leader Dick Armey of Texas announced, "I've been to Europe once; I don't have to go again." Such disdain for other cultures among some American political leaders dismayed U.S. allies overseas.

Most Americans got used to having more immigrants around. Americans cheered for the one in four major league baseball players who were born in Latin America or had parents from there, and they became accustomed to the high number of Asian Americans in college classrooms. Many churches worked to help new arrivals adjust to life in the United States. Above all, American employers depended on immigrant workers to keep the nation's powerful economy afloat—to pick its fruits and vegetables, tend its young children, and work in its factories. Nearly all-white Iowa even began an immigrant recruitment drive to sustain a vibrant state economy that lacked sufficient workers. If the estimated 6 million mostly Latino undocumented workers in the United States were expelled, thousands of hotels, restaurants, meatpacking plants, landscaping companies, and garment manufacturers would be forced to close.

Conclusion

What held Americans together as they set off into the twenty-first century was a common loyalty to a set of ideas about economic opportunities and individual liberties. Unlike such nations as Germany and Israel, where citizenship was extended automatically to people of a certain ethnicity, the United States awarded citizenship to those who were born within its borders, regardless of ethnicity or race. Those born elsewhere became citizens on the basis not of their past lineage but of their future commitments—of their newly sworn loyalty to the U.S. Constitution, with its guarantees of freedom and its responsibilities of citizenship. In a vast society of multiple political and cultural beliefs, the scope of specific freedoms and the nature of individual responsibilities inevitably remained matters of ongoing tension and conflict. Nonetheless, the United States continued to address most of its problems through an orderly legal system, in contrast to the ethnic and religious strife marking so many of the world's nations.

That strife from abroad impinged on Americans in a shocking new way on September 11, 2001. On a sunny Tuesday morning, 19 hijackers—four of them trained as pilots—seized control simultaneously of four large commercial jets and turned them into suicidal missiles. At 8:48 A.M., one flew into the 110-story north tower of New York City's World Trade Center, igniting an enormous fireball. Fifteen minutes later, the second plane flew into the south tower. In less than two hours, both towers collapsed, trapping hundreds of firefighters, police officers, and other rescue workers who had raced into the building to evacuate the thousands of occupants. The third plane flew into the Pentagon. The fourth was also being directed towards Washington, apparently to destroy the White House or the Capital Building, when the passengers rushed the hijackers in the cockpit. In the ensuing struggle, the plane crashed in a field 75 miles southeast of Pittsburgh.

The carefully coordinated assaults killed some 3000 people, destroyed the two tallest buildings in the country's largest city, and left a gaping hole in the headquarters of the nation's military command. Not since the Japanese assault on Pearl Harbor 60 years earlier had the United States experienced such a devastating attack on its soil. During the intervening half-century of the Cold War, the Soviet Union and other Communist forces had never attempted direct aggression against the American homeland. Who was responsible for the most horrific act of terrorism against civilians in U.S. history?

The 19 perpetrators were self-styled holy warriors of a secretive, extremist Islamic organization known as Al Qaeda, organized by wealthy, charismatic Saudi Arabian expatriate Osama bin Laden. The rage of bin Laden and other Islamic terrorists against the United States had been building throughout the 1990s, fueled by the presence of "infidel" American troops in Saudi Arabia since the Gulf War, by American support for Israel, and by the rapid spread of secular American popular culture around the globe. At odds with moderate Islamic mainstream thought throughout the world, bin Laden announced in 1998, "To kill Americans and their allies, is an individual duty of every Muslim who is able."

Al Qaeda worked out of Afghanistan. It was hosted by the most repressive Islamic government on Earth, the Taliban, which came to power in 1996 out of the chaos that followed the withdrawal of the Soviet army in 1989. U.S. aid had helped in the anti-Soviet struggle, but the American government had ignored Afghanistan after the Soviets left. Four weeks after the attacks on New York City and Washington in 2001, U.S. planes began bombing Taliban and Al Qaeda positions in Afghanistan. Meanwhile, U.S. special operations forces worked on the ground with anti-Taliban Afghan forces. By December, the Taliban had been driven from power throughout the country, and U.S. forces had captured hundreds of Taliban and Al Qaeda fighters. President Bush warned of a long struggle still ahead against remaining forces of anti-American terrorism, regardless of bin Laden's fate.

The terrorist attacks of September 11, 2001 tested—and often strengthened—ties across religious and ethnic lines as Americans shared a renewed sense of national unity and pride. Anti-government sentiments dropped sharply and flag sales soared. Traditional social divisions ebbed at least temporarily as citizens contemplated the assault on their nation. New Yorker Louis Johnson, the son of immigrants from Trinidad, said that previously, "I just thought of myself as black. But now I feel like I'm an American, more than ever." The Bush administration's subsequent restrictions on the civil liberties of young Arab men, part of an effort to prevent further attacks while the United States was at war in Afghanistan, riled defenders of American constitutional freedoms on both the left and the right, as well as such influential mainstream leaders as Democratic Senate Judiciary Committee chair Patrick Leahy from Vermont. But the president and his attorney general, John Ashcroft, maintained broad public support for their actions a year after 9-11.

Following September 11, national unity was threatened by sporadic hostility and vengeful assaults against Muslims and others of Middle Eastern appearance. A handful of deaths and hundreds of incidents of harassment and vandalism revealed the difficulty some citizens had in distinguishing between a few Islamic terrorists and several million Muslim Americans. But Muslims also encountered a powerful trend of support for them and curiosity about their faith. President Bush set the tone in highly publicized meetings with Muslim leaders in which he emphasized that "this is not a war against Islam" but only against terrorists, a point underlined by the close U.S. cooperation with the Islamic Republic of Pakistan and with Muslim anti-Taliban fighters in the war in Afghanistan. Within a few hours of the September 11 attacks, the leadership of the Ford Motor Company reached out to Detroit's large Arab American community (including several hundred of its own workers) and began a series of interfaith meetings to promote dialogue and tolerance. And the Coca-Cola Company hired Muhammad Ali, one of most famous figures on the planet, to do publicity work. "I am a Muslim," declared the former Olympic and world boxing champion from Louisville, Kentucky. "I am an American."

Average Americans also sought to improve communication and understanding between Muslims and non-Muslims. Fearful of possible vandalism, the handful of Muslims in Laramie,

Wyoming, stayed home after September 11. "And then our neighbors called up," homemaker Zubaida Husain said, and promised to help protect homes and property. "That made me feel very good." The unfortunately named "Osama's Place," a restaurant owned by a Jordanian American right near the entrance to Fort Bragg in Spring Lake, North Carolina, did not change its name and experienced little loss of business. Indeed, several thousand Muslims served in the U.S. armed forces, where the number of Islamic chaplains was increasing rapidly. In Cary, North Carolina, conservative Christian Yvonne Young-Capece and Muslim immigrant Mona el-Ramly were neighbors who had become so close that Young-Capece traveled to Egypt for the wedding of Ramly's son. After the terrorist attacks, Young-Capece hosted a get-together for 16 of her friends along with Ramly and a few other Muslim friends to combat prejudice.

At the heart of American society remained a common assumption that this was a democratic country. The events on United Airlines Flight 93, one of the four doomed planes on September 11, 2001, revealed the tenacity of the belief in majority rule. After the hijackers seized control and herded the passengers into the rear of the cabin, a few passengers were able to communicate by cell phone with loved ones on the ground. They learned that two other planes had already crashed into the World Trade Center towers in New York City, and they realized that

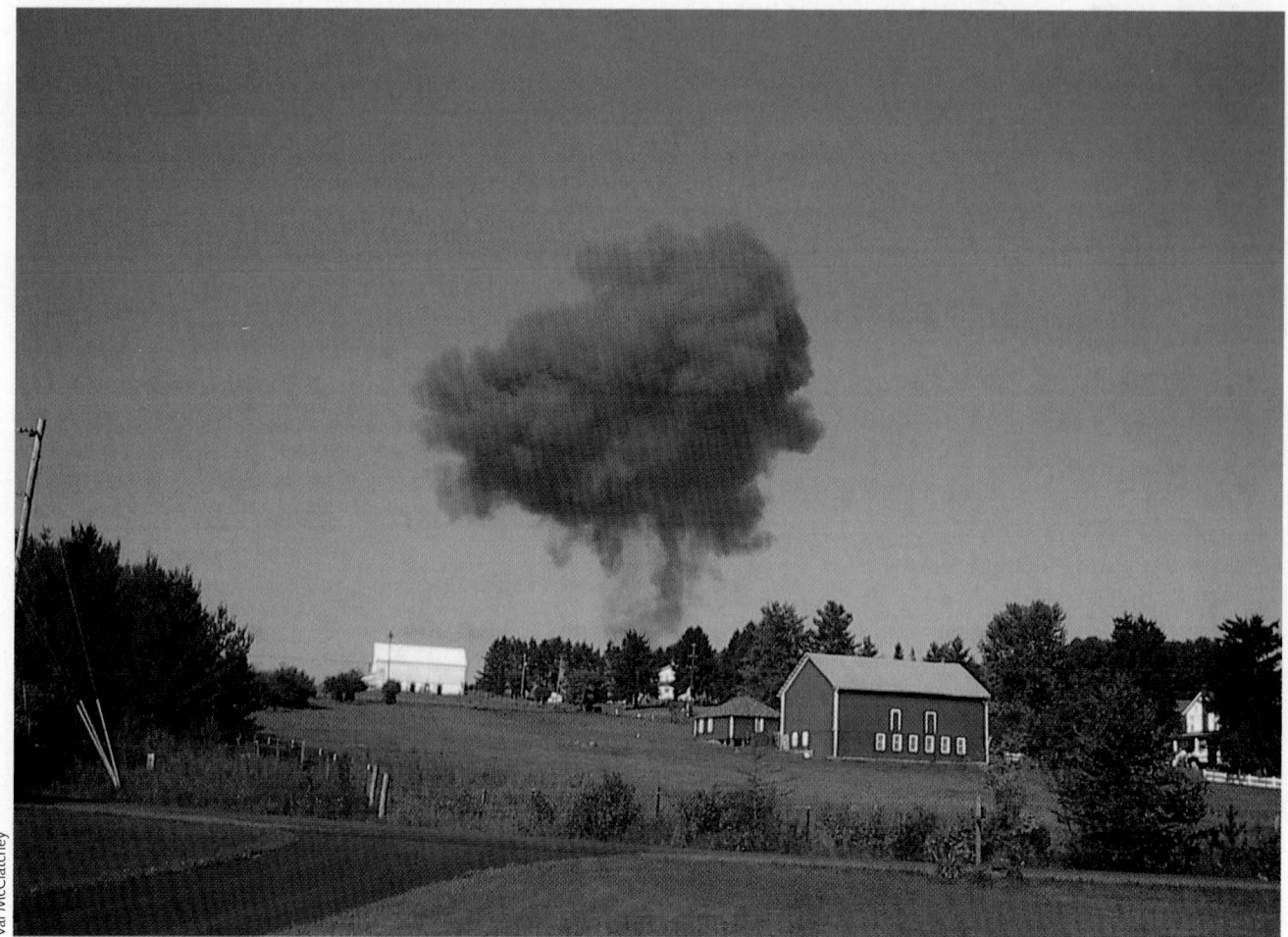

Val McClatchey

■ Smoke rises from the crash of United Airlines Flight 93 near Shanksville, Pennsylvania. For almost all Americans, the hijackings and destruction of September 11, 2001 came indeed out of a clear blue sky. Anti-American actions of the previous decade by Islamic terrorists had created little anxiety in a powerful nation that had imagined itself safe from major attack.

these hijackers—unlike previous ones who sought concrete gains and an escape—planned only destruction for them all. Face-to-face with imminent death and the certainty that many others would perish if they failed to act, the passengers discussed what to do. They made a plan to rush the hijackers, led by several large, athletic passengers, including Mark Bingham, a prominent gay businessperson and rugby player from San Francisco. Should they proceed? Quintessential Americans, they took a vote. GTE Airfone operator Lisa Jefferson heard the rest: "Are you guys ready?" asked Todd Beamer, a tall father of two from Cranbury, New Jersey. Pause. "Let's roll." Screams and a scuffle followed before the line went dead. The plane, headed for the heart of Washington, crashed minutes later in an unpopulated part of western Pennsylvania with no casualties on the ground.

Sites to Visit

Smithsonian Center for Latino Initiatives

latino.si.edu/

This site offers an array of links to information on Latino culture and history.

How Race Is Lived in America

www.nytimes.com/library/national/race/most-recent.html

This is a collection of revealing articles from the *New York Times* in 2000 on race relations and racial identities in contemporary America.

Islam in the United States

usinfo.state.gov/usa/islam/

Here, researchers can find information on Muslims in modern America and links to other sources for research.

History Link: The History of Seattle and King County

www.historylink.org/welcome.htm

This site provides an array of historical information about one of the fastest growing areas in the country.

The September 11 Digital Archive

911digitalarchive.org/stories/

Created by the Center for History and New Media and George Mason University and the American Social History Project at City University of New York Graduate Center, this site offers a large collection of stories and images from September 11, 2001, when terrorists attacked New York City and Washington, D.C.

Native Americans

www.americanwest.com/pages/indians.htm

This site contains information about American Indian history and culture, along with links to the home pages of many Indian nations.

The National Security Archive at George Washington University

www.gwu.edu/~nsarchiv/

This extraordinary site includes the most recent declassified documents on the making of U.S. foreign policy.

The Natural Resources Defense Council

www.nrdc.org/

This site contains considerable information and links about an array of current environmental issues.

For Further Reading

General

Harvard Sitkoff, ed., *Perspectives on Modern America: Making Sense of the Twentieth Century* (2001).

The American Place in a Global Economy

William M. Adler, *Mollie's Job: A Story of Life and Work on the Global Assembly Line* (2000).

Richard J. Barnet and John Cavanagh, *Global Dreams: Imperial Corporations and the New World Order* (1994).

Jefferson Cowie, *Capital Moves: RCA's Seventy-Year Quest for Cheap Labor* (1999).

Thomas L. Friedman, *The Lexus and the Olive Tree: Understanding Globalization* (1999).

William Greider, *One World, Ready or Not: The Manic Logic of Global Capitalism* (1997).

Robert Kuttner, *Everything for Sale: The Virtues and Limits of Markets* (1996).

The Stewardship of Natural Resources

Lester R. Brown, Michael Renner, and Brian Halweil, *Vital Signs 2000: The Environmental Trends That Are Shaping Our Future* (2000).

J. R. McNeill, *Something New Under the Sun: An Environmental History of the Twentieth-Century World* (2000).

David Quammen, *The Song of the Dodo: Island Biogeography in an Age of Extinction* (1996).

Hal K. Rothman, *Saving the Planet: The American Response to the Environment in the Twentieth Century* (2000).

The Expansion of American Popular Culture Abroad

Benjamin R. Barber, *Jihad vs. McWorld: How the Planet Is Both Falling Apart and Coming Together and What This Means for Democracy* (1995).

Chalmers Johnson, *Blowback: The Costs and Consequences of American Empire* (2000).

Richard F. Kuisel, *Seducing the French: The Dilemma of Americanization* (1993).

Richard Pells, *Not Like Us: How Europeans Have Loved, Hated, and Transformed American Culture Since World War II* (1997).

Ronald Steel, *Temptations of a Superpower* (1995).

Reinhold Wagnleitner and Elaine Tyler May, eds., *"Here, There and Everywhere": The Foreign Politics of American Popular Culture* (2000).

Identity in Contemporary America

Gary Gerstle, *American Crucible: Race and Nation in the Twentieth Century* (2001).

Charles Hirshman and Philip Kasinitz, eds., *The Handbook of International Migration: The American Experience* (1999).

David A. Hollinger, *Postethnic America: Beyond Multiculturalism*, rev. ed. (2000).

Gary Y. Okihiro, *Common Ground: Reimagining American History* (2001).

Robert D. Putnam, *Bowling Alone: The Collapse and Revival of American Community* (2000).

Ruth Rosen, *The World Split Open: How the Modern Women's Movement Changed America* (2000).

Alan Wolfe, *One Nation After All: What Americans Really Think About God, Country, Family, Racism, Welfare, Immigration, Homosexuality, Work, the Right, the Left and Each Other* (1998).

Online Practice Test

Test your understanding of this chapter with interactive review quizzes at

www.ablongman.com/jonescreatedequal/chapter30

Additional Photo Credits

Page 1003: PhotoDisc
Page 1004: W. Cody/CORBIS
Page 1007: Courtesy, Samsung Corporation
Page 1018: Photofest
Page 1019: Courtesy, Newstream.com
Page 1022: Permission to reproduce logo provided courtesy of Slow Food U.S.A.

Appendix

The Declaration of Independence

The Articles of Confederation

The Constitution of the United States of America

Amendments to the Constitution

Presidential Elections

For additional reference material, go to
www.ablongman.com/jonescreatedequal/appendix
The online appendix includes the following:

The Declaration of Independence

In Congress, July 4, 1776

The Unanimous Declaration of the Thirteen United States of America

When, in the course of human events, it becomes necessary for one people to dissolve the political bonds which have connected them with another, and to assume, among the powers of the earth, the separate and equal station to which the laws of nature and of nature's God entitle them, a decent respect to the opinions of mankind requires that they should declare the causes which impel them to the separation.

We hold these truths to be self-evident: That all men are created equal; that they are endowed by their Creator with certain unalienable rights; that among these are life, liberty, and the pursuit of happiness; that, to secure these rights, governments are instituted among men, deriving their just powers from the consent of the governed; that whenever any form of government becomes destructive of these ends, it is the right of the people to alter or to abolish it, and to institute new government, laying its foundation on such principles, and organizing its powers in such form, as to them shall seem most likely to effect their safety and happiness. Prudence, indeed, will dictate that governments long established should not be changed for light and transient causes; and accordingly all experience hath shown that mankind are more disposed to suffer, while evils are sufferable, than to right themselves by abolishing the forms to which they are accustomed. But when a long train of abuses and usurpations, pursuing invariably the same object, evinces a design to reduce them under absolute despotism, it is their right, it is their duty, to throw off such government, and to provide new guards for their future security. Such has been the patient sufferance of these colonies; and such is now the necessity which constrains them to alter their former systems of government. The history of the present King of Great Britain is a history of repeated injuries and usurpations, all having in direct object the establishment of an absolute tyranny over these states. To prove this, let facts be submitted to a candid world.

He has refused his assent to laws, the most wholesome and necessary for the public good.

He has forbidden his governors to pass laws of immediate and pressing importance, unless suspended in their operation till his assent should be obtained; and, when so suspended, he has utterly neglected to attend to them.

He has refused to pass other laws for the accommodation of large districts of people, unless those people would relinquish the right of representation in the legislature, a right inestimable to them, and formidable to tyrants only.

He has called together legislative bodies at places unusual, uncomfortable, and distant from the depository of their public records, for the sole purpose of fatiguing them into compliance with his measures.

He has dissolved representative houses repeatedly, for opposing, with manly firmness, his invasions on the rights of the people.

He has refused for a long time, after such dissolutions, to cause others to be elected; whereby the legislative powers, incapable of annihilation, have returned to the people at large for their exercise; the state remaining, in the mean time, exposed to all the dangers of invasions from without and convulsions within.

He has endeavored to prevent the population of these states; for that purpose obstructing the laws for naturalization of foreigners; refusing to pass others to encourage their migration hither, and raising the conditions of new appropriations of lands.

He has obstructed the administration of justice, by refusing his assent to laws for establishing judiciary powers.

He has made judges dependent on his will alone, for the tenure of their offices, and the amount and payment of their salaries.

He has erected a multitude of new offices, and sent hither swarms of officers to harass our people and eat out their substance.

He has kept among us, in times of peace, standing armies, without the consent of our legislatures.

He has affected to render the military independent of, and superior to, the civil power.

He has combined with others to subject us to a jurisdiction foreign to our constitution, and unacknowledged by our laws, giving his assent to their acts of pretended legislation:

For quartering large bodies of armed troops among us;

For protecting them, by a mock trial, from punishment for any murder which they should commit on the inhabitants of these states;

For cutting off our trade with all parts of the world;

For imposing taxes on us without our consent;

For depriving us, in many cases, of the benefits of trial by jury;

For transporting us beyond seas, to be tried for pretended offenses;

For abolishing the free system of English laws in a neighboring province, establishing therein an arbitrary government, and enlarging its boundaries, so as to render it at once an example and fit instrument for introducing the same absolute rule into these colonies;

For taking away our charters, abolishing our most valuable laws, and altering fundamentally the forms of our governments;

For suspending our own legislatures, and declaring themselves invested with power to legislate for us in all cases whatsoever.

He has abdicated government here, by declaring us out of his protection and waging war against us.

He has plundered our seas, ravaged our coasts, burned our towns, and destroyed the lives of our people.

He is at this time transporting large armies of foreign mercenaries to complete the works of death, desolation, and tyranny already begun with circumstances of cruelty and perfidy scarcely paralleled in the most barbarous ages, and totally unworthy the head of a civilized nation.

He has constrained our fellow-citizens, taken captive on the high seas, to bear arms against their country, to become the executioners of their friends and brethren, or to fall themselves by their hands.

He has excited domestic insurrection among us, and has endeavored to bring on the inhabitants of our frontiers the merciless Indian savages, whose known rule of warfare is an undistinguished destruction of all ages, sexes, and conditions.

In every stage of these oppressions we have petitioned for redress in the most humble terms; our repeated petitions have been answered only by repeated injury. A prince, whose character is thus marked by every act which may define a tyrant, is unfit to be the ruler of a free people.

Nor have we been wanting in our attentions to our British brethren. We have warned them, from time to time, of attempts by their legislature to extend an unwarrantable jurisdiction over us. We have reminded them of the circumstances of our emigration and settlement here. We have appealed to their native justice and magnanimity; and we have conjured them, by the ties of our common kindred, to disavow these usurpations, which would inevitably interrupt our connections and correspondence. They,

too, have been deaf to the voice of justice and of consanguinity. We must, therefore, acquiesce in the necessity which denounces our separation, and hold them, as we hold the rest of mankind, enemies in war, in peace friends.

We, therefore, the representatives of the United States of America, in General Congress assembled, appealing to the Supreme Judge of the world for the rectitude of our intentions, do, in the name and by the authority of the good people of these colonies, solemnly publish and declare, that these United Colonies are, and of right ought to be, FREE AND INDEPENDENT STATES; that they are absolved from all allegiance to the British crown, and that all political connection between them and the state of Great Britain is, and ought to be, totally dissolved; and that, as free and independent states, they have full power to levy war, conclude peace, contract alliances, establish commerce, and do all other acts and things which independent states may of right do. And for the support of this declaration, with a firm reliance on the protection of Divine Providence, we mutually pledge to each other our lives, our fortunes, and our sacred honor.

JOHN HANCOCK

New Hampshire
Josiah Bartlett
William Whipple
Matthew Thornton

Massachusetts
John Adams
Samuel Adams
Robert Treat Paine
Elbridge Gerry

New York
William Floyd
Philip Livingston
Francis Lewis
Lewis Morris

Rhode Island
Stephen Hopkins
William Ellery

New Jersey
Richard Stockton
John Witherspoon
Francis Hopkinson
John Hart
Abraham Clark

Pennsylvania
Robert Morris
Benjamin Rush
Benjamin Franklin
John Morton
George Clymer
James Smith
George Taylor
James Wilson
George Ross

Delaware
Caeser Rodney
George Read
Thomas McKean

Maryland
Samuel Chase
William Paca
Thomas Stone
Charles Carroll of Carrollton

North Carolina
William Hooper
Joseph Hewes
John Penn

Virginia
George Wythe
Richard Henry Lee
Thomas Jefferson
Benjamin Harrison
Thomas Nelson, Jr.
Francis Lightfoot Lee
Carter Braxton

South Carolina
Edward Rutledge
Thomas Heyward, Jr.
Thomas Lynch, Jr.
Arthur Middleton

Connecticut
Roger Sherman
Samuel Huntington
William Williams
Oliver Wolcott

Georgia
Button Gwinnett
Lyman Hall
George Walton

The Articles of Confederation

Between the States of New Hampshire, Massachusetts Bay, Rhode Island and Providence Plantations, Connecticut, New York, New Jersey, Pennsylvania, Delaware, Maryland, Virginia, North Carolina, South Carolina, Georgia

Article 1

The stile of this confederacy shall be "The United States of America."

Article 2

Each State retains its sovereignty, freedom and independence, and every power, jurisdiction, and right, which is not by this confederation expressly delegated to the United States, in Congress assembled.

Article 3

The said states hereby severally enter into a firm league of friendship with each other for their common defence, the security of their liberties and their mutual and general welfare; binding themselves to assist each other against all force offered to, or attacks made upon them, or any of them, on account of religion, sovereignty, trade, or any other pretence whatever.

Article 4

The better to secure and perpetuate mutual friendship and intercourse among the people of the different states in this union, the free inhabitants of each of these states, paupers, vagabonds, and fugitives from justice excepted, shall be entitled to all privileges and immunities of free citizens in the several states; and the people of each State shall have free ingress and regress to and from any other State, and shall enjoy therein all the privileges of trade and commerce, subject to the same duties, impositions, and restrictions, as the inhabitants thereof respectively; provided, that such restrictions shall not extend so far as to prevent the removal of property, imported into any State, to any other State of which the owner is an inhabitant; provided also, that no imposition, duties, or restriction, shall be laid by any State on the property of the United States, or either of them.

If any person guilty of, or charged with treason, felony, or other high misdemeanor in any State, shall flee from justice and be found in any of the United States, he shall, upon demand of the governor or executive power of the State from which he fled, be delivered up and removed to the State having jurisdiction of his offence.

Full faith and credit shall be given in each of these states to the records, acts, and judicial proceedings of the courts and magistrates of every other State.

Article 5

For the more convenient management of the general interests of the United States, delegates shall be annually appointed, in such manner as the legislature of each State shall direct, to meet in Congress, on the 1st Monday in November in every year, with a power reserved to each State to recall its delegates, or any of them, at any time within the year, and to send others in their stead for the remainder of the year.

No State shall be represented in Congress by less than two, nor by more than seven members; and no person shall be capable of being a delegate for more than three years in any term of six years; nor shall any person, being a delegate, be capable of holding any office under the United States, for which he, or any other for his benefit, receives any salary, fees, or emolument of any kind.

Each State shall maintain its own delegates in a meeting of the states, and while they act as members of the committee of the states.

In determining questions in the United States, in Congress assembled, each State shall have one vote.

Freedom of speech and debate in Congress shall not be impeached or questioned in any court or place out of Congress: and the members of Congress shall be protected in their persons from arrests and imprisonments, during the time of their going to and from, and attendance on Congress, except for treason, felony, or breach of the peace.

Article 6

No State, without the consent of the United States, in Congress assembled, shall send any embassy to, or receive any embassy from, or enter into any conference, agreement, alliance, or treaty with any king, prince, or state; nor shall any person, holding any office of profit or trust under the United States, or any of them, accept of any present, emolument, office or title, of any kind whatever, from any king, prince, or foreign state; nor shall the United States, in Congress assembled, or any of them, grant any title of nobility.

No two or more states shall enter into any treaty, confederation, or alliance, whatever, between them, without the consent of the United States, in Congress assembled, specifying accurately the purposes for which the same is to be entered into, and how long it shall continue.

No State shall lay any imposts or duties which may interfere with any stipulations in treaties entered into by the United States, in Congress assembled, with any king, prince, or state, in pursuance of any treaties already proposed by Congress to the courts of France and Spain.

No vessels of war shall be kept up in time of peace by any State, except such number only as shall be deemed necessary by the United States, in Congress assembled, for the defence of such State or its trade; nor shall any body of forces be kept up by any State, in time of peace, except such number only as, in the judgment of the United States, in Congress assembled, shall be deemed requisite to garrison the forts necessary for the defence of such State; but every State shall always keep up a well regulated and disciplined militia, sufficiently armed and accoutred, and shall provide, and constantly have ready for use, in public stores, a due number of field pieces and tents, and a proper quantity of arms, ammunition and camp equipage.

No State shall engage in any war without the consent of the United States, in Congress assembled, unless such State be actually invaded by enemies, or shall have received certain advice of a resolution being formed by some nation of Indians to invade such State, and the danger is so imminent as not to admit of a delay till the United States, in Congress assembled, can be consulted; nor shall any State grant commissions to any ships or vessels of war, nor letters of marque or reprisal, except it be after a declaration of war by the United States, in Congress assembled, and then only against the kingdom or state, and the subjects thereof, against which war has been so declared, and under such regulations as shall be established by the United States, in Congress assembled, unless such States be infested by pirates, in which case vessels of war may be fitted out for that occasion, and kept so long as the danger shall continue, or until the United States, in Congress assembled, shall determine otherwise.

Article 7

When land forces are raised by any State for the common defence, all officers of or under the rank of colonel, shall be appointed by the legislature of each State respectively, by whom such forces shall be raised, or in such manner as such State shall direct; and all vacancies shall be filled up by the State which first made the appointment.

Article 8

All charges of war and all other expences, that shall be incurred for the common defence or general welfare, and allowed by the United States, in Congress assembled, shall be defrayed out of a common treasury, which shall be supplied by the several states, in proportion to the value of all land within each State, granted to or surveyed for any person, as such land and the buildings and improvements thereon shall be estimated according to such mode as the United States, in Congress assembled, shall, from time to time, direct and appoint.

The taxes for paying that proportion shall be laid and levied by the authority and direction of the legislatures of the several states, within the time agreed upon by the United States, in Congress assembled.

Article 9

The United States, in Congress assembled, shall have the sole and exclusive right and power of determining on peace and war, except in the cases mentioned in the 6th article; of sending and receiving ambassadors; entering into treaties and alliances, provided that no treaty of commerce shall be made, whereby the legislative power of the respective states shall be restrained from imposing such imposts and duties on foreigners as their own people are subjected to, or from prohibiting the exportation or importation of any species of goods or commodities whatsoever; of establishing rules for deciding, in all cases, what captures on land or water shall be legal, and in what manner prizes, taken by land or naval forces in the service of the United States, shall be divided or appropriated; of granting letters of marque and reprisal in times of peace; appointing courts for the trial of piracies and felonies committed on the high seas, and establishing

courts for receiving and determining, finally, appeals in all cases of captures; provided, that no member of Congress shall be appointed a judge of any of the said courts.

The United States, in Congress assembled, shall also be the last resort on appeal in all disputes and differences now subsisting, or that hereafter may arise between two or more states concerning boundary, jurisdiction or any other cause whatever; which authority shall always be exercised in the manner following: whenever the legislative or executive authority, or lawful agent of any State, in controversy with another, shall present a petition to Congress, stating the matter in question, and praying for a hearing, notice thereof shall be given, by order of Congress, to the legislative or executive authority of the other State in controversy, and a day assigned for the appearance of the parties by their lawful agents, who shall then be directed to appoint, by joint consent, commissioners or judges to constitute a court for hearing and determining the matter in question; but, if they cannot agree, Congress shall name three persons out of each of the United States, and from the list of such persons each party shall alternately strike out one, the petitioners beginning, until the number shall be reduced to thirteen; and from that number not less than seven, nor more than nine names, as Congress shall direct, shall, in the presence of Congress, be drawn out by lot; and the persons whose names shall be drawn, or any five of them, shall be commissioners or judges to hear and finally determine the controversy, so always as a major part of the judges who shall hear the cause shall agree in the determination; and if either party shall neglect to attend at the day appointed, without shewing reasons which Congress shall judge sufficient, or, being present, shall refuse to strike, the Congress shall proceed to nominate three persons out of each State, and the secretary of Congress shall strike in behalf of such party absent or refusing; and the judgment and sentence of the court to be appointed, in the manner before prescribed, shall be final and conclusive; and if any of the parties shall refuse to submit to the authority of such court, or to appear or defend their claim or cause, the court shall nevertheless proceed to pronounce sentence or judgment, which shall, in like manner, be final and decisive, the judgment or sentence and other proceedings being, in either case, transmitted to Congress, and lodged among the acts of Congress for the security of the parties concerned: provided, that every commissioner, before he sits in judgment, shall take an oath, to be administered by one of the judges of the supreme or superior court of the State where the cause shall be tried, "well and truly to hear and determine the matter in question, according to the best of his judgment, without favour, affection, or hope of reward": provided, also, that no State shall be deprived of territory for the benefit of the United States.

All controversies concerning the private right of soil, claimed under different grants of two or more states, whose jurisdictions, as they may respect such lands and the states which passed such grants, are adjusted, the said grants, or either of them, being at the same time claimed to have originated antecedent to such settlement of jurisdiction, shall, on the petition of either party to the Congress of the United States, be finally determined, as near as may be, in the same manner as is before prescribed for deciding disputes respecting territorial jurisdiction between different states.

The United States, in Congress assembled, shall also have the sole and exclusive right and power of regulating the alloy and value of coin struck by their own authority, or by that of the respective states; fixing the standard of weights and measures throughout the United States; regulating the trade and managing all affairs with the Indians not members of any of the states; provided that the legislative right of any State within its own limits be not infringed or violated; establishing and regulating post offices from one State to another throughout all the United States, and exacting such postage on the papers passing through the same as may be requisite to defray the expences of the said office; appointing all officers of the land forces in the service of the United States, excepting regimental officers; appointing all the officers of the naval forces, and commissioning all officers whatever in the service of the United States; making rules for the government and regulation of the said land and naval forces, and directing their operations.

The United States, in Congress assembled, shall have authority to appoint a committee to sit in the recess of Congress, to be denominated "a Committee of the States," and to consist of one delegate from each State, and to appoint such other committees and civil officers as may be necessary for managing the general affairs of the United States, under their direction; to appoint one of their number to preside; provided that no person be allowed to serve in the office of president more than one year in any term of three years; to ascertain the necessary sums of money to be raised for the service of the United States, and to appropriate and apply the same for defraying the public expences; to borrow money or emit bills on the credit of the United States, transmitting, every half year, to the respective states, an account of the sums of money so borrowed or emitted; to build and equip a navy; to agree upon the number of land forces, and to make requisitions from each State for its quota, in proportion to the number of white inhabitants in such State; which requisitions shall be binding; and, thereupon, the legislature of each State shall appoint the regimental officers, raise the men, and cloathe, arm, and equip them in a soldier-like manner, at the expence of the United States; and the officers and men so cloathed, armed, and equipped, shall march to the place appointed and within the time agreed on by the United States, in Congress assembled; but if the United States, in Congress assembled, shall, on consideration of circumstances, judge proper that any State should not raise men, or should raise a smaller number than its quota, and that any other State should raise a greater number of men than the quota thereof, such extra number shall be raised, officered, cloathed, armed, and equipped in the same manner as the quota of such State, unless the legislature of such State shall judge that such extra number cannot be safely spared out of the same, in which case they shall raise, officer, cloathe, arm, and equip as many of such extra number as they judge can be safely spared. And the officers and men so cloathed, armed, and equipped, shall march to the place appointed and within the time agreed on by the United States, in Congress assembled.

The United States, in Congress assembled, shall never engage in a war, nor grant letters of marque and reprisal in time of peace, nor enter into any treaties or alliances, nor coin money, nor regulate the value thereof, nor ascertain the sums and expences necessary for the defence and welfare of the United States, or any of them: nor emit bills, nor borrow money on the credit of the United States, nor appropriate money, nor agree upon the number of vessels of war to be built or purchased, or the number of land or sea forces to be raised, nor appoint a commander in chief of the army or navy, unless nine states assent to the same; nor shall a question on any other point, except for adjourning from day to day, be determined, unless by the votes of a majority of the United States, in Congress assembled.

The Congress of the United States shall have power to adjourn to any time within the year, and to any place within the United States, so that no period of adjournment be for a longer duration than the space of six months, and shall publish the journal of their proceedings monthly, except such parts thereof, relating to treaties, alliances or military operations, as, in their judgment, require secrecy; and the yeas and nays of the delegates of each State on any question shall be entered on the journal, when it is desired by any delegate; and the delegates of a State, or any of them, at his, or their request, shall be furnished with a transcript of the said journal, except such parts as are above excepted, to lay before the legislatures of the several states.

Article 10

The committee of the states, or any nine of them, shall be authorized to execute, in the recess of Congress, such of the powers of Congress as the United States, in Congress assembled, by the consent of nine states, shall, from time to time, think expedient to vest them with; provided, that no power be delegated to the said committee for the exercise of which, by the articles of confederation, the voice of nine states, in the Congress of the United States assembled, is requisite.

Article 11

Canada acceding to this confederation, and joining in the measures of the United States, shall be admitted into and entitled to all the advantages of this union; but no other colony shall be admitted into the same, unless such admission be agreed to by nine states.

Article 12

All bills of credit emitted, monies borrowed and debts contracted by, or under the authority of Congress before the assembling of the United States, in pursuance of the present confederation, shall be deemed and considered as a charge against the United States, for payment and satisfaction whereof the said United States and the public faith are hereby solemnly pledged.

Article 13

Every State shall abide by the determinations of the United States, in Congress assembled, on all questions which, by this confederation, are submitted to them. And the articles of this confederation shall be inviolably observed by every State, and the union shall be perpetual; nor shall any alteration at any time hereafter be made in any of them, unless such alteration be agreed to in a Congress of the United States, and be afterwards confirmed by the legislatures of every State.

These articles shall be proposed to the legislatures of all the United States, to be considered, and if approved of by them, they are advised to authorize their delegates to ratify the same in the Congress of the United States; which being done, the same shall become conclusive.

The Constitution of the United States of America

Preamble

We the People of the United States, in Order to form a more perfect Union, establish Justice, insure domestic Tranquility, provide for the common defence, promote the general Welfare, and secure the Blessings of Liberty to ourselves and our Posterity, do ordain and establish this Constitution for the United States of America.

Article I

Section 1

All legislative Powers herein granted shall be vested in a Congress of the United States, which shall consist of a Senate and House of Representatives.

Section 2

The House of Representatives shall be composed of Members chosen every second Year by the People of the several States, and the Electors in each State shall have the Qualifications requisite for Electors of the most numerous Branch of the State Legislature.

No Person shall be a Representative who shall not have attained to the Age of twenty five Years, and been seven Years a Citizen of the United States, and who shall not, when elected, be an inhabitant of that State in which he shall be chosen.

Representatives and direct Taxes shall be apportioned among the several States which may be included within this Union, according to their respective Numbers, *which shall be determined by adding to the whole Number of free Persons, including those bound to Service for a Term of Years, and excluding Indians not taxed, three fifths of all other Persons.** The actual Enumeration shall be made within three Years after the first Meeting of the Congress of the United States, and within every subsequent Term of ten Years, in such Manner as they shall by Law direct. The Number of Representatives shall not exceed one for every thirty Thousand, but each State shall have at Least one Representative; *and until such enumeration shall be made, the State of New Hampshire shall be entitled to chuse three, Massachusetts eight, Rhode-Island and Providence Plantations one, Connecticut five, New York six, New Jersey four, Pennsylvania eight, Delaware one, Maryland six, Virginia ten, North Carolina five, South Carolina five, and Georgia three.*

When vacancies happen in the Representation from any State, the Executive Authority thereof shall issue Writs of Election to fill such Vacancies.

The House of Representatives shall chuse their Speaker and other Officers; and shall have the sole Power of Impeachment.

Section 3

The Senate of the United States shall be composed of two Senators from each State, *chosen by the Legislature thereof,* for six Years; and each Senator shall have one Vote.

Immediately after they shall be assembled in Consequence of the first Election, they shall be divided as equally as may be into three Classes. The Seats of the Senators of the first Class shall be vacated at the Expiration of the second Year, of the second Class at the Expiration of the fourth Year, and of the third Class at the Expiration of the sixth Year so that one third may be chosen every second Year; and if Vacancies happen by Resignation, or otherwise, during the Recess of the Legislature of any state, the Executive thereof may make temporary Appointments until the next Meeting of the Legislature, which shall then fill such Vacancies.

No Person shall be a Senator who shall not have attained to the Age of thirty Years, and been nine Years a Citizen of the United States, and who shall not, when elected, be an Inhabitant of that State for which he shall be chosen.

The Vice President of the United States shall be President of the Senate, but shall have no Vote, unless they be equally divided.

The Senate shall chuse their other Officers, and also a President *pro tempore,* in the Absence of the Vice President, or when he shall exercise the Office of President of the United States.

The Senate shall have the sole Power to try all Impeachments. When sitting for that Purpose, they shall be on Oath or Affirmation. When the President of the United States is tried the Chief Justice shall preside: And no Person shall be convicted without the Concurrence of two thirds of the Members present.

Judgment in Cases of Impeachment shall not extend further than to removal from Office, and disqualification to hold and enjoy any Office of honor, Trust or Profit under the United States: but the Party convicted shall nevertheless be liable and subject to Indictment, Trial, Judgment and Punishment, according to Law.

Section 4

The Times, Places and Manner of holding Elections for Senators and Representatives, shall be prescribed in each State by the Legislature thereof; but the Congress may at any time by Law make or alter such Regulations, except as to the Places of chusing Senators.

The Congress shall assemble at least once in every Year, *and such Meeting shall be on the first Monday in December, unless they shall by Law appoint a different Day.*

Section 5

Each House shall be the Judge of the Elections, Returns and Qualifications of its own Members, and a Majority of each shall constitute a Quorum to do Business; but a smaller Number may adjourn from day to day, and may be authorized to compel the Attendance of absent Members, in such Manner, and under such Penalties as each House may provide.

---

*Passages no longer in effect are printed in italic type.

Each House may determine the Rules of its Proceedings, punish its Members for disorderly Behaviour, and, with the Concurrence of two thirds, expel a Member.

Each House shall keep a Journal of its Proceedings, and from time to time publish the same, excepting such Parts as may in their Judgment require Secrecy; and the Yeas and Nays of the Members of either House on any question shall, at the Desire of one fifth of those Present, be entered on the Journal.

Neither House, during the Session of Congress, shall, without the Consent of the other, adjourn for more than three days, nor to any other Place than that in which the two Houses shall be sitting.

Section 6

The Senators and Representatives shall receive a Compensation for their Services, to be ascertained by Law, and paid out of the Treasury of the United States. They shall in all Cases, except Treason, Felony and Breach of the Peace, be privileged from Arrest during their Attendance at the Session of their respective Houses, and in going to and returning from the same; and for any Speech or Debate in either House, they shall not be questioned in any other Place.

No Senator or Representative shall, during the Time for which he was elected, be appointed to any civil Office under the Authority of the United States, which shall have been created, or the Emoluments whereof shall have been encreased during such time, and no Person holding any Office under the United States, shall be a Member of either House during his Continuance in Office.

Section 7

All Bills for raising Revenue shall originate in the House of Representatives; but the Senate may propose or concur with Amendments as on other Bills.

Every Bill which shall have passed the House of Representatives and the Senate, shall, before it become a Law, be presented to the President of the United States; If he approve he shall sign it, but if not he shall return it, with his Objections to the House in which it shall have originated, who shall enter the Objections at large on their Journal, and proceed to reconsider it. If after such Reconsideration two thirds of that House shall agree to pass the Bill, it shall be sent, together with the Objections, to the other House, by which it shall likewise be reconsidered, and if approved by two thirds of that House, it shall become a Law. But in all such Cases the Votes of both Houses shall be determined by yeas and Nays, and the Names of the Persons voting for and against the Bill shall be entered on the Journal of each House respectively. If any Bill shall not be returned by the President within ten Days (Sundays excepted) after it shall have been presented to him, the Same shall be a Law, in like Manner as if he had signed it, unless the Congress by their Adjournment prevent its Return, in which Case it shall not be a Law.

Every Order, Resolution, or Vote to which the Concurrence of the Senate and House of Representatives may be necessary (except on a question of Adjournment) shall be presented to the President of the United States; and before the Same shall take Effect, shall be approved by him, or being disapproved by him, shall be repassed by two thirds of the Senate and House of Representatives, according to the Rules and Limitations prescribed in the Case of a Bill.

Section 8

The Congress shall have Power To lay and collect Taxes, Duties, Imposts and Excises, to pay the Debts and provide for the common Defence and general Welfare of the United States; but all Duties, Imposts and Excises shall be uniform throughout the United States;

To borrow Money on the credit of the United States;

To regulate Commerce with foreign Nations, and among the several States, and with the Indian Tribes;

To establish an uniform Rule of Naturalization, and uniform Laws on the subject of Bankruptcies throughout the United States;

To coin Money, regulate the Value thereof, and of foreign Coin, and fix the Standard of Weights and Measures;

To provide for the Punishment of counterfeiting the Securities and current Coin of the United States;

To establish Post Offices and post Roads;

To promote the Progress of Science and useful Arts, by securing for limited Times to Authors and Inventors the exclusive Right to their respective Writings and Discoveries;

To constitute Tribunals inferior to the supreme Court;

To define and punish Piracies and Felonies committed on the high Seas, and Offences against the Law of Nations;

To declare War, grant Letters of Marque and Reprisal, and make Rules concerning Captures on Land and Water;

To raise and support Armies, but no Appropriation of Money to that Use shall be for a longer Term than two Years;

To provide and maintain a Navy;

To make Rules for the Government and Regulation of the land and naval Forces;

To provide for calling forth the Militia to execute the Laws of the Union, suppress Insurrections and repel Invasions;

To provide for organizing, arming, and disciplining, the Militia, and for governing such Part of them as may be employed in the Service of the United States, reserving to the States respectively, the Appointment of the Officers, and the Authority of training the Militia according to the discipline prescribed by Congress;

To exercise exclusive Legislation in all Cases whatsoever, over such District (not exceeding ten Miles square) as may, by Cession of particular States, and the Acceptance of Congress, become the Seat of the Government of the United States, and to exercise like Authority over all Places purchased by the Consent of the Legislature of the State in which the Same shall be, for the Erection of Forts, Magazines, Arsenals, dock-Yards, and other needful Buildings;—And

To make all Laws which shall be necessary and proper for carrying into Execution the foregoing Powers, and all other Powers vested by this Constitution in the Government of the United States, or in any Department of Officer thereof.

Section 9

The Migration or Importation of such Persons as any of the States now existing shall think proper to admit, shall not be prohibited by the Congress prior to the Year one thousand eight hundred and

eight, but a Tax or duty may be imposed on such Importation, not exceeding ten dollars for each Person.

The Privilege of the Writ of Habeas Corpus shall not be suspended, unless when in Cases of Rebellion or Invasion the public Safety may require it.

No Bill of Attainder or ex post facto Law shall be passed.

No Capitation, or other direct, Tax shall be laid, unless in Proportion to the Census or Enumeration herein before directed to be taken.

No Tax or Duty shall be laid on Articles exported from any State.

No Preference shall be given by any Regulation of Commerce or Revenue to the Ports of one State over those of another: nor shall Vessels bound to, or from, one State, be obliged to enter, clear, or pay Duties in another.

No Money shall be drawn from the Treasury, but in Consequence of Appropriations made by Law; and a regular Statement and Account of the Receipts and Expenditures of all public Money shall be published from time to time.

No Title of Nobility shall be granted by the United States: And no Person holding any Office of Profit or Trust under them, shall, without the Consent of the Congress, accept of any present, Emolument, Office, or Title, of any kind whatever, from any King, Prince, or foreign State.

Section 10

No State shall enter into any Treaty, Alliance, or Confederation; grant Letters of Marque and Reprisal; coin Money; emit Bills of Credit; make any Thing but gold and silver Coin a Tender in Payment of Debts; pass any Bill of Attainder, ex post facto Law, or Law impairing the obligation of Contracts, or grant any Title of Nobility.

No State shall, without the Consent of the Congress, lay any Imposts or Duties on Imports or Exports, except what may be absolutely necessary for executing its inspection Laws: and the net Produce of all Duties and Imposts, laid by any State on Imports or Exports, shall be for the Use of the Treasury of the United States; and all such Laws shall be subject to the Revision and Controul of the Congress.

No State shall, without the Consent of Congress, lay any Duty of Tonnage, keep Troops, or Ships of War in time of Peace, enter into any Agreement or Compact with another State, or with a foreign Power, or engage in War, unless actually invaded, or in such imminent Danger as will not admit of delay.

Article II

Section 1

The executive Power shall be vested in a President of the United States of America. He shall hold his Office during the Term of four Years, and, together with the Vice President, chosen for the same Term, be elected, as follows:

Each State shall appoint, in such Manner as the Legislature thereof may direct, a Number of Electors, equal to the whole Number of Senators and Representatives to which the State may be entitled in the Congress: but no Senator or Representative, or Person holding an Office of Trust or Profit under the United States, shall be appointed an Elector.

The Electors shall meet in their respective States, and vote by Ballot for two Persons, of whom one at least shall not be an Inhabitant of the same State with themselves. And they shall make a List of all the Persons voted for, and of the Number of Votes for each; which List they shall sign and certify, and transmit sealed to the Seat of the Government of the United States, directed to the President of the Senate. The President of the Senate shall, in the Presence of the Senate and House of Representatives, open all the Certificates, and the Votes shall then be counted. The Person having the greatest Number of Votes shall be the President, if such Number be a Majority of the whole number of Electors appointed; and if there be more than one who have such Majority, and have an equal Number of Votes, then the House of Representatives shall immediately chuse by Ballot one of them for President; and if no Person have a Majority, then from the five highest on the List the said House shall in like Manner chuse the President. But in chusing the President, the Votes shall be taken by States, the Representation from each State having one Vote; A quorum for this Purpose shall consist of a Member or Members from two thirds of the States, and a Majority of all the States shall be necessary to a Choice. In every Case, after the Choice of the President, the Person having the greatest Number of Votes of the Electors shall be the Vice President. But if there should remain two or more who have equal Votes, the Senate shall chuse from them by Ballot the Vice President.

The Congress may determine the time of chusing the Electors, and the Day on which they shall give their Votes; which Day shall be the same throughout the United States.

No person except a natural born Citizen, *or a Citizen of the United States, at the time of the Adoption of this Constitution,* shall be eligible to the Office of President; neither shall any Person be eligible to that Office who shall not have attained to the Age of thirty five Years, and been fourteen Years a Resident within the United States.

In Case of the Removal of the President from Office, or of his Death, Resignation, or Inability to discharge the Powers and Duties of the said Office, the Same shall devolve on the Vice President, and the Congress may by Law provide for the Case of Removal, Death, Resignation or Inability, both of the President and Vice President, declaring what Officer shall then act as President, and such Officer shall act accordingly, until the Disability be removed, or a President shall be elected.

The President shall, at stated Times, receive for his Services, a Compensation, which shall neither be encreased nor diminished during the Period for which he shall have been elected, and he shall not receive within that period any other Emolument from the United States, or any of them.

Before he enter on the Execution of his Office, he shall take the following Oath or Affirmation:—"I do solemnly swear (or affirm) that I will faithfully execute the Office of President of the United States, and will to the best of my Ability, preserve, protect and defend the Constitution of the United States."

Section 2

The President shall be Commander in Chief of the Army and Navy of the United States, and of the Militia of the several States, when called into the actual Service of the United States; he may require the Opinion, in writing, of the principal Officer in each of the executive Departments, upon any Subject relating to the Duties of their respective Offices, and he shall have

Power to grant Reprieves and Pardons for Offences against the United States, except in Cases of Impeachment.

He shall have Power, by and with the Advice and Consent of the Senate, to make Treaties, provided two thirds of the Senators present concur; and he shall nominate, and by and with the Advice and Consent of the Senate, shall appoint Ambassadors, other public Ministers and Consuls, Judges of the supreme Court, and all other Officers of the United States, whose Appointments are not herein otherwise provided for, and which shall be established by Law: but the Congress may by Law vest the Appointment of such inferior Officers, as they think proper in the President alone, in the Courts of Law, or in the Heads of Departments.

The President shall have Power to fill up all Vacancies that may happen during the Recess of the Senate, by granting Commissions which shall expire at the End of their next Session.

Section 3

He shall from time to time give to the Congress Information of the State of the Union, and recommend to their Consideration such Measures as he shall judge necessary and expedient; he may, on extraordinary Occasions, convene both Houses, or either of them, and in Case of disagreement between them, with Respect to the Time of Adjournment, he may adjourn them to such Time as he shall think proper; he shall receive Ambassadors and other public Ministers; he shall take Care that the Laws be faithfully executed, and shall Commission all the officers of the United States.

Section 4

The President, Vice President and all civil Officers of the United States, shall be removed from Office on Impeachment for, and Conviction of, Treason, Bribery or other high Crimes and Misdemeanors.

Article III

Section 1

The judicial Power of the United States, shall be vested in one supreme Court, and in such inferior Courts as the Congress may from time to time ordain and establish. The Judges, both of the supreme and inferior Courts, shall hold their offices during good Behaviour, and shall, at stated Times, receive for their Services, a Compensation, which shall not be diminished during their Continuance in Office.

Section 2

The judicial Power shall extend to all Cases, in Law and Equity, arising under this Constitution, the Laws of the United States, and Treaties made, or which shall be made, under their Authority;—to all Cases affecting Ambassadors, other public Ministers and Consuls;—to all Cases of admiralty and maritime Jurisdiction;—to Controversies to which the United States shall be a Party;—to Controversies between two or more States;— *between a State and Citizens of another State;*—between Citizens of different States;—between Citizens of the same State claiming Lands under Grants of different States, and between a State, or the Citizens thereof, and foreign States, Citizens or Subjects.

In all Cases affecting Ambassadors, other public Ministers and Consuls, and those in which a State shall be Party, the supreme Court shall have original Jurisdiction. In all the other Cases before mentioned, the supreme Court shall have appellate Jurisdiction, both as to Law and Fact, with such Exceptions, and under such Regulations as the Congress shall make.

The Trial of all Crimes, except in Cases of Impeachment, shall be by Jury; and such Trial shall be held in the State where the said Crimes shall have been committed; but when not committed within any State, the Trial shall be at such Place or Places as the Congress may by Law have directed.

Section 3

Treason against the United States, shall consist only in levying War against them, or in adhering to their Enemies, giving them Aid and Comfort. No person shall be convicted of Treason unless on the Testimony of two Witnesses to the same overt Act, or on Confession in open Court.

The Congress shall have Power to declare the Punishment of Treason, but no Attainder of Treason shall work Corruption of Blood, or Forfeiture except during the Life of the Person attainted.

Article IV

Section 1

Full Faith and Credit shall be given in each State to the public Acts, Records, and judicial Proceedings of every other State. And the Congress may by general Laws prescribe the Manner in which such Acts, Records and Proceedings shall be proved, and the Effect thereof.

Section 2

The Citizens of each State shall be entitled to all Privileges and Immunities of Citizens in the several States.

A Person charged in any State with Treason, Felony, or other Crime, who shall flee from Justice, and be found in another State, shall on Demand of the executive Authority of the State from which he fled, be delivered up, to be removed to the State having Jurisdiction of the Crime.

No Person held to Service or Labour in one State, under the Laws thereof, escaping into another, shall, in Consequence of any Law or Regulation therein, be discharged from such Service or Labour, but shall be delivered up on Claim of the Party to whom such Service or Labour may be due.

Section 3

New States may be admitted by the Congress into this Union; but no new State shall be formed or erected within the Jurisdiction of any other State; nor any State be formed by the Junction of two or more States, or Parts of States, without the Consent of the Legislatures of the States concerned as well as of the Congress.

The Congress shall have Power to dispose of and make all needful Rules and Regulations respecting the Territory or other Property belonging to the United States; and nothing in this Constitution shall be so construed as to Prejudice any Claims of the United States, or of any particular States.

Section 4

The United States shall guarantee to every State in this Union a Republican Form of Government, and shall protect each of them against Invasion; and on Application of the Legislature, or of the Executive (when the Legislature cannot be convened) against domestic violence.

Article V

The Congress, whenever two thirds of both Houses shall deem it necessary, shall propose Amendments to this Constitution, or, on the Application of the Legislatures of two thirds of the several States, shall call a Convention for proposing Amendments, which, in either Case, shall be valid to all Intents and Purposes, as Part of this Constitution, when ratified by the Legislatures of three fourths of the several States, or by Conventions in three fourths thereof, as the one or the other Mode of Ratification may be proposed by the Congress; Provided *that no Amendment which may be made prior to the Year One thousand eight hundred and eight shall in any Manner affect the first and fourth Clauses in the Ninth Section of the first Article;* and that no State, without its Consent, shall be deprived of its equal Suffrage in the Senate.

Article VI

All Debts contracted and Engagements entered into, before the Adoption of this Constitution, shall be as valid against the United States under this Constitution, as under the Confederation.

This Constitution, and Laws of the United States which shall be made in Pursuance thereof; and all Treaties made, or which shall be made, under the Authority of the United States, shall be the supreme Law of the Land; and the Judges in every State shall be bound thereby, any Thing in the Constitution or Laws of any State to the Contrary notwithstanding.

The Senators and Representatives before mentioned, and the Members of the several State Legislatures, and all executive and Judicial Officers, both of the United States and of the several States, shall be bound by Oath or Affirmation, to support this Constitution; but no religious Test shall ever be required as a Qualification to any Office of public Trust under the United States.

Article VII

The Ratification of the Conventions of nine States, shall be sufficient for the Establishment of this Constitution between the States so ratifying the Same.

Done in Convention by the Unanimous Consent of the States present the Seventeenth Day of September in the Year of our Lord one thousand seven hundred and Eighty seven and of the Independence of the United States of America the Twelfth* IN WITNESS whereof We have hereunto subscribed our Names,

George Washington
President and Deputy from Virginia

Delaware	*South Carolina*	*New York*
George Read	John Rutledge	Alexander Hamilton
Gunning Bedford, Jr.	Charles Cotesworth Pinckney	
John Dickinson	Charles Pinckney	*New Jersey*
Richard Bassett	Pierce Butler	William Livingston
Jacob Broom		David Brearley
	Georgia	William Paterson
Maryland	William Few	Jonathan Dayton
James McHenry	Abraham Baldwin	
Daniel of St. Thomas Jenifer		*Pennsylvania*
Daniel Carroll	*New Hampshire*	Benjamin Franklin
	John Langdon	Thomas Mifflin
Virginia	Nicholas Gilman	Robert Morris
John Blair		George Clymer
James Madison, Jr.	*Massachusetts*	Thomas FitzSimons
	Nathaniel Gorham	Jared Ingersoll
North Carolina	Rufus King	James Wilson
William Blount		Gouverneur Morris
Richard Dobbs Spraight	*Connecticut*	
Hugh Williamson	William Samuel Johnson	
	Roger Sherman	

---

*The Constitution was submitted on September 17, 1787, by the Constitutional Convention, was ratified by conventions of the several states at various dates up to May 29, 1790, and became effective on March 4, 1789.

Amendments to the Constitution

Amendment I

Congress shall make no law respecting an establishment of religion, or prohibiting the free exercise thereof; or abridging the freedom of speech, or of the press; or the right of the people peaceably to assemble, and to petition the Government for a redress of grievances.

Amendment II

A well regulated Militia being necessary to the security of a free State, the right of the people to keep and bear Arms, shall not be infringed.

Amendment III

No Soldier shall, in time of peace be quartered in any house, without the consent of the Owner, nor in time of war, but in a manner to be prescribed by law.

Amendment IV

The right of the people to be secure in their persons, houses, papers, and effects, against unreasonable searches and seizures, shall not be violated, and no Warrants shall issue, but upon probable cause, supported by Oath or affirmation, and particularly describing the place to be searched, and the persons or things to be seized.

Amendment V

No person shall be held to answer for a capital, or otherwise infamous crime, unless on a presentment or indictment of a Grand Jury, except in cases arising in the land or naval forces, or in the Militia, when in actual service in time of War or public danger; nor shall any person be subject for the same offense to be twice put in jeopardy of life or limb; nor shall be compelled in any criminal case to be a witness against himself, nor be deprived of life, liberty, or property, without due process of law; nor shall private property be taken for public use, without just compensation.

Amendment VI

In all criminal prosecutions, the accused shall enjoy the right to a speedy and public trial, by an impartial jury of the State and district wherein the crime shall have been committed, which district shall have been previously ascertained by law, and to be informed of the nature and cause of the accusation; to be confronted with the witnesses against him; to have compulsory process for obtaining witnesses in his favor, and to have the Assistance of Counsel for his defence.

Amendment VII

In Suits at common law, where the value in controversy shall exceed twenty dollars, the right of trial by jury shall be preserved, and no fact tried by a jury, shall be otherwise re-examined in any Court of the United States, than according to the rules of the common law.

Amendment VIII

Excessive bail shall not be required, nor excessive fines imposed, nor cruel and unusual punishments inflicted.

Amendment IX

The enumeration in the Constitution, of certain rights, shall not be construed to deny or disparage others retained by the people.

Amendment X*

The powers not delegated to the United States by the Constitution, nor prohibited by it to the States, are reserved to the States respectively, or to the people.

Amendment XI
[Adopted 1798]

The Judicial power of the United States shall not be construed to extend to any suit in law or equity, commenced or prosecuted against one of the United States by Citizens of another State, or by Citizens or Subjects of any Foreign State.

Amendment XII
[Adopted 1804]

The Electors shall meet in their respective states, and vote by ballot for President and Vice President, one of whom, at least, shall not be an inhabitant of the same state with themselves; they shall name in their ballots the person voted for as President, and in distinct ballots the person voted for as Vice President, and they shall make distinct lists of all persons voted for as President, and of all persons voted for as Vice President, and of the number of votes for each, which lists they shall sign and certify, and transmit sealed to the seat of the government of the United States, directed to the President of the Senate;—The President of the Senate shall, in the presence of the Senate and House of Representatives, open all the certificates and the votes shall then be counted;—The person having the greatest number of votes for President, shall be the President, if such number be a majority of the whole number of Electors appointed; and if no person have such majority, then from the persons having the highest numbers not exceeding three on the list of those voted for as President, the House of Representatives shall choose immediately, by ballot, the President. But in choosing the President, the votes shall be taken by states, the representation from each state having one vote; a quorum for this purpose shall consist of a

---

*The first ten amendments (the Bill of Rights) were ratified and their adoption was certified on December 15, 1791.

member or members from two-thirds of the states, and a majority of all the states shall be necessary to a choice. And if the House of Representatives shall not choose a President whenever the right of choice shall devolve upon them, before *the fourth day of March* next following, then the Vice President shall act as President, as in the case of the death or other constitutional disability of the President.—The person having the greatest number of votes as Vice President, shall be the Vice President, if such number be a majority of the whole number of Electors appointed, and if no person have a majority, then from the two highest numbers on the list, the Senate shall choose the Vice President; a quorum for the purpose shall consist of two-thirds of the whole number of Senators, and a majority of the whole number shall be necessary to a choice. But no person constitutionally ineligible to the office of President shall be eligible to that of Vice President of the United States.

Amendment XIII
[Adopted 1865]

Section 1

Neither slavery nor involuntary servitude, except as a punishment for crime whereof the party shall have been duly convicted, shall exist within the United States, or any place subject to their jurisdiction.

Section 2

Congress shall have power to enforce this article by appropriate legislation.

Amendment XIV
[Adopted 1868]

Section 1

All persons born or naturalized in the United States, and subject to the jurisdiction thereof, are citizens of the United States and of the State wherein they reside. No State shall make or enforce any law which shall abridge the privileges or immunities of citizens of the United States; nor shall any State deprive any person of life, liberty, or property, without due process of law; nor deny to any person within its jurisdiction the equal protection of the laws.

Section 2

Representatives shall be apportioned among the several States according to their respective numbers, counting the whole number of persons in each State, excluding Indians not taxed. But when the right to vote at any election for the choice of electors for President and Vice President of the United States, Representatives in Congress, the Executive and Judicial officers of a State, or the members of the Legislature thereof, is denied to any of the male inhabitants of such State, being twenty-one years of age, and citizens of the United States, or in any way abridged, except for participation in rebellion, or other crime, the basis of representation therein shall be reduced in the proportion which the number of such male citizens shall bear to the whole number of male citizens twenty-one years of age in such State.

Section 3

No person shall be a Senator or Representative in Congress, or elector of President and Vice President, or hold any office, civil or military, under the United States, or under any State, who, having previously taken an oath, as a member of Congress, or as an officer of the United States, or as a member of any State legislature, or as an executive or judicial officer of any State, to support the Constitution of the United States, shall have engaged in insurrection or rebellion against the same, or given aid or comfort to the enemies thereof. But Congress may by a vote of two-thirds of each House, remove such disability.

Section 4

The validity of the public debt of the United States, authorized by law, including debts incurred for payment of pensions and bounties for services in suppressing insurrection or rebellion, shall not be questioned. But neither the United States nor any State shall assume or pay any debt or obligation incurred in aid of insurrection or rebellion against the United States, or any claim for the loss or emancipation of any slave; but all such debts, obligations and claims shall be held illegal and void.

Section 5

The Congress shall have power to enforce, by appropriate legislation, the provisions of this article.

Amendment XV
[Adopted 1870]

Section 1

The right of citizens of the United States to vote shall not be denied or abridged by the United States or by any State on account of race, color, or previous condition of servitude.

Section 2

The Congress shall have power to enforce this article by appropriate legislation.

Amendment XVI
[Adopted 1913]

The Congress shall have power to lay and collect taxes on incomes, from whatever source derived, without apportionment among the several States, and without regard to any census or enumeration.

Amendment XVII
[Adopted 1913]

The Senate of the United States shall be composed of two Senators from each State, elected by the people thereof, for six years; and each Senator shall have one vote. The electors in each State shall have the qualifications requisite for electors of the most numerous branch of the State legislatures.

When vacancies happen in the representation of any State in the Senate, the executive authority of such State shall issue writs of election to fill such vacancies: *Provided,* That the legislature of any State may empower the executive thereof to make temporary appointments until the people fill the vacancies by election as the legislature may direct.

This amendment shall not be so construed as to affect the election or term of any Senator chosen before it becomes valid as part of the Constitution.

Amendment XVIII
[Adopted 1919, repealed 1933]

Section 1

After one year from the ratification of this article the manufacture, sale, or transportation of intoxicating liquors within, the importation thereof into, or the exportation thereof from the United States and all territory subject to the jurisdiction thereof for beverage purposes is hereby prohibited.

Section 2

The Congress and the several States shall have concurrent power to enforce this article by appropriate legislation.

Section 3

This article shall be inoperative unless it shall have been ratified as an amendment to the Constitution by the legislatures of the several States, as provided in the Constitution, within seven years from the date of the submission hereof to the States by the Congress.

Amendment XIX
[Adopted 1920]

The right of citizens of the United States to vote shall not be denied or abridged by the United States or by any State on account of sex.

Congress shall have power to enforce this article by appropriate legislation.

Amendment XX
[Adopted 1933]

Section 1

The terms of the President and Vice President shall end at noon on the 20th day of January, and the terms of Senators and Representatives at noon on the 3d day of January, of the years in which such terms would have ended if this article had not been ratified and the terms of their successors shall then begin.

Section 2

The Congress shall assemble at least once in every year, and such meeting shall begin at noon on the 3d day of January, unless they shall by law appoint a different day.

Section 3

If, at the time fixed for the beginning of the term of the President, the President elect shall have died, the Vice President elect shall become President. If a President shall not have been chosen before the time fixed for the beginning of his term, or if the President elect shall have failed to qualify, then the Vice President elect shall act as President until a President shall have qualified; and the Congress may by law provide for the case wherein neither a President elect nor a Vice President elect shall have qualified, declaring who shall then act as President, or the manner in which one who is to act shall be selected, and such person shall act accordingly until a President or Vice President shall have qualified.

Section 4

The Congress may by law provide for the case of the death of any of the persons from whom the House of Representatives may choose a President whenever the right of choice shall have devolved upon them, and for the case of the death of any of the persons from whom the Senate may choose a Vice President whenever the right of choice shall have devolved upon them.

Section 5

Sections 1 and 2 shall take effect on the 15th day of October following the ratification of this article.

Section 6

This article shall be inoperative unless it shall have been ratified as an amendment to the Constitution by the legislatures of three fourths of the several States within seven years from the date of its submission.

Amendment XXI
[Adopted 1933]

Section 1

The eighteenth article of amendment to the Constitution of the United States is hereby repealed.

Section 2

The transportation or importation into any State, Territory, or possession of the United States for delivery or use therein of intoxicating liquors in violation of the laws thereof, is hereby prohibited.

Section 3

This article shall be inoperative unless it shall have been ratified as an amendment to the Constitution by conventions in the several States, as provided in the Constitution, within seven years from the date of the submission hereof to the States by the Congress.

Amendment XXII
[Adopted 1951]

Section 1

No person shall be elected to the office of the President more than twice, and no person who has held the office of President, or acted as President, for more than two years of a term to which some other person was elected President shall be elected to the office of the President more than once. But this Article shall not apply to any person holding the office of President when this Article was proposed by the Congress, and shall not prevent any person who may be holding the office of President, or acting as President, during the term within which this Article becomes operative from holding the office of President or acting as President during the remainder of such term.

Section 2

This article shall be inoperative unless it shall have been ratified as an amendment to the Constitution by the legislatures of three-fourths of the several States within seven years from the date of its submission to the States by the Congress.

Amendment XXIII
[Adopted 1961]

Section 1

The District constituting the seat of Government of the United States shall appoint in such manner as the Congress shall direct:

A number of electors of President and Vice President equal to the whole number of Senators and Representatives in Congress to which the District would be entitled if it were a State, but in no event more than the least populous State; they shall be in addition to those appointed by the States, but they shall be considered, for the purposes of the election of President and Vice President, to be electors appointed by a State; and they shall meet in the District and perform such duties as provided by the twelfth article of amendment.

Section 2

The Congress shall have power to enforce this article by appropriate legislation.

Amendment XXIV
[Adopted 1964]

Poll tax

Section 1

The right of citizens of the United States to vote in any primary or other election for President or Vice President, for electors for President or Vice President, or for Senator or Representative in Congress, shall not be denied or abridged by the United States or any state by reason of failure to pay any poll tax or other tax.

Section 2

The Congress shall have the power to enforce this article by appropriate legislation.

Amendment XXV
[Adopted 1967]

Section 1

In case of the removal of the President from office or his death or resignation, the Vice President shall become President.

Section 2

Whenever there is a vacancy in the office of the Vice President, the President shall nominate a Vice President who shall take the office upon confirmation by a majority vote of both houses of Congress.

Section 3

Whenever the President transmits to the President pro tempore of the Senate and the Speaker of the House of Representatives his written declaration that he is unable to discharge the powers and duties of his office, and until he transmits to them a written declaration to the contrary, such powers and duties shall be discharged by the Vice President as Acting President.

Section 4

Whenever the Vice President and a majority of either the principal officers of the executive departments or of such other body as Congress may by law provide, transmit to the President pro tempore of the Senate and the Speaker of the House of Representatives their written declaration that the President is unable to discharge the powers and duties of his office, the Vice President shall immediately assume the powers and duties of the office as Acting President.

Thereafter, when the President transmits to the President pro tempore of the Senate and the Speaker of the House of Representatives his written declaration that no inability exists, he shall resume the powers and duties of his office unless the Vice President and a majority of either the principal officers of the executive department or of such other body as Congress may by law provide, transmit within four days to the President pro tempore of the Senate and the Speaker of the House of Representatives their written declaration that the President is unable to discharge the powers and duties of his office. Thereupon Congress shall decide the issue, assembling within 48 hours for that purpose if not in session. If the Congress, within 21 days after receipt of the latter written declaration, or, if Congress is not in session, within 21 days after Congress is required to assemble, determines by two-thirds vote of both houses that the President is unable to discharge the powers and duties of his office, the Vice President shall continue to discharge the same as Acting President; otherwise, the President shall resume the powers and duties of his office.

Amendment XXVI
[Adopted 1971]

Section 1

The right of citizens of the United States, who are 18 years of age or older, to vote shall not be denied or abridged by the United States or any state on account of age.

Section 2

The Congress shall have the power to enforce this article by appropriate legislation.

Amendment XXVII
[Adopted 1992]

No law, varying the compensation for the services of the Senators and Representatives shall take effect, until an election of Representatives shall have intervened.

Presidential Elections

Year	Candidates	Parties	Popular Vote	Electoral Vote	Voter Participation
1789	**George Washington**		*	69	
	John Adams			34	
	Others			35	
1792	**George Washington**		*	132	
	John Adams			77	
	George Clinton			50	
	Others			5	
1796	**John Adams**	Federalist	*	71	
	Thomas Jefferson	Democratic-Republican		68	
	Thomas Pinckney	Federalist		59	
	Aaron Burr	Dem.-Rep.		30	
	Others			48	
1800	**Thomas Jefferson**	Dem.-Rep.	*	73	
	Aaron Burr	Dem.-Rep.		73	
	John Adams	Federalist		65	
	C. C. Pinckney	Federalist		64	
	John Jay	Federalist		1	
1804	**Thomas Jefferson**	Dem.-Rep.	*	162	
	C. C. Pinckney	Federalist		14	
1808	**James Madison**	Dem.-Rep.	*	122	
	C. C. Pinckney	Federalist		47	
	George Clinton	Dem.-Rep.		6	
1812	**James Madison**	Dem.-Rep.	*	128	
	De Witt Clinton	Federalist		89	
1816	**James Monroe**	Dem.-Rep.	*	183	
	Rufus King	Federalist		34	
1820	**James Monroe**	Dem.-Rep.	*	231	
	John Quincy Adams	Dem.-Rep.		1	
1824	**John Quincy Adams**	Dem.-Rep.	108,740 (30.5%)	84	26.9%
	Andrew Jackson	Dem.-Rep.	153,544 (43.1%)	99	
	William H. Crawford	Dem.-Rep.	46,618 (13.1%)	41	
	Henry Clay	Dem.-Rep.	47,136 (13.2%)	37	
1828	**Andrew Jackson**	Democratic	647,286 (56.0%)	178	57.6%
	John Quincy Adams	National Republican	508,064 (44.0%)	83	
1832	**Andrew Jackson**	Democratic	687,502 (55.0%)	219	55.4%
	Henry Clay	National Republican	530,189 (42.4%)	49	
	John Floyd	Independent		11	
	William Wirt	Anti-Mason	33,108 (2.6%)	7	
1836	**Martin Van Buren**	Democratic	765,483 (50.9%)	170	57.8%
	William Henry Harrison	Whig		73	
	Hugh L. White	Whig	739,795 (49.1%)	26	
	Daniel Webster	Whig		14	
	W. P. Magnum	Independent		11	
1840	**William Henry Harrison**	Whig	1,274,624 (53.1%)	234	80.2%
	Martin Van Buren	Democratic	1,127,781 (46.9%)	60	
	J. G. Birney	Liberty	7069	—	

*Electors selected by state legislatures.

Year	Candidates	Parties	Popular Vote	Electoral Vote	Voter Participation
1844	James K. Polk	Democratic	1,338,464 (49.6%)	170	78.9%
	Henry Clay	Whig	1,300,097 (48.1%)	105	
	J. G. Birney	Liberty	62,300 (2.3%)	—	
1848	Zachary Taylor	Whig	1,360,967 (47.4%)	163	72.7%
	Lewis Cass	Democratic	1,222,342 (42.5%)	127	
	Martin Van Buren	Free-Soil	291,263 (10.1%)	—	
1852	Franklin Pierce	Democratic	1,601,117 (50.9%)	254	69.6%
	Winfield Scott	Whig	1,385,453 (44.1%)	42	
	John P. Hale	Free-Soil	155,825 (5.0%)	—	
1856	James Buchanan	Democratic	1,832,955 (45.3%)	174	78.9%
	John C. Frémont	Republican	1,339,932 (33.1%)	114	
	Millard Fillmore	American	871,731 (21.6%)	8	
1860	Abraham Lincoln	Republican	1,865,593 (39.8%)	180	81.2%
	Stephen A. Douglas	Democratic	1,382,713 (29.5%)	12	
	John C. Breckinridge	Democratic	848,356 (18.1%)	72	
	John Bell	Union	592,906 (12.6%)	39	
1864	Abraham Lincoln	Republican	2,213,655 (55.0%)	212[*]	73.8%
	George B. McClellan	Democratic	1,805,237 (45.0%)	21	
1868	Ulysses S. Grant	Republican	3,012,833 (52.7%)	214	78.1%
	Horatio Seymour	Democratic	2,703,249 (47.3%)	80	
1872	Ulysses S. Grant	Republican	3,597,132 (55.6%)	286	71.3%
	Horace Greeley	Dem.; Liberal Republican	2,834,125 (43.9%)	66[†]	
1876	Rutherford B. Hayes ‡	Republican	4,036,298 (48.0%)	185	81.8%
	Samuel J. Tilden	Democratic	4,300,590 (51.0%)	184	
1880	James A. Garfield	Republican	4,454,416 (48.5%)	214	79.4%
	Winfield S. Hancock	Democratic	4,444,952 (48.1%)	155	
1884	Grover Cleveland	Democratic	4,874,986 (48.5%)	219	77.5%
	James G. Blaine	Republican	4,851,981 (48.2%)	182	
1888	Benjamin Harrison	Republican	5,439,853 (47.9%)	233	79.3%
	Grover Cleveland	Democratic	5,540,309 (48.6%)	168	
1892	Grover Cleveland	Democratic	5,556,918 (46.1%)	277	74.7%
	Benjamin Harrison	Republican	5,176,108 (43.0%)	145	
	James B. Weaver	People's	1,041,028 (8.5%)	22	
1896	William McKinley	Republican	7,104,779 (51.1%)	271	79.3%
	William Jennings Bryan	Democratic People's	6,502,925 (47.7%)	176	
1900	William McKinley	Republican	7,207,923 (51.7%)	292	73.2%
	William Jennings Bryan	Dem.-Populist	6,358,133 (45.5%)	155	
1904	Theodore Roosevelt	Republican	7,623,486 (57.9%)	336	65.2%
	Alton B. Parker	Democratic	5,077,911 (37.6%)	140	
	Eugene V. Debs	Socialist	402,283 (3.0%)	—	
1908	William H. Taft	Republican	7,678,908 (51.6%)	321	65.4%
	William Jennings Bryan	Democratic	6,409,104 (43.1%)	162	
	Eugene V. Debs	Socialist	420,793 (2.8%)	—	
1912	Woodrow Wilson	Democratic	6,293,454 (41.9%)	435	58.8%
	Theodore Roosevelt	Progressive	4,119,538 (27.4%)	88	
	William H. Taft	Republican	3,484,980 (23.2%)	8	
	Eugene V. Debs	Socialist	900,672 (6.0%)	—	
1916	Woodrow Wilson	Democratic	9,129,606 (49.4%)	277	61.6%
	Charles E. Hughes	Republican	8,538,221 (46.2%)	254	
	A. L. Benson	Socialist	585,113 (3.2%)	—	
1920	Warren G. Harding	Republican	16,152,200 (60.4%)	404	49.2%
	James M. Cox	Democratic	9,147,353 (34.2%)	127	
	Eugene V. Debs	Socialist	919,799 (3.4%)	—	

[*]Eleven secessionist states did not participate.
[†]Greeley died before the electoral college met. His electoral votes were divided among the four minor candidates.
[‡]Contested result settled by special election.

Year	Candidates	Parties	Popular Vote		Electoral Vote	Voter Participation
1924	**Calvin Coolidge**	Republican	15,725,016	(54.0%)	382	48.9%
	John W. Davis	Democratic	8,386,503	(28.8%)	136	
	Robert M. La Follette	Progressive	4,822,856	(16.6%)	13	
1928	**Herbert Hoover**	Republican	21,391,381	(58.2%)	444	56.9%
	Alfred E. Smith	Democratic	15,016,443	(40.9%)	87	
	Norman Thomas	Socialist	267,835	(0.7%)	—	
1932	**Franklin D. Roosevelt**	Democratic	22,821,857	(57.4%)	472	56.9%
	Herbert Hoover	Republican	15,761,841	(39.7%)	59	
	Norman Thomas	Socialist	881,951	(2.2%)	—	
1936	**Franklin D. Roosevelt**	Democratic	27,751,597	(60.8%)	523	61.0%
	Alfred M. Landon	Republican	16,679,583	(36.5%)	8	
	William Lemke	Union	882,479	(1.9%)	—	
1940	**Franklin D. Roosevelt**	Democratic	27,244,160	(54.8%)	449	62.5%
	Wendell L. Willkie	Republican	22,305,198	(44.8%)	82	
1944	**Franklin D. Roosevelt**	Democratic	25,602,504	(53.5%)	432	55.9%
	Thomas E. Dewey	Republican	22,006,285	(46.0%)	99	
1948	**Harry S Truman**	Democratic	24,105,695	(49.5%)	304	53.0%
	Thomas E. Dewey	Republican	21,969,170	(45.1%)	189	
	J. Strom Thurmond	State-Rights Democratic	1,169,021	(2.4%)	38	
	Henry A. Wallace	Progressive	1,156,103	(2.4%)	—	
1952	**Dwight D. Eisenhower**	Republican	33,936,252	(55.1%)	442	63.3%
	Adlai E. Stevenson	Democratic	27,314,992	(44.4%)	89	
1956	**Dwight D. Eisenhower**	Republican	35,575,420	(57.6%)	457	60.6%
	Adlai E. Stevenson	Democratic	26,033,066	(42.1%)	73	
	Other	—	—		1	
1960	**John F. Kennedy**	Democratic	34,227,096	(49.9%)	303	62.8%
	Richard M. Nixon	Republican	34,108,546	(49.6%)	219	
	Other	—	—		15	
1964	**Lyndon B. Johnson**	Democratic	43,126,506	(61.1%)	486	61.7%
	Barry M. Goldwater	Republican	27,176,799	(38.5%)	52	
1968	**Richard M. Nixon**	Republican	31,770,237	(43.4%)	301	60.6%
	Hubert H. Humphrey	Democratic	31,270,533	(42.7%)	191	
	George Wallace	American Indep.	9,906,141	(13.5%)	46	
1972	**Richard M. Nixon**	Republican	47,169,911	(60.7%)	520	55.2%
	George S. McGovern	Democratic	29,170,383	(37.5%)	17	
	Other	—	—		1	
1976	**Jimmy Carter**	Democratic	40,828,587	(50.0%)	297	53.5%
	Gerald R. Ford	Republican	39,147,613	(47.9%)	241	
	Other	—	1,575,459	(2.1%)	—	
1980	**Ronald Reagan**	Republican	43,901,812	(50.7%)	489	52.6%
	Jimmy Carter	Democratic	35,483,820	(41.0%)	49	
	John B. Anderson	Independent	5,719,722	(6.6%)	—	
	Ed Clark	Libertarian	921,188	(1.1%)	—	
1984	**Ronald Reagan**	Republican	54,455,075	(59.0%)	525	53.3%
	Walter Mondale	Democratic	37,577,185	(41.0%)	13	
1988	**George H. W. Bush**	Republican	48,886,000	(53.4%)	426	57.4%
	Michael S. Dukakis	Democratic	41,809,000	(45.6%)	111	
1992	**William J. Clinton**	Democratic	43,728,375	(43%)	370	55.0%
	George H. W. Bush	Republican	38,167,416	(38%)	168	
	H. Ross Perot	Independent	19,237,247	(19%)	—	
1996	**William J. Clinton**	Democratic	45,590,703	(50%)	379	48.8%
	Robert Dole	Republican	37,816,307	(41%)	159	
	H. Ross Perot	Reform	7,866,284			
2000	**George W. Bush**	Republican	50,456,167	(47.88%)	271	51.2%
	Al Gore	Democratic	50,996,064	(48.39%)	266*	
	Ralph Nader	Green	2,864,810	(2.72%)	—	
	Other	—	834,774	(< 1%)	—	

*One District of Columbia Gore elector abstained.

Credits

Part One Timeline

Page 1: (Top) Lee Boltin Picture Library; (middle) The Ohio Historical Society; (bottom) Museum of the History of Science, Oxford, Oxfordshire, UK/Bridgeman Art Library.

Page 2: (Top) Nettie Lee Benson Latin American Collection, University of Texas, Austin; (bottom) The Granger Collection, New York.

Chapter 1

Page 22 (Map 1.3): From *Columbus* by Bjorn Landstrom. Copyright © 1966 by Bjorn Landstrom. Copyright © 1967 by Bokforlaget Forum AB. Reprinted with the permission of Simon & Schuster, Inc.

Pages 26–27 (Figure 1.1): Adapted from "The Columbian Exchange" by Jeff Glick with Celeste Schaefer from *U.S. News and World Report*, July 8, 1991.

Page 31: From *Colonial Spanish America: A Documentary History* by Kenneth Mills and William B. Taylor. Wilmington, DE: Scholarly Resources, 1998.

Chapter 2

Page 66 (Figure 2.1): From *Founding of Massachusetts* by Edmund S. Morgan, © 1964. Reprinted by permission of Pearson Education, Inc., Upper Saddle River, NJ.

Page 69: From "Verses upon the Burning of Our House," July 18th, 1666 by Anne Bradstreet.

Part Two Timeline

Page 112: (Top) Chicago Historical Society, ICHi-x.1354; (middle) The Historical Society of Pennsylvania; (bottom) Courtesy, Reading Public Museum, Reading, Pennsylvania (44-132-1).

Page 113: (Top) Peabody Essex Museum. Photograph by Mark Sexton. (Bottom) Library of Congress.

Chapter 4

Page 136 (Figure 4.2): From *Blacks Who Stole Themselves: Advertisements for Runaways in The* Pennsylvania Gazette, *1728–1790* by Billy G. Smith and Richard Wojtowicz.

Page 139: From "Releese us out of this Cruell Bondegg: An Appeal from Virginia in 1723."

Chapter 5

Page 158 (Figure 5.1): Adapted from "Gender and Age Structure of Population: British Mainland Colonies, 1760s" and "Gender and Age Structure of Population: United States, 1980s" in *Mapping America's Past: A Historical Reference Book* by Mark C. Carnes and John A. Garraty with Patrick Williams, © 1996 by Arcadia Editions Limited. Reprinted by permission of Henry Holt and Company, LLC.

Chapter 6

Page 204: From a petition signed by thirty North Carolina Regulators, October 4, 1768.

Part Three Timeline

Page 216: (Top) The Bostonian Society; (bottom) Courtesy, Janice L and David Frent

Page 217: (Top) Abby Aldrich Rockefeller Folk Art Center, Williamsburg, VA; (bottom) The National Archives

Chapter 7

Pages 224–225: From a declaration signed by 15 grand jury members in South Carolina, May 1776.

Page 236 (Figure 7.1): From *British Historical Statistics,* Mitchell, 579.

Chapter 8

Page 259: From narratives by Joseph Plumb Martin, 1830.

Chapter 9

Page 312 (Figure 9.3): From Robert J. Dinkin, *Voting in Revolutionary America: A Study of Elections in the Original Thirteen States, 1776–1789* (1982), 36–39.

Pages 314–315: From *Means for the Preservation of Public Liberty* by Georges James Warner (New York, 1797).

Page 321 (Figure 9.4): From *Distribution of Wealth and Income in the United States, 1798* by Lee Soltow (1989).

Part Four Timeline

Page 326: (Top) Courtesy, Missouri Historical Society; (bottom) The American Numismatic Society, New York.

Page 327: (Top) Massachusetts Historical Society, MHS image #0031; (bottom) Samuel J. Miller, *Frederick Douglass,* 1847–52. Major Acquisitions Centennial Endowment, 1996.433. ©The Art Institute of Chicago. All Rights Reserved

Chapter 10

Page 343: From Cherokee Women to Cherokee Council, May 2, 1817, series 1, Andrew Jackson Presidential Papers, Library of Congress Manuscripts Division, Washington, D.C.

Page 348 (Figure 10.1): From *Transatlantic Industrial Revolution: The Diffusion of Textile Technologies Between Britain and America, 1790–1830s* by David J. Jeremy. Copyright © 1981 by The MIT Press. Reprinted by permission of MIT Press.

Chapter 11

Pages 366 (Map 11.4) and 373 (Map 11.5): Adapted from *The Mexican Frontier 1821–1846: The American Southwest Under Mexico* by David J. Weber.

Page 372 (Figure 11.1): Table "Cherokee Nation Intercensus Changes, 1809–24" from *Cherokee Removal Before and After* edited by William L. Anderson. Reprinted by permission of The University of Georgia Press.

Page 375: From "Jose Agustin de Escudero Describes New Mexico as a Land of Opportunity, 1827" in H. Bailey Carroll and J. Villasana Haggard, trans. and ed., *Three New Mexico Chronicles* (Albuquerque, 1942)

Chapter 12

Page 395 (Map 12.2): Adapted from *Mapping America's Past: A Historical Reference Book* by Mark C. Carnes and John A.

Garraty with Patrick Williams, © 1996 by Arcadia Editions Limited. Reprinted by permission of Henry Holt and Company, LLC.

Page 397 (Map 12.3): "The Grand Migration" from *The Penguin Atlas of Diasporas* by Gerard Chaliand and Jean-Pierre Rageau. New York: Viking Press, 1995.

Page 399 (Map 12.4): Adapted from "Expansion of the Cotton Belt" in *Mapping America's Past: A Historical Reference Book* by Mark C. Carnes and John A. Garraty with Patrick Williams, © 1996 by Arcadia Editions Limited. Reprinted by permission of Henry Holt and Company, LLC.

Page 402 (Map 12.5): Adapted from "Indian Removal from the Old Southeast" in *Mapping America's Past: A Historical Reference Book* by Mark C. Carnes and John A. Garraty with Patrick Williams, © 1996 by Arcadia Editions Limited. Reprinted by permission of Henry Holt and Company, LLC.

Page 403 (Table 12-1): From *Women and Men on the Overland Trail* by John Mack Faragher. Copyright 1979 by Yale University Press. Reprinted by permission.

Pages 424–425: From a speech by Senator John C. Calhoun, January 1848.

Part Five Timeline

Page 428: (Top) Michael Freeman/CORBIS; (middle) Harriet Beecher Stowe Center, Hartford, CT; (bottom) The Ohio Historical Society

Page 429: (Top) Antique Textile Resource, Bethesda MD; (bottom) William T. Garrell Foundry, San Francisco, *The Golden Spike*. The Iris & B. Gerald Cantor Center for Visual Arts at Stanford University (1998.115). Gift of David Hewes

Chapter 13

Pages 442–443: From *The Endowments, Position and Education of Woman. An Address Delivered Before the Hemans and Sigourney Societies of the Female High School at Limestone Springs*, July 23, 1850 (Columbia, SC: I.C. Morgan, 1850.)

Chapter 14

Page 468 (Figure 14.1): From "Alabama Secession Convention Occupations" and "Alabama Convention Property Holding" in Ralph Wooster, *The Secession Conventions of the South.* Copyright © 1962 by Princeton University Press. Reprinted by permission of Princeton University Press.

Pages 472–473: From a letter by John B. Spiece to the Confederate Attorney General, December 4, 1861.

Pages 475 (Figure 14.2) and 492 (Figure 14.3): From *Battle Cry of Freedom* by James McPherson. Oxford University Press, 1988.

Page 480 (Map 14.3): Adapted from Confederates Battle Southwestern Indians, Central New Mexico, 1861 by Jerry Thompson from *New Mexico Historical Review*, April 1998.

Page 489 (Map 14.4): From *Battle Cry of Freedom* by James McPherson. Oxford University Press, 1988.

Page 493 (Map 14.5): Adapted from Major African American Battle Sites in *The Atlas of African-American History and Politics: From the Slave Trade to Modern Times* by Arwin D. Smallwood with Jeffrey M. Elliot. McGraw Hill, 1998.

Page 496 (Map 14.6): Adapted from *The Atlas of African-American History and Politics: From the Slave Trade to Modern Times* by Arwin D. Smallwood with Jeffrey M. Elliot. McGraw-Hill, 1998.

Chapter 15

Page 510: From "Post-Bellum Southern Rental Contracts" by Rosser H. Taylor from *Agricultural History*, Volume 17, Number 2, April 1943. Published by The Agricultural History Society.

Page 523 (Table 15-3): From *Americans and Their Forests: A Historical Review* by Michael Williams. Copyright © 1989 by Cambridge University Press. Reprinted by permission of Cambridge University Press.

Page 530 (Table 15-4): From *Beyond Equality: Labor and the Radical Republicans, 1862–1872* by David Montgomery. New York: Alfred Knopf, 1967.

Part Six Timeline

Page 536: (Top) Michael Freeman Photography; (bottom) Courtesy, Janice L. and David Frent

Page 537: (Top) From the HUC Skirball Cultural Center, Museum Collection, Los Angeles, CA. Gift of Brenda Grossman Spivack in memory of Godina Eisenstein Schwartz. Clothes and Textiles: Gift of Harold Brill and Regina Starr Brill. HUCSM 31.194. Photography by Susan Einstein; (bottom) Fair Street Pictures

Chapter 16

Page 545 (Table 16-1): From *Americans and Their Forests: A Historical Review* by Michael Williams. Copyright © 1989 by Cambridge University Press. Reprinted by permission of Cambridge University Press.

Page 547 (Table 16-2): From "How Indians Used the Buffalo" adapted from *The Native American Almanac* by Arlene B. Hirschfelder and Martha Kreipe de Montano. Copyright © 1998. Reprinted by permission of Hungry Minds.

Page 549 (Map 16.2): Adapted from "Population of Foreign Birth by Region, 1880" in *Historical Atlas of the United States* by Clifford L. Lord & Elizabeth H. Lord. New York: Holt, 1953.

Page 551 (Map 16.3): From *Chinese in the Post–Civil War South* by Lucy Cohen. Copyright © 1984 by Louisiana State University Press. Reprinted by permission of Louisiana State University Press.

Page 568: From "The Gospel of Wealth" by Andrew Carnegie from *North American Review*, No. CCCXCL (June 1889).

Chapter 17

Page 579 (Map 17.1): From "Farm Tenancy, by Counties, 1880" in *Historical Atlas of the United States* by Clifford L. Lord & Elizabeth H. Lord. New York: Holt, 1953.

Page 582 (Map 17.2): From *The Atlas of African-American History and Politics: From the Slave Trade to Modern Times* by Arwin D. Smallwood with Jeffrey M. Elliot. McGraw-Hill, 1998.

Page 585 (Map 17.3): From *American History Atlas*, revised edition by Martin Gilbert. London: Weidenfeld & Nicolson, 1969.

Chapter 18

Page 609 (Map 18.1): From *Atlas of American History* by Kenneth T. Jackson and James T. Adams. New York: Charles Scribner's Sons. 1985.

Page 610 (Map 18.2): From "Population Density, 1890" in *Historical Atlas of the United States* by Clifford L. Lord & Elizabeth H. Lord. New York: Holt, 1953.

Page 613 (Map 18.3): From Paullin and Wright, *Atlas of the Historical Geography of the United States,* 1932.

Page 616 (Map 18.4): From "Compulsory School Attendance, 1890" and Compulsory School Attendance, 1900" in *Historical Atlas of the United States* by Clifford L. Lord & Elizabeth H. Lord. New York: Holt, 1953.

Pages 632–633 (Map 18.6): Adapted from Spanish-American War in the Pacific and Spanish-American War in the Caribbean in Kenneth T. Jackson and James T. Adams, *Atlas of American History.* New York: Charles Scribner's Sons. 1985.

Pages 634–635: From Proceedings of the Congressional Committee on the Philippines—Testimony of Robert P. Hughes and Charles S. Riley, 1902.

Part Seven Timeline

Page 638: (Top) From the Collections of Henry Ford Museum & Greenfield Village; (middle) Courtesy, The Lilly Library, Indiana University, Bloomington, Indiana; (bottom) Courtesy, Military Antiques & Museum, Petaluma, CA

Page 639: (Top) Fair Street Pictures; (middle) Courtesy, Janice L. and David Frent; (bottom) From the Collections of Ford Museum & Greenfield Village

Chapter 19

Page 645 (Map 19.1): From *Historical Atlas of the United States* by Clifford L. Lord & Elizabeth H. Lord. New York: Holt, 1953.

Page 646 (Figure 19.1): "Immigration by Decade, 1821–1990 from Immigration and Naturalization Service.

Page 648 (Map 19.2): Adapted from "Areas Restricted by Chinese Exclusion Acts" in *Atlas of American Migration* by Stephen A. Flanders. New York: Facts on File, 1998.

Page 651 (Map 19.3): Adapted from "Italian and Russian Immigrants in the United States, 1910" in *Atlas of American Migration* by Stephen A. Flanders. New York: Facts on File, 1998.

Chapter 20

Page 693: From Addie W. Hunton & Kathryn M. Johnson, *Two Colored Women with the American Expeditionary Forces.* Brooklyn, NY: Brooklyn Eagle Press, 1920.

Chapter 21

Page 706 (Figure 21.1): From *Brought to Bed: Childbearing in America, 1750–1950* by Judith Walzer Leavitt, copyright © 1986 by Judith Walzer Leavitt. Used by permission of Oxford University Press, Inc.

Page 708 (Figure 21.2): From U.S. Immigration, 1891–1940.

Page 712 (Figure 21.4): "Changes in Farm and Nonfarm Populations: 1880–1980" from *America's Northern Heartland: An Economic and Historical Geography of the Upper Midwest* by John R. Borchert. Copyright © 1987, published by the University of Minnesota Press. Used by permission.

Page 730: From *The Fortunate Pilgrim* by Mario Puzo. New York: Antheneum, 1965.

Part Eight Timeline

Page 734: (Top) Courtesy, Janice L. and David Frent; (middle) Nationalmuseet, Copenhagen/The Bridgeman Art Library International Ltd.; (bottom) Gift of Mr. and Mrs. Jim Kawaminami, Japanese American National Museum. Photo by Norman Sugimoto

Page 735: (Top) Fair Street Pictures; (middle) Courtesy, The United Nations; (bottom) Joseph Sohm; ChromoSohm Inc./CORBIS

Chapter 23

Page 789: Interview with Zelda Anderson in R. T. King, ed., from *War Stories: Veterans Remember World War II.* Published by the University of Nevada Oral History Program, 1995. Used by permission of Zelda Anderson and the University of Nevada Oral History Program.)

Chapter 24

Page 825: From NSC-68: United States Objectives and Programs for National Security (April 14, 1950).

Part Nine Timeline

Page 832: (Top) Library of Congress; (bottom) Roger Ressmeyer/CORBIS

Page 833: (Top) Library of Congress; (middle) Tamiment/Wagner Poster and Broadside Collection, Tamiment Library, New York University; (bottom) TimePix

Chapter 25

Page 857: From *Silent Spring* by Rachel Carson. Boston: Houghton Mifflin, 1962.

Page 863: Martin Luther King, Jr., "I Have a Dream" (speech delivered August 28, 1963, Washington, D.C.) Reprinted by arrangement with The Heirs to the Estate of Martin Luther King Jr., c/o Writers House, Inc as agent for the proprietor. Copyright 1963 by Martin Luther King Jr., copyright renewed 1991 by Coretta Scott King.

Chapter 26

Page 882: "A Time to Break Silence" by Martin Luther King, Jr. Reprinted by arrangement with the Estate of Martin Luther King Jr., c/o Writers House as agent of the proprietor. Copyright 1963 by Martin Luther King Jr., copyright renewed 1991 by Coretta Scott King.

Chapter 27

Page 920: Interim Report of the U.S. Senate Select Committee to Study Government Operations (November 20, 1975).

Part Ten Timeline

Page 934: (Top) Courtesy, Janice L and David Frent; (bottom) W. Cody/CORBIS

Page 935: (Top) Justin Sullivan/AP/Wide World; (bottom) Amy E. Conn/AP/Wide World

Chapter 28

Pages 954–955: From *Listen America* by Jerry Falwell, copyright © 1980 by Jerry Falwell. Used by permission of Doubleday, a division of Random House.

Page 955: "The Need for a Moral Minority" by Robert McAfee Brown. Reprinted by permission of the estate of Robert McAfee Brown.

Chapter 29

Pages 976 (Map 29.1) and 983 (Map 29.2): From *Atlas of American Migration* by Stephen A. Flanders. New York: Facts on File, 1998.

Page 980: From the Vermont Civil Union Law (April 26, 2000.)

Chapter 30

Page 1022: The Slow Food Manifesto (Nov. 9, 1989) of The Slow Food Movement (http://www.slowfood.com)

Index

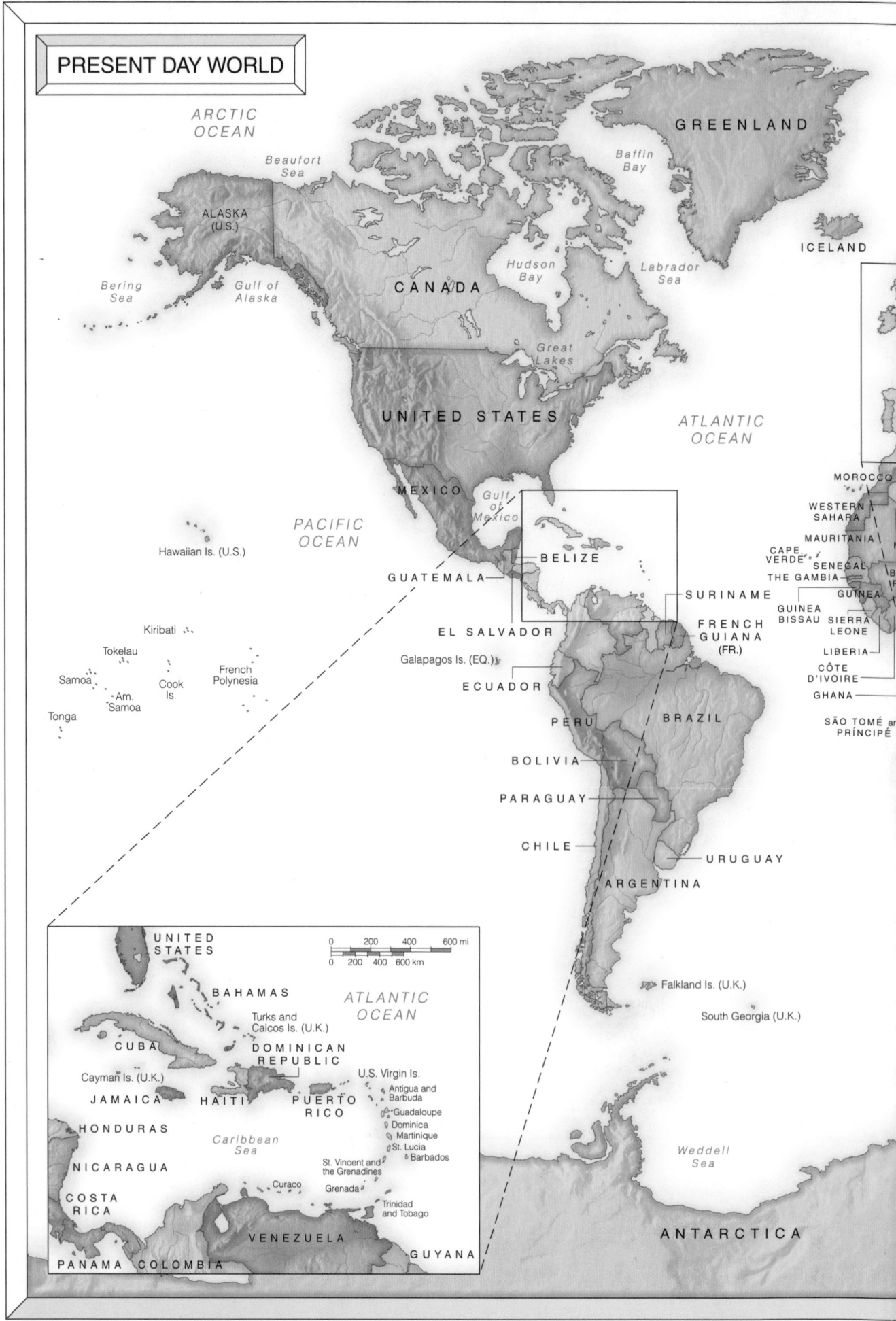

PRESENT DAY WORLD